AIIMS

MedE@sy™

(Nov 2018–May 2015)

Subject-wise cum Year-wise approach

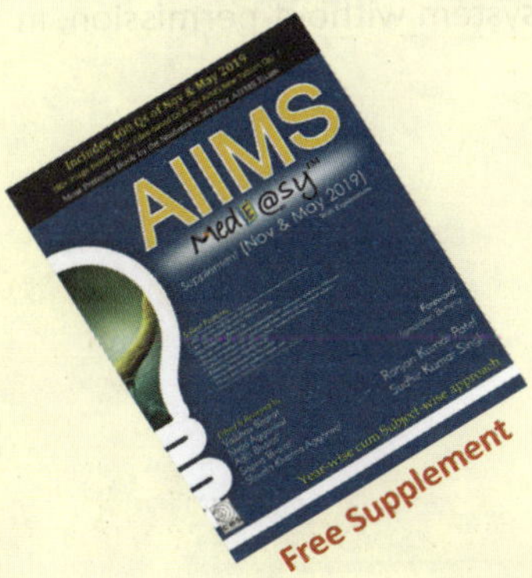

4th Edition

Editor-in-Chief

Vaibhav Bharat (DNB/MS General Surgery)
Director, MedE@sy

Authors

Ishad Aggarwal MD Dermatology
IPGIMER, Kolkata

Aditi Bharat MD Anesthesia
TATA Memorial Hospital, Mumbai

Sapna Bharat DNB OBG
SRV Hospital, Mumbai

Shweta Khanna Aggarwal MD Radiodiagnosis
IGMC, Shimla

Associate Authors

Gaurav Bharat MD Pathology
Diagno Labs, Mumbai

Manoj Gupta DNB General Medicine, DNB Nephrology
RTIICS, Kolkata

Vivek Dudeja MS ENT, DNB, MNAMS
AIIMS, Bhopal

Rohit Katre (MD PSM)

Nikhil Lohiya DNB Pediatrics, Fellow Pediatric Endocrinology
BVP, Pune

CBS Publishers & Distributors Pvt Ltd

• New Delhi • Bengaluru • Chennai • Kochi • Mumbai
• Hyderabad • Kolkata • Patna • Vijayawada

SET ISBN: 978-81-940256-4-1

Fourth Edition: 2020
Third Edition: 2019
Second Edition: 2018
First Edition: 2017

Published by **Satish Kumar Jain** and produced by **Varun Jain** for
CBS Publishers and Distributors Pvt Ltd

4819/XI Prahlad Street, 24 Ansari Road, Daryaganj, New Delhi 110 002, India.
Ph: +91-11-23289259, 23266861, 23266867 Website: www.cbspd.com
Fax: 011-23243014
e-mail: delhi@cbspd.com; cbspubs@airtelmail.in.

Corporate Office: 204 FIE, Industrial Area, Patparganj, Delhi 110 092
Ph: +91-11-4934 4934 Fax: 4934 4935
e-mail: feedback@cbspd.com; bhupesharora@cbspd.com

Branches

- **Bengaluru:** Seema House 2975, 17th Cross, K.R. Road, Banasankari 2nd Stage, Bengaluru 560 070, Karnataka
  Ph: +91-80-26771678/79 Fax: +91-80-26771680 e-mail: bangalore@cbspd.com
- **Chennai:** 7, Subbaraya Street, Shenoy Nagar, Chennai 600 030, Tamil Nadu
  Ph: +91-44-26680620, 26681266 Fax: +91-44-42032115 e-mail: chennai@cbspd.com
- **Kochi:** 68/1534, 35, 36-Power House Road, Opp. KSEB, Cochin-682018, Kochi, Kerala
  Ph: +91-484-4059061-65 Fax: +91-484-4059065 e-mail: kochi@cbspd.com
- **Kolkata:** 6/B, Ground Floor, Rameswar Shaw Road, Kolkata-700 014, West Bengal
  Ph: +91-33-22891126, 22891127, 22891128 e-mail: kolkata@cbspd.com
- **Mumbai:** 83-C, Dr E Moses Road, Worli, Mumbai-400018, Maharashtra
  Ph: +91-22-24902340/41 Fax: +91-22-24902342 e-mail: mumbai@cbspd.com

Representatives

- **Hyderabad** +91-9885175004
- **Pune** +91-9623451994
- **Patna** +91-9334159340
- **Vijayawada** +91-9000660880

Printed at: Magic International Pvt. Ltd. Greater Noida, UP, India

MEDE@SY REVIEW BOARD

Subject	Subject Authors and Reviewers
Anatomy	Dr Aprajita Awasthi
Physiology	Dr Vishal Goel
Biochemistry	Dr Ashutosh Saxena
Microbiology	Dr Swati Gupta
Pathology	Dr Gaurav Bharat
Pharmacology	Dr Pratik Shrivastava
Forensic Medicine	Dr Shashank Sharma
Preventive & Social Medicine	Dr Madhur Verma, Dr Rohit Katre
Ear, Nose & Throat	Dr Vivek Dudeja, Dr Deepti Singh
Ophthalmology	Dr Vineet Sehgal
Medicine	Dr Manoj Gupta
Pediatrics	Dr Nikhil Lohiya, Dr Ruby Singh
Obstetrics & Gynecology	Dr Sapna Bharat
General Surgery	Dr Vaibhav Bharat, Dr Mayank Porwal
Orthopedics	Dr Anurag Tiwari
Dermatology	Dr Ishad Aggarwal
Psychiatry	Dr Tanay Maiti, Dr Arvind Gautam
Radiodiagnosis & Radiotherapy	Dr Shweta Khanna Aggarwal, Dr Vaibhav Bharat
Anesthesia	Dr Aditi Bharat, Dr Harshvardhan Bharadwaj

MEDEASY ONLINE RESOURCE

Visit our dedicated web portal for errata, free downloads and feedback
http://www.medeasyindia.com/
Join our Facebook Page for Updates and Notifications
Join Subject-wise MedE@sy Groups for Discussions
https://www.facebook.com/MedEasyindia/

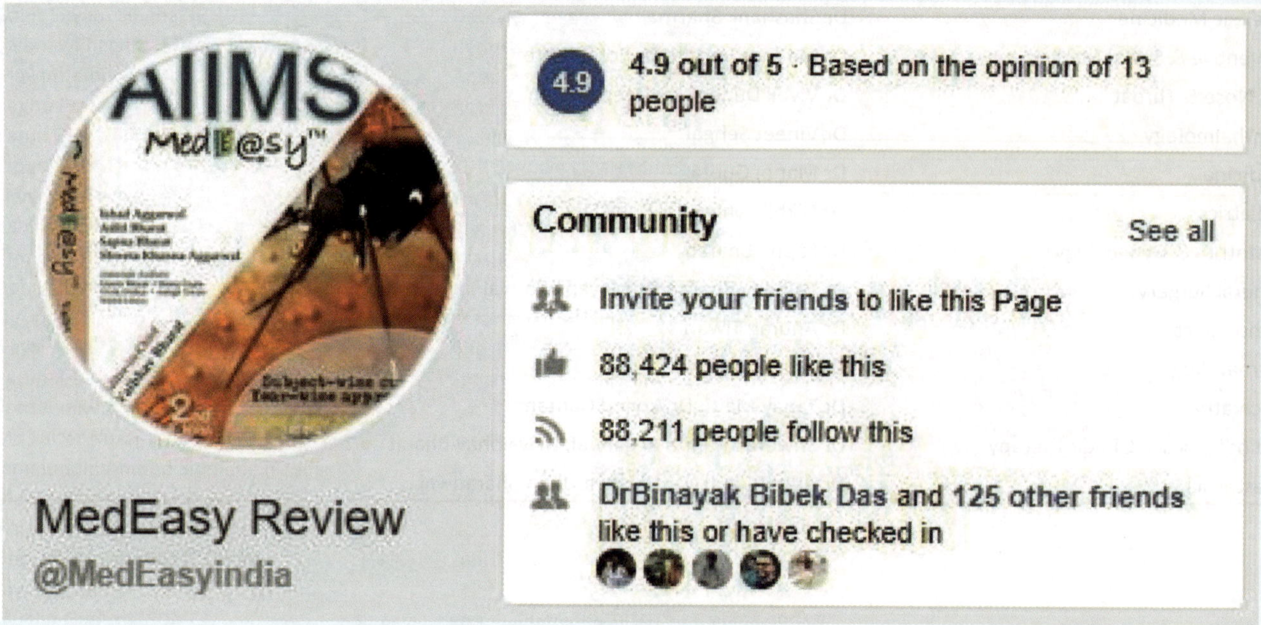

Preface

First of all it is our pleasure and duty to thank all our readers, who have time and again shown faith in our endeavors. It is always encouraging if your work is appreciated and we are grateful to all our readers. With the success of AIIMS MedE@sy, it gives us immense pleasure to present to you the 3rd edition of this book.

AIIMS is the most prestigious medical exam of our country and we have tried our best to present to you a book which does justice to its repute. We have taken utmost care of each and every question, new or old. The questions in each subject have been dealt separately with an expert in the subject and have been checked and counter checked. Views and counter views have been acknowledged. A section of "**RECALL BIAS**" has also been included, for the first time in any PGMEE entrance book. It took us almost one and a half year to finalize its contents. As they say, all good things take time!

Also with changing pattern of online Computer-Based Test (CBT) exams we have made this book a fully colored book and comprehensively covered "**COLOR PLATES**", relevant to the topics with each question. Also we have decided to give **access to mobile application** especially designed for this purpose. With new changed pattern of AIIMS PG we have tried our best to include a new mock section of new pattern questions and tricks of how to attempt them.

We have done our level best to come up with right answers, but to err is human, and we are humans too. However, we constantly keep in touch with our readers through our website **www.medeasyindia.com,** and our Facebook fan page **https://www.facebook.com/MedEasyindia/** to keep them updated with any correction, change or improvement in our book. We are also operating subject-wise groups by the name of MedE@sy followed by respective subject name.

We heartily invite any suggestions, corrections or discussions of PG medical entrance MCQs on our mail id **info.medeasy@gmail.com**

Thanks!

Editor-in-Chief/Authors
AIIMS MedE@sy

Dedications and Acknowledgements

I would also like to take this opportunity to dedicate this work and to thank people who directly contributed or indirectly inspired this book.

Almighty, Our Parents and Grandparents

- Almighty
- Our Parents and Grandparents
- Ishan Agarwal
- Saurabh Bharat (MPCD, NYFA)
- Anuj Shrivastava
- Harshvardhan Bharadwaj (SRMC, DMIM)
- Saket Kumar (SRMC)
- Pankul Mangla (SRMC)
- Rohit Shyam Singhal (BHU)
- Vaibhav Chachra (SRMC, SMC Gaziabad)
- Mayank Goel (SRMC, ISB Hyderabad)
- Raghu Prakash (SRMC, CNMC, LHMC)
- Varun Gupta (SRMC, ASCOMS, Gangaram)
- Vipan Bhandari (SRMC)
- Siaram Sharan Kushwah (SRMC)
- Ashish Kumar Gupta (KIMS Hubli)
- Prashant Bharadwaj (SRMC, LLRM)
- Abhay Kumar Singh (SRMC, VMMC)
- Nirupam Sharan (SRMC, Patel Chest)
- Naval Asija (SRMC, NIHFW)
- Parimal Tara (SRMC)
- Pradeep Kumar (SRMC)
- Md Faizer Nazer (SRMC, RPGMC, MAMC)
- Jamaluddin Ahmed Siddique (Medanta)
- Mankeshwar Kumar (SRMC)
- Brajesh Kumar (SRMC, AMC)
- Deepak Ranjan (SRMC, AMC)
- Diwakar Kumar (SRMC, INS Ashvini)
- Harsha Guduru (SRMC)
- Ranjeet Jha (SRMC)
- Swanay Mondal (SRMC, Bombay Hospital)
- Sandip Singh (SRMC, Mission Hospital)
- Vinish Agarwal (KMC, GRMC, HIHT)
- Mayank Porwal (GRMC Gwalior)
- Vikram Singh Rathore (GRMC)
- Aprajita Pandey (GRMC)
- Savyasanchi Tiwari (RDGMC)
- Triloki Nath Soni (RDGMC, People's Bhopal)
- Jorawar Singh Bhatia (RDGMC)
- Ankush Sharma (RDGMC)
- Rakesh Soni (RDGMC)
- Nandeep Kushwah (RDGMC)
- Surjeet Shukla (RDGMC)
- Ruby Singh (RDGMC, SAIMS Indore)
- Malvika Tripathi (RDGMC)
- Jyotsna Khatri (RDGMC)
- Shubha Jaggi (RDGMC)
- Aditi Damle (RDGMC)
- Shravan Patidar (RDGMC, SAIMS)
- Ashvini Natu (RCSM, TMH Mumbai)
- Rasika Thosar (RCSM, TMH Mumbai)
- Tineesh Mathew (TMH Mumbai)
- Deepika Menon (TMH Mumbai)
- Renuka Purohit (TMH Mumbai)
- Anupama Zade (TMH Mumbai)
- Rishi Shankar (TMH Mumbai)
- Sanika Patil (TMH Mumbai)
- Kirti Salunke (TMH Mumbai)
- Shreyas Bhor (TMH Mumbai)
- Raghvendra Gowda (TMH Mumbai)
- Prashant Kumar Yadav (TMH Mumbai)
- Amit Yadav (TMH Mumbai)
- Meera Metha (TMH Mumbai)
- Ritesh Patil (TMH Mumbai)
- Satish Sarode (TMH Mumbai)
- A K Singh (Director I/C M&HS, HOD DSP)
- N Kulshreshta (Director M&HS, DSP)
- A K Sahay (MCh DNB Plastic Surgery DSP)
- Ravitej Golive (DSP)
- Noor Ain Khan (DSP)
- Zahid Zahiri (DSP)
- Parthasarthi Buniya (DSP)
- Prof. G. Chatterjee, HOD Dermatology IPGMER
- Arghya Prasun Ghosh (Assoc. Prof IPGMER)
- Abhishek De (Asst. Prof IPGMER)
- Sumit Sen (Assoc. Prof IPGMER)
- Trupti Surana (IPGMER)
- S. Biswas (IPGMER)
- Rakesh Patel (IPGMER)
- Keshab Sil (IPGMER)
- Nandini (IPGMER)
- Nidhi Chaudhary (IPGMER)
- Sampriti Sendur (IPGMER)
- Neha Sori (IPGMER)
- Rakibul Hasan (IPGMER)
- Shatabdi (IPGMER)
- Vivek Sharma (IPGMER)
- Tony (IPGMER)
- Atanu Chakraborty (IPGMER)
- Arindam (IPGMER)
- Shagun Gupta (IPGMER)
- Bhavika Sen (IPGMER)
- Amit Varma (Prof & HOD Pathology SAIMS)
- S. S. Nandedkar (Prof Pathology SAIMS)
- Kamal Malukaani (SAIMS)
- Mallika Kinger (SIAMS)
- Mukul Raj Jain (SAIMS)
- Shilpi Dosi (SAIMS)
- Preeti Rihal Chakraborty (SAIMS)
- Gaurav Pawar (SAIMS)
- Surabhi Sharma (SAIMS)
- Isha Bansal (SAIMS)
- Aparna Khandelwal (SAIMS)
- Kapil Gupta (SAIMS)
- Priyanka Kiyawat (SAIMS)
- Monal Dixit (SAIMS)
- Garima Gupta (SAIMS)
- Prashant Yashwante (SAIMS)
- Brig. Ashok Hooda (AMC)
- Kunal Mahajan (PGI Rohtak)
- Sharada Datar (RCSM)
- Anuradha Dhawal (RCSM)
- Hrishikesh Wagholikar (RCSM, GMC Miraj)
- Freni Shah (RCSM)
- Priyanka Iyangar (RCSM)
- Chhanvar Lal Mali (RCSM)
- Chinmay Inamdar (RCSM)
- Md Sadat Wasim (IPGIMER)
- Nikhat Ara (CNCI Kolkata)
- Rita Hansa (HOD OBG BGH Bokaro)
- Roopam Singh (BGH Bokaro)
- Kusum Dash (BGH Bokaro)
- Snehil Sharma (SKMCH)
- Tulika Joshi (Index Medical college)
- Nazia Noor (Index Medical college)
- Anjali Patil (Index Medical college)
- Pooja Jain (Index Medical college)
- Hardik Seth
- Vikas Mathur

Contents

AIIMS New Pattern 2019 Model Questions

Volume I

(Nov 2018 – May 2015)

Subject-wise MCQs and Answers with Explanations

Special Thanks

We extend our heartfelt gratitude to all our student reviewers whose feedbacks and suggestions helped us in authenticating and strengthening the content of 2nd edition.

- Ekta Mishra, Government Medical College and Hospital, Chandigarh
- Haneef Shaik, Fathima Institute of Medical Sciences, Kadapa, Andhra Pradesh
- Karthick Raja, Government Villupuram Medical College, Villupuram, Tamil Nadu
- Shubham Jain, Netaji Subhash Chandra Bose Medical College, Jabalpur, Madhya Pradesh
- Shivam Sabharwal, Dr SN Medical College, Jodhpur, Rajasthan
- Theeran R, Government Villupuram Medical College, Villupuram, Tamil Nadu
- Vatsal Sampat, Pandit Deendayal Upadhyay Medical College, Rajkot, Gujarat

Video Questions

1. A patient who had undergone renal transplant 3 months back presented with complaints of dysentery. No parasitic ova/cysts are found on fecal examination. Video showing larva was shown and asked what is incorrect about this organism? *(For explanation see page 246)*

   a. Organism shown is filiform larva which is responsible for diarrhea
   b. Organism may cause Loeffler's pneumonia
   c. Organism is monoecious in nature so able to reproduce by using parthenogenesis
   d. It is caused due to food/water contamination

2. A video of sick neonate is shown in the video. What is the most likely diagnosis? (Scan the given QR code from your mobile to watch the video. Install a QR code scanner if not done already). *(For explanation see page 798)*

   a. Focal clonic seizure
   b. Multifocal clonic seizure
   c. Multifocal tonic clonic seizure
   d. Focal tonic seizure

3. Video of a child having respiratory distress is shown in the video. The Silverman score is? (Scan the given QR code from your mobile to watch the video. Install a QR code scanner if not done already). *(For explanation see page 800)*

   a. 7
   b. 8
   c. 9
   d. 10

4. What is the method of breast examination depicted in the video? *(For explanation see page 925)*

   a. Vertical strip method
   b. Concentric method
   c. Clockwise method
   d. Quadrant method

For Detail Refer Respective Chapters.

Ans
1.
2.
3.
4.

AIIMS New Pattern 2019 Model Questions

Scheme of Marking

- Please see the individual explanations above and the table below.
- No credit will be given for the questions not answered or marked for review *(Questions marked for review shall be considered as unanswered).*
- Percentile scores are generated for the entire examination separately for MD/MS and for MDS.

Type of MCQ	Correct	Wrong	For review	Not answered
Single best response	+1	−1/3	0	0
Multiple true false*	+1/5	−1/5	0	0
Match the following*	+1/4	−1/4	0	0
Sequential arrangement	+1	−1	0	0
Multiple completion	+1/4	−1/4	0	0
Reason assertion	+1/4	−1/4	0	0
Extended matching**	+1/2	−1/2	0	0

*For each alternative/response in the MCQ
**If two scenarios in each question

Majority of the MCQs for the July 2019 MD/MS/MDS examination shall be of the Single best response type.

VARIANT 1. SINGLE BEST ANSWER TYPE

Each question/statement shall have four alternatives/statements of which only and one best response is to be selected/marked. **Majority of MCQs for July 2019 MD/MS/MDS examination shall be of the SBA type.** *This is the conventional MCQ type which is well covered in 3rd edition of AIIMS MEDEASY.*

VARIANT 2. MULTIPLE TRUE-FALSE TYPE

Each question shall have a stem followed by five alternatives/statements and every alternative/statement will have to be marked as either True or False

1. A child presents with blue eyes, White patch of hair and fair skin. Guthrie test is positive. The following statements are true/false:

1. Due to Phenyl alanine hydroxylase enzyme defect
2. White patch of hair due to tryptophan
3. Phenyl acetate positive in urine
4. Mental retardation is present
5. Guthrie's test is negative

Ans. True: 1, 3, 4; False: 2, 5

Ref: Nelson 20th Ed Pg 368

1. Due to Phenyl alanine hydroxylase enzyme defect → ***TRUE***
2. White patch of hair due to tryptophan → ***FALSE***
3. Phenyl acetate positive in urine → ***TRUE***
4. Mental retardation is present → ***TRUE***
5. Guthrie's test is negative → ***FALSE***

Phenylketonuria:

- The affected infant is normal at birth. Profound intellectual disability develops gradually if the infant remains untreated. Cognitive delay may not be evident for the first few months. In untreated patients, 50-70% will have an IQ below 35, and 88-90% will have an IQ below 65. Only 2-5% of untreated patients will have normal intelligence. Many patients require institutional care if the condition remains untreated. Vomiting, sometimes severe enough to be misdiagnosed as pyloric stenosis, may be an early symptom. Older untreated children become hyperactive with autistic behaviors, including purposeless hand movements, rhythmic rocking, and athetosis.
- **Guthrie's test** is positive in Phenylketonuria (PKU), and hence, diagnosis in the child described is PKU.
- Deficiency of the enzyme phenylalanine hydroxylase (PAH) or of its cofactor tetrahydrobiopterin (BH4) causes accumulation of **phenylalanine.**
- In affected infants with plasma concentrations >20 mg/dL, excess phenylalanine is metabolized to phenylketones (phenylpyruvate and **phenylacetate)** that are excreted in the urine, giving rise to the term phenylketonuria (PKU).
- Infants with **PKU** tend to have fair skin, blond **hair**, and blue eyes, because the inability to convert ***phenylalanine to tyrosine.***
- Profound intellectual disability develops gradually if the infant remains untreated. Cognitive delay may not be evident for the first few months. In untreated patients, 50-70% will have an IQ below 35, and 88-90% will have an IQ below 65.

2. The following statements are true/false about γδ T cells?

1. A first line defense for bacterial peptide
2. Contain CD5
3. Contain CD4
4. Contain CD8
5. Do not require specialized antigen presentation

Ans. True: 1, 5; False: 2, 3, 4

Ref: Cell Signaling in Host-Pathogen Interactions by Diana Bahia 1st Ed Pg 113

1. A first line defense for bacterial peptide → ***TRUE***
2. Contain CD5 → ***FALSE***
3. Contain CD4 → ***FALSE***
4. Contain CD8 → ***FALSE***
5. Do not require specialized antigen presentation → ***TRUE***

- Gamma delta (γδ) T cells are the prototype of 'unconventional' T cells and represent a relatively small subset of T cells in peripheral blood.
- They are defined by expression of heterodimeric T-cell receptors (TCRs) composed of γ and δ chains. This sets them apart from the classical CD4+ helper T cells and CD8+ cytotoxic T cells that express αβ TCRs.
- Gamma-delta TCR binds directly to the antigens and does not require specialized antigen processing and presentation, as alpha-beta T cells do.
- These cells do not have a thymic differentiation phase and are derived directly from bone marrow precursors. They are positive for CD3, CD2, and CD7 but negative for CD4 and CD8, and they express cytotoxic granules in the cytoplasm.
- They are present primarily in mucocutaneous sites (skin, genital tract, GIT) where they serve as first responders to commonly encountered bacteria.
- Many antigens recognized by gamma delta T-cell are unconventional nonpeptide phosphoantigens, endogenous metabolites of cholesterol biosynthesis that are produced by bacteria.
- They participate in innate immune responses and also in tissue repair by expressing epithelial growth factors

3. Identify the following statements as true/false with respect to screening tests done in series:

1. Sensitivity increases specificity decreases
2. Sensitivity decreases specificity increases
3. Sensitivity and specificity increases
4. Sensitivity and specificity decreases
5. Both remain the same

Ans. True: 2; False: 1, 3, 4, 5

Ref: Park 24th ed page 149, Lecture Notes on Epidemiology By Professor Dr Abdul Rashid Khan, Professor K.A. Narayan 2nd ed page 149

1. Sensitivity increases specificity decreases → *FALSE*
2. Sensitivity decreases specificity increases → *TRUE*
3. Sensitivity and specificity increases → *FALSE*
4. Sensitivity and specificity decreases → *FALSE*
5. Both remain the same → *FALSE*

Two screening tests done in series increase specificity and decrease sensitivity

Two screening tests done in parallel increase sensitivity and decrease specificity

4. Identify true/false statements regarding IgE antibodies?

1. It mediates release of histamine and other chemical mediators
2. It is the primary antibody involved in allergic reactions
3. It is involved in anti-parasitic immune responses
4. May cross the placenta and fix complement
5. They are heat stable

Ans. True: 1, 2, 3; False: 4, 5

Ref: Ananthanarayan 9th ed page 98-99

1. It mediates release of histamine and other chemical mediators → *TRUE*
2. It is the primary antibody involved in allergic reactions → *TRUE*
3. It is involved in anti-parasitic immune responses → *TRUE*
4. May cross the placenta and fix complement → *FALSE*
5. They are heat stable → *FALSE*

Immunoglobulins

	IgG	IgA	IgM	IgD	IgE
Heavy chain	γ	A	μ	δ	ε
Percentage	75-85 (max)	7-15	5-10	0.3	0.019 (min)
Carbohydrate %	4	10	10.7	12	12
Serum half-life (days)	21 (max)	6	5	3	2 (min)
Concentration	12 mg/mL	2 mg/mL	1.2 mg/mL	0.03 mg/mL	0.00004 mg/mL
Molecular form	Monomer	Serum IgA= monomer Secretory IgA = Dimer	Pentamer	Monomer	Monomer
Molecular weight	150,000 (lightest)	Serum IgA= 160,000 Secretory IgA= 400,000	950,000 (heaviest)	175,000	190,000
Subclasses	IgG1> IgG2> IgG3> IgG4	IgA1= circulatory, IgA2= secretory	M1, M2	none	none
Complement activation	Classical ++ G4 subclass= alternate	Alternate (only IgA1 fixes complement)	Classical +++	Alternate	Alternate or None
Sedimentation coefficient	7S	Monomer=7S Dimer= 15S	7S	7S	8S
Placental crossing	Yes	No	No	No	No
Presence in milk	Present	Present	Absent	Absent	Absent
Compartment	Equal in intravascular (45%) and extravascular (55%) compartment	Mostly extravascular (Minimum intravascular distribution)	mostly intravascular		Mostly extravascular
Heat stability	Stable	Stable	Stable	Stable	Heat labile

Contd...

Immunoglobulins					
	IgG	IgA	IgM	IgD	IgE
Comments	→ Produces secondary (A.K.A Anamnestic) response → Enhances phagocytosis of microbes → IgG2 most useful against encapsulated bacteria → 2-mercapto ethanol does not destroy IgG → Most opsonins are IgG	→ Only Ig secreted by seromucinous glands	→ First to appear in fetus(20wk) → Produces primary response → 2-mercapto ethanol selectively destroys IgM → Monomeric IgM is the major antibody receptor on surface of B cell for antigen recognititon		→ Homocytotropic → Cannot be demonstrated by conventional serological reactions. → Detected by RAST, ELISA, Passive agglutination

Footnote:
- Of the IgGs, only IgG subclasses 1, 2, and 3 fix complement; IgG4 does not. IgG1 and IgG3 react most readily with C1q, the first component of complement, and therefore activate complement most efficiently. IgG2 is less reactive, and intact IgG4 proteins are completely unreactive.
- C1, which is bound to a site in the Fc region, is composed of three proteins: C1q, C1r, and C1s. C1q is an aggregate of polypeptides that bind to the Fc portion of IgG and IgM.
- Secretory IgA does not activate complement by the classic pathway, but chemically aggregated IgA has been shown to have activity in the alternate complement
- The **anamnestic response** refers to the immune response of the body to a pathogen it recognize i.e. Secondary response. Anamnestic reaction is seen in persons who have had past typhoid/enteric fever or who have had immunization against typhoid.

5. Identify True/ False statements with respect to Glomerular Filtration Rate

1. Increases with increased renal blood flow
2. Decreases with decreased plasma oncotic pressure
3. Increases with increased efferent arteriole resistance
4. Increases with ureter obstruction with stone
5. Decreases with afferent arteriolar constriction

Ans. True: 1, 3, 5; False: 2, 4

Ref: Guyton 13th Ed Pg 337-341; Ganong 24th Ed Table 37-4

1. Increases with increased renal blood flow → ***TRUE***
2. Decreases with decreased plasma oncotic pressure → ***FALSE***
3. Increases with increased efferent arteriole resistance → ***TRUE***
4. Increases with ureter obstruction with stone → ***FALSE***
5. Decreases with afferent arteriolar constriction → ***TRUE***

The basic factors that affect GFR are:
- Net filtration (The sum of the hydrostatic and plasma oncotic forces in the glomerular capsule and Bowman's capsule respectively).
- Capillary filtration coefficient determined by permeability and filtering surface area of the capillary.

Changes seen in Factors Affecting GFR		
Factor	Increased GFR	Decreased GFR
Renal blood flow	↓	↓
Glomerular capillary hydrostatic pressure	↑	↓

Contd...

Changes seen in Factors Affecting GFR		
Factor	Increased GFR	Decreased GFR
Afferent arteriolar constriction	↓	↑
Efferent arteriolar constriction	↑	↓
Hydrostatic pressure in Bowman's capsule	↑	↓
Plasma oncotic pressure	↓	↑
Filtration coefficient (K_f)	↑	↓
Glomerular capillary permeability	↑	↓
Effective filtration surface area	↑	↓
Ureteral obstruction	–	GFR decreases

6. Identify as True/False with respect to autonomic nervous system

1. Sympathetic system stimulation decreases blood flow to kidneys
2. Sympathetic system stimulation decreases blood flow to coronaries
3. Parasympathetic stimulation decreases heart rate
4. Sympathetic system stimulation can cause mydriasis
5. Detrusor muscle contracts due to parasympathetic stimulation

Ans. True: 1, 3, 4, 5; False: 2

Ref: Guyton 11th Ed page 754, Ganong 23rd Ed Pg 702

1. Sympathetic system stimulation decreases blood flow to kidneys → ***TRUE***
2. Sympathetic system stimulation decreases blood flow to coronaries → ***FALSE***
3. Parasympathetic stimulation decreases heart rate → ***TRUE***
4. Sympathetic system stimulation can cause mydriasis → ***TRUE***
5. Detrusor muscle contracts due to parasympathetic stimulation → ***TRUE***

Most systemic blood vessels, especially those of the abdominal viscera and skin of the limbs, are constricted by sympathetic stimulation except coronaries and skeletal muscles which are dilated by Beta receptor stimulation. Parasympathetic stimulation has almost no effects on most blood vessels except to dilate vessels in certain restricted areas, such as in the blush area of the face. Thus Sympathetic stimulation can decrease blood flow to all organs except coronaries and skeletal muscles

Autonomic Effects on Various Organs of the Body

Effector organ	Adrenergic response	Receptor involved	Cholinergic response	Dominant response (A or C)
Heart				
Rate of contraction	Increase	β_1	Decrease	C
Force of contraction	Increase	β_1	Decrease	C
Blood vessels				
Arteries (most)	Vasoconstriction	α_1		A
Skeletal muscle	Vasodilation	β_2		A
Veins	Vasoconstriction	α_2		A
Bronchial tree	Bronchodilation	β_2	Bronchoconstriction	C
Splenic capsule	Contraction	α_1		A
Uterus	Contraction	α_1	Variable	A
Vas deferens	Contraction	α_1		A
Prostatic capsule	Contraction	α_1		A
Gastrointestinal tract	Relaxation	α_2	Contraction	C
Eye				
Radial muscle, iris	Contraction (mydriasis)	α1		A
Circular muscle, iris			Contraction (miosis)	C
Ciliary muscle	Relaxation	B	Contraction (accommodation)	C
Kidney	Renin secretion	β_1		A
Urinary bladder				
Detrusor	Relaxation	B	Contraction	C
Trigone and sphincter	Contraction	α_1	Relaxation	A, C
Ureter	Contraction	α_1	Relaxation	A
Insulin release from pancreas	Decrease	α_2		A
Fat cells	Lipolysis	β_1 (β_3)		A
Liver glycogenolysis	Increase	α_1		A
Hair follicles, smooth muscle	Contraction (piloerection)	α_1		A
Nasal secretion			Increase	C
Salivary glands	Increase secretion	α_1	Increase secretion	C
Sweat glands	Increase secretion	α_1	Increase secretion	C

Footnote:

The adrenergic pathway is otherwise known as the SNS or sympathetic nervous system. While cholinergic pathway is also known as the parasympathetic nervous system (PNS). i.e. Adrenergic receptors respond to sympathetic stimulation and Cholinergic receptor responds to Parasympathetic stimulation

7. Identify as true/false regarding Transfusion related acute lung injury (TRALI):

1. Self-resolving in 2-3 weeks
2. Role of corticosteroids not clear
3. Morality < 10%
4. Symptoms start after 72 hours
5. Supportive care is the mainstay of treatment

Ans. True: 2, 3, 5; False: 1, 4

Ref: Wintrobe's 12th ed page 699, Harrison 19th ed page 138 e5.

1. Self-resolving in 2-3 weeks → ***FALSE***
2. Role of corticosteroids not clear → ***TRUE***
3. Morality < 10% → ***TRUE***
4. Symptoms start after 72 hours → ***FALSE***
5. Supportive care is the mainstay of treatment → ***TRUE***

Transfusion-Related Acute Lung Injury	
Transfusion-Related Acute Lung Injury Transfusion-related acute lung injury (TRALI) is the most common cause of transfusion related fatalities	
Definition	Transfusion-related acute lung injury (TRALI) most commonly presents as severe respiratory distress of sudden onset, caused by a **syndrome of noncardiogenic pulmonary edema resembling the adult respiratory distress syndrome.** Chills, fever, chest pain, hypotension, and cyanosis, as well as the usual manifestations of pulmonary edema, may be seen.
Incidence	TRALI is reported by the FDA as the number-one cause of transfusion-associated fatality. The incidence of TRALI being reported varies greatly, from **1 in 5,000 to 1 in 13,000**
Events	It is hypothesized that TRALI reactions may be the result of two cumulative events: the first event is linked to the patient (i.e., **underlying sepsis, hematologic disease, and/or postsurgical status**), and the second event is related to the transfusion of potential granulocyte primers such as inflammatory cytokines, active lipids, and/ or alloantibodies.
Clinical course	• Initial descriptions detailing the clinical course for TRALI suggested quick resolution of hypoxemia, generally within **24 to 48 hours** of symptom onset. • However, the majority of patients who develop TRALI will require ICU admission and ventilator support. • For those requiring mechanical ventilation, these early reports described a mean duration of ventilatory support lasting approximately 40 hours. • In contrast, subsequent evidence suggests that most cases will require respiratory support for a longer period (eg, approximately 3 to 10 days). • These more contemporary data frequently report composite outcomes from cases of TRALI and possible TRALI/ transfused ARDS and limit the study population to the critically ill. • Such cases are likely to represent the more severe end of the clinical spectrum. In contrast, milder cases of TRALI and/ or possible TRALI/transfused ARDS may go undiagnosed or unreported.
Mortality	5–10% in general 40–50% in critically ill patients
Risk factors	• Testing the donor's plasma for anti-HLA antibodies can support this diagnosis. • The implicated donors are frequently **multiparous women.** • The transfusion of plasma from male and nulliparous women donors reduces the risk of TRALI. • Recipient factors that are associated with increased risk of TRALI include smoking, chronic alcohol use, shock, liver surgery (transplantation), mechanical ventilation with >30 cmH2O pressure support and positive fluid balance treatment is supportive, and patients usually recover without sequelae If TRALI or possible TRALI/transfused ARDS are suspected, the transfusion should be discontinued immediately.
Diagnosis	The diagnosis of a TRALI reaction is based on the onset of acute lung injury (ALI) **within/ up to 6 hours of transfusion.** ALI is characterized by an acute onset of hypoxemia (oxygen saturation <90% by pulse oximetry for a patient breathing room air or a PaO_2/FiO_2 ≤300 mmHg), bilateral infiltrates on frontal chest radiograph, and no evidence of circulatory overload. Based on studies of adult respiratory distress syndrome, which has similar pulmonary manifestations, it has been suggested that agglutination of granulocytes and complement activation occur in the pulmonary vascular bed, leading to capillary endothelial damage with consequent fluid leak into the alveoli.

Contd...

Transfusion-Related Acute Lung Injury	
Prevention	The AABB requires evaluation of donors implicated in TRALI. Donors whose plasma is implicated in such reactions should be examined for the presence of granulocyte specific and HLA antibodies that react with recipient leukocytes. It is recommended to avoid further transfusion of plasma-containing products from implicated donors found to have anti-HLA or antigranulocyte antibodies. **Recently, the AABB recommended that blood banks minimize the production of high-plasma-content components** (such as FFP and pheresis platelets) from donors at risk for alloimmunization (e.g., women with a history of pregnancy) . Ultimately, criteria for TRALI susceptibility will have to be clarified in order to prevent it effectively .
Management	**Management** of the patient with either TRALI or possible TRALI/transfused ARDS is supportive, with oxygen supplementation for the correction of hypoxemia being the cornerstone of treatment. Hemodynamic monitoring may be required to determine whether fluid overload is a factor; if not, diuretics are of no proven value . Very high doses of corticosteroids may be of benefit in transfusion-related acute lung injury, probably by blocking granulocyte aggregation and consequent vascular damage. Non-invasive respiratory support with continuous positive airway pressure (CPAP) or bilevel positive airway pressure (BiPAP) may be sufficient in less severe cases, but endotracheal intubation with invasive mechanical ventilation is often required . The available evidence suggests that most patients who develop either TRALI or possible TRALI/transfused ARDS will require ventilatory support (approximately 70 to 80 percent. **Steroids** — the routine use of corticosteroids when TRALI is suspected is not recommended .

8. Mark the following statements as True/ False:

1. Weight in Kgs is a continuous variable
2. Blood group (A, B, AB, O) is a categorical variable
3. Age in years and months is a continuous variable
4. Height in cms is a discrete variable
5. Number of children is a continuous variable

Ans. True: 1, 2, 3; False: 4, 5

Ref: Medical Statistics Made easy by M Harris and G Taylor page 98, Medical Statistics from A to Z 2nd ed by B.S. Everitt page 39

1. Weight in Kgs is a continuous variable → ***TRUE***
2. Blood group (A, B, AB, O) is a categorical variable → ***TRUE***
3. Age in years and months is a continuous variable → ***TRUE***
4. Height in cms is a discrete variable → ***FALSE***
5. Number of children is a continuous variable → ***FALSE***

Types of Variables	
Continuous variable: (AKA Interval variable)	A variable which can take any value within a given range, for examples include weight, height, temperature and blood pressure. For such a variable, equal-sized differences on different parts of the scale are equivalent
Covariate	A covariate is a continuous variable that is not of primary interest but is measured because it may affect the outcome and may therefore need to be included in the analysis.
Discrete variable	A variable where the data can only be certain values, usually whole numbers, for example the number of children in families. Compare this with continuous variable

Contd...

Types of Variables	
Categorical variable	A variable that gives the appropriate label of an observation after allocation to one of several possible categories, for example gender: male or female; marital status: married, single or divorced; blood group: A, B, AB or O. Categorical variables separate observations into groups. The categories are often given numerical labels, but for this type of data these have no numerical significance
Categorizing continuous variables	A procedure common in medical research in which continuous variables are converted into categorical variables by grouping values into two or more categories, for example age might become 'young' (<40) and 'old' (≥40)

9. Mark the following as True/false regarding Meckel's diverticulum:

1. Occurs in 3% of population
2. 3 inch long
3. Remnant of distal part of vitello intestinal duct
4. Found on Anti mesenteric border
5. 2 Feet from iliocaecal valve

Ans. True: 4, 5; False: 1, 2, 3

REF: Maingot 11th ed ch , Bailey 26th ed page 1169, Sabiston 19th ed page 1268 -1270, Schwartz 9th Ed Ch 28, Sutton 7th Ed Pg 631

1. Occurs in 3% of population → ***FALSE***
2. 3 inch long → ***FALSE***
3. Remnant of distal part of vitello intestinal duct → ***FALSE***
4. Found on Anti mesenteric border → ***TRUE***
5. 2 Feet from iliocaecal valve → ***TRUE***

Meckel's Diverticulum	
Definition	A Meckel's diverticulum is a persistent remnant of the vitellointestinal duct and is present in about 2% of the population. It is the most common congenital anomaly of the alimentary tract
Embryology	In fetal life the umbilicus is connected to the gut by the vitellointestinal duct. Further duct becomes totally obliterated and vanishes. The bowel end (Proximal end) of the duct may persist as a Meckel's diverticulum.
Epidemiology	Present in 2% population
Anatomy	• It is found on the antimesenteric side of the ileum, commonly at 60 cm **(2 foot) from the ileocaecal valve** and is classically 5 cm long **(2 Inches)** • A Meckel's diverticulum contains all three coats of the bowel wall and has its own blood supply.
Clinical features	In around **20% of cases**, the mucosa of a Meckel's diverticulum contains heterotopic epithelium of gastric, colonic or pancreatic type. • Vast majority of Meckel's diverticula are **asymptomatic** unless associated complications • **Haemorrhage**. If gastric mucosa is present, peptic ulceration can occur and present as painless maroon rectal bleeding or melaena. Most common presentation in children • **Diverticulitis**. Present in 20% of patients with symptomatic Meckel's diverticula, is associated with a clinical syndrome that is indistinguishable from acute appendicitis, although if perforation occurs the presentation may resemble a perforated duodenal ulcer. • **Intussusception**. A Meckel's can be the lead point for ileoileal or ileocolic intussusception. • **Chronic ulceration**. Pain is felt around the umbilicus, as the site of the diverticulum is midgut in origin. • **Intestinal obstruction**. A band between the apex of the diverticulum and the umbilicus. Most common presentation in adults • **Perforation**. • **Neoplasms,** most commonly carcinoid tumors, are present in 0.5 to 3.2% of symptomatic Meckel's diverticula that are resected.
Diagnosis	Most Meckel's diverticula are discovered incidentally on radiographic imaging, during endoscopy, or at the time of surgery. In the absence of bleeding, Meckel's diverticula rarely are diagnosed before the time of surgical intervention. **Meckel's diverticulum is infrequently visualised on contrast studies, even when carefully sought, and scintigraphic techniques are more useful for diagnosis."** • Plain radiography, barium studies, angiography, computed tomography (CT), ultrasonography, and scintigraphy all play complementary roles in the diagnosis of the complications of Meckel diverticulum. • **Radionuclide scans (99mTc-pertechnetate) can be helpful in the diagnosis of Meckel's diverticulum; this test is, however, positive only when the diverticulum contains associated ectopic gastric mucosa that is capable of uptake of the tracer . The accuracy of radionuclide scanning is reported to be 90% in pediatric patients but less than 50% in adults.** • The diagnosis is notoriously difficult and remains a continuing challenge for the radiologist. • In all imaging modalities, findings of Meckel diverticulum are nonspecific. • **Most Meckel diverticula are diagnosed during surgery or autopsy, with imaging playing a secondary role.** • **The most sensitive technique is scintigraphy, and various modifications to imaging techniques have been devised to improve sensitivity**. Ultrasonography and CT are improving and can help in making an anatomic diagnosis. • **Diagnosis of ectopic gastric mucosa using $^{99}Tc^{m}$-pertechnetate:** Meckel's diverticulum. $^{99}Tc^{m}$-pertechnetate scintigraphy images showing focal area of intense abnormal tracer accumulation in the hypogastrium appearing at the same time as gastric mucosal uptake, this pattern is characteristic of Meckel's diverticulum. The Tc-99 is taken up by gastric mucosa (hence positive in the region of stomach-black areas in the picture). A black area is also seen in the region of the intestines.it signifies **ectopic gastric mucosa, suggestive of Meckel's diverticulum.**
Management	When found in the course of abdominal surgery, a Meckel's can safely be left alone provided it has a wide mouth and is not thickened. **Meckel's diverticulectomy**: A broad-based Meckel's diverticulum should not be amputated at its base and invaginated (as for an appendix), as there is the risk of stricture and of leaving heterotopic epithelium behind. It is safer simply to excise the diverticulum, either by resecting it and suturing the defect at its base, or with a linear stapler-cutter.
RULE OF 2 = Occurs in 2 percent of patients, 2 inches (5 cm long), 2 feet (60 cm) from the ileocaecal valve, 20 percent heterotopic epithelium	

10. Classify the following features as true/false about HELLP syndrome?

1. Retroplacental hemorrhage is always present
2. Hemolysis
3. Liver enzymes are elevated
4. Thrombocytopenia
5. Nausea may be present
6. Retroplacental hemorrhage is always present

Ans. True: 2, 3, 4, 5; False: 1

Ref: Williams Obstetrics 24th ed ch 40, Dutta 7th ed page 222

1. Retroplacental hemorrhage is always present → ***FALSE***
2. Hemolysis → ***TRUE***
3. Liver enzymes are elevated → ***TRUE***
4. Thrombocytopenia → ***TRUE***
5. Nausea may be present → ***TRUE***

HELLP Syndrome:

This is an acronym for Hemolysis (H), Elevated Liver enzymes (EL) and Low Platelet count (LP) (<100,000/mm3).

- This is a rare complication of pre-eclampsia (10–15%). HELLP syndrome may develop even without maternal hypertension.
- **Clinical features:** Nausea, vomiting, epigastric or right upper quadrant pain, along with biochemical, and hematological changes.
- Parenchymal necrosis of liver causes elevation in hepatic enzymes (AST and ALT >70 IU/L, LDH >600 IU/L) and bilirubin (>1.2 mg/dL).
- Subcapsular hematoma formation (which is diagnosed by CT scanning) and abnormal peripheral blood smear. Eventually liver may rupture to cause sudden hypotension, due to hemoperitoneum.
- Recurrence risk of HELLP syndrome is **3–19%**.
- In HELLP syndrome perinatal mortality ranges between **5 and 60%** and maternal mortality may be up to **25%**.

VARIANT 3. MATCH THE FOLLOWING TYPE

Each question shall have two columns with four items in one column (A) that need to be matched appropriately with the best alternative available in the next column(B). Note: Column A will always have 4 options while Column B might have more than 4 options.

11. Match the gastrointestinal content at each site with its appropriate ionic composition (mEq/L).

	Column A		Column B
1	Salivary	A	Na = 140, K = 5, Cl = 104, HCO$_3$ = 30
2	Stomach	B	Na = 140, K = 5, Cl = 75, HCO$_3$ = 115
3	Small bowel	C	Na = 60, K = 10, Cl = 130, HCO$_3$ = 0
		D	Na = 10, K = 26, Cl = 10, HCO$_3$ = 30
		E	Na = 60, K = 30, Cl = 40, HCO$_3$ = 50

Ans. 1-D, 2-C, 3-A

Ref: Schwartz 7th ed page 56

Composition of Gastrointestinal Secretions

Source	Vol (mL/24 hr)	Na$^+$ (mmol/L)	K$^+$ (mmol/L)	Cl$^-$ (mmol/L)	HCO$_3^-$ (mmol/L)
Salivary	1,500 (500–2,000)	10 (2–10)	26 (20–30)	10 (8–18)	30
Stomach	1,500 (100–4,000)	60 (9–116)	10 (0–32)	130 (8–154)	0
Duodenum	(100–2,000)	140	5	80	0
Ileum	3,000	140 (80–150)	5 (2–8)	104 (43–137)	30
Colon	(100–9,000)	60	30	40	0
Pancreas	(100–800)	140 (113–185)	5 (3–7)	75 (54–95)	115
Bile	(50–800)	145 (131–164)	5 (312)	100 (89–180)	35

12. Match the following correctly?

	Column A		Column B
1	Abrus precatorius	a	Blue rocket
2	Spanish fly	b	Brown sugar
3	Aconite	c	Foxglove
4	Heroin	d	Kaner
		e	Gunchi
		f	Blister beetle

Ans. 1-e, 2-f, 3-c, 4-b

Ref: Review of Forensic Medicine and Toxicology by Gautam Biswas 3rd ed Pg 519

The table indicates the local vernacular names of certain poisons:

Scientific and Vernacular Names of Certain Poisons		
Poison	**Name**	**Image**
Abrus precatorius	Rati, Gunchi, Jequirity	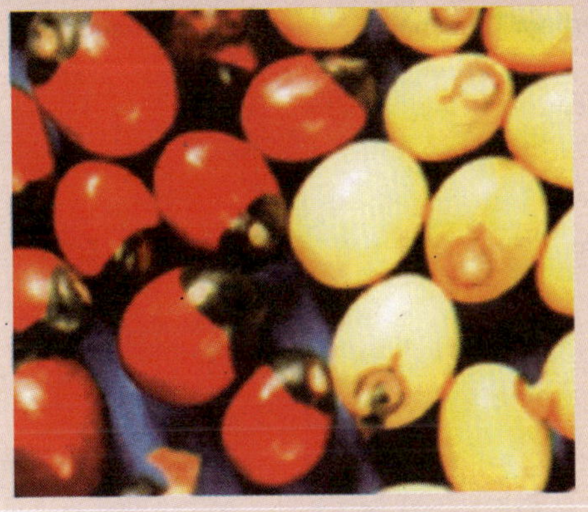
Spanish fly	Blister beetle	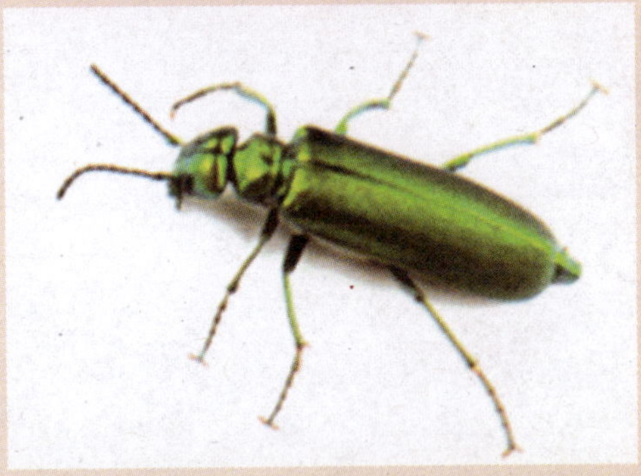
Aconite	Monk's hood, mitha zaher, bish, wolf's bane, women's bane, devil's helmet or blue rocket	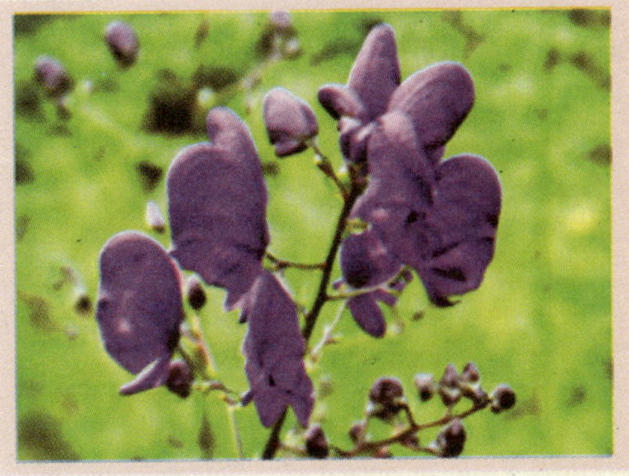

Contd...

Scientific and Vernacular Names of Certain Poisons		
Poison	**Name**	**Image**
Heroin (derived from Papaver somniferum)	Brown sugar, smack	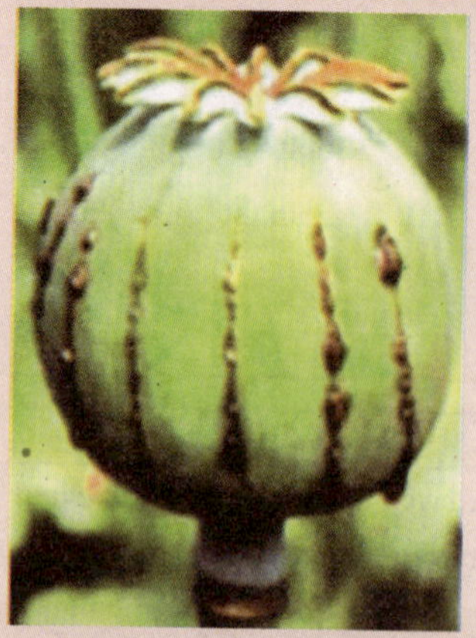 Papaver somniferum
Nerium Odorum Cerbera Thevetia	White Oleander Yellow Oleander Kaner	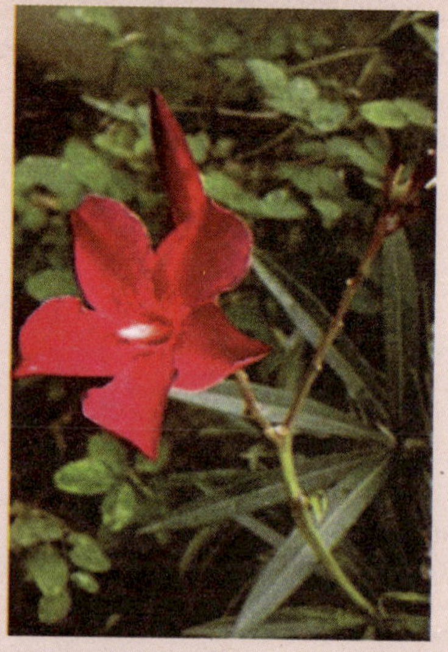 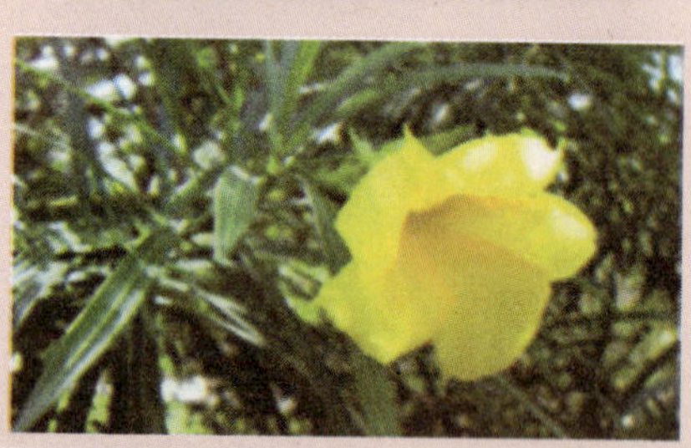
Digitalis	Foxglove	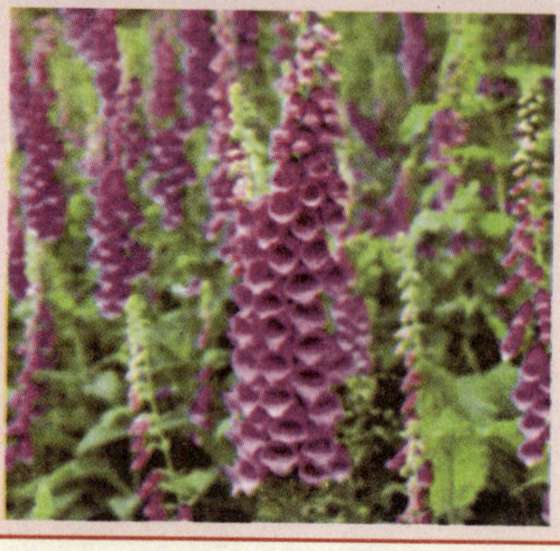

13. Match the following blood components with their storage temperatures

	Column A		Column B
1	Whole blood	a	–30°C
2	Platelets	b	20–24°C
3	FFP	c	–80°C
4	Frozen RBCs	d	2–6°C

Ans. 1-d, 2-b, 3-a, 4-c

Ref: Essentials of Haematology by Shirish Kawathalkar 2nd Ed Pg 396

Blood Components and Indications for Use				
Component	**Composition**	**Volume**	**Storage**	**Indications and expected benefit**
Whole blood	RBC and plasma (approx. HCT, 40%); WBCs; platelets	500 mL	2-6°C	To increase red cell mass and plasma volume (plasma deficient in labile clotting factors V and VIII); for hypovolemic anemia, massive transfusion, or exchange transfusion in neonates
Packed RBCs	RBC and reduced plasma (approx. Hct, 75%); WBCs; platelets	250 mL	2-6°C	To increase red cell mass in symptomatic anemia; 10 mL/kg raises Hct by 10%
RBCs, adenine-saline added	RBC and 100 mL of additive solution (approx. Hct, 60%); WBCs; platelets; little plasma	330 mL	2-6°C	To increase red cell mass in symptomatic anemia; 10 mL/kg raises Hct by 8%
RBCs, leukocytes reduced (prepared by filtration)	>85% original volume of RBCs; <5 × 10^6 WBCs	>85% of original volume	2-6°C	To increase red cell mass; <5 × 10^6 WBCs to decrease the likelihood of febrile reactions, immunization to leukocytes (HLA antigens), or CMV transmission
RBCs, washed	RBCs (approx. Hct, 75%); reduced WBCs; no plasma	225 mL	2-6°C	To increase red cell mass; reduce risk of allergic reactions to plasma proteins; or reduce free potassium dose
RBCs, frozen	RBCs (approx. Hct, 75%);	225 mL	–80°C (–176°F)	To increase red cell mass; minimize febrile or allergic transfusion reactions; use for prolonged RBC blood storage
Granulocytes, pheresis	> 1 × 10^{10} granulocytes per unit 10-30 mL of RBC 1-6 × 10^6 platelet	220 mL	20-24°C	To provide granulocytes for selected patients with sepsis and severe neutropenia (Absolute neutrophil count <0.5 × 10^9/L i.e. <500/µl). Dose: Generally ≥ 4x10^{10} once daily either until significant clinical improvement or ANC > 500/µl or 42 days, whichever comes earlier
RDP- Random donor platelet (Platelet concentrates)	Platelets (>5.5 × 10^{10}/unit); RBCs; WBCs; plasma	50 mL	20-24°C in platelet agitator	Bleeding due to thrombocytopenia or thrombocytopathy; 1 unit/10 kg raises platelet count by 17–50 × 10^9/L
SDP- Single donor platelet (Platelets pheresis)	Platelets (>3 × 10^{11}/unit); RBCs; WBCs; plasma	300 mL	20-24°C in platelet agitator	Same as platelets; sometimes HLA matched; benefit is equivalent to 6 platelet concentrates
Platelets, leukocytes reduced	Platelets (as above); <5 × 10^6 WBCs/final dose of pooled or pheresis platelets	300 mL	20-24°C	Same as platelets; <5 × 10^6 WBCs to decrease the likelihood of febrile reactions, alloimmunization to leukocytes (HLA antigens), or CMV transmission
FFP; thawed plasma	FFP: all coagulation factors; thawed plasma: reduced factors V and VIII	200 mL	–30°C thawed just before use	Best for multiple clotting factor deficiency. Treatment of some coagulation disorders; 10 mL/kg of FFP raises factor levels by a maximum of 25%

Contd...

Blood Components and Indications for Use				
Component	Composition	Volume	Storage	Indications and expected benefit
Cryoprecipitate (antihemophilic factor)	Fibrinogen; factors VIII and XIII; von Willebrand factor	15 mL	-30 °C	MC use in Hypofibrinogenemia (<100 mg/dl) (1 unit/5 kg raises fibrinogen 70 mg/dl). Also used for factor XIII replacement (now not first-choice therapy for hemophilia A), von Willebrand disease, topical fibrin sealant

14. Match the following anti-fungal drugs with their mechanism of action

	Column A		Column B
1	Flucytosine	a	Inhibit glycan synthesis by inhibiting beta 1,3 glycan synthase
2	Azoles	b	Impair barrier mechanism in cell membrane
3	Polyenes	c	Inhibit lanosterol alpha demethylase thereby preventing ergosterol synthesis
4	Echinocandins	d	Competitive inhibitor of squalene epoxidase
		e	Antimetabolite

Ans. 1-e, 2-c, 3-b, 4-a

Ref: KDT 7th Ed Pg 790

Mechanism of Action of Anti Fungals

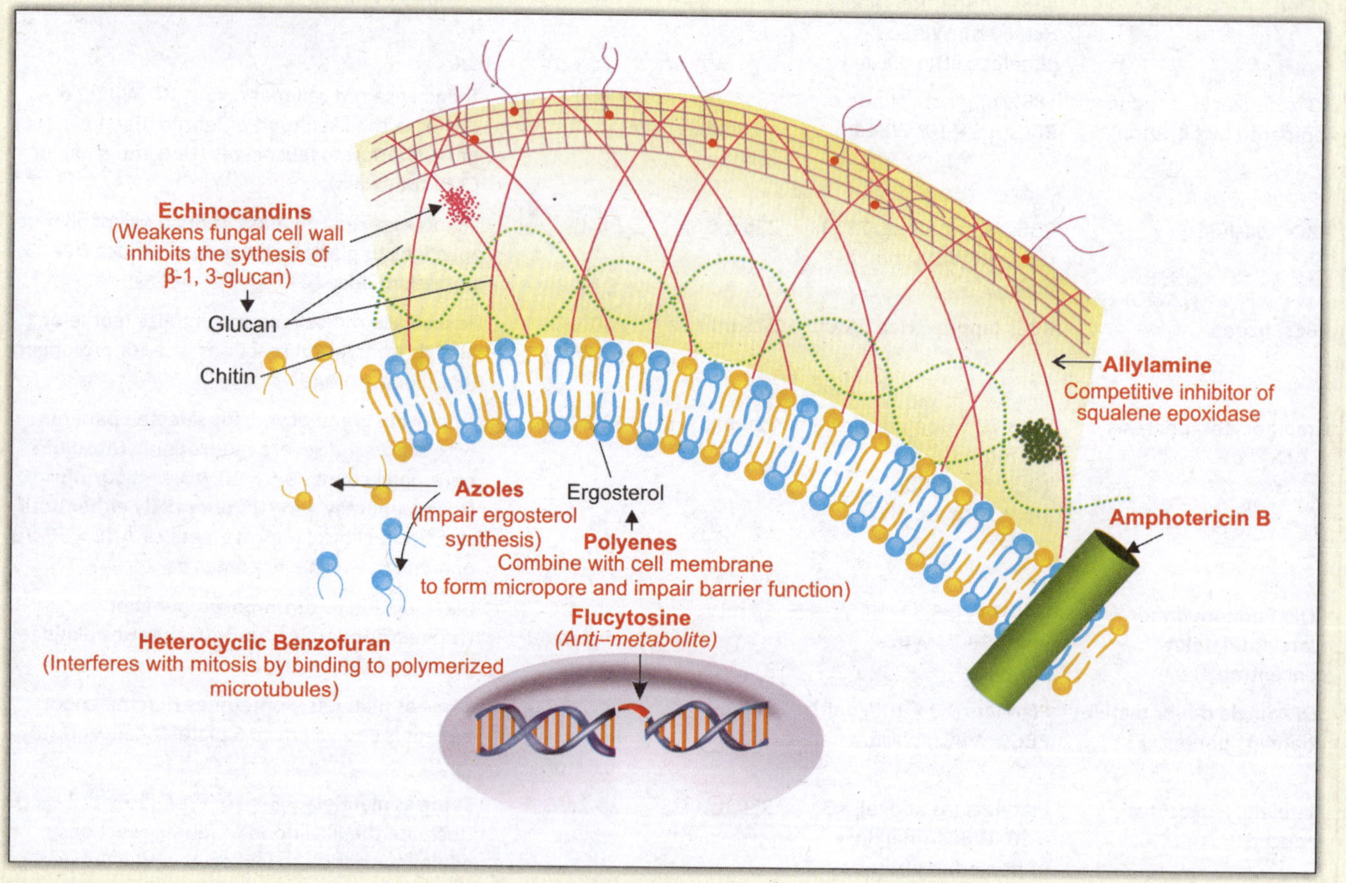

15. Match the following:

1	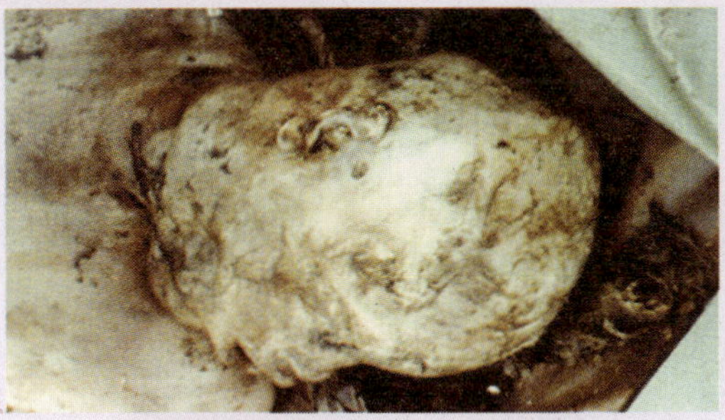	a	Marbling
2	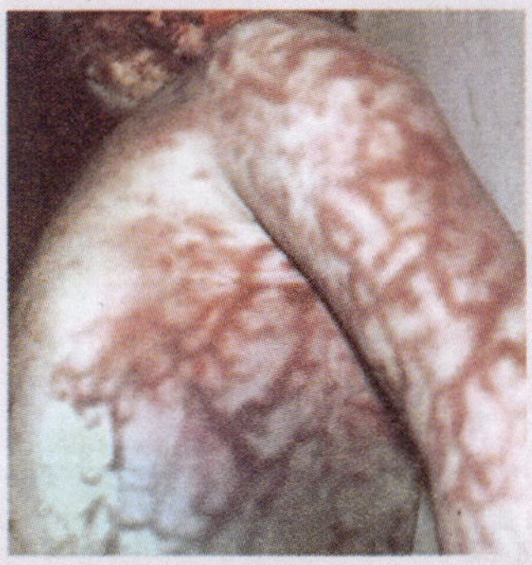	b	Mummification
3	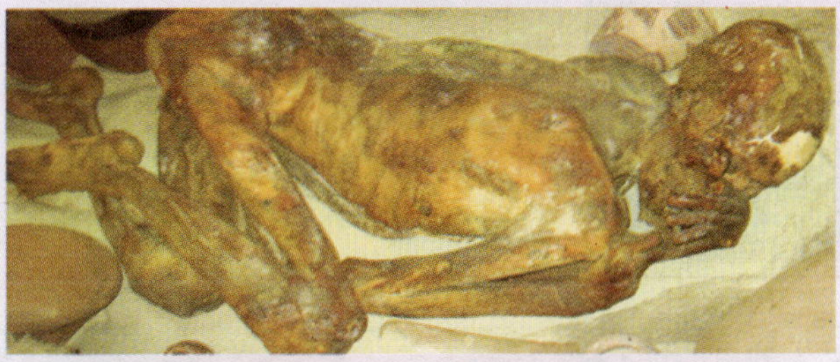	c	Postmortem Lividity
4	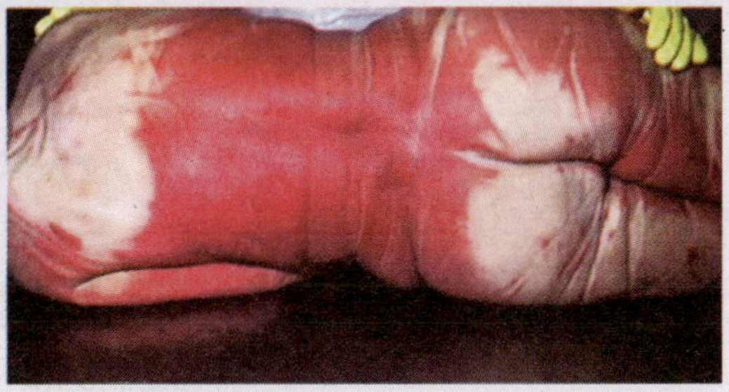	d	Adipocere
		e	Rigor mortis

Ans. 1-d, 2-a, 3-b, 4-c

Ref: Gautam Biswas 3rd Ed Pg 151

1	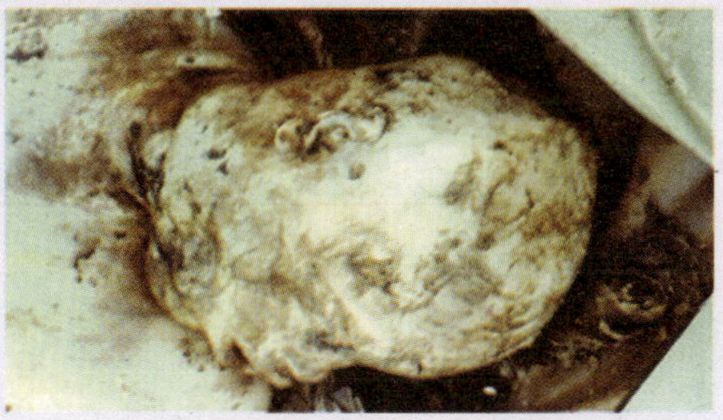	d	**Adipocere**

Contd...

2	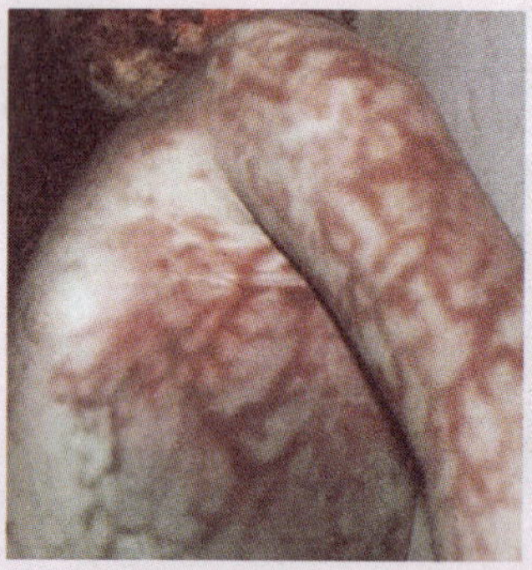	a	Marbling
3	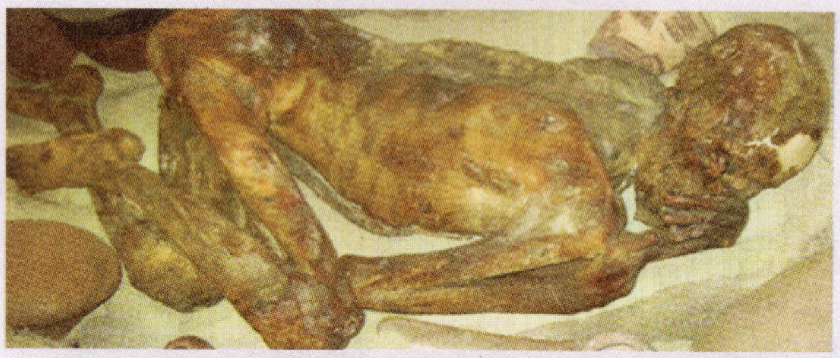	b	Mummification
4	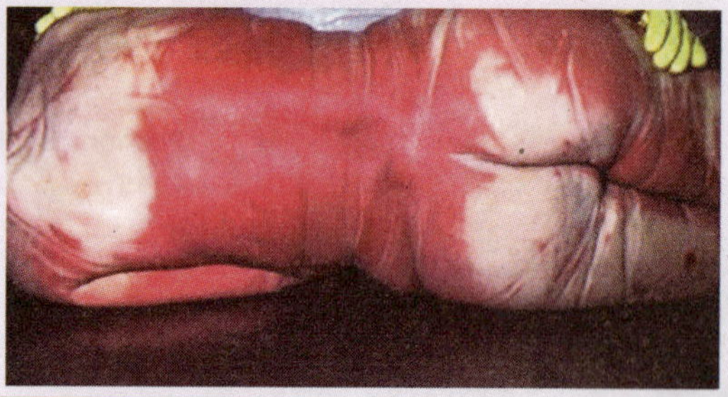	c	Postmortem Lividity

- **Adipocere:** Conversion of fatty tissues into fatty acids. Rancid smell. Gains moisture and undergo hydrolysis. Ideal conditions are warm temperature, moisture, (hot and humid) less air, bacteria, and fat splitting enzymes. Time required = 1 week (5-15 days)
- **Marbling:** Decomposition of hemoglobin to sulphmethemoglobin in the blood vessels causes a greenish or reddish-brown staining of the inner walls of the superficial vessels. This is seen as linear branching patterns, which gives a **'marbled' ('road map')** appearance of the skin. Marbling commences after 24 hours. In summers, 'marbling' is seen in 36–48 hours after death.
- **Mummification:** Dehydration or desiccation. Odorless. Ideal conditions are High temperature, dry condition, and free circulation of air 3–12 months.
- **Postmortem Lividity:** Livor mortis has been variously named as postmortem hypostasis, postmortem lividity, postmortem staining, suggillations, vibices, and so on.
- **Rigor mortis:** Rigor mortis (Latin, stiffness of death) is that state of the muscles in a dead body when they become stiff or rigid with some degree of shortening.

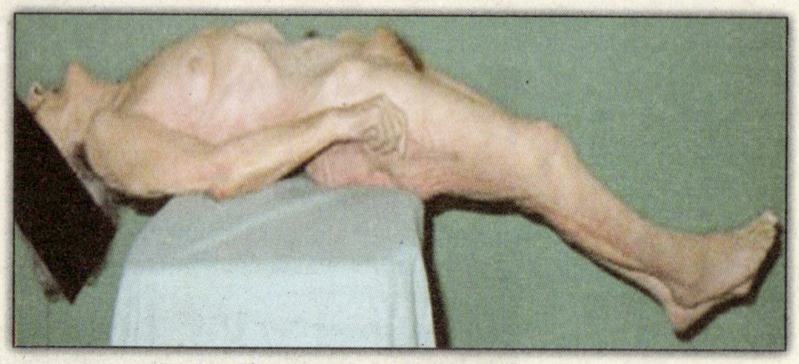

Fig: Rigor mortis

16. Match the techniques of tonsillectomy with their basic classification:

	Column A		Column B
1.	Hot intracapsular	a.	Megadebrider
2.	Hot extracapsular	b.	Laser
3.	Cold Intracapsular	c.	Bipolar cautery
4.	Cold extracapsular	d.	Microdebrider
		e.	Cold knife

Ans. 1- b, 2- c, 3 - d, 4 - e

Ref: Scott Brown 7th ed page 3576, Dhingra 6th ed page 430

Types And Techniques of Tonsillectomy

- The techniques of Tonsillectomy can be broadly divided into 2 major categories: extracapsular (total tonsillectomy, subcapsular) and intracapsular (partial tonsillectomy). Intracapsular is also known as "subtotal,"
- The traditional technique of 'cold' dissection/ Cold steel dissection was introduced about one hundred years ago. In this technique, the tonsils are dissected with metal instruments by blunt dissection. Any subsequent bleeding may be controlled by packing the tonsillar fossae with gauze dressings or ligating bleeding vessels.
- About 40 years ago, diathermy techniques were first introduced. In the last two decades, use of these 'hot' techniques has increased dramatically in routine practice and diathermy is now the most frequently used method
- Extracapsular tonsillectomy involves dissecting lateral to the tonsil in the plane between the tonsillar capsule and the pharyngeal musculature, and the tonsil is generally removed as a single unit. Partial tonsillectomy, or tonsillotomy, involves removal of most of the tonsil, while preserving a rim of lymphoid tissue and tonsillar capsule in the most recent iteration of this older technique. Preservation of this margin of tissue, this "biologic dressing," may promote an easier recovery, with lower hemorrhage rates and better recovery of diet and activity reported in comparison with traditional monopolar tonsillectomy techniques

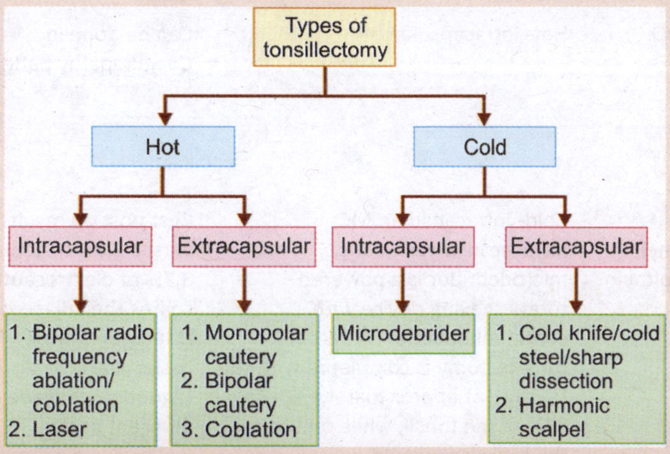

Technique	Type	Advantages	Disadvantages
Cold knife/Cold steel/Sharp dissection (with ligature or cautery) Historically most commonly used method, Gold standard (6 fold increase in use from 2002–2007 (2.7– 15.9%) by ASPO survey (84% academic settings)	Cold- Extracapsular: In this technique, the tonsil and capsule are dissected from surrounding tissue using scissors, knife, or t dissector and the inferior pole is amputated with a tonsil snare.	Low post OP pain (Higher side with cautery) , Low secondary hemorrhage risk (Higher side with cautery)	Higher intraop blood loss (lesser in cautery) Long operative time (shorter in cautery)
Monopolar electrocautery (53% use Cumming's)	Hot- Extracapsular: Lately Most common and most popular technique worldwide	Quick operative time , Minimal intraoperative bleeding	High risk of secondary hemorrhage, Longer recovery, Higher Post OP pain
Bipolar electrocautery (6% use Cumming's)	Hot- Extracapsular	Minimal intraoperative bleeding, Limited post OP morbidity	Longer operative time, Higher secondary hemorrhage rate.

Contd...

Harmonic scalpel (ASPO survey: 1/113 respondents, i.e.< 1% use)	Cold-Extracapsular: uses ultrasonic energy to vibrate its blade at 55 kHz/second. The vibration transfers energy to the tissue, providing simultaneous cutting and coagulation	Less tissue damage, Less postoperative pain compared to cautery, No additional instrument is needed for haemostasis	Long operative time, Variable intraoperative hemostasis
Bipolar radiofrequency ablation (AKA- Cold ablation or Coblation or coagulation wand or conduction wand, PlasmaBlade). 2nd most common method (16% use Cumming's)	Hot- Intracapsular (MC)> Extracapsular: Radiofrequency bipolar current is conducted across the electrodes across the tip of the conduction wand. Conductive saline solution is converted into an ionized plasma layer, resulting in molecular dissociation with minimal thermal energy transfer. Best technique in terms of results	The heat generated varies from 40-80°C, much lower than that of electro cautery 400-600°C Relatively quick operative time, Minimal intraoperative bleeding, mixed post op morbidity results. Haemostasis can usually be performed with the coblation wand alone. Suction is built in the want itself.	Mixed post op morbidity results, High secondary hemorrhage rates
Laser KTP 512 > CO_2 (ASPO survey 2007: Use 0/120 respondents)	Hot- Intracapsular:	Can be done in Coagulopathy patient	Anterior pillar must be sacrificed. Use is practically limited to patients with coagulopathies or hypertension
Microdebrider (Powered intracapsular tonsillectomy) introduced by Dr Peter Koltai in 2003 ASPO survey 2007: –27% use for obstructive indication –11% use for infection as primary indication	Cold- Intracapsular: MC intracapsular technique. microdebrider is a powered rotary shaving device with continuous suction, A partial tonsillectomy is completed with the removal of approximately 90% to 95% of the tonsil, while preserving the tonsillar capsule.	Best post op results (0.7% versus 2.8% of coblation and 3.1% of electrocautery, It spares the adjacent mucosa (Mucosal sparing), Removes tissue real fast, Visualization is good since blade comes in different angles	Technically more difficult.

Footnote:

- Either extracapsular or intracapsular tonsillectomy can be performed for the pediatric patient with obstructive sleep apnea, but intracapsular tonsillectomy is preferred in debulking in OSA and only extracapsular techniques should be used for patients undergoing tonsillectomy as a result of tonsillitis or peritonsillar abscess.
- Intracapsular approach is superior to Extracapsular approach in terms of superior recovery outcomes. Intracapsular approach causes less intraoperative and Secondary hemorrhage because intracapsular resection is being performed distal to the arborization of primary tonsillar blood vessel, exposing only its branches.
- Hot technique had a postoperative haemorrhage rate that was at least three times as high as cold steel tonsillectomy without the use of a 'hot' technique, however intraoperative blood loss was far less compared to cold technique
- Extracapsular (also known as total tonsillectomy) best technique is coblation
- Most commonly used technique is Monopolar cautery (53%) > Coblation (16%) > Cold dissection combined with electrocautery (10%) > Bipolar electrocautery (6%)
- Least commonly used techniques are: Laser > Harmonic scalpel
- Frequency of use of Intracapsular also known as subtotal tonsillectomy: Microdebrider or powered instrument or shaver> bipolar radiofrequency ablation > Carbon dioxide laser

17. Match the types of collagen with the location of their occurrence:

	Column A		Column B
1	Type II	a.	Skin
2	Type VII	b.	Hyaline cartilage
3	Type I	c.	Basal lamina of glomeruli
4	Type IV	d.	Anchoring of eye fibrils
		e.	Placenta

Ans. **1-b, 2- d, 3-a, 4-c**

Ref: Ross's Histology 6th Edition pg 165, 166

Types of Collagen and Their Location

Type of collagen	Location
I	Skin, Bone, Tendon, Ligaments, Dentin, sclera, Fascia and organ capsules
II	Cartilage (hyaline and elastic) , Notochord, Intervertebral disc
III	Loose connective tissue and organs , Smooth muscle , Endometrium, Blood vessels , foetal skin
IV	Basal lamina of epithelia, kidney glomeruli, Lung capsule
V	Distributed uniformly throughout connective tissue stroma
VI	Cartilage matrix immediately surrounding the chondrocytes
VII	Anchoring fibrils of skin, eye, uterus, and esophagus
VIII	Product of endothelial cells
IX	Cartilage associated with type II collagen fibrils
X	Chondrocytes in the zone of hypertrophy of normal growth plate
XI	Produced by chondrocytes; associated with type II collagen fibrils, forms core of type I collagen fibrils
XII	Skin and placenta
XIII	An unusual transmembrane collagen detected in bone, cartilage, intestine, skin, placenta, and striated muscles

Contd...

18. Match the following:

	Column A		Column B
1	Protein	a	Northern blot
2	RNA	b	Eastern- Western blot
3	DNA	c	Southern blot
4	Post-translational modification	d	Far Eastern blot
		e	Eastern blot
		f	Western blot

Ans. **1-f, 2-a, 3-c, 4-e**

Ref: Harper's 30th Ed page 457

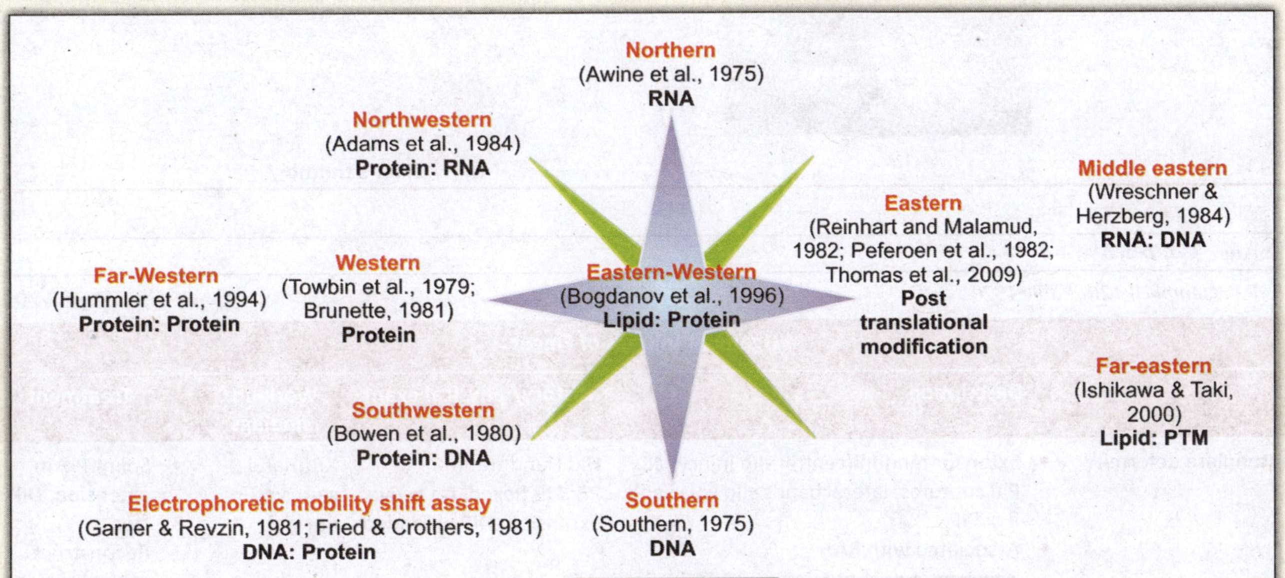

Blotting compass

19. Match the deformities with their image

Column A		Column B	
1	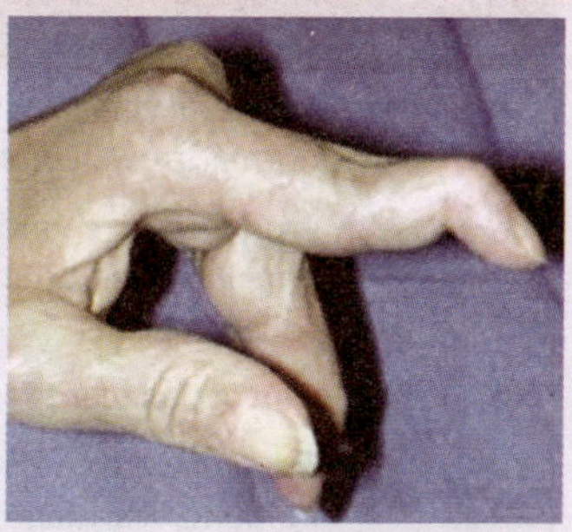	a	**Boutonniere Deformity**
2	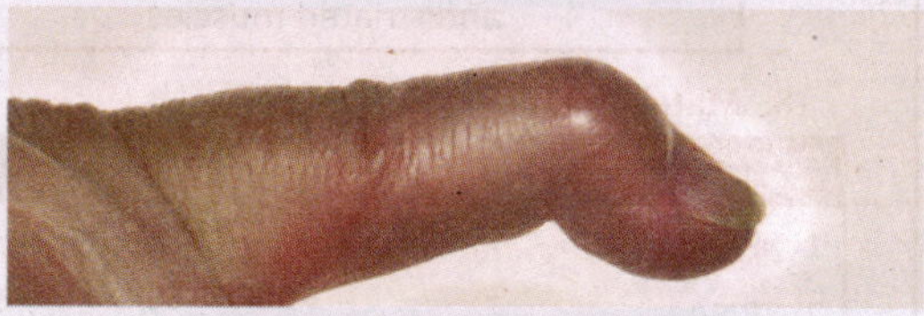	b	**Mallet finger**
3	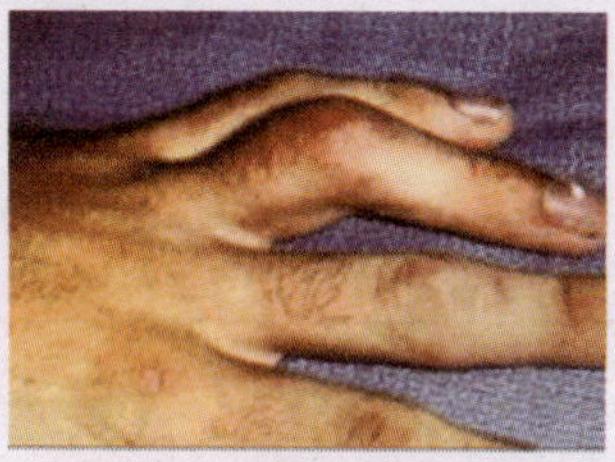	c	**Jersey Finger**
4	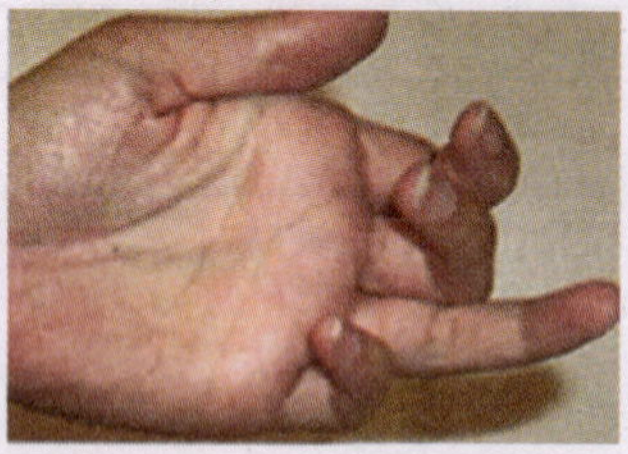	d	**Swan neck deformity**
		e	**Skier's thumb**

Ans. 1-d, 2-b, 3-a, 4-c

Ref: Campbell 12th Ed Pg 1370

Ligament Injuries of Finger				
	Description	History/ physical exam	Work-up/ findings	Treatment
Boutonniere deformity	• Extensor tendon (central slip injury) at PIP ruptures, lateral bands slip volar and flex PIP • Associated with RA 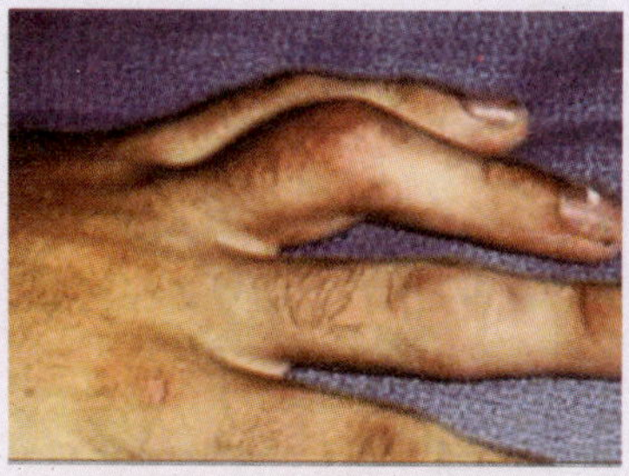	**Hx:** Hand trauma PE: PIP flexed, no active extension, DIP extended	**XR:** Hand series: normal	• Splint PIP in extension, DIP free • Reconstruct central slip and bands • **Severe:** fusion or arthroplasty

Contd...

Ligament Injuries of Finger

	Description	History/ physical exam	Work-up/ findings	Treatment
Jersey finger	Flexor digitorum profundus (FDP) tendon injury by forceful extension on a flexed digit, typically in an athlete grabbing opponent's jersey. (also called a Zone 1 Flexor tendon injury). Occur mostly in rugby/ football. Occurs most commonly in the ring finger (75%). 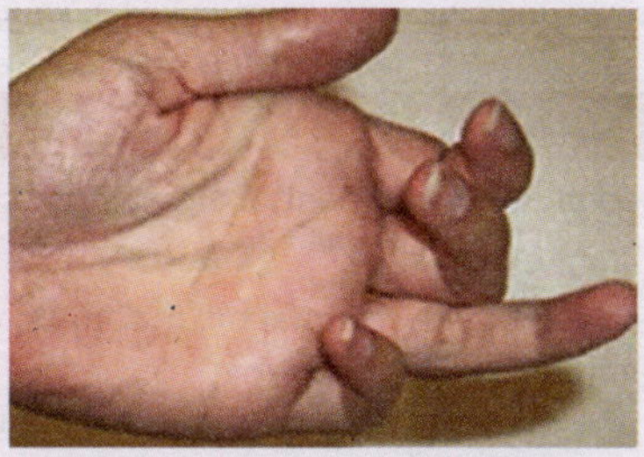	**Hx:** Extension injury, 1/2 pain. PE: FDS: 1 sublimus test FDP: 1 profundus test	**XR:** Rule out fracture (1/2 avulsion fracture)	• Primary repair • Older patient: DIP fusion
Mallet finger	**AKA: baseball, dropped, dolphin finger** • Hyperflexion Extensor digitorum tendon injury of the fingers at DIP • FDP unopposed so DIP flexes	**H/O:** Hyperflexion injury of Extensor digitorum, usually occurs when a ball, while being caught, hits an outstretched finger **Exm:** Cannot extend DIP, minimal pain and swelling, hyperextended PIP Jt	X Ray: 1/2 avulsion fracture	• **Constant splint** (DIP only) for 8 weeks followed by 4 wks night only splint • Operative treatment is considered only if there is a large fragment (>50%) and subluxation of DIP.
Swan neck deformity	• FDS rupture/volar plate injury • Lateral bands subluxes dorsally, PIP hyperextends and DIP flexes 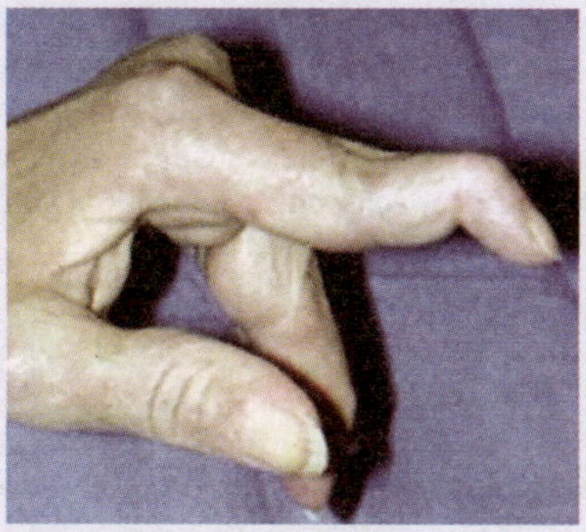	**Hx:** Trauma, RA, spastic **PE:** PIP hyperextended, DIP flexed	XR: Hand series	• **Early:** Splint • **Late:** Surgical repair (individualize each case)
Gamekeeper's thumb	• **AKA; SKIER'S THUMB** • Ulnar collateral ligament tear of the thumb metacarpo phalangeal joint • **Mechanism:** forceful radial deviation or fall on extended thumb causing hyperabduction 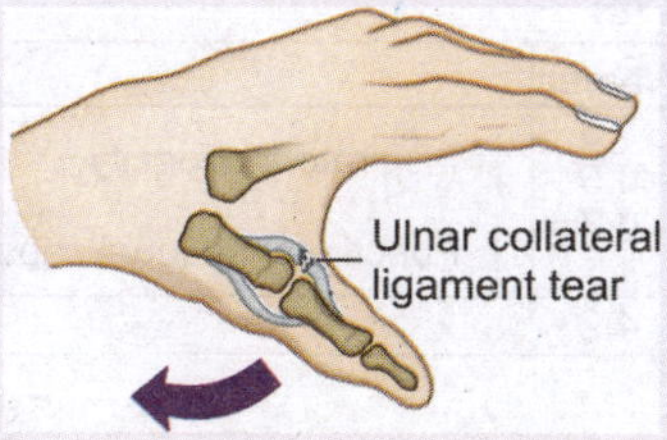	**H/O:** Trauma. Pain and swelling. EXM: partial rupture: only the ligament proper is torn and the thumb is unstable in flexion but stable in full extension because the palmar plate is intact. complete rupture, both ligament proper and palmar plate are torn and thumb is unstable in all positions	**XR:** 1/2 avulsion fracture. Stress view shows injury	• **Incomplete:** splint 2-4 weeks, avoid pinch for 6-8 weeks • **Complete:** surgical repair (treat Stener lesion; proximal end of torn ligament gets trapped in front of the adductor pollicis aponeurosis)

20. Match the lung capacities with their components

	Column A		Column B
1	Inspiratory capacity	a	Expiratory reserve volume + Residual volume
2	Vital capacity	b	Inspiratory reserve volume + tidal volume + expiratory reserve volume + residual volume.
3	Functional residual capacity	c	Tidal volume + Inspiratory reserve volume
4	Total lung capacity	d	inspiratory reserve volume + tidal volume + expiratory reserve volume
		e	Volume of gas that can be moved into and out of the lungs in 1 min

Ans. 1- c, 2- d, 3- a, 4- b

Ref: Ganong 24th ed page 629

Pulmonary Volumes and Capacities

A simple method for studying pulmonary ventilation is to record the volume movement of air into and out of the lungs, a process called **spirometry.**

Pulmonary Volumes	There are four pulmonary lung volumes that, when added together, equal the maximum volume to which the lungs can be expanded. The significance of each of these volumes is the following: • **The tidal volume** is the volume of air inspired or expired with each normal breath; it amounts to about 500 milliliters in the adult male. • **The inspiratory reserve volume** is the extra volume of air that can be inspired over and above the normal tidal volume when the person inspires with full force; it is usually equal to about 3000 milliliters. • **The expiratory reserve volume** is the maximum extra volume of air that can be expired by forceful expiration after the end of a normal tidal expiration; this normally amounts to about 1100 milliliters. • **The residual volume** is the volume of air remaining in the lungs after the most forceful expiration; this volume averages about 1200 milliliters.
Pulmonary Capacities	In describing events in the pulmonary cycle, it is sometimes desirable to consider two or more of the volumes together. Such combinations are called pulmonary capacities. Important pulmonary capacities can be described as follows: • **The inspiratory capacity** equals the tidal volume plus the inspiratory reserve volume. This is the amount of air (about 3500 milliliters) a person can breathe in, beginning at the normal expiratory level and distending the lungs to the maximum amount. • **The functional residual capacity** equals the expiratory reserve volume plus the residual volume. This is the amount of air that remains in the lungs at the end of normal expiration (about 2300 milliliters). • **The vital capacity** equals the inspiratory reserve volume plus the tidal volume plus the expiratory reserve volume. This is the maximum amount of air a person can expel from the lungs after first filling the lungs to their maximum extent and then expiring to the maximum extent (about 4600 milliliters). • **The total lung capacity** is the maximum volume to which the lungs can be expanded with the greatest possible effort (about 5800 milliliters); it is equal to the vital capacity plus the residual volume.

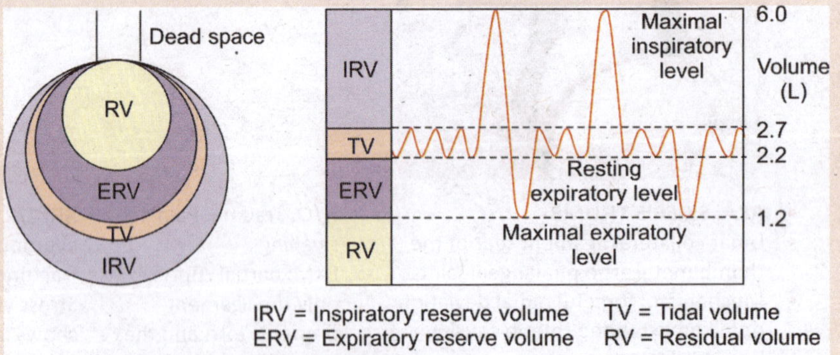

		Volume (L) Men	Women	
Vital capacity	IRV	3.3	1.9	Inspiratory capacity
	TV	0.5	0.5	
	ERV	1.0	0.7	Functional residual capacity
	RV	1.2	1.1	
Total lung capacity		6.0	4.2	

Contd...

Pulmonary Volumes and Capacities

Footnote:

- All pulmonary volumes and capacities are about 20 to 25 percent less in women than in men
- The amount of air inspired per minute **(pulmonary ventilation, respiratory minute volume)** is normally about 6 L (500 mL/ breath x 12 breaths/min).
- The **maximal voluntary ventilation (MVV)** is the largest volume of gas that can be moved into and out of the lungs in 1 min by voluntary effort. The normal MVV is 125 to 170 L/min
- The **spirometer cannot be used in a direct way to measure the functional residual capacity**, because the air in the residual volume of the lungs cannot be expired into the spirometer, and this volume constitutes about one half of the functional residual capacity. To measure functional residual capacity, the spirometer must be used in an indirect manner, usually by means of a **helium dilution method**

VARIANT 4. SEQUENTIAL ARRANGEMENT TYPE

Each question shall have a list of items that need to be arranged sequentially or in order as indicated.

21. Arrange the following events in leukocyte migration in order of occurrence.

a. Rolling
b. Stable adhesion
c. Activation of integrins
d. Transmigration

Ans. (a) Rolling, (c) Activation of Integrins, (b) Stable Adhesion, (d) Transmigration

Ref: Robin's 9th Ed Pg 35

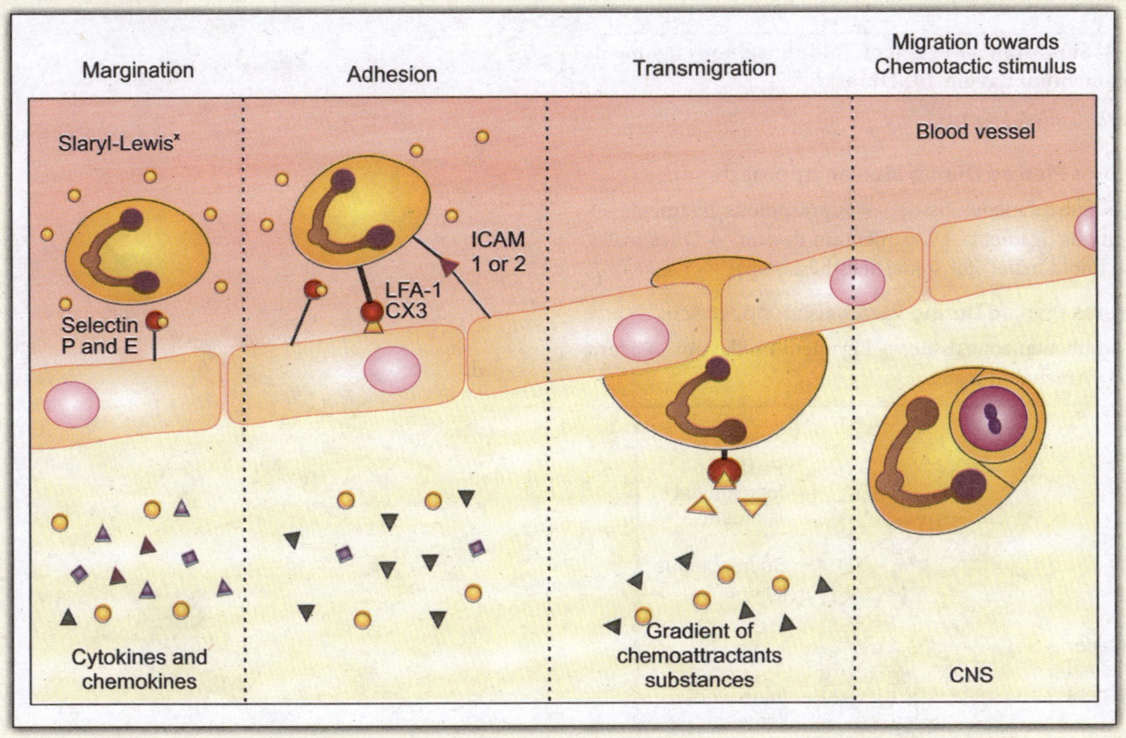

Leukocyte migration

22. Arrange the following symptoms of Lignocaine toxicity in order of appearance with increasing serum level of lignocaine

a. Muscular twitching
b. Perioral numbness
c. Tinnitus
d. Coma
e. Respiratory depression

Ans. (b) Perioral numbness, (c) Tinnitus, (a) Muscular twitching, (d) Coma, (e) Respiratory depression

Ref: Miller's 8th Ed Pg 1047

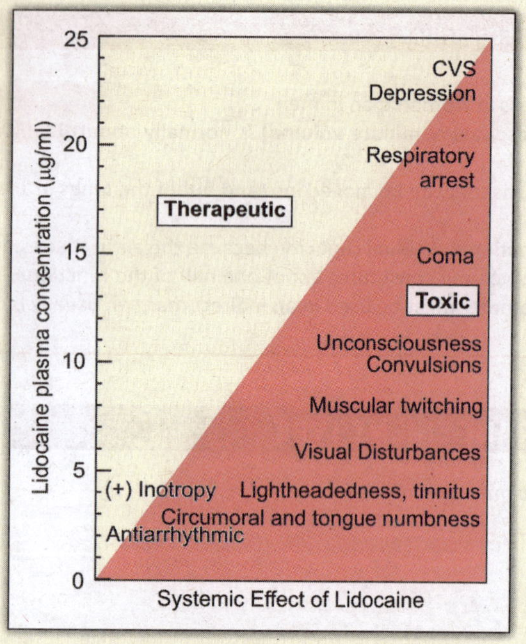

23. Arrange the following structures in order of penetration while inserting a spinal needle by median approach.

a. Ligamentum flavum b. Interspinous ligament
c. Supraspinous ligament d. Dura

Ans. (c) Supraspinous ligament, (b) Interspinous ligament, (a) Ligamentum flavum, (d) Dura

Ref: Miller's 8th Ed Pg 1685

Structures Pierced During Median Approach:

Skin → Subcutaneous tissue → Supraspinous ligaments → Interspinous ligament → Ligamentum flavum → Dura mater → Arachnoid mater (for spinal anesthesia/tap)

Structures Pierced During Paramedian Approach:

Skin → Subcutaneous tissue → Ligamentum flavum → Dura mater → Arachnoid mater

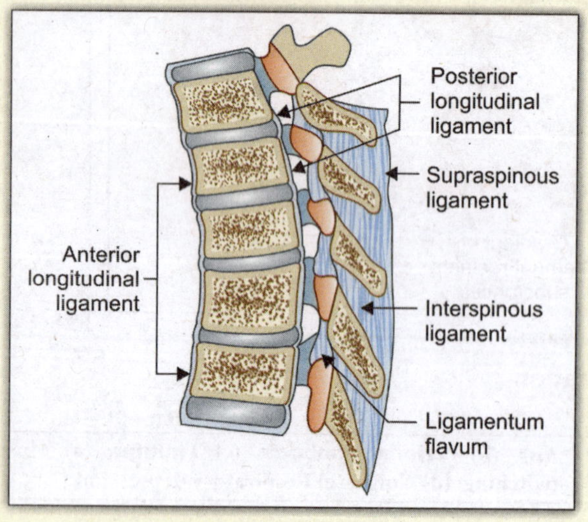

24. Arrange the following cannulae in order of increasing size of the lumen from smallest to largest lumen.

a.

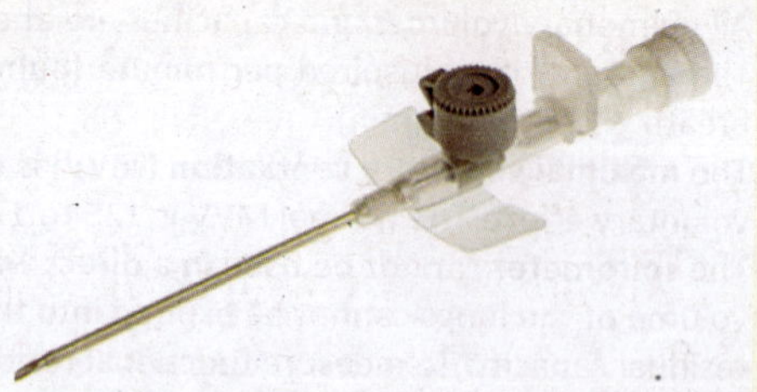

b.

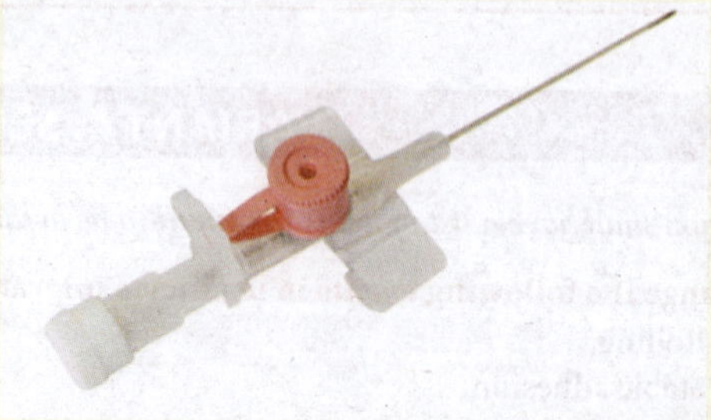

c.

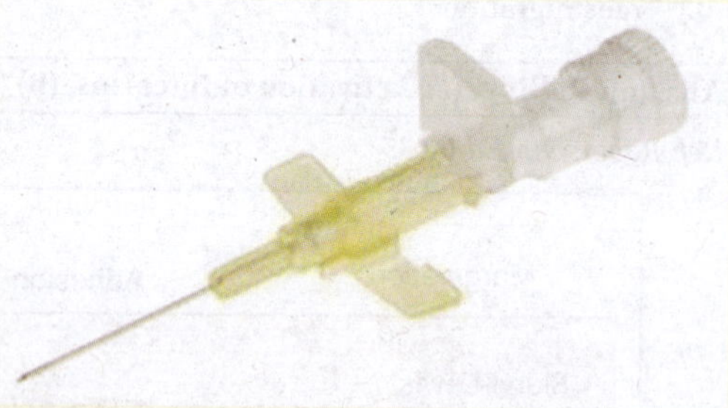

d.

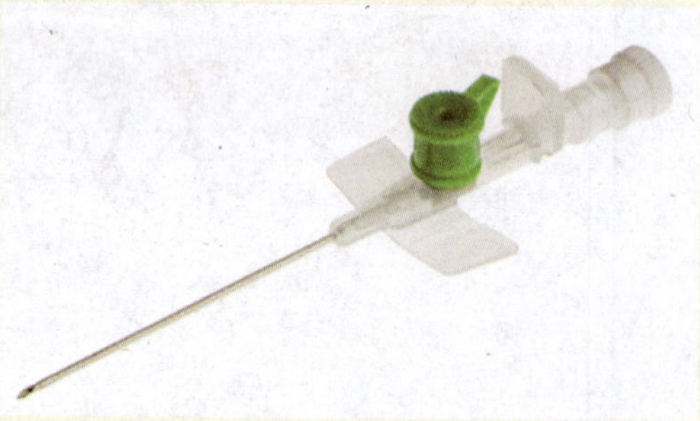

e.

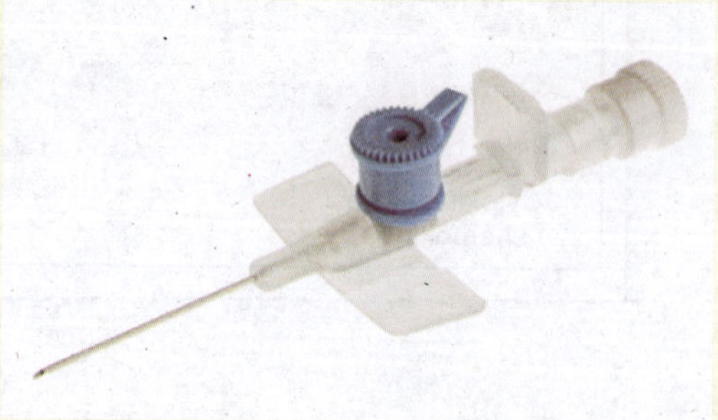

Ans. c, e, b, d, a

Cannula Sizes And Color Codes					
Color code	**Gauge (G)**	**External Dia (mm)**	**Length (mm)**	**Flow rate (mL/min)**	**Uses**
Red	14	2.2	32	325	For emergency use (e.g: shock)
Grey	16	1.7	50	196	For use in large blood transfusions and emergency use (Shock)
Green	18	1.3	45	96	Suitable for IV fluids and smaller blood transfusions
Pink	20	1.1	33	61	Suitable for the majority of patients that require IV fluids
Blue	22	0.9	25	36	For difficult hand veins - elderly patients with fragile veins. May be used in slightly older children
Yellow	24	0.7	19	22	Used commonly in pediatric patients

Size and flow data may vary to some extent with the manufacturer

25. Arrange the following muscles in order of appearance of rigor mortis:

a. Neck
b. Eyelids
c. Abdomen
d. Fingers
e. Facial muscles

Ans. (b) Eyelids, (e) Facial muscles, (a) Neck, (c) Abdomen, (d) Fingers

Ref: Gautam Biswas 3rd ed page 143, APC Essentials of Forensic Medicine and Toxicology By Anil Aggrawal 1st ed page 124

Nysten's law: After French Pathologist Pierre Hubert Nysten who proposed the law in 1811. It is applicable to voluntary muscles only. It states that the muscles closest to the brain goes into Rigor mortis first and those which are farthest goes into Rigor mortis last. Hence it is also known as *Proximodistal progression of Rigor Mortis*. This it appears in the order of (Mnemonic- in the multiples of 3)

- Eyelids (orbicularis oculi) [2 hrs]
- *Jaw first and then facial muscles* [3 hrs] (since temporalis and masseter are placed high on face but effect is seen on jaw so jaw shows RM first and then facial muscles)
- Neck, Thorax [4-5 hrs]
- Upper limb (from shoulder to the hand) [6 hrs]
- Abdomen, lower limb (from the hip to the foot) [9 hrs]
- Small muscles of fingers and toes [12 hrs]

26. Arrange the following Colors of vacutainers in order of draw during blood collection:

a. Red
b. Black
c. Light blue
d. Grey
e. Lavender
f. Pink

Ans. (c) Light blue, (b) Black, (a) Red, (e) Lavender, (f) Pink, (d) Grey

Ref: Wintrobe's 12th ed page 1, Dacie and lewis practical hematology 10th ed page 7

MNEMONIC Order of draw (Brackets): Blood culture packs (Read Sterile for Mnemonic), Followed by Light blue, Black, Red, Yellow, Green, Lavender, Pink, Grey

(Stupid Boys Bravely Read, Yet Get Low and Poor Grades)

Blood Collection System (Vacutainer System)					
	Color code	**Additive**	**Blood draw**	**Mixing**	**Clinical use**
Serum blood collection tubes	Yellow/ Golden (4)	Plain, No additive, Serum Separator Tube (SST) contains clot activator with gel separator at the bottom to separate blood from serum on centrifugation	4 mL 6 mL	5 times	Serum biochemistry, Dug monitoring, Serum immunology
	Red	Plain, No additive, clot activator (Blood clots and serum is separated by centrifugation)	4 mL 4 mL 6 mL	5 times for plastic tubes, no mixing for glass tubes	Serum biochemistry, Dug monitoring, Serum immunology Blood bank profiles
Whole blood collection tubes	Lavender (6)	EDTA Liquid (Form calcium salts to remove calcium)	2 mL	8-10 times	Haematology (FBC), Blood Bank (Cross Match); gently invert bottle after filling to prevent clotting and platelet clumping

Contd...

Blood Collection System (Vacutainer System)					
	Color code	Additive	Blood draw	Mixing	Clinical use
	Pink (7)	EDTA	2 mL	8-10 times	Blood grouping, cross matching, Direct combs test, Antenatal grouping
	Black (2)	Sodium citrate ESR	2 mL	8-10 times gently	Erythrocyte sedimentation rates
Plasma blood collection tubes	Grey (8)	Sodium Fluoride + potassium oxalate (Antiglycolytic agent preserves glucose up to 5 days)	2 mL	8- 10 times	For Glucose levels (Blood sugar)
	Light blue (1)	Buffered Sodium Citrate 3.2% (Form calcium salts to remove calcium) studies (9 volume of blood added to 1 volume of 10^9 mmol/L sodium citrate solution)	2 mL	3-4 times	Coagulation test (INR), Full draw required
	Green (5)	Plasma Separating Tube (PST) with Lithium Heparin (Anticoagulates with lithium heparin; Plasma is separated with PST gel at the bottom of the tube)	2 mL	8 10 times	Cytogenetics (chromosome studies), carboxy Hb, MethHb

MNEMONIC Order of draw (Brackets): Blood culture packs (Read Sterile for Mnemonic), Followed by Light blue, Black, Red, Yellow, Green, Lavender, Pink, Grey
(Stupid Boys Bravely Read, Yet Get Low and Poor Grades)

Anticoagulants Used for Blood and their Uses	
Sodium fluoride	Estimation of glucose since it inhibits enolase
Double oxalate	Used where vol of RBC is preserved like ESR , PCV
Sodium citrate	Coagulation studies and ESR by westergren's method
EDTA	EDTA is the preferred anticoagulant for blood counts because it produces complete anticoagulation with minimal morphologic and physical effects on cells
Heparin	Heparin is often used for red cell testing, osmotic fragility testing, and functional or immunologic analysis of leukocytes
ESR	All except coagulation studies

27. Arrange the following layers of retina from vitreous to sclera:
  a. Rods and cones
  b. Outer plexiform layer
  c. Inner plexiform layer
  d. Outer limiting membrane
  e. Inner limiting membrane
  f. Ganglion cell layer

Ans. (e) Inner limiting membrane, (f) Ganglion cell layer, (c) Inner plexiform layer, (b) Outer plexiform layer, (d) Outer limiting membrane, (a) Rods and cones

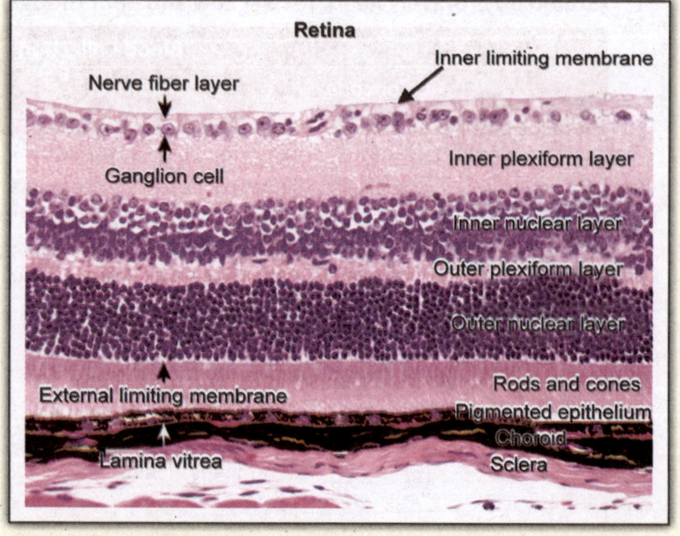

Fig: Layers of Retina (labelled). Retina consists of 3 types of cells and their synapses arranged in ten layers.

Layers of Retina		
1	Inner limiting membrane	Innermost layer of retina and is essentially a basement membrane. It separates the retina from vitreous and is formed by the union of terminal expansions of the Muller's fibers
2	Nerve fiber layer (Stratum Opticum)	Consists of axons of the ganglion cells, which pass through the lamina cribrosa to form the optic nerve.
3	Ganglion cell layer	Consists of cell bodies of ganglion cells (2nd order neurons of visual pathway). There are two types of ganglion cells. • **Midget ganglion cells** are present in the macular region and the dendrite of each such cell synapses with the axon of single bipolar cell. • **Polysynaptic ganglion cells** lie mainly in the peripheral retina and each cell may synapse with up to a hundred bipolar cells.
4	Inner Plexiform layer	Consists of connections between the axons of bipolar cells and dendrites of the ganglion cells, and processes of amacrine cells.
5	Inner Nuclear Layer	Contains cell bodies of bipolar cells (majorly), cell bodies of horizontal amacrine and Muller's cells and capillaries of central artery of retina. *The bipolar cells is the 1st order neurons of visual pathway.*
6	Outer Plexiform Layer	Consists of connections of rod spherules and cone pedicles with the dendrites of bipolar cells and horizontal cells.
7	Outer Nuclear Layer	Contains nuclei of rods and cones
8	External Limiting membrane	Fenestrated membrane, through which passes the processes of rods and cones.
9	Inner/outer segment Junction (Photoreceptor layer- Rods and Cones)	Rods and cones (photoreceptors) arranged in a palisade manner.

Photoreceptors		
	Rods	Cones
Number	120 millions	6.5 millions.
Photosensitive substance	Rhodopsin	Photopsin
Responsible for	Peripheral vision and vision of low illumination (scotopic vision).	Central vision (photopic vision) and color vision.

10	Retinal Pigment Epithelium	Outermost layer of retina. Consists of a single layer of pigment cells. Firmly adherent to the underlying basal lamina (Bruch's membrane) of choroid

Mnemonic = In New Generation Improved Interns Opt Only Externship to Rule PGME
In (Inner limiting) New (Nerve fiber layer) Generation (Ganglion layer) Improved (Inner plexiform) Interns (Inner Nuclear) Opt (Outer Plexiform) Only (Outer Nuclear) Externship (External limiting) to Rule (Rods and Cones) PGME (Pigment epithelium layer)

28. Arrange the following structures from medial to lateral:

a. Brachial artery
b. Median nerve
c. Radial nerve- deep branch
d. Biceps brachii tendon

Ans. (b) Median nerve, (a) Brachial artery, (d) Biceps brachii tendon, (c) Biceps brachii tendon

Ref: Gray's 41st Ed Pg 837

Contents of Cubital fossa

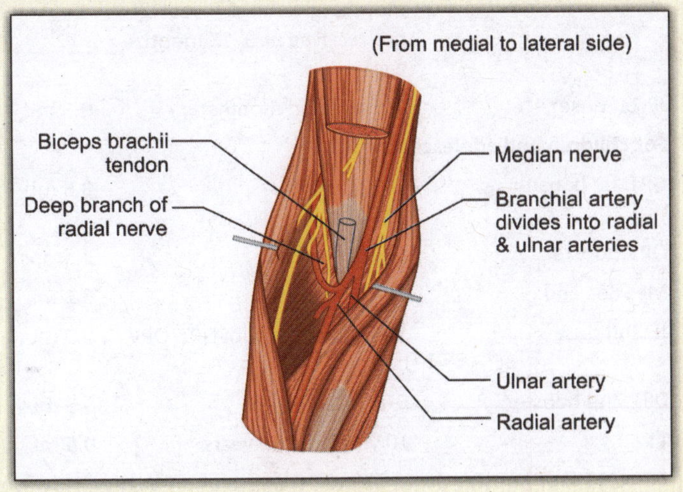

29. Arrange the following vaccines according to the recommended age of their administration:

a. MMR 1st dose b. BCG
c. HPV d. OPV 1
e. DPT 2nd booster

Ans. (b) BCG, (d) OPV 1, (a) MMR 1st dose, (e) DPT 2nd booster, (c) HPV

Ref: WHO guidelines for UIP in India, 2014

BCG → AT birth
OPV1 → 6 weeks
MMR 1st dose → 9 months
DPT 2nd booster → 5–6 years
HPV ≥ 9 years

Vaccine	When to give	Dose	Route	Site
For pregnant woman				
TT-1	Early in pregnancy	0.5 mL	Intramuscular	Upper arm
TT-2	4 weeks after TT-1*	0.5 mL	Intramuscular	Upper arm
TT-booster	If received 2 TT doses in a pregnancy within the last 3 years	0.5 mL	Intramuscular	Upper arm
For infants				
BCG	At birth or as early as possible till one year of age	0.1 mL (0.05 mL until 1 month of age)	Intra-dermal	Left upper arm
Hepatitis B birth dose	At birth or as early as possible within 24 hours	0.5 mL	Intramuscular	Anterolateral side of mid-thing
OPV zero dose	At birth as early as possible within the first 15 days	2 drops	Oral	Oral
OPV 1, 2, and 3	At 6 weeks, 10 weeks and 14 weeks	2 drops	Oral	Oral
DPT 1, 2, and 3		0.5 mL	Intramuscular	Anterolateral side of mid-thing
Hepatitis B 1, 2 and 3		0.5 mL	Intramuscular	Anterolateral side of mid-thing
Hib containing pentavalent 1, 2, and 3**		0.5	Intramuscular	Anterolateral side of mid-thing
Measles 1st dose	9 completed months 12 months (give up to 5 years if not received at 9–12 months age)	0.5 mL	Subcutaneous	Right upper arm
JE 1st dose***	9 completed months	0.5 mL	Subcutaneous	Left upper arm
For children and adolescents				
DPT 1st booster	16–24 months	0.5 mL	Intramuscular	Anterolateral side of mid-thing
OPV booster	16–24 months	2 drops	Oral	Oral
Measles 2nd	16–24 months	0.5 mL	Subcutaneous	Right upper arm
JE 2nd dose	16–24 months with DPT/OPV booster	0.5 mL	Subcutaneous	Left upper arm
DPT 2nd booster	5–6 years	0.5 mL	Intramuscular	Upper arm
TT	10 years and 16 years	0.5 mL	Intramuscular	Upper arm

*Give TT-2 or booster doses before 36 weeks of pregnancy. However, give these even if more than 36 weeks have passed. Give TT to a woman in labor, if she has not previously received TT.
**Pentavalent vaccines contains a combination of DPT, HepB and Hib. In the states where it has been introduced. It will replace DPT 1, 2 and 3 and Hepatitis B 1, 2 and 3. Hepatitis B birth dose and booster doses of DPT will continue as before.
***JE vaccine (SA 14–14–2) is given in select endemic districts, after the campaign is over in that district.
****The 2nd to 9th doses of vitamin A can be administered to children 1–5 years old during biannual rounds, in collaboration with ICDS.

30. Arrange the following clotting factors according to the number assigned to them:

a. Proaccelerin
b. Stuart- Prower factor
c. Fibrinogen
d. Proconvertin
e. Christmas factor

Ans. (c) Fibrinogen, (a) Proaccelerin, (d) Proconvertin, (e) Christmas factor, (b) Stuart- Prower factor

Ref: Robbin's 8th Ed, Ch: 4

Clotting Factors Participating in Coagulation Cascade

- Factor I - fibrinogen
- Factor II - prothrombin
- Factor III - tissue thromboplastin (tissue factor)
- Factor IV - ionized calcium (Ca^{++})
- Factor V - labile factor or proaccelerin
- Factor VI - unassigned
- Factor VII - stable factor or proconvertin
- Factor VIII - antihemophilic factor
- Factor IX - plasma thromboplastin component, Christmas factor
- Factor X - Stuart-Prower factor
- Factor XI - plasma thromboplastin antecedent
- Factor XII - Hageman factor
- Factor XIII - fibrin-stabilizing factor
- Prekallikrein - Fletcher factor
- High-molecular-weight Fitzgerald factor; HMWK kininogen (high-molecular-weight) kininogen

VARIANT 5. MULTIPLE COMPLETION TYPE

Each question/statement shall have four alternatives/statements of which one or more may be correct

31. Treatment options for a patient who developed post cataract surgery endophthalmitis after 5 days are:

1. Topical antibiotics
2. Intravenous antibiotics
3. Intravitreal antibiotics
4. Pars Plana Vitrectomy

A. Only (1) is correct
B. (1), (3), (4) are correct
C. (1), (2), (3) are correct
D. All are correct

Ans. B. (1), (3), (4) are correct

Ref: Parson 22nd ed page 235, Khurana 6th ed page 170-172

Intravenous antibiotics have no role in management of endophthalmitis. All clinical trials have shown the results are not superior of adding intravenous antibiotics in the management of Endophthalmitis.

Endophthalmitis	
Definition	Infection of uveal tissue with involvement of vitreous
Most common cause	Postoperative endophthalmitis
Postoperative Endophthalmitis	Delayed/ Post Yag: MC cause- P. acnes > Fungal MC in total- Coagulase Negative Staphylococci MC-Post traumatic- Bacillus Cereus MC cause in AIDS Patients: Candida

Contd...

Endophthalmitis	
Clinical features	• Hypopyon and anterior segment inflammation • USG posterior segment suggestive of mild to moderate amplitude spikes • Exudates and associated corneal edema can be noted • Lids and conjunctiva may be swollen • Amaurotic cat's eye reflex (yellowish white reflex) can be seen through pupil
Treatment	• Intravitreal Antibiotics • Pars plana vitrectomy • Topical Fortified Antibiotics • Cycloplegics • Antiglaucoma medications
Prevention	• Hand Scrub • Sterilization of instruments

32. Laboratory features in iron deficiency anaemia:

1. Serum Ferritin is reduced
2. Serum Iron is increased
3. Transferrin saturation is reduced
4. TIBC is reduced

A. (1) and (2) are correct
B. (3) and (4) are correct
C. (1) and (3) are correct
D. (2) and (4) are correct

Ans. C. (1) and (3) are correct

Ref: Harrison 19th ed page 628, Robbins 9th ed page 455

Total Iron binding capacity is Increased not reduced in Iron deficiency anemia. Serum Iron, Serum Ferritin and Transferrin saturation all are reduced in iron deficiency anemia

Types of Microcytic Anemia

	Iron deficiency (Sideropenic anemia)	Thalassemia	Sideroblastic anemia	Anemia of chronic disease
Peripheral smear	Microcytic hypochromic	Microcytic hypochromic	Microcytic hypochromic	Normocytic normochromic (Microcytic hypochromic can be seen)
Serum iron	Low	Normal	Normal	Low
TIBC	High	Normal	Normal	Low
Transferrin Saturation %	↓ (< 20%)	N/↑	N/↑	↓
Serum Ferritin (μg/l)	↓ (Best/most specific and sensitive marker of Fe deficiency anemia)	↑	↑ (reflects degree of iron overload)	N/↑
Hemoglobin pattern on electrophoresis	Normal	Abnormal with β thalassemia; can be normal with α thalassemia	Normal	Normal
RDW	High	Normal	High	
MCV	Normal (pre latent and latent) or low (stage 3)	Low	Low	
Bone marrow	Normoblastic		Prussian blue stain of RBC in marrow shows ringed sideroblasts.	

Footnote:

- Transferrin saturation, which is normally 25–50%, is obtained by the following formula: **serum iron x 100 ÷ TIBC**
- The serum iron level represents the amount of circulating iron bound to transferrin
- TIBC is an indirect measure of the circulating transferrin. (Hence plasma transferrin is increased in Iron deficiency anemia)
- **RDW = Red cell distribution width** is a quantitative measure of the variation in red cell size, and the higher the values, the more heterogeneous the RBC population size (i.e., anisocytosis). The upper limit of normal values for RDW is 14.6%.
- ***RDW is particularly useful in characterizing microcytic anemia***, allowing to distinguish between uncomplicated iron deficiency anemia (high RDW, normal to low MCV) and uncomplicated heterozygous thalassemia (normal RDW, low MCV)

33. Following are features of Pyrexia of unknown origin:

1. Fever persisting for more than 4 weeks
2. Two fever spikes more than 39°C
3. Undiagnosed after one week of investigation
4. No history of immunocompromised state
5. Fever persisting for more than 3 weeks

A. (1), (2), (3) are correct
B. (1), (4), (5) are correct
C. (3), (4), (5) are correct
D. All are correct

Ans. C. (3), (4), (5) are correct

REF: Harrison 19th ed page no 135

Accordingly, FUO is Now Defined as:

- Fever >38.3°C (101°F) on at least two occasions
- Illness duration of ≥3 weeks
- No known immunocompromised state
- Diagnosis that remains uncertain after a thorough history-taking, physical examination, and the following obligatory investigations:
  - Determination of erythrocyte sedimentation rate (ESR) and C-reactive protein (CRP) level
  - Platelet count
  - Leukocyte count and differential
  - Measurement of levels of hemoglobin, electrolytes, creatinine, total protein, alkaline phosphatase, alanine aminotransferase, aspartate aminotransferase, lactate dehydrogenase, creatine kinase, ferritin, antinuclear antibodies, and rheumatoid factor
  - Protein electrophoresis
  - Urinalysis
  - Blood cultures and Urine culture
  - Chest X-ray
  - Abdominal ultrasonography
  - Tuberculin skin test (TST)

34. Identify dimorphic fungi:

1. Histoplasma capsulatum
2. Penicillium marneffei
3. Pneumocystis jiroveci
4. Sporothrix schenckii

A. (1), (2), (3) are correct
B. (2), (3), (4) are correct
C. (1), (2), (4) are correct
D. (1) and (2) are correct

Ans. C. (1), (2), (4) are correct

Ref: Ananthnarayan 9th Ed Page 593

Dimorphic fungi: Fungi that have two growth forms, such as a mold and a yeast. All dimorphic fungi are yeasts in humans (molds in dirt). Human infection is by spore inhalation, so no Person-Person transmission for dimorphic fungi; **HB PSC** (use **HB** pencil in **PSC** exam)

- Histoplasma capsulatum
- Blastomycosis dermatitidis
- Paracoccidioides brasiliensis
- Penicillium marneffei
- Sporothrix schenckii
- Coccidioides immitis
- Candida albicans

35. Factors affecting fertility:

1. Vegetarian diet
2. Loss of weight
3. Gain of weight
4. Less exercise
5. Spicy food

A. All affect fertility
B. None affect fertility
C. (1), (2) (3) (4) affect fertility
D. (1) and (5) do not affect fertility

Ans. D. (1) and (5) do not affect fertility

Ref: Speroff 8th ed ch 27

Obesity decreases ovarian function. Hence loss or gain of weight affects fertility and exercise affects weight. There is no relation established between type of diet and fertility.

Lifestyle choices and environmental factors that influence fertility

- In women, obesity is associated with menstrual dysfunction, decreased fertility, and increased risks of miscarriage and obstetric and neonatal complications.
- Smoking has well-known adverse impact on pregnancy outcome, and evidence strongly suggests that fertility is lower in both men and women who smoke.
- Substance abuse such as Marijuana, Cocaine, Heavy alcohol consumption and higher levels of caffeine consumption may delay conception.
- Exposures to perchlorethylene in the dry cleaning industry, toluene in the printing business, ethylene oxide, and mixed solvents have been associated with decreased fecundity. Semen abnormalities have been described in men exposed to radiant heat or heavy metals.

Environmental exposure to herbicides or fungicides has been associated with decreased fertility in women, and exposure to pesticides and other chlorinated hydrocarbons with an increased risk of miscarriage.

36. Identify the correct statements amongst the following, regarding Antidiuretic hormone (ADH)

1. Post-operative increase in secretion
2. Neurosecretion
3. Increased secretion when plasma osmolality is low
4. Act on distal tubule and increase permeability
5. Stress decreases ADH secretion

A. (1), (2), (3) are correct
B. (1), (2), (4) are correct
C. (3) and (5) are correct
D. All are correct

Ans. B. (1), (2), (4) are correct

Ref: Ganong 24/e, p 313,698, Guyton 12/e, p 357, 375-376, 904-905

Synthesis of ADH

ADH is synthesised in the cell bodies of the supraoptic and paraventricular nuclei of hypothalamus.

The hormone is transported by supraoptic-paraventricular hypophyseal tract to the posterior pituitary. It is stored along with specific neurophysin.

Release

When a specific stimulus reaches SON and PVN, The two nuclei get excited. Impulses are conducted to terminals. Hormone along with specific neurophysin is released into the blood by exocytosis. This is preceded by Ca^{++} entry to nerve terminals. The hormone is transported to the target tissue by blood. Neurophysin acts as transport protein in the tracts.

Regulation

ADH secretion is primarily controlled by two important stimuli

1. *Plasma osmolality*
   Increased plasma osmolality above 285 mOsm/kg increase ADH proportionate to the osmolality rise. The increased osmolality is sensed by hypothalamic osmoreceptors that increases the synthesis of ADH in supraoptic and paraventricular nuclei and increases the releases of ADH from posterior pituitary.
   ADH causes water retention and brings osmolality back to normal.
2. *Blood Volume and Pressure*
   Decrease in blood pressure and blood volume stimulates ADH secretion.

Factors Affecting ADH Secretion

Factors that increase ADH secretion	Factors that decrease ADH secretion
Increased plasma osmolality	Decreased plasma osmolality
Decreased ECF Volume	Increased ECF volume
Decreased blood pressure	Decreased temperature
Angiotensin II	Cortisol
Pain, Postsurgical phase	ANP
Nausea	Thyroxine
Vomiting	α-adrenergic agonist decreases ADH secretion.
Emotion	
Hypoglycaemia	
Standing	
Increased temperature	
Stress	

Actions

- ADH acts mainly on DCT and Collecting duct of renal tubule to increase water reabsorption.
  It is secreted in case of hypovolemia, hypotension, and hyperosmolality
- Acting on blood vessels, ADH causes vasoconstriction. Thus, in higher concentration it increases blood pressure.
- ADH increases CRH release and therefore increases ACTH secretion.
- It causes glycogenolysis in liver.
- It facilitates memory by acting as neurotransmitter in memory area of brain.

37. Consider the following statements regarding Angiotensin II:

1. Decreases the release of norepinephrine
2. Causes Stimulation of thirst
3. Causes Aldosterone secretion
4. Increased ADH secretion
5. Vasodilation

A. Only (1) is correct
B. (1) and (5) are correct
C. (2), (3) (4) are correct
D. All are correct

Ans. C. (2), (3) (4) are correct

Ref: Ganong 24 ed page 704

Physiological function of Angiotensin II

Peripheral Action

- It is one of the most potent vasoconstrictors. Vasoconstriction potency is about eight times more than that of nor epinephrine.
- It increases the synthesis and secretion of aldosterone from adrenal cortex. The RAS is also called Renin – Angiotensin – Aldosterone Axis. The aldosterone increases sodium and water reabsorption from kidney that increases ECF volume
- It directly increases the release of nor epinephrine from post ganglionic sympathetic neurons. Thus, it also potentiates vasoconstriction through nor epinephrine release.
- It also causes contraction of mesangial cells. Hence decreases GFR.
- It increases sodium and water reabsorption from PCT of kidney.

Central Action

- Angiotensin II act on brain centers to decrease sensitivity of barorreflex. This potentiates the pressure effect of Angiotensin II.
- It stimulates thirst centres in the brain to increase water intake.
- It increases secretion of ADH from posterior pituitary.
- It increases the secretion of ACTH from anterior Pituitary

38. Consider the following statements:

1. **Isolation:** Splitting or separating an idea from the affect that accompanies it but is repressed
2. **Dissociation:** Temporarily but drastically modifying a person's character or one's sense of personal identity to avoid emotional distress
3. **Suppression:** Expelling or withholding from consciousness an idea or feeling.
4. **Primary repression:** Curbing of ideas and feelings before they have attained consciousness
5. **Dissociation:** Temporarily but drastically modifying a person's character or one's sense of personal identity to avoid emotional distress

A. (1), (2), (3) are correct
B. (1), (2), (4), (5) are correct
C. (3), (4), (5) are correct
D. None is correct

Ans. B. (1), (2), (4), (5) are correct

Ref: Kaplan 10th edition page 206

- **Isolation:** Splitting or separating an idea from the affect that accompanies it but is repressed
- **Repression:** Expelling or withholding from consciousness an idea or feeling. Primary repression refers to the curbing of ideas and feelings before they have attained consciousness: Secondary repression excludes from awareness what was once experienced at a conscious level. The repressed is not really forgotten in that symbolic behavior may be present. This defense differs from suppression by effecting conscious inhibition of impulses to the point of losing and not just postponing cherished goals. Conscious perception of instincts and feelings is blocked in repression.
- **Dissociation:** Temporarily but drastically modifying a person's character or one's sense of personal identity to avoid emotional distress
- **Suppression:** Consciously or semiconsciously postponing attention to a conscious impulse or conflict. Issues may be deliberately cut off, but they are not avoided. Discomfort is acknowledged but minimized.

39. Identify correct statements regarding opioid receptors:

1. Mu (μ) receptors cause analgesia by spinal and supraspinal pathways
2. Kappa receptors can cause dysphoria
3. Delta receptors are responsible for euphoria
4. All 3 receptors cause respiratory depression

A. All are correct
B. None of these statements is correct
C. (1), (2) and (4) are correct
D. (2), (3), (4) are correct

Ans. (C) (1), (2) and (4) are correct

Ref: KDT 7th ed page 479

Actions Ascribed to Different Types of Opioid Receptors

Mu (μ)	Kappa (K)	Delta (Δ)
Analgesia (supraspinal μ1 + spinal μ2) Respiratory depression μ2) Sedation Euphoria Miosis Muscular rigidity Reduced GI motility (μ2) Physical dependence (morphine type)	Analgesia (spinal K1) (Supraspinal- K3) Respiratory depression (lower ceiling) Dysphoria, psychotomimetic Miosis (lower ceiling) Sedation Physical dependence (nalorphine type) Reduced g.i. motility	Analgesia (Spinal + Affective component of supraspinal) Respiratory depression Affective behaviour Reinforcing actions Reduced g.i. motility Proconvulsant

40. Following are Unfavourable interaction of drug and substrate in human beings. Identify the correct ones:

1. Omeprazole-reducing acid secretion
2. Methotrexate inhibiting folate
3. Barbiturates-vitamin B12 absorption
4. Retinoic acid inhibits vitamin E
5. Anticonvulsant drugs inhibit hepatic microsomal enzymes

A. (1), (2),(3) are correct
B. (3), (4), (5) are correct
C. (1), (2), (4) are correct
D. (1), (2), (3) (4) are correct

Ans. C. (1), (2), (4) are correct

Ref: Medical Biochemistry - By N. V. Bhagavan 4th ed Page 904

Some examples of unfavorable drug—nutrient interactions are

- Drugs that inhibit stomach acid production (e.g., omeprazole);
- Drugs that reduce vitamin B12 absorption;
- Anticonvulsant drugs (e.g., barbiturates, phenytoin, primidone) that act by inducing hepatic microsomal enzymes which accelerate inactivation of vitamin d metabolites and aggravate osteoporosis
- Interference with folate metabolism by antifolate drugs (methotrexate) used in the treatment of some neoplastic diseases;
- And vitamin B6 metabolism affected by isoniazid, hydralazine, and d-penicillamine.

Vitamin E absorption decreases with large intake of retinoic acid

VARIANT 6. REASON ASSERTION TYPE

Each question shall have two statements: Assertion (A) and Reason (B) connected by the term "because". The appropriate answer should be marked using the following key:

1. Both Assertion and Reasons are independently true/correct statements and the Reason is the correct explanation for the Assertion
2. Both Assertion and Reasons are independently true/correct statements, but the Reason is not the correct explanation for the Assertion
3. Assertion is independently a true/correct statement, but the Reasons is independently a false/incorrect statement
4. Assertion is independently a false/incorrect statement, but the Reasons is independently a true/correct statement
5. Both Assertion and Reasons are independently false/incorrect statements

41. A patient from North eastern region comes with history of fever and body ache. Antigen test is positive for falciparum malaria.

Assertion: The presently recommended ACT in national drug policy is fixed dose combination (FDC) of Artemether-lumefantrine (AL) in north eastern states.

Reasoning: North eastern states have reported late treatment failures to combination of artesunate + sulfadoxine-pyrimethamine in P. falciparum malaria

a. Both Assertion and Reasons are independently true/ correct statements and the Reason is the correct explanation for the Assertion
b. Both Assertion and Reasons are independently true/ correct statements, but the Reason is not the correct explanation for the Assertion
c. Assertion is independently a true/correct statement, but the Reasons is independently a false/incorrect statement
d. Assertion is independently a false/incorrect statement, but the Reasons is independently a true/correct statement

Ans. a. Both Assertion and Reasons are independently true / correct statements and the Reason is the correct explanation for the Assertion

REF: Guidelines for Diagnosis and Treatment of Malaria in India 3rd Edition (National Vector Borne Disease Control Programme Delhi)

- Artemisinin Combination Therapy (ACT) should be given to all the confirmed P. falciparum cases found positive by microscopy or RDT. ACT consists of an artemisinin derivative combined with a long-acting antimalarial (amodiaquine, lumefantrine, mefloquine, piperaquine or sulfadoxine-pyrimethamine).
- In the **northeastern states** (Arunachal Pradesh, Assam, Manipur, Meghalaya, Mizoram, Nagaland, and Tripura), due to the recent reports of late treatment failures to the current combination of artesunate + sulfadoxine-pyrimethamine in P. falciparum malaria, the presently recommended ACT in national drug policy is fixed dose combination (FDC) of Artemether-lumefantrine (AL).

42. A term woman presents with non progress of labour for 15 hours and posted for C-Section.

Assertion: The woman is to be placed in a head low position on the operation table

Reasoning: By placing a wedge under the right hip, the gravid uterus will not compress the IVC

a. Both Assertion and Reasons are independently true/ correct statements and the Reason is the correct explanation for the Assertion
b. Both Assertion and Reasons are independently true/ correct statements, but the Reason is not the correct explanation for the Assertion
c. Assertion is independently a true/correct statement, but the Reasons is independently a false/incorrect statement
d. Assertion is independently a false/incorrect statement, but the Reasons is independently a true/correct statement

Ans. (d) Assertion is independently a false/incorrect statement, but the Reasons is independently a true/correct statement

Ref: Miller's 8th Ed page 2344

- The gravid uterus compresses the Inferior Vena Cava in supine position. This decreases venous return to the heart. The mother is going to be taken up for a C-section, and will require Spinal anaesthesia for conduction of the surgery.

- After administration of spinal anaesthesia, due to vasodilatation, the venous return will further fall. Moreover, there has been non progress of labor so the patient is likely to be dehydrated and exhausted.
- Under such circumstances, there will be a profound fall in BP, and decreased venous return due to gravid uterus will further complicate the above situation.
- By placing a wedge under the right hip, the gravid uterus will not compress the IVC and hypotension will not be compounded.

43. Consider the following statements about Endometriotic lesions:

Assertion: Pregnancy causes atrophy of endometriosis

Reasoning: The course of endometriosis is predominantly dependent on progesterone

a. Both Assertion and Reasons are independently true/ correct statements and the Reason is the correct explanation for the Assertion
b. Both Assertion and Reasons are independently true/ correct statements, but the Reason is not the correct explanation for the Assertion
c. Assertion is independently a true/correct statement, but the Reason is independently a false/incorrect statement
d. Both Assertion and Reasons are independently false/ incorrect statements

Ans. c. Assertion is independently a true/correct statement, but the Reason is independently a false/incorrect statement

Ref: Robbin Basic Pathology 10th edition. Page. 721, Shaw's gynaec 15th ed pg 466

Whatever the initial genesis of endometriosis, its further development depends on the presence of hormones, mainly oestrogen. Various facts proving it are

- Pregnancy causes atrophy of endometriosis chiefly through high progesterone level.
- Regression follows oophorectomy and irradiation.
- Rarely seen before puberty and it regresses after menopause.
- Hormones with antioestrogenic activity also suppress endometriosis and are used therapeutically.

44. In thyroid surgery $ETCO_2$ suddenly falls from 38 to 14. Consider the following statements:

Assertion: Venous air embolism may occur during thyroid surgery

Reasoning: Release of thyroid hormones is common during handling of thyroid gland during surgery

a. Both Assertion and Reasons are independently true/ correct statements and the Reason is the correct explanation for the Assertion
b. Both Assertion and Reasons are independently true/ correct statements, but the Reason is not the correct explanation for the Assertion
c. Assertion is independently a true/correct statement, but the Reason is independently a false/incorrect statement
d. Both Assertion and Reasons are independently false/ incorrect statements

Ans. (b) Both Assertion and Reasons are independently true/correct statements, but the Reason is not the correct explanation for the Assertion

Ref: SRB's Surgical Operations: Text and Atlas 2nd Ed By Sriram Bhat Pg 499

In the above question, there is a sudden drastic fall in ET CO_2.

- During thyroid surgery, the head end of the table is elevated to improve venous return. This reduces venous congestion in the neck and decreases oozing in the surgical field. Around 15 degree head up position can be achieved by placing pillows or towel rolls beneath the shoulder. Neck is extended.
- However, as the neck is at a higher level than the heart, there is a chance of air embolism.
- Thus, veins should be ligated securely and then cut.
- Any doubtful air in internal jugular vein should be aspirated immediately.

Changes in End-tidal Carbon Dioxide ($ETCO_2$)

Increased $ETCO_2$	Reduced $ETCO_2$
Decreased alveolar ventilation	**Increased alveolar ventilation**
• Reduced respiratory rate	• Increased respiratory rate
• Reduced tidal volume	• Increased tidal volume
• Increased equipment dead space	
Increased CO_2 production	**Reduced CO_2 production**
• Fever	• Hypothermia
• Hypercatabolic state	• Hypocatabolic state
Increased inspired pCO_2	**Increased alveolar dead space**
• Rebreathing	• Reduced cardiac output
• CO_2 absorber exhausted	• Pulmonary embolism
• External source of CO_2	• High positive end-expiratory pressure during intermittent positive-pressure ventilation
	Sampling error
	• Inadequate tidal volume
	• Water blocking sampling line
	• Air entrainment into sampling line

45. Consider the following statements about Endrin poisoning:

Assertion: Atropine can be used as an antidote

Reason: Endrin is an organophosphate

a. Both Assertion and Reasons are independently true/ correct statements and the Reason is the correct explanation for the Assertion
b. Both Assertion and Reasons are independently true/ correct statements, but the Reason is not the correct explanation for the Assertion
c. Assertion is independently a true/correct statement, but the Reason is independently a false/incorrect statement
d. Both Assertion and Reasons are independently false/ incorrect statements

Ans. (d) Both Assertion and Reasons are independently false / incorrect statements

Ref: Gautam Biswas 3rd ed page 601, KDT 7th ed page 111

Endrin is an Organochlorine Pesticide with no antidote available. Treatment is symptomatic. Parathion and TIK20 are Organophosphates. Baygon is a Carbamate. For both Organophosphate and Carbamates Atropine is the Antidote.

Pesticides Classification

Insecticides are classified into three groups: Contact poisons, stomach poisons and fumigants.

- **Contact Poisons** are those which kill insects primarily by contact e.g., pyrethrum, DDT, HCH, dieldrin.
- **Stomach Poisons** are those which when ingested cause the death of the insects, e.g., paris green, sodium fluoride.
- **Fumigants** are those which give off vapours which have a lethal effect on the insects, e.g., sulfur dioxide. This classification is by no means a rigid one, because a poison can also be a stomach poison.

Most of the present-day insecticides available for vector control (excluding inorganic chemicals and larvicidal oils) may be classified conveniently into 3 groups based on their chemical composition

- Group I: Organochlorine compounds
- Group II: Organophosphorous compounds
- Group III: Carbamates

Organophosphorous	Alkyl phosphates	TEPP: Tetra ethyl pyrophosphate HETP: Hexa ethyl tetraphosphate OMPA: Octa methyl pyrophoramide MALATHION: Killbug, Bugsoline Dimefox Isopestox
	Aryl phosphates	PARATHION: Follidol, Killphos, Ekato METHYLPARATHION: Metacide CHLORTHION DIAZION: **Tik 20** CHLORPYRIPHOS
Carbamates	ALDICARB: Temik AMINOCARB: Matacil APPROCARB: **Baygon** CARBARYL: Sevin CARBOFURAN: Furaxdan	
Organochlorides	DDT	
	BHC	GBH: Gamma benzene hexachloride LINDANE: Gamma hexa chloro cyclo hexane
	Cyclodienes	ALDRIN DIELDRIN ENDOSULFAN: Thiodan ENDRIN **(most toxic organochloride)** HEPTACHLOR: ISOBENZAN: CHLORDANE: CHLORDECONE: Kepone DECHLORANE: Mirex
	Toxaphene	
Pyrethroids	ALLETHRIN: Active ingredient of Raid IMIPROTHRIN: active ingredient of Raid Ant and Roach Killer BIFENTHRIN: Active ingredient of *Talstar, Capture, Ortho Home Defense Max* BETA-CYFLUTHRIN: Active ingredient in Baygon TRANSFLUTHRIN: Active ingredient in Baygon CYPHENOTHRIN: active ingredient of K2000 Insect spray sold in Israel	

46. Following statements about angina:

Assertion: Nitrates relieve Prinzmetal angina

Reasoning: Nitrates reduce preload

a. Both Assertion and Reasons are independently true/ correct statements and the Reason is the correct explanation for the Assertion

b. Both Assertion and Reasons are independently true/ correct statements, but the Reason is not the correct explanation for the Assertion

c. Assertion is independently a true/correct statement, but the Reason is independently a false/incorrect statement

d. Both Assertion and Reasons are independently false/ incorrect statements

Ans. (b) Both Assertion and Reasons are independently true/correct statements but the Reason is not the correct explanation for the Assertion

Ref: KDT 7th Ed Pg 541, Kaplan's Cardiac Anesthesia 6th Ed Pg 236

Nitrates relieve Prinzmetal angina primarily by causing coronary vasodilatation.

Effect Of Nitrates		
Preload	**Intracardiac**	**After load**
Preferential action at comparatively lower doses **Main mechanism of action** Venodilation → peripheral pooling of blood → decreased venous return → preload on heart is reduced → end diastolic size and pressure are reduced → decreased cardiac work according to Laplace's law → reduction in ventricular radius decreases the tension that must be generated in the ventricular Wall → decreased O2 consumption. Decrease in end diastolic pressure abolishes the subendocardial crunch by restoring the pressure gradient across ventricular wall due to which subendocardial perfusion occurs during diastole.	Main mechanism of relief **in Prinzmetal angina.** Preferentially relaxation of bigger conducting coronary arteries than arterioles or resistance vessels → Favourable redistribution of blood flow to ischaemic areas[a]	At slightly higher doses: Arteriolar dilatation → slight decrease in total peripheral resistance (t.p.r.) or afterload on heart → BP falls → contributes to the reduction in cardiac work which is directly proportional to aortic impedance
Note: [a]In ischemic zones, dilatation of autoregulatory resistance vessels increases blood flow, while in the non-ischaemic zones, resistance vessels maintain their tone → flow does not increase, or may decrease to compensate for increased flow to ischaemic zone.		

47. Following are statements regarding Antiretroviral drugs
Assertion: Zidovudine is an integrase inhibitor
Reasoning: Some drugs bind to integrase enzyme and prevent viral DNA strand transfer to host DNA

a. Both Assertion and Reasons are independently true/correct statements and the Reason is the correct explanation for the Assertion
b. Both Assertion and Reasons are independently true/correct statements, but the Reason is not the correct explanation for the Assertion
c. Assertion is independently a true/correct statement, but the Reason is independently a false/ incorrect statement
d. Assertion is independently a false/incorrect statement, but the Reasons is independently a true/correct statement

Ans. (d) Assertion is independently a false/incorrect statement, but the Reasons is independently a true/correct statement

Ref: Goodman and Gilman's 12th ed pg 1628 to 1659; KDT 7th ed pg 805, Harrison's 19th Ed Pg 1274

Zidovudine is an NRTI

Targets and Mechanism of Antiretroviral Drugs			
Target	**Normal function in virus**	**Drug class**	**Mechanism of action**
gp41	HIV attaches through gp 160 (which includes gp120 and gp41) ==> gp 41 fuses viral envelop to host membrane==> entry of virus	Enfuvirtide (Entry inhibitor)	Binds to gp41==> does not allow conformational changes that allow fusion of virus blocks entry of virus into host cell.
CCR5		Maraviroc (Entry inhibitor)	Binds specifically to host protein ccr5 ==> blocks entry
RT (Reverse transcriptase)	RT then converts viral RNA to DNA	NRTI [Nucleoside/ Nucleotide (tenofovir)] e.g. zidovudine, lamivudine, etc.	These drugs are purine or pyrimidine analogues that enter cells get phosphorylated and then blocks replication by 2 ways: 1) Competitively inhibits incorporation of native nucleotides. 2) once incorporated terminates elongation of nascent DNA because NRTI lack 3' hydroxyl group
		NNRTI (Non-nucleoside) e.g. nevirapine	Bind to NNRTI binding pocket in enzyme RT which is separate from catalytic site and cause change in 3D structure of the enzyme reducing its activity.

Contd...

Targets and Mechanism of Antiretroviral Drugs			
Target	**Normal function in virus**	**Drug class**	**Mechanism of action**
Integrase	Incorporates viral DNA into host DNA.	Integrase inhibitor e.g. Raltegravir	These drugs bind to integrase enzyme and prevent viral DNA strand transfer to host DNA
Protease	Proteolytic cleavage of gag and pol precursor polypeptides and other precursor proteins to final structural proteins of mature virion	Protease inhibitors e.g. ritonavir, saquinavir, etc.	HIV protease inhibitors are peptide-like chemicals that competitively inhibit the action of the viral protease thereby blocking formation of mature virions.

48. Consider the following assertion and reason.

Assertion: NSAID's cause inhibition of platelet function

Reasoning: NSAID's inhibit Prostaglandin pathway

a. Both Assertion and Reasons are independently true/correct statements and the Reason is the correct explanation for the Assertion
b. Both Assertion and Reasons are independently true/correct statements, but the Reason is not the correct explanation for the Assertion
c. Assertion is independently a true/correct statement, but the Reason is independently a false/incorrect statement
d. Assertion is independently a false/incorrect statement, but the Reasons is independently a true/correct statement

Ans. (a) Both Assertion and Reasons are independently true/correct statements and the Reason is the correct explanation for the Assertion

Ref: KDT 7th Ed Pg 183

Aspirin acetylates COX in prostaglandin synthesis at a serine residue and causes irreversible inhibition while other NSAIDs are competitive and reversible inhibitors.

Drugs Affecting Platlet Function and Mechanism of Action			
Interfering with platelet membrane	**Inhibition of prostaglandin pathways**	**Inhibition of platelet phosphodiesterase**	**Unknown mechanism of action**
Tricyclic antidepressant; Amitriptyline, Imipramine	Antiplatelet: Aspirin, clopidogrel	Caffeine	Acetazolamide
SSRI; citalopram, Escitalopram, fluoxetine Fluvoxamine, paroxetine Sertraline	NSAID (Indomethacin, ibuprofen, naproxen, diclofenac, ketorolac)	Dipyridamole Cilostazol	Ethacrynic acid
Antipsycotic; Chlorpromazine	Furosemide	Aminophylline	Hydroxychloroquine
Anesthetic; Cocaine, Lidocaine	Calcium channel blockers; Verapamil	Theophylline	Nitroprusside
Antihistamine; Promethazine, Diphenhydramine	Hydralazine	Vinblastine	Cyproheptadine
Isoproterenol	Cyclosporine	Vincristine	Nitroglycerin
Beta blockers; Propranolol	Hydrocortisone	Colchicine	Famotidine
Antibiotics: Penicillin Ampicillin, Cephalothin, Carbenicillin		Papaverine	Cimetidine

49. Consider the following reason-assertion:

Assertion: Thinking about food increases gastric acid production

Reasoning: This is an example of positive feedback mechanism

a. Both Assertion and Reasons are independently true/correct statements and the Reason is the correct explanation for the Assertion
b. Both Assertion and Reasons are independently true/correct statements, but the Reason is not the correct explanation for the Assertion
c. Assertion is independently a true/correct statement, but the Reason is independently a false/incorrect statement
d. Assertion is independently a false/incorrect statement, but the Reasons is independently a true/correct statement

Ans. (c) Assertion is independently a true/correct statement, but the Reason is independently a false/incorrect statement

Ref: Guyton 12th ed page 9

The increased gastric acid production while thinking about food is due to feed forward or adaptive control.

Feed forward or Anticipatory or Adaptive Control

Some are simple feedback systems but many are not. For instance, some movements of the body occur so rapidly that there is not enough time for nerve signals to travel from the peripheral parts of the body all the way to the brain and then back to the periphery again to control the movement. Therefore, the brain uses a principle called **feed-forward control** to cause required muscle contractions. That is, sensory nerve signals from the moving parts apprise the brain whether the movement is performed correctly. If not, the brain corrects the feed-forward signals that it sends to the muscles the next time the movement is required. Then, if still further correction is necessary, this will be done again for subsequent movements. This is called **adaptive control.** Adaptive control, in a sense, is delayed negative feedback.

Examples of Feed Forward Control

- Temperature control: Thermoregulatory responses are initiated by hypothalamus BEFORE the changes in environmental temperature have succeeded in changing the body's core body temperature
- Cephalic phase of gastric secretion- Just thinking about food increases gastric acid production
- Thinking about exercise itself increases heart rate and respiratory rate
- Role of cerebellum in motor coordination

50. Following are statements regarding Minimum alveolar concentration (MAC)

Assertion: Adults have a greater MAC requirement than paediatric patients

Reasoning: MAC requirement is directly proportional to age

a. Both Assertion and Reasons are independently true/ correct statements and the Reason is the correct explanation for the Assertion
b. Both Assertion and Reasons are independently true/ correct statements, but the Reason is not the correct explanation for the Assertion
c. Assertion is independently a true/correct statement, but the Reason is independently a false/incorrect statement
d. Both Assertion and Reasons are independently false/ incorrect statements

Ans. (d) Both Assertion and Reasons are independently false / incorrect statements

Ref: Miller's anaesthesia 8th Ed Pg 2764

MAC requirement is higher for paediatric patients than adult patients.

Anesthetic requirement is smaller for preterm than for term neonates and smaller for term neonates than for 3 month olds. Infants have a higher MAC than that of older children or adults; the reasons for these age-related differences in MAC are not known.

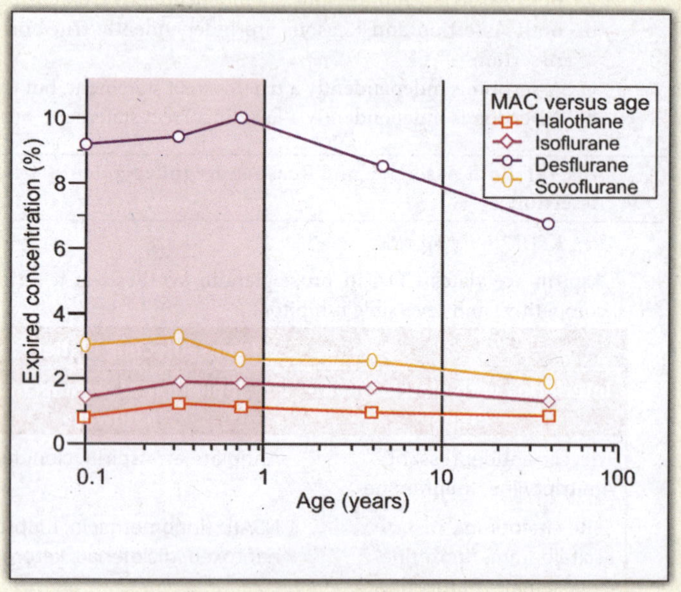

Fig: The minimum alveolar concentrations (MACs) of four commonly used inhaled anesthetics are plotted versus age. MAC is highest in infants 3 to 6 months of age

VARIANT 7. EXTENDED MATCHING ITEMS/QUESTIONS (EMI/EMQ)

Each EMI /EMQ will broadly have the following components.
Theme and Focus
Answer option list
Lead in question
Scenarios or Vignettes
There will be two or more scenario/vignette related to the overall Theme and Focus of the question
The candidate should select the best possible answer from the Answer Option List.

Theme: Diaphragmatic Hernia

51. Match each description with the correct abnormality.

a. Rupture of the diaphragm
b. Paraesophageal hiatal hernia
c. Sliding hiatal hernia
d. Foramen of Bochdalek hernia
e. Foramen of Morgagni hernia

Scenario 1: The most common congenital diaphragmatic hernia in infants

Ans. (d) Foramen of Bochdalek hernia

Scenario 2: The hernia most likely to cause acute respiratory distress in infants

Ans. (d) Foramen of Bochdalek hernia

Scenario 3 A congenital hernia that is most frequently discovered as an incidental finding in adults

Ans. (e) Foramen of Morgagni hernia

Ref: Schwartz 7th ed page 1161–1167

Paraesophageal hernias, is generally acquired, involve herniation of any portion or all of the stomach into the thoracic cavity via the esophageal hiatus. These hernias are usually repaired electively because of a high incidence of complications. Diaphragmatic ruptures usually affect adults and result from blunt trauma to the abdomen. Unless such ruptures are repaired, the negative intrathoracic pressure associated with each respiratory effort tends to such the abdominal contents into the chest with consequent loss of necessary space for lung expansion and substantial risk of damage to the intrathoracic bowel.

Sliding hiatal hernias, the most frequent type of hernia found in adults, are generally acquired. The significance of this type of hernia rests in its association with gastroesophageal reflux, a condition that may lead to reflux esophagitis. Because sliding hiatal hernias frequently do not exhibit significant gastroesophageal reflux, it is likely that other factors may be more important in the pathophysiology of that disorder.

Foramen of Bochdalek hernia is a congenital hernia of the posterolateral aspect of the diaphragm in which abdominal viscera enter the thorax and cause acute respiratory distress in infants. This hernia requires emergency repair.

Foramen of Morgagni hernia, although also congenital, is not usually detected until adulthood. It is usually an incidental finding on chest X-ray, where it appears as a low anterior mediastinal mass. However, on rare occasions it can produce acute respiratory distress in infants.

52. Match the appropriate pharmacologic agent with each description.

a. Epinephrine b. Norepinephrine
c. Isoproterenol d. Dopamine
e. Dobutamine f. Amrinone
g. Digitalis h. Nitroprusside
i. Nitroglycerin j. Milrinone

Balanced arterial and venous dilation

Ans. (h) Nitroprusside

Pure beta agonist with profound chronotropic properties

Ans. (c) Isoproterenol

Inotropic and antiarrhythmic properties

Ans. (g) Digitalis

Ref: Schwartz 7th ed page 103–105, 114

Epinephrine is a circulating endogenous catecholamine, released mainly from the adrenal medulla, whose effects are mediated by binding of free circulating hormone to β1- and β2-receptors, with lesser effects on α-adrenoreceptors.

Norepinephrine is also endogenously produced, but acts locally through release at nerve synapses.

Isoproterenol is a synthetic sympathomimetic that acts as a pure beta agonist, resulting in profound vasodilator and chronotropic effects.

Dopamine is an endogenous catecholamine that is released into the circulation and acts by binding to β1-receptors as well as specific dopamine receptors in the renal, mesenteric, coronary, and intracerebral vascular beds, causing vasodilation.

Dobutamine is a synthetic sympathomimetic structurally related to dopamine and is a potent inotrope but possesses only small chronotropic properties.

Amrinone and milrinone are bipyridine derivatives that induce vasodilation and inotropy via inhibition of phosphodiesterase, thereby enhancing intracellular concentrations of cyclic AMP.

Digitalis exerts positive inotropic effects by inhibition of Na-K-activated ATPase, resulting in increased intracellular sodium concentrations, which lead to increased intracellular calcium concentrations. Digitalis is also used in the management of arrhythmias, most commonly atrial fibrillation.

Nitroprusside and nitroglycerin are systemic vasodilators, and while nitroprusside causes balanced arterial and venous dilation, the effects of nitroglycerin are less pronounced in the arterial than the venous system, often resulting in venous pooling.

53. Theme and focus: BLS and ACLS

Answer option list:

a. Give shock b. Give chest compressions
c. Intubate d. Give adrenaline
e. Verify scene safety f. Give atropine
g. Administer amiodarone h. Give vasopressin

Case 1: You are travelling by train and suddenly you are informed by fellow passengers that a fellow traveller has collapsed. You find the patient unresponsive, and ask to inform authorities. There is no pulse or respiration. What is the next step?

Ans. (b) Give chest compressions

Case 2: You are called by the attendant of a patient on ventilator in the ICU that the monitor's alarm is beeping. On arrival you find that the patient's BP is 60/40 mm Hg. The ECG shows following pattern. Which is the most effective treatment option?

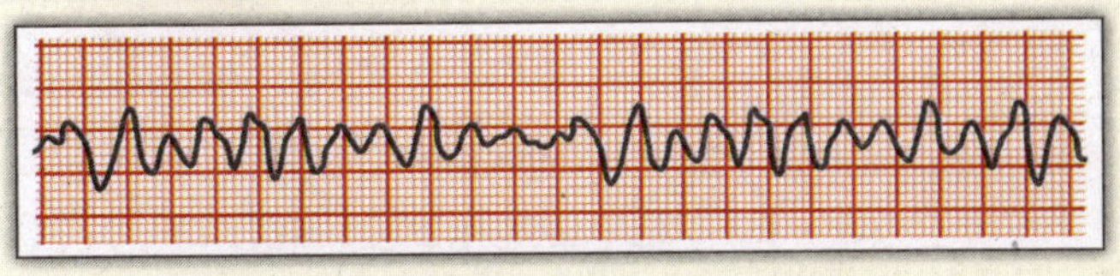

Ans. (a) Give Shock

The ECG shows Ventricular fibrillation, which is a shockable rhythm.

Case 3: You are called in for code blue in your hospital. During CPR cycles you observe the following pattern on ECG. What will you do along with CPR cycles?

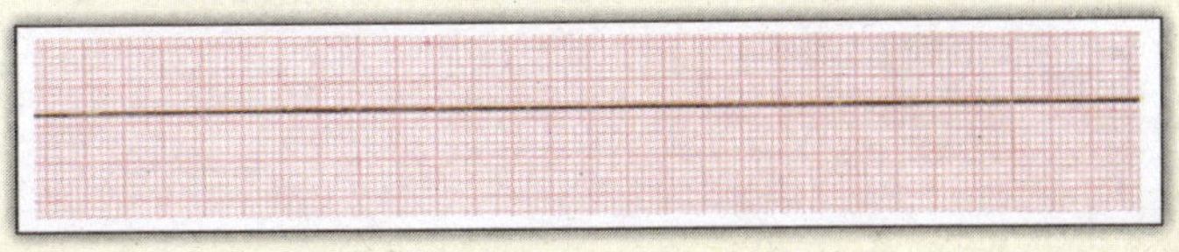

Ans. (d) Give adrenaline

Case 4: You are performing CPCR in the ICU. Which instruction is NOT to be given to your assistant, in accordance with the recent CPCR guidelines?

Ans. (f) Give atropine

Adult Cardiac Arrest -basic Cardiac Life Support (BCLS) Algorithm 2015 Update

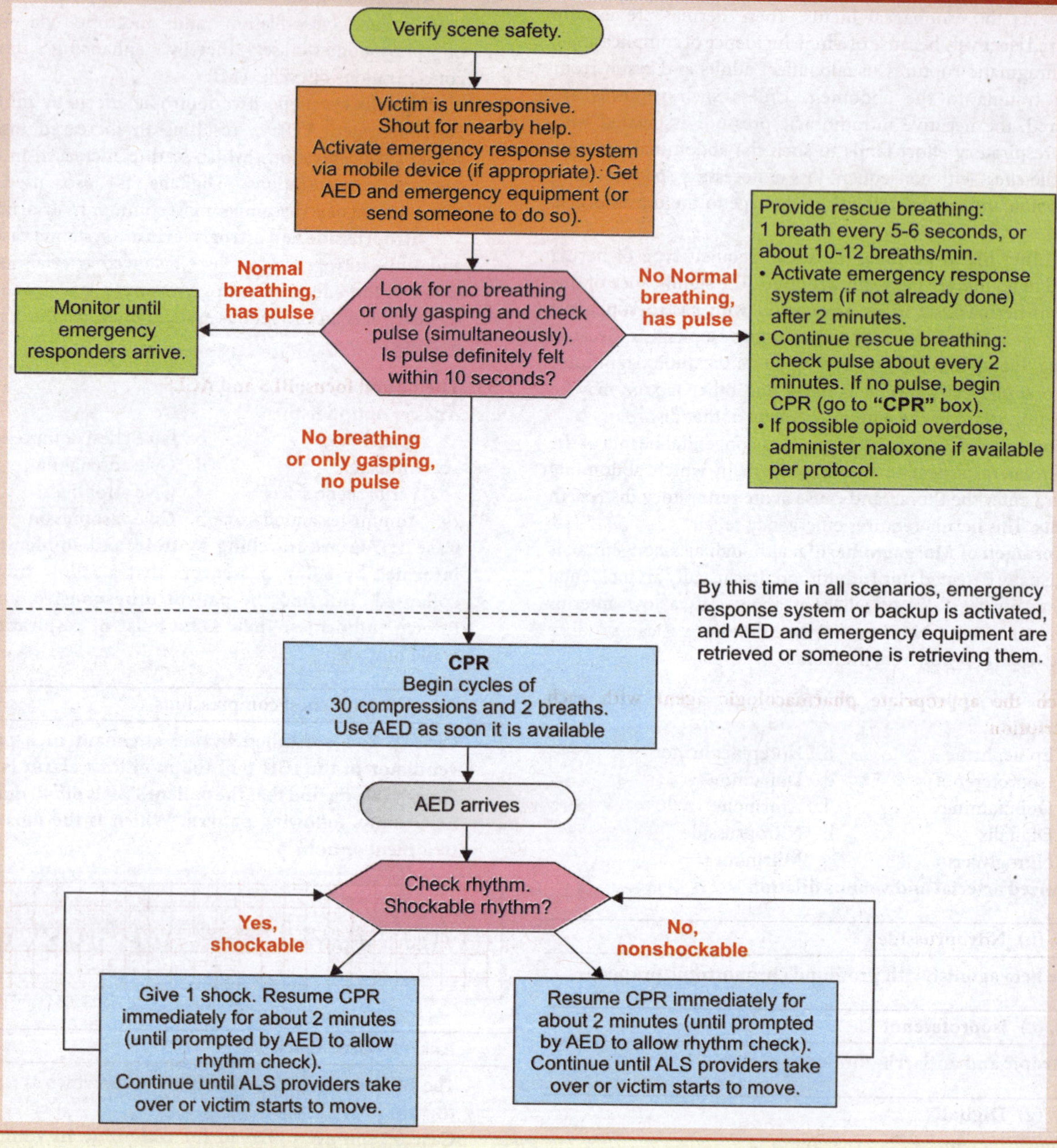

Anesthesia Appendix 35: Adult Cardiac Arrest-Advanced Cardiac Life Support (ACLS) Algorithm 2015 Update

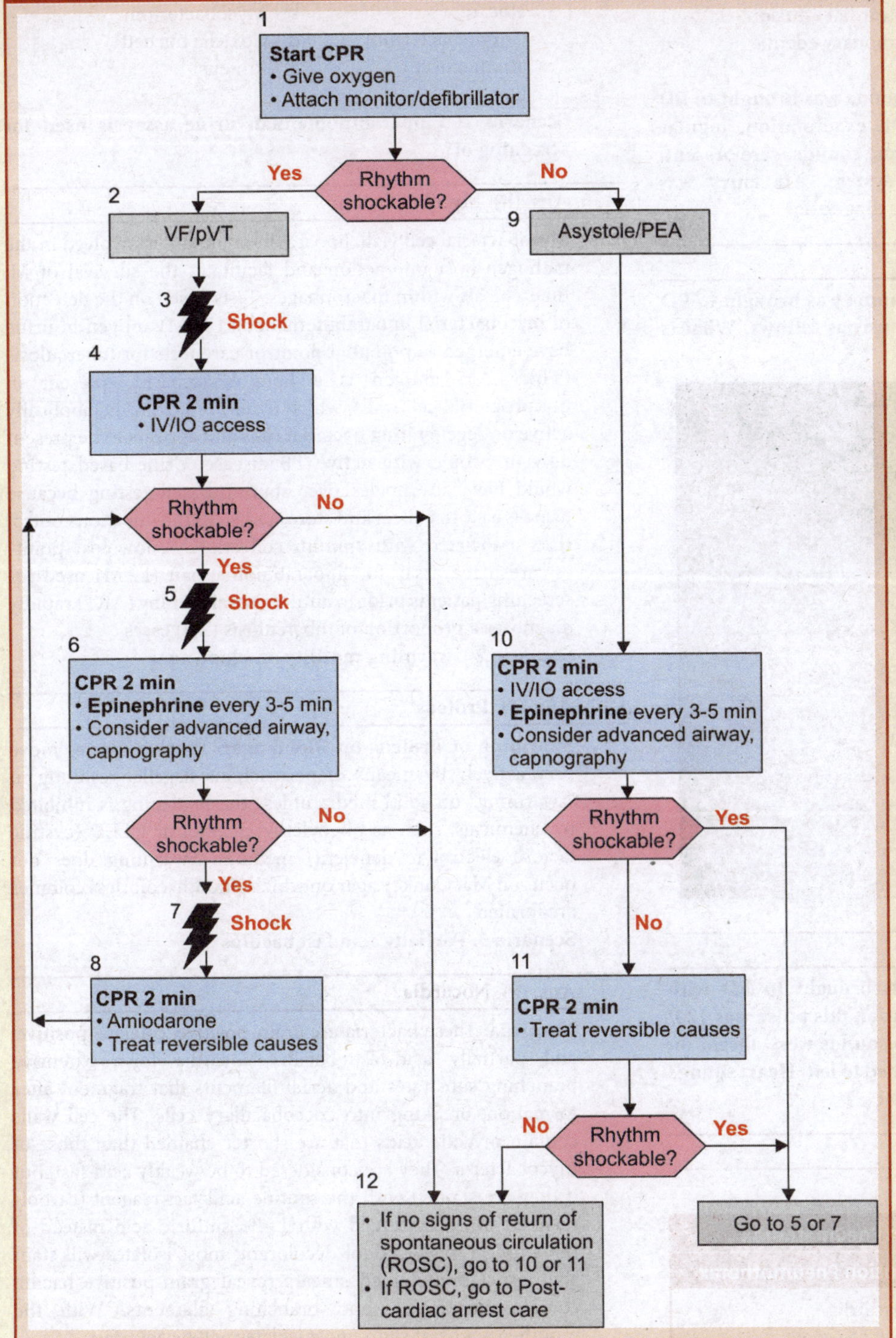

CPR Quality

- Push hard (at least 2 inches [5 cm]) and fast (100-120/min) and allow complete chest recoil.
- Minimize interruptions in compressions.
- Avoid excessive ventilation.
- Rotate compressor every 2 minutes, or sooner if fatigued.
- If no advanced airway, 30:2 compression-ventilation ratio.
- Quantitative waveform capnography
  - If $PEtCO_2$ <10 mm Hg, attempt to improve CPR quality.
- Intra-arterial pressure
  - If relaxation phase (diastolic) pressure <20 mm Hg, attempt to improve CPR quality.

Shock Energy for Defibrillation

- **Biphasic:** Manufacturer recommendation (e.g. initial dose of 120-200 J); if unknown, use maximum available. Second and subsequent doses should be equivalent and higher doses may be considered.
- **Monophasic:** 360 J

Drug Therapy

- **Epinephrine IV/IO dose:** 1 mg every 3-5 minutes
- **Amiodarone IV/IO dose:** First dose: 300 mg bolus, Second dose: 150 mg.

Advanced Airway

- Endotracheal intubation or supraglottic advanced airway
- Waveform capnography or capnometry to confirm and monitor ET tube placement
- Once advanced airway in place, give 1 breath every 6 seconds (10 breaths/min) with continuous chest compressions

Return of Spontaneous Circulation (ROSC)

- Pulse and blood pressure
- Abrupt sustained increase in $PETCO_2$ (typically ≥40 mm Hg)
- Spontaneous arterial pressure waves with intra-arterial monitoring

Reversible Causes

- **H**ypovolemia
- **H**ypoxia
- **H**ydrogen ion (acidosis)
- **H**ypo-/hyperkalemia
- **H**ypothermia
- **T**ension pneumothorax
- **T**amponade, cardiac
- **T**oxins
- **T**hrombosis, pulmonary
- **T**hrombosis, coronary

54. Theme and focus: Chest trauma and surgery

Answer option list:

a. Tension pneumothorax b. Closed pneumothorax
c. Cardiac tamponade d. Pericardial effusion
e. Haemothorax f. Pulmonary edema
g. Pericardial tapping

Scenario 1: A patient with chest trauma was brought to ED with hypotension, tachycardia. On examination, jugular vein was distended and muffled heart sounds were present. On examination of respiratory system, Air entry was present. What is the most probable diagnosis?

Ans. (c) Cardiac tamponade

Scenario 2: A patient with chest trauma was brought to ED with difficulty in breathing. X ray was as follows. What is your most probable diagnosis?

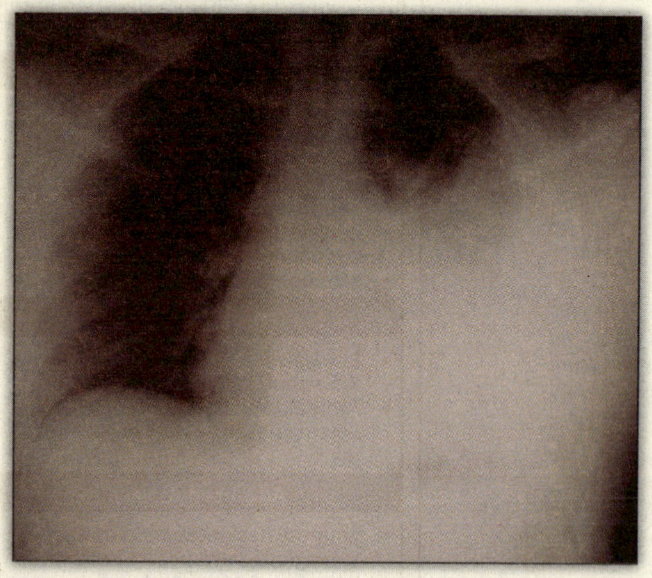

Ans. (e) Haemothorax

Scenario 3: A patient of RTA was brought to ED with difficulty in breathing. On examination, his pulse was 120/min, BP was 70/50 mm Hg. Breath sounds were absent on the right side, and trachea was deviated to left. Heart sounds were present. What is your diagnosis?

Ans. (a) Tension Pneumothorax

Ref: Harrison's 19th Ed Pg 1719

Cardiac Tamponade Versus Tension Pneumothorax

Feature	Tamponade	Tension Pneumothorax
Pulse	Tachycardia	Tachycardia
Blood Pressure	Hypotension	Hypotension
Pulsus Paradoxus	Yes	Yes
Jugular vein	Distended	Distended
Trachea	Midline	Deviated to opposite side
Percussion	Normal	Hyperresonant note
Heart sounds	Muffled	Yes
Breath sounds	Present	Absent

Theme: Microbes

55. Answer option list:

a. Nocardia b. Mycobacterium
c. Corynebacterium d. Coxiella burnetti
e. Streptococcus f. Proteus
g. E coli

Scenario 1: Lipoarabinomannan urine assay is used for screening of?

Ans. (b) Mycobacterium

Mycobacterial cell wall, lipoarabinomannan, is involved in the pathogen-host interaction and facilitates the survival of M. tuberculosis within macrophages. Tests based on the detection of mycobacterial lipoarabinomannan (LAM) antigen in urine have emerged as potential point-of-care tests for tuberculosis (TB). LAM antigen is a lipopolysaccharide present in mycobacterial cell walls, which is released from metabolically active or degenerating bacterial cells and appears to be present only in people with active TB disease. Urine-based testing would have advantages over sputum-based testing because urine is easy to collect and store, and lacks the infection control risks associated with sputum collection. A low-cost point-of-care urine assay for lipoarabinomannan (LAM) used for screening patients prior to antiretroviral therapy (ART) rapidly diagnoses a proportion of tuberculosis (TB) cases.

Scenario 2: Swarming motility on blood agar

Ans. (f) Proteus

Swarming of Proteus on Blood agar: Proteus species move very actively by means of peritrichous flagella, resulting in "swarming" on solid media unless the swarming is inhibited by chemicals, such as phenylethyl alcohol or CLED (cystine lactose electrolyte deficient) medium. Swarming does not occur on MacConkey agar on which smooth, colorless colonies are formed.

Scenario 3: Partially acid fast bacillus

Ans. (a) Nocardia

Nocardia: These bacteria are gram-positive, catalase-positive, and partially acid-fast bacilli. Nocardia form extensive branching substrates and aerial filaments that fragment after formation, breaking into coccobacillary cells. The cell walls contain mycolic acids that are shorter chained than those of Mycobacteria. They are considered to be weakly acid-fast, but if they are stained with the routine acid-fast reagent (carbol-fuchsin) but decolorized with 1–4% sulfuric acid instead of the stronger acid-alcohol decolorant, most isolates will stain acid-fast. Gram-stained smears reveal gram-positive bacilli, coccobacillary cells, and branching filaments. With the modified acid-fast stain, most isolates will be acid-fast

Scenario 4: Obligate intracellular pathogen

Ans. (d) Coxiella burnetti

Coxiella is pleomorphic coccobacilli with a Gram negative wall. It is an obligate intracellular pathogen infecting monocyte-macrophage cells. However Omsland et al 2009 discovered the milestone advance of Coxiella host cell-free (axenic) growth. After Omsland many researchers proved host free growth of Coxiella

Scenario 5: Enterohemorrhagic, enterotoxic and enteroinvasive are types of?

Ans. (g) E coli

Ref: Ananthanarayan 9th ed page 279

Types of E. Coli	
Enteropathogenic E coli (EPEC)	Attaches to enterocytes (enteroadherent) and destroy brush border microvilli. Causes *infantile diarrhea* (remember EPEC affects pediatric population) and *sporadic diarrhea in adult*
Enterotoxigenic E coli (ETEC)	Acute watery diarrhea in infant and *Traveler's diarrhea* in adult. Heat stable toxin- Tc-GMP Heat stable toxin- Tc-AMP Produces cholera like enterotoxin (Cholera infantum), Biken test ++
Enteroinvasive E coli (EIEC)	*Dysentery like disease in all ages.* Only E-coli which invades G.I. Mucosa (enteroinvasive) and produces dysentery like disease (toxin resembles shigella). Sereny test+ (invasive test for shigella), growth in HeLa cell culture or HEP-2 cells.
Enterohemorrhagic E coli (EHEC/ VTEC)	Produces verotoxin or verocytotoxin (VTEC) (shiga like toxin) which acts on vascular endothelium and causes *hemorrhagic colitis + HUS* (Strain 0157). Does not ferment sorbitol (sorbitol")
Enteroaggregative E coli (EAEC)	Form a heat stable enterotoxin EAST1. It causes *persistent diarrhoea in developing countries* Most are "O" untypable but "H" typable

56. Theme and focus: Neurological Side Effects of Neuroleptic Drugs

Answer option list:

a. Anaphylaxis b. Akathisia
c. Tardive dyskinesia
d. Neuroleptic malignant syndrome
e. Acute dystonia f. Parkinsonism
g. Alzheimer's disease

Scenario 1: A patient was started on antipsychotic drugs. 3 months later, patient developed abnormal, involuntary, irregular choreoathetoid movements of the muscles of the head, arms, legs and trunk. What is your diagnosis?

Ans. (c) Tardive dyskinesia

Scenario 2: A young male patient was started on antipsychotic drugs. 2 days later, he started developing tilting of neck, stiffness, abnormal posturing. What is your diagnosis?

Ans. (e) Acute dystonia

Scenario 3: An elderly woman was started on antipsychotic medication. She developed perioral tremors and rigidity. What is your diagnosis?

Ans. (f) Parkinsonism

Scenario 4: An elderly woman on antipsychotic medication was taken to the psychiatrist. After evaluation, the psychiatrist increased the dosage of the medications she was on. 2 weeks, later, she started pacing around the house restlessly, and did not stop even when she was asked to. What could be the probable cause?

Ans. (b) Akathisia

Neurological Side Effects of Neuroleptic Drugs

	Acute dystonia	Akathisia	Parkinsonism	Tardive dyskinesia	Neuroleptic malignant syndrome
	Early	Intermediate	Intermediate	Late (tardive)	Any
Onset	Within 7 days of therapy or ↑ dose	Within 3 months of therapy or ↑ dose	Within 3 months of therapy or ↑ dose	>3-6 months (↓dose may unmask dyskinesia)	Anytime during therapy (↑ dose or high potency drugs)
Incidence	15-20% with typical neuroleptics, 5% with atypical	20%	30%	5% per year of therapy i.e. 50% in 10 years	0.5% (20-30% mortality)

Contd...

Neurological Side Effects of Neuroleptic Drugs					
	Acute dystonia	Akathisia	Parkinsonism	Tardive dyskinesia	Neuroleptic malignant syndrome
Mechanism	Unclear, dopamine hypofunction at basal ganglia	D2 receptor blockage in mesocortical pathway	D2 receptor blockage at striatum	D2 receptor blockage at striatum	Idiosyncratic, Relative depletion of dopamine in CNS
Risk factors	Male , young, mental retardation, h/o ECT, dose elevation	Elderly, female, mental retardation, Iron deficiency, Affective disorders, dose elevation	Elderly ,Females , dementia, underlying parkinsonism, AIDS, dose elevation	Elderly, female, h/o ECT, substance abuse, iron deficiency, Mental retardation, Mood disorder, Organic brain damage, Anticholinergic Dose decrease	Male, young, dose elevation
Symptoms	Slow, irregular, continuous contractions, oculogyric movements of tongue, torticollis, trismus, abnormal posture, blepherospasm	Uncontrolled restlessness, pacing, compulsive foot taping, rocking movement, adversity to stand still, rapid alternation of standing and sitting	R = rigidity A = akinesia (mc) T = tremor (atypical-coarse, not pill rolling, late) RABBIT SYNDROME= Lip and perioral tremors.	Most serious adverse effect. Rapid, irregular, continuous or intermittent contractions, or fasciolingual or limb/ trunkal, ↑by stress activity,	Life threatening F = fever E = Encephalopathy V = Vitals unstable E = Elevated CPK, WBC R = Rigidity
Treatment	Antiparkinsonian agents are diagnostic and curative Anti- cholinergics: Benztropine, promethazine or hydroxyzine i.m. clears the reaction within 10-15 min. Antihistaminics: Diphenhydramine	Reduce dose and/or change antipsychotic. Propranolol= doc, central anticholinergic may reduce the intensity in some cases	Antiparkinsonian agents Anticholinergics may be useful as monotherapy in early, untreated Parkinson's or as adjunct therapy to patients already on levodopa Antihistaminics: Amantadine, Diphenhydramine	No established treatment, discontinue or replace the antipsychotic agent and then eliminate all drugs with central anticholinergic Action, lithium and carbamazepine for psychosis, BZD: buspirone for dyskinesia	Stop neuroleptic immediately; dantrolene or bromocriptine may help; antiparkinsonian agents not effective anticholinergics are of no help.

57. Theme and focus: Differential Diagnosis of steatorrhea

a. Celiac disease
b. Chronic Pancreatitis
c. Bacterial overgrowth syndrome
d. Intestinal lymphangiectasia
e. Ileal disease

Following are laboratory features of patients with steatorrhea. Choose the correct diagnosis from the above list.

Scenario 1: Laboratory features: Stool test- Steatorrhea, D-xylose test: Normal , Schilling test: Abnormal , Duodenal biopsy: Normal. There was no improvement in Schilling test after administration of pancreatic enzymes.

Ans. (e) Ileal disease

Scenario 2: Laboratory features: Stool test- Steatorrhea, D-xylose test: Normal, Schilling test: Abnormal, Duodenal biopsy: Normal. There was an improvement in Schilling test results after administration of pancreatic enzymes.

Ans. (b) Chronic pancreatitis

Scenario 3 : Laboratory features: Stool test- Steatorrhea, D-xylose: Decreased, Schilling test:Normal , Duodenal biopsy: Flat mucosa

Ans. (a) Celiac disease

Scenario 4: Laboratory features: Stool test-Steatorrhea, D-xylose: Normal, Schilling test: Normal, Duodenal biopsy: dilated lymphatics

Ans. (d) Intestinal lymphangiectasia

Ref: Harrison's 19th Ed Pg 1941

Diagnostic Studies in Various Etiologies of Steatorrhea and their Results					
Test	**Chronic pancreatitis**	**Ileal disease**	**Celiac disease**	**Bacterial overgrowth syndromes**	**Intestinal lymphangiectasia**
D-Xylose	Normal	Normal	Decreased	Normal or slightly abnormal	Normal
Schilling test	50% abnormal	Abnormal	Normal	Often abnormal	Normal
Duodenal mucosal biopsy	Normal	Normal	Abnormal (flat)	Normal	Abnormal : "dilated lymphatics"

Note:
- Abnormal Schilling test in chronic pancreatitis gives a normal result with pancreatic enzyme treatment
- Abnormal Schilling test in Bacterial overgrowth syndromes gives a normal result after antibiotic treatment.

58. Theme and focus: Fractures and inflammation in wrist and hand

a. De Quervain's disease
b. Carpometacarpal osteoarthritis
c. Triangular fibrocartilage complex
d. Kienböck's disease
e. Scaphoid fracture
f. Lunate fracture

Identify the most probable diagnosis on the basis of sites of tenderness:

Scenario 1 : Tenderness in Base of first metacarpal:

Ans. (b) Carpometacarpal osteoarthritis

Scenario 2: Tenderness in anatomical snuffbox

Ans. (e) Scaphoid fracture

Scenario 3: Tenderness just distal to the head of the ulna

Ans. (c) Triangular fibrocartilage complex

Scenario 4: Tenderness over the lunate

Ans. (d) Kienböck's disease

Diagnosis Based on Site of Tenderness in Orthopedics	
Site	**Diagnosis**
Tip of radial Styloid	De Quervain's disease
Anatomical snuffbox	Scaphoid fracture
Base of first metacarpal	Carpometacarpal osteoarthritis
Over the lunate	Kienböck's disease
Just distal to the head of the ulna	Triangular fibrocartilage complex

59. Theme and focus : Malingering in orthopedics

a. Mannkopf's test
b. McBride's test
c. Hoover's test
d. O'Donoghue maneuver
e. Burn's test
f. Drawers test

A patient is being examined and is suspected to be malingering. Identify the following tests:

Scenario 1: A student complains of pain in the leg. On examination you find that there is no increase in heart rate on touching the leg. Which test is being done?

Ans. (a) Mannkopf's test

Scenario 2: A young lady is complaining of back pain and is asking for sickness certificate to submit in the school. You ask her to stand on one leg while raising the opposite knee to the chest. On doing so, she starts complaining of increased back pain. Identify the test.

Ans. (b) McBride's test

Scenario 3: A patient of a minor bike accident is brought to ED complaining of lower limb weakness and wants a certificate to sue the car driver who hit him. Examiner places one hand under the patient heel and patient is then asked to raise his other leg against downward resistance. What is the test being performed?

Ans. (c) Hoover's test

Ref: Neurologic Emergencies edited by Latha Ganti, Joshua N. Goldstein page 198, Neurology and Trauma by Randolph W. Evans 2nd ed page 648

- Hoover's test is used to check for malingering in patients presenting with lower limb weakness. It relies on the fact that all individuals, extend their hip when flexing the contralateral hip against resistance. Hold the supine patient's heels off the table and ask them to raise one leg. If this is easy, the test is negative, if difficult, the patient will push the contralateral leg towards the table to assist raising the leg. Lack of downward pressure from the contralateral leg is a positive sign of malingering.
- Mannkopf's test: palpation of a painful area should increase the pulse rate by at least 5 per cent and absence of this finding is a positive behavioural sign.
- O'Donoghue's maneuver: Patients with true physiological pain have a greater passive range of motion than active so, it is a positive behavioural sign if the patient's active range of motion is greater.
- McBride's test: Ask the patient to stand on one leg while raising the opposite knee to the chest. This should lessen low back pain. A reported increase in pain, or a refusal to do the test, is a positive behavioural sign.

- Burn's test: Ask the patient to kneel on a chair and touch the floor - those with true back pain or sciatica should be able to do this but those with non-organic back pain usually cannot.

60. Theme and focus: Organisms causing food poisoning.

Answer option list:

a. Bacillus cereus
b. Salmonella
c. Shigella
d. Listeria
e. E. coli
f. Vibrio parahaemolyticus

Following are food items which can cause food poisoning. Identify the causative microbe.

Case 1: Fried rice

Ans. (a) Bacillus cereus

Case 2: Chicken

Ans. (c) Shigella

Case 3: Eggs

Ans. (b) Salmonella

Case 4: Mayonnaise

Ans. (b) Salmonella

NOTE

Answers from the option list may be applicable to one or more questions.

Ref: Jawetz 24th ed ch 18, Harrison 19th Ed Pg 266,856

Common Causative Organisms for Food Poisoning

Food item	Organism
Chicken	Shigella
Undercooked hamburger	E. coli (01 57:H7)
Fried rice or other reheated food	Bacillus cereus
Mayonnaise or creams	Staphylococcus aureus or Salmonella
Eggs	Salmonella
Uncooked foods or soft cheeses	Listeria
Shellfish	V. parahaemolyticus

AIIMS
Nov 2018–May 2015
Subject-wise MCQs and Answers with Explanations

Anatomy
Physiology
Biochemistry
Microbiology
Pathology
Pharmacology
Forensic Medicine
Preventive and Social Medicine
Ear, Nose and Throat
Ophthalmology

11. Medicine
12. Pediatrics
13. Obstetrics and Gynecology
14. General Surgery
15. Orthopedics
16. Dermatology
17. Psychiatry
18. Radiodiagnosis and Radiotherapy
19. Anesthesia

Anatomy

1

AIIMS NOVEMBER 2018

1. **Ligamentum flavum contains:**
   a. Elastin b. Reticulin
   c. Type 1 Collagen d. Type 2 Collagen
2. **Which of the following bone does not take part in wrist joint formation is:**
   a. Ulna b. Radius
   c. Scaphoid d. Triquetral
3. **All of the following muscles help in inversion of foot EXCEPT:**
   a. Tibialis anterior b. Tibialis posterior
   c. Peroneus longus d. Extensor hallucis longus
4. **Normal curvature of lumbar spine is:**
   a. Recurvatum b. Scoliosis
   c. Kyphosis d. Lordosis
5. **Left Superior intercostal vein drains into?**
   a. Azygos vein b. Hemiazygos vein
   c. Internal thoracic vein d. Left brachiocephalic vein
6. **Which of the following nerve is not associated with olfaction?**
   a. Trigeminal b. Hypoglossal
   c. Vagus d. Glossopharyngeal
7. **Golgi apparatus in serous acinar cell is at:**
   a. Basal b. Apical
   c. Supranuclear d. Adjacent to nucleus
8. **Occlusion of artery supplying marked area in the given picture will cause all of the following EXCEPT:**

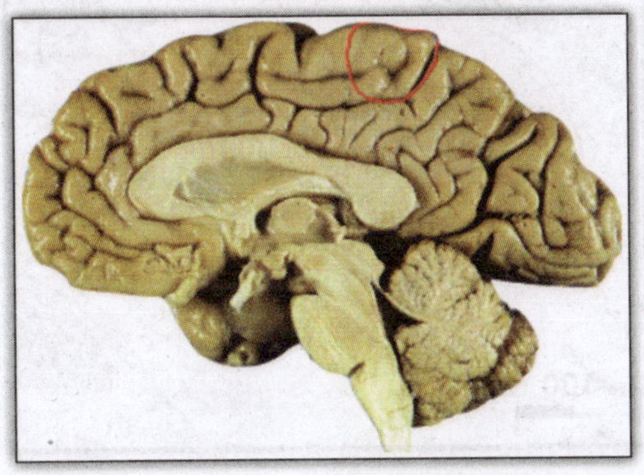

   a. Apraxia b. Urinary incontinence
   c. Anal incontinence d. Perineal anesthesia
9. **Identify the nerve marked in given image:**

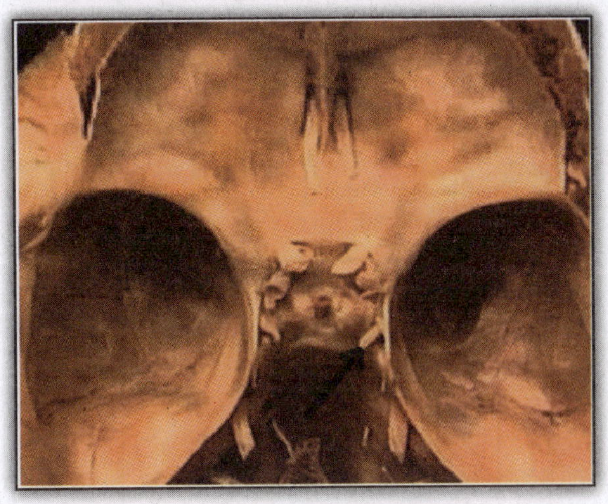

   a. Optic b. Oculomotor nerve
   c. Trochlear d. Abducent
10. **Main action of muscle marked in the given image is:**

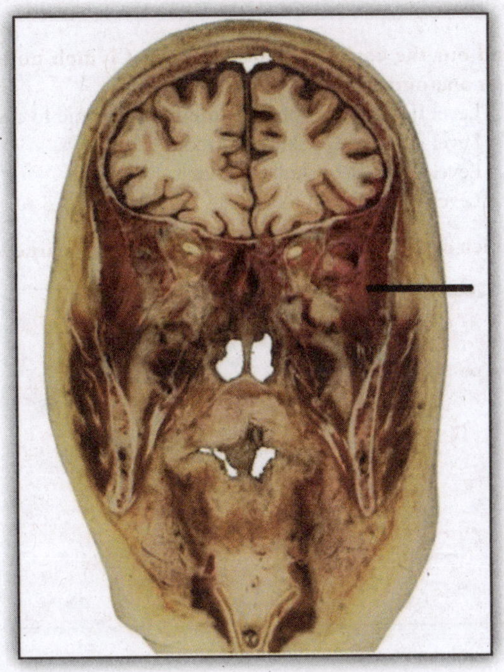

   a. Elevation b. Depression
   c. Retraction d. Protrusion

11. Identify the connective tissue marked in the image:

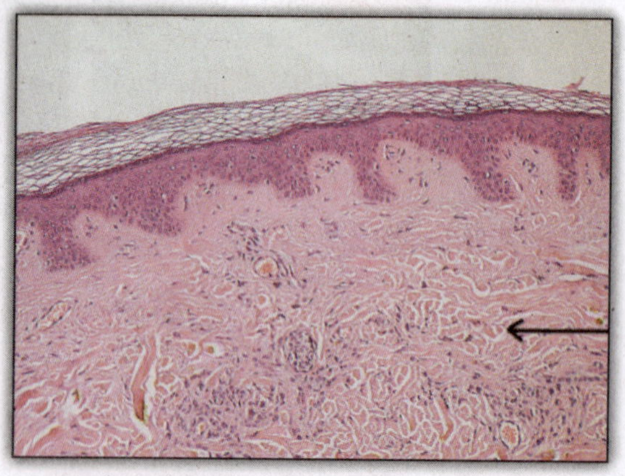

a. Dense regular connective tissue
b. Loose irregular connective tissue
c. Dense irregular connective tissue
d. Specialized connective tissue

12. Transverse section of spinal cord showing four marked areas. Identify area which is involved in decreased sensation of pain on massaging?

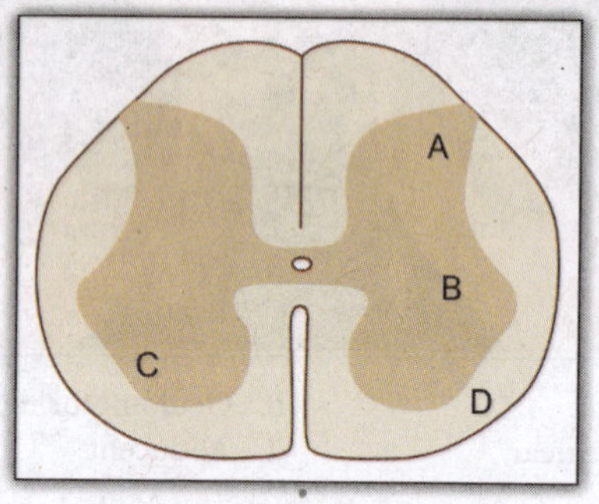

a. A   b. B
c. C   d. D

13. Find out the correctly matched pair of lymph nodes with their anatomical boundaries:

a. Level II—Caudal border of medial pterygoid to clavicle
b. Level III—base of skull to cricoid
c. Level V—base of skull to clavicle
d. Level VI—Cricoid to clavicle

14. Which of the following organelle is absent at marked site?

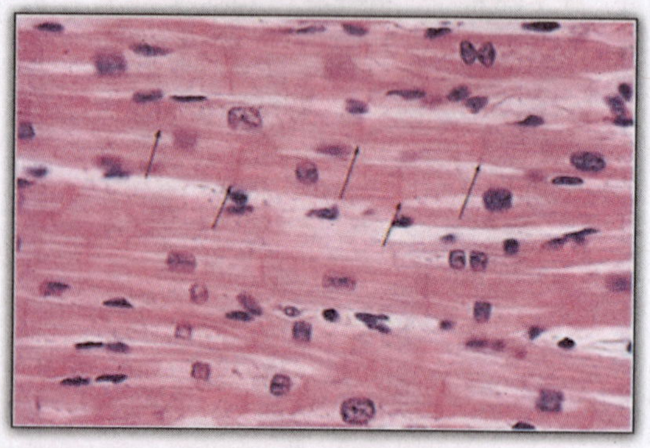

a. Golgi apparatus   b. SER
c. Mitochondria   d. Lysosomes

15. Glycogen rich cells as shown in the given picture are connected to each other by:

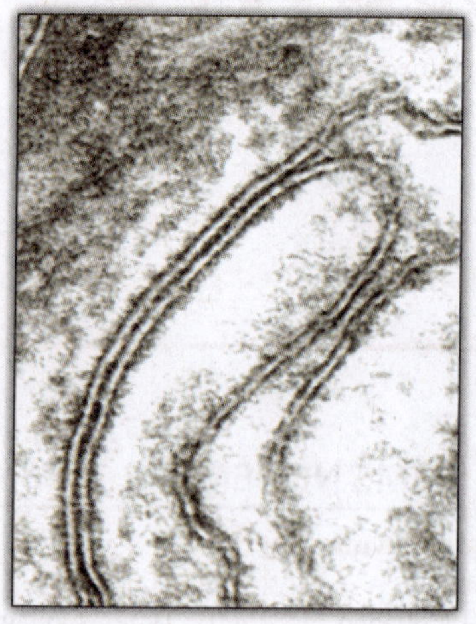

a. Tight junction   b. Desmosomes
c. Gap junction   d. Adherens junction

16. Following electron microscopic picture shows:
(AIIMS Nov 2018, May 2018)

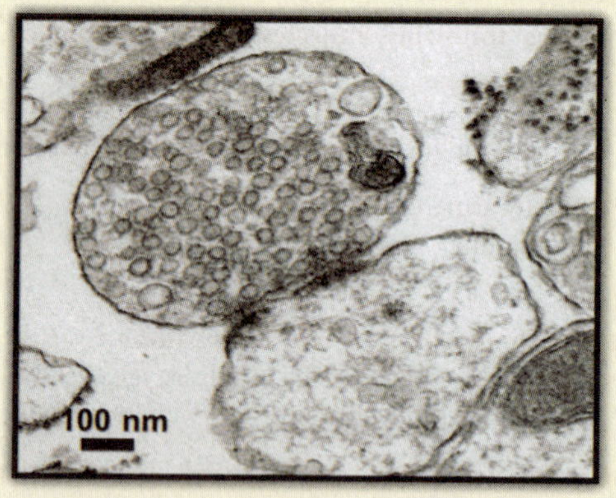

a. Microtubules   b. Collagen fibers
c. Neurosecretory vesicles   d. Golgi bodies

AIIMS MAY 2018

17. Following electron microscopic picture shows?
(AIIMS Nov 2018, May 2018)

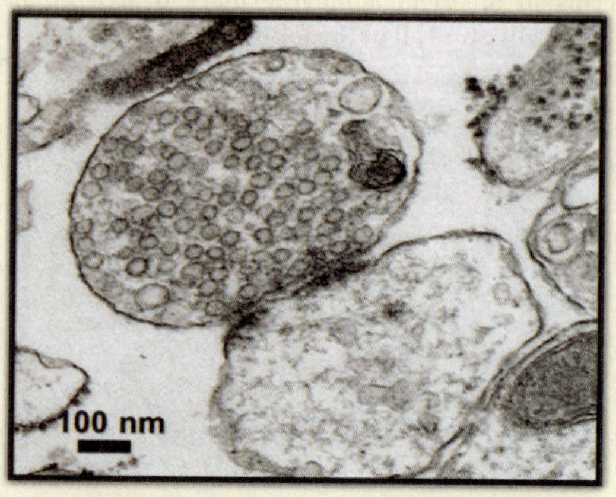

a. Microtubules   b. Collagen fibers
c. Neurosecretory vesicles   d. Golgi bodies

18. True statement about nerve supply of adrenals is?

a. Preganglionic fibers from lower dorsal and upper lumbar spine relay in sympathetic chain to supply adrenal cortex
b. Adrenal medulla is devoid of nerve supply
c. Adrenal cortex is devoid of nerve supply
d. Stress hormone secretions are not under nervous control

19. All of the sensation are carried to spinal nucleus from face EXCEPT:

a. Pain
b. Temperature
c. Proprioception
d. Touch

20. Type 1 collagen is present in all EXCEPT:

a. Bone
b. Hyaline cartilage
c. Ligament
d. Aponeurosis

21. Axons of Purkinje cells ends in:

a. Caudate nucleus
b. Dentate nucleus
c. Basal ganglia
d. Amygdala

22. Which of the following arteries does not supply the endosteal dural layer of meninges:

a. Middle meningeal artery
b. Accessory meningeal artery in middle cranial fossa
c. Meningeal branches of anterior and posterior ethmoidal arteries
d. Branches of ICA in posterior cranial fossa

23. Inferior thyroid artery is a branch of:

a. External carotid artery
b. Internal carotid artery
c. Thyrocervical trunk
d. Vertebral artery

24. Which of the following is wrongly labeled in the given picture?

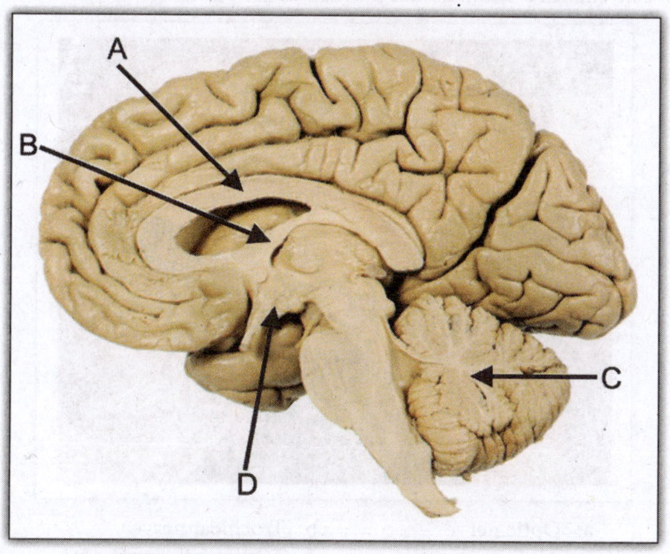

a. A = Corpus callosum
b. B = Fornix
c. C = Cerebellum
d. D = Hypothalamus

25. The arrow marked structure in the given picture is:

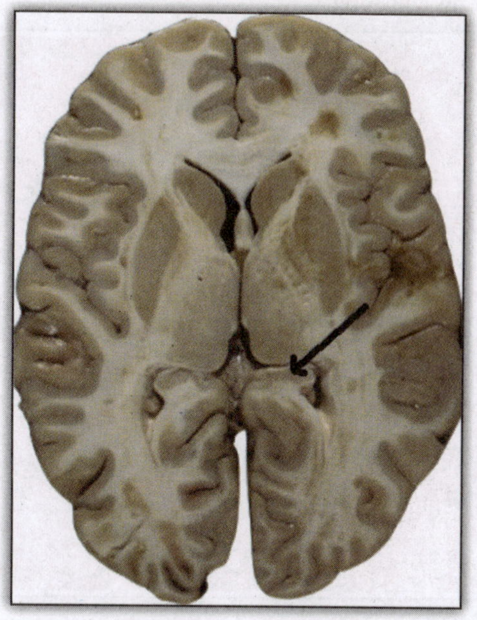

a. Amygdala
b. Mammillary body
c. Hippocampus
d. Caudate nucleus

26. Spinal cord in adults ends at which vertebral level?

a. D_{12}
b. L_1
c. L_3
d. L_4

27. Neurovascular bundle is absent in which compartment of lower leg?

a. Anterior compartment
b. Lateral compartment
c. Superficial posterior compartment
d. Deep posterior compartment

AIIMS NOVEMBER 2017

28. In the following picture identify the structure that gives rise to heart:

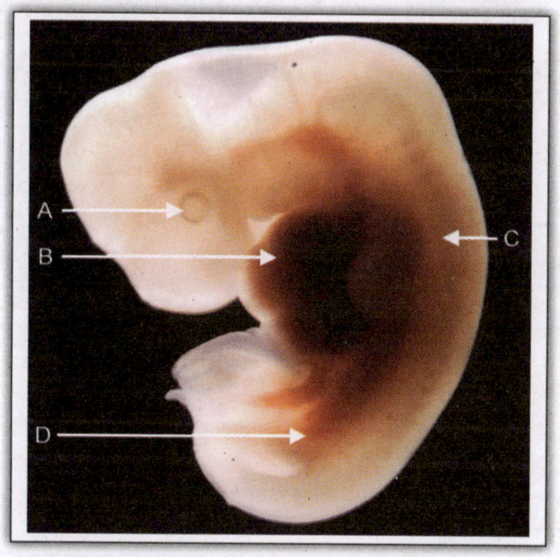

a. A
b. B
c. C
d. D

29. **Which of the following structure shows holocrine gland in the given picture?**

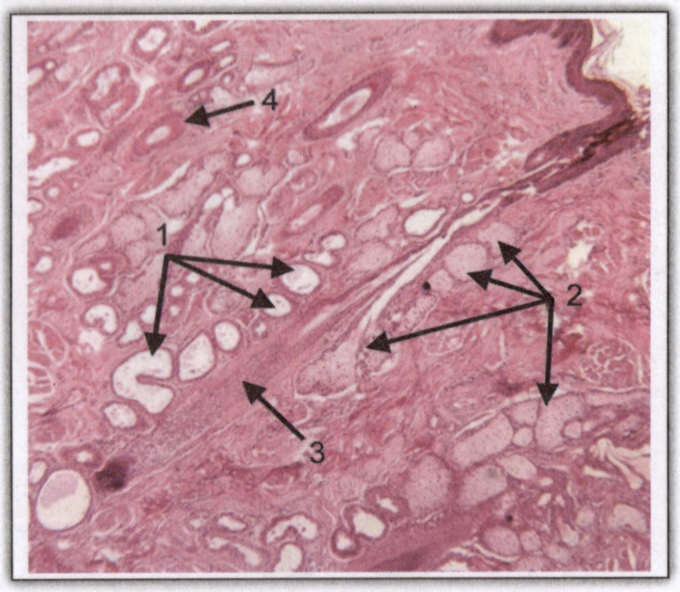

a. 1
b. 2
c. 3
d. 4

30. **Dense irregular connective tissues are seen in:**

a. Tendon
b. Ligament
c. Dermis
d. Lamina propria

31. **The marked structure in the given picture is made up of all EXCEPT:** (AIIMS Nov 2017, 2016)

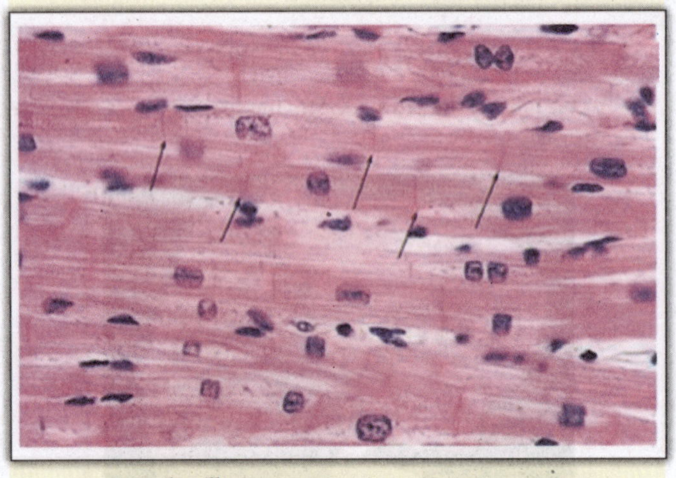

a. Macula adherens
b. Zonaula occludens
c. Gap junction
d. Fascia adherens

32. **In the given picture which muscle is responsible for opening of the Jaw?**

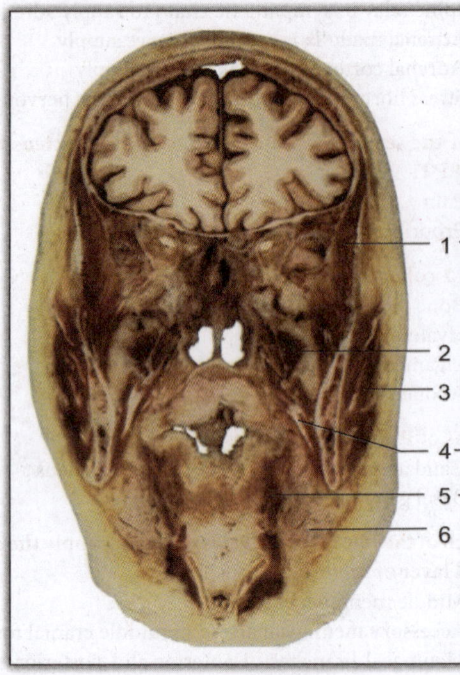

a. 1 b. 2
c. 3 d. 4

33. **Talocalcaneonavicular joint is an example of:**

a. Pivot joint b. Ellipsoid joint
c. Ball and socket joint d. Saddle joint

34. **First carpal bone to ossify is:**

a. Capitate b. Hamate
c. Pisciform d. Lunate

35. **Identify the structure marked in the picture:**

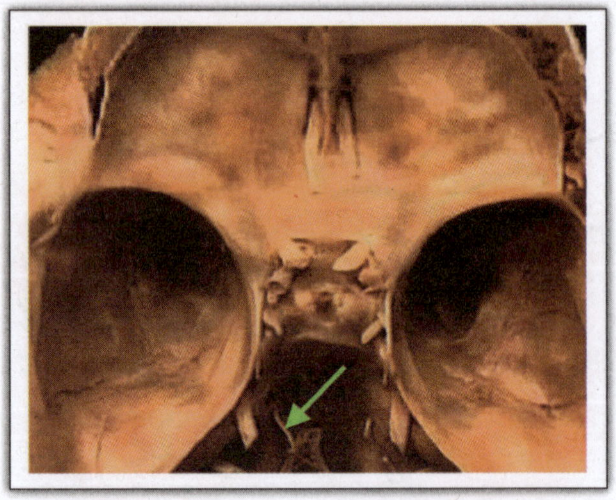

a. Optic nerve b. Trochlear nerve
c. Abducens nerve d. Trigeminal nerve

36. Deepest part of perineal body injury to which causes both urethral and anal incontinence?
a. Pubococcygeus
b. Ischiocavernosus
c. Bulbospongiosus
d. Sphincter of urethra and anus

37. Shape of trapezius muscle is:
a. Strap
b. Triangular
c. Quadrilateral
d. Rhomboid

38. Root value of cremasteric reflex is:
a. L1 L2
b. S2 S3
c. L3 L4
d. L4 S1

39. Which of the following Structure passes through central tendon of diaphragm?
a. Aorta
b. Esophagus
c. Thoracic duct
d. Inferior vena cava

40. The structure marked in the given picture connects to:

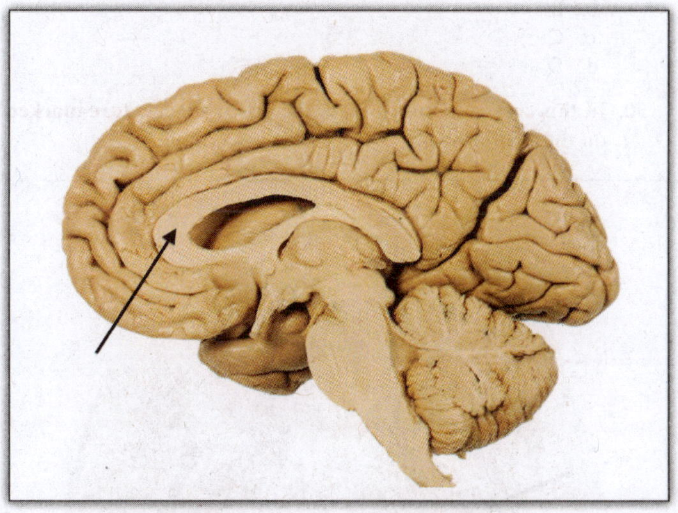

a. Hypothalamus
b. Striate cortex
c. Orbital cortex
d. Dentate nucleus

41. True about grey rami communicantes to all EXCEPT:
a. Unmyelinated nerve fibers
b. Connects to spinal nerves
c. Preganglionic sympathetic supply
d. Present medial to white fibers

42. All are true about posterior cruciate ligament EXCEPT:
a. It is extrasynovial
b. Inserts on anterolateral aspect of medial condyle of femur in intercondylar region
c. Primary restraint to posterior movement of leg
d. Primary restraint to internal rotation of knee

AIIMS MAY 2017

43. A 5-year-old child presented with absence of thymus, hypoparathyroidism and tetany. Which of the following marked area is defective in this case?

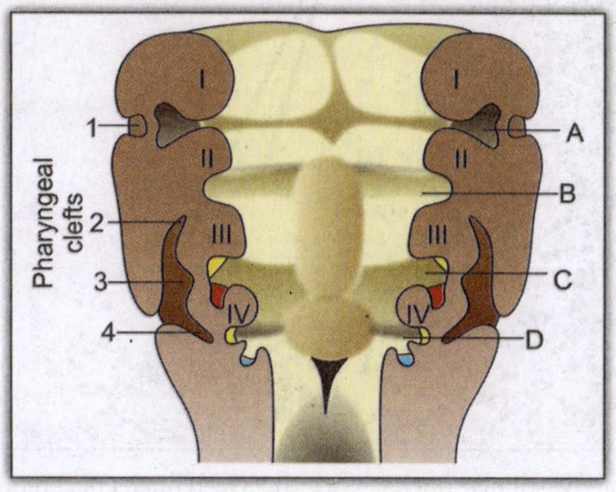

a. A
b. B
c. C
d. D

44. Nucleus pulposus originate from which of the following marked area?

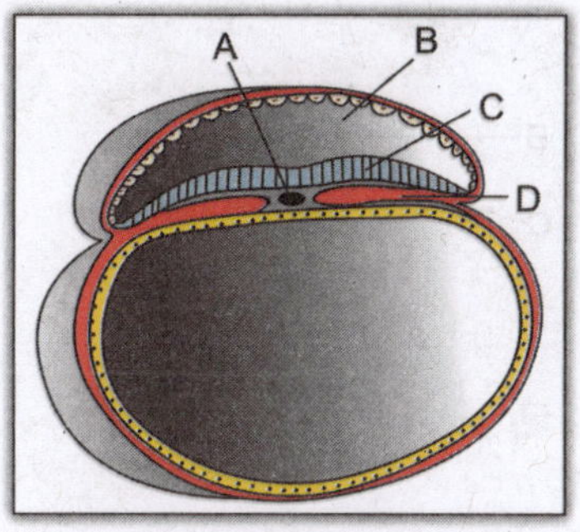

a. A
b. B
c. C
d. D

45. The area marked in the following picture of cut section of lymphatic follicle:

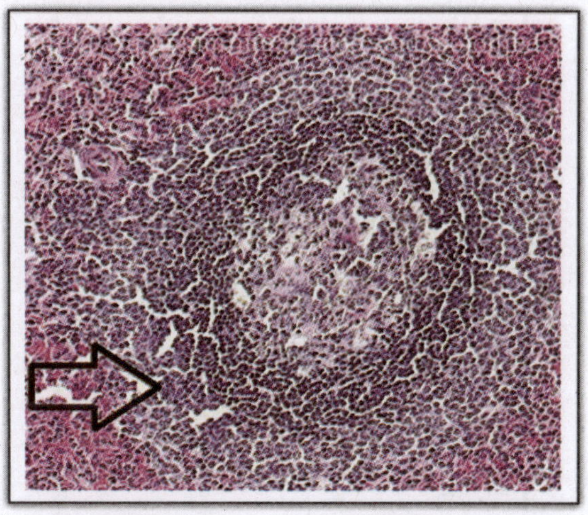

a. Germinal center
b. Mantle zone
c. Paracortical area
d. Marginal zone

46. Which cell is inhibited by the cell given in the slide?

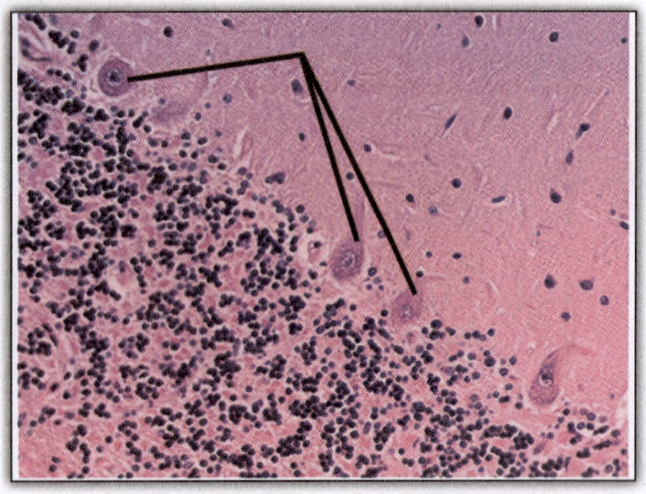

a. Vestibular nuclei
b. Deep nuclei of cerebellum
c. Anterior horn of spinal
d. Basal ganglia

47. Which of the following marked structure can be palpated in the infraclavicular fossa?

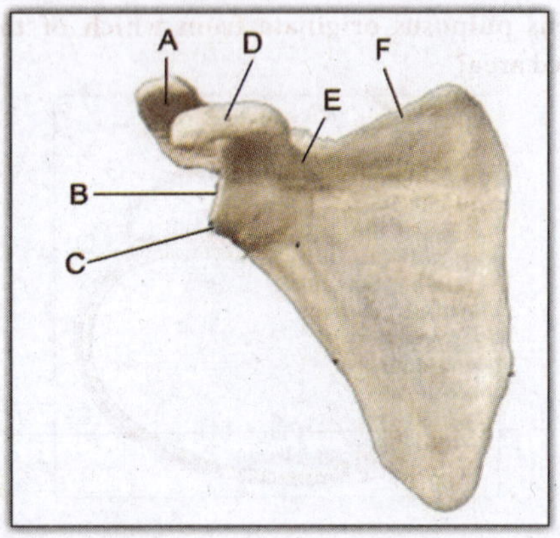

a. A
b. B
c. C
d. D

48. Which of the following marked structure is pelvic diaphragm?

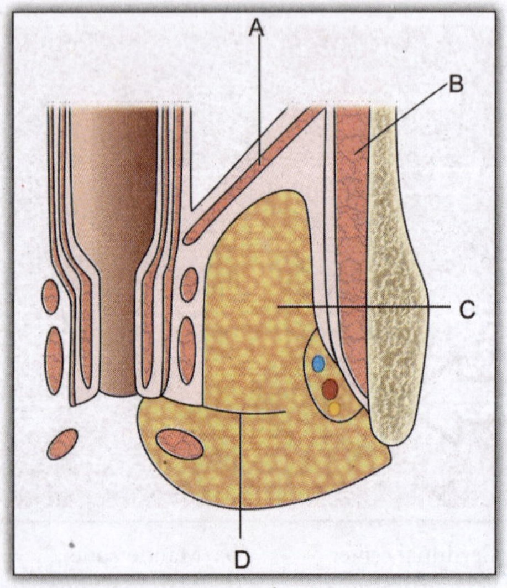

a. A
b. B
c. C
d. D

49. In the following image of transversus abdominis, which label denotes conjoint tendon?

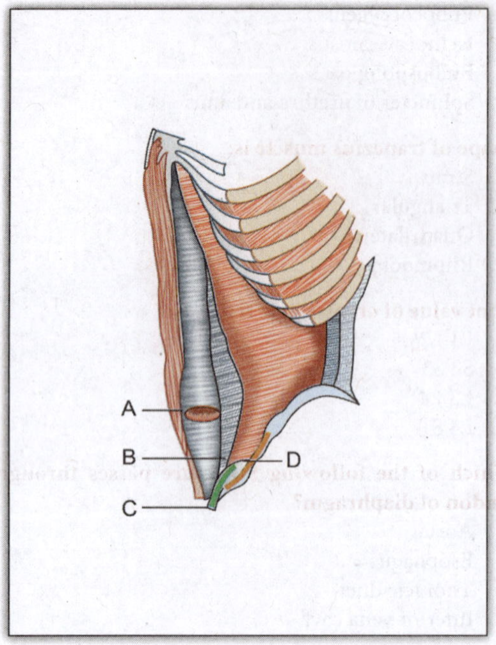

a. A
b. B
c. C
d. D

50. In this cross section of head, the action of structure marked on the mandible is:

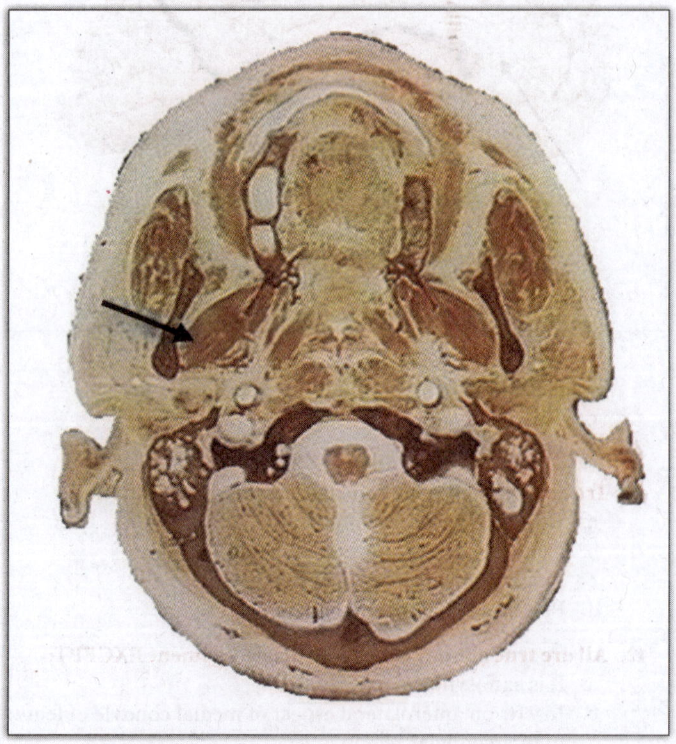

a. Protraction
b. Retraction
c. Elevation
d. Depression

Subject-wise MCQs and Answers with Explanations

51. **Which of the following forms the superior boundary of epiploic foramen?**

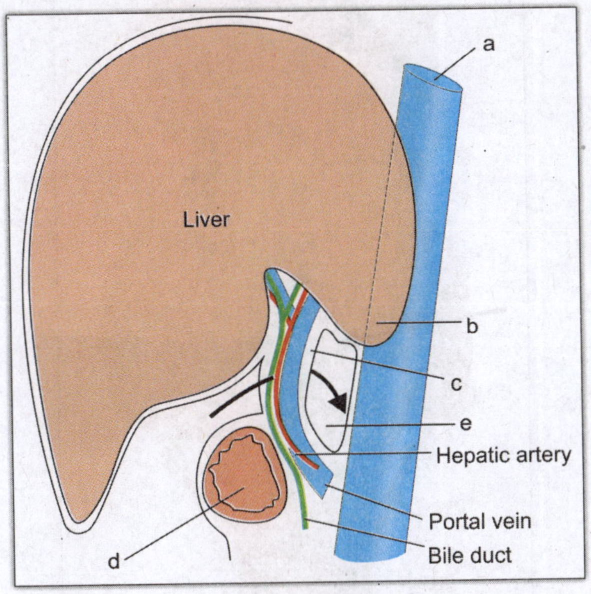

a. a
b. b
c. c
d. d

52. **The arrow marked structure in the given picture connects which of the following structure?**
a. Amygdala
b. Mammillary body
c. Habenular nuclei
d. Hippocampus

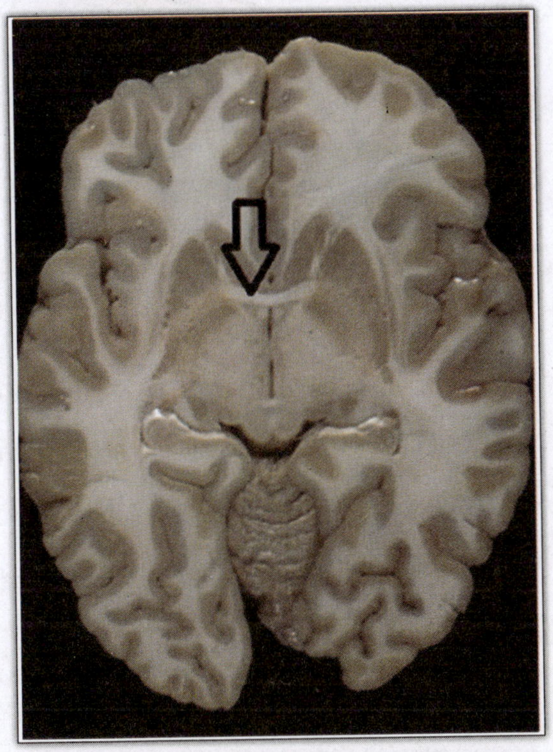

53. **Mandibular branch of trigeminal nerve passes through which of the following marked structure?**

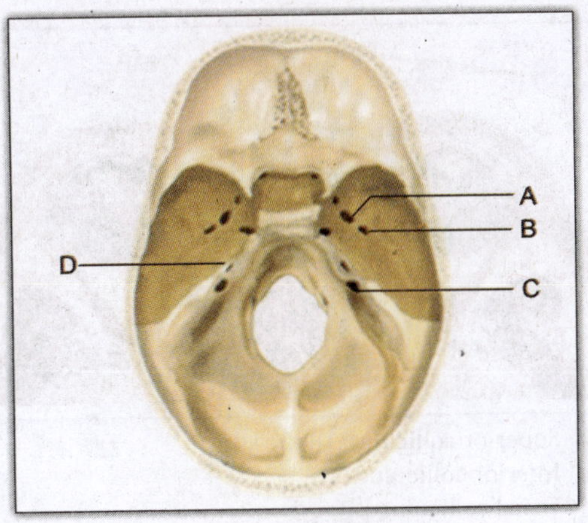

a. A
b. B
c. C
d. D

54. **Disease caused by the structure marked in the picture below is:**

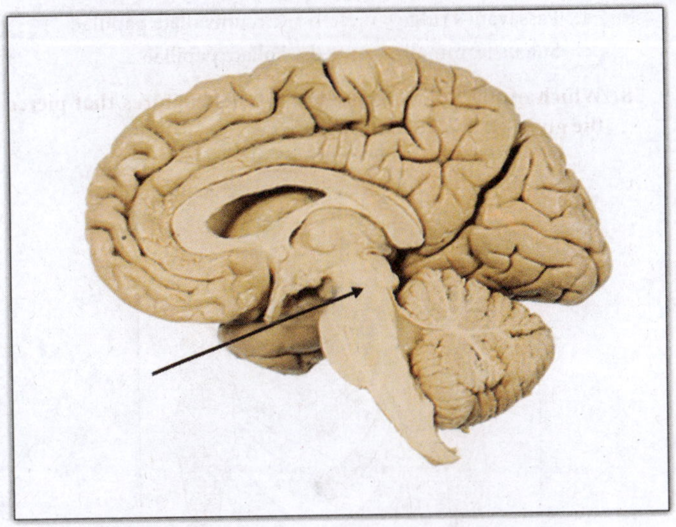

a. Paralysis agitans
b. Huntington's Chorea
c. Alzheimer's disease
d. Dementia

55. **Third part of vertebral artery is related to which of the marked structure in the given picture?**

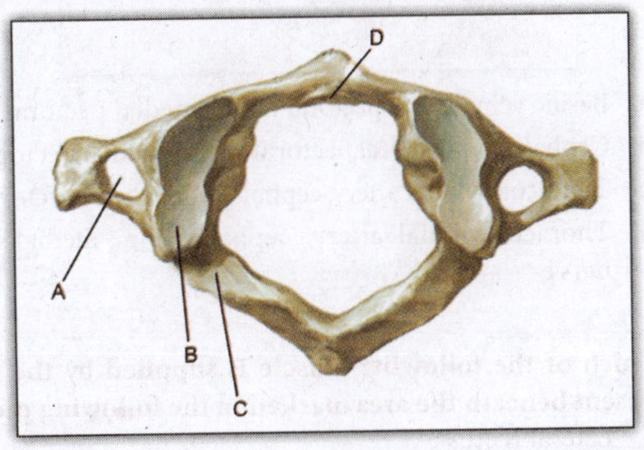

a. A
b. B
c. C
d. D

56. Location of the nucleus supplying the muscle marked in the picture is:

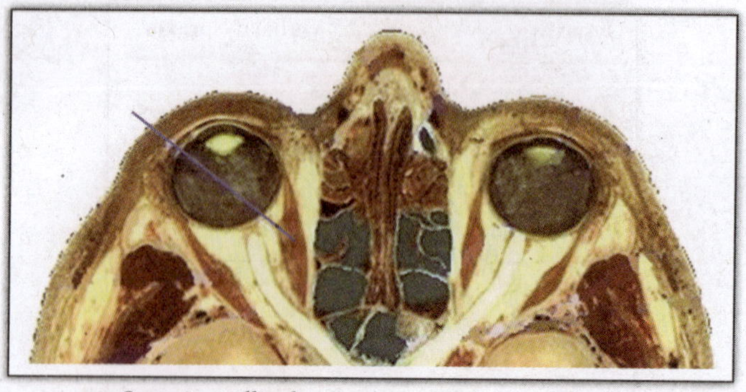

a. Superior colliculus
b. Inferior colliculus
c. Facial colliculus
d. Inferior salivatory nucleus

AIIMS NOVEMBER 2016

57. Anterior 2/3rd of the tongue demarcated by:

a. Passavant's ridge
b. Circumvallate papillae
c. Sulcus terminalis
d. Foliate papillae

58. Which of the following are the set of structures that pierce the given structure in the picture?

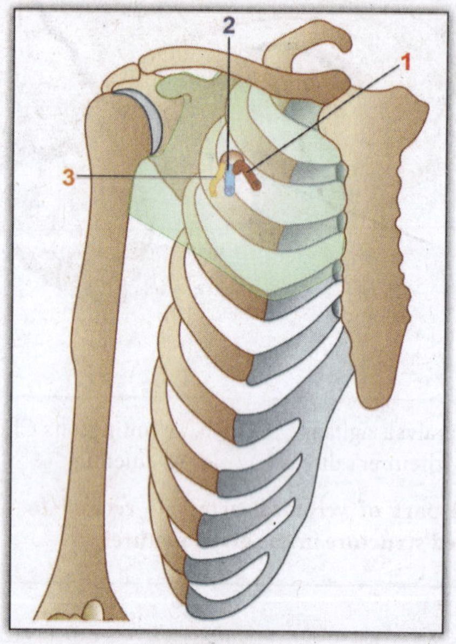

a. Basilic vein, lateral pectoral nerve, medial pectoral nerve
b. Cephalic vein, lateral pectoral nerve, medial pectoral nerve
c. Thoracoacromial artery, cephalic vein, lateral pectoral nerve
d. Thoracoacromial artery, cephalic vein, medial pectoral nerve

59. Which of the following muscle is supplied by the nucleus present beneath the area marked in the following picture?

a. Lateral rectus
b. Risorius
c. Superior oblique
d. Levator palpebrae superioris

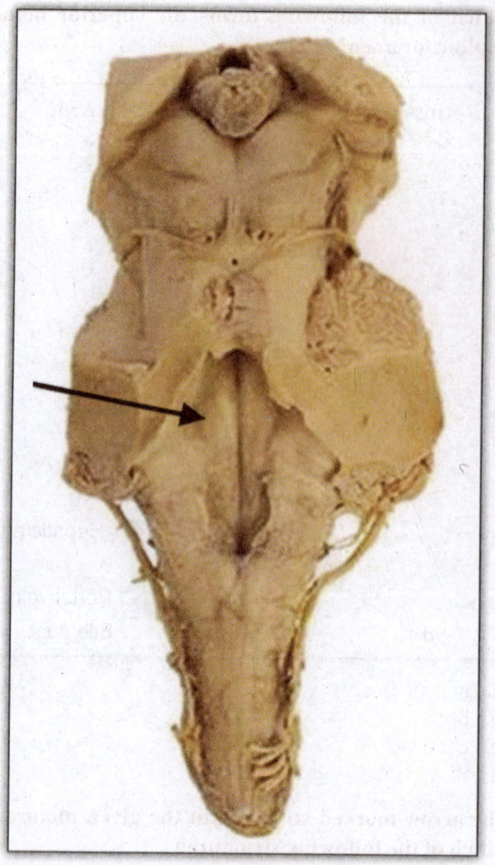

60. In the given cross section of axilla, the structures marked are:

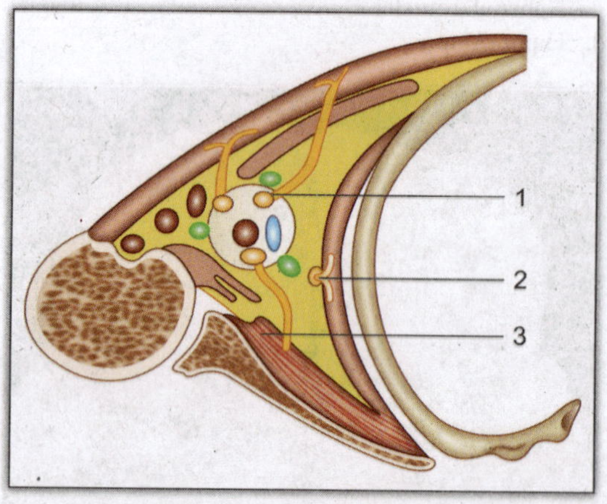

a. 1- Lateral cord of brachial plexus, 2- Long thoracic nerve, 3- Serratus anterior
b. 1- Medial cord of brachial plexus, 2- Long thoracic nerve, 3- Subscapularis
c. 1- Posterior cord of brachial plexus, 2- Nerve to serratus anterior, 3- Subscapularis
d. 1- Lateral cord of brachial plexus, 2- Long thoracic nerve, 3- Subscapularis

61. Relations of left ureter are all EXCEPT:

a. Sigmoid mesentery ***(AIIMS Nov 2016, DNB June 2010)***
b. Bifurcation of common iliac artery
c. Quadratus lumborum
d. Gonadal vessels

62. **All are example of muscle in which fibers are arranged parallel EXCEPT:**
a. Sternohyoid
b. Sartorius
c. Rectus abdominis
d. Tibialis anterior

63. **In the following image of anterior abdominal wall, the correct matching of markings is:**

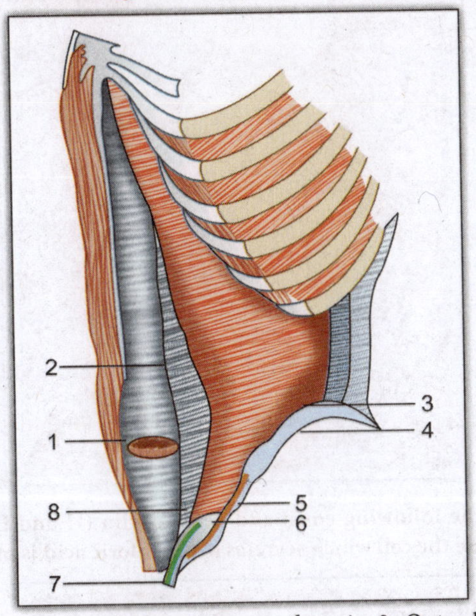

a. 1. Linea alba, 2. Linea semilunaris, 3. Outer lip of iliac crest, 4. Inner lip of iliac crest, 5. Inguinal ligament, 6. Superficial inguinal ring
b. 1. Linea alba, 2. Linea semilunaris, 3. Inner lip of iliac crest, 4. Outer lip of iliac crest, 5. Inguinal ligament, 6. Deep inguinal ring
c. 1. Linea semilunaris, 2. Linea alba, 3. Outer lip of iliac crest 4. Inner lip of iliac crest 5. Inguinal ligament, 6. Superficial inguinal ring
d. 1. Linea semilunaris, 2. Linea alba, 3. Inner lip of iliac crest 4. Outer lip of iliac crest 5. Inguinal ligament, 6. Deep inguinal ring

64. **Extraembryonic mesoderm develops from:**
a. Hypoblast
b. Epiblast
c. Primary yolk sac
d. Secondary yolk sac

65. **Injury to the area marked by the arrow in the given picture will lead to:**

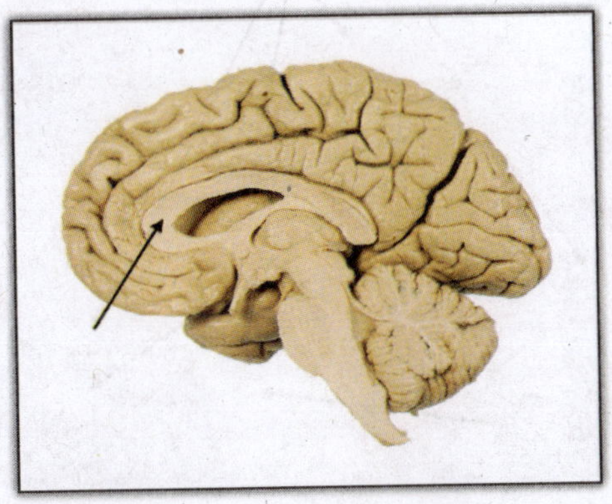

a. Lower limb paralysis
b. Apraxia
c. Aphasia
d. Visual disturbance

66. **Defect in the structure, the histology of which is shown in the figure, will lead to which of the following speech disorder?**
a. Apraxia
b. Aphasia
c. Dysarthria
d. Verbal dyspraxia

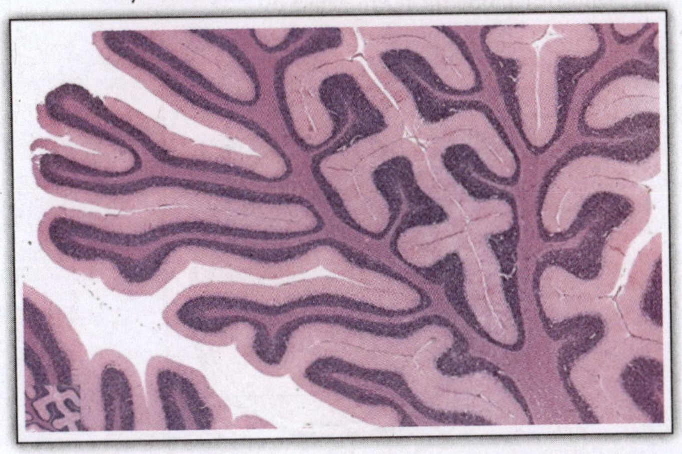

67. **Histology image of epithelium shown in the picture is of which organ?**

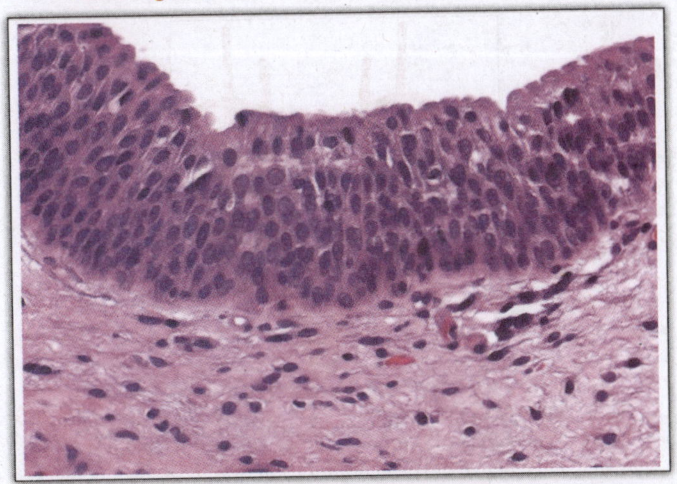

a. Skin
b. Urinary bladder
c. Common bile duct
d. Bile duct

68. **The marked structure in the given picture is made up of all EXCEPT:** *(AIIMS Nov 2017, 2016)*

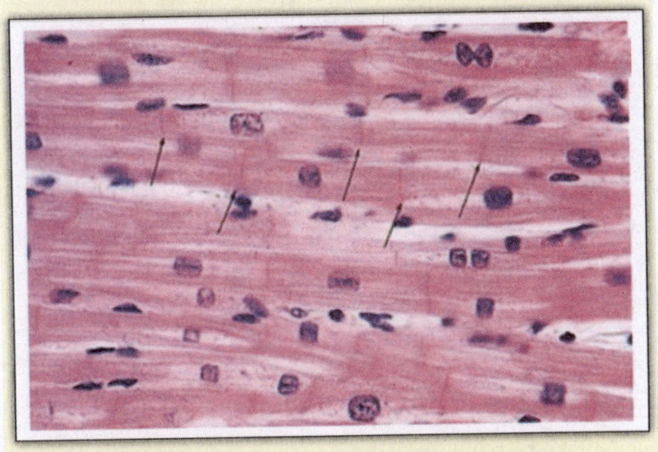

a. Macula adherens
b. Zonula occludens
c. Gap junction
d. Fascia Adherens

AIIMS MAY 2016

69. The below figure depicts various parts from which diaphragm develops. Congenital diaphragmatic hernia is mostly commonly due to defect in:

a. A b. B
c. C d. D

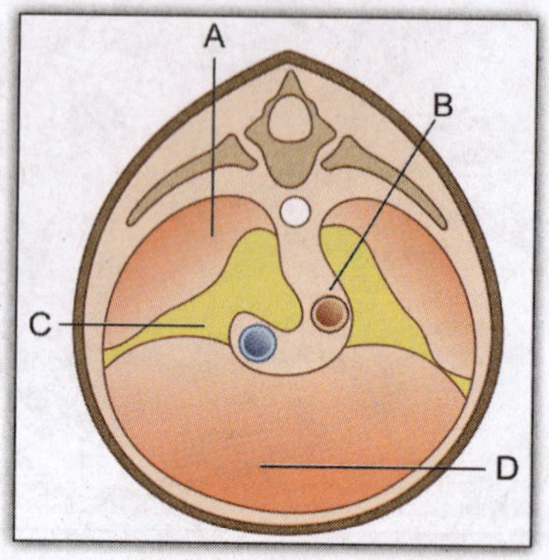

70. The figure below represents a stage of development of aortic arches. Abnormal subclavian artery results due to:

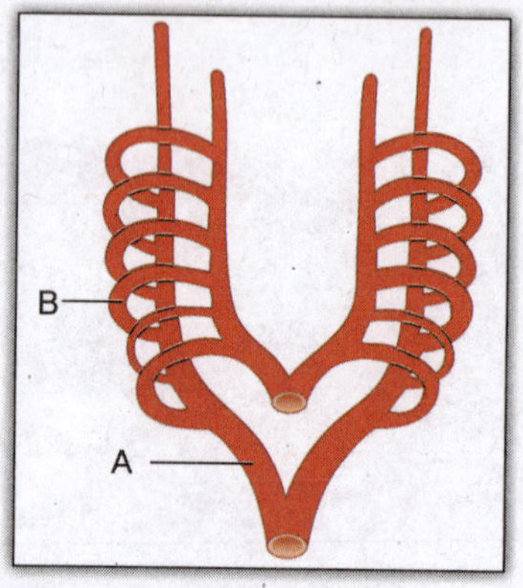

a. Persistence of A only
b. Persistence of B only
c. Persistence of B and obliteration of A
d. Persistence of A and obliteration of B

71. Portal vein develops from which structure shown in the following picture?

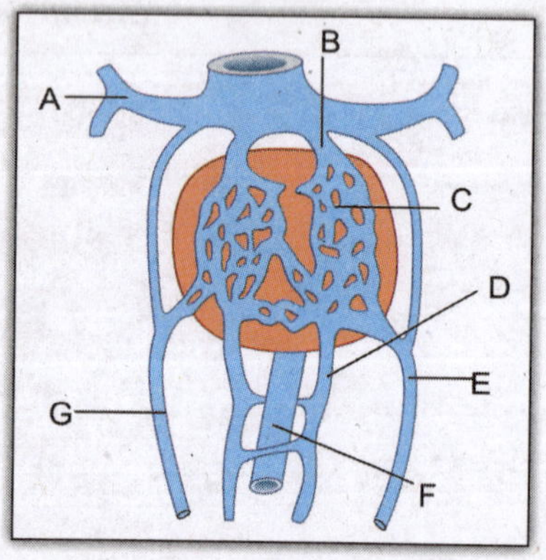

a. A
b. B
c. C
d. D

72. An image of H and E stained section of a tissue is given below. The glands shown in this image is:

a. Holocrine gland b. Paracrine gland
c. Endocrine gland d. Apocrine gland

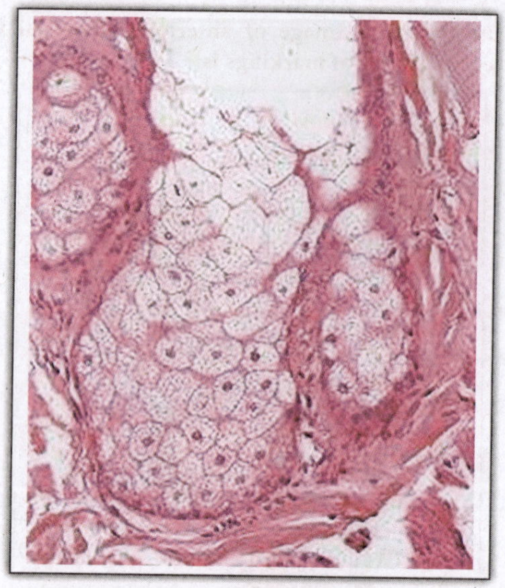

73. In the following eosin and hematoxylin (H and E) stained tissue the cell which secretes hydrochloric acid is marked as:

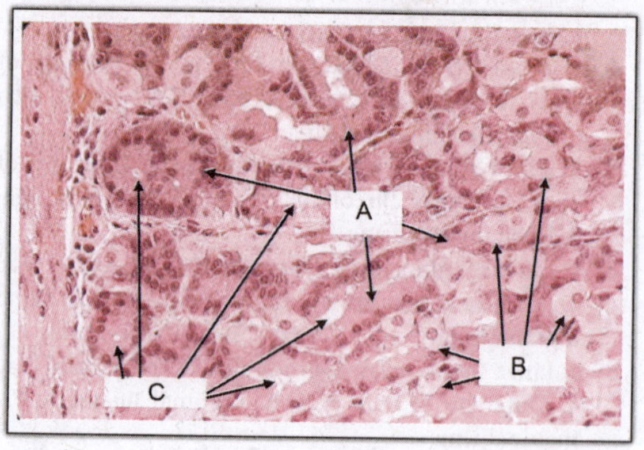

a. A b. B
c. C d. D

74. Image of H and E section of stained tissue is provided below. Identify the organ?

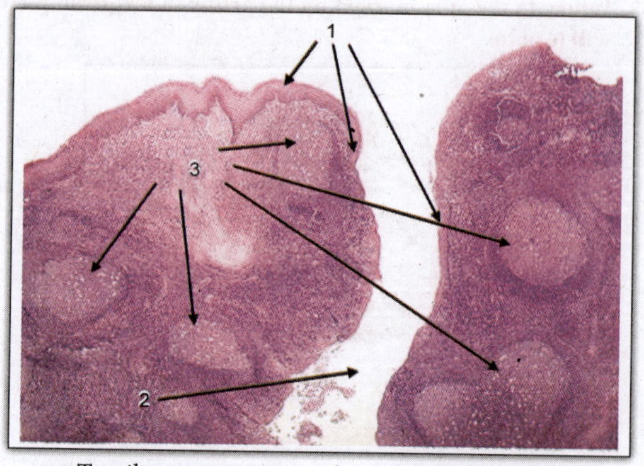

a. Tonsil b. Spleen
c. Lymph node d. Peyers patches

75. The tissue shown in lower 2/3 of this picture Eosin (H and E) stained section of a tissue is shown below is found in:

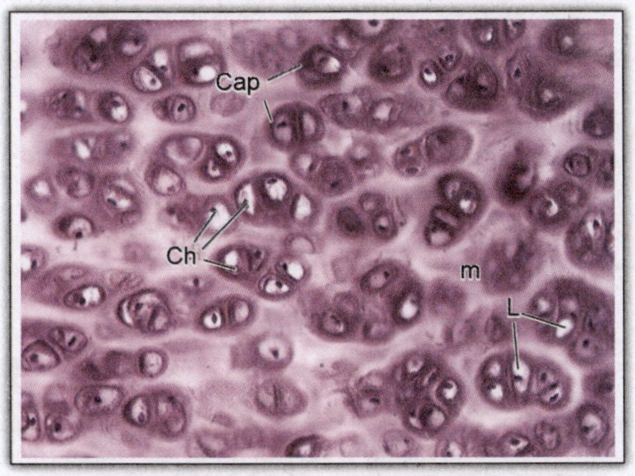

a. Articular disc
b. Intervertebral discs
c. Epiphyseal growth plates
d. Pinna of ear

76. In the diagram given below, different muscles of larynx are marked by labelled arrows. Abduction of vocal cord is done by the muscle marked by:

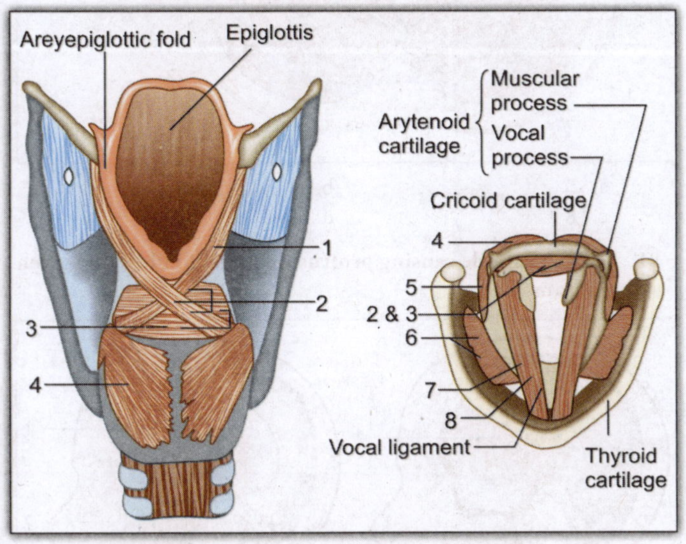

a. 1
b. 2
c. 3
d. 4

77. The following system of depiction of the 32 teeth is in accordance with which system?

a. Palmar notation
b. Haderup system
c. Universal system
d. Diagram chart

Upper right								Upper left							
1	2	3	4	5	6	7	8	9	10	11	12	13	14	15	16
32	31	30	29	28	27	26	25	24	23	22	21	20	19	18	17
Lower right								Lower left							

78. In the image given below, the structure marked with the arrow 1 is an important area related to motor function. All of the following gives afferent fibers to this structure EXCEPT:

a. Substantia nigra
b. Spinal cord
c. Thalamus
d. Cerebral cortex

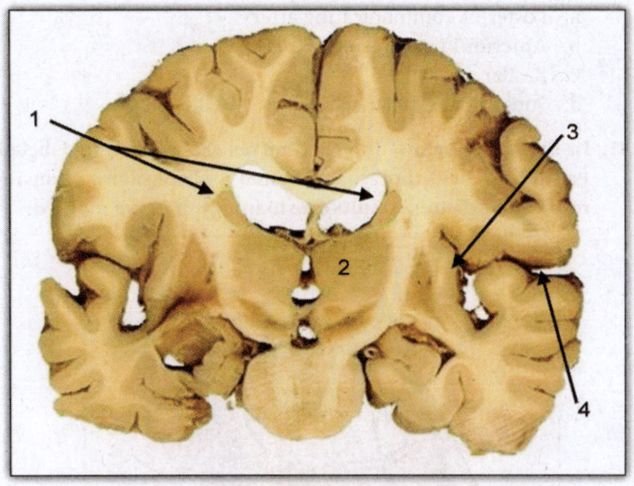

79. In this coronal section of brain, insula is marked as:

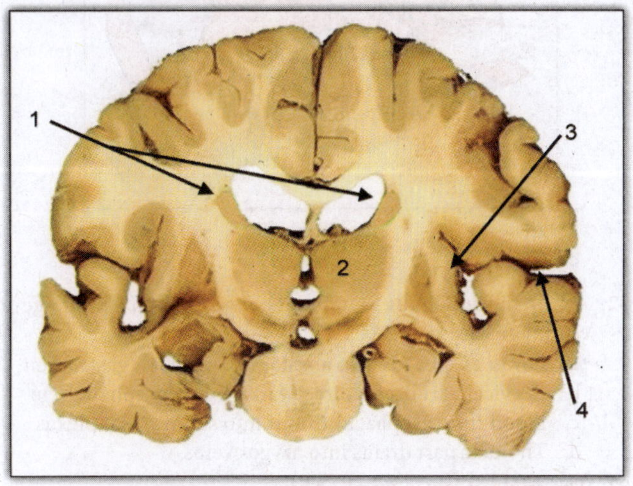

a. 1
b. 2
c. 3
d. 4

80. In the image given below, artery pointed with an arrow marked 3 is:

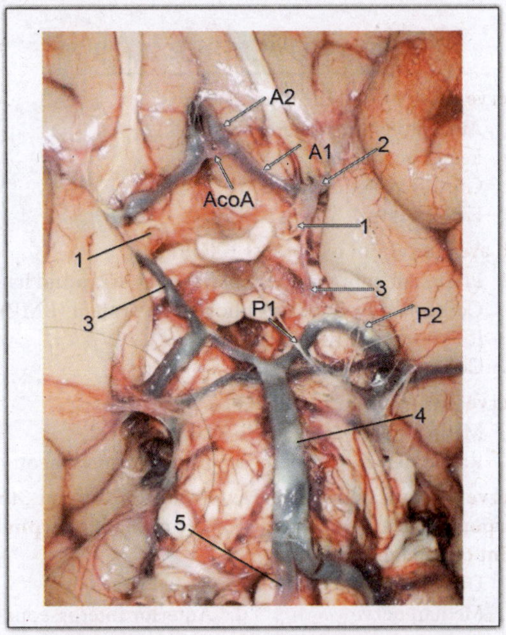

ANATOMY • Questions

a. Posterior communicating artery
b. Anterior inferior cerebellar artery
c. Basilar artery
d. Superior cerebellar artery

81. In the figure below, different nerves are marked by labeled. Paralysis of thoracoabdominal diaphragm causing respiratory distress results due to injury to nerve marked:

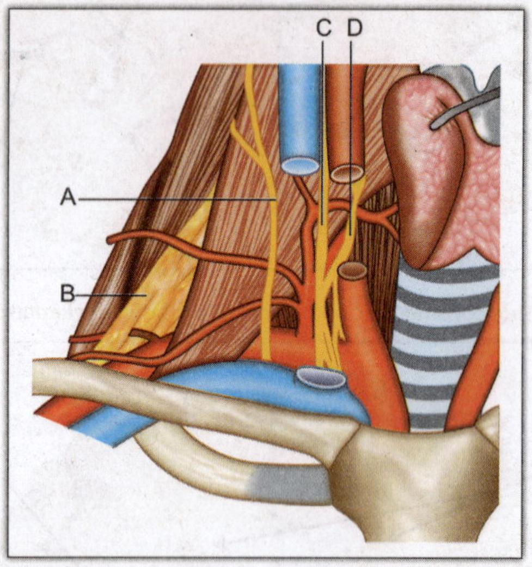

a. A
b. B
c. C
d. D

82. All of the following statements about venous drainage of esopahgus are true EXCEPT:
a. Lower esophagus vein anastomose with left gastric vein
b. Cervical part drains directly into brachiocephalic vein
c. Blood from esophagus drains into submucosal plexus
d. Thoracic part drains into azygos veins

83. The angle of jaw is supplied by:
a. Greater auricular nerve
b. Lesser occipital nerve
c. Mandibular division of trigeminal nerve
d. Maxillary division of trigeminal nerve

AIIMS NOVEMBER 2015

84. Nerve supply of lobule of ear is by:
a. Auriculotemporal nerve
b. Lesser occipital nerve
c. Greater auricular nerve
d. Facial nerve

85. All are true about osteoblast EXCEPT:
a. Plasma membrane does not have dendrites and its smooth
b. Controlled by bone morphogenetic protein (BMP)
c. It has neuropeptide receptors
d. Contains actin and myosin

86. Nerve involved in Pronator teres syndrome is:
a. Median nerve
b. Ulnar nerve
c. Radial nerve
d. Anterior interosseous nerve

87. Nerve injury causing hyperextension of 4th and 5th metacarpophalageal joint and flexion at proximal interphalangeal joint of ring and little finger is:
a. Ulnar nerve
b. Radial nerve
c. Median nerve
d. Anterior interosseous nerve

88. Anal canal is supplied by all vessels EXCEPT:
a. Superior rectal artery
b. Middle rectal artery
c. Inferior rectal artery
d. Median sacral artery

89. All are involved in development of diaphragm EXCEPT:
a. Pleuroperitoneal membrane
b. Pleuropericardial membrane
c. Septum transversum
d. Body wall

90. Identify vagus nerve in the given transverse section of neck:

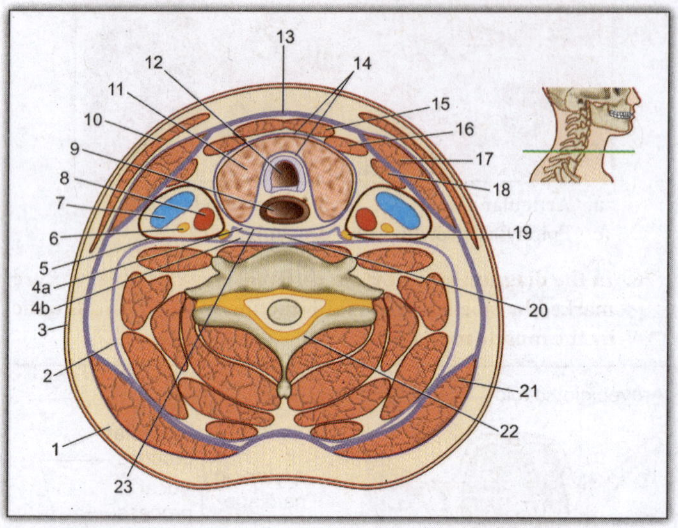

a. 5
b. 6
c. 8
d. 19

91. Identify muscle causing protrusion of mandible in the given diagram:

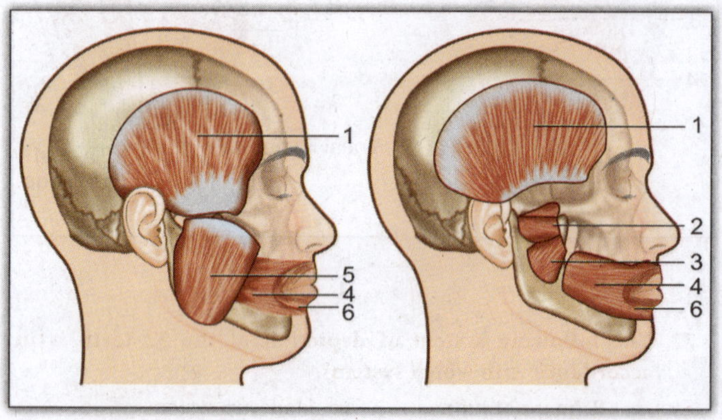

a. 1
b. 2
c. 3
d. 4

92. Which of the following is false about location of otic ganglion?
a. Anterior to middle meningeal artery
b. Lateral to mandibular nerve
c. Lateral to tensor veli palatini
d. Inferior to foramen ovale

93. All of the following articulates with maxilla EXCEPT:
a. Lacrimal bone
b. Ethmoid bone
c. Sphenoid bone
d. Zygomatic bone

94. All the following form craniovertebral junction EXCEPT:

a. Atlas b. Axis
c. Basiocciput d. Wings of sphenoid

95. Identify the nerve causing convergent strabismus in the diagram shown:

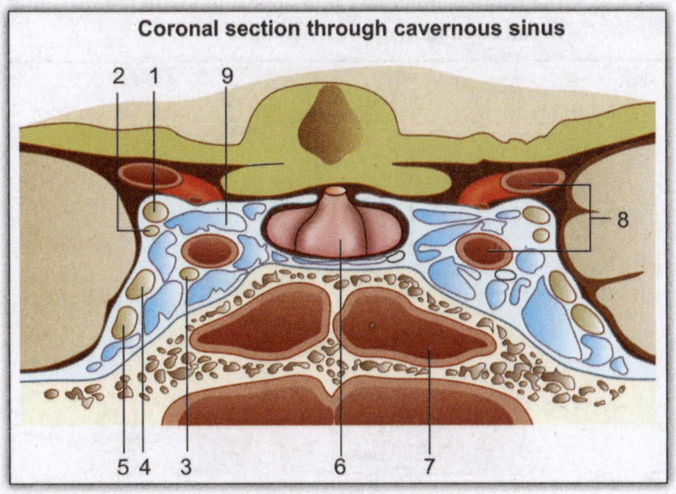

a. 1 b. 2
c. 3 d. 4

96. In the following picture identify the nerve supplying superior oblique muscle?

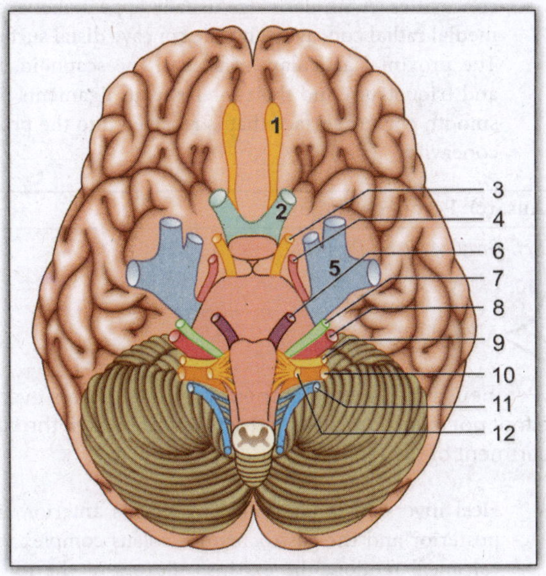

a. 1 b. 2
c. 3 d. 4

97. Meralgia paresthetica is caused due to involvement of:

a. Genitofemoral nerve
b. Ilioinguinal nerve
c. Lateral cutaneous nerve of thigh
d. Popliteal nerve

98. Buccinator is pierced by all EXCEPT: *(AIIMS Nov 2015, 2008)*

a. Parotid duct
b. Buccal branch of mandibular nerve
c. Buccal branch of facial nerve
d. Mucous glands of molars

AIIMS MAY 2015

99. Independent assortment of maternal and paternal chromosome occurs at which stage of spermatocyte maturation? *(AIIMS May 2015, Nov 2013)*

a. Spermatogonia to primary spermatocyte
b. Primary to secondary spermatocyte
c. Secondary spermatocyte to spermatids
d. Spermatid to spermatogonia

100. At what stage of meiosis are oogonia in ovaries present at birth?

a. Telophase I b. Prophase I
c. Anaphase d. Metaphase

101. All structures are derived from mesonephros EXCEPT:

a. Glomerulus b. Paroophoron
c. Vas deferens d. Epididymis

102. Muscle not inserted on greater tubercle is:

a. Teres minor b. Supraspinatus
c. Infraspinatus d. Subscapularis

103. Reticular fibers of collagen tissues are present in all EXCEPT:

a. Thymus b. Bone marrow
c. Spleen d. Lymph node

104. Which of the following is not a branch of external carotid artery?

a. Transverse cervical artery
b. Lingual
c. Superior thyroid artery
d. Ascending pharyngeal

105. Most metabolically active layer in the bone is:

a. Periosteum b. Endosteum
c. Cancellous bone d. Cortical bone

106. Microvilli are not present in:

a. Duodenum
b. Gallbladder
c. Proximal convoluted tubule
d. Collecting duct

107. Which of the following cranial nerve nucleus is located beneath the facial colliculus? *(AIIMS May 2015, Nov 2014)*

a. Facial b. Abducent
c. Glossopharyngeal d. Trigeminal

108. Card test done for:

a. Lumbricals
b. Dorsal interossei
c. Palmar interossei
d. Adductor pollicis

109. Mesorectal fascia contains all of the following structures EXCEPT: *(AIIMS May 2015, 2014, Nov 2013)*

a. Interior rectal vein b. Pararectal node
c. Superior rectal vein d. Inferior mesenteric plexus

110. All have general visceral efferent fibers EXCEPT:

a. Olfactory nerve
b. Facial nerve
c. Oculomotor nerve
d. Glossopharyngeal nerve

ANSWERS WITH EXPLANATIONS

AIIMS NOVEMBER 2018

1. Ans. (a) Elastins

Ref: Gray's 41st Ed Pg 745

Ligamentum Flavum

The ligamenta flava connect laminae of adjacent vertebrae in the vertebral canal.

Extent: From facet joint capsules to the point where laminae fuse to form spines, where their posterior margins are partially united; the intervals between them admit veins that connect the internal and posterior external vertebral venous plexuses.

Variation: Thin, broad and long in the cervical region, thicker in the thoracic and thickest at lumbar levels.

Function: Arrest separation of the laminae in spinal flexion, preventing abrupt limitation, assist restoration to an erect posture after flexion, protecting discs from injury.

Composition: The ligamentum flavum has such a high content of elastin that it is always under tension and can be stretched by 80% without damage. This ligament probably functions to provide a constant smooth lining to the vertebral canal, which is never overstretched in flexion and which never goes slack in extension.

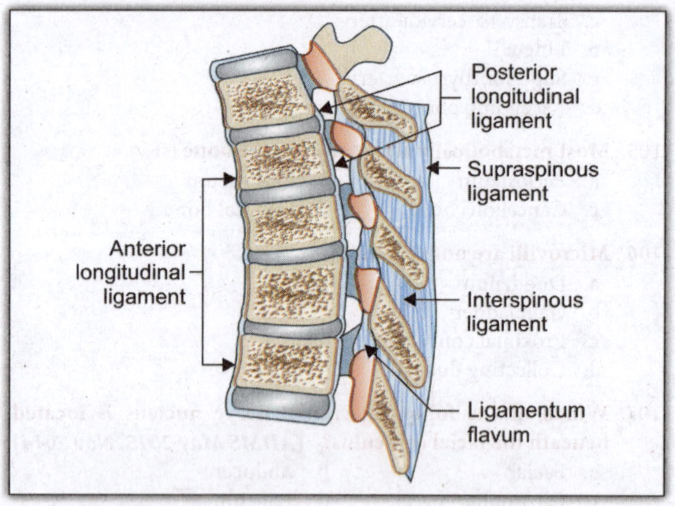

2. Ans. (a) Ulna

Ref: Gray's Anatomy 41st Ed page 872

Summary: Wrist joint is composed of radiocarpal and intercarpal joints. There is no articulation between ulna and carpal bones and distal radioulnar joint is not a part of Wrist joint.

- The radiocarpal joint is a synovial, biaxial and ellipsoid joint formed by articulation of the **distal end of the radius and the articular disc of the triangular fibrocartilage with the scaphoid, lunate and triquetrum.**
- In the neutral position of the wrist, only the scaphoid and lunate are in contact with the radius and articular disc; the triquetrum comes into apposition with the disc only in full adduction of the wrist joint.

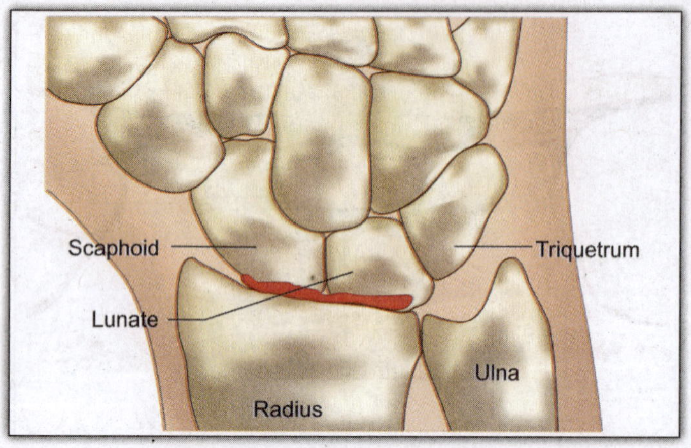

- The radial articular surface and distal surface form an almost elliptical, concave surface with a transverse long axis.
- The radial surface is bisected by a low ridge into two concavities. A similar ridge usually appears between the medial radial concavity and the concave distal surface.
- The proximal articular surfaces of the scaphoid, lunate and triquetrum and their interosseous ligaments form a smooth convex surface that is received into the proximal concavity.

3. Ans. (c) Peroneus longus

Ref: Gray's 41st Ed Pg 1435

NOTE

Both Peroneus longus and Peroneus brevis facilitates eversion of the foot not inversion. Both of them are muscles of the lateral compartment of the leg.

- Heel inversion is controlled by tibialis anterior, tibialis posterior and the gastrocnemius soleus complex via the calcaneal tendon; the extrinsic flexors of the toes also contribute.
- Eversion of the foot results from the pull of peroneus longus, brevis and tertius in addition to the extrinsic muscles that extend the toes.

4. Ans. (d) Lordosis

Ref: Gray's 41st ed Pg 716

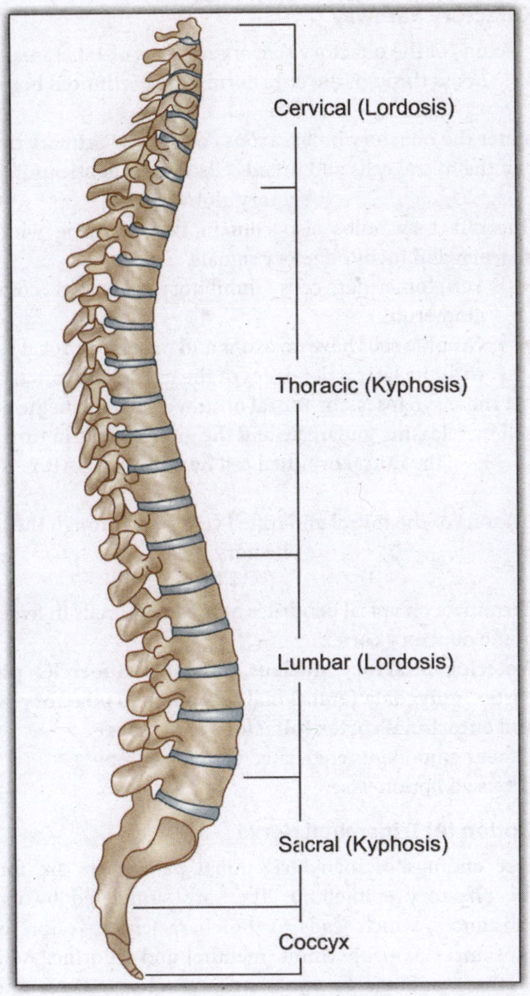

Fig: Curvatures of spine

Vertebral column and its curvature		
Region	**Curvature**	**Extent**
Cervical	Lordosis	Atlas to 2nd thoracic vertebra
Thoracic	Kyphosis	2nd to 12th thoracic vertebrae, apex between 6th and 9th vertebrae
Lumbar	Lordosis	Lumbosacral junction to the apex of the coccyx.
Sacral	Kyphosis	Lumbosacral junction to the apex of the coccyx.

Footnote:

- In the normal vertebral column, there are well-marked curvatures in the sagittal plane and no lateral curvatures other than in the upper thoracic region, where there is often a slight lateral curvature, convex to the right in right-handed persons and to the left in the left-handed.
- **Embryonic and fetal curvatures:** Embryonic body is flexed. Thoracic and pelvic curves, which are primary and convex dorsally. Functional muscle development leads to the early appearance of secondary cervical and lumbar spinal curvatures in the sagittal plane. The cervical curvature appears at the end of the embryonic period.
- **Neonatal curvatures:** In the neonate, the vertebral column has no fixed curvatures. The thoracic part of the column is the first to develop a relatively fixed curvature (concave anteriorly). Developmental changes like sitting, walking exert major influences on secondary curvatures.

5. **Ans. (d) Left brachiocephalic vein**

Ref: Gray's 41st Ed Pg 937, 1027

Left Superior Intercostal Vein

Course: It ascends obliquely forwards across the left aspect of the aortic arch, lateral to the left vagus and medial to the left phrenic nerve, to open into the left brachiocephalic vein.

It usually receives the left bronchial veins, sometimes the left pericardiacophrenic vein and connects inferiorly with the accessory hemiazygos vein. **It drains into the brachiocephalic vein and the anterior intercostal veins, which drain into the internal thoracic vein.**

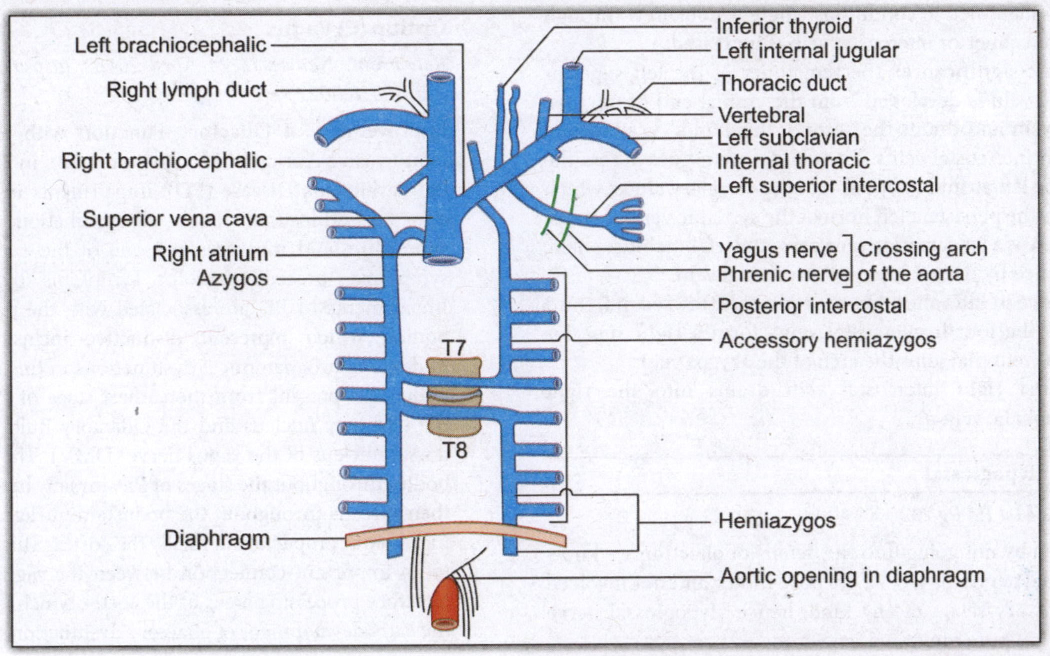

Radiological significance: It may be seen on a chest X-ray as the 'aortic nipple', not to be confused with a small lung nodule. (Note: Aortic arch forms the aortic "knuckle")

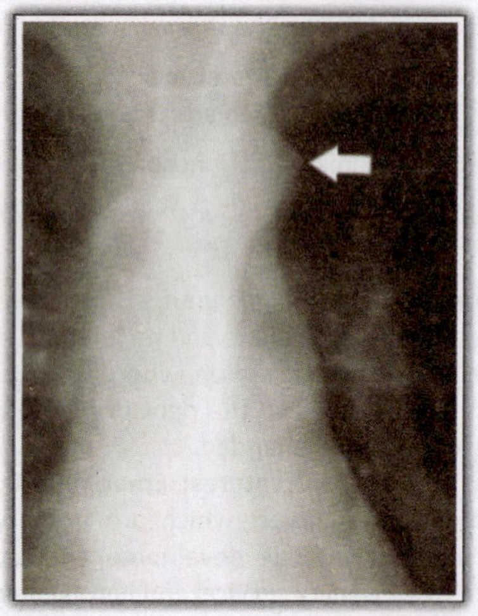

Fig: Aortic nipple—Left superior intercostal vein

Aortic Nipple

- The 'aortic nipple' is the radiographic term used to describe a lateral nipple-like projection from the aortic knuckle seen in a small number of individuals that corresponds to the end-on appearance of the left superior intercostal vein coursing anteriorly.
- It may be mistaken radiologically for lymphadenopathy or an intrapulmonary nodule/neoplasm.
- Despite their relative independence, the aortic nipple is defined by new contours in cases of pneumomediastinum, taking on an 'inverted aortic nipple' appearance.
- In this position, the inverted aortic nipple may facilitate radiographic discrimination of pneumomediastinum from similar conditions.
- An aortic nipple has been shown to precede pathological conditions such as venous obstruction in the superior and inferior vena cavae or left brachiocephalic vein and has been identified in conditions where venous flow through the left superior intercostal vein is increased.

Embryonic significance: The remainder of the left superior intercostal vein is developed from the cranial end of the post cardinal vein and drains the second, third and, on occasion, the fourth intercostal veins. The oblique vein goes across the back of the left atrium to opens into the coronary sinus, which represents the persistent left horn of the systemic venous sinus. When there is a left superior vena cava, the left brachiocephalic vein is joined by the left superior intercostal vein.

Significance of laterality: On the right side, the second, third and often the fourth intercostal veins form a right superior intercostal vein that joins the arch of the azygos vein.

The first right intercostal vein drains into the right brachiocephalic vein.

6. Ans. (b) Hypoglossal

Ref: Gray's 41st Ed Pg 232

Note: Even by not going into the details of olfaction we know that Cranial nerves 3, 4, 6, 12 are pure motor and not involved in any sensory relays of any kind, hence Hypoglossal nerve (CN XII) is a pure motor nerve.

Olfactory Pathway

Axons of the olfactory sensory neurons of 1st cranial nerve pass through the cribriform figure (ethmoid bone)

↓

Enter the olfactory bulbs, axons contact the primary dendrites of the mitral cells and tufted cells form synaptic units called olfactory glomeruli

The olfactory bulbs also contain the following which help sharpen and focus olfactory signals.

- Periglomerular cells (inhibitory neurons) connecting glomeruli
- Granule cells have no axons and make reciprocal synapses with the lateral dendrites of the mitral and tufted cells

At these synapses, the mitral or tufted cells excite the granule cell by releasing glutamate and the granule cells in turn inhibit the mitral or tufted cell by releasing GABA.

↓

Axons of the mitral and tufted cells pass through the lateral olfactory stria

↓

Terminate on apical dendrites of pyramidal cells in five regions of the olfactory cortex:

Anterior olfactory nucleus, olfactory tubercle, piriform cortex, amygdala (emotional responses to olfactory stimuli) and entorhinal cortex (olfactory memories)

Other components associated with Olfaction:

Let us go option wise:

Option (A) Trigeminal Nerve

Free endings of many trigeminal pain fibers are found in the olfactory epithelium. They are stimulated by irritating substances, which leads to the characteristic "odor" of such substances as peppermint, menthol and chlorine. Activation of these endings by nasal irritants also initiates sneezing, lacrimation, respiratory inhibition and other reflexes.

Option (B) Hypoglossal

Hypoglossal nerve is a purely motor nerve and is not associated with sense of olfaction.

Option (C) Vagus

Ref: Front. Neurosci., 24 April 2018 | https://doi.org/10.3389/fnins.2018.00225

Improvement of Olfactory Function with High Frequency Noninvasive Auricular Electrostimulation in Healthy Humans "In Parkinson's Disease (PD), impairments in odor detection, odor identification, odor discrimination and olfactory supra-threshold measures, are one of the earliest non-motor symptoms, preceding motor symptoms by several years. Impairments in PD are associated with the presence of Lewy bodies, which represent distinctive inclusion bodies that underlie neuroanatomical dysfunctions in this condition. Lewy bodies are present from the earliest stage of PD, identified in the olfactory nucleus and the Olfactory Bulb, but also in the dorsal nucleus of the vagus nerve (DMV). The spread of Lewy bodies throughout the stages of PD, initially begins at the DMV, then spreads throughout the brainstem nuclei to the substantia nigra-pars compacta and finally the cortex. This evidence points to an important connection between the vagus nerve and the olfactory processing areas of the cortex which is responsible for the early development of olfactory dysfunction in PD."

Option (D) Glossopharyngeal

Fibers from the olfactory system project via the dorsal longitudinal fasciculus to influence the output of the inferior salivatory nucleus. This can cause salivation in response to smelling food (mediated by the olfactory system)

7. Ans. (c) Supranuclear

Ref: Gray's anatomy 41st ed page

NOTE

If supranuclear is not provided in the option, then Adjacent to nucleus will become next best possible answer.

Serous Secretory Cells/Acinus (Unit)

Tubuloveolar; small lumen, round nuclei and well stained cytoplasm

The cytoplasm is divided into:

- **Basal cytoplasm** is basophilic due Ribosomes on rough endoplasmic reticulum. It also contains basal nucleus.
- **Supranuclear region:** The Golgi apparatus is usually located midway along the cell, typically in a supranuclear position. Supranuclear Golgi complex is surrounded by large, membrane bound granules containing the proteinaceous constituents of secretions, including enzymes which are only active after release.
- **Apical cytoplasm:** Dense secretory zymogen granules stain deeply with eosin in the apical region.

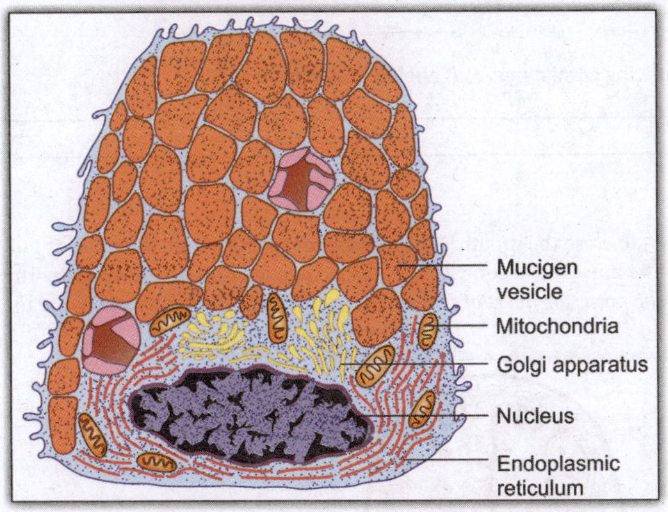

Fig: Secretory acinar unit showing basal, supranuclear and apical cytoplasm. Note supranuclear Golgi apparatus

8. Ans. (d) Perineal anesthesia

Ref: Differential Diagnosis in Neurology By Robert J. Schwartzman page 678

NOTE

Similar question on function of Paracentral lobule was asked in AIIMS MAY 2010 with different options and the question was not in the format of "All EXCEPT". Answer to that question was "Contralateral foot weakness"

The marked area in the given picture is of Paracentral lobule which is supplied by anterior cerebral artery. Leg and foot of motor homunculus is represented on the medial surface of the hemisphere in the paracentral lobule. ***Paracentral lobule is also responsible for control of defecation and urination.***

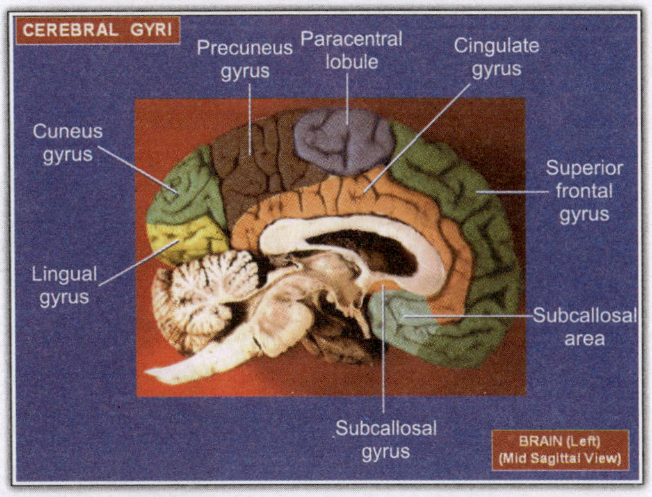

Apraxia's are the inability to perform an individual or sequential function with intact motor, sensory and coordinative abilities. Different areas of brain are specific for specific forms of apraxia. **ACA occlusion causes infarction of the paracentral lobule and, as a result, weakness and sensory loss in the contralateral leg. Hence, the lesion of paracentral lobule causes Gait apraxia, Urinary Incontinence and Fecal incontinence.**

9. Ans. (b) Oculomotor nerve

Ref: Grant's Atlas of Anatomy 12th Ed page 814, Gray's 41st ed page 272, 320

Recall Bias

Some recallers believe that Trochlear nerve was asked

The cranial nerve marked in the given picture is culomotor nerve. See following labeled picture for details.

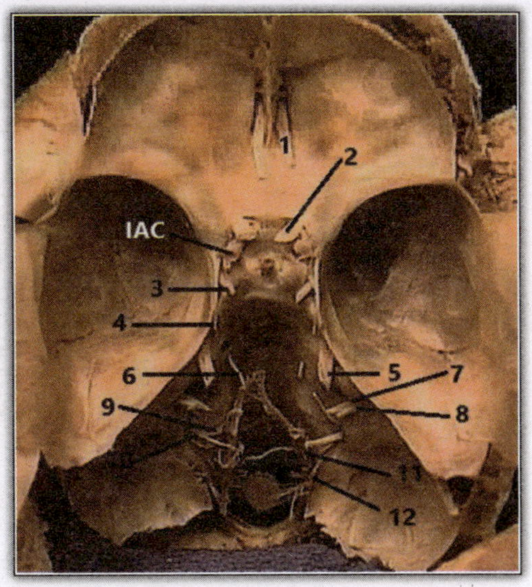

Fig: Superior view of the base of the skull showing cranial nerves. The posterior fossa contains the brainstem, cerebellum and cranial nerves IV-XII

Figure Legend

1. Olfactory nerve (CN I)
2. Optic nerve (CN II)
3. Oculomotor nerve (CN III)
4. Trochlear nerve (CN IV)
5. Trigeminal nerve (CN V)
6. Abducens nerve (CN VI): Abducens nerve located between pons and the clivus in the way to the cavernous sinus.
7. Facial nerve (CN VII)
8. Vestibulocochlear nerve (CN VIII)
9. Glossopharyngeal nerve (CN IX)
10. Vagus nerve (CN X)
11. Spinal accessory nerve (CN XI)
12. Hypoglossal nerve (CN XII)

IAC = Internal carotid artery

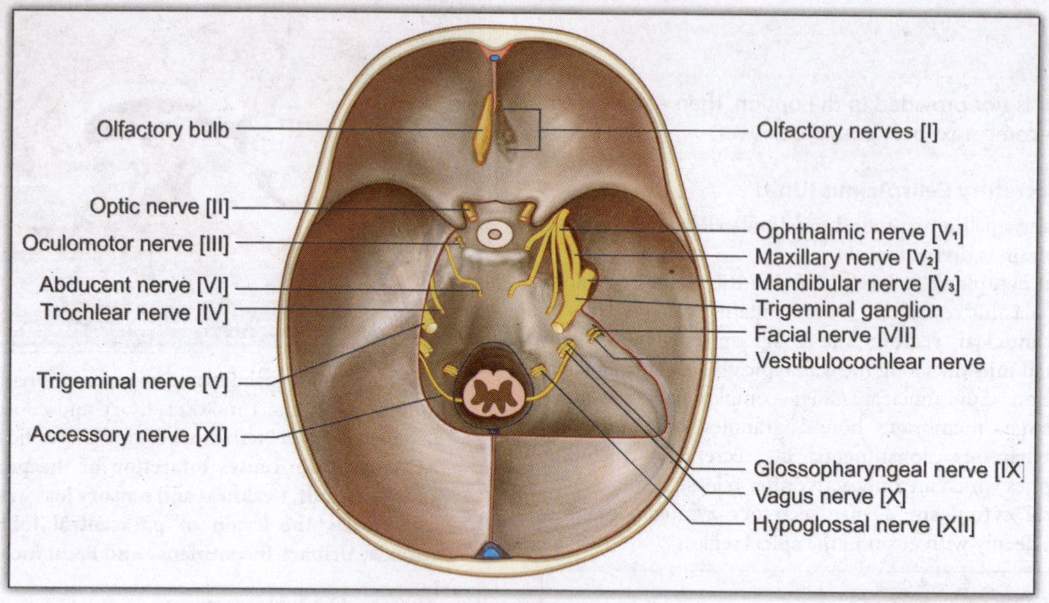

Fig: Superior view of the base of the skull showing cranial nerves (Labeled illustration)

10. Ans. (a) Elevation

Ref: Gray's anatomy 41st ed page 498

The muscle marked in the given figure is Temporalis.

Temporalis muscle main action is **Elevation of mandible** (all fibers) to close the mouth. This movement requires both the upward pull of the anterior fibers and the backward pull of the posterior fibers. The muscle also contributes to side-to-side grinding movements. The posterior fibers retract the mandible after it has been protruded. *The posterior fibers of temporalis, which are almost horizontal, are the only source of mandibular retrusion.*

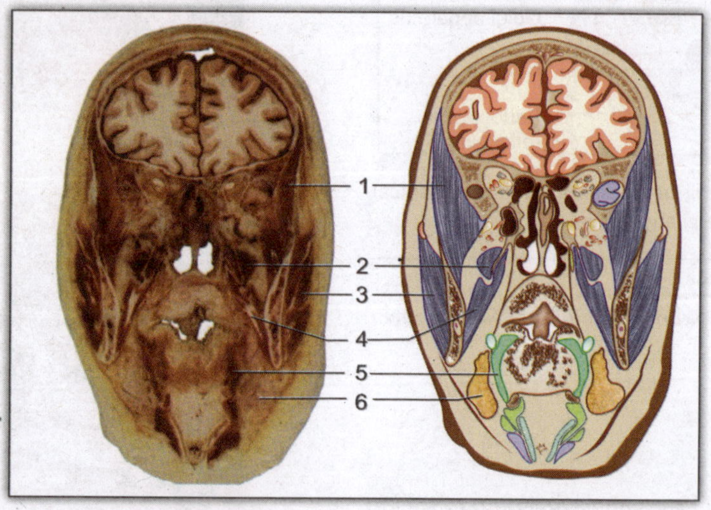

Fig: Coronal section of head with muscles of mastication and comparative illustration

Legends: 1. Temporalis, 2. Lateral pterygoid, 3. Masseter muscle, 4. Medial pterygoid, 5. Hypoglossal muscle, 6. Submandibular gland

Muscles of mastication (acting on temporomandibular joint)				
Muscle	**Origin**	**Insertion**	**Innervation**	**Main Action**
Temporalis (Fan shaped; anterior, intermediate and posterior fibers)	Floor of temporal fossa and deep surface of temporal fascia	Tip and medial surface of coronoid process and anterior border of ramus of mandible	Deep temporal branches of *mandibular nerve* (CN V^3)	**Elevates mandible** (all fibers), Retrudes mandible (posterior fibers)
Masseter (superficial, middle and deep layers) (superficial layer is the largest)	Inferior border and medial surface of zygomatic arch	Lateral surface of ramus of mandible and coronoid process	Anterior trunk of *Mandibular nerve* (CN V^3) through masseteric nerve	**Elevates mandible**, minor actions are: protrudes mandible (superficial fibers), retrudes mandible (deep fibers)
Lateral pterygoid (Upper head and Lower head)	*Superior head:* infratemporal surface and infratemporal crest of greater wing of sphenoid bone *Inferior head: lateral surface of lateral pterygoid figure*	Neck of mandible, articular disc and capsule of temporomandibular joint	*Mandibular nerve* (CN V^3) through lateral pterygoid nerve which enters its deep surface	*Acting bilaterally,* protrude mandible and depress chin; *Acting unilaterally* alternately, they produce side-to-side movements of mandible (pulled medially towards the opposite side)
Medial pterygoid (small superficial head and major Deep head)	*Deep head:* medial surface of lateral pterygoid figure and pyramidal process of palatine bone *Superficial head:* tuberosity of maxilla	Medial surface of ramus of mandible, inferior to mandibular foramen	*Mandibular nerve* (CN V^3) through medial pterygoid nerve	**Acts Synergistically with masseter** to elevate mandible, contributes to protrude mandible; *acting unilaterally* produce small grinding movements
# Unlike the other muscles of mastication, lateral pterygoid is not pennate, nor does it have a significant number of Golgi tendon organs associated with its attachments				

11. Ans. (c) Dense irregular connective tissue

Ref: Gray's 41st Ed Pg 39

- Dense irregular connective tissue is found in regions that are under considerable mechanical stress and where protection is given to ensheathed organs.
- The matrix is relatively acellular and contains a high proportion of collagen fibers organized into thick bundles interweaving in three dimensions and imparting considerable strength.
- There are few active fibroblasts, which are usually flattened with heterochromatin nuclei.
- Dense irregular connective tissue occurs in: the reticular layer of the dermis; the superficial connective tissue sheaths of muscle and nerves and the adventitia of large blood vessels; and the capsules of various glands and organs (e.g. testis, sclera of the eye, periosteum and perichondrium).

Marked area is of Reticular dermis which is composed of Dense irregular connective tissue.

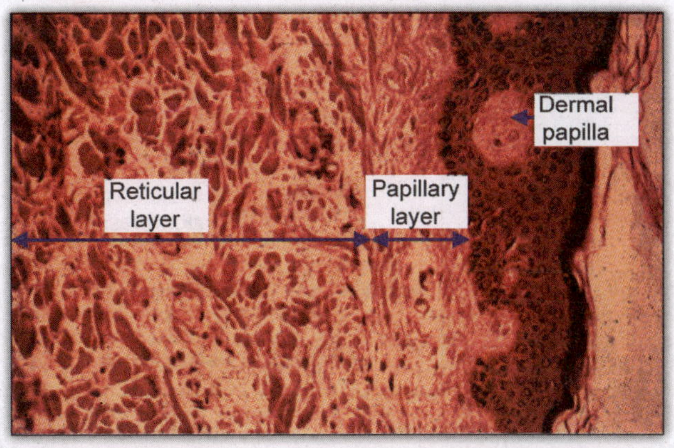

Fig: Note demarcation of reticular and papillary layers of dermis. Papillary layer interdigitates with basal surface of epithelium. Reticular layer is the major portion of the dermis and is composed of dense bundles of collagen fibers and thick elastic fibers.

12. Ans. (a) A

Ref: Morgan 5th Ed Pg 1037

https://nba.uth.tmc.edu/neuroscience/m/s2/chapter08.html

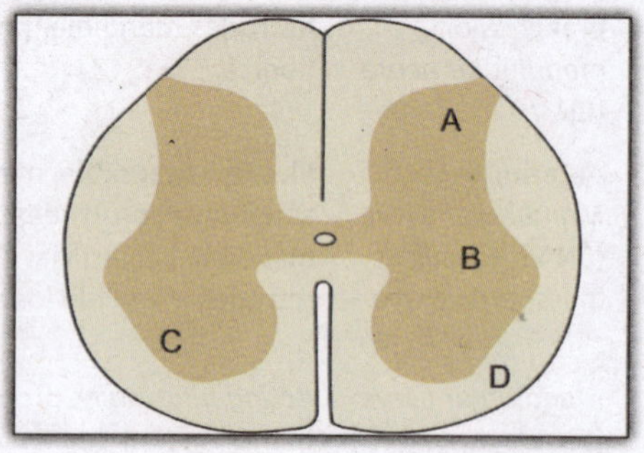

Figure Legends

A = Dorsal Horn

B = Lateral horn or Intermediate column

C = Ventral horn

D = Anterior spinothalamic tract

This question is based on the **gate control theory of pain.**

To understand this fully, we must first understand the pain pathway.

Pain Pathway

- Pain impulses passes through a gate to reach the **lateral spinothalamic system.**
- The pain pathway consists of the following major steps:

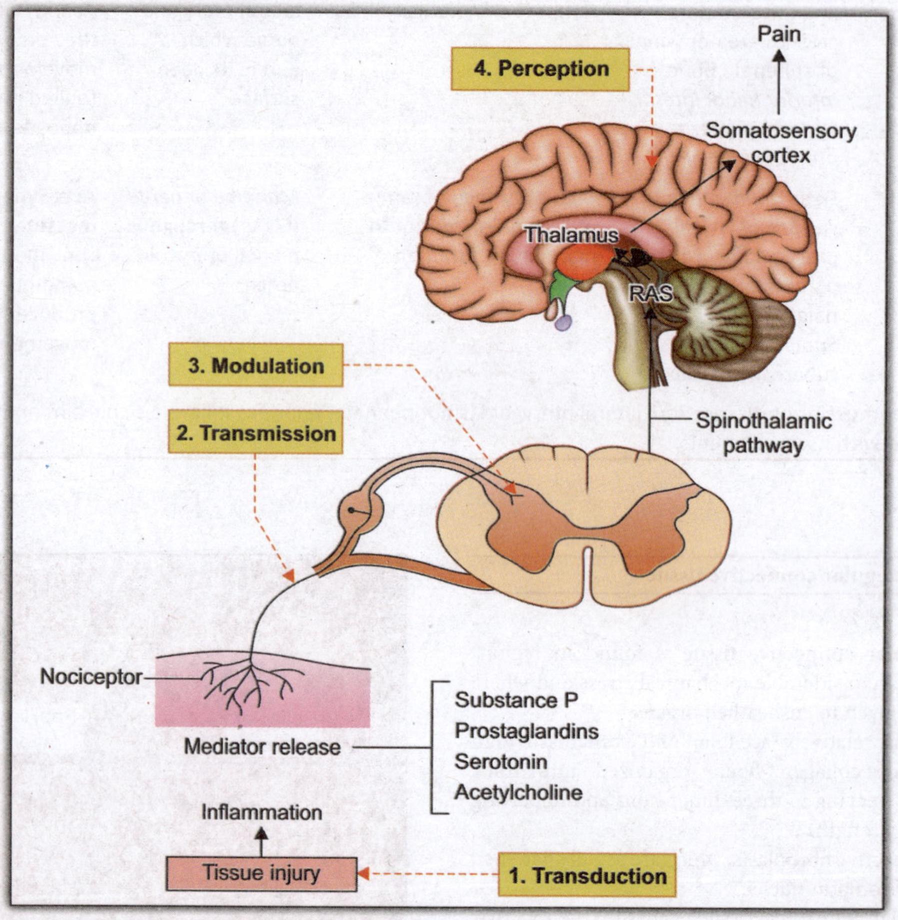

Fig: Pain pathway

1. **Transduction:** Primary afferent fibers (Aβ-, Aδ- and C-fibers) generate action potential in response to stimuli from the periphery. Aδ- and C-fibers generate action potential in response to nociceptive stimuli, while Aβ transmits touch.
2. **Transmission:** Transmission of action potential to the dorsal root ganglion. Aß fibers also modulate C and Að activity within the **dorsal horn** (Gate control).

Fiber type		What they transmit	Characteristics	Effect on gate
Small fibers	A-δ	Sharp, prickly pain	Thin, myelinated, slow	Opens
	C-fiber	Dull, aching pain	Thin, unmyelinated, slow	Opens
Large fibers	A-β	Non-painful stimuli	Thick, myclinated, fast	Closes

- Nociceptive specific (NS) cells are mainly found in the superficial dorsal horn (laminae I–II), whereas most wide dynamic ranges are located deeper (lamina V).

- **Lamina II, also called the substantia gelatinosa, contains many interneurons and is believed to play a major role in processing and modulating nociceptive input from cutaneous nociceptors.**

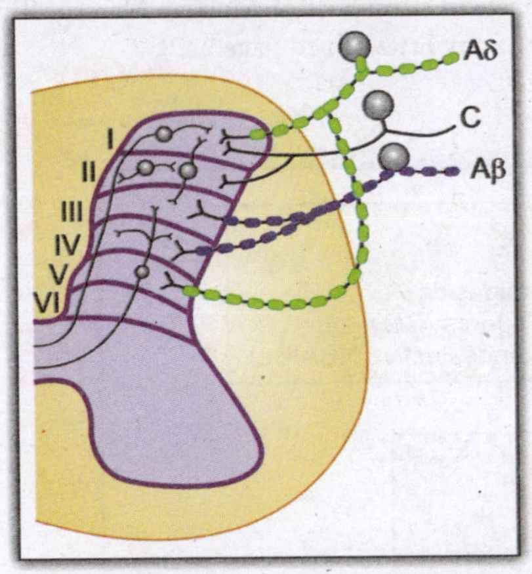

Fig: Diagrammatic representation of laminae in spinal cord with respect to pain pathway

- Lamina V neurons mainly project to the thalamus (spinothalamic tract) and from here the various cortical regions forming the 'pain matrix' (primary and secondary somatosensory, insular, anterior cingulate and prefrontal cortices) are activated

3. **Modulation:**
   - Modulation of pain occurs peripherally at the nociceptor, in the spinal cord and in supraspinal structures. This modulation can either inhibit (suppress) or facilitate (intensify) pain. Facilitation leads to conditions like hyperalgesia. Transmission of nociceptive input in the spinal cord can be inhibited by segmental activity in the cord itself, as well as by descending neural activity from supraspinal centers.
   - One of the mechanisms of segmental inhibition is **stimulating the large fast Aβ fibers in the area of injury, which can induce interneurons in the dorsal horn to release GABA and glycine, which inhibit the release of glutamate from the primary afferent terminal, thereby preventing depolarization of the second order neuron.**
   - The axons of most second-order neurons cross the midline close to their dermatomal level of origin (at the anterior commissure) to the contralateral side of the spinal cord before they form the spinothalamic tract
4. **Perception:** Perception of nociceptive pain is dependeant upon neural processing in the spinal cord and several brain regions. It is the integration of sensations, emotions and cognition that result in our perception of pain.

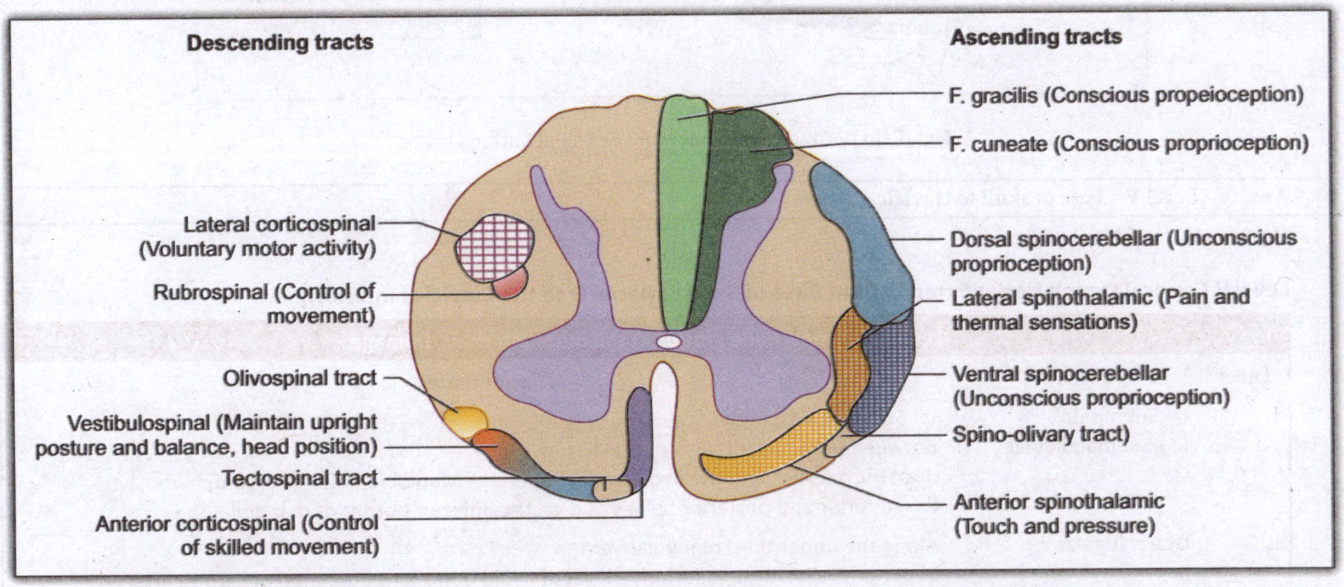

Fig: Cross section of spinal cord showing different areas and tracts

Gate Control Theory of Pain

- According to the gate control theory, pain signals are not free to reach the brain as soon as they are generated at the injured tissues or sites. They need to encounter certain '*neurological gates*' at the spinal cord level and these gates determine whether the pain signals should reach the brain or not.
- In other words, pain is perceived when the gate gives way to the pain signals and it is less intense or not at all perceived when the gate closes for the signals to pass through. This theory gives the explanation for why someone finds relief by rubbing or massaging an injured or a painful area.
- ***The gate is formed from the Dorsal Root Ganglion*** going into the Dorsal Horns that will control whether the signal transmitted from the receptor is allowed to pass up the spine to the brainstem or not.
- Stimulation of large diameter fibers prevents the small diameter fibers from transmitting signals because they

travel to the gate of the spinal cord first. Stimulation of large fibers (e.g. rubbing, massaging) helps to suppress the sensation of pain especially sharp or visceral pain.

- One of the tremendous advances in pain management research is the advent of Transcutaneous Electrical Nerve Stimulation (TENS). The gate control theory forms the basis of TENS.
- The gate control theory has brought about a drastic revolution in the field of pain management. The theory suggested that pain management can be achieved by selectively influencing the larger nerve fibers that carry non-pain stimuli. (Ref: Mosby's Massage Therapy Review by Sandy Fritz 4th ed page 229)

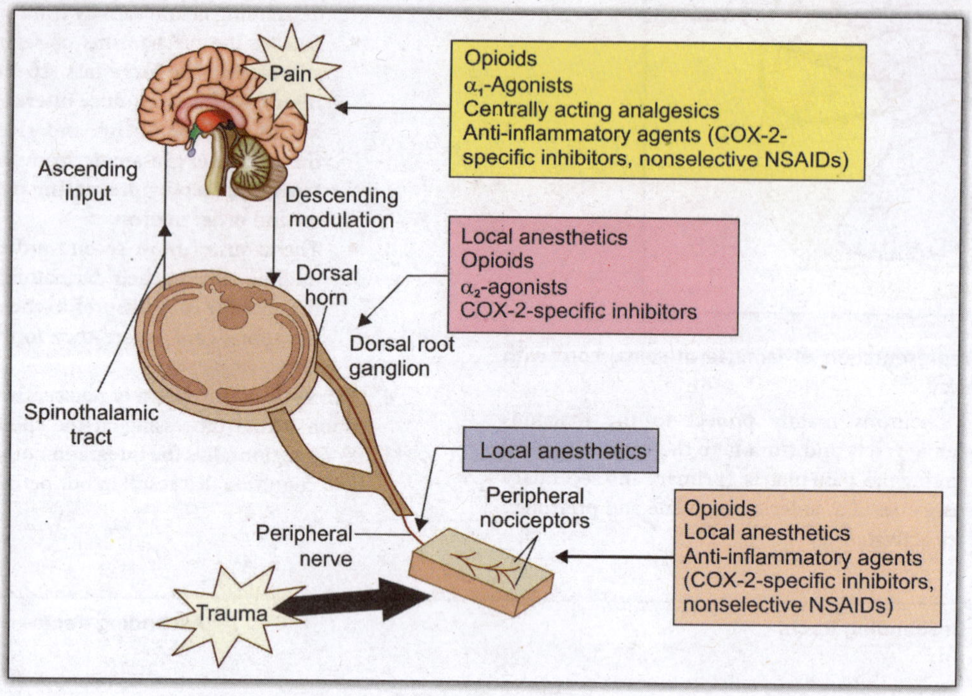

Fig: Pain pathway and analgesics acting at various levels

13. Ans. (c) Level V—base of skull to clavicle

Ref: Gray's 41st Ed Pg 362

Level V Cervical Lymph Nodes Extends from Base of Skull Superiorly to the Clavicles Inferiorly

Levels of lymph node groups in the neck and their drainage		
Level	**Content**	**Boundaries**
I	Ia- Submental Ib - Submandibular	**Ia** -Submental triangle Between right and left anterior bellies of digastric muscles and the hyoid bone, Superior - Mandible, Inferior- Hyoid **Ib** - Anterior and posterior bellies of digastric, Inferior border of mandible
II	Upper jugular IIa IIb	Along the upper third of jugular vein Superiorly- skull base, Inferiorly - level of hyoid bone (or bifurcation of carotid artery) IIa - anterior to spinal accessory nerve IIb - posterior to spinal accessory nerve
III	Mid jugular	Inferior border of hyoid to inferior border of cricoid, anterior- sternohyoid muscle, posterior - sternocleidomastoid muscle
IV	Lower Jugular	From cricoid cartilage to clavicle
V	Posterior triangle	Triangle formed by anterior border of trapezius, posterior border of sternocleidomastoid, inferiorly clavicle
VI	Anterior compartment	Hyoid to suprasternal notch inferiorly. Lateral- sternohyoid muscle, medial border of common carotid artery

Contd...

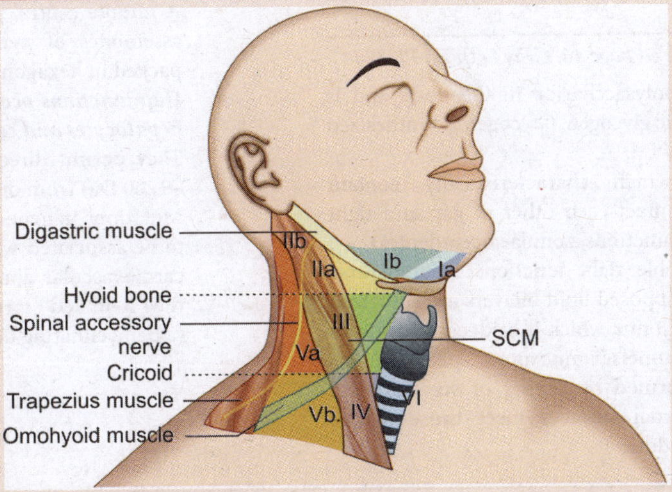

Note:

Level VII: They are located below the suprasternal notch and include nodes of the upper mediastinum.

- **Classic radical neck dissection**—clearance of levels I–V, including the sacrifice of sternocleidomastoid, the internal jugular vein and the accessory nerve.
- **Modified radical neck dissections** (functional neck dissections): Remove level I–V
- Nodes, spare either or all of sternocleidomastoid, the internal jugular vein and the accessory nerve.
- **Selective neck dissections** remove selected groups of nodes.
  - **Supraomohyoid neck dissection** removes level I–III nodes
  - **Lateral neck dissection** removes level II–IV nodes
  - **Posterolateral neck dissection** removes level II–V nodes.

14. Ans. (d) Lysosome

Ref: Wolfgang histology 4th ed page 172

NOTE

Similar question was asked in AIIMS NOV 2017 (Anatomy). Intercalated disc was marked and question about gap junction was asked.

The given image is of Cardiac myocyte and the arrow shows intercalated disc. Lysosome is the best possible answer.

Because of the low levels of lysosomal enzymes detected in the cardiac muscle homogenates, myocytes were thought to be totally devoid of lysosomes and lysosomal enzymes in heart muscle tissue were believed to be of interstitial origin. The first electron microscopic identifications of lysosomes were performed in 1966 by Hibbs and co-workers among others (Hibbs et al., 1966). They found, in perinuclear areas, acid phosphatase positive ovoid granules, which were relatively few compared to similar bodies in other tissues such as liver.

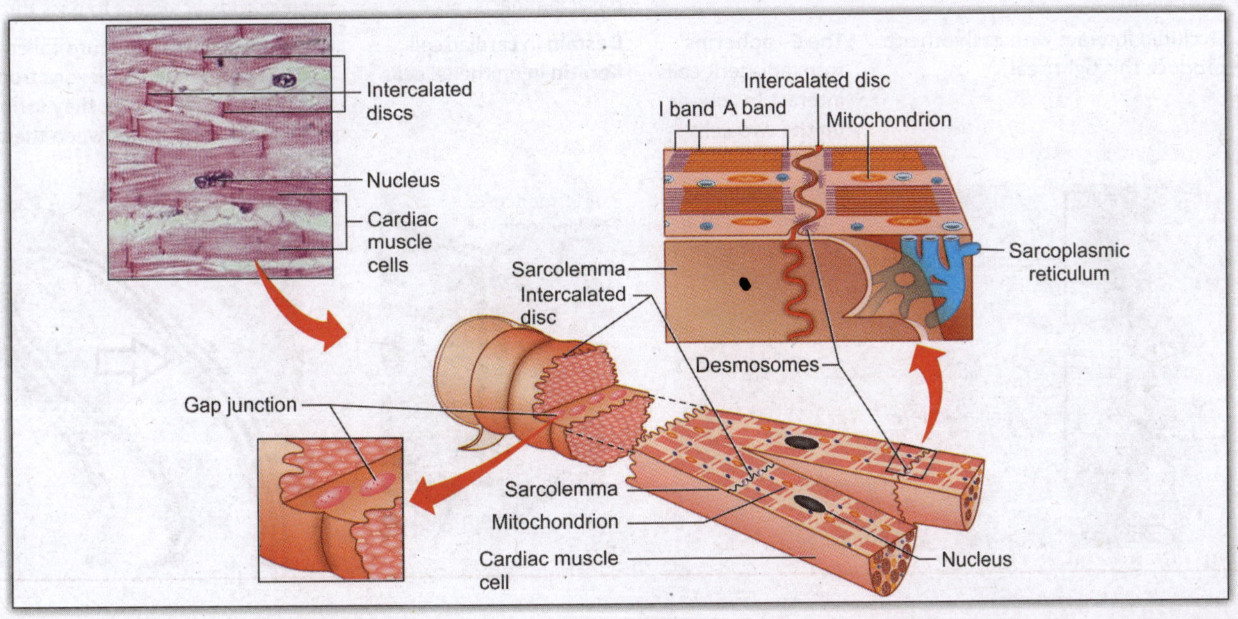

15. Ans. (c) Gap junction

Ref: Wolfgang Histology 4th ed page 46, Gray's 4th Ed Ph 154

Glycogen is the reserve polysaccharide in the body and is mainly comprised of hepatic glycogen. Glycogen is synthesized in the liver and muscles.

- Ectodermal cells, which characteristically contain glycogen deposits, contact each other at gap and tight junctions (occluding junctions, zonulae occludentes).
- Gap junctions resemble tight junctions in transverse section, but the two opposed lipid bilayers are separated by an apparent gap of 3 nm, which is bridged by a cluster of transmembrane channels (connexons).
- Each connexon is formed by a ring of six connexin proteins whose external surfaces meet those of the adjacent cell in the middle.
- A minute central pore links one cell to the next. Larger assemblies of many thousands of channels are often packed in hexagonal arrays.
- ***Gap junctions occur between numerous cells, including hepatocytes and cardiac myocytes.***
- They permit direct transfer of small molecules (up to ~1200 Da) from one cell to its neighbor.
- Mutations in genes encoding connexins have been found to be associated with a number of conditions, including cardiovascular abnormalities, one type of deafness and the X-linked form of Charcot-Marie-Tooth disease (a demyelinating neurologic disorder)

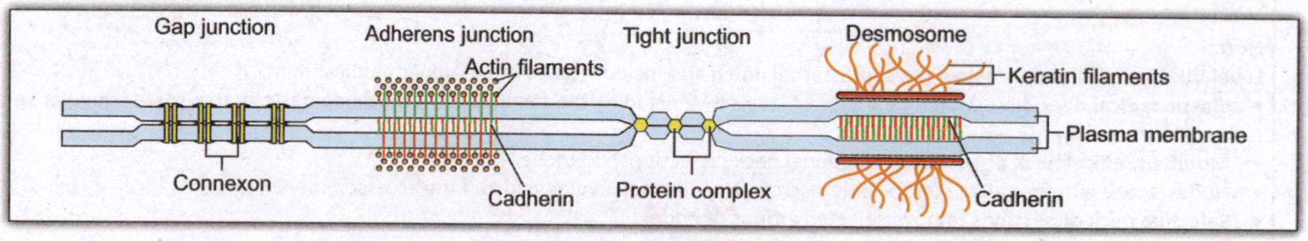

Fig: Types of cell junctions

Types of cell junction			
Occluding junctions	**Anchoring junctions**		**Communicating junctions**
Zonula occludens or Tight junctions	Adhering junctions (zonula adherens)	Desmosomes (macula adherens)	Gap junctions (septate junction)
A continuous **belt like junction,** these regions of cell are very tightly connected together, such that the adjacent plasma membranes are sealed together. It greatly restricts the passage of water, electrolytes and other small molecules across the epithelium	Analogous to **Fascia adherans** of non-epithelial cells. Adherens junction lies below the tight junction (occluding junction)	It is circular or **spot like** in outline and not belt- or band shaped. There are also **'hemidesmosomes'** that lie on the basal membrane, to help stick the cells to the underlying basal lamina	These are communicating junctions. This channel is big enough to allow small molecules such as inorganic ions and other small water-soluble molecules (smaller than 1000 kDa) to pass between the cells. However, the channel is too small for proteins, nucleic acids or sugars to pass through
Occludin interact with each other to produce this tight seal	The **E-cadherins** from adjacent cells interact to 'zipper' up the two cells together	**Desmin** in cardiac cell **Keratin** in epithelial cells	**Connexins** form a structure called a connexon. When connexons from two adjacent cells align, they form a continuous channel between them

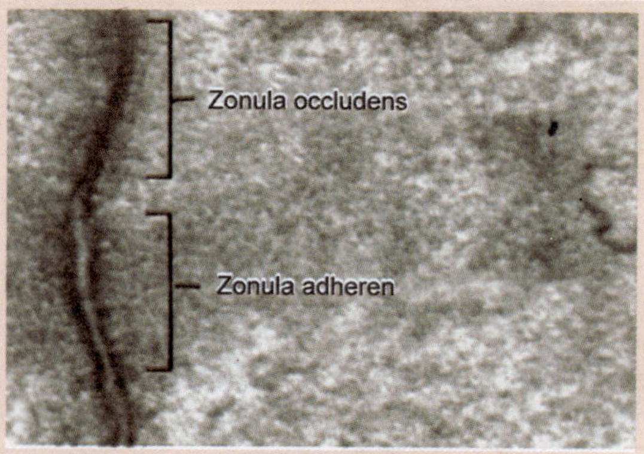

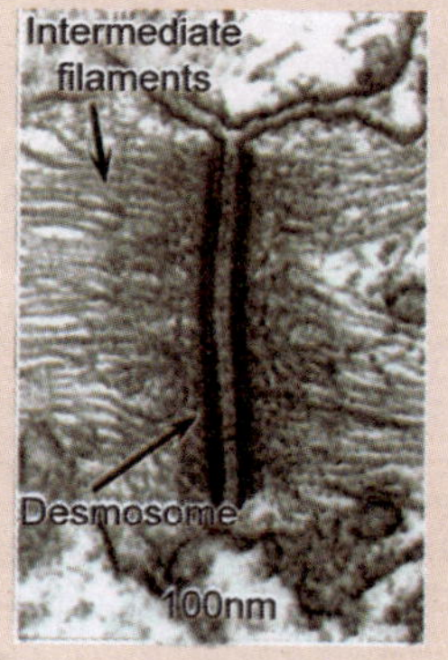

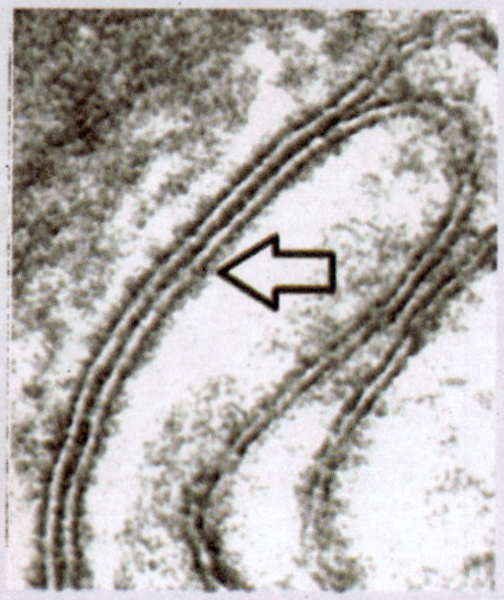

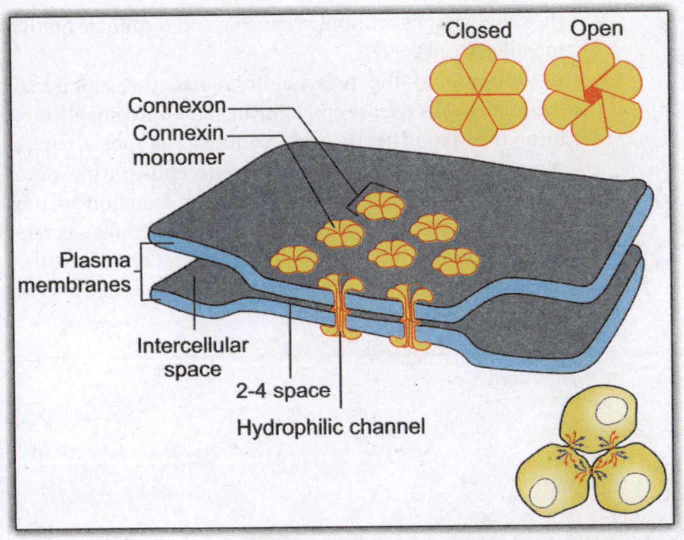

Fig: Gap junction

16. Ans. (c) Neurosecretory vesicles

Ref: Stevens and Lowe's Human Histology - Page 87, Wheater's Functional Histology: A Text and Color Atlas page 332

Neurosecretory Granules (A.K.A Substantia Neurosecretoria)

Neurons and related cell types often contain two major classes of neurosecretory vesicles, synaptic vesicles (SVs) and dense-core granules (DCGs), which store and release distinct cargo. SVs store and release classic neurotransmitters, which facilitate propagation of action potentials across the synaptic cleft, whereas DCGs transport, store and release hormones, proteins and neuropeptides, which facilitate neuronal survival, synaptic transmission and learning.

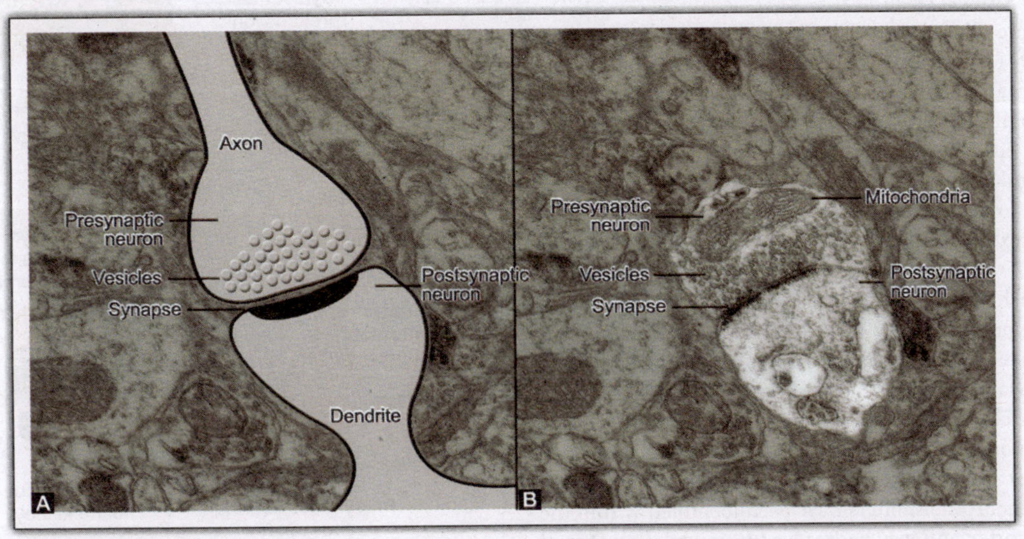

Figs A and B: Synaptic vesicles are small, electron-lucent vesicles that are clustered at presynaptic terminals. They store neurotransmitters and release them by calcium-triggered exocytosis

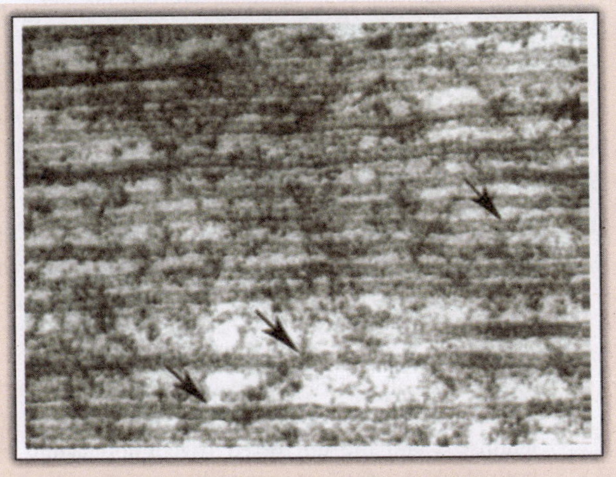

Fig: Microtubules in longitudinal section

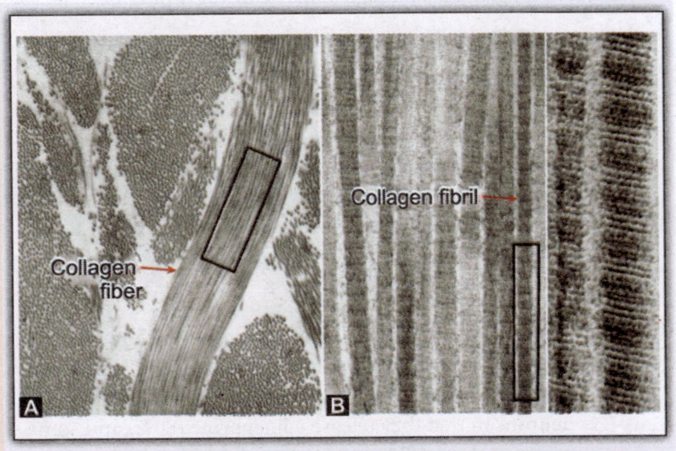

Figs A and B: Collagen fibers EM

This specimen shows the appearance of type I collagen fibers under the electron microscope at three different magnifications. Individual fibrils show a characteristic banding pattern which results from the overlap of the tropocollagen constituents. The periodicity of this pattern is typically 64 nanometers.

AIIMS MAY 2018

17. Ans. (c) Neurosecretory vesicles (see page 27)

Ref: Stevens and Lowe's Human Histology - Page 87, Wheater's Functional Histology: A Text and Color Atlas page 332

Repeat AIIMS Nov 2018 Anatomy (See for explanation)

18. Ans. (c) Adrenal cortex is devoid of nerve supply

Ref: Grays Anatomy 41st edition page 1197, Keith L Moore 4th ed page 180

Option (A) and (B) False

Preganglionic fibers supplies adrenal medulla not cortex. Hence both (A) and (B) are false. Sympathetic innervation to the adrenal medulla is via myelinated presynaptic fibers, mainly from the T10 to L1 spinal cord segments. The nerves are distributed throughout the gland: around blood vessels (regulating blood flow), in the medulla (stimulating the release of catecholamines from chromaffin cells) and in the cortex (where they may influence steroid hormone production). A suprarenal plexus lies between the medial aspect of each gland and the coeliac and aorticorenal ganglia. It contains predominantly preganglionic sympathetic fibres that originate in the lower thoracic spinal segments, reach the plexus via branches of the greater splanchnic nerves and synapse on clusters of large medullary chromaffin cells. A smaller proportion of postganglionic sympathetic nerve fibres innervate cortical blood vessels. Other nerve fibres containing a variety of neurotransmitters have been identified within the suprarenal cortex and may be involved in modulating steroid hormone secretion. The cell bodies of afferent nerve fibres arising in the suprarenal medulla are almost all located in dorsal root ganglia, although some lie in vagal ganglia.

Option (C) True

The suprarenal glands have a rich nerve supply from the celiac plexus and abdominopelvic (greater, lesser and least) splanchnic nerves. The nerves are mainly myelinated presynaptic sympathetic fibers that derive from the lateral horn of the spinal cord and traverse the paravertebral and prevertebral ganglia, without synapse, to be distributed to the chromaffin cells in the suprarenal medulla.

Option (D) False

- The suprarenal/adrenal gland is unique in its innervation and function. The cells in the medulla of the suprarenal gland behave like a collection of postsynaptic sympathetic neurons in that they release epinephrine (80%) and some norepinephrine (20%) upon stimulation by a presynaptic sympathetic nerve.
- Presynaptic sympathetic fibers to the suprarenal medulla pass from the greater thoracic splanchnic nerves through the celiac ganglia without synapsing and terminate on the medullary cells.
- In response to the presynaptic signal, the suprarenal medullary cells release epinephrine (and norepinephrine) into the bloodstream. In contrast to postsynaptic sympathetic neurons that release norepinephrine onto specific organs resulting in a change of function within that organ, the cells of the suprarenal medulla secrete epinephrine (80%) and norepinephrine (20%) into the bloodstream producing a systemic, or whole-body, fight or flight response.

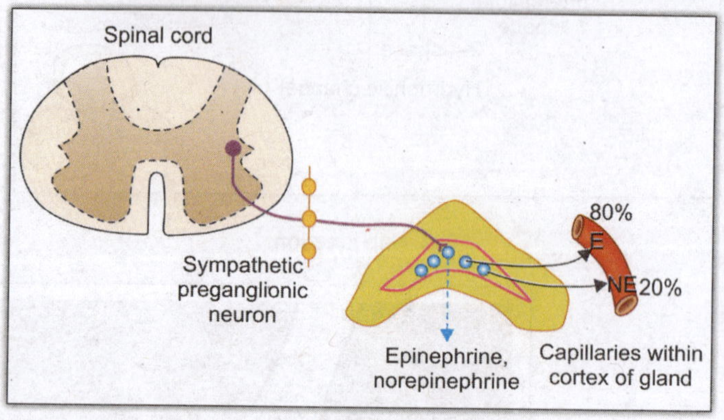

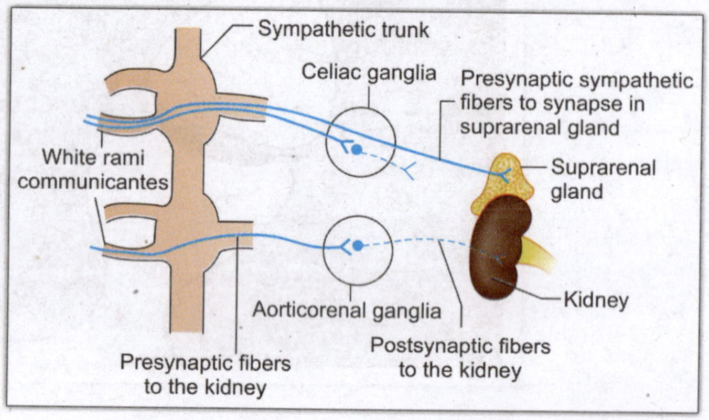

19. Ans. (c) Proprioception

Ref: Netter's Cranial Nerve Collection E-Book By Frank H. Netter Pg 23

- The central processes of trigeminal nerve form a sensory root to terminate in one of the major nuclear complexes - spinal (inferior) trigeminal nucleus, principal (pontine) and mesencephalic nucleus.
- The spinal nucleus receives pain, temperature, soft touch sensations from the face, from where, fibers ascend ipsilaterally to trigeminothalamic tract to ventral posteromedial (VPM) and intralaminar nucleus of thalamus. Projections further ascend to primary sensory cortex.
- The principal sensory nucleus receives tactile and proprioceptive impulses. These, through trigeminal lemniscus and the uncrossed trigeminothalamic tract, both of which terminate in the VPM nucleus of thalamus. It is represented bilaterally in the cortex.
- The mesencephalic nucleus receives proprioceptive input from extraocular muscle spindles and

masticatory muscles. It is the only place in the CNS where cell bodies of primary sensory afferents are found in the CNS and not sensory ganglia.

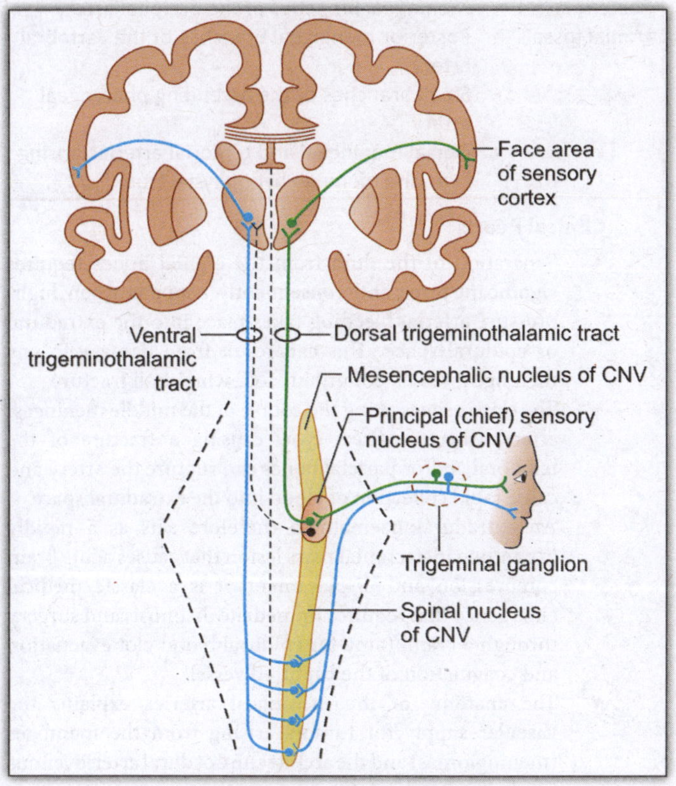

Fig: Trigeminal sensory nuclei

20. Ans. (b) Hyaline cartilage

Ref: Ross's Histology 6th Edition pg 165, 166

Hyaline Cartilage Contains Type II Collagen

Types of Collagen and their Location

Type of collagen	Location
I	Skin, Bone, Tendon, Ligaments, Dentin, sclera, Fascia and organ capsules
II	Cartilage (hyaline and elastic), Notochord, Intervertebral disc
III	Loose connective tissue and organs, Smooth muscle, Endometrium, Blood vessels, foetal skin
IV	Basal lamina of epithelia, kidney glomeruli, Lung capsule
V	Distributed uniformly throughout connective tissue stroma
VI	Cartilage matrix immediately surrounding the chondrocytes
VII	Anchoring fibrils of skin, eye, uterus and esophagus
VIII	Product of endothelial cells
IX	Cartilage associated with type II collagen fibrils

Contd...

Types of Collagen and their Location

Type of collagen	Location
X	Chondrocytes in the zone of hypertrophy of normal growth figure
XI	Produced by chondrocytes; associated with type II collagen fibrils, forms core of type I collagen fibrils
XII	Skin and placenta
XIII	An unusual transmembrane collagen detected in bone, cartilage, intestine, skin, placenta and striated muscles

21. Ans. (b) Dentate nucleus

Ref: Grays 41st ed page 256, 335, Ganong 24th Ed, pg 249, Guyton 12th ed page 684

The cerebellar cortex possess three layers are distinguished in the cerebellar cortex - **Molecular layer, Purkinje layer and Granular layer.** Purkinje cell axons pass into the white matter and form inhibitory synaptic connections with neurons of the deep cerebellar nuclei, releasing GABA as the neurotransmitter. GABA is the main inhibitory transmitter and Glutamate is the main excitatory transmitter of Purkinje cells

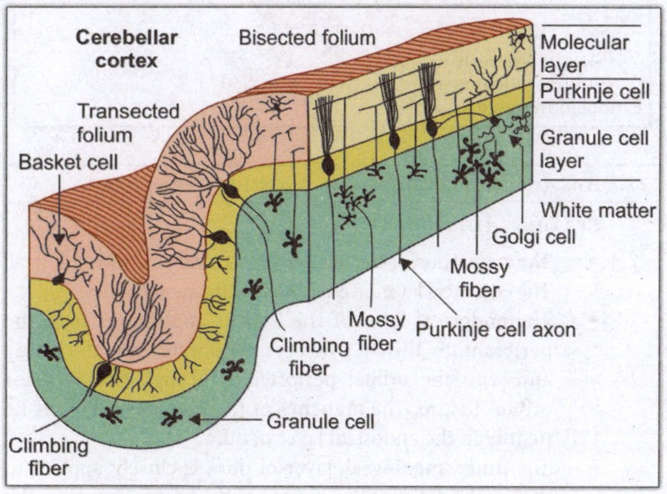

Functional Unit of the Cerebellar Cortex—the Purkinje Cell and the Deep Nuclear Cell

The cerebellum has about 30 million nearly identical functional units, one of which is shown in the figure. This functional unit centers on a single, very large **Purkinje cell and on a corresponding deep nuclear cell**. To the top and right in figure, the three major layers of the *cerebellar cortex are shown: the molecular layer, Purkinje cell layer and granule cell layer.* Beneath these cortical layers, in the center of the cerebellar mass, are the deep cerebellar nuclei that send output signals to other parts of the nervous system.

Neuronal Circuit of the Functional Unit: The output from the functional unit is from a **deep nuclear cell**. This cell is continually under *both excitatory and inhibitory influences.*

Deep cerebellar nuclei: *From lateral to medial, the four deep cerebellar nuclei are the* ***Dentate, Emboliform, Globose and Fastigial*** *(Mnemonic: "Don't Eat Greasy Food").* The globose and the emboliform nuclei are sometimes lumped together as the **Interpositus nucleus** in lower species; the emboliform and globose nuclei may sometimes be referred to as the anterior and posterior interposed nuclei, respectively. *The dentate nucleus, which is located most laterally and is by far the largest, is the only nucleus easily visible to the naked eye.*

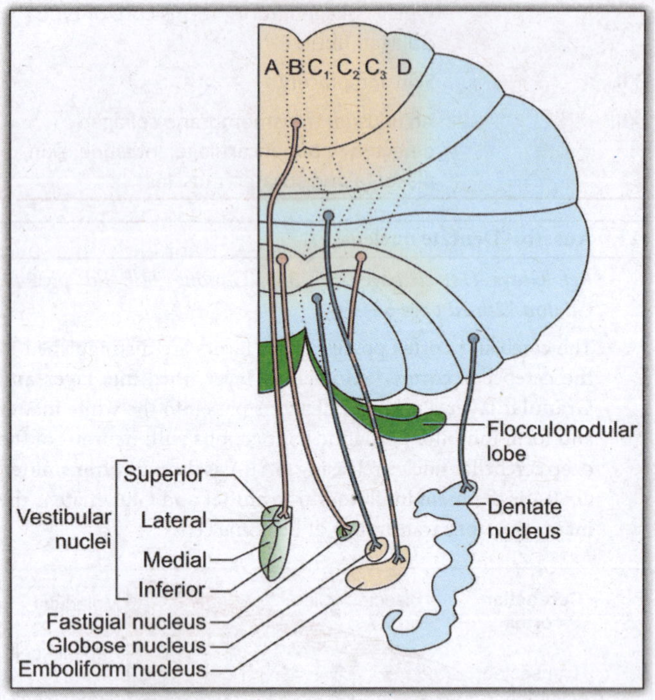

22. Ans. (d) Branches of ICA in posterior cranial fossa

Ref: Gray's 41st Ed Pg 439

- The cranial dura mater has 2 layers—meningeal and endosteal. The endosteal layer invests closely with cranial bones.
- The endosteal layer of the dura is continuous with the pericranium through the cranial sutures and foramina and with the orbital periosteum through the superior orbital fissure. The branches of the meningeal vessels lie mainly in the endosteal layer of dura.
- The inner, meningeal, layer of dura is closely applied to the arachnoid over the surface of the brain. However, the two membranes are physically joined only at sites where veins pass from the brain into venous sinuses, e.g. the superior sagittal sinus.

Blood Supply of Meninges

Area	Artery
Anterior cranial fossa	• Anterior meningeal branches of the anterior and posterior ethmoidal • Internal carotid arteries and a branch of the middle meningeal artery.
Middle cranial fossa	• Middle and accessory meningeal branches of the maxillary artery • A branch of the ascending pharyngeal artery • Branches of the internal carotid artery • Recurrent branch of the lacrimal artery.

Contd...

Blood Supply of Meninges

Area	Artery
Posterior cranial fossa	• Meningeal branches of the occipital artery • Posterior meningeal branches of the vertebral artery • Small branches of the ascending pharyngeal artery • Dorsal meningeal and tentorial arteries arising from the meningo hypophysial trunk

Clinical Pearls

- Separation of the dura from the cranial bones requires significant force and consequently happens when high-pressure arterial bleeding takes place into the extradural or epidural space. This can result from damage to any meningeal vessel, commonly following skull fracture.
- The classic site is along the course of the middle meningeal artery, where a direct blow causing a fracture of the temporal and/or parietal bones can rupture the artery and cause rapid collection of blood into the extradural space.
- An extradural haematoma therefore acts as a rapidly expanding intracranial mass lesion that causes acute brain compression and displacement; it is a classic medical emergency that requires immediate diagnosis and surgery through a craniotomy for epidural blood clot evacuation and coagulation of the ruptured vessel.
- The anatomy of the meningeal arteries explains the vascular supply for tumors arising from the meninges (meningiomas) and the architecture of dural arteriovenous fistulae and malformations.

23. Ans. (c) Thyrocervical trunk

Ref: Gray's Anatomy 41st Ed Pg 458

The thyrocervical trunk is a short, wide artery that arises from the front of the first part of the subclavian artery near the medial border of scalenus anterior and divides almost at once into the inferior thyroid, suprascapular and superficial cervical arteries.

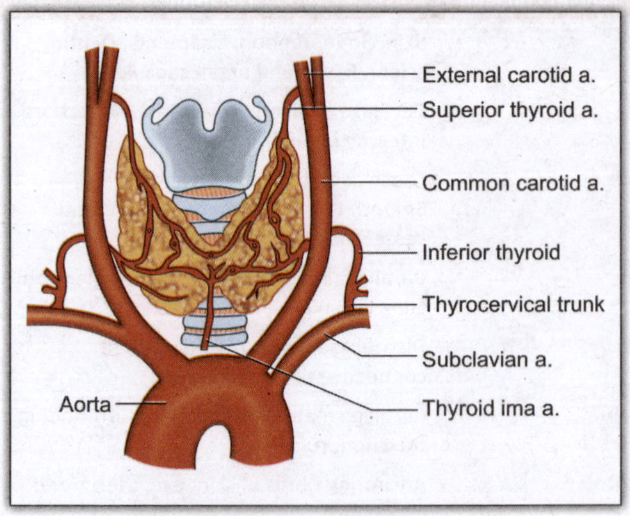

Fig: Arterial supply of thyroid gland

24. Ans. (d) Hypothalamus

Ref: Grays 41st edition page 274

Sagittal section of Brain is covered in AIIMS NOV 2017 Anatomy

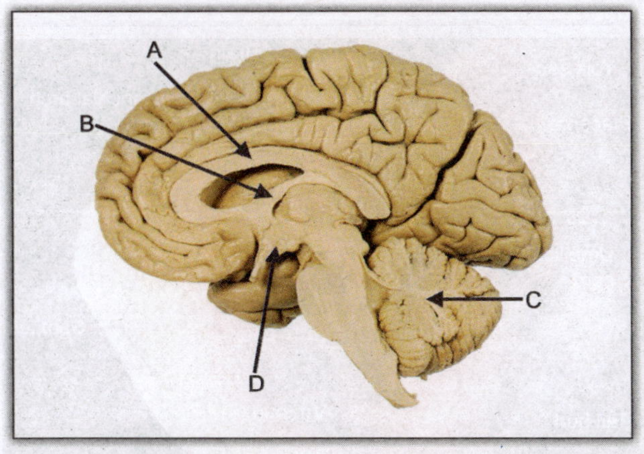

Figure Legend

A = Corpus callosum
B = Fornix
C = Cerebellum
D = Pituitary gland

25. Ans. (c) Hippocampus

Ref: High Yield Neuroanatomy 4th ed page 138, Gray's 41st Ed Pg 348-355

Structure marked in the given image is Hippocampus

Hippocampal Formation

The hippocampal formation includes the dentate gyrus, hippocampus, subicular complex and entorhinal cortex. The hippocampus lies above the subiculum and medial parahippocampal gyrus, forming a curved elevation, approximately 5 cm long, along the floor of the inferior horn of the lateral ventricle.

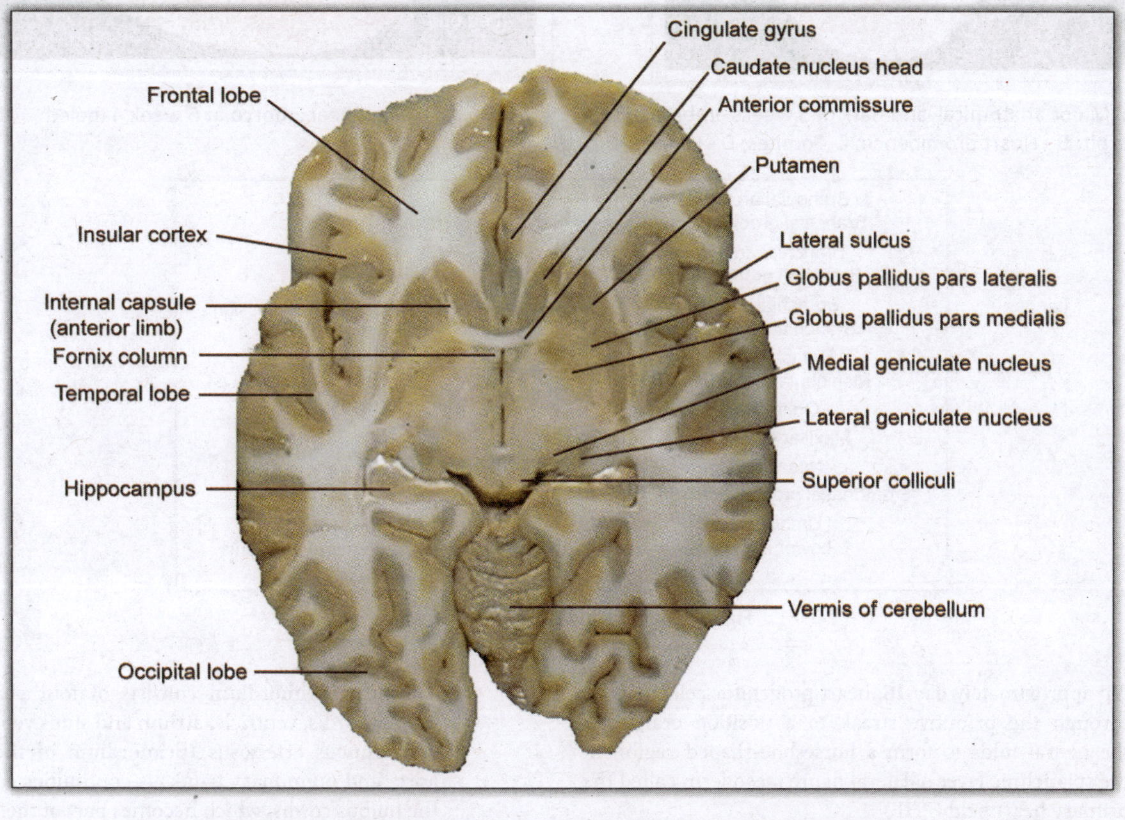

Fig: Transverse section of brain at the level of cerebellum (Labeled)

26. Ans. (b) L1

Ref: Gray's Anatomy 41st Ed Pg 748

- The spinal cord ends at L_1 in adults.
- **Clinical significance**: Spinal needle is inserted for administration of subdural block at L_{3-4}/L_{4-5} space so as to avoid injury to the spinal cord.
- Note: The spinal cord ends at L_3 in children

27. Ans. (c) Superficial posterior compartment

Ref: Keith L Moore's 7th edition pg 587, Grays 41st edition page 1412

Posterior compartment of the leg is divided into a superficial part and deep part by a transverse intermuscular septa. The tibial nerve and posterior tibial and fibular vessels (neurovascular bundle) supply both parts of the posterior compartment but run in the deep subcompartment deep (anterior) to the transverse intermuscular septum.

Hence, the neurovascular bundle is absent in the superficial posterior compartment.

28. Ans. (b) B

Ref: The Developing Human Keith and Moore 10th ed page 82

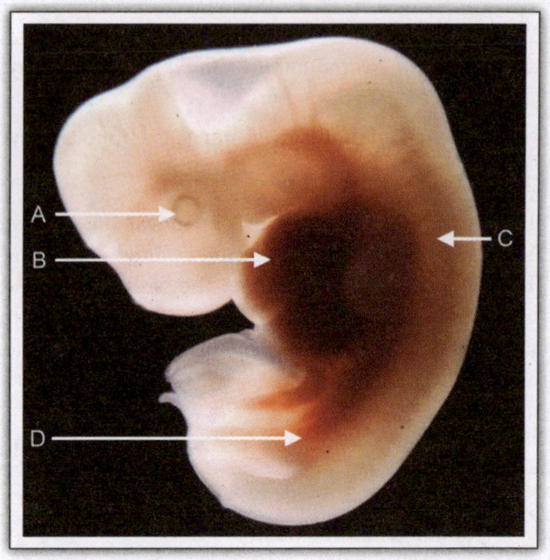

Fig: Major anatomical landmark of 5 weeks embryo; A - Lens pit; B - Heart prominence; C- Somites; D - Limb bud

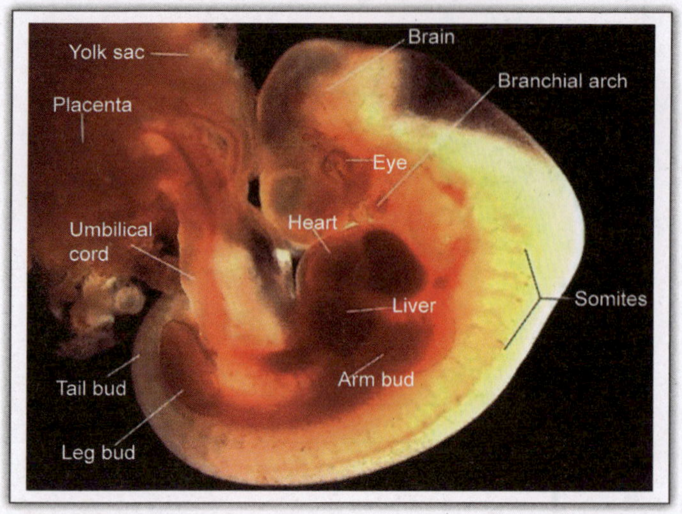

Fig: Real Embryo at 5 week, labeled

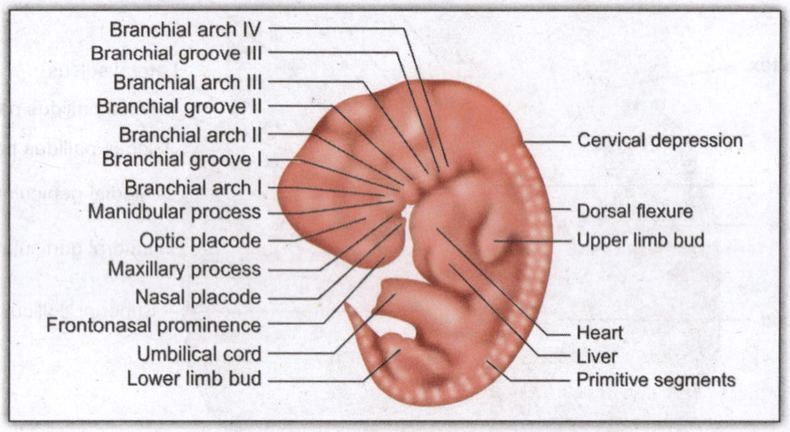

Fig: A 5-weeks-old embryo illustration

- On approximately **day 16,** heart progenitor cells migrate through the primitive streak to a position cranial to the neural folds to form a horseshoe-shaped region in the splanchnic layer of lateral figure mesoderm called the primary heart field (PHF)
- The cardiovascular system begins to develop at the **end of the third week.**
- By the **22nd day** of development, lateral body wall folds bring the two sides of the horseshoe toward the midline where they fuse (except for their caudal [atrial] ends to form a single, slightly bent heart tube
- The primordial heart starts to beat at the beginning of the **fourth week.**
- Splanchnic mesoderm surrounding the heart tube forms the primordial myocardium.
- The heart primordium consists of four chambers: the bulbus cordis, ventricle, atrium and sinus venosus.
- The truncus arteriosus (primordium of the ascending aorta and pulmonary trunk) is continuous caudally with the bulbus cordis, which becomes part of the ventricles.
- As the heart grows, it bends to the right and soon acquires the general external appearance of the adult heart. This bending is called cardiac loop in and happens during the **fourth week.**
- The heart becomes partitioned into four chambers **between the fourth and seventh weeks.**

29. Ans. (b) 2

Ref: Wolfgang Histology 4th ed page 98

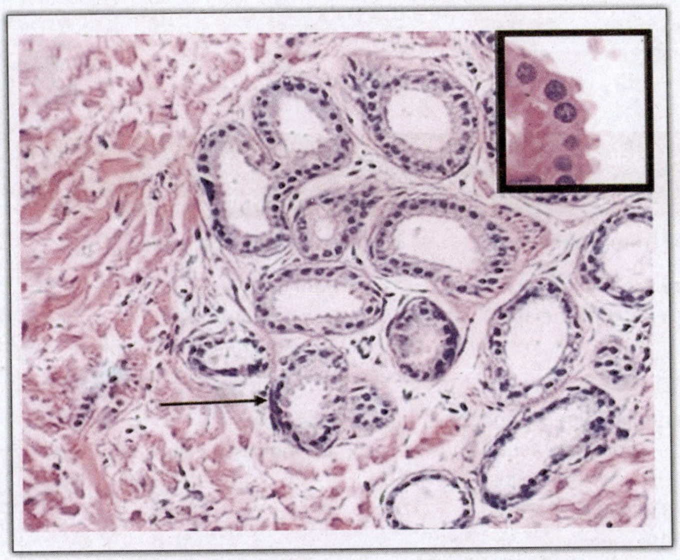

Fig: Apocrine gland: Apocrine sweat glands are typically larger and more productive than merocrine (eccrine) glands. They are characterized by a simple cuboidal epithelium and widely dilated lumen that stores the secretory product. Secretion from apocrine glands contains protein, lipid, carbohydrate, ammonium and other organic compounds. The ducts of the glands empty into an adjacent hair follicle. The bleb (insat) on the apical surface of the secretory cells suggested that the cell underwent apocrine secretion

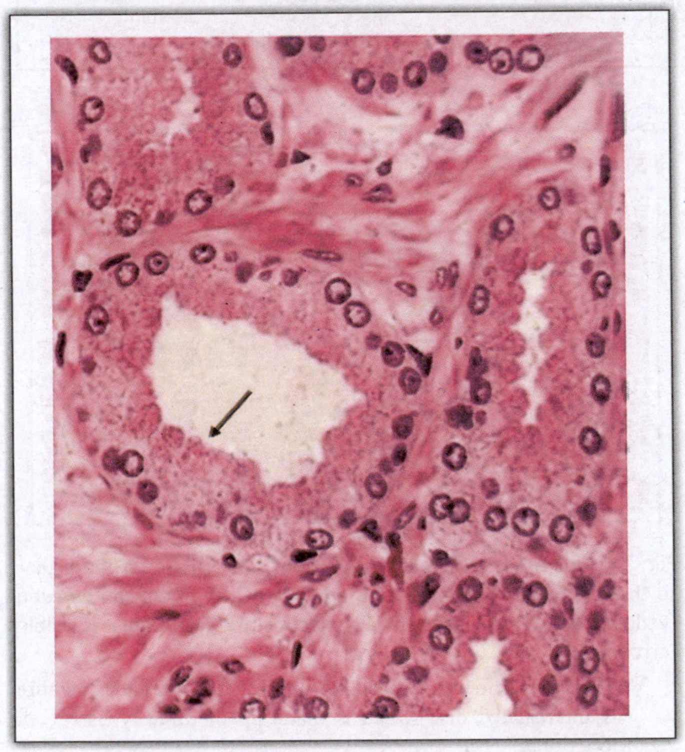

Fig: Merocrine (Eccrine) gland: Merocrine sweat glands are simple tubular glands. However the secretory units and the beginnings of the duct are coiled. The coiled mass is seen as numerous closely arranged tubular sections. Most merocrine glands have their main portions in the dermis, but some may reach even the hypodermis. In this picture note the dense connective tissue of the reticular dermis around the gland

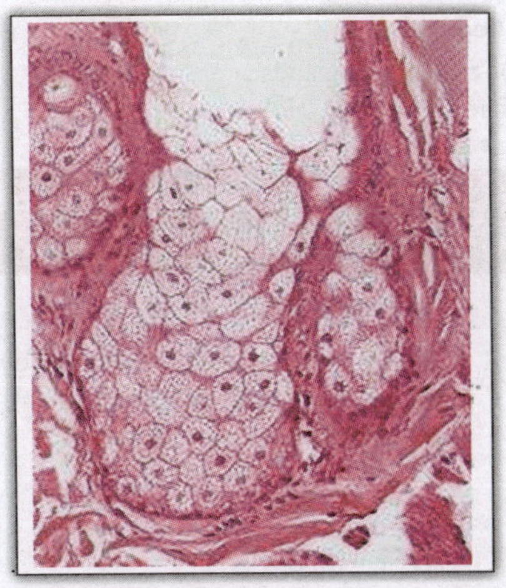

Fig: Holocrine gland: Sebaceous glands are holocrine glands. Their secretion, sebum, is an oily material. In this picture, note the outer cells comparable to the basal layer. As the cells grow they move inwards and accumulate their secretion. The fatty secretion is lost in processing leaving behind a spongy framework of other cytoplasmic elements. The cells are very similar to brown fat cells in appearance. In the deepest part of the gland you can see cells without nuclei disintegrating. The entire cell dies in releasing the sebum. Sebum travels to the surface along a hair shaft

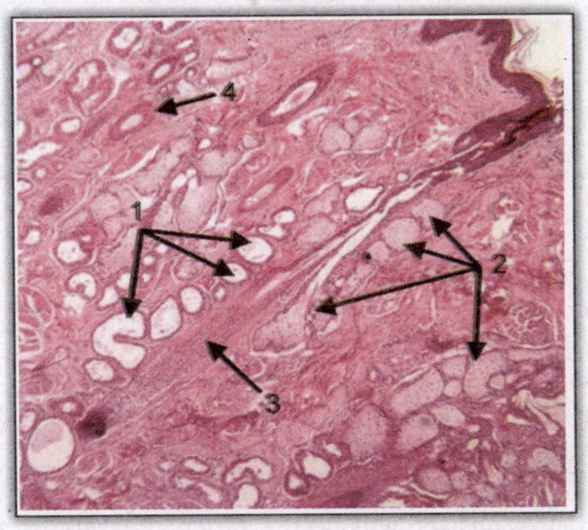

Fig: 40X magnification; sweat and sebaceous gland

Figure Legends:

1. Apocrine sweat glands
2. Sebaceous glands (Holocrine)
3. Hair follicle
4. Duct of sweat gland

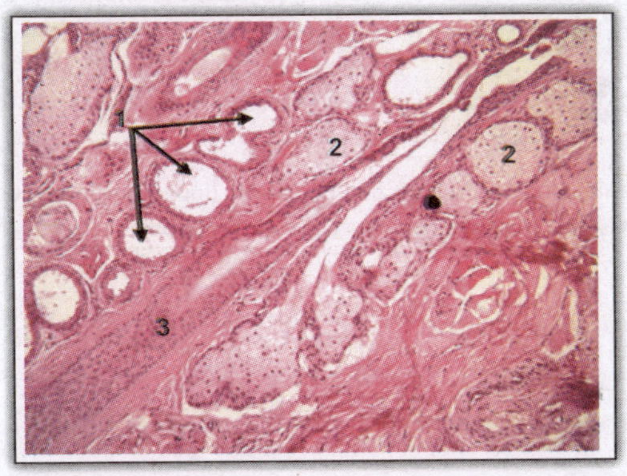

Fig: 100X magnification; sweat and sebaceous gland

Figure Legends

1. Apocrine Sweat glands
2. Sebaceous glands (Holocrine)
3. Hair follicle

Classification of Exocrine Glands on the Basis of Mechanism of Secretion

	Merocrine	Apocrine	Holocrine
Greek	Gr. meros, part, + krinein	Gr. apo, away from, + krinein	Gr. holos, whole, + krinein
Mode of secretion	The secretory granules leave the cell by exocytosis with no loss of other cellular material most common mechanism of secretion	The secretory product is discharged together with parts of the apical cytoplasm	The product of secretion is shed with the whole cell, a process that involves destruction of the secretion filled cells
Example	Pancreas Eccrine sweat gland	Lactating mammary glands, Apocrine glands of skin, Apocrine sweat glands, Ciliary (Moll's) glands of eyelids Ceruminous glands of external auditory meatus	Sebaceous glands Tarsal (Meibomian) glands of eyelids
Representative diagram	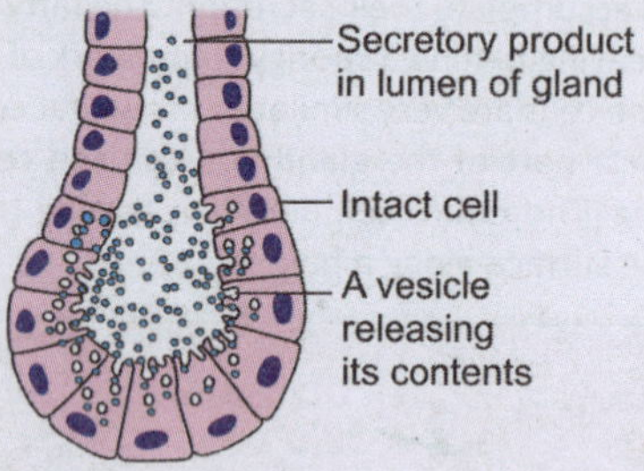 Merocrine gland	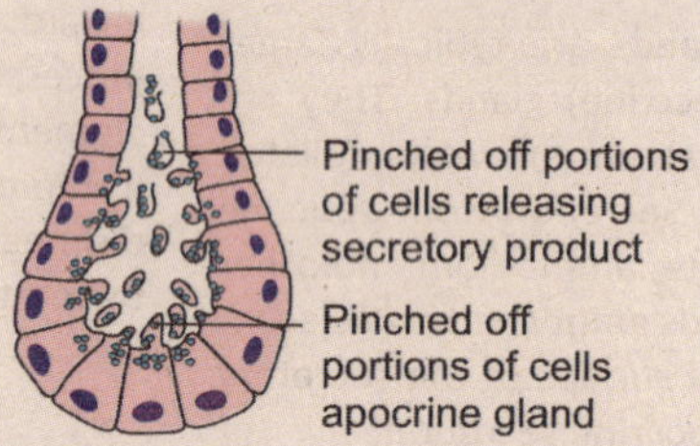 Apocrine gland	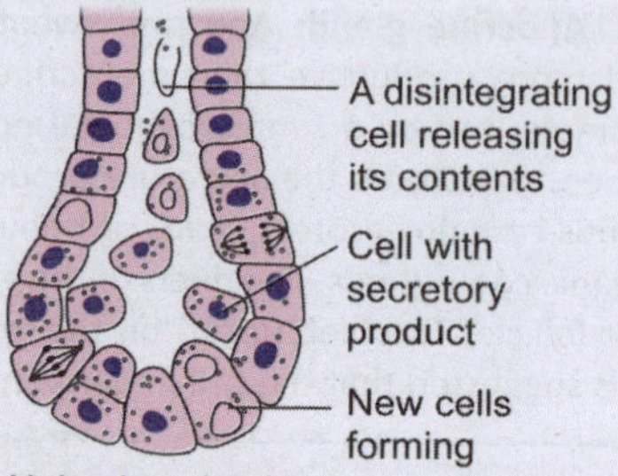 Holocrine gland

30. Ans. (c) Dermis

Ref: Ross's Histology 6th ed page 161

See table of Connective Tissues (see page no 110) in Anatomy AIIMS MAY 2015

The better answer will be the reticular layer/ deep layer of dermis. Dense Irregular connective tissue gets its name due to high proportion of collagen fiber in it (hence dense) and orientation of collagen bundles in different directions (hence) irregular. Tendon and ligament have dense regular connective tissue whereas Lamina propria has loose connective tissue.

31. Ans. (b) Zonula occludens

Ref: Ross Histology 6th ed page 328-329

Recall Bias

Some students believe that Connexins (found in gap Junction) was one of the option. This won't change the answer.

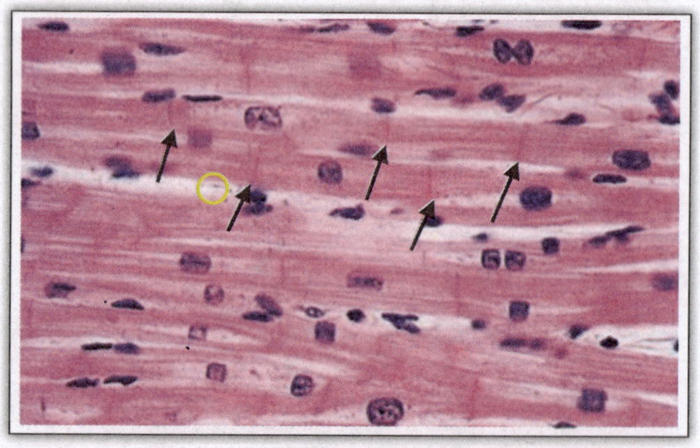

Fig: Cardiac muscle histology: Striations are visible perpendicular to the length of muscle fibers. Branching of the fibers can be seen (yellow circle). Nuclei are centrally placed. Intercalated disc is visible (arrows).

The given slide is of cardiac muscle. The marked structure is Intercalated disc which is made up of three types of cell junctions.

- Fascia adherens (Analogous to Zonula adherens of non-muscle cell)
- Gap junction
- Desmosomes (Macula adherens)

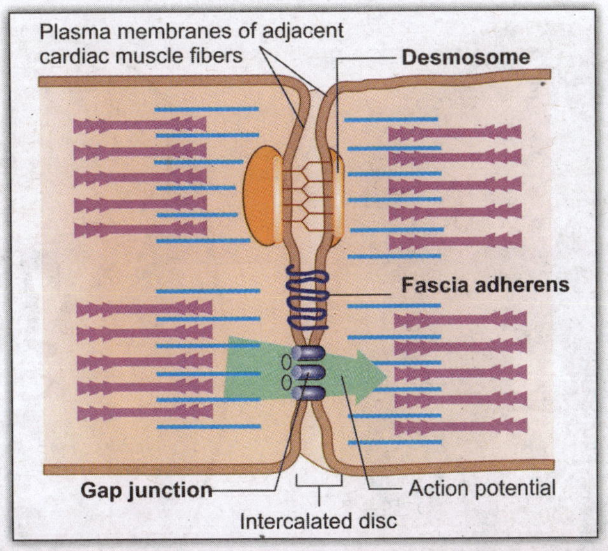

Types of cell junction			
Occluding junctions	Anchoring junctions		Communicating junctions
Occluding junctions (zonula occludens or tight junctions)	**Adhering junctions (zonula adherens)**	**Desmosomes (macula adherens)**	**Gap junctions (septate junction)**
A continuous **belt like junction**, these regions of cell are very tightly connected together, such that the adjacent plasma membranes are sealed together. It greatly restricts the passage of water, electrolytes and other small molecules across the epithelium	Analogous to **Fascia adherans** of non-epithelial cells. Adherens junction lies below the tight junction (occluding junction)	It is circular or **spot like** in outline and not belt- or band shaped. There are also **'hemidesmosomes'** that lie on the basal membrane, to help stick the cells to the underlying basal lamina.	These are communicating junctions. This channel is big enough to allow small molecules such as inorganic ions and other small water soluble molecules (smaller than 1000 kDa) to pass between the cells. However the channel is too small for proteins, nucleic acids or sugars to pass through.
Occludin interact with each other to produce this tight seal.	The **E- cadherins** from adjacent cells interact to 'zipper' up the two cells together	**Desmin** in cardiac cell **Keratin** in epithelial cells	**Connexins** form a structure called a connexon. When connexons from two adjacent cells align, they form a continuous channel between them

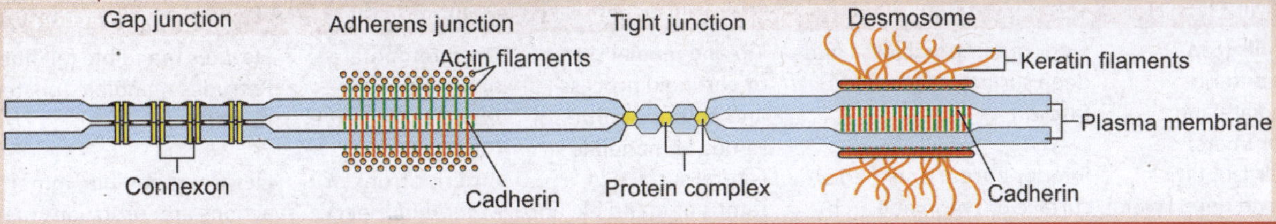

32. Ans. (b) **2**

Ref: Grays 41st ed page 547, Grant's Atlas of Anatomy 12th Ed page 672 Table 7.9

Opening of jaw is done by lateral pterygoid muscle marked as 2, in the given diagram.

Muscles of mastication are the new Love of AIIMS exams. All possible cut sections are asked in past few papers.

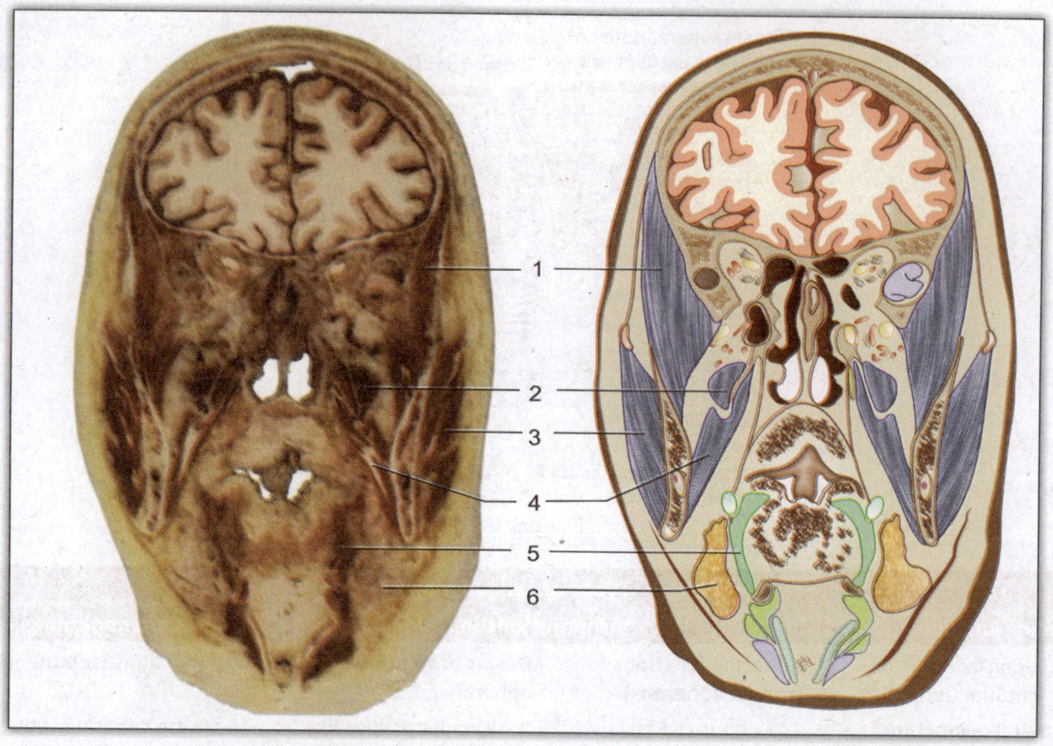

Fig: Coronal section of head with muscles of mastication and comparative illustration

Figure Legends

1. Temporalis
2. Lateral pterygoid
3. Masseter muscle
4. Medial pterygoid
5. Hypoglossal muscle
6. Submandibular gland

Muscles of Mastication (Acting on Temporomandibular Joint)				
Muscle	**Origin**	**Insertion**	**Innervation**	**Main action**
Temporails (Fan shaped; anterior, intermediate and posterior fibers)	Floor of temporal fossa and deep surface of temporal fascia	Tip and medial surface of coronoid process and anterior border of ramus of mandible	Deep temporal branches of ***mandibular nerve*** (CN V_3)	Elevates mandible (all fibers), Retrudes mandible (posterior fibers)
Masseter (superficial, middle and deep layers) (superficial layer is the largest)	Inferior border and medial surface of zygomatic arch	Lateral surface of ramus of mandible and coronoid process	Anterior trunk of ***Mandibular nerve*** (CN V_3) through masseteric nerve	Elevates mandible, minor actions are: protrudes mandible (superficial fibers), retrudes mandible (deep fibers)
Lateral pterygoid (Upper head and lower head)	**Superior head:** Infratemporal surface and infratemporal crest of greater wing of sphenoid bone **Inferior head:** *Lateral surface of lateral pterygoid figure*	Neck of mandible, articular disc and capsule of temporomandibular joint	***Mandibular nerve*** (CN V_3) through lateral pterygoid nerve which enters its deep surface	*Acting bilaterally,* protrude mandible and depress chin; *Acting unilaterally* alternately, they produce side-to-side movements of mandible (pulled medially towards the opposite side)
Medial pterygoid (small superficial head and major deep head)	**Deep head:** Medial surface of lateral pterygoid figure and pyramidal process of palatine bone **Superficial head:** Tuberosity of maxilla	Medial surface of ramus of mandible, inferior to mandibular foramen	***Mandibular nerve*** (CN V_3) through medial pterygoid nerve	Acts synergistically with masseter to elevate mandible, contributes to protrude mandible; *acting unilaterally* produce small grinding movements

Unlike the other muscles of mastication, lateral pterygoid is not pennate, nor does it have a significant number of Golgi tendon organs associated with its attachments

33. Ans. (c) Ball and socket joint

Ref: Grant's atlas 12th ed ch 5.82

Types of synovial joints

Type of joint	Axis	Movements	Examples
Plane/ Gliding joint	Uniaxial	Gliding	Intercarpal joints Intertarsal joints Between articular processes of vertebrae
Hinge joints	Uniaxial	Flexion, Extension	Elbow joints Ankle joints Interphalangeal joints
Pivot joints	Uniaxial	Rotation	Median Atlantoaxial joint Superior and inferior radioulnar joints
Condylar joints	Biaxial	Flexion, Extension, Limited rotation	Knee joints Joints between condyles of mandible and temporal bone
Ellipsoid joints	Biaxial	Flexion, Extension, Abduction, Adduction, Circumduction	Wrist Joint Metacarpophalangeal joint Atlantoaxial joints (lateral)
Saddle joints	Multiaxial	Flexion, Extension, Abduction, Adduction, Conjunct Rotation	Sternoclavicular joint First carpometacarpal joint Calcaneocuboid joint Incudomalleolar
Ball and socket joints	Multiaxial	Flexion, Extension, Abduction, Adduction, Circumduction, Rotation	**Mnemonic: SHIT** Shoulder joint Hip Joint Incudostapedial joint Talocalcaneonavicular joint

34. Ans. (a) Capitate

Ref: Grays 41st ed page 869

Carpal Bones Osteology

- Carpal bones are cartilaginous at birth
- Each Carpal bone ossified from one center
- The capitate is the first and the pisiform is the last carpal to ossify.
- Capitate- 2nd month, Hamate - End of the 3rd month, Triquetrum - 3rd year
- Lunate, Scaphoid, Trapezium and Trapezoid- 4th year
- Pisiform- 9th year

35. Ans. (c) Abducens nerve

Ref: Grant's Atlas of Anatomy 12th Ed page 814, Gray's 41st ed page 272, 320

The marked structure is abducens nerve see following labeled picture for details.

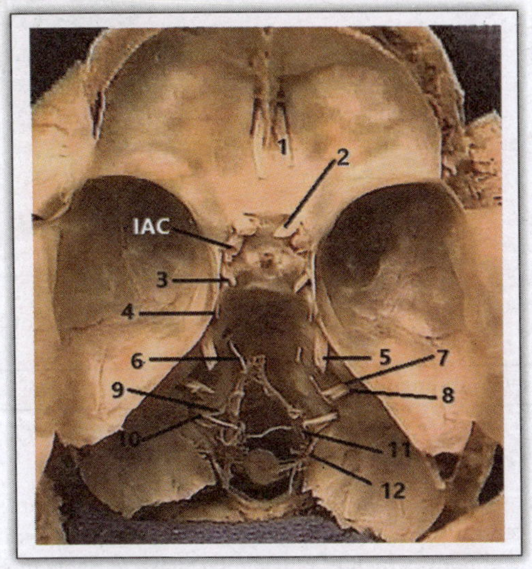

Fig: Superior view of the base of the skull showing cranial nerves. The posterior fossa contains the brainstem, cerebellum and cranial nerves IV-XII

Figure Legend

1. Olfactory nerve (CN I)
2. Optic nerve (CN II)
3. Oculomotor nerve (CN III)
4. Trochlear nerve (CN IV)
5. Trigeminal Nerve (CN V)
6. Abducens nerve (CN VI): Abducens nerve located between pons and the clivus in the way to the cavernous sinus.
7. Facial nerve (CN VII)
8. Vestibulocochlear nerve (CN VIII)
9. Glossopharyngeal nerve (CN IX)
10. Vagus nerve (CN X)
11. Spinal accessory nerve (CN XI)
12. Hypoglossal nerve (CN XII)

IAC = Internal carotid artery

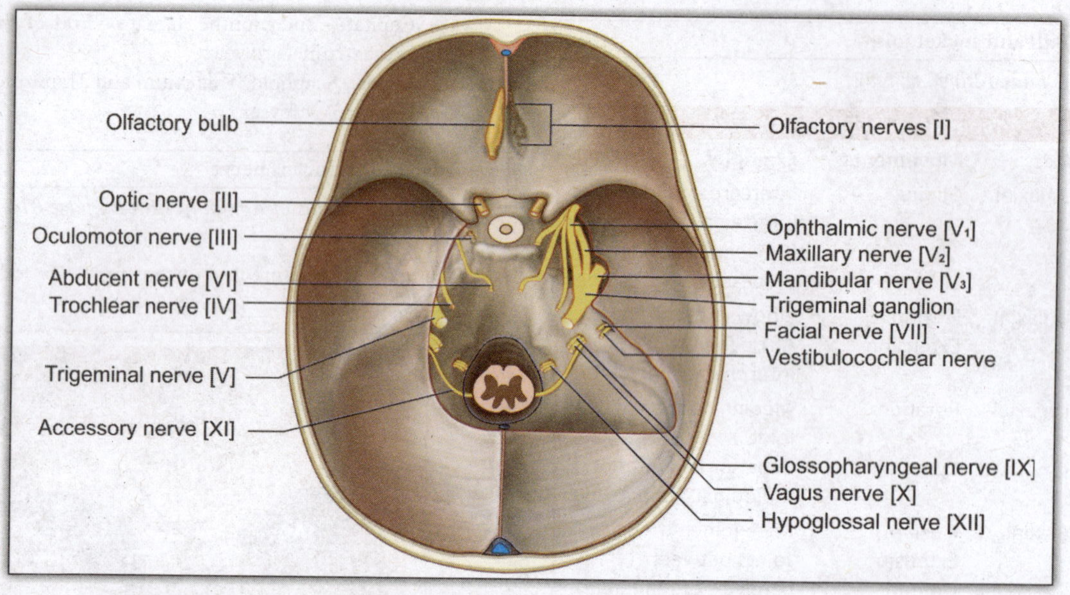

Fig: Superior view of the base of the skull showing cranial nerves (Labeled illustration)

36. Ans. (a) Pubococcygeus

Ref: Gray's 41st ed page 1222, Shaw's 16th ed page 493, Novak's 15th ed page 861

The midpoint of the line joining the ischial tuberosities is the central point of the perineum. This is the location of the perineal body, which is an irregular mass, variable in size and consistency and containing collagenous and elastic fibers and both skeletal and smooth muscle. The perineal body lies deep to the skin, with relatively little overlying subcutaneous tissue, posterior to the vestibule of the vagina or bulb of the penis and anterior to the anus and anal canal.

The perineal body is the site of convergence and interlacing of fibers of several muscles, including the:

- Bulbospongiosus.
- External anal sphincter.
- Superficial and deep transverse perineal muscles.
- Smooth and voluntary slips of muscle from the external urethral sphincter, levator ani and muscular coats of the rectum.

Anteriorly, the perineal body blends with the posterior border of the perineal membrane and superiorly with the recto-vesical or rectovaginal septum.

Pubococcygeus originates from the posterior aspect of the body of the pubis and passes back almost horizontally. The most medial fibres run directly lateral to the urethra and its sphincter as it passes through the pelvic floor; here, the muscle is correctly called **puboperinealis**, although, because of its close relationship to the upper half of the urethra in both sexes, it is often referred to as **pubourethralis**; despite this, no direct connection with the urethra is present.

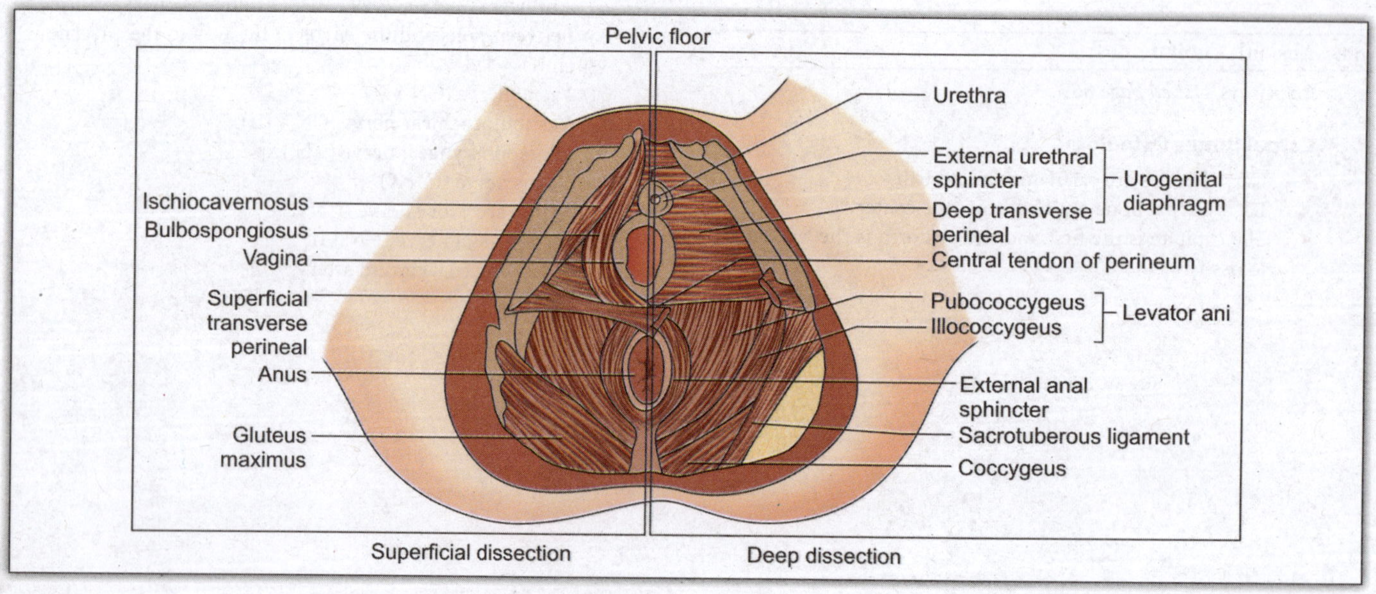

	Ischiococcygeus (sometime separately named as coccygeus)		Tip of ischial spine and obturator fascia	Lateral margins of the coccyx and the fifth sacral segment	Direct branches of sacral plexus from 3rd and 4th sacral spinal segments	Forms **small part of pelvic diaphragm** that supports pelvic viscera; flexes coccyx
Levator ani	**Pubococcygeus**	Puboperinealis (AKA Pubo urethralis)	Back of the body of the pubis	Pulls the perineal body ventrally. Forms part of **urethral sphincter**	2nd and 3rd sacral spinal segments via the **pudendal nerve**	Forms most of **pelvic diaphragm** that helps support pelvic viscera and resists increases in intra-abdominal pressure
		Puboprostaticus or pubovaginalis	Back of the body of the pubis	Slings around prostate or vagina		
		Puboanalis	Back of the body of the pubis	Slings around anal canal		
		Puborectalis	Back of the body of the pubis	Slings around rectum		
	Iliococcygeus		Inner surface of ischial spine and obturator fascia	Sacrum and coccyx but most join with opposite side to form raphe	Direct branches of sacral plexus from 3rd and 4th sacral spinal segments	

37. Ans. (b) Triangular

Ref: Gray's Anatomy 41st edition page 749

Trapezius is a **flat triangular muscle** that covers the back of neck and shoulder. The two trapezius resemble a trapezium in which the two angles correspond to the shoulders, third to the external occipital protuberance and the fourth to the spine of twelfth thoracic vertebra.

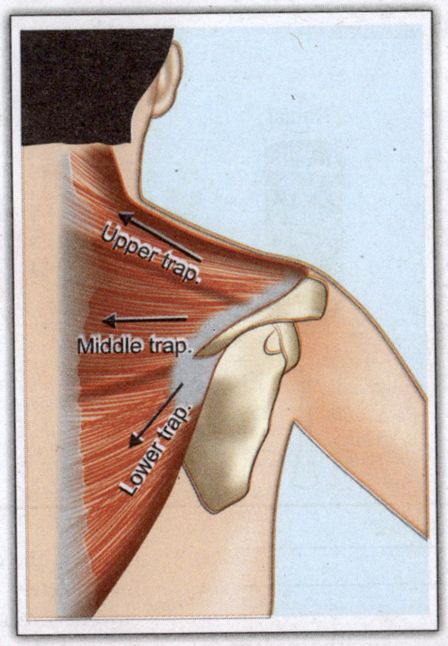

Muscles Classification According to Shape and Orientation of fibers		
Type	**Subtype**	**Example**
Parallel fibers (fibers that are largely parallel to the line of pull)	Quadrilateral (flat and short)	Thyrohyoid Quadratus Lumborum
	Long strap like	Sternohyoid, sartorius Rectus Abdominis (Strap like with tendinous intersections)
	Fusiform (parallel in the belly)	Biceps

Contd...

Muscles Classification According to Shape and Orientation of fibers

Type	Subtype		Example
Oblique Fibers (fibers are oblique to the line of pull	Triangular		Temporalis, Trapezius, Adductor longus
	Pennate (feather-like)	Unipennate	Flexor pollicis longus, Soleus, Extensor digitorum longus, Peroneus tertius
		Bipennate	Rectus femoris, dorsal interossei, Tibialis posterior
		Multipennate	Deltoid
		Circumpinnate	Tibialis anterior
Spiral (spiral or twisted arrangement)	180° twist between their median and lateral attachments		Sternocostal fibers of pectoralis major and latissimus dorsi
	Spiral around a bone		Supinator
	Cruciate- contain 2 or more planes of fibers arranged in differing directions		Sternocleidomastoid, masseter and adductor magnus

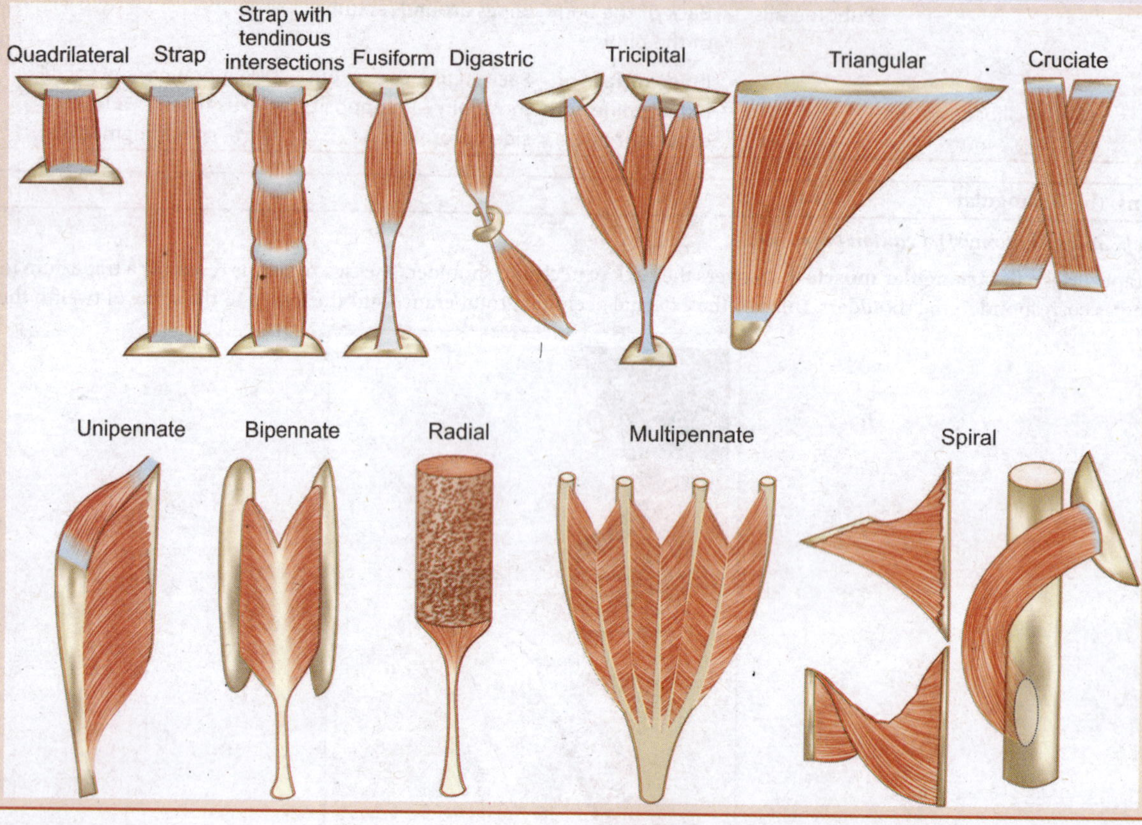

38. Ans. (a) L1 L2

Ref: Grays Anatomy 41st edition page 1045

The cremaster is reflex is brought about by stroking the medial side of the thigh. This leads to contraction of cremaster muscle which elevates the ipsilateral testes. This reflex is mediated by **genitofemoral nerve** with root value L_1 **and** L_2. The reflex is absent if there is torsion of the testicle

39. Ans. (d) Inferior vena cava

Ref: Clinically Oriented Anatomy Keith and Moore 7th ed page 306

The central teandon is the central aponeurotic part where the muscular peripheral fibers converge in a trifoliate manner. The central tendon has no bony attachments and is incompletely divided into three leaves, resembling a wide cloverleaf. Although it lies near the center of the diaphragm, the central tendon is closer to the anterior part of the thorax. The caval opening (vena caval foramen), through which the terminal part of the IVC passes to enter the heart, perforates the central tendon.

Extra Edge

- Inferior vana cava (IVC) hiatus is in the central tendon of the diaphragm
- Esophageal hiatus is between the left and right bundles of the right crus of the diaphragm
- Aortic hiatus is between the right and left crus of the diaphragm

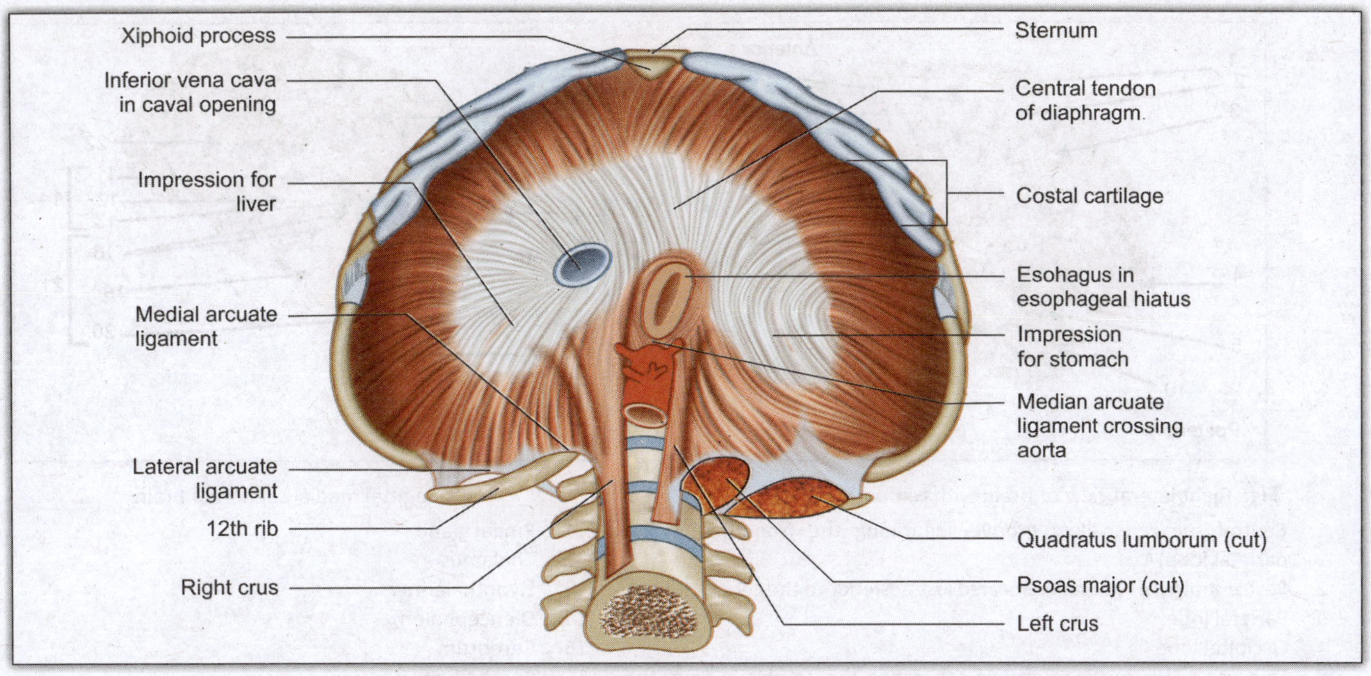

40. Ans. (c) Orbital cortex

Ref: Gray's Anatomy 41st ed page 393

Structure marked in the figure is Corpus callosum

Corpus callosum is the largest set of interhemispheric connecting fibers. It lies inferior to the longitudinal fissure and superior to the diencephalon. It connects homologous neocortical areas.

Axons of the corpus callosum radiate into the white matter core of each hemisphere, thereafter dispersing to the cerebral cortex.

- Commissural fibers forming the rostrum extend laterally, below the anterior horn of the lateral ventricle, connecting the orbital surfaces of the frontal lobes.
- Fibers in the genu curve forwards, as the forceps minor, to connect the lateral and medial surfaces of the frontal lobes.
- Fibers of the trunk pass laterally, intersecting with the projection fibers of the corona radiata to connect wide neocortical areas of the hemispheres.
- Fibers of the trunk and splenium, which form the roof and lateral wall of the atrium and the lateral wall of the inferior horn of the lateral ventricle, constitute the tapetum, which runs underneath the optic radiation within the sagittal stratum.
- The remaining fibers of the splenium curve back into the occipital lobes as the forceps major.
- Interhemispheric connections through the corpus callosum do not all represent a simple linking of loci in one hemisphere with the same loci in the other. In areas containing a clear representation of a contralateral sensorium (e.g. body surface, visual field), only those areas that are functionally related to midline representation are linked to the contralateral hemisphere.
- Connections that link the same, or similar, areas on each side are termed homotopic connections. The corpus callosum also interconnects heterogeneous cortical areas on the two sides (heterotopic connections).
- These may serve to connect functionally similar, but anatomically different, loci in the two hemispheres and/or to connect functional areas in one hemisphere with regions that are specialized for a unilaterally confined function in the other.

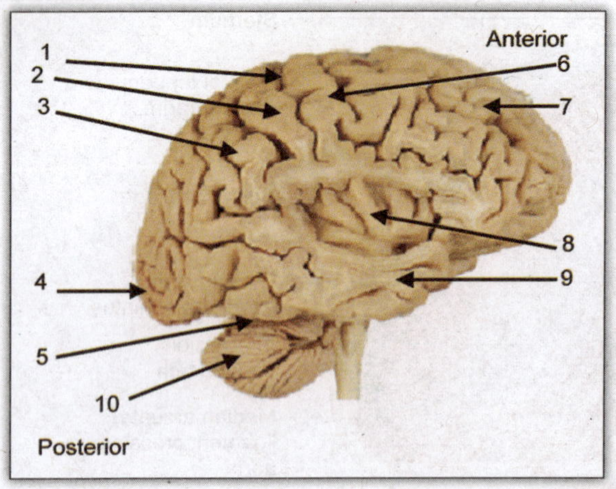

Fig: Right lateral view of brain with temporal lobe cut away

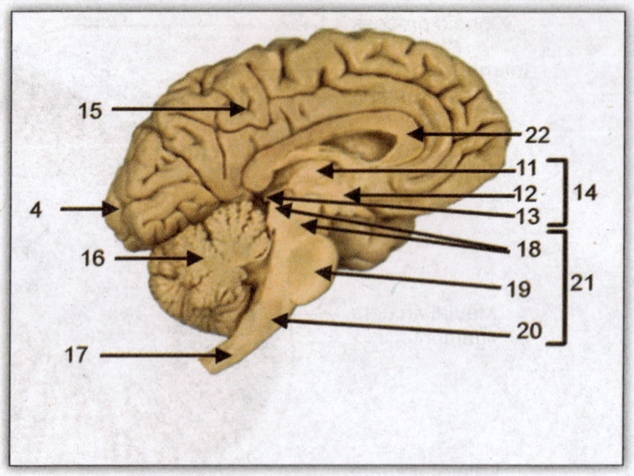

Fig: Sagittal medial section of brain

1. Central sulcus (shallow groove separating the frontal lobe and parietal lobe)
2. Postcentral gyrus (elevation located just posterior to the central sulcus)
3. Parietal lobe
4. Occipital lobe
5. Transverse fissure (deep groove separating the cerebrum from the cerebellum in the posterior/inferior part of the brain)
6. Precentral gyrus (elevation located just anterior to the central sulcus)
7. Frontal lobe
8. Insula (inner lobe deep to the lateral cerebral fissure)
9. Temporal lobe (cut)
10. Cerebellum
11. Pineal gland
12. Thalamus
13. Hypothalamus
14. Diencephalon
15. Cerebrum
16. Cerebellum
17. Spinal cord
18. Midbrain
19. Pons
20. Medulla oblongata
21. Brainstem
22. Corpus callosum

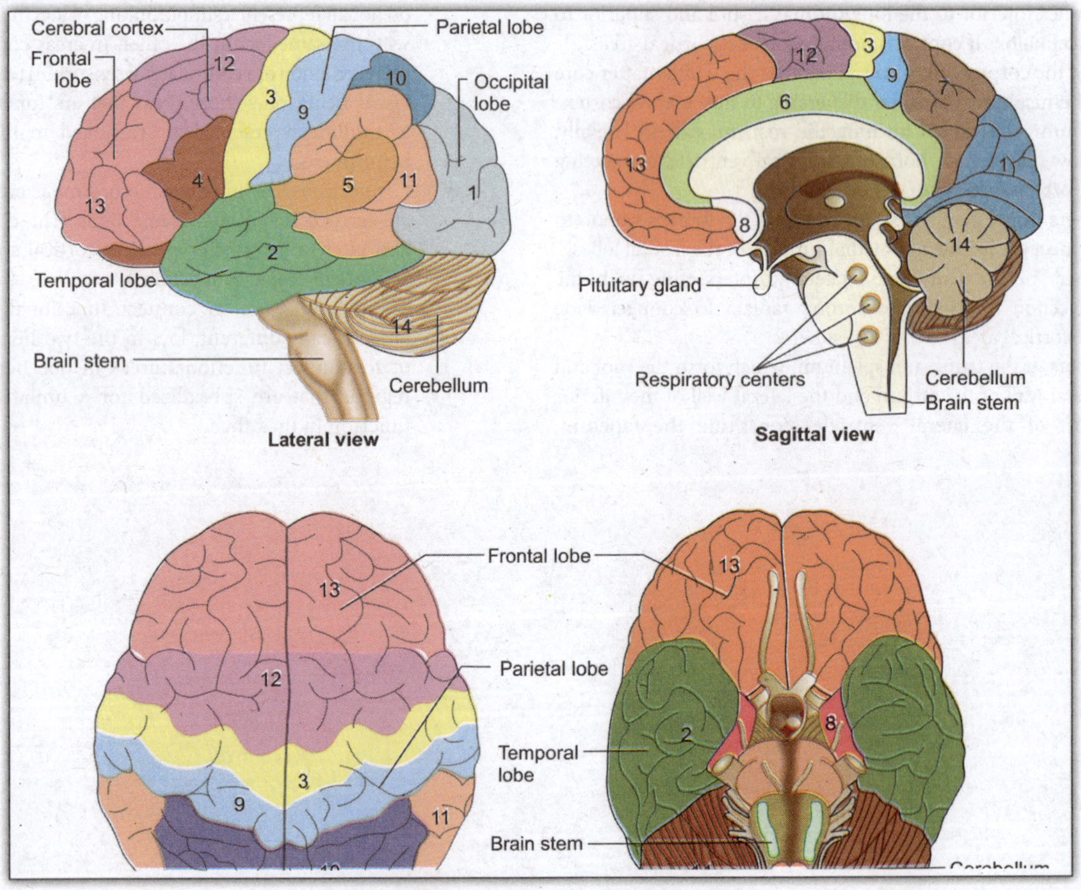

Fig: Functional areas of cerebral cortex

Area No.	Area name	Area function
1.	Visual area	Sight, image recognition, image perception
2.	Association area	Short-term memory, equilibrium, emotion
3.	Motor function area	Initiation of voluntary muscles
4.	Broca's area	Muscles of speech
5.	Auditory area	Hearing
6.	Emotional area	Pain, hunger, flight or fight response
7.	Sensory association area	
8.	Olfactory area	Smelling
9.	Sensory area	Sensation from muscle and skin
10.	Somatosensory association area	Evaluation of weight, texture, temperature etc. for object recognition
11.	Wernicke's area	Written and spoken comprehension
12.	Motor function area	Eye movement and orientation
13.	Higher mental function	Concentration, planning, judgment, emotional expression, creativity
14	Cerebellar motor area	Coordination of movement, balance, equilibrium, inhibition

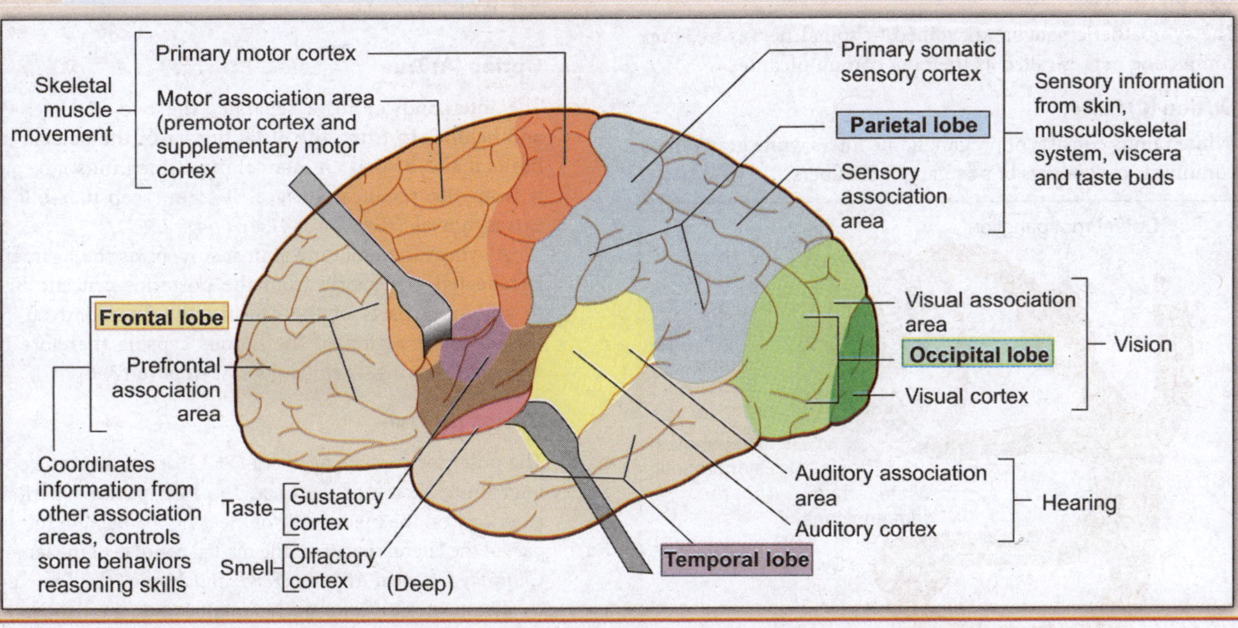

Note: The above area numbers are arbitrary numbers and does not represents Brodmann area

41. Ans. (c) Preganglionic sympathetic supply

Ref: Grays Anatomy 41st edition page 235, Last's Anatomy: Regional and Applied by Mcminn 9th ed page 31, General Anatomy 2nd ed by Vishram Singh page 181

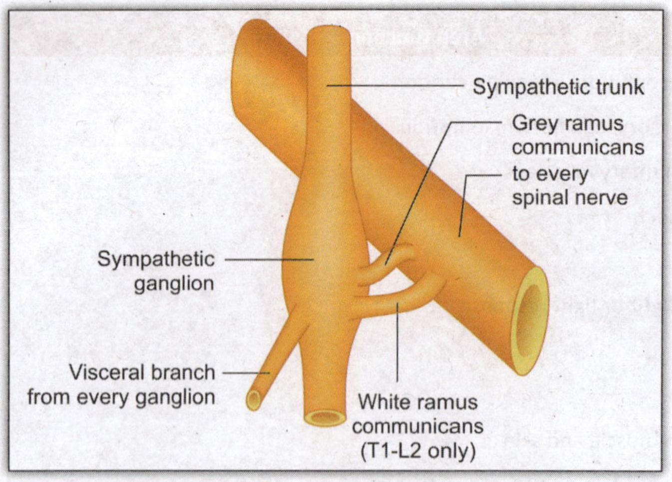

Fig: Typical sympathetic trunk ganglion. Every ganglio have grey ramus while only T1 to L2 have white ramus

Option (A) True:

The white rami are myelinated hence appear whitish in color whereas grey rami are nonmyelinated.

Option (B) True:

The sympathetic ganglia are joined to spinal nerves by short connecting nerves called as the rami communicantes.

Option (C) False:

White ramus consists of preganglionic fibers while gray ramus communicans consists of postganglionic fibers.

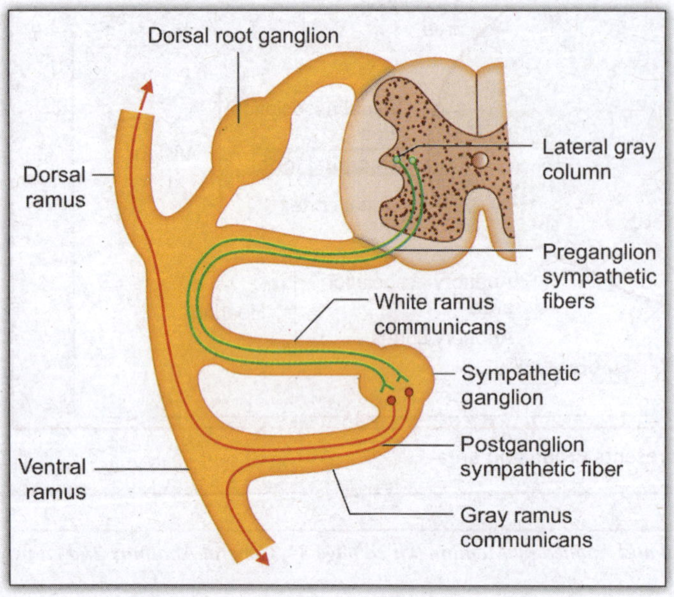

Option (D) True

The gray ramus communicans is positioned medial to the white ramus communicans. *(Ref: Gray's Anatomy for Students 2nd ed page 44)*

Difference between white and grey rami communication		
	White ramus communication	**Grey ramus communication**
Types of fibers	Myelinated	Non-myelinated
Source of origin	Lateral Horn cells of spinal cord	Cells of sympathetic ganglion
Destination	Relay in sympathetic ganglion (Preganglionic fibers and Afferent fibers)	Efferent postganglionic. Distributed to blood vessels, hair and sweat glands through branches of anterior and posterior rami of spinal nerves

42. Ans. (d) Primary restraint to internal rotation of knee

Ref: With Text

Option (A) True

The intercondylar fossa separates the two condyles distally and behind. In front, the distal border of the patellar surface limits it and behind an intercondylar line limits it, separating it from the popliteal surface. It is intracapsular but largely extrasynovial. *(Ref: Gray's 41st ed page 1351)*

A synovial membrane almost surrounds the ligaments but is reflected posteriorly from the posterior cruciate ligament to adjoining parts of the capsule; the intercondylar part of the posterior region of the fibrous capsule therefore has no synovial covering. *(Ref: Gray's 41st ed page 1390)*

Option (B) True

The posterior cruciate ligament (PCL), arises from the posterior intercondylar area of the tibia. The PCL passes superiorly and anteriorly on the medial side of the ACL to attach to the anterior part of the lateral surface of the medial condyle of the femur. *(Ref: Clinically Oriented Anatomy Keith and Moore 7th ed page 640)*

The posterior cruciate ligament is attached to the lateral surface of the medial femoral condyle and extends up on to the anterior part of the roof of the intercondylar fossa, where its attachment is extensive in the anteroposterior direction. Anterolateral and posteromedial bundles have been defined; they are named (against convention) according to their femoral attachments. The anterolateral bundle tightens in flexion while the posteromedial bundle is tight in extension of the knee. Each bundle slackens as the other tightens. Unlike the anterior cruciate ligament, it is not isometric during knee motion, i.e. the distance between attachments varies with knee position. *(Ref: Gray's 41st ed page 1391)*

Option (C) True

PCL prevents anterior displacement of the femur on the tibia or posterior displacement of the tibia on the femur and helps prevent hyperflexion of the knee joint. In the weight-bearing flexed knee, the PCL is the main stabilizing factor for the femur (e.g., when walking downhill). (*Ref: Clinically oriented Anatomy Keith and Moore 7th ed page 640*)

The meniscofemoral ligaments are believed to act as secondary restraints, supporting the posterior cruciate ligament in minimizing displacement caused by posteriorly directed forces on the tibia. (*Ref: Gray's 41st ed page 1389*)

There are two types of restraints which work to stabilize a joint. Some of these are better aligned to resist the applied load or displacement and are termed **primary restraints,** e.g. the cruciate ligaments and the tibial and fibular collateral ligaments. **Secondary restraints** are less well aligned but still have a significant restraining effect, e.g. the menisci and the meniscofemoral ligaments. **The anterior cruciate ligament is well aligned to resist the applied anterior force whereas the posterior cruciate resists the posterior force.**

Option (D) False

The posterior cruciate ligament is the primary restraint to the posterior displacement of the tibia and along with the posterior capsule, it also resists internal rotation of the tibia. During internal rotation of the knee, the anterior and posterior cruciate ligaments develop functional synergism by coiling around each other, becoming taut, pulling the articular surfaces together and checking excessive internal rotation.

Recent studies have also identified the PCL as a secondary restraint to internal rotation, particularly between 90° and 120° of flexion. (*Ref: R. Papannagari, L.E. DeFrate, K.W. Nha, et al. Function of posterior cruciate ligament bundles during in vivo knee flexion Am J Sports Med, 35 (2007), pp. 1507-1512*)

Structures limiting movements of knee joint

Movement	Limiting structures
Flexion (femoropatellar and femorotibial)	• Soft tissue apposition posteriorly • Tension of vastus lateralis, medialis and intermedius • Tension of rectus femoris (especially with hip joint extended)
Extension (femoropatellar and femorotibial)	Ligaments: Anterior cruciate and posterior cruciate, fibular and tibial collateral, posterior joint capsule and oblique popliteal ligament
Internal rotation (femorotibial with knee flexed)	Ligaments: Anterior cruciate and posterior cruciate
External rotation (femorotibial with knee flexed)	Ligaments: Fibular and tibial collateral

Some rotation occurs when the knee is flexed

Extra Edge

- The posterior cruciate ligament is thicker and stronger than the anterior cruciate ligament
- The posterior cruciate ligament ruptures less commonly than the anterior cruciate ligament and rupture is usually better
- Many synovial joints also contain **accessory ligaments** called extracapsular ligaments and intracapsular ligaments. Extracapsular ligaments lie outside the articular capsule. Examples are the fibular and tibial collateral ligaments of the knee joint. Intracapsular ligaments occur within the articular capsule but are excluded from the synovial cavity by folds of the synovial membrane. Examples are the anterior and posterior cruciate ligaments of the knee joint
- The **Anterior cruciate ligament (ACL),** the weaker of the two cruciate ligaments, arises from the anterior intercondylar area of the tibia, just posterior to the attachment of the medial meniscus. It extends superiorly, posteriorly and laterally to attach to the posterior part of the medial side of the lateral condyle of the femur. The ACL has a relatively poor blood supply. ACL limits posterior rolling of the femoral condyles on the tibial plateau during flexion and prevents posterior displacement of the femur on the tibia and hyperextension of the knee joint.

AIIMS MAY 2017

43. Ans. (c) C

Ref: Gray's 41st ed page 618, 619

The patient presents with DiGeorge syndrome caused due to defective development of 3rd and 4th pharyngeal pouches. But since thymus develops from 3rd pharyngeal pouch and there is absence of thymus in this patient, the better answer is 3rd pouch.

DiGeorge Syndrome

A congenital disorder in which defective development of the 3rd and 4th pharyngeal pouches results in hypoplasia or aplasia of the thymus and parathyroid glands.

Branchial Arches

There are six pharyngeal arches, but in humans the fifth arch only exists transiently during embryologic growth and development. Since no human structures result from the fifth arch, the arches in humans are I, II, III, IV and VI. The first three contribute to structures above the larynx, while the last two contribute to the larynx and trachea

Contd...

Pharyngeal arch	Muscular contributions	Skeletal contributions	Nerve	Artery	Corrosponding pouch structures	Corrosponding cleft structures
1st (mandibular arch)	Muscles of mastication, Anterior belly of the digastric, Mylohyoid, Tensor tympani, Tensor veli palatini	Maxilla, mandible (only as a model for mandible not actual formation of mandible), Incus and Malleus, Meckel's cartilage, Ant. ligament of malleus, Sphenomandibular ligament	Trigeminal nerve (V_2 and V_3)	Maxillary artery, external carotid artery	Eustachian tube, Tympanic (Middle ear) cavity, mastoid antrum and inner layer of the tympanic membrane	External auditory canal, External auditory meatus
2nd (hyoid arch)	Muscles of facial expression, Buccinator, Platysma, Stapedius, Stylohyoid, Posterior belly of the digastric	Stapes, Styloid process, hyoid (lesser horn and upper part of body), Reichert's cartilage, Stylohyoid ligament	Facial nerve (VII)	Stapedial Artery	Palatine tonsils, Tonsillar fossa	Second, third and fourth clefts form a cavity lined with ectodermal epithelium, the cervical sinus, but with further development, this sinus disappears
3rd	Stylopharyngeus	Hyoid (greater horn and lower part of body)	Glossopharyngeal nerve (IX)	Common carotid/ Internal carotid	Inferior parathyroid, Thymus	
4th	Cricothyroid muscle, all intrinsic muscles of soft palate including levator veli palatini	Thyroid cartilage, epiglottic cartilage	Vagus nerve (X) Superior laryngeal nerve	Right 4th aortic arch: subclavian artery Left 4th aortic arch: aortic arch	Superior parathyroid, ultimobranchial body (which forms the Para follicular C-Cells of thyroid gland)	
6th	All intrinsic muscles of larynx except the cricothyroid muscle	Cricoid cartilage, arytenoid cartilages, corniculate cartilage	Vagus nerve (X) Recurrent laryngeal nerve	Right 6th aortic arch: pulmonary artery Left 6th aortic arch: Pulmonary artery and ductus arteriosus	Rudimentary structure, becomes part of the fourth pouch contributing to thyroid C-cells.	

Footnote

- **Ultimobranchial body** is the most caudal endodermal invaginations of the pharynx are the fourth pharyngeal pouch and elements of the transitory fifth pharyngeal pouch
- **Pharyngeal arches cut section:** In addition to mesenchyme derived from paraxial and lateral figure mesoderm, the core of each arch receives substantial numbers of **Neural crest cells**, which migrate into the arches to contribute to skeletal components of the face. Each arch consists of a mesenchymal core derived from mesoderm and neural crest cells and each is lined internally by endoderm and externally by ectoderm
- **Parafollicular C cells** are derived from the Neural crest component of Ultimobanchial body, so if neural crest is provided in the options, it is a better answer

Contd...

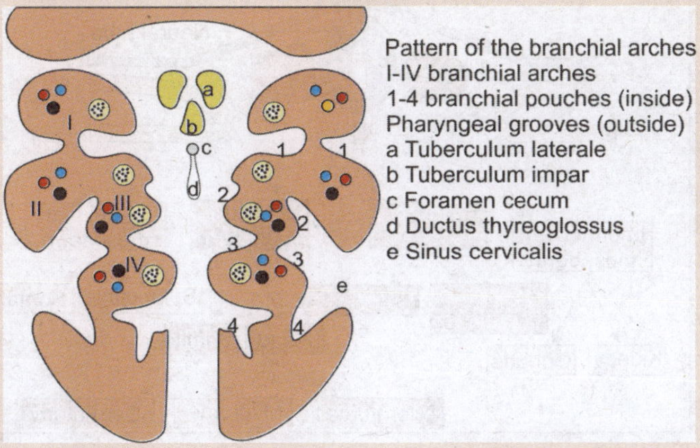

44. Ans. (a) A

Ref: Grays 41st ed page 756, Langman's Embryology 10th ed page 140, 352

The notochord expands between the developing vertebrae as localized aggregates of cells and matrix that form the nucleus pulposus of the intervertebral disc

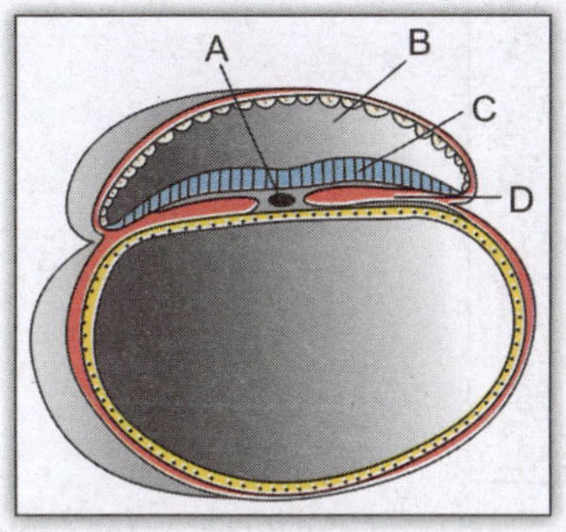

Figure Legends

A = Notochord

B = Amniotic cavity

C = Ectoderm

D = Mesoderm

Nucleus pulposus is central gelatinous portion of an intervertebral disc derived from proliferation of notochord cells.

Mesenchymal cells between cephalic and caudal parts of the original sclerotome segment do not proliferate but fill the space between two precartilaginous vertebral bodies. In this way, they contribute to formation of the intervertebral disc. Although the notochord regresses entirely in the region of the vertebral bodies, it persists and enlarges in the region of the intervertebral disc. Here it contributes to the nucleus pulposus, which is later surrounded by circular fibers of the annulus fibrosus. Combined, these two structures, form the intervertebral disc.

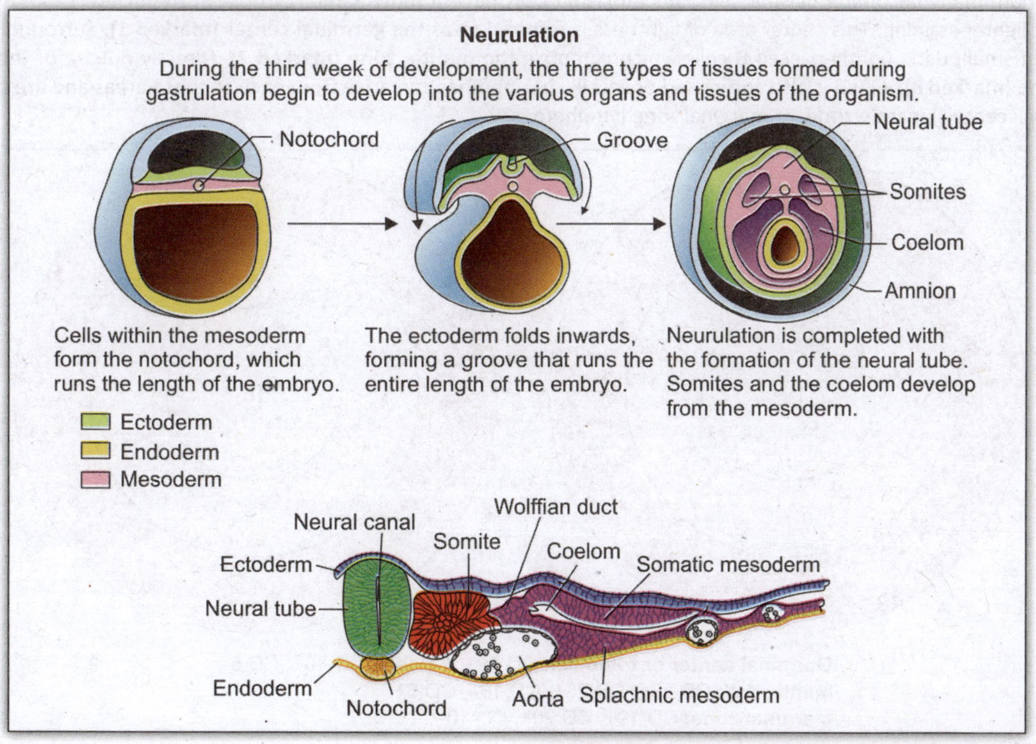

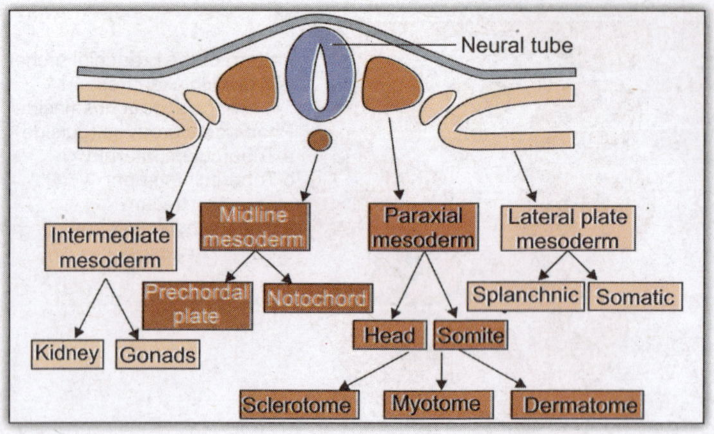

45. Ans. (d) Marginal zone

Ref: Wolfgang 4th ed page 320, 323

The area marked in the picture is marginal zone.

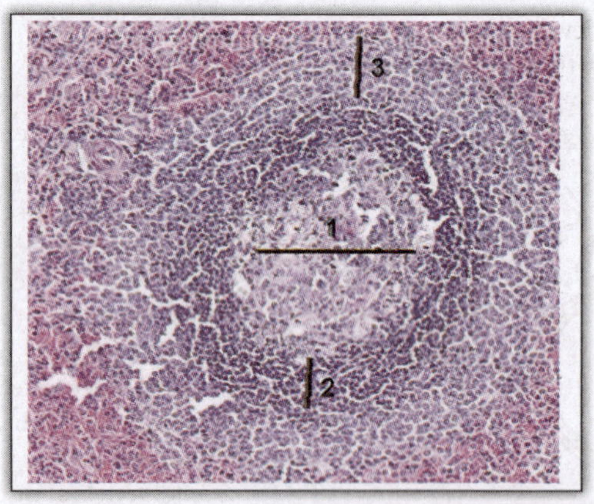

Fig: Lymphatic follicle: It is common to all lymphatic organs. When these nodules become activated, the B-cells in the center of the nodule undergo maturation, many becoming plasma cells. Since plasma cells have a much larger cytoplasm-to-nucleus ratio, the center of the nodule becomes lighter-staining. This center area of lightness is referred to as the **germinal center (marked 1)**. Surrounding the germinal center is a ring of small, dark, tightly-packed B cells which comprise the **mantle zone (marked 2)**. Directly outsize of the mantle zone is the **marginal zone (marked 3)**, which is also comprised of B-cells. Lymphomas can arise from each of these areas and are thus classified as follicular (germinal center), mantle zone, or marginal zone lymphomas.

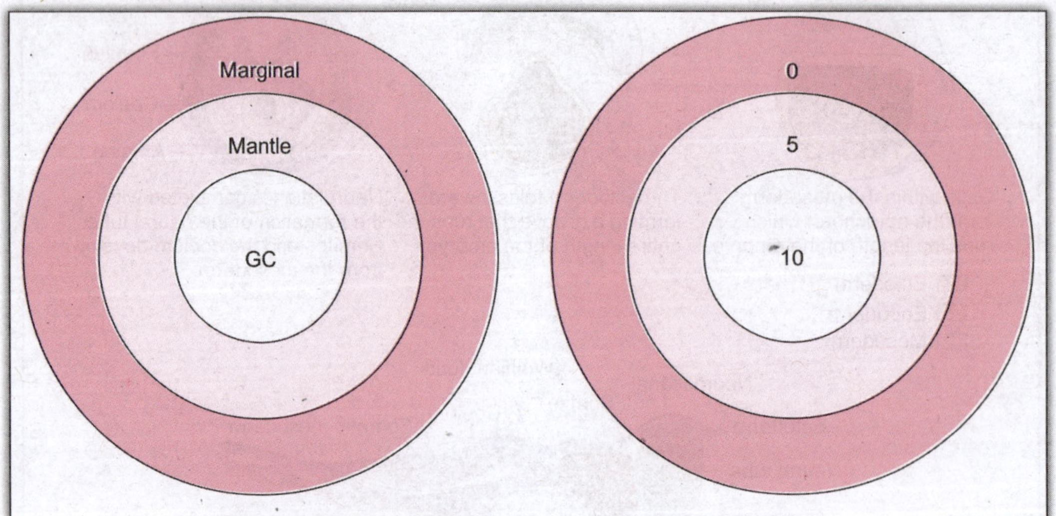

Germinal center or follicular. CD 19+, CD 20+, CD 10+, CD 5–
Mantle cell: CD 19+, CD 20+, CD 10–, CD 5+
Marginal zone: CD 19+, CD 20+, CD 10–, CD 5–

Lymphatic Organs: Distinctive Morphological Features				
Organ	Capsule and connective tissue septa	Parenchyma	Vessels	Other features
Lymph node	Well-developed capsule, clearly visible trabeculae	Lymphoreticular, compact cortex with lymph follicles, lighter medulla with medullary cords	Afferent vessel, marginal sinus, intermediary sinus, medullary sinus, efferent vessel; in the lumina of all sinuses: a bow-net (weir) system of reticular fibers & reticular cells, no blood cells	Surrounded by loosely organized connective tissue and adipose tissue; lymph vessels with valves often exist in the vicinity; no surface epithelium
Spleen	Very well developed capsule, strong trabeculae	Lymph nodes & lymphoreticular sheaths around the central artery = **white pulp.** The **red pulp** is not part of the lymphatic system	Characteristic blood vessels (laminar vessels, central artery, penicillary arteriolae, splenic sinus with gaps, muscle-free pulp and laminar veins); blood cells in the lumen of the splenic sinus	Single layered flat peritoneal epithelium forms a sheath around the capsule
Tonsils	Well-developed capsule, weak trabeculae (palatine tonsils), Not developed capsule, thin or no trabeculae (Pharyngeal and Lingual tonsil)	Lymphoreticular nodes (lymph follicles) surround 10–15 branched, Narrow epithelial invaginations (fossulae tonsillares with tonsillar crypts)	–	–
Thymus	Well-developed capsule, partitioning into lobes by connective tissue septa	Lymphoepithelial; no lymph follicles; denser cortex, more loosely organized medulla with interspersed lymphocytes; epithelial **Hassall bodies** in the medulla	–	Involution after puberty; adipose tissue Gradually replaces the parenchyma; in senescence: adipose tissue with parenchyma islets
Peyer's patches	No capsule or onnective tissue septa	The patches are regions of concentrated B lymphocyte follicles covered in a 'dome' of a specialized follicle associated epithelium (FAE) which consists of follicle associated enterocytes and M (microfold or multifold) cells. M-cells are a specialized epithelial cell that reside above Peyer's patches and take up antigen from the lumen of the intestine		Peyer's patches are lymphoid tissues found in the wall of the small intestine. They are part of the mucosal associated lymphoid tissues (MALT) and more specifically gut associated lymphoid tissue (GALT)

46. Ans. (b) Deep nuclei of cerebellum

Ref: Grays 41st ed page 256, 335, Ganong 24th Ed, pg 249, Guyton 12th ed page 684

NOTE

A question on low power histology of cerebellum was asked in AIIMS Nov 2016.

Marked cells in the figure are Purkinje cells of cerebellum. Purkinje cell is inhibitory to deep cerebellar nuclei.

The developed cerebellar cortex contains three layers: namely, the molecular layer, the Purkinje layer and the granular layer. **Purkinje cell axons pass into the white matter and form inhibitory synaptic connections with neurons of the deep cerebellar nuclei, releasing GABA as the neurotransmitter.** GABA is the main inhibitory transmitter and glutamate is the main excitatory transmitter of Purkinje cells.

Functional Unit of the Cerebellar Cortex—The Purkinje Cell and the Deep Nuclear Cell

The cerebellum has about 30 million nearly identical functional units, one of which is shown in the figure. This functional unit centers on a single, very large **Purkinje cell and on a corresponding deep nuclear cell**. To the top and right in figure, the three major layers of the *cerebellar cortex are shown: the molecular layer, Purkinje cell layer and granule cell layer.*

Beneath these cortical layers, in the center of the cerebellar mass, are the deep cerebellar nuclei that send output signals to other parts of the nervous system.

Neuronal Circuit of the Functional Unit

The output from the functional unit is from a **deep nuclear cell**. This cell is continually under *both excitatory and inhibitory influences*.

- **Deep cerebellar nuclei:** *From lateral to medial, the four deep cerebellar nuclei are the* ***Dentate, Emboliform, Globose and Fastigial*** *(Mnemonic: "Don't Eat Greasy Food").* The globose and the emboliform nuclei are sometimes lumped together as the **interpositus nucleus** in lower species; the emboliform and globose nuclei may sometimes be referred to as the anterior and posterior interposed nuclei, respectively. *The dentate nucleus, which is located most laterally and is by far the largest, is the only nucleus easily visible to the naked eye.*

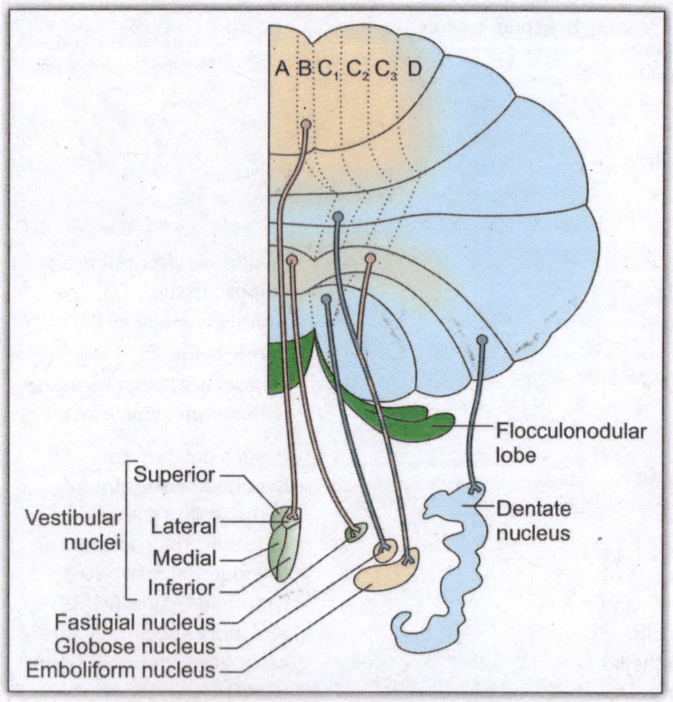

- **The excitatory influences** arise from direct connections with afferent fibers that enter the cerebellum from the brain or the periphery. **Primary afferent inputs**: The afferent inputs to the cerebellum are mainly of two types, one called the climbing fiber type and the other called the mossy fiber type. They send collaterals to the deep nuclei and pass to the cortex. *The two main inputs to the cerebellar cortex are climbing fibers and mossy fibers.*
- **The inhibitory influence** arises entirely from the Purkinje cell in the cortex of the cerebellum.
- **Balance between excitation and inhibition:** Direct stimulation of the deep nuclear cells by both the climbing and the mossy fibers excites them. By contrast, signals arriving from the Purkinje cells inhibit them. Normally, the balance between these two effects is slightly in favor of excitation so that under quiet conditions, output from the deep nuclear cell remains relatively constant at a moderate level of continuous stimulation.

Primary Afferent Inputs of Cerebellum		
	Climbing fibers	**Mossy fibers**
Type	Excitatory (strong)	Excitatory (week)
Type of input	Indirect	Direct
Signal from (source of input)	Single source (inferior olivary nuclei of medulla). Proprioceptive input to the inferior olivary nuclei comes from all over the body	Direct proprioceptive input from all parts of the body plus input from the cerebral cortex via the pontine nuclei to the cerebellar cortex
Signal to	Single Purkinje cells (5–10 climbing fibers per Purkinje cells)	Many Purkinje cells via parallel fibers of the granule cells. (500–1000 granule cells, 80,000-200,000 parallel fibers per Purkinje cell)
Synapse with Purkinje cells	300 synapse with soma and dendrite of Purkinje cell	Mossy fibers synapse to hundred to thousands of granule cell
Resultant Purkinje cell action potential	Complex spike; strong primary spike followed by trail of week secondary spike	Simple spike

- **Other inhibitory cells in the cerebellum:** In addition to the deep nuclear cells, granule cells and Purkinje cells, two other types of neurons are located in the cerebellum: **basket cells and stellate cells and Golgi cells.**
  - **Basket cells** are located in the **molecular layer**. They receive input from the parallel fibers and each projects to many Purkinje cells. Their axons form a basket around the cell body and axon hillock of each Purkinje cell they innervate. They end their axons at right angles across the parallel fibers and cause lateral inhibition of adjacent Purkinje cells
  - **Stellate cells** are similar to the basket cells but more **superficial in location**. They end their axons at right angles across the parallel fibers and cause lateral inhibition of adjacent Purkinje cells
  - **Golgi cells** are located in the **granular layer**. Their dendrites, which project into the molecular layer, receive input from the parallel fibers. Their cell bodies receive input via collaterals from the incoming mossy fibers and the Purkinje cells. Their axons project to the dendrites of the granule cells.

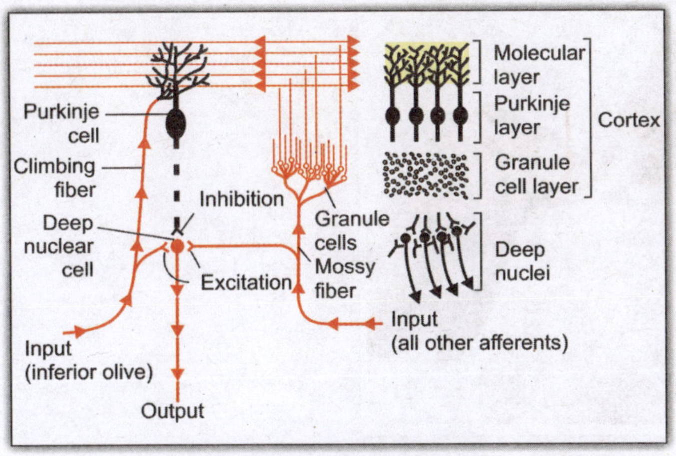

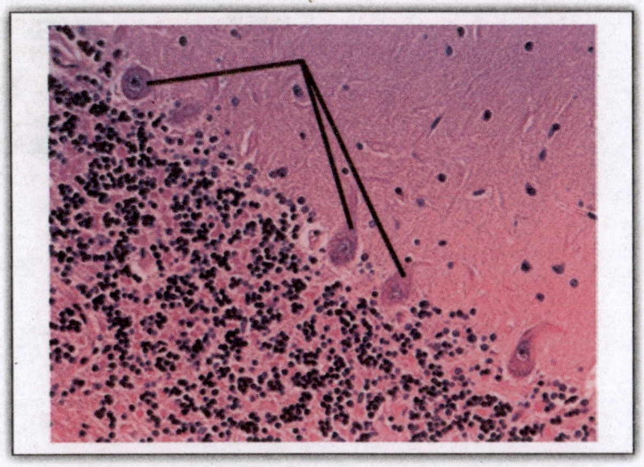

Fig: Histology of cerebellum H&E staining 100 X view: Arrow marked structures are Purkinje cells between dense Granular cell layer (left inferior) and Molecular cell layer (Right anterior)

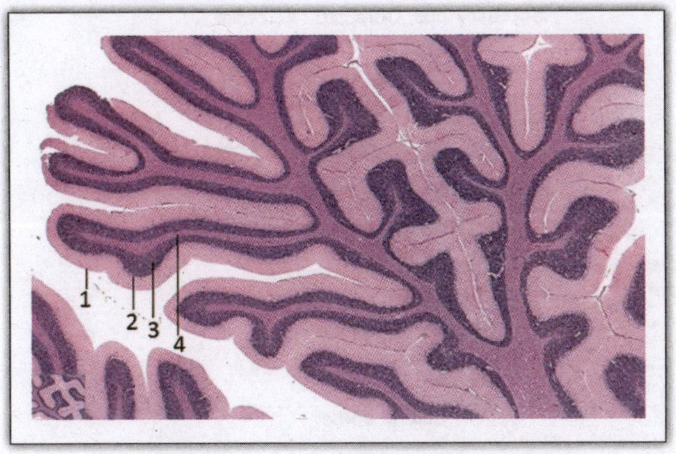

Fig: Histology of cerebellum H&E staining 4X view

1. Molecular layer
2. Purkinje cell layer
3. Granular cell layer
4. White matter

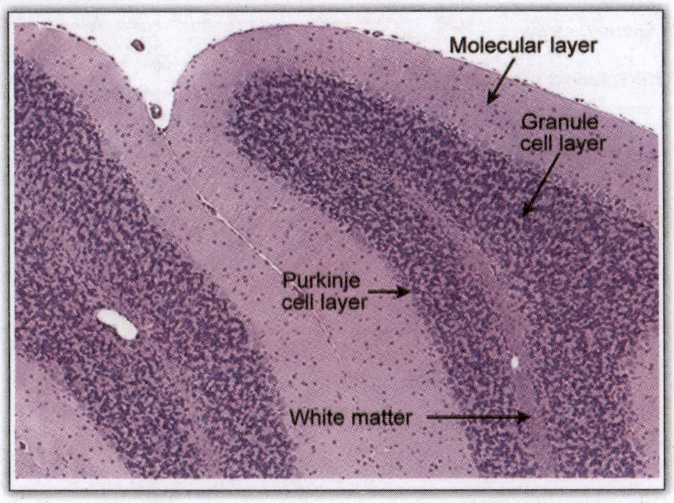

Fig: Histology of cerebellum H&E staining 10 X view

47. Ans. (d) D

Ref: Gray's 41st ed page 787, 803, McMinn's Clinical Atlas of Human Anatomy 6th ed ch 5

Gray's anatomy states ***"When the arm is by the side, the coracoid process points almost straight forwards. Its tip can be felt through the skin and is covered by the anterior fibers of deltoid, about 2.5 cm below the clavicle at the junction of the lateral fifth with the rest of the bone, at the lateral border of the infraclavicular fossa.***

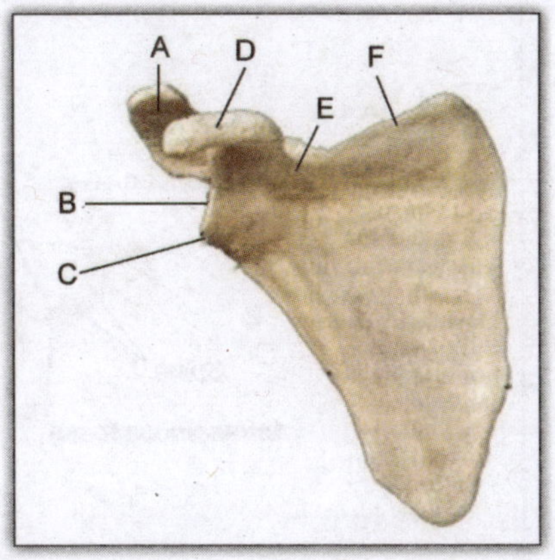

Figure Legends

Anterior Surface/View of scapula
A = Acromion process
B = Glenoid cavity
C = Glenoid tubercle
D = Coracoid process
E = Scapular notch
F = Superior border
Infraclavicular fossa is an indentation (fossa) just below the clavicle. The spine of scapula divides the dorsal surface into supraspinous and infraspinous fossae.

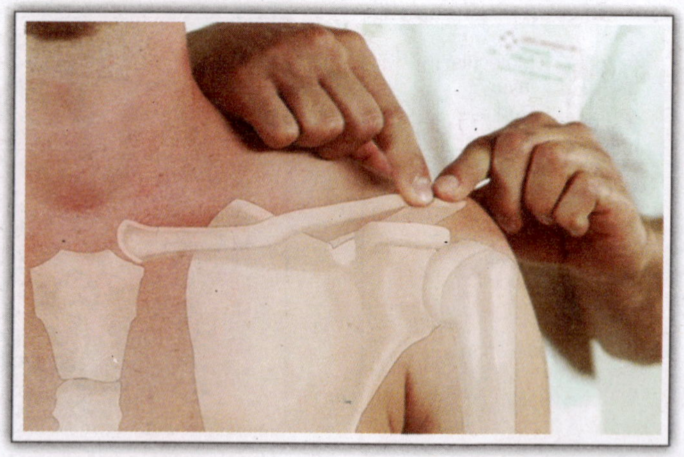

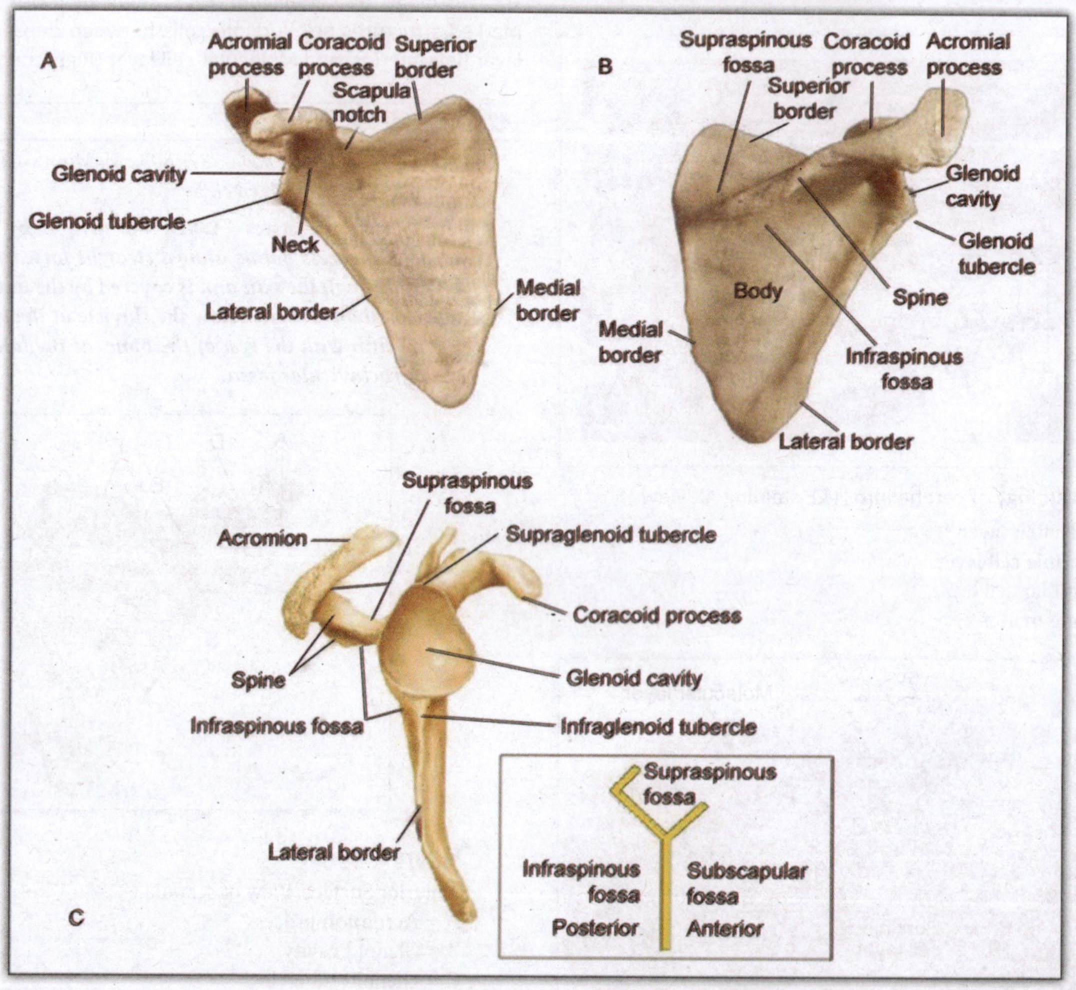

Scapula Bone

The scapula is a large, flat, triangular bone which lies on the posterolateral aspect of the chest wall, covering parts of the 2nd to 7th ribs. It has 2 surfaces; costal and dorsal, 3 borders; superior, lateral and medial and 3 angles; inferior, superior and lateral angles and 3 processes, the spine, its continuation the acromion and the coracoid process

(A) Costal surface of scapula (labeled): Costal surface can easily be distinguished from the dorsal surface, which is interrupted by the shelf-like projection of the spine

(B) Dorsal surface of scapula (labeled)

(C) Lateral border of scapula showing Glenoid cavity (labeled)

Palpable Parts of Scapula

- The tip of the coracoid process is palpable in the infraclavicular fossa around 2.5 cm below the clavicle. Deltopectoral groove is the location through which cephalic vein passes and coracoid process is easily palpable
- Crest of spine and Acromion are palpable
- Inferior angle of scapula is a palpable landmark
- Medial border of scapula is palpable below the spine of scapula

48. Ans. (a) A

Ref: Gray's 41st ed page 1222

Levator ani is a broad muscular sheet of variable thickness attached to the internal surface of the pelvis. It forms a large portion of the pelvic floor. The muscle is subdivided into named portions according to their attachments and the pelvic viscera to which they are related (pubococcygeus, iliococcygeus and puborectalis). These parts are often referred to as separate muscles but the boundaries between each part cannot be easily distinguished and, moreover, they perform many similar physiological functions.

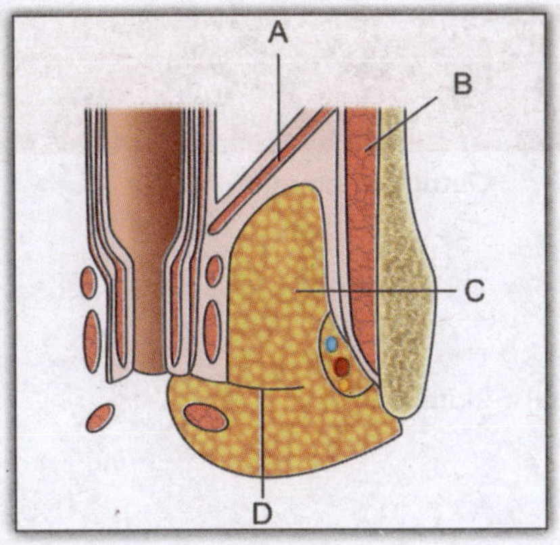

Figure Legends

A = Pelvic diaphragm (Levator ani)
B = Obturator internus
C = Ischiorectal space filled with fat
D = Perianal fascia

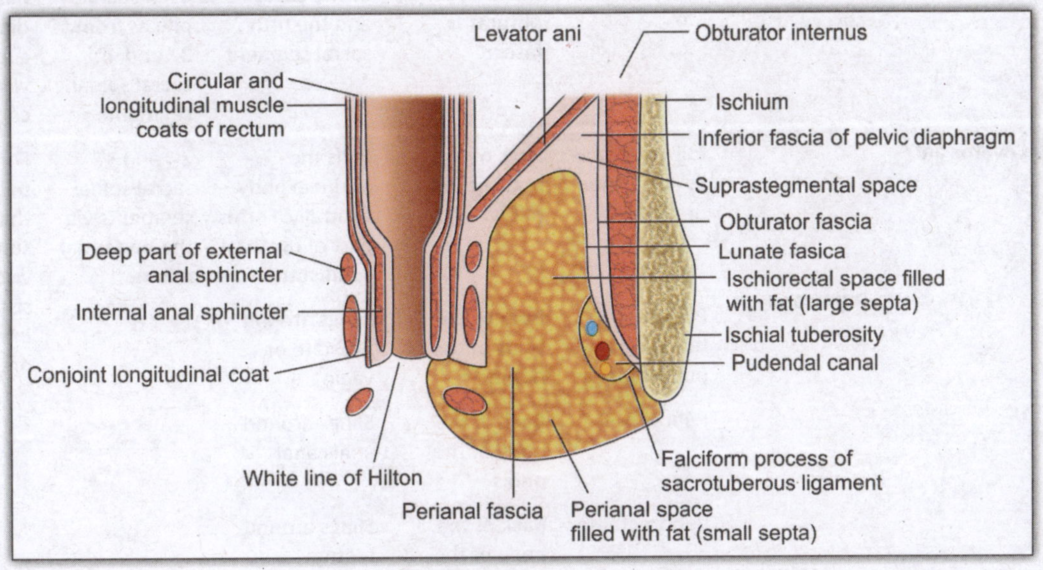

Fig: Coronal section of ischiorectal fossa

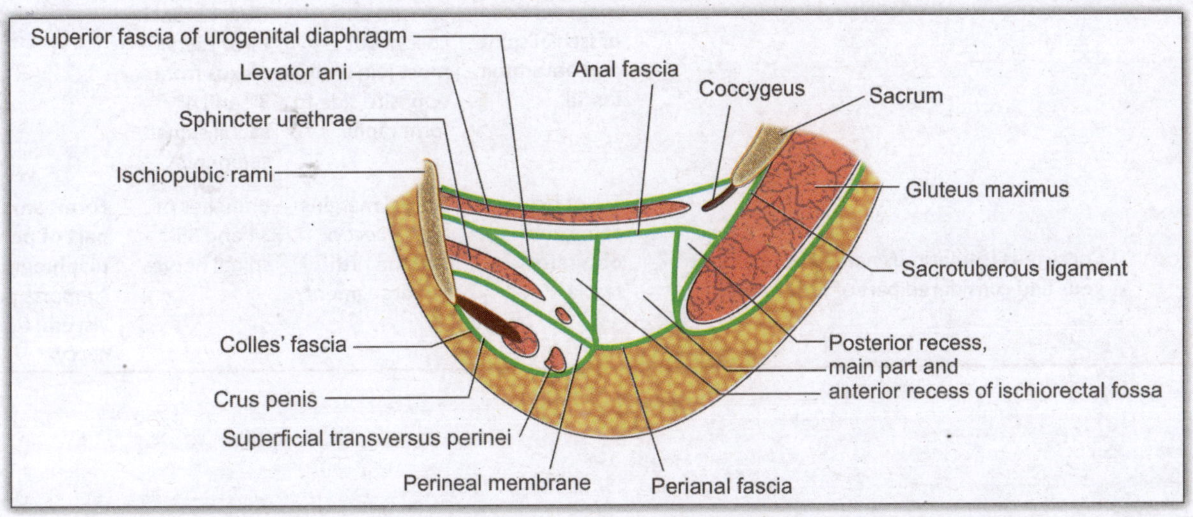

Fig: Parasagittal section of ischiorectal fossa

Muscles of Pelvic Walls and Floor								
Muscle				Proximal attachment	Distal attachment	Innervation	Main action
Lateral wall	Obturator internus			Pelvic surfaces of ilium and ischium, obturator membrane	Greater trochanter of femur	Nerve to obturator internus (L5, S1, S2)	Rotates thigh laterally; assists in holding head of femur in acetabulum
Posterolateral wall	Piriformis			Pelvic surface of S2–S4 segments, superior margin of greater sciatic notch, sacrotuberous ligament	Greater trochanter of femur	Anterior rami of S1 and S2	Rotates thigh laterally; abducts thigh; assists in holding head of femur in acetabulum
		Ischiococcygeus (sometime separately named as coccygeus)		Tip of ischial spine and obturator fascia	Lateral margins of the coccyx and the fifth sacral segment	Direct branches of sacral plexus from 3rd and 4th sacral spinal segments	Forms **small part of pelvic diaphragm** that supports pelvic viscera; flexes coccyx
Floor or outlet (**pelvic diaphragm**)	**Levator ani**	**Pubococcygeus**	Puboperinealis (AKA Pubo urethralis)	Back of the body of the pubis	Pulls the perineal body ventrally. Forms part of **urethral sphincter**	2nd and 3rd sacral spinal segments via the **pudendal nerve**	Forms most of **pelvic diaphragm** that helps support pelvic viscera and resists increases in intra-abdominal pressure
			Puboprostaticus or pubovaginalis	Back of the body of the pubis	Slings around prostate or vagina		
			Puboanalis	Back of the body of the pubis	Slings around anal canal		
			Puborectalis	Back of the body of the pubis	Slings around rectum		
		Iliococcygeus		Inner surface of ischial spine and obturator fascia	Sacrum and coccyx but most join with opposite side to form raphe	Direct branches of sacral plexus from 3rd and 4th sacral spinal segments	
	Coccygeus (sometimes named as ischiococcygeus and considered part of levator ani)			Tip of ischial spine and obturator fascia	Lateral margins of the coccyx and the fifth sacral segment	Branches of S4 and S5 spinal nerves	Forms **small part of pelvic diaphragm** that supports pelvic viscera; flexes coccyx

Contd...

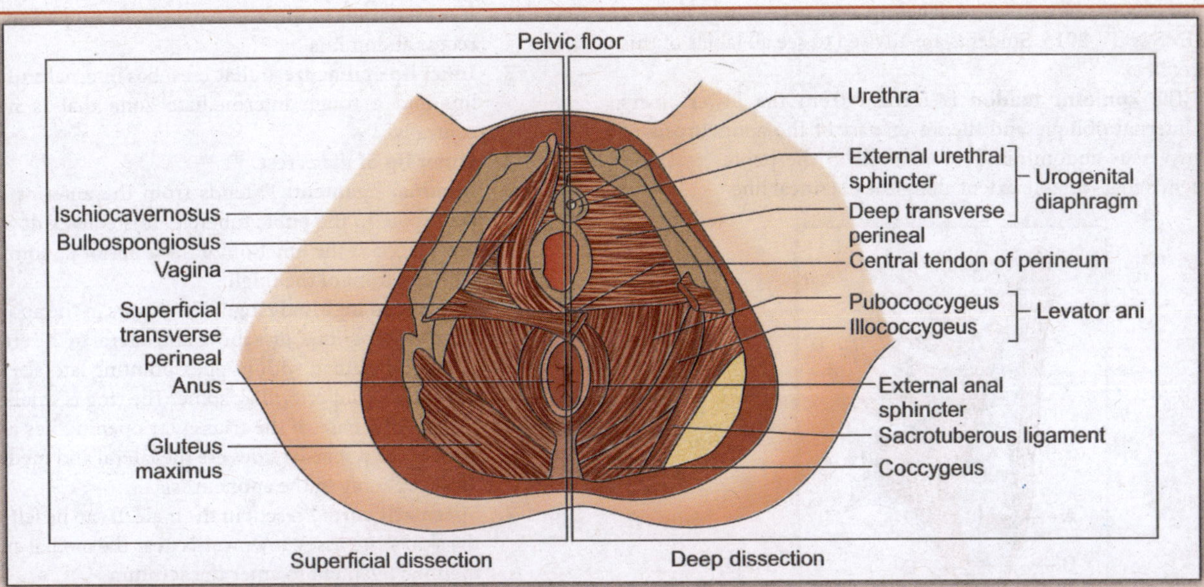

Note:

- Whereas the anal sphincters are responsible for the closure of the anal canal to retain gas and liquid stool, the **puborectalis muscle** and the anorectal angle are designed to maintain gross **fecal continence"**.
- **Anorectal ring:** This is a muscular ring present at the anorectal junction. It is formed by the fusion of the puborectalis, deep external sphincter and the internal sphincter. It is easily felt by a finger in the anal canal. Surgical division of this ring results in rectal incontinence. The ring is less marked anteriorly where the fibers of the puborectalis are absent. Rectal continence depends solely on the anorectal ring. Damage to the ring results in rectal incontinence. The surgeon has to carefully protect the anorectal ring in operating on the region.

Pelvic Diaphragm

- Forms the **pelvic floor** and **supports all of the pelvic viscera.**
- **Levator ani and coccygeus** form the pelvic diaphragm and delineate the lower limit of the true pelvis.
- The fasciae investing the muscles are continuous with visceral pelvic fascia above, perineal fascia below and obturator fascia laterally.
- Lies posterior and deep to the urogenital diaphragm and medial and deep to the ischiorectal fossa.
- On contraction, **raises the entire pelvic floor.**
- Flexes the anorectal canal during defecation and helps the voluntary control of micturition.
- Helps direct the fetal head toward the birth canal at **parturition.**

Urogenital Diaphragm

- The term **"perineal membrane"** replaces the old term **"urogenital diaphragm"**, reflecting the fact that this layer is not a single muscle layer with a double layer of fascia ("diaphragm"), but rather a set of connective tissues that surround the urethra *formed by deep transverse perineal muscle, sphincter urethra muscle and transverse perineal ligament*.
- Traditionally, a trilaminar UG diaphragm was described as making up the deep perineal pouch. The long-held concept of a flat, essentially two-dimensional UG diaphragm is erroneous (Wendell-Smith, 1995). According to this concept, the *UG diaphragm consisted of the* ***perineal membrane (inferior fascia of UG diaphragm) inferiorly and a superior fascia of the UG diaphragm superiorly,*** *between which was a flat muscular sheet composed of a disc-like sphincter urethra and the transversely oriented deep transverse perineal muscle.*

Structures Pearcing Urogenital Diaphragm

In males	In females
• Urethra, 2–3 cm behind the inferior border of the symphysis pubis • Vessels and nerves to the bulb of the penis • Ducts of the bulbourethral glands, posterolateral to the urethral orifice • Deep dorsal vessels and dorsal nerves of the penis, behind the pubic arch in the midline • Posterior scrotal vessels and nerves, anterior to the transverse perinei	• Urethra, 2–3 cm behind the inferior border of the symphysis pubis • Vagina, centrally • Ducts of Bartholin's glands, posterolateral to the urethral orifice • Deep dorsal vessels and dorsal nerves of the clitoris, behind the pubic arch in the midline • Posterior labial vessels and nerves, anterior to the transverse perinei

49. Ans. (b) B

Ref: Grays 41st ed page 1071, 1079, 1343

Same figure, but different labeling was asked in Anatomy AIIMS NOV 2016. Students are advised to see all labels of this carefully.

The **conjoint tendon** is formed from the lower fibers of internal oblique and the lower part of the aponeurosis of transversus abdominis. It is attached to the pubic crest and extends to a variable extent along the pectineal line

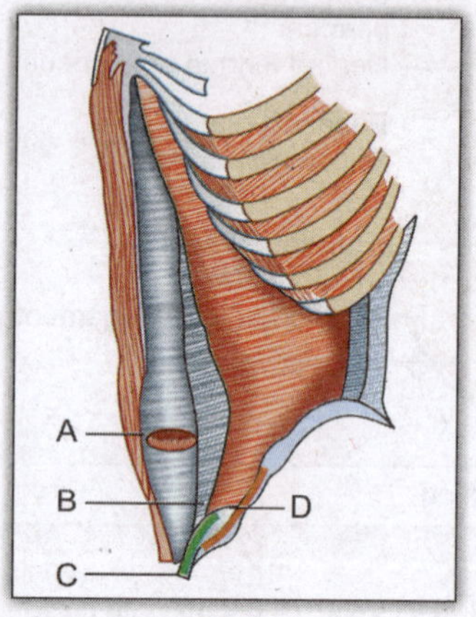

Figure Legend

A = Linea alba
B = Conjoint tendon
C = Spermatic cord
D = Deep inguinal ring

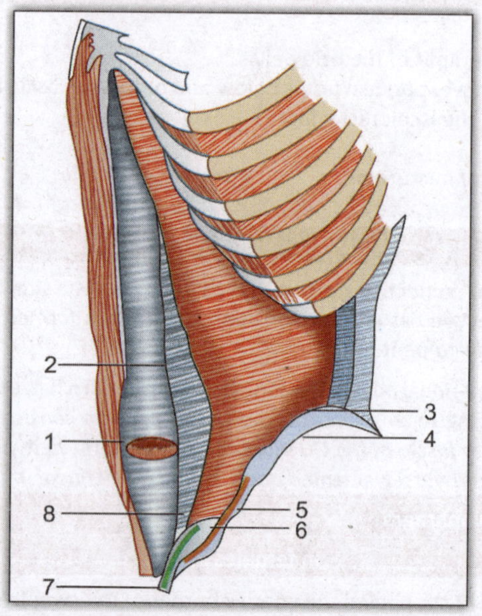

Figure Legends

1. **Linea alba:** It is a tendinous raphe extending from xiphoid process to pubic symphysis and pubic crest. It lies between the two recti and is formed by the interlacing and decussating aponeurotic fibers of external oblique, internal oblique and transversus abdominis.
2. **Linea semilunaris:** A few centimeters lateral to the median furrow, the abdominal wall shows a curved vertical groove. Its upper end reaches the costal margin at the tip of I the ninth costal cartilage. Interiorly it reaches the pubic tubercle. This line is called the linea semilunaris. It corresponds to the lateral margin of a muscle called the rectus abdominis.
3. **Inner lip of iliac crest:** Iliac crest has internal and external lips and a rough intermediate zone that is narrowest centrally.
4. **Outer lip of iliac crest.**
5. **Inguinal ligament:** Extends from the anterior superior iliac spine to the pubic tubercle. It is convex downwards. It is placed at the junction of the anterior abdominal wall with the front of the thigh.
6. **Superficial inguinal ring:** It is a hiatus in the aponeurosis of external oblique, just above and lateral to the crest of the pubis. Triangular, with its apex pointing laterally towards the anterior superior iliac spine. The ring is smaller in the female. The base of the triangular opening lies along the crest of the pubis. Its sides are the lateral and medial crura of the opening in the aponeurosis.
7. **Spermatic cord:** Present in the male. It can be felt through the skin as it passes downwards near the medial end of the inguinal ligament to enter the scrotum.
8. **Conjoint tendon:** It is a structure formed from the lower part of the common aponeurosis of the internal abdominal oblique and the transverse abdominal as it inserts into the crest of the pubis and pectineal line immediately behind the superficial inguinal ring. It forms the medial part of the posterior wall of the inguinal canal.

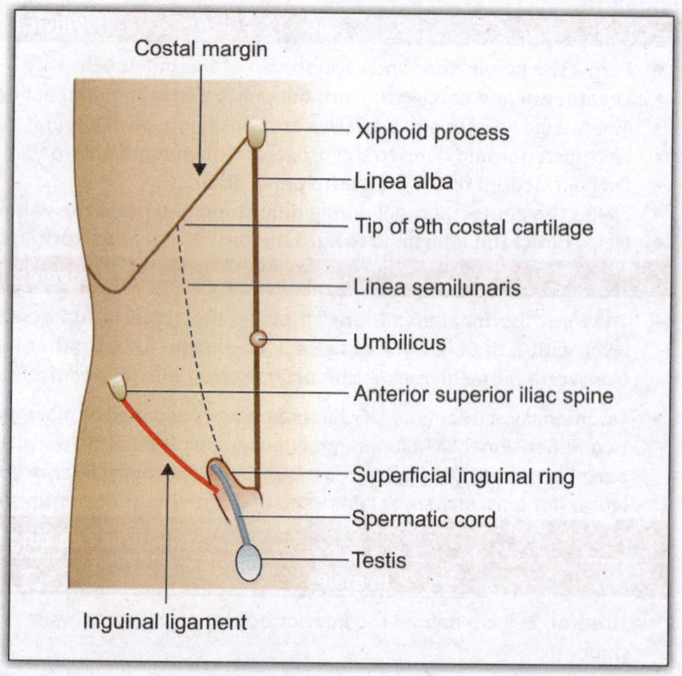

50. Ans. (a) Protraction

Ref: Grays 41st ed page 547, Grant's Atlas of Anatomy 12th Ed page 672 Table 7.9

The muscle marked in the picture is lateral pterygoid which is the major protruder of the mandible.

Similar Question on Lateral Pterygoid was asked in Anatomy AIIMS NOVEMBER 2015 with plain dissection diagram of face and now the examiner have given a cross section of head pointing on lateral pterygoid.

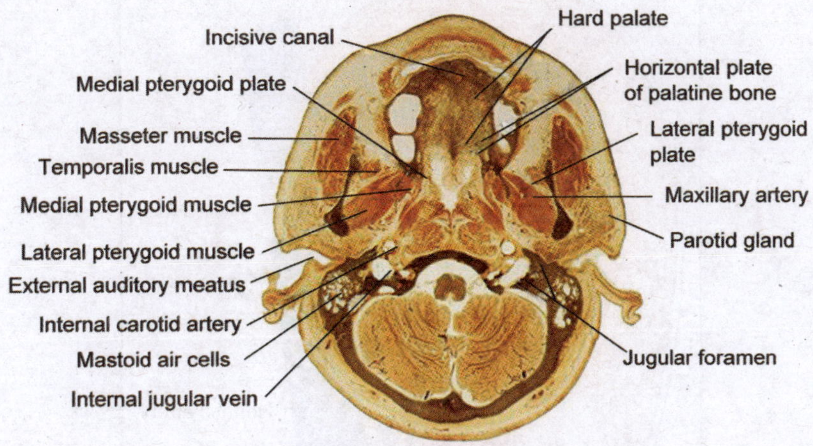

Fig: Muscles of mastication in transverse/cross section of head (Labeled)

Muscles of Mastication (Acting on Temporomandibular Joint)				
Muscle	**Origin**	**Insertion**	**Innervation**	**Main action**
Temporalis (Fan shaped; anterior, intermediate and posterior fibers)	Floor of temporal fossa and deep surface of temporal fascia	Tip and medial surface of coronoid process and anterior border of ramus of mandible	Deep temporal branches of ***mandibular nerve*** (CN V_3)	Elevates mandible (all fibers), Retrudes mandible (posterior fibers)
Masseter (superficial, middle and deep layers) (superficial layer is the largest)	Inferior border and medial surface of zygomatic arch	Lateral surface of ramus of mandible and coronoid process	Anterior trunk of ***mandibular nerve*** (CN V_3) through masseteric nerve	Elevates mandible, minor actions are: protrudes mandible (superficial fibers), retrudes mandible (deep fibers)
Lateral pterygoid (Upper head and lower head)	**Superior head:** Infratemporal surface and infratemporal crest of greater wing of sphenoid bone **Inferior head:** *Lateral surface of lateral pterygoid figure*	Neck of mandible, articular disc and capsule of temporomandibular joint	***Mandibular nerve*** (CN V_3) through lateral pterygoid nerve which enters its deep surface	*Acting bilaterally,* protrude mandible and depress chin; *Acting unilaterally* alternately, they produce side-to-side movements of mandible (pulled medially towards the opposite side)
Medial pterygoid (small superficial head and major deep head)	**Deep head:** Medial surface of lateral pterygoid figure and pyramidal process of palatine bone **Superficial head:** Tuberosity of maxilla	Medial surface of ramus of mandible, inferior to mandibular foramen	***Mandibular nerve*** (CN V_3) through medial pterygoid nerve	Acts synergistically with masseter to elevate mandible, contributes to protrude mandible; *acting unilaterally* produce small grinding movements
# Unlike the other muscles of mastication, lateral pterygoid is not pennate, nor does it have a significant number of Golgi tendon organs associated with its attachments				

51. Ans. (b) b

Ref: Gray's 41st ed page 1107

Superior boundary of epiploic foramen is formed by caudate lobe of liver.

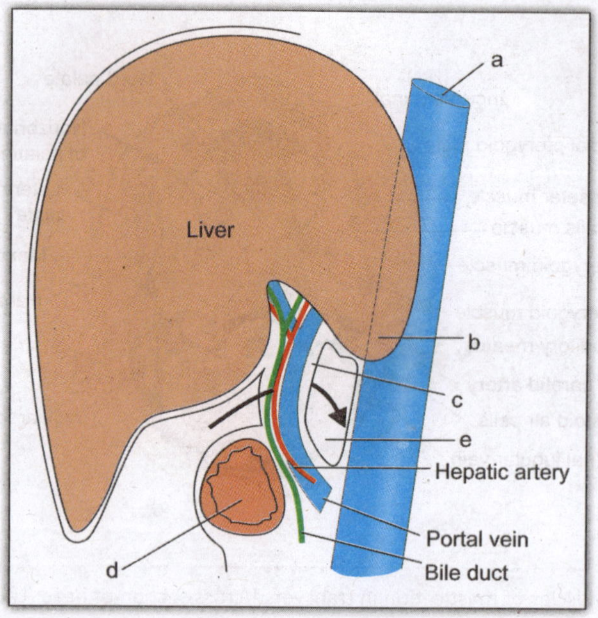

Fig: Sagittal section of abdomen showing epiploic foramen (Arrow)

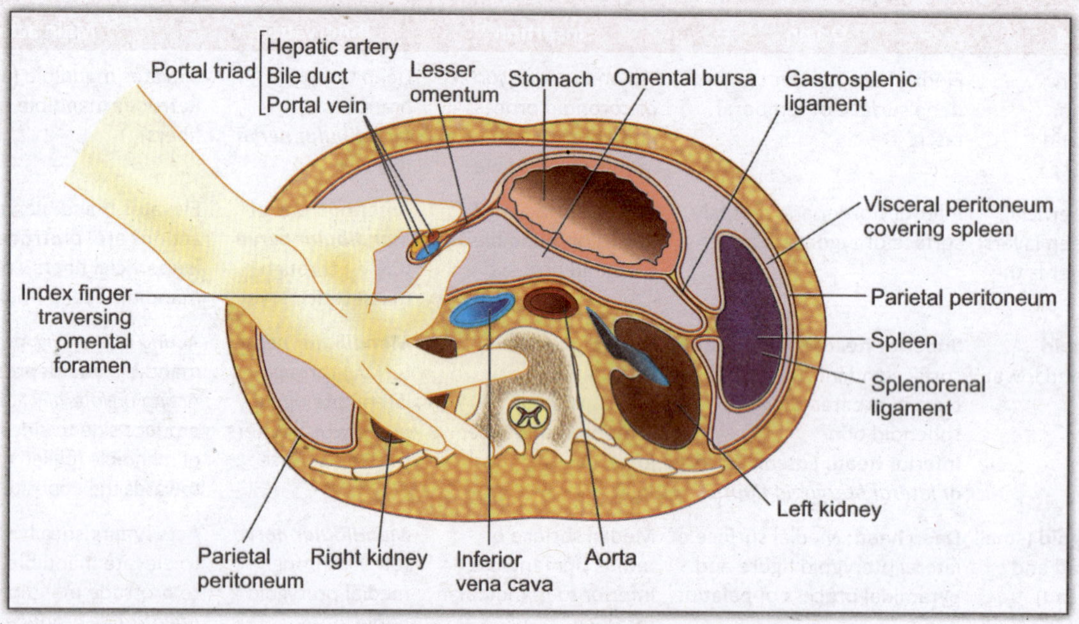

Fig: Transverse section of abdomen showing epiploic foramen (Index finger inserted in epiploic formamen) a = Inferior vena cava, b = Caudate lobe of liver, c = Lesser sac, d = First part of duodenum, e = Epiploic foramen

In human anatomy, the **omental foramen (Epiploic foramen, foramen of Winslow**, or uncommonly aditus) is the passage of communication, or foramen, between the greater sac (general cavity of the abdomen) and the lesser sac.

Borders of Epiploic Foramen

It has the following borders:

1. **Anterior:** The free border of the lesser omentum, known as the hepatoduodenal ligament. This has two layers and within these layers are common bile duct (on the right), portal vein (posteriorly) and hepatic artery (on the left).
2. **Posterior:** IVC and right crus of diaphragm, covered with parietal peritoneum. (They are retroperitoneal). The anterior and posterior walls of the foramen are normally apposed.
3. **Superior:** The peritoneum covering the caudate lobe of the liver.
4. **Inferior:** The peritoneum covering the commencement of the duodenum (superior or first part of the duodenum).
5. **Left lateral:** Gastrosplenic ligament and splenorenal ligament.

52. Ans. (a) Amygdala

Ref: High Yield Neuroanatomy 4th ed page 138

The structure shown by the arrow in the given figures is anterior commissure.

NOTE

In transverse section, Fornix are seen as the rounded cut structures of fornix columns

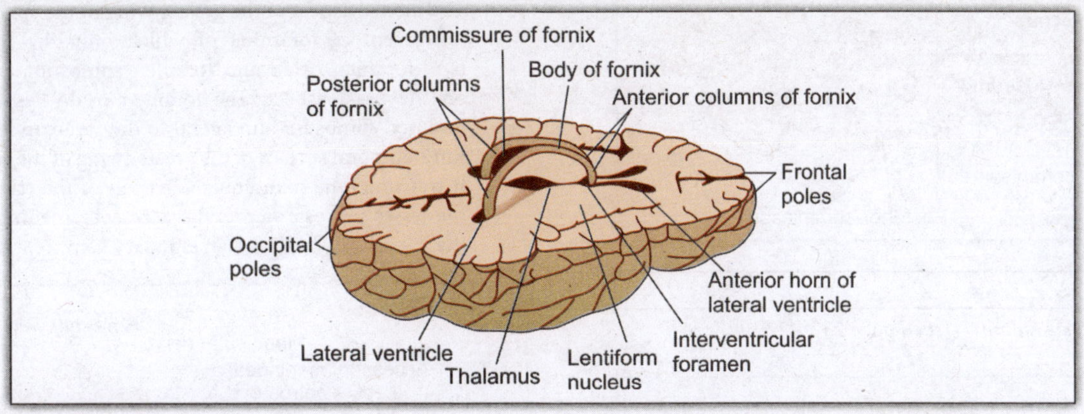

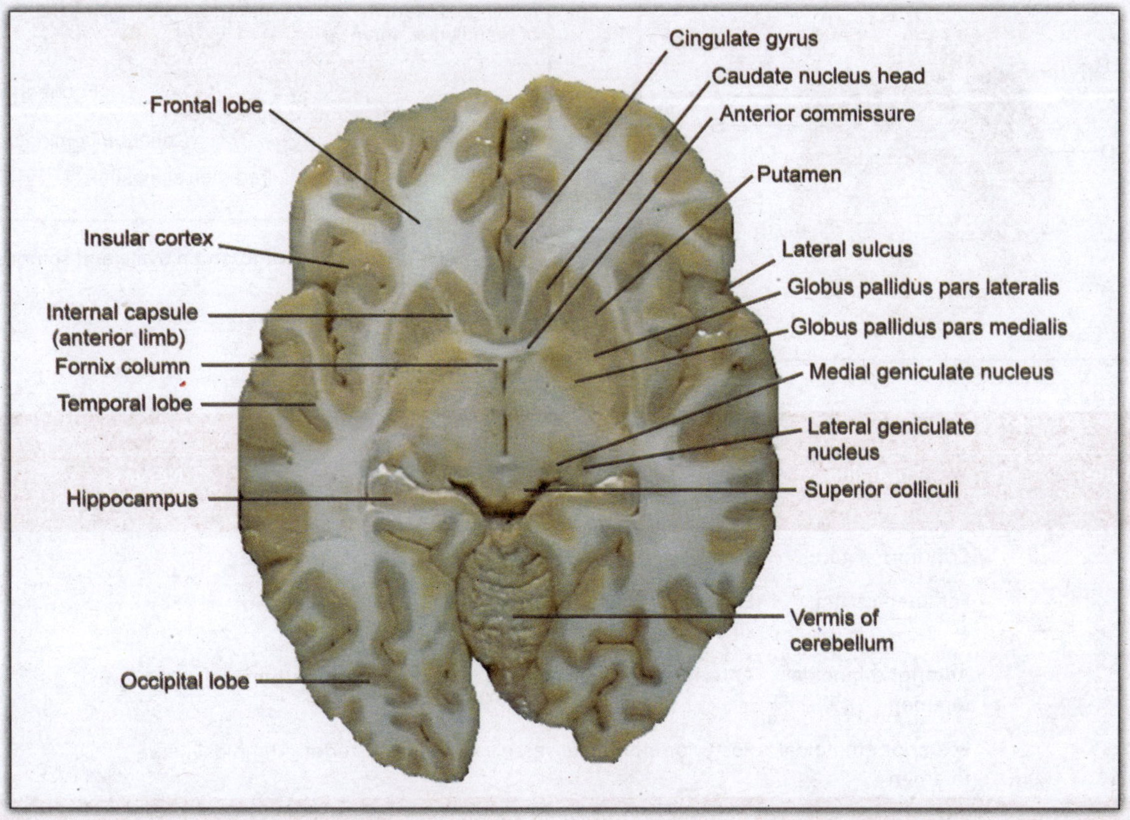

Fig: Transverse section of brain at the level of cerebellum (Labeled)

The anterior commissure arose phylogenetically as part of the rhinencephalon; it connects the olfactory bulbs (of temporal lobes), amygdala and basal forebrain region of the two sides. It lies in the lamina terminalis forming part of anterior part of third ventricle, above the optic chiasm, behind and below the rostrum of the corpus callosum. **(DeJong's The Neurologic Examination by William W. Campbell 7th ed page 58)**

Fibers of the olfactory tracts cross in the ventral or lower part of the lamina terminalis and, together with fibers from the piriform and prepiriform areas and the amygdaloid bodies, form the rostral part of the anterior commissure **(Gray's 41st ed page 262)**

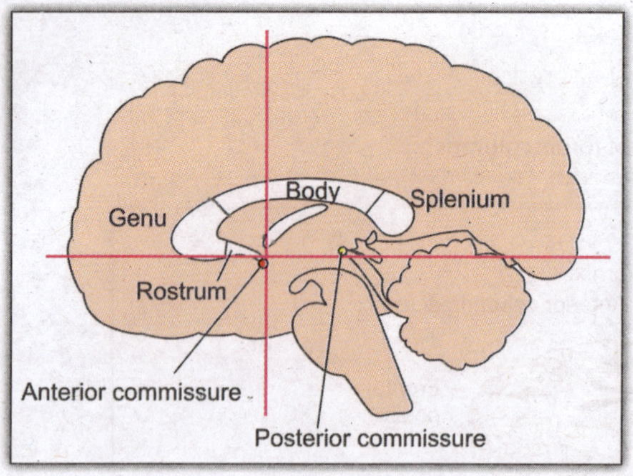

Figure Legends

A = Foramen ovale
B = Foramen spinosum
C = Jugular Foramen
D = Internal acoustic meatus

The medial aspect of the greater wing of the sphenoid presents a crescent of foramina of which only the most posterior two, foramen ovale and foramen spinosum, can be viewed on the basal aspect. The foramen ovale lies medial to the foramen spinosum and lateral to the foramen lacerum on the infratemporal surface of the greater wing of the sphenoid bone. It transmits the mandibular division of the trigeminal nerve, the lesser petrosal nerve, the accessory meningeal branch of the maxillary artery and an emissary vein.

53. Ans. (a) A

Ref: Gray's Anatomy 41st ed page 232, 422

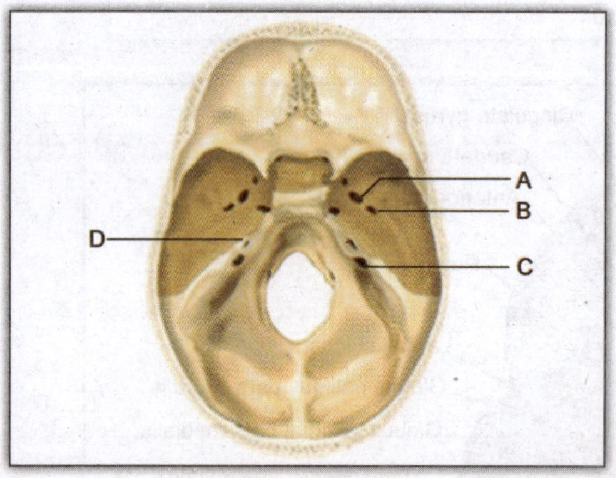

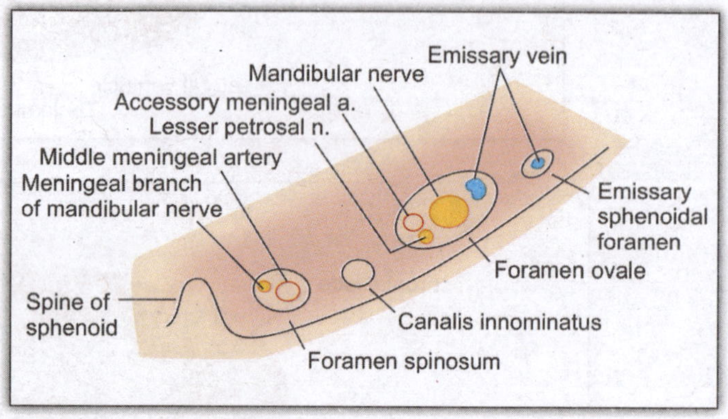

Fig: Line diagram of foramen ovale and spinosum

Foramina of The Skull			
Bone	**Foramina**	**Vessels**	**Nerves**
Foramina in the Anterior Cranial Fossa			
Ethmoid	Cribriform figure		Olfactory nerve
Frontal	Foramen cecum	Emissary veins to superior sagittal sinus	-
Ethmoid	Anterior ethmoidal foramen	Anterior ethmoidal vessels	Anterior ethmoidal nerve
Ethmoid	Posterior ethmoidal foramen	Posterior ethmoidal vessels	Posterior ethmoidal nerve
Foramina in the Middle Cranial Fossa			
Sphenoid	Optic canal	Ophthalmic artery Central retinal artery and vein	Optic nerve (II)
Sphenoid	Superior orbital fissure	Superior ophthalmic vein	Oculomotor nerve (III), trochlear nerve (IV), lacrimal, frontal and nasociliary branches of ophthalmic nerve (V_1), abducent nerve (VI)
Sphenoid and maxilla	Inferior orbital fissure	Inferior ophthalmic veins, infraorbital vessels	Zygomatic nerve, infraorbital branch of maxillary nerve (V_2), orbital branches of pterygopalatine ganglion
Sphenoid	Foramen rotundum	—	Maxillary division of trigeminal nerve (CN V_2)

Contd...

Sphenoid	Foramen ovale **(Mnemonic: OVALE)**	Accessory meningeal artery, Emissary veins	Otic ganglion, mandibular division of trigeminal nerve (V_3) Lesser petrosal nerve (Occasionally)
Sphenoid	Foramen spinosum	Middle meningeal artery	Meningeal branch of the mandibular nerve (V_3)
Sphenoid	Foramen lacerum	Internal carotid artery, artery of pterygoid canal	Nerve of pterygoid canal, greater and deep petrosal nerve
	Carotid canal	Internal carotid artery	Sympathetic carotid plexus
	Hiatus of facial canal		Greater petrosal nerve
Foramina in the Posterior Cranial Fossa			
Temporal	**Internal acoustic meatus/canal:** [Vertical crest (AKA- **Bill's bar**) divides the superior compartment of IAC into anterior and posterior compartment. The transverse crest (AKA- **crista falciformis**) divides upper 2 quadrants from lower 2 quadrants	Labyrinthine artery, occasionally by branches of the anterior inferior cerebellar artery (AICA) or a loop of the AICA itself	Five nerves pass through the internal auditory canal (IAC): • **Anterosuperior quadrant:** Facial (motor root), nervus intermedius (sensory component of facial nerve) • **Anteroinferior quadrant:** Cochlear nerve • **Posterosuperior quadrant:** Superior vestibular nerve • **Posteroinferior quadrant:** Inferior vestibular nerve **(Mnemonic:** 7up- 7th cranial nerve is Up/superior, Coke - Cochlear nerve is down/inferior)
			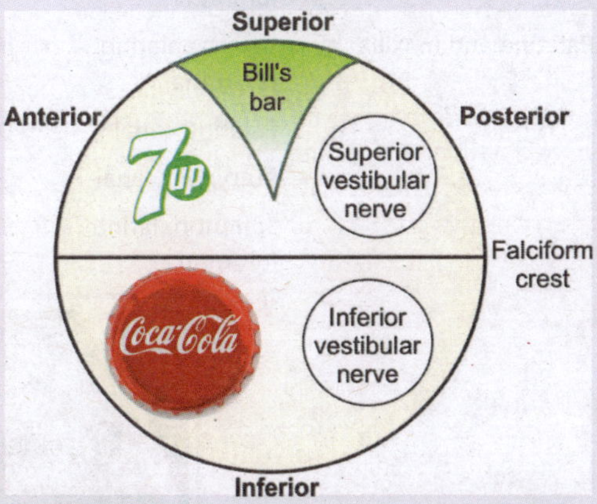
Temporal	Jugular Foramen **(Mnemonic:** *Juggles with three cranial nerves; 9, 10, 11*)	Anterior part: Inferior petrosal sinus **Middle part:** Meningeal branch of ascending pharyngeal artery **Posterior part:** Internal jugular vein, inferior petrosal sinus, sigmoid sinus	**Middle part:** Glossopharyngeal nerve (IX), Vagus nerve (X), Spinal accessory nerve (XI) 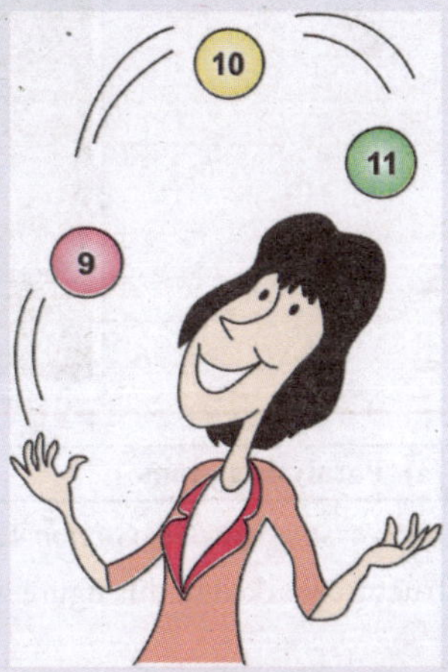

Occipital	Hypoglossal canal	Meningeal artery	Hypoglossal nerve (XII)
Occipital	Foramen magnum	Anterior and posterior spinal arteries, vertebral arteries, venous plexus of vertebral canal	Medulla oblongata, ascending spinal fibers of accessory nerve (XI)
	Condyloid foramen	Condyloid emissary vein	
	Mastoid foramen	Branch of occipital artery to dura mater, mastoid emissary vein	
Foramina in the Front of the Skull			
Frontal	Supraorbital foramen	Supraorbital vessels	Supraorbital nerve
Maxilla	Infraorbital foramen	Infraorbital vessels	Infraorbital nerve
	Mental foramen	Mental vessels	Mental nerve
	Zygomaticofacial foramen		Zygomaticofacial nerve
Foramina in the Base of the Skull			
Temporal	Stylomastoid foramen	Stylomastoid artery	Facial nerve
Temporal	Petrotympanic fissure	Anterior tympanic artery (often)	Chorda tympani
Maxilla	Incisive foramen/ Incisive canal	Terminal part of sphenopalatine or greater palatine vessels	Nasopalatine nerve (V_2)
Palatine	Greater palatine foramen	Greater palatine vessels	Greater palatine nerve
Palatine and maxilla	Lesser palatine foramina	Lesser palatine vessels	Lesser palatine nerve
	Palatine canal	Descending palatine vessels	Greater and lesser palatine nerves
	Pterygoid canal		Nerve of the pterygoid canal (Vidian nerve)
	Sphenopalatine foramen	Sphenopalatine vessels	Nasopalatine nerve

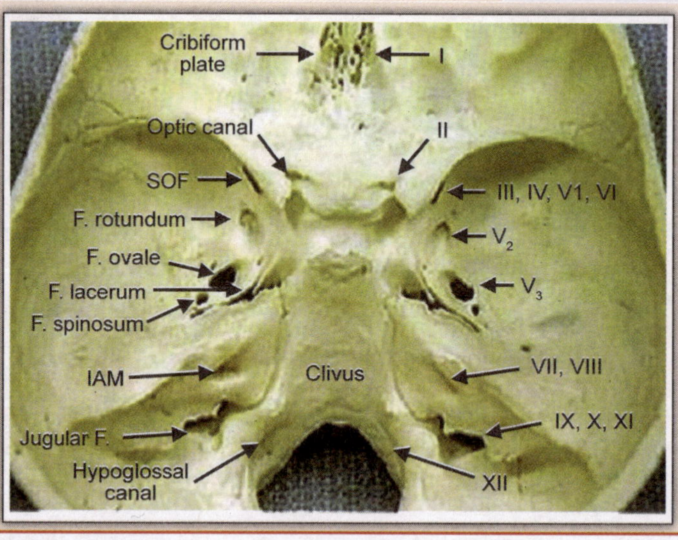

54. Ans. (a) Paralysis agitans

Ref: Gray's 41st ed age 370, Guyton 12th ed page 693

The structure marked in this figure is Midbrain.

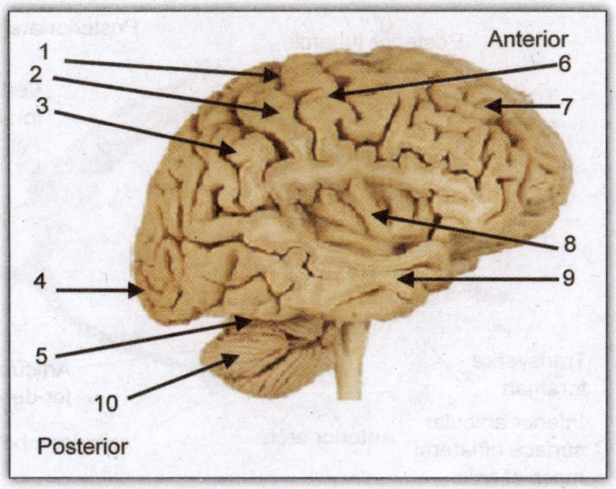

Fig: Right lateral view of brain with temporal lobe cut away

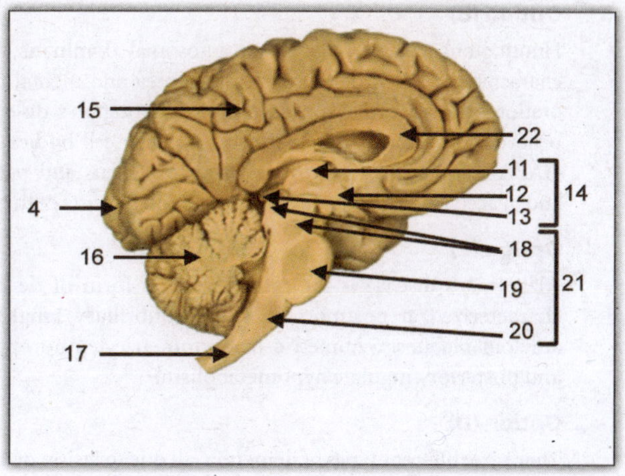

Fig: Sagittal medial section of brain

1. Central sulcus (shallow groove separating the frontal lobe and parietal lobe)
2. Postcentral gyrus (elevation located just posterior to the central sulcus)
3. Parietal lobe
4. Occipital lobe
5. Transverse fissure (deep groove separating the cerebrum from the cerebellum in the posterior/inferior part of the brain)
6. Precentral gyrus (elevation located just anterior to the central sulcus)
7. Frontal lobe
8. Insula (inner lobe deep to the lateral cerebral fissure)
9. Temporal lobe (cut)
10. Cerebellum
11. Pineal gland
12. Thalamus
13. Hypothalamus
14. Diencephalon
15. Cerebrum
16. Cerebellum
17. Spinal cord
18. Midbrain
19. Pons
20. Medulla oblongata
21. Brainstem
22. Corpus callosum

Option (A)

Parkinson suggested the name 'paralysis agitans' but it was "Parkinson's disease" that stuck, a name suggested by neurologist Jean-Martin Charcot after Parkinson's death.

Disorders of the basal ganglia are characterized, depending on the underlying pathology, by an inability to initiate and execute wanted movements (as in Parkinson's disease) or an inability to prevent unwanted movements (as in Huntington's disease).

Parkinson's disease is the most common pathological condition affecting the basal ganglia. It is characterized by akinesia, muscular rigidity and tremor due to degeneration of the dopaminergic neurones of the substantia nigra pars compacta (which project to the striatum in the **nigrostriatal pathway**).

The core pathology of Parkinson's disease is from widespread destruction of that portion of the substantia nigra (the pars compacta) that sends dopamine-secreting nerve fibers to the caudate nucleus and putamen. The **triad of rigidity, akinesia/bradykinesia and tremor at rest (Mnemonic RAT),** correlates with degeneration of the dopaminergic nigrostriatal pathway and DA depletion in the striatum. In advanced PD, loss of these neurons results in depigmentation of the SN (A) and in loss of the DA synthesizing enzyme tyrosine-hydroxylase (TH)

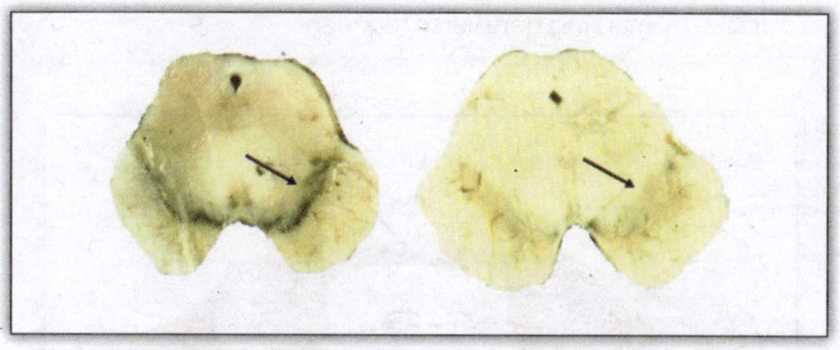

Fig: Left—normal midbrain in which dark pigmentation appears in the region of the substantia nigra above the cerebral peduncles. Right—loss of pigmentation in the substantia nigra of the midbrain in a patient with Parkinson disease

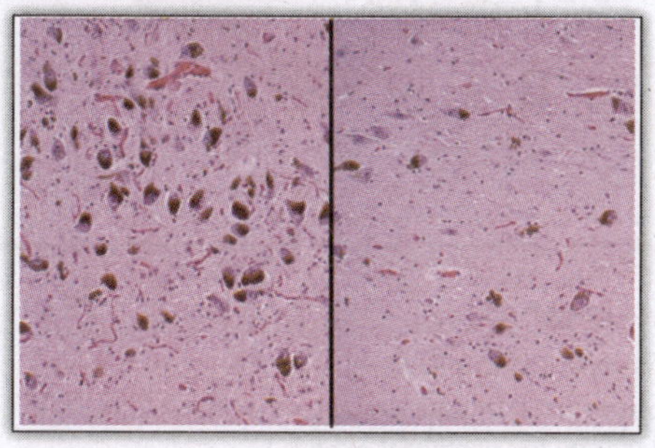

Fig: Left—normal numbers of neurons in the subtantia nigra are pigmented. Right—loss of neurons and loss of pigmentation with Parkinson's disease

Option (B)

Huntington's disease, chorea: an autosomal dominant disease characterized by chronic progressive chorea and mental deterioration. The abnormal movements of Huntington's disease are believed to be caused by loss of most of the cell bodies of the GABA-secreting neurons in the caudate nucleus and putamen and of acetylcholine-secreting neurons in many parts of the brain.

Option (C)

Alzheimer's disease is the most common form of dementia, characterized at postmortem by neurofibrillary tangles and amyloid plaques. Symmetric or asymmetric temporoparietal and posterior cingulate hypometabolism.

Option (D)

There are different types of dementia, all due to lesion of cortex. Alzheimer's is the most common dementia which is provided separately in option C.

Bilateral lesion of anterior temporal neocortex (middle and inferior temporal gyri) (e.g. in semantic dementia) lead to loss of recognition of words and percepts. Bilateral in frontotemporal dementia lead to the 'frontal lobe syndrome'.

55. Ans. (c) C

Ref: Grays 41st ed page 283, 722, Keith L Moore 7th ed page 1015

NOTE

Conventionally we remember that vertebral artery transmits through transverse foramen. The examiner cleverly asked for 3rd part of vertebral artery and here most of the students made a mistake by marking transverse foramen.

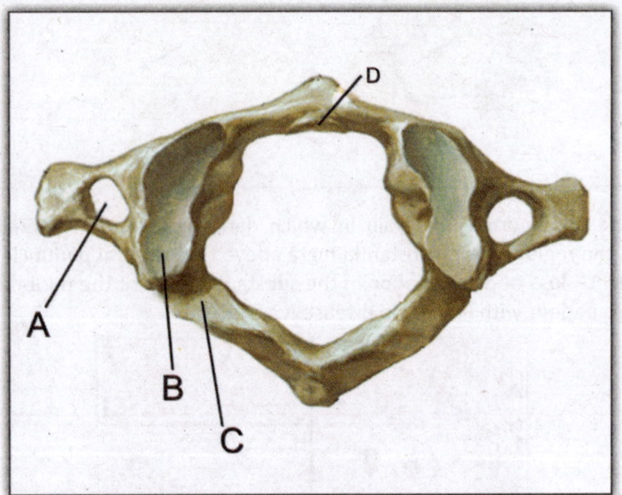

Figure Legends

A = Transverse foramen
B = Superior articular surface or occipital condyle
C = Groove for vertebral artery
D = Articular facet of dens

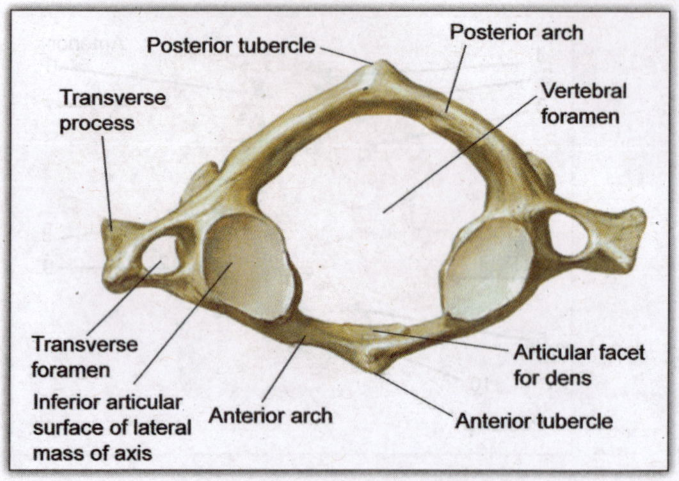

Fig: Atlas (C1) inferior view (Labeled)

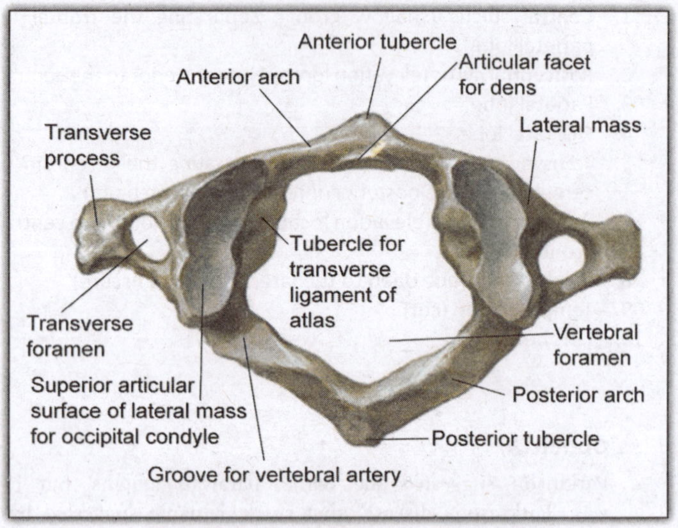

Fig: Atlas (C1) superior view (Labeled)

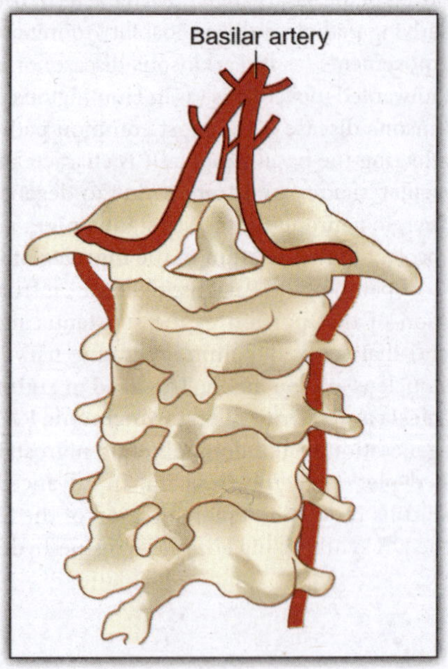

Parts of Vertebral Artery		
Cervical part	1st part	Arises from 1st part of subclavian artery Ascends in pyramidal space between scalene and longus muscle
	2nd part	Through transverse foramen of transverse process of C1-C6
Suboccipital part	3rd part	Courses in the groove of posterior arch of atlas before it enters the cranial cavity It enters the vertebral canal below the inferior border of the posterior atlanto-occipital membrane. This part of the artery, covered by semispinalis capitis, lies in the suboccipital triangle. The first cervical dorsal spinal ramus separates the artery from the posterior arch.
Cranial part	4th part	Pierces the dura and arachnoid mater and ascends anterior to the hypoglossal roots. Supplies branches to spinal cord, medulla, part of cerebellum and dura of posterior cranial fossa. Unites with its contralateral vertebral artery to form the basilar artery at the lower border of the pons

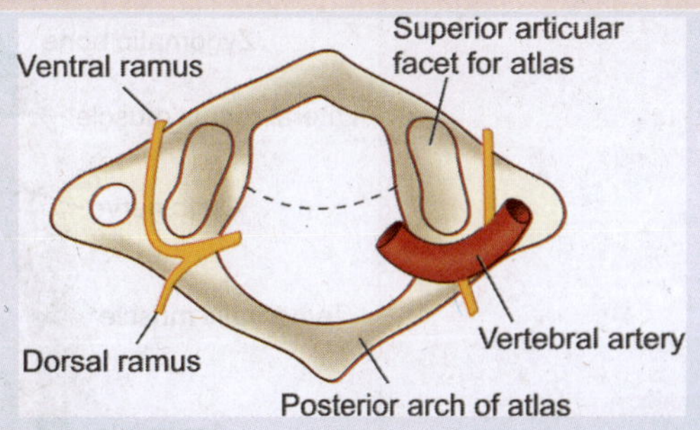

Relationship of the artery to the atlas vertebra and to the first cervical nerve, as seen from above

Branches of Vertebral Artery

The vertebral arteries and their major branches (sometimes referred to as the 'vertebrobasilar system') essentially supply blood to the upper spinal cord, the brain stem, cerebellum and occipital lobe of the cerebrum.

- **Posterior inferior cerebellar artery:** The largest branch of the vertebral artery is the posterior inferior cerebellar artery. It arises near the lower end of the olive, which it curves back around and then ascends behind the roots of the glossopharyngeal and vagus nerves to reach the inferior border of the pons. Here it curves and descends along the inferolateral border of the fourth ventricle before it turns laterally into the cerebellar vallecula between the hemispheres and divides into medial and lateral branches. The medial branch runs back between the cerebellar hemisphere and inferior vermis and supplies both.
- **Basilar artery:** This large median vessel is formed by the union of the vertebral arteries at the mid-medullary level and extends to the upper border of the pons. The basilar artery terminates by dividing into two posterior cerebral arteries at a variable level but most frequently in the interpeduncular cistern, behind the dorsum sellae.
- The **anterior inferior cerebellar artery** is given off from the lower part of the basilar artery and runs posterolaterally, usually ventral to the abducens, facial and vestibulocochlear nerves. It commonly exhibits a loop into the internal acoustic meatus below the nerves and when this occurs, the labyrinthine artery may arise from the loop. The anterior inferior cerebellar artery supplies the inferior cerebellar surface anterolaterally and anastomoses with the posterior inferior cerebellar branch of the vertebral artery.
- The **superior cerebellar artery** arises near the distal portion of the basilar artery, immediately before the formation of the posterior cerebral arteries. It passes laterally below the oculomotor nerve, which separates it from the posterior cerebral artery and curves round the cerebral peduncle below the trochlear nerve to gain the superior cerebellar surface.

The **posterior cerebral artery** is a terminal branch of the basilar artery. The posterior cerebral artery is larger than the superior cerebellar artery, from which it is separated near its origin by the oculomotor nerve and, lateral to the midbrain, by the trochlear nerve. It passes laterally, parallel with the superior cerebellar artery and receives the posterior communicating artery. It then winds round the cerebral peduncle and reaches the tentorial cerebral surface, where it supplies the temporal and occipital lobes.

56. Ans. (a) Superior colliculus

Ref: Grays 41st ed page 312, 325, Khurana 4th ed page 313

NOTE

In exam only half of the figure was given.

Structure marked in the picture is Medial rectus muscle. Medial rectus is supplied by oculomotor nerve [CN-III] which lies on superior colliculus.

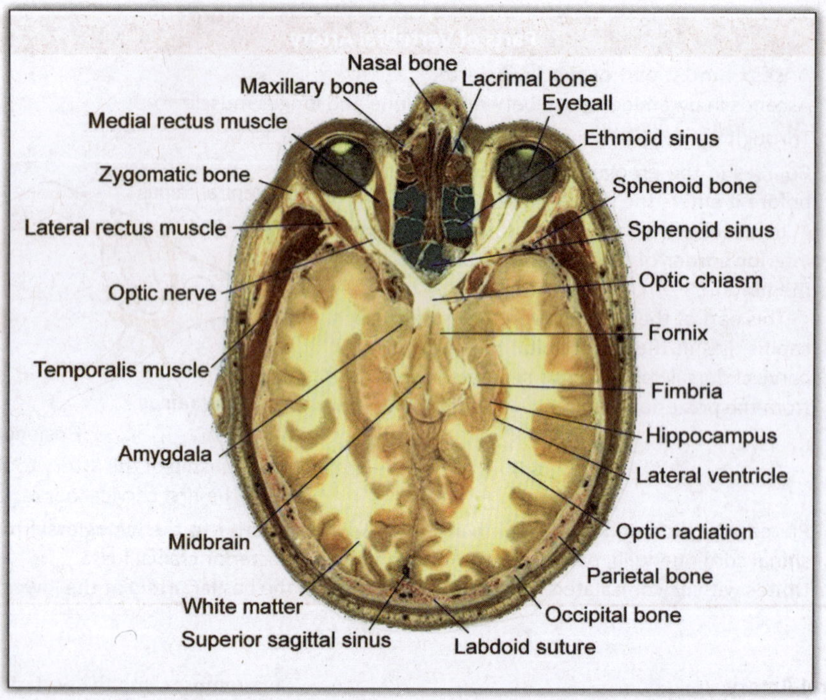

Fig: Transverse section of brain at the level of eyes (Labeled)

Nerve Supply of Extraocular Muscle

The extraocular muscles are supplied by third, fourth and sixth cranial nerves. The third cranial nerve (oculomotor) supplies the superior, medial and inferior recti and inferior oblique muscles. The fourth cranial nerve (trochlear) supplies the superior oblique and the sixth nerve (abducent) supplies the lateral rectus muscle.

> **NOTE**
>
> Remember this Mnemonic for intraocular muscles nerve supply
> SO4 -LR6- Rest all by 3rd (Oculomotor nerve)

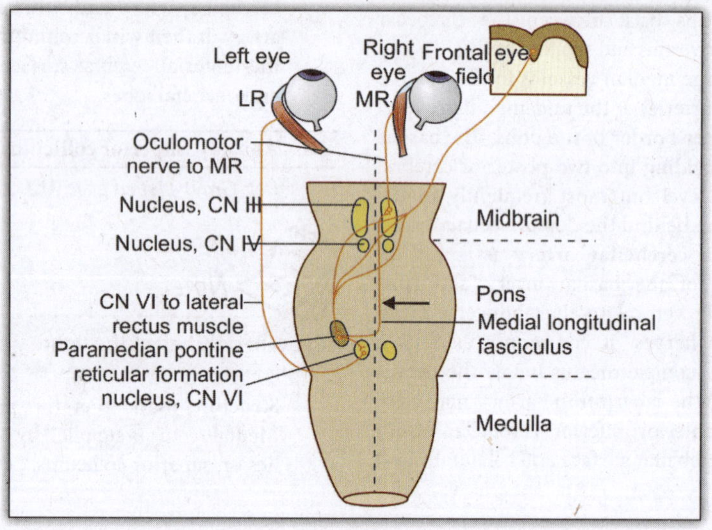

57. Ans. (c) Sulcus terminalis

Ref: Gray's 41st ed page 511, Moore - Clinically Oriented Anatomy 7th edition page 940

The dorsum (posterosuperior surface) is generally convex in all directions at rest. It is divided by a V-shaped **sulcus terminalis** into an anterior, oral (presulcal) part that faces upwards and a posterior, pharyngeal (postsulcal) part that faces posteriorly.

Anatomy of Tongue	
Parts	Root, Tip and Body, which has (a) a curved upper surface or dorsum and (b) an inferior surface.
Dorsum	The dorsum is divided into oral and pharyngeal parts. The inferior surface is confined to the oral part only. The dorsum of the tongue is convex in all directions. It is divided into: • An oral part or anterior two-thirds • A pharyngeal part or posterior one-third, by a faint V-shaped groove, the **sulcus terminalis**. The two limbs of the 'V meet at a median pit, named the **foramen caecum.** They run laterally and forwards up to the palatoglossal arches. The foramen caecum represents the site from which the thyroid diverticulum grows down in the embryo.
Root	The root is attached to the mandible and soft palate above and to the hyoid bone below. Because of these attachments we are not able to swallow the tongue itself. In between the two bones, it is related to the geniohyoid and mylohyoid muscles.
Tip	The tip of the tongue forms the anterior free end which, at rest, lies behind the upper incisor teeth.

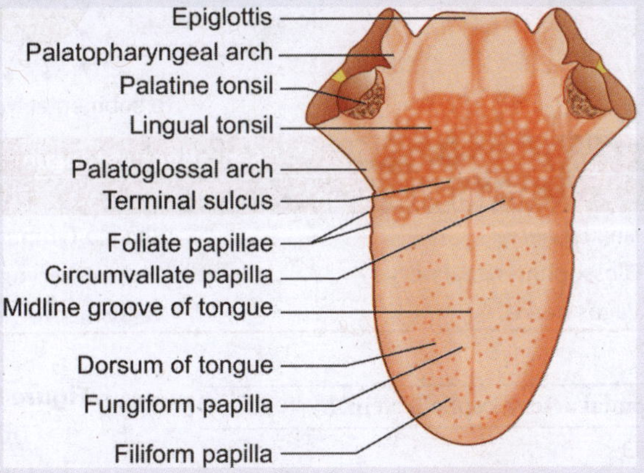

Papillae of the Tongue	
These are projections of mucous membrane or corium which give the anterior two-thirds of the tongue its characteristic roughness. These are of the following three types.	
Vallate or circumvallate papillae	They are large in size 1–2 mm in diameter and are 8–12 in number. They are situated immediately in front of the sulcus terminalis.
Fungiform papillae	The fungiform papillae are numerous near the tip and margins of the tongue, but some of them are also scattered over the dorsum
Filiform papillae	The filiform papillae or conical papillae cover the presulcal area of the dorsum of the tongue and give it a characteristic velvety appearance. They are the smallest and most numerous of the lingual papillae. Each is pointed and covered with keratin; the apex is often split into filamentous processes

Artery, Vein and Lymphatics of Tongue	
Arterial supply	It is chiefly derived from the lingual artery, a branch of the external carotid artery. The root of the tongue is also supplied by the tonsillar and ascending pharyngeal arteries
Venous drainage	The arrangement of the vena comitantes veins of the tongue is variable. Two venae comitantes accompany the lingual artery and one vena comitantes accompanies the hypoglossal nerve. The deep lingual vein is the largest and principal vein of the tongue. It is visible on the inferior surface of the tongue. It runs backwards and crosses the genioglossus and the hyoglossus below the hypoglossal nerve. These veins unite at the posterior border of the hyoglossus to form the lingual vein which ends either in the common facial vein or in the internal jugular vein.

Contd...

Lymphatics	• The tip of the tongue drains bilaterally to the submental nodes. • The right and left halves of the remaining part of the anterior two-thirds of the tongue drain unilaterally to the submandibular nodes. • The posterior one-third of the tongue drains bilaterally to the jugulo-omohyoid nodes, these are known as the lymph nodes of the tongue.

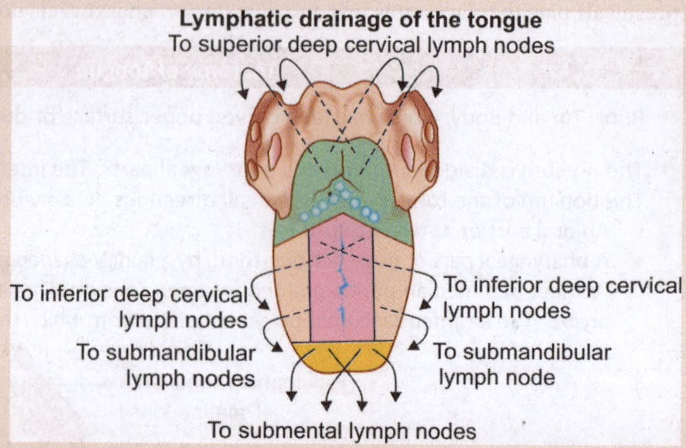

Sensations of tongue

	General sensation	Taste sensation
Anterior 2/3rd	Lingual nerve	Chorda tympani (branch of facial)
Posterior 1/3rd	Glossopharyngeal nerve	Glossopharyngeal nerve
Posterior most	Vagus nerve	Vagus nerve

58. Ans. (c) Thoracoacromial artery, cephalic vein...

Ref: BDC 4th ed page 83

NOTE

It was a handmade line diagram in the examination

The structure in the picture is clavipectoral fascia

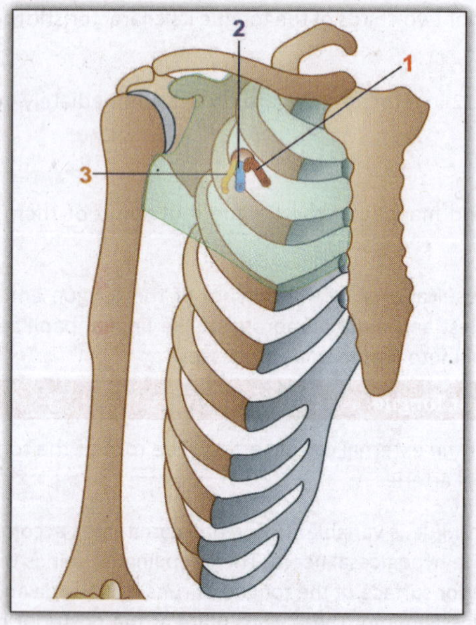

Fig: Clavipectoral Fascia (Shaded)

Figure Legend

1. Thoraco acromial artery
2. Cephalic vein draining in axillary vein
3. Lateral pectoral nerve

Clavipectoral Fascia

- Extent: from clavicle above to axillary fascia below.
- Upper part splits to enclose subclavius muscle while lower part splits to enclose pectoralis minor muscle.
- It helps to pull up axillary fascia.
- Upper thickened part is called the costocoracoidal ligament.

Clavipectoral fascia is a fibrous sheet situated deep to the clavicular portion of the pectoralis major muscle. It extends from the clavicle above to the axillary fascia below. **Its upper part splits to enclose the subclavius muscle**. The posterior lamina is fused to the investing layer of the deep cervical fascia and to the axillary sheath. Inferiorly, the clavipectoral fascia splits to enclose the pectoralis minor muscle. Below this muscle it continues as the suspensory ligament which is attached to the dome of the axillary fascia and helps to keep it pulled up.

The clavipectoral fascia is pierced by the following structures:

- Cephalic vein
- Lateral pectoral nerve
- Thoracoacromial vessels
- Lymphatics passing from the breast and pectoral region to the apical group of axillary lymph nodes.

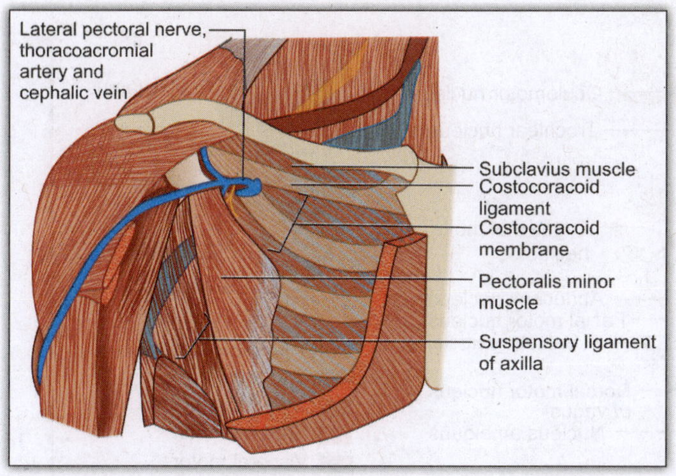

59. Ans. (a) Lateral rectus

Ref: Gray's 41st ed page 275, Last's Anatomy: Regional and Applied 4th ed Page 615

Facial colliculus is marked in the given picture. Facial colliculus is formed by motor fibers of facial nerve around abducens nucleus, hence deeper structure beneath the facial colliculus is abducent nucleus.

Abducents nucleus is motor, somatic, near midline in pons deep to facial colliculus in floor of fourth ventricle, for **lateral rectus**.

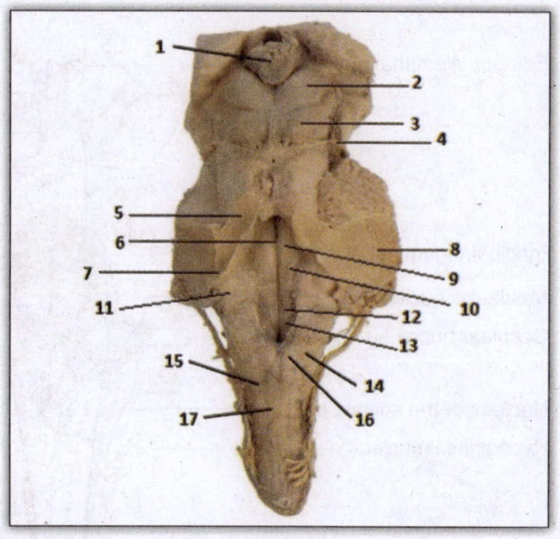

Fig: Brain stem dissected—Legends

1. Pineal gland
2. Superior colliculus
3. Inferior colliculus
4. Trochlear nerve
5. Superior cerebellar peduncle
6. Dorsal median sulcus
7. Inferior cerebellar peduncle
8. Middle cerebellar peduncle
9. Medial eminence
10. Facial colliculus
11. Striae medullares
12. HHypoglossal trigone
13. Vagal trigone
14. Cuneate tubercle
15. Fasciculus cuneatus
16. Gracilis tubercle
17. Fasciculus gracilis

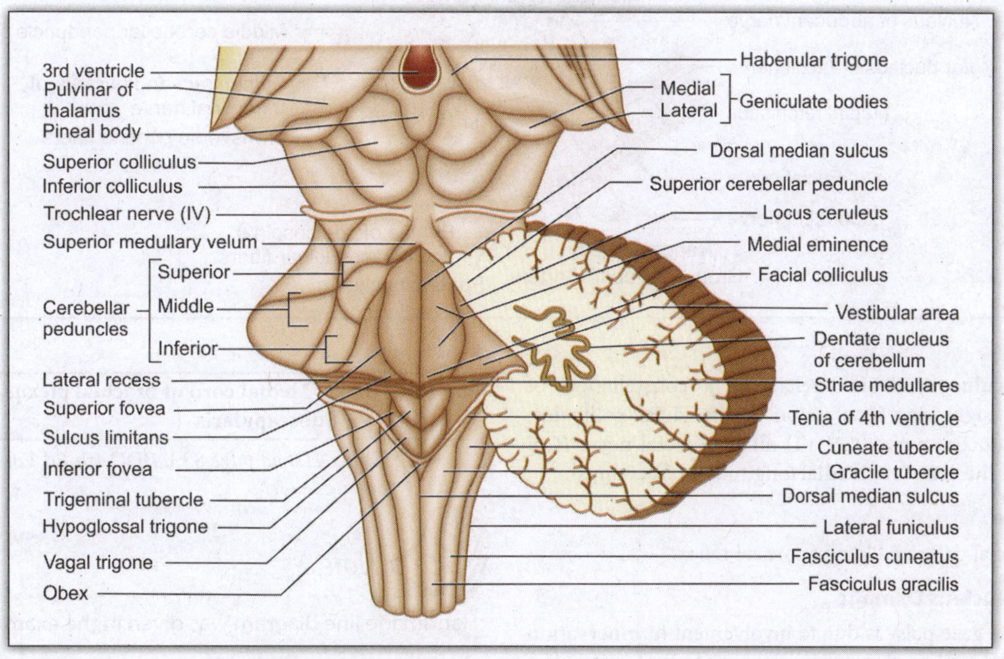

Fig: Brain stem illustration: Self-explanatory labeling of structures

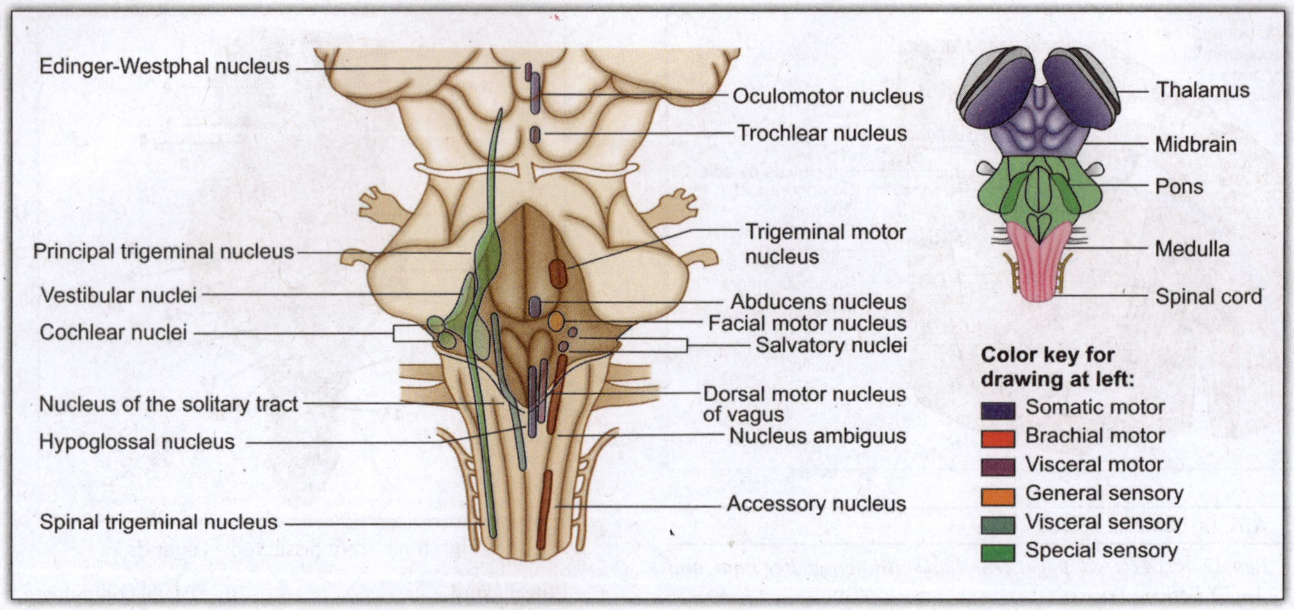

Fig: Brain stem illustrations: with emphasis of different nucleus

Section of Pons at the level of Facial Colliculus

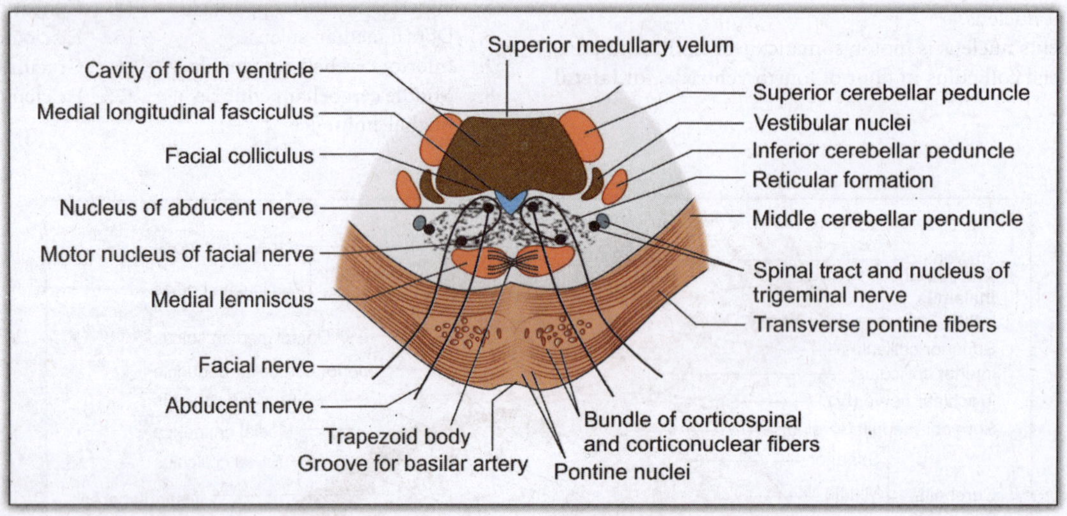

Facial colliculus syndrome refers to a constellation of neurological signs due to a lesion at the facial colliculus, involving abducens nerve (CN VI) nucleus, facial nerve (CN VII) fibers at the genu and medial longitudinal fasciculus

Facial Nerve

Ipsilateral facial palsy and loss of corneal reflex.

Abducent Nucleus Damage

The conjugate gaze palsy is due to involvement of innervation not only to the ipsilateral abducens nerve to **lateral rectus**, but also to the interneurons projecting into the medial longitudinal fasciculus which contribute innervation of the contralateral **medial rectus** (thus internuclear ophthalmoplegia).

60. Ans. (b) 1- Medial cord of brachial plexus, 2- Long thoracic nerve, 3- Subscapularis

Ref: Gray's 41st ed page 833, BDC 4th Ed Vol 1 page 89

NOTE

Handmade line diagram was given in the exam

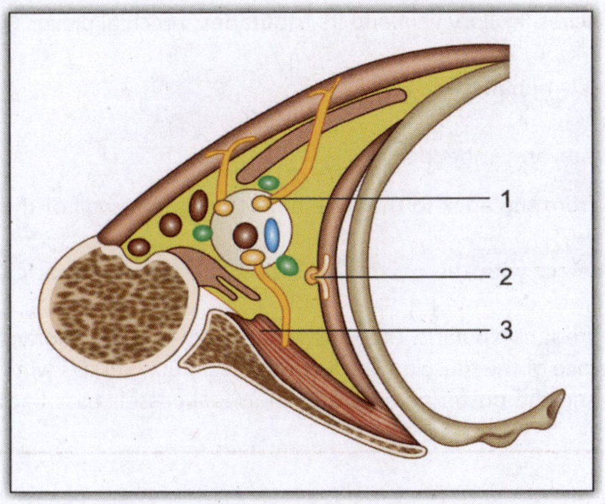

Fig: Cross section of axilla (Unlabeled)

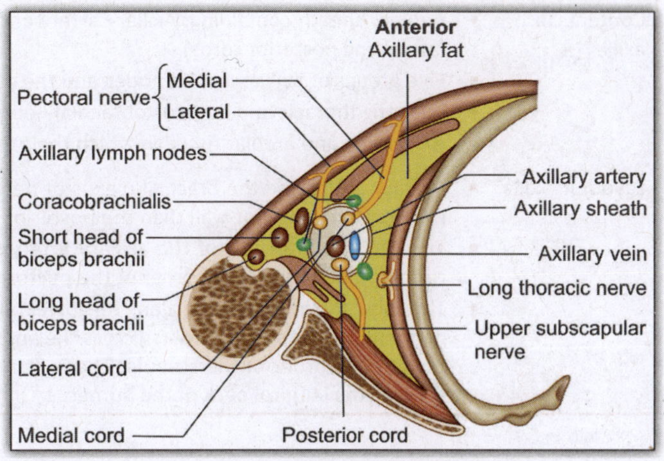

Fig: Cross section of axilla (Labelled)

Figure Legends: 1. Medial cord of brachial plexus (Towards the rib, contrary to lateral cord which is towards the head of humerus); **2.** Long thoracic nerve (supplying the Serratus anterior muscle of the medical wall of axilla); **3.** Subscapularis muscle

Axilla

The axilla or armpit is a pyramidal space situated between the upper part of the arm and the chest wall. It resembles a four-sided pyramid and has (i) an apex, (ii) a base and (iii) 4 walls—anterior, posterior, medial and lateral.

The axilla is disposed obliquely in such a way that the apex is directed upwards and medially towards the root of the neck and the base is directed downwards.

- **Apex:** It is directed upwards and medially towards the root of the neck. It is truncated (not pointed) and corresponds to a triangular interval bounded anteriorly by the clavicle, posteriorly by the superior border of the scapula and medially by the outer border of the first rib. This passage is called the **cervicoaxillary canal**. The axillary artery and the brachial plexus enter the axilla through this canal.
- **Base or floor:** It is directed downwards and is formed by skin and fasciae
- **Anterior wall:** It is formed by the following:
  - The pectoralis major in front and
  - The clavipectoral fascia enclosing the pectoralis minor and the subclavius; all deep to the pectoralis major
- **Posterior wall:** It is formed by : (i) Subscapularis above (ii) Teres major and latissimus dorsi below
- **Medial wall:** It is formed by : (i) Upper four ribs with their intercostal muscles, (ii) Upper part of the serratus anterior muscle
- **Lateral wall:** It is very narrow because the anterior and posterior walls converge on it. It is formed by: (i) Upper part of the shaft of the humerus in the region of the bicipital groove and (ii) Coracobrachialis and short head of the biceps.

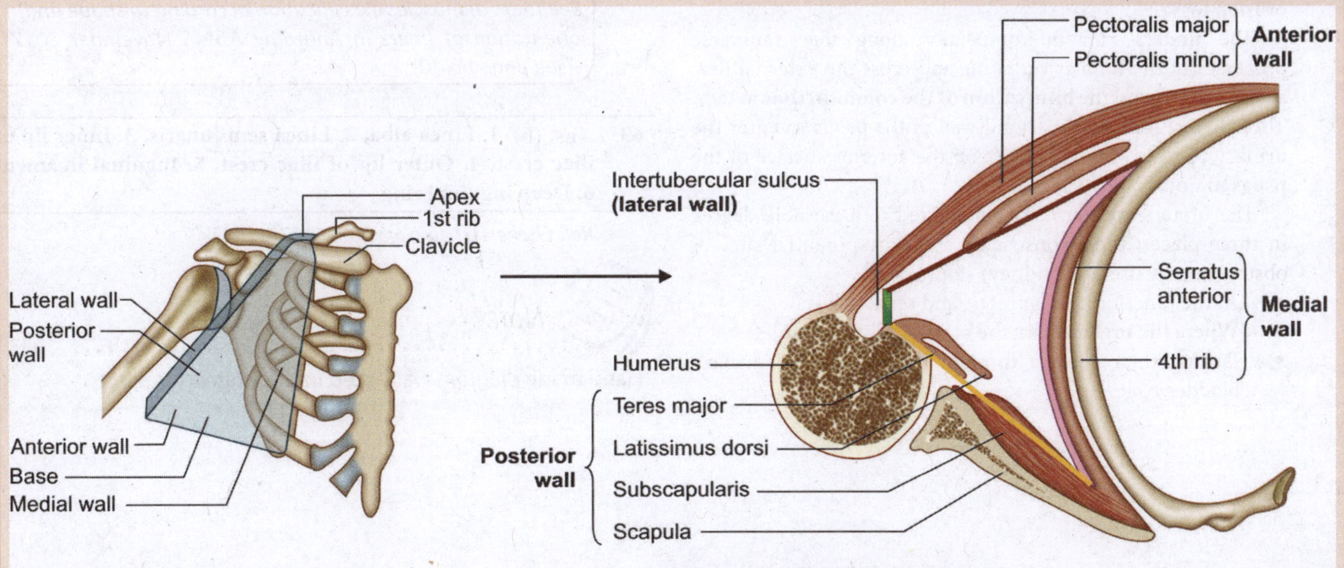

Inferior view of transverse section

Contd...

Contents in axilla	• **Axillary sheath** containing: Axillary artery and its branches, axillary vein and its tributaries, brachial plexus (Medial, lateral and posterior cords) • Five groups of axillary lymph nodes and the associated lymphatics. • The long thoracic and intercostobrachial nerves. • Axillary fat and areolar tissue in which the other contents are embedded.
Layout in axilla	• Axillary artery and the brachial plexus of nerves run from the apex to the base along the lateral wall of the axilla, nearer to the anterior wall than the posterior wall. • The thoracic branches of the axillary artery lie in contact with the pectoral muscles, the lateral thoracic vessels running along the lower border of the pectoralis minor. • The subscapular vessels run along the lower border of the subscapularis. The subscapular nerve and the thoracodorsal nerve (nerve to latissimus dorsi) cross the anterior surface of the muscle. The circumflex scapular vessels wind round the lateral border of the scapula. The axillary nerve and the posterior circumflex humeral vessels pass backwards close to the surgical neck of the humerus.

61. Ans. (c) Quadratus lumborum

Ref: Gray's Anatomy 41st edition page 1251, Keith L. Moore, 4th ed page 117

"The Ureter Lies Over Psoas Major Muscle not Quadratus Lumborum"

Grays anatomy states that: The left ureter is crossed by the **gonadal and left colic vessels.** It passes posterior to loops of jejunum and **sigmoid colon and its mesentery** in the posterior wall of the inter sigmoid recess. On the pelvic side wall, it is anterior to the internal iliac artery and the *beginning of its anterior trunk*, posterior to which are the internal iliac vein, lumbosacral nerve and sacroiliac joint. Laterally, it lies on the fascia of **obturator internus**. It progressively crosses to become medial to the umbilical, inferior vesical and middle rectal arteries. In males, the pelvic ureter hooks under the vas deferens, it then passes anterior and slightly superior to the upper pole of the seminal vesicle to traverse the bladder wall obliquely before opening at the ipsilateral trigonal angle. Its terminal part is surrounded by tributaries of the vesical veins. In females, the pelvic part initially has the same relations as in males but, anterior to the internal iliac artery, it is immediately **behind the ovary,** forming the posterior boundary of the ovarian fossa.

The ureters run inferomedially along the transverse processes of the lumbar vertebrae and cross the external iliac artery just beyond the **bifurcation of the common iliac artery.** They then run along the lateral wall of the pelvis to enter the urinary bladder. The ureter lies on the anterior surface of the **psoas major.**

The ureters are normally constricted to a variable degree in three places; these constricted areas are potential sites of obstruction by ureteric (kidney) stones:

- At the junction of the ureters and renal pelvis
- Where the ureters cross the brim of the pelvic inlet
- During their passage through the wall of the urinary bladder.

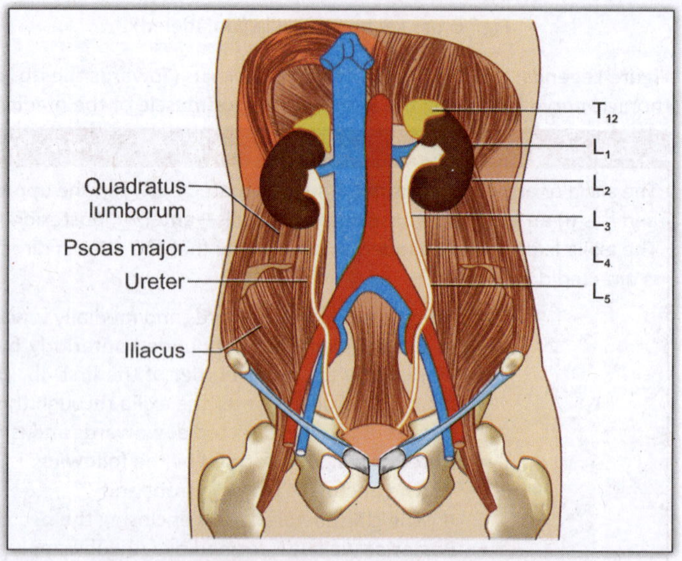

62. Ans. (d) Tibialis anterior

Ref: Gray's Anatomy 41st ed page 112

See table of muscles classification according to shape and orientation of fibers in Anatomy AIIMS November 2017 (see page no 40)

63. Ans. (b) 1. Linea alba, 2. Linea semilunaris, 3. Inner lip of iliac crest, 4. Outer lip of iliac crest, 5. Inguinal ligament 6. Deep inguinal ring

Ref: Grays 41st ed page 1071, 1079, 1343

NOTE

Hand made diagram was asked in the exam

Subject-wise MCQs and Answers with Explanations

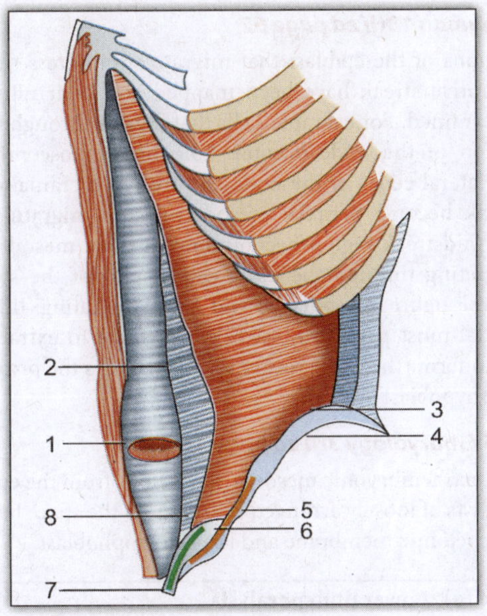

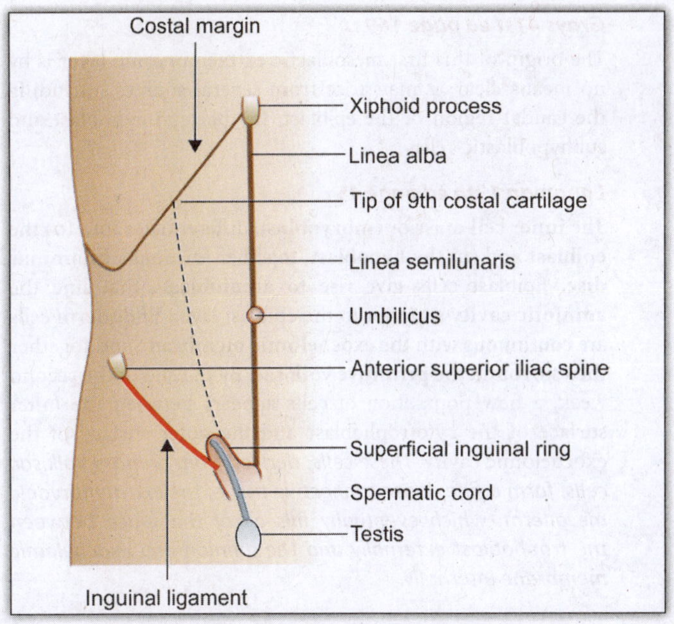

Figure Legends

1. **Linea alba:** It is a tendinous raphe extending from xiphoid process to pubic symphysis and pubic crest. It lies between the two recti and is formed by the interlacing and decussating aponeurotic fibers of external oblique, internal oblique and transversus abdominis.
2. **Linea semilunaris:** A few centimeters lateral to the median furrow, the abdominal wall shows a curved vertical groove. Its upper end reaches the costal margin at the tip of I the ninth costal cartilage. Interiorly it reaches the pubic tubercle. This line is called the linea semilunaris. It corresponds to the lateral margin of a muscle called the rectus abdominis.
3. **Inner lip of iliac crest:** Iliac crest has internal and external lips and a rough intermediate zone that is narrowest centrally.
4. **Outer lip of iliac crest.**
5. **Inguinal ligament:** Extends from the anterior superior iliac spine to the pubic tubercle. It is convex downwards. It is placed at the junction of the anterior abdominal wall with the front of the thigh.
6. **Superficial inguinal ring:** It is a hiatus in the aponeurosis of external oblique, just above and lateral to the crest of the pubis. Triangular, with its apex pointing laterally towards the anterior superior iliac spine. The ring is smaller in the female. The base of the triangular opening lies along the crest of the pubis. Its sides are the lateral and medial crura of the opening in the aponeurosis.
7. **Spermatic cord:** Present in the male. It can be felt through the skin as it passes downwards near the medial end of the inguinal ligament to enter the scrotum.
8. **Conjoint tendon:** It is a structure formed from the lower part of the common aponeurosis of the internal abdominal oblique and the transverse abdominal as it inserts into the crest of the pubis and pectineal line immediately behind the superficial inguinal ring. It forms the medial part of the posterior wall of the inguinal canal.

64. Ans. (c) Primary yolk sac

Ref: With text

Summary

Extraembryonic mesoderm have multiple origins and for the purpose of exams the best possible answer in order of priority should be; ***Epiblast + Hypoblast + Primary yolk sac > Hypoblast + Primary yolk sac > Primary yolk sac > Hypoblast > Epiblast***

NOTE

Earlier knowledge of devlopment were largely based on animal (avian) models.

Scott F. Gilbert Developmental Biology 10th ed **"Studies of human and rhesus monkey embryos have suggested that the yolk sac (and hence the hypoblast) is the source of this extraembryonic mesoderm** (Bianchi et al. 1993).

One adaptation of a flow chart by Gray's 41st ed is shown below to clarify the concept better. From this picture the Hierarchy is dearcated and it can be seen that primary yolk sac is the immediate precursor of extraembryonic mesoderm hence if given, it is to be preferred over hypoblast.

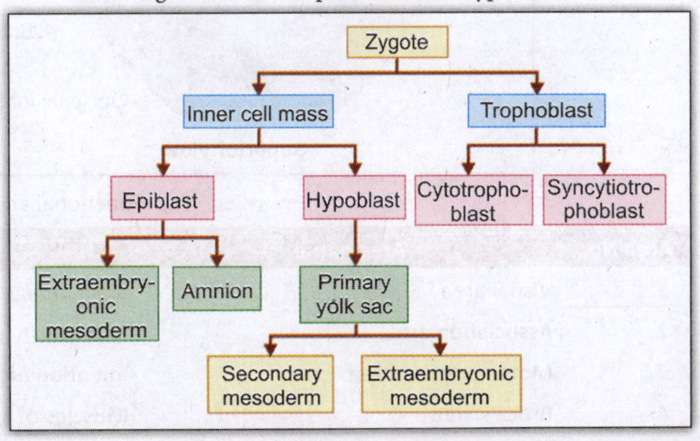

Grays 41st ed page 169

The origin of this first mesoblastic extraembryonic layer is by no means clear; it may arise from several sources, including the caudal region of the epiblast, the parietal hypoblast and subhypoblastic cells.

Langman 13th ed page 45

The **inner cell mass** or **embryoblast**, differentiates into (*a*) the **epiblast** and (*b*) the **hypoblast**, together forming a **bilaminar disc**. Epiblast cells give rise to **amnioblasts** that line the **amniotic cavity** superior to the epiblast layer. Endoderm cells are continuous with the **exocoelomic membrane** and together they surround the **primitive yolk sac**. By the end of the second week, a new population of cells appears between the inner surface of the cytotrophoblast and the outer surface of the exocoelomic cavity. *These cells, derived from primary yolk sac cells, form a fine, loose connective tissue, the extraembryonic mesoderm, which eventually fills all of the space between the trophoblast externally and the amnion and exocoelomic membrane internally.*

Langman 13th ed page 62

Regions of the epiblast that migrate and ingress through the primitive streak have been mapped and their ultimate fates determined. For example, cells that ingress through the cranial region of the node become notochord; those migrating at the lateral edges of the node and from the cranial end of the streak become paraxial mesoderm; cells migrating through the midstreak region become intermediate mesoderm; those migrating through the more caudal part of the streak form lateral figure mesoderm; and cells migrating through the caudal-most part of the streak contribute to extraembryonic mesoderm (the other source of this tissue is the primitive yolk sac [hypoblast].

BRS Embryology 3rd ed page 14

The extraembryonic mesoderm develops from the epiblast and consists of loosely arranged cells that fill the space between the exocoelomic membrane and the cytotrophoblast.

65. Ans. (a) Lower limb paralysis

Ref: Harrison 19th ed page 156, 178, 2574

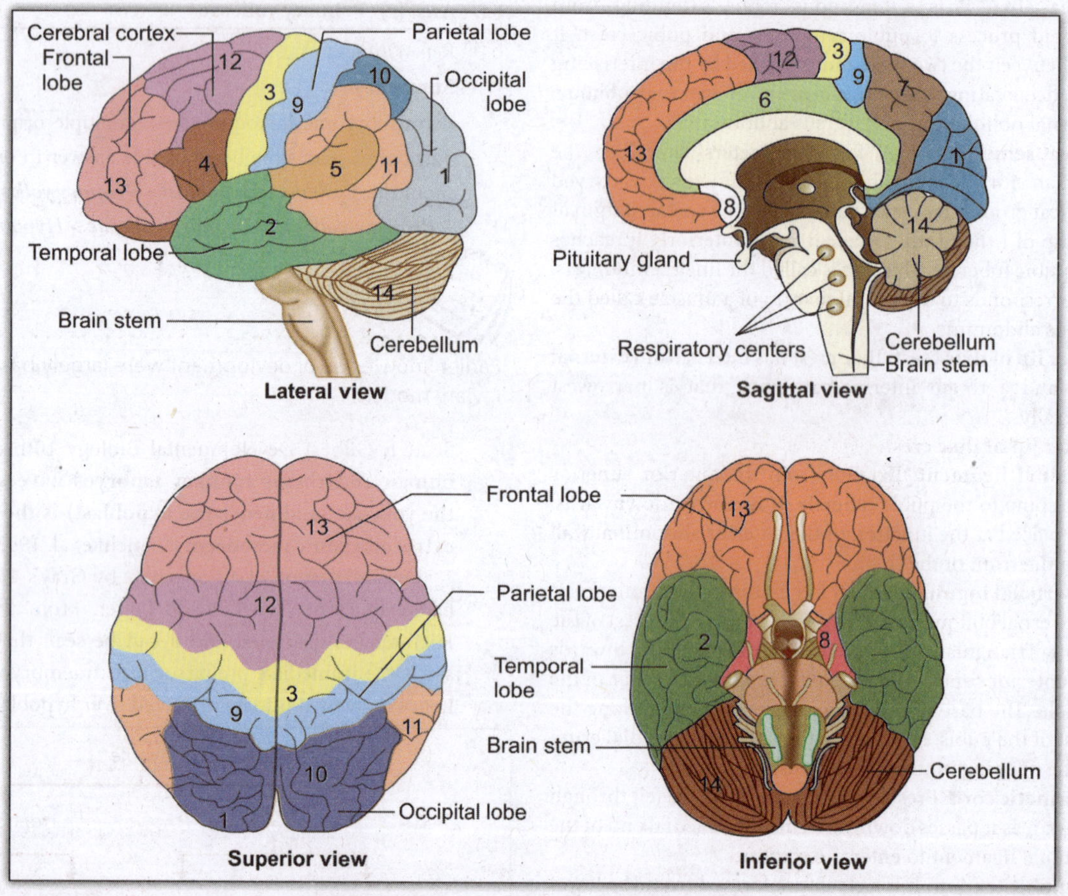

Fig: Functional areas of cerebral cortex

Area No.	Area name	Area function
1.	Visual area	Sight, image recognition, image perception
2.	Association area	Short term memory, equilibrium, emotion
3.	Motor function area	Initiation of voluntary muscles
4.	Broca's area	Muscles of speech

Contd...

Area No.	Area name	Area function
5.	Auditory area	Hearing
6.	Emotional area	Pain, hunger, flight or fight response
7.	Sensory association area	
8.	Olfactory area	Smelling
9.	Sensory area	Sensation from muscle and skin
10.	Somatosensory association area	Evaluation of weight, texture, temperature etc. for object recognition
11.	Wernicke's area	Written and spoken comprehension
12.	Motor function area	Eye movement and orientation
13.	Higher mental function	Concentration, planning, judgment, emotional expression, creativity
14	Cerebellar motor area	Coordination of movement, balance, equilibrium, inhibition

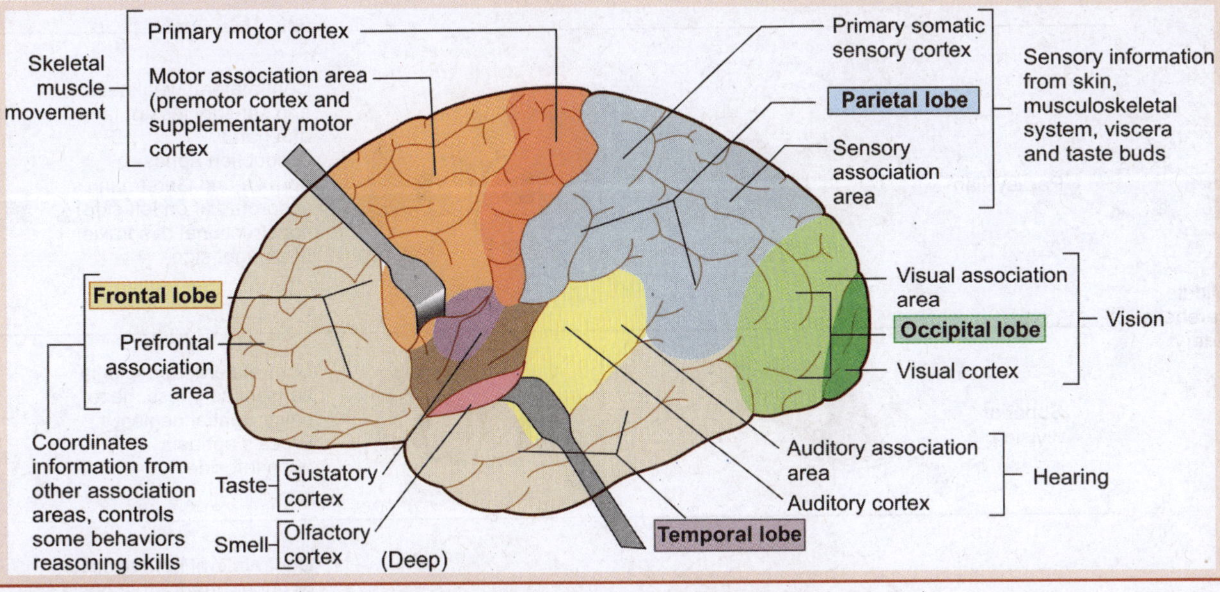

Note: The above area numbers are arbitrary numbers and does not represents Brodmann area

Option (A)

The area marked in the picture is frontal lobe area of the medial surface of the brain supplied by the anterior cerebral artery. Although anterior cerebral artery is not marked in the picture but that does not rule our frontal lobe injury. Injury to this area causes contralateral hemiplagia (Half-side of body including both upper and lower limb). Paraplagia is apralysis of both lower limbs, it is caused by spinal cord lesion or brainstem lesion or parasagittal frontal lobe lesion. Also, the lower limb representation of the of the homunculus is on the medical surface of the brain shown in the picture.

	Lesion	Infarct, surface	Infarct, coronal section	Clinical manifestations
Middle cerebellar artery	Entire territory	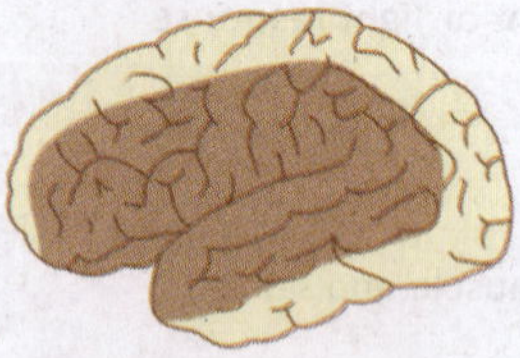	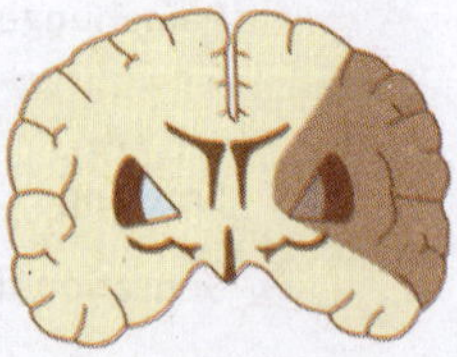	Contralateral gaze palsy, hemiplegia, hemisensory loss, global aphasia (if on left side) may lead to coma
	Deep	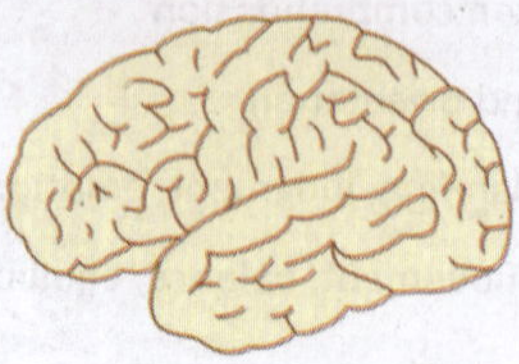	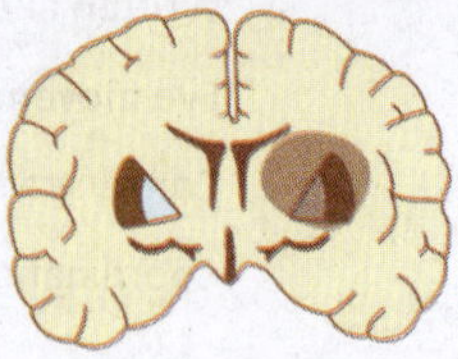	Contralateral hemiplegia hemisensory loss transcortical motor and/or sensory aphasia (if on left side)
	Parasylvian	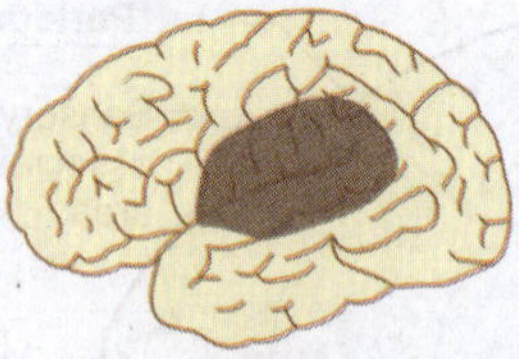	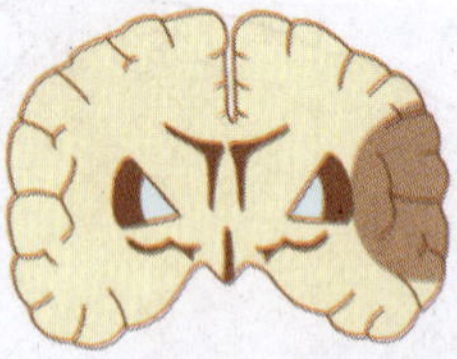	Contralateral weakness and sensory loss of face and hand conduction aphasia, apraxia and Gerstmann's syndrome (if on left side) constructional dyspraxia (if on right side)
	Superior division	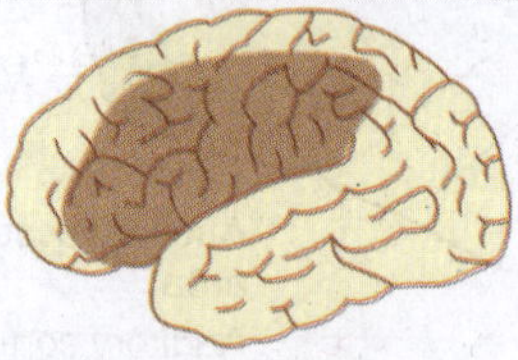	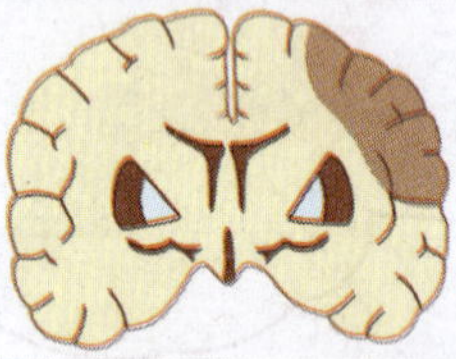	Contralateral hemiplegia, hemisensory loss, gaze palsy, spatial neglect Broca's aphasia (if on left side)
	Inferior division	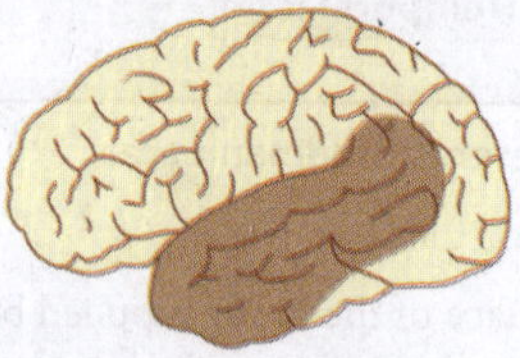	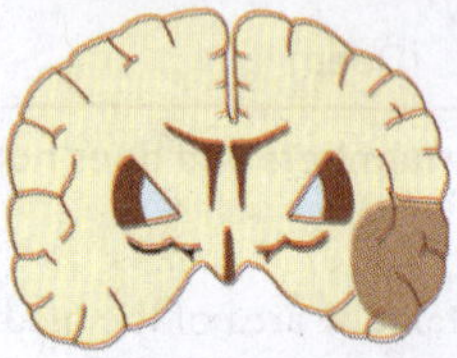	Contralateral hemianopsia or upper quadrant anopsia Wernicke's aphasia (if on left side) Constructional dyspraxia (if on right side)
Anterior cerebellar artery	Entire territory	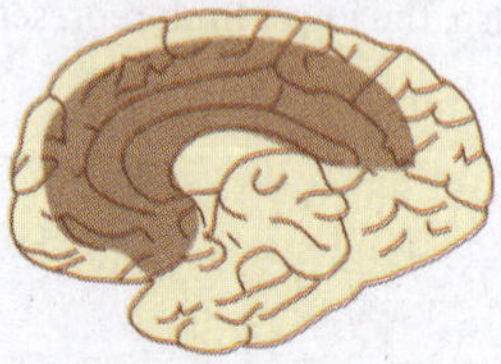	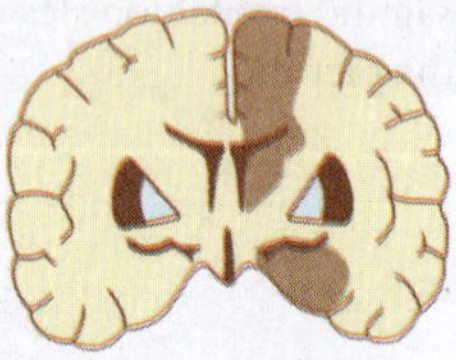	Incontinence contralateral hemiplegia Abulia Transcortical motor aphasia or motor and sensory aphasia left limb dyspraxia
	Distal	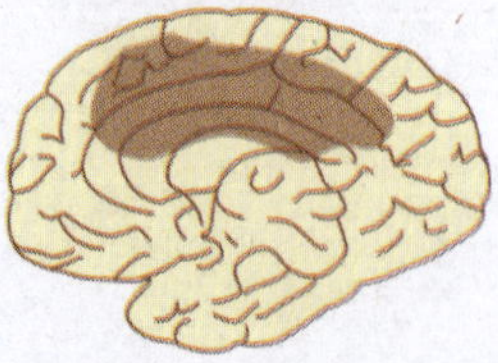	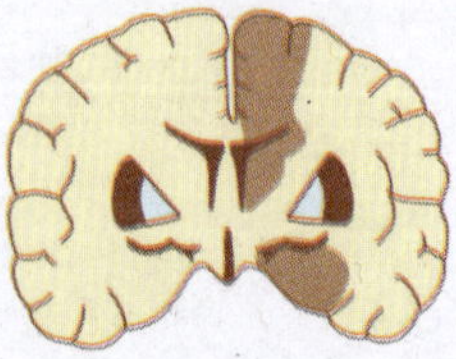	Contralateral weakness of leg, hip, foot and shoulder sensory loss in foot transcortical motor aphasia or motor and sensory aphasia left limb dyspraxia

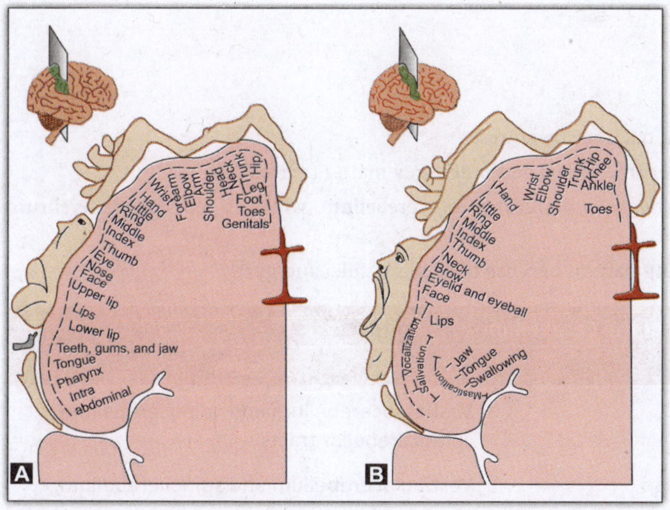

Figs A and B: Somatosenson contex in right cerebral hemisphere

Option (B)

Apraxia is a disorder of planning and initiating a skilled or learned movement unrelated to a significant motor or sensory deficit. The most frequent cause of apraxia is a lesion of the parietal lobes of the brain and sometimes a frontal lobe disease (Gait apraxia). In patients with left hemisphere damage, apraxia and aphasia frequently coexist. Ref: Dejong's Neurologic Examination page 303

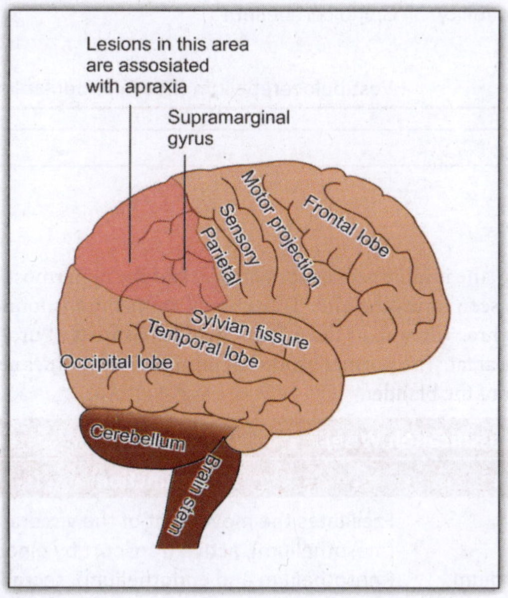

Option (C)

The most confusing option was aphasia. Students marked it thinking of Broca's area. But looking into the given picture carefully one can see that the medial cut section is given in the picture and Broca's area is on the lateral surface. Also note that Broca's area does not reach the medial surface in any possible way.

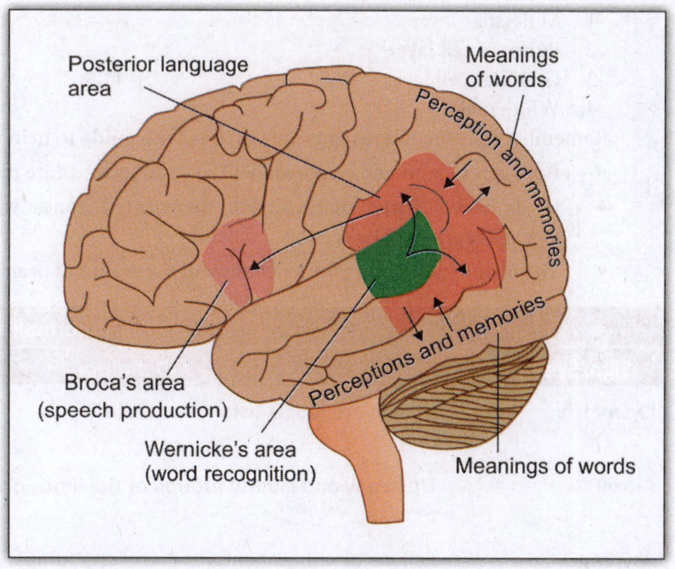

Fig: GB: Motor cortex in right cerebral hemisphere

Option (D)

Visual disturbances are seen in the lesion of occipital lobe.

66. Ans. (c) Dysarthria

Ref: Inderbir Singh Histology 6th Ed page 370, Wolfgang 4th ed page 498, Harrison 19th ed page 2579

Cerebellar lesion is related to two speech disorders: Dysarthria and scanning speech. Therefore, the answer here is dysarthria.

Even if in the first look you are unable to pin down which organ it is in the given histology slide, if you take a look at the options, you will understand that the options are mainly pertaining to the speech defects which generally arise in disorders of central nervous system.

So the first clue is: The histology is of a structure of CNS

Two main histologies from the CNS that we should be aware of are cerebral cortex and of cerebellum.

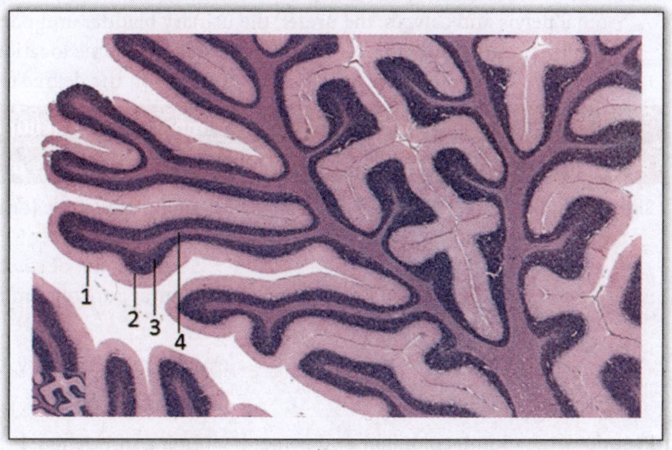

Fig: Histology of cerebellum H&E staining 4X view

1. Molecular layer
2. Purkinje cell layer
3. Granular cell layer
4. White matter

Remember that the following points shall serve a guide to help you nail the structures.

- Both cerebellum and cerebrum will have an inner white matter (medullar) and outer grey matter (cortex).
- In 4x view: Three characteristic demarcated zones will be seen in cortex of cerebellum while in cortex of cerebrum 6 zones/layers will be seen
- The histological slide of cerebellum will show a lot of branching pattern because of so many sulci and gyri.

Clinical Abnormalities of the Cerebellum

Sign/Symptom	Definition	Lesion
Dysmetria	Inability to judge distance or scale	Vestibulocerebellum and spinocerebellum, spinocerebellar tracts
Ataxia	Unsteady and clumsy motion of the limbs or torso	Vestibulocerebellum and spinocerebellum, spinocerebellar tracts
Asynergia	Failure of components of complex multiple joint movements in coordinated fashion	Cerebrocerebellum
Past pointing	Pointing beyond the finger in the finger-nose test	Cerebrocerebellum
Intention tremor	Inability to coordinate fine motor activities, tremor is slow (at 2–4 cycles per second) and is present only during movement	Cerebrocerebellum ipsilateral to symptomatic limb
Dysarthria	Motor speech disorder due to lack of coordination of muscles of speech	Cerebrocerebellum
Dysdiadochokinesis	Inability to perform rapid alternating movements, e.g. inability to rapidly flip the hands	Spino cerebellum
Nystagmus	Involuntary left-right eye movements	Vestibulocerebellum (flocculonodular lobes)

67. Ans. (b) Urinary bladder

Ref: Inderbir singh 6th Ed page 288

Transitional Epithelium

It is a multilayered epithelium, the lowermost cells are columnar or cuboidal, the middle cells are polyhedral and the uppermost cells are almost umbrella shaped. This is typical of transitional epithelium which is seen in urothelium. Transitional epithelium is found in the renal pelvis and calyces, the ureter, the urinary bladder and part of the urethra. The wall of the urinary bladder consists of urothelium, lamina propria, muscularis propria, serosa and, in some locations, perivesical fat. The normal urothelial lining varies in thickness from two layers to seven layers of cells, depending upon the degree of distension of the bladder.

Some Important Epithelium Linings (Classification Wise)

Type	Cell form	Examples of distribution	Main function
Simple	Squamous	Lining of vessels (endothelium)	Facilitates the movement of the viscera (mesothelium), active transport by pinocytosis (mesothelium and endothelium), secretion of biologically active molecules (mesothelium)
		Serous lining of cavities; pericardium, pleura, peritoneum (mesothelium)	
	Cuboidal	Covering the ovary, thyroid	Covering, secretion
	Columnar	Lining of intestine, gallbladder	Protection, lubrication, absorption, secretion
Pseudo-stratified	Some columnar and some cuboidal	Lining of trachea, bronchi, nasal cavity	Protection, secretion; cilia-mediated transport of particles trapped in mucus
Stratified	Surface layer squamous keratinized (dry)	Epidermis	Protection; prevents water loss
	Surface layer squamous nonkeratinized (moist)	Mouth, esophagus, larynx, vagina, anal canal	Protection, secretion; prevents water loss

Contd...

Some Important Epithelium Linings (Classification Wise)			
Type	**Cell form**	**Examples of distribution**	**Main function**
	Cuboidal	Sweat glands, developing ovarian follicles.	Protection, secretion.
	Transitional: domelike to flattened, depending on the functional state of the organ	Urinary bladder, ureters, renal calyces.	Protection, distensibility.
	Columnar	Conjunctiva	Protection
	Simple	**Stratified**	
Squamous	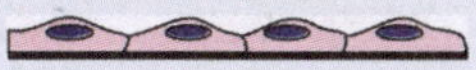 Simple squamous epithelium	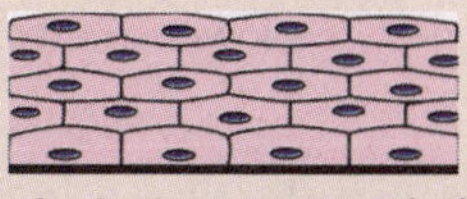 Stratified squamous epithelium	
Cuboidal	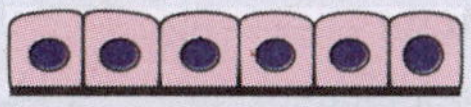 Simple cuboidal epithelium	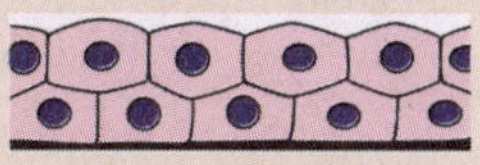 Stratified cuboidal epithelium	**Pseudostratified**
Columnar	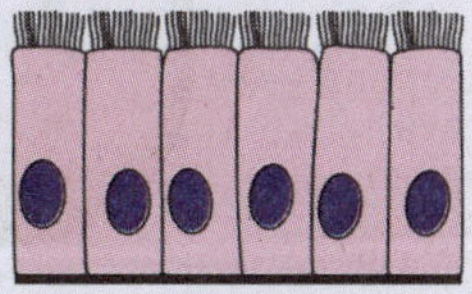 Simple columnar epithelium	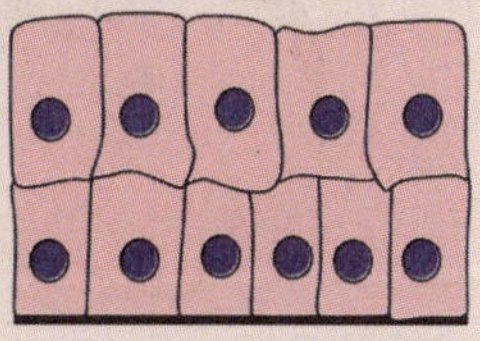 Stratified columnar epithelium	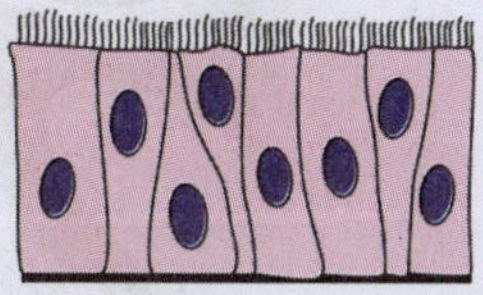 Pseudostratified columnar epithelium

68. Ans. (b) Zonula occludens

REF: Ross Histology 6th ed page 328-329

Repeat AIIMS NOV 2017 (See for explanation [see page no. 34])

AIIMS MAY 2016

69. Ans. (a) A

Ref: Langman's Embryology 11th ed page 161

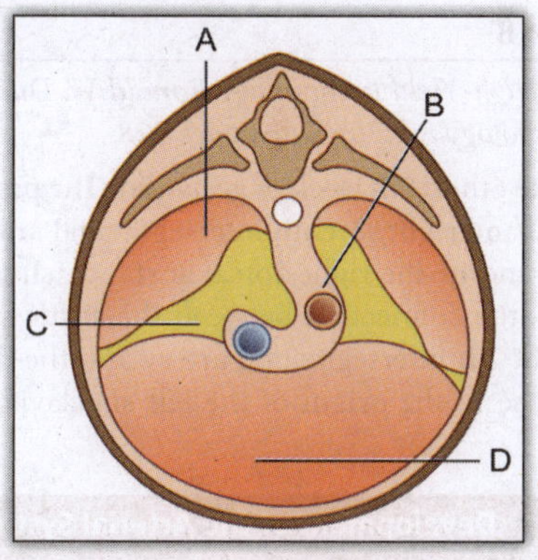

Figure Key

A = Pleuroperitoneal membrane
B = Dorsal mesentery of esophagus
C = Intraembryonic coelom
D = Septum transversum

Development of Diaphragm
Diaphragm is derived from cervical **somites 3, 4, 5.** (Hence, its innervation is by phrenic nerve-C3, 4, 5). The diaphragm is formed through the fusion of tissue from four different sources:

Contd...

Development of Diaphragm
• **Septum transversum** is the unpaired ventral portion. It is a thick mass of mesoderm located between the primitive heart tube and the developing liver. The septum transversum is the primordium of the central tendon of the diaphragm in the adult. Initially, the septum transversum lies opposite cervical somites and nerve components of the third, fourth and fifth cervical segments of the spinal cord grow into the septum. • **Paired pleuroperitoneal membranes** are sheets of somatic mesoderm that appear to develop from the dorsal and dorsolateral body wall by an unknown mechanism. • **Dorsal mesentery of the esophagus** is invaded by myoblasts and forms the crura of the diaphragm in the adult. • **Body wall** contributes muscle to the peripheral portions of the definitive diaphragm. The phrenic nerves supply the diaphragm with its motor and sensory innervation. Since the most peripheral part of the diaphragm is derived from mesenchyme of the thoracic wall, it is generally accepted that some of the lower intercostal (thoracic) nerves contribute sensory fibers to the peripheral part of the diaphragm.

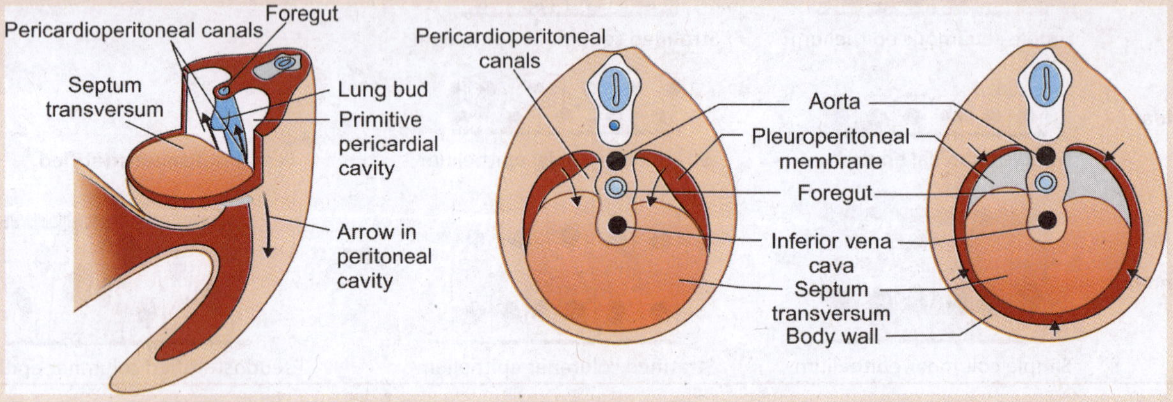

NOTE

- Diaphragm develops during 8th week of fetal life
- Right dome closes first
- Congenital diaphragmatic hernia is a herniation of abdominal contents into the pleural cavity caused by a failure of the pleuroperitoneal membrane to develop or fuse with the other components of the diaphragm.

70. Ans. (d) Persistence of A and obliteration of B

Ref: Langman's Embryology 11th ed page 191, High-Yield Embryology Ronald W. Dudek 4th ed page 41, Embryology for Medical Students By Sudhir Sant 2nd ed page 121, Human Embryology 8 Ed by Singh page 228

The right subclavian artery develops during the 6th to 8th week of gestation. The proximal part originates from the right 4th aortic arch artery and the distal part from the right dorsal and right seventh intersegmental arteries.

In ARSA, the right 4th aortic arch artery and/or the right dorsal aorta which is denoted by B in the picture, involute (obliterate) cranial to the seventh intersegmental artery—the connection between the aortic sac and the right subclavian artery disappears. The right subclavian artery develops from the right 7th intersegmental artery and the distal segment of the right dorsal aorta. Differential growth shifts the origin cranially and lies close to the origin of the left subclavian artery. It originates dorsally and therefore has a retroesophageal course.

Development of the Arterial System

Embryonic structure	Adult structure
	Aortic arches
1st	Maxillary arteries
2nd	Hyoid and stapedial arteries
3rd	Right and left common carotid arteries Right and left first part of internal carotid arteries, i.e. point of bifurcation of internal and external carotids (Remainder of the internal carotid arteries are derived from the dorsal aorta) External carotid artery is a sprout of the third aortic arch
4th left side	Arch of the aorta from the left common carotid to the left subclavian arteries

Contd...

4th right side	Right subclavian artery (proximal portion)
6th left side	Left pulmonary artery and ductus arteriosus
6th right side	Right pulmonary artery
7th intersegmental arteries	The distal portion of the right subclavian artery, as well as the left subclavian artery
	Ventral aorta
Cranial to 3rd arch	External carotid artery (part of)
Between 3rd and 4th arch	Common carotid arteries (part of)
Aortic sac (Between 4th and 6th arch)	Right brachiocephalic artery (on right) Proximal segment of aortic arch (on left)
	Dorsal aorta
Cranial portion	Internal carotid artery
Posterolateral branches	Arteries to upper and lower extremity Intercostal, lumbar and lateral sacral arteries
Lateral branches	Renal, suprarenal and gonadal arteries
Ventral branches — **Vitelline arteries** (paired ventral branches supplying the yolk sac)	Celiac, superior mesenteric and inferior mesenteric arteries
Umbilical arteries (initially paired ventral branches of the dorsal aorta to the placenta, close to allantois)	Proximal portions of the umbilical arteries persist as the internal iliac and superior vesical arteries and the distal parts are obliterated to form the medial umbilical ligaments

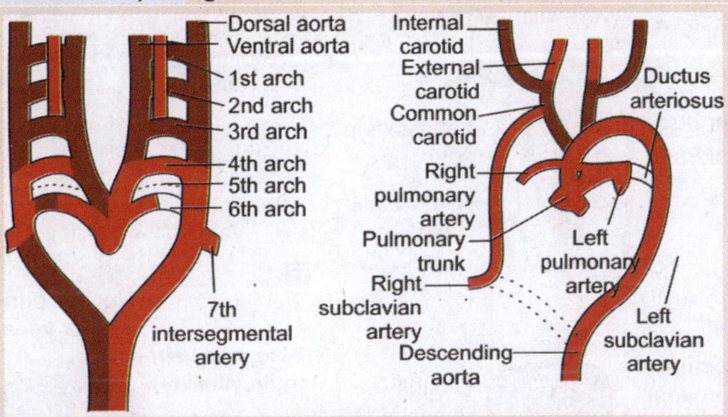

Anomalies of Aortic Arches	
Left aortic arch with retroesophageal right subclavian artery	The incidence of **ARSA** (Aberrant right subclavian artery) varies between **0.4% and 1.8%** of the population and is probably the **most common aortic arch anomaly.** Higher incidence in Down's syndrome with CHD – 38%, mostly asymptomatic 1st arch—no bifurcation, goes to right 2nd, 3rd—no bifurcation, goes to left 4th—towards right, disappear behind trachea **Dysphagia lusoria** is dysphagia secondary to an ARSA (Aberrant right subclavian artery) that has a retroesophageal course. The term "dysphagia lusoria" was coined by Bayford in 1794. **The Adachi Williams Classification** • In about 80% of individuals, three branches arise from the aortic arch: the brachiocephalic trunk, the left subclavian artery and the left common carotid artery. This Adachi described as **Type A** • 11% of individuals have an Adachi **type B** pattern, which consists of a common trunk for the left common carotid and the brachiocephalic artery and therefore has only two aortic arch branches • The next most common **type C**, has a vertebral artery originating proximal to the left subclavian artery as a 4th branch of the arch • The origin of the retroesophageal right subclavian artery as the last branch occurs in between 0.4 and 2% of individuals
Right aortic arch	Loss of Left 6th arch and persistence of right 6th arch
Cervical aortic arch	Persistence of ductus caroticus + involution of 4th arch → 3rd arch becomes aortic arch (int and ext carotid arising separately)
Double aortic arch	Both R and L arches persist Both 4th arches and dorsal aortae persist But usually only one 6th arch (ductus)

71. Ans. (d) D

Ref: High-Yield Embryology Ronald W. Dudek 4th ed page 41, Embryology for Medical Students by Sudhir Sant 2nd ed page 121, Langmann's 11th ed page 193, Human Embryology 8 Ed by Singh page 228

Portal vein develops from left vitelline vein

Key of the picture

A. Cardinal vein
B. Left hepatocardiac channel
C. Hepatic sinusoids
D. Left vitelline vein
E. Left umbilical vein
F. Duodenum
G. Right umbilical vein

Development of the Venous System

Vitelline veins
(The proximal part of the left vitelline vein and distal part of right vitelline vein disappears)

Right vitelline vein	Hepatocardiac/superior/terminal portion of the IVC, superior mesenteric vein
Left vitelline vein	Proximal part disappears The anastomotic network around the duodenum develops into a single vessel, the portal vein

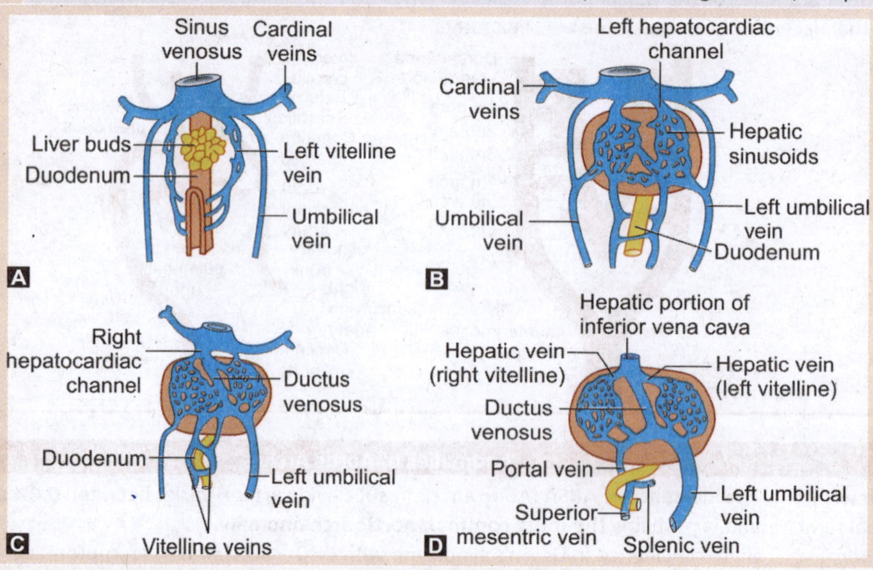

Umbilical veins
(The right umbilical vein and the part of the left between the liver and the sinus venosus degenerate)

Right umbilical vein	Hepatic sinusoids (degenerates early in fetal life)
Left umbilical vein	Hepatic sinusoids Ligamentum teres Communication between the left umbilical vein and the right hepatocardiac channel, the ductus venosus obliterates to form **ligamentum venosum**

Cardinal veins

Common cardinal (Duct of cuvier)	Right	SVC
	Left	Oblique vein of left atrium and coronary sinus
Anterior cardinal	Right	SVC, internal jugular veins
	Left	Vanishes
	Lt-Rt Anastomosis	Left brachiocephalic vein
Posterior cardinal	Right	Lowest portion of IVC Right common iliac vein
	Left	Left common iliac vein

Contd...

Subcardinal	Renal segment of IVC, renal veins, adrenal veins, gonadal veins
Supracardinal	Post renal portion of IVC, intercostal veins, hemiazygos vein, azygos vein

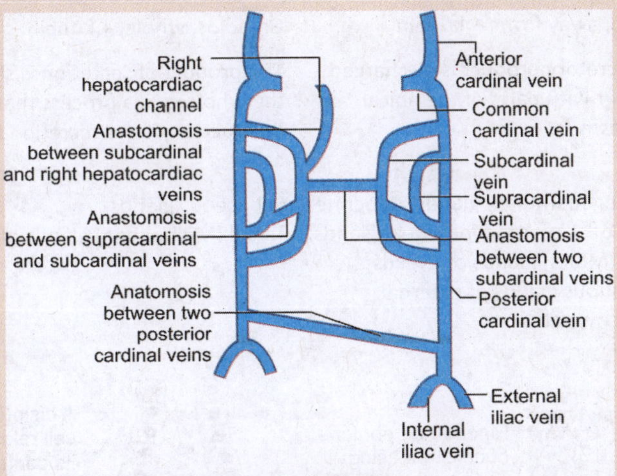

Cardinal veins

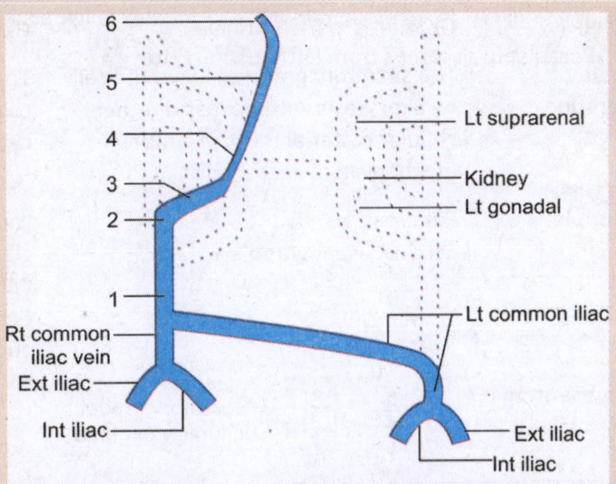

Six segments of IVC (1) part of post. cardinal vein (2) part of Rt supracardinal vein (3) Supracardinal-Subcardinal anastomosis (4) Part of Rt subcardinal vein (5) Rt subcardinal Rt vitelline anastomosis (6) Rt vitelline vein

Abnormal Venous Drainage	
Double IVC	Left supracardinal vein retains connection with left subcardinal vein
Absent IVC	Right subcardinal vein fails to connect to right hepatocardiac segment
Left SVC	Left common cardinal and anterior cardinal veins persists with concomitant loss of right common and right anterior cardinal vein
Double SVC	Left brachiocephalic does not forms, hence entire left common and left anterior cardinal vein persists

72. Ans. (a) Holocrine gland

Ref: Wolfgang Histology 4th ed page 98

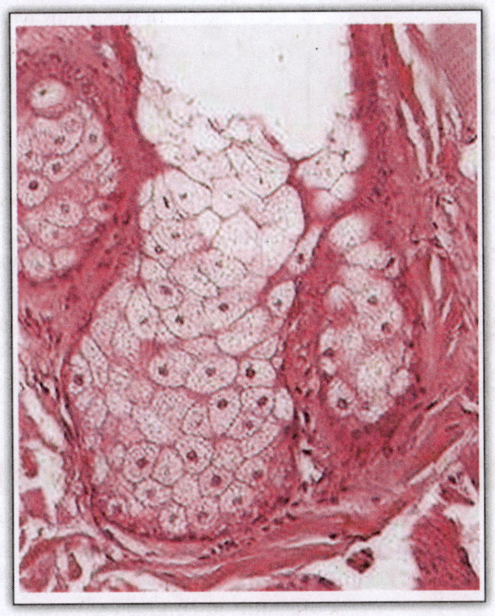

Fig: Holocrine gland: Sebaceous glands are holocrine glands. Their secretion, sebum, is an oily material. In this picture, note the outer cells comparable to the basal layer. As the cells grow they move inwards and accumulate their secretion. The fatty secretion is lost in processing leaving behind a spongy framework of other cytoplasmic elements. The cells are very similar to brown fat cells in appearance. In the deepest part of the gland you can see cells without nuclei disintegrating. The entire cell dies in releasing the sebum. Sebum travels to the surface along a hair shaft.

Classification of Exocrine Glands on the Basis of Mechanism of Secretion	Merocrine	Apocrine	Holocrine
Greek	Gr. meros, part, + krinein	Gr. apo, away from, + krinein	Gr. holos, whole, + krinein
Mode of secretion	The secretory granules leave the cell by exocytosis with no loss of other cellular material most common mechanism of secretion	The secretory product is discharged together with parts of the apical cytoplasm	The product of secretion is shed with the whole cell, a process that involves destruction of the secretion filled cells
Example	Pancreas Eccrine sweat gland	Lactating mammary glands, Apocrine glands of skin, Apocrine sweat glands, Ciliary (Moll's) glands of eyelids Ceruminous glands of external auditory meatus	Sebaceous glands Tarsal (Meibomian) glands of eyelids
Representative diagram	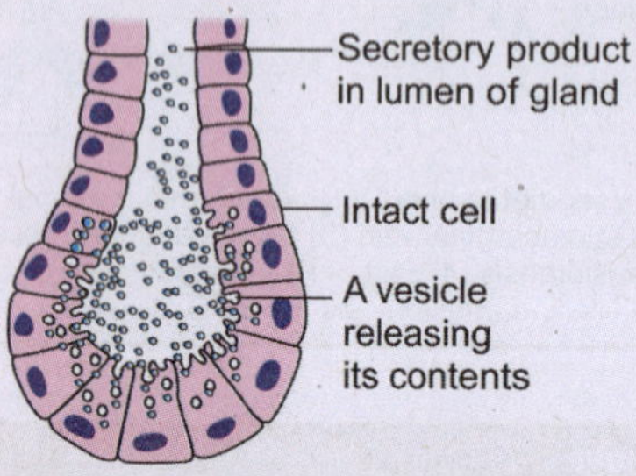 Merocrine gland	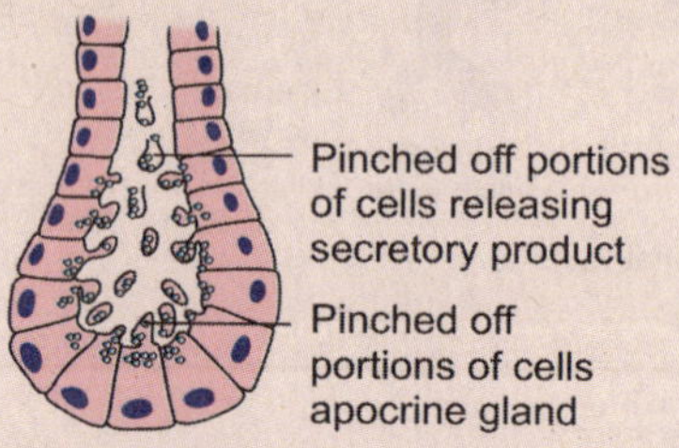 Apocrine gland	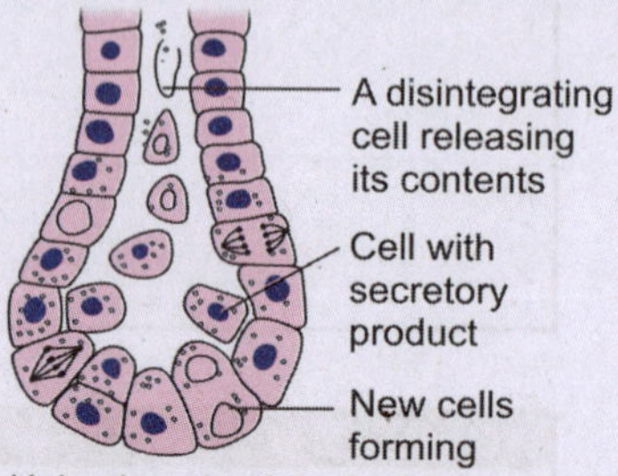 Holocrine gland

Classification of Exocrine Glands

Exocrine glands may be classified according to their structure, secretory product, or mode of secretion.

73. Ans. (b) B

Ref: Sternberg's Diagnostic Surgical Pathology, 5th Edition page 1279

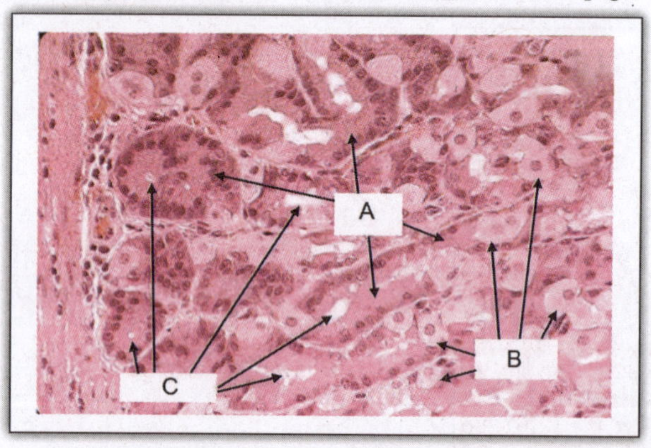

Figure Key: Gastric Mucosa High power

(A) Chief cells

(B) Parietal cells

(C) Glandular lumen

The parietal cells (acid-producing) have a light eosinophilic cytoplasm and the chief cells (enzyme-producing) have a bluish or amphophilic cytoplasm. Generally, chief cells occupy the basal half of the glands whereas parietal cells occupy the superficial half. At the midpoint of the mucosa, the two types of cells gradually mingle

Most of the bulk of the gastric mucosa is occupied by secretory cells of the gastric glands, primarily parietal cells and chief cells, together with lamina propria. In routine sections, the secretory cells often appear rather jumbled together. Sometimes, however, tubular organization is more evident, especially deep in the gastric glands near the muscularis mucosae, as in the figure above. Cells with conspicuous eosinophilic cytoplasm and centrally located nuclei (sometimes paired) are the parietal cells. Cells with basal nuclei, basally basophilic cytoplasm and apical vesicles are the chief cells. The glands are separated by thinner strands of lamina propria, visible as strands of denser, flattened or irregular nuclei.

Gastric Mucosa Cells

Name	Location	Secretion	Appearance
Mucous neck cell	Common to all type of gastric glands specially neck of glands at Fundus and Body	Gastric mucous (Mucin)	Lightly eosinophilic or clear cytoplasm and bubbly PAS positive neutral mucin
Zymogenic, or chief	Gastric glands of body and fundus	Pepsinogen and Gastric lipase	Basophilic cytoplasm due to abundant rough endoplasmic reticulum

Contd...

Parietal (oxyntic) cells		Gastric glands of body and fundus	HCl and Intrinsic factor	Eosinophilic due to abundant mitochondria
Endocrine (APUD) cells	Gastrin cells or G cells (60%)	Antrum only	Gastrin, GABA	Small condensed nucleus with clear cytoplasm
	D cell (20%)	Antrum and Fundus	Somatostatin	
	Enterochromaffin (EC) cells	Antrum and Fundus	Enterostatin, serotonin	
	Enterochromaffin-like (ECL) cells	Fundus only	Histamine	

74. Ans. (a) Tonsil

Ref: Wolfgang 4th ed page 248, 512

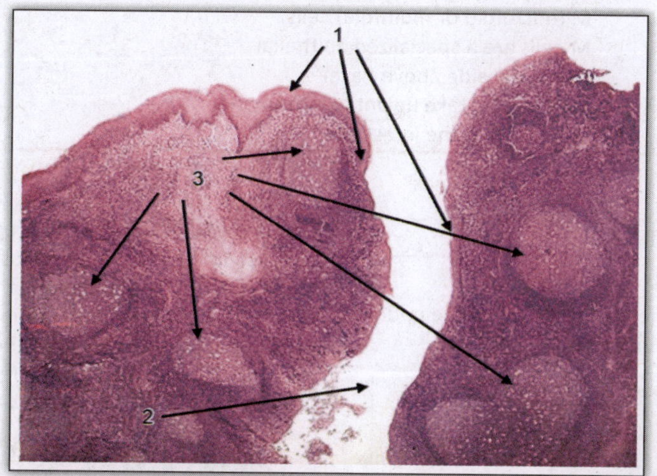

Fig: Tonsil histology: stratified squamous epithelium lining (marked as 1), tonsillar crypt (marked as 2), Lymph nodules (marked as 3)

Lymphatic Organs: Distinctive Morphological Features

Organ	Capsule and connective tissue septa	Parenchyma	Vessels	Other features
Lymph node	Well-developed capsule, clearly visible trabeculae	Lymphoreticular, compact cortex with lymph follicles, lighter medulla with medullary cords	Afferent vessel, marginal sinus, intermediary sinus, medullary sinus, efferent vessel; in the lumina of all sinuses: a bow-net (weir) system of reticular fibers & reticular cells, no blood cells	Surrounded by loosely organized connective tissue and adipose tissue; lymph vessels with valves often exist in the vicinity; no surface epithelium
Spleen	Very well-developed capsule, strong trabeculae	Lymph nodes & lymphoreticular sheaths around the central artery = **white pulp.** The **red pulp** is not part of the lymphatic system	Characteristic blood vessels (laminar vessels, central artery, penicillary arteriolae, splenic sinus with gaps, muscle-free pulp and laminar veins); blood cells in the lumen of the splenic sinus	Single layered flat peritoneal epithelium forms a sheath around the capsule
Tonsils	Well-developed capsule, weak trabeculae (palatine tonsils), Not developed capsule, thin or no trabeculae (Pharyngeal and Lingual tonsil)	Lymphoreticular nodes (lymph follicles) surround 10–15 branched, Narrow epithelial invaginations (fossulae tonsillares with tonsillar crypts)	–	–
Thymus	Well-developed capsule, partitioning into lobes by connective tissue septa	Lymphoepithelial; no lymph follicles; denser cortex, more loosely organized medulla with interspersed lymphocytes; epithelial **Hassall bodies** in the medulla	–	Involution after puberty; adipose tissue Gradually replaces the parenchyma; in senescence: adipose tissue with parenchyma islets

Contd...

Lymphatic Organs: Distinctive Morphological Features				
Organ	Capsule and connective tissue septa	Parenchyma	Vessels	Other features
Peyer's patches	No capsule or connective tissue septa	The patches are regions of concentrated B lymphocyte follicles covered in a 'dome' of a specialized follicle associated epithelium (FAE) which consists of follicle associated enterocytes and M (microfold or multifold) cells. M-cells are a specialized epithelial cell that reside above Peyer's patches and take up antigen from the lumen of the intestine		Peyer's patches are lymphoid tissues found in the wall of the small intestine. They are part of the mucosal associated lymphoid tissues (MALT) and more specifically gut associated lymphoid tissue (GALT)

75. Ans. (c) Epiphyseal growth plates

Ref: Ross's Histology 6th Ed page 206

The picture shown is of hyaline cartilage. Out of the options provided only epiphysis is hyaline cartilage.

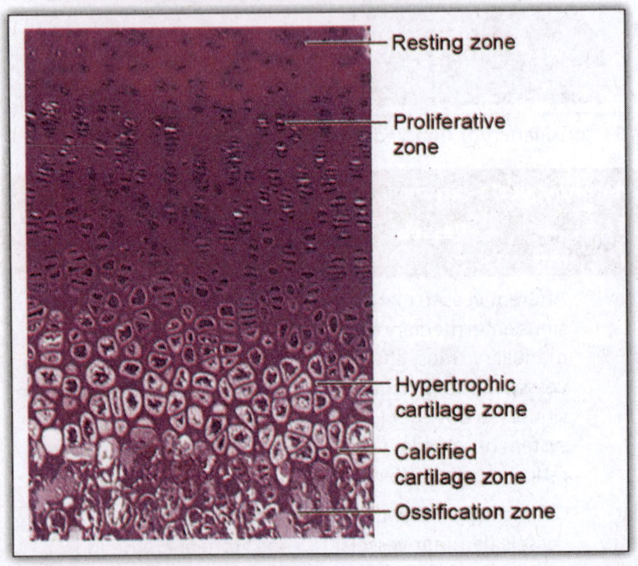

Fig: Hyaline Cartilage (Low Power; Epiphysis): Meta-epiphyseal cartilage is divided into five zones, starting from the epiphyseal side of cartilage: (1) The resting zone consists of hyaline cartilage without morphologic changes in the cells. (2) In the proliferative zone (columnar), chondrocytes divide rapidly and form columns of stacked cells parallel to the long axis of the bone. (3) The hypertrophic cartilage zone contains large chondrocytes whose cytoplasm has accumulated glycogen. The resorted matrix is reduced to thin septa between the chondrocytes. (4) Simultaneous with the death of chondrocytes in the calcified cartilage zone, the thin septa of cartilage matrix become calcified by the deposit of hydroxyapatite. (5) In the ossification zone, endochondral bone tissue appears. Blood capillaries and osteoprogenitor cells formed by mitosis of cells originating from the periosteum invade the cavities left by the chondrocytes. The osteoprogenitor cells form osteoblasts, which are distributed in a discontinuous layer over the septa of calcified cartilage matrix. Ultimately, the osteoblasts deposit bone matrix over the three-dimensional calcified cartilage matrix.

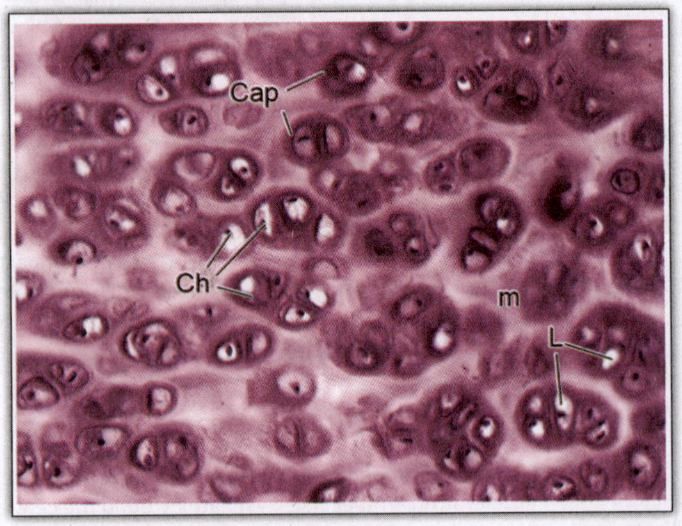

Fig: Hyaline cartilage (high power): The word hyaline is derived from the Greek word "hyalos" which means glass. Enzymatic digestion of the ground substances in the cartilage matrix can unmask the collagen fibrils and render them visible. Cap = capsule, Ch = chondrocytes, L = lacuna, m = avascular matrix.

76. Ans. (d) 4

Ref: Grays 41st ed page 571, BDC 5th ed page 242

Posterior cricoarytenoid muscle denoted by arrow 4, is an abductor of vocal cord.

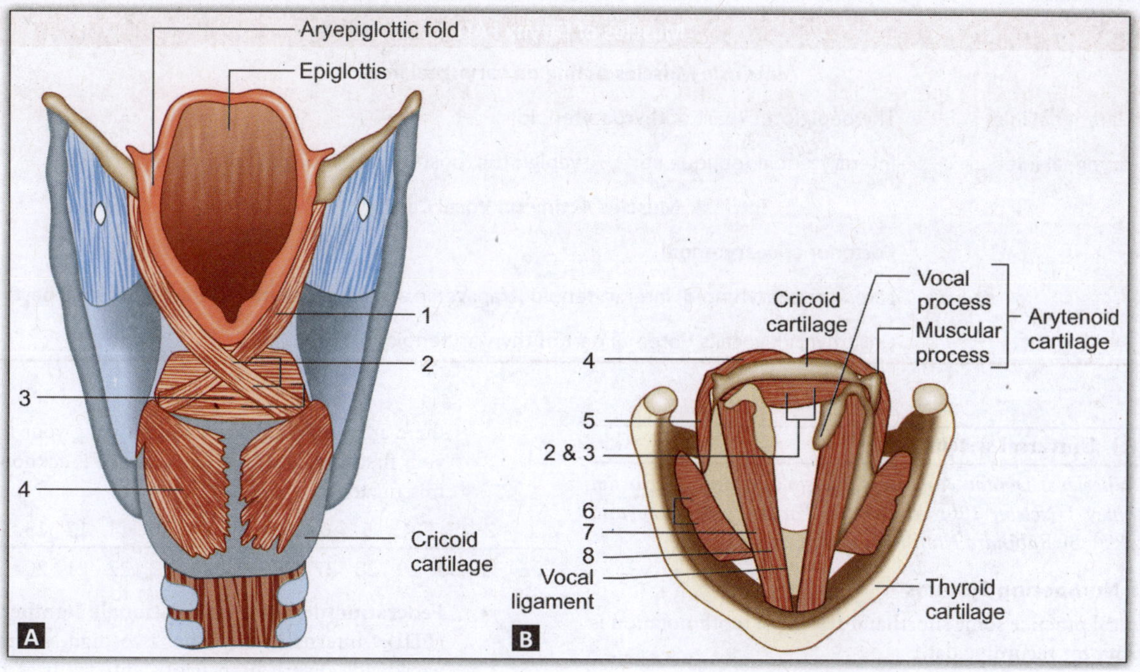

Fig: Intrinsic muscles of larynx (Posterior view and internal view)

1. Aryepiglottic muscle
2. Oblique arytenoid muscle
3. Transverse arytenoid muscle
4. Posterior cricoarytenoid muscle
5. Lateral cricoarytenoid muscle
6. Cricothyroid muscle
7. Thyroarytenoid muscle
8. Vocalis muscle

Muscles of Larynx				
Muscle	**Origin**	**Insertion**	**Innervation**	**Main action(s)**
Cricothyroid	Anterolateral part of cricoid cartilage	Inferior margin and inferior horn of thyroid cartilage	External branch of superior laryngeal nerve (CN X)	Tenses vocal fold
Posterior cricoarytenoid	Posterior surface of laminae of cricoid cartilage	Muscular process of arytenoid cartilage	Recurrent laryngeal nerve (CN X)	Abducts vocal fold
Lateral cricoarytenoid	Arch of cricoid cartilage			Adducts vocal fold
Thyroarytenoid[a]	Posterior surface of thyroid cartilage			Relaxes vocal fold
Transverse and oblique arytenoids[b]	One arytenoid cartilage	Opposite arytenoid cartilage		Close inlet of larynx by approximating arytenoid cartilages
Vocalis[c]	Angle between laminae of thyroid cartilage	Vocal ligament, between origin and vocal process of arytenoid cartilage		Alters vocal fold during phonation

[a] Superior fibers of the thyroarytenoid muscle pass into the aryepiglottic fold and some of them reach the epiglottic cartilage. These fibers constitute the **thyroepiglottic muscle**, which widens the inlet of the larynx.
[b] Some fibers of the oblique arytenoid muscle continue as the aryepiglottic muscle.
[c] This slender muscular slip is derived from inferior ***deeper fibers of the thyroarytenoid musc***le.

Muscles of Larynx FAQ	
Intrinsic Muscles Acting on Laryngeal Inlet	
Openers of laryngeal inlet	Thyroepiglottic (part of thyroarytenoid)
Closers of laryngeal inlet	Interarytenoid (oblique part), Aryepiglottic (posterior oblique part of interarytenoids)
Intrinsic Muscles Acting on Vocal Cords	
Abductors	Posterior cricoarytenoid
Adductors	Lateral cricoarytenoid, interarytenoid (transverse arytenoid) thyroarytenoid (external part)
Tensors	Cricothyroid, vocalis (internal part of thyroarytenoid)

77. Ans. (c) Universal system

Ref: Wheeler's Dental Anatomy, Physiology and Occlusion by Stanley J Nelson 10th ed Page 4, Forensic Medicine and Toxicology By Rabindra Nath Karmakar 5th ed page 10

Tooth Numbering Systems

In clinical practice some shorthand system of tooth notation is necessary for recording data.

- **Zsigmondy/palmer notation:** The symbolic system of permanent dentition was introduced by Adolf Zsigmondy of Vienna in 1861 and then modified for the primary dentition in 1874. Independently Ohio dentist Dr. Corydon Palmer also published the symbolic system in 1870. The symbolic system is most often referred to as Palmer notation and less often as Zsigmondy/palmer notation. In this system, the arches are divided into quadrants, with entire dentition being noted as:

EDCBA	ABCDE
EDCBA	ABCDE

  Thus for single tooth such as maxillary central incisor the designation is A. Hence, this numbering system presents difficulty when appropriate font is not available for Keyboard recording.

- **Universal system:** Number 1 is the tooth farthest back on the right side of your mouth in the upper (maxillary) jaw. Numbering continues along your upper teeth toward the front and across to the tooth farthest back on the top left side number 16. The numbers continue by dropping down to the lower (mandibular) jaw. Number 17 is the tooth farthest back on the left side of your mouth on the bottom. Numbering continues again toward the front and across to the tooth farthest back on the bottom right side of you mouth number 32. In this system, the teeth that should be there are numbered. If you are missing your third molars, your first number will be 2 instead of 1, acknowledging the missing tooth.

1	2	3	4	5	6	7	8	9	10	11	12	13	14	15	16
32	31	30	29	28	27	26	25	24	23	22	21	20	19	18	17

- **Federation dentaire internationale numbering system (FDI):** Internationally the two-digit system is used worldwide. Every branch of dentistry uses this system. Each quadrant is assigned a number. The maxillary right quadrant is assigned the number 1, the maxillary left quadrant is assigned the number 2, the mandibular left quadrant is assigned the number 3 and the mandibular right quadrant is assigned the number 4.The teeth within each quadrant are assigned a number from 1 through 8 with 1 being the central incisor and 8 being the third molar. It is important to note that 11 is not pronounced as Eleven but One.

For the permanent teeth:

Upper right								Upper left							
18	17	16	15	14	13	12	11	21	22	23	24	25	26	27	28
48	47	46	45	44	43	42	41	31	32	33	34	35	36	37	38
Lower right								Lower left							

For the permanent teeth

Upper right					Upper left				
55	54	53	52	51	61	62	63	64	65
85	84	83	82	81	71	72	73	74	75
Lower right					Lower left				

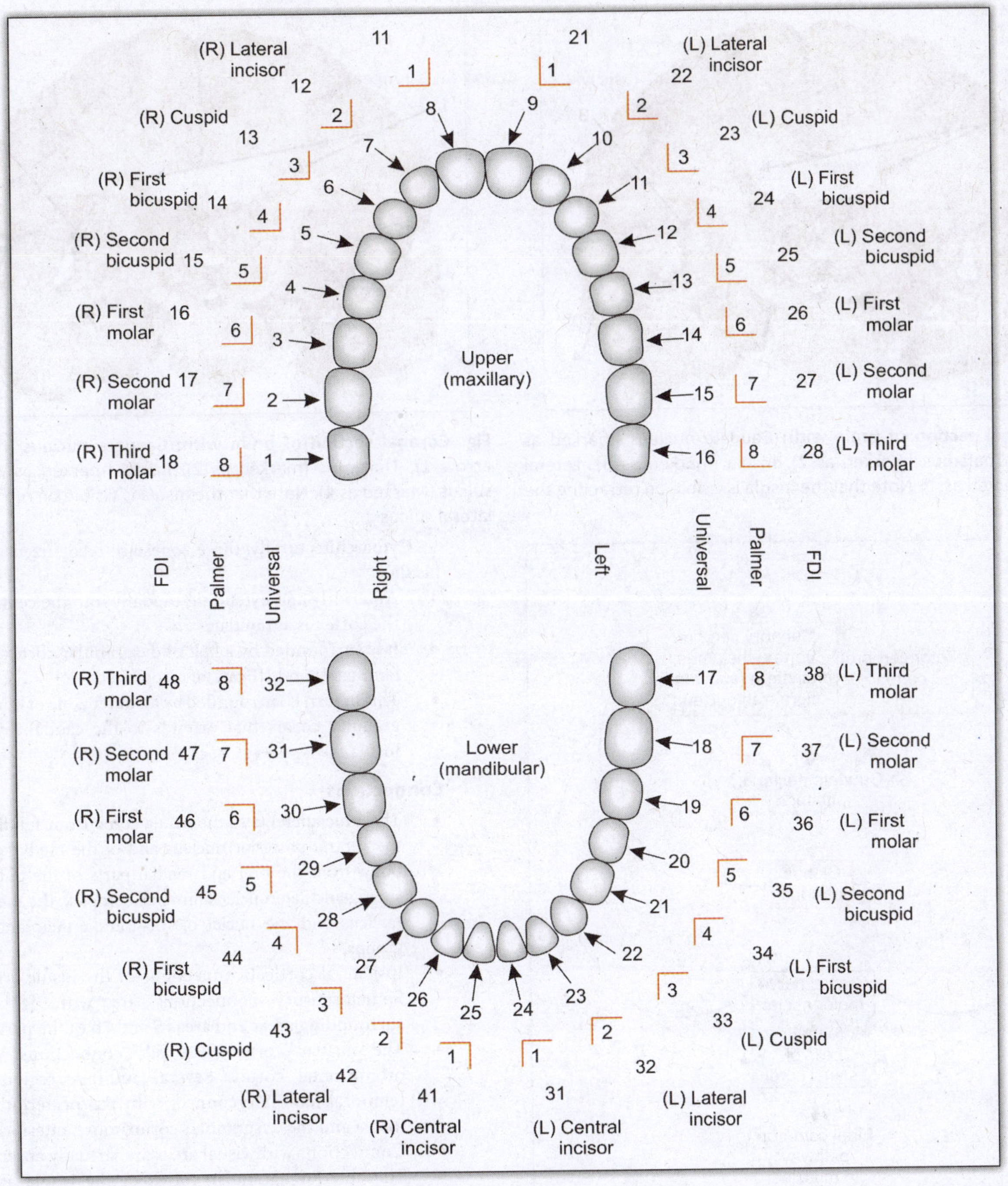

78. Ans. (b) Spinal cord

Ref: Gray's 41st ed page 230, Snell's Clinical Neuroanatomy 7th ed figure 10-2. BDC 5th ed page 417

Marked area is caudate nucleus of basal ganglia. Afferent and efferent connections are shown in the diagrammatic representation below:

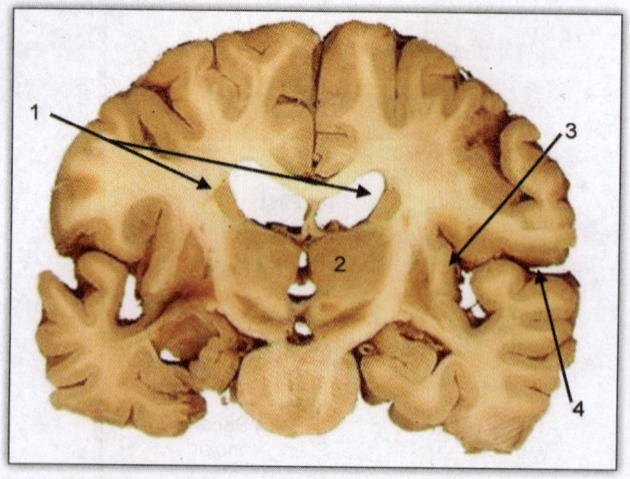

Fig: Coronal section of brain with: Caudate nucleus (marked as arrow 1), Thalamus (marked as 2), Insula (marked as 3), Lateral sulcus (Marked as 4). Note that the Insula is visible on retracting the lateral sulcus.

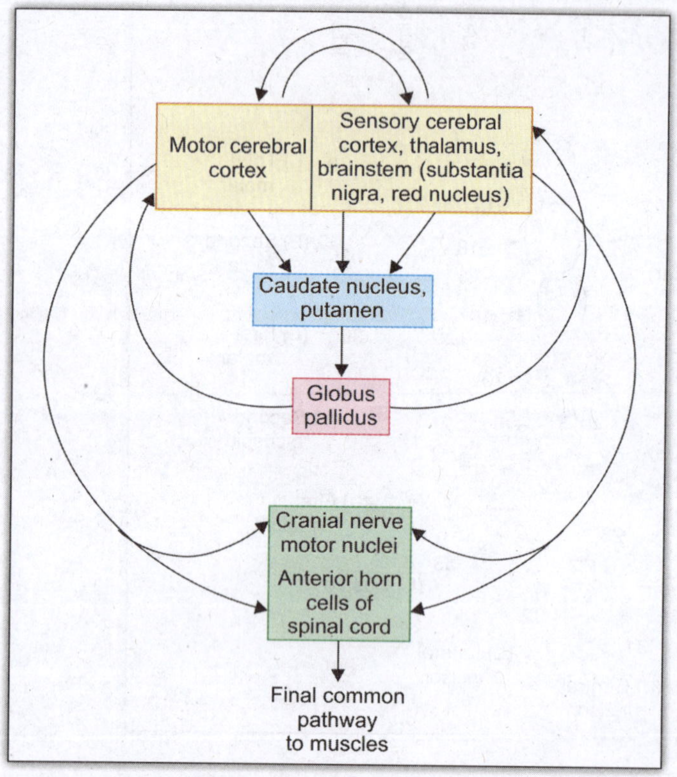

79. Ans. (c) 3

Ref: Grays 41st ed page 383

The insula forms the base of the sylvian cistern and lies between the frontal and temporal lobes.

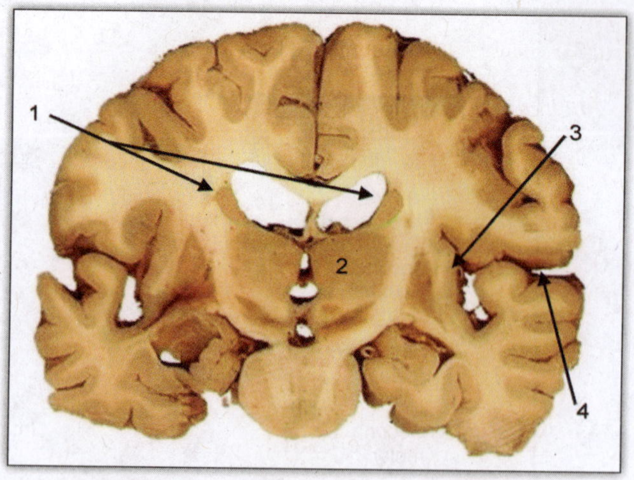

Fig: Coronal section of brain with: Caudate nucleus (marked as arrow 1), Thalamus (marked as 2), Insula (marked as 3), Lateral sulcus (Marked as 4). Note that the Insula is visible on retracting the lateral sulcus.

Cytoarchitecturally, three zones are recognized within the insula.

- Anteriorly and extending caudally into the central insula, the cortex is agranular.
- It is surrounded by a belt of dysgranular cortex, in which laminae II and III can be recognized
- This in turn is surrounded by an outer zone of homotypical granular cortex that extends to the caudal limit of the insula.

Connections

- Thalamic afferents to the insula come from subdivisions of the ventral posterior nucleus and of the medial geniculate body, from the oral and medial parts of the pulvinar, the suprageniculate/nucleus limitans complex, the mediodorsal nucleus and the nuclei of the intralaminar and midline groups.
- Ipsilateral cortical connections of the insula are diverse. Somatosensory connections are with SI, SII and surrounding areas and areas 5 and 7b of the parietal lobe.
- The insular cortex also has connections with the orbitofrontal cortex. Several auditory regions in the temporal lobe interconnect with the posterior granular insula and the dysgranular cortex more anteriorly.
- Connections with visual areas are virtually absent.
- The anterior agranular cortex of the insula appears to have connections primarily with olfactory, limbic and paralimbic structures, including, most prominently, the amygdala.
- The insula receives somatosensory, viscerosensory, homeostatic and nociceptive information from the entire body.

80. Ans. (a) Posterior communicating artery

Ref: Gray's 41st ed page 285, BDC 5th ed page 446, Grant's Atlas 12th ed page 647, High Yield Neuroanatomy by James D Fix 4th ed page 38

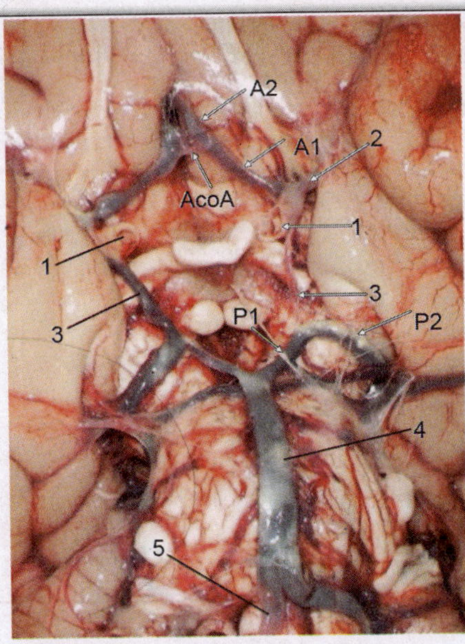

Fig: This image shows a normal cerebral arterial circle of Willis

1 = Internal carotid artery (cut lumen)
2 = Middle cerebral artery
3 = Posterior communicating artery
4 = Basilar artery
5 = Vertebral artery
A1 = A1 segment of anterior cerebral artery
A2 = A2 segment of anterior cerebral artery
P1 = P1 segment of posterior cerebral artery
P2 = P2 segment of posterior cerebral artery

At 16 weeks' gestation, the anterior, middle and posterior cerebral arteries that contribute to the formation of the **circle of Willis** are well established. The posterior communicating artery originates from the cerebral part of the internal carotid artery and courses caudally to join the posterior cerebral artery (PCA). The part of the PCA medial to this intersection is the P1 segment and the part of the PCA immediately lateral to this junction is the P2 segment. The posterior communicating artery irrigates the hypothalamus and ventral thalamus. An aneurysm of this artery is the second most common aneurysm of the circle of Willis. It commonly results in third-nerve palsy. The posterior cerebral artery is connected to the carotid artery through the posterior communicating artery.

Arterial Supply to Brain

Artery	Origin	Distribution
Vertebral	Subclavian artery	Cranial meninges and cerebellum
Posterior inferior cerebellar	Vertebral artery	Posteroinferior aspect of cerebellum
Basilar	Formed by junction of vertebral arteries	Brainstem, cerebellum and cerebrum
Pontine	Basilar artery	Numerous branches to brainstem
Anterior inferior cerebellar		Inferior aspect of cerebellum
Superior cerebellar		Superior aspect of cerebellum
Internal carotid	Common carotid artery at superior border of thyroid cartilage	Gives branches in cavernous sinus and provides supply to brain
Anterior cerebral	Internal carotid artery	Cerebral hemispheres, except for occipital lobes
Middle cerebral	Continuation of the internal carotid artery distal to anterior cerebral artery	Most of lateral surface of cerebral hemispheres
Posterior cerebral	Terminal branch of basilar artery	Inferior aspect of cerebral hemisphere and occipital lobe
Anterior communicating	Anterior cerebral artery	Cerebral arterial circle
Posterior communicating	Internal carotid artery	

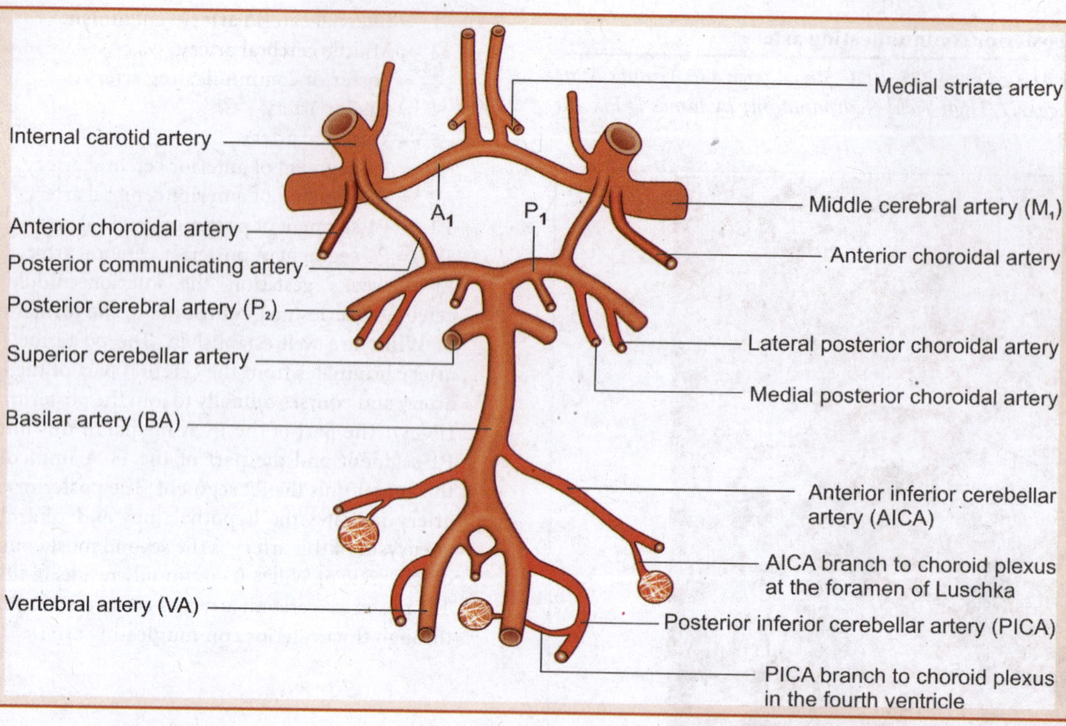

81. Ans. (a) A

Ref: Grays 41st ed page 970, Grant's Atlas of Anatomy 12th Ed page 758

Phrenic Nerve in Neck

Muscular (deep) branches of cervical plexus distribute to several groups of muscles. A major branch is the phrenic nerve, which supplies the diaphragm with both sensory and motor innervation. It arises from the anterior rami of cervical nerves C3 to C5. Hooking around the upper lateral border of the anterior scalene within the prevertebral fascia to enter the thorax. As the nerve descends in the neck, it is pinned to the anterior scalene muscle by the transverse cervical and suprascapular arteries.

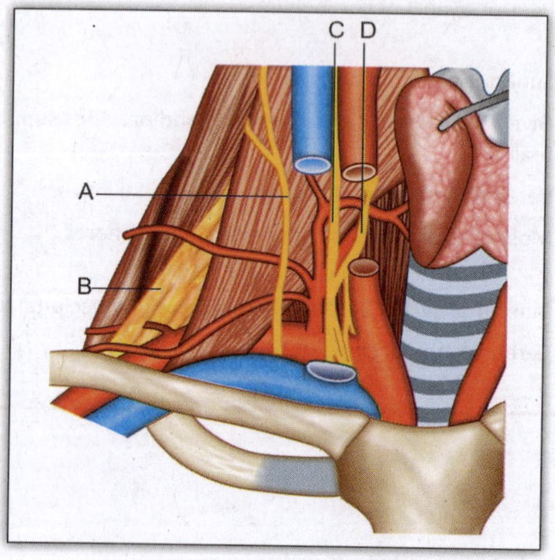

Fig: Legends: A = Phrenic nerve; B = Brachial plexus; C = Vagus nerve; D = Sympathetic trunk

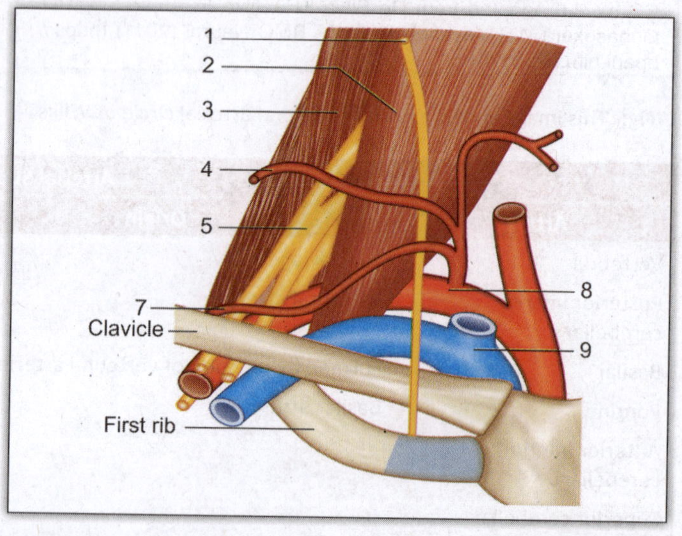

Fig: Legend: 1. Phrenic nerve; 2. Scalenus anterior; 3. Scalenus medius; 4. Transverse cervical artery; 5. Brachial plexus; 7. Suprascapular artery; 8. Thyrocervical trunk originating from the subclavian artery; 9. Subclavian vein

82. Ans. (b) Cervical part drains directly into brachiocephalic vein

Ref: Gray's 41st edition page 1111, Snell's Clinical Anatomy 9th ed page 185

Blood from the esophagus drains into a **submucous plexus** and thence into a perioesophageal venous plexus from which oesophageal veins arise.

- Those from the upper/cervical esophagus drain into the brachiocephalic or inferior thyroid veins
- Those from the middle/thoracic esophagus drain predominantly into the azygos veins and, to a lesser extent, the hemiazygos, intercostal and bronchial veins.

- Those from the lower end it goes to the left gastric vein. The lower end of the esophagus is one of the sites of portosystemic anastomoses.

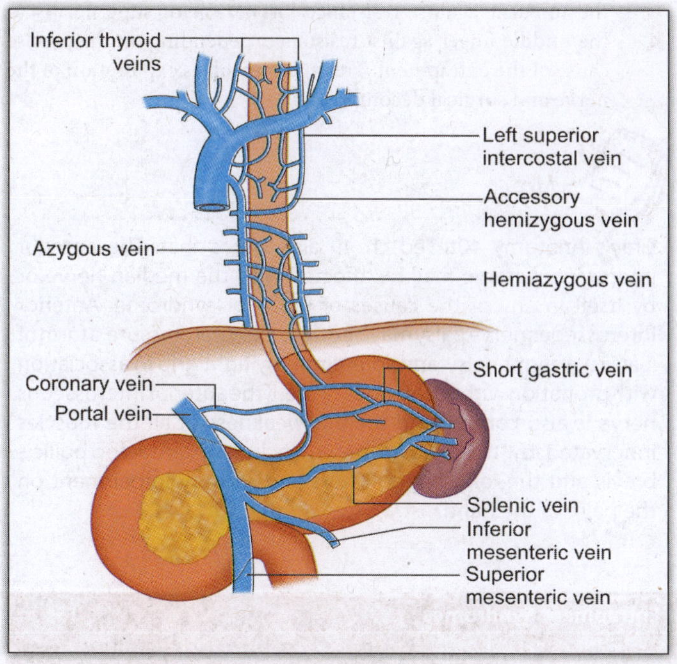

83. Ans. (a) Greater auricular nerve

Ref: With text

Gray's 41st ed page 407

The upper four cervical ventral rami form the cervical plexus, whose branches collectively innervate the infrahyoid strap muscles and the diaphragm and the skin covering the lateral and anterior parts of the neck and the angle of the mandible.

Gray's 41st ed page 413

The dermatomes of the face arise mainly from cutaneous branches of the three major divisions of the trigeminal nerve. The skin covering the front and sides of the neck and over the angle of the mandible and over the lateral scalp and posterior aspect of the pinna is supplied by branches of the cervical plexus (C_2–C_4) and the skin over the back of the head is supplied by the greater occipital nerve (C_2, posterior primary ramus)

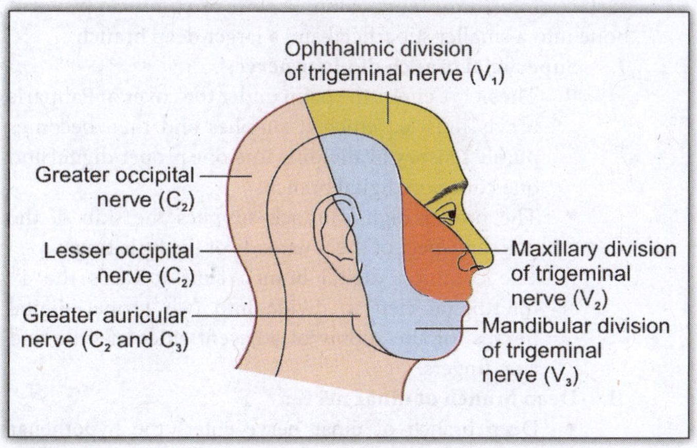

AIIMS NOVEMBER 2015

84. Ans. (c) Greater auricular nerve

Ref: Gray's 41st ed page 627

Nerve supply of Pinna

- **Auriculotemporal nerve** supplies the anterior upper part of the auricle and the adjacent temporal skin, it is a branch of the trigeminal mandibular.
- **Lesser occipital nerve** supplies the posterior upper part of the auricle and the adjacent cranial surface, it originates from C_2 spinal nerves.
- **Greater auricular nerve** supplies the lower half anteriorly and posteriorly, it originates from C_2, C_3 spinal nerves.
- External auditory meatus is supplied by the auriculotemporal nerve anteriorly and the auricular branch of the vagus posteriorly.

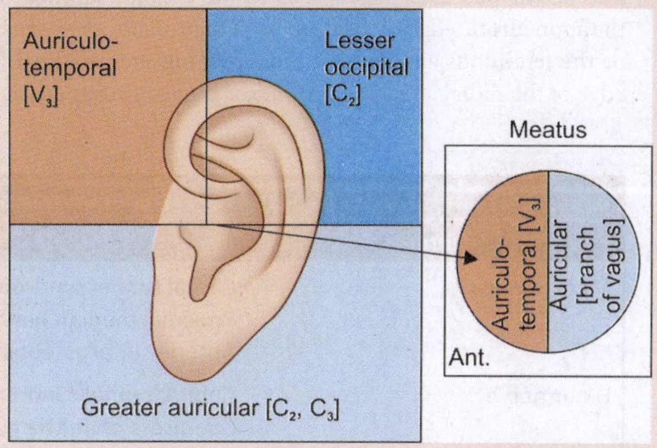

85. Ans. (a) Plasma membrane does not have dendrites and its smooth

Ref: IB Singh Histology 7th ed page 90, Ross's Histology 6th ed page 225

Option (A)

Osteoblasts have irregular shapes. They are branched and may contain as many as 50 or more nuclei. Numerous slender cytoplasmic processes radiate from each cell and come into contact with similar processes of neighboring cells.

Option (B)

Bone morphogenic protein (BMP) 7 has major role in osteoblast differentiation, osteocytes formation and fracture healing. BMP 12 is also known is cartilage derived morphogenic protein (CDMP) 3 has role in tendon and ligament formation.

Option (C)

Neuropeptide VIP receptors have been found in osteoblasts and neuropeptide SP receptors found in osteoclasts.

Option (D)

Osteoblasts also contain prominent bundles of actin, myosin and cytoskeletal proteins which are associated with maintenance of cell shape, attachment and motility.

The bone matrix proteins produced by the osteoblast include calcium-binding proteins such as **osteocalcin and osteonectin**;

multiadhesive glycoproteins such as bone sialoproteins I and II, osteopontin and throsbospondin, various proteoglycans and their aggregates and alkaline phosphatase (ALP). Circulating levels of ALP and osteocalcin are used clinically as markers of osteoblast activity.

86. Ans. (a) Median nerve >> (D) Anterior interosseous nerve

Ref: Gray's 41st ed page 784-86

Pronator Syndrome

This is an uncommon entrapment neuropathy of the ***median nerve*** occurring in the elbow region. Entrapment can occur typically at four sites. The first occurs at the site of the ***ligament of Struthers***. This ligament represents an anatomical variant and when present connects a small supracondylar spur of bone to an accessory origin of pronator teres. *The median nerve can be compressed as it passes under this ligament.* The nerve may also be trapped as it passes deep to the bicipital aponeurosis; the aponeurotic edge of the deep head of pronator teres muscle; or the tendinous aponeurotic arch forming the proximal free edge of the radial attachment of flexor digitorum superficialis.

The syndrome presents with pain on the volar aspect of the distal arm and proximal forearm. The symptoms may be aggravated by flexing the elbow against resistance, pronating the forearm against resistance, or flexion of superficialis to the middle finger against resistance, depending on the precise cause of the entrapment. Treatment involves exploration of the nerve and surgical decompression.

NOTE

Gray's Anatomy 40th ed ch 49 also states that: The anterior interosseous nerve may be affected with the median nerve or by itself in any of the causes of Pronator syndrome. Anterior interosseous nerve palsy may be due to external pressure, a form of 'Saturday night palsy' and sometimes by tight grip in association with pronation without obvious cause. If the anterior interosseous nerve is also compressed there is weakness of all the muscles innervated by the median nerve, including abductor pollicis brevis and the long finger flexors and sensory impairment on the palm of the hand.

Nerve Compression or Entrapment Syndromes

Nerve	Syndrome
Median nerve	Carpal tunnel syndrome (most common) Proximal median nerve compression (Pronator syndrome) Anterior interosseous compression syndrome
Ulnar nerve	Cubital tunnel syndrome Compression in the guyon's canal
Radial nerve	Posterior interosseous nerve compression Radial tunnel syndrome or resistant tennis elbow syndrome
Supraclavicular nerve	Supraclavicular nerve compression syndrome
Lateral cutaneous nerve of thigh	Meralgia paresthetica
Posterior tibial nerve	Tarsal tunnel syndrome
Lower limb digital nerves	Morton's metatarsalgia
Structures of neck	Thoracic outlet syndrome

87. Ans. (a) Ulnar nerve

Ref: Gray's 41th ed page 784, 866, BDC 5th Vol 1 page 55, Clinical Anatomy for Students: Problem Solving Approach by Neeta V. Kulkarni page 97

The given case is of Ulnar claw hand; also known as intrinsic minus hand.

Motor Branches of Ulnar Nerve

Branches in the forearm: In the anterior forearm, the muscular branch of the ulnar nerve supplies two muscles. The remaining muscles in the anterior forearm are innervated by the median nerve.

- Flexor carpi ulnaris – Flexes and adducts the hand at the wrist.
- Flexor digitorum profundus (medial half) – Flexes the fingers.

Branches in the Palm: Ulnar nerve terminates on the anterior surface of the flexor retinaculum in close proximity to pisiform bone into a smaller superficial and a larger deep branch.

I. Superficial branch of ulnar nerve:

- The nerve enters the palm under the cover of Palmaris brevis muscle, which it supplies and then becomes purely sensory by dividing into one proper digital and one common digital branch.
- The proper digital branch supplies the skin of the palmar aspect of the ulnar side of the little finger
- The common digital branch runs towards the 4th interdigital cleft to divide into two proper digital nerves for the supply of adjacent sides of little and ring fingers.

II. Deep branch of ulnar nerve:

- Deep branch of ulnar nerve enters the hypothenar compartment of the palm where it gives motor twigs to

1. Abductor digiti minimi
2. Flexor digiti minimi
3. Opponens digiti minimi

- The nerve turns laterally on the hook of hamate and croses the palm where it supplies

1. All interossei
2. Medial 2 lumbricals
3. Deep head of flexor pollicis brevis
4. Adductor pollicis (terminal)

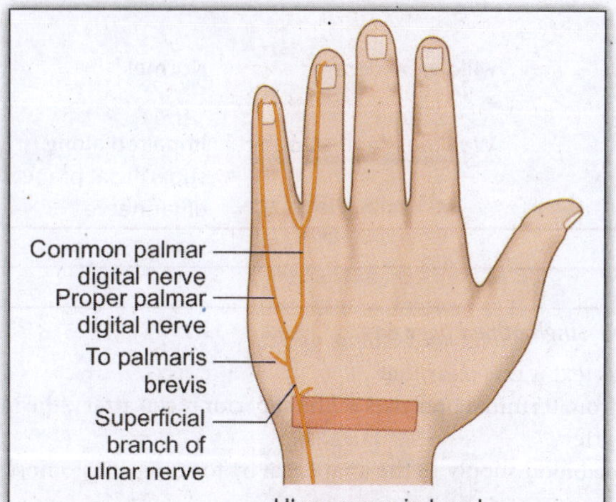

Ulnar nerve in hand

Sensory Branches of Ulnar Nerve

- **Superficial cutaneous branch:** Innervates the palmar surface of the medial one and a half fingers.
- **Deep cutaneous branches:** The palmar and dorsal cutaneous sensory branches leave the ulnar nerve within the lower forearm.
  - **Palmar cutaneous branch:** Innervates the skin of the medial half of the palm.
  - **Dorsal cutaneous branch:** Innervates the skin of the medial 1 and 1/2 fingers and the associated palm area.

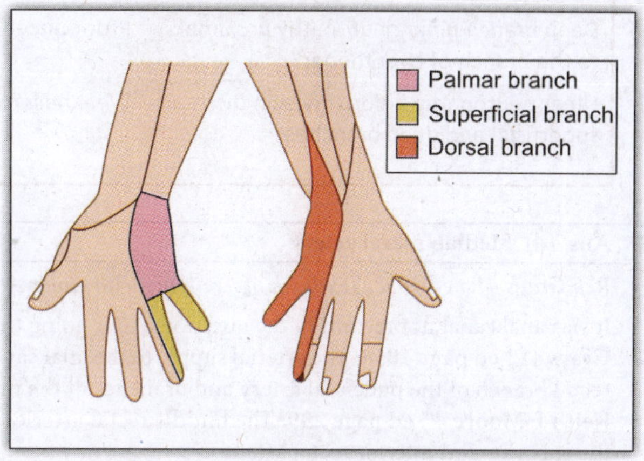

Ulnar (C_8, T_1) at elbow	**"Ulnar Claw hand" (AKA 'intrinsic minus' hand)**- Loss of flexion/hyperextension of 4th and 5th MCP joints and loss of extension (i.e. Flexion) of IP joints. Due to paralysis of palmar and dorsal interossei and medial 2 lumbricals. Typical presentation at rest. Wasted hypothenar eminence and loss of adduction of thumb. Similar to the hand of benediction except that ulnar claw is seen at rest while benediction hand is seen while trying to make fist 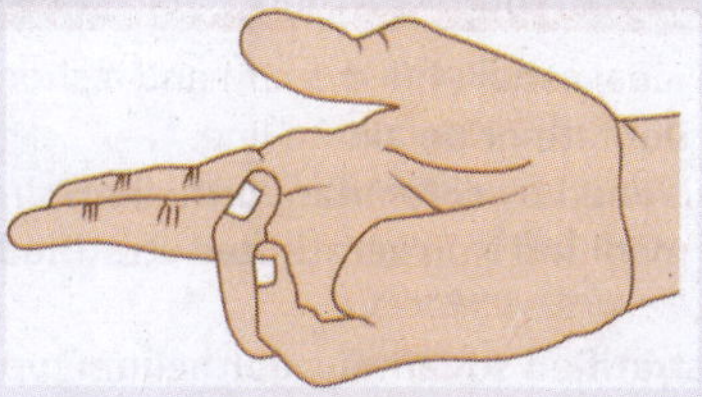 **Ulnar paradox:** In lesion of the ulnar nerve at the elbow, in addition to the muscles of the hand medial half of flexor digitorum profundus (FDP) and flexor carpi ulnaris are also paralyzed. The ulnar claw will develop as before, but with one key difference. There will not be any flexion of the ring and little fingers. Now the ulnar claw only consists of hyperextension at the MCP joints, giving a less evident claw hand. This is known as the 'ulnar paradox'. The worse injury, lesion at elbow, looks less serious than a lesion at the wrist. Ulnar nerve injury of elbow is more prominent when patient is asked to make a fist.	Sensory supply = Ulnar and dorsal aspect of palm and of ulnar 1½ digits
Ulnar (C_8, T_1) at wrist	**"Ulnar Claw hand" (AKA 'intrinsic minus' hand)**- Loss of flexion/hyperextension of 4th and 5th MCP joints and loss of extension (i.e. Flexion) of IP joints. Due to paralysis of palmar and dorsal interossei and medial 2 lumbricals. Typical presentation at rest. Wasted hypothenar eminence and loss of adduction of thumb. Unlike ulnar nerve injury at elbow, the FDP is spared and hence clawing is more prominent **NOTE** Dupuytren's contracture: This typically involves the little and ring fingers and can mimic a claw hand, but the metacarpophalangeal joint is flexed and the contracted fingers cannot passively be extended. Palpation of the Dupuytren's tissue in the palm confirms the diagnosis.	

Contd...

Combined median and ulnar nerve palsy at wrist	**Full claw hand** with thenar and hypothenar flattening and thumb adduction and flexion. **[AKA- Simian hand or Ape Hand (true)]**	Palm and digits

Lower Ulnar Nerve Neuropathy			
Location	**Lumbricals and interossei**	**Hypothenar muscles**	**Sensation**
Deep branch ulnar neuropathy distal to the branch of hypothenar	Weakness	No weakness	Normal
Deep branch ulnar neuropathy proximal to the branch of hypothenar	Pronounced weakness	Mild weakness	Normal
Ulnar neuropathy before division of superficial and deep branches	Weakness	Weakness and atrophy	Impaired along superificial branch of ulnar nerve

88. Ans. (d) Median sacral artery

Ref: Gray's 41st ed 1058, Textbook of Anatomy with Color Atlas by Inderbir Singh 4th ed page 644

It was anal canal not rectum in the question. After going through various text it was clear that

Grays 41th ed page 1058: The arterial supply to the anal canal is derived from terminal branches of the superior rectal artery, the inferior rectal branch of the pudendal artery and branches of the median sacral artery.

Keith L Moore 4th ed page 259: The middle rectal arteries assist with the blood supply to the anal canal by forming anastomoses with the superior and inferior rectal arteries.

From the references above, the answer is not clear as all 4 are involved in blood supply of anal canal, however on reading following reference it will be clear that median sacral artery is only involved occasionally, hence is the answer of choice.

Manual of Total Mesorectal Excision edited by Brendan Moran, Richard John Heald CRS Press 2013 page 40; Blood Supply of the Rectum and Anal Canal: As the rectum derives from the hindgut, the rectum, including the upper anal canal, is supplied mainly by the inferior mesenteric artery via the superior rectal artery. The middle and inferior rectal arteries originate from the internal iliac vessels and contribute to the blood supply of the lower anal canal and minor parts of the rectum via intramural anastomoses. Occasionally, the posterior part of the anal canal and internal anal sphincter are additionally supplied by the median sacral artery.

Anal Canal

The literature describes a longer "surgical" anal canal (4.0–4.5 cm) and a shorter "anatomical" or "embryological" canal. Anatomists the distinction is made by the Dentate or pectinate line.

- **The proximal 1.5 cm of the anal canal** is lined by **columnar epithelium** similar to that of rectum
- The **middle 1.5 cm (pecten)** is lined by modified Non **keratinized stratified squamous epithelium** without sweat glands, sebaceous glands and hairs
- **Distal 0.8-1 cm** is lined by **Keratinized stratified squamous epithelium** typical of skin

	Above Pectinate Line	**Below Pectinate Line**
Embryological origin	Endoderm (Cloaca)	Ectoderm
Nerve supply	Visceral afferent nerves: an incision or a needle insertion in this region is **painless**). Sensitive only to stretching	**Inferior rectal nerves—S2, S3, S4** (AKA inferior anal nerves, inferior hemorrhoidal nerve) a branch of Pudendal nerve containing **somatic sensory fibers.** Quite sensitive to pain, touch and temperature
Arterial supply	**Superior rectal (Hemorrhoidal) artery** (Br of inferior mesenteric)	Middle rectal artery (Br of internal iliac artery), Inferior rectal artery (Br of internal pudendal)
Venous drainage (internal rectal venous plexus drains in both directions from the level of the pectinate line)	Internal rectal venous plexus drains into **superior rectal vein** (tributary of inferior mesenteric vein) and the **portal system**	Internal rectal venous plexus drains into **inferior rectal veins** and **middle rectal vein** (tributaries of the caval venous system) around the margin of the external anal sphincter
Lymphatic drainage	Internal iliac nodes	Superficial inguinal nodes
Epithelium	Simple columnar	Stratified squamous (Non keratinized above line of Hilton, Keratinized below line of Hilton)

Contd...

The Dentate Line is also called as Pectinate Line
Internal hemorrhoids ("piles") are prolapses of the rectal mucosa containing the normally dilated veins of the internal rectal venous plexus

External hemorrhoids are thrombosed (blood clots) in the veins of the external rectal venous plexus and are covered by skin.

The anastomoses among the superior, middle and inferior rectal veins form clinically important communications between the portal and the systemic venous systems. The superior rectal vein drains into the inferior mesenteric vein, whereas the middle and inferior rectal veins drain through the systemic system into the inferior vena cava

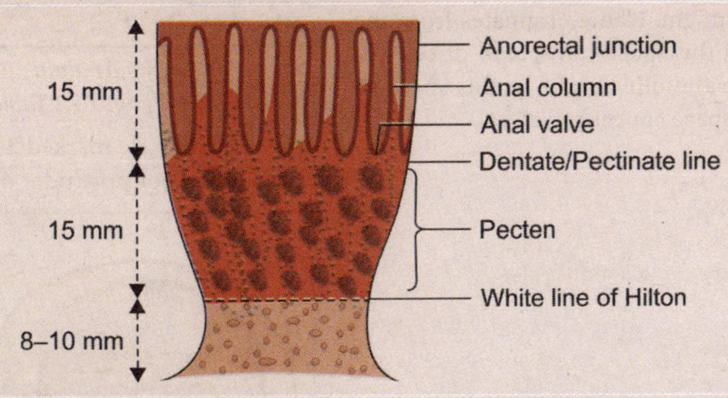

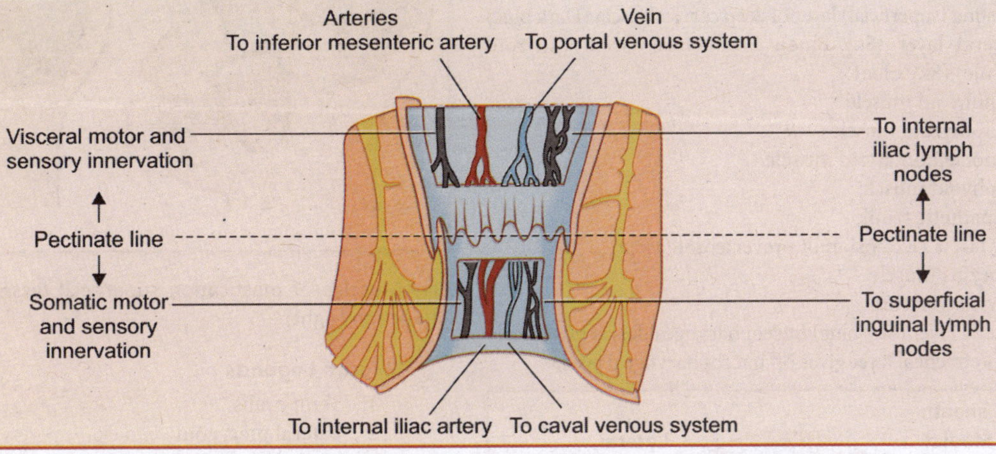

89. Ans. (b) Pleuropericardial membrane

Ref: High-Yield Embryology Ronald W. Dudek 4th ed page 124, Langman's Embryology 11th ed page 161

See table of Development of Diaphragm in Anatomy AIIMS May 2016 (see page no. 79)

90. Ans. (b) 6

Ref: Gray's 41th ed page 982, Keith L Moore 4th ed page 105, 596

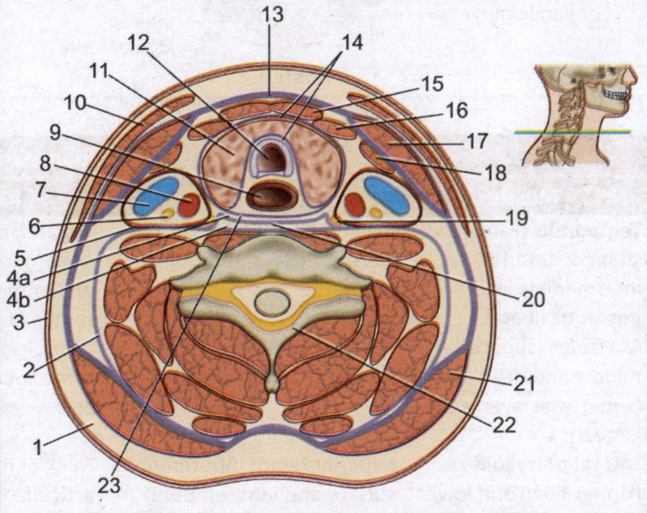

Fig: Cross section of neck

1. Superficial fascia
2. Prevertebral fascia (Parrot green)
3. Skin

4A. Retropharyngeal space (Between buccopharyngeal fascia anteriorly and alar layer of prevertebral fascia posteriorly)

4B. Danger space/Alar space/Space 4 (Grodinsky and Holyoke). Between alar fascia anteriorly and prevertebral fascia posteriorly and extends from the cranial base above to the level of the diaphragm. Name originates from the risk that an infection in this space can spread directly to the thorax. There exists a midline raphe in this space so some infections of this space appear unilateral.

5. Carotid sheath
6. Vagus nerve
7. Internal jugular vein
8. Common carotid artery
9. Esophagus
10. Platysma muscle
11. Thyroid gland
12. Trachea
13. Investing (superficial) layer of deep cervical fascia (Dark blue)
14. Visceral layer (Sky blue); Pretracheal fascia (Thyroid capsule) (Sky blue)
15. Sternohyoid muscle
16. Sternothyroid muscle
17. Sternocleidomastoid muscle
18. Omohyoid muscle
19. Sympathetic trunk
20. Alar fascia (Extension of prevertebral fascia)
21. Trapezius muscle
22. Cervical vertebra
23. Visceral layer (Sky-blue) buccopharyngeal fascia posteriorly the pretracheal layer gives off buccopharyngeal fascia

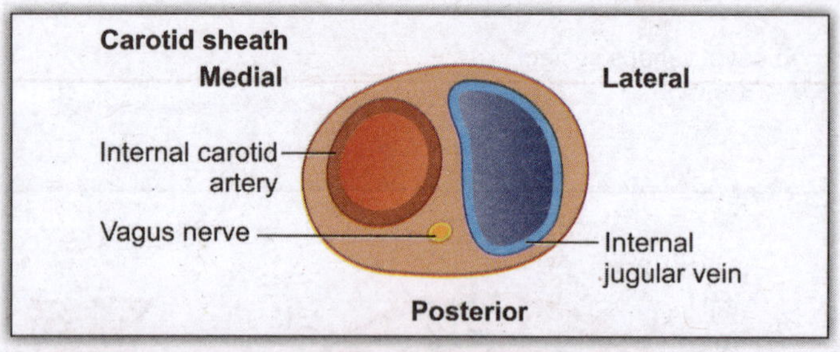

The carotid sheath contains:

1. The common and internal carotid arteries.
2. The internal jugular vein (IJV).
3. The vagus nerve (CN X).
4. Some deep cervical lymph nodes.
5. The carotid sinus nerve.
6. Sympathetic nerve fibers (carotid periarterial plexuses).

91. Ans. (b) 2

Ref: Gray's Anatomy 41st ed page 547, Grant's Atlas of Anatomy 12th Ed page 672 Table 7.9

The muscle marked 2 in the figure is lateral pterygoid which is the major protruder of the mandible.

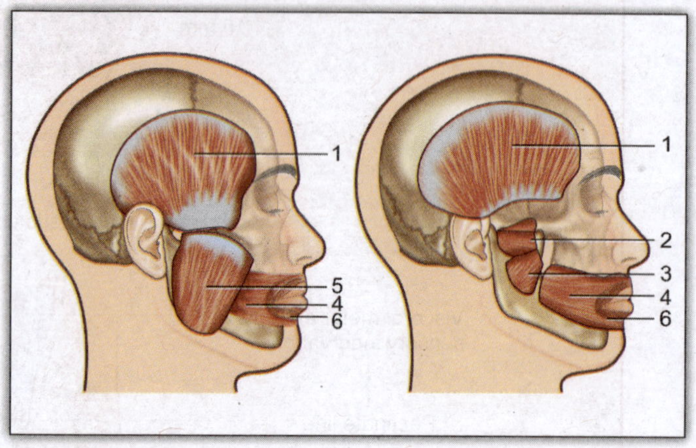

Fig: Muscles of mastication superficial dissection (left) and deep dissection (right)

Figure Legends

1. Temporalis
2. Lateral pterygoid
3. Medial pterygoid
4. Buccinator
5. Masseter
6. Orbicularis oris

Muscles of Mastication (Acting on Temporomandibular Joint)				
Muscle	**Origin**	**Insertion**	**Innervation**	**Main action**
Temporalis (Fan shaped; anterior, intermediate and posterior fibers)	Floor of temporal fossa and deep surface of temporal fascia	Tip and medial surface of coronoid process and anterior border of ramus of mandible	Deep temporal branches of ***mandibular nerve*** (CN V_3)	Elevates mandible (all fibers), Retrudes mandible (posterior fibers)
Masseter (superficial, middle and deep layers) (superficial layer is the largest)	Inferior border and medial surface of zygomatic arch	Lateral surface of ramus of mandible and coronoid process	Anterior trunk of ***Mandibular nerve*** (CN V_3) through masseteric nerve	Elevates mandible, minor actions are: protrudes mandible (superficial fibers), retrudes mandible (deep fibers)
Lateral pterygoid (Upper head and lower head)	**Superior head:** Infratemporal surface and infratemporal crest of greater wing of sphenoid bone **Inferior head:** *Lateral surface of lateral pterygoid figure*	Neck of mandible, articular disc and capsule of temporomandibular joint	***Mandibular nerve*** (CN V_3) through lateral pterygoid nerve which enters its deep surface	*Acting bilaterally,* protrude mandible and depress chin; *Acting unilaterally* alternately, they produce side-to-side movements of mandible (pulled medially towards the opposite side)

Contd...

Muscles of Mastication (Acting on Temporomandibular Joint)				
Muscle	**Origin**	**Insertion**	**Innervation**	**Main action**
Medial pterygoid (small superficial head and major deep head)	**Deep head:** Medial surface of lateral pterygoid figure and pyramidal process of palatine bone **Superficial head:** Tuberosity of maxilla	Medial surface of ramus of mandible, inferior to mandibular foramen	***Mandibular nerve*** (CN V_3) through medial pterygoid nerve	Acts synergistically with masseter to elevate mandible, contributes to protrude mandible; *acting unilaterally* produce small grinding movements
# Unlike the other muscles of mastication, lateral pterygoid is not pennate, nor does it have a significant number of Golgi tendon organs associated with its attachments				

92. Ans. (b) Lateral to mandibular nerve

Ref: Gray's 41st ed page 552

"Mandibular nerve lies lateral to otic ganglion, i.e. otic ganglion is not lateral to mandibular nerve"

Otic Ganglion

It is a peripheral parasympathetic ganglion related topographically to the mandibular nerve, but connected functionally with the glossopharyngeal nerve.

Relations

- Superiorly: Foramen ovale
- Laterally: Mandibular nerve
- Medially: Tensor veli palatini
- Posteriorly: Middle meningeal artery
- The otic ganglion usually surrounds the origin of the nerve to medial pterygoid

Roots

- Like all parasympathetic ganglia, there are **three roots**, motor, sympathetic and sensory. Only the parasympathetic fibers relay in the ganglion.
- The motor, parasympathetic, root of the otic ganglion is **the lesser petrosal nerve**, conveying preganglionic fibers from the glossopharyngeal nerve which originate from neurones in the inferior salivatory nucleus.
- The nerve synapses in the otic ganglion and postganglionic fibers pass by a communicating branch to the **auriculotemporal nerve and so to the parotid gland**.
- The sympathetic root is from a plexus on the middle meningeal artery. It contains postganglionic fibers from the superior cervical sympathetic ganglion which traverse the otic ganglion without relay and emerge with parasympathetic fibers in the connection with the auriculotemporal nerve to supply blood vessels in the parotid gland.
- The sensory fibers from the gland are derived from the auriculotemporal nerve. Clinical observations suggest that in humans the gland also receives secretomotor fibers through the chorda tympani.

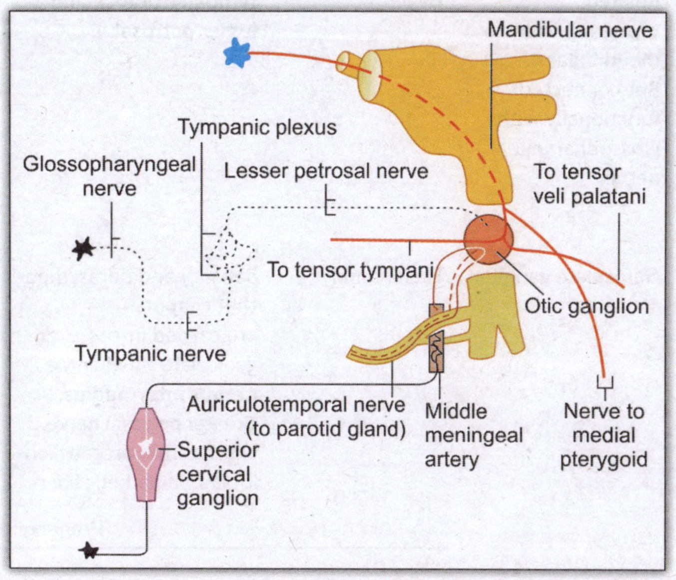

Parasympathetic Ganglions in Head and Neck				
Ganglion	**Location**	**Parasympathetic fibers**	**Sympathetic fibers**	**Chief distribution**
Ciliary concerned with the innervation of certain intraocular muscles	Lateral to optic nerve	**Oculomotor n.** and its inferior division, consists of preganglionic fibers from the **Edinger–Westphal nucleus**	Internal carotid plexus	**Via short ciliary nerves to ciliary muscle and sphincter pupillae** (parasympathetic); **dilator pupillae** and tarsal mm. (sympathetic)
Pterygopalatine a.k.a **sphenopalatine ganglion** Largest of the peripheral parasympathetic ganglia	Pterygopalatine fossa	**Greater petrosal branch of the facial nerve** and then in the nerve of the pterygoid canal **(Vidian nerve)**, after the greater petrosal unites with the deep petrosal nerve.	Internal carotid plexus	• Postganglionic parasympathetic fibers leave the ganglion and join the **maxillary nerve via a ganglionic branch**, then travel via the zygomatic and zygomatico temporal branches of the maxillary nerve to the **lacrimal gland** • Preganglionic secretomotor fibers of uncertain origin also travel in the nerve of the pterygoid canal. They synapse in the pterygopalatine ganglion and postganglionic

Contd...

Parasympathetic Ganglions in Head and Neck				
Ganglion	**Location**	**Parasympathetic fibers**	**Sympathetic fibers**	**Chief distribution**
				fibers are distributed to **palatine, pharyngeal and nasal mucous glands via palatine and nasal branches of the maxillary nerve.** Hence it supplies both **nasal mucosa and conjunctiva.** • The greater and lesser palatine nerves pass downwards from the pterygopalatine ganglion through the greater palatine canal, **Greater palatine nerve supplies the gingivae, mucosa and glands of the hard palate** The lesser (middle and posterior) palatine nerves innervate the **uvula, tonsil and soft palate**
Submandibular ganglion	On hyoglossus	Facial n., chorda tympani and lingual n.	Plexus on facial a.	**Chorda tympani branch of the facial nerve** which synapses in the submandibular ganglion: postganglionic branches are distributed to the lingual mucosa via the **lingual nerve** to **Submandibular and sublingual glands**
Otic ganglion Related topographically to mandibular n. But connected functionally with glossopharyngeal nerve.	Below foramen ovale	Glossopharyngeal n., its tympanic branch and lesser petrosal n.	Plexus on middle meningeal a.	**Only the parasympathetic fibers relay in the ganglion.** The motor, parasympathetic, root of the otic ganglion is the **lesser petrosal nerve,** conveying preganglionic fibers from the **glossopharyngeal nerve** which originate from neurones in the inferior salivatory nucleus. The nerve synapses in the otic ganglion and postganglionic fibers pass by a communicating branch to the **auriculotemporal nerve** and so to the **parotid gland.**
Geniculate ganglion	Facial canal	Sensory and parasympathetic inputs are carried into geniculate ganglion via **nervus intermedius. Greater petrosal nerve,** which carries preganglionic parasympathetic fibers		**Secretometer nerve supply to lacrimal gland:** Lacrimatory nucleus—nervus intermedius—geniculate ganglion of facial nerve—greater petrosal nerve—nerve of pterygoid canal—pterygopalatine ganglion—relay—Zygomatic nerve—zygomaticotemporal nerve—lacrimal nerve—lacrimal gland Motor fibers are carried via the facial nerve proper

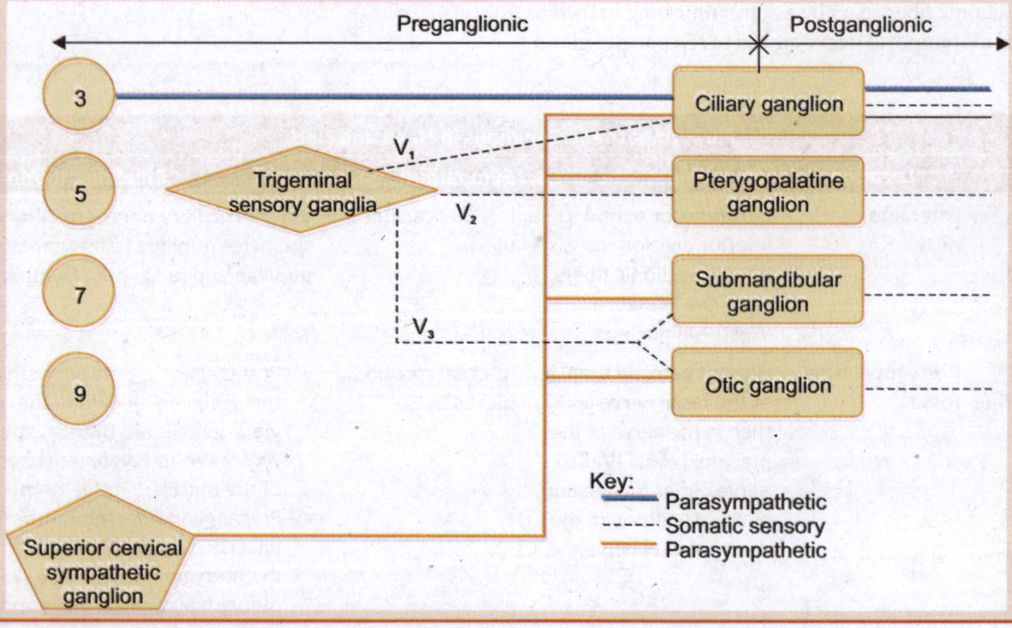

93. Ans. (c) Sphenoid bone

Ref: Gray's Anatomy 41st ed page 484

Some say frontal was there in options in place of zygomatic, in both the cases the answer will be same i.e. Sphenoid

Each **maxilla articulates** with nine bones

- Frontal
- Ethmoid
- Nasal
- Zygomatic
- Lacrimal
- Inferior nasal concha
- Palatine
- Vomer
- Adjacent fused maxilla

Important Anatomical Points about Maxilla

- Each maxilla forms the greater part of the floor and lateral wall of the nasal cavity and of the floor of the orbit.
- Maxilla contributes to the infratemporal and pterygopalatine fossa and bounds the inferior orbital and pterygomaxillary fissures.
- The maxilla has a body and four processes, namely the **zygomatic, frontal, alveolar and palatine** processes.

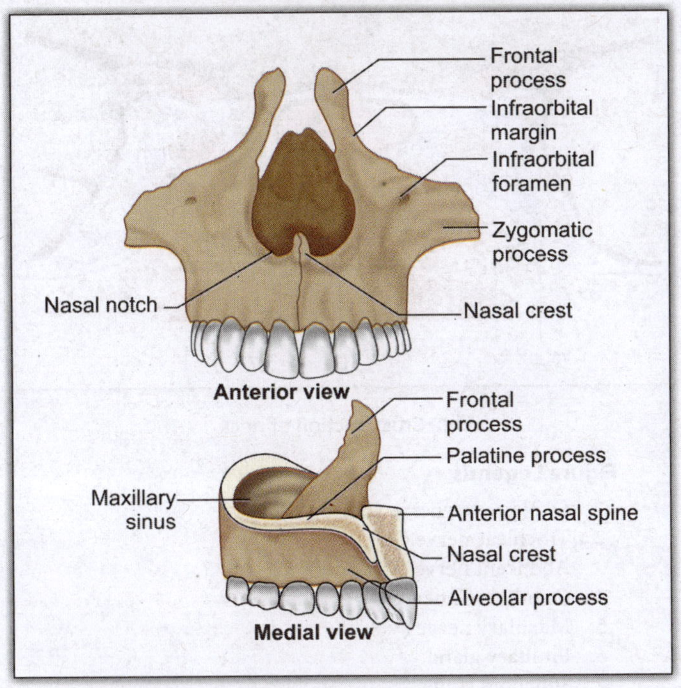

94. Ans. (d) Wings of sphenoid

Ref: Gray's Anatomy 40th ed page 733, Reconstruction of Upper Cervical Spine and Craniovertebral Junction By Petr Suchomel, Ondrej Choutka Page: 2

In humans, the junction between the head and neck (termed **occipitocervical, craniovertebral or spinomedullary**) is placed at the boundary between the fourth and fifth somites

The **craniovertebral junction (CVJ)** is a collective term that refers to the occiput (posterior skull base), atlas, axis and supporting ligaments. It encloses the soft tissue structures of the cervicomedullary junction (medulla, spinal cord and lower cranial nerves)

Bony Structures seen in the Craniovertebral Junction

Upper surfaces of C1 lateral masses are cup-like or concave which fit into the ball and socket configuration, united by articular capsules surrounding the atlantooccipital joint and by the anterior and posterior atlantooccipital membranes.

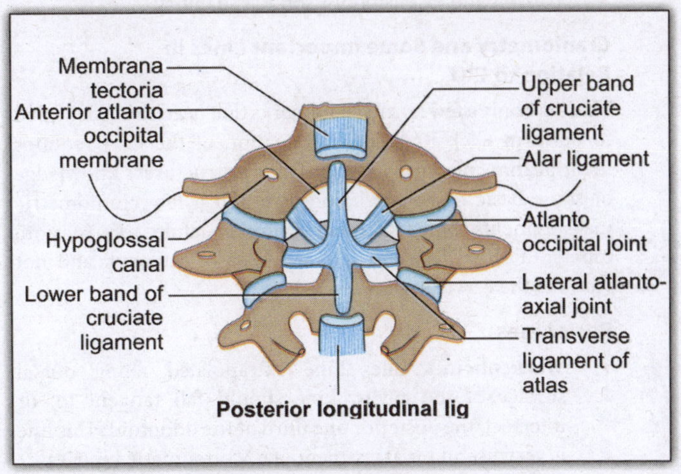

Ligaments of the Craniovertebral Junction

Principal stabilizing ligaments of C1

- Transverse atlantal ligament
- Alar ligaments

Secondary stabilizing ligaments of CVJ: These are more elastic and weaker than the primary ligaments.

- Apical ligament
- Anterior and posterior atlantal occipital membrane
- Tectorial membrane
- Ligamentum flavum
- Capsular ligaments

Neural Structures Related to the Cranio Vertebral Junction are:

- Caudal portion of brainstem (Medulla)
- Cerebellum: Only the tonsils, biventral lobules and the lower part of the vermis (nodule, uvula and pyramid)
- Fourth ventricle
- Rostral part of spinal cord
- Lower cranial nerves (9th, 10th, 11th, 12th)
- Upper cervical nerves (c1, c2, c3)

Arterial Structures Related to CVJ

- The major arteries related to CVJ are vertebral, posteroinferior cerebellar arteries (PICA) and the meningeal branches of the vertebral and external and internal carotid arteries.

Radiological Assessement of CVJ

- **Lateral view**: 85-90% of cervical injuries are evident in lateral view. Following parameters are seen.
  - Atlantodental interval: <3 mm adult, <5 mm child. Suspect transverse ligament disruption if these limits are exceeded.
  - Prevertebral space. At level C2 < 7 mm. If widened suspect hematoma secondary to a fracture.
  - Spinal fanning
  - Abrupt change in angulation

- **Odontoid/Open mouth view:** To evaluate an area that is difficult to visualize in the lateral view. Alignment of the lateral masses of C_1 with respect to the odontoid process.
- **Oblique view:** It is considered laminar view
- **Anteroposterior view:** Least useful view
- Flexion and extension for soft tissue injury

Craniometry and Some Important Lines in Relation to CVJ

There are only a few normal landmarks that need to be identified to perform CVJ. Radiologic evaluation of the CVJ requires identification of only a few anatomic structures, knowledge of some basic osseous relationships and a few craniometric measurements. Some of these anatomic landmarks (nasion, tuberculum, hard palate) require views of the skull and not views of the cervical spine.

Basic Lines

- **Wackenheim's line**: Line extrapolated along dorsal surface of the clivus. Line should fall tangent to, or intersect, the posterior one third of the odontoid. This line is very useful for assessment of CVJ traumatic injuries.
- **Chamberlain's line:** Posterior margin of hard palate to the posterior margin of foramen magnum (opisthion). Normal: over 5 mm of odontoid apex, anterior arch of C1 typically lies below.
- **McGregor's line:** Posterior margin of hard palate undersuface of occipital squamosal surface. Normal: greater than 7 mm odontoid apex. The odontoid projecting above is diagnostic of BASILAR IMPRESSION
- **Digastric line**: Line between incisurae mastoidae. Normal: 11 mm (± 4) above atlanto-occipital joint.
- **McRae's line:** Drawn from the basion, which corresponds to the anterior contour of the foramen magnum to the posterior contour opisthion. It is used to assess the decrease in content injury.
- **Bimastoid line:** Line connecting the tips of both mastoid processes to tip of odontoid.

Basic Angles

- **Basal Welcher angle:** Is drawn from the nasion and basion tuberculum. Must be between 123° and 143°. When this angle is less than 123° is called kyphotic skull. If the angle is greater than 143° is called platybasia. Angle subtendend by the junction of the nasion-tuberculum and tuberculum-basion tangents. Average = 134° – 135° Minimum = 121° Maximum = 148°–149°. Platybasia if >150°.
- **Clivus-canal angle:** Angle formed at junction of Wackenheim's line and posterior vertebral body line, along the posterior margin of the dens and axis body. Should be between 150° and 180° (in extension). When less than 150° can be ventral compression of the CVJ, between the medulla oblongata and spinal cord, which is optimal evaluation with MRI.
- **Atlanto-occipital joint axis angle**: Is formed at the intersection of tangents drawn parallel to the atlanto-occipital joints. These tangents typically intersect at the center of the odontoid process when the condyles are symmetric. The average angle measures 124° to 127°. Angle becomes more obtuse in occipital condylar hypoplasia.

95. Ans. (c) 3

Ref: Gray's Anatomy 41st ed page 437, 664, 670, Khurana 4th ed page 357

Convergent squint is due to paralysis of lateral rectus which is supplied by 6th cranial nerve (Abducens). "Abducent nerve is the content of cavernous sinus not the component of lateral wall"

Coronal section through cavernous sinus

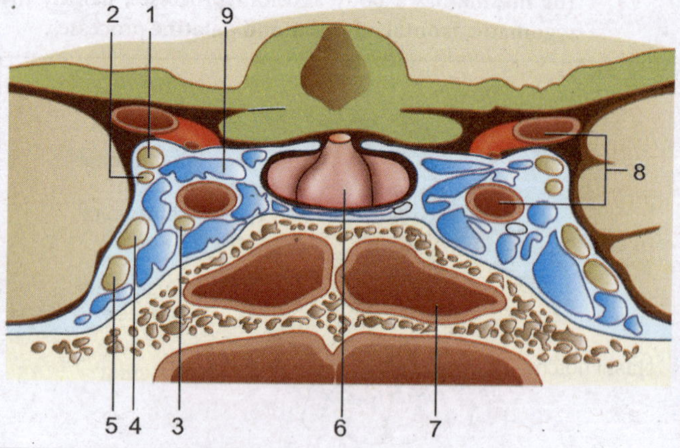

Fig: Cross section of neck

Figure Legends

1. Oculomotor nerve (III)
2. Trochlear nerve (IV)
3. Abducent nerve (VI)
4. Ophthalmic nerve (V_1)
5. Maxillary nerve (V_2)
6. Pituitary gland
7. Sphenoid sinus
8. Carotid artery
9. Cavernous sinus

Cavernous Sinus	
The cavernous sinus is a large venous plexus that lies on both sides of the body of the sphenoid bone. The sinus extends from the superior orbital fissure to the apex of the petrous temporal bone, with an average length of 2 cm and width of 1 cm.	
Relationship	**Superiorly:** Optic tract, optic chiasma, olfactory tract, internal carotid artery and anterior perforated substance **Inferiorly:** Foramen lacerum and the junction of the body and greater wing of the sphenoid bone **Medially:** Hypophysis cerebri and sphenoidal air sinus **Laterally:** Temporal lobe with uncus **Anteriorly:** Superior orbital fissure and the apex of the orbit **Posteriorly:** Apex of the petrous temporal and the crus cerebri of the midbrain.

Contd...

Cavernous Sinus	
Tributaries or incomming channels	**From the orbit:** (a) The superior ophthalmic vein; (b) a branch of the inferior ophthalmic vein or sometimes the vein itself; (c) the central vein of the retina may drain either into the superior ophthalmic vein or into the cavernous sinus. **From the brain:** (a) Superficial middle cerebral vein and (b) inferior cerebral veins from the temporal lobe **From the meninges:** (a) Sphenoparietal sinus (b) the frontal trunk of the middle meningeal vein may drain either into the pterygoid plexus through the foramen ovale or into the sphenoparietal or cavernous sinus
Draining channels or communications	The cavernous sinus drains: • Into the transverse sinus through the superior petrosal sinus • Into the internal jugular vein through the inferior petrosal sinus and through a plexus around the internal carotid artery • Into the pterygoid plexus of veins through the emissary veins passing through the foramen ovale, the foramen lacerum and the emissary sphenoidal foramen and • Into the facial vein through the superior ophthalmic vein • The right and left cavernous sinuses communicate with each other through the anterior and posterior intercavernous sinuses and through the basilar plexus of veins. All these communications are valveless and blood can flow through them in either direction.
Contents	• Internal carotid artery • Sympathetic chain around the ICA • Abducens nerve (inferolateral to ICA)
Lateral wall	• Uncus of the temporal lobe • **Oculomotor nerve:** In the anterior part of the sinus, it divides into superior and inferior divisions which leave the sinus by passing through the superior orbital fissure • **Trochlear nerve:** In the anterior part of the sinus, it crosses superficial to the oculomotor nerve and enters the orbit through the superior orbital fissure • **Ophthalmic nerve (V1):** In the anterior part of the sinus, it divides into the lacrimal, frontal and nasociliary nerves • **Maxillary nerve (V2):** It leaves the sinus by passing through the foramen rotundum on its way to the pterygopalatine fossa • **Trigeminal ganglion:** The ganglion and its dural cave project into the posterior part of the lateral wall of the sinus

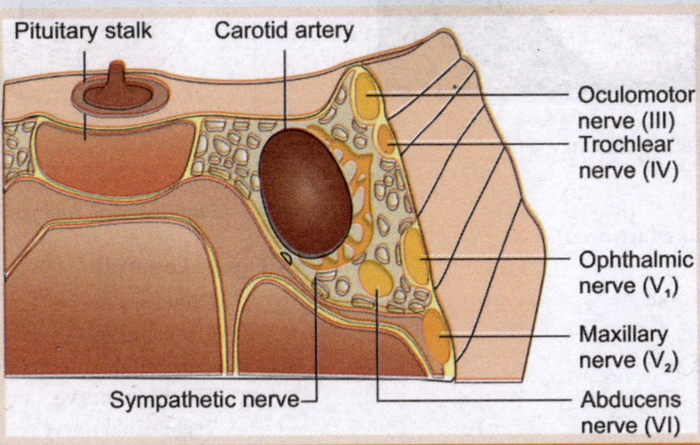

Clinical Features of Cavernous Sinus Thrombosis

- The most common signs of CST are related to anatomical structures affected within the cavernous sinus, notably cranial nerves III–VI, as well as symptoms resulting from impaired venous drainage from the orbit and eye.
- Classic presentations are abrupt onset of unilateral periorbital edema, headache, photophobia and bulging of the eye (proptosis).
- Ptosis, chemosis, cranial nerve palsies (III, IV, V, VI).
- Sixth nerve palsy is the most common.
- Sensory deficits of the ophthalmic and maxillary branch of the fifth nerve are common.
- V_1 ophthalmic division of trigeminal is afferent of corneal reflex while CN 7 is the efferent. Hence, corneal sensations are affected and corneal reflex is lost.
- Meandibular division (V_3) of trigeminal nerve does not passes through cavernous sinus wall hence jaw jerk is intact.
- Papilledema, retinal hemorrhages and decreased visual acuity and blindness may occur from venous congestion within the retina.
- Fever, tachycardia and sepsis may be present.
- Headache with nuchal rigidity may occur. Pupil may be dilated and sluggishly reactive.

- Infection can spread to contralateral cavernous sinus within 24–48 hours of initial presentation.

96. Ans. (d) 4

Ref: Gray's Anatomy 41st ed page 664, 670

Superior oblique is supplied by 4th cranial nerve, i.e. trochlear nerve—The only cranial nerve that exit the brainstem from the dorsal/posterior aspect (lateral most)

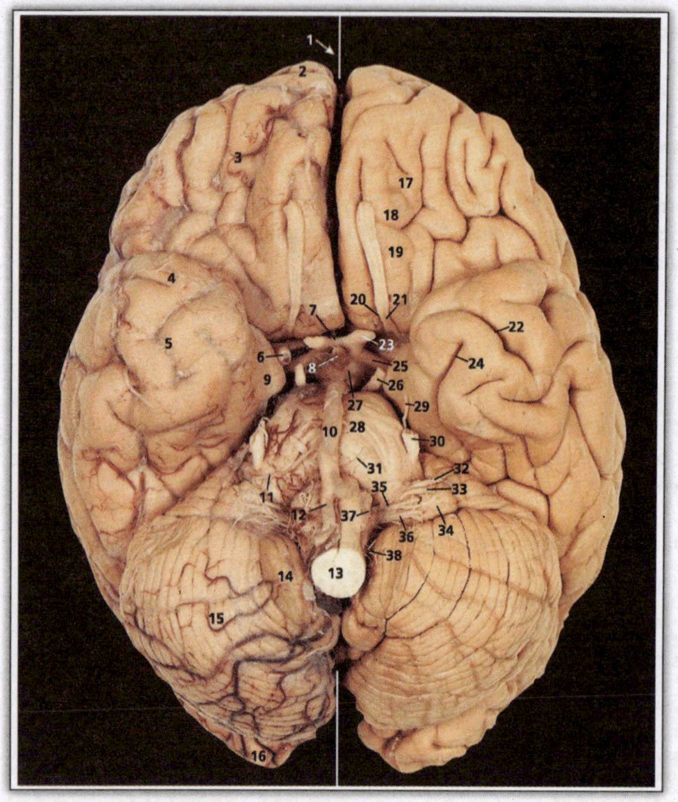

Fig: Inferior surface of Brain

Figure Legends

1. Longitudinal cerebral fissure (arrowed)
2. Frontal pole
3. Inferior surface of frontal pole
4. Temporal pole
5. Inferior surface of temporal pole
6. Internal carotid artery
7. Optic chiasma
8. Infundibulum
9. Parahippocampal gyrus
10. Basilar artery
11. Labyrinthine artery
12. Right vertebral artery
13. Medulla oblongata
14. Tonsil of cerebellum
15. Cerebellar hemisphere
16. Occipital pole
17. Orbital gyri
18. Olfactory bulb
19. Olfactory tract (I)
20. Medial olfactory stria
21. Lateral olfactory stria
22. Inferior temporal sulcus
23. Optic nerve (II)
24. Collateral sulcus
25. Optic tract
26. Oculomotor nerve (III)
27. Mammillary body
28. Pons
29. Trochlear nerve (IV)
30. Trigeminal nerve (V)
31. Abducent nerve (VI)
32. Facial nerve (VII)
33. Vestibulocochlear nerve (VIII)
34. Flocculus
35. Glossopharyngeal nerve (IX)
36. Vagus nerve (X)
37. Hypoglossal nerve (XII)
38. Accessory nerve (XI)

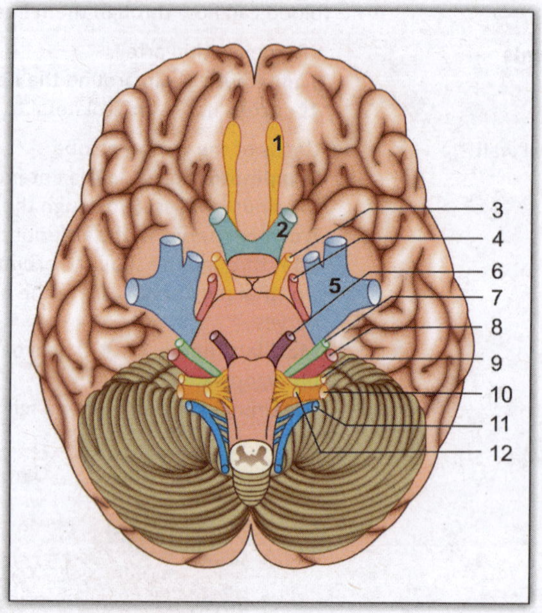

Fig: Inferior surface of brain representational

Figure Legends

1. Olfactory nerve
2. Optic nerve
3. Oculomotor nerve
4. Trochlear nerve
5. Trigeminal nerve
6. Abducens nerve
7. Facial nerve
8. Vestuibulocochlear nerve
9. Glossopharyngeal nerve
10. Vagus nerve
11. Accessory spinal nerve
12. Hypoglossal nerve

97. Ans. (c) Lateral cutaneous nerve of thigh

Ref: Gray's Anatomy 41st ed page 1371, BDC 5th Ed Vol 2 Page 47

Meralgia Paresthetica

- Lateral cutaneous nerve of thigh is a purely sensory branch of lumbar plexus—L_2 L_3 as it passes through the opening between inguinal ligament and its attachment 1-2 cm medial to the anterior superior iliac spine.

- Entrapment of lateral cutaneous nerve of thigh causes **Meralgia paresthetica** as it passes through the opening between inguinal ligament and its attachment 1-2 cm medial to the anterior superior iliac spine.
- Numbness is the earliest and most common symptom
- Pain, paresthesia, hyposthesia over the anteriolateral aspect of thigh.
- Particularly common in obese and in abdominal distension.

98. Ans. (c) Buccal branch of facial nerve

Ref: With Test

We are sorry to inform you that your conventional knowledge of this question is wrong, due to some wrong reference. **"Buccal branch of facial nerve supplies buccinator but does not pierce it".** Kindly note the following texts, option wise.

"Buccinator motor innervation is from the buccal branch of the facial nerve and sensory innervation is by the buccal branch (one of the muscular branches) of the mandibular part of the trigeminal".

Option (A)

The parotid duct pierces buccinator opposite the third upper molar tooth and lies on the deep surface of the muscle before opening into the mouth opposite the maxillary second molar tooth (Grays Anatomy 41st ed page 495)

NOTE

Structures pierced by Parotid duct are:
1. Buccal pad of fat
2. Buccopharyngeal fascia
3. Buccinator muscle
4. Mucous membrane

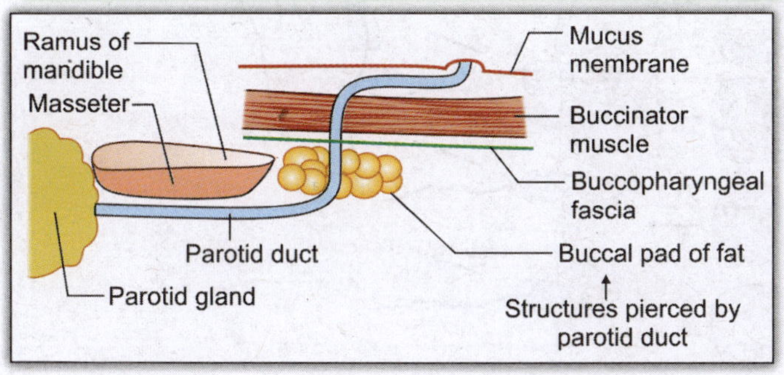

Option (B)

Buccal branch (sensory branch) of mandibular nerve sends branches to skin of the cheek before piercing the buccinator to supply the mucous membrane of the cheek. (Ref: Plastic Surgery: Volume 3 Plastic surgery 3rd ed By Eduardo D Rodriguez, Joseph E Losee, Peter C. Neligan page 19)

Now Read Following Reference

Ref: Grant's Dissector by Patrick W. Tank, John Charles Boileau Grant 15th ed page 224

There are two nerves with names buccal, associated with Buccinator muscle:
1. Buccal branch of facial nerve crosses superficial to the masseter muscle and provides motor innervation to the buccinator muscle.
2. Buccal branch of mandibular division of trigeminal nerve emerges from deep to the masseter muscle. It is sensory nerve and do not gives motor innervation to masseter. It pierces buccinator muscle to provide sensory innervation to the mucosa of cheek. It also provides sensory innervation to the skin of the cheek.

NOTE

The mandibular division of trigeminal nerve (the largest of 3 divisions) gives following branches:
1. **From main trunk:** Meningeal branch, Nerve to medial pterygoid
2. **From anterior trunk:** Buccal nerve, masseteric nerve, Deep temporal nerve, Nerve to lateral pterygoid
3. **From posterior trunk:** Auriculotemporal nerve, lingual nerve, inferior alveolar nerve

Option (D)

Near the end of the parotid duct are found 4-5 molar mucous gland of buccopharyngeal fascia, their ducts pierce the cheek/buccinator to reach the oral cavity opposite to third upper molar (Ref: Cunningham's textbook of anatomy By Daniel John Cunningham page 1109, Last's Anatomy: Regional and Applied By Mcminn 9th ed page 448)

AIIMS MAY 2015

99. Ans. (b) Primary to secondary spermatocyte

Ref: Gray's Anatomy 41st ed page 1275, I.B. Singh Embryology 8th Ed page 7, Langman 12th ed page 26, Principles of Genetics by Tamarin 4th Ed page 63

Independent assortments of chromosomes occur when the primary spermatocyte completes meiosis I and divides into two secondary spermatocytes. It increases genetic diversity in genes. Through the process of independent assortment, cross over happens between homologous chromosomes during pachytene stage of meiosis I, which allows genetic variations to happen.

Male Gametogenesis (Spermatogenesis)

Spermatogenesis is classically divided into three phases: spermatocytogenesis, meiosis and spermiogenesis.

A. Spermatocytogenesis

- **Primordial germ cells (46, 2N)** from the wall of the yolk sac arrive in the testes at week 4 of embryonic development and remain dormant until puberty.
- At puberty, primordial germ cells differentiate into **type A spermatogonia (46, 2N)**.
- Type A spermatogonia undergo **mitosis** to provide a continuous supply of stem cells throughout the reproductive life of the male (called spermatocytogenesis).
- Some type A spermatogonia differentiate into **type B spermatogonia (46, 2N)**.

B. Meiosis

- Type B spermatogonia enter meiosis I and undergo DNA replication to form **primary spermatocytes (46, 4N)**. Primary spermatocytes have a diploid chromosome number but duplicated sister chromatids (DNA content is thus 4N, where N is the DNA content of haploid spermatozoa) and are all at some stage of a long meiotic prophase of approximately 3 weeks.
- Primary spermatocytes complete meiosis I to form two **secondary spermatocytes (23, 2N)**. Secondary spermatocytes have a haploid chromosome complement (but 2N DNA content); the reduction division is designated as meiosis I. Independent assortment of chromosomes occur when the primary spermatocyte completes meiosis I and divides into two secondary spermatocytes. It increases genetic diversity in genes. Through the process of independent assortment, cross over happens between homologous chromosomes during pachytene stage of meiosis I, which allows genetic variations to happen.
- Secondary spermatocytes complete meiosis II to form four haploid **spermatids (23, 1N)**.

C. SPERMIOGENESIS

1. Spermatids undergo a **postmeiotic series of morphological changes** (called spermiogenesis) to form **sperm (23, 1N)**.
2. Newly ejaculated sperm are incapable of fertilization until they undergo **capacitation**, which occurs in the female reproductive tract and involves the unmasking of sperm glycosyltransferases and removal of proteins coating the surface of the sperm.

Note:

Small n is denotes the haploid or diploid nature (haploid being n and diploid being 2n)

Capital N denotes the DNA content of the cells (primary spermatocytes contains 4 copies of DNA 4N, secondary spermatocytes after 1st meiotic division has 2 copies of DNA 2N and after they undergo 2nd meiotic division, they have a single copy of DNA, N)

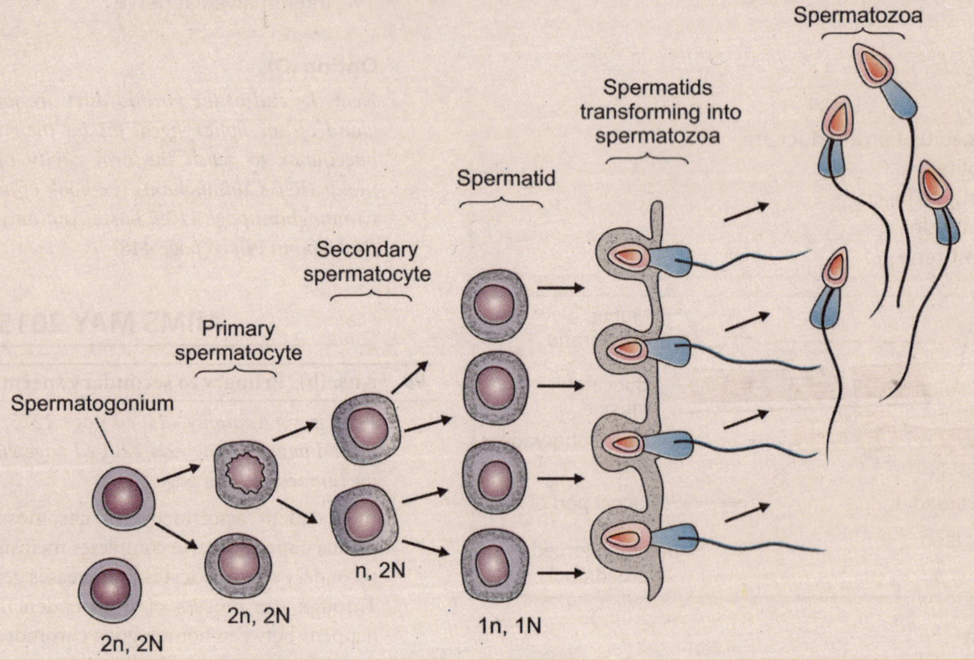

100. Ans. (B) Prophase I

Ref: Gray's 41st ed page 19, I.B. Singh embryology 8th Ed page 7

Female Gametogenesis (Oogenesis)

Maturation of Oocytes begins before Birth

- Once primordial germ cells have arrived in the gonad of a genetic female, they differentiate into **oogonia**.
- These cells undergo a number of mitotic divisions and by the end of the third month are arranged in clusters surrounded by a layer of flat epithelial cells.
- The majority of oogonia continue to divide by mitosis, but some of them arrest their cell division in **prophase of meiosis I** and form **primary oocytes**.
- During the next few months, oogonia increase rapidly in number and by the **fifth month** of prenatal development, the total number of germ cells in the ovary reaches its **maximum, estimated at 7 million**.
- At this time, cell death begins and many oogonia as well as primary oocytes become atretic.
- **By the seventh month**, the majority of oogonia have degenerated except for a few near the surface.
- All surviving **primary oocytes** have entered **prophase of meiosis I** and most of them are individually surrounded by a layer of flat epithelial cells. A primary oocyte, together with its surrounding flat epithelial cells, is known as a **primordial follicle**.

Maturation of Oocytes Continues at Puberty

- Near the time of birth, all primary oocytes have started prophase of meiosis I, but instead of proceeding into metaphase, they enter the **diplotene stage,** a resting stage during prophase that is characterized by a lacy network of chromatin.
- Primary oocytes remain arrested in prophase and do not finish their first meiotic division before puberty is reached.

At puberty in under the influence of pituitary hormones Meiosis I is completed, resulting in formation of two daughter cells of unequal size, each with 23 double-structured chromosomes. One cell, the secondary oocyte, receives most of the cytoplasm; the other, the first polar body, receives practically none. The first polar body lies between the zona pellucida and the cell membrane of the secondary oocyte in the perivitelline space.

The cell then enters meiosis II but arrests in metaphase approximately 3 hours before ovulation. Meiosis II is completed only if the oocyte is fertilized; otherwise, the cell degenerates approximately 24 hours after ovulation. The product of second meiotic division is ovum and second polar body. The first polar body either degenerates to undergoes second division to form two more polar bodies.

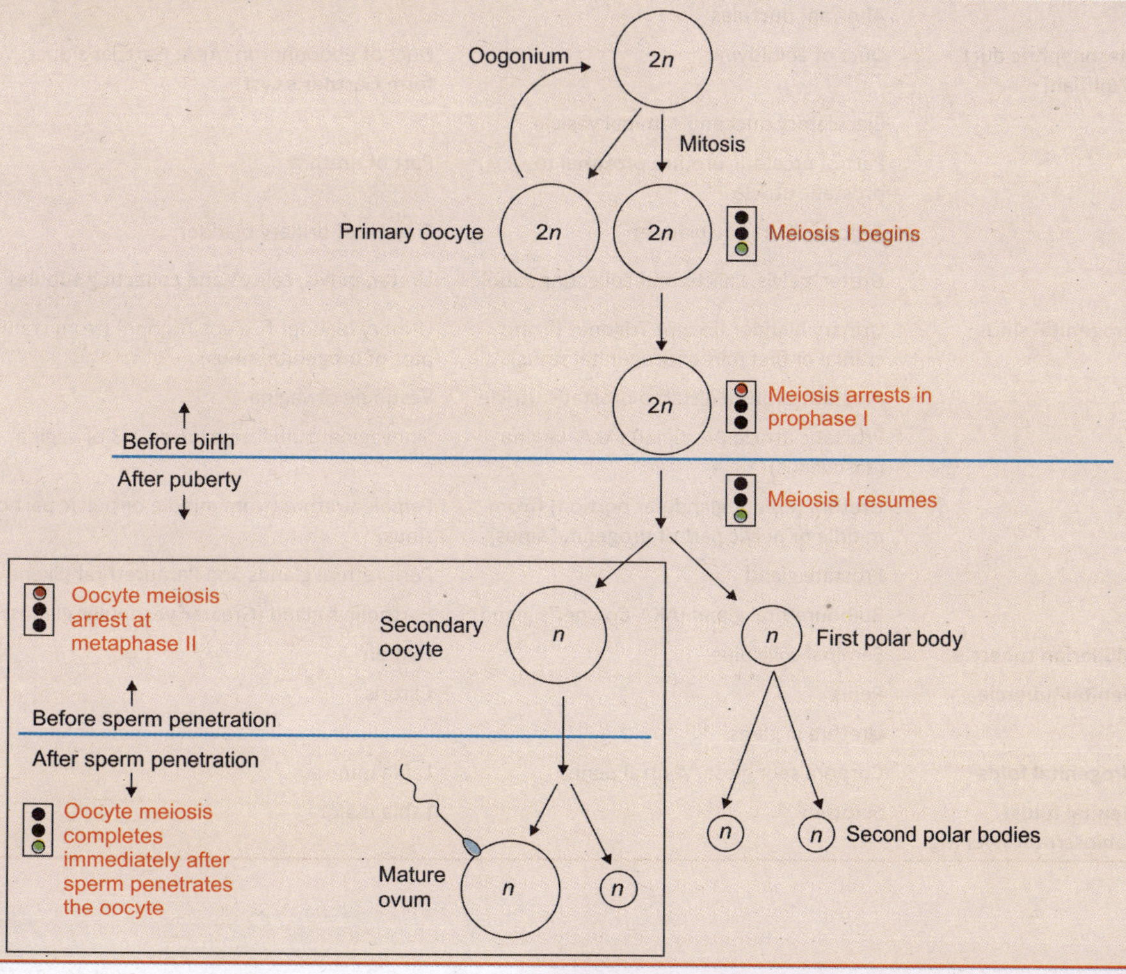

101. Ans. (a) Glomerulus

Ref: I.B. Singh Embryology 8th ed page 237-241

Glomerulus is formed from metanephros and not mesonephros

Adult Derivatives and Vestigial Remains of Embryonic Urogenital Structures/ Structural Homologues in Males and Females		
	Male	**Female**
Gubernacular cord	Gubernaculum testis	Ovarian and round ligaments
Gonadal ridge	Testis	Ovary
Cortex	Seminiferous tubules	Ovarian follicles
Medulla	Rete testis	Rete ovarii
Gonadal cells		
Germ cells	Spermatozoa	Oogonia
Coelomic epithelium	Sertoli cells	Granulosa cells
Mesenchyme	Interstitial Leydig cells	Theca cells/Hilus cells
Paramesonephric duct (Mullerian)	Appendix of testis (Vestigial)	Hydatid of Morgagni (Vestigial; can form **Hydatid cyst of Morgagni**), Uterine/fallopian tubes
		Uterovaginal primordium forms uterus, cervix and upper 1/3 of vagina
Mesonephros (Wolffian body)	Appendix of epididymis	Appendices vesiculosa (can form **Kobelt's cyst**)
	Efferent ductules	Epoophoron (organ of Rosenmuller)
	Lobules of epididymis	
	Paradidymis (vestigial) (organ of Giraldes)	Paroophoron
	Aberrant ductules	
Mesonephric duct (Wolffian)	Duct of epididymis	Duct of epoöphoron (AKA; Gartner's duct; Vestigial; can form **Gartner's cyst**)
	Ejaculatory duct and seminal vesicle	
	Part of prostatic urethra proximal to prostatic utricle	Part of urethra
	Trigone of urinary bladder	Trigone of urinary bladder
	Ureter, pelvis, calices and collecting tubules	Ureter, pelvis, calices and collecting tubules
Urogenital sinus	Urinary bladder (Except Trigone) (from cranial or first part of urogenital sinus)	Urinary bladder (Except Trigone) (from cranial or first part of urogenital sinus)
	Prostatic urethra distal to prostatic utricle	Vestibule of vagina
	Prostatic utricle (Vestigial) (AKA- vagina masculinus)	Sinovaginal bulb forms lower 2/3 of vagina
	Urethra (except glandular portion) (from middle or pelvic part of urogenital sinus)	Female urethra (from middle or pelvic part of urogenital sinus)
	Prostate gland	Periurethral glands and Paraurethral (Skene's) gland
	Bulbourethral gland (AKA-Cowper's gland)	Bartholin's gland (Greater vestibular glands)
Müllerian tubercle	Seminal colliculus	Hymen
Genital tubercle	Penis	Clitoris
	Urethra in glans	
Urogenital folds	Corpora spongiosa/Ventral penis	Labia minora
Genital folds/ Labioscrotal swelling	Scrotum	Labia majora

102. Ans. (d) Subscapularis

Ref: Gray's Anatomy 41st ed page 823

Subscapularis is attached to the lesser tubercle of the humerus not greater tubercle (Read following lines from Gray's)

Subscapularis is a bulky, triangular muscle which fills the subscapular fossa. In its medial two-thirds, the fibers are attached to the periosteum of the costal surface of the scapula. Other fibers arise from tendinous intramuscular septa, which are attached to ridges on the bone and from the aponeurosis which covers the muscle and separates it from teres major and the long head of triceps. The fibers converge laterally into a broad tendon which is attached to the *lesser tubercle of the humerus* and the front of the articular capsule. The tendon is separated from the neck of the scapula by the large subscapular bursa, which communicates with the shoulder joint.

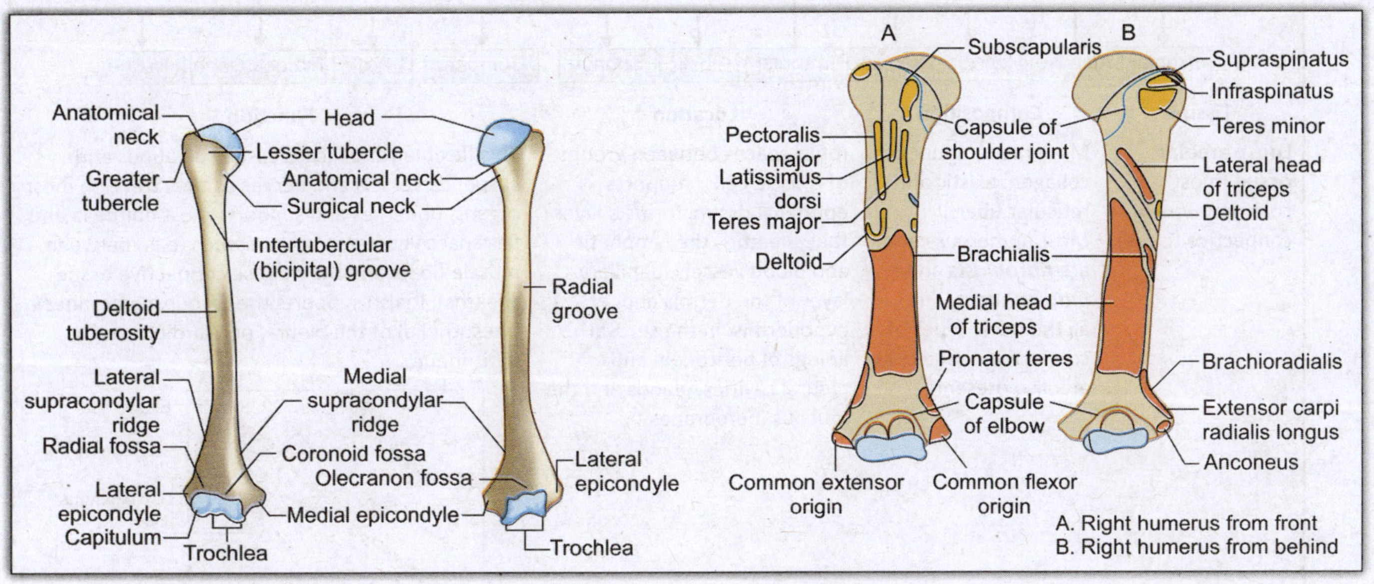

A. Right humerus from front
B. Right humerus from behind

Greater Tubercle

- The greater tubercle is the most lateral part of the proximal end of the humerus.
- Its posterosuperior aspect, near the anatomical neck, bears three smooth flattened impressions for the attachment of **(Mnemonic: SIT)**
  - Supraspinatus (uppermost)
  - Infraspinatus (middle)
  - Teres minor (lowest and placed on the posterior surface of the tubercle)

The Lesser Tubercle

- It has a smooth, muscular impression on its upper part palpable through the thickness of deltoid 3 cm below the acromial apex.
- The bony prominence slips away from the examining finger when the humerus is rotated.
- The lateral edge of the lesser tubercle is sharp and forms the medial border of the intertuberous sulcus.
- Subscapularis is attached to the lesser tubercle
- The transverse ligament of the shoulder joint is attached to the lateral margin.

The Intertuberous Sulcus (Bicipital Groove)

- It lies between the tubercles.
- It contains the long tendon of biceps, its synovial sheath and an ascending branch from the anterior circumflex humeral artery.
- The rough lateral lip of the groove is marked by the bilaminar tendon of pectoralis major, its floor by the tendon of latissimus dorsi and its medial lip by the tendon of teres major; the attachment of pectoralis major extends beyond that of teres major, that of latissimus dorsi is least extensive.

103. Ans. (a) Thymus

Ref: Gray's 41st ed page 38

Connective Tissues

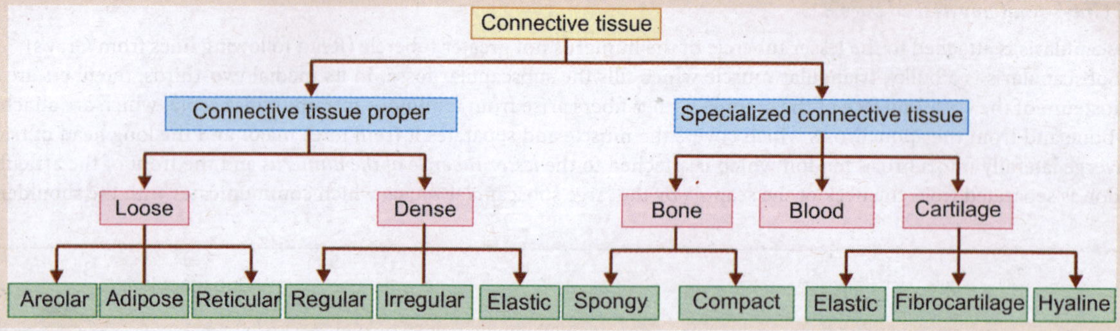

Tissue	Composition	Location	Function
Loose areolar tissue (most common type of connective tissue)	Moderate amount of collagen, elastic and reticular fibers. Most numerous cells are ***fibroblasts*** and ***macrophages***, but all the other types of connective tissue cells are also present.	It fills spaces between groups of muscle cells, supports epithelial tissue, forms a layer that sheathes the lymphatic and blood vessels, papillary layer of the dermis and hypodermis, in the serosal linings of peritoneal and pleural cavities, glands and the mucous membranes	This flexible yet delicate tissue surrounds and suspends vessels and nerves as they traverse most organs, underlies and supports most epithelia and fills spaces between other tissues (e.g., between muscle fibers and their dense connective tissue sheaths). It also supports the serous membranes (mesothelia) of the pleura, pericardium and peritoneum. 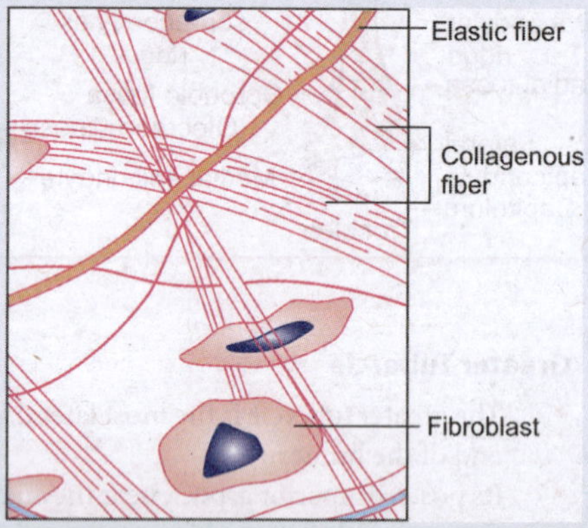 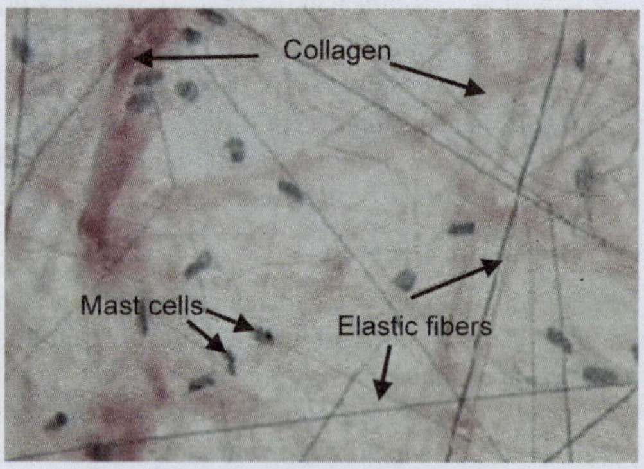
Reticular tissue	Special form of connective tissue, with few fibers. Type III collagen, macrophages and dendritic cells	Support structure for lymphoreticular system like **bone marrow, spleen, lymph nodes**	This tissue form delicate 3-dimensional, netlike scaffolding upon which cells, the predominant element, are suspended. Nuclei appear **deep blue** and the reticular fibers are stained **light blue**

Contd...

White Adipose tissue	**Unilocular** Adipocytes	Subcutaneous tissue all throughout the body in adults	It **stores and releases lipids** as follows: • Adipose cells synthesize the enzyme **lipoprotein lipase** • Dietary fat is transported to adipose tissue VLDLs and **chylomicrons.** • Free fatty acids enters and stored as triglycerides adipose tissue. Adipose cells also synthesize fatty acids from glucose. • **Insulin,** ↑ses the rate of synthesis of lipoprotein lipase and the uptake of glucose by adipose cells. • Release of lipids is affected by neural impulses and/or adrenaline. Stored triglycerides are hydrolyzed by **hormone sensitive lipase** (which is activated by cAMP). The free fatty acids are released into the extracellular matrix and then enter the capillary lumen.

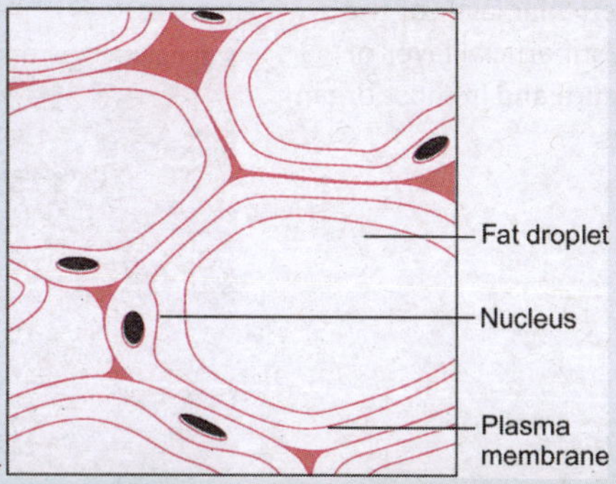

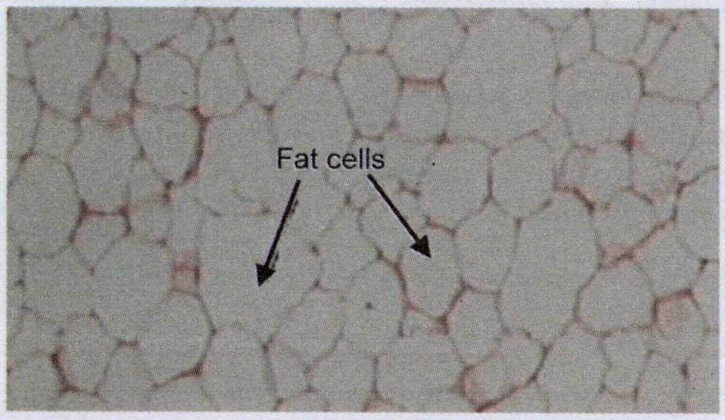

Brown adipose tissue	**Multilocular** adipocytes which contain many large mitochondria	This tissue is found in ***infants*** (also in hibernating animals) and is much reduced in adults	**Thermogenin,** a transmembrane protein located in mitochondria, causes the release of protons away from ATP synthesis, resulting in heat production.
Dense (regular)	Contents are same as Loose areolar tissue, but having fewer cells and more collagen fibers. Densely packed collagen type 1 bundles in uniform parallel fashion and fibroblasts	Tendon, ligament, aponeurosis and some organ capsules	Strength, resistance and protection

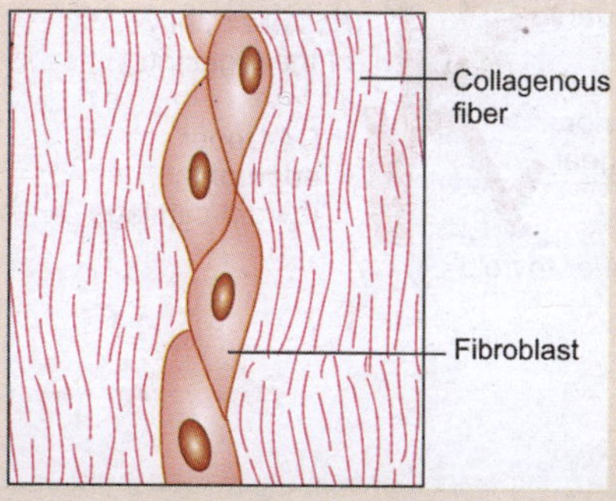

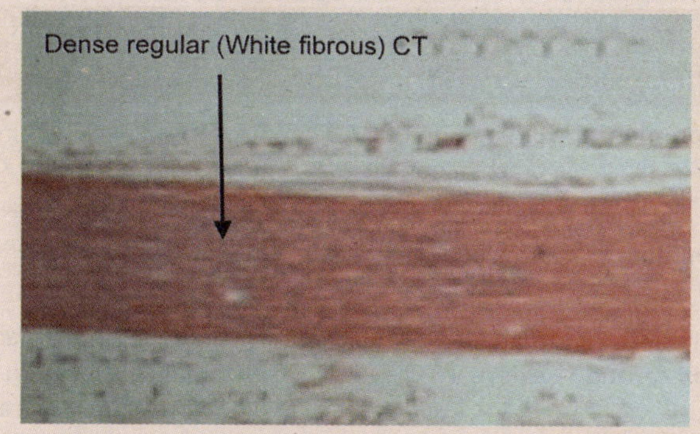

Fig: Dense regular (white fibrous) connective tissue

Contd...

Dense (irregular)	Contents are same as loose areolar tissue, but having fewer cells and more collagen fibers Collagen bundles have a complex irregular, woven pattern that provides resistance to tensile stress from any direction	Most common dense connective tissue. It is found in the reticular layer of the dermis, superficial layer of periosteum and in most organ capsules.	Covering the more fragile tissues and organs and protecting them from multidirectional mechanical stresses. 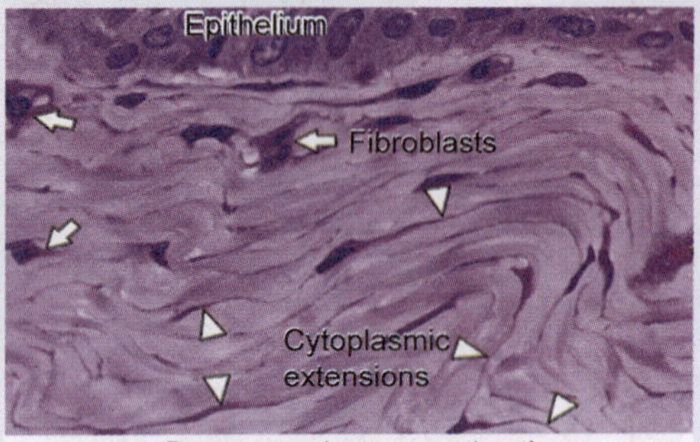 Dense regular connective tissue
Elastic	Bundles of thick, parallel **elastic fibers**. Space between elastic fibers is occupied by thin collagen fibers and flattened **fibroblasts**	Arteries, larynx, trachea, bronchus, yellow ligaments of vertebral column, suspensory ligament of penis	Typical yellow color, elasticity, flexibility and distensibility

104. Ans. (a) Transverse cervical artery

Ref: Gray's Anatomy 41st ed page 453, 797, Grants 12th ed page 765

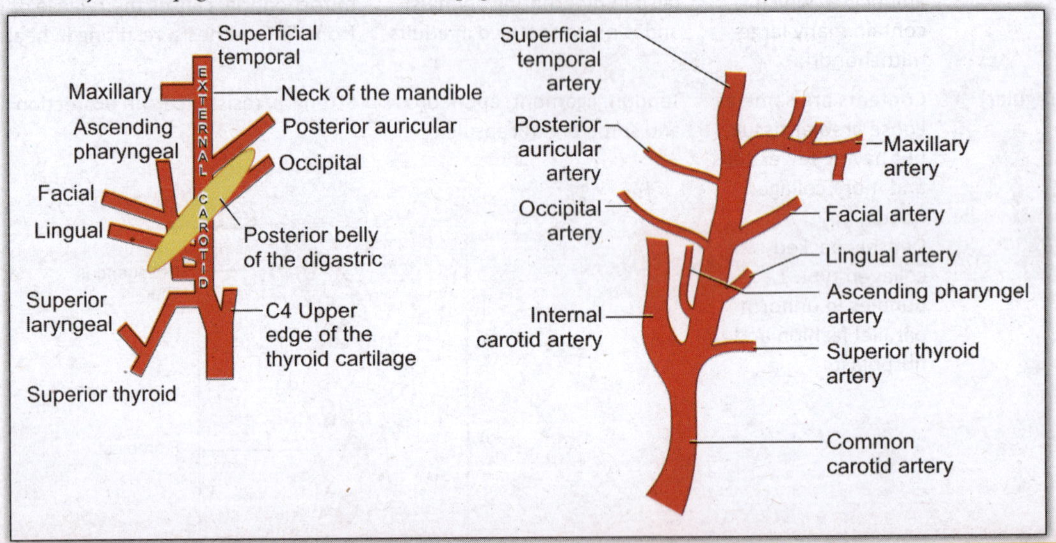

Arteries of the Neck		
Artery	**Origin**	**Course and Distribution**
Right common carotid	Bifurcation of brachiocephalic trunk	Ascends in neck within carotid sheath with the internal jugular vein and vagus nerve (CN X). Terminates at superior border of thyroid cartilage (C4 vertebral level) by dividing into internal and external carotid arteries
Left common carotid	Arch of aorta	
Right and left common carotid	Right and left external	No branches in the neck. Enters cranium via carotid canal to supply brain and orbits. Proximal part location of carotid sinus, a baroreceptor that reacts to change in arterial blood pressure. The carotid body, a chemoreceptor that monitors oxygen level in blood, is located in bifurcation of common carotid
Right and left internal carotid		Supplies most structures external to cranium; the orbit, part of forehead and scalp are major exceptions (supplied by ophthalmic artery from intracranial internal carotid)

Contd...

Arteries of the Neck		
Artery	**Origin**	**Course and Distribution**
Ascending pharyngeal	External carotid	Ascends on pharynx to supply pharynx, prevertebral muscles, middle ear and cranial meninges
Occipital		Passes posteriorly, medial and parallel to the posterior belly of digastric, ending in the posterior scalp
Posterior auricular		Ascends posteriorly between external acoustic meatus and mastoid process to supply adjacent muscles, parotid gland, facial nerve, auricle and scalp
Superior thyroid		Runs anteroinferiorly deep to infrahyoid muscles to reach thyroid gland. Supplies thyroid gland, infrahyoid muscles, SCM and larynx via *superior laryngeal artery*
Lingual		Lies on middle constrictor muscle of pharynx; arches superoanteriorly and passes deep to CN XIII, stylohyoid muscle and posterior belly of digastric then passes deep to hyoglossus, giving branches to the posterior tongue and bifurcating into *deep lingual* and *sublingual arteries*
Facial		After giving rise to *ascending palatine artery* and a tonsillar branch, it passes superiorly under cover of the angle of the mandible. It then loops anteriorly to supply the submandibular gland and give rise to the *submental artery* to the floor of the mouth before entering the face
Maxillary	Terminal branches of external carotid	Passes posterior to neck of mandible, enters infratemporal fossa then pterygopalatine fossa to supply teeth, nose, ear and face
Superficial temporal		Ascends anterior to auricle to temporal region and ends in scalp
Vertebral	Subclavian	Passes through the transverse foramina of the transverse processes of vertebrae C1–C6, runs in a groove on the posterior arch of the atlas and enters the cranial cavity through the foramen magnum
Internal thoracic		No branches in neck; enters thorax
Thyrocervical trunk		Has two branches: the *inferior thyroid artery*, the main visceral artery of the neck; the cervicodorsal trunk sending branches to the lateral cervical region, trapezius and medial scapular arteries
Costocervical trunk		Trunk passes posterosuperiorly and divides into *superior intercostal* and *deep cervical arteries* to supply the 1st and 2nd intercostal spaces and posterior deep cervical muscles, respectively

105. Ans. (a) Periosteum

Ref: Essentials of Skeletal Radiology 3rd ed Volume 1 by Yochum page 717, Textbook of Human Histology by I. Singh 7th ed page 88-102

- Trabecular bone is more metabolically active than compact bone.
- Metabolically most active part of bone is Metaphysis
- Periosteum has an inner metabolically active layer that can lay down or take away cortical bones.

106. Ans. (d) Collecting duct

Ref: Textbook of Human Histology by I. Singh 7th Ed page 43, Krause's Essential Histology 3rd Ed page 37

"In kidney Microvilli are present in PCT not collecting duct"

Specializations of Epithelial membranes: Cells of the epithelial sheets show special adaptations of the apical or basolateral surfaces that aid in increasing the surface area of the cell or constitute the motile appendag. These are Microvilli, Cilia and Basal lateral infoldings

Microvilli: These are small apical projections of the epithelial plasma membrane which enclose a core of cytoplasm. They perform the function of absorption, secretion, mechanotransduction, cellular adhesion. They are present in:

- Brush border of proximal convoluted tubule of kidney
- Striated border of small intestinal cells and gall bladder: Microvilli of small intestine may contain digestive enzymes such as glucosidase
- Stereocilia of inner ear
- Taste hair of taste buds
- Lining of epididymis
- Surface of the ovum
- Surface of WBC's

Diseases Caused by Microvillus Damage

- Celiac sprue
- Enteropathogenic E. coli
- Microvillus inclusion disease

107. Ans. (b) Abducent

Ref: Gray's 41st ed page 318, BRS Neuroanatomy 2nd ed page 14-15, The Neurosurgeon's Handbook by George Samandouras Oxford University Press page 13

This question is modified into an image-based question in AIIMS Nov 2016

The sixth nerve nucleus is located on the floor of rhomboid fossa, beneath facial colliculus in the pons. It is surrounded by geniculum of the facial nerve. The abducent nucleus and the facial nerve fibers looping around it together form a surface elevation, the facial colliculus, in the floor of the fourth ventricle.

Structures of Brainstem

	Ventral surface	Dorsal surface
Midbrain	Cerebral peduncle Interpediuncular fossa *Oculomotor nerve CN3* Posterior perforated substance created by posterior cerebral and posterior communicating arteries	Superior colliculus (Visual system) Inferior colliculus (Auditory system) *Trochlear nerve CN 4* (Only cranial nerve that exits from dorsal aspect)
Pons	*Trigeminal nerve CN5* *Abducens nerve CN 6* *Facial nerve CN 7* *Vestibulocochlear nerve CN 8* Ventral cochlear nuclei Facial nucleus	Motor and sensory nucleus of trigeminal Vestibular nuclei Dorsal cochlear nuclei Superficially pontine portion of **Rhomboid fossa** containing Locus coeruleus (Largest collection of norepinephrinergic neurons in CNS) Sulcus limitans Stria medullaris **Facial colliculus** (contains *Abduscent nucleus* and internal genu of facial nerve
Medulla	Pyramid (Corticospinal tract) Olive (Superior and inferior olivary nucleus) *Glossopharyngeal nerve CN 9* *Vagus nerve CN 10* *Accessory nerve CN 11* *Hypoglossal nerve CN 12*	Nucleus gracilis Nucleus cuneatus Medullary **Rhomboid fossa** containing Stria medullaris Dorsal motor nucleus of vagus CN10 (Vagal trigone) Hypoglossal nucleus CN12 (Hypoglossal trigone) Sulcus limitans Area postrema (Vomiting center)

Note: Stria medullaris divides rhomboid fossa into pontine and medullary parts

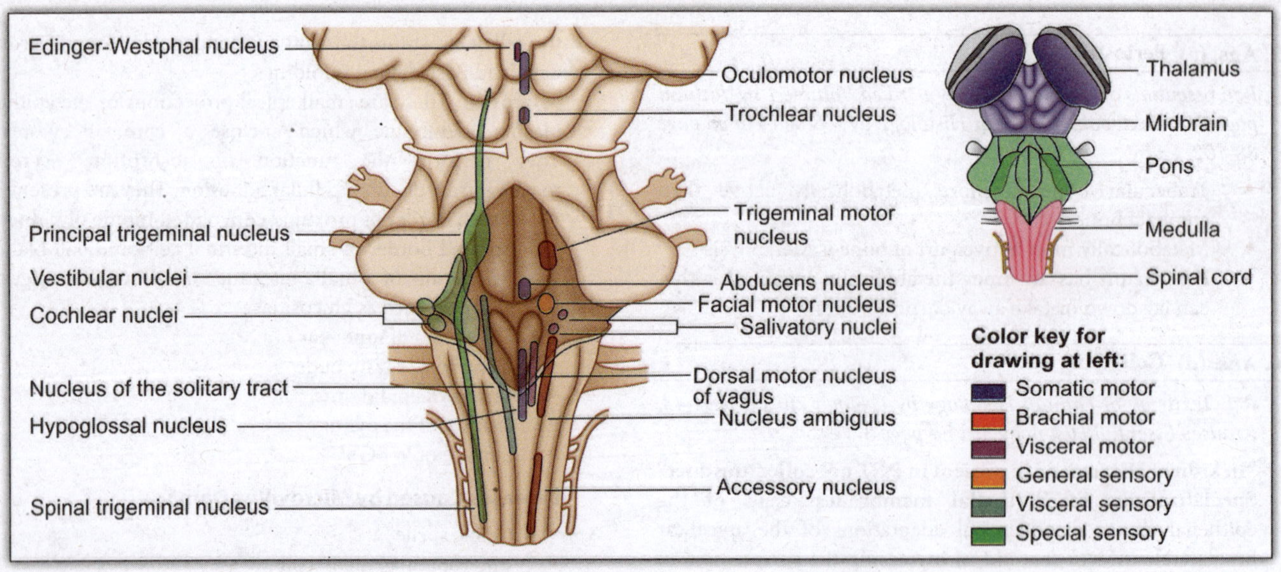

Fig: Brain Stem illustrations: with emphasis of different nucleus

108. Ans. (c) Palmar interossei

Ref: Apley's Orthopedics 9th ed page 291

Card test: Palmar interossei are adductors (Pad), tested by asking the patient to hold a card between the extended fingers and assess resistance against pulling

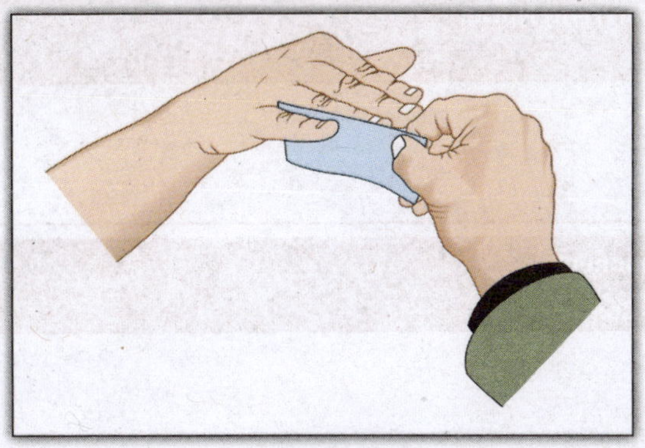

Book test and Froment's Sign

It is a test employed to test the adductor pollicis muscle. Patient is asked to hold a book in first web space. The examiner holds the book in similar manner and tries to pull. When adductor pollices is paralyzed the patient uses flexors of the thumb to hold back the book and the thumb lies in flexion.

IGAWA Test

To access both palmar and dorsal interossei. The patient is made to place the hand on the table and asked to raise the middle finger and move it side to side. If the interossei are paralysed he will not be able to do so.

109. Ans. (a) Inferior rectal vein

Ref: Grays 41st ed page 1147

The mesorectum (mesentery of the rectum) and its contents are intimately related to the rectum down to the level of levator ani. The mesorectum is a distinct compartment that derives from the embryological hindgut. The mesorectum is enclosed by the mesorectal fascia which is a distinct covering derived from the visceral peritoneum. It is also known as the **visceral fascia of the mesorectum**, fascia propria of the rectum or the presacral wing of the hypogastric sheath. The fascia bounds the mesorectum posteriorly and thus lies anterior to the retrorectal space and the presacral fascia. The mesorectum and its fascia are surrounded by loose areolar tissue which separates them from the posterior and lateral walls of the true pelvis.

Contents

- Superior rectal artery and its branches
- Superior rectal vein and tributaries
- Superior rectal and pararectal nodes and lymphatic along the superior rectal artery
- Branches from the inferior mesenteric plexus which descend to innervate the rectum and loose adipose connective tissue.

110. Ans. (a) Olfactory nerve

Ref: Gray's Anatomy 41st ed page 390, 562, BDC 6th ed vol 3 page 351

Olfactory nerve is sensory visceral afferent (SVA)

Parasympathetic (general visceral motor/efferent) involuntary are cranial nerves 3, 7, 9, 10

Cranial Nerve Nuclei			
Cranial Nerve Motor (Efferent) Nuclei			
Nucleus	Position	Cranial nerve	Function
General Somatic motor/Efferent - voluntary *(Mnemonic: 3, 4, 6, 12 = supplies eye ball and tongue)*			
Oculomotor	Upper midbrain	Oculomotor III	Eyeball movements: extrinsic ocular muscles
Trochlear	Lower midbrain	Trochlear IV	Eyeball movements: extrinsic ocular muscles
Abducens	Pons	Abducens VI	Eyeball movements: extrinsic ocular muscles
Hypoglossal	Medulla	Hypoglossal XII	Tongue muscles and movements
Branchiomotor (special visceral motor/efferent) – voluntary# *(Mnemonic = cranial nerves dervied from branchial arches = 5, 7, 9, 10)*			
Trigeminal	Pons	Mandibular Vc (1st arch)	Chewing, tensor tympani
Facial	Pons	Facial VII (2nd arch)	Facial expression, buccinator, stapedius
Nucleus ambiguus	Medulla	Glossopharyngeal IX (3rd arch) Vagus X, various branches (4th arch) Vagus (X), recurrent laryngeal (6th arch)	Muscles of swallowing and phonation
Cervical accessory nucleus	Upper cervical spinal cord	Spinal accessory XI	Sternocleidomastoid, trapezius
Parasympathetic (General visceral motor/efferent) – involuntary *(3, 7, 9, 10)*			
Edinger–Westphal	Midbrain	Oculomotor III	Ciliary muscle: Lens accommodation, iris muscle: Pupilloconstriction

Contd...

Salivatory: Superior	Pons	Facial VII	Secretomotor: Lacrimal, nasal, palate, submandibular, sublingual glands
Salivatory: Inferior	Upper medulla	Glossopharyngeal IX	Secretomotor: Parotid gland
Dorsal motor of vagus	Medulla	Vagus X	Heart, foregut and midgut derivatives

Cranial Nerves Sensory (Afferent) Nuclei	
Afferent (Mnemonic = 7, 9, 10 are common)	**Nerve**
General somatic afferent (GSA)	5, 7, 9, 10
Special visceral afferent (SVA)	1, 7, 9, 10
General visceral afferent (GVA)	7, 9, 10

Cranial Nerve Components

Nerve	Component
Olfactory nerve	SVA
Optic nerve	SSA
Oculomotor nerve	GSE Component: Inferior oblique, levator palpabre superiorous, inferior rectus, superior rectus, medial rectus GVE component: Ciliary ganglion (supplies ciliary muscle, sphincter pupilae)
Trochlear nerve	GSE: Superior oblique
Trigeminal	GSA Spinal nucleus – nociceptors, thermoreceptors and some mechanoreceptors Chief sensory nucleus – mechanoreceptors Mesencephalic nucleus – proprioceptors SVE: Motor nucleus
Abducens	GSE – Lateral rectus
Facial	SVA – Geniculate ganglion via Nucleus tractus solitarius to taste buds SVE – Facial nucleus GSA – Geniculate ganglion GVA – Solitary tract GVE – Preganglionic – superior salivatory nucleus Postganglionic: Submandibular and sphenopalatine ganglion
Glossopharyngeal	SVA- preganglionic: Solitary nucleus Postganglionic – inferior petrosal ganglion SVE: Nucleus ambiguus supplying stylopharyngeus GSA – Superior ganglion of 9th nerve, supplying taste buds GVA – Inferior ganglion of 9th nerve, supplying Mechanoreceptors – pharynx, tonsils, palate; baroreceptors – carotid sinus; chemoreceptors – carotid body GVE component – parasympathetic to otic ganglion
Vagus	**SVA component** – nodose ganglion or inferior ganglion X to taste buds **SVE component** – nucleus ambiguous supplying larynx and pharynx **GSA component** – superior ganglion of X nerve **GVA component** – nodose ganglion or inferior ganglion X, supplying Larynx, abdominal viscera, baroreceptors and chemoreceptors **GVE component** – dorsal motor nucleus supplying to abdominal and thoracic viscera
Hypoglossal	GSE component: Through hypoglossal nucleus to tongue

Footnote:
General (G) - distributed throughout body
Special (S) - restricted area of the body
Visceral (V)
Somatic – soma, bones, muscles, joints
Afferent (A); sensory
Efferent (E); motor

Physiology

2

AIIMS NOVEMBER 2018

1. How glucose is absorbed into intestine?
a. By simple diffusion
b. By counter transport
c. By primary active transport
d. By secondary active transport

2. Meissner's corpuscles are located in:
a. Papillary dermis
b. Reticular dermis
c. Stratum basale
d. Stratum spinosum

3. Fibers from which nucleus reach to Purkinje cells directly?
a. Inferior olivary nucleus
b. Vestibular nucleus
c. Locus coeruleus
d. Raphe nucleus

4. The hormone which has 'permissive' role in puberty?
a. Leptin b. Growth hormone
c. Insulin d. GnRH

5. Hypothalamus has inhibitory action on which hormone?
a. Prolactin
b. Growth hormone and prolactin
c. Growth hormone
d. Only prolactin

6. Calculate net filtration pressure using plasma pressure in glomerular capillary = 42 mm Hg, oncotic pressure in glomerular capillary = 18 mm Hg, plasma pressure in bowman's capsule = 10 mm Hg assuming no protein has filtered across the membrane.
a. 14 mm Hg b. 24 mm Hg
c. 34 mm Hg d. Data insufficient

7. Thyroid hormones, T_3 and T_4 acts through thyroid hormone receptor (THR). What is THR?
a. It is tyrosine kinase receptor
b. It acts as a transcription factor
c. It acts by increasing cAMP
d. It acts through activation of phospholipase A

8. Erythropoietin acts on which stage of red blood cells?
a. Colony forming units
b. Blast forming unit
c. Late erythroblast
d. Normoblast

9. Most effective way to increase blood supply in a tissue bed is:
a. Increase diameter of blood vessel
b. Increase venous pressure
c. Increasing viscosity of blood
d. Decreasing diameter of blood vessel

10. Weber Fechner law implies that strength of stimulus is directly related to: ***(AIIMS Nov 2018, 2008, May 2016)***
a. Intensity of stimulus
b. Duration of stimulus
c. Number of muscle fibers
d. Number of nerve fibers

11. Larger representation of any area of body in motor homunculus signifies:
a. Lower control but more skilled movements
b. More number of muscle fibers are involved
c. Better precision of movements
d. More control but less skilled movements

12. Nobel Prize for Medicine and Physiology in the year 2018 was given for which work?
a. Circadian rhythm b. CRISPR pathway
c. Autophagy d. Negative immune regulation

13. Integrin binds mainly to which component of extracellular matrix (ECM)?
a. Laminin b. Fibronectin
c. Vimentin d. Collagen

AIIMS MAY 2018

14. Which of following is true regarding the image given below?
a. B has both preload and afterload added to it
b. B has done more work than A
c. A has undergone maximum tension
d. B has undergone maximum tension

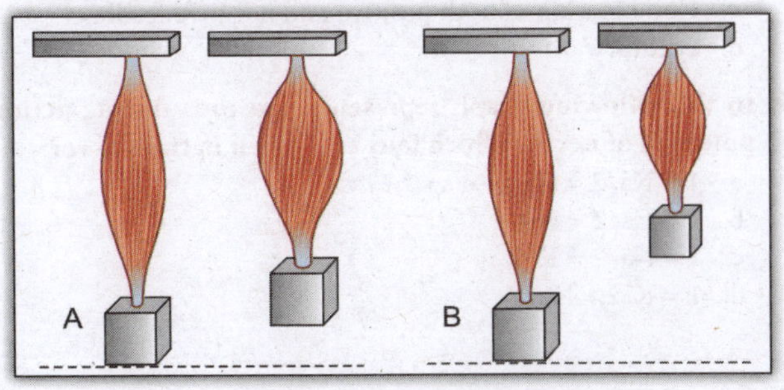

15. A and B graphs represent length - tension relationship of which muscle:

a. A- skeletal muscle, B- cardiac muscle
b. A- cardiac muscle, B- skeletal muscle
c. A - smooth muscle, B - cardiac muscle
d. A - cardiac muscle , B- Smooth muscle

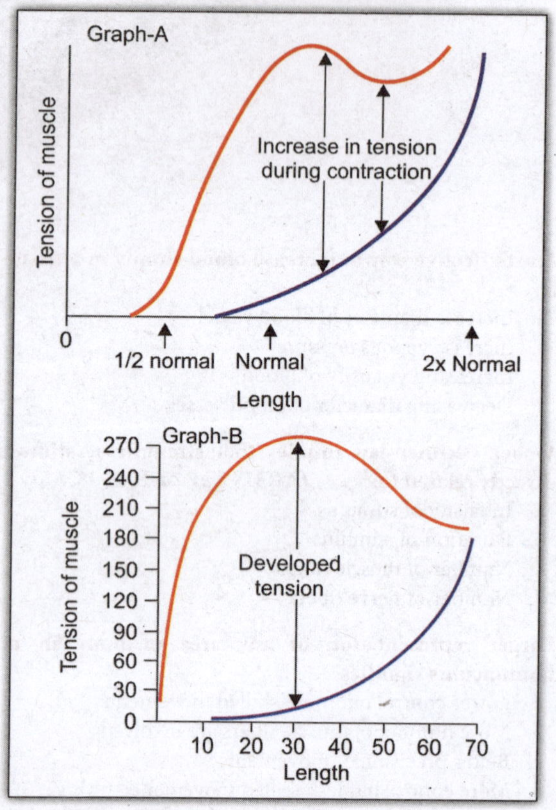

16. Which of the following statement about electric synapse is true compared to chemical synapse?

a. No cytoplasmic continuity between presynaptic and postsynaptic neurons
b. Has more latent period than chemical synapse
c. Bidirectional transmission
d. More vulnerable to repeated stimulus

17. Which of the following condition GFR increases EXCEPT:

a. Increased renal blood flow
b. Decreased plasma oncotic pressure
c. Increased efferent arteriole resistance
d. Ureter obstruction with stone

18. Baroreceptor reflex is:

a. Negative feedback
b. Positive feedback
c. Combination of both positive and negative feedback
d. Feedforward

19. In the following graph represents two ions during action potential of nerve. Which ions are shown in this curve?

a. 1 = Na, 2 = Ca
b. 1 = Ca, 2 = Na
c. 1 = Na, 2 = K
d. 1 = K, 2 = Na

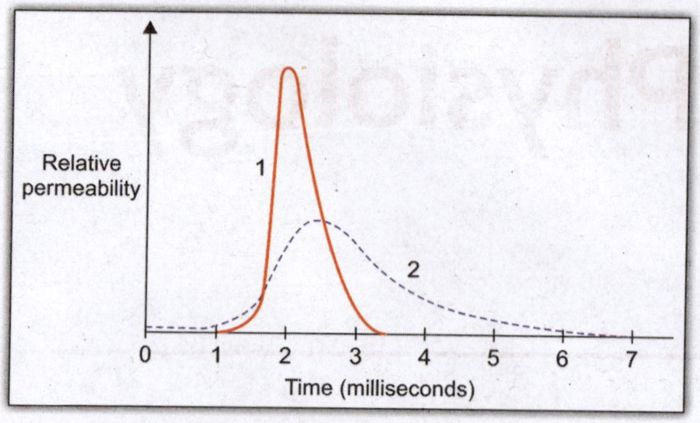

20. End systolic volume of a person doing exercise within his physiological range:

a. Increases with every alternating beat
b. Fluctuates with degree of exercise
c. Decreases
d. No change

21. Which of the following is a G protein coupled receptors?

a. Muscarinic receptors
b. Insulin receptors
c. Nicotinic receptors
d. GABA receptors

22. In JVP 'a' wave is due to? ***(AIIMS May 2018, 2017)***

a. Atrial contraction
b. Passive atrial filling
c. Ventricular contraction
d. Ventricular relaxation

23. Which of the following is the diluting segment of nephron?

a. Proximal convoluted tubule
b. Thick limb of ascending loop of Henle
c. Descending limb of Loop of Henle
d. Distal convoluted tubule

24. A person met with an accident. He is unable to speak but can understand & write things to describe what he want to tell. Which of the following marked area in the given image is most likely to be damaged?

a. 1 b. 2
c. 3 d. 4

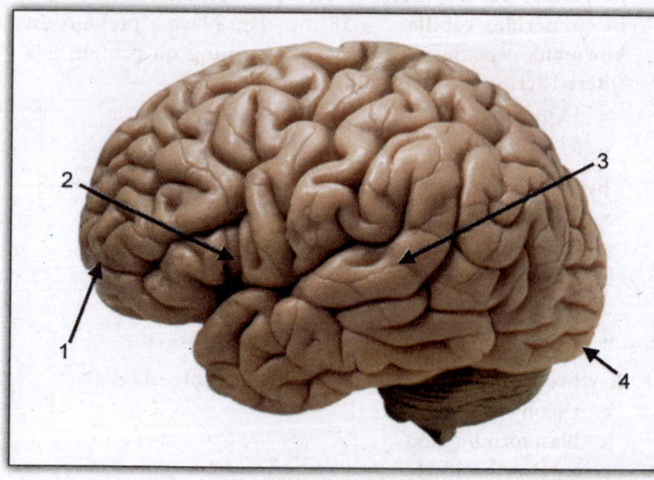

25. **In a nonexcitable cell X, Y & Z are three ions in cell whose permeability is different for different ions. At RMP, X & Y had potential of –30mV & –50mV respectively. If experimentally, conductance of Z is blocked what would be effect on RMP?**
   a. Hyperpolarization of membrane
   b. Depolarization
   c. Repolarization
   d. Maintains RMP

AIIMS NOVEMBER 2017

26. **Difference in trajectory between inspiratory loop and the expiratory loop in the curve is due to?**

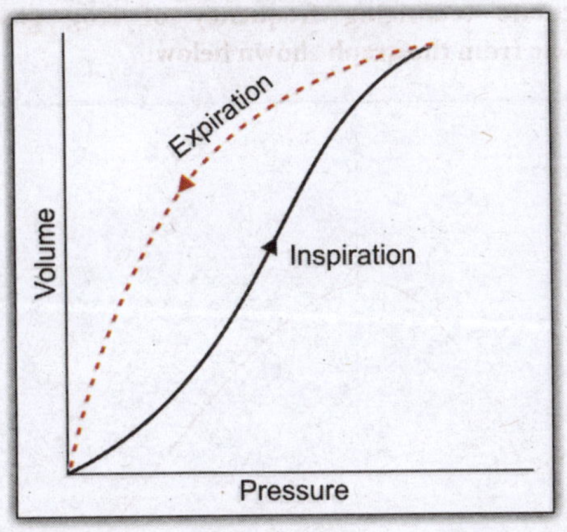

   a. Difference in alveolar pressure during inspiration and expiration
   b. Difference in concentration of surfactant during inspiration and expiration
   c. Difference in airway resistance during inspiration and expiration
   d. Inspiration is active and expiration is passive

27. **All the following are involved in K^+ homeostasis EXCEPT:**
   a. Catecholamine induced working of Na/K^+ ATPase pump
   b. Aldosterone induced K^+ excretion
   c. Insulin induced cellular shift of K^+
   d. Change in plasma osmolarity

28. **Absolute refractory period is due to:**
   a. Opening of calcium channels
   b. Closure of potassium channels
   c. Closure of active gates of sodium channel
   d. Closure of inactive gates of sodium channel

29. **X, Y, Z are the three permeable ions. X = –50 and Y = –30. If at RMP, when there is no net electrogenic transfer, what is the value of Z?**
   a. +20
   b. –20
   c. +80
   d. –80

30. **Identify the stage of sleep from the given picture:**
   a. Stage I NREM
   b. Stage II NREM
   c. Stage III NREM
   d. REM

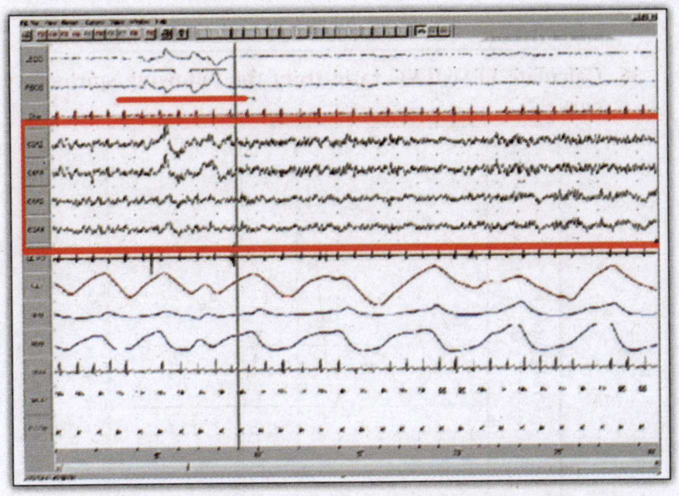

31. **A graphic variation of hormone was shown asked to identify. Graph showed elevation of hormone during exercise and at night time (during sleep).**

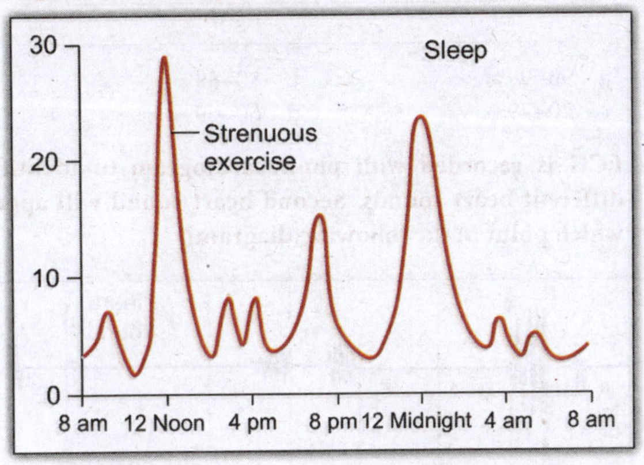

   a. Insulin
   b. Cortisol
   c. Estrogen
   d. Growth hormone

32. **Feed forward mechanism of regulation is employed in regulation of:**
   a. pH
   b. Temperature
   c. Blood volume
   d. Blood pressure

33. **Reflex responsible for tachycardia during right atrial distension is:**
   a. Bainbridge reflex
   b. Bezold-Jarisch reflex
   c. Frank Starling law
   d. J reflex

34. **Efferent arteriolar constriction causes all EXCEPT:**
   a. Decrease in GFR
   b. Decreases renal blood flow
   c. Decreases oncotic pressure in peritubular capillaries
   d. Increases hydrostatic pressure in glomerular capillaries

35. **Slow waves are generated by:**
   a. Myenteric neurons
   b. Smooth muscles
   c. Interstitial cells of Cajal
   d. Parasympathetic neurons

AIIMS MAY 2017

36. Calculate FEV1/FVC ratio from the following spirometry curve:

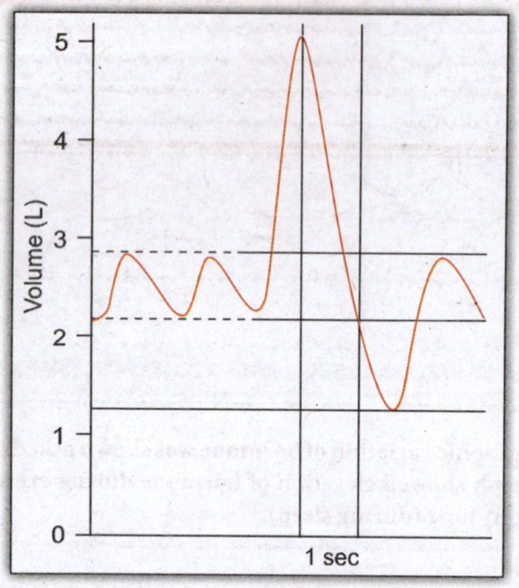

a. 90–99% b. 80–89%
c. 70–79% d. 60–69%

37. ECG is recorded with phonocardiogram to identify the different heart sounds. Second heart sound will appear at which point in the following diagram?

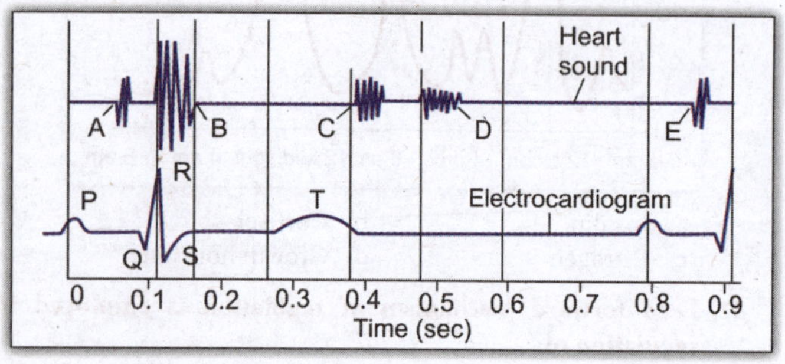

a. Point A
b. Point B
c. Point C
d. Point D

38. The oxygen carrying capacity of a 18-year-old boy with hemoglobin of 14 g/dL is:

a. 14
b. 16
c. 18
d. 22

39. Bezold-Jarisch reflex is mediated by:

a. Angiotensin
b. Histamine
c. Serotonin
d. Prostaglandin

40. In JVP 'a wave' is due to: ***(AIIMS May 2018, 2017)***

a. Atrial contraction
b. Passive atrial filling
c. Ventricular contraction
d. Ventricular relaxation

41. Which of the following is the constituent of the marked area in the electron microscopic picture of muscle?

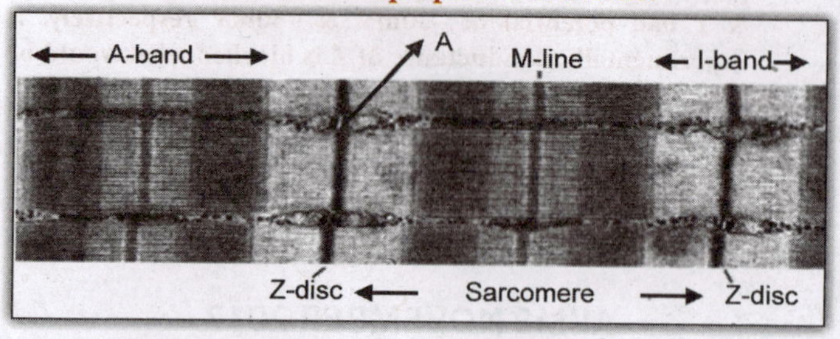

a. Alpha actinin b. Titin
c. Nebulin d. Calmodulin

42. Calculate tetanizing frequency of frog gastrocnemius muscle from the graph shown below:

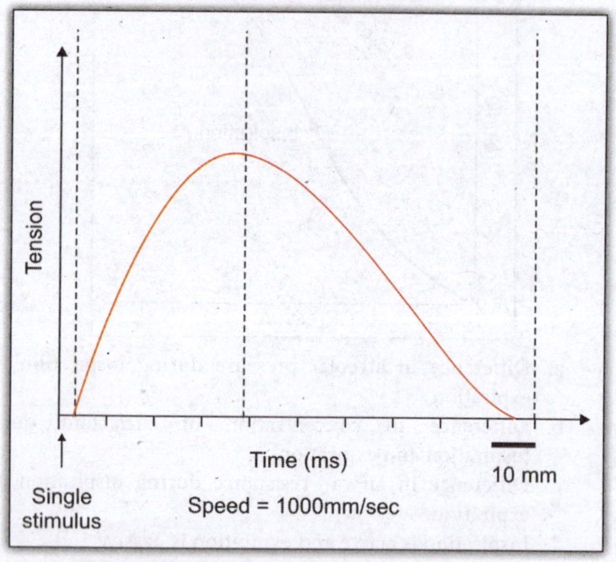

a. 25–30 Hz b. 30–35 Hz
c. 35–40 Hz d. 40–50 Hz

43. Below are two vessels shown. Assuming the pressure along both the vessels is the same and both of them follow linear flow pattern. What will the amount of blood flow in vessel A compared to vessel B?

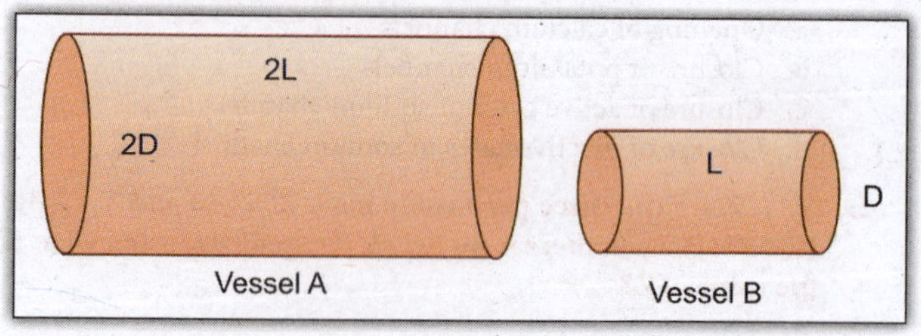

a. 4 times b. 8 times
c. 16 times d. 32 times

44. In a diseased person intrapleural pressure measured –4 mm Hg & –9 mm Hg at the start and end of inspiration having tidal volume 500 mL. Calculate pulmonary compliance in Lit/mm Hg?

a. 0.1 b. 0.2
c. 0.5 d. 0.7

45. **A diabetic patient having blood glucose of 200 mg/dL and GFR of 90 mL/min. Transport maximum of glucose = 150 mg/min. What is the amount of glucose excreted in urine?**

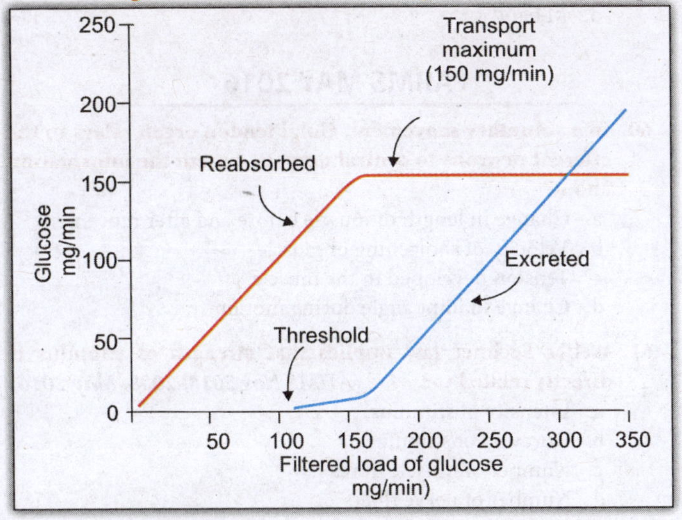

a. 10 mg/min
b. 20 mg/min
c. 30 mg/min
d. 40 mg/min

AIIMS NOVEMBER 2016

46. **Which of the following graph represents normal glucose tolerance test?**

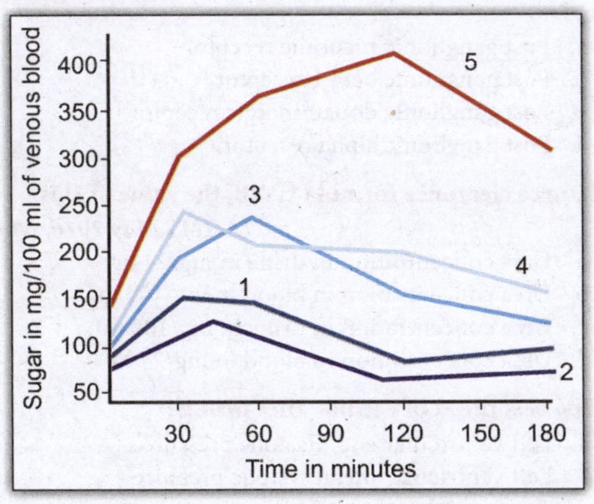

a. 1
b. 2
c. 3
d. 4

47. **Parasympathetic outflow involves:**
a. Cranial nerves 3, 7, 9, 10 and S2, S3, S4
b. Cranial nerves 5, 7, 9, 10 and S2, S3, S4
c. Cranial nerves 3, 7, 9, 10 and S3, S4, S5
d. Cranial nerves 5, 7, 9, 10 and S3, S4, S5

48. **Which of the following inhibits calcium absorption?**
a. Vitamin D
b. Phytates
c. Proteins in diet
d. Alkaline pH in GIT

49. **The following diagram is from adrenal gland. Hormone produced by the marked area A in the following image is:**

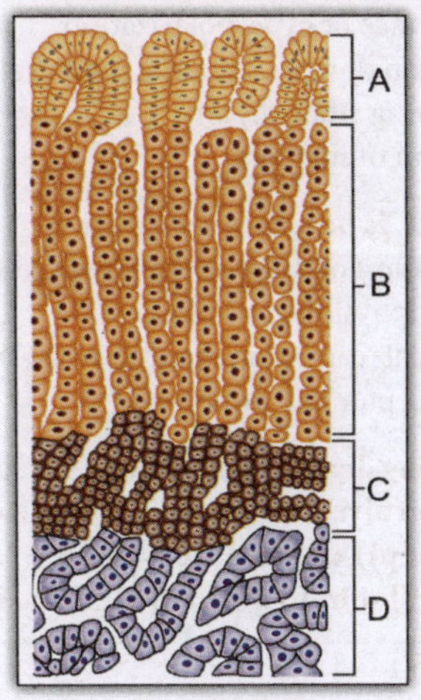

a. Aldosterone
b. Cortisol
c. Epinephrine
d. Androgen

50. **The effect of different thyroid hormones in plasma during starvation is shown in the following curve. Curve C indicate which of the following?**

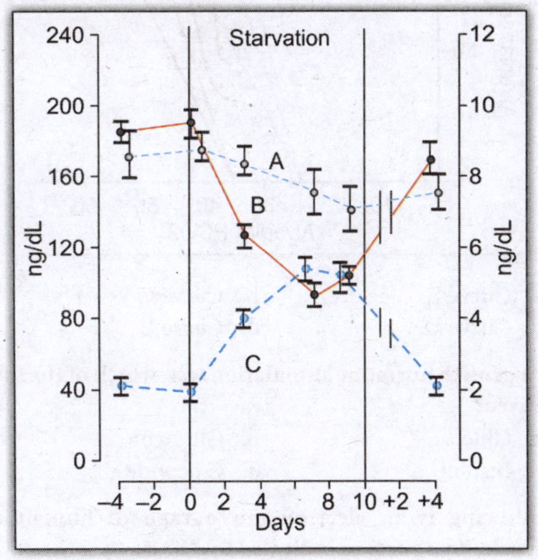

a. DIT
b. rT3
c. T3
d. T4

51. **Countercurrent mechanism is seen in all EXCEPT:**
a. Eye
b. Kidney
c. GIT
d. Testes

52. **Migratory motor complex reappears after an interval of:**
a. 60 min
b. 90 min
c. 120 min
d. 150 min

53. **Which will have maximum effect due to decrease in SHBG?**
a. DHEA
b. Testosterone
c. Progesterone
d. Estrogen

54. **Potential developed due to free movement of a diffusible ion is calculated by:**
a. Nernst equation
b. Gibb's equation
c. Fick's Equation
d. Goldman-Katz equation

55. Which of the following is the function of hyperpolarizing cyclic nucleotide (HCN) channel?

a. Maintenance of hyperpolarization
b. Generation of mitochondrial potential
c. Maintaining sinus rhythm
d. Formation of memory

56. HCO_3^-/H_2CO_3 is best buffer because?

a. Combination of weak acid and weak base
b. pKa near physiological pH
c. Components can be increased or decreased in body as needed
d. Good acceptor and donor of H^+

57. In the following diagram, the curve "X" represents the normal relationship of alveolar ventilation with $PaCO_2$, when PaO_2 is 100 mmHg. If pH changed from 7.4 to 7.3, change in alveolar ventilation will shift to which of the curve?

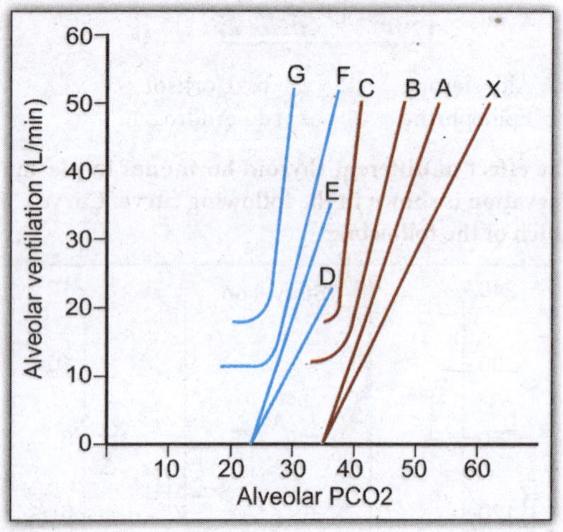

a. Curve B
b. Curve C
c. Curve D
d. Curve E

58. For growth hormone stimulation test, which of the following is used?

a. Glucose
b. Glucagon
c. Insulin
d. C peptide

59. Following is an electron micrograph of human skeletal muscle. The portion indicated by "E" is:

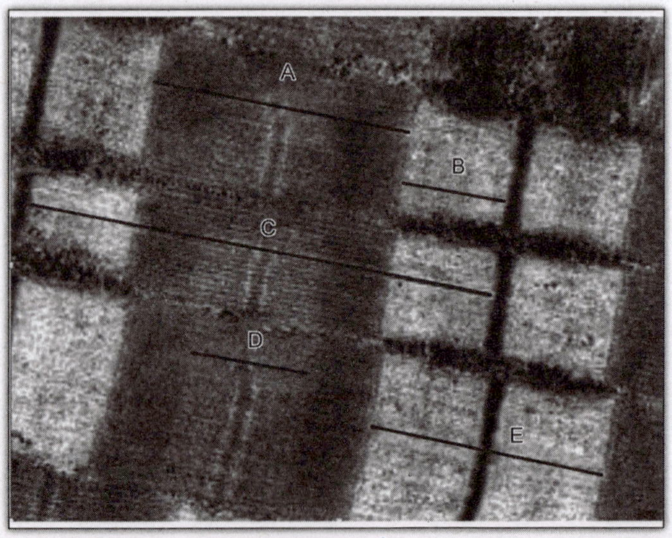

a. I band
b. A band
c. G band
d. M band

AIIMS MAY 2016

60. In a voluntary movement, Golgi tendon organ relays to the efferent neurons to central nervous system the information about?

a. Change in length of muscle before and after movement
b. Velocity of shortening of muscle
c. Tension developed in the muscle
d. Change in joint angle during motion

61. Weber Fechner law implies that strength of stimulus is directly related to? ***(AIIMS Nov 2018, 2008, May 2016)***

a. Intensity of stimulus
b. Duration of stimulus
c. Number of muscle fibres
d. Number of nerve fibers

62. Extracellular concentration of ion is 100 mmol/L and its intracellular concentration is 10 mmol/L. The action potential across the membrane using Nernst equation is?

a. –60 mV ***(AIIMS May 2016, Nov 2015)***
b. –10 mV
c. 60 mV
d. 10 mV

63. The ganglionic transmission of nerve impulse is mediated by?

a. Post ganglionic nicotinic receptor
b. Post ganglionic beta 1 receptor
c. Post ganglionic dopaminergic receptor
d. Post ganglionic alpha receptor

64. In urea clearance formula UV/B, the value of U is? ***(AIIMS May 2016, Nov 2015)***

a. Urea concentration in urine in mg/24 hr
b. Urea concentration in blood in mg/100 mL
c. Urea concentration in urine in mg/100 mL
d. Urea concentration in blood in mg/24 hr

65. The best index of cardiac after load is?

a. Left ventricular end diastolic pressure
b. Left ventricular mean systolic pressure
c. Total peripheral resistance
d. Mean arterial pressure

66. In relaxed state, the recoil of chest wall and lungs are balanced at:

a. Functional residual capacity
b. Residual volume
c. Total lung capacity
d. Minute volume

67. In the electron micrographic picture given below, identify the organ marked as 2 with the arrow?

a. Cis Golgi complex
b. Trans Golgi complex
c. Smooth endoplasmic reticulum
d. Medial Golgi complex

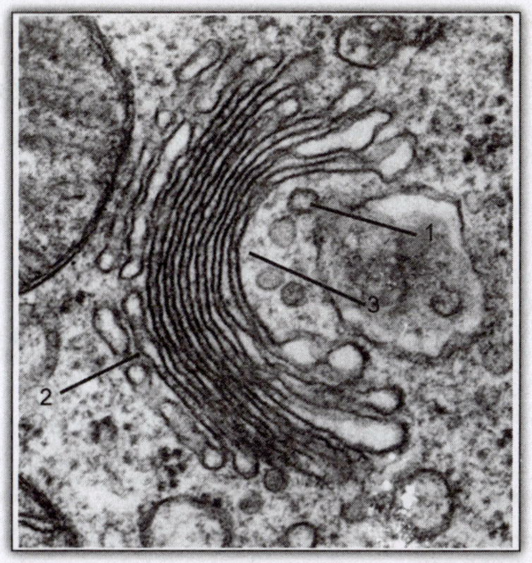

68. **On changing position from lying down to standing there is fall in BP of 10 mm Hg. Immediately he recovered by 8 mm Hg leaving behind 2 mm Hg. The gain for baroreceptor system for the control of BP is:**
   a. 2 b. 4
   c. 8 d. 10

69. **Respiratory rhythm generation center is located at:**
   a. Pneumotactic center b. Pre-botzinger complex
   c. Dorsal respiratory group d. Ventral respiratory neuron

70. **Cellular location of receptors of hormone X is mapped to the nucleus. Which of the following is hormone X?**
   a. Thyroxine b. Insulin
   c. Norepinephrine d. FSH

71. **Nitric oxide produces smooth muscle relaxation using second messenger:**
   a. Calcium b. cAMP
   c. cGMP d. Magnesium

72. **The hormone that plays permissive role in the attainment of puberty is:**
   a. GnRH b. Leptin
   c. Insulin d. Growth hormone

AIIMS NOVEMBER 2015

73. **Dye used for interstitial fluid volume determination:**
   a. Radioactive sodium and radioiodine labeled albumin
   b. Radioactive water and radioiodine labeled albumin
   c. Radioactive water and radioactive sodium
   d. Radioactive iodine labeled iothalamate

74. **In Urea clearance formula UV/P, the value of U is?** ***(AIIMS May 2016, Nov 2015)***
   a. Urea concentration in urine in mg/24 hr
   b. Urea concentration in blood in mg/100 mL
   c. Urea concentration in urine in mg/100 mL
   d. Urea concentration in blood in mg/24 hr

75. **Anatomical dead space is measured with:**
   a. Spirometer
   b. Bohr's method
   c. Xenon isotope inhalation
   d. Single breath nitrogen test

76. **False about atrial natriuretic peptide is:**
   a. Dilatation of afferent arterioles
   b. Mesangial cell constriction
   c. Inhibition of Na+ reabsorption at PCT.
   d. Inhibition of Na+ reabsorption at collecting duct

77. **Coagulation and clumping of plasma protein is favored by all EXCEPT:**
   a. Factor 2 b. Factor 7
   c. Factor C d. Factor 9

78. **If extracellular potassium is 100 mEq/mmol and intracellular potassium is 10 mEq/mmol. What will be Nernst equilibrium potential for potassium?** ***(AIIMS May 2016, Nov 2015)***
   a. –90 V b. 0 V
   c. –60 V d. –30 V

79. **Skeletal muscle twitch with latent period 10 milli sec, contraction period 40 milli sec and relaxation period 50 milli sec, what is tetanic contraction frequency?**
   a. 25 Hz b. 40 Hz
   c. 50 Hz d. 100 Hz

80. **Na$^+$ iodide transporter is present in all EXCEPT:**
   a. Pituitary b. Thyroid
   c. Salivary d. Placenta

81. **Gastric smooth muscle was isolated, put in dales broth and electrical, mechanical recording was done. All are true about following graph EXCEPT:**

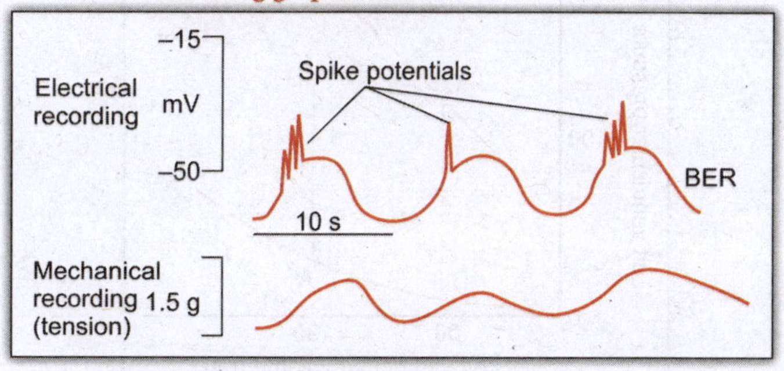

   a. Threshold voltage is –50 mV
   b. Frequency = 6/min
   c. Muscle contraction is related to amplitude of BER
   d. Tension is directly proportional to frequency of spike potential

82. **Part of smooth muscle of intestine was put in dales broth and electrical, mechanical recording were done. After addition of a compound at point Y in the following graph, the amplitude of contraction decreases, what is added at point X?**

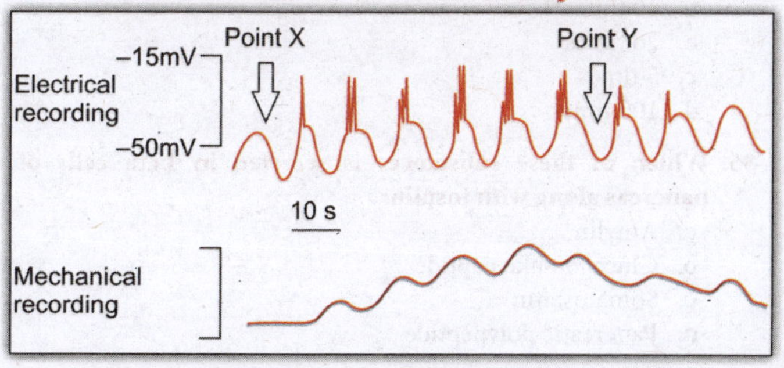

   a. Adrenaline b. Acetylcholine
   c. KCl d. $BaCl_2$

83. **Calculate left ventricular ejection fraction from the given diagram:**

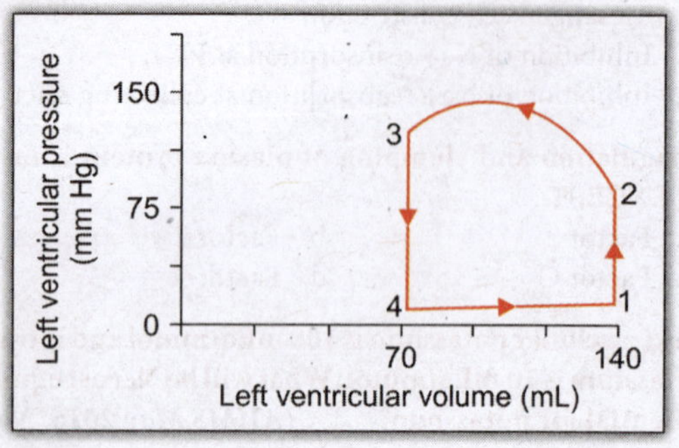

a. 50%
b. 60%
c. 67%
d. 70%

AIIMS MAY 2015

84. **In the following diagram left ventricular pressure is equal to diastolic blood pressure at which point?**

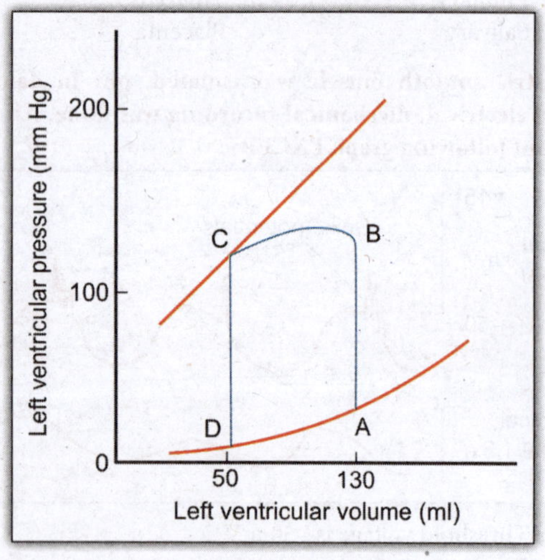

a. A
b. B
c. C
d. D

85. **If the radius of an artery increases by 50%, blood flow increases by:**
a. 10 times
b. 20 times
c. 5 times
d. 100 times

86. **Which of these substances is secreted by beta cells of pancreas along with insulin:**
a. Amylin
b. Glucagon like peptide
c. Somatostatin
d. Pancreatic polypeptide

87. **Wave patterns of EEG, EOG and EMG are shown in the following graph. What does C in the following set of picture represents?** *(AIIMS May 2015, 2014)*

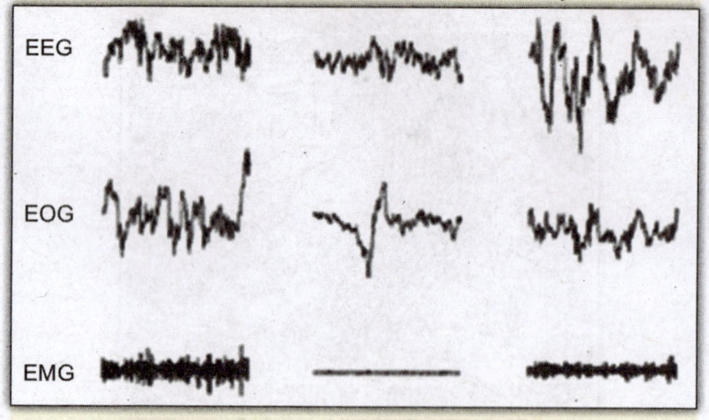

a. REM sleep
b. NREM sleep
c. Quiet wakefulness
d. Awake state

88. **If the interstitial hydrostatic pressure is 2 mm Hg, interstitial oncotic pressure is 7 mm Hg and capillary hydrostatic pressure is 25 mm Hg, What would be the capillary oncotic pressure to allow a net filtration pressure of 3 mm Hg?**
a. 21 mm Hg
b. 27 mm Hg
c. 20 mm Hg
d. 23 mm Hg

89. **In a study to detect extracellular fluid volume, 10g Mannitol is injected intravenous by and after waiting for adequate time for equilibration of levels, concentration was measured as 50 mg/100 mL. In this time 10% of mannitol was excreted. What is the calculated volume of the ECF?**
a. 18 L
b. 42 L
c. 50 L
d. 10 L

90. **During initiation of voluntary movement, which of the following is a true statement regarding alpha and gamma neuron activation?**
a. Alpha motor neuron gets activated first followed by gamma motor neuron
b. Gamma motor neurons are activated before alpha motor neuron
c. Both alpha and gamma motor neurons are activated together
d. Only alpha motor neurons get activated

91. **Brown fat is absent in:**
a. Scapular region
b. Mesentery
c. Subcutaneous tissue
d. Adrenal cortex

92. **Adrenergic receptor responsible for lipolysis in fat cells is:**
a. Alpha 1
b. Alpha 2
c. Beta 1
d. Beta 3

93. **The clot formed is not stable unless extensive cross linking occurs. This is done by:**
a. Plasmin
b. Thrombin
c. Factor XIII
d. HMWK

AIIMS NOVEMBER 2018

1. Ans. (d) By secondary active transport

Ref: Ganong's 24th Ed page 480

- The transport of glucose and galactose is dependent on Na^+ in the intestinal lumen; a high concentration of Na^+ on the mucosal surface of the cells facilitates and a low concentration inhibits sugar influx into the epithelial cells.
- This is because these sugars and Na^+ share the same cotransporter, or symport, the sodium-dependent glucose transporter (SGLT, Na^+ glucose cotransporter).
- SGLT-1 is responsible for uptake of dietary glucose from the gut.
- Because the intracellular Na^+ concentration is low in intestinal cells (as it is in other cells), Na^+ moves into the cell along its concentration gradient. Glucose moves with the Na^+ and is released in the cell.
- The Na^+ is transported into the lateral intercellular spaces and the glucose is transported by GLUT2 into the interstitium and thence to the capillaries. Thus, glucose transport is an example of secondary active transport.

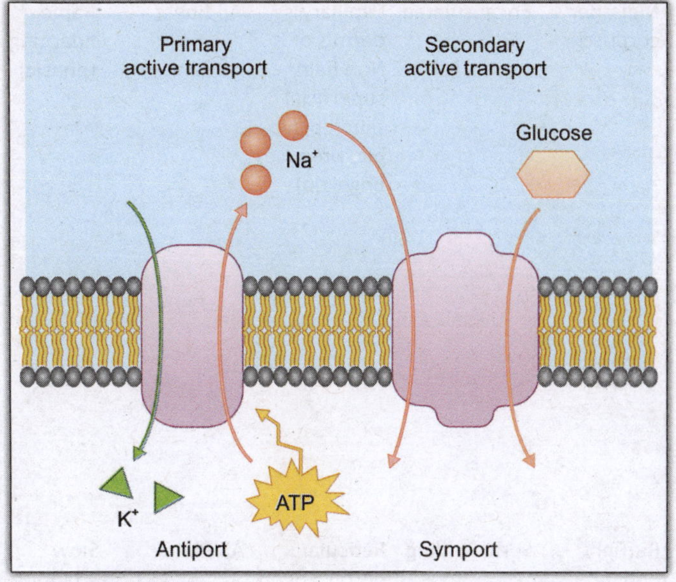

2. Ans. (a) Papillary dermis

Ref: Andrew's Diseases of the Skin 11th ed Pg 10

Touch and pressure are mediated by Meissner corpuscles found in dermal papillae, particularly on digits of palms and soles and by Vater-Pacini corpuscles located in the reticular portion of the dermis.

Mechanoreceptors						
Receptor	**Ending**	**Site**	**Fiber**	**Type**	**Sensation**	**Figure**
Pacinian corpuscle	Encapsulated (onion like)	Reticular dermis, deep fibrous tissue	Aβ fibers	Rapid adapting (phasic)	Pressure, vibration (200–300 Hz), touch	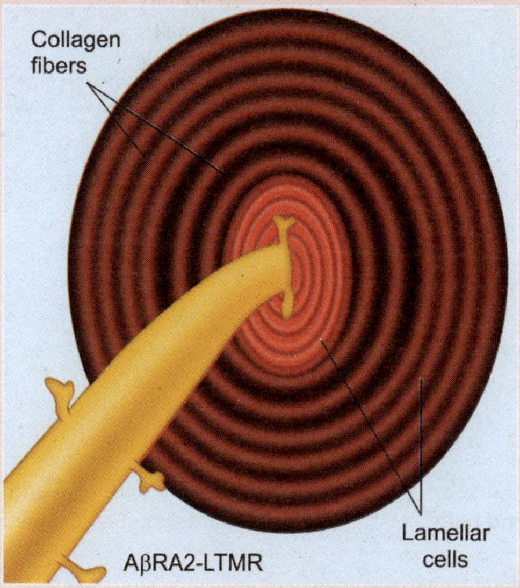

Contd...

Mechanoreceptors						
Receptor	Ending	Site	Fiber	Type	Sensation	Figure
Meissner's corpuscle	Encapsulated	Papillary dermis of Non hairy superficial skin (lip, nipple, prepuce, fingertip)	Aβ fibers	Rapid adapting (phasic)	Pressure, vibration (50 Hz), touch	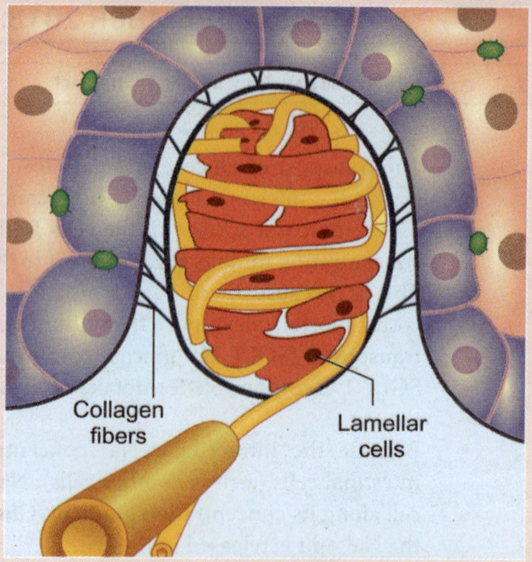
Ruffini's Ending	Spray ending	Reticular dermis, deep fibrous tissue	Aβ fibers	Slow adapting (tonic)	Heat, pressure, touch	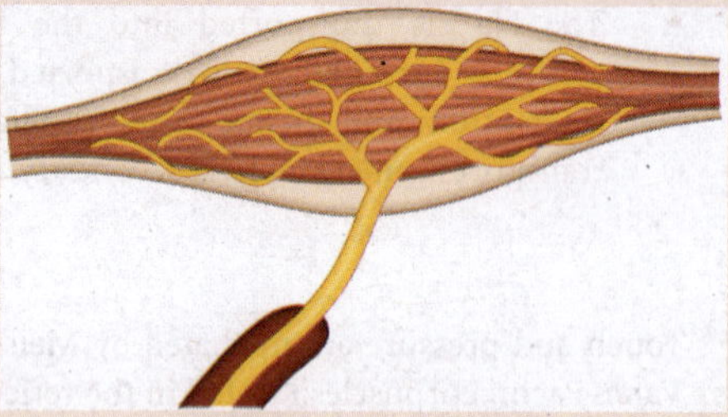
Merkel's disc	Expanded	Hairy superficial skin (Papillary dermis)	Aβ fibers	Slow adapting (tonic)	Tactile localization, continuous touch	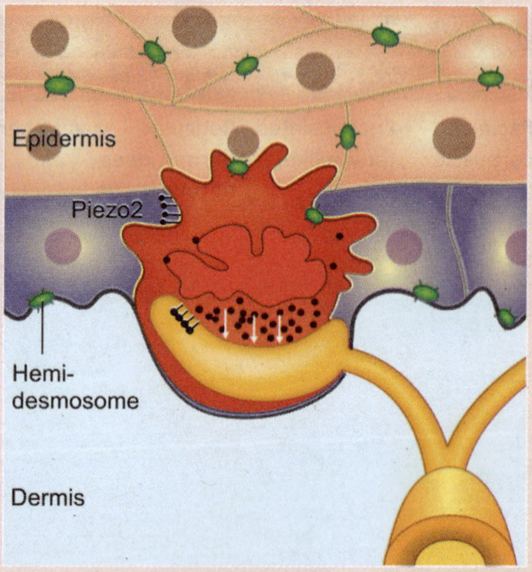
Krause's end bulb	Encapsulated	Skin (Reticular dermis)	Aδ and C-fibers	Slow adapting (tonic)	Cold	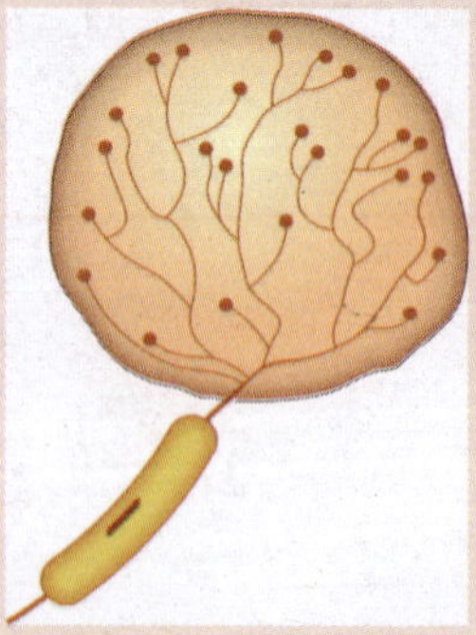

Contd...

Mechanoreceptors						
Receptor	**Ending**	**Site**	**Fiber**	**Type**	**Sensation**	**Figure**
Free nerve ending	Uncapsulated	Skin (Papillary dermis), muscle, viscera	Aδ (Fast-pricking pain) C-fiber (slow-aching pain)	Non adapting	Nociception-pain	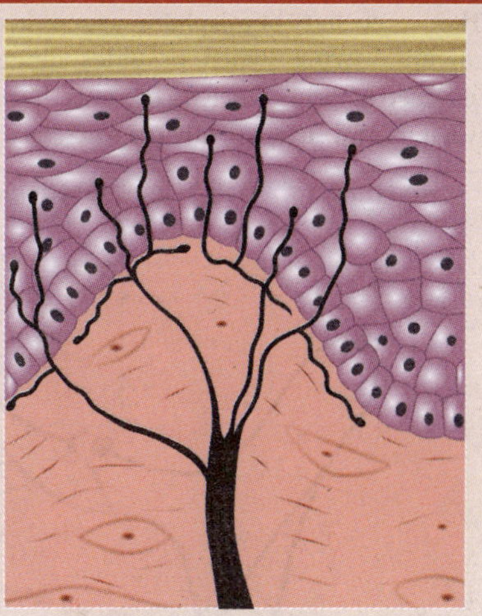
Golgi tendon organ	Muscle ending	Joint space, muscle	Aα fiber	Slow adapting (tonic)	Proprioception, position sense	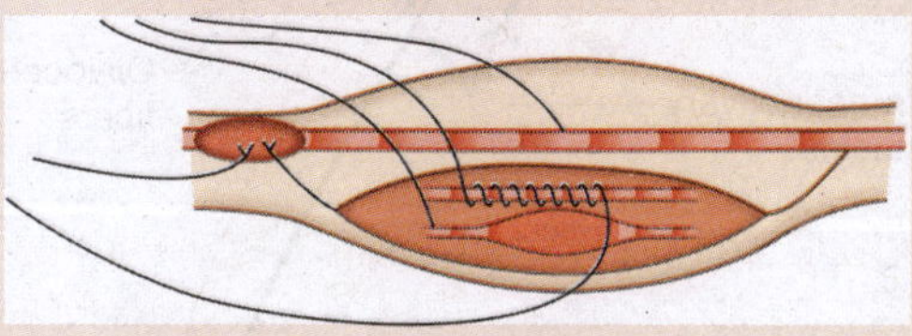
Muscle spindle	Muscle ending	Muscle	Aα fiber	Slow adapting (tonic)	Stretch	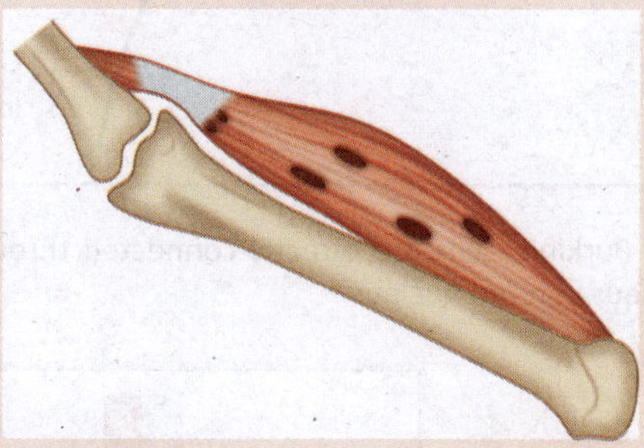

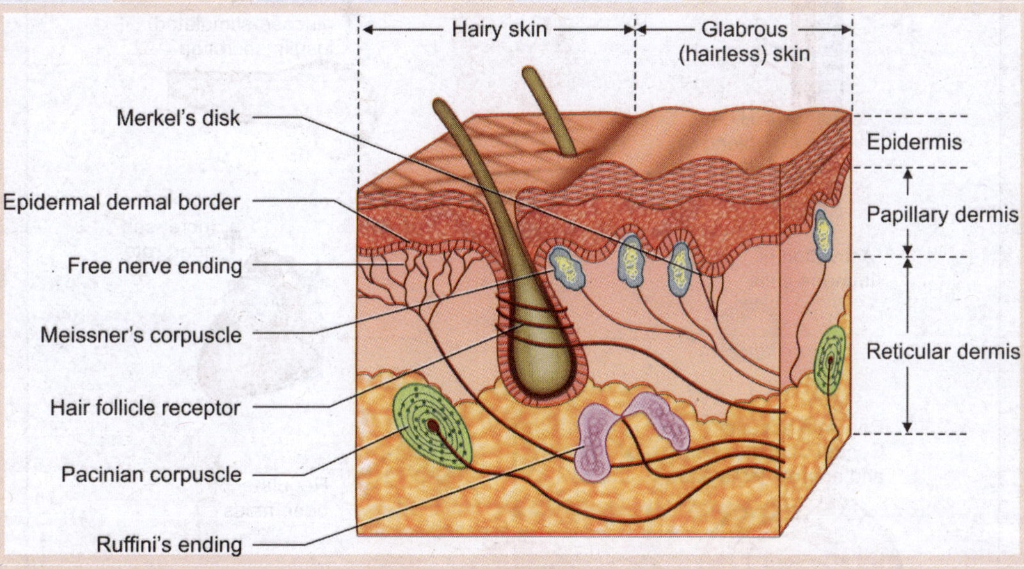

Footnote:
- Slowly adapting receptors (Tonic) detect continuous stimulus strength
- Rapidly adapting receptors detect change in stimulus strength—The "Rate Receptors," "Movement Receptors," or "Phasic Receptors." Receptors that adapt rapidly cannot be used to transmit a continuous signal because these receptors are stimulated only when the stimulus strength changes. Yet they react strongly while a change is actually taking place

3. **Ans. (a) Inferior olivary nucleus**

Ref: Ganong 24th ed page 249, 253

The cerebellar hemisphere are linked functionally to the cerebral cortex which provides inputs to the hemispheres via deep pontine nucleus or more indirectly through the **red nucleus and inferior olivary nucleus**

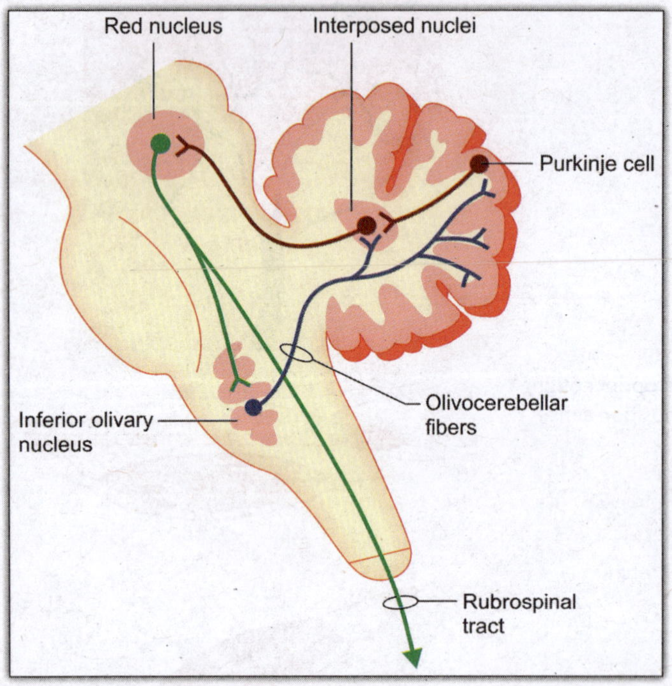

Fig: Purkinje cells are directly connected through inferior olivary nucleus and red nucleus

The cerebellar cortex contains five types of neurons: Purkinje, granule, basket, stellate and Golgi cells. The two main inputs to the cerebellar cortex are climbing fibers and mossy fibers; both are excitatory. Purkinje cells are the only output from the cerebellar cortex and they generally project to the deep nuclei. **Climbing fibers from contralateral Inferior olivary nucleus ends directly to the Purkinje cells. The Purkinje cells are among the biggest neurons in the CNS.**

4. **Ans. (a) Leptin**

Ref: Ganong 24th ed page 399, 450

White fat depots are actually endocrine tissues that secrete not only leptin but also other hormones that affect fat metabolism. These adipose derived hormones are commonly termed adipokines as they are cytokines secreted by adipose tissue. Known adipokines are leptin, adiponectin and resistin.

Leptin

Critical body weight must normally be reached for puberty to occur.

- Young women who engage in strenuous athletics lose weight and stop menstruating, as do girls with anorexia nervosa. If these girls start to eat and gain weight, they menstruate again, that is, they **"go back through puberty."**
- **It appears that leptin, the satiety-producing hormone secreted by fat cells, may be the link between body weight and puberty.**
- Obese ob/ob mice that cannot make leptin are infertile and their fertility is restored by injections of leptin.
- Leptin treatment also induces precocious puberty in immature female mice.

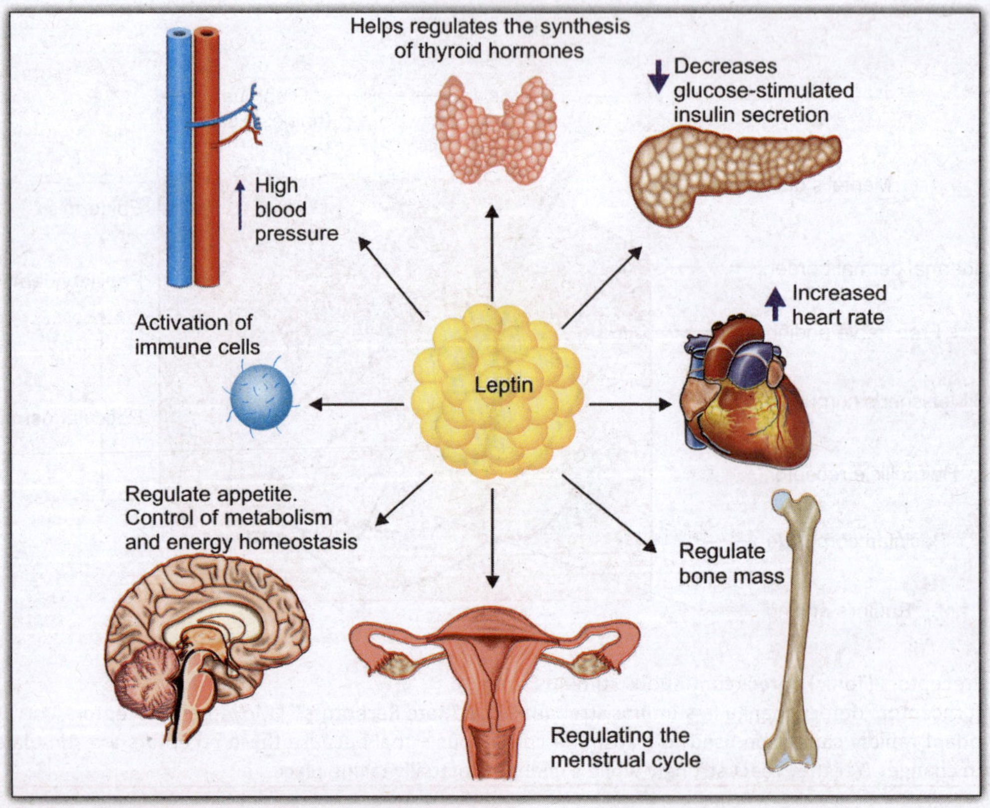

5. Ans. (b) Growth hormone and prolactin

Ref: Ganong 24th Ed Pg 334

Secretion of prolactin is tonically inhibited by the hypothalamus. Prolactin facilitates the secretion of dopamine in the median eminence. Thus, prolactin acts in the hypothalamus in a negative feedback fashion to inhibit its own secretion.

Effect of Hypothalamus on Anterior Pituitary	
Hypothalamic hormone	**Effect on anterior pituitary**
Thyrotropin releasing hormone (TRH)	Stimulates release of TSH and prolactin
Corticotropin releasing hormone (CRH)	Stimulates release of ACTH (corticotropin)
Gonadotropin releasing hormone (GnRH)	Stimulates release of growth hormone
Growth hormone releasing hormone (GHRH)	Stimulates release of growth hormone
Growth hormone release inhibiting hormone (GHRIH)	Inhibits release of growth hormone
Prolactin releasing hormone (PRH)	Stimulates release of prolactin
Prolactin release inhibitory hormone (PRIH) dopamine	Inhibits release of prolactin

6. Ans. (a) 14 mm Hg

Ref: Guyton's 13th Ed Pg 337

1. The four primary forces called "Starling forces" determine whether fluid will move out of the blood into the interstitial fluid or in the opposite direction.
2. The *capillary pressure* (Pc), which tends to force fluid *outward* through the capillary membrane.
3. The *interstitial fluid pressure* (Pif) → forces fluid *inward* through the capillary membrane when Pif is positive but outward when Pif is negative.
4. The capillary *plasma colloid osmotic pressure* (Πp), → osmosis of fluid *inward* through the capillary membrane.

The *interstitial fluid colloid osmotic pressure* (Πif), → causes osmosis of fluid *outward* through the capillary membrane.

Note that under normal circumstances, the concentration of protein in Bowman's space is so low that the colloid osmotic pressure of Bowman's capsule fluid is considered to be zero.

The net filtration pressure (NFP) is calculated as:

$$NFP = Pc - Pif - \Pi p + \Pi if$$

Thus, in the above case, since it has been specifically mentioned that no protein has filtered across the membrane, we shall assume that the colloid oncotic pressure in Bowman's capsule is zero.

Hence,

Net Filtration Pressure = 42 – 10 – 18 + 0 = 14 mm Hg

So, the answer is (A) 14 mm Hg

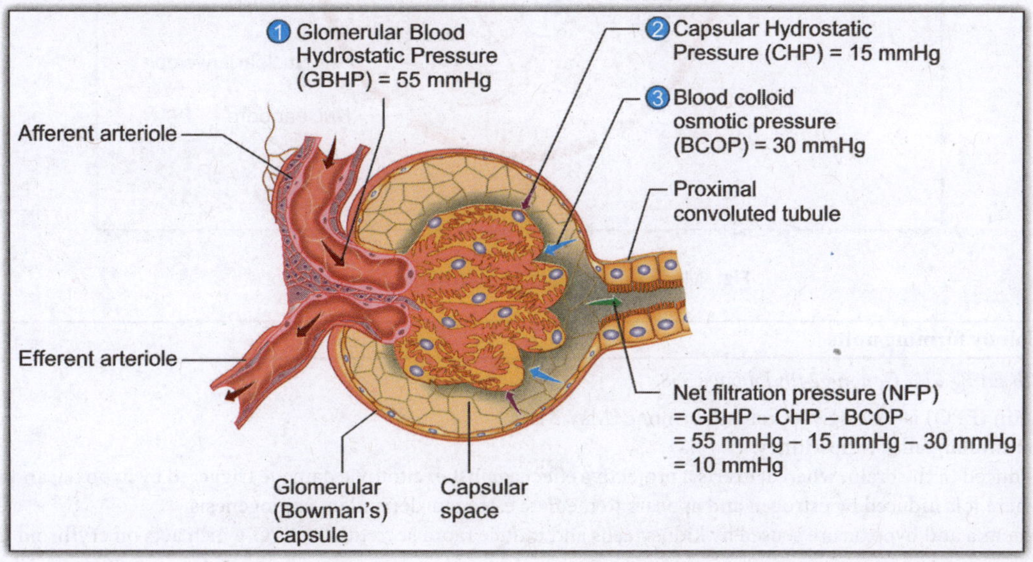

7. Ans. (b) It acts as a transcription factor

Ref: Ganong 24th ed page 300, Guyton 12th ed page 910

Guyton states that: "The **thyroid hormone receptors** are either attached to the DNA genetic strands or located in proximity to them. The thyroid hormone receptor usually forms a heterodimer with **retinoid X receptor (RXR)** at specific thyroid hormone response elements on the DNA. On binding with thyroid hormone, the receptors become activated and initiate the transcription process. Then large numbers of different types of messenger RNA are formed, followed within another few minutes or hours by RNA translation on the cytoplasmic ribosomes to form hundreds of new intracellular proteins. However, not all the proteins are increased by similar percentages-some only slightly and others at least as much as six fold. It is believed that most of the actions of thyroid hormone result from the subsequent enzymatic and other functions of these new proteins"

- T_3 modulates gene expression through ligand dependent transcription factors through ligand dependent transcription factors, the thyroid hormone receptors.

- Both T_3 and T_4 penetrate cells by active transport and produce majority of their actions by combining with a nuclear thyroid hormone receptor (TR) which belongs to the steroid and retinoid superfamily of intracellular receptors.
- ***There are two TR isoform families (TRα and TRβ).*** Both bind T_3 and function in similar manner, but their tissue distribution differs, which may account for quantitative differences in the sensitivity of different tissues to T_3.
- In contrast to the steroid receptor, the TR resides in the nucleus even in the unliganded inactive state. It is bound to the 'thyroid hormone response element' (TRE) in the enhancer region of the target genes along with corepressors. This keeps gene transcription suppressed.
- When T_3 binds to the ligand-binding domain of TR, it heterodimerizes with retinoid X receptor (RXR) and undergoes a conformation change releasing the corepressor and binding the coactivator. This induces gene transcription → production of specific mRNA and a specific pattern of protein synthesis → various metabolic and anatomic effects.
- The expression of certain genes is repressed by T_3. In their case, the unliganded TR allows gene transcription, while binding of T_3 to TR halts the process.

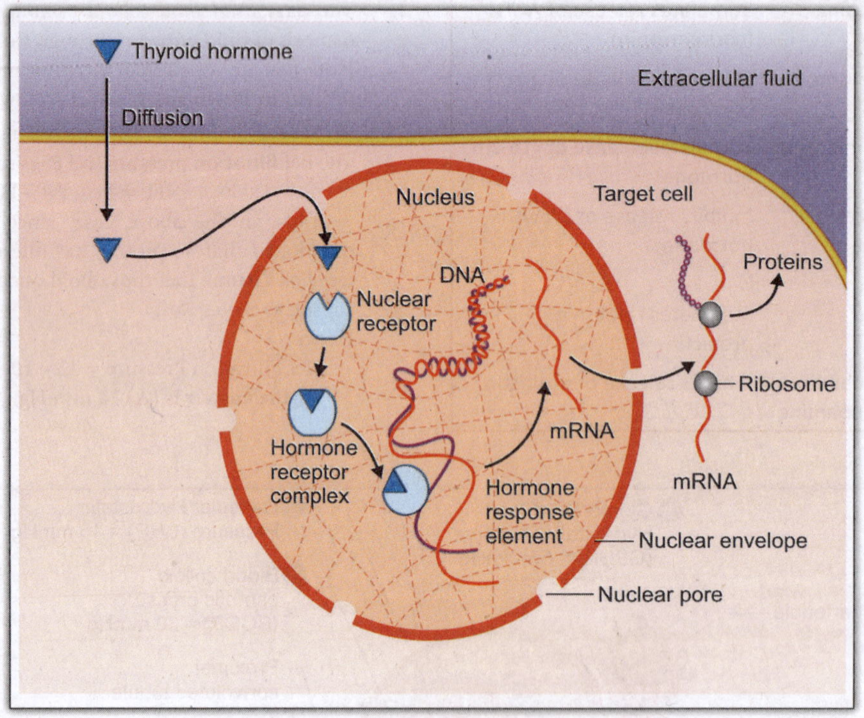

Fig: Mechanism of action of thyroid hormones

8. Ans. (a) Colony forming units

Ref: KDT 7th Ed Pg 611, Ganong 24th Ed page 558

Erythropoietin (EPO) is a sialoglycoprotein hormone (MW 34000)

Source: Peritubular cells of the kidney.

It is also produced in the brain, where it exerts a protective effect against excitotoxic damage triggered by hypoxia; and in the uterus and oviducts, where it is induced by estrogen and appears to mediate estrogen-dependent angiogenesis.

Triggers: Anemia and hypoxia are sensed by kidney cells and induce rapid secretion of EPO which acts on erythroid marrow.

Mechanism of Action

a. **Principal action:** Stimulates proliferation of colony forming cells of the erythroid series.
b. Induces hemoglobin formation and erythroblast maturation.
c. Releases reticulocytes in the circulation.

EPO binds to specific receptors on the surface of its target cells. The EPO receptor is a JAK-STAT-binding receptor that alters phosphorylation of intracellular proteins and activates transcription factors to regulate gene expression.

It induces erythropoiesis in a dose dependent manner, but has no effect on RBC lifespan.

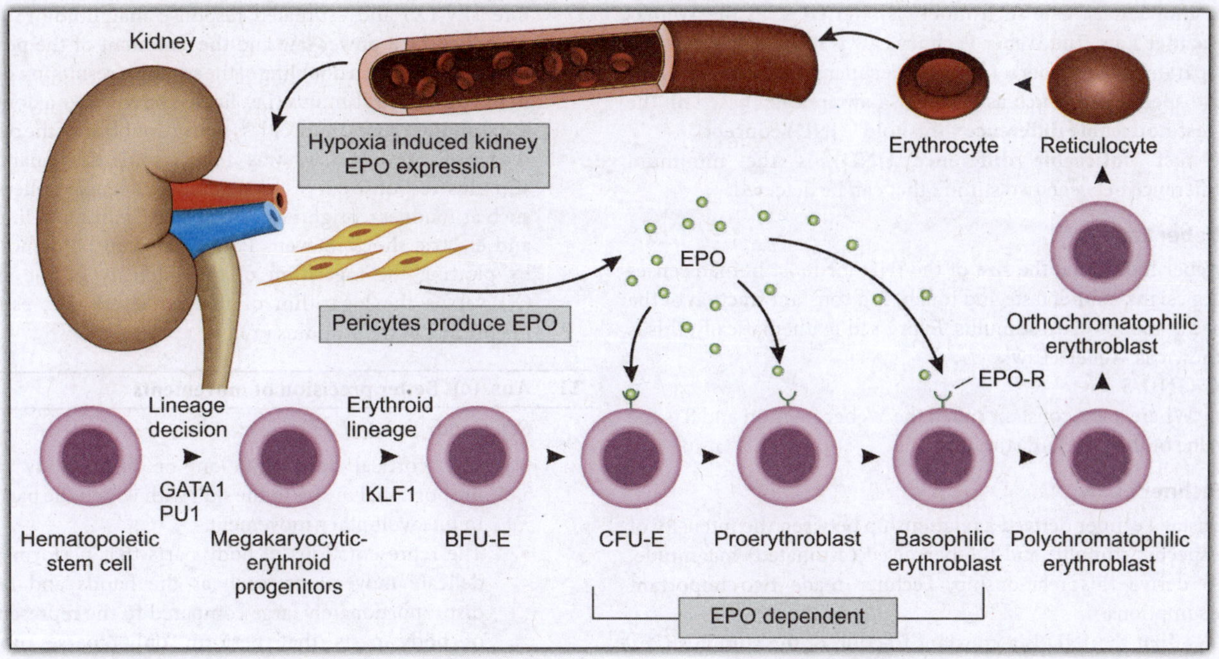

9. Ans. (a) Increase diameter of blood vessel

Ref: Guyton's 12th Ed Pg 163

- In a blood vessel, blood is divided into concentric rings due to difference in velocity in each ring. The velocity in the central lamina is relatively highest, while it is minimum in the lamina near the walls of the vessel. This is called laminar flow.

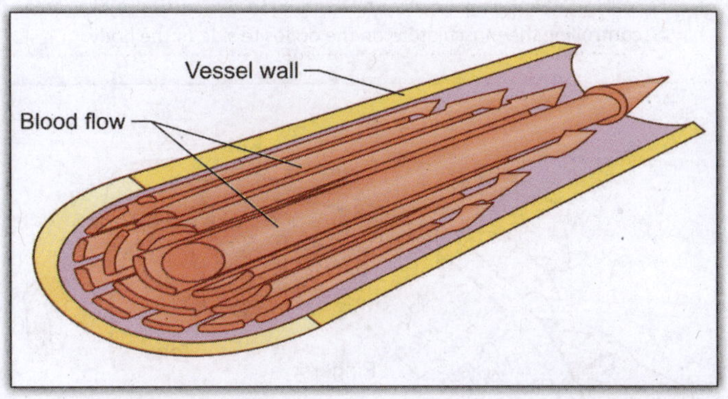

Fig: Laminar flow in blood vessels—blood moves in concentric rings at various velocities

- However, in a small vessel, essentially all the blood is near the wall, so the extremely rapidly flowing central stream of blood simply does not exist By integrating the velocities of all the concentric rings of flowing blood and multiplying them by the areas of the rings, **Poiseuille's law** has been derived as follows:

$F = \pi \Delta P r^4/\eta L$

Where

$F \rightarrow$ rate of blood flow

$\Delta P \rightarrow$ pressure difference between the ends of the vessel

$r \rightarrow$ radius of the vessel

$l \rightarrow$ length of the vessel

$\eta \rightarrow$ viscosity of the blood

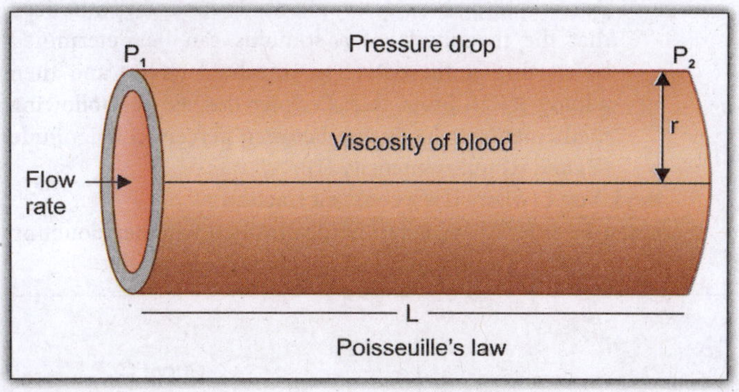

Note

In· this equation that the rate of blood flow is directly proportional to the fourth power of the radius of the vessel, which demonstrates that the diameter of a blood vessel (2 times radius) plays the greatest role of all factors in determining the rate of blood flow through a vessel.

- As for the other options, an increase in venous pressure will decrease the ΔP and hence, will decrease the flow rate.
- Since viscosity of blood is inversely proportional to blood flow, increasing the viscosity will lead to a fall in blood flow.

10. Ans. (a) Intensity of stimulus

Ref: Ganong 24th ed page 153, Guyton 12th Ed Pg 579

Several models have been proposed in the field of psychophysics to quantify relationships between any stimulus (e.g., touch, sound, light and smell) and the perceived response by individuals. One such model is referred to as the **Weber-Fechner Law.** The Weber Fechner Law is not one law, but two separate laws: Weber's Law and Fechner's Law. Weber's Law and special cases such as Fechner's Law are each based on the **"just noticeable difference threshold"** (JND) concept.

Just noticeable difference (JND) is the minimum difference between two stimuli that can be detected.

Weber Law

Weber found that the size of the JND for most human senses (e.g., sight, sound, taste and touch) is a constant fraction of the size of the standard stimulus. Expressed mathematically, this is known as Weber's Law:

K = JND/S

Where k is a constant called the Weber fraction and S is the value of the standard stimulus.

Fechner's Law

Gustav Fechner derived a relationship between the intensity of a specific stimulus and the perceived (estimated) magnitude. To derive this relationship, Fechner made two important assumptions:

1. That the JND is a constant fraction of the stimulus (i.e., Weber's Law holds)
2. That the JND is the basic unit of perceived magnitude, so that one JND is perceptually equal to another JND. By accepting these assumptions, Fechner hypothesized that the magnitude of a stimulus can be determined by starting at the detection threshold (JND) and then adding JNDs. From this, Fechner derived the following mathematical relationship between perceived magnitude (P) and stimulus intensity (I):

P = k Log I (where k is a constant fraction)

Using Fechner's Law, it can be determined whether doubling the intensity of a light makes it appear twice as bright.

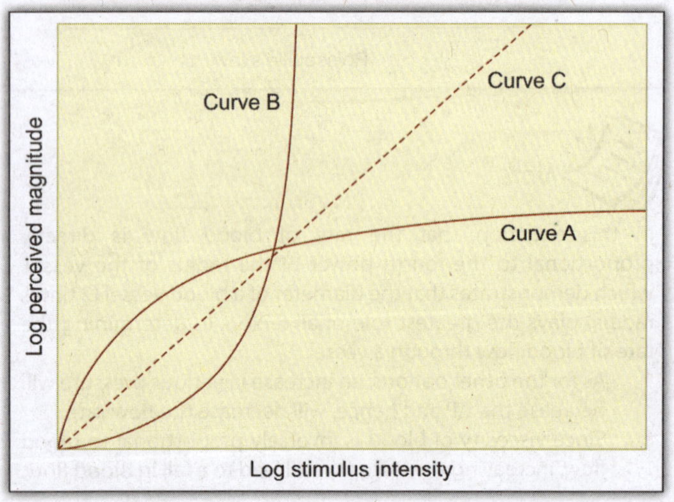

Fig: Curves showing the relationship between perceived magnitude (Y) and stimulus intensity (X) for curve A (brightness), curve B (electric shock) and curve C (line length)

Stevens's Power Law

Stanley Smith Stevens proposed that the perceived magnitude of a stimulus (P) equals a constant (k) times the stimulus intensity (S), raised to a power (n). Stevens found that for all senses (in general), the relationship between any stimulus intensity (X) and estimated response magnitude (Y) is best described by a power law and the exponent of the power law indicates whether a doubling of the stimulus results in a doubling in the perceived stimulus (i.e., linear) or whether a doubling of the stimulus causes more or less than a doubling of the perceived response. Stevens Law was found to better quantify the stimulus-response curves for a number of sensory phenomena, such as loudness, brightness, smell, taste, vibration, line length and electric shock. Stevens Power Law can be demonstrated by plotting the logarithm of the intensity of the stimulus (X) versus the logarithm of the perceived (i.e., estimated) magnitude of the stimulus (Y).

11. Ans. (c) Better precision of movements

Ref: Ganong's 24th Ed Pg 237

- The cortical representation of each body part is proportional in size to the skill with which the part is used in fine, voluntary movement.
- The representations of body parts that perform precise, delicate movements, such as the hands and face, are disproportionately large compared to the representations of body parts that perform only coarse, unrefined movements, such as the trunk or legs.
- The areas involved in speech and hand movements are especially large in the cortex; use of the pharynx, lips and tongue to form words and of the fingers and opposable thumbs to manipulate the environment are activities in which humans are especially skilled.

Also Know

The facial area is represented bilaterally, but the rest of the representation is generally unilateral, with the cortical motor area controlling the musculature on the opposite side of the body.

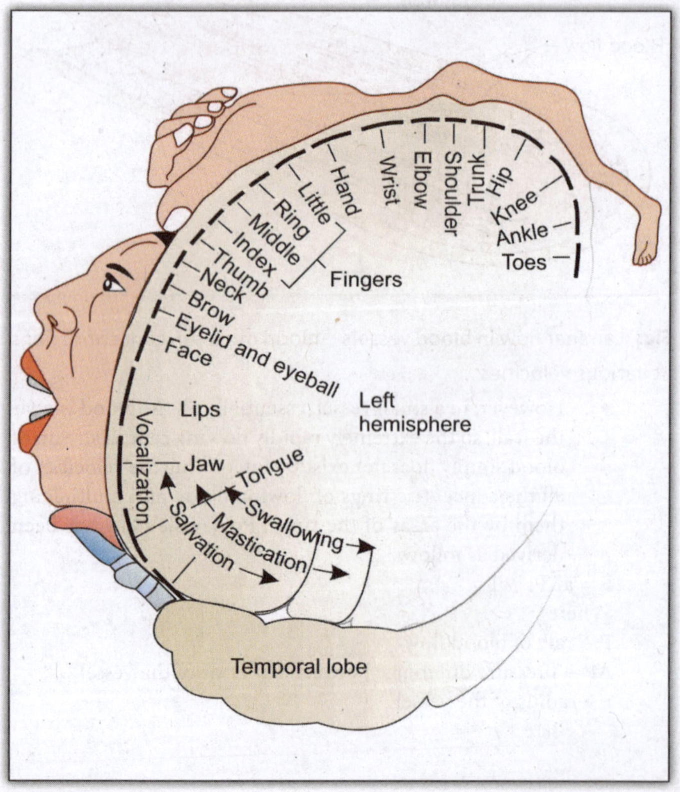

12. Ans. (d) Negative immune regulation

Ref: https://www.nobelprize.org/nobel-prizes-2018/

- The Nobel Prize in Physiology or Medicine 2018 was awarded to **James P. Allison and Tasuku Honjo** "for their discovery of cancer therapy by inhibition of negative immune regulation." i.e. **Immune checkpoints in Cancer.**
- James P. Allison studied a known protein that functions as a brake on the immune system. He realized the potential of releasing the brake and thereby unleashing our immune cells to attack tumors. He then developed this concept into a brand new approach for treating patients.
- In parallel, Tasuku Honjo discovered a protein on immune cells and, after careful exploration of its function, eventually revealed that it also operates as a brake, but with a different mechanism of action. Therapies based on his discovery proved to be strikingly effective in the fight against cancer.

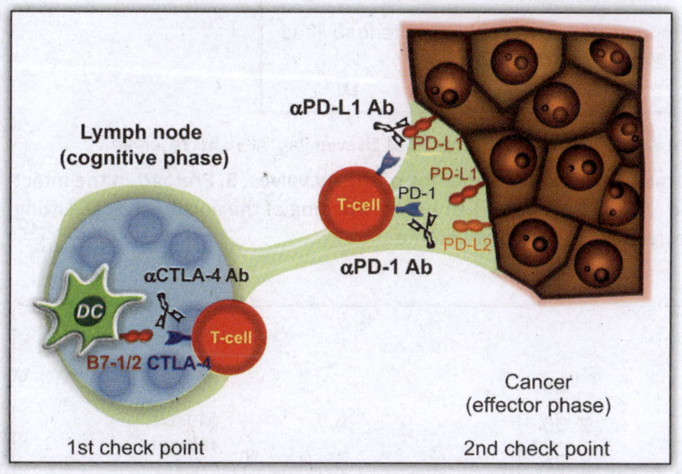

Fig: Immune checkpoints in cancer

13. Ans. (b) Fibronectin

Ref: Gray's 41st Ed Pg 24, 188

Integrins mediate cell extracellular matrix and cell–cell interactions and integrate extracellular signals with the cytoskeleton and cellular signaling pathways. Because integrins can be activated by proteins binding to their extracellular or their intracellular domains, they can function in a bidirectional fashion by transmitting information outside in (cues from the extracellular environment) and inside-out (cues from the intracellular environment) of the cell. The integrin family of proteins consists of α subunits and β subunits forming transmembrane heterodimers. The amino-acid sequence arginine glycine aspartic acid, or RGD motif, on target ligands (such as fibronectin, laminin and other extracellular matrix proteins) has binding affinity to the extracellular binding head of integrins.

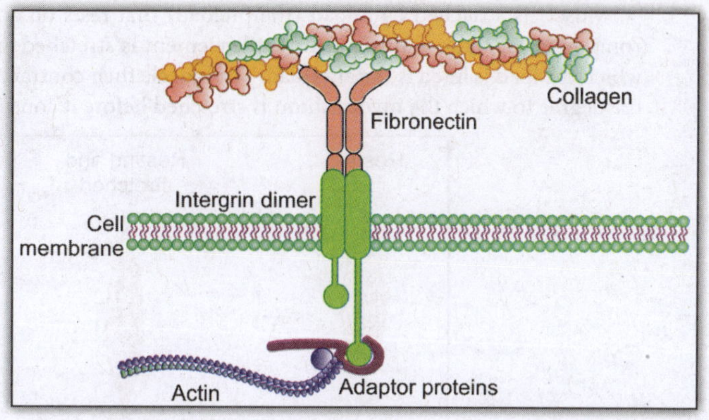

Fig: Integrin connects the extracellular matrix with the actin cytoskeleton inside the cell by crossing a cell membrane. Above the cell membrane is the extracellular environment and below the cell membrane is the cytoplasm within the cell. Embedded in the membrane is an integrin dimer, which is shown in green. The integrin dimer is composed of two different subunits, which are shown side by side, each with a similar hot dog-shaped segment. ***On the extracellular side of the membrane, integrin binds to fibronectin and fibronectin in turn binds to collagen.*** Fibronectin is a dimer made up of two monomers that each look likes a string of four orange hot dogs; each of the fibronectin monomers interacts with one of the integrin subunits. Collagen is shown as a triple-helical structure made up of three different collagen chains, colored orange, green and pink, wrapped around each other in a triple-helical manner; the last two hot dog-like segments of each fibronectin monomer branch out and appear to wrap around each side of the collagen triple helix. Inside the cell, the head of the lollipop from the intracellular segment of the integrin subunit on the right binds to an adaptor protein, which in turn binds to actin. 32

AIIMS MAY 2018

14. Ans. (b) B has done more work than A

Ref: Ganong 24th ed page 547

NOTE

Both A and B are isotonic contractions. Displacement of B is more than A and hence work done is more in B than A.

Preload is the force that stretches the muscle before contraction. In the left ventricle, for example, the blood filling and thus stretching the wall during diastole represents the preload.

Afterload is the force that stretches the muscle after contraction. In the left ventricle, afterload is the pressure in the aorta that must be overcome by the contracting left ventricular muscle to open the aortic valve and eject the blood.

Muscle is stretched by a load (the preload) that rests on a platform. The initial phase of the contraction is isometric; the elastic component in series with the contractile element is stretched and tension increases until it is sufficient to lift the load. The tension at which the load is lifted is the afterload. The muscle then contracts isotonically without developing further tension. In vivo, the preload is the degree to which the myocardium is stretched before it contracts and the afterload is the resistance against which blood is expelled.

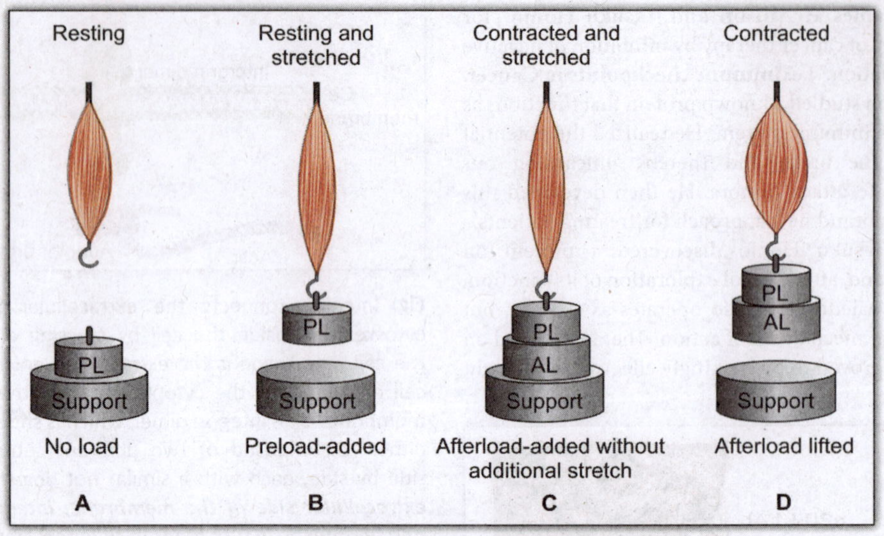

Fig: Preload and afterload of cardiac muscle. **A.** Resting stage of cardiac muscle just before opening of the AV valves. **B.** Preload-in the intact heart at the end of ventricular filling. **C.** Supported preload plus afterload-in the intact heart just before opening of the aortic valve. **D.** Lifting preload plus afterload-in the intact heart, ventricular ejection with a decrease in ventricular volume

Abbreviations: AL, afterload; PL, preload; PL + AL, total load.

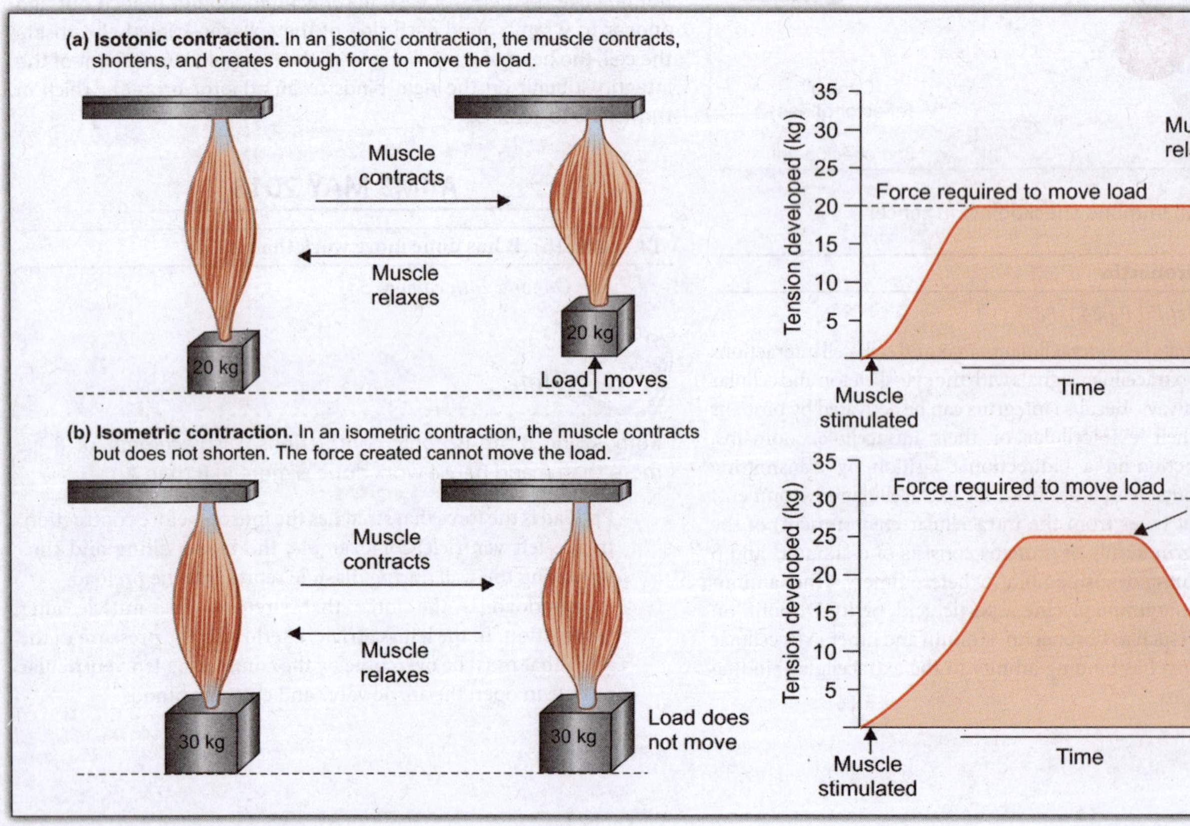

Fig: Isotonic contraction: The muscle contracts and shortens and creates enough force to displace the load. Hence, work done is not zero

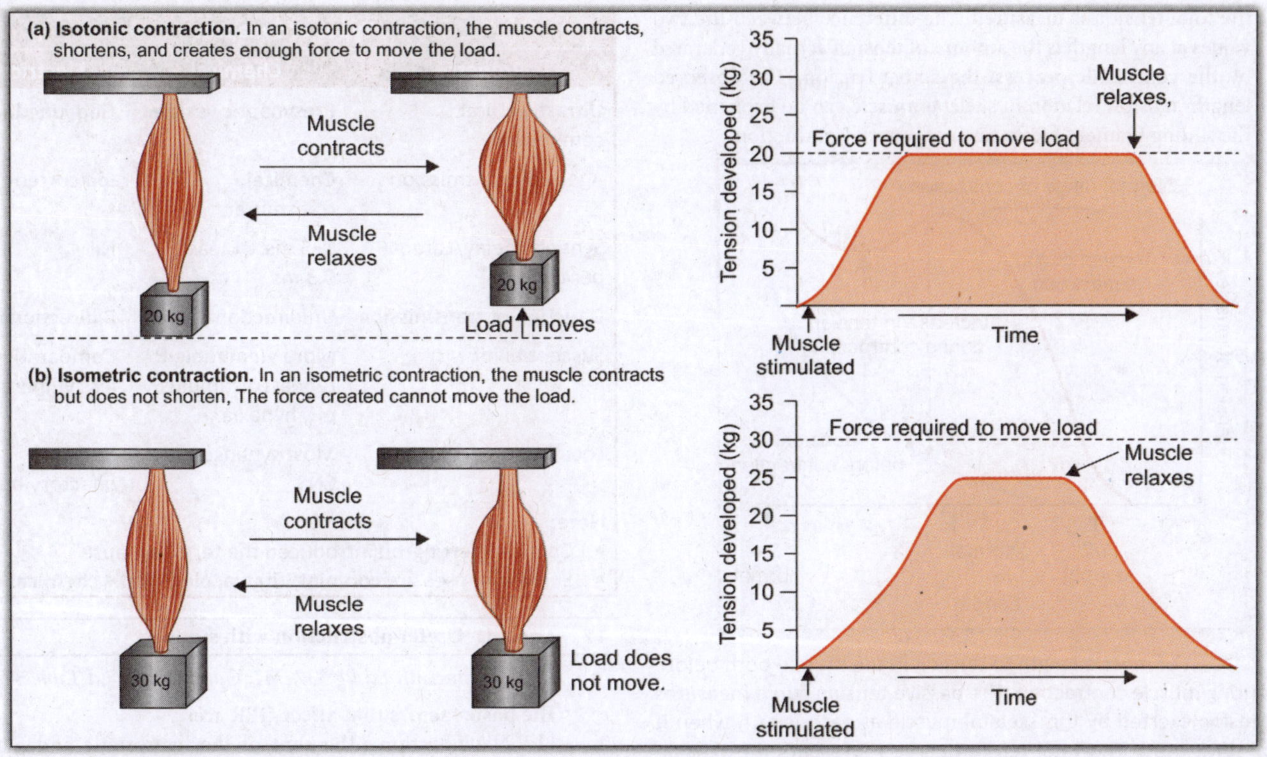

Fig: Isometric contraction: The muscle contracts but does not shorten and the force created does not move the load. Since work done is W = F × D (Force x displacement) and displacement is nil, the work done will be zero

Now let us discuss the options:

Option (A) False

B has both preload and afterload added to it

In the figure given, we can see that the load is unchanged both, before and after contraction. In other words, it is only preload that has been added to the muscle. The muscle B is first under maximum stretch, however, it generates enough pressure to lift the load. Hence, only preload has been added in figure B. This option is false.

Option (B) True

B has done more work than A

The work done is given by Force × Distance. Since in Figure B, the muscle has covered more distance, the work done is more in Figure B. This option is true.

Option (C) and (D) False

Force (Tension) required to lift the load is same in both A and B since the load is same in both A and B. The only difference in A and B is displacement which is function of time. Once the plateau of Force (Tension) is reached there is no additional force (Tension) required. The more displacement in B is due to more time spent on the displacement.

From the above explanation, it is clear that this is an example of isotonic contraction, since the force acting on the muscles is constant, while the length of the muscle changes. Now, we note that the force acting on both muscles in the form of load is the same with respect to magnitude. When a muscle is subjected to a load in isotonic contraction, the muscle first builds up internal tension in order to overcome the resistance (load in this case). During this time, the actin myosin cross-bridges develop. After this, as the internal tension overcomes the external resistance, the muscle undergoes contraction. Since both the muscles are subjected to the same amount of external resistance, obviously, the tension in both of them is equal.

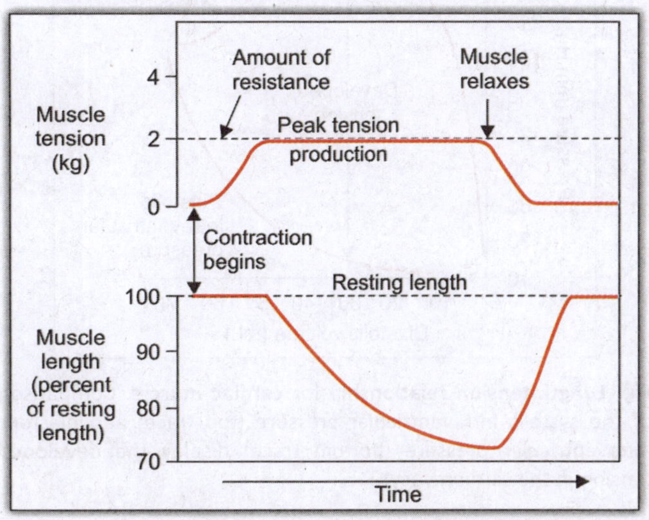

Fig: Relationship between tensions developed and muscle length in isotonic contraction

15. Ans. (a) A- skeletal muscle, B- cardiac muscle

Ref: Guyton 12th ed page 77, Guyton 24th ed page 113

Both the tension that a muscle develops when stimulated to contract isometrically (the total tension) and the passive tension exerted by the unstimulated muscle vary with the length of the muscle fiber. At each length, the passive tension is measured, the muscle is then stimulated electrically and the total tension is measured. The difference between the two values at any length is the amount of tension actually generated by the contractile process, the active tension. The observed length–tension relation in skeletal muscle can be explained by the sliding filament mechanism of muscle contraction.

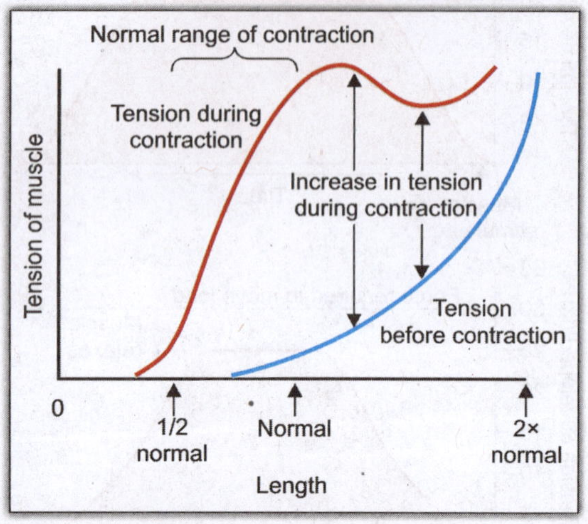

Fig: Relation of muscle length to tension in the muscle both before and during muscle contraction. The passive tension curve measures the tension exerted by this skeletal muscle at each length when it is not stimulated. The total tension curve represents the tension developed when the muscle contracts isometrically in response to a maximal stimulus. The active tension is the difference between the two.

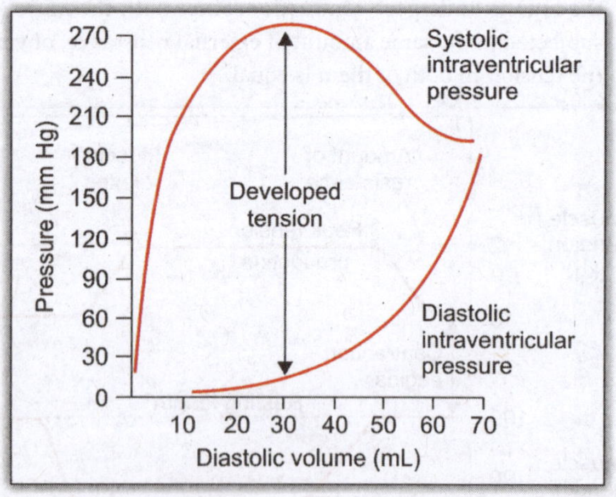

Fig: Length-tension relationship for cardiac muscle. Comparison of the systolic intraventricular pressure (top trace) and diastolic intraventricular pressure (bottom trace) display the developed tension in the cardiomyocyte

16. Ans. (c) Bidirectional transmission

Ref: Textbook of Medical Physiology By Khurana 2nd Ed Pg 1011

Types of Synapses		
Property	**Chemical**	**Electrical**
Synaptic cleft	20–40 nm	4 nm
Cytoplasmic continuity between neurons	No	Yes
Ultrastructural component	Presynaptic vesicle	Gap junction
Agent of transmission	Chemical transmitter	Ion current
Synaptic delay/Latent period	1–5 ms. At least 0.3 ms	Nil
Direction of transmission	Unidirectional	Bidirectional
Susceptibility	More vulnerable to repeated stimulus, pH, hypoxia	Comparatively less vulnerable
Location	Most synapses in CNS	Retina, olfactory bulb

Contd...

Note:
- Charles Sherrington introduced the term "synapse"
- Some synapses are **conjoint, that is, electrical + chemical**

17. Ans. (d) Ureter obstruction with stone

Ref: Guyton 13th Ed Pg 337-341; Ganong 24th Ed Table 37-4

The basic factors that affect GFR are:

1. Net filtration (The sum of the hydrostatic and plasma oncotic forces in the glomerular capsule and Bowman's capsule respectively).
2. Capillary filtration coefficient determined by permeability and filtering surface area of the capillary.

Changes Seen in Factors Affecting GFR		
Factor	**Increased GFR**	**Decreased GFR**
Renal blood flow	↑	↓
Glomerular capillary hydrostatic pressure	↑	↓
Afferent arteriolar constriction	↓	↑
Efferent arteriolar constriction	↑	↓
Hydrostatic pressure in Bowman's capsule	↑	↓
Plasma Oncotic pressure	↓	↑
Filtration Coefficient (K_f)	↑	↓
Glomerular capillary permeability	↑	↓
Effective filtration surface area	↑	↓
Ureteral obstruction	-	GFR decreases

18. Ans. (a) Negative feedback

Ref: Guyton 13th/ed Pg 219, Ganong 24th Ed Pg 589

- Baroreceptor reflex is a nervous mechanism for arterial pressure control.
- The reflex is initiated by stretch receptors or pressoreceptors located in specific points in large systemic arteries.
- A rise in arterial pressure **stretches** the baroreceptors and causes them to transmit signals into brainstem through Hering's nerve. Thus, the baroreceptors are **activated by stretch.**

- Increased baroreceptor discharge inhibits the tonic discharge of sympathetic nerves and excites the vagal innervation of the heart. These neural changes produce vasodilation, venodilation, hypotension, bradycardia and a decrease in cardiac output.
- Baroreceptors act as buffers. Any drop in systemic arterial pressure decreases the discharge in the buffer nerves and there is a compensatory rise in blood pressure and cardiac output. Any rise in pressure produces dilation of the arterioles and decreases cardiac output until the blood pressure returns to its previous baseline level.
- Thus, it is a negative feedback mechanism.

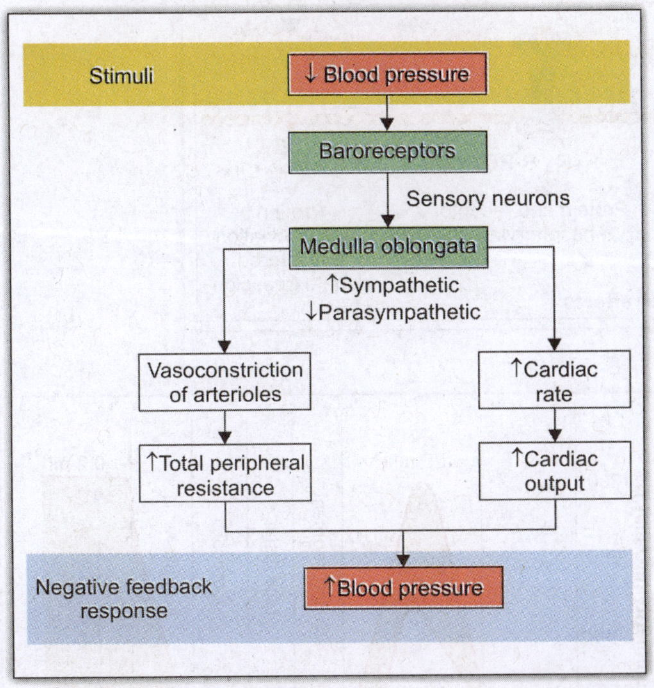

Fig: Negative feedback in baroreceptor reflex. Any drop in systemic arterial pressure decreases the discharge in the buffer nerves and there is a compensatory rise in blood pressure and cardiac output

19. Ans. (c) 1 = Na, 2 = K

Ref: Ganong 24th Ed Pg 88

(See table of "Ionic Basis of Nerve Action Potential" in AIIMS May 2014 Physiology)

Keys to the Answer

Graph 1: Prompt overshoot, rapid upstroke → inward Na channel

Graph 2: Overshoot starts slowly, reaches a lower peak and settles down much later → K channel

- Depolarization causes rapid opening of the activation gates of Na^+ channels and thus Na^+ conductance promptly increases Thus the membrane potential is driven towards the equilibrium potential of Na^+ ion (+65 mV)
- Thus the rapid depolarization during upstroke is due to inward Na^+ current
- Depolarization slowly opens K^+ channels and increases K^+ conductance to even higher levels than at rest.

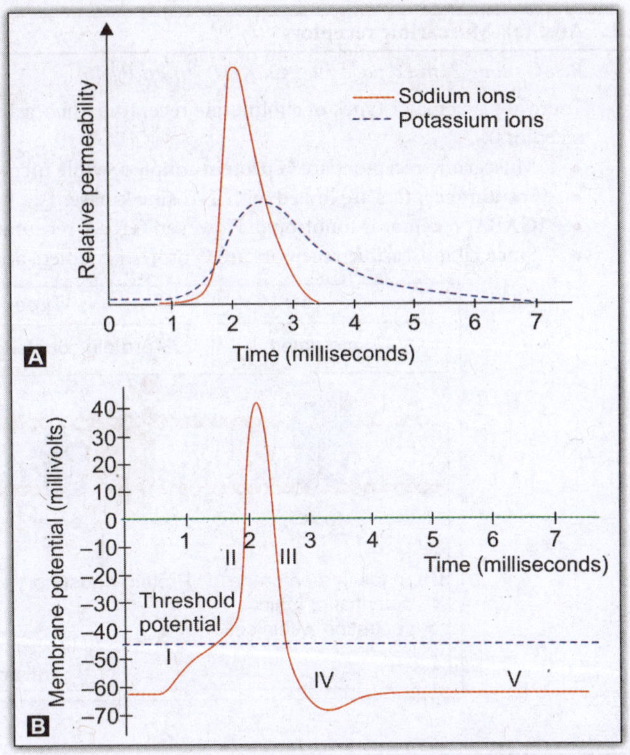

Figs A and B: A. Membrane permeability to sodium and potassium ions during an actions potential; **B.** Membrane potential an action potential

- The combined effect of closing Na^+ channels and greater opening of K^+ channels make the K^+ conductance higher than the Na^+ conductance and membrane potential is repolarized. Thus repolarization is caused by outward K^+ current.
- The K^+ conductance remains higher than at rest for some time after closure of Na^+ channel and the membrane potential is driven more closer to K^+ equilibrium potential than at rest. This is called as undershoot

20. Ans. (c) Decreases

Ref: Anatomy & Physiology 8th Ed by Seeley Stephens Tate Publisher McGraw-Hill page 704

During normal exercise, end-diastolic volume increases because of an increase in venous return and End systolic volume decreases because the heart contracts more forcefully.

- Exercise causes an increase in cardiac output by increasing heart rate, venous return and stroke volume.
- During exercise, there is enhanced diastolic filling due to increased venous return.
- The sympathetic system is activated which causes positive inotropic effect on the heart and increases the force of systole.
- Also, as per Frank-Starling's law, there is more complete systolic ejection due to increased end diastolic volume. The myocardium pumps more optimally due to an increase in length of muscle fibers due to increased end diastolic volume.
- Thus, the residual volume left inside the heart at the end of systole (end-systolic volume) is less as compared to that at rest, mainly because of better emptying of the ventricle during systole.

21. Ans. (a) Muscarinic receptors

Ref: Ganong 24th Ed page 59, 143, KDT 7th Ed Pg 46

There are two major types of cholinergic receptors: muscarinic (G protein-coupled receptors) and nicotinic (ligand-gated ion channel receptors).

- Muscarinic receptors are G protein coupled, while nicotinic are ionotropic.
- Insulin receptors are linked with Tyrosine kinase.
- $GABA_A$ receptor is ionotropic. However, $GABA_B$ receptor is G protein coupled.
- Since all muscarinic receptors are G protein coupled, answer is (A) Muscarinic.

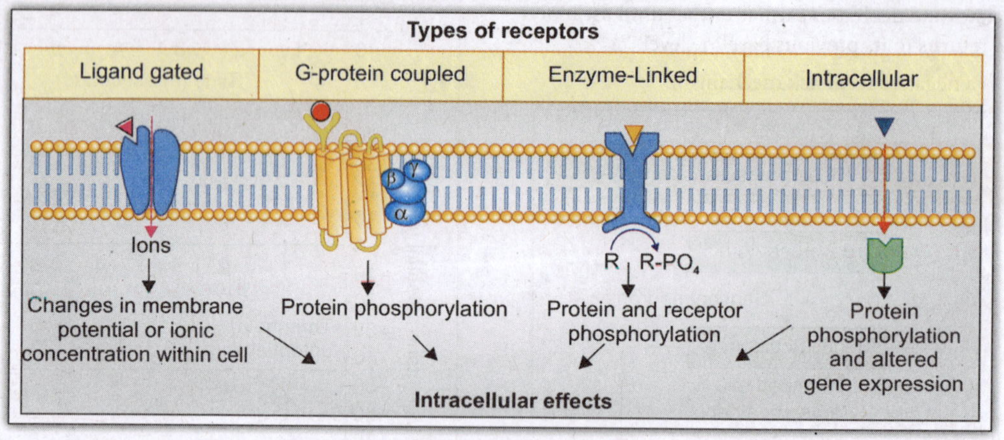

22. Ans. (a) Atrial contraction

Ref: Ganong 24th ed page 544

(See table of JVP Waveforms in Physiology AIIMS May 2014 "a wave" of JVP is due to atrial contraction)

23. Ans. (b) Thick ascending limb of Loop of Henle

Ref: Ganong 24th Ed Pg 686, Essential Medical Physiology by Leonard R. Johnson 3rd Ed Pg 396

- In the ascending limb tubular becomes more dilute because of the movement of Na^+ and Cl^- out of the tubular lumen and when fluid reaches the top of the ascending limb (**called the diluting segment**) it is now hypotonic to plasma.
- The cortical part of thick ascending limb of loop of Henle is often called as the diluting segment as it produces dilute tubular fluid with respect to plasma, **regardless of the osmolality of urine.**

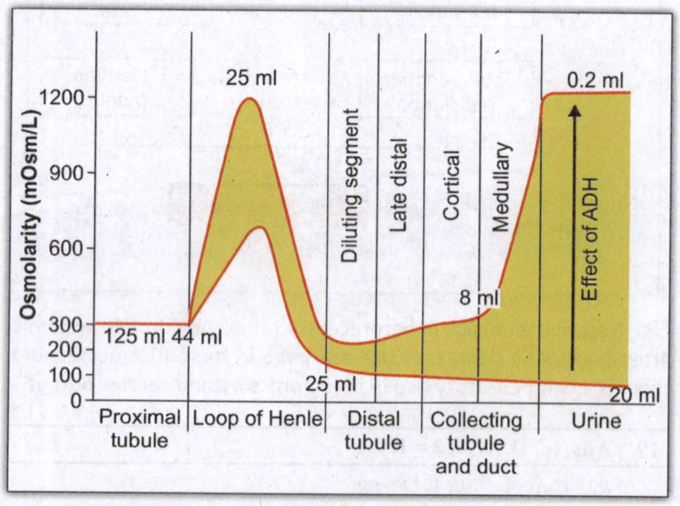

Renal Physiology					
Substance	**Description**	**Proximal tubule**	**Loop of Henle**	**Distal tubule**	**Collecting duct**
Glucose (100% reabsorption)	If glucose is not reabsorbed by the kidney, it appears in the urine, in a condition known as glucosuria. This is associated with diabetes mellitus.	Reabsorption (almost 100%) via sodium-glucose transport proteins (apical) and GLUT (basolateral).			
Oligopeptides, proteins and amino acids	All are reabsorbed nearly completely.	Reabsorption			

Contd...

Subject-wise MCQs and Answers with Explanations

Renal Physiology					
Substance	**Description**	**Proximal tubule**	**Loop of Henle**	**Distal tubule**	**Collecting duct**
Urea (53%/ minimum reabsorption)	Regulation of osmolality. Varies with ADH	Reabsorption (50%) via passive transport	Secretion		Reabsorption in medullary collecting ducts
Sodium (99.4 % reabsorbs)	Uses Na-H antiport, Na-glucose symport, sodium ion channels (minor)	Reabsorption (65%, isosmotic)	Reabsorption (25%, thick ascending, Na-K-2Cl symporter)	Reabsorption (5%, NaCl symporter)	Reabsorption (5%, principal cells), stimulated by aldosterone via ENaC
Chloride (99.2% reabsorption)	Usually follows sodium. Active (transcellular) and passive (paracellular)	Reabsorption	Reabsorption (thin ascending, thick ascending, Na-K-2Cl symporter)	reabsorption (sodium-chloride symporter)	
Water (99.4% reabsorption)	Uses aquaporin water channels	Absorbed osmotically along with solutes	Reabsorption (descending)		Reabsorption (regulated by ADH, via arginine vasopressin receptor 2)
Bicarbonate (100% reabsorption)	Helps maintain acid-base balance	Reabsorption (80-90%)	Reabsorption (thick ascending)		Reabsorption (intercalated cells, via band 3 and pendrin)
Protons	Uses vacuolar H + ATPase				Secretion (intercalated cells)
Potassium (93.3% reabsorbs)	Varies upon dietary needs	Reabsorption (65%)	Reabsorption (20%, thick ascending, Na-K-2Cl symporter)		Secretion (common, via Na+/K+-ATPase, increased by aldosterone), or reabsorption (rare, hydrogen potassium ATPase)
Calcium	Uses calcium ATPase, sodium-calcium exchanger	Reabsorption	Reabsorption (thick ascending) via passive transport		
Magnesium	Calcium and magnesium compete and an excess of one can lead to excretion of the other	Reabsorption	Reabsorption (thick ascending)	reabsorption	
Phosphate	Excreted as titratable acid.	Reabsorption (85%) via sodium/ phosphate cotransporter. Inhibited by parathyroid hormone			
Carboxylate		Reabsorption (100%) via carboxylate transporters			

Contd...

Renal Physiology					
Substance	Description	Proximal tubule	Loop of Henle	Distal tubule	Collecting duct

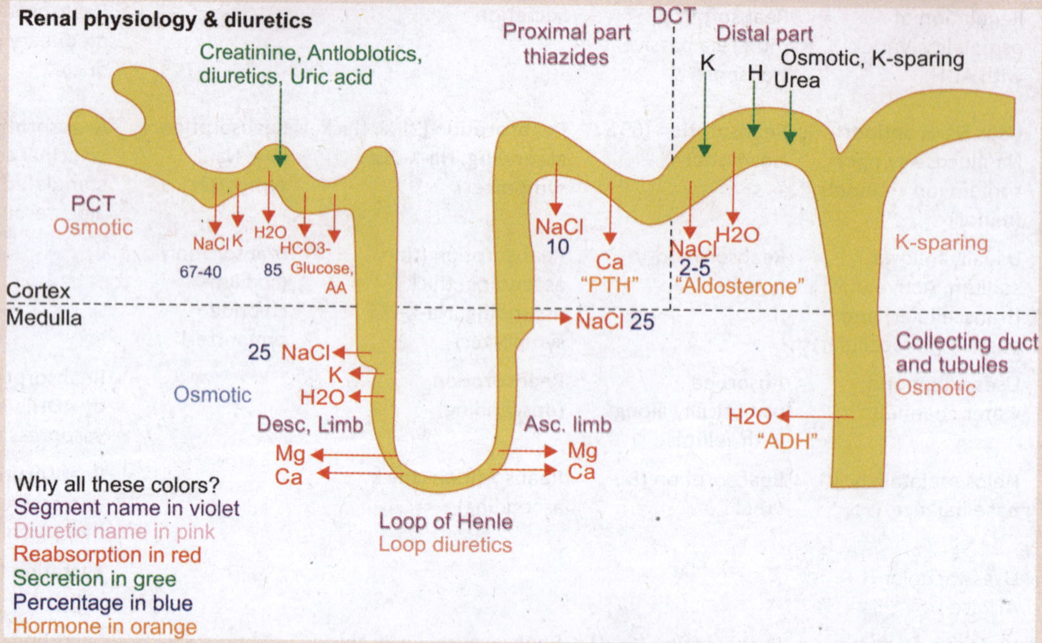

24. Ans. (b) 2

Ref: Ganong 24th ed page 168, 293

The patient is suffering from Broca's Aphasia. Since the patient hos no difficulty in understanding the language Wernicke's area is intact.

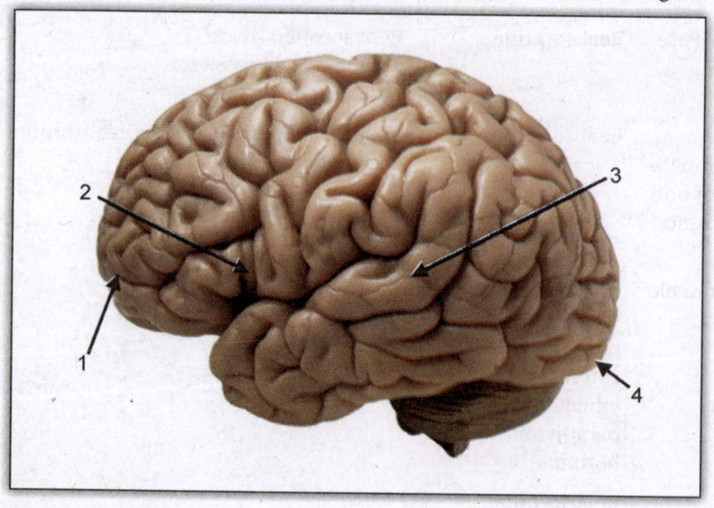

Figure Legends

1. Prefrontal association area of frontal lobe
2. Broca's area- Brodmann area 44 at inferior frontal gyrus
3. Wernicke's area Brodmann area 22 at superior temporal gyrus
4. Visual association area at occipital lobe

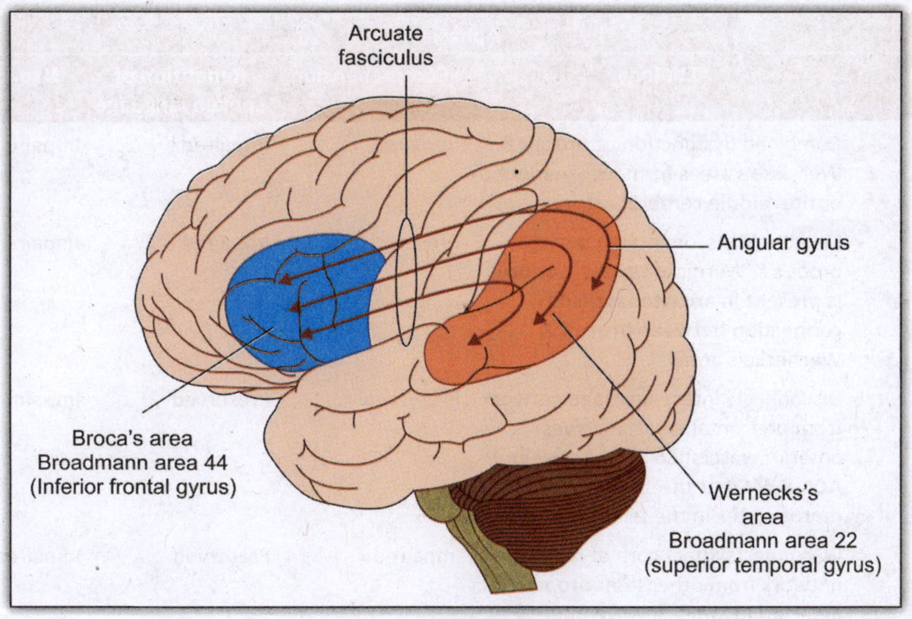

Fig: Broca's and Wernicke's area

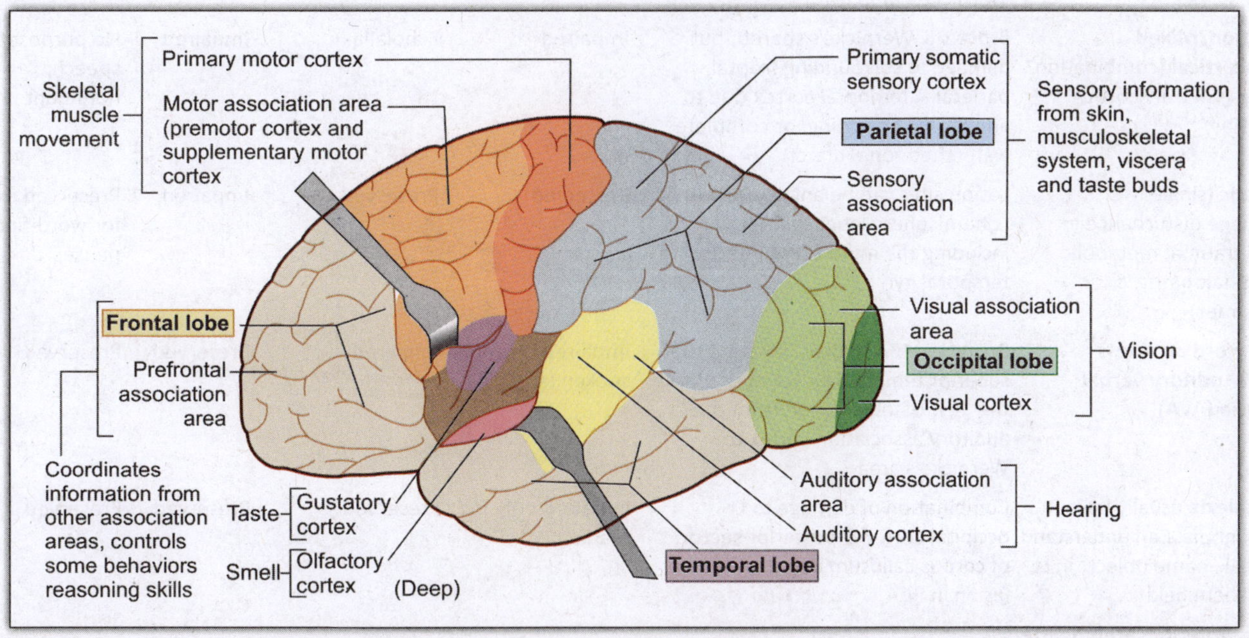

Fig: The above area numbers are arbitrary numbers and does not represents Brodmann area

Aphasias					
Type of aphasia	**Etiology**	**Comprehension**	**Repetition of spoken language**	**Naming**	**Fluency**
Wernicke's (AKA- fluent or jargon aphasia) (Mnemonic: Wernicke is wordy but nonsense)	Infarction of Wernicke's area due to **inferior division of the middle cerebral artery**	Impaired (without meaningful content)	Impaired (Mild to severe)	Impaired	Preserved or increased (paraphasic)
Broca's (Mnemonic: Broca is broken)	Infarction of Broca's area due to **superior division of the middle cerebral artery**	Preserved (except grammar)	Impaired (Moderate to severe)	Impaired	Decreased, Non-fluent, effortful, slow

Contd...

Aphasias					
Type of aphasia	**Etiology**	**Comprehension**	**Repetition of spoken language**	**Naming**	**Fluency**
Global	Combined dysfunction of Broca's & Wernicke's areas from involvement of **entire middle cerebral artery**	Impaired	Impaired	Impaired	Decreased, nonfluent
Conduction	Functional disconnection between Broca's & Wernicke's areas. **Lesion is present in arcuate fasciculus, connection between broca's & Wernecke's areas.**	Preserve	Impaired	Impaired	Preserved, Fluent
Nonfluent (motor) transcortical	Disconnects intact language network from prefrontal areas, involves anterior **watershed zone between ACA & MCA** or the supplementary motor cortex in the territory of ACA	Preserved	Preserved	Impaired	Impaired, nonfluent
Fluent (sensory) transcortical	Disconnects intact core of language network from other temporoparietal association areas. Involve temporoparietal cortex posterior to Wernicke's area (MC)	Impaired	Preserved	Impaired	Preserved, fluent
Isolation/Mixed transcortical (combination of the two transcortical aphasias)	Broca's & Wernicke's spared, but damage to surrounding frontal, parietal & temporal cortex due to anoxia, CO poisoning, or complete watershed zone infarct	Impaired	Echolalia	Impaired	No purposeful speech, nonfluent
Anomic (single MC language disturbance in head trauma, metabolic encephalopathy, & Alzheimer)	Lesion sites can be anywhere within Lt hemisphere language network, including the middle and inferior temporal gyri	Preserved	Preserved	Impaired	Preserved except for word-finding pauses
Pure word deafness A.K.A **Auditory verbal agnosia (AVA)**	B/L or Lt-MCA strokes affecting the superior temporal gyrus interrupting the flow of information from the auditory association cortex to Wernicke's area	Impaired only for spoken language	Impaired	Preserved	Preserved
Pure alexia usually have Rt hemianopia. Can understand & speak, name objects in Lt visual hemifield	Combination of damage to Lt occipital cortex & posterior sector of corpus callosum due to vascular lesion in PCA	Impaired only for reading	Preserved	Preserved	Preserved

ACA = Anterior cerebral artery
MCA = Middle cerebral artery
PCA = Posterior cerebral artery

Footnote:

- The neural substrate of language is composed of a distributed network centered in the **perisylvian region of the *left* hemisphere.**
- **Wernicke's area:** The posterior pole of this network is located at the temporoparietal junction (**Superior temporal gyrus**) and includes a region known as *Wernicke's area*. An essential function of Wernicke's area is to transform sensory inputs into their neural word representations so that they can establish the distributed associations that give a word its meaning.
- **Broca's area:** The anterior pole of the language network is located in the **inferior frontal gyrus** and includes a region known as *Broca's area*. An essential function of this area is to transform neural word representations into their articulatory sequences so that the words can be uttered in the form of spoken language. The sequencing function of Broca's area also appears to involve the ordering of words into sentences that contain a meaning-appropriate *syntax* (grammar).
- Wernicke's and Broca's areas are interconnected with each other and with additional perisylvian, temporal, prefrontal and posterior parietal regions, making up a neural network that subserves the various aspects of language function. Damage to any one of these components or to their interconnections can give rise to language disturbances (*aphasia*)
- *In approximately 90% of right-handers and 60% of left-handers, aphasia occurs only after lesions of the left hemisphere.*

25. Ans. (d) Maintains RMP

Ref: Ganong's 23rd ed page 87

(See table of" Ionic Basis of Nerve Action Potential" in Physiology AIIMS Nov 2014) (see Volume II)

No net electrogenic transfer at RMP means X + Y + Z = 0

Since X = –50 and Y = –30, then Z must be +80 since (–80 +80 = 0)

AIIMS NOVEMBER 2017

26. Ans. (b) Difference in concentration of surfactant during inspiration and expiration

Ref: Guyton f 12th ed page 468

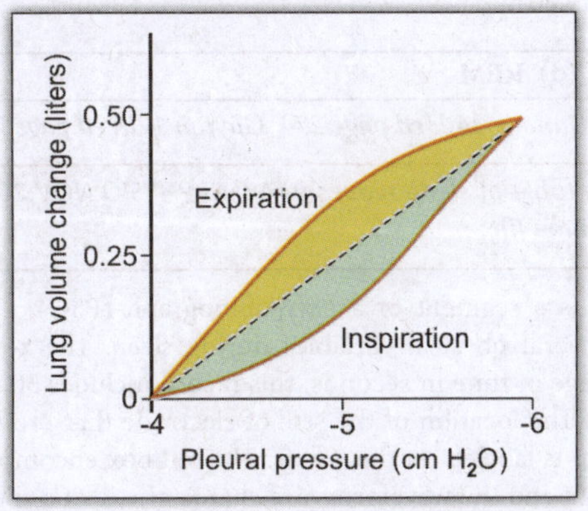

Fig: This a diagram relating lung volume changes to changes in transpulmonary pressure. Note that the relation is different for inspiration and expiration. Each curve is recorded by changing the transpulmonary pressure in small steps and allowing the lung volume to come to a steady level between successive steps. The two curves are called, respectively, the inspiratory compliance curve and the expiratory compliance curve and the entire diagram is called the compliance diagram of the lungs

The characteristics of the compliance diagram are determined by the elastic forces of the lungs. These can be divided into two parts:

1. **Elastic forces of the lung tissue:** Tissue elastic forces tending to cause collapse of the air-filled lung represent only about 1/3 of the total lung elasticity.
2. **Elastic forces caused by surface tension** of the fluid that lines the inside walls of the alveoli and other lung air spaces. Fluid-air surface tension forces in the alveoli represent about 2/3 of Lung elasticity. The fluid-air surface tension elastic forces of the lungs also increase tremendously when the substance called surfactant is not present in the alveolar fluid. Surfactant is a surface active agent in water, which means that it greatly reduces the surface tension of water. It is secreted by special surfactant-secreting epithelial cells called type II alveolar epithelial cells, which constitute about 10 percent of the surface area of the alveoli.

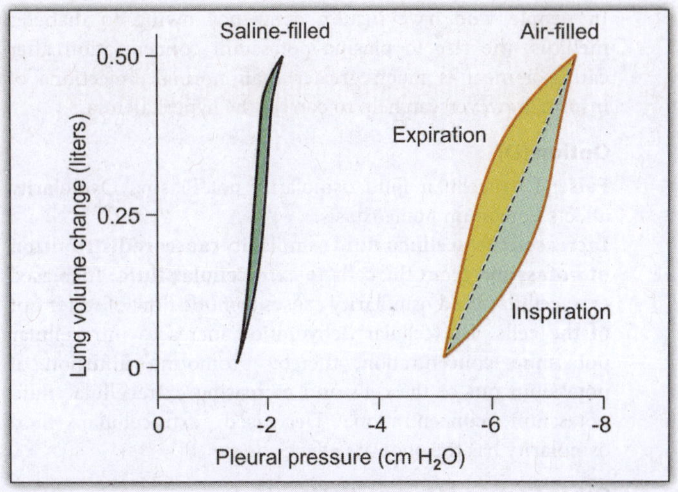

Fig: When the lungs are filled with air, there is an interface between the alveolar fluid and the air in the alveoli. In the case of the saline solution-filled lungs, there is no air-fluid interface; therefore, the surface tension effect is not present-only tissue elastic forces are operative in the saline solution-filled lung

27. Ans. (d) Change in plasma osmolarity

Ref: Guyton 12th ed page 361-362

Extracellular fluid potassium concentration normally is regulated precisely at about 4.2 mEq/L, seldom rising or falling more than ±0.3 mEq/L. This precise control is necessary because many cell functions are very sensitive to changes in extracellular fluid potassium concentration.

Option (A)

True: β-Adrenergic stimulation increases cellular uptake of potassium: Increased secretion of catecholamines, especially epinephrine, can cause movement of potassium from the extracellular to the intracellular fluid, mainly by activation of β2-adrenergic receptors. Conversely, treatment of hypertension with β-adrenergic receptor blockers, such as propranolol, causes potassium to move out of the cells and creates a tendency toward hyperkalemia.

Option (B)

True: Aldosterone increases potassium uptake into cells: Increased potassium intake also stimulates secretion of aldosterone, which increases cell potassium uptake. Excess aldosterone secretion (Conn's syndrome) is almost invariably associated with hypokalemia, due in part to movement of extracellular potassium into the cells. Conversely, patients with deficient aldosterone production (Addison's disease) often have clinically significant hyperkalemia due to accumulation of potassium in the extracellular space, as well as to renal retention of potassium.

Option (C)

True: Insulin stimulates potassium uptake into cells: Insulin is important for increasing cell potassium uptake after a meal.

In people who have insulin deficiency owing to diabetes mellitus, the rise in plasma potassium concentration after eating a meal is much greater than normal. Injections of insulin, however, can help to correct the hyperkalemia.

Option (D)

False: Extracellular fluid osmolarity not Plasma Osmolarity affects Potassium homeostasis.

Increased extracellular fluid osmolarity causes redistribution of potassium from the cells to extracellular fluid: Increased extracellular fluid osmolarity causes osmotic flow of water out of the cells. The cellular dehydration increases intracellular potassium concentration, thereby promoting diffusion of potassium out of the cells and increasing extracellular fluid potassium concentration. Decreased extracellular fluid osmolarity has the opposite effect.

Other Factors Affecting K^+ Homeostasis

- **Acid-base abnormalities can cause changes in Potassium Distribution:** Metabolic acidosis increases extracellular potassium concentration, in part by causing loss of potassium from the cells, whereas metabolic alkalosis decreases extracellular fluid potassium concentration. Although the mechanisms responsible for the effect of hydrogen ion concentration on potassium internal distribution are not completely understood, one effect of increased hydrogen ion concentration is to reduce the activity of the sodium-potassium adenosine triphosphatase (ATPase) pump. This in turn decreases cellular uptake of potassium and raises extracellular potassium concentration.
- **Cell lysis causes increased extracellular potassium concentration:** As cells are destroyed, the large amounts of potassium contained in the cells are released into the extracellular compartment. This can cause significant hyperkalemia if large amounts of tissue are destroyed, as occurs with severe muscle injury or with red blood cell lysis.
- **Strenuous exercise can cause hyperkalemia by releasing potassium from skeletal muscle:** During prolonged exercise, potassium is released from skeletal muscle into the ECF. Usually the hyperkalemia is mild, but it may be clinically significant after heavy exercise, especially in patients treated with β-adrenergic blockers or in individuals with insulin deficiency. Rarely hyperkalemia after exercise may be severe enough to cause cardiac arrhythmias and sudden death.

Factors that can Alter Potassium Distribution Between the Intracellular and Extracellular Fluid

Factors that shift K^+ into cells (decrease extracellular [K^+])	Factors that shift K^+ Out of cells (increase extracellular [K^+])
• Insulin • Aldosterone • β-adrenergic stimulation • Alkalosis	• Insulin deficiency (diabetes mellitus) • Aldosterone deficiency (Addison's disease) • β-adrenergic blockade • Acidosis • Cell lysis • Strenuous exercise • Increased extracellular fluid osmolarity

28. Ans. (d) Closure of inactive gates of sodium channel

Ref: Ganong's 23rd ed page 87

See table of "IONIC Basis of Nerve Action Potential" in Physiology AIIMS Nov 2014 (see Volume II)

29. Ans. (c) +80

Ref: Ganong's 23rd ed page 87

See table of "IONIC Basis of Nerve Action Potential" in Physiology AIIMS Nov 2014 (see Volume II)

No net electrogenic transfer at RMP means X + Y + Z = 0

Since X = –50 and Y = –30, then Z must be + 80 since (–80 + 80 = 0)

30. Ans. (d) REM

Ref: Ganong 24th ed page 274, Guyton 12th ed page 764

See table of sleep waves in AIIMS PHYSIO NOV 2014 (see Volume II)

This is a segment of a polysomnograph (PSG), a recording of several physical variables during sleep. The x-axis shows passage of time in seconds; this record includes 30 seconds of data. The location of the sets of electrode that produced each signal is labeled on the y-axis. The red box encompasses EEG output and the waveforms are characteristic of a specific stage of sleep. Other curves show other sleep-related data, such as body temperature, muscle activity and heartbeat.

31. Ans. (d) Growth hormone

Ref: Guyton 13th ed page 945

The graph in the examination was directly taken from Guyton

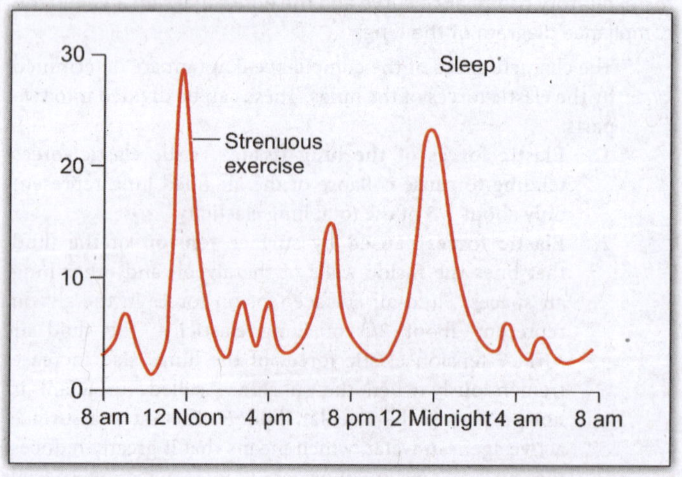

Fig: Typical variations in growth hormone secretion throughout the day, demonstrating the especially powerful effect of strenuous exercise and also the high rate of growth hormone secretion that occurs during the first few hours of deep sleep

Factors That Stimulate or Inhibit Secretion of Growth Hormone	
Stimulate growth hormone secretion	**Inhibit growth hormone secretion**
Decreased blood glucose Decreased blood free fatty acids Increased blood amino acids (arginine) Starvation or fasting, protein deficiency Trauma, stress, excitement Exercise Testosterone, estrogen Deep sleep (stages II and IV) Growth hormone-releasing hormone Ghrelin	Increased blood glucose Increased blood free fatty acids Aging Obesity Growth hormone inhibitory hormone (somatostatin) Growth hormone (exogenous) Somatomedins (insulin-like growth factors)

32. Ans. (b) Temperature

Ref: Guyton 12th ed page 9

Feed Forward or Anticipatory or Adaptive Control

Some are simple feedback systems but many are not. For instance, some movements of the body occur so rapidly that there is not enough time for nerve signals to travel from the peripheral parts of the body all the way to the brain and then back to the periphery again to control the movement. Therefore, the brain uses a principle called **feed-forward control** to cause required muscle contractions. That is, sensory nerve signals from the moving parts appraise the brain whether the movement is performed correctly. If not, the brain corrects the feed-forward signals that it sends to the muscles the next time the movement is required. Then, if still further correction is necessary, this will be done again for subsequent movements. This is called **adaptive control.** Adaptive control, in a sense, is delayed negative feedback.

Examples of Feedforward Control

- Temperature control: Thermoregulatory responses are initiated by hypothalamus BEFORE the changes in environmental temperature have succeeded in changing the body's core body temperature
- Cephalic phase of gastric secretion- Just thinking about food increases gastric acid production
- Thinking about exercise itself increases heart rate and respiratory rate
- Role of cerebellum in motor coordination

33. Ans. (a) Bainbridge reflex

Ref: Ganong 25th ed page 591

Option (A)

Bainbridge reflex: The Bainbridge reflex is elicited by stretch receptors located in the right atrial wall and the cavoatrial junction. An increase in right-sided filling pressure sends vagal afferent signals to the cardiovascular center in the medulla. These afferent signals inhibit parasympathetic activity, thereby increasing the heart rate. Acceleration of the heart rate also results from a direct effect on the SA node by stretching the atrium. The changes in heart rate are dependent on the underlying heart rate before stimulation. **(Guyton 12th ed page 110)**

Option (B)

Bezold-Jarisch reflex: The concept of depressor reflexes originating in the heart was introduced by von Bezold in 1867 and was later revived by Jarisch. The Bezold–Jarisch reflex overlaps with vasovagal syncope. It was initially described as a bradycardic response to injection of various alkaloid compounds and later found to be mediated by chemoreceptors in the heart. The term has now come to include reactions triggered by cardiac mechanoreceptor activation and it has been used to describe perioperative bradycardia with hypotension. **(Ref: Oxford Journals medicine and health BJA Volume 86, Issue 6Pp. 859-868)**

The Bezold-Jarisch reflex (BJR) has been implicated as a cause of bradycardia, hypotension and cardiovascular collapse after central neuraxial anesthesia and in particular spinal anesthesia. The BJR is a cardio-inhibitory reflex and consists of the triad of symptoms, bradycardia, hypotension and coronary vasodilatation, seen after intravenous injection of Veratrum alkaloids in animals.

Option (C)

Frank starling law: The intrinsic ability of the heart to adapt to increasing volumes of inflowing blood is called the Frank-Starling mechanism of the heart, in honor of Otto Frank and Ernest Starling. Frank-Starling mechanism means that the greater the heart muscle is stretched during filling, the greater is the force of contraction and the greater the quantity of blood pumped into the aorta. Or, stated another way: Within physiological limits, the heart pumps all the blood that returns to it by the way of the veins.

Option (D)

The J-receptors were discovered by an Indian physiologist A. S. Paintal in 1954. J receptors are basically unmyelinated vagal afferent nerve endings (type C Fibers). The name J receptors (Juxtapulmonary capillary receptor) was given to them because of close proximity to pulmonary capillaries. J receptors are sensitive to any increase in interstitial fluid between capillary endothelium and alveolar epithelium. J receptor response is characterized by Apnea followed by Tachypnea, Bradycardia, Hypotension.

34. Ans. (c) Decreases oncotic pressure in peritubular capillaries

Ref: Guyton 12th Ed page 314, Ganong 24th ed page 679

Option (A)

True: Efferent arteriole constriction causes decrease in GFR. However, the effect of efferent arteriolar constriction depends on the severity of the constriction; modest efferent constriction raises GFR, but severe efferent constriction (more than a threefold increase in resistance) tends to reduce GFR.

Option (B)

True: Modest Efferent arteriole constriction causes increase in renal Blood flow while severe Efferent arteriole constriction causes decrease in renal blood flow

Option (C)

False: Renal circulation is unique in that it has two capillary beds; the glomerular and peritubular capillaries which are arranged in series and separated by efferent arterioles that help regulate the hydrostatic pressures in both sets of capillaries. High hydrostatic pressure in glomerular capillaries (about 60 mm Hg) causes rapid fluid filtration, lower hydrostatic pressure in peritubular capillaries (about 13 mm Hg) permits rapid fluid reabsorption. By adjusting the resistances of afferent and efferent arterioles, kidneys regulate the hydrostatic pressures in both glomerular and peritubular capillaries. Hence, When the efferent arteriole constricts, pressure proximal to it (Glomerular hydrostatic pressure) will increase while pressure distal to it (Peritubular capillary pressure) will decrease.

NOTE

Pericapillary Oncotic pressure is different from Pericapillary hydrostatic pressure which works in opposite directions.

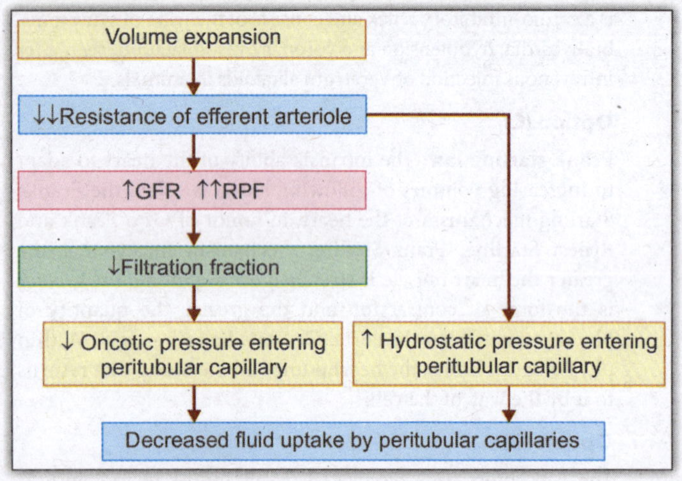

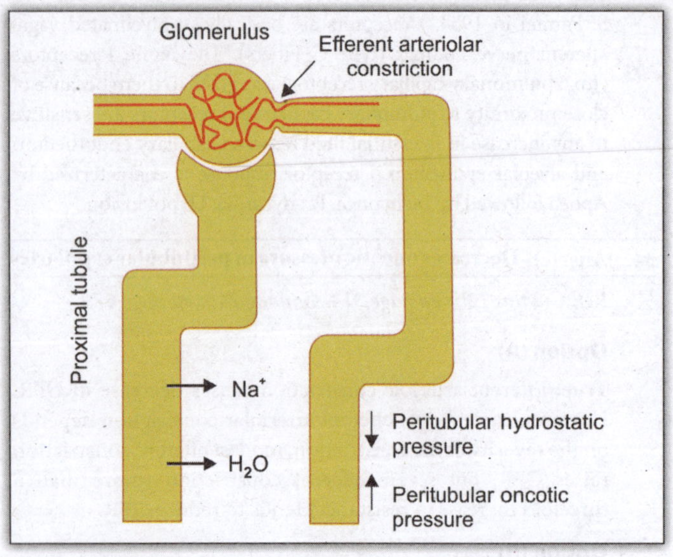

Option (D)

True: Constriction of afferent arteriole decreases glomerular hydrostatic pressure while constriction of efferent arteriole increases glomerular hydrostatic pressure.

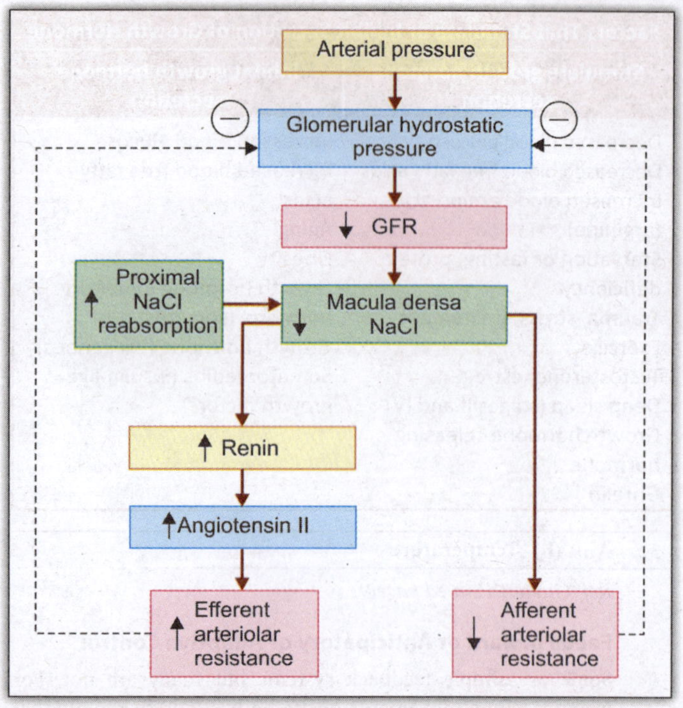

Effect of Afferent and Efferent Arteriole on GFR and Renal Blood Flow

	GFR	Renal blood flow
Dilatation of afferent arteriole	↑	↑
Constriction of afferent arteriole	↓	↓
Dilatation of efferent arteriole	↑	↑
Modest Constriction of efferent arteriole	↑	↓
Severe Constriction of efferent arteriole	↓	↓

Constriction of afferent arterioles reduces GFR. However, the effect of efferent arteriolar constriction depends on the severity of the constriction; modest efferent constriction raises GFR, but severe efferent constriction (more than a threefold increase in resistance) tends to reduce GFR.

35. Ans. (c) Interstitial cells of Cajal

Ref: Ganong 25th ed page 496, Guyton 12th ed page 754, Physiology by Indu Khurana 2012 ed page 473

Electrical Activity of Gastrointestinal Smooth Muscle

The smooth muscle of the gastrointestinal tract is excited by almost continual slow, intrinsic electrical activity along the membranes of the muscle fibers. This activity has two basic types of electrical waves: **(1) slow waves and (2) spikes.** In addition, the voltage of the resting membrane potential of the gastrointestinal smooth muscle can be made to change to different levels and this, too, can have important effects in controlling motor activity of the gastrointestinal tract Slow Waves/BER: The smooth muscles of GIT shows spontaneous rhythmic fluctuations in their membrane potentials (between –65 mV to –45 mV), this is called Basic electrical rhythm.

- BER is present throughout the GIT except esophagus and proximal stomach
- BER (Basal Electric Rhythm) is first observed in the body of stomach, which becomes faster distally.
- BER is caused by the pacemaker cells of GIT AKA **"Interstitial cells of Cajal"** located near the fundus on the greater curvature of stomach.
- Slow waves are produced due to opening of Na^+ channels
- Normally slow waves on their own are unable to cause smooth muscle contraction, rather they act as pacemaker that excite the spike potentials
- Rate of BER is different for different parts of the GIT; Stomach = 4/min, Duodenum = 12/min, Terminal Ileum = 8/min, Caecum = 8/min, Sigmoid colon = 16/min

AIIMS MAY 2017

36. Ans. (c) 70–79%

Ref: Ganong 24th ed page 629

Recall Bias

In the given graph of examination the Tidal volume was from 2300 to 2700 (approximately). The values and calculations are as per the most closely recalled graph. Also the options were in range not the exact numbers.

Step 1

Determine the "start of expiration" and "end of maximum expiration" points. Volume between these two points is FVC (in the given graph 5000 – 1300 = 3700)

Step 2

Determine how much volume has been expired within one second (FEV1 = 5000 – 2300 = 2700).

Step 3

Calculate FEV1/FVC = 2700/3700 × 100 = 72.9%

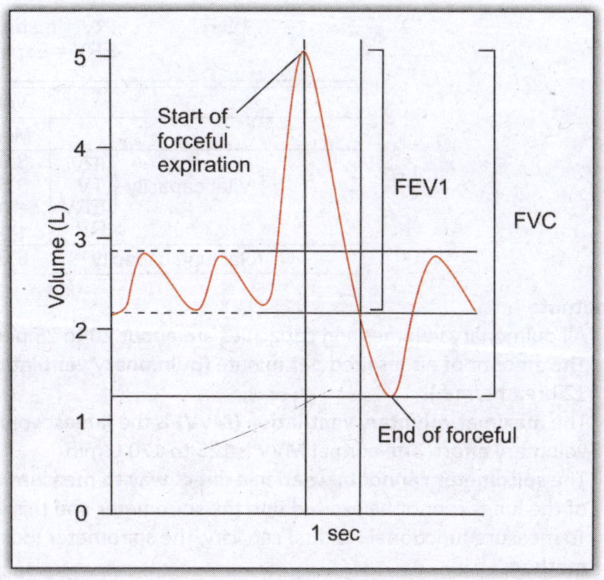

Pulmonary Volumes and Capacities

A simple method for studying pulmonary ventilation is to record the volume movement of air into and out of the lungs, a process called **spirometry.**

Pulmonary volumes	There are four pulmonary lung volumes that, when added together, equal the maximum volume to which the lungs can be expanded. The significance of each of these volumes is the following: • **The tidal volume** is the volume of air inspired or expired with each normal breath; it amounts to about 500 mL in the adult male. • **The inspiratory reserve volume** is the extra volume of air that can be inspired over and above the normal tidal volume when the person inspires with full force; it is usually equal to about 3000 mL. • **The expiratory reserve volume** is the maximum extra volume of air that can be expired by forceful expiration after the end of a normal tidal expiration; this normally amounts to about 1100 mL. • **The residual volume** is the volume of air remaining in the lungs after the most forceful expiration; this volume averages about 1200 mL.
Pulmonary capacities	In describing events in the pulmonary cycle, it is sometimes desirable to consider two or more of the volumes together. Such combinations are called pulmonary capacities. Important pulmonary capacities can be described as follows: • **The inspiratory capacity** equals the tidal volume plus the inspiratory reserve volume. This is the amount of air (about 3500 mL) a person can breathe in, beginning at the normal expiratory level and distending the lungs to the maximum amount. • **The functional residual capacity** equals the expiratory reserve volume plus the residual volume. This is the amount of air that remains in the lungs at the end of normal expiration (about 2300 mL). • **The vital capacity** equals the inspiratory reserve volume plus the tidal volume plus the expiratory reserve volume. This is the maximum amount of air a person can expel from the lungs after first filling the lungs to their maximum extent and then expiring to the maximum extent (about 4600 mL). • **The total lung capacity** is the maximum volume to which the lungs can be expanded with the greatest possible effort (about 5800 mL); it is equal to the vital capacity plus the residual volume.

Contd...

Pulmonary Volumes and Capacities

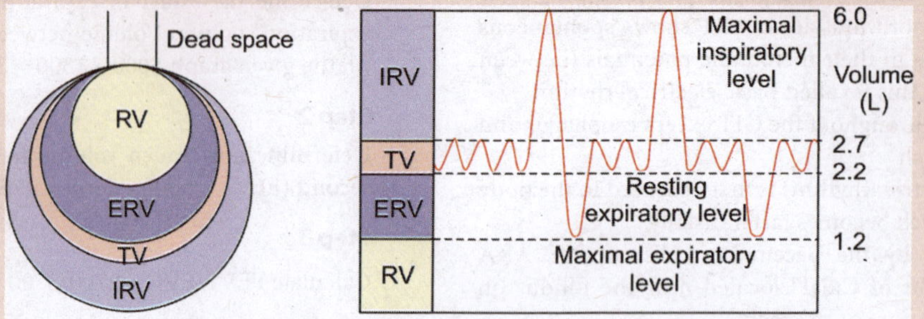

IRV = Inspiratory reserve volume TV = Tidal volume
ERV = Expiratory reserve volume RV = Residual volume

	Volume (L) Men	Volume (L) Women	
Vital capacity: IRV	3.3	1.9	Inspiratory capacity
Vital capacity: TV	0.5	0.5	Inspiratory capacity
Vital capacity: ERV	1.0	0.7	Functional residual capacity
RV	1.2	1.1	Functional residual capacity
Total lung capacity	6.0	4.2	

Footnote

- All pulmonary volumes and capacities are about 20 to 25 percent less in women than in men
- The amount of air inspired per minute **(pulmonary ventilation, respiratory minute volume)** is normally about 6 L (500 mL/breath × 12 breaths/min).
- The **maximal voluntary ventilation (MVV)** is the largest volume of gas that can be moved into and out of the lungs in 1 minute by voluntary effort. The normal MVV is 125 to 170 L/min
- The **spirometer cannot be used in a direct way to measure the functional residual capacity**, because the air in the residual volume of the lungs cannot be expired into the spirometer and this volume constitutes about one half of the functional residual capacity. To measure functional residual capacity, the spirometer must be used in an indirect manner, usually by means of a **helium dilution method**

37. Ans. (c) Point C

Ref: Ganong, 25th ed page 542

Second heart sound precedes or appears 0.09 sec after summit of 'T' wave

In the given Figure A = E = S4, B = S1, C = S2, D = S3

Heart Sounds

Heart sounds	Occurs during	Cause	Characteristics	Pitch or frequency	Duration (sec)	Relation to ECG
First	Isometric contraction & ejection period, start of ventricular systole	Sudden closure of mitral & tricuspid (AV) valves	Long, soft, & low pitched. Resembles the word 'LUBB'	25 to 45 Hz	0.15 (0.10 – 0.17)	'R' wave
Second	Protodiastole & part of isometric relaxation, just after end of ventricular systole	Closure of aortic or pulmonary (semilunar) valves	Short, sharp, & high pitched. Resembles the word 'DUBB'	50 Hz	0.10 – 0.14	Precedes or appears 0.09 sec after summit of 'T' wave
Third	Rapid filling, beginning of middle third of diastole	Rushing of blood into ventricles	Low pitched	-	0.07 – 0.1	B/W 'P' wave & 'Q' wave.
Fourth	Atrial systole, just before 1st sound	Contraction of atrial musculature	Inaudible sound	<20 Hz	0.02 – 0.04	B/W 'P' wave & 'Q' wave

Note: S3 and S4 are usually not well heard by stethoscope and require phonocardiogram. However, they are better appreciated with the bell of the stethoscope.

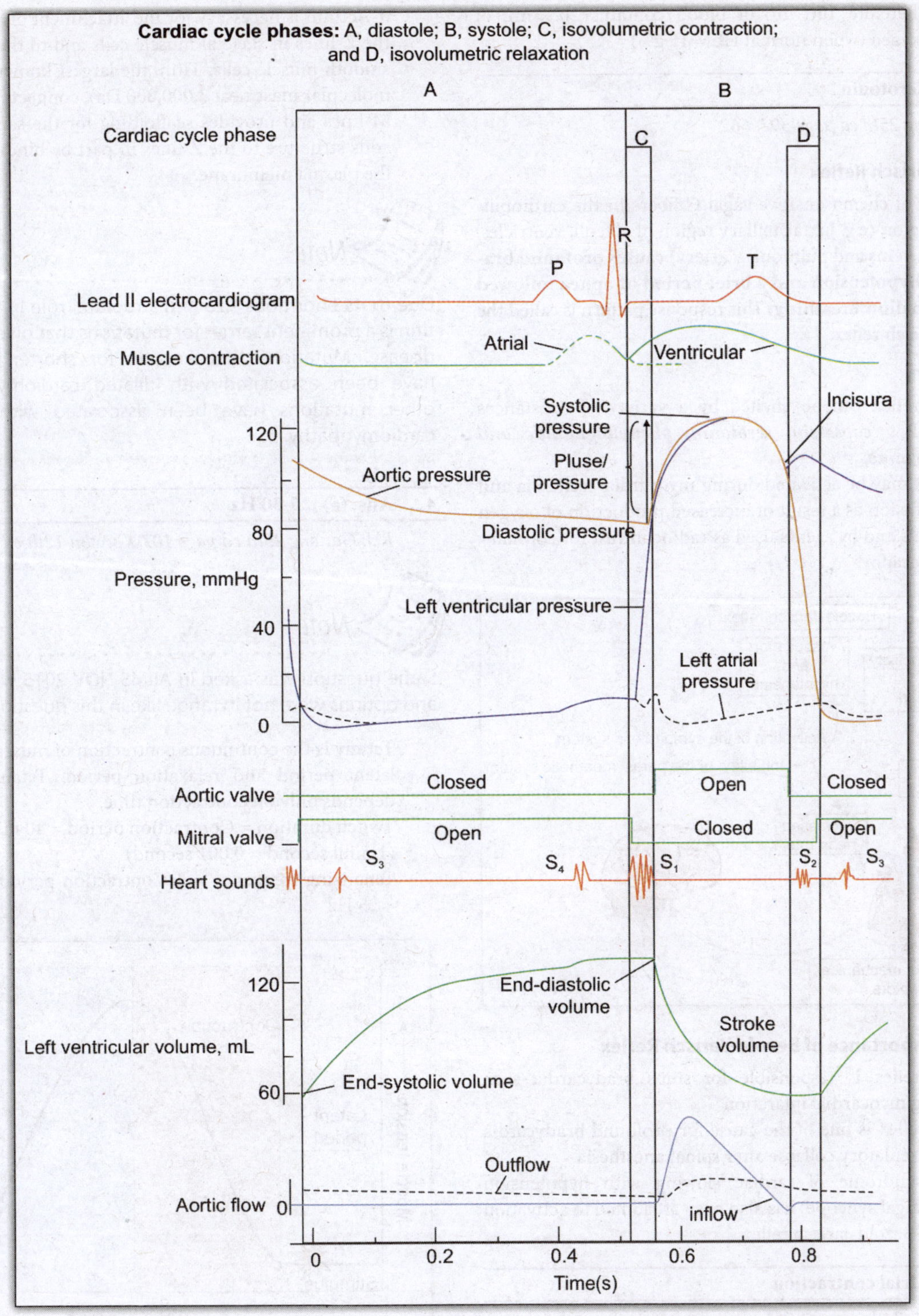

Cardiac cycle phases: A, diastole; B, systole; C, isovolumetric contraction; and D, isovolumetric relaxation

38. Ans. (c) 18

Ref: Ganong, 25th ed page 640

If hemoglobin saturation is normal: **1g Hb contains 1.34 mL oxygen.**

So, total oxygen carried by 14 g of Hb = (1.34 × 14) = 18.76 mL. (19 would have been a better answer considering the rounding off rules)

Calculation of Hb-bound O_2

This depends on saturation of Hb (SaO_2/SpO_2) with oxygen. SaO_2 depends on PaO_2

- **In arterial blood:**
  - At PaO_2 of 95 mm Hg, 97% hemoglobin is saturated with oxygen.
  - With this saturation, 1 g of Hb, contains 1.34 mL of O_2.

- Therefore 100 mL of blood contains 20.1 mL of oxygen (when normal Hb = 15 g%)

39. Ans. (c) Serotonin

Ref: Ganong 25th ed page 592, 662

Bezold-Jarisch Reflex

Activation of chemosensitive vagal C fibers in the cardiopulmonary region (e.g. juxtacapillary region of alveoli, ventricles, atria, great veins and pulmonary artery) causes **profound bradycardia, hypotension and a brief period of apnea followed by rapid shallow breathing.** This response pattern is called the Bezold-Jarisch reflex.

Activation

- This reflex can be elicited by a variety of substances including ***capsaicin, serotonin, phenylbiguanide and veratridine.***
- Reflex may be activated during myocardial ischemia and reperfusion as a result of increased production of oxygen radicals and by agents used as radiocontrast for coronary angiography.

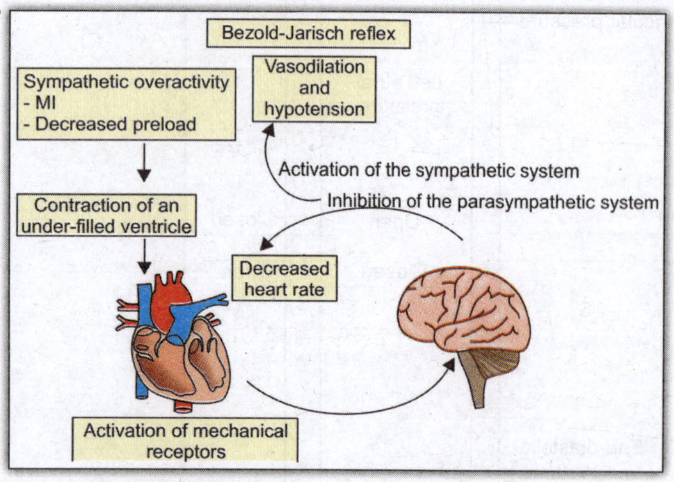

Clinical Importance of Bezold-Jarisch Reflex

- This reflex is responsible for sinus bradycardia seen during myocardial infarction
- This reflex is one of the cause for profound bradycardia and circulatory collapse after spinal anesthesia
- The syndrome of cardiac slowing with hypotension (vasovagal syncope) has also been attributed to activation of the Bezold-Jarisch reflex.

40. Ans. (a) Atrial contraction

Ref: Ganong 24th ed page 544

See table of JVP Waveforms in Physiology AIIMS May 2014 (see Volume II)

"a wave" of JVP is due to atrial contraction

41. Ans. (a) Alpha actinin

Ref: Ganong 25th ed page 101

(See table of Contractile Apparatus in Physiology AIIMS NOV 2016) (see page no. 160)

α-Actinin is necessary for the attachment of actin filaments to the Z-lines in skeletal muscle cells and to the dense bodies in smooth muscle cells. Titin, the largest known protein (with a molecular mass near 3,000,000 Da), connects the Z lines to the M lines and provides scaffolding for the sarcomere. Desmin adds structure to the Z lines in part by binding the Z lines to the plasma membrane.

NOTE

Due to its enormous size and structural role in the sarcomere, titin is a prominent target for mutations that give rise to muscle disease. Mutations that encode for shorter titin structure have been associated with dilated cardiomyopathy, while other mutations have been associated with hypertrophic cardiomyopathy.

42. Ans. (a) 25-30 Hz

Ref: Ganong 25th ed page 107, Guyton 12th ed page 80

NOTE

Same question was asked in AIIMS NOV 2015 without a graph and options were not in range like in this question.

Tetany is the continuous contraction of muscle fibers, without latent period and relaxation period. Tetanizing frequency depends only on contraction time.

Twitch duration = Contraction period = 40 milli sec = 0.04 sec (1 milli second = 0.001 second)

Tetanizing frequency = 1/Contraction period in sec = 1/0.04 = 25 Hz

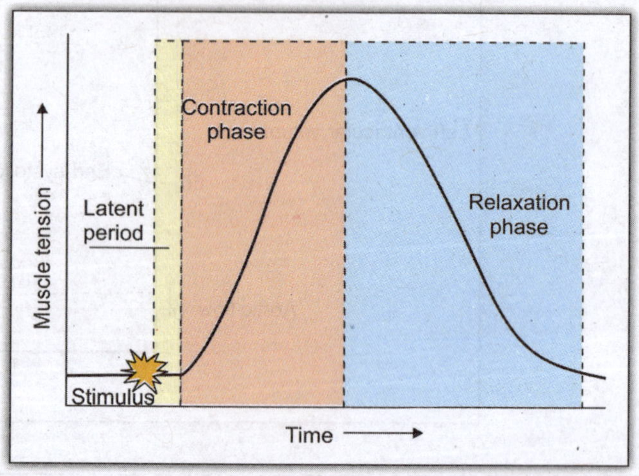

43. Ans. (b) 8 times

Ref: Ganong 25th ed page 573, 575

Indirect repeat Physiology AIIMS MAY 2015

Blood flow in a vessel is determined by the **Poiseuille's law** which states that "In the case of smooth flow (laminar flow), the volume flow rate is given by the pressure difference divided by the viscous resistance. This resistance depends linearly upon the viscosity and the length, but the fourth power dependence upon the radius is dramatically different".

Therefore blood flow is directly proportional to fourth power of radius.

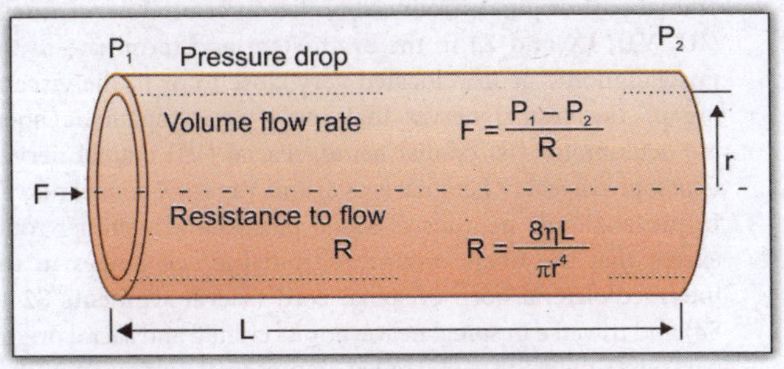

Flow inversely proportional to resistance (R).

R calculated based on **Poiseuille-Hagen formula**

($R = 8\eta L/\pi r^4$)

Using the above two: A will have 8 times more blood flow.

$$\text{Volume flow rate} = F = \frac{P_1 - P_2}{R} = \frac{\pi(\text{Pressure difference})(\text{radius})^4}{8(\text{viscosity length})}$$

$$\text{Resistance to flow} = R = \frac{8\eta L}{\pi r^4} = \frac{\pi(\text{Pressure difference})(\text{radius})^4}{8(\text{viscosity length})}$$

44. Ans. (a) 0.1

Ref: Guyton 12th ed page 467

Pulmonary Compliance = Change in volume (Tidal volume) divided by change in pressure

= 500 mL/5 mm Hg = 100 mL/mm Hg or 0.1 L/mm Hg

Pulmonary compliance refers to the relationship between the volume of the lungs and the transmural pressure across the lungs. At low lung volumes the pulmonary compliance is high; however, as the lungs expand their compliance progressively decreases. This reflects progressive stretching of elastin fibers to their physical limits as well as increasing surface tension as alveoli expand.

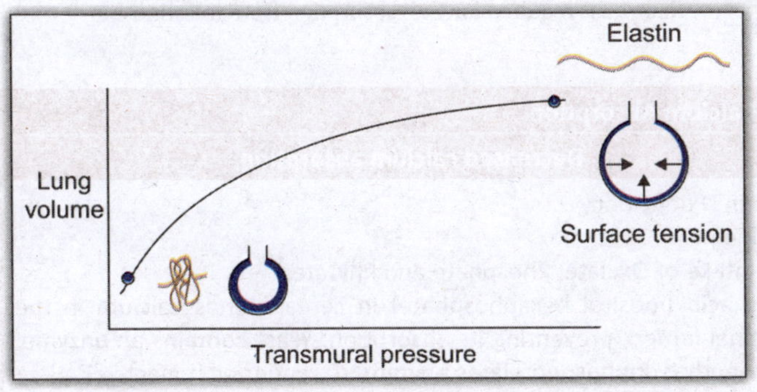

45. (c) 30 mg/min

Ref: Ganong 25th ed page 681

Step 1

Calculate the tubular filtration load of the substance (Glucose here)

GFR × plasma concentration of the substance (in mg/mL) = 90 × 2 = 180 (use 200 mg/dL = 2 mg/mL)

Step 2

Determine T_{max} (resorption of glucose) = 150.

Step 3

Excretion of glucose in urine = Filtration – Absorption = 180 – 150 = 30 mg/min

AIIMS NOVEMBER 2016

46. Ans. (a) 1

Ref: Ganong 24th ed page 438

– Curve 1 is a normal oral glucose tolerance test, Curve 5 is a diabetic.

Oral glucose tolerance test: Adults are given 75 g of glucose in 300 mL of water. In normal individuals, the fasting venous plasma glucose is less than 115 mg/dL, the 2-hour value is less than 140 mg/dL and no value is greater than 200 mg/dL. Diabetes mellitus is present if the 2-hour value and one other value are greater than 200 mg/dL. Impaired glucose tolerance is diagnosed when the values are above the upper limits of normal but below the values diagnostic of diabetes.

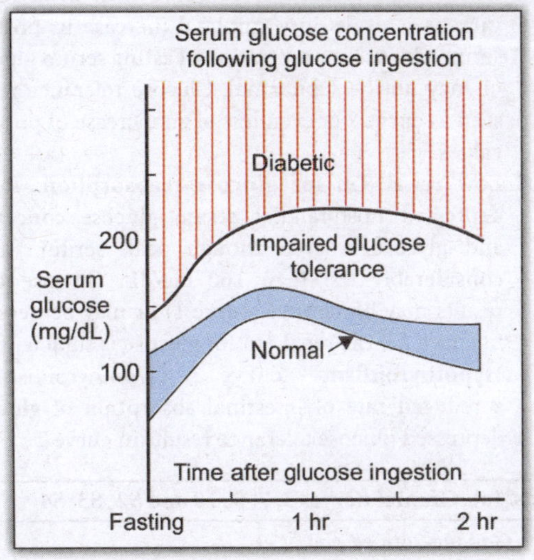

Pathologic Conditions Causing Impaired, or Diabetic, Glucose Tolerance Results

- **Hypercorticism - curve 4:** Hypercorticism increases the rate of intestinal glucose absorption to produce an early and elevated postprandial peak serum glucose concentration. The additional effects of increased gluconeogenesis and inhibition of glucose uptake in peripheral tissue generally causes an elevated 2 hours postprandial value and an elevated fasting serum glucose. Glucose tolerance results are seen as curve 4
- **Acromegaly - between curves 3 and 4:** Increased growth hormone stimulates glycogenolysis and inhibits the uptake of glucose in peripheral tissue causing elevated fasting and postprandial serum glucose concentrations. Glucose tolerance results are typically between curves 4 and 5.
- **Hyperthyroidism - curve 3:** Hyperthyroidism increases the rate of intestinal glucose absorption to produce an early and elevated peak postprandial serum glucose concentration. The effect of thyroid hormone on peripheral

tissue causing increased glucose utilization is generally greater than the effect of increased glycogenolysis on the liver so that the 2 hours postprandial value is usually normal as is the fasting serum glucose concentration. Typical glucose tolerance results are represented by curve 3

- **Pheochromacytoma (or "emotional hyperglycemia") - between curves 3 and 4:** Increased epinephrine increases glycogenolysis resulting in increased fasting and postprandial serum glucose concentrations. Glucose tolerance results are typically between curves 3 and 4.

Pathologic Conditions Causing Flat or Depressed Glucose Tolerance Results

- **Insulinoma - Curve 2 or even more depressed:** Insulinoma causes rapid uptake of glucose by peripheral tissue resulting in fasting hypoglycemia and a minimal increase in postprandial serum glucose concentrations. Curve 2 or even more depressed glucose tolerance results are typical.
- **Intestinal malabsorption; curve 2 or even less of an increase:** results in a minimal increase in postprandial serum glucose concentrations. Fasting serum glucose may or may not be subnormal. Glucose tolerance results are seen as curve 2 or even less of an increase of postprandial values.
- **Low renal Tm for glucose reabsorption**: Results in depressed postprandial serum glucose concentrations and glycosuria even though peak serum values are considerably less than 160 mg/dL. Glucose tolerance results may be normal (curve 1) or may be depressed as in curve 2 if the renal Tm for glucose is sufficiently low.
- **Hypothyroidism - curve 2:** Hypothyroidism causes a reduced rate of intestinal absorption of glucose and depressed glucose tolerance results in curve 2

47. Ans. (a) Cranial nerves 3, 7, 9, 10 and S2, S3, S4

Ref: Ganong 24th ed page 259

Parasympathetic Nuclei

The cranial outflow of parasympathetic system originates from cranial nerve nuclei that are located in the brain stem. In parasympathetic system, the preganglionic neurons of cranial part originate from cell bodies in **cranial nerve nuclei (III, VII, IX and X)** in the brain stem and terminate in the postganglionic neuron located very close to or in the visceral organ. The cranial nerves that carry parasympathetic fibers are oculomotor (III cranial nerve), Facial (VII cranial nerve), Glossopharngeal (XI cranial nerve) and Vagus (X cranial nerve). In preganglionic neurons of sacral part follow a similar route except that the fibers originates from the cell bodies in the intermediolateral horn of spinal cord **(sacral segments S2 to S4)** and traverse in spinal nerve. For its cranial and sacral origin, parasympathetic system is called craniosacral outflow of ANS.

48. Ans. (d) Alkaline pH in GIT > (b) Phytates

Ref: Guyton 12th ed page 956, Ganong 24 edition page 485, Harper 27th ed ch 43

Both Phytate and Alkaline pH inhibits calcium absorption, however Calcium oxalate/phosphate/phytate are particularly insoluble at neutral or alkaline pH, whereas it readily dissolves in acid medium. Hence pH is the primary effector of the Calcium absorption

Absorption and excretion of calcium and phosphate: Calcium ions are actively absorbed into the blood, especially from the duodenum and the amount of calcium ion absorption is exactly controlled to supply the daily need of the body for calcium. The usual rates of intake are about **1000 mg/day** each for calcium and phosphorus, about the amounts in 1 liter of milk. Normally, divalent cations such as calcium ions are poorly absorbed from the intestines. However, as discussed later, vitamin D promotes calcium absorption by the intestines and about *35 percent (350 mg/day) of the ingested calcium is usually absorbed*; the calcium remaining in the intestine is excreted in the feces. An additional 250 mg/day of calcium enters the intestines via secreted gastrointestinal juices and sloughed mucosal cells. Thus, about 90 percent (900 mg/day) of the daily intake of calcium is excreted in the feces Ca: P ratio: Ideal ratio is 1:1 for absorption. A ratio of Ca:P not more than 2:1 and not less than 1:2 is required for Ca^{++} absorption from intestine

Factors Affecting Calcium Absorption

Increased calcium absorption	Decreased calcium absorption
Parathormone (PTH): Parathyroid hormone activates vitamin D and the activated vitamin D in turn greatly enhances calcium absorption Vitamin D Body need: Growth, Pregnancy, Lactation, old age High protein diet Acidic pH Lactose; through the action of lactobacillus produces Lactic acid and hence acidic pH	Vitamin D deficiency Alkaline pH High intake of Oxalate, Phosphate and Phytates Phytic acid (inositol hexaphosphate) in cereals binds calcium in the intestinal lumen, preventing its absorption. Yeast contains an enzyme, phytase, that dephosphorylates phytate, so rendering it inactive. High concentrations of fatty acids in the intestinal lumen, as a result of impaired fat absorption, can also reduce calcium absorption, by forming insoluble calcium salts (soap) Dietary fibers can bind calcium and hinders absorption

49. Ans. (a) Aldosterone

Ref: Ganong 24 ed page 355, Guyton 12th ed page 921

Zona Glomerulosa is marked as A and mainly secretes Aldosterone.

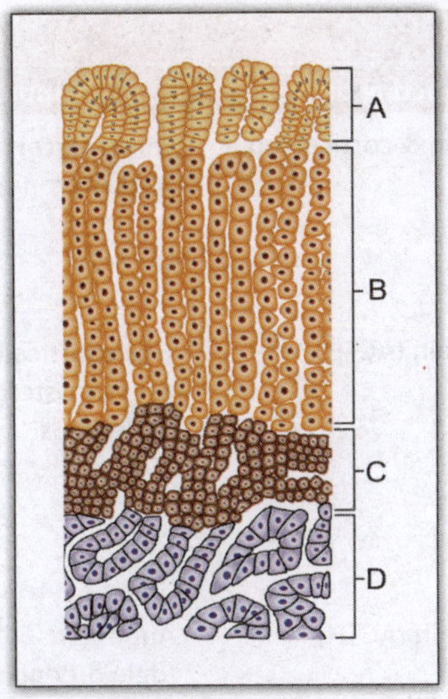

The slide shown is of Adrenal gland
A = Zona glomerulosa
B = Zona fasciculata
C = Zona reticularis
D = Medulla

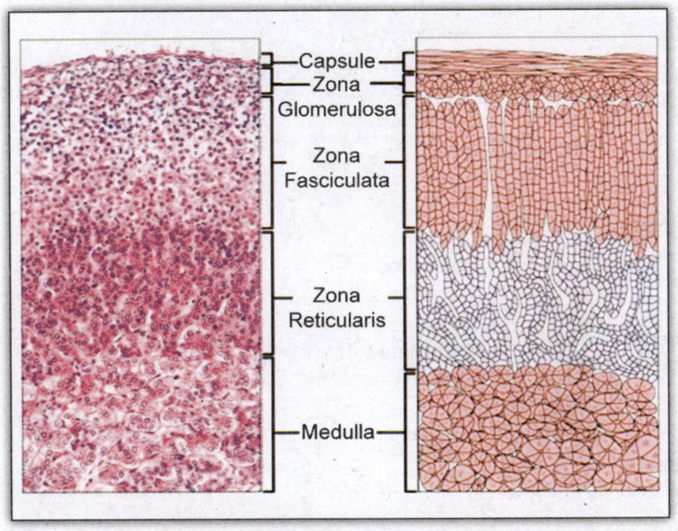

Fig: Histology of adrenal gland (low power): Labeled, with representative illustration along with

1. **Zona glomerulosa:** Capsule is visible in right upper quadrant; cells are arranged in rounded clusters like glomeruli (arrowhead). Minimal or no vaculation
2. **Zona fasciculata:** Cells are arranged in long cords that run perpendicular to capsule. Abundant lipid vacuoles (containing mainly glucocorticoids), round uniform nuclei
3. **Zona reticularis:** Small cells with anastomosing network, Some ageing cells contain the yellow-brown pigment lipofuscin (brown, see Insat), Blood capillaries run between cell plates (Arrow)
4. **Adrenal medulla:** The medulla consists of anastomosing cords and trabecuale of groups of cells (arrow) separated by venous sinusoids. Minimal or no vacuolation. In addition to pheochromocytes, medulla contains single or groups of sympathetic ganglions (Visible in High HD)

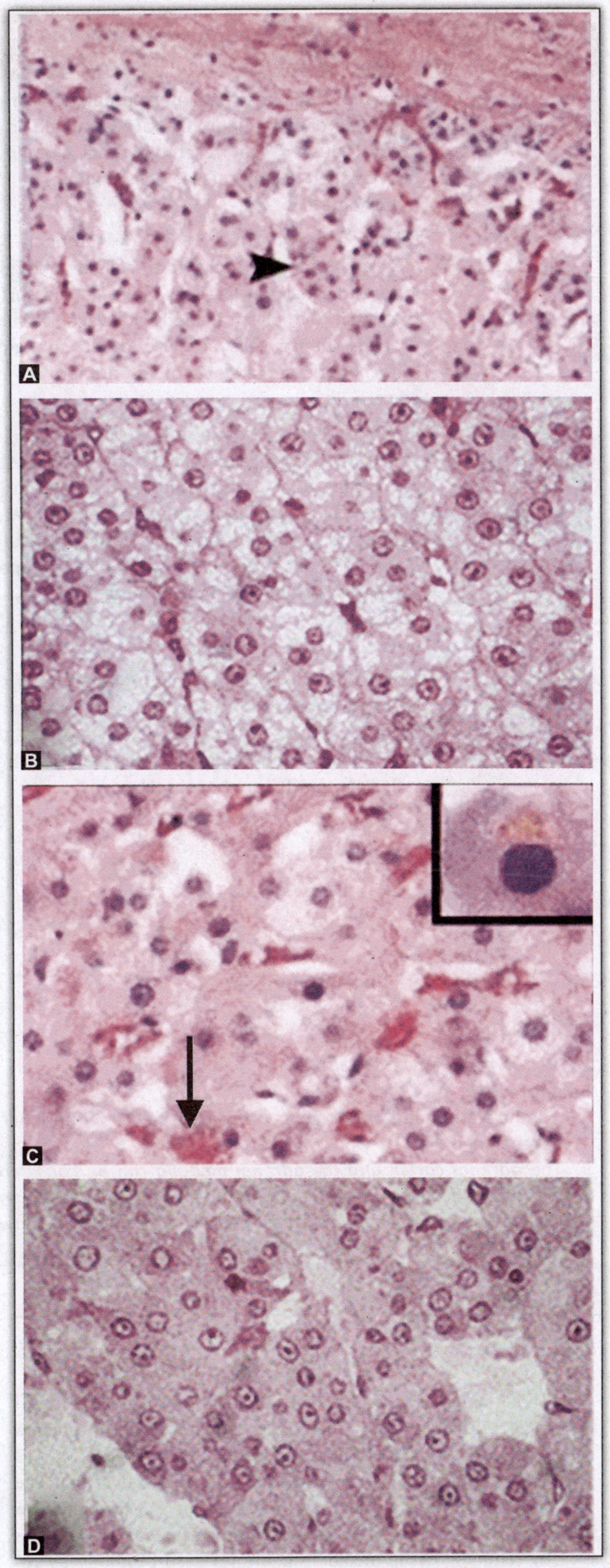

Fig: Histology of adrenal zones (high power)

Adrenal Gland			
Part	**Comments**	**Factors acting on gland**	**Hormone secreted**
Cortex: Zona glomerulosa	Outermost, thinnest, 15% of adrenal, 20% of cortex, columnar or pyramidal cells are arranged in round to oval clusters that resemble renal glomeruli and hence called "glomerulosa. Cells contains numerous mitochondria	Angiotensin & corticotropin (ACTH)	Mineralocorticoids (Aldosterone)
Cortex: Zona fasciculata	Middle and widest layer, 65% of adrenal, 80% of cortex, columnar or polyhedral cells in 1–2 cell thick long cords that run at right angles to the surface of the organ, Cytoplasm loaded with vacuoles and lipid droplets, hence cells are also called **spongiocytes**. Mitochondria are large & contain numerous vesicular cristae	Corticotropin (ACTH)	Glucocorticoids (Cortisol & corticosterone), some androgens
Cortex: Zona reticularis	Innermost layer, 7% of adrenal, 10% of cortex, Irregularly shaped cells smaller than other layers forming irregular cords that form an anastomosing network, blood capillaries run between cell plates, mitochondria are large and have vesicular cristae, no vacuoles and fat droplets in cytoplasm. Some aged cells have **lipofuscin pigment** granules **pyknotic nuclei** suggesting cell death are often found in this layer	Corticotropin (ACTH)	Androgens (dehydroepiandrosterone-DHEA), Some glucocorticoids
Medulla	13% of adrenal, polygonal cells (pheochromocytes) nests are arranged in anastomosing cords separated by large venous sinusoids/muscular veins. Due to their affinity to chromium salts, the cells are often called **chromaffin or pheochrome cells.**		Catecholamines (adrenaline or noradrenaline)

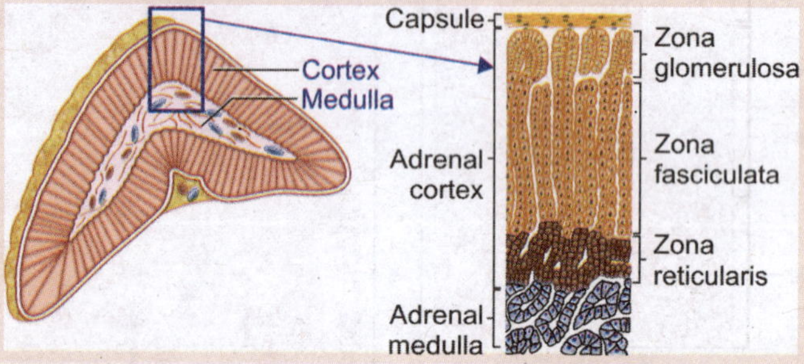

Footnote:

- Adrenals are made of two concentric layers: a yellow peripheral layer, the adrenal cortex; and a reddish-brown central layer, the adrenal medulla
- The ***adrenal cortex and the adrenal medulla can be considered two organs with distinct origins, functions and morphological characteristics*** that became united during embryonic development. They arise from different germ layers. The cortex arises from the coelomic epithelium, whereas the cells of the medulla derive from the neural crest, from which sympathetic ganglion cells also originate.

50. Ans. (b) rT3

Ref: Ganong 24 ed page 344-345

This graph was taken by the examiner from Ganong 24th ed page 345 figure 199-9 titled **"Effect of starvation on plasma levels of T 4, T 3 and RT 3 in humans"** - The scale for T 3 and RT 3 is on the left and the scale for T 4 is on the right. **The most pronounced effect is a reduction in T 3 levels with a reciprocal rise in RT 3.** The changes, which conserve calories by reducing tissue metabolism, are reversed promptly by re-feeding. Similar changes occur in wasting diseases.

Much more RT3 and much less T3 are formed during fetal life and the ratio shifts to that of adults about 6 weeks after birth. Various drugs inhibit deiodinase, producing a fall in plasma T3 levels and a reciprocal rise in RT3. A wide variety of nonthyroidal illnesses also suppress deiodinase. These include burns, trauma, advanced cancer, cirrhosis, renal failure, myocardial infarction and febrile states. The low-T3 state produced by these conditions disappears with recovery. It is difficult to decide whether individuals with low-T3 state produced by drugs and illness have mild hypothyroidism.

Diet also has a clear-cut effect on conversion of T4 to T3. In fasted individuals, plasma T3 is reduced by 10-20% within 24 hours and by about 50% in 3-7 days, with a corresponding rise in RT3. Free and bound T4 levels remain essentially normal. During more prolonged starvation, RT3 returns to normal but T3 remains depressed. At the same time, the basal metabolic rate (BMR) falls and urinary nitrogen excretion, an index of protein breakdown, is decreased. Thus, the decline in T3 conserves calories and protein. Conversely, overfeeding increases T3 and reduces RT3.

51. Ans. (a) Eye

Ref: Guyton 13th ed page 805 Principles and Practice of Endo. and Metabolism, by K. L. Becker page 957

Countercurrent Mechanism is not Seen in Eye

Option (B)

The countercurrent mechanism depends on the special anatomical arrangement of the loops of Henle and the vasa recta, the specialized peritubular capillaries of the renal medulla. In the human, about 25 percent of the nephrons are juxtamedullary nephrons, with loops of Henle and vasa recta that go deeply into the medulla before returning to the cortex. Some of the loops of Henle dip all the way to the tips of the renal papillae that project from the medulla into the renal pelvis. Paralleling the long loops of Henle are the vasa recta, which also loop down into the medulla before returning to the renal cortex. And finally, the collecting ducts, which carry urine through the hyperosmotic renal medulla before it is excreted, also play a critical role in the countercurrent mechanism. Ref: Guyton 12th ed page 348

Option (C)

"Countercurrent" blood flow in the villi: The arterial flow into the villus and the venous flow out of the villus are in directions opposite to each other and that the vessels lie in close apposition to each other. Because of this vascular arrangement, much of the blood oxygen diffuses out of the arterioles directly into the adjacent venules without ever being carried in the blood to the tips of the villi. As much as 80 percent of the oxygen may take this short-circuit route and therefore not be available for local metabolic functions of the villi. The reader will recognize that this type of countercurrent mechanism in the villi is analogous to the countercurrent mechanism in the vasa recta of the kidney medulla. Ref: Guyton 12th ed page 761

Option (D)

The spermatic arteries to the testes are tortuous and blood in them runs parallel but in the opposite direction to blood in the pampiniform plexus of spermatic veins. Th is anatomic arrangement may permit countercurrent exchange of heat and testosterone. (Ref Ganong 24th ed page 419)

> **NOTE**
>
> The deep veins (venae comitantes) run alongside the arteries supplying the limbs and heat is transferred from the warm arterial blood going to the limbs to the cold venous blood coming from the extremities by countercurrent exchange (Ref: Ganong 24th ed page 319)

52. Ans. (b) 90 min

Ref: Ganong 24th ed page 498

Migrating Motor Complex

- During fasting between periods of digestion, the pattern of electrical and motor activity in gastrointestinal smooth muscle becomes modified so that cycles of motor activity migrate from the stomach to the distal ileum.
- Each cycle, or **migrating motor complex (MMC),** starts with a quiescent period (phase I), continues with a period of irregular electrical and mechanical activity (phase II) and ends with a burst of regular activity (phase III).
- The MMCs migrate aborally at a rate of about 5 cm/min and they occur at intervals of approximately 90 minutes. Their function is unsettled, although gastric secretion, bile flow and pancreatic secretion increase during each MMC. They may clear the stomach and small intestine of luminal contents in preparation for the next meal.
- They are immediately stopped by ingestion of food, with a return to peristalsis and the other forms of BER and spike potentials.

53. Ans. (b) Testosterone

Ref: With Text

Option (A)

Zona reticularis secretes androgens dehydroepiandrosterone (DHEA). Most of the dehydroepiandrosterone that is formed is converted to dehydroepi-androsterone sulfate (DHEAS) by adrenal sulfokinase and this enzyme is localized in the zona reticularis as well. All but about 0.3% of the circulating DHEA is conjugated to sulfate (DHEAS). Dehydroepiandrosterone (DHEA) values peak at about age 25 (Ganong 24th ed page 361)

Option (B)

Sex hormone-binding globulin (SHBG) is a glycoprotein that binds to the sex hormones, testosterone and 17β-estradiol. Progesterone, cortisol and other corticosteroids are bound by transcortin. *(Ref: Ganong 24th ed page 302)*

In a pathophysiological setting, some medications can alter levels of binding proteins or displace hormones that are bound to them. In addition, some binding proteins are promiscuous and bind multiple hormones (e.g. SHBG). *(Ref: Ganong 24th ed page 302)*

After secretion by the testes, about 97 percent of the testosterone becomes either loosely bound with plasma albumin or more tightly bound with a beta globulin called sex hormone-binding globulin and circulates in the blood in these states for 30 minutes to several hours *(Ref: Guyton 12th ed page 980)*

Option (C) and (D)

Both estrogens and progesterone are transported in the blood bound mainly with plasma albumin and with specific estrogen- and progesterone-binding globulins. The binding between these hormones and the plasma proteins is loose enough that they are rapidly released to the tissues over a period of 30 minutes or so *(Ref: Guyton 12th ed page 993)*

54. Ans. (a) Nernst equation

Ref: Ganong 24 ed page 9

Membrane Potential

In living cells, the resting membrane potential (V_m) is seldom governed by only one ion such as K^+, Na^+, Cl^-, etc. If this were the case, the membrane potential could be predicted by the equilibrium potential ($V_{Eq.}$) for that ion and could be easily calculated by using the **Nernst equation (Is a mathematical equation applied in physiology, to calculate equilibrium potentials for certain ions).** Instead, the membrane potential is generally established as a result of the relative contributions of several ions. In many cells, K^+, Na^+ and Cl^- are the main contributors to the membrane potential.

Nernst equation	The diffusion potential level across a membrane that exactly opposes the net diffusion of a particular ion through the membrane is called the Nernst potential for that ion. ***The Nernst equation can be considered a special case of the Goldman equation for only one ion.*** Degree of importance of each of the ions in determining the voltage is proportional to the membrane permeability for that particular ion. That is, if the membrane has zero permeability to both potassium and chloride ions, the membrane potential becomes entirely dominated by the concentration gradient of sodium ions alone and the resulting potential will be equal to the Nernst potential for sodium. In general the membrane potential will be closest to the equilibrium potential of the ion (ions) with the greatest membrane permeability.
Goldman equation, or Goldman Hodgkin Katz equation	It gives the calculated membrane potential on the inside of the membrane when two univalent positive ions, sodium (Na^+) and potassium (K^+) and one univalent negative ion, chloride (Cl^-), are involved.

$$A.\ V = \frac{2.3\ RT}{zF} \log \frac{[K^+]_{outside}}{[K^+]_{inside}} = 61.5 \log \frac{[K^+]_{outside}}{[K^+]_{inside}} \text{ (at 37°C)}$$

$$B.\ V = \frac{2.3\ RT}{zF} \log \frac{p_k[K^+]_0 + p_{Na}[Na^+]_0 + p_{cl}[Cl^-]_1}{p_k[K^+]_1 + p_{Na}[Na^+]_1 + p_{cl}[Cl^-]_0} = 61.5 \log \frac{p_k[K^+]_0 + p_{Na}[Na^+]_0 + p_{cl}[Cl^-]_1}{p_k[K^+]_1 + p_{Na}[Na^+]_1 + p_{cl}[Cl^-]_0}$$

R = Gas constant (8.316 joules/degree)

T = Absolute temperature

F = Faraday constant

z = Charge on the ion (+1 for Na, +2 for Ca, –1 for Cl)

Also, the sign of the potential is positive (+) if the ion diffusing from inside to outside is a negative ion and it is negative (–) if the ion is positive.

A = Nernst equation: At body temperature, the potassium equilibrium potential (which represents the great majority of resting membrane potential) is a constant times the logarithm of the ratio of concentrations of potassium outside and inside the cell.

B = Goldman-Hodgkins-Katz equation: This is similar to the Nernst equation except that it adds a factor for permeability. If an ion is impermeable, its contribution to the membrane potential (V) is nil. The higher the relative permeability, the closer the membrane will be to the equilibrium potential for that ion.

Nernst equation deals with chloride shift. Chloride shift (also known as the Hamburger shift or Hamburger's phenomenon, named after Hartog Jacob Hamburger (1859–1924), Dutch physiologist) is a process which occurs in a cardiovascular system and refers to the exchange of bicarbonate (HCO_3^-) and chloride (Cl^-) across the membrane of red blood cells (RBCs)

55. Ans. (c) Maintaining sinus rhythm

Ref: Ganong 24 ed page 523, Signaling at the Cell Surface in the Circulatory and Ventilatory Systems by Marc Thiriet 137

NOTE

Myocardial potential is different from Pacemaker potential. Myocardial potential is the action potential of the nonpacemaker cells of the heart.

Hyperpolarization activated cyclic nucleotide-gated (HCN) channels are expressed in pacemaker cells found in the heart and the nervous system.

- HCN channel belongs to the cyclic nucleotide gated (CNG) channel to the K^+ channel superfamily
- Unlike voltage gated channels the HCN channels are activated by Hyperpolarization when V_m is below –50 mV to –70 mV
- HCN channel are activated by Hyperpolarized rather than depolarized potentials.
- HCN channels are permeable to both monovalent (Na^+, K^+) and bivalent (Ca^{++}) cations.
- HCN channels are activated by cAMP and cGMP
- The HCN channels generate pacemaker currents in many excitable cells such as cardiac nodal cells and neurons. **The pacemaker current is found in SA and AV nodal cells. The channel underlying this current is a nonspecific cation channel called HCN (Hyperpolarization-activated Cyclic Nucleotide-gated) channel.**
- There are 4 known HCN subunit isoforms; HCN 1-4, which combine to form tetrameric channel
- HCN channels are not implicated in increased heart rate. They are required to maintain the stable cardiac rhythm
- **Sinus rhythm is dictated by hyperpolarization activated cyclic nucleotide gated monovalent cation channels known as HCN or pacemaker channels** (and to a greater or lesser extent, Ca^{2+} oscillations, a matter of current debate).

Pacemaker Action Potential	
SA nodal action potentials are divided into three phases. Cells within the sinoatrial (SA) node are the primary pacemaker site within the heart, characterized as having no true resting potential, but instead generate regular, **spontaneous action potentials.** Unlike non-pacemaker action potentials in the heart and most other cells that elicit action potentials (e.g., nerve cells, muscle cells), the depolarizing current is carried into the cell primarily by relatively **slow Ca^{++} currents** instead of by fast Na^+ currents.	
Phase 4: Pacemaker potential	• Phase 4 is the spontaneous depolarization (pacemaker potential) that triggers the action potential once the membrane potential reaches threshold between –40 and –30 mV). • At the end of repolarization, when the membrane potential is very negative (about **–60 mV**), ion channels open that conduct slow, inward (depolarizing) Na^+ currents. A channel permeable to both Na^+ and K^+ is activated. Because this channel is activated following **hyperpolarization**, it is referred to as an **"h" channel**; however, because of its unusual (funny) activation it has also been dubbed an **"f" channel** and the current produced as **"funny current"** and abbreviated as "I_f". These depolarizing currents cause the membrane potential to begin to spontaneously depolarize, thereby initiating **Phase 4**. As the membrane potential reaches about –50 mV, another type of channel opens. This channel is called transient or **T-type Ca^{++} channel**.
Phase 0: Depolarization	• Phase 0 is the depolarization phase of the action potential • Primarily caused by increased Ca^{++} conductance (gCa^{++}) through the **L-type Ca^{++} channels** that began to open toward the end of Phase 4 • When the membrane depolarizes to about –40 mV, a second type of Ca^{++} channel opens. These are the so-called long-lasting, or L-type Ca^{++} channels. Opening of these channels causes more Ca^{++} to enter the cell and to further depolarize the cell until an action potential threshold is reached (usually between –40 and –30 mV). It should be noted that a hyperpolarized state is necessary for pacemaker channels to become activated. • Because the movement of Ca^{++} through these channels into the cell is not rapid, the rate of depolarization (slope of Phase 0) is much slower than found in other cardiac cells (e.g., Purkinje cells) • Closure of Funny Na^+ channel and T-type Ca^{++} channels. • During depolarization, the membrane potential (Em) moves toward the equilibrium potential for Ca++, which is about +134 mV.
Phase 3: Repolarization	• Repolarization occurs (**Phase 3**) as K^+ channels open (increased gK^+) thereby increasing the outward directed, hyperpolarizing K^+ currents. At the same time, the L-type Ca^{++} channels become inactivated and close, which decreases gCa^{++} and the inward depolarizing Ca^{++} currents. • Once the cell is completely repolarized at about –60 mV, the cycle is spontaneously repeated • During repolarization, $g'Ca^{++}$ (relative Ca^{++} conductance) decreases and $g'K^+$ (relative K^+ conductance) increases, which brings E_m closer toward the equilibrium potential for K^+, which is about –96 mV).
Therefore, the action potential in SA nodal cells is primarily dependent upon changes in Ca^{++} and K^+ conductances as: **$E_m = g'K^+ (-96\ mV) + g'Ca^{++} (+134\ mV)$**	

56. Ans. (c) Components can be increased or decreased as needed

Ref: Guyton 13th ed page 413, Nelson 20th ed page 370

The best buffers are weak acids and bases. This is because a buffer works best when it is 50% dissociated (half HA and half A-). The pH at which a buffer is 50% dissociated is its pK. The best physiologic buffers have a pK close to 7.40. The concentration of a buffer and its pK determine the buffer's effectiveness (buffering capacity). When the pH is lower than the pK of a buffer, there is more HA than A-. When the pH is higher than the pK, there is more A- than HA.

The bicarbonate buffer system is very effective as a result of the high concentration of bicarbonate in the body (24 mEq/L) and the fact that it is an open system. The remaining body buffers are in a closed system. The bicarbonate buffer system is an open system because the lungs increase carbon dioxide excretion when the blood carbon dioxide concentration increases. When acid is added to the body, the following reaction occurs:

$$H^+ + HCO_3^- \rightarrow CO_2 + H_2O$$

In a closed system, the CO2 would increase. The higher CO_2 concentration would lead to an increase in the reverse reaction: $CO_2 + H_2O \rightarrow H^+ + HCO_3^-$. This would increase the concentration of hydrogen ions, limiting the buffering capacity of bicarbonate. However, because the lungs excrete the excess carbon dioxide, the reverse reaction does not increase; this enhances the buffering capacity of bicarbonate. The same principle holds with the addition of base because the lungs decrease carbon dioxide excretion and prevent the level of carbon dioxide from falling. The lack of change in carbon dioxide concentration dramatically increases the buffering capacity of bicarbonate.

Carbonic acid-bicarbonate system is one of the most effective buffer systems in the body, because the H_2CO_3 level in plasma is in equilibrium with the dissolved CO_2 ($H_2CO_3 \rightarrow CO_2 + H_2O$); and the amount of dissolved CO_2 is controlled by respiration. In addition, the plasma concentration of HCO_3^- is regulated by kidneys.

Compartment-wise Buffer Systems			
Compartment			Major buffer
ECF	Blood	Plasma	Plasma proteins
		RBC	Hemoglobin
	Interstitial fluid		Bicarbonate
ICF			Imidazole and Proteins (52%) Bicarbonate (42%) Phosphate (6%)

- Bicarbonate is the predominant and most abundant buffer of ECF as a whole (95%)
- Bicarbonate buffer is very effective as a result of the high concentration of bicarbonate in the body (24 mEq/L) and it is an **open system.** This is an open ended system, because CO_2 can be adjusted immediately by ventilation through lungs and HCO_3^- by kidney in long run. Rest all are closed systems
- Hemoglobin is the predominant buffer of blood as a whole because hemoglobin is present in large amounts the **hemoglobin in blood has six times the buffering capacity of the plasma proteins**
- Although hemoglobin is intracellular (inside RBC), it is often considered ECF buffer because RBC is a cellular component of ECF and because of the cellular permeability of RBC membrane.
- As with ***hemoglobin***, the most important ***buffering*** sites of the plasma proteins are the side groups of ***histidine***. Thus, conceptually, it would not be wrong to consider ***hemoglobin*** and plasma proteins as a single class of ***"histidine buffers"***

57. Ans. (c) Curve D

Ref: Guyton 12 ed page 510

This figure is directly taken from Guyton by the examiner

Composite Effects of PCO_2, pH and PO_2 on Alveolar Ventilation

Figure gives a quick overview of the manner in which the chemical factors PO_2, PCO_2, and pH together affect alveolar ventilation.

- To understand this diagram, first observe the four red curves. These curves were recorded at different levels of arterial PO_2-40 mm Hg, 50 mm Hg, 60 mm Hg and 100 mm Hg.
- For each of these curves, the PCO_2 was changed from lower to higher levels. Thus, this "family" of red curves represents the combined effects of alveolar PCO_2 and PO_2 on ventilation. The red curves were measured at a blood pH of 7.4
- Now observe the green curves. The green curves were measured at a pH of 7.3.
- We now have two families of curves representing the combined effects of PCO_2 and PO_2 on ventilation at two different pH values.
- **Still other families of curves would be displaced to the right at higher pHs and displaced to left at lower pHs.** Thus, using this diagram, one can predict the level of alveolar ventilation for most combinations of alveolar PCO_2, alveolar PO_2 and arterial pH

By comparing the graph provided in the question from that of the explanation, it is clear when PaO_2 is 100 mm Hg. If pH changed from 7.4 to 7.3, change in alveolar ventilation will shift to curve D.

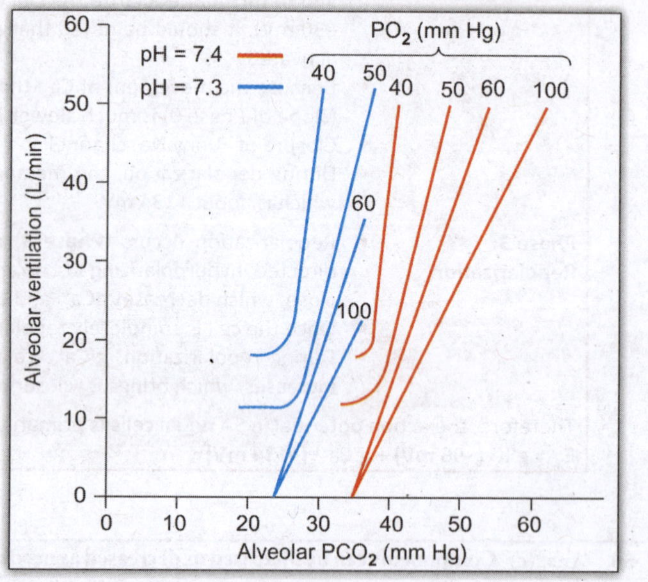

58. Ans. (c) Insulin > (b) Glucagon

Ref: Ganong 24 ed page 330, Brook's Clinical Pediatric Endocrinology By Charles G. D. Brook, Peter Clayton, Rosalind Brown 6th ed page 141, A K Jain 6 edition page no 662

While Both Insulin and Glucagon can be used in Growth Hormone Stimulation test, Glucagon is only an alternative to Insulin.

Because of the unavailability of the GHRH analog, the glucagon stimulation test (GST) is currently the accepted alternative test to the insulin tolerance test (ITT)

Stimulation tests are classified into:

- Screening tests: Exercise, Fasting, Levodopa, Clonidine
- Definitive tests: Arginine, Insulin, Glucagon

To improve specificity, provocative tests are often combined.

Tests of Pituitary Insufficiency

Hormone	Test	Blood Samples	Interpretation
Growth Hormone	**Insulin tolerance test:** Regular insulin (0.05–0.15 U/kg IV)	–30, 0, 30, 60, 120 min for glucose and GH	Glucose < 40 mg/dL; GH should be >3 g/L. Additionally it is a test of HPA integrity. Most reliable provocative test.
	GHRH test: 1 g/kg IV	0, 15, 30, 45, 60, 120 min for GH	Normal response is GH >3 g/L. Used to differentiate Hypothalamic from Pituitary causes and those who gives subnormal response to standard provocative test.
	L-Arginine test: 30 g IV over 30 min	0, 30, 60, 120 min for GH	Normal response is GH >3 g/L
	L-Dopa test: 500 mg PO	0, 30, 60, 120 min for GH	Normal response is GH >3 g/L
	Prolactin	TRH test: 200–500 g IV	0, 20 and 60 min for TSH and PRL Normal prolactin is >2 g/L and increase >200% of baseline
	Glucagon Stimulation test	Glucagon 30 µg/kg (max 1 mg) IV, SC, IM. 60, 80, 120, 150, 180 Min. Normal response serum cortisol >18 µg/dL in any sample	Used in children < 2 years and if Insulin tolerance is contraindicated
ACTH	Insulin tolerance test: regular insulin (0.05–0.15 U/kg IV)	–30, 0, 30, 60, 90 min for glucose and cortisol	Glucose <40 mg/dL Cortisol should increase by >7 g/dL or to >20 g/dL
	CRH test: 1 g/kg ovine CRH IV at 8 A.M.	0, 15, 30, 60, 90, 120 min for ACTH and cortisol	Basal ACTH increases 2- to 4-fold and peaks at 20–100 pg/mL Cortisol levels >20–25 g/dL
	Metyrapone test: Metyrapone (30 mg/kg) at midnight	Plasma 11-deoxycortisol and cortisol at 8 A.M.; ACTH can also be measured	Plasma cortisol should be <4 g/dL to assure an adequate response Normal response is 11-deoxycortisol >7.5 g/dL or ACTH >75 pg/mL
	Standard ACTH Stimulation test: ACTH 1-24 (cosyntropin), 0.25 mg IM or IV	0, 30, 60 min for cortisol and aldosterone	Normal response is cortisol >21 g/dL and aldosterone response of >4 ng/dL above baseline
	Low-dose ACTH test: ACTH 1-24 (cosyntropin), 1 g IV	0, 30, 60 min for cortisol	Cortisol should be >21 g/dL
	3-day ACTH stimulation test consists of 0.25 mg ACTH 1-24 given IV over 8 hours each day	?	Cortisol >21 g/dL
TSH	Basal thyroid function test: T4, T_3, TSH	Basal measurements	Low free thyroid hormone levels in the setting of TSH levels that are not appropriately increased indicate pituitary insufficiency
	TRH test: 200–500 g IV	0, 20, 60 min for TSH and PRL	TSH should increase by >5 mU/L unless thyroid hormone levels are increased
LH, FSH	LH, FSH, testosterone, estrogen	Basal measurements	Basal LH and FSH should be increased in postmenopausal women Low testosterone levels in the setting of low LH and FSH indicate pituitary insufficiency
	GnRH test: GnRH (100 g) IV	0, 30, 60 min for LH and FSH	In most adults, LH should increase by 10 IU/L and FSH by 2 IU/L Normal responses are variable
Multiple hormone	Combined anterior pituitary test: GHRH (1 g/kg), CRH (1 g/kg), GnRH (100 g), TRH (200 g) are given IV	–30, 0, 15, 30, 60, 90, 120 min for GH, ACTH, cortisol, LH, FSH and TSH	Combined or individual releasing hormone responses must be elevated in the context of basal target gland hormone values and may not be uniformly diagnostic

59. Ans. (a) I band

Ref: Ganong 24 ed page 99

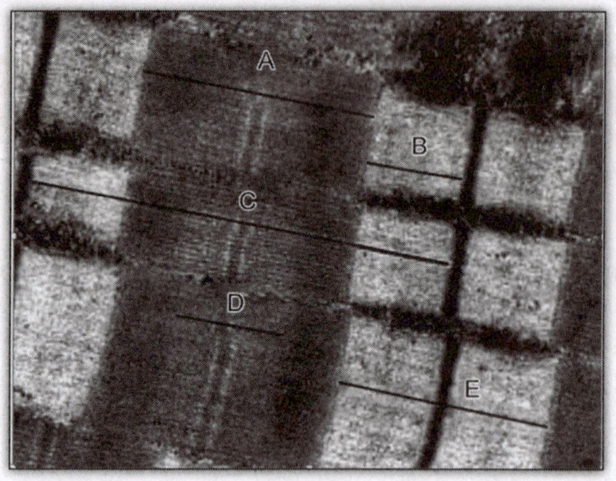

Figure Key

Portion indicated by A = A band
Portion indicated by B = ½ I band
Portion indicated by C = Sarcomere
Portion indicated by D = H zone
Portion indicated by E = I band

Contractile Apparatus		
Contractile proteins	**Regulatory proteins**	**Anchoring protein**
Interacts to generate contractile force in a muscle	Regulate the interaction between actin and myosin	Anchors different protein to each other and to sarcolemma and extracellular matrix
Actin Myosin	Tropomyosin Troponin	α-actinin, titin, nebulin, dystrophin

Sarcomere: The *area between two adjacent Z lines is called a sarcomere* ***(contractile unit of muscle)***. Differences in the refractive indexes of the various parts of the muscle fiber are responsible for the characteristic cross-striations seen in skeletal muscle when viewed under the microscope. ***Sarcomere = ½ I band + A band + ½ I band and is about 2.5 micrometer in length at rest.*** During muscle contraction the sarcomere reduced in length to 1.5 micrometer and during stretching of the muscle it increases in length to 3.5 micrometer

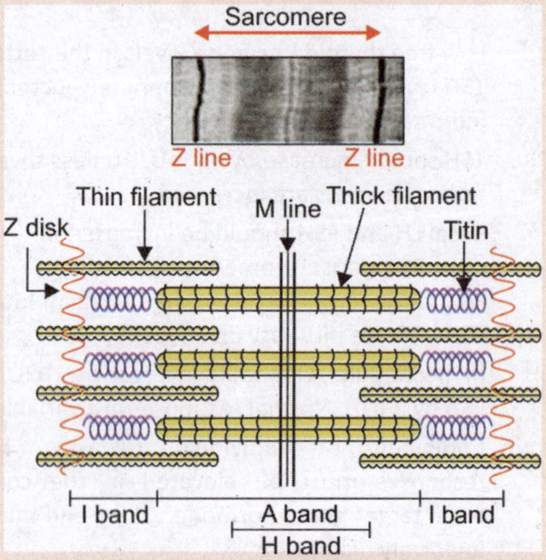

Proteins in Sarcomere	
1. The thick filaments	• Twice the diameter of the thin filaments • Made up of **myosin** • The thick filaments are lined up to form the **A bands.** • The form of myosin found in muscle is myosin-II, with two globular heads and a long tail. • The **dark band** is called A band (anisometropic to polarised light). It is 1.5 micrometer in length. In the area of A band the thick (myosin) filament line up the thin filaments. • In the center of each A band there is a lighter **H band** where thin filaments do not overlap the thick filaments. The lighter **H bands** in the center of the A bands are the regions where, when the muscle is relaxed, the thin filaments do not overlap the thick filaments. • In the center of each H zone is seen **M line,** which is more pronounced during muscle contraction. **The M line** is the site of the reversal of polarity of the myosin molecules in each of the thick filaments. At these points, there are slender cross-connections that hold the thick filaments in proper array. Each thick filament contains several hundred myosin molecules. • If a transverse section through the A band is examined under the electron microscope, *each thick filament is seen to be surrounded by six thin filaments in a regular hexagonal pattern.* The heads of the myosin molecules form cross-bridges with actin. *Myosin contains heavy chains and light chains* and its heads are made up of the light chains and the amino terminal portions of the heavy chains. These heads contain an actin-binding site and a catalytic site that hydrolyzes ATP. The myosin molecules are arranged symmetrically on either side of the center of the sarcomere and it is this arrangement that creates the light areas in the **pseudo-H zone.** • The **Z lines** transect the fibrils and connect to the thin filaments. If a transverse section through the A band is examined under the electron microscope, each thick filament is seen to be surrounded by six thin filaments in a regular hexagonal pattern.
2. The thin filaments	• Each thin filament is made up of *contractile protein actin and two regulatory proteins; troponin and tropomyosin*. The thin filaments are polymers made up of two chains of actin that form a long double helix. • Array of thin filaments forms the less dense **I bands.** The **light band** is called I band, because it is isotropic to polarized light. It is about 1 micrometer in length • At the center of I band, the dark color line is Z line. *The ends of actin filaments are attached to a Z disc.* The Z lines allow for anchoring of the thin filaments.

Contd...

- **Tropomyosin:** The actin filament also contains another protein, tropomyosin. Tropomyosin molecules are long filaments located in the groove between the two chains in the actin. Each thin filament contains *300 to 400 actin molecules and 40 to 60 tropomyosin molecules*
- **Troponin:** Attached intermittently along the sides of the tropomyosin molecules are still other protein molecules called troponin. These are actually complexes of three loosely bound protein subunits, each of which plays a specific role in controlling muscle contraction. This complex is believed to attach the tropomyosin to the actin.

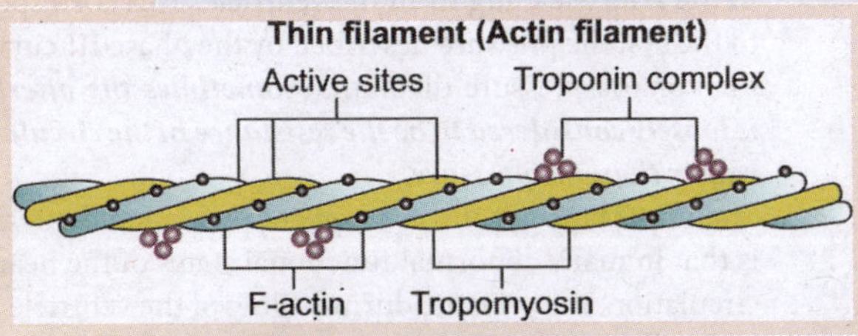

a. **Troponin I** – has an affinity for actin
b. **Troponin T** – has an affinity for tropmyosin
c. **Troponin C**- has an affinity for calcium ions

- An actin filament without the tropnin–tropomyosin complex can instantly bind with the heads of myosin molecules. Hence it is believed that the active sites on the action filament are kept covered by the troponin- tropomyosin complex. Before contraction can take place, the inhibitory effect of the complex itself must be inhibited.
- In place of troponin, smooth muscle cells contain a large amount of another regulatory protein called ***calmodulin.***

Footnote:
- The troponin-tropomyosin complex so-called relaxing proteins which inhibit the interaction between actin and myosin
- **Actinin** binds actin to the Z lines.
- **Desmin** adds structure to the Z lines in part by binding the Z lines to the plasma membrane.
- **TITIN:** The side by side relationship between the myosin and actin filaments is difficult to maintain. This is achieved by large number of filamentous molecules of a protein called titin. It is filamentous and very springy. It acts as the framework that hold actins and myosin in place so that the contractile machinery of the sarcomere will work. ***Titin plays a major role in muscle elasticity.*** The elastic portion of titin has an affinity for calcium ion and has binding sites for calcium

AIIMS MAY 2016

60. Ans. (c) Tension developed in the muscle

Ref: Ganong 24th ed page 229, 232, Guyton 11th ed page 673-76

See table of Stretch Reflex VS Inverse Stretch Reflex in Physiology AIIMS NOV 2014 for details of Inverse stretch reflex. In the same question also see table of Muscle Sensory Receptor.

61. Ans. (a) Intensity of stimulus

Ref: Ganong 24th ed page 153, Guyton 12th Ed Pg 579

Repeat AIIMS NOV 2018 Physiology (See for explanation) *(see page no. 131)*

62. Ans. (a) –60 mV

Ref: Guyton 12th ed page 100, Ganong 24th ed page 6

See Details of Membrane Potential (Nernst Equation) in Physiology AIIMS NOV 2016 *(see page no. 151)*

$$\text{EMF (millivolts)} = \pm 61 \log \frac{\text{Concentration inside}}{\text{Concentration outside}}$$

- When using this formula, it is usually assumed that the potential in the extracellular fluid outside the membrane remains at zero potential and the Nernst potential is the potential inside the membrane.
- Thus, when the concentration of positive potassium ions on the inside is 10 times that on the outside, the log of 10 is 1, so that the Nernst potential calculates to be –61 mV inside the membrane.

Replacing the Values given in Question

Electron potential of ion across membrane = 61.5 log (10/100) mmol/lit = 61.5 log 0.1
= 61.5 × –1 = –61.5 mV (remember log 10 = 1, log 0.1 = –1, log 100 = 2)

63. Ans. (a) Post-ganglionic nicotine receptor

Ref: Ganong 24th ed page 257, KDT 6th ed page 115

The question can be answered by basic understanding of the autonomic receptors

- Cholinergic receptors: muscarinic and nicotinic
  - Muscarinic receptors (M_1, M_2, M_3) are predominantly located on the effector organs and are activated by Acetylcholine.
  - Nicotinic receptors: They are located post junctionally (N_1 or N_n in autonomic nerves and N_2 or N_m in skeletal muscle end plate) and are involved with nerve transmission across a ganglion
- **Adrenoreceptors**: They are stimulated by epinephrine, norepinephrine, dopamine. Beta (β_1, β_2, β_3) and α1 receptors are located on target effector organs. α-2 receptors are located post junctionally and are called autoreceptors

64. Ans. (c) Urea concentration in urine in mg/100 mL

Ref: Guyton 12th ed page 663, Ganong 24th ed page 300, 678

Renal Clearance

- The rates at which different substances are "cleared" from the plasma provide a useful way of quantitating the effectiveness with which the kidneys excrete various substances. **By definition, the renal clearance of a substance is the volume of plasma that is completely cleared of the substance by the kidneys per unit time.**
- To illustrate the clearance principle, consider the following example: If the plasma passing through the kidneys contains 1 milligram of a substance in each milliliter and if 1 milligram of this substance is also excreted into the urine each minute, then **1 mL/min** of the plasma is "cleared" of the substance.

Contd...

Renal Clearance

- Thus, clearance refers to the volume of plasma that would be necessary to supply the amount of substance excreted in the urine per unit time

Clearance is the volume of plasma per unit time for which all of a specific substance is removed. Renal clearance of a substance is calculated from the urinary excretion rate (Us x V) of that substance divided by its plasma concentration.

Formula of Clearance; **C = UV/P** = Amount of urine/plasma concentration

Where C = Clearance

U = concentration of the substance in the urine in mg/dL (mg/100 mL)

V = Urine flow in mL/min

P = concentration of the substance in plasma mg/dL

If the Clearance is measured for a substance, which is not absorbed or, not secreted in tubules (e.g., Inulin), then: Clearance = Amount of urine/Plasma concentration = Filtration amount/Plasma concentration = Filtration rate = GFR

Footnote

- **Determination of GFR (glomerular filtration rate)**: If a substance is freely filtered but not reabsorbed or secreted (nor metabolized or synthesized) by the kidney, then its clearance must equal GFR. Substances which are only filtered include inulin and (more-or-less) creatinine. **Clearance = GFR for Inulin**, hence inulin clearance is gold standard test of GFR measurement. Other substances that have been used clinically to estimate GFR include **radioactive iothalamate** and **creatinine.**
- Because measurement of creatinine clearance does not require intravenous infusion into the patient, this method is much more widely used than inulin clearance for estimating GFR clinically
- If there is secretion of a substance in renal tubules, but no absorption, then: Clearance of a substance >> GFR
- If there is absorption of substance in renal tubule, but no secretion, then: Clearance of the substance << GFR.
- **Determination of RPF (renal plasma flow):** If a substance is completely cleared from the renal blood (combination of filtration and secretion) in one pass through the kidney, then its clearance is equal to RPF. A substance which fulfills this criteria is PAH (Para Amino Hippuric acid)

For urea clearance, U = urea concentration in urine in mg/dL, V= Urine flow rate in mL/min, Ps = BUN = Blood urea nitrogen in mg/dL

NOTE

10^{-1} L	Deciliter	Dl	dL
10^{-2} L	Centiliter	Cl	cL
10^{-3} L	Milliliter	Ml	mL
10^{-6} L	Microliter	µl	µL

I.e. dL = 100 mL

65. Ans. (c) Total peripheral resistance

Ref: Ganong 24th ed page 546, Guyton 11th ed page 122

Concepts of Preload and Afterload

- In assessing the contractile properties of muscle, it is important to specify the degree of tension on the muscle when it begins to contract, which is called the preload and to specify the load against which the muscle exerts its contractile force, which is called the afterload.
- For cardiac contraction, the preload is usually considered to be the end-diastolic pressure when the ventricle has become filled. The afterload of the ventricle is the pressure in the artery leading from the ventricle. This corresponds to the systolic pressure described by the phase III curve of the volume-pressure diagram. (***Sometimes the afterload is loosely considered to be the resistance in the circulation rather than the pressure.)***
- The importance of the concepts of preload and afterload is that in many abnormal functional states of the heart or circulation, the pressure during filling of the ventricle (the preload), the arterial pressure against which the ventricle must contract (the afterload), or both are severely altered from normal.
- One must be clear with the concept of total peripheral resistance and mean arterial pressure.
- Systemic vascular resistance (SVR) refers to the resistance to blood flow offered by *all* of the systemic vasculature, excluding the pulmonary vasculature. This is sometimes referred as total peripheral resistance (TPR). SVR is therefore determined by factors that influence vascular resistance in individual vascular beds. Mechanisms that cause vasoconstriction increase SVR and those mechanisms that cause vasodilation decrease SVR. Afterload is increased when aortic pressure and systemic vascular resistance are increased, by aortic valve stenosis and by ventricular dilation. When afterload increases, there is an increase in end-systolic volume and a decrease in stroke volume.
- MAP, or **mean arterial pressure**, is **defined** as the average **pressure** in a patient's **arteries** during one cardiac cycle. It is considered a better indicator of perfusion to vital organs than systolic blood **pressure** (SBP).

66. Ans. (a) Functional residual capacity

Ref: Ganong 24th ed page 630

Harrison's 19th ed page 306 e5 states ***"There is a passive resting point of the respiratory system, attained when alveolar gas pressure equals body surface pressure (i.e., the transrespiratory system pressure is zero). At this volume [called functional residual capacity (FRC)], the outward recoil of the chest wall is balanced exactly by the inward recoil of the lung.***

Let us Understand Compliance of Lung in Greater Detail

The forces required to actuate the cyclical motion of breathing are in large part determined by the interrelationship between the mechanical compliances of the lung and chest wall.

Although not physically attached, the lung and chest wall are intimately opposed to one another across the intrapleural space. Importantly, the intrapleural space acts as a sealed compartment which can maintain large variations in pressure; consequently, the forces generated by the lung and chest wall can be communicated to one another by changing the pressure within the intrapleural space.

Lung Compliance

- The compliance of the lung describes the relationship between the transmural pressures across the lung compared with organ's volume. By transmural pressure we mean the relative pressure between the alveoli compared with that in the intrapleural space. Positive transmural pressures mean greater alveolar pressures than intrapleural pressures.
- Lung is most contracted when there is no transmural pressure (i.e. the transmural pressure is zero). As the lung encounters positive transmural pressure, meaning greater pressure in the alveolar air compared with that in the intrapleural space, the lung expands. These properties stem from the lung›s inherent elastic recoil which renders the organ similar to a rubber balloon that expands when progressively blown into. Consequently, progressively greater transmural pressures must be achieved in order to generate increasing lung volumes.
- However, it is important to note the non-linear nature of the compliance curve which displays the greatest slope at smaller volumes and largely plateaus at large volumes. This indicates that the lung is most compliant, that is easiest to expand, at lower volumes as compared to larger volumes where greater changes in transmural pressure are required to achieve the same value of expansion.

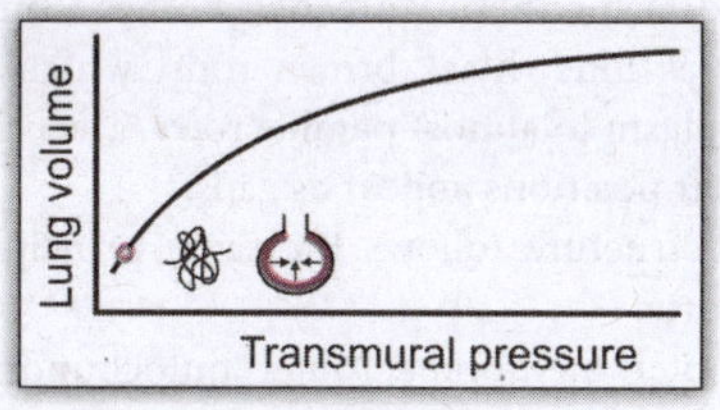

Although positive transmural pressures are required to expand the lung, they are not achieved by generating positive alveolar air pressures. Rather, lung expansion is achieved by generating progressively negative pressures within the intrapleural space.

Compliance in the Chest Wall

- The compliance of the chest wall describes the relationship between the transmural pressures across the chest wall compared with the chest cavity's volume. By transmural pressure we mean the relative pressure between the atmospheric pressure compared with that in the intrapleural space. Positive transmural pressures mean greater intrapleural pressures than atmospheric pressures.
- The chest cavity has a large volume when there is no transmural pressure (i.e. the transmural pressure is zero). This is the result of the natural tendency of the chest wall to spring outward, likely due to its skeletal and muscular anatomy. Consequently, in order to reduce the chest cavity volume, progressively large negative intrapleural pressures must be generated. However, the outward springing tendency of the chest wall does have limits and past a certain threshold, greater chest cavity volumes can only be achieved by applying positive intrapleural pressures. Consequently, at extremely large chest cavity volumes, even the chest wall displays a natural tendency to recoil toward smaller volumes.

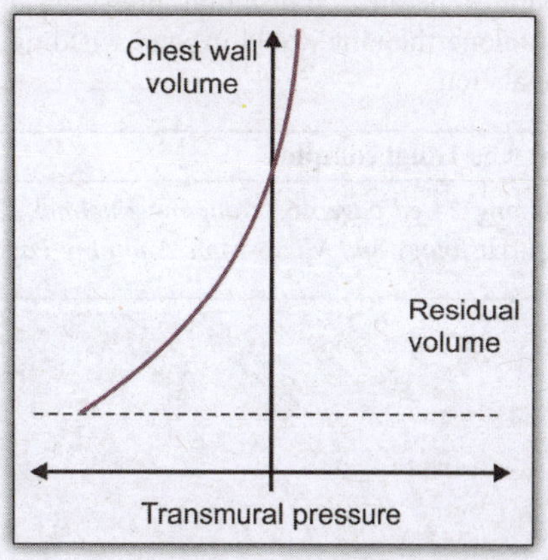

Chest wall compliance refers to the relationship between the volume of the chest cavity and the transmural pressure across it. As can be seen, negative transmural pressures are required to reduce the chest cavities size to the lung's residual volume. This demonstrates the chest wall's natural tendency to spring outward and expand. However, at large volumes the chest cavity begins to resist further expansion as shown by the positive transmural pressures required to generate more expansion.

Integrated pulmonary compliance and ventilation: The forces required to actuate the cyclical motion of breathing are in large part determined by the interrelationship between the mechanical compliances of the lung and chest wall.

The Integrated Compliance Curve

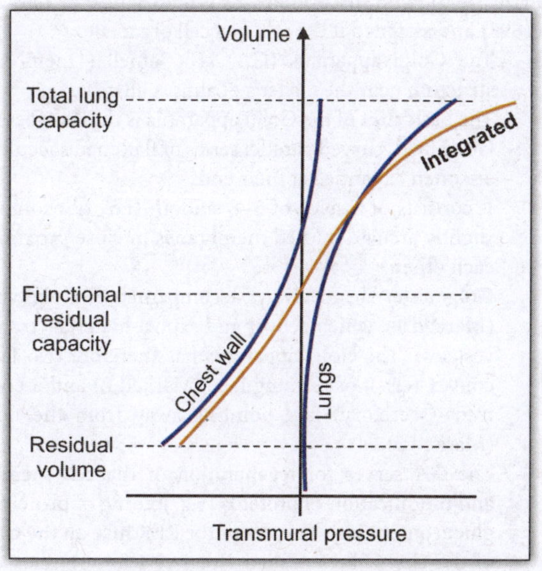

- The compliance curves of the isolated chest wall and lungs are plotted in black while the integrated compliance curve of the chest wall-lung unit is shown in blue.
- This blue curve represents the summation of the transmural pressures of the isolated chest wall and lungs at a given volume.
- When these pressures are precisely equal and opposing, the chest wall-lung unit is at equilibrium and, as seen, this

occurs at the Functional Residual Capacity. Expansion of the lung-chest wall unit beyond the FRC requires positive transmural pressures, meaning that left alone the unit would collapse, yielding exhalation.

- Contraction of the lung-chest wall unit below the FRC requires negative transmural pressures, meaning that left alone the unit would expand, yielding spontaneous inhalation.

67. Ans. (a) Cis-Golgi complex

Ref: Ganong 24 ed page 46, Wolfgang Kuehnel, Color Atlas of Cytology, Histology and Microscopic Anatomy Page 26

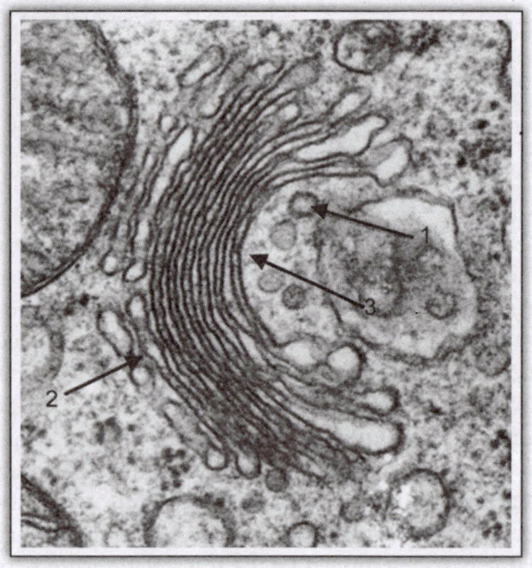

Fig: Electron microscopic picture of golgi apparatus

The Golgi apparatus was named after Camillo Golgi (Nobel Prize 1906), who discovered this cell structure in nerve cells (1898) and assigned it the role of a cell organelle.

- The Golgi apparatus (GA) is a lamellar membranous structure near the nucleus of almost all cells.
- The basic unit of the Golgi apparatus is the dictyosome or Golgi field; curved parallel series of flattened saccules that are often expanded at their ends
- It consists of a stack of 3–8 smooth (i.e., ribosome-free) slightly arcuate stacked membranes in close proximity to each other.
- Golgi cisternae are always accompanied by Golgi vesicles (Marked 1), which deliver and export material (transport vesicles). The Golgi apparatus has therefore two faces, a convex (cis-), or forming face (Marked 2) and a concave trans-(secretory) face pointing away from the nucleus (Marked 3).
- The GA serves for regeneration of the cell membrane and modification of proteins (e.g. joining of proteins and glucuronic acids). Vesicles of the RER fuse on the cis-part of the GA while so called Golgi-vesicles are released on its trans-part.

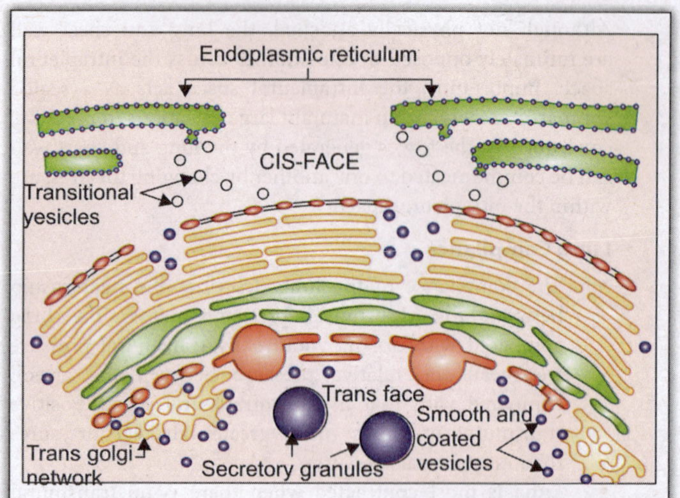

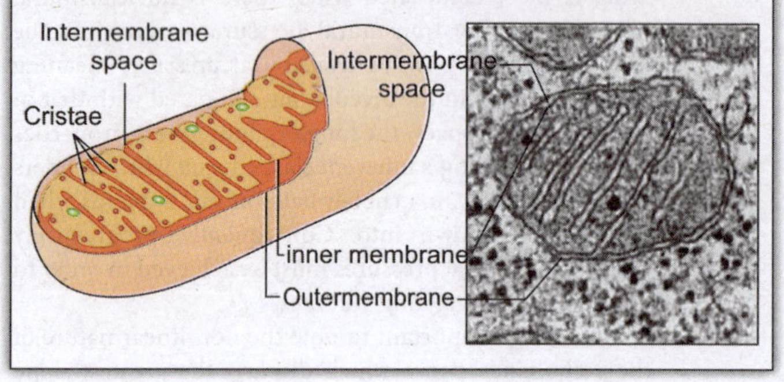

Fig: Electron microscopic picture of mitochondria

Altmann discovered and described mitochondria, the power plant organelle of cells, as granular, rod-like stringy cell components. In 1898, C. Benda introduced the term mitochondria for these "threaded bodies" The mitochondria stand out as long, black-brown rods, which line up in the basal cytoplasm to almost parallel rows. The cell nuclei are not visible; their positions appear as gaps.

The basic structure follows the same principle layout in all mitochondria.

- An outer membrane (outer mitochondrial membrane) separates the mitochondrion from the cytoplasm.
- Inside this outer membrane (border) lays the inner membrane. It forms septum-like folds (cristae mitochondriales), which extend to various lengths across the organelle (crista-type mitochondria).
- The inner and outer membranes separate two cell compartments. Between the outer and inner membrane, separated by about 8 nm, lies the outer compartment (outer metabolic compartment, intermembrane space), which extends into the crevices of the cristae.
- The inner membrane and its cristae form the border around the inner compartment (inner metabolic space). It contains a homogeneous or granular matrix of variable density.

- The inner mitochondrial matrix often contains granules, the granula mitochondrialia or matrix granules, which have a size of 30–50 nm and are rich in Ca^{2+} and other ions.

Cell Organelle			
Name	**Prokaryotic/Plant/ Animal**	**Description**	**Function**
Cell membrane	Pro, A, P	Flexible boundary that surrounds the cell, Bi-layer of proteins & lipids	Separates the cell from outside environment, Selectively permeable
Cell wall	Pro, P	Rigid Structure outside plasma membrane, Made of cellulose	Additional support, protection, Gives cell its shape
Nucleus	A, P	Contains DNA, Surrounded by double membrane, visible on light microscopy	Controls the cell activities
Nuclear membrane/ envelope	A, P	Double membrane layer that surrounds nucleus	Allows material to move into & out of Nucleus (RNA pass through pores)
Nuclear pores	A, P	1000s of pores in nuclear envelope	Allow material to move into & out of Nucleus
Chromatin	A, P	Granular material within nucleus, DNA bound to protein	Condenses to form chromosome at the time of cell division
Chromosome	A, P	Distinct thread like Contains genetic info	Blueprint - controls cell activity Pass on genetic info to next generation
Nucleolus	A, P	Small dense dark stained region inside in nucleus	Site of transcription of RNA, Assembly of ribosomes take place here
Cytoplasm	Pro, A, P	Clear Gelatinous (jelly) fluid inside the cell	Chemical reactions take place here
Cytoskeleton	A, P	Network of protein filaments	Helps the cell to maintain its shape & 3 D structure, Cell movement
Cilia/Flagella	A	Short/long projections of microtubules	Cell Movement
Microtubule	A, P	Hollow tubes of protein	Maintain cell shape, Form cilia/flagella, Separate chromosomes in cell division
Microfilament	A, P	Long thin fibers	Maintain cell shape Cell movement & support
Ribosome	Pro, A, P	Tiny round structures found on the surface of the RER or free in the cytoplasm, Made of RNA & Protein	Translation of RNA and protein synthesis
Endoplasmic reticulum	A, P	Highly folded membrane in cytoplasm. Internal membrane surrounding a lumen • Rough E.R. (ribosome) • Smooth E.R. (no ribosomes)	RER – protein synthesis SER – lipid biosynthesis
Golgi apparatus	A, P	Pancake like stacks of membrane bound sacs called cisternae. Found near cell membrane. Has a cis and a trans face	Collects, sorts, packages and secretes proteins. Proteins are taken in by the cis side & exit from the trans side
Lysosome	A	Tiny round vesicles containing digestive enzymes	Digests food, bacteria, worn out organelle
Vacuole	P, A (small or none)	Sac (membrane bound)	• Stores food, enzyme and other material • Support
Mitochondrion	A, P	Double membrane bound organelle. The inner membrane has folds called cristae	Power house of cell – produces energy for growth, development and movement
Centrioles/Basal bodies	A	Small structure outside nucleus formed from microtubules	• Helps in cell division (mitosis) • Helps in forming flagella and cilia

Contd…

Cell Organelle			
Name	**Prokaryotic/Plant/ Animal**	**Description**	**Function**
Chloroplast	P	• Double membrane bound organelle • Pigment chlorophyll is present in inner menbrane	• Captures light & converts it into chemical energy • Pigment chlorophyll (photosynthesis)

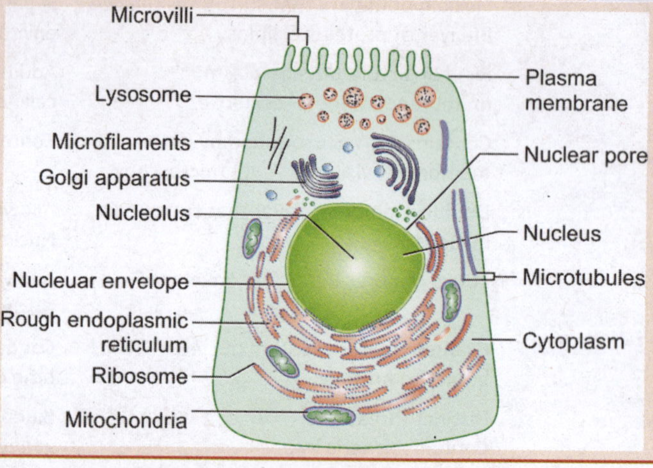

68. Ans. (b) 4

Ref: Guyton 12 th ed page 9, 10

This question is based upon the gain of a negative feedback system "Gain" of a Control System. The degree of effectiveness with which a control system maintains constant conditions is determined by the gain of the negative feedback.

For instance, let us assume that a large volume of blood is transfused into a person whose baroreceptor pressure control system is not functioning and the arterial pressure rises from the normal level of 100 mm Hg up to 175 mm Hg. Then, let us assume that the same volume of blood is injected into the same person when the baroreceptor system is functioning and this time the pressure increases only 25 mm Hg.

Thus, the feedback control system has caused a "correction" of –50 mm Hg—that is, from 175 mm Hg to 125 mm Hg. There remains an increase in pressure of +25 mm Hg, called the "error," which means that the control system is not 100% effective in preventing change. The gain of the system is then calculated by the following formula:

Gain = Correction/Error

- Thus, in the baroreceptor system example, the correction is –50 mm Hg and the error persisting is +25 mm Hg. Therefore, the gain of the person's baroreceptor system for control of arterial pressure is –50 divided by +25, or –2. That is, a disturbance that increases or decreases the arterial pressure does so only one third as much as would occur if this control system were not present.
- The gains of some other physiologic control systems are much greater than that of the baroreceptor system. For instance, the gain of the system controlling internal body temperature when a person is exposed to moderately cold weather is about –33. Therefore, one can see that the temperature control system is much more effective than the baroreceptor pressure control system.
- Let us see our question now

The person had a fall of BP of 10 mm Hg, but because of baroreceptors he only had a correction of 8 mm of BP and had a fall of 2 mm Hg of BP. Had his baroreceptors been able to maintain normal BP, he wouldn't have fall of 2 mm Hg.

Therefore correction in our question is of 8 mm Hg, error is of 2 mm Hg

Gain = 8/2 = 4

69. Ans. (b) Pre-Botzinger complex

Ref: Ganong 24th ed page 658

Respiratory Centers
The respiratory center is composed of several groups of neurons located bilaterally in the medulla oblongata and pons of the brain stem. It is divided into collections of neurons: Neural control of respiration involves three distinct components. • Factors that generate alternating inspiratory and expiratory rhythm • Factors that regulate the magnitude of ventilation (rate and depth of breathing) to match body needs • Factors that modify respiratory activity to serve other purposes.

Contd...

Center	Location	Function
Dorsal respiratory center	Dorsal portion of the medulla	• Most fundamental role in the control of respiration • Responsible for the basic rhythm of respiration.
Ventral respiratory center	Located in each side of medulla, about 5 mm anterior and lateral to the dorsal respiratory group of neurons, found in the *nucleus ambiguus* rostrally and *nucleus retroambiguus* caudally.	Totally *inactive* during normal quiet respiration. Contributes extra respiratory drive. However contributes to both inspiration and expiration, mainly causes expiration during heavy exercise.
Pneumotaxic center	Located dorsally in the *nucleus parabrachialis* of the upper pons	Primarily to limit inspiration. Secondarily inhibits apneustic center to cause shallow and rapid inspiration
Apneustic center	Inhibitory neurons located bilaterally in the lower part of pons	Increases the tidal volume and duration of inspiration resulting in deeper and prolonged inspiratory efforts called apneusis

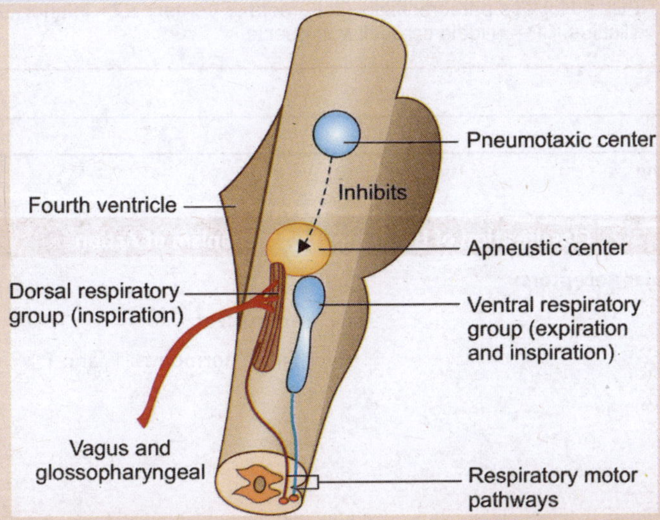

Lesions of the respiratory center

- Neurons in the **pre-Bötzinger complex** discharge rhythmically in brain slice preparations in vitro and if the slices become hypoxic, discharge changes to one associated with gasping.
- Addition of cadmium to the slices causes occasional sigh-like discharge patterns. There are NK1 receptors and μ-opioid receptors on these neurons, and, in vivo, substance P stimulates and opioids inhibit respiration
- Depression of respiration is a side effect that limits the use of opioids in the treatment of pain. However, it is now known that $5HT_4$ receptors are present in the pre-Bötzinger complex and treatment with $5HT_4$ agonists blocks the inhibitory effect of opiates on respiration in experimental animals, without inhibiting their analgesic effect.
- In addition, dorsal and ventral groups of respiratory neurons are present in the medulla. However, lesions of these neurons do not abolish respiratory activity and they apparently project to the pre-Bötzinger pacemaker neurons

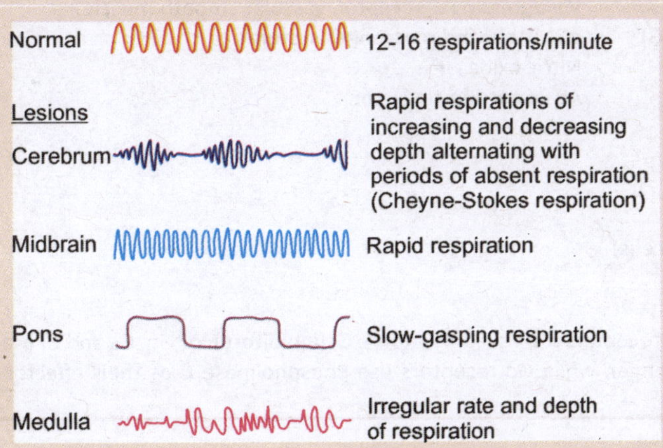

Contd...

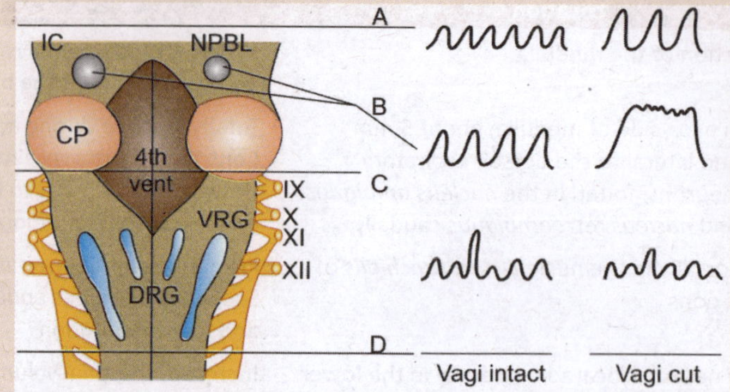

DRG = Dorsal group of respiratory neurons; VRG = Ventral group of respiratory neurons;
NPBL = Nucleus parabrachialis (pneumotaxic center); IC = Inferior colliculus; CP = middle cerebellar peduncle

70. Ans. (a) Thyroxine

Ref: Ganong 24th ed page 56, 300

Classification of Hormones by Mechanism of Action

I. Hormones that Bind to Intercellular Receptors	
Intracytoplasmic	**Intranuclear**
Androgens Estrogen Calcitriol (1,25[OH]$_2$-D$_3$) Glucocorticoids Mineralocorticoids Progestins Retinoic acid	Thyroid hormones (T$_3$ and T$_4$)

II. Hormones that Bind to cell Surface Receptors/Hormones Using Second Messenger Systems		
Adenylyl Cyclase–Camp Second Messenger System	**Ip3-Dag System Or Phospholipase C Second Messenger System**	**Calcium Calmodulin System**
Adrenocorticotropic hormone (ACTH) Angiotensin II (epithelial cells) Calcitonin Catecholamines (b receptors) Corticotropin-releasing hormone (CRH) Follicle-stimulating hormone (FSH) Glucagon Human chorionic gonadotropin (hCG) Luteinizing hormone (LH) Parathyroid hormone (PTH) Secretin Somatostatin Thyroid-stimulating hormone (TSH) Melanocyte-stimulating hormone Vasopressin (V$_2$ receptor, epithelial cells)	Angiotensin II (vascular smooth muscles) Catecholamines (α receptors) Gonadotropin-releasing hormone (GnRH) Growth hormone–releasing hormone (GHRH) Oxytocin Thyroid-releasing hormone (TRH) Vasopressin (V$_1$ receptor, vascular smooth muscle) **cGMP second messenger system** Nitric oxide Atrial natriuretic factor	Adenylyl cyclase Phosphodiesterase Ca^{2+}/calmodulin dependent protein kinases. Phosphoprotein phosphatases Phospholipase A$_2$ and Troponin C cGMP second messenger system Nitric oxide atrial natriuretic factor

G proteins that are coupled to the receptors are Gs (stimulatory), Gi (inhibitory), or Gq. Gs and Gi use Adenylate Cyclase as their effector and Calcium as their second messenger, while Gq receptors use Phospholipase C as their effector and IP3 and DAG as their second messengers.

71. Ans. (c) cGMP

Ref: Ganong 24th ed page 56, 300

See table of previous question (see page no. 168)

72. Ans. (b) Leptin

Ref: Ganong 24th ed page 399, William's endocrinology 13th ed page 1117

According To William's Textbook of Endocrinology

Leptin only has a permissive (tonic) role in onset of puberty and not a triggering (phasic) role. Onset of puberty is due to pulsatile release of GnRH.

According to Ganong

- It has been argued for some time that a critical body weight must normally be reached for puberty to occur.
- Thus, for example, young women who engage in strenuous athletics lose weight and stop menstruating, as do girls with anorexia nervosa. If these girls start to eat and gain weight, they menstruate again, that is, they "go back through puberty."
- It now appears that leptin, the satiety-producing hormone secreted by fat cells, may be the link between body weight and puberty. Obese ob/ob mice that cannot make leptin are infertile and their fertility is restored by injections of leptin.
- Leptin treatment also induces precocious puberty in immature female mice. However, the way that leptin fits into the overall control of puberty remains to be determined.

AIIMS NOVEMBER 2015

73. Ans. (a) Radioactive sodium and radioiodine labeled albumin

Ref: Guyton 12th ed page 289, Ganong 23rd ed page 2-6

Sodium has two radioactive cosmogenic isotopes (^{22}Na, half-life = 2.605 years; and ^{24}Na, half-life ≈ 15 hours)

Body Fluid Compartments Volume Measurements

Body fluid compartment	% of body weight	Fraction of total body water (TBW)	Markers used to measure volume	Major cation	Major anion
Total body water (TBW)	100%	1.0	^3H_2O, ^2H_2O, antipyrine		
Extracellular fluid (ECF)	20%	1/3	^{22}Na, ^{125}I-iothalamate, thiosulfate, inulin	Na^+	Cl^- HCO_3^-
Plasma	5%	1/12 (1/4 of ECF)	Evans blue (T-1824), RISA- Radio iodinated serum albumin (^{125}I-albumin)	Na^+	Cl^- HCO_3^- Plasma proteins
Interstitial fluid	15%	1/4 (3/4 of ECF)	ECF – Plasma volume (indirect)	Na^+	Cl^- HCO_3^-
Intracellular fluid (ICF)	40%	2/3	TBW – ECF (indirect)	K^+	Organic phosphates, Proteins

Total Body Water Composition in Children

Age	Body water%	ECF%	ICF%
Term neonate	75	40	35
Pre-term	90	60	30

Footnote

- Blood volume is calculated by 51Cr-labeled red blood cells, or calculated as blood volume = Plasma volume/(1 - Hematocrit)
- Total blood volume is measured by formula **100/(100 – hematocrit)**
- Red cell volume is measured by formula **Total body volume – plasma volume or by 51Cr**

74. Ans. (c) Urea concentration in urine in mg/100 mL

Ref: Guyton 12th ed page 663, Ganong 24th ed page 300, 678

Repeat (See AIIMS May 2016 Physiology for explanation) (see page no. 131)

75. Ans. (d) Single breath nitrogen test

Ref: Guyton 12th ed page 885, Oxford Textbook of Cardiothoracic Anaesthesia by Marco Ranucci page 50

Anatomical dead space may be measured by rapid analysis of exhaled gas for nitrogen using Fowler's method which is single breath nitrogen concentration test.

Dead Space	
"The normal dead space air in a young adult man is about 150 milliliters. This increases slightly with age" Some of the air a person breathes never reaches the gas exchange areas but simply fills respiratory passages where gas exchange does not occur, such as the nose, pharynx and trachea. This air is called dead space air because it is not useful for gas exchange. **TOTAL DEAD SPACE** (also known as "PHYSIOLOGICAL" DEAD SPACE) can be divided into anatomical dead space and alveolar dead space.	
Anatomical dead space	**Alveolar dead space**
Anatomical dead space is the gas in the conducting areas of the respiratory system, such as the mouth and trachea, where air does not come into contact with the alveoli of the lungs. Birds, which, relatively, have a far longer and wider trachea than mammals, have a higher proportion of dead space. It is normally equal in milliliters to your body weight in pounds. **A 150 lb (68 kg) male would have an anatomical dead space of about 150 mL.** 1 mL per lb or 2.2 mL per kilogram of body weight. This is the same conversion of kilograms to pounds, except the final unit is in mL. **This is about a third of the resting tidal volume (450-500 mL).** Anatomic dead space is the volume of the conducting airways. It may be measured by Fowler's method, a nitrogen washout technique.	Alveolar dead space is caused by air contacting alveoli without blood flow in their adjacent pulmonary capillaries, i.e. ventilation without perfusion. As a result, no gas exchange can occur. **Alveolar dead space is negligible in healthy individuals, but can increase dramatically in some lung diseases.**
Fowler method for measurement of anatomical dead space: The patient takes a single breath of 100% oxygen and then exhales into a tube that continuously measures the concentration of gas like Nitrogen, in the exhaled gas. As the subject exhales, the anatomical dead space empties first. This volume contains 100% oxygen and 0% indicator gas, because it has not participated in any gas exchange. As the alveoli begin to empty, the oxygen falls and the nitrogen begins to rise. Finally, the concentration of nitrogen is almost uniform and it represents alveolar gas almost entirely. This phase of expired air exhalation is called the alveolar plateau. The volume with initially 0% nitrogen plus half of the rising nitrogen volume is equal to the anatomical dead space.	**Bohr's method for physiological dead space:** Based on the fact that "all expired CO_2 comes from ventilated alveolar gas" and dead space eliminates negligible CO_2. Total tidal volume (V_t) is made up of $V_a + V_d$ (alveolar volume + dead space volume), $V_t = V_d + V_a$ Defining Fe as the fraction of expired CO_2 and Fa as the fraction of expired alveolar CO_2 and Fd as fraction of expired dead space volume CO_2, we can say **$V_t \times Fe = (V_d \times F_d) + (V_a \times F_a)$** Since the expiration for CO_2 from dead space is negligible we can count it as zero. Therefore **Vt x Fe = Va x Fa.** Referring to Vt = Va + Vd, Va = Vt – Vd, substituting it in the above equation $V_t \times Fe = (V_t - V_d) \times Fa = V_t \times Fa - V_d \times Fa$ $V_d \times Fa = V_t \times Fa - V_t \times Fe = V_t\,(Fa - Fe)$ $V_d/V_t = Fa - Fe/Fa$ Since fraction of expired gas x total pressure = Pa of that gas $FeCO_2$ x total pressure = $PeCO_2$ $FaCO_2$ x total pressure = $PaCO_2$ **$V_d/V_t = Pa\,CO_2 - Pe\,CO_2/Pa\,CO_2$**

76. Ans. (b) Mesangial cell constriction

Ref: Guyton 12th ed page 339, 374, Ganong 23rd ed page 674

Types of Natriuretic Peptides

- The first natriuretic hormone isolated from the heart was **atrial natriuretic peptide (ANP). ANP was subsequently isolated from other tissues, including the brain, where it exists in two forms that are smaller than circulating ANP**
- A second natriuretic polypeptide was isolated from porcine brain and named **brain natriuretic peptide (BNP**; also known as **B-type natriuretic peptide**). It is also present in the brain in humans, but more is present in the human heart, including the ventricles
- Third naturetic peptide has been named **C-type natriuretic peptide (CNP)** because it was the third in the sequence to be isolated. CNP is present in the brain, the pituitary, the kidneys and vascular endothelial cells. However, very little is present in the heart and the circulation and it appears to be primarily a paracrine mediator.

Action

- ANP and BNP in the circulation act on the kidneys to increase Na^+ excretion and injected CNP has a similar effect. They appear to produce this effect by **dilating afferent arterioles and relaxing mesangial cells**. Both of these actions increase glomerular filtration.
- In addition, they act on the renal tubules to inhibit Na^+ reabsorption.
- Other actions include an increase in capillary permeability, leading to extravasation of fluid and a decline in blood pressure.
- In addition, they relax vascular smooth muscle in arterioles and venules.
- CNP has a greater dilator effect on veins than ANP and BNP.
- These peptides also inhibit renin secretion and counteract the pressor effects of catecholamines and angiotensin II.

- In the brain, ANP is present in neurons and an ANP-containing neural pathway projects from the anteromedial part of the hypothalamus to the areas in the lower brain stem that are concerned with neural regulation of the cardiovascular system. In general, the effects of ANP in the brain are opposite to those of angiotensin II and ANP-containing neural circuits appear to be involved in lowering blood pressure and promoting natriuresis.
- CNP and BNP in the brain probably have functions similar to those of ANP.

Factors Affecting Secretion of ANP and BNP

ANP secretion is increased when the ECF volume is increased by infusion of isotonic saline and when the atria are stretched. BNP secretion is increased when the ventricles are stretched. ANP secretion is also increased by immersion in water up to the neck, a procedure that counteracts the effect of gravity on the circulation and increases central venous and consequently atrial pressure. Conversely, a small but measurable decrease in plasma ANP occurs in association with a decrease in central venous pressure on rising from the supine to the standing position. Thus, it seems clear that the atria respond directly to stretch in vivo and that the rate of ANP secretion is proportional to the degree to which the atria are stretched by increases in central venous pressure. Similarly, BNP secretion is proportional to the degree to which the ventricles are stretched. Plasma levels of both hormones are elevated in congestive heart failure and their measurement is seeing increasing use in the diagnosis of this condition.

77. Ans. (c) Factor C

Ref: Ganong 24th ed page 567

Factor C is anticoagulant not procoagulant

Anticoagulant Mechanisms

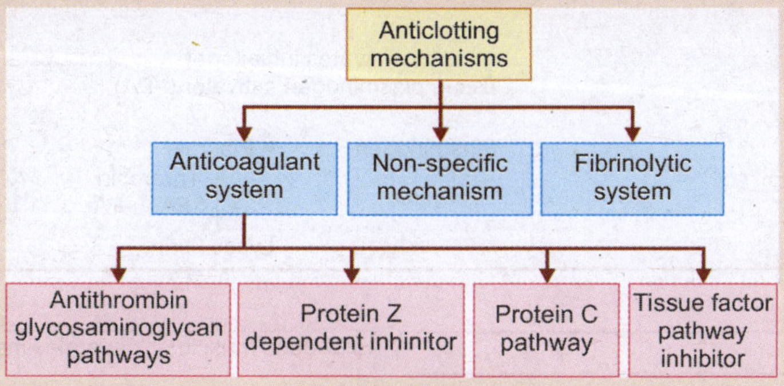

Physiological anticoagulation mechanisms act to reduce thrombin production or reduce the effects of thrombin.

Antithrombin	Antithrombin (AT), previously known as AT III is the main inhibitor of thrombin. It is a serine protease inhibitor, which binds and inactivates thrombin, factor IXa, Xa, XIa and XIIa. The enzymatic activity of AT is enhanced in the presence of heparin. However, the plasma concentration of heparin is low and does not contribute significantly to the in vivo activation of AT. AT is activated by binding of heparin sulphate present on endothelial cell surface. Other thrombin inhibitors are heparin cofactor II, α2 macroglobulin and α1-antitrypsin.
Tissue factor plasminogen inhibitor	It is a polypeptide produced by endothelial cells. It acts as a natural inhibitor of the extrinsic pathway by inhibiting TF-VIIa complex. Protein S enhances the interaction of factor Xa in the presence of calcium and phospholipids.
Protein C pathway	The propagation phase of the coagulation is inhibited by the Protein C pathway that primarily consist of four key elements: • Protein C is a serine protease with potent anticoagulant, profibrinolytic and anti-inflammatory properties. It is activated by thrombin to form activated protein C (APC) and acts by inhibiting activated factors V and VIII (with Protein S and phospholipids acting as cofactors) • Thrombomodulin - A transmembrane receptor on the endothelial cells, it prevents the formation of the clot in the undamaged endothelium by binding to the thrombin • Endothelial protein C receptor is another transmembrane receptor that helps in the activation of Protein C • Protein S is a vitamin K-dependent glycoprotein, synthesized by endothelial cells and hepatocytes. It exists in plasma as both free (40%) and bound (60%) forms (bound to C4b-binding protein). The anticoagulant activity is by virtue of free form while the bound form acts as an inhibitor of the complement system and is up regulated in the inflammatory states, which reduce the Protein S levels thus resulting in procoagulant state. It functions as a cofactor to APC in the inactivation of FVa and FVIIIa. It also causes direct reversible inhibition of the prothrombinase (FVa-FXa) complex
Protein Z dependent protease inhibitor/protein Z (PZI)	It is a recently described component of the anticoagulant system that is produced in the liver. It inhibits Factor Xa in reaction requiring PZ and calcium.

Contd...

Anticoagulant Mechanisms

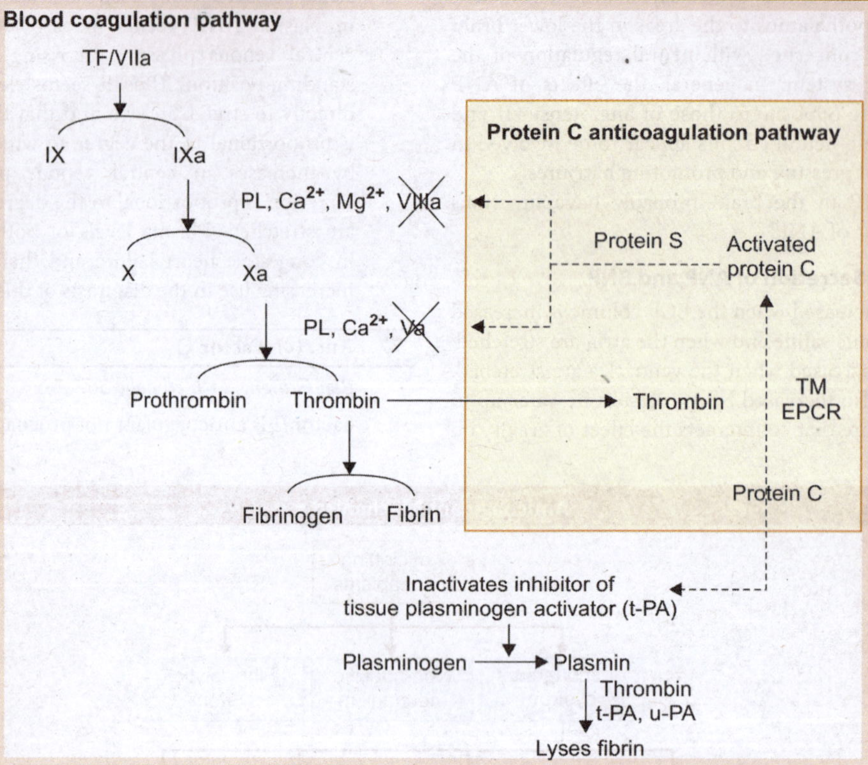

78. Ans. (c) –60 mV

Ref: Guyton 12th ed page 100, Ganong 24th ed page 6

Repeat AIIMS May 2016 (Different Options)
(see page no. 161)

79. Ans. (a) 25 Hz

Ref: Guyton 12th ed page 80, Ganong 24th ed page 104

Tetany is the continuous contraction of muscle fibers, without latent period and relaxation period. Tetanizing frequency depends only on contraction time.

Twitch duration = Contraction period = 40 milli sec = 0.04 sec

(1 milli second = 0.001 second)

Tetanizing frequency = 1/0.04 = 25 Hz

Summation means the adding together of individual twitch contractions to increase the intensity of overall muscle contraction. Summation occurs in two ways:

- By increasing the number of motor units contracting simultaneously, which is called multiple fiber summation
- By increasing the frequency of contraction, which is called frequency summation and can lead to tetanization.

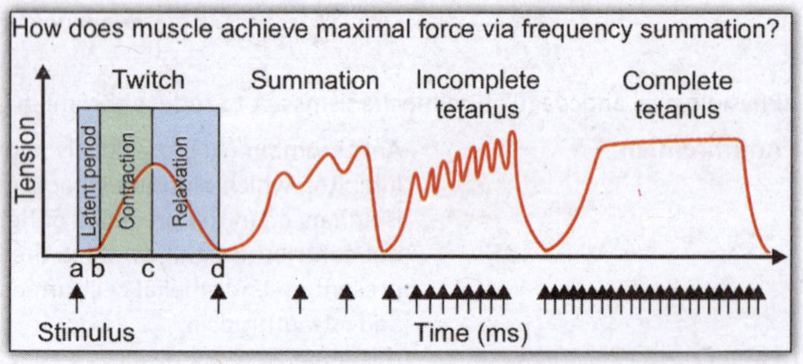

Twitch: A single contraction-relaxation cycle invoked by a single action potential.

Frequency of stimulation at which tetanus will occur is determined by the twitch duration of particular muscle.

4 Points

a – stimulus
b – beginning of contraction
c – maximum contraction and beginning of relaxation
d – end of relaxation

3 Phases

a-b – Latent period
b-c – Contraction
c-d – Relaxation

80. Ans. (a) Pituitary

Ref: Ganong 23rd ed page 303

Option (B)

The basolateral membranes of thyrocytes facing the capillaries contain a **symporter** that transports **two Na^+ ions and one I ion into the cell with each cycle**, against the electrochemical gradient for I^-. This Na^+/I^- symporter (**NIS**) is capable of producing intracellular I concentrations that are 20 to 40 times as great as the concentration in plasma. The process involved is secondary active transport, with the energy provided by active transport of Na^+ out of thyroid cells by Na, K ATPase. NIS is regulated both by transcriptional means and by active trafficking into and out of the thyrocyte basolateral membrane; in particular, thyroid stimulating hormone (TSH) induces both NIS expression and the retention of NIS in the basolateral membrane where it can mediate sustained iodide uptake.

Option (C) and (D)

The salivary glands, the gastric mucosa, the placenta, the ciliary body of the eye, the choroid plexus, the mammary glands and certain cancers derived from these tissues also express NIS and can transport iodide against a concentration gradient, but the transporter in these tissues is not affected by TSH. The physiologic significance of all these extrathyroidal iodide-concentrating mechanisms is obscure, but they may provide pathways for radioablation of NIS-expressing cancer cells using iodide radioisotopes. This approach is also useful for the ablation of thyroid cancers.

NOTE

- Also it is important to know about another iodide transporter called Pendrin. Iodide must also exit the thyrocyte across the apical membrane to access the colloid, where the initial steps of thyroid hormone synthesis occur. This transport step is believed to be mediated, at least in part, by a Cl/I exchanger known as pendrin.
- This protein was first identified as the product of the gene responsible for the Pendred syndrome, whose patients suffer from thyroid dysfunction and deafness.

81. Ans. (c) Muscle contraction is related to amplitude of BER

Ref: Guyton 12th ed page 754, Physiology by Indu Khurana 2012 ed page 473

Recall Bias

Some recalls also say that one option was (E) "It is produced in body of stomach", however it will not change the answer.

Electrical Activity of Gastrointestinal Smooth Muscle

The smooth muscle of the gastrointestinal tract is excited by almost continual slow, intrinsic electrical activity along the membranes of the muscle fibers. This activity has two basic types of electrical waves: (1) slow waves and (2) spikes. In addition, the voltage of the resting membrane potential of the gastrointestinal smooth muscle can be made to change to different levels and this, too, can have important effects in controlling motor activity of the gastrointestinal tract

Slow Waves/BER: The smooth muscles of GIT shows spontaneous rhythmic fluctuations in their membrane potentials (between –65 mV to –45 mV), this is called Basic electrical rhythm.

- BER is present throughout the GIT except esophagus and proximal stomach
- BER (Basal Electric Rhythm) is first observed in the body of stomach, which becomes faster distally.
- BER is caused by the pacemaker cells of GIT AKA **"Interstitial cells of Cajal"** located near the fundus on the greater curvature of stomach.
- Slow waves are produced due to opening of Na^+ channels
- Normally slow waves on their own are unable to cause smooth muscle contraction, rather they act as pacemaker that excite the spike potentials
- Rate of BER is different for different parts of the GIT; Stomach = 4/min, Duodenum = 12/min, Terminal Ileum = 8/min, Cecum = 8/min, Sigmoid colon = 16/min

Spike potentials are caused by opening of Ca^{++} channels and corresponds with peak of slow waves

- Slow wave potentials results in spike potential (true action potential) only when they reach the threshold value
- Spike potentials are superimposed on the slow waves
- The higher the amplitude of slow wave, higher is the amplitude of Spike potential
- Amount of tension developed by muscle is directly proportional to the number of spikes.

82. Ans. (a) Adrenaline

Ref: Guyton 12th ed page 754, Ganong 23rd ed page 471

The frequency of the slow wave is constant in each segment of the tract where it occurs and is not significantly affected by either humoral or neural factors. Although the frequency of the slow wave is fixed, its amplitude and duration may be influenced by humoral or neural factors. **Acetylcholine, for example, will increase the amplitude and the duration of the plateau.** This increases the frequency of spike potentials associated with each slow wave plateau and increases contraction. **Adrenaline/ Norepinephrine have the opposite effect.**

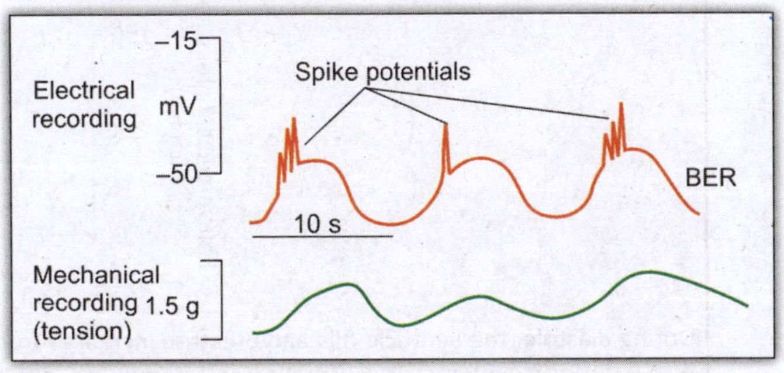

83. Ans. (a) 50%

Ref: Ganong 24th ed page 542

See Normal pressure–volume loop of the left ventricle in Physiology AIIMS MAY 2015

Ejection fraction can be calculated by the formula

$$E_f(\%) = \frac{SV}{EDV} \times 100$$

SV = Stroke volume = EDV – ESV
EDV = End diastolic volume

Therefore EF = (150 – 75)/150 × 100 = 50%

Ganong 23rd ed page 510: The end-diastolic ventricular volume is about 130 mL. Thus, about 50 mL of blood remains in each ventricle at the end of systole (end-systolic ventricular volume) and the ejection fraction, the percent of the end-diastolic ventricular volume that is ejected with each stroke, is about 65%.

Guyton 12th ed page 106: During diastole, normal filling of the ventricles increases the volume of each ventricle to about 110 to 120 mL. This volume is called the end-diastolic volume. Then, as the ventricles empty during systole, the volume decreases about 70 mL, which is called the stroke volume output. The remaining volume in each ventricle, about 40 to 50 mL, is called the end-systolic volume. The fraction of the end-diastolic volume that is ejected is called the ejection fraction-usually equal to about 60 percent.

AIIMS MAY 2015

84. Ans. (d) D

Ref: Ganong 24th ed page 542, Gayton 12th ed page 108

Recall Bias.....................................

Some recallers think that Beginning of Systole (Point A) was asked

DA segment in the given graph is diastolic pressure curve representing diastolic filling period from D to A. The left ventricular pressure is lowest at point D, while A represents the end diastolic point.

Volume-Pressure Diagram during the Cardiac Cycle

Phase I: Period of filling	This phase in the volume-pressure diagram begins at a ventricular volume of about 50 mL and a diastolic pressure of 2 to 3 mm Hg. The amount of blood that remains in the ventricle after the previous heartbeat, 50 mL, is called the end-systolic volume. As venous blood flows into the ventricle from the left atrium, the ventricular volume normally increases to about 120 mL, called the end-diastolic volume, an increase of 70 mL. Therefore, the volume-pressure diagram during phase I extends along the line labeled "I," from point A to point B, with the volume increasing to 120 mL and the diastolic pressure rising to about 5 to 7 mm Hg.
Phase II: Period of isovolumic contraction	During isovolumic contraction, the volume of the ventricle does not change because all valves are closed. However, the pressure inside the ventricle increases to equal the pressure in the aorta, at a pressure value of about 80 mm Hg, as depicted by point C.
Phase III: Period of ejection	During ejection, the systolic pressure rises even higher because of still more contraction of the ventricle. At the same time, the volume of the ventricle decreases because the aortic valve has now opened and blood flows out of the ventricle into the aorta. Therefore, the curve labeled "III," or "period of ejection," traces the changes in volume and systolic pressure during this period of ejection.
Phase IV: Period of isovolumic relaxation	At the end of the period of ejection (point D), the aortic valve closes and the ventricular pressure falls back to the diastolic pressure level. The line labeled "IV" traces this decrease in intraventricular pressure without any change in volume. Thus, the ventricle returns to its starting point, with about 50 mL of blood left in the ventricle and at an atrial pressure of 2 to 3 mm Hg.

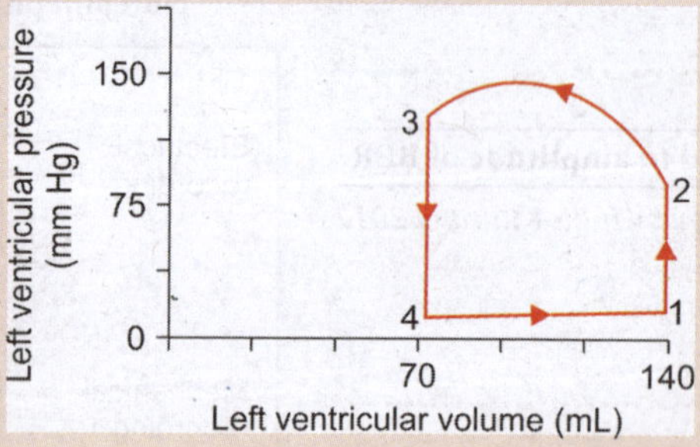

During diastole, the ventricle fills and pressure increases from D to A (A represents End diastolic point). Pressure then rises from A to B during isovolumetric contraction and from B to C during ventricular ejection. At C, the aortic valves close and pressure falls during isovolumetric relaxation from C to D.

85. Ans. (c) 5 times

Ref: Ganong 24th ed page 575

Blood flow in a vessel is determined by the **Poiseuille's law** which states that "In the case of smooth flow (laminar flow), the volume flow rate is given by the pressure difference divided by the viscous resistance. This resistance depends linearly upon the viscosity and the length, but the fourth power dependence upon the radius is dramatically different"

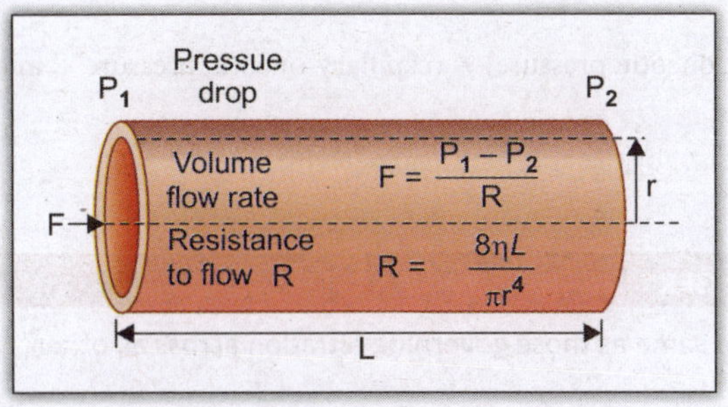

Volume flow rate $= F = \dfrac{P_1 - P_2}{R}$

$$= \frac{\pi \text{ (Pressure difference) (radius)}^4}{8\text{(viscosity)(length)}}$$

Resistance to flow $R = \dfrac{8\eta L}{\pi r^4}$

Therefore, blood flow is directly proportional to fourth power of radius. Now coming to our question:

If radius is increased by 50% the new radius would become 1.5 r as follows:

$$r + 50/100 \times r = 1.5\ r$$

If F_1 is flow of blood before and F_2 is flow of blood after increasing the radius and all the parameter being constant

$$F_2/F_1 = (1.5\ r)^4/r^4$$
$$F_2/F_1 = 5.0625 \text{ (round off to 5)}$$
$$F_2 = 5\ F_1$$

86. Ans. (a) Amylin

Ref: Guyton's 11th Ed page 961

The beta cells, constituting about 60% of all the cells of the islets, lie mainly in the middle of each islet and secrete **insulin and amylin**, a hormone that is often secreted in parallel with insulin, although its function is unclear.

Endocrine Pancreas (1 to 2 million islets of Langerhans)	Insulin and Amylin (β cells = 60%)	Promotes glucose entry in many cells and in this way controls carbohydrate metabolism	Peptide
	Glucagon (α cells = 25%)	Increases synthesis and release of glucose from the liver into the body fluids	Peptide
	Somatostatin (Delta cells = 10%)	Inhibit the release of growth hormone, suppresses the release of gastrointestinal hormones	Peptide
	Pancreatic polypeptide (PP cell = small number)	Uncertain function	Peptide

87. Ans. (b) NREM sleep

Ref: Ganong 24th ed page 274, Guyton 12th ed page 764

The graph shown in the question is of Polysomnography. **Polysomnography (PSG)**, a type of sleep study, is a multiparametric test used in the study of sleep and as a diagnostic tool in sleep medicine. The PSG monitors many body functions including brain (EEG), eye movements (EOG), muscle activity or skeletal muscle activation (EMG) and heart rhythm (ECG) during sleep. After the identification of the sleep apnea, the breathing functions such as respiratory airflow and respiratory effort indicators were added along with peripheral pulse oximetry.

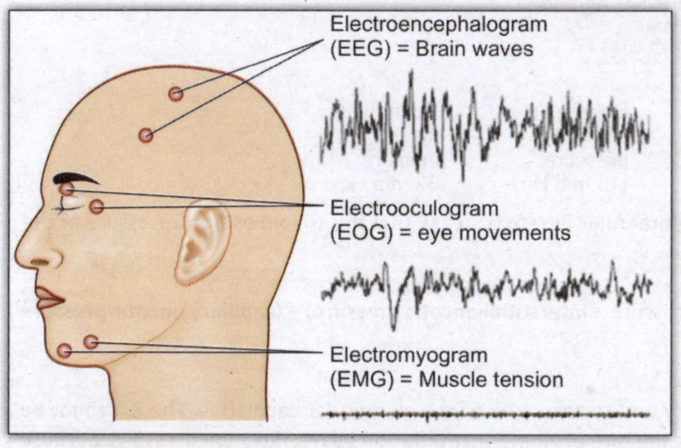

The present graph shows: Characteristic EEG, EOG and EMG patterns for wakefulness, REM sleep and NREM sleep. Each of the nine patterns was made over a period of about three seconds.

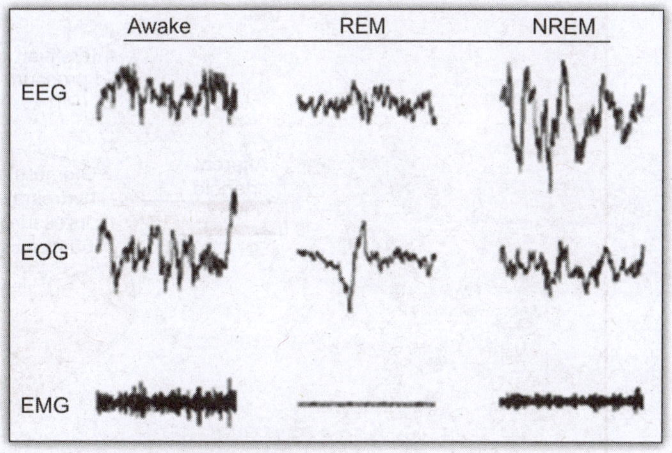

Points of Identification

- ***Lack of muscular activity (EMG) during REM*** as compared with activity during NREM or wakefulness is the key for determining that this individual is in REM-stage sleep
- **Increased amplitude and decreased frequency of brain waves during NREM** compared with the pattern during REM and wakefulness
- Large eye movements during wakefulness, **Rapid eye movement in REM as compared with little or no eye movements during NREM.**

88. Ans. (b) 27 mm Hg

Ref: Ganong 24th ed page 679

This question is based upon renal physiology of net filtration pressure.

Net filtration pressure = (capillary hydrostatic pressure + interstitial oncotic pressure) – (capillary oncotic pressure + interstitial hydrostatic pressure). Putting values in the equation

$$3 = (25 + 7) - (COP + 2)$$
$$COP + 2 = 32 - 3$$
$$COP = 27$$

Determinants of GFR

The factors governing filtration across the glomerular capillaries are the same as those governing filtration across all other capillaries. The GFR is determined by:

- The sum of the hydrostatic and colloid osmotic forces across the glomerular membrane, which gives the net filtration pressure and
- Glomerular capillary filtration coefficient, K_f.

Expressed mathematically, the GFR equals the product of Kf and the net filtration pressure:

GFR = K_f x Net filtration pressure

The net filtration pressure represents the sum of the hydrostatic and colloid osmotic forces that either favor or oppose filtration across the glomerular capillaries. Let us understand that certain forces push fluid out and certain forces try to retain it. These forces include:

- Capillary pressure of normal capillary translates into **Glomerular capillary hydrostatic pressure**, which promotes filtration (Normal **60 mm Hg**)
- Plasma colloidal osmotic pressure of capillary translates into **Glomerular colloidal osmotic pressure**, which opposes filtration (Normal **32 mm Hg**)
- Hydrostatic pressure (interstitial) in Bowman's capsule (PB) outside the capillaries, which opposes filtration (Normal **18 mm Hg**)
- Interstitial Colloid osmotic pressure of the proteins in Bowman's capsule (πB), which promotes filtration. (Normal 0 m Hg)

Note: 3 and 4 combines forms the Bowman's capsule pressure

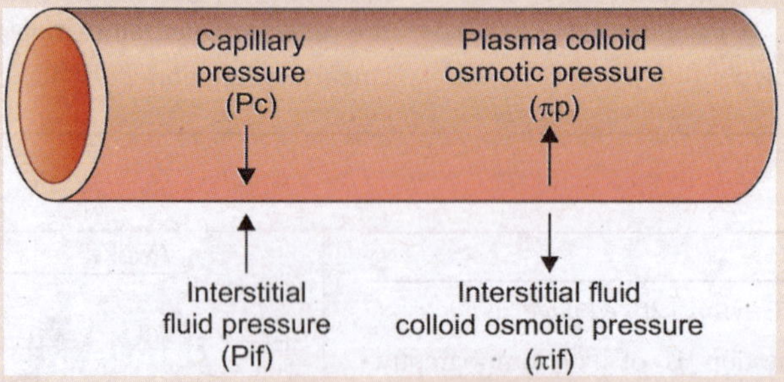

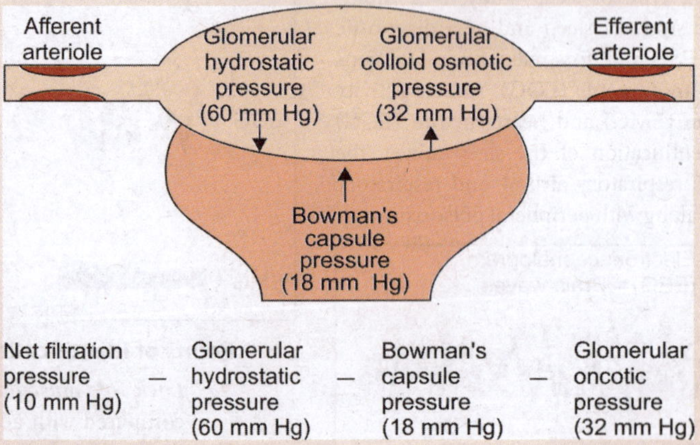

(Under normal conditions, the concentration of protein in the glomerular filtrate is so low that the colloid osmotic pressure of the Bowman's capsule fluid is considered to be zero.)

The GFR can therefore be expressed as

GFR = Kf × Net filtration pressure = Kf × (capillary hydrostatic pressure + interstitial oncotic pressure) – (capillary oncotic pressure + interstitial hydrostatic pressure).

Net filtration pressure = 60 – 18 – 32 = **10 mm Hg**

The K_f is a measure of the product of the hydraulic conductivity and surface area of the glomerular capillaries. The K_f cannot be measured directly, but it is estimated experimentally by dividing the rate of glomerular filtration by net filtration pressure: Because total GFR for both kidneys is about 125 mL/min and the net filtration pressure is 10 mm Hg, the normal K_f is calculated to be about **12.5 mL/min/mm Hg** of filtration pressure

89. Ans. (a) 18 L

Ref: Guyton 11th ed page 296

To measure the volume of any fluid compartment within the body you must inject or infuse a marker substance that will equilibrate (diffuse freely to a uniform concentration) throughout this compartment. To be a perfect marker a substance must also not be metabolized. Furthermore, it must be possible to measure the concentration of the marker once equilibration is complete.

Given that concentration (C) = mass (M)/volume (V) it should be obvious that:

$$V = M/C$$

Therefore: if you know the mass of marker injected into the body and are able to measure the marker concentration once equilibration is complete, you can calculate the volume of the compartment occupied by the marker. To be an absolutely perfect marker, the substance should also not be excreted. As this is not possible (the kidney will excrete everything dissolved in the bloodstream) the calculation must correct for excretion. Thus:

$$V = (M - M_U)/C$$

Where V is the volume of the body fluid compartment, M is the mass of marker injected, M_U is the mass of marker lost in the urine during equilibration and C is the measured concentration of the marker. M_U is usually calculated from C_U, the concentration of marker lost in the urine and V_U, the volume of the urine thus: $M_U = C_U \cdot V_U$. Therefore, to measure the volume of the blood plasma fluid compartment, you need a marker which equilibrates throughout the blood supply and nowhere else.

Now putting our question's values

$$V = M - M_u/C$$

Mass of mannitol (M) = 10 g = 10000 mg

M_u = 10% of 10 g = 1 g = 1000 mg

C = 50 mg/100 mL = 0.5 mg/mL

Therefore

V = 10000–1000/0.5 = 9000/0.5 = 18000 mL = 18 L

90. Ans. (c) Both alpha and gamma motor neurons are activated together

Ref: Guyton's 11th Ed page 678

Whenever signals are transmitted from the motor cortex or from any other area of the brain to the alpha motor neurons, in most instances the gamma motor neurons are stimulated simultaneously, an effect called coactivation of the alpha and gamma motor neurons. This causes both the extrafusal skeletal muscle fibers and the muscle spindle intrafusal muscle fibers to contract at the same time.

The purpose of contracting the muscle spindle intrafusal fibers at the same time that the large skeletal muscle fibers contract is twofold:

- First, it keeps the length of the receptor portion of the muscle spindle from changing during the course of the whole muscle contraction. Therefore, coactivation keeps the muscle spindle reflex from opposing the muscle contraction.
- Second, it maintains the proper damping function of the muscle spindle, regardless of any change in muscle length. For instance, if the muscle spindle did not contract and relax along with the large muscle fibers, the receptor portion of the spindle would sometimes be flail and sometimes be overstretched, in neither instance operating under optimal conditions for spindle function

91. Ans. (c) Subcutaneous tissue

Ref: Ganong 24th ed page 24, Human Physiology By Gillian Pocock, Christopher D. Richards, David Richards 4th ed page 723

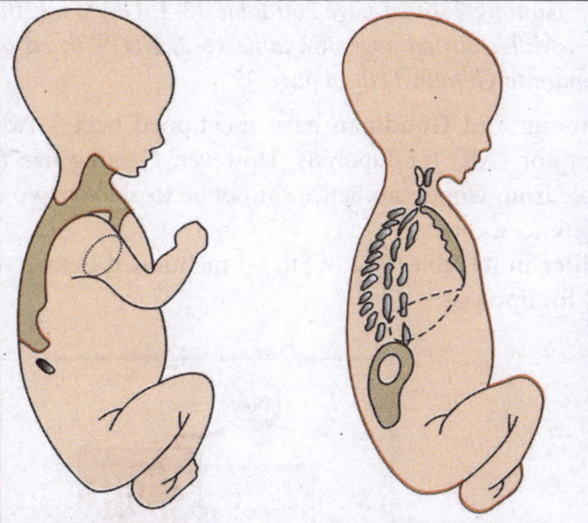

Interscapular pad of brown fat　　Thoracic and abdominal depots of brown fat

Cellular Lipid		
Structural lipid	**Neutral Lipid (WAT- White adipocyte tissue)**	**Brown fat (BAT-brown adipocyte tissue)**
Part of cell membrane lipid bilayer)	Stored in the adipose cells of the fat depots scattered throughout	Makes up a small percentage of total body fat. More abundant in infants but is present in adults as well. Located • Between the scapulas • Axilla • Supraclavicular • Nape of the neck • Along the great vessels in the thorax and abdomen • Between trachea and esophagus • Around the kidney and adrenals

Cellular Lipid		
Structural lipid	**Neutral Lipid (WAT- White adipocyte tissue)**	**Brown fat (BAT-brown adipocyte tissue)**
Fat droplets are not seen	Ordinary lipocytes have only a single large droplet of white fat	Brown fat cells contain several small droplets of fat
As it is intramembranous lipid, there is no mitochondria	Contains mitochondria but not as abundant as Brown fat	Brown fat cells also contain many mitochondria.
Serve as progenitors for cellular signaling molecules. Preserved during starvation	Neutral fat is mobilized during starvation. Broken down and free fatty acids (FFAs) are released into the circulation. Calorigenesis but no nonshivering thermogenesis	A source of considerable heat, particularly in infants. This fat has a high rate of metabolism No calorigenesis. Exclusively nonshivering thermogenesis
No sympathetic innervation hence no effect on sympathetic stimulation	White fat depots, in which some fat cells may be innervated but the principal sympathetic innervation is solely on blood vessels.	In brown fat depots, the fat cells as well as the blood vessels have an extensive sympathetic innervation. When the cells are stimulated by the sympathetic nerves, the mitochondria produce a large amount of heat but almost no ATP, so almost all the released oxidative energy immediately becomes heat.

Beige fat cells are those brown cells that can emerge in white fat depots under certain conditions.

92. Ans. (c) Beta 1 > (d) Beta 3

Ref: Ganong 24th ed page 260 table 13-1, Guyton 12th ed page 733, Miller 8th ed page 362 table 16-2, KDT 7th ed page 128, Goodman Gilman 11th ed page 93

Ganong and Goodman have mentioned beta 3 Adrenergic receptor (AR) for Lipolysis. However, Ganong has taken its table from Goodman hence cannot be treated as two different references.

Miller in its table 16-2 of 8th ed mentioned Beta 1 AR (Beta -3) for lipolysis.

Guyton in its table have mentioned β1 AR for Lipolysis and β3 AR for thermogenesis

KDT states: Beta 3 (atypical beta) have very low affinity for the standard β blockers. These are located on adipocytes, mediate lipolysis and induce thermogenesis. Selective β3 agonists have the potential to be used as antiobesity drugs.

Goodman states: All three β adrenergic receptors have been found in human fat cells. Activation of β3 adrenergic receptors produces a vigorous thermogenic response as well as lipolysis. The significance is unclear.

After reading all these statements we were forced to do more R and D on the topic. This is a big time research topic since decades and hence is out of scope of this book. However, we will try to summarize the points in short.

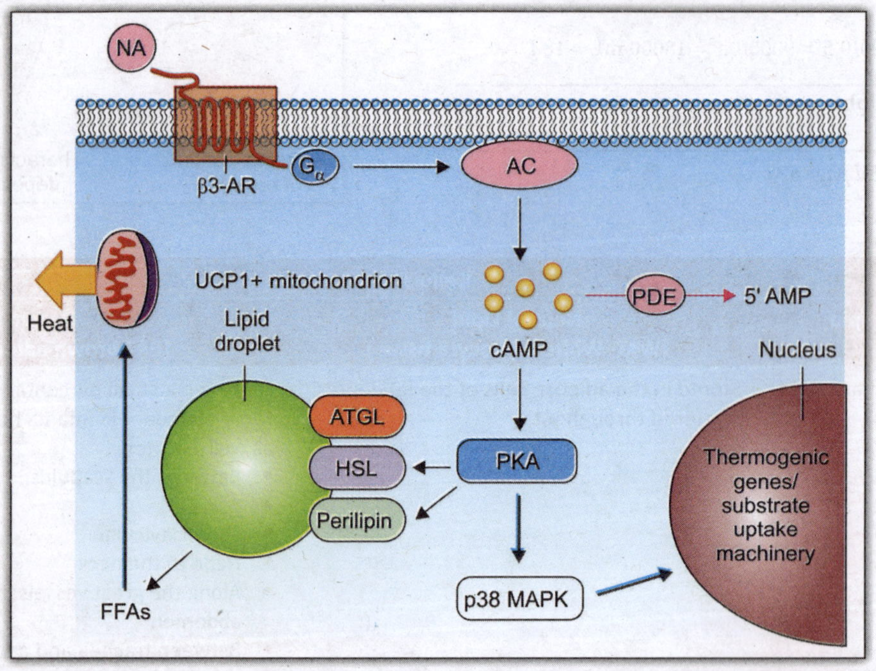

Fig: The sympathetic nervous system triggers intracellular signaling events that lead to lipolysis (black arrows). Noradrenaline (NA) released by sympathetic nerve endings binds to β-ARs, which couple to Gα G-proteins that activate adenylate cyclase (AC), increasing the cellular

concentration of cAMP. This activates protein kinase A (PKA), which phosphorylates lipid droplet proteins including hormone sensitive lipase (HSL) and perilipin, allowing activation of adipose triglyceride lipase (ATGL). The net result is the hydrolysis of triglycerides stored in the lipid droplet to free fatty acids (FFAs), which are released. This response can be attenuated by the activation of phosphodiesterases (PDE), which hydrolyze cAMP. In the case of recruitment and activation of beige adipocytes and the activation of brown adipocytes, this signaling pathway also leads to increased expression of UCP1 and other thermogenic genes through the p38 MAPK cascade. FFAs released by lipolysis activate existing UCP1 in the mitochondria and their oxidation produces heat

Summary

- Adipose tissue can be grossly divided into two major depots, white adipose tissue (WAT) and brown adipose tissue (BAT). WAT stores excess energy as triglycerides (TGs), which can be mobilized by lipolysis to generate free fatty acids (FFAs) for use by other tissues. BAT, on the other hand, is the main site of nonshivering thermogenesis (NST), which requires a brown adipocyte-specific protein called uncoupling protein 1 (UCP1).
- Rodent and human adipose tissue display different β-AR expression profiles. In mouse, the β3-AR is highly expressed in both BAT and WAT with several-fold higher abundance than the β1-AR, whereas in the adult human, the β3-AR is only expressed in BAT. In human WAT, β1-AR has been reported to be 50-fold more abundant than β3-AR
- There are also two major types of adrenergic receptors, alpha receptors and beta receptors. The alpha receptors are divided into. The beta receptors in turn are divided into beta1, beta2 and beta3 receptors each of which is coupled to the G-alpha subunit of the Gs protein.
- All three β adrenergic receptors have been found in human fat cells. Activation of β3 adrenergic receptors produces a vigorous thermogenic response as well as lipolysis.
- Fat cells Lipolysis-thermogenesis α1, β1, β2, β3 and Inhibition of lipolysis α2
- There are three beta-adrenergic receptor subtypes (beta 1, beta 1 and beta 3), each of which is coupled to the G-alpha subunit of the Gs protein. Their stimulation increases intracellular cAMP levels in fat cells of various species although considerable species-specific differences exist. In human white fat cells, both beta1 and beta 2 are known to stimulate lipolysis in vitro and in vivo (Langin 2006). The physiological role of the beta 3 in human remains questionable, but, importantly, this receptor does not contribute to catecholamine-induced lipolysis in human subcutaneous adipocytes (Langin 2006). (Ref: Physiology and Physiopathology of Adipose Tissue edited by Jean-Philippe Bastard, Bruno Fève Springer 2013 page 143)

Conclusion

- Beta 1, 2, 3, all are present in adipocytes but
- Beta 1 is seen in White adipocyte tissue (WAT- abundant in adults) and triggered by catecholamines and sympathetic stimuli for lipolysis which is then used for calorigenesis, but not for nonshivering thermogenesis
- Beta 3 AR is limited to Brown adipocyte tissue (BAT) which is not absent but very limited in adults. Its triggered by catecholamines and sympathetic stimuli for lipolysis which is used majorly for nonshivering thermogenesis (NST)
- Hence, if both Beta 1 and 3 are provided in the options it is a better answer, otherwise Beta 1> Beta 3

Adrenergic Receptors and Function

Alpha receptor	Beta receptor
Vasoconstriction	Cardioacceleration (β_1)
Iris dilation	Vasodilation (β_2)
Intestinal relaxation	Increased myocardial strength (β_1)
Intestinal sphincter contraction	Intestinal relaxation (β_2)
	Uterus relaxation (β_2)
Pilomotor contraction	Bronchodilation (β_2)
	Calorigenesis (β_2)
Bladder sphincter contraction	Glycogenolysis (β_2)
	Lipolysis (β_1)
	Bladder wall relaxation (β_2)
	Thermogenesis (β_3)

93. Ans. (c) Factor XIII

Ref: Guyton 11th ed page 454, Robbin's 9th ed page 83

In the early stages of polymerization, the fibrin monomer molecules are held together by weak noncovalent hydrogen bonding and the newly forming fibers are not cross-linked with one another; therefore, the resultant clot is weak and can be broken apart with ease. But another process occurs during the next few minutes that greatly strengthens the fibrin reticulum. This involves a substance called **fibrin-stabilizing factor (Factor XIII)** that is present in small amounts in normal plasma globulins but is also released from platelets entrapped in the clot. Before fibrin-stabilizing factor can have an effect on the fibrin fibers, it must itself be activated. The same thrombin that causes fibrin formation also activates the fibrin-stabilizing factor. Then this activated substance operates as an enzyme to cause covalent bonds between more and more of the fibrin monomer molecules, as well as multiple cross-linkages between adjacent fibrin fibers, thus adding tremendously to the three-dimensional strength of the fibrin meshwork.

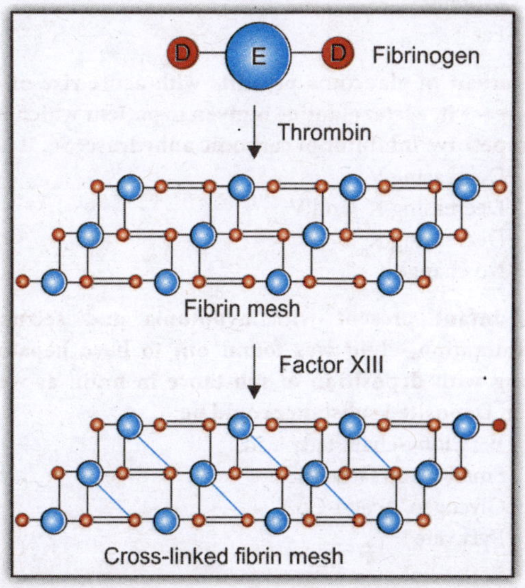

Biochemistry 3

AIIMS NOVEMBER 2018

1. **Respiratory quotient after an exclusive carbohydrate meal is:** ***(AIIMS Nov 2018, 2016)***
   a. 0.7
   b. 0.8
   c. 1
   d. 1.2

2. **The fastest way to "resynthesize" ATP during exercise is:** ***(AIIMS Nov 2018, 2016)***
   a. Phosphocreatine breakdown
   b. Glycogenolysis
   c. Glycolysis
   d. TCA cycle

3. **A 25-year-old male who is type I diabetic patient presents to OPD with complaints of increased thirst, increased urine frequency and increased appetite. Which of following metabolically will be most commonly occurring inside his body?**
   a. Decreased de novo synthesis of cholesterol
   b. Increased conversion of fatty acids into acetyl-CoA
   c. Glycogenesis in muscle
   d. Increased protein synthesis

4. **Northern blot is used for?**
   a. DNA
   b. RNA
   c. Proteins
   d. Fat

5. **A patient of glaucoma presents with acute rise of IOP. To decrease it, acetazolamide is given to patient which is a non-competitive inhibitor of carbonic anhydrase. So, it acts by:**
   a. Decreasing V_{max}
   b. Decreasing K_m and V_{max}
   c. Decreasing K_m
   d. No change

6. **An infant present with hypotonia and seizures. On examination, child was found out to have hepatomegaly along with deposition of substance in brain as well as in liver. Deposited substance could be:**
   a. Very long-chain fatty acids
   b. Small-chain fatty acids
   c. Glycogen/Acetyl-CoA
   d. Pyruvate

AIIMS MAY 2018

7. **In a reaction, substrate is available in a concentration that is 1000 times the K_m value of the enzyme. After 9 minutes of the reaction, 1% substrate is converted into product (12 mcg/mL). If the concentration of the enzyme is changed to ⅓ and concentration of substrate is doubled, what is the time taken to convert the substrate into the same amount of product, i.e, 12 mcg/mL?**
   a. 9 min
   b. 12 min
   c. 18 min
   d. 27 min

8. **A child presents with blue eyes, white patch of hair and fair skin. Guthrie test is positive. All are true EXCEPT:**
   a. Due to phenylalanine hydroxylase enzyme defect
   b. White patch of hair due to tryptophan
   c. Phenyl acetate positive in urine
   d. Mental retardation is present

9. **A middle-aged man comes to you after having muscle cramps after strenuous exercise. On examination muscle glycogen was found to be higher than normal. What could be deficient enzyme in this individual?**
   a. Phosphofructokinase 1
   b. Debranching enzyme
   c. Glycogen phosphorylase
   d. Glucose 6 phosphatase
   e. Glycogen phosphorylase

10. **All are true about Klenow fragment EXCEPT:**
    a. 3′ → 5′ exonuclease activity
    b. 5′ → 3′ exonuclease activity
    c. Both 3′ & 5′ exonuclease activity
    d. DNA polymerase activity

11. **In which RNA 5′ end is uncapped?**
    a. tRNA of Alanine
    b. mRNA for Histones
    c. pri-mi-RNA
    d. U6 Sn RNA

12. **Middle aged female presents with complaints of fatigue & tiredness. On examination she has red fissured tongue, fissures at angle of lip. Glutathione reductase activity in RBC is found to be reduced. What could be deficient?**
    a. Vitamin B_1
    b. Vitamin B_2
    c. Vitamin B_6
    d. Vitamin B_{12}

13. Best investigation for metabolic disorders is?
a. Western blot
b. Tandem mass spectrometry
c. Ion chromatography
d. ELISA

14. Which enzyme activity decreases in fasting state?
a. PFK-1
b. Hormone sensitive lipase
c. Glycogen phosphorylase
d. Acetyl CoA carboxylase

15. A 25-year-old comes to you who has been diagnosed with lactase deficiency. What would you advise to him to have out of following?
a. Yoghurt
b. Ice cream
c. Condensed milk
d. Skimmed milk

16. Fluoride released from fluoroacetate inhibit which metabolic pathway?
a. ETC
b. Glycolytic pathway
c. Oxidative phosphorylation
d. TCA cycle

17. Which of the following techniques is based on RNA?
a. Sanger's technique
b. RT PCR
c. Western Blot
d. ELISA

18. In which of the following, viral load done by Real Time PCR is of no role in investigative procedures?
a. Person with hepatitis B on Tenofovir therapy
b. HSV causing temporal encephalitis
c. BK virus in patient of allograft renal transplant
d. CMV PCR in blood of patient of liver transplant

19. Vitamin K as coenzyme form is regenerated by:
a. Epoxide reductase
b. Glutathione reductase
c. Pyruvate decarboxylase
d. Dihydrofolate reductase

20. Vitamin C is not produced in human because of deficiency of?
a. L-gluconolactone oxidase
b. Xyltitol reductase
c. Pyruvate dehydrogenase
d. UDP glucose dehydrogenase

21. Which of the following vitamins helps in increasing iron absorption?
a. Thiamine
b. Niacin
c. Vitamin C
d. Riboflavin

22. Which of the following does not favour permissive euchromatin due to changes at cytosine residues at CpG islands in DNA?
a. Methylation
b. Phosphorylation
c. Alkylation
d. Sumoylation

AIIMS NOVEMBER 2017

23. SCID is due to defect in what type of DNA repair?
a. Base excision repair
b. Nucleotide excision repair
c. Nonhomologous disjunction repair
d. Homologous disjunction repair

24. A 4-year-old boy comes with complaints of getting early fatigue while playing. On investigation Blood pH was 7.3, Fasting blood sugar = 60 mg/dL with hypertriglyceridemia, Ketosis and Lactic acidosis. On examination he had hepatomegaly. Biopsy of liver and kidney showed increased glycogen content. On USG liver and kidney was enlarged. What is your diagnosis?
a. Mc Ardle disease
b. Cori's disease
c. Von Gierke disease
d. Pompe disease

25. All of the following are results of post transcriptional modification EXCEPT:
a. Selenocysteine
b. Hydroxyproline
c. Triiodothyronine
d. Hydroxylysine

26. Which of the following is cofactor for glycogen phosphorylase?
a. Thiamine
b. Pyridoxal phosphate
c. Biotin
d. Pantothenic acid

27. Which of the following test is positive for the substance increased in prolonged starvation?

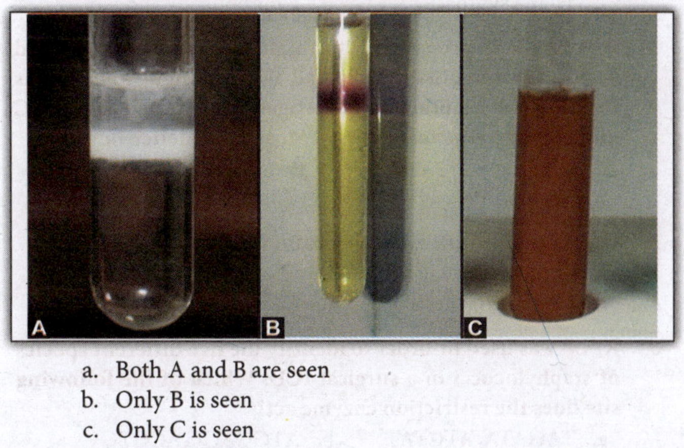

a. Both A and B are seen
b. Only B is seen
c. Only C is seen
d. All A, B and C are seen

28. Which bond is maked in the following picture?

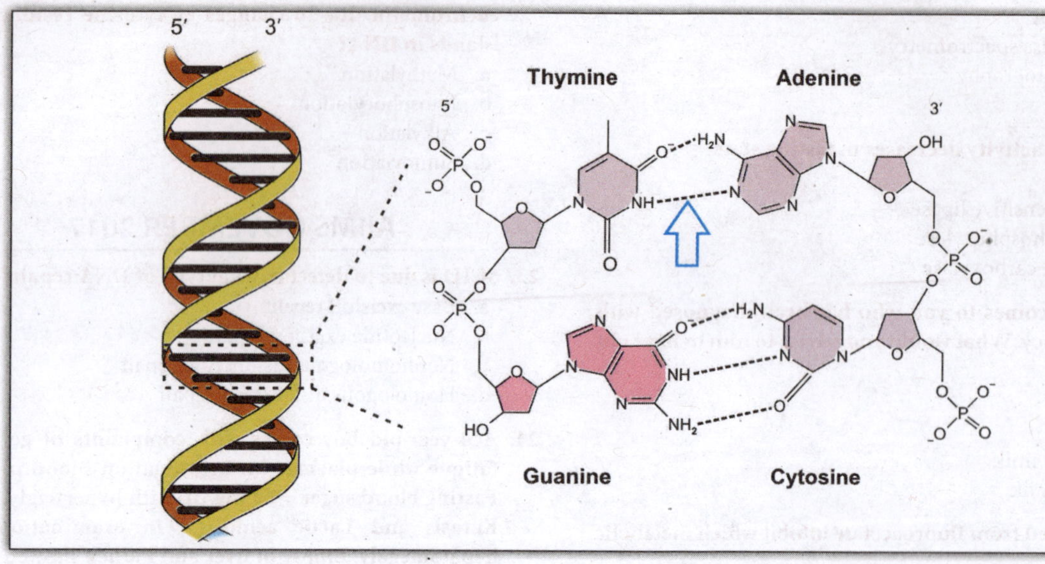

a. 2′5′ Phosphodiester bond
b. 3′5′ Phosphodiester bond
c. Hydrogen bond
d. Covalent bond

AIIMS MAY 2017

29. Maximum Thermic energy is seen in:

a. Fat metabolism
b. Carbohydrate metabolism
c. Proteins metabolism
d. Not dependent on macronutrient

30. A girl with habit of eating paint from the wall complaints of acute abdominal pain on and off and tingling sensation of limbs and at times weakness of limbs. She had a history of eating paint from the wall of newly built house. Which of the following enzyme deficiency will be the cause of her condition?

a. ALA synthase
b. ALA dehydratase
c. Heme synthase
d. Coproporphyrinogen

31. A young lady presented with tingling sensation in legs and hands. On examination she had fissure tongue and lesions in angle of mouth. On investigation, she had low RBC glutathione reductase activity. Most likely deficiency is of:

a. Vitamin B_1
b. Vitamin B_2
c. Vitamin B_6
d. Vitamin B_{12}

32. Decreased Insulin-Glucagon ratio is seen in all EXCEPT:

a. Glycogen storage
b. Glycogen breakdown
c. Gluconeogenesis
d. Ketogenesis

33. RFLP was used in-order to identify the five different species of staphylococci in a surgical ICU. Which of the following site does the restriction enzyme act?

a. TAGATA/ATCTAT
b. ATGGAC/TACGTG
c. AATATA/TATAAT
d. GATTAC/CATTAG

34. Which of the following is true regarding Mitochondrial DNA?

a. It has 3×10^9 base pairs
b. It has less mutations than human DNA
c. 23 pairs inherited from each parent
d. Less than 20% respiratory chain proteins codes from mDNA

35. Thiamine deficiency results in decreased energy production, because TPP interferes with?

(AIIMS May 2017, AI PGMEE 2010)

a. Alcohol metabolism
b. Transketolase activity
c. Its coenzyme for pyruvate and alpha ketoglutarate dehydrogenase
d. Energy production from amino acids

36. 3 ATPs for each sugar, will be generated if the following substrate is used for anaerobic glycolysis?

a. Fructose
b. Glucose
c. Galactose
d. Glycogen

37. Which of the following is an example of anapleurotic reaction?

a. Pyruvate to oxaloacetate
b. Pyruvate to Acetyl CoA
c. Pyruvate to lactic acid
d. Pyruvate to acetaldehyde

38. Phenylbutyrate is used in urea cycle disorders because it:

a. Activates enzymes
b. Maintains renal output
c. Maintains energy level
d. Increases renal excretion of ammonia

39. In uncontrolled diabetes, VLDL and triglycerides are high because of:

a. Increased in activity of hepatic lipase
b. Increase in peripheral function of LDL receptors
c. Increased activity of lipoprotein lipase and decreased activity of hormone sensitive lipase
d. Increased activity of hormone sensitive lipase and decreased activity of lipoprotein lipase

AIIMS NOVEMBER 2016

40. The fastest way to "resynthesize" ATP during exercise is? ***(AIIMS Nov 2018, 2016)***

a. Phosphocreatine breakdown
b. Glycogenolysis
c. Glycolysis
d. TCA cycle

41. Respiratory quotient after an exclusive carbohydrate meal is: ***(AIIMS Nov 2018, 2016)***

a. 0.7 b. 0.8
c. 1 d. 1.2

42. HDL has maximum concentration of:

a. Triglyceride
b. Cholesterol
c. Apoprotein
d. Saturated fatty acid

43. Vitamin synthesized De novo by metabolism in the body is:

a. Niacin
b. Pantothenic acid
c. Vitamin B_{12}
d. Folic acid

44. Glucose oxidase test is negative, but Benedict's test is positive for reducing sugar in which of the following?

a. Fructose
b. Galactose
c. Latent DM
d. Sucrose

45. In starvation, for gluconeogenesis the most effective pathway is? ***(AIIMS Nov 2016, May 2012)***

a. Citrate activates acetyl-CoA carboxylase
b. Acetyl-CoA activates pyruvate carboxylase
c. Fructose 2,6 bisphosphate activates phosphofructokinase
d. Fructose 1,6 bisphosphate activates phosphofructokinase

46. All of the following processes are seen in mitochondria EXCEPT:

a. Fatty acid synthesis b. Proteins synthesis
c. DNA synthesis d. Beta oxidation fatty acids

47. CG Island sequence in human genome is for:

a. DNA acetylation b. DNA methylation
c. tRNA synthesis d. Origin of replication

48. A child who was normal at birth, at 4 years age he developed delayed motor development and involuntary movements. CT brain was done and was normal. The child has self-mutilating behavior of head banging, biting of lip and fingers and Arthritis and later on he dies of renal failure. Enzyme responsible for this is:

a. Phenylalanine hydroxylase
b. HGPRTase
c. Hexosaminidase A
d. Adenine deaminase

49. Ammonia in brain is trapped as:

a. Glutamate
b. Glutamine
c. Urea
d. Glycine

50. What is the pH when H^+ ion concentration is 5 mmol/litre?

a. 1.7 b. 2.3
c. 3.7 d. 6.4

51. Common intermediate of steroid hormone synthesis from cholesterol is:

a. 7-dehydrocholesterol
b. 7-hydroxycholesterol
c. Pregnenolone
d. Corticosterone

52. At normal physiological pH amino acid having positive charge is:

a. Arginine b. Aspartic acid
c. Valine d. Isoleucine

AIIMS MAY 2016

53. The graph shown below is the titration curve of a biochemical compound. Which of the following statement is true?

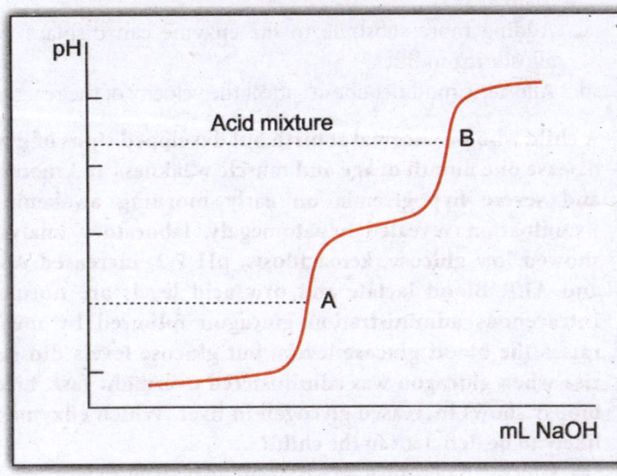

a. The maximum buffering capacity of the compound is represented by points A and B
b. The points A and B represent the range of ionization of the amine and carboxyl group
c. The compound has three ionizable side chains
d. The compound has one ionizable group

54. The graph given below denotes the transport kinetics across the cell membrane. The solute is:

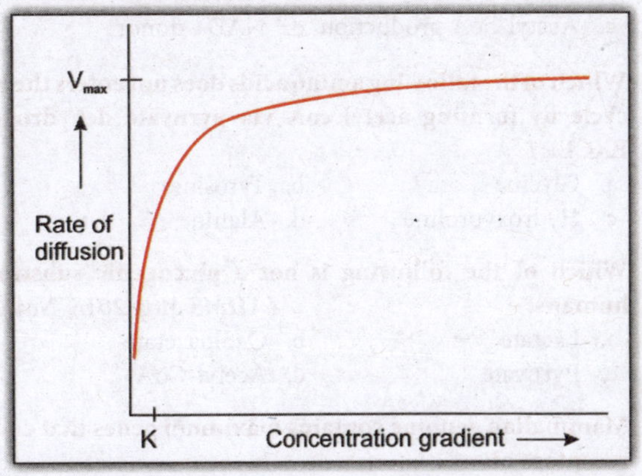

a. O_2 b. Na
c. Cl^- d. Glucose

55. True about the Michaelis Menten curve below is:

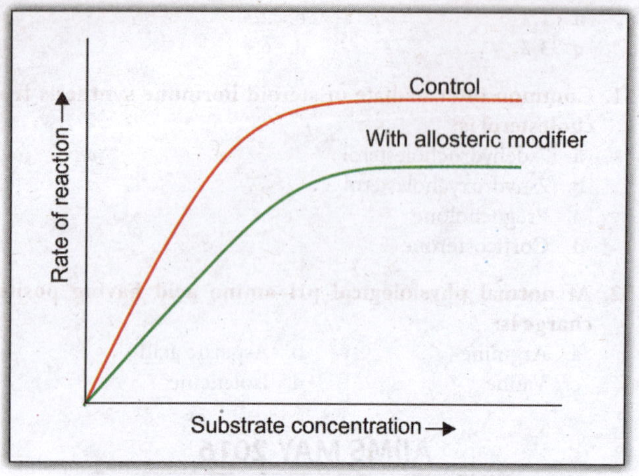

a. Allosteric modifier can affect the catalytic site too
b. Allosteric modifier binds in concentration dependent manner
c. Adding more substrate to the enzyme can displace the allosteric modifier
d. Allosteric modifier doesn't affect the velocity of the reaction

56. A child who was normal at birth but developed signs of liver disease one month of age and muscle weakness at 3 months and severe hypoglcemia on early morning awakening. Examination revealed hepatomegaly, laboratory analysis showed low glucose, ketoacidosis, pH 7.2, increased AST and ALT. Blood lactate and uric acid levels are normal. Intravenous administration glucagon followed by meals raises the blood glucose levels, but glucose levels did not rise when glucagon was administered overnight fast. Liver biopsy shows increased glycogen in liver. Which enzyme is likely to be deficient in the child?

a. Glucose 6 phosphatase b. Muscle phosphorylase
c. Branching enzyme d. Debranching enzyme

57. Which type of Lipase is controlled by Glucagon?

a. Lipoprotein lipase b. Hormone sensitive lipase
c. Gastric lipase d. Pancreatic lipase

58. A child ingested cyanide and rushed to the emergency room. Which of the following enzymes of citric acid cycle is inhibited?

a. Citrate synthase b. Aconitase
c. Acetyl CoA production d. NAD+ donor

59. Which of the following amino acids does not enters the Kreb's cycle by forming acetyl coA via pyruvate dehydrogenase EXCEPT:

a. Glycine b. Tyrosine
c. Hydroxyproline d. Alanine

60. Which of the following is not a glucogenic substrate in humans? ***(AIIMS May 2016, Nov 2015)***

a. Lactate b. Oxaloacetate
c. Pyruvate d. Acetyl-CoA

61. Mammalian genome contains maximum genes that code for receptors of:

a. Odorants b. Interleukins
c. Immunoglobulins d. Growth factors

62. All of the following can be used to precipitate protein EXCEPT:

a. Salts of heavy metals
b. Alcohol and acetone
c. Precipitate at pH other than isoelectric pH
d. Trichloroacetic acid

AIIMS NOVEMBER 2015

63. Which of the following is not a technique for protein precipitation?

a. Trichloroacetic acid
b. Heat precipitation
c. Isoelectric point method
d. Titration with reducing sugar

64. Which of the following is not a glucogenic substrate in humans? ***(AIIMS May 2016, Nov 2015)***

a. Lactate b. Oxaloacetate
c. Pyruvate d. Acetyl-CoA

65. Codon for transcription of Selenocysteine is:

a. UAA b. UGA
c. UAG d. GUA

66. Cofactor Vitamin-B_{12} is required for all EXCEPT:

a. Glycogen phosphorylase
b. Methionine synthase
c. Leucine amino mutase
d. Methyl malonyl CoA mutase

67. Biotin has role in all of the following reactions EXCEPT:

a. Gamma carboxylation of glutamate
b. Propionyl CoA to methyl malonyl CoA
c. Acyl CoA to methyl malonyl CoA
d. Pyruvate to oxaloacetate

68. Glycogen synthesis and breakdown takes place in the same cell, having enzymes necessary for both pathways. Why is Glucose-6-phosphate produced during glycogenesis in the cytoplasm of liver cells, not acted upon by Glucose-6-phosphatase enzyme?

a. Steric inhibition of phosphatase by albumin
b. Glucose-6-phosphatase is present in endoplasmic reticulum while glycogen is in the cytoplasm
c. It is thermodynamically viable only when gluconeogenesis has stated
d. Require protein kinase for activation

69. Which of the following is not a glucogenic substrate in humans? ***(AIIMS May 2016, Nov 2015)***

a. Lactate b. Oxaloacetate
c. Pyruvate d. Acetyl-CoA

70. In genomic imprinting DNA is modified by?

a. Acetylation
b. Methylation
c. Phosphorylation
d. Deamination

71. Thiamine is a cofactor for all the following enzymes EXCEPT:

a. Alpha ketoglutarate dehydrogenase
b. Branched chain ketoacid dehydrogenase
c. Succinate dehydrogenase
d. Pyruvate dehydrogenase

72. **Glycogen phosphorylase is regulated by all EXCEPT:**
   a. Protein kinase A b. Calmodulin
   c. C-AMP d. Glycogenin

73. **Sickle cell Hemoglobin is formed when glutamic acid is replaced by valine. Mobility of HbS on electrophoresis as compared to HbA will be?**
   a. Decreased
   b. Increased
   c. Dependent on HbS concentration
   d. Unchanged

74. **Heme biosynthesis occur in all EXCEPT:**
   a. Hepatocytes
   b. RBC
   c. Osteocytes
   d. Erythroid cells of Bone marrow

75. **In a patient with lead poisoning, which heme pathway intermediate will increase in urine?**
   a. ALA
   b. Porphobilinogen
   c. Protoporphyrin
   d. Coproporphyrinogen III

AIIMS MAY 2015

76. **A 10-year-old boy presented with abdominal pain, muscle weakness and fatigue. On investigations, serum lead levels were found increased. Activity of which of following enzyme in the liver is increased?**
   a. ALA synthase
   b. Ferrochelatase
   c. PBG deaminase
   d. Heme oxygenase

77. **Enzyme involved in both glycogenesis and glycogenolysis is?** ***(AIIMS May 2015, 2014)***
   a. Glycogen synthase b. Phosphoglucomutase
   c. Phosphorylase d. Glycogen transferase

78. **If in a person, total Cholesterol = 300 mg/dL, HDL = 25 mg/dL and Triglycerides = 150 mg/dL, what will be the LDL levels?**
   a. 245 b. 125
   c. 95 d. 55

79. **Which of the following is used by RBCs for metabolism during fasting state?**
   a. Glucose b. Alanine
   c. Ketone body d. Fatty acid

80. **In a person, serum LDL levels are highly elevated but the number of LDL receptors is normal. What could be the probable cause?**
   a. Phosphorylation of LDL receptors
   b. ApoB-100 mutation
   c. Lipoprotein lipase deficiency
   d. Cholesterol acyl CoA transferase deficiency

81. **A 7-year-old boy presents with severe abdominal pain. On examination he has xanthomas. Blood drawn for work up has milky appearance of plasma. Which lipoprotein is increased?**
   a. Chylomicron b. Chylomicron remnants
   c. LDL d. HDL

82. **What is forward scatter in flow cytometry used to assess?**
   a. Cell death b. Cell size
   c. Cell granules d. Cell fluorescence

83. **Thiamine deficiency can cause lactic acidosis due to which enzyme dysfunction?**
   a. PEP carboxykinase b. Pyruvate dehydrogenase
   c. Pyruvate carboxylase d. Citrate synthase

84. **RNAi causes the following to a gene:**
   a. Knock in b. Knock out
   c. Knock down d. Knock up

85. **Specific site to which the CRE recombinase binds?**
   a. RE site b. LoxP site
   c. Int site d. FRT site

AIIMS NOVEMBER 2018

1. Ans. (c) 1

Ref: Harper 30th ed page 148, Guyton's 11th ed page 867

Repeat (See Biochemistry Nov 2016 for explanation) (see page no. 205)

2. Ans. (a) Phosphocreatine breakdown

Ref: Harper 30th ed chapter 30, Guyton 12th ed page 1033

Repeat AIIMS Nov 2016 Biochemistry (see page no. 204)

3. Ans. (b) Increased conversion of fatty acids into Acetyl-CoA

Ref: Harper 29th ed Ch 57

- The patient has Type-I diabetes and symptoms are suggestive of Diabetic Ketoacidosis.
- In Type-I diabetes mellitus, there is a deficiency of insulin, due to which tissues are unable to take up glucose as their energy source. As a result, the body enters a catalytic state and tries to utilize lipids and proteins as a source of energy, along with increased gluconeogenesis and protein catabolism.
- Due to increased lipolysis, there is an increase in fatty acids. In the liver, these fatty acids are converted into Acetyl-CoA which then enters the TCA cycle for production of ATP (less common pathway). Two Acetyl-CoA molecules form Acetoacetyl-CoA which in turn causes formation of ketone bodies (main pathway in liver).
- The liver is the only organ to add significant quantities of ketone bodies to the blood. Extrahepatic tissues utilize them as respiratory substrates.
- The net flow of ketone bodies from the liver to the extrahepatic tissues result from active hepatic synthesis coupled with very low utilization. The reverse situation occurs in extrahepatic tissues.

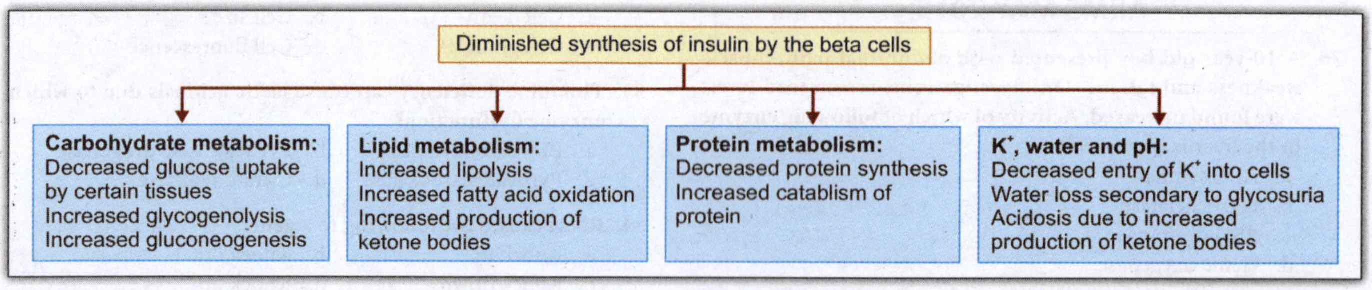

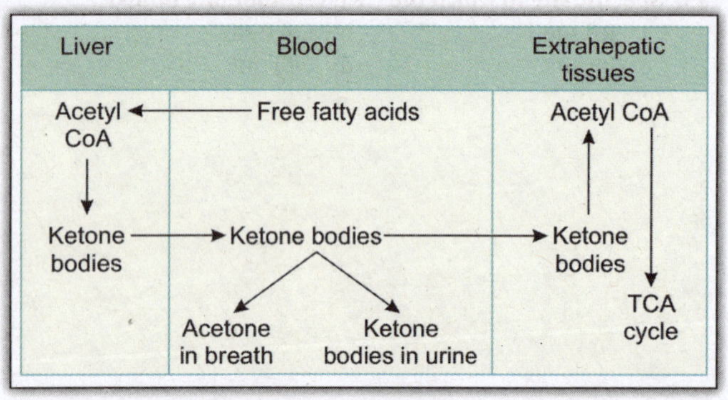

Fig: Formation, excretion and utilization of ketone bodies

4. Ans. (b) RNA

Ref: Harper's 30th Ed page 457

- Visualization of a specific DNA or RNA fragment among the many thousands of "contaminating" molecules in a complex sample requires the convergence of a number of techniques, collectively termed blot transfer.
- These are Southern (DNA), Northern (RNA) and Western (protein) blot transfer procedures. (The first is named for the person who devised the technique [Edward Southern] and the other names began as laboratory jargon but are now accepted terms.)
- These procedures are useful in determining how many copies of a gene are in a given tissue or whether there are any alterations in a gene (deletions, insertions, or rearrangements) because the requisite electrophoresis step separates the molecules on the basis of size.
- Occasionally, if a specific base is changed and a restriction site is altered, these procedures can detect a point mutation.
- The Northern and Western blot transfer techniques are used to size and quantitate specific RNA and protein molecules, respectively.
- A fourth hybridization technique, the Southwestern blot, examines protein–DNA interactions. In this method, proteins are separated by electrophoresis, blotted to a membrane, renatured and analyzed for an interaction with a particular sequence by incubation with a specific labeled nucleic acid probe.

Blotting Compass

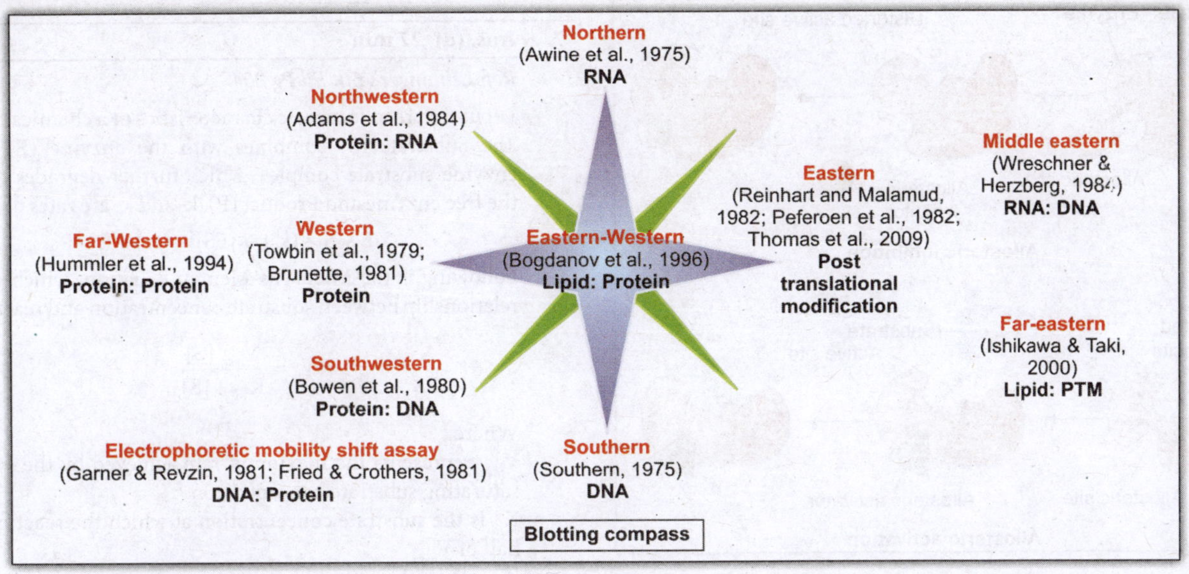

5. **Ans. (a) Decreasing V_{max}**

Ref: Harper 30th ed page 82, 91

This question is basically designed to test your knowledge of competitive and noncompetitive inhibitors.

Summary

1. In competitive inhibition K_m is raised without an effect on V_{max}.
2. In noncompetitive inhibition V_{max} decreases without affecting the K_m.

There are three different ways by which the action of an enzyme can be inhibited:

- **Competitive inhibition:** A competitive inhibitor has a close structural resemblance to the substrate of an enzyme. It competes with the substrate molecules for the active site of an enzyme. The inhibitor may remain bound to the enzyme and excludes substrate molecules from the active site of the enzyme while it remains attached.

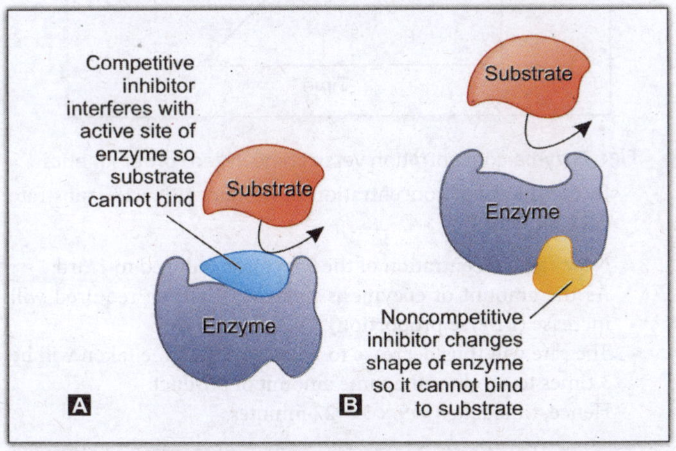

Fig: A. Competitive inhibition; **B.** Noncompetitive inhibition

- **Noncompetitive inhibition:** Noncompetitive inhibitors have no structural resemblance to the substrates of enzymes. A noncompetitive inhibitor combines with the enzyme at a region other than at its active site. This results in a change in the conformation of the enzyme molecule, including the configuration of its active site.
- **Allosteric or feedback inhibition:**

Allosteric modifier: The prefix 'allo' of allosteric enzymes means 'other' and stereos means 'shape'. Allosteric regulation (or allosteric control) is the regulation of an enzyme by binding an effector molecule at a site other than the enzyme's active site. Allosteric enzyme is one whose activity can be altered by molecules acting at a site other than the active site. This site is called the allosteric site. The active site is the region of an enzyme where substrate molecules bind and undergo a chemical reaction. The active site consists of residues that form temporary bonds with the substrate (**binding site**) and residues that catalyze a reaction of that substrate (**catalytic site**). The binding of a regulatory molecule to the allosteric site changes the overall shape of the enzyme. This can either enable or prevent the binding of substrate to the active site.

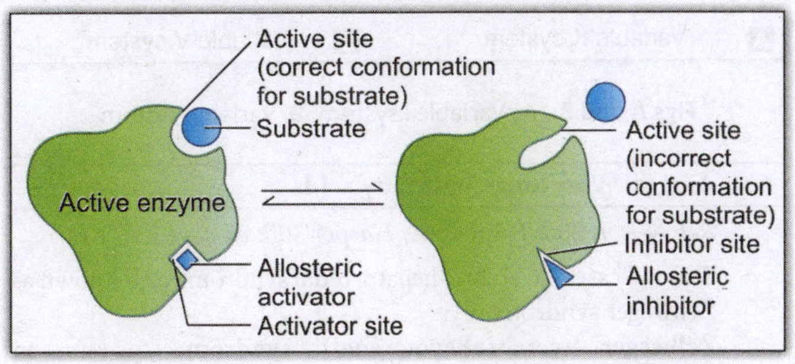

Fig: Schematic representation of allosteric enzyme activity

There are two types of regulatory molecules, namely **allosteric activators** and **allosteric inhibitors.** Allosteric activators enable the substrate to bind to the active site and thus increase the rate of reaction. In contrast, allosteric inhibitors prevent the binding of the substrate to the active site and therefore decrease the rate of reaction.

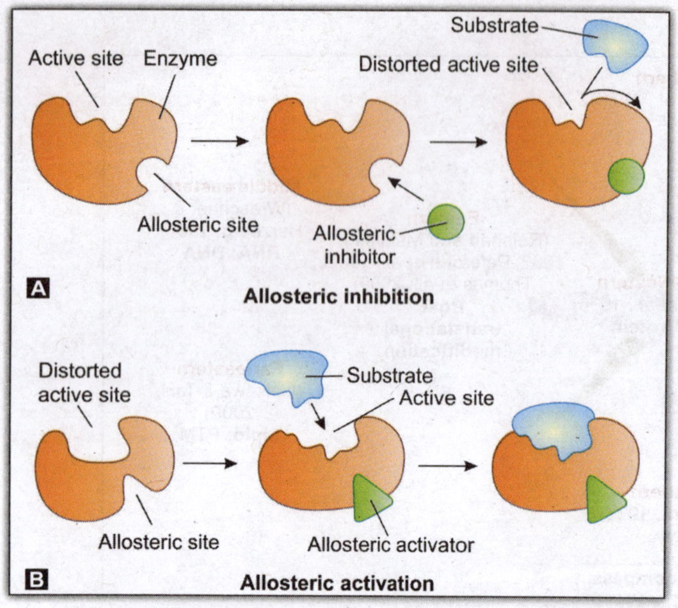

Figs A and B: **A.** Allosteric inhibition; **B.** Allosteric activation

To refer to the kinetics of allosteric inhibition as "competitive" or "noncompetitive" with substrate carries misleading mechanistic implications. Instead to two classes of allosterically regulated enzymes: K-series and V-series enzymes.

- For **K-series allosteric enzymes (Competitive inhibition)**, the substrate saturation kinetics is competitive in the sense that K_m is raised without an effect on V_{max}.
- For **V-series allosteric enzymes (Noncompetitive inhibition)**, the allosteric inhibitor lowers V_{max} without affecting the K_m.

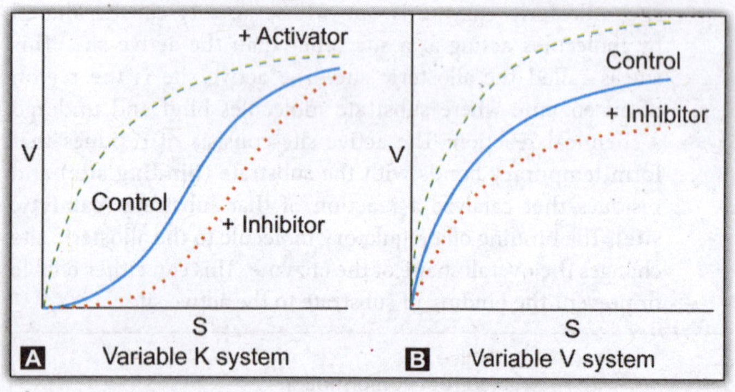

Figs A and B: **A.** Variable ksystem; **B.** Variable system

6. Ans. (a) Very long-chain fatty acids

Ref: Nelson 20th Ed pg 2989, Harper 30th ed page 231, 614

This is a case of Cerebro-hepato-renal syndrome also known as Zellweger syndrome.

Zellweger (cerebrohepatorenal) syndrome occurs in individuals with a rare inherited absence of peroxisomes in all tissues. They accumulate C26–C38 polyenoic acids in brain tissue and also exhibit a generalized loss of peroxisomal functions. The disease causes severe neurological symptoms and most patients die in the first year of life. ***Elevated levels of very long-chain polyenoic acids have been found in the brains of patients with Zellweger syndrome.***

7. Ans. (d) 27 min

Ref: Lehninger's 6th Ed Pg 204

Let us first recollect basic characteristics of a chemical reaction. The Substrate (S) combines with the enzyme (E) to form enzyme-substrate complex, which further degrades to release the free enzyme and Product (P). k_1 and k_2 are rates of reaction.

$$E + S - (k_1) \rightarrow [ES] - (k_2) \rightarrow E + P$$

Following is the Michaelis-Menten equation, which gives the relationship between substrate concentration and reaction rate.

$$V_0 = \frac{V_{max}\,[S]}{K_m + [S]}$$

Where,

V_{max} represents the maximum rate achieved by the system, at saturating substrate concentration

K_m is the substrate concentration at which the reaction rate is half of V_{max}

[S] is the substrate concentration.

Now,

$[S] = 1000 \times K_m$ that is, substrate concentration $[S] >> K_m$

Thus, the substrate is present in an excess amount; i.e., the reaction is independent of the substrate concentration since all enzyme active sites are occupied. Any change in the amount of product formed over a specified period of time will be dependent upon the level of enzyme present. This also means that the rate is equal to the maximum velocity and is independent of the substrate concentration. The reaction thus follows zero-order kinetics.

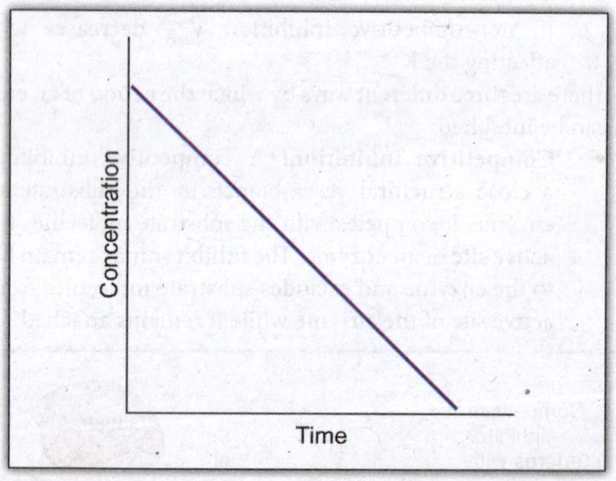

Fig: Enzyme concentration versus time in zero order kinetics

In the question, concentration of product [P] = 1% substrate = 12 mcg/mL.

Now, the concentration of the enzyme is reduced to 1/3rd.

As the amount of enzyme is reduced, the time required will increase (inverse proportion).

The rate will thus decrease to 1/3rd and the time taken will be 3 times to produce the same amount of product.

Hence, time taken = 9 × 3 = 27 minutes.

8. Ans. (b) White patch of hair due to tryptophan

Ref: Nelson 20th Ed Pg 368

Phenylketoneuria

- The affected infant is normal at birth. Profound intellectual disability develops gradually if the infant remains untreated. Cognitive delay may not be evident for the first few months. In untreated patients, 50-70% will have an IQ below 35 and 88-90% will have an IQ below 65. Only 2-5% of untreated patients will have normal intelligence. Many patients require institutional care if the condition remains untreated. Vomiting, sometimes severe enough to be misdiagnosed as pyloric stenosis, may be an early symptom. Older untreated children become hyperactive with autistic behaviors, including purposeless hand movements, rhythmic rocking and athetosis.
- Guthrie's test is positive in Phenylketonuria (PKU) and hence, diagnosis in the child described is PKU.
- Deficiency of the enzyme phenylalanine hydroxylase (PAH) or of its cofactor tetrahydrobiopterin (BH4) causes accumulation of **phenylalanine**.
- In affected infants with plasma concentrations >20 mg/dL, excess phenylalanine is metabolized to phenylketones (phenylpyruvate and **phenylacetate**) that are excreted in the urine, giving rise to the term phenylketonuria (PKU).
- Infants with **PKU** tend to have fair skin, blond hair and blue eyes, because the inability to convert ***phenylalanine to tyrosine.***
- Profound intellectual disability develops gradually if the infant remains untreated. Cognitive delay may not be evident for the first few months. In untreated patients, 50-70% will have an IQ below 35 and 88-90% will have an IQ below 65.

9. Ans. (e) Glycogen phosphorylase > (a) Phosphofructokinase 1

Ref: Harper 30th ed page 179

(See table of "Glycogen Storage Disorders" in AIIMS May 2016) (see page no. 218)

Recall Bias

Some students believe that Glycogen Phosphorylase was provided in the options.

Hint to Diagnosis

- Exercise-induced cramps, Rhabdomyolysis is seen in McArdle disease or glycogen storage disorder (GSD) type V and Tarui's disease (GSD type VII)
- If muscle phosphorylase is given in place of Glycogen Phosphorylase then it is the best answer as McArdles is most common glycogen storage disorder in adolescent age. If it is not there then PFK-1 is the answer.
- High muscle glycogen points towards glycogen storage disorder.

Option (B)

Debranching enzyme deficiency is seen in Cori's disease or Forbes' disease (Type III GSD) in which hypoglycemia, hepatomegaly and hyperlipidemia is seen but exercise induced cramps are not seen.

Option (D)

Glucose-6-phosphatase deficiency is seen in von Gierke's disease (GSD Type I) in which hypoglycemia, hepatomegaly and hyperlipidemia is seen but exercise induced cramps are not seen.

10. Ans. (b) 5′ → 3′ exonuclease activity

Ref: Lehringer biochemistry 7th Ed Pg 994

DNA polymerase I protein is a single polypeptide chain, it is folded into 3-D structure that resembles a palm, where the fingers can be closed and opened. The enzyme 928aa long can dimerize in the presence of Hg2+ and the dimerized protein exhibits very high enzyme activity. The NH2-terminal region, nearly at 1/3rd of the polypeptide chain possesses 5′ to 3′ exonuclease activity; it accounts to about 35 KD. This property is unique among known polymerases including both DNA and RNA polymerases. The rest of the fragment (68 KD) is called large fragment or **Klenow fragment.** The NH2 terminal part of the Klenow has 3′ to 5′ exonuclease activity and the rest has 5′ > 3′ polymerase activity. **The Klenow fragment of DNA polymerase I has both the DNA polymerase and 3′ → 5′ exonuclease activities.** Hence, it is widely used in molecular biology.

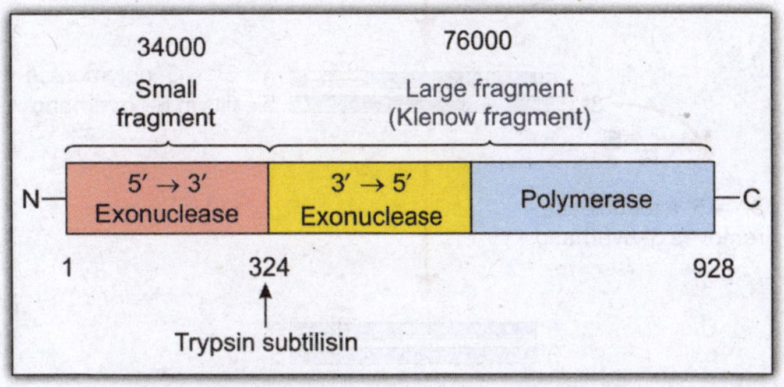

Large **(Klenow) Fragment** is a proteolytic product of E. coli DNA Polymerase I after treatment with protease subtilisin, which retains 5' → 3' polymerase and 3'→ 5' exonuclease activity, but has lost 5'→ 3' exonuclease activity.

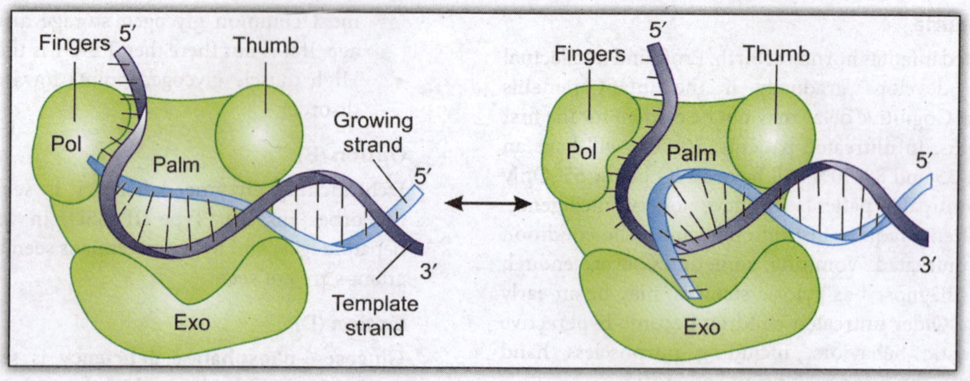

Fig: DNA polymerase I (3D model): Palm, thumb and fingers having specific functions

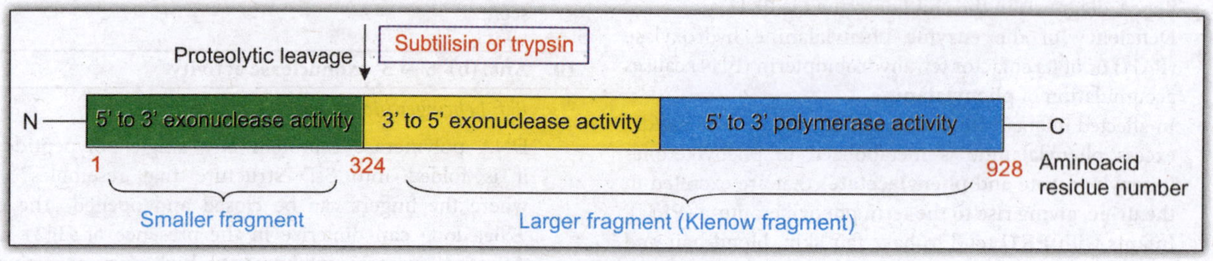

Fig: Smaller larger (Klenow) fragment

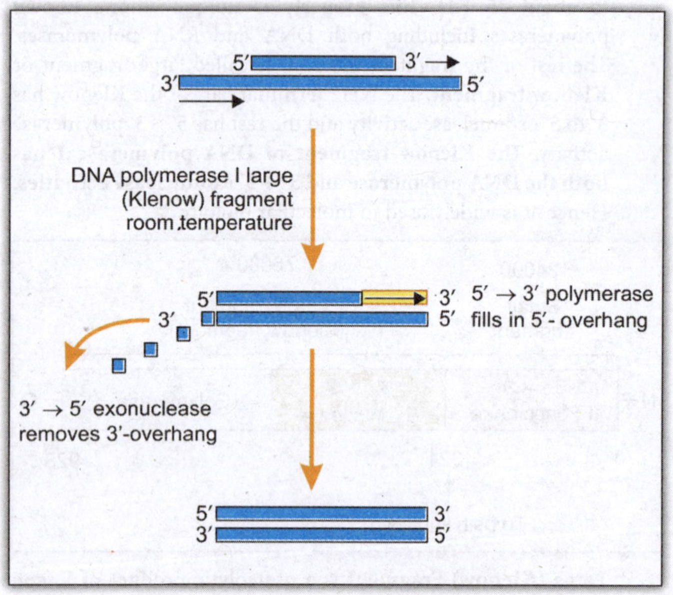

Fig: Applications of Klenow fragment

NOTE

Generally, the products of RNA polymerase II undergo capping. *U6 RNA, though capped on its 5′-end, is transcribed by RNA polymerase III; this is the first report of a capped RNA molecule synthesized by RNA polymerase III.*

(*Ref: https://www.ncbi.nlm.nih.gov/pubmed/3793736*)

Types of RNA Polymerase

RNA polymerase	Synonym	Product
RNA polymerase I	Pol-I	Ribosomal RNA (but not 5S rRNA, which is synthesized by RNA polymerase III)
RNA polymerase II	Pol-II	hnRNA, pri-mRNA, pri-mi-RNA and snRNA
RNA polymerase III	Pol-III	tRNA, U6-snRNA and 5S rRNA

11. Ans. (b) tRNA of Alanine

Ref: With text

In molecular biology, the five-prime cap (5′ cap) is a specially altered nucleotide on the 5′ end of some primary transcripts such as precursor messenger RNA. This process, known as mRNA capping, is highly regulated and vital in the creation of stable and mature messenger RNA able to undergo translation during protein synthesis. Mitochondrial mRNA and chloroplastic mRNA are not capped.

Option (A)

tRNAs typically do not carry any modified 5′-ends or cap structure, as the mature 5-end

Option (B)

The 5′ terminal of mRNA is "capped" by a 7-methylguanosine triphosphate that is linked to an adjacent 2′-O-methyl ribonucleoside at its 5′-hydroxyl through the three phosphates (*Ref: Harper 30th ed page 365*)

Option (C)

miRNA precursors, which are 5′-capped and 3′-polyadenylated, usually range in size from about 500 to 1000 nucleotides.

The majority of miRNAs are transcribed by RNA pol II into primary transcripts termed pri-miRNAs. pri-miRNAs are 5'-capped and 3'-polyadenylated (Harper 30th ed page 409)

Option (D)

The small RNA can be broadly divided into two classes. The 5' end capped small nuclear RNA (sn RNA or U-sn RNA) which is synthesised by RNA polymerase II and 5' ed non capped small cytoplasmic RNA (sc RNA) which is synthesised by RNA polymerase III. The U-snRNAs contain a cap structure on their 5'-ends; except for U6 snRNA, the cap structure contains trimethylguanosine

Flow chart 1: RNA flow chart

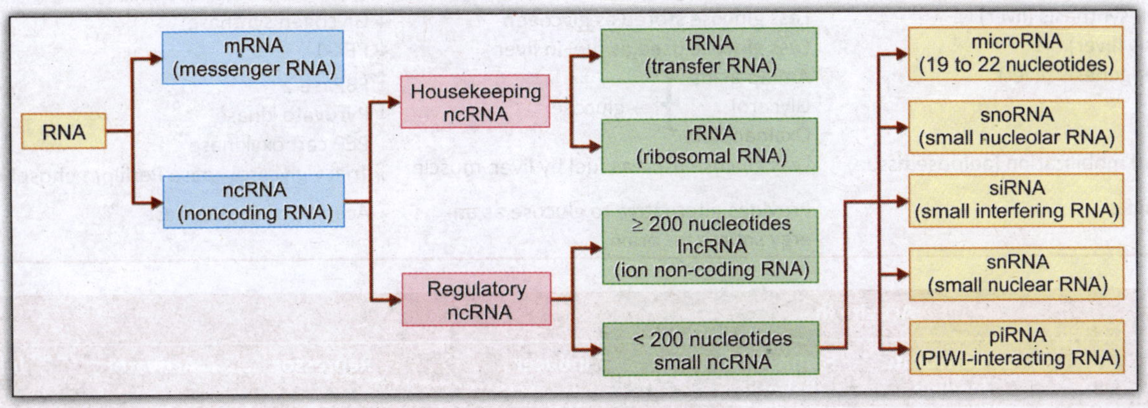

12. Ans. (b) Vitamin B_2

Ref: Harper's 30th Ed Pg 556

- Measurement of erythrocyte glutathione reductase and its activation by FAD is used to assess vitamin B_2 nutritional status.
- Glutathione reductase catalyzes the reduction of glutathione disulfide to the sulfhydryl form glutathione (GSH), which is a critical molecule in resisting oxidative stress and maintaining the reducing environment of the cell.
- Riboflavin is a precursor for FAD, whose reduced form donates two electrons to the disulfide bond which is present in the oxidized form of glutathione reductase in order to begin the enzyme's catalytic cycle.
- Deficiency of Riboflavin is characterized by cheilosis, desquamation and inflammation of the tongue and a seborrheic dermatitis.
- Riboflavin nutritional status is assessed by measurement of the activation of erythrocyte glutathione reductase by FAD added in vitro.

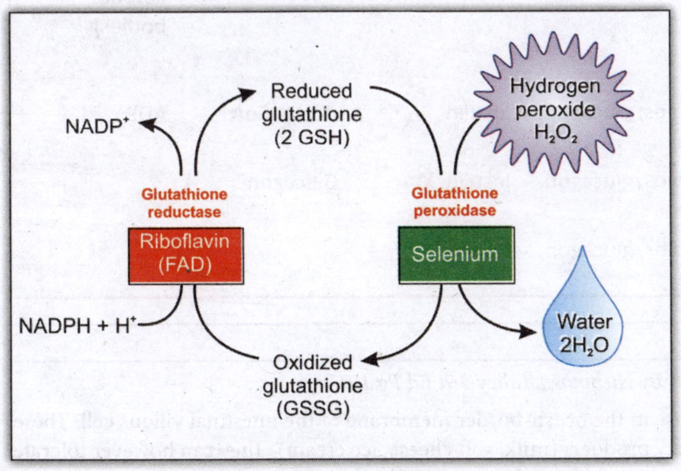

Fig: Role of riboflavin in glutathione cycle

13. Ans. (b) Tandem mass spectrometry

Ref: Tietz 5th Ed Pg 2052

- Metabolic diseases caused by the absence or functional impairment of metabolic enzymes can be devastating.
- Early dietary intervention, however, can in many instances ameliorate the otherwise inevitable dire effects.
- The early detection of such metabolic diseases is of primary importance.
- The powerful and sensitive technique of tandem mass spectrometry can in a few minutes detect over 40 analytes of significance in the detection of metabolic disorders.
- Tandem MS can be used to screen blood samples from newborns for the presence and concentrations of amino acids, fatty acids and other metabolites. Abnormalities in metabolite levels can serve as diagnostic indicators for a variety of genetic disorders, such as phenylketonuria, ethylmalonic encephalopathy and glutaric acidemia type 1.
- With the advent of tandem mass spectrometry, it is now possible to rule out inborn errors of metabolism, especially presymptomatic identification of conditions that cause acute illness in a newborn.
- It is a sensitive technique in which samples can be collected earlier in a newborn (48–72 hours) allowing for diagnosis of many disorders before initial decompensation.

14. Ans. (a) PFK-1

Ref: Lehringer 4th Ed Pg 634, Vasudevan 7th Ed Pg 159

The activity of the enzyme Phosphofructokinase 1 decreases during the fasting state.

Fasting State

- The fuel reserves of a healthy adult human are of three types: glycogen stored in the liver and, in relatively small quantities, in muscles; large quantities of triacylglycerols in adipose tissues; and tissue proteins, which can be degraded when necessary to provide fuel.

- In the first few hours after a meal, the blood glucose level is diminished slightly and tissues receive glucose released from liver glycogen. There is little or no synthesis of lipids.
- By 24 hours after a meal, blood glucose has fallen further, insulin secretion has slowed and glucagon secretion has increased.

Following table depicts the effect of increased glucagon on various enzymes:

Effects of Glucagon on Blood Glucose: Production and Release of Glucose by the Liver		
Metabolic effect	**Effect on glucose metabolism**	**Target enzyme**
↑ Glycogen breakdown (liver) ↓ Glycogen synthesis (liver) ↓ Glycolysis (liver) ↑ Gluconeogenesis (liver)	Glycogen → glucose Less glucose stored as glycogen Less glucose used as fuel in liver Amino acids, Glycerol, Oxaloacetate } → glucose	↑ Glycogen phosphorylase ↓ Glycogen synthase ↓ PFK-1 ↑ FBPase-2 ↓ Pyruvate kinase ↑ PEP carboxykinase
↑ Fatty acid mobilization (adipose tissue)	Less glucose used as fuel by liver, muscle	↑ Triacylglycerol lipase Perilipin phosphorylation
↑ Ketogenesis	Provides alternative to glucose as energy source for brain	↑ Acetyl-CoA carboxylase

	Activity In					
	Carbohydrate feeding	Fasting and diabetes	Inducer	Repressor	Activator	Inhibitor
Glycogenolysis, glycolysis and pyruvate oxidation						
Glycogen synthase	↑	↓			Insulin, glucose 6-phosphate	Glucagon
Hexokinase						Glucagon 6-phosphate
Glucokinase	↑	↓	Insulin	Glucagon		
Phosphofructokinase-1	↑	↓	Insulin	Glucagon	5' AMP, fructose 6-phosphate, fructose 2, 6-bisphosphate, P_1	Citrate, ATP, glucagon
Pyruvate kinase	↑	↓	Insulin, fructose	Glucagon	Fructose 1,6-bisphosphate, insulin	ATP, alanine, glucagon, norepinephrine
Pyruvate dehydrogenase	↑	↓			CoA, NAD^+, Insulin, ADP, pyruvate	Acetyl-CoA, NADH, ATP (fatty acids, ketone bodies)
Gluconeogenesis						
Pyruvate carboxylase	↓	↑	Glucocorticoids, glucagon, epinephrine	Insulin	Acetyl-CoA	ADP
Phosphoenolpyruvate carboxykinase	↓	↑	Glucocorticoids, glucagon, epinephrine	Insulin	Glucagon?	
Glucose 6-phosphatase	↓	↑	Glucocorticoids, glucagon, epinephrine	Insulin		

15. Ans. (a) Yoghurt

Ref: Clinical Gastroenterology: A Practical Problem-Based Approach By Nicholas J Talley 3rd Ed Pg 101

- Lactose intolerance is due to a deficiency of the enzyme lactase in the brush-border membrane of the intestinal villous cell. These patients are not able to digest lactose containing food like dairy products (milk, soft cheese, ice cream). They can however tolerate products like yogurt. Some even tolerate hard cheese which contains minimal amounts of lactose.

- It is manifested by abdominal cramps, borborygmi, bloating, excessive flatus (bacterial fermentation) and diarrhea (osmotic effect) following milk ingestion.
- Primary lactase deficiency is genetically determined and lactose intolerance occurs from late childhood. Secondary lactase deficiency occurs in association with small-intestinal mucosal disease, with abnormalities in both structure and function of other brush border enzymes and transport processes.
- Secondary lactase deficiency is often seen in celiac disease.

16. Ans. (d) TCA cycle

Ref: Harper's 30th Ed Pg 162, 171

- Fluoride released from fluoroacetate inhibits conversion of citrate to cis-aconitate.
- The poison fluorcetate is found in some of plants and their consumption can be fatal to grazing animals.
- Some fluorinated compounds used as anticancer agents and industrial chemicals (including pesticides) are metabolized to fluoroacetate.
- It is toxic because fluoroacetyl-CoA condenses with oxaloacetate to form fluorocitrate, which inhibits aconitase, causing citrate to accumulate.

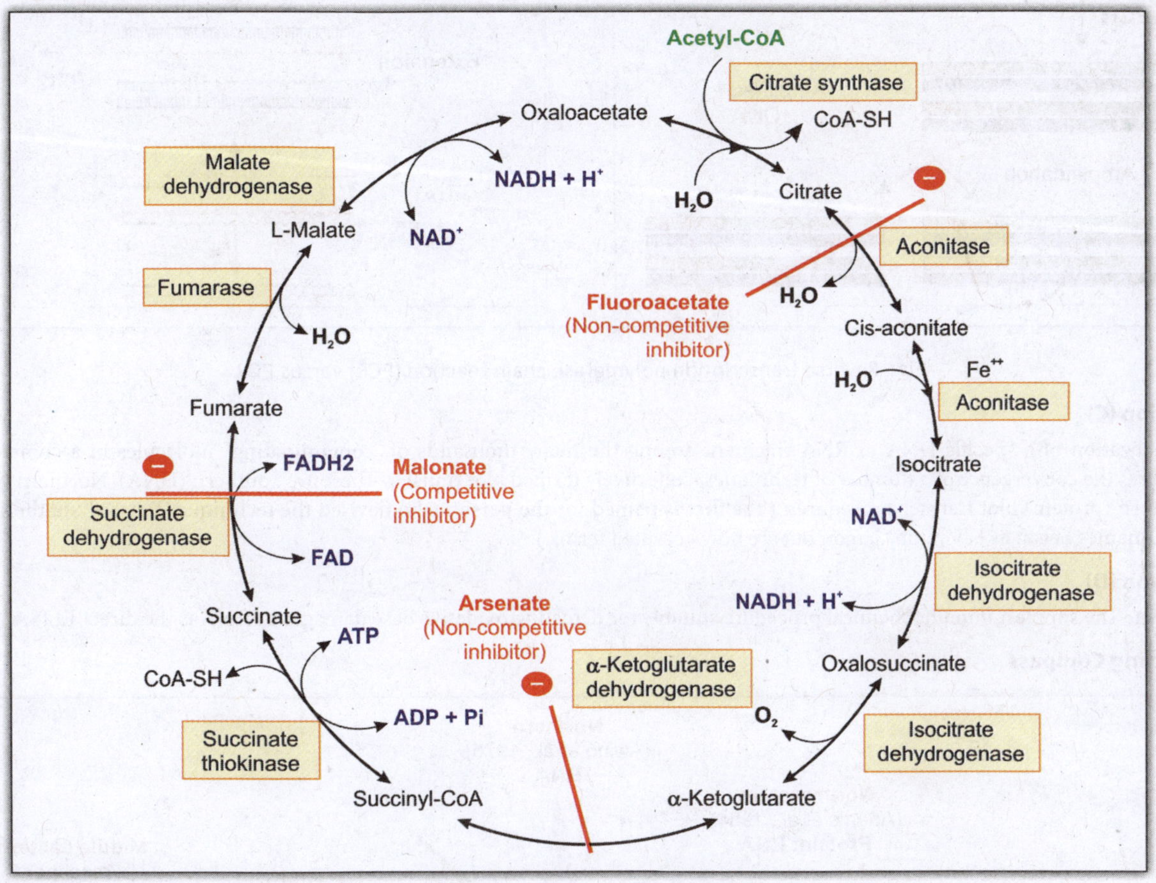

Fig: Inhibitors of citric acid cycle

17. Ans. (b) RT PCR

Ref: Harper's 30th Ed Pg 29, 457, Molecular Pathology in Clinical Practice edited by Debra G.B. Leonard page 26

NOTE

Reverse transcription PCR (RT-PCR) should not be confused with Real time PCR

Option (A)

Sanger sequencing, also known as the chain-termination method, is a technique for DNA sequencing based upon the selective incorporation of chain-terminating dideoxynucleotides (ddNTPs) by DNA polymerase during in vitro DNA replication.

Option (B)

Reverse transcription PCR (RT-PCR) is used when the starting material is RNA. In this method, RNA is first transcribed into complementary DNA (cDNA) by reverse transcriptase from total RNA or messenger RNA (mRNA). Reverse transcription PCR (RT-qPCR) is used when the starting material is RNA. In this method, RNA is first transcribed into complementary DNA (cDNA) by reverse transcriptase from total RNA or messenger RNA (mRNA).

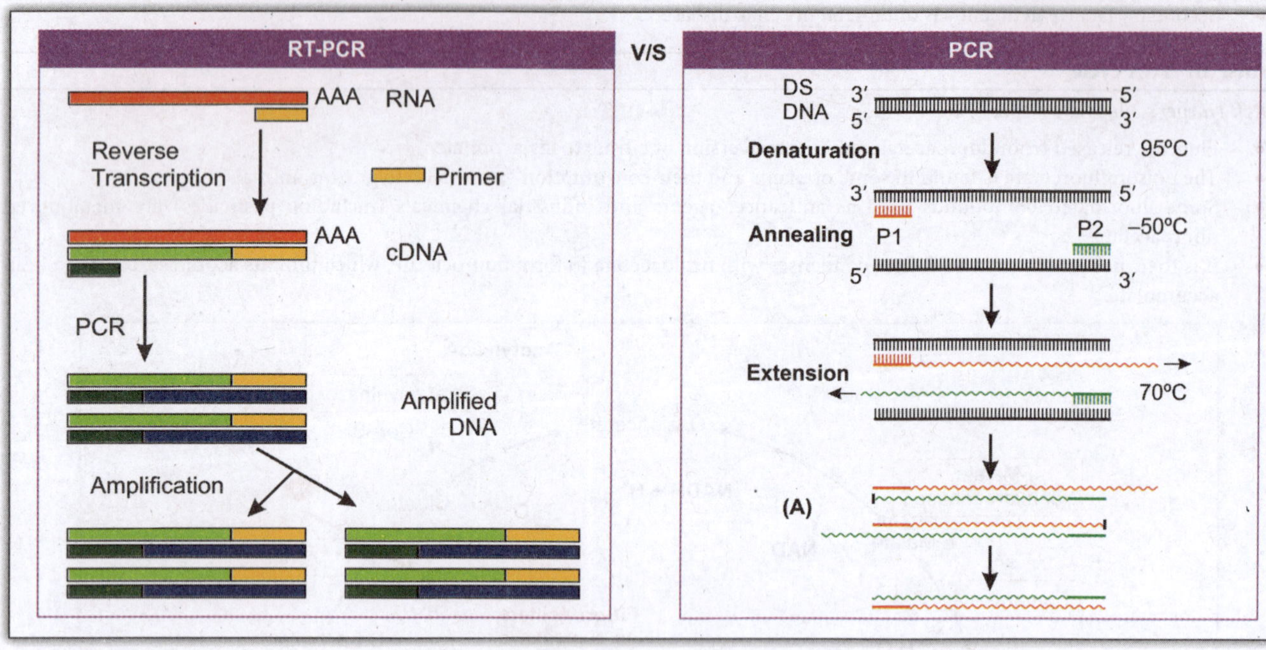

Fig: Reverse transcription polymerase chain reaction (PCR) versus PCR

Option (C)

Visualization of a specific DNA or RNA fragment among the many thousands of "contaminating" molecules in a complex sample requires the convergence of a number of techniques, collectively termed blot transfer. These are Southern (DNA), Northern (RNA) and Western (protein) blot transfer procedures. (The first is named for the person who devised the technique [Edward Southern] and the other names began as laboratory jargon but are now accepted terms.)

Option (D)

ELISA: The simplest immunochemical procedure suitable for detecting oxidative base damages in DNA is the direct ELISA

Blotting Compass

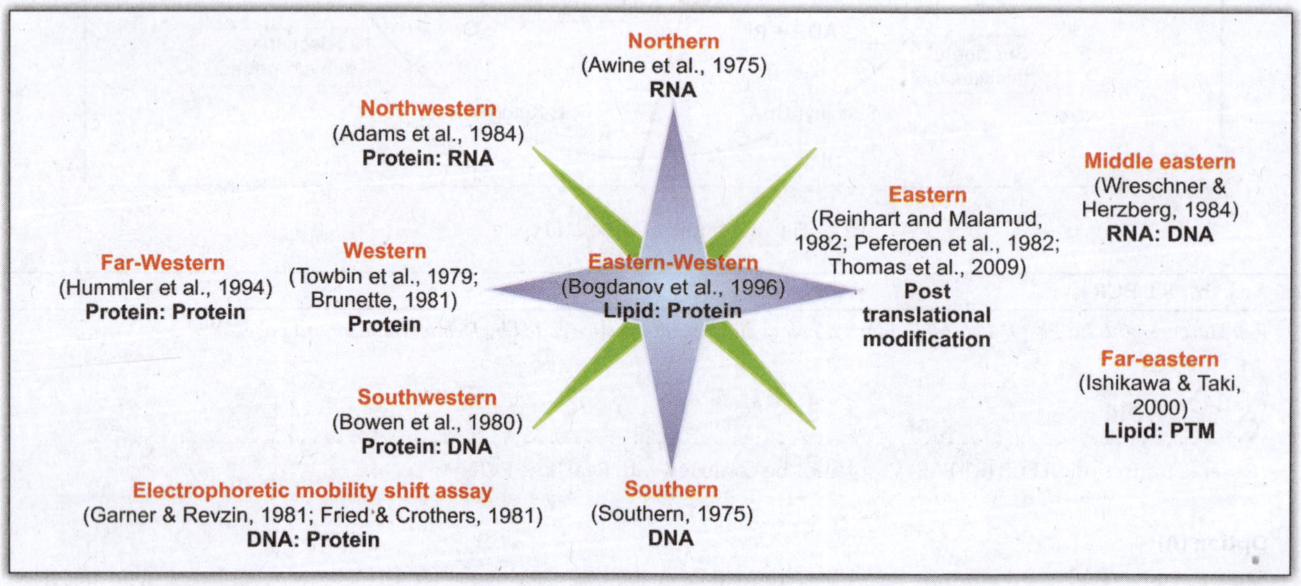

Fig: Blotting compass

18. Ans. (b) HSV causing temporal encephalitis

Ref: Real-Time PCR edited by M Tevfik Dorak page 239

Real-time PCR assays can provide HSV viral load measurements, but their utility in patient management is undefined at present. (*Ref: Clinical Pediatric Dermatology by DM Thappa Page 197*)

Real-time PCR amplification techniques are currently used to determine the viral load in clinical samples for an increasing number of targets and in a short-time.

- Real-time PCR is commonly used for viral load of blood borne viruses like HBV, HCV, HIV
- EBV, CMV and BK virus in transplant patients

19. Ans. (a) Epoxide reductase

Ref: Harper's 30th Ed Pg 555

- Vitamin K is a factor essential for coagulation. About 70% of vitamin K absorbed from the diet is lost to excretion. Therefore, the body's stores of vitamin K are recycled in a process known as the vitamin K cycle.
- In the vitamin K cycle, an endoplasmic reticulum (ER) membrane protein called vitamin K epoxide reductase (VKOR) reduces vitamin K 2,3-epoxide (KO) to vitamin K (K); VKOR is the target of the popular vitamin K antagonist (VKA) drug warfarin, which is widely used to treat thrombosis.

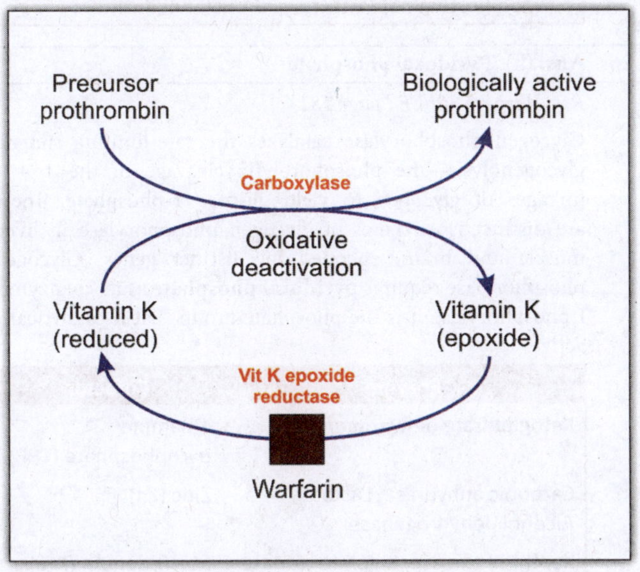

Fig: Vitamin K cycle

20. Ans. (a) L-gluconolactone oxidase

Ref: Vasudevan 7th Ed Pg 135

- Ascorbic acid is produced in some animals by the uronic acid pathway due to the presence of the enzyme L-gluconolactone oxidase.
- However, humans lack this enzyme and cannot synthesize vitamin C.
- Hence, vitamin C is an essential vitamin.

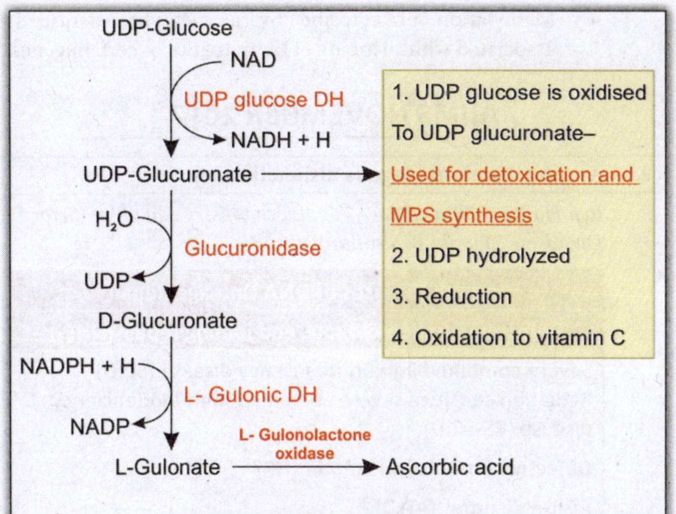

Oxidation of glucose

21. Ans. (c) Vitamin C

Ref: Harper's 30th Ed Pg 541, Davidson's Principles and Practice of Medicine by Brian R. Walke 22nd Ed Pg 24

Gastric acidity, Vitamin C, Amino acids aid the absorption of iron form the gut, while phytates, tannins and phosphate containing foods inhibit iron absorption.

Gastric acidity is required to release iron from food and helps to keep iron in the soluble ferrous state.

Factors Affecting IRON Absorption

Enhancers:	Inhibitors:
Vitamin C	Tannins
Cooking in iron vessels	Phosphates
Gastric acid	Oxalates
Cysteine	Milk
Sugar	Antacids
Amino acid	Calcium
Lactate	Tetracyclines
Pyruvate	Phytates

22. Ans. (a) Methylation

Ref: Harper's biochemistry 30th Ed Pg 560

Let us first go through a few terms that have been used in and related to the above question:

- Euchromatin: ***Transcriptionally active*** chromatin stains less densely and is referred to as euchromatin.
- Heterochromatin: ***transcriptionally inactive*** chromatin which is densely packed during interphase
- A CpG Island is a stretch of DNA with a high quantity of the nucleotides G and C next to one another. CpG islands typically occur at or near the transcription start site of genes, particularly housekeeping genes.
- Epigenetic changes are biochemical changes that affect chromatin structure and thereby gene expression without actually altering the DNA sequence itself. DNA methylation is one such epigenetic change. It causes methylation of Cytosine residues in CpG islands.
- Methylation of cytosine forms 5' methylcytosine.

- Methylation of cytosine by a methyltransferase is associated with silencing of the activities of certain genes.

AIIMS NOVEMBER 2017

23. Ans. (c) Nonhomologous disjunction repair

Ref: Harper's 30th ed page 762, Biochemistry edited by Victor L. Davidson, Donald B. Sittman page 135

Human Diseases of DNA Damage Repair
Defective nonhomologous end joining repair (NHEJ)
Severe combined immunodeficiency disease (SCID) Radiation sensitive severe combined immunodeficiency disease (RS-SCID)
Defective homologous repair (HR)
AT-like disorder (ATLD) Nijmegen breakage syndrome (NBS) Bloom syndrome (BS) Werner syndrome (WS) Rothmund-Thomson syndrome (RTS) Breast cancer susceptibility 1 and 2 (BRCA1, BRCA2)
Defective DNA nucleotide excision repair (NER)
Xeroderma pigmentosum (XP) Cockayne syndrome (CS) Trichothiodystrophy (TTD)
Defective DNA base excision repair (BER)
MUTYH-associated polyposis (MAP) Defective DNA Mismatch Repair (MMR) Hereditary non-polyposis colorectal cancer (HNPCC)

24. Ans. (c) Von Gierke disease

Ref: Harper 30th ed page 179, 355

Triad of Hypoglycemia, Hyperlipidemia and Hepatomegaly along with Lactic acidosis is suggestive of Von Gierke's disease. Cori's disease also has triad of Hypoglycemia, Hyperlipidemia and Hepatomegaly but without lactic acidosis.

(See Table of "Glycogen Storage Disorders" Biochemistry AIIMS May 2016) (see page no. 218)

25. Ans. (a) Selenocysteine

Ref: Harper 30th ed page 16, 18, 286

Selenocysteine (21st Amino acid- encoded by UGA) and Pyrrolysine (22nd Amino acid-encoded by UAG) are encoded by stop codons by Co Translational modification not Post translational modification.

Selenocysteine the 21st AMINO Acid

- It is an L-α-amino acid found in a handful of proteins called selenoproteins
- Selenocysteine has a structure similar to that of cysteine, but with an atom of selenium taking the place of the usual sulfur, forming a selenol group which is deprotonated at physiological pH. The pK_3 of selenocysteine, 5.2, is 3 units lower than that of cysteine.

Contd...

Selenocysteine the 21st AMINO Acid

- Unlike other amino acids present in biological proteins, selenocysteine is not coded for directly in the genetic code. Instead, it is encoded in a special way by a **UGA codon**, which is normally a stop codon. Such a mechanism is called translational recoding and its efficiency depends on the selenoprotein being synthesized and on translation initiation factors. Since selenocysteine is inserted into polypeptides during translation, it is commonly referred to as the "21st amino acid."
- The UGA codon is made to encode selenocysteine by the presence of aSECIS element (**SElenoCysteine Insertion Sequence**) in the mRNA.
- Selenocysteine is present in several enzymes (for example **glutathione peroxidases, tetraiodothyronine 5' deiodinases, thioredoxin reductases, formate dehydrogenases, glycine reductases, selenophosphate synthetase 1, methionine-R-sulfoxide reductase B1 (SEPX1)** and some hydrogenases

Footnote:

- **Pyrrolysine,** sometimes considered **"the 22nd amino acid"** is encoded in a special way by a UAG codon, which is normally a stop codon. It is not used by humans
- Selenocysteine (21st Amino acid- encoded by UGA) and Pyrrolysine (22nd Amino acid-encoded by UAG) are encoded by stop codons by Co Translational modification not Post translational modification.

26. Ans. (b) Pyridoxal phosphate

Ref: Harper's 30th Ed page 181

Glycogen phosphorylase catalyzes the rate-limiting step in glycogenolysis—the phosphorolytic cleavage of the 1 – 4 linkages of glycogen to yield glucose 1-phosphate. There are distinct isoenzymes of glycogen phosphorylase in liver, muscle and brain, encoded by distinct genes. Glycogen phosphorylase requires **pyridoxal phosphate** as its coenzyme. I phosphorylase it is the phosphate group that it catalytically active.

Enzyme	Cofactor
Ketoglutarate dehydrogenase	Thiamine pyrophosphate (TPP)
Carbonic anhydrase, Lactate/ Alcohol dehydrogenase	Zinc (Zn)
Xanthine oxidase, Sulphite oxidase	Molybdenum (Mo)
Glutathione peroxidase	Selenium (Se)
Amine oxidase, Superoxide dismutase, Cytochrome oxidase, Tyrosinase	Copper (Cu)
Kinase, peptidase	Magnesium (Mg)
Hydrolase, decarboxylase, transferase	Manganese (Mn)
Hb and cytochrome	Iron (Fe)
Carboxylation	Biotin
Transamination	Pyridoxine
Glycogen Phosphorylase	Pyridoxal Phosphate

27. Ans. (b) Only B is seen

Ref: Harper 30th ed page 207, 230, Textbook of Biochemistry for Medical Students By Vasudevan- 8th ed Page 209

Free fatty acid and Ketone bodies rises on starvation. Hence (B) Rothera's test for ketone bodies will be positive. Acetoacetate is the primary ketone body. Beta hydroxy butyric acid and acetone are secondary ketone bodies. Ketosis is seen in diabetes mellitus and starvation. During prolonged starvation, ketone bodies are the major fuel source for the brain and other parts of central nervous system.

Plasma Concentrations of Metabolic Fuels (mmol/L) in the Fed and Fasting States			
	Fed	40 hours fasting	7 Days starvation
Glucose	5.5	3.6	3.5
Free fatty acids	0.30	1.15	1.19
Ketone bodies	Negligible	2.9	4.5

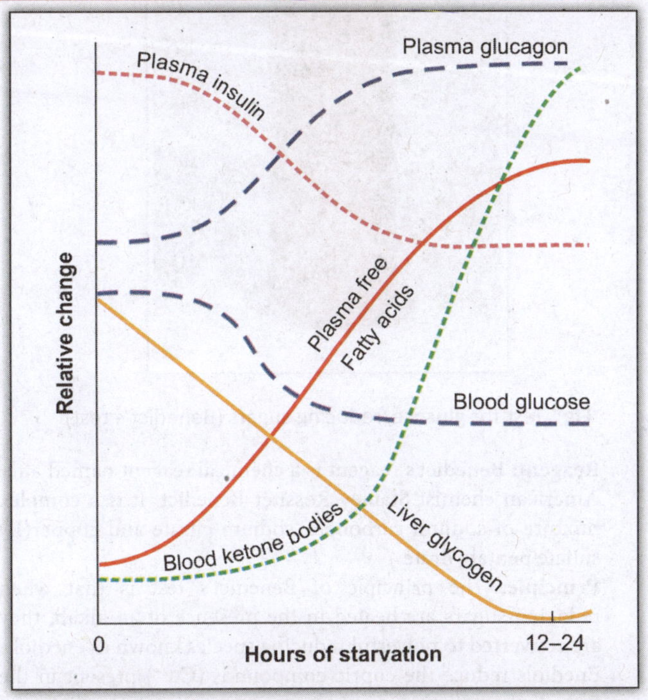

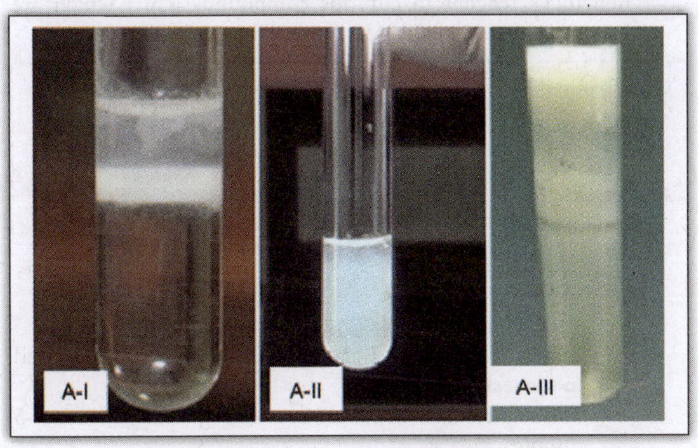

Fig: (A) Urine protein test

It can be done by several methods.

- **Heller's ring test reagent:** Concentrated nitric acid is taken in a test tube and few drops of Urine sample is added to the test tube by sliding down through an angle along the inner side of the test tube. A white ring is formed at the point of contact (white ring of denatured protein) indicating the presence of albumin in the sample
- **Urine protein sulfosalicylic acid precipitation test (SSA):** This technique provides a more quantitative estimate of all the proteins present in the urine, including both albumin and the low molecular weight proteins.
  - **Principle:** This test is performed by mixing one-part urine supernatant with three parts 30% sulfosalicylic acid. The acidification causes precipitation of protein in the sample (seen as increasing turbidity), which is subjectively graded as trace, 1+, 2+, 3+ or 4+. Unlike the routine urine protein chemistry dipstick pad, the SSA reaction will detect globulin and Bence-Jones proteins, in addition to albumin and essentially detects all urinary proteins. (although it is more sensitive to albumin).
  - **Procedure:** 1. Pour a small amount of urine into a test tube 2. Add 30% SSA into the tube directly on top of the urine drop by drop 3. Shake tube gently with a quick flick and read for turbidity immediately indicating presence of protein
- **Heating and acetic acid test:** Proteins are coagulated by heat in acidic urine and do not dissolve on acidification. Whereas, phosphates and carbonates which are also precipitated by heating are dissolved in acid. Heated upper half shows precipitate and lower half is used as control for comparison.

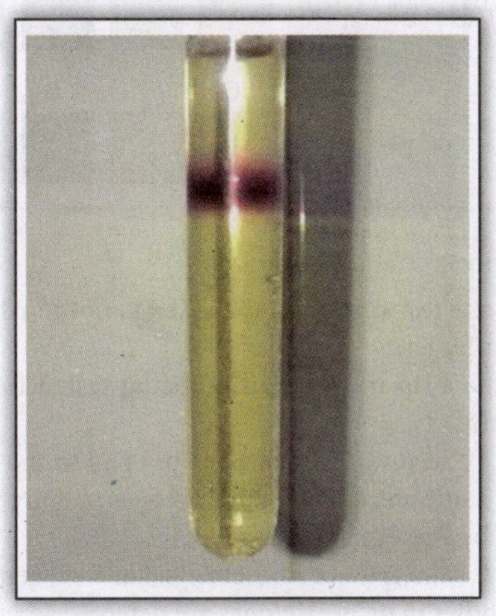

Fig: (B) Test for ketone bodies (Rothera's test)

Method

- Take 5 mL of urine in a test tube and saturate it with ammonium sulfate.
- Add a small crystal of sodium nitroprusside. Mix well.
- Slowly run along the side of the test tube liquor ammonia to form a layer.
- Immediate formation of a purple permanganate colored ring at the junction of the two fluids indicates a positive test

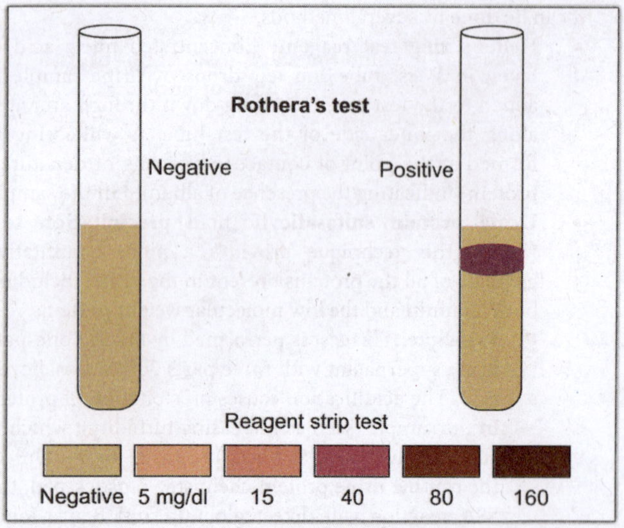

Fig: Rothera's tube test and reagent strip test for ketone bodies in urine. Rothera's test is sensitive to 1-5 mg/dL of acetoacetate and to 10-25 mg/dL of acetone. Reagent strips tests are modifications of nitroprusside test with sensitivity of 5-10 mg/dL of acetoacetate

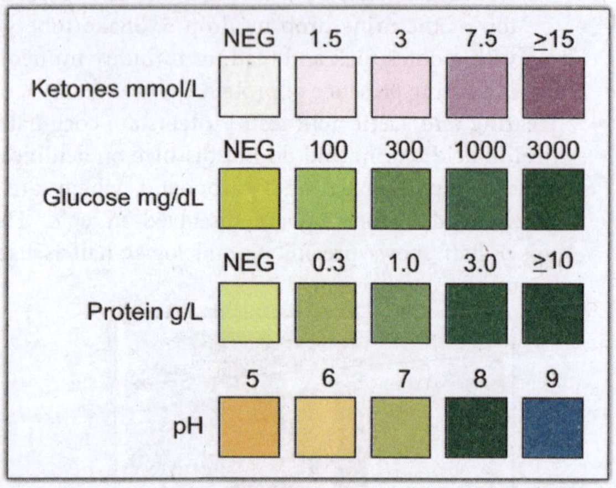

Instructions

Remove one test strip from the vial. Do not touch the test pads with your fingers.

Dip the strip in to the urine being tested for 1-2 seconds and remove.

After 10 seconds, compare the pH pad to the color chart.

After 1 minute, compare the Ketones pad to the color chart, followed by Protein and Glucose.

Principle: Principles of Rothera's test and reagent strip test for ketone bodies in urine. Ketones are detected as acetoacetic acid and acetone but not β-hydroxybutyric acid. Acetoacetic acid or acetone reacts with nitroprusside in alkaline solution to form a purple-colored complex.

Rothera's test

Acetoacetate + Sodium nitroprusside $\xrightarrow{\text{Alkaline pH}}$ Purple color

Reagent strip test

Acetoacetate + Sodium nitroprusside + Glycine $\xrightarrow{\text{Alkaline pH}}$ Purple color

NOTE

Ketone bodies in urine = β-hydroxybutyric acid 78%, acetoacetic acid 20% and acetone 2%. No method for detection of ketonuria reacts with all the three ketone bodies because β-hydroxybutyric acid is not detected by any of the screening tests. Rothera's test and Dipstick test (Modified Rothera) and detect acetoacetic acid and acetone (the test is 10-20 times more sensitive to acetoacetic acid than acetone). Ferric chloride test detects acetoacetic acid only.

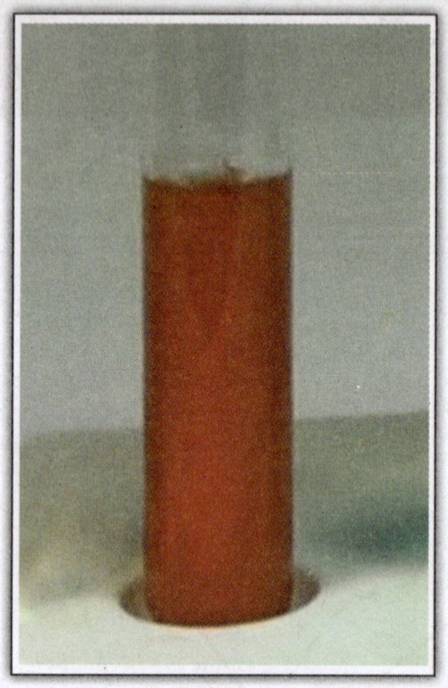

Fig: Test for glucose/reducing sugars (Benedict's test)

Reagent: Benedict's reagent is a chemical reagent named after American chemist Stanley Rossiter Benedict. It is a complex mixture of sodium carbonate, sodium citrate and copper(II) sulfate pentahydrate

Principle: The principle of Benedict's test is that when reducing sugars are heated in the presence of an alkali, they are converted to powerful reducing species known as enediols. Enediols reduce the cupric compounds (Cu^{2+}) present in the Benedict's reagent to cuprous compounds (Cu^{+}) which are precipitated as insoluble red copper(I) oxide(Cu_2O).

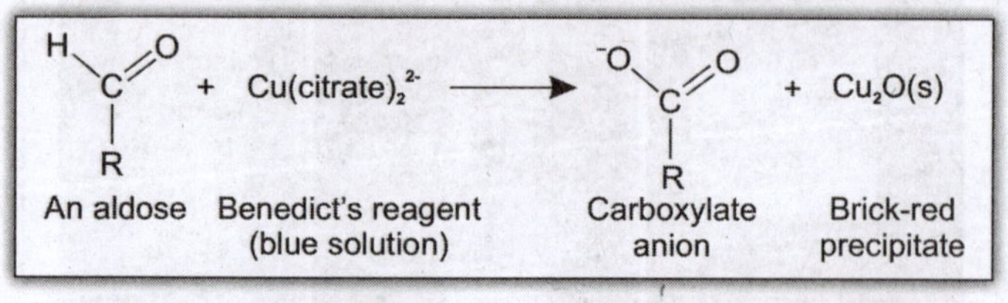

Procedure

- 1 mL of urine sample is placed into a test tube.
- 2 mL (10 drops) of Benedict's reagent ($CuSO_4$) is added in the test tube.
- The solution is then heated in a boiling water bath for 3–5 minutes.
- Observe for color change in the solution of test tubes or precipitate formation.

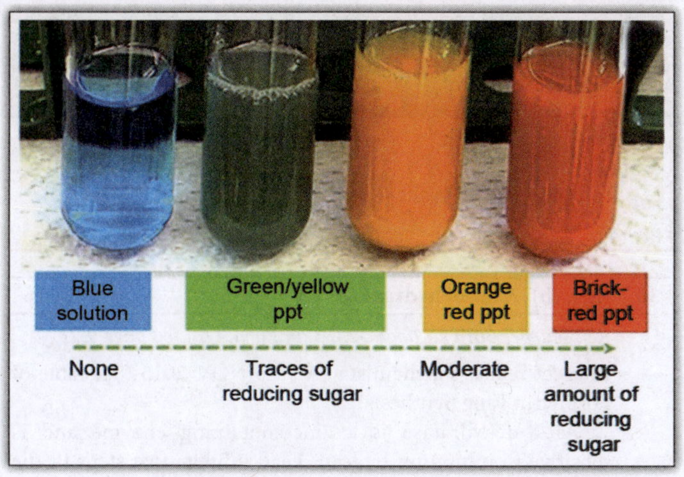

Fig: Interpretation of Benedict's test:

The color of the obtained precipitate gives an idea about the quantity of sugar present in the solution, hence the test is semi-quantitative.

- Greenish precipitate = 0.1 to 0.5 g% sugar in solution
- Yellow precipitate = 0.5 to 1 g% sugar in solution
- Orange precipitate = 1 to 1.5 g% sugar in solution
- Red precipitate = 1.5 to 2.0 g% sugar in solution
- Brick red means > 2 g% sugar in solution

28. Ans. (c) Hydrogen bond

Ref: Harper 30th ed page 360-361

Summary

Backbone of DNA is connected by Covalent 3' 5' Phosphodiester bond

Bases are connected by weak Hydrogen Bonds

DNA Structure

In 1953 Watson and Crick postulated a three-dimensional model of DNA structure. It is in the form of a right-handed double helix, the shape of which is maintained by hydrogen bonding between organic bases Nucleic acids (DNA and RNA) are polymers of nucleotides, joined together by phosphodiester linkages between the 5-hydroxyl group of one pentose and the 3-hydroxyl group of the next. There are two types of nucleic acid: RNA and DNA. The nucleotides in RNA contain ribose and the common pyrimidine bases are uracil and cytosine. In DNA, the nucleotides contain 2-deoxyribose and the common pyrimidine bases are thymine and cytosine. The primary purines are adenine and guanine in both RNA and DNA. A nucleotide consists of a nitrogenous base (purine or pyrimidine), a pentose sugar and one or more phosphate groups. The four types of nitrogen bases are adenine (A), thymine (T), guanine (G) and cytosine (C). The purine and pyrimidine bases of both strands are stacked inside the double helix, with their hydrophobic and nearly planar ring structures very close together and perpendicular to the long axis. The offset pairing of the two strands creates a major groove and minor groove on the surface of the duplex.

Watson and Crick found that the hydrogen-bonded base pairs, G with C and A with T (or U), are those that fit best within the structure, providing a rationale for Chargaff's rule that in any DNA, G = C and A = T. Hydrogen bonds between bases permit a complementary association of two (and occasionally three or four) strands of nucleic acid. ***Between cytosine and guanine bases there are three hydrogen bonds. Between adenine and thymine bases there are only two hydrogen bonds.***

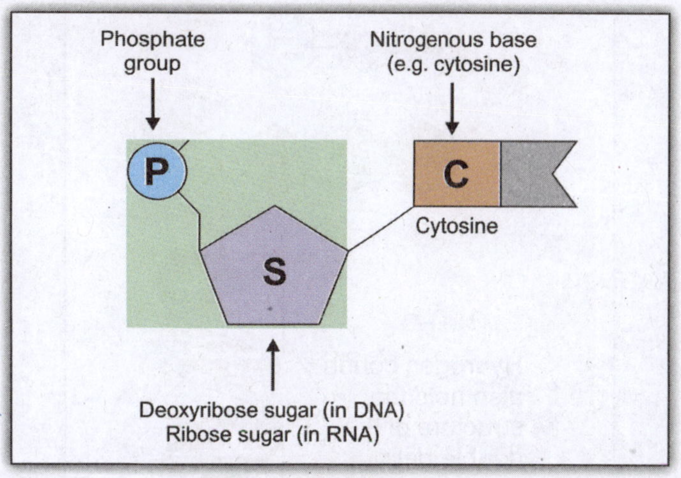

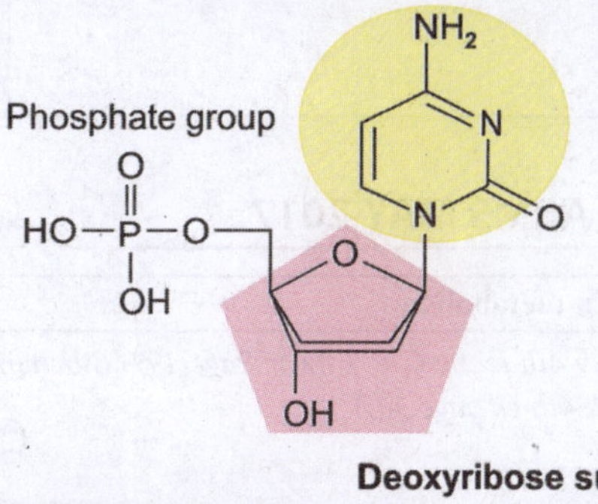

Molecular structure
A nucleotide with cytosine as the nitrogenous base. You do not need to be able to draw this molecular structure, it is here for reference only

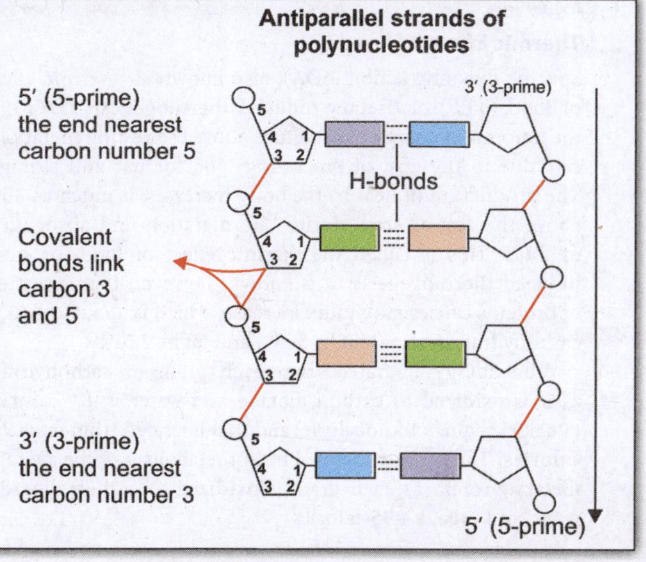

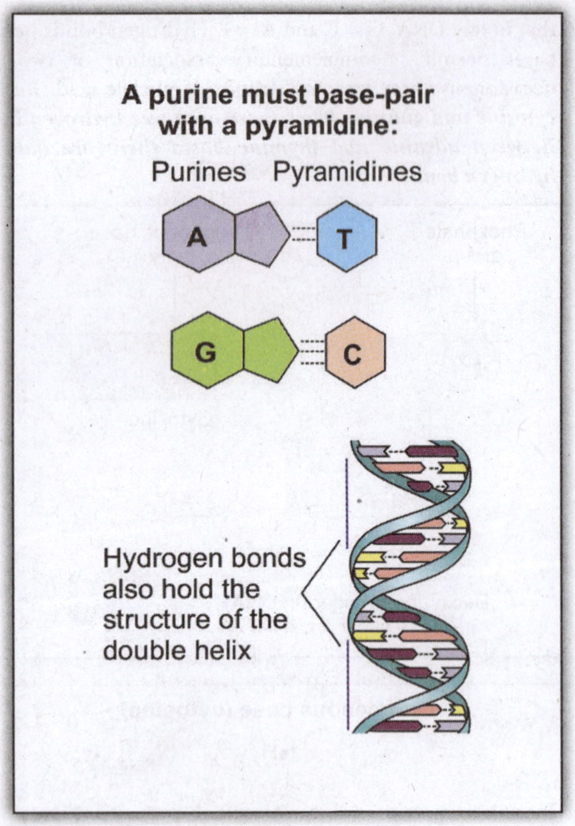

AIIMS MAY 2017

29. Ans. (c) Protein metabolism

Ref: Biochemistry 4th ed By G P Talwar Page 497, Biochemistry By Pankaja Naik 4th ed page 347

NOTE

Diet induced Thermogenesis (DIT) is different from Respiratory Quotient. Question of Respiratory Quotient was asked in Biochemistry AIIMS NOV 2016. (Q. 41 for exp. see page no. 205)

Thermic Effect of Food

Specific dynamic action (SDA), also known as Thermic effect of food (TEF) or **dietary induced thermogenesis (DIT)**, is the amount of energy expenditure above the resting metabolic rate due to the cost of processing food for use and storage. The production of heat by the body increases as much as 30% above the resting level during the digestion and absorption of food. This is called the thermic effect of food, or diet-induced thermogenesis. It is known, however, that ingestion of proteins causes maximum increase, which is about 20–30%, carbohydrates increase it by 5–6% and fat by 2.5–4%.

The energy liberated from each gram of carbohydrate as it is oxidized to carbon dioxide and water is 4.1 calories (1 calorie equals 1 kilocalorie) and that liberated from fat is **9.3 calories.** The energy liberated from metabolism of the average dietary protein as each gram is oxidized to carbon dioxide, water and urea is 4.35 calories.

Calories of Food Components

Food	Average absorption	Respiratory quotient	Calories	Diet induced thermogenesis
Carbohydrate	98%	1	4	5–6%
Fat	95%	0.7	9	2.5–4%
Protein	92%	0.8	4	20–30%

30. Ans. (b) ALA dehydratase

Ref: Harper 30th ed page 325, 329, Parikh 6th ed page 9.22

Indirect repeat Biochemistry AIIMS NOV 2015 (See table of Porphyrin Ring Synthesis)

ALA dehydratase is a zinc-containing enzyme and is sensitive to inhibition by lead. Lead inhibits two steps in the heme synthetic pathway. ALA dehydratase and ferrochelatase. Ferrochelatase sensitivity to lead is the greatest and thus the most significant in lead poisoning.

31. Ans. (b) Vitamin B_2

Ref: Harper's 30th ed page 346, Harrison's 18th Ed, Ch: 74

NOTE

Although peripheral neuropathy (tingling etc) is not characteristic of B_2-Riboflavin deficiency it can be seen. Low glutathione reductase points to riboflavin deficiency.

Glutathione reductase is one of two RBC enzymes requiring riboflavin for its activation. Erythrocyte glutathione is present in at least two forms, an active form associated with flavin adenine dinucleotide (FAD) and an inactive form not bound to FAD, which can be activated in vitro by additional extraneous FAD. The FAD is derived from riboflavin via flavin mononucleotide (FMN). It has been demonstrated that measurement of both active and inactive forms of glutathione reductase may have a clinical value in the assessment of nutritional status of riboflavin.

Riboflavin

- Biologically active forms: FAD, FMN
- FMN and FAD are bound tightly, sometimes covalently, to flavoenzymes (for example, NADH dehydrogenase [FMN] and succinate dehydrogenase [FAD]) that catalyze the oxidation or reduction of a substrate.
- Enzymes that contain flavin adenine dinucleotide (FAD) or flavin mononucleotide (FMN) as prosthetic groups are known as flavoenzymes (e.g., succinic acid dehydrogenase, monoamine oxidase, glutathione reductase). FAD is a cofactor for methyl tetrahydrofolate reductase and therefore, modulates homocysteine metabolism. The vitamin also plays a role in drug and steroid metabolism, including detoxification reactions.
- **Riboflavin deficiency** is manifested principally by lesions of the mucocutaneous surfaces of the mouth and skin. Magenta tongue, angular stomatitis, seborrhea, cheilosis. In addition to the mucocutaneous lesions, corneal vascularization, anemia, personality changes

and peripheral neuropathy have been described with riboflavin deficiency.
- Riboflavin deficiency almost always is due to dietary deficiency.
- **Sources**: Milk, other dairy products and enriched breads and cereals are the most important dietary sources of riboflavin. Lean meat, fish, eggs, broccoli and legumes are also good sources.
- **Storage:** Riboflavin is extremely sensitive to light and milk should be stored in containers that protect against photodegradation.
- **Laboratory diagnosis** of riboflavin deficiency can be made by measurement of red blood cell or urinary riboflavin concentrations or by measurement of erythrocyte glutathione reductase activity, with and without added FAD. Because the capacity of the gastrointestinal tract to absorb riboflavin is limited (20 mg if given in one oral dose), riboflavin toxicity has not been described.

32. Ans. (a) Glycogen storage

Ref: Harper 30th Ed page 230

Indirect Repeat Biochemistry AIIMS Nov 2013

Elevated insulin level results in overall increased glycogenesis and decreased glycogenolysis, whereas an elevated glucagon, or epinephrine, level causes increased glycogenolysis and decreased glycogenesis.

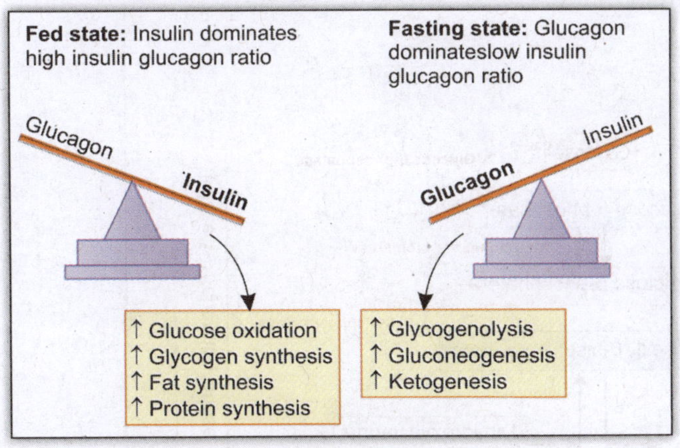

33. Ans. (d) GATTAC/CATTAG

Ref: Lippincott 6th Ed page 840

Restriction enzymes act on **palindromic sequences.** To be a palindrome, both strands must have the same sequence when read in the 5 → 3 direction. Of the options given only option D GATTAC/CATTAG is a palindrome.

Restriction endonucleases are bacterial enzymes that cleave double-stranded DNA (dsDNA) into smaller fragments. Each enzyme cleaves at a specific four to eight–base pair sequence (a restriction site), producing DNA segments called restriction fragments. The sequences that are recognized are palindromic. Restriction enzymes form either staggered cuts (sticky ends) or blunt-end cuts on the DNA.

34. Ans. (d) Less than 20% respiratory chain proteins codes from mDNA

Ref: Harper's 29th Ed page 609

Mitochondrial DNA

- The majority of the polypeptides in mitochondria (about 54 out of 67) are coded by nuclear genes, while the rest are coded by genes found in mitochondrial (mt) DNA.
- Human mitochondria contain 2–10 copies of a small circular dsDNA molecule that makes up approximately 1% of total cellular DNA. This mtDNA codes for mt-specific ribosomal and transfer RNAs and for 13 proteins that play key roles in the respiratory chain
- It is circular, double-stranded and composed of heavy (H) and light (L) chains or strands
- Contains 16,569 bp
- Encodes 13 protein subunits of the respiratory chain (of a total of about 67)
  - Seven subunits of NADH dehydrogenase (complex I)
  - Cytochrome b of complex III
  - Three subunits of cytochrome oxidase (complex IV)
  - Two subunits of ATP synthase
- Encodes large (16S) and small (12S) mt ribosomal RNAs
- Encodes 22 mt tRNA molecules
- Genetic code differs slightly from the standard code
  - UGA (standard stop codon) is read as Trp
  - AGA and AGG (standard codons for Arg) are read as stop codons
- Contains very few untranslated sequences
- **High mutation rate** (5 to 10 times that of nuclear DNA)
- Comparisons of mtDNA sequences provide evidence about evolutionary origins of primates and other species
- An important feature of human mitochondrial mtDNA is that—because all mitochondria are contributed by the ovum during zygote formation—it is transmitted by maternal non-mendelian inheritance

Let us review the options now.

Option (A) False

mDNA contains 16569 base pairs

Option (B) False

Mitochondrial DNA has high mutation rates.

Option (C) False

It is only inherited from mother

Option (D) True

Mitochondrial DNA codes 13/67 = 19.4% of respiratory chain proteins.

35. Ans. (c) Its coenzyme for pyruvate and alpha ketoglutarate dehydrogenase.

Ref: Harper 30th ed Page 555

Thiamine has a central role in energy-yielding metabolism and especially the metabolism of carbohydrates. Thiamine diphosphate is the coenzyme for three multienzyme complexes that catalyze oxidative decarboxylation reactions:

- Pyruvate dehydrogenase in carbohydrate metabolism
- Ketoglutarate dehydrogenase in the citric acid cycle
- Branched-chain keto-acid dehydrogenase involved in the metabolism of leucine, isoleucine and valine
- In each case, the thiamine diphosphate provides a reactive carbon on the thiazole moiety that forms a carbanion, which then adds to the carbonyl group, e.g. pyruvate. The

addition compound is then decarboxylated, eliminating CO_2. Thiamine diphosphate is also the coenzyme for transketolase, in the pentose phosphate pathway.

- Thiamine pyrophosphate (TPP) is the biologically active form of the vitamin, formed by the transfer of a pyrophosphate group from adenosine triphosphate (ATP) to thiamine. TPP serves as a coenzyme in the formation or degradation of α-ketols by transketolase and in the oxidative decarboxylation of α-keto acids.
- The oxidative decarboxylation of pyruvate and α-ketoglutarate, which plays a key role in energy metabolism of most cells, is particularly important in tissues of the CNS. In thiamine deficiency, the activity of these two dehydrogenase-catalyzed reactions is decreased, resulting in decreased production of ATP and, therefore, impaired cellular function. TPP is also required by branched-chain α-keto acid dehydrogenase of muscle. It is the decarboxylase of each of these α-keto acid dehydrogenase multienzyme complexes that requires TPP.
- Thiamine deficiency is diagnosed by an increase in erythrocyte transketolase activity observed on addition of TPP.

36. Ans. (d) Glycogen > (a) Fructose

Ref: Medical Biochemistry at a Glance 3rd ed By J. G. Salway page 42

Anaerobic Glycolysis Yield of ATP

Reaction	Glucose ATP yield	Glycogen ATP yield	Fructose (F1P pathway)-Major	Fructose (F6P pathway)
Hexokinase	−1 ATP	NA	NA	NA
Phosphofructokinase 1	−1 ATP	−1 ATP	NA	−1 ATP
Fructokinase	NA	NA	−1 ATP	NA
Triose kinase	NA	NA	−1 ATP	NA
Phosphoglycerate kinase	+2 ATP	+2 ATP	+2 ATP	+2 ATP
Pyruvate kinase	+2 ATP	+2 ATP	+2 ATP	+2 ATP
Net ATP	+2 ATP	+3 ATP	+2 ATP	+3 ATP

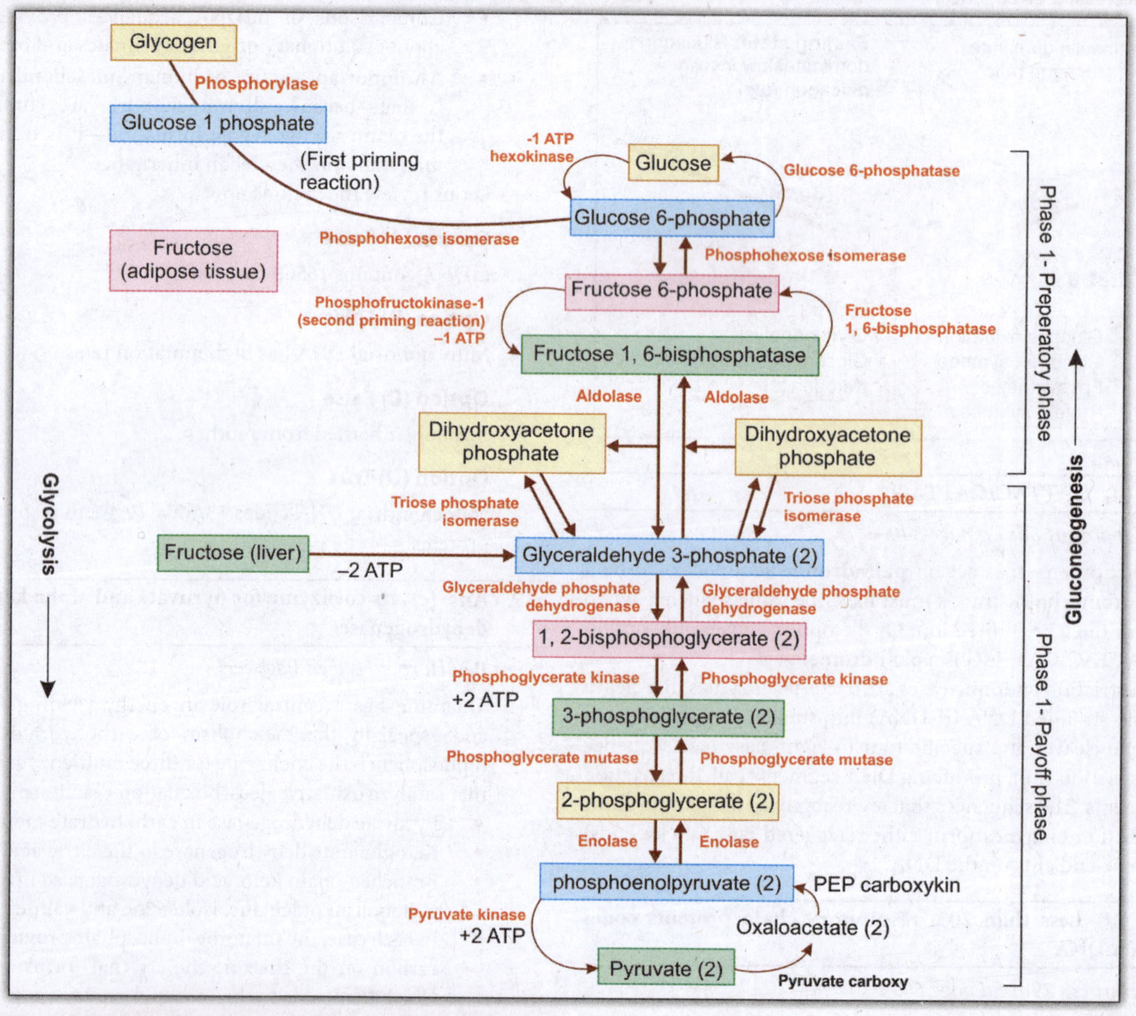

Anaerobic glycolysis, in which lactic acid is the end product, occurs in cells that lack mitochondria and in cells deprived of sufficient oxygen.

- Glucose can be metabolised to generate a net total of two molecules of ATP in the absence of oxygen, i.e. anaerobically. This initially needs the investment of ATP for each of the hexokinase and phosphofructokinase reactions. Fructose 6-phosphate is eventually split into two molecules of glyceraldehyde 3-phosphate, which when oxidised by glyceraldehyde 3-phosphate dehydrogenase yields 2 NADH. Two molecules of ATP are produced by 3-phosphoglycerate kinase and another two molecules of ATP are made in the pyruvate kinase reaction. Under aerobic conditions, NADH is oxidised by the respiratory chain to recycle RAU for the glyceraldehyde 3-phosphate dehydrogenase reaction. However, under anaerobic conditions lactate dehydrogenase causes NADH to reduce pyruvate and NAD is recycled for glyceraldehyde 3-phosphate dehydrogenase. The lactate goes to the liver and forms glucose by gluconeogenesis in the Cori cycle.
- When glycogen is the source of glucose 6-phosphate, the net yield is 3 molecules of ATP.
- Fructose can follow two pathways.

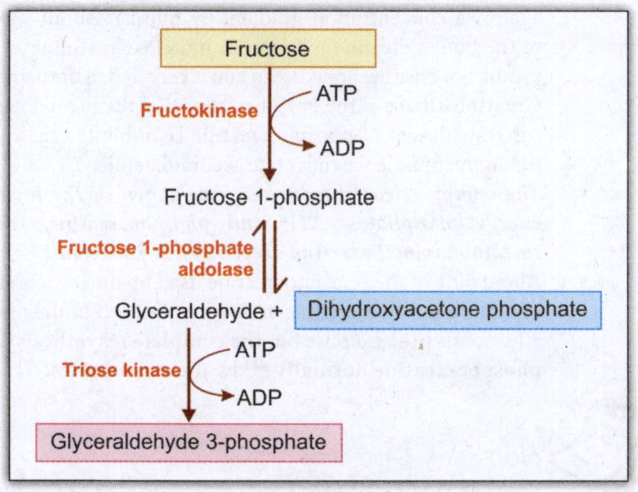

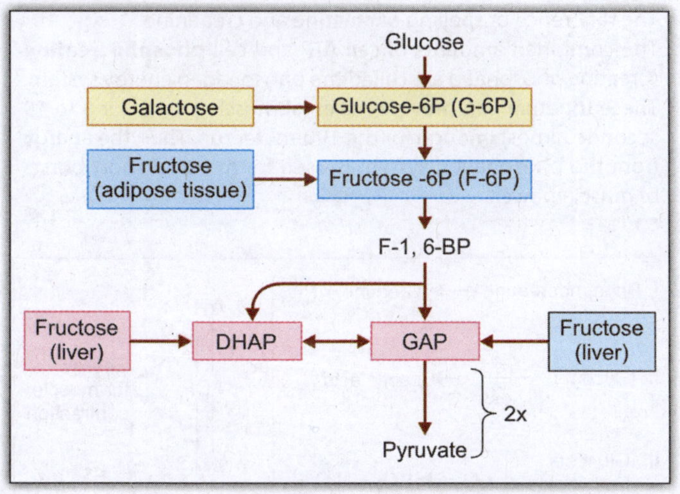

1. Much of the ingested fructose is metabolized by the liver, using the fructose 1-phosphate pathway. The first step is the phosphorylation of fructose to fructose 1-phosphate by fructokinase. Fructose 1-phosphate is then split into glyceraldehyde and dihydroxyacetone phosphate, an intermediate in glycolysis. This aldol cleavage is catalyzed by a specific fructose 1-phosphate aldolase. Glyceraldehyde is then phosphorylated to glyceraldehyde 3-phosphate, a glycolytic intermediate, by triose kinase.
2. Alternatively, fructose can be phosphorylated to fructose 6-phosphate by hexokinase

37. Ans. (a) Pyruvate to oxaloacetate

Ref: Vasudevan Biochemistry 7th ed page 253

Reactions such as the catabolism of some amino acids generate intermediates of TCA cycle and are called anaplerotic ("filling up") reactions.

Four reactions are classed as anaplerotic, although the production of oxaloacetate from pyruvate is probably the most important physiologically. The anaplerotic reactions are:

- Carboxylation of pyruvate to oxaloacetate (malate can be formed similarly, though thermodynamics favor the reaction malate to pyruvate)
  pyruvate + CO_2 + H_2O + ATP → pyruvate carboxylase → oxaloacetate + ADP + P_i + 2H+
- Transamination of aspartate to oxaloacetate by aspartate aminotransferase, which allows incorporation of acetyl CoA into citrate via citrate synthase in glyoxysomes.
- Hydration of glutamate to α-ketoglutarate glutamate + NAD + H_2O → glutamate-dehydrogenase → NH_4^+ + α-ketoglutarate + NADH + H+
- β-oxidation of fatty acids to succinyl-CoA

38. Ans. (d) Increases renal excretion of ammonia

Ref: Lippincott 6th Ed page 471

Phenylbutyrate and sodium benzoate are orphan drugs approved for the treatment of hyperammonemia in patients with urea cycle disorders. Phenylbutyrate is a prodrug that is metabolized to phenylacetate, which is the active molecule that combines with glutamine to form phenylacetylglutamine which is rapidly excreted by the kidneys and does not require metabolism via the urea cycle. Phenylbutyrate thus provides an **"ammonia sink"**, an alternative pathway for excretion of excess nitrogen and ammonia. The active metabolite phenylacetate is also effective therapeutically, but has a disagreeable odor and taste that affect compliance and acceptability.

Congenital Hyperammonemia

- Genetic deficiencies of each of the five enzymes of the urea cycle have been described, with an overall incidence estimated to be 1:25,000 live births. X-linked **ornithine transcarbamoylase deficiency** is the most common of these disorders, predominantly affecting males, although female carriers may become symptomatic.
- All of the other urea cycle disorders follow an autosomal recessive inheritance pattern. In each case, the failure to synthesize urea leads to hyperammonemia during the first weeks following birth.
- Treatment included restriction of dietary protein in the presence of sufficient calories to prevent catabolism. Administration of compounds that bind covalently to amino acids, producing nitrogen-containing molecules that are excreted in the urine, has improved survival. For example, phenylbutyrate given orally is converted to

phenylacetate. This condenses with glutamine to form phenylacetylglutamine, which is excreted.

39. Ans. (d) Increased activity of hormone sensitive lipase and decreased activity of lipoprotein lipase

Ref: Clinical Biochemistry Metabolic and Clinical Aspects By William J. Marshall, Márta Lapsley, Andrew Day, Ruth Ayling 3rd ed page 290

Diabetes is strongly associated with abnormalities of lipid metabolism and several mechanisms are postulated

- Obesity and body fat distribution linked to DM in itself is a cause of dyslipidemias.
- Nonenzymatic glycation of apolipoprotein impairs lipoprotein clearance.
- Insulin is the principal antilipolytic regulator, through its inhibition of **hormone-sensitive lipase.** HSL breaks down Triglycerides TG) and mobilizes fat stores. HSL is regulated by insulin, its most active in fasting state and least active in fed state. In DM this regulation is decreased or lost and stored fat breakdown is carried out even if food is available (This leads to body fat loss). ***Free fatty acid are metabolised by Beta oxidation but once it exceeds the capacity of oxidation its re-esterified to TG and VLDL.***
- **Lipoprotein lipase** levels are low in diabetes because of low insulin. This leads to low lipoprotein degradation in adipose tissue. This leads to increased levels of plasma chylomicrons and VLDL levels.

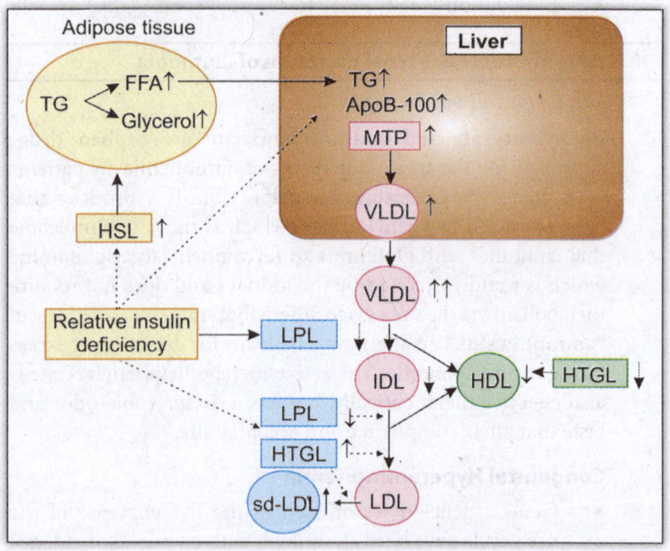

AIIMS NOVEMBER 2016

40. Ans. (a) Phosphocreatine breakdown

Ref: Harper 30th ed chapter 30, Guyton 12th ed page 1033,

Creatinine is formed in muscle from creatine phosphate by irreversible, nonenzymatic dehydration and loss of phosphate Phosphocreatine can easily provide enough energy to reconstitute the high-energy bond of ATP. Furthermore, most muscle cells have two to four times as much phosphocreatine as ATP

- The ATP store in muscle is limited and can only supply energy in high intensity exercise (which has a high demand for ATP) for about ***2 seconds***. Thus, means of resynthesizing ATP must be activated very rapidly after the onset of exercise.
- ***Phosphocreatine breakdown is the most rapid method*** available to resynthesize ATP. The *next fastest is glycolysis* followed by aerobic metabolism in the tricarboxylic acid cycle (Krebs' cycle). Glycogenolysis is the breakdown of glycogen to glucose phosphates and does not generate ATP directly.
- In general, the higher the intensity of exercise, the greater the proportional contribution of **anaerobic energy production** (ATP resynthesis via phosphocreatine breakdown and glycolysis that does not involve the use of oxygen). The TCA cycle and electron transport are components of the aerobic metabolism that takes place in the mitochondria and requires the presence of oxygen.
- Phosphocreatine in the muscle cell is found only in the cytoplasm (also known as the cytosol or sarcoplasm).
- Creatine is synthesized from the amino acids ***glycine, arginine and methionine (energy for playing GAMe)*** in the liver. It is released into the circulation and taken up against a concentration gradient by muscle. About 95% of the body's creatine is found in muscle. Creatinine is a product of creatine breakdown and is excreted in the urine. **Creatine kinase** is the enzyme catalyzing the breakdown (or resynthesis) of phosphocreatine (is inhibited by low pH in the muscle when lactate accumulate!!!!!)
- ***The energy released from the breakdown of the high-energy phosphates, ATP and phosphocreatine, can sustain maximal exertion exercise for 5-10 seconds.***
- About 50% of the phosphocreatine used up during a bout of high intensity exercise can be resynthesized in the first 30 seconds post-exercise but **the complete resynthesis of phosphocreatine normally takes about 4 minutes.**

NOTE

The difference of spelling of creatine and creatinine

The combined amounts of cell ATP and cell **phosphocreatine** (Creatine phosphate) are called the phosphagen energy system. These together can provide maximal muscle power for 8 to 10 seconds, almost enough for the 100-meter run. Thus, the energy from the phosphagen system is used for maximal short bursts of muscle power.

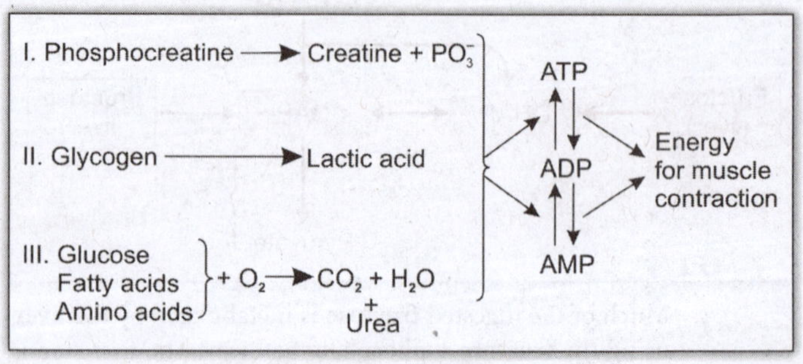

Moles of ATP/min	
Phosphagen system	4
Glycogen-lactic acid system	2.5
Aerobic system	1

41. Ans. (c) 1

Ref: Harper 30th ed page 148, Guyton's 11th ed page 867

"Respiratory quotient" is the ratio of CO_2 production to O_2 utilization and can be used to estimate fat and carbohydrate utilization.

Respiratory Quotient	
Carbohydrate	1
Fat	0.70
Protein	0.80

The RQ of carbohydrate is 1.00 and that of fat is about 0.70. For a person on a normal diet consuming average amounts of carbohydrates, fats and proteins, the average value for R.Q = 0.825. The RQ of the brain is regularly 0.97–0.99, indicating that its principal but not its only fuel is carbohydrate

- ***In a healthy adult, on a mixed diet, it is 0.85.***
- ***In case of carbohydrate diet, RQ is 1 (one).***

Because in carbohydrate diet, the volume of CO_2 produced is the same as the volume of O_2 consumed.

Explanation

This is due to the fact that in carbohydrate molecule, the amount of O_2 present is just sufficient to oxidise the H present in the same molecule. Hence, external O_2 is necessary only to convert the C of the molecule to CO_2 so that the volume of O_2 consumed and the volume of CO_2 produced will be same.

$C_6H_{12}O_6 + \mathbf{6\,O_2} = \mathbf{6\,CO_2} + 6\,H_2O$

RQ for carbohydrate = CO_2 produced/O_2 consumed = 6/ 6 = 1

- ***More than 1 (here1.2) of RQ*** value is seen in heavy carb diets as excess carb is converted to fats in liver (lipogenesis via acetyl coA generated from pyruvate)*(overfeeding syndromes)*
- ***When carbohydrates are converted into fats in the body, RQ will rise.***

Explanation

In this process, an O_2-rich substance is converted into an O_2-poor compound, so that some amount of O_2 liberated from carbohydrates will be utilised for purposes of oxidation. Consequently, less O_2 will be needed from outside. ***Hence, the amount of CO_2 produced will be more than the amount of O_2 consumed.*** So that RQ will rise and will be considerably elevated.

- A reversal of the above process, i.e. conversion of fats to carbohydrate, would lower the RQ below 0.7. This has been reported but has not been generally confirmed. It is, therefore, evident that RQ value will indicate the following:
- ***The type of foodstuffs burning in the body, or***
- ***The nature of conversion of one foodstuff into another in the body.***

Other causes of RQ > 1

Clinical Aspects

- **In acidosis:** During acidosis, CO_2 output is greater than O_2 consumption, hence RQ increases in acidosis.
- **In alkalosis:** In this RQ will fall, because respiration is depressed and CO_2 will be retained in the body, i.e. less CO_2 is produced.
- **In febrile conditions:** It may increase RQ. Rise of body temperature such as in high fever, will cause increased breathing and thereby will wash out more CO_2, hence CO_2 production increases.
- **In diabetes mellitus:**
  - In advanced cases of Diabetes mellitus, when little carbohydrate is burning, energy is supplied mainly by oxidation of fats. Hence RQ will fall.
  - In such cases, when Insulin is administered, carbohydrates will start burning and RQ will rise.
- **In starvation:** Here the subject has to live on its own body tissues.
  - In the first stages (initial 1 to 2 days), energy is derived mainly from the stored glycogen so that the RQ although it falls below normal 0.85, is proportionately high 0.78.
  - But later on, when energy is derived chiefly from the combustion of fats, RQ will fall still further and will be about 0.7.
- ***With violent exercise:*** Lactic acid enters blood and produces acidosis, as a result pulmonary ventilation will be increased, washing out more CO_2. Consequently, RQ rises and **may go above 2 even**.
  - During recovery from violent exercise: RQ falls, because less CO_2 is evolved. Gradually it goes back to normal.

42. Ans. (c) Apoprotein

Ref: Harper 30th Ed page 254, Lehninger 4th ed page 821

Highest amount of TG- chylomicron, VLDL
Highest amount of cholesterol - LDL
Highest amount of protein- HDL

Major Classes of Human Plasma Lipoproteins: Some Properties						
		Composition (wt %)				
Lipoprotein	Density (g/mL)	Protein	Phospholipids	Free cholesterol	Cholestery esters	Triacylglycerols
Chylomicrons	<1.006	2	9	7	3	85
VLDL	0.95–1.006	10	18	7	12	50
LDL	1.006–1.063	23	20	8	37	10
HDL	1.063–1.210	55	24	2	15	4

Remember

Points to remember about HDL

- Smallest of all lipoproteins (5 nm)
- Most dense of all lipoproteins
- Made of 50% proteins (Two major apoproteins of HDL are designated as **apo-A-I** and **apo-A-II**. In addition to above, HDL also contains apo-C-I, C-II and C-III.
- HDL is synthesized and secreted from both liver and intestine
- A major function of HDL is to act as a repository for the apo C and apo E required in the metabolism of chylomicrons and VLDL
- Nascent HDL consists of discoid phospholipid bilayers containing apo A and free cholesterol. These lipoproteins are similar to the particles found in the plasma of patients with a deficiency of the plasma enzyme lecithin: cholesterol acyltransferase (LCAT) and in the plasma of patients with obstructive jaundice.
- LCAT—and the LCAT activator apo A-I—bind to the discoidal particles and the surface phospholipid and free cholesterol are converted into cholesteryl esters and lysolecithin. The nonpolar cholesteryl esters move into the hydrophobic interior of the bilayer, whereas lysolecithin is transferred to plasma albumin. Thus, a nonpolar core is generated, forming a spherical, pseudomicellar HDL covered by a surface film of polar lipids and apolipoproteins. This aids the removal of excess unesterified cholesterol from lipoproteins and tissues.
- **Reverse cholesterol transport:** The class B scavenger receptor B1 (SR-B1) has been identified as an HDL receptor with a dual role in HDL metabolism. In the liver and in steroidogenic tissues, it binds HDL via apo A-I and cholesteryl ester is selectively delivered to the cells, although the particle itself, including apo A-I, is not taken up. In the tissues, on the other hand, SR-B1 mediates the acceptance of cholesterol effluxed from the cells by HDL, which then transports it to the liver for excretion via the bile (either as cholesterol or after conversion to bile acids) in the process known as reverse cholesterol transport.
- **HDL cycle**: HDL3, generated from discoidal HDL by the action of LCAT, accepts cholesterol from the tissues via the SR-B1 and the cholesterol is then esterified by LCAT, increasing the size of the particles to form the less dense HDL2. HDL3 is then reformed, either after selective delivery of cholesteryl ester to the liver via the SR-B1 or by hydrolysis of HDL2 phospholipid and triacylglycerol by hepatic lipase and endothelial lipase. This interchange of HDL2 and HDL3 is called the HDL cycle
- Pre BETA-HDL is the most potent form of HDL inducing cholesterol efflux from the tissues.

Reverse Cholesterol Transport

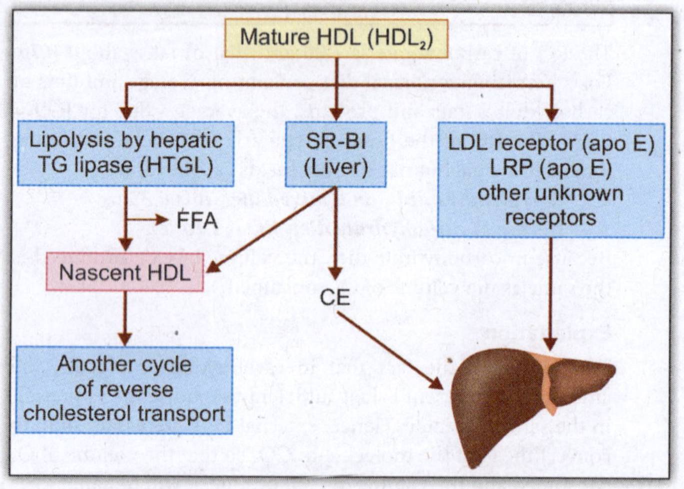

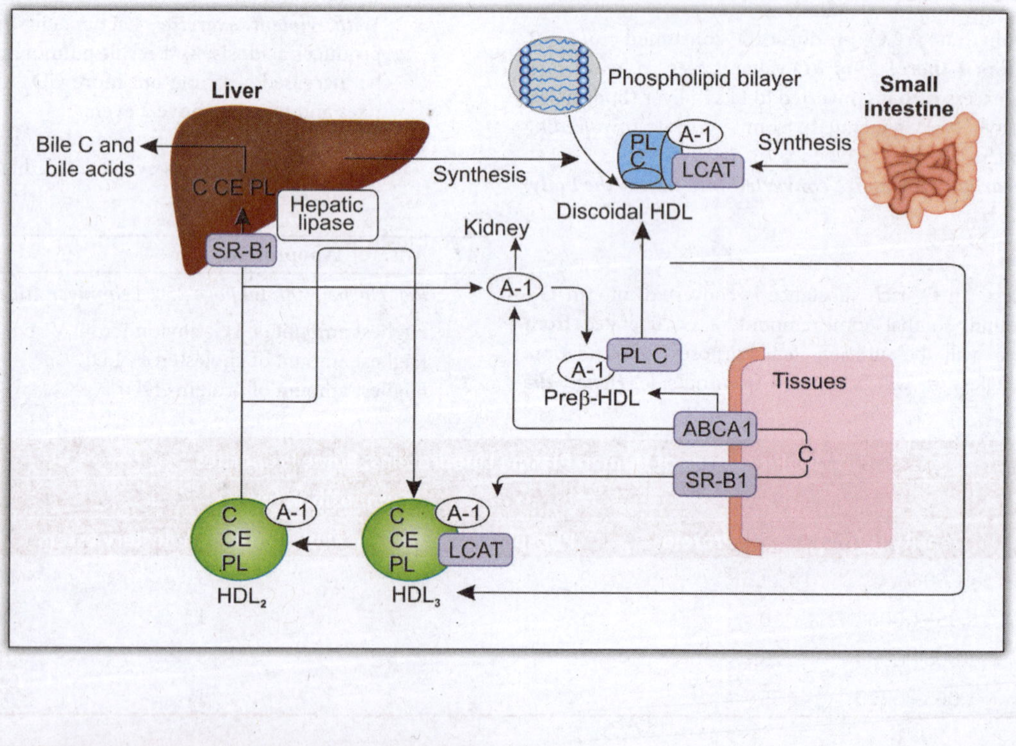

43. Ans. (a) Niacin

Ref: Harper 30th ed page 556, Lippincott 6th Ed page 695

Harper says, ***"Niacin was discovered as a nutrient during studies of pellagra. It is not strictly a vitamin since it can be synthesized in the body from the essential amino acid tryptophan"***

Points to remember about Niacin

- 60 mg of tryptophan = 1 mg of niacin
- Nicotinic acid (niacin) has long been used for the treatment of lipid disorders and cardiovascular disease. Niacin directly and noncompetitively ***inhibits hepatocyte diacylglycerol acyltransferase-2***, a key enzyme for triglyceride synthesis. The inhibition of triglyceride (TG) synthesis by niacin results in accelerated intracellular hepatic Apo B degradation and the decreased secretion of VLDL and LDL particles. Inhibition of TG synthesis by niacin results in reversal of fatty liver.
- Pellagra 3D order is dermatitis à diarrhea à dementia.
- Niacin is found in unrefined and enriched grains and cereal; milk; and lean meats, especially liver.
- Two compounds, nicotinic acid and nicotinamide, have the biologic activity of niacin; its metabolic function is as the nicotinamide ring of the coenzymes NAD and NADP in oxidation/reduction reactions.

Remember

Vitamin K_2, Biotin and Pantothenic acid are synthesized by intestinal bacteria.

44. Ans. (b) Galactose

Ref: Nelson's 20th Ed Ch 87

Benedict's test is used as a simple test for reducing sugars. A reducing sugar is a carbohydrate possessing either a free aldehyde or free ketone functional group as part of its molecular structure. This includes all monosaccharides (eg. glucose, fructose, galactose) and many disaccharides, including lactose and maltose. Reducing sugars under alkaline condition tautomerise and form enediols. Enediols are powerful reducing agents. They can reduce cupric ions (Cu^{2+}) to cuprous form (Cu^{+}), which is responsible for the change in color of the reaction mixture. This is the basis of Benedict's test. When the conditions are carefully controlled, the colorations developed and the amount of precipitate formed (Cuprous oxide) depends upon the amount of reducing sugars present.

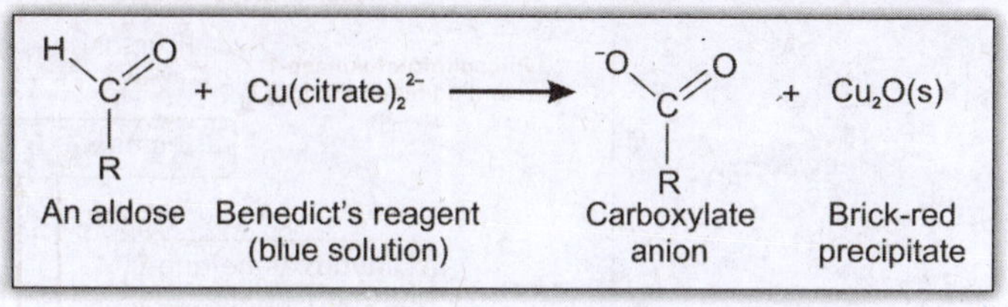

Principle of Glucose Oxidase Test

- Glucose turns into gluconic acid and hydrogen peroxide in the presence of glucose oxidase enzyme.
- Second reaction is: Gluconic acid + 4-aminoantipyrene + 4 - hydroxy benzoic acid → Quinone-imine dye+ water
- The reaction is catalyzed by peroxidase. Glucose oxidase test is specific for glucose, while Benedict's test gives only the presence of reducing sugars.
- **"Test materials relying on the action of glucose oxidase give a negative test for galactose, since glucose oxidase is specific for glucose and is nonreactive with galactose."**

45. Ans. (b) Acetyl-CoA activates pyruvate carboxylase

Ref: Harper 30th ed page 185, Lehninger 4th Ed page 906

Gluconeogenesis is the process of synthesizing glucose from noncarbohydrate precursors such as, lactate, amino acids and glycerol.

During starvation: *Due to excess lipolysis in the adipose tissue, Acetyl-CoA accumulates in the liver. Acetyl-CoA allosterically activates Pyruvate carboxylase resulting in enhanced glucose production. (Ref: Satyanarayana 4th ed page 263)*

Regulation of gluconeogenesis: Hormone glucagon and availability of substrate mainly regulate Gluconeogenesis. The key controlling effect of gluconeogenesis is exerted by the first enzyme of the pathway, Pyruvate carboxylase. This enzyme is allosterically activated by Acetyl CoA.

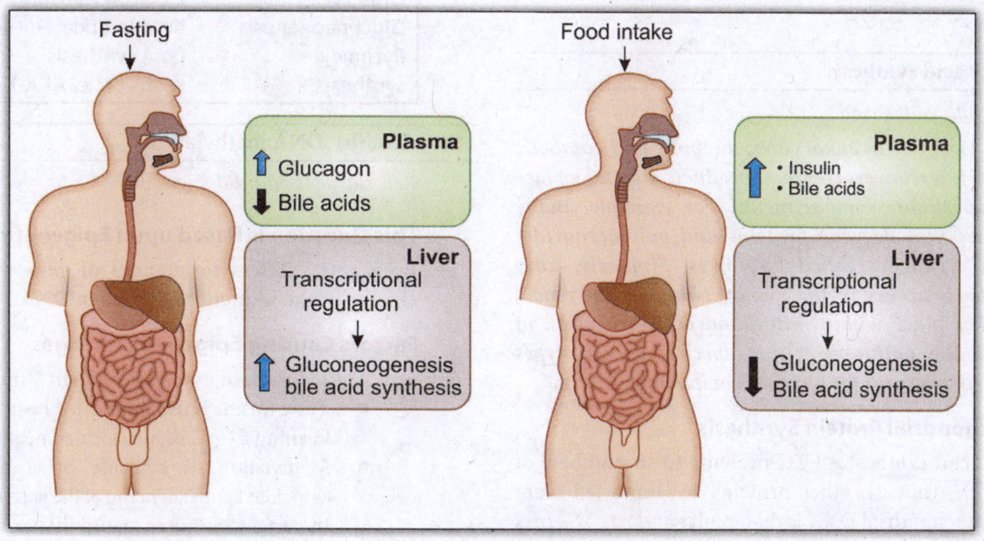

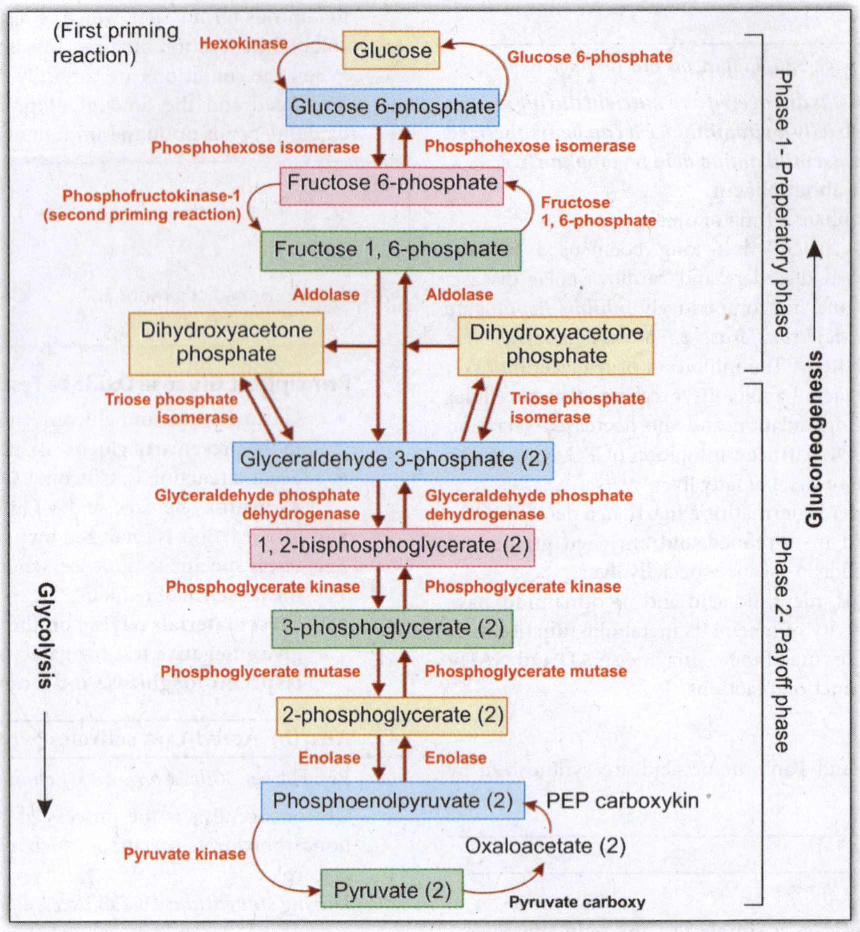

NOTE

- Always mark hormonal control as primary mechanism of regulation of any pathway (Glucagon/Cortisol)
- Rate limitng enzymes are important site of regulation/ modification by hormones

46. Ans. (a) Fatty acid synthesis

Ref: Harper's 30th ed page 88

According to Harper, "***In eukaryotes, anabolic and catabolic pathways that interconvert common products may take place in specific subcellular compartments. For example, many of the enzymes that degrade proteins and polysaccharides reside inside organelles called lysosomes. Similarly, fatty acid biosynthesis occurs in the cytosol, whereas fatty acid oxidation takes place within mitochondria. Segregation of certain metabolic pathways within specialized cell types provides a further means for physical compartmentation.***"

About Mitochondrial Protein Synthesis

Mitochondria can synthesize ETC proteins 13 in numbers of complex 1/3/4/5 (not 2), other proteins are imported from cytoplasm. Mitochondrial DNA is ds-circular and has 37 genes with 16569 base pairs

Sites of Pathways of Protein Synthesis	
Both mitochondria and cytoplasm	**Exclusively in the mitochondria**
(Mnemonic: Hug-Pyramid) Heme synth Urea cycle Gluconeogenesis Pyrimidine synthesis	**(Mnemonic: Bekk)** Fatty acid oxidation (**Beta-oxidation)** Oxidative phosphorylation and Electron transport chain Ketone body synthesis, AKA Acetyl Co A synthesis Krebs cycle, AKA TCA cycle

47. Ans. (b) DNA methylation

Ref: Harper's 30th Ed page 735

This Question is Based upon Epigenetics

Epigenetic: Refers to changes of gene expression without change of the sequence of bases in DNA.

Factors Causing Epigenetic Changes

- **Methylation of cytosine to form 5'methylcytosine**
  - The cytosine is usually located next to a guanine residue, forming a CpG island (located near promotor region).
  - Methylation of cytosine by a methyltransferase is associated with silencing of the activities of certain genes. In certain instances, genes that are methylated are less readily transcribed than those that are not methylated.

- For example, globin genes are more extensively methylated in nonerythroid cells (cells that are not a part of the erythroid, or red blood cell, lineage) than in cells, in which these genes are expressed (such as erythroblasts and reticulocytes).
- Methylation is a mechanism for regulating gene expression during differentiation, particularly in fetal development. Methylation has been implicated in ***genomic imprinting***, a process that occurs during the formation of eggs or sperm that blocks the expression of the gene in the fertilized egg. (around 30 genes show imprinting).
- Males methylate a different set of genes than females. This sex-dependent differential methylation has been studied most extensively in two human disorders, Prader Willi syndrome and Angelman syndrome.

- **Post-translational modifications of various histones:**
  - Posttranslational modifications of histones, such as acetylation, methylation, phosphorylation and ubiquitination, also affect gene expression.
  - Changes in acetylation of histones H3 and H4, affecting gene transcription, have been found in cancer cells.
  - For example, acetylation of N-terminal lysines in certain histones are associated with opening up of chromatin and with increased transcription of certain genes.
- **Chromatin remodeling:**
  - Mutations affecting the structures of protein complexes (e.g., the SW1/SNF complexes) involved in chromatin remodeling can also affect gene transcription.
  - Indeed, several of the components of the SW1/SNF complexes may act as tumor suppressor genes.
  - The complexes contain domains homologous to ATP-dependent helicase; these are involved in the changes of conformation.

48. Ans. (b) HGPRTase

Ref: Lippincott 6th Ed page 536, Nelson 19th Ed Ch 78

This is a typical case of Lesch Nyhan syndrome. Before we understand the syndrome, let us quickly review Purine metabolism.

Purine synthesis occurs mainly by two methods

- **De novo:** De novo synthesis of nucleotides begins with their metabolic precursors: amino acids, ribose 5-phosphate, CO_2 and NH_3. The purine ring is constructed primarily in the liver by a series of reactions that add the donated carbons and nitrogens to a preformed ribose 5-phosphate.
- Salvage pathways recycle the free bases and nucleoside released from nucleic acid breakdown. The de-novo synthesis does not occur in all the cells. Brain cells and leukocytes lack this mechanism. In these cells purine synthesis occurs by salvage pathway. Salvage pathway involves synthesis of purine nucleotides from free purine bases, which are salvaged from dietary sources and tissue breakdown.

Summary of Steps in De novo Synthesis of Purines

- Activated form of D-ribose-5-phosphate serves as the starting material on which purine ring is build up step by step.
- Synthesis of inosine monophosphate, the "parent" purine nucleotide is the most important intermediary step
- Synthesis of Adenosine monophosphate (AMP) and guanine monophosphate (GMP) from inosine monophosphate (IMP) required energy

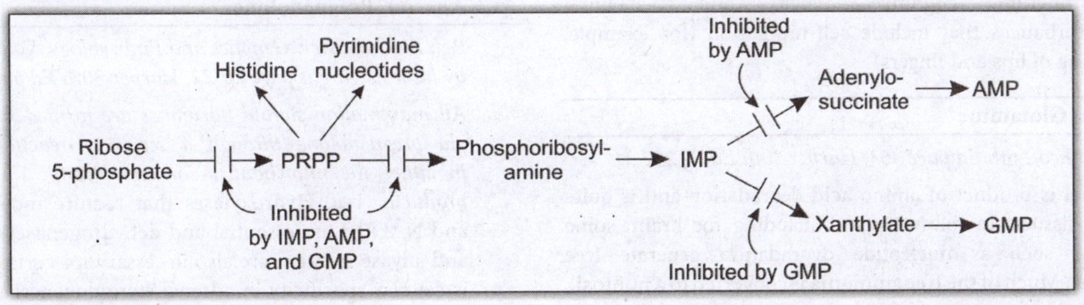

Summary of Steps of Salvage Pathway

The enzymes are:

- Adenine phosphoribosyl transferase and
- Hypoxanthine guanine phosphoribosyl transferase (HGPRT).

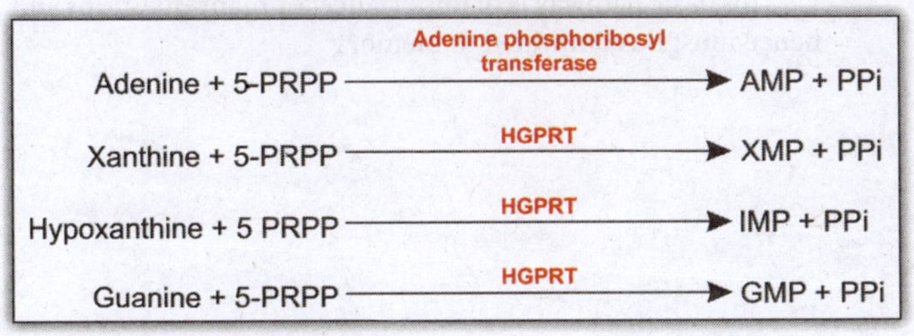

A note about PRPP

5-Phosphoribosyl-1-pyrophosphate (PRPP) is an "activated pentose" that participates in the synthesis and salvage of purines and pyrimidines. Synthesis of PRPP from ATP and ribose 5-phosphate is catalyzed by PRPP synthetase

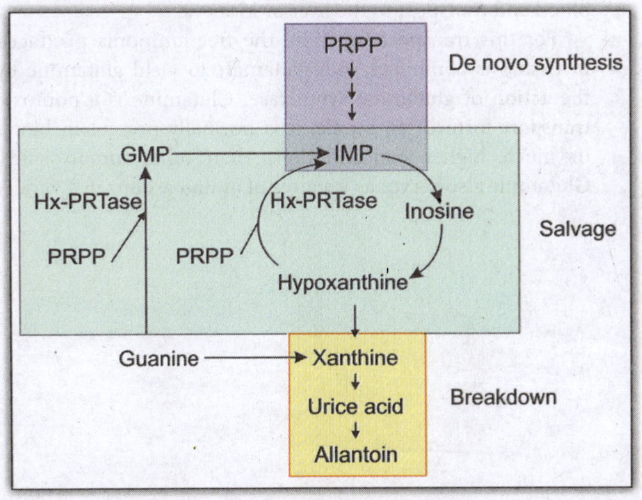

Lesch Neyhan syndrome

Pathogenesis

- **A genetic lack of hypoxanthine-guanine phosphoribosyl transferase activity, seen almost exclusively in male children, results in a bizarre set of symptoms called Lesch-Nyhan syndrome.**
- Lesch-Nyhan is a rare, X-linked recessive disorder. The deficiency results in an inability to salvage hypoxanthine or guanine, from which excessive amounts of uric acid, the end product of purine degradation, are then produced.
- In addition, the lack of this salvage pathway causes increased PRPP levels and decreased IMP and GMP levels.
- **As a result, glutamine:** Phosphoribosyl pyrophosphate amidotransferase (the regulated step in purine synthesis) has excess substrate and decreased inhibitors available and de novo purine synthesis is increased.
- The combination of decreased purine reutilization and increased purine synthesis results in increased degradation of purines and the production of large amounts of uric acid, making Lesch-Nyhan a heritable cause of hyperuricemia.

Clinical Features

- In patients with Lesch-Nyhan syndrome, the hyperuricemia frequently results in the formation of uric acid stones in the kidneys (urolithiasis) and the deposition of urate crystals in the joints
- (Gouty arthritis) and soft tissues.
- In addition, the syndrome is characterized by motor dysfunction, cognitive deficits and behavioral disturbances that include self-mutilation (for example, biting of lips and fingers)

49. Ans. (b) Glutamine

Ref: Lippincott 6th Ed page 463, Harper 30th Ed Pg 292

Ammonia is product of amino acid degradation and is quite toxic to tissues. In many tissues, including the brain, some processes such as nucleotide degradation generate free ammonia. Much of the free ammonia is converted to a nontoxic compound before export from the extrahepatic tissues into the blood and transport to the liver or kidneys.

For this transport function, the free ammonia produced in tissues is combined with glutamate to yield glutamine by the action of glutamine synthetase. Glutamine is a nontoxic transport form of ammonia; it is normally present in blood in much higher concentrations than other amino acids. Glutamine also serves as a source of amino groups in a variety of biosynthetic reactions. Glutaminase enzyme in liver then remove ammonia to synthesize urea. Remember that enzymes of urea cycle required to form urea are present only in liver.

Points to Remember

- Glutamine is major transport and temporary storage form of toxic ammonia
- Brain can also excrete ammonia as **asparagine** (less significant)
- Muscles excrete ammonia as **alanine via glutamate-alanine cycle**

50. Ans. (b) 2.3

Ref: Harper 30th Ed page 10

pH is the negative log of the hydrogen ion concentration

The term pH was introduced in 1909 by Sörensen, who defined pH as the negative log of the hydrogen ion concentration

$pH = -\log [H^+]$

to calculate pH

- Calculate the hydrogen ion concentration $[H^+]$ in mol/L
- Calculate the base 10 logarithm of $[H^+]$.
- pH is the negative of the value found in step 2.

H^+ ion concentration = 5 mmol/l = 5×10^{-3}

$$pH = -\log [5 \times 10^{-3}]$$
$$= -\log [5] - \log [10^{-3}]$$
$$= -0.6989 - (-3)$$
$$= -0.6989 + 3$$
$$= -0.7 \text{ (rounding off)} + 3$$
$$= 2.3$$

51. Ans. (c) Pregnenolone

Ref: Biochemistry, Genetics and Embryology, Volume 297 edited by Juan E. Vargas page 20-22, Harper 30th Ed page 503

All mammalian steroid hormones are formed from cholesterol via pregnenolone through a series of reactions that occur in either the mitochondria or endoplasmic reticulum of the producing cell. Hydroxylases that require molecular oxygen and NADPH are essential and dehydrogenases, an isomerase and a lyase reaction are also necessary for certain steps. There is cellular specificity in adrenal steroidogenesis. For instance, 18-hydroxylase and 19-hydroxysteroid dehydrogenises, which are required for aldosterone synthesis, are found only in the zona glomerulosa cells (the outer region of the adrenal cortex), so that the biosynthesis of this mineralocorticoid is confined to this region.

This basic pathway is of importance for many questions and hence must be committed to memory

Steroid Hormone Synthesis Pathway

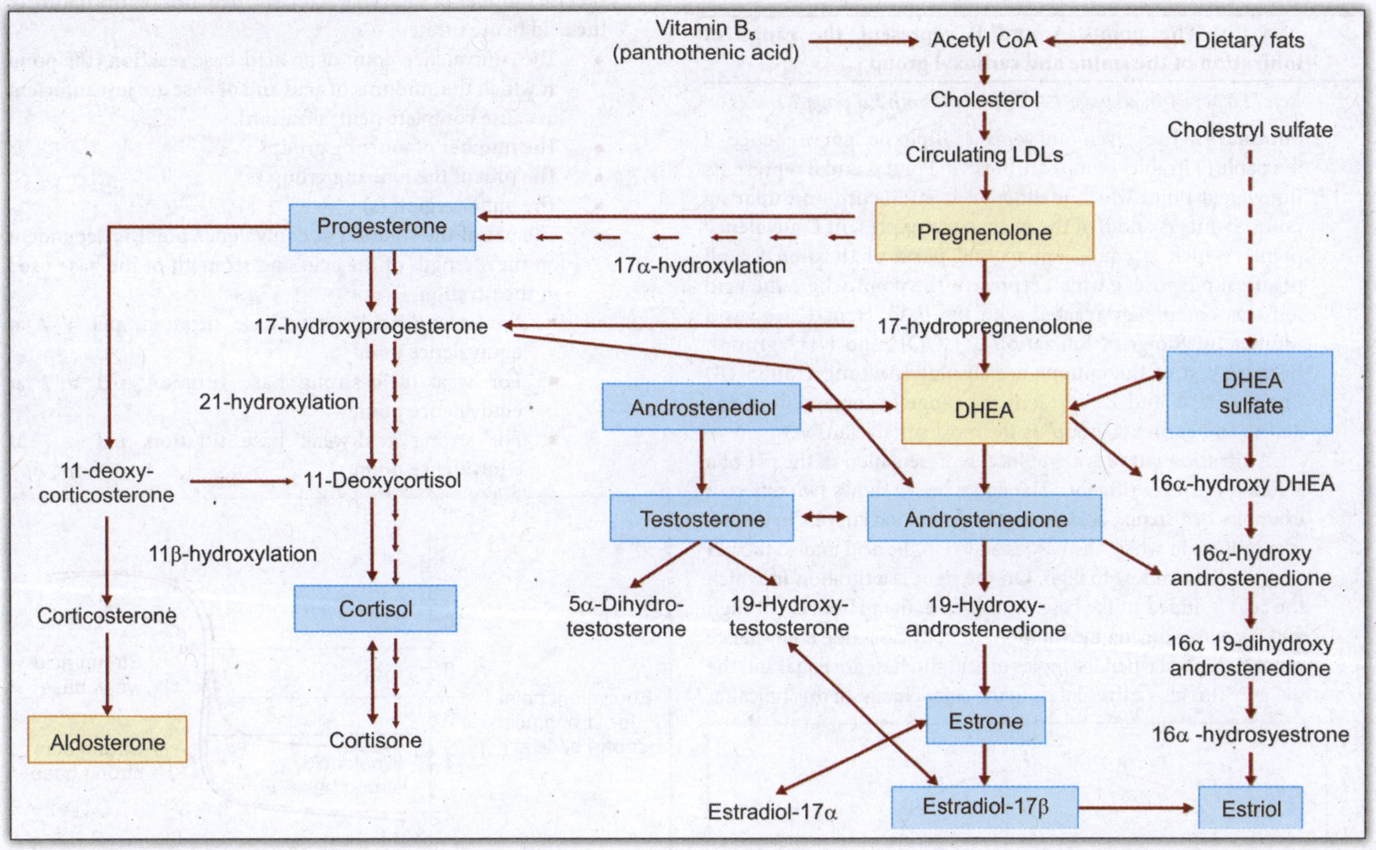

52. Ans. (a) Arginine

Ref: Lippincott 6th Ed page 13, Harper 30th Ed page 21

Among the 20 **common** amino acids, five have a side chain which can be **charged**. At **pH** = 7, two are negatively **charged**: **aspartic acid** (Asp, D) and **glutamic acid** (Glu, E) (acidic side chains) and three are positive **charged**: lysine (Lys, K), **arginine** (Arg, R) and histidine (His, H) (basic side chains)

Amino Acid Polarity and Charge

Amino acid	3-Letter	1-Letter	Side-chain polarity	Side-chain charge (pH 7.4)
Alanine	Ala	A	Nonpolar	Neutral
Arginine	Arg	R	Basic polar	Positive
Asparagine	Asn	N	Polar	Neutral
Aspartic acid	Asp	D	Acidic polar	N
Cysteine	Cys	C	Nonpolar	Neutral
Glutamic acid	Glu	E	Acidic polar	Negative
Glutamine	Gln	Q	Polar	Neutral
Glycine	Gly	G	Nonpolar	Neutral
Histidine	His	H	Basic polar	Positive (10%), neutral (90%)
Isoleucine	Ile	I	Nonpolar/ Branched chain	Neutral
Leucine	Leu	L	Nonpolar / Branched chain	Neutral
Lysine	Lys	K	Basic polar	Positive
Methionine	Met	M	Nonpolar	Neutral
Phenylalanine	Phe	F	Nonpolar	Neutral
Proline	Pro	P	Nonpolar	Neutral
Serine	Ser	S	Polar	Neutral
Threonine	Thr	T	Polar	Neutral
Tryptophan	Trp	W	Nonpolar	Neutral
Tyrosine	Tyr	Y	Polar	Neutral
Valine	Val	V	Nonpolar/ Branched chain	Neutral

The pH at which the net charge on the molecules in solution is zero is called the *isoelectric point* (**pI**). At this pH, the molecules will not migrate in an electric field toward either a positive pole (cathode) or a negative pole (anode), because the number of negative charges on each molecule is equal to the number of positive charges.

The ***hydropathic index*** is a scale used to denote the hydrophobicity of the side chain; the more positive the hydropathic index, the greater is the tendency to cluster with other nonpolar molecules and exclude water in the hydrophobic effect. The more negative the hydropathic index of an amino acid, the more hydrophilic is its side chain.

53. Ans. (b) The points A and B represent the range of ionization of the amine and carboxyl group

Ref: Harper 30th ed page 12, Lippincott's 6th Ed page 20

Summary: The given curve is a Biphasic curve hence 2 ionisable (Titrable) groups are present. Point A and B represents Equivalent point which is different from Maximum Buffering point. Points A and B of the given curve represent Equivalence point (Which is equivalent to End point of titration for all practical purposes), which represent the point where the acid ion was completely reacted with the base, Hence, it gives a estimate of Range of Ionization of COOH and NH_3^- groups. Because rest of the options are absolutely wrong Option (B) The points A and B represent the range of ionization of the amine and carboxyl group" is the most suitable answer.

A **titration curve** is a graphical representation of the pH of a solution during a titration. The figure below shows two different examples of a **strong acid-strong base** titration curve. On the left is a titration in which the base is added to the acid and so the pH progresses from low to high. On the right is a titration in which the acid is added to the base. In this case, the pH starts out high and decreases during the titration. In both cases, the equivalence point is reached when the moles of acid and base are equal and the pH is 7. This also corresponds to the color change of the indicator.

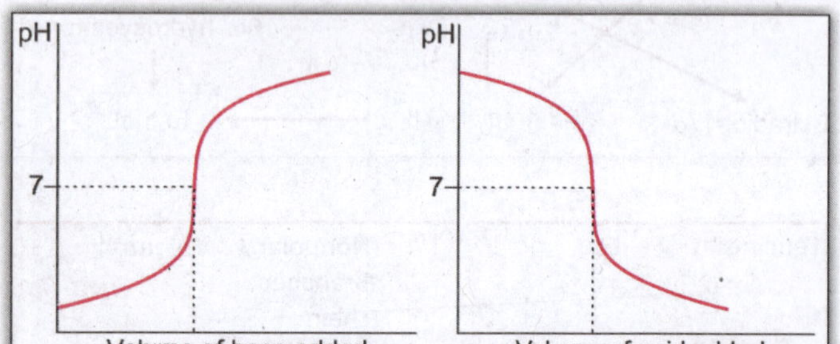

Titration curve of a strong acid (HCl) with a strong base (NaOH)

Titration curve of a strong base (NaOH) with a strong acid (HCl)

Titration curves can also be generated in the case of a weak acid-strong base titration or a strong acid-weak base titration. The general shape of the titration curve is the same, but the pH at the equivalence point is different. In a weak acid-strong base titration, the pH is greater than 7 at the equivalence point. In a strong acid-weak base titration, the pH is less than 7 at the equivalence point.

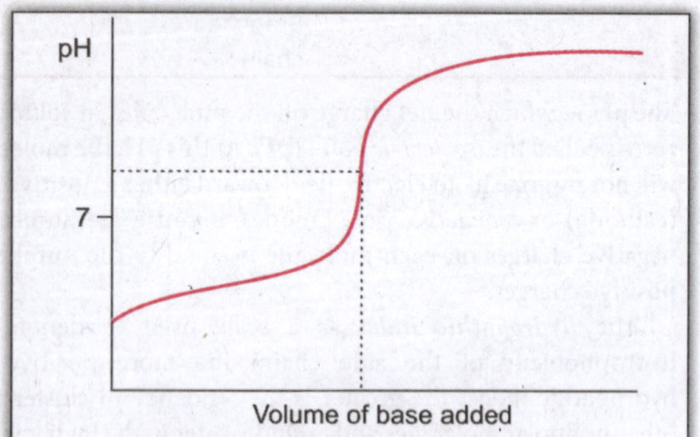

Titration curve of a weak acid (HC_3COOH) with a strong base (NaOH)

This curve empirically defines several characteristics. The precise number of each characteristic depends on the nature of the acid being titrated:

- The equivalence point of an acid-base reaction (the point at which the amounts of acid and of base are just sufficient to cause complete neutralization).
- The number of ionizing groups
- The pKa of the ionizing group (s)
- The buffer region (s)
- The pH of the solution at equivalence point is dependent on the strength of the acid and strength of the base used in the titration.
  - For strong acid-strong base titration, pH = 7 at equivalence point
  - For weak acid-strong base titration, pH > 7 at equivalence point
  - For strong acid-weak base titration, pH < 7 at equivalence point

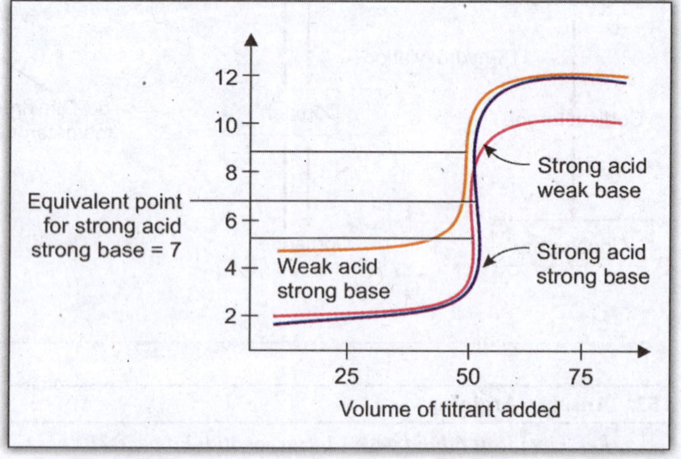

Equivalence point: In acid–base titrations, the equivalence point is reached when the number of acid equivalents present in the original solution equals the number of base equivalents added, or vice-versa.

Concept of indicator: Indicators change color as they shift between their conjugate acid and base forms:

$$\underset{\text{(color 1)}}{\text{H–Indicator}} \rightleftharpoons H^+ + \underset{\text{(color 2)}}{\text{Indicator}^-}$$

Because this is an equilibrium process, we can apply **Le Chatelier's principle**. Adding H^+ shifts the equilibrium to the left. Adding OH^- removes H^+ and therefore shifts the equilibrium to the right.

End point of titration: In the early part of the curve when little base has been added, the acidic species predominates, so the addition of small amounts of base will not appreciably change either the $[OH^-]$ or the pH. Similarly, in the last part of the titration curve when an excess of base has been added, the addition of small amounts of base will not change the $[OH^-]$ significantly and the pH will remain relatively constant. ***Endpoint is close to, but not exactly equal to, the equivalence point;*** selection of a better indicator would have given a better approximation. Still, the amount of error introduced by the use of an indicator is not especially significant

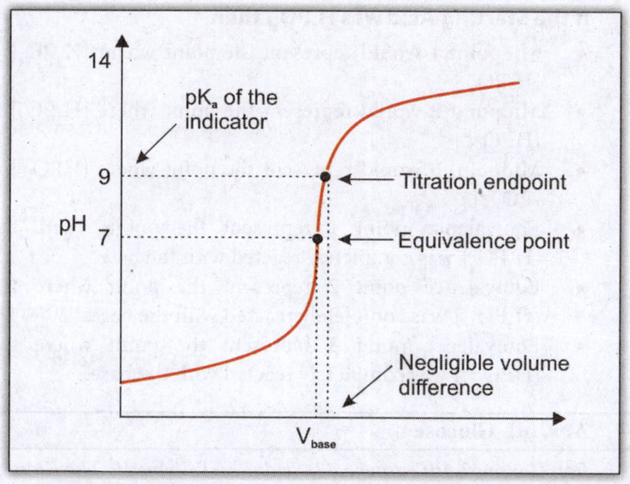

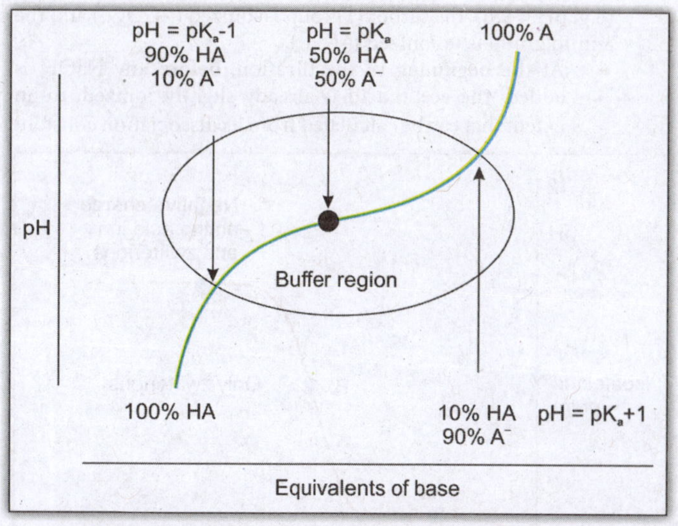

Buffer capacity (β) is defined as the moles of an acid or base necessary to change the pH of a solution by 1, divided by the pH changes and the volume of buffer in liters; it is a unitless number. When determining buffer capacity through a titration experiment, the flat region of the titration curve before the equivalence point is the buffer region.

Maximum buffering: The buffering strength is maximum when [HA] = [A-]. The point where $pH = pK_a1$ is halfway to the first equivalence point. Where $pH = pK_a2$ is halfway between the first and second equivalence points, etc. The solution has maximum buffer capacity at these points. In other words, there is maximum resistance to changes in pH.

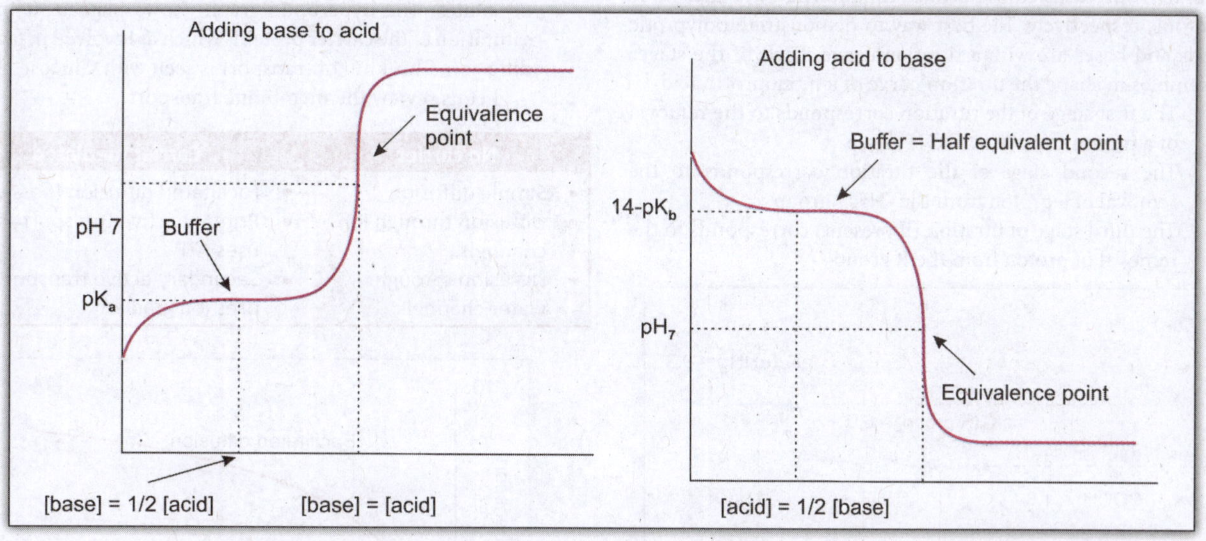

Amino acid titration: An α amino acid consists of an amino group, a carboxyl group, a hydrogen atom and a distinctive R group, all of which bind to an α – carbon atom. This carbon atom is named as α because it is adjacent to the carboxyl (acidic) group.

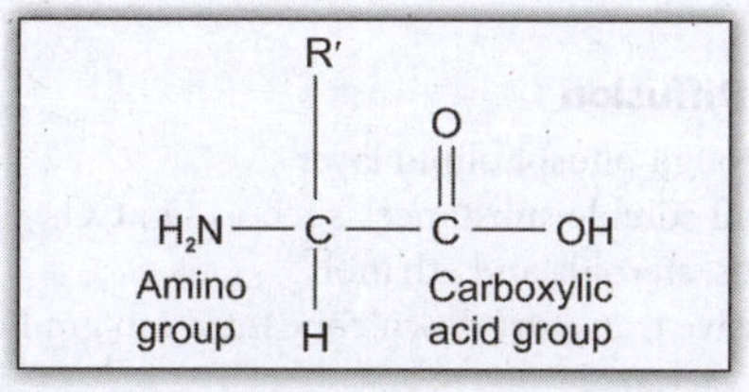

Fig: Unionized form of an amino acid

Amino acids in solution at neutral pH are predominantly dipolar ions, or zwitterions, rather than un-ionized molecules.

The point at which the zwitterions formed is called the isoelectric point (pI) of an amino acid. At the isoelectric point, the amine group shows a positive charge and the carboxyl group has a negative charge, therefore, the overall zwitterionic form is neutral.

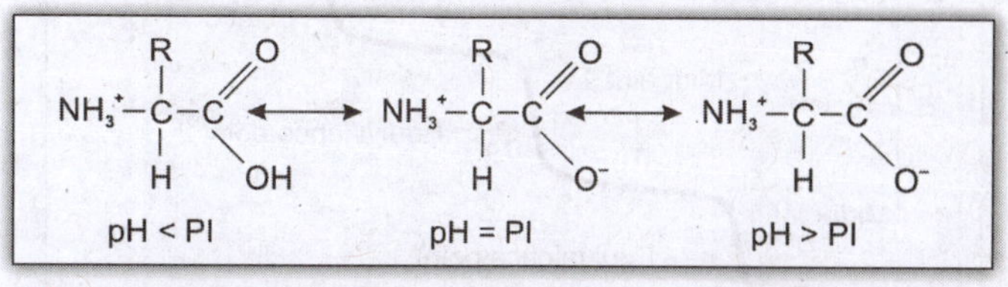

Fig: The zwitterionic form of an amino acid at different pH values

Titration curve of Amino acids: In acidic solution, (e.g. pH = 3.0), the carboxyl group is unionized (–COOH) and the amino group is ionized ($-NH_3^+$). Whereas, in an alkaline solution, (e.g. pH = 9.0), the carboxyl group is ionized (–COO^-) and the amino group is unionized (–NH_2).

- At the beginning of the titration, before any NaOH is added, the acetic acid is already slightly ionized, to an extent that can be calculated from its dissociation constant

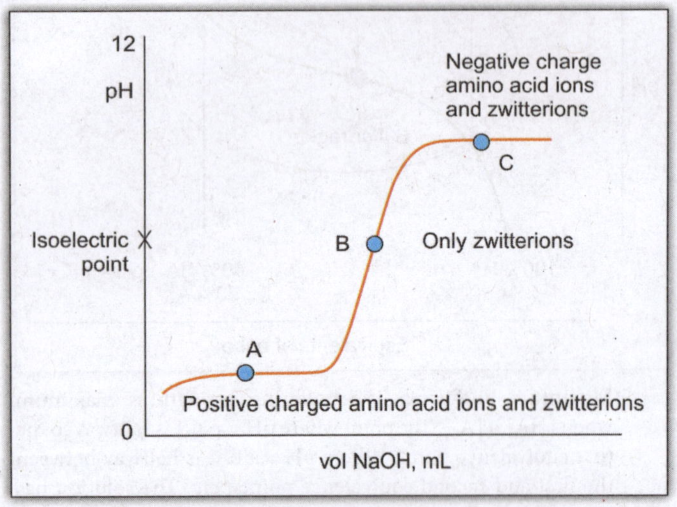

Polyprotic acids are acids that can lose several protons per molecule. They can be further categorized into *diprotic acids* and *triprotic acids*, those which can donate two and three protons, respectively. The best way to demonstrate polyprotic acids and bases are with a titration curve. Each of the stages resembles in shape the titration curve of a monoprotic acid.

- The first stage of the titration corresponds to the removal of a proton from the COOH group
- The second stage of the titration corresponds to the removal of a proton from the -NH_3^- group
- The third stage of titration (if present) corresponds to the removal of proton from the R group.

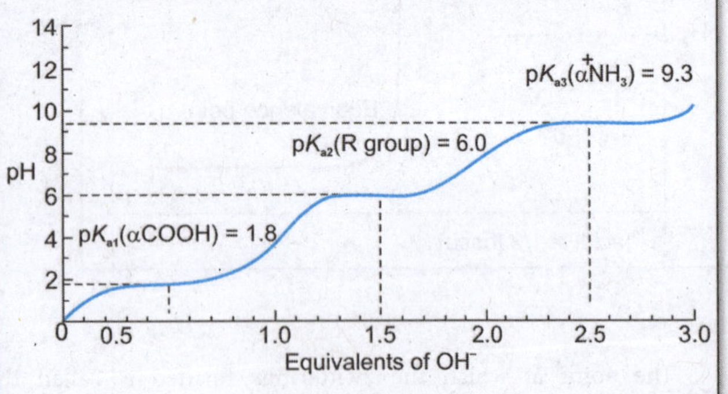

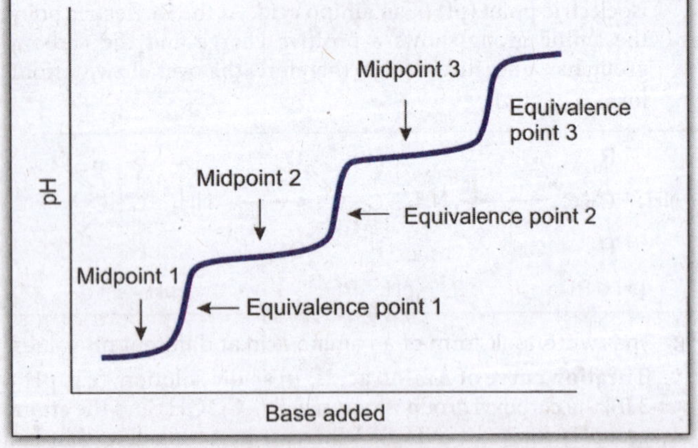

If the Starting Acid was H_3PO_4, then

- Midpoint 1 would represent the point where [H_3PO_4] = [$H_2PO_4^-$]
- Midpoint 2 would represent the point where [H_2PO_4] = [HPO_4^{2-}]
- Midpoint 3 would represent the point where [HPO_4^2] = [PO_4^{3-}]
- Equivalence point 1 represent the point where the [H_3PO_4] was completely reacted with the base.
- Equivalence point 2 represent the point where the [$H_2PO_4^-$] was completely reacted with the base.
- Equivalence point 3 represent the point where the [HPO_4^{2-}] was completely reacted with the base.

54. Ans. (d) Glucose

Ref: Ganong 24th ed page 47, Seldin and Giebisch's The Kidney: Physiology and Pathophysiology page 41, Harper 30th ed page 486

Let us first examine the graphs of passive diffusion of a solute vs facilitated diffusion. Both the graphs show the solute flux (rate of transport) as a function of solute concentration. The linear curve indicates that solute flux or rate of transportation of solute across the membrane is only dependent upon on concentration of solute, thus it is the graph of passive diffusion of solutes. The hyperbolic graph shows plateau. It indicates saturation of the carrier proteins which as involved in facilitated diffusion. This kind of transport is seen with Glucose.

Let us review the membrane transport

No carrier	Carrier mediated
• Simple diffusion • Diffusion through ion channels • Diffusion through water channels	• Facilitated diffusion (passive) • Primary active transport that uses ATP • Secondary active transport that uses ion gradient

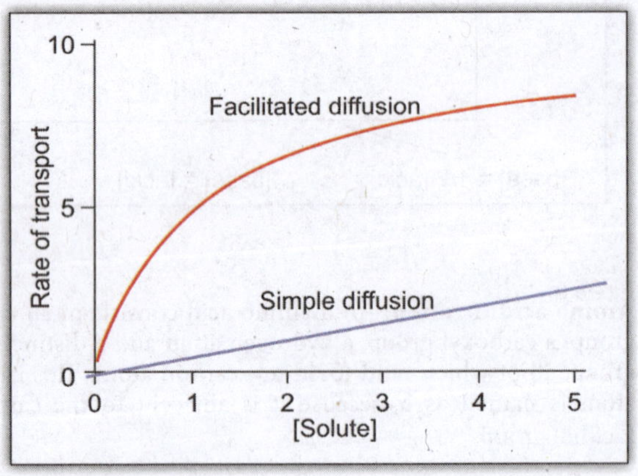

Simple Diffusion

- Through phospholipid layer
- Lipid soluble substances such as O_2, CO_2, NH_3, N_2, Fatty acids, steroids and ethanol
- Passive transport down concentration gradient
- No carrier

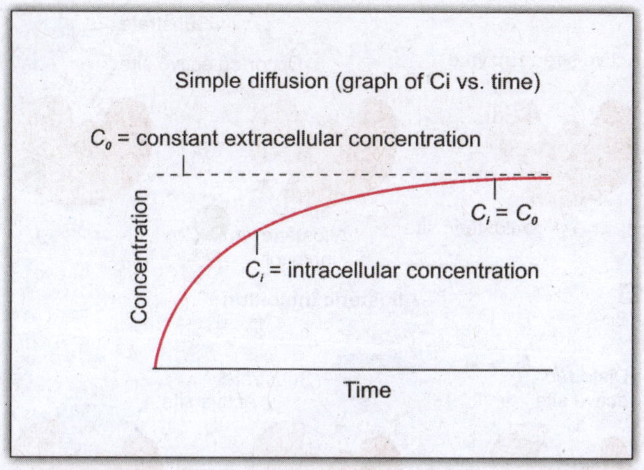

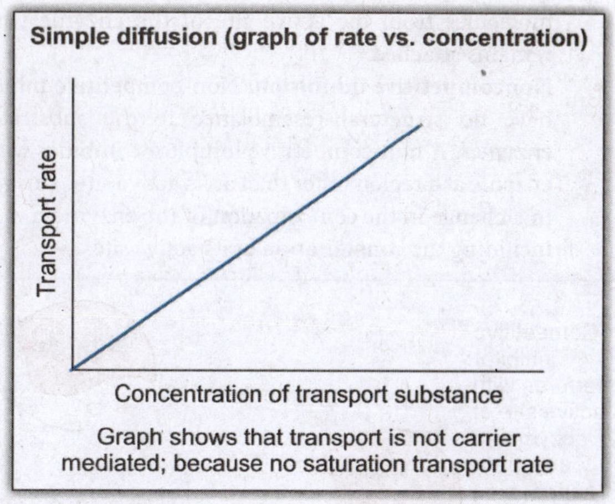

Properties of Ion Channels

- Usually highly specific for the ion
- Ion transport is passive
- Depends upon electrochemical gradient
- Channels open and close spontaneously
- Open time depends upon gating which can be ligand gated (binding by ligand), voltage gated, mechanically gated or covalently gated

Facilitated Diffusion

- Passive, carrier mediated
- Glucose in most cells except luminal membrane of kidney and intestine, urea and some amino acids

Primary Active Transport

- Uses ATP
- Carrier mediated
- Na/K pump, Ca ATPase pump in muscle, H/ATPase pump in stomach, H/ATPase pump in kidney

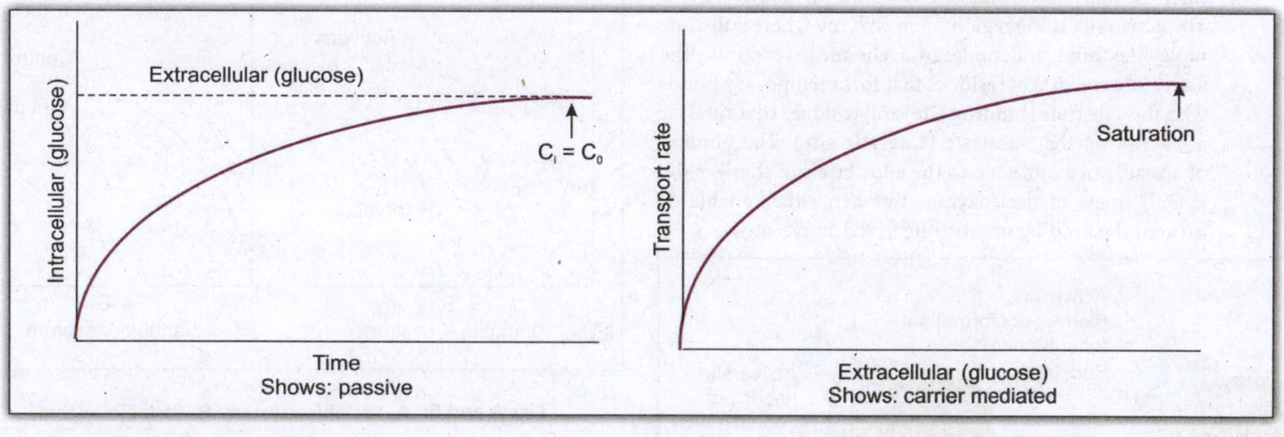

Secondary Active Transport

- Active transport of one substance coupled by transport of another.
- **Symport:** If both substances move in same direction. E.g. Na and glucose in luminal membrane of intestine
- **Antiport:** If both substances move in opposite direction. E.g. Na and Ca in heart muscle.

55. Ans. (a) Allosteric modifier can affect the catalytic site too

Ref: Harper 30th ed page 82, 91

The given graph is V-series allosteric enzymes which looks like noncompetitive inhibition type on Michaelis Menten curve (hence option C is wrong), the allosteric inhibitor lowers V_{max} without affecting the K_m. (Hence option D is wrong)

There are three different ways by which the action of an enzyme can be inhibited

- **Competitive inhibition:** A competitive inhibitor has a close structural resemblance to the substrate of an enzyme. It competes with the substrate molecules for the active site of an enzyme. The inhibitor may remain bound to the enzyme and excludes substrate molecules from the active site of the enzyme while it remains attached.

- **Noncompetitive inhibition:** Non-competitive inhibitors have no structural resemblance to the substrates of enzymes. A non-competitive inhibitor combines with the enzyme at a region other than at its active site. This results in a change in the conformation of the enzyme molecule, including the configuration of its active site.

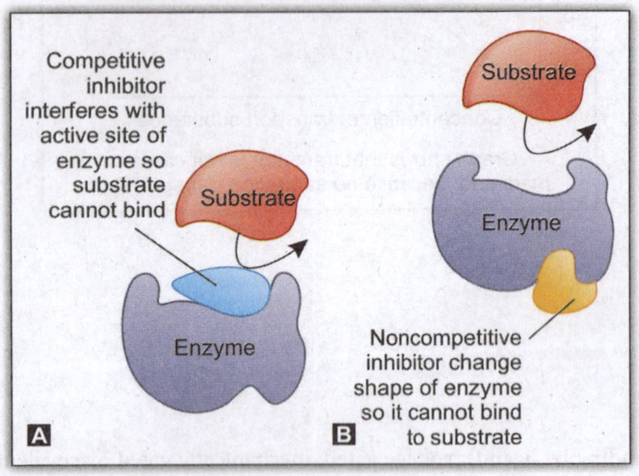

Figs A and B: A. Competitive inhibition; **B.** Noncompetitive inhibition

- **Allosteric or feedback inhibition:**
  Allosteric modifier: The prefix 'allo' of allosteric enzymes means 'other' and stereos means 'shape'. allosteric regulation (or allosteric control) is the regulation of an enzyme by binding an effector molecule at a site other than the enzyme's active site. Allosteric enzyme is one whose activity can be altered by molecules acting at a site other than the active site. This site is called the allosteric site. The active site is the region of an enzyme where substrate molecules bind and undergo a chemical reaction. The active site consists of residues that form temporary bonds with the substrate (**binding site**) and residues that catalyse a reaction of that substrate (**catalytic site**). The binding of a regulatory molecule to the allosteric site changes the overall shape of the enzyme. This can either enable or prevent the binding of substrate to the active site.

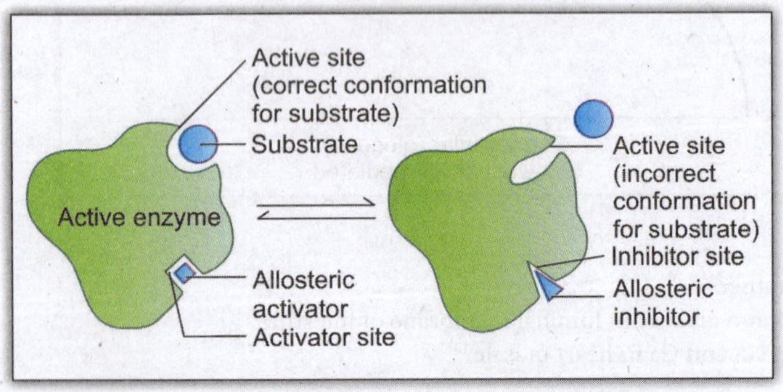

Fig: Schematic representation of allosteric enzyme activity

There are two types of regulatory molecules, namely **allosteric activators** and **allosteric inhibitors.** Allosteric activators enable the substrate to bind to the active site and thus increase the rate of reaction. In contrast, allosteric inhibitors prevent the binding of the substrate to the active site and therefore decrease the rate of reaction.

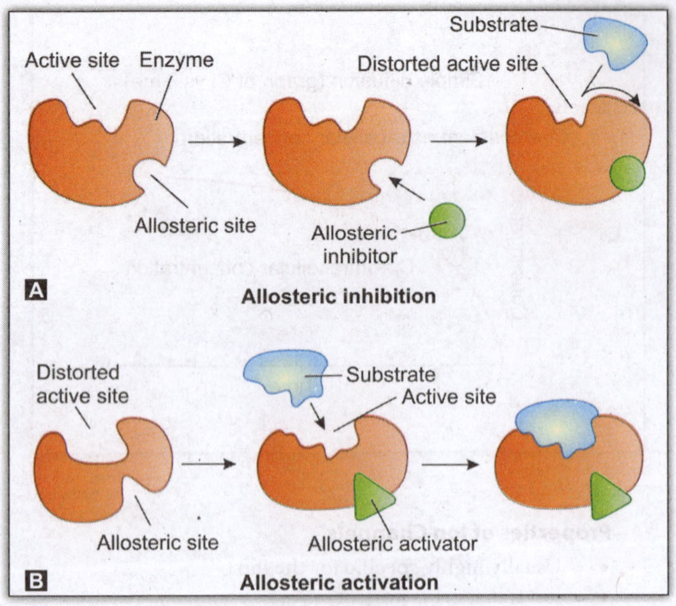

Figs A and B: A. Allosteric inhibition; **B.** Allosteric activation

To refer to the kinetics of allosteric inhibition as "competitive" or "noncompetitive" with substrate carries misleading mechanistic implications. Instead to two classes of allosterically regulated enzymes: K-series and V-series enzymes.

- For **K-series allosteric enzymes (Competitive inhibition),** the substrate saturation kinetics is competitive in the sense that Km is raised without an effect on V_{max}.
- For **V-series allosteric enzymes spinocerebellar (Noncompetitive inhibition),** the allosteric inhibitor lowers V_{max} without affecting the Km.

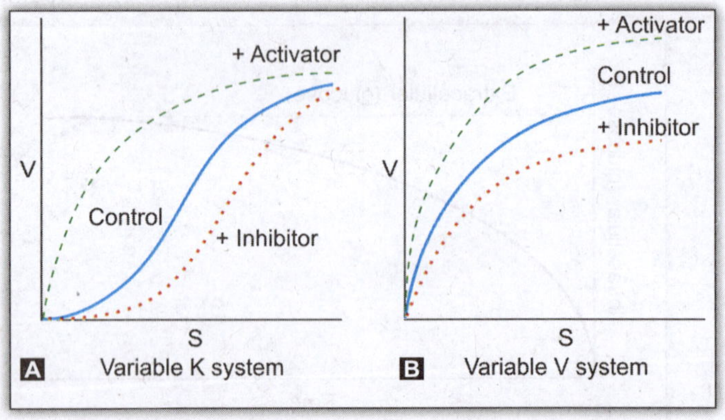

Figs A and B: A. Variable ksystem; **B.** Variable system

The Michaelis-Menten Equation

The Michaelis-Menten equation illustrates in mathematical terms the relationship between initial reaction velocity V_i and substrate concentration [S]. The Michaelis constant K_m is the substrate concentration at which vi is half the maximal velocity ($V_{max}/2$) attainable at a particular concentration of enzyme. K_m thus has the dimensions of substrate concentration.

$$V_1 = \frac{V_{max}\,[S]}{\{K_m + [S]\}}$$

- When [S] <<< K_m, [S] becomes negligible and can be ignored in denominator $V_i = V_{max}\,[S]/K_m$

- When [S]>>>> K_m, K_m becomes negligible and can be ignored in denominator $V_i = V_{max}$ [S]/[S] i.e. $V_i = V_{max}$
- When [S] = K_m, $V_i = V_{max}$ [S]/2[S] i.e. $V_i = V_{max}/2$

Characteristics of K_m: K_m, the Michaelis constant, is characteristic of an enzymeand its particular substrate and reflects the affinity of the enzyme for that substrate. K_m is numerically equal to the substrate concentration at which the reaction velocity is equal to $1/2 V_{max}$. K_m does not vary with enzyme concentration.

- **Small K_m:** A numerically small (low) K_m reflects a high affinity of the enzyme for substrate, because a low concentration of substrate is needed to half-saturate the enzyme—that is, to reach a velocity that is $1/2 V_{max}$
- **Large K_m:** A numerically large (high) K_m reflects a low affinity of enzyme for substrate because a high concentration of substrate is needed to half-saturate the enzyme

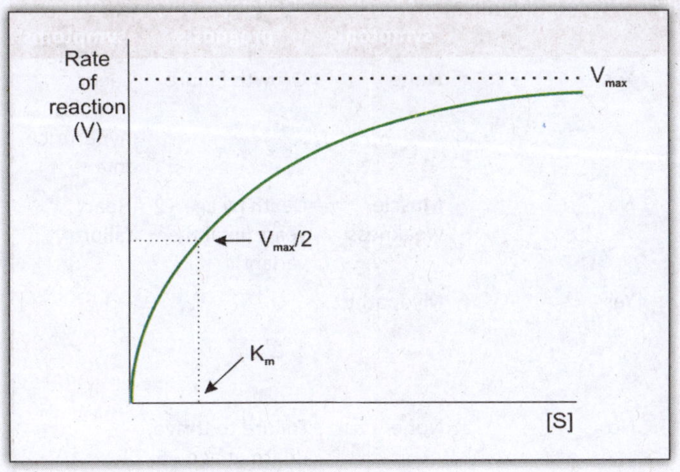

A Linear form of the Michaelis-Menten Equation is used to Determine K_M and V_{MAX}

The direct measurement of the numeric value of V_{max} and therefore the calculation of K_m often requires impractically high concentrations of substrate to achieve saturating conditions. A linear form of the Michaelis-Menten equation circumvents this difficulty and permits V_{max} and K_m to be extrapolated from initial velocity data obtained at less than saturating concentrations of substrate. Equation is the equation for a straight line, $y = ax + b$.

where $y = 1/V_i$ and $x = 1/[S]$. A plot of $1/V_i$ as y as a function of $1/[S]$ as x therefore gives a straight line whose y intercept is $1/V_{max}$ and whose slope is K_m/V_{max}. Such a plot is called a **double reciprocal** or **Lineweaver-Burk plot**

$$\frac{1}{V_i} = \left(\frac{K_m}{V_{max}}\right)\frac{1}{[S]} + \frac{1}{V_{max}}$$

Double reciprocal plots distinguish between competitive and noncompetitive inhibitors and simplify evaluation of inhibition constants. V_i is determined at several substrate concentrations both in the presence and in the absence of inhibitor. For classic competitive inhibition, the lines that connect the experimental data points meet at the y axis. Since the y intercept is equal to $1/V_{max}$, this pattern indicates that when 1/[S] approaches 0, vi is independent of the presence of inhibitor. Note, however, that the intercept on the x axis does vary with *inhibitor* concentration—and that since $-1/K_m$ is smaller than $1/K_m$, K_m, (the "apparent K_m") becomes larger in the presence of increasing concentrations of inhibitor.

- **Competitive inhibitor has no effect on V_{max} but raises K'_m, the apparent K_m for the substrate.**
- **Noncompetitive Inhibitors Lower V_{max} but do not affect K_m**

Lineweaver Burk Plot

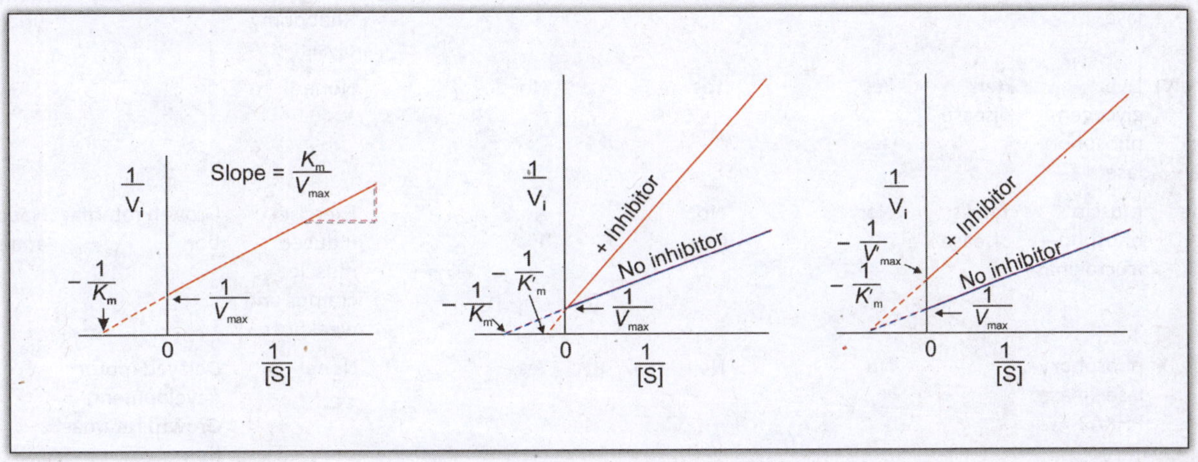

However, in using a double-reciprocal plot to determine kinetic constants, it is important to avoid the introduction of bias through the clustering of data at low values of 1/[S]. To achieve this, prepare a solution of substrate whose dilution into an assay will produce the maximum desired concentration of substrate. Now use the same volume of solutions prepared by diluting the stock solution by factors of 1:2, 1:3, 1:4, 1:5, etc. The data will then fall on the 1/[S] axis at intervals of 1, 2, 3, 4, 5, etc. Alternatively, a **single-reciprocal plot such as the Eadie-Hofstee** (V_i versus V_i/[S]) or **Hanes-Woolf** ([S]/V_i versus [S]) plot can be used to minimize clustering.

56. Ans. (d) Debranching enzyme

Ref: Harper 30th ed page 178-179, Nelson 20th Ed Ch 76

This question is based upon knowledge of glycogenoses or diseases of glycogen metabolism. The disorders of glycogen metabolism, the glycogen storage diseases (GSDs), result from deficiencies of various enzymes or transport proteins in the pathways of glycogen metabolism. The glycogen found in these disorders is abnormal in quantity, quality, or both.

Lets Review the Options

Option (A)

Glucose 6 phosphatase: It causes Von gierke's disease. Normal lactic acid levels rule out the disease

Option (B)

Muscle phosphorylase: Exercise intolerance and fatiguability are major symptoms. Hence ruled out

Option (C)

Branching enzyme: It causes amylopectinosis. Liver, cardiomegaly and heart failure are major symptoms. Hence ruled out

Option (D)

Debranching enzyme: Causes forbe's disease. Clinical picture of both liver and muscle symptoms clinches the diagnosis.

Glycogen Storage Disorders

Number	Enzyme deficiency	Eponym	Hypoglycemia	Hepatomegaly	Hyperlipidemia	Muscle symptoms	Development/ prognosis	Other symptoms
GSD type I	Glucose-6-phosphatase	Von Gierke's disease	Yes	Yes	Yes	None	Growth failure	Lactic acidosis, hyperuricemia
GSD type II	Acid maltase	Pompe's disease	No	Yes	No	Muscle weakness	Death by age ~2 years (infantile variant)	Heart failure
GSD type III	Liver and muscle debranching enzyme	Cori's disease or Forbes' disease	Yes	Yes	Yes	Myopathy		
GSD type IV	Glycogen branching enzyme	Andersen disease	No	Yes, also cirrhosis	No	None	Failure to thrive, death at age ~5 years	
GSD type V	Muscle glycogen phosphorylase	McArdle disease	No	No	No	Exercise-induced cramps, Rhabdomyolysis		Renal failure by myoglobinuria
GSD type VI	Liver glycogen phosphorylase	Hers' disease	Yes	Yes	No	None		
GSD type VII	Muscle phosphofructokinase	Tarui's disease	No	No	No	Exercise-induced muscle cramps and weakness	Growth retardation	Haemolytic anaemia
GSD type IX	phosphorylase kinase, PHKA2	-	No	No	Yes	None	Delayed motor development, Growth retardation	
GSD type XI	Glucose transporter, GLUT2	Fanconi-Bickel syndrome	Yes	Yes	No	None		
GSD type XII	Aldolase A	Red cell aldolase deficiency	?	?	?	Exercise intolerance, cramps		

Contd...

Glycogen Storage Disorders								
Number	Enzyme deficiency	Eponym	Hypoglycemia	Hepatomegaly	Hyperlipidemia	Muscle symptoms	Development/ prognosis	Other symptoms
GSD type XIII	β-enolase	-	?	?	?	Exercise intolerance, cramps	Increasing intensity of myalgias over decades	Serum CK: Episodic elevations; Reduced with rest
GSD type 0	Glycogen synthase	-	Yes	No	No	Occasional muscle cramping		

Although Traditionally Glycogen storage disorders are given roman numerals on the basis of the chronological order of their discovery, however they are also classified according to the organ type they affect the most.

- Liver forms: Hypoglycemia is the major feature
- Myopathic forms: Lactic acidosis and muscle pains are major features
- Others: Organomegaly like cardiomegaly is a major feature

Glycogen Metabolism

Glycogen is a storage form of glucose. Glycogen synthesis begins with the conversion of glucose to glucose-6-phosphate by the action of a hexokinase (glucokinase). A phosphoglucomutase then transforms the glucose-6-phosphate to glucose-1-phosphate, which, in turn, is converted to uridine diphosphoglucose. A highly branched, large polymer is then built (molecular weight as high as 100 million), containing as many as 10,000 glucose molecules linked together by α- 1,4-glucoside bonds. The glycogen chain and branches continue to be elongated by the addition of glucose molecules mediated by glycogen synthetases. During degradation, distinct phosphorylases in the liver and muscle split glucose-1-phosphate from the glycogen until about four glucose residues remain on each branch, leaving a branched oligosaccharide called limit dextrin. This can be further degraded only by the debranching enzyme. In addition to these major pathways, glycogen is also degraded in the lysosomes by acid maltase. If the lysosomes are deficient in this enzyme, the glycogen contained within them is not accessible to degradation by cytoplasmic enzymes such as phosphorylases.

57. Ans. (b) Hormone sensitive lipase

Ref: Harper 30th ed page 262

Let's understand the function and regulation of lipoprotein lipase and hormone sensitive

Lipoprotein Lipase

Chylomicrons deliver triacylglycerols to tissues, where lipoprotein lipase in capillaries releases free fatty acids for entry into cells. Dietary lipids are packaged into chylomicrons; much of their triacylglycerol content is released by lipoprotein lipase to adipose and muscle tissues during transport through capillaries. Apo C-II activates lipoprotein lipase and insulin upregulates it

Hormone Sensitive Lipase

Neutral lipids are stored in adipocytes (and in steroid synthesizing cells of the adrenal cortex, ovary and testes) in the form of lipid droplets, with a core of sterol esters and triacylglycerols surrounded by a monolayer of phospholipids. The surface of these droplets is coated with perilipins, a family of proteins that restrict access to lipid droplets, preventing untimely lipid mobilization.

When hormones signal the need for metabolic energy, triacylglycerols stored in adipose tissue are mobilized (brought out of storage) and transported to tissues (skeletal muscle, heart and renal cortex) in which fatty acids can be oxidized for energy production.

The hormones epinephrine and glucagon, secreted in response to low blood glucose levels, activate the enzyme adenylyl cyclase in the adipocyte plasma membrane. which produces the intracellular second messenger cyclic AMP. Cyclic AMP– dependent protein kinase (PKA) phosphorylates perilipin A and the phosphorylated perilipin causes hormone-sensitive lipase in the cytosol to move to the lipid droplet surface, where it can begin hydrolyzing triacylglycerols to free fatty acids and glycerol. PKA also phosphorylates hormone-sensitive lipase, doubling or tripling its activity, but the more than 50-fold increase in fat mobilization triggered by epinephrine is due primarily to perilipin phosphorylation.

Hormones affecting hormone sensitive lipase	
Stimulators	Inhibitors
• Epinephrine (most important) • Glucagon • Growth hormone	Insulin

58. Ans. (d) NAD+ donor

Ref: Harper 30th ed page 132

Cyanide inhibits Complex IV - (Inhibit cytochrome a3) of Electron transport chain. If electron transport chain is blocked NADH will not be converted to NAD^+

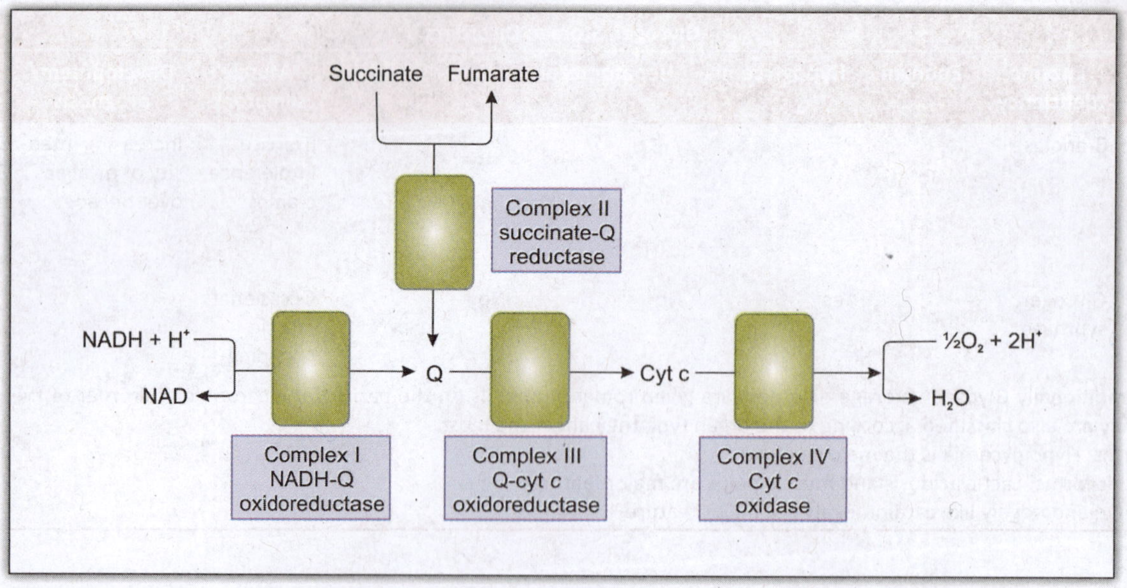

Fig: Overview of electron flow through the respiratory chain

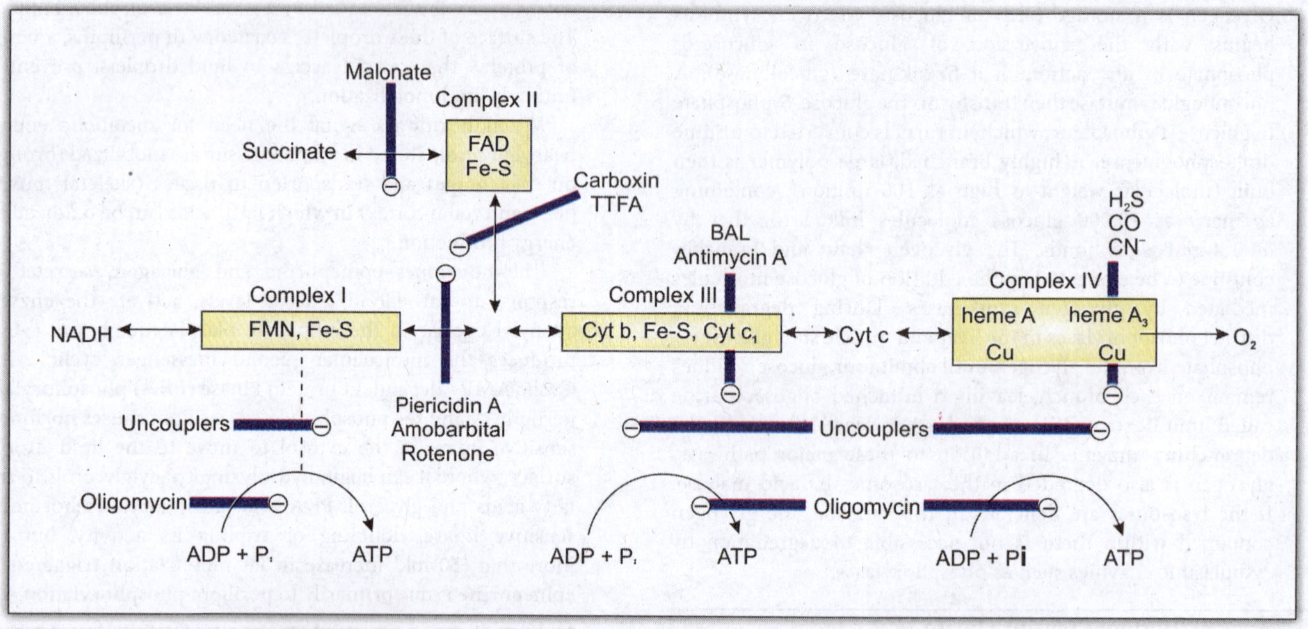

Fig: Sites of inhibition (–) of the respiratory chain by specific drugs, chemical and antibiotics

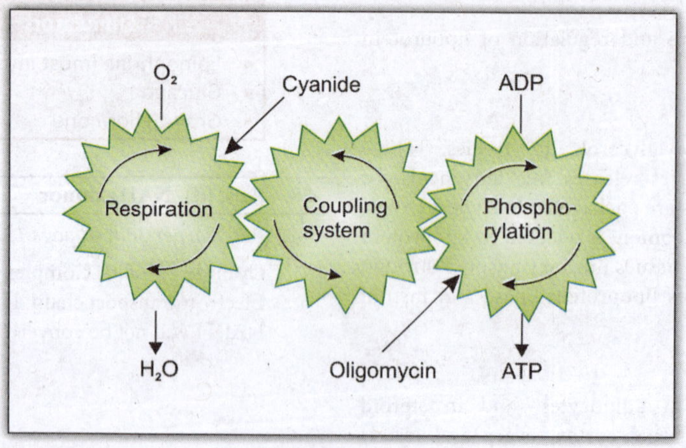

Respiratory Poisons, Inhibitors and Uncouplers			
Type of Effector	**Example**	**Electron Transport Chain**	**Phosphorylation**
Electron transport (respiratory) inhibitors	**Complex I inhibitors-** by blocking the transfer from Fe-S to Q. • Rotenone (insecticide) • Amytal (barbiturate) • Demerol (painkiller) **Complex II inhibitors** • 2-Thenoyltrifluoroacetone (TTFA) • Carboxin • Malonate is a competitive inhibitor of Complex II **Complex III inhibitors-(Inhibit Cytochrome C1)** • Antimycin A1 • Dimercaprol **Complex IV inhibitors- (Inhibit cytochrome a3)** • H_2S, carbon monoxide, azide and cyanide	Inhibition	Inhibition
Phosphorylation inhibitor	**Phosphate transporter inhibitor:** *N*-Ethylmaleimide **Pyruvate symport inhibitor:** *N*-Ethylmaleimide, hydroxycinnamate **Adenine nucleotide transporter inhibitor** • Atractyloside **ATP synthase inhibitors:** • DCCD (Di-clyclohexyl-carbo-diimide) • Oligomycin	Inhibition (secondary to inhibition of ATP synthesis)	Inhibition
Uncouplers (dissociate oxidation in the respiratory chain from phosphorylation)	**Synthetic uncouplers-** 2,4-Dinitrophenol, dicumarol and carbonyl cyanidep-trifluorocarbonyl-cyanide methoxyphenyl hydrazone (FCCP), **Physiological uncoupler**-Thermogenin, Thyroxine in high doses,	Stimulation	Inhibition (secondary to dissipating proton gradient thus bypassing ATP synthesis)

59. Ans. (b) Tyrosine

Ref: Harper 30th ed page 165

Pyruvate is oxidatively decarboxylated by pyruvate dehydrogenase (PDH) complex, producing acetyl coenzyme A (CoA), which is the major fuel for the tricarboxylic acid cycle [TCA cycle]

Amino acids whose catabolism yields pyruvate or one of the intermediates of the TCA cycle are termed glucogenic. These intermediates are substrates for gluconeogenesis

Transamination	
Products formed by amino acids	**Amino acids**
Amino acids that form oxaloacetate	Asparagine, Aspartate
Amino acids that form α-ketoglutarate	Glutamine, Proline, Arginine, Histidine
Amino acids that form pyruvate	Alanine, Serine, Glycine, Cystine, Hydroxyproline, Threonine (minor pathway)
Amino acids that form fumarate	Phenylalanine and tyrosine
Amino acids that form succinyl CoA	Methionine, Valine and isoleucine, Threonine
Amino acids that form acetyl CoA or acetoacetyl CoA	Leucine, Isoleucine, Lysine, Tryptophan

Contd...

Transamination

Products formed by amino acids	Amino acids

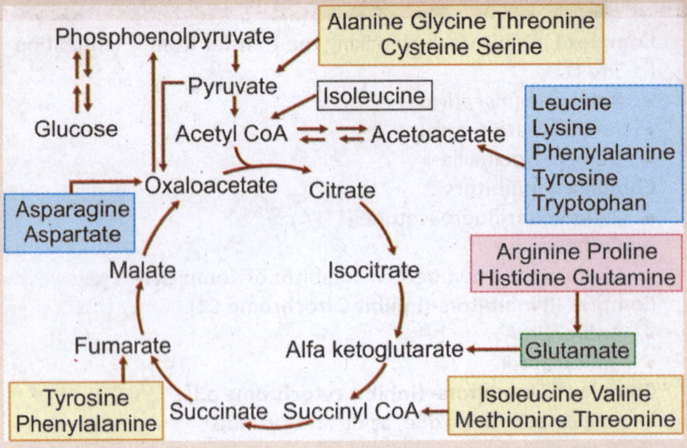

60. Ans. (d) Acetyl-CoA

Ref: Harper 30th ed page 185

Harper's States

- **Fatty acids (and ketone bodies formed from them) cannot be used for the synthesis of glucose.** The reaction of pyruvate dehydrogenase, forming acetyl-CoA, is irreversible and for every two-carbon unit from acetyl-CoA that enters the citric acid cycle, there is a loss of two carbon atoms as carbon dioxide before oxaloacetate is reformed. **This means that acetyl-CoA (and hence any substrates that yield acetyl-CoA) can never be used for gluconeogenesis.**
- The (relatively rare) fatty acids with an odd number of carbon atoms yield propionyl-CoA as the product of the final cycle of oxidation and this can be a substrate for gluconeogenesis, as can the glycerol released by lipolysis of adipose tissue triacylglycerol reserves.

Gluconeogenesis is the process of synthesizing glucose or glycogen from noncarbohydrate precursors. The major substrates are:

- Glucogenic amino acids
- Lactate
- Glycerol
- Propionate
- Intermediates of TCA cycle

Ketogenic and Glucogenic Amino Acids

Purely ketogenic	Leucine, Lysine
Both ketogenic and glucogenic	Tyrosine, tryptophan, isoleucine and phenylalanine
Purely glucogenic	Alanine, serine, glycine, cysteine, aspartic acid, asparagine, glutamic acid, glutamine, arginine, histidine, valine, threonine, methionine, proline

Those amino acids that give rise to acetyl-CoA are referred to as ketogenic, because in prolonged fasting and starvation much of the acetyl-CoA is used for synthesis of ketone bodies in the liver.

61. Ans. (a) Odorants

Ref: Mammalian Genomics edited by Anatoly Ruvinsky, Jennifer A. Marshall Graves page 273

Odorant receptors are the first dedicated molecules with which an odorant first comes in contact. They constitute the largest gene family in mammals of 900 genes in humans and 1100 genes in mouse.

62. Ans. (c) Precipitate at pH other than isoelectric pH

Ref: Harper 30th ed page 26, Vasudevan 7th ed page 42

Indirect repeat Biochemistry AIIMS NOV 2015 (Next Question, See for explanation)

AIIMS NOVEMBER 2015

63. Ans. (d) Titration with reducing sugar

Ref: Harper 30th ed page 26, Vasudevan 7th ed page 42

Agents of Denaturation

Disruption of higher order structure without splitting peptide linkage i.e. Primary structure is not altered in denaturation. However denaturation is almost always associated with loss of biological function.

- Heat (50-80°C)
- Detergents and Organic solvents (Disrupt hydrophobic amino acids)
- Strong acids and bases (disrupts the intermolecular salt bond)
- 8M Urea or 6M Guanidine hydrochloride (hydrophilic agents with high hydrogen binding potentials. Denatures protein by disrupting hydrogen bond between protein and surrounding water molecule)
- Potent precipitating agent like Trichlorocetic acid (10% v/v). Is of special use for laboratories because it can rapidly denature and precipitate proteins
- Physical agents like X-ray, UV rays, High pressure
- Heavy metal ion (they have affinity to carboxylate group and for Sulfhydryl group in many proteins)

Agents of Precipitation

Precipitation of proteins occurs when its solubility decreases. Unlike denaturation, precipitation is reversible and does not cause permanent loss of protein function.

- Precipitation by heat coagulation
- Salting in and out: salt at moderate concentration cause increase protein solubility (Salting in) and at higher concentration may decrease the solubility of protein resulting in protein precipitation (salting out). Ammonium chloride is one of the most soluble salt and is most commonly used agent for salting out.
- Precipitation by organic solvent such as ethanol or acetone (high affinity to water)
- Precipitation by altering the pH: At the isoelectric point, the precipitation of protein is maximum, i.e. in other words the solubility of proteins is minimum.
- Precipitation by heavy metals

64. Ans. (d) Acetyl CoA

Ref: Harper 30th ed page 185

Repeat Biochemistry AIIMS May 2016 (See for explanation) (see page no. 222)

65. Ans. (b) UGA

Ref: Harper 30th ed page 18, 286

Selenocysteine the 21st Amino Acid

- It is an L-α-amino acid found in a handful of proteins called selenoproteins
- Selenocysteine has a structure similar to that of cysteine, but with an atom of selenium taking the place of the usual sulfur, forming a selenol group which is deprotonated at physiological pH. The pK_3 of selenocysteine, 5.2, is 3 units lower than that of cysteine.
- Unlike other amino acids present in biological proteins, selenocysteine is not coded for directly in the genetic code. Instead, it is encoded in a special way by a **UGA codon**, which is normally a stop codon. Such a mechanism is called translational recoding and its efficiency depend on the selenoprotein being synthesized and on translation initiation factors. Since selenocysteine is inserted into polypeptides during translation, it is commonly referred to as the "21st amino acid."
- The UGA codon is made to encode selenocysteine by the presence of aSECIS element **(SElenoCysteine Insertion Sequence)** in the mRNA.
- Selenocysteine is present in several enzymes (for example **glutathione peroxidases, tetraiodothyronine 5' deiodinases, thioredoxin reductases, formate dehydrogenases, glycine reductases, selenophosphate synthetase 1, methionine-R-sulfoxide reductase B1 (SEPX1)** and some hydrogenases

Pyrrolysine, sometimes considered "the **22nd amino acid**", is not listed here as it is not used by humans

66. Ans. (a) Glycogen phosphorylase

Ref: Harper's 30th Ed page 550, Katzung 12th ed page 587

Recall Bias

Some students think that options were different and question was not "all except".

Vitamin B_{12} is Required for the conversion of:

- Dopamine to norepinephrine
- Propionyl CoA to methyl malonyl CoA
- **Methyl malonyl CoA to Succinyl CoA**
- Cysteine to homocysteine

There are three Vitamin B_{12} Dependent Enzymes

- **Methylmalonyl CoA mutase**: Reaction that requires vitamin B_{12} is isomerization of methylmalonyl-CoA to succinyl-CoA by the enzyme methylmalonyl-CoA mutase
- **Methionine synthase:** Methylcobalamin is a coenzyme for methionine synthase, which transfers methyl-tetrahydrofolate and homocysteine to methionine
- **Leucine aminomutase:** B_{12} is required for the interconversion of β leucine and leucine catalysed by 2–3 Aminomutase enzyme (No human disease)

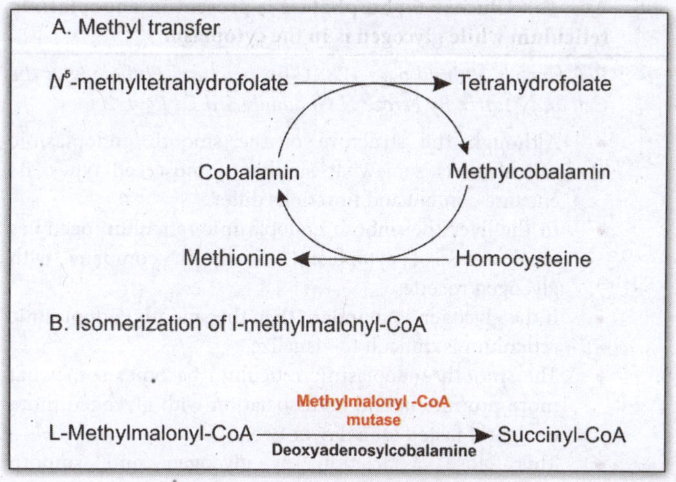

67. Ans. (a) Gamma carboxylation of glutamate

Ref: Harper's 30th Ed page 550

Biotin is a cofactor responsible for carbon dioxide transfer in several carboxylase enzymes

- **Acetyl-CoA carboxylase:** Carboxylation of acetyl-CoA to malonyl-CoA in the presence of ATP and acetyl-CoA carboxylase require Biotin

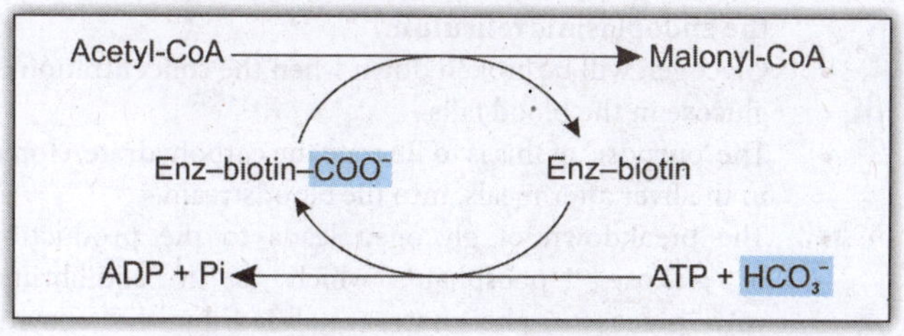

- **Methylcrotonyl-CoA carboxylase:** is a biotin-requiring enzyme located in the mitochondria which catalyze the carboxylation of a carbon adjacent to a carbonyl group performing the fourth step in processing leucine

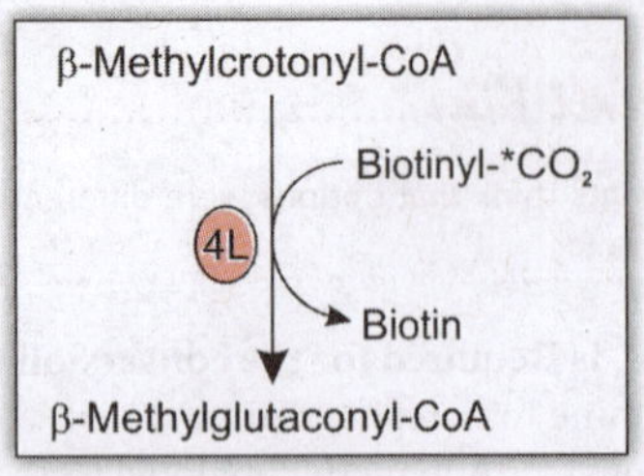

- **Propionyl-CoA carboxylase:** Catalyses the carboxylation reaction of propionyl CoA to Methylmalonyl CoA

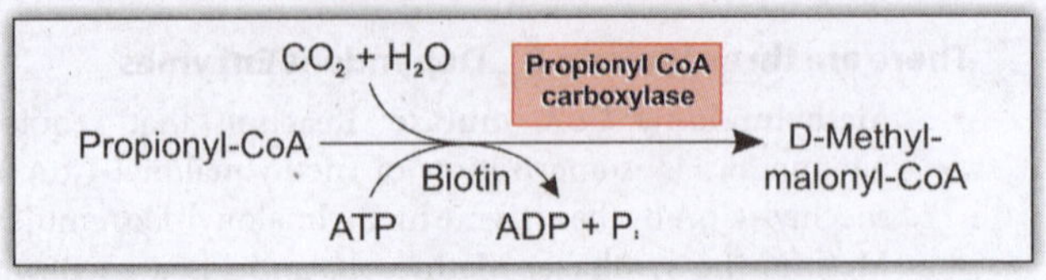

- **Pyruvate carboxylase:** Mitochondrial pyruvate carboxylase catalyzes the carboxylation of pyruvate to oxaloacetate, an ATP-requiring reaction in which the vitamin biotin is the coenzyme.

68. Ans. (b) Glucose-6-phosphatase is present in endoplasmic reticulum while glycogen is in the cytoplasm

Ref: Harper 30th ed page 178, Ultrastructural Pathology of the Cell and Matrix By Feroze N.Ghadially 3rd Ed Pg 422

- Although the structure of the smooth endoplasmic reticulum is somewhat similar in most cell types, its enzyme content and functions differ.
- In the liver the smooth endoplasmic reticulum occupies focal areas of cytoplasm, usually in company with glycogen rosettes.
- If the glycogen is abundant then the smooth endoplasmic reticulum is difficult to visualize.
- The smooth endoplasmic reticulum becomes somewhat more prominent and its association with glycogen more evident if fasted for a day or two.
- This close association of glycogen and smooth endoplasmic reticulum led to the suggestion that the smooth endoplasmic reticulum was perhaps involved in glycogenesis or glycogenolysis. Biochemical studies on microsomal fractions have, however, failed to support this idea.
- It would appear that the main enzymes of glycogen metabolism lie in the cytoplasmic matrix or elsewhere, but not in the endoplasmic reticulum. (**An exception to this is glucose-6- phosphatase, which is associated with the endoplasmic reticulum)**
- Glycogen will be broken down when the concentration of glucose in the blood falls.
- The 'purpose' of this is to liberate the carbohydrate, stored in the liver after meals, into the bloodstream.
- The breakdown of glycogen leads to the production of glucose 1-phosphate, which is in equilibrium with glucose 6-phosphate (catalysed by the enzyme phosphoglucomutase).
- Glucose 6-phosphate cannot be converted to glucose by the enzyme glucokinase, which catalyses an essentially irreversible reaction and the formation of glucose from glucose 6-phosphate is instead brought about by glucose-6-phosphatase.
- Like glucokinase, the Km of glucose-6-phosphatase is high relative to normal concentrations of its substrate, glucose 6-phosphate.
- Glucose-6-phosphatase is not free in the cytoplasm: it is a membrane-bound enzyme present in the membranes of the endoplasmic reticulum Is complex of membranes enclosing a compartment separate from the cell cytoplasm).
- Its catalytic site faces into the lumen of the endoplasmic reticulum and the enzyme is associated with subunits that act as specific transporters for the facilitated diffusion of glucose 6-phosphate (from the cytosol into the lumen) and glucose (from lumen to cytosol); the latter is a member of the GLUT family, possibly GLUT9.

69. Ans. (d) Acetyl-CoA

Ref: Harper 30th ed page 185

Repeat (See Biochemistry AIIMS May 2016 for explanation) (see page no. 222)

70. Ans. (b) Methylation

Ref: Harper 29th ed page 709

- We all inherit two copies of each autosomal gene, carried on homologous maternal and paternal chromosomes. Studies over the past two decades have provided definite evidence that, at least with respect to some genes, important functional differences exist between the paternal allele and the maternal allele.
- These differences result from an epigenetic process called imprinting. In most cases, imprinting selectively inactivates either the maternal or paternal allele.
- Thus, maternal imprinting refers to transcriptional silencing of the maternal allele, whereas paternal imprinting implies that the paternal allele is inactivated. Imprinting occurs in the ovum or the sperm, before fertilization and then is stably transmitted to all somatic cells through mitosis.
- As with other instances of epigenetic regulation, imprinting is associated with differential patterns of **DNA methylation at CG nucleotides**. Other mechanisms include histone H4 deacetylation and methylation.

The best examples of genomic imprinting are:

- Angelman syndrome
- Prader-Willi syndrome

Prader-Willi Syndrome (PWS)

- Characterized by mental retardation, short stature, hypotonia, profound hyperphagia, obesity, small hands and feet and hypogonadism. In 65% to 70% of cases, an interstitial deletion of band q12 in the long arm of chromosome 15, del (15)(q11.2q13), can be detected.
- In most cases the breakpoints are the same, causing a 5-Mb deletion. It is striking that in all cases the deletion affects the paternally derived chromosome 15.

Angelman Syndrome (AS)

- Patients with the phenotypically distinct Angelman syndrome are born with a deletion of the same chromosomal region as PWS, derived from their mothers.
- Patients with Angelman syndrome are also mentally retarded, but in addition they present with ataxic gait, seizures and inappropriate laughter.

- Because of their laughter and ataxia, they have been referred to as happy puppets.
  - The molecular basis of these two syndromes lies in the genomic imprinting.
  - It is known that a gene or set of genes on maternal chromosome 15q12 is imprinted (and hence silenced) and thus, the only functional allele(s) are provided by the paternal chromosome.
  - When these are lost as a result of a deletion, the person develops Prader-Willi syndrome.
  - Conversely, a distinct gene that also maps to the same region of chromosome 15 is imprinted on the paternal chromosome.
  - Only the maternally derived allele of this gene is normally active. Deletion of this maternal gene on chromosome 15 gives rise to the Angelman syndrome.

Concept of Uniparental Disomy

- Inheritance of both chromosomes of a pair from one parent is called uniparental disomy.
- Not all individuals with PWS or AS carry the chromosome 15 deletion. For such individuals, the parental origin of the chromosome 15 region is again the important determinant. In PWS, for example, nondeletion patients invariably have two maternal and no paternal chromosomes 15 [maternal uniparental disomy (UPD)], whereas for some nondeletion AS patients the reverse is true (paternal UPD). The net effect is the same (i.e., the person does not have a functional set of genes from the [nonimprinted] paternal chromosomes 15).
- In the Angelman syndrome, the affected gene is a ubiquitin ligase that is involved in catalyzing the transfer of activated ubiquitin to target protein substrates. **The gene, called UBE3A,** maps within the 15q12 region, is imprinted on the paternal chromosome and is expressed from the maternal allele primarily in specific regions of the brain.

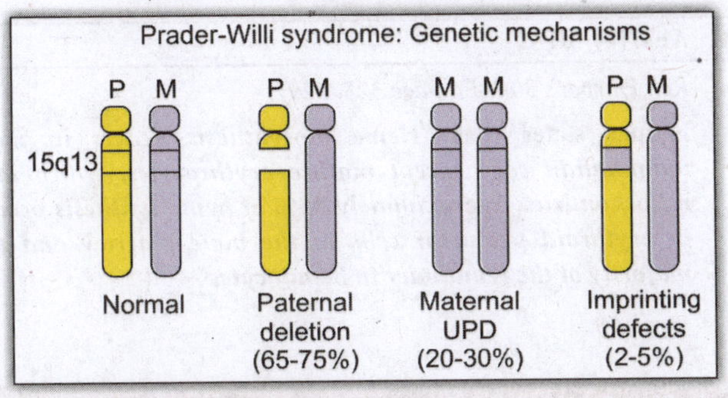

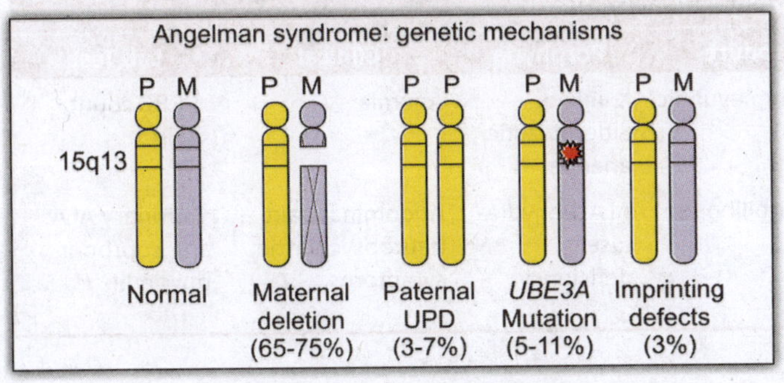

Molecular diagnosis of these syndromes is based on assessment of methylation status of marker genes and FISH

71. Ans. (c) Succinate dehydrogenase

Ref: Harper 30th Ed page 555, Rapid Review Biochemistry By John W. Pelley, Edward F. Goljan 3rd ed page 41

Thiamine Acts as Coenzyme in

- Pyruvate dehydrogenase in carbohydrate metabolism
- α-ketoglutarate dehydrogenases in the citric acid cycle
- Branched-chain keto-acid dehydrogenase involved in the metabolism of leucine, isoleucine and valine

72. Ans. (d) Glycogenin

Ref: Harper's 30th Ed page 181

Glycogen phosphorylase catalyzes the rate-limiting step in glycogenolysis— the phosphorolytic cleavage of the 1–4 linkages of glycogen to yield glucose 1-phosphate.

- There are distinct isoenzymes of glycogen phosphorylase in liver, muscle and brain, encoded by distinct genes. Glycogen phosphorylase requires **pyridoxal phosphate** as its coenzyme. I phosphorylase it is the phosphate group that it catalytically active.
- The principal enzymes controlling glycogen metabolism—glycogen phosphorylase and glycogen synthase—are regulated in opposite directions by **allosteric mechanisms and covalent modification** by reversible phosphorylation and dephosphorylation of enzyme protein in response to hormone action.
- **Phosphorylation of glycogen phosphorylase increases its activity; phosphorylation of glycogen synthase reduces its activity.**
- Phosphorylation is increased in response to cyclic AMP (cAMP) formed from ATP by adenylyl cyclase at the inner surface of cell membranes in response to hormones such as epinephrine norepinephrine and glucagon. cAMP is hydrolyzed by phosphodiesterase, so terminating hormone action; in liver insulin increases the activity of phosphodiesterase.

Factors Affecting Phosphorylase

Factors causing activation	Factors causing deactivation
• cAMP	• Phosphodiesterase
• Adenyl Cyclase	• Insulin In Liver
• Epinephrine In Muscle	• Phosphoprotien Phosphatase
• Norepinephrine	• Glucose 6P
• Glucagon	• ATP
• Phosphorylase Kinase	• Glucose In Liver
• 5-AMP In Muscle	
• Calcium In Muscle	

In both muscle and liver, the enzyme is activated by phosphorylation catalyzed by phosphorylase kinase (to yield phosphorylase a) and inactivated by dephosphorylation catalyzed by phosphoprotein phosphatase (to yield phosphorylase b), in response to hormonal and other signals.

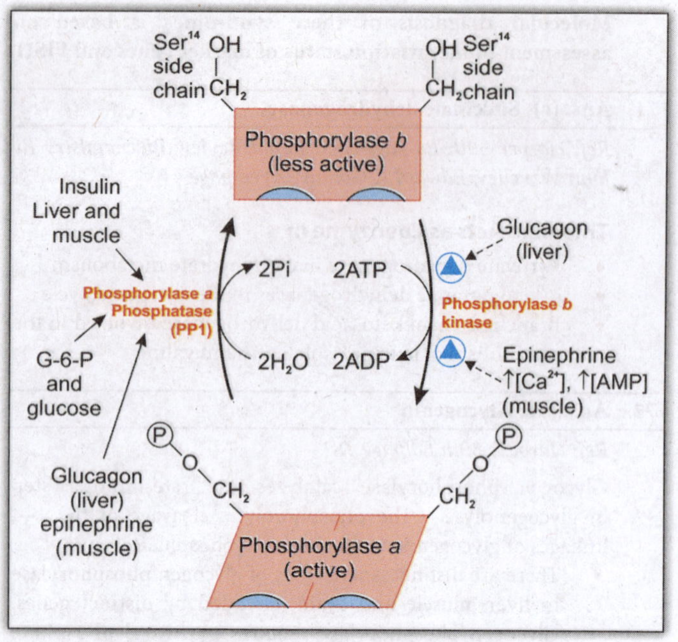

Active phosphorylase a in both tissues is allosterically inhibited by ATP and glucose 6-phosphate; in liver, but not muscle, free glucose is also an inhibitor. Muscle phosphorylase differs from the liver isoenzyme in having a binding site for 5' AMP, which acts as an allosteric activator of the (inactive) dephosphorylated b-form of the enzyme.

- Increasing the concentration of cAMP activates cAMP-dependent protein kinase, which catalyzes the phosphorylation by ATP of inactive phosphorylase kinase b to active phosphorylase kinase a, which in turn, phosphorylates phosphorylase b to phosphorylase a. In the liver, cAMP is formed in response to glucagon, which is secreted in response to falling blood glucose.
- Muscle is insensitive to glucagon; in muscle, the signal for increased cAMP formation is the action of norepinephrine, which is secreted in response to fear or fright, when there is a need for increased glycogenolysis to permit rapid muscle activity.
- Glycogenolysis in muscle increases several 100-fold at the onset of contraction; the same signal (increased cytosolic Ca^{2+} ion concentration) is responsible for initiation of both contraction and glycogenolysis.
- Muscle phosphorylase kinase has a subunit which is identical to the Ca^{2+}-binding protein calmodulin and binds four Ca^{2+}. The binding of Ca^{2+} activates the catalytic site of the subunit even while the enzyme is in the dephosphorylated b state; the phosphorylated a form is only fully

73. Ans. (a) Decreased

Ref: Harper 30th Ed page 460, Lippincott 5th Ed Pg 475

Hemoglobin electrophoresis is used as a screening test to evaluate for and identify variant and abnormal hemoglobins. Alkaline and/or citrate agar electrophoresis is the commonly used method. Separation of hemoglobins is based on variable rates of migration of charged hemoglobin molecules in an electrical field. Hemoglobin is negatively charged and move towards Anode (Positive charge)

In the case of Sickle Cell hemoglobin, replacement of a negatively-charged Glu in the standard HbA beta-globin by a neutral Val in HbS results in a protein with a slightly reduced negative charge. Hence mobility of HbS is decreased compared to HbA.

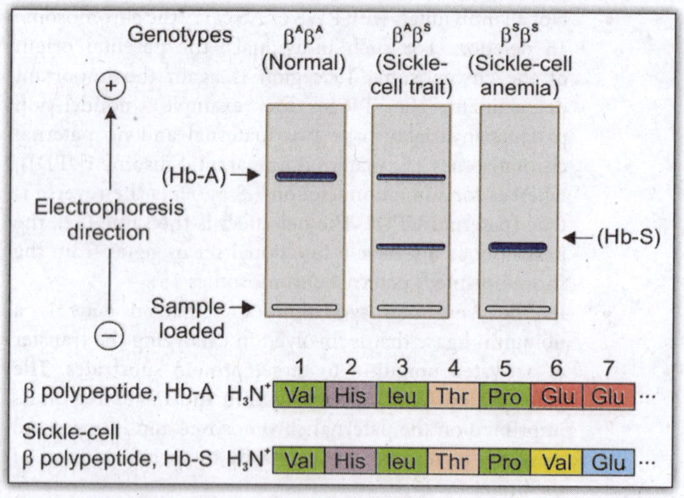

74. Ans. (b) RBC

Ref: Harper's 30th Ed page 325, 329

Harper states that ***"Heme biosynthesis occurs in most mammalian cells except mature erythrocytes, which lack mitochondria. Approximately 85% of heme synthesis occurs in erythroid precursor cells in the bone marrow and the majority of the remainder in hepatocytes"***

Steps of Heme/ Porphyrin Ring Synthesis

Enzyme	Location	Substrate	Product	Porphyria	Clinical	Lab Test
ALA synthase ***(Rate limiting)***	Mitochondrion	Glycine, succinyl CoA	D-Aminolevulinic acid	X linked Sideroblastic anemia	Anemia	↓RBC count, ↓Hb
ALA dehydratase (Zinc containing, Sensitive to lead poisoning)	Cytosol	D-Aminolevulinic acid	Porphobilinogen	ALA-Dehydratase deficiency	Abdominal pain, neuropsychiatric symptoms	↑Urinary ALA and coproporphyrin III

Contd...

Steps of Heme/ Porphyrin Ring Synthesis						
Enzyme	**Location**	**Substrate**	**Product**	**Porphyria**	**Clinical**	**Lab Test**
PBG deaminase/ HMB synthase/ **Uroporphyrinogen I synthase**	Cytosol	Porphobilinogen	Hydroxymethyl bilane	Acute intermittent porphyria	Abdominal pain, neuropsychiatric symptoms	↑Urinary ALA and PBG
Uroporphyrinogen III synthase	Cytosol	Hydroxymethyl bilane	Uroporphyrinogen III	Congenital erythropoietic porphyria	No photosensitivity	↑Urinary, fecal and RBC uroporphyrin I
Uroporphyrinogen III decarboxylase	Cytosol	Uroporphyrinogen III	Coproporphyrinogen III	Porphyria cutanea tarda	Photosensitivity	↑Urinaryuroporphyrin I
Coproporphyrinogen III oxidase	Mitochondrion	Coproporphyrinogen III	Protoporphyrinogen IX	Coproporphyria	Photosensitivity, abdominal pain, neuropsychiatric symptoms	↑Urinary ALA, PBG and coproporphyrin III and fecal coproporphyrin III
Protoporphyrinogen oxidase	Mitochondrion	Protoporphyrinogen IX	Protoporphyrin IX	Variegate porphyria	Photosensitivity, abdominal pain, neuropsychiatric symptoms	↑Urinary ALA, PBG and coproporphyrin III and fecal protoporphyrin IX
Ferrochelatase (Sensitive to Lead poisoning)	Mitochondrion	Protoporphyrin IX	Heme	Erythropoietic protoporphyria	Photosensitivity	↑Fecal and RBC protoporphyrin IX

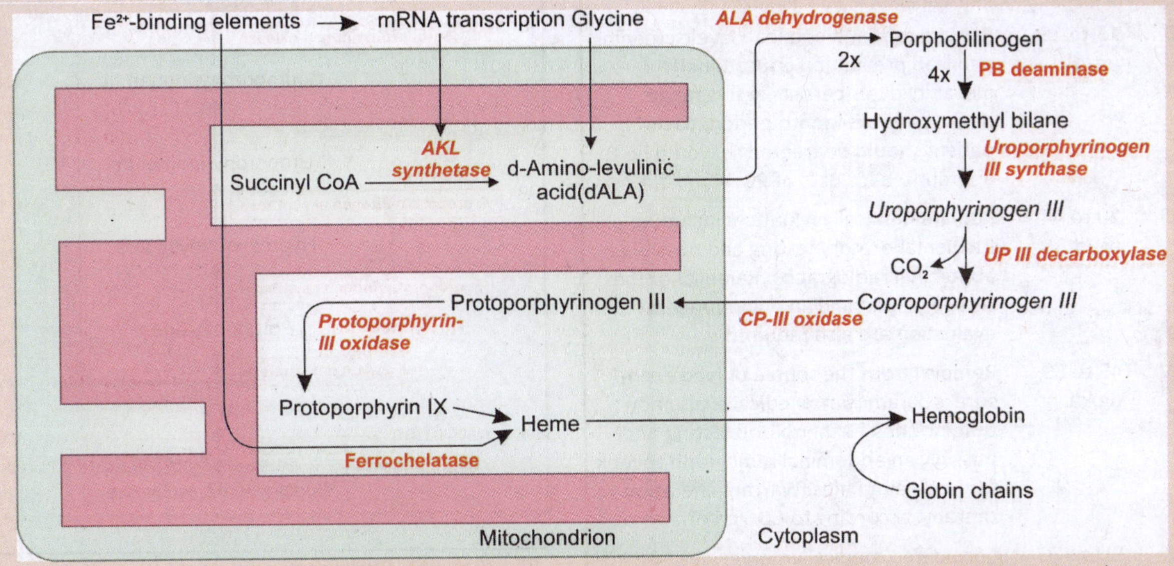

Fig: Heme synthesis—note that some reactions occur in the cytoplasm and some in the mitochondrion

Footnote

- Approximately 85% of heme synthesis occurs in erythroid precursor cells in the bone marrow and the majority of the remainder in hepatocytes
- The last three enzymes in the pathway and ALA synthase are located in the mitochondrion, whereas the other enzymes are cytosolic. Both erythroid and nonerythroid ("housekeeping") forms of ALA synthase are found.
- Humans express two isozymes of ALA synthase. ALAS1 is ubiquitously expressed throughout the body, whereas ALAS2 is expressed in erythrocyte precursor cells.
- ALA Synthase is the **Rate Limiting enzyme** of Heme synthesis and **Pyridoxal phosphate** is the cofactor
- **ALA dehydratase** is a zinc-containing enzyme and is sensitive to inhibition by lead, as can occur in lead poisoning.
- Lead inhibits two steps in the heme synthetic pathway: **ALA dehydratase and ferrochelatase**. This affects porphyrin metabolism. Elevated levels of protoporphyrin are found in RBC and elevated levels of ALA and coproporphyrin are found in urine.
- Ferrochelatase sensitivity to lead is the greatest and thus the most significant in lead poisoning.

75. Ans. (a) ALA

Ref: Harper 30th ed page 325, 329, Parikh 6th ed page 9.22

(See previous question for details of Heme Synthesis) (see page no. 227)

Lead inhibits two steps in the heme synthetic pathway: **ALA dehydratase and ferrochelatase**. This affects porphyrin metabolism. Elevated levels of protoporphyrin are found in RBC and elevated levels of ALA and coproporphyrin are found in urine.

Ferrochelatase sensitivity to lead is the greatest and thus the most significant in lead poisoning.

Lab Investigations for Lead Poisoning

The criterion standard is a whole blood lead level (BLL). Any BLL higher than 10 µg/dL is considered positive and consequential. Patients with BLLs between 10 and 20 µg/dL require removal from the exposure, repeated testing and follow-up. A free erythrocyte protoporphyrin (FEP) level may be useful in demonstrating the degree of biological abnormalities that exists.

Class	Lead levels	Management
Class I	10 to 14 µg/dL	Require no further treatment other than lead prevention education, but periodic screening in young children should continue
Class II	15 to 19 µg/dL	Require repeat blood lead level screening and lead prevention education. If elevated levels persists in this range or rise over a 3-month period, the patient should be treated as would be appropriate for BLLs of 20-44 µg/dL)
Class III	20 to 44 µg/dL	Require medical evaluation, including further laboratory testing and possible abdominal radiographs. Removal of the source of lead and an environmental evaluation are also required
Class IV	45 to 69 µg/dL	Removal from the source of lead exposure is paramount. Medical evaluation that includes further blood testing and possibly an abdominal radiograph to look for lead paint chips. Warrant **chelation therapy**, according to CDC criteria
Class V	BLLs >70 µg/dL	Considered medical emergencies, regardless of whether neurologic symptoms are present The risk of encephalopathy is high and treatment is required.

NOTE

Here the enzyme not the Product or substrate which is increases is asked. We know the enzymes that are inhibited by lead are ALA dehydrogenase and Ferrochelatase. But here the enzyme that is increases is asked.

Harper states "It appears that heme, probably acting through an aporepressor molecule, acts as a negative regulator of the synthesis of ALAS1. The rate of synthesis of ALAS1 thus increases greatly in the absence of heme, but diminishes in its presence"

Hence in lead poisoning Heme production is decreased and this feedback inhibition is also decreased resulting in increased levels of ALA synthase.

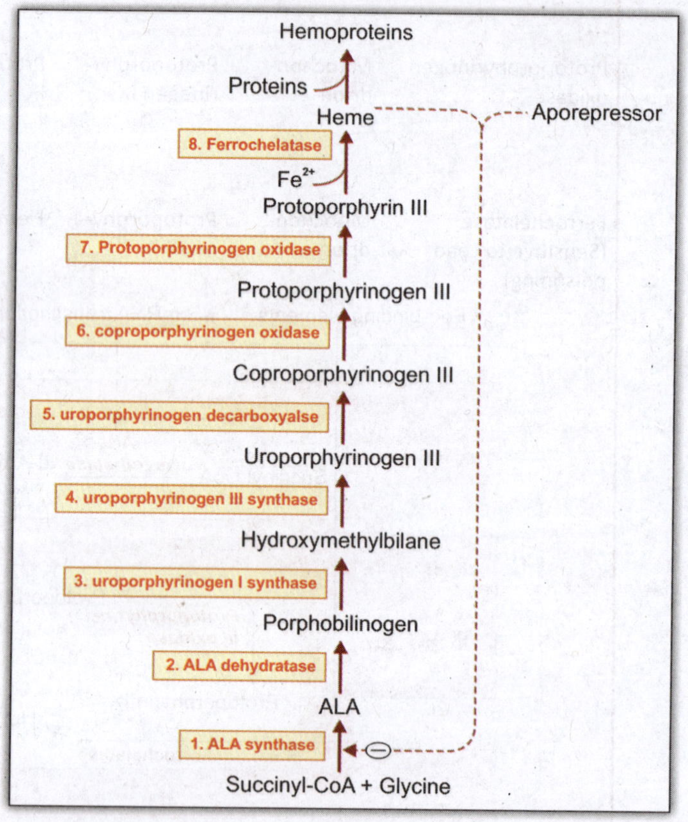

AIIMS MAY 2015

76. Ans. (a) ALA synthase

Ref: Harper 30th ed page 327

(See previous question Biochemistry AIIMS Nov 2015 for details of Lead poisoning)

77. Ans. (b) Phosphoglucomutase

Ref: Harper 29th Ed page 180, 190

Phosphoglucomutase is the enzyme used in both glycogenesis and glycogenolysis

Glycogenesis	
Step	**Enzyme**
Formation of glucose 1 phosphate from glucose 6 phosphate Glucose 6P → Glucose 1P	Phosphoglucomutase
Synthesis of uridine diphosphate glucose Glucose 1 P + UTP → UDP Glucose	Pyrophosphate
UDP Glucose + Glycogenin → Primer glycogen	Autocatalysis by glycogenin

Contd...

Glycogenesis	
Step	**Enzyme**
Elongation of a glycogen chain: It involves the transfer of glucose from UDP-glucose to the nonreducing end of the growing chain, forming a new glycosidic bond between the anomeric hydroxyl group of carbon 1 of the activated glucose and carbon 4 of the accepting glucosyl residue	Glycogen synthetase
Branching Branches are made by the action of the branching enzyme, amylo-α(1→4)→α(1→6)-transglucosidase. This enzyme removes a set of six to eight glucosyl residues from the nonreducing end of the glycogen chain, breaking an α(1→4) bond to another residue on the chain and attaches it to a nonterminal glucosyl residue by an α(1→6) linkage, thus functioning as a 4:6 transferase.	Amylo-α (1→4) → α(1→6)-transglucosidase

Steps and Enzymes in Degeneration of Glycogen

When glycogen is degraded, the primary product is glucose 1-phosphate, obtained by breaking α(1→4) glycosidic bonds. In addition, free glucose is released from each α(1→6)–linked glucosyl residue

Glycogenolysis	
Steps	**Enzymes**
Shortening of chains Glycogen phosphorylase sequentially cleaves the α(1→4) glycosidic bonds between the glucosyl residues at the nonreducing ends of the glycogen chains by simple phosphorolysis (producing glucose 1-phosphate) until four glucosyl units remain on each chain before a branch point	Glycogen phosphorylase
Debranching Branches are removed by the two enzymic activities of a single bifunctional protein, the debranching. First, oligo-α(1→4)→α(1→4)- glucantransferase activity removes the outer three of the four glucosyl residues attached at a branch. It next transfers them to the nonreducing end of another chain, lengthening it accordingly. Thus, an α(1→4) bond is broken and an α(1→4) bond is made and the enzyme functions as a 4:4 transferase. Next, the remaining glucose residue attached in an α(1→6) linkage is removed hydrolytically by amylo-α(1→6)-glucosidase activity, releasing free glucose. The glucosyl chain is now available again for degradation by glycogen phosphorylase until four glucosyl units in the next branch are reached.	Debranching enzyme α (1→ 4) → α(1→4)-glucan-transferase, 4:4 transferase
Glucose 1-phosphate, produced by glycogen phosphorylase, is converted in the cytosol to glucose 6-phosphate ; Glucose IP → Glucose 6 P	Phosphoglucomutase

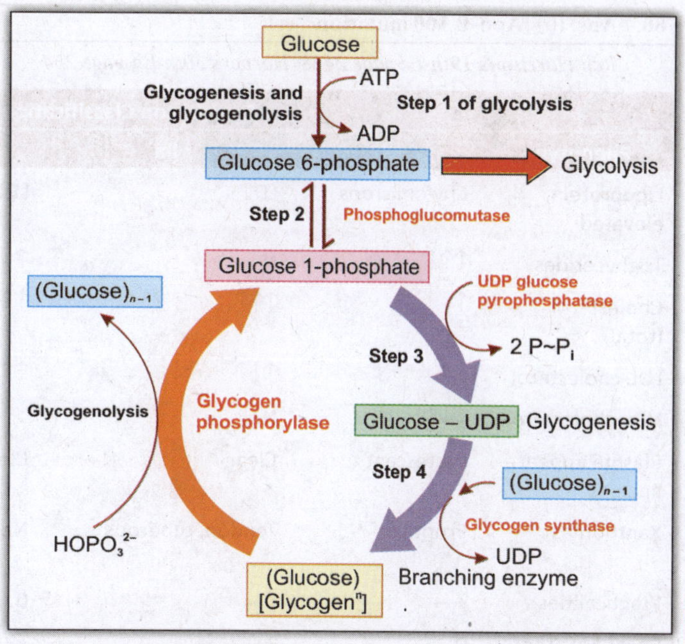

Thus the common enzyme is phosphoglucomutase.

78. Ans. (a) 245

Ref: Lippincott's 6th Ed page 420, Harrison's 19th ed page 2446

The cholesterol (C) content of plasma lipoproteins is now routinely measured in fasting blood. Total C = LDL + HDL + VLDL, where VLDL is calculated by dividing TAG by 5 because TAG represent 20% of the volume of VLDL. The goal value for total cholesterol is less than 200 mg/dL.

Thus, putting down values in equation

300 = LDL + 25 + 150/5

300 = LDL + 25 + 30

300 = LDL + 55

LDL = 300 -55

LDL = 245

79. Ans. (a) Glucose

Ref: Harper's 28th Ed, P- 141,612

Glucose is Always Required by the Central Nervous System and Erythrocytes

- Erythrocytes lack mitochondria and hence are wholly reliant on (anaerobic) glycolysis and the pentose phosphate pathway at all times.
- The brain can metabolize ketone bodies to meet about 20% of its energy requirements; the remainder must be supplied by glucose.
- The metabolic changes that occur in the fasting state and starvation are the consequences of the need to preserve glucose and the limited reserves of glycogen in liver and muscle for use by the brain and red blood cells and to ensure the provision of alternative metabolic fuels for other tissues.

80. Ans. (b) Apo-B 100 mutation

Ref: Harrison's 19th Ed page 2438, Harper's 30th Ed page 254

Fredrickson Classification of Hyperlipoproteinemias

Phenotype	I	IIa	IIb	II	IV	V
Lipoprotein, elevated	Chylomicrons	LDL	LDL and VLDL	Chylomicron and VLDL remnants	VLDL	Chylomicrons and VLDL
Trighycerides	↑↑↑	N	↑	↑↑	↑↑	↑↑↑
Cholesterol (total)	↑	↑↑↑	↑↑	↑↑	N/↑	↑↑
LDL-cholesterol	↓	↑↑↑	↑↑	↓	↓	↓
HDL-cholesterol	↓↓↓	N/↓	↓	N	↓↓	↓↓↓
Plasma appearance	Lactescent	Clear	Clear	Turbid	Turbid	Lactescent
Xanthomas	Eruptive	Tendon, tuberous	None	Palmar, tubero-eruptive	None	Eruptive
Practicalities	+++	0	0	0	0	+++
Coronary atherosclerosis	0	+++	+++	+++	+/–	+/–
Peripheral atherosclerosis	0	+	+	++	+/–	+/–
Molecular defects	*LPL and ApoC-II*	*LDL receptor, ApoB–100, PCSk9, LDLRAP, ABCG5 and ABCG 8*		*ApoE*	*ApoA–V*	*ApoA–V and GPIHBP1*
Genetic nomenclature	*FCS*	*FH, FDB, ADH, ARH, Sitosterolemia*	*FCHL*	*FDBL*	*FHTG*	*FHTG*

81. Ans. (a) Chylomicron

Ref: Harrison's 19th Ed page 2438, Harper's 30th Ed page 254

See table in previous question.

Xanthomas are present in hyperlipoproteinemias I, IIa, III, V. Amongst these, I, III, V show turbid appearance of plasma. In each of these 3, chylomicrons are elevated.

82. Ans. (b) Cell size

Ref: Haematology: Clinical Principles and Application Pg 456; Introduction to Flow Cytometry: A Learning Guide Pg 10

- Light scattering occurs when a particle deflects incident laser light. The extent to which this occurs depends on the physical properties of a particle, namely its size and internal complexity.
- Factors that affect light scattering are the cell's membrane, nucleus and any granular material inside the cell.
- Cell shape and surface topography also contribute to the total light scatter. Forward-scattered light (FSC) is proportional to cell-surface area or size.
- FSC is a measurement of mostly diffracted light and is detected just off the axis of the incident laser beam in the forward direction by a photodiode.
- FSC provides a suitable method of detecting particles greater than a given size independent of their fluorescence and is therefore often used in immunophenotyping to trigger signal processing. Side-scattered light (SSC) is proportional to cell granularity or internal complexity. SSC is a measurement of mostly refracted and reflected light that occurs at any interface within the cell where there is a change in refractive index.
- SSC is collected at approximately 90 degrees to the laser beam by a collection lens and then redirected by a beam splitter to the appropriate detector.

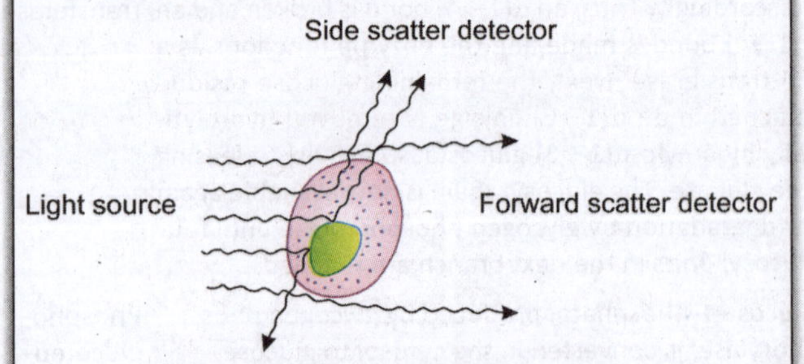

Light-scattering properties of a cell

- Correlated measurements of FSC and SSC can allow for differentiation of cell types in a heterogeneous cell population. Major leucocyte subpopulations can be differentiated using FSC and SSC.

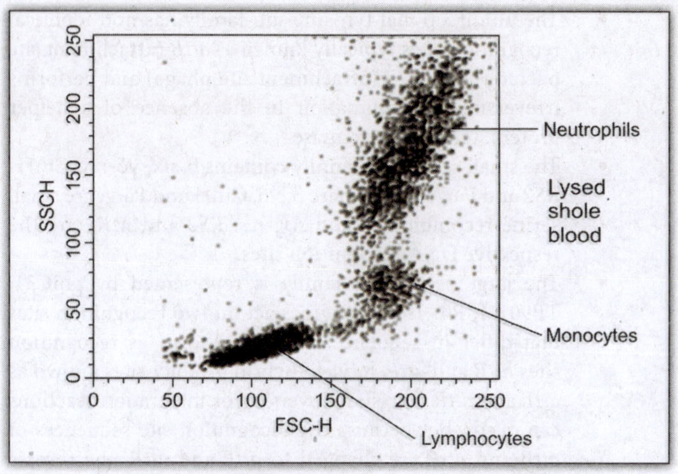

Fig: Cell subpopulation based on FSC vs SSS

83. Ans. (b) Pyruvate dehydrogenase

Ref: Harper's 30th ed page 165, 172, 555

- In the mitochondrial matrix, pyruvate is converted to acetyl CoA by the pyruvate dehydrogenase complex (PDH complex), which is a multienzyme complex. The PDH complex is a protein aggregate of multiple copies of three enzymes, pyruvate carboxylase (E1, sometimes called pyruvate dehydrogenase), dihydrolipoyl transacetylase (E2) and dihydrolipoyl dehydrogenase E3). Each catalyzes a part of the overall reaction.
- The PDH complex contains five coenzymes that act as carriers or oxidants for the intermediates of the reactions. E1 requires thiamine pyrophosphate (TPP), E2 requires lipoic acid and CoA and E3 requires flavin adenine dinucleotide (FAD) and nicotinamide adenine dinucleotide (NAD+).
- Therefore, in absence of thiamine, E1 of Pyruvate dehydrogenase complex will not work, Hence pyruvate will not be able to get converted into Acetyl CoA and will be shunted to form lactate by lactate dehydrogenase.
- *Pyruvate dehydrogenase complex deficiency: A deficiency in the activity of the α subunit of the dimeric E1 component of the PDH complex, although rare, is the most common biochemical cause of congenital lactic acidosis. This enzyme deficiency results in an inability to convert pyruvate to acetyl CoA, causing pyruvate to be shunted to lactate via lactate dehydrogenase.*

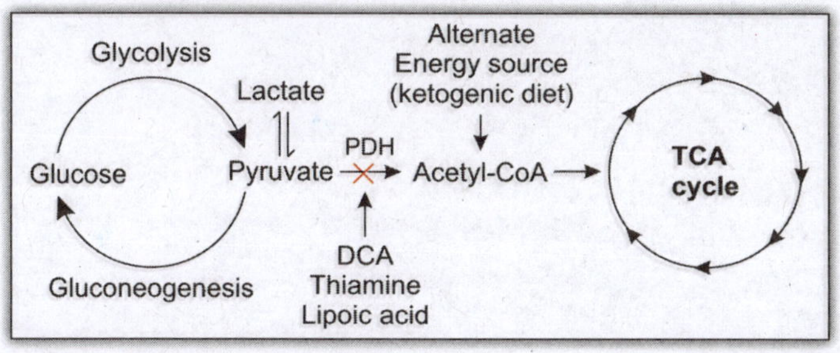

84. Ans. (c) Knock down

Ref: Advanced Delivery and Therapeutic Applications of RNAi edited by Kun Cheng page 9

- **RNA interference** (**RNAi**) is an important set of pathways that are used to regulate gene expression. **RNAi** is a blanket term which can refer to both small interfering RNAs (**siRNAs**) and microRNAs (miRNAs).
- Small interfering RNA (siRNA), which is a group of double-stranded RNA molecules of approximately 21 nucleotides in length, plays an important role in messenger RNA (mRNA) degradation, where it prevents the expression of a specific gene.
- Given the ability to knock down any gene of interest, siRNA has been widely used as an experimental tool that is now becoming a progressive field of research due to its large medicinal potential in the pharmaceutical industry.
- Therapeutic siRNA, which is a group of new pharmaceutically active molecules, provides a potent and selective gene-inhibition mechanism that can be used to achieve targeted therapeutics at a transcriptional level.
- Compared to existing molecular targeting technologies, such as antibody-mediated therapy, siRNA therapy can easily be adapted and applied to virtually any target of interest, including the key factors that govern gene expression, signalling cascades, intracellular factors and transcription factors.
- In addition to the advanced synthetic techniques of nucleic acids, the affordability of siRNA therapy further facilitates its translation into clinical trials for disease treatment.

85. Ans. (b) LoxP site

Ref: Harper 30th ed page 454

- *As an adjunct to the use of restriction endonucleases scientists have recently begun utilizing specific prokaryotic or eukaryotic recombinases (such as bacterial lox P sites, which are recognized by the CRE recombinase, or yeast FRT sites recognized by the Flp recombinase) to catalyze specific incorporation of two DNA fragments that carry the appropriate recognition sequences. These enzymes catalyze homologous recombination between the relevant recognition sites.*
- Site-specific recombinase systems were discovered in bacteria and yeast and found to facilitate a number of biological functions, including the phase variation of certain bacterial virulence factors and the integration of bacteriophage into the host genome. Site-specific recombination occurs at a specific sequence or recognition site and involves cleavage and reunion leading to integration, deletion or inversion of a DNA fragment without the gain or loss of nucleotides. Whether its integration, deletion or inversion of a DNA fragment, orientation of the recognition sites determines the mode of action.
- The recombinase super family can be split into two fundamental groups, the tyrosine and serine recombinases. This division is based on the active amino acid (Tyr or Ser) within the catalytic domain of the enzymes in each family. Both families can be further subdivided into unique members based on either size or mode of recombinase action.

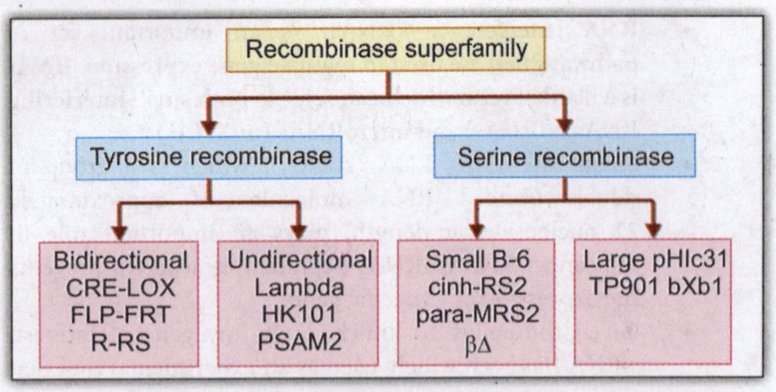

- Within this bidirectional tyrosine sub-family, the recombinase-mediated genetic cross-over occurs between the two identical recognition sites. Because of the identical nature of the recognition sites the recombination reaction is fully reversible, although intra-molecular recombination (excision) is highly favored over intermolecular reactions (integration).
- The unidirectional tyrosine sub-family has non-identical recognition sites typically known as *attB* (**att**achment site **b**acteria) and *attP* (**att**achment site **p**hage) and performs irreversible recombination in the absence of a helper protein, termed an excinase.
- The small serine sub-family contains β-*six*, γδ-*res*, CinH-*RS2* and ParA-*MRS* where β, γδ, CinH and ParA are small serine recombinases and *six, res, RS2* and *MRS* are the respective DNA recognition sites.
- The large serine sub-family is represented by phiC31, TP901-1, R4. These enzymes act on two recognition sites that differ in sequence, typically known as recognition sites *attB* and *attP*, to yield hybrid product sites known as *attL* and *attR*. Excision, inversion or integration reactions can occur, but because the recognition site sequences of *attB* and *attP* are changed to *attL* and *attR*, the reverse reaction cannot occur.

Microbiology

4

AIIMS NOVEMBER 2018

1. The Most common causative agent of Bacterial meningitis in a 1 year child is?

a. Pneumococcus
b. H. influenzae
c. Neisseria meningitidis
d. Listeria

2. Interferon beta production is stimulated by?

a. Virus
b. Bacteria
c. Fungus
d. Mycoplasma

3. A party was organised in which 200 people attended it. Few of them developed food poisoning after 24 hrs of party in which they consumed following items. Identify causative agent from the data given below?

40 ill from 50 who consumed oyster
50 ill from 135 who consumed hamburger
60 ill from 140 who consumed salad
49 ill from 115 who consumed ice cream

a. Staphylococcus aureus
b. Yersinia enterocolitica
c. Vibrio parahemolyticus
d. Salmonella enteritidis

4. The picture below indicates the Life cycle of?

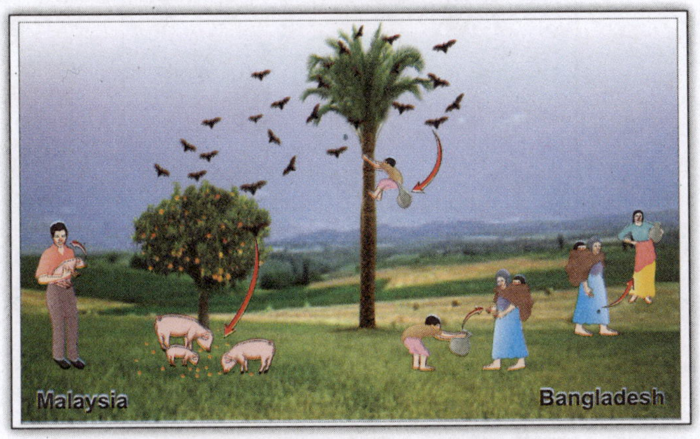

a. Nipah virus
b. Chandipura virus
c. Influenza virus
d. Japanese encephalitis

5. A patient who had undergone renal transplant 3 months back presented with complaints of dysentery. No parasitic ova/cysts are found on fecal examination. Video showing larva was shown and asked what is incorrect about this organism?

a. Organism shown is filiform larva which is responsible for diarrhea
b. Organism may cause Loeffler's pneumonia
c. Organism is monoecious in nature so able to reproduce by using parthenogenesis
d. It is caused due to food/water contamination

6. A HIV/AIDS patient presents with complaint of diarrhea. No parasitic cysts/ovas are found on fecal examination. On Kinyoun stain, 2-6 μm organism are seen as shown in the slide. What could be the causative agent?

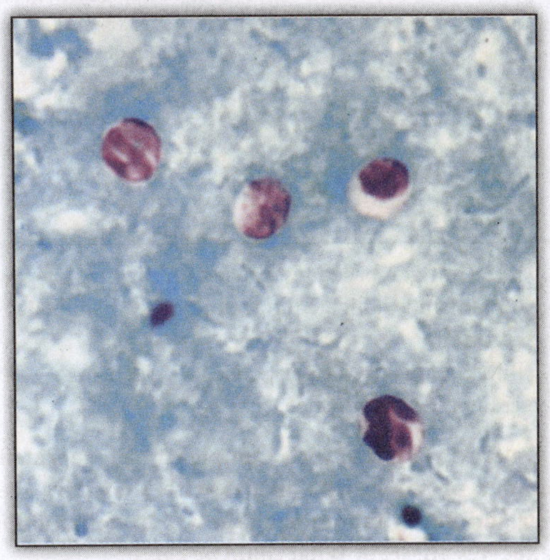

a. Cystoisospora
b. Cryptosporidium
c. Giardia
d. Balantidium coli

7. **A child presents with greyish membrane over pharyngeal wall. On stripping it bleeds. A throat swab was taken and stained which showed following. Components of stain are**

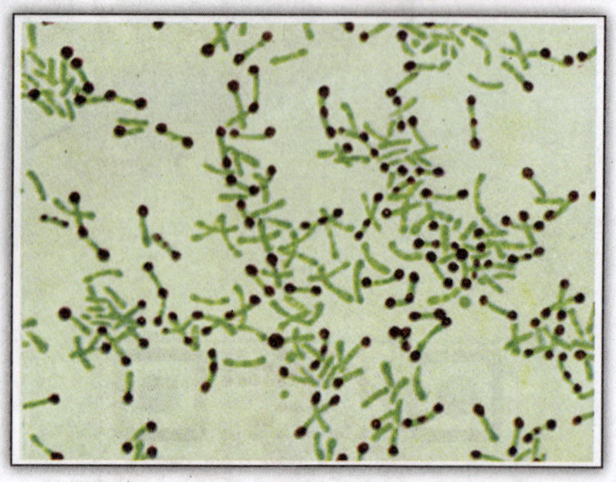

a. Gram's iodine, acetone and safranin
b. Toluidine blue, acetone and malachite green
c. Toluidine blue, glacial acetic acid and malachite green
d. Gram's iodine, acetone and methylene blue

8. **Tuberculosis is transmitted through droplets mode of transmission; which other disease also has similar mode of transmission in which isolation is done?**
a. Pertussis
b. Atypical pneumonia
c. Faucial diphtheria
d. Hepatitis B

9. **25 yr old male presents with hepatosplenomegaly associated with fever. Bone marrow biopsy revealed following findings. Which of the following is Correct about this?**

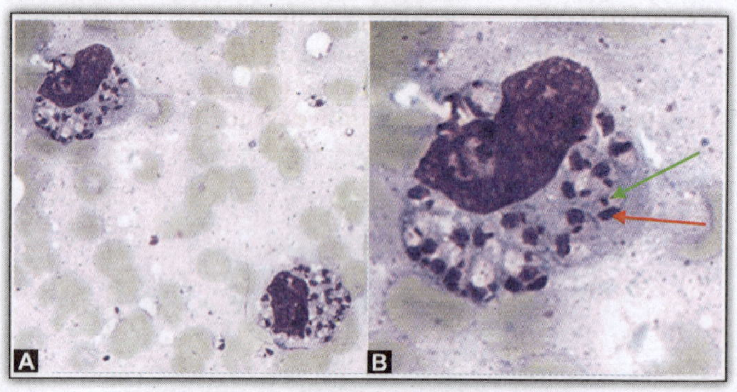

a. Rk39 antigen based test is used for diagnosis
b. Organism is obligate intracellular organism hence can't be cultured
c. Buffy coat is used to diagnose the organism
d. Transmitted from sheep

10. **A patient presents with complaints of repeated small amounts of stools with mucus with subjective feeling of fever and lower abdominal pain. On examination of stool leukocytes are seen. What could be cause?**
a. Giardia
b. Entamoeba histolytica
c. Clostridium perfringens
d. Staphylococcus

AIIMS MAY 2018

11. **A patient presented with complaints of dysphagia. On Upper GI endoscopy, a diagnosis of esophageal candidiasis was made. The organism obtained from the sample was cultured on special media and the below findings were visible on microscopy of the culture. What phenomenon is shown below?**

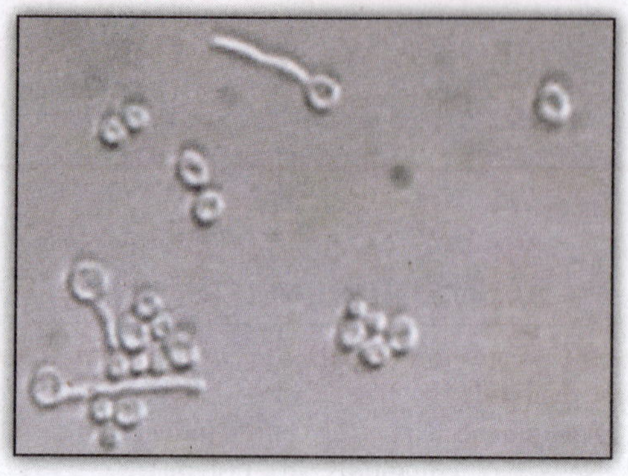

a. Germ tube formation
b. Spore formation
c. Mould to yeast formation
d. Budding

12. **A HIV/AIDS patient presents with complaint of diarrhea. No parasitic cysts/ovas are found on fecal examination. On Kinyoun stain, 2-6 μm organism are seen as shown in the slide. What could be the causative agent?**
(AIIMS Nov 2018, May 2018)

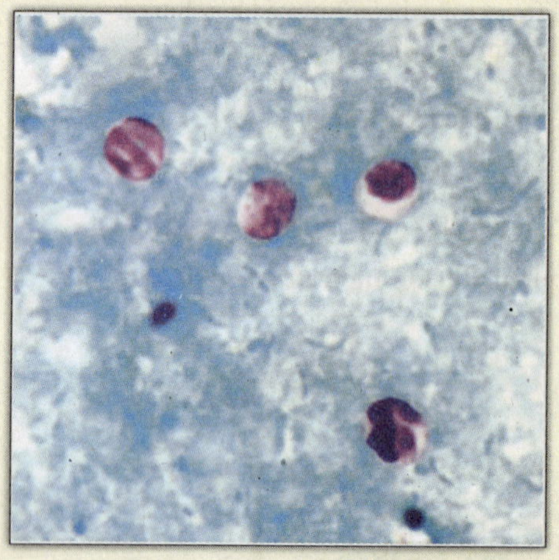

a. Cystoisospora
b. Cryptosporidium
c. Giardia
d. Balantidium coli

13. **A patient is suffering from acute hepatitis. LFT is done. Which test is to be done next?**
a. IgM HAV
b. IgM HDV
c. IgM HEV
d. HBsAg

14. **Single donor plasma destroys enveloped viruses. Which of the following viral infection is still possible with single donor plasma transfusion?**
a. HAV
b. HBV
c. HCV
d. HIV

15. **Which of the following gas is used in plasma sterilization?**
a. Hydrogen peroxide
b. Ethylene Oxide
c. Carbon dioxide
d. Nitrous oxide

16. Identify the microscopic technique and the bacteria in the given picture?

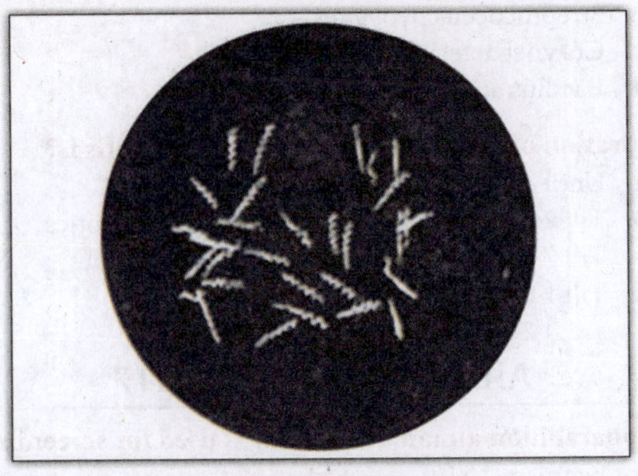

a. Dark field microscopy for T. Pallidum
b. Negative staining for Borrelia
c. Fluorescent staining for T Pallidum
d. Treponema Pallidum-particle Agglutination (TP-PA) Test

17. The process shown in the given picture is of?

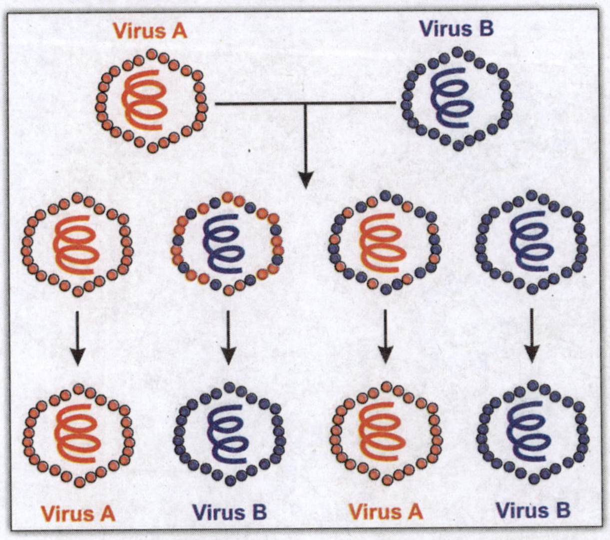

a. Conjugation
b. Transformation
c. Complementation
d. Translation

18. Identify the organism in the following image?

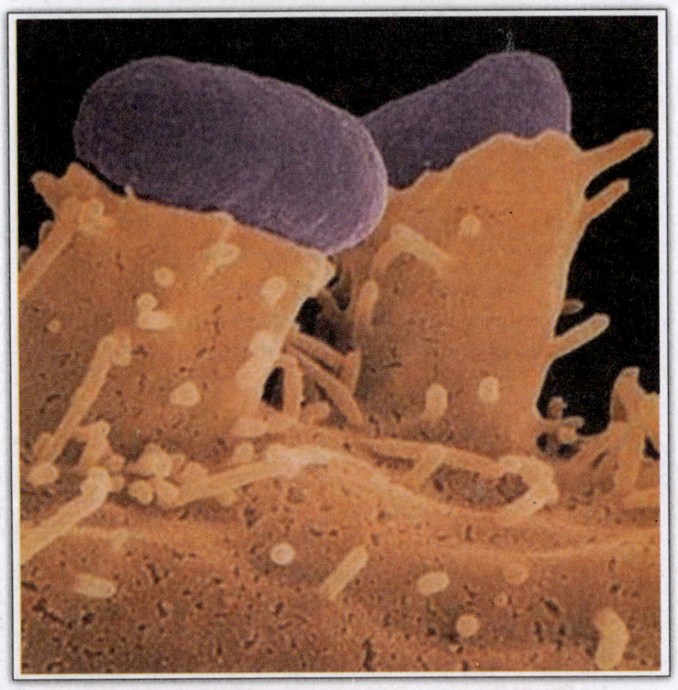

a. Enterotoxigenic E coli
b. Enteroinvasive E coli
c. Enteropathogenic E coli
d. Shigella

19. Identify the Organism from life cycle shown in the picture?

a. SARS
b. Influenza A
c. Parainfluenza virus
d. Respiratory Syncytial virus

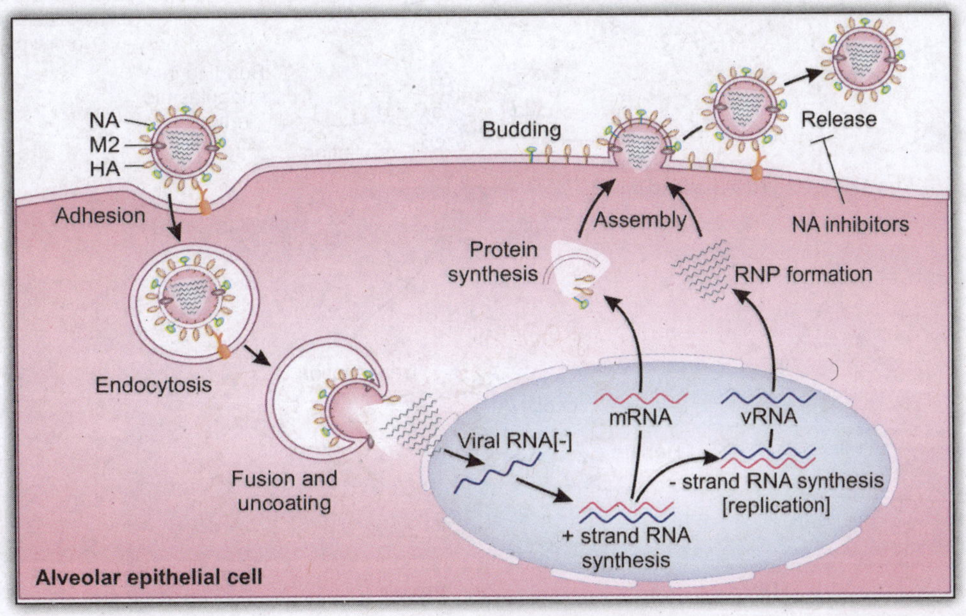

20. A child presented with upper GI pain and nausea. Stool examination was done and following picture was seen. What treatment will be given for this condition?

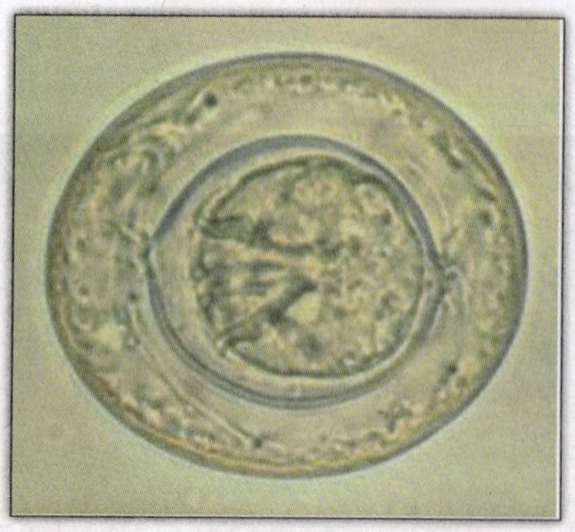

a. Praziquantel
b. Mebendazole
c. Albendazole
d. Pyrantel pamoate

21. Which of the following is bacitracin sensitive?

a. Staphylococcus aureus
b. Streptococcus pyogenes
c. Corynebacterium diphtheriae
d. Bacillus anthracis

22. Duration of isolation for bacterial meningitis is?

a. Until cultures become negative
b. Till 24 hour after administration of antibiotics
c. Till 7 days post administration of antibiotics
d. Till 1 month after giving antibiotics

AIIMS NOVEMBER 2017

23. Lipoarabinomannan urine assay is used for screening of?

a. Leprosy
b. Tuberculosis
c. Corynebacterium
d. Streptococcus

24. Replication cycle of which virus is shown in the Picture Below?

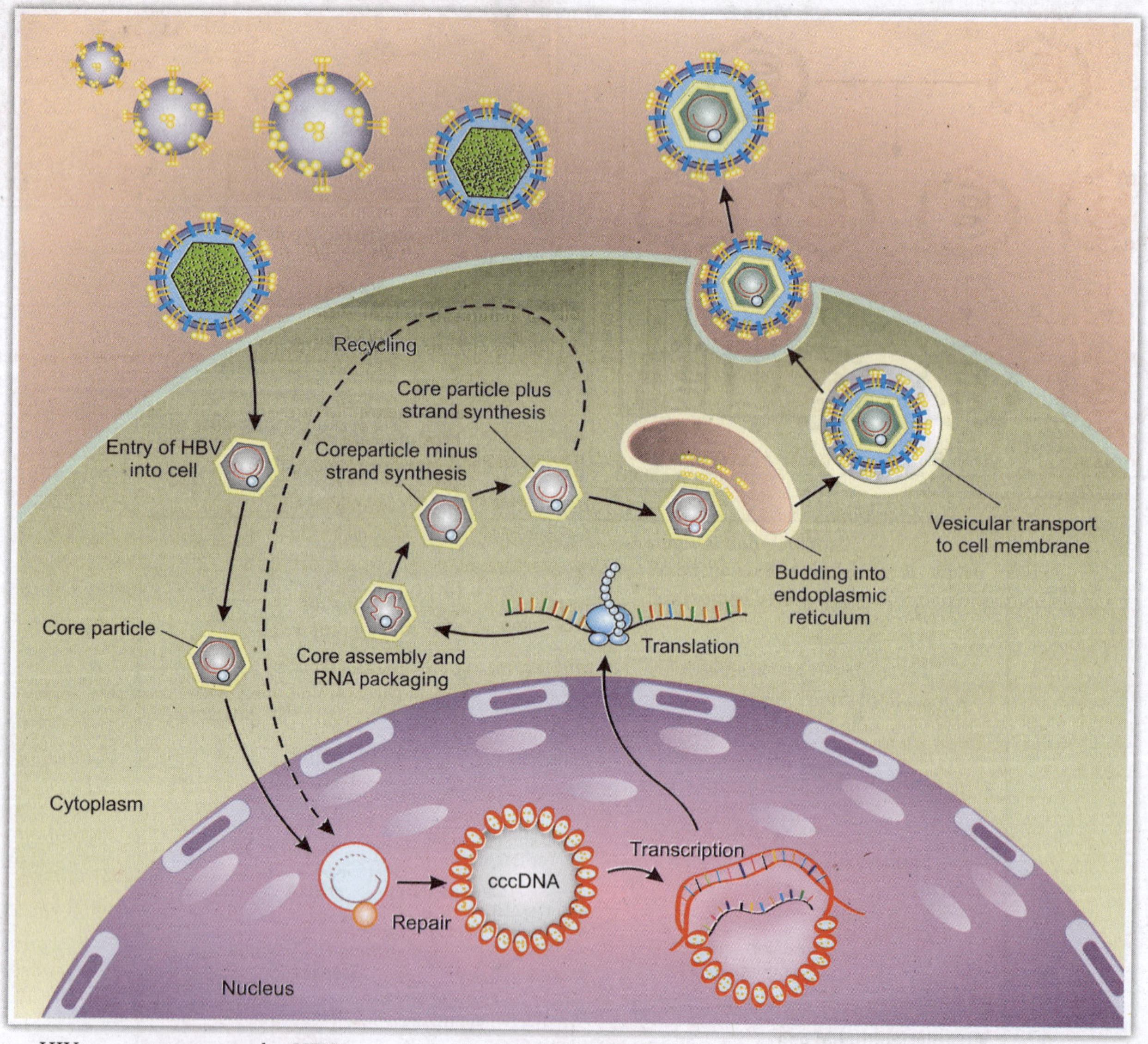

a. HIV
b. HBV
c. EBV
d. Polio

25. Identify the parasite in fecal smear picture?

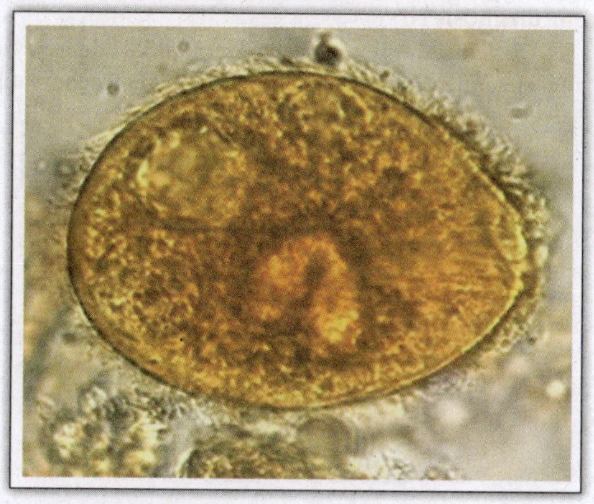

a. Entamoeba dyspar b. Balantidium coli
c. Cryptosporidium d. Giardia

26. Best method of diagnosis of clostridium difficile is?

a. Toxin assay by ELISA
b. Pure strain Isolation by culture
c. Gene detection by PCR
d. Colonoscopy

27. Identify the Bacteria with structure shown in the picture?

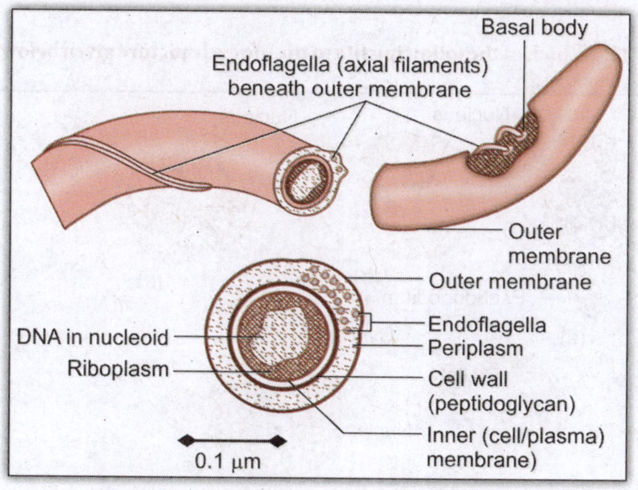

a. Vibrio
b. Leptospira
c. Helicobacter pylori
d. Campylobacter

28. All of following are dimorphic fungi EXCEPT:

a. Histoplasma capsulatum
b. Penicillium marneffei
c. Pneumocystis jiroveci
d. Sporothrix schenckii

29. A lady presented with verrucous growth as show in the picture. She gives history of thorn prick 6 months back. What is the most likely causative agent?

a. Mycetoma
b. Sporotrichosis
c. Chromoblastomycosis
d. Tinea nigra

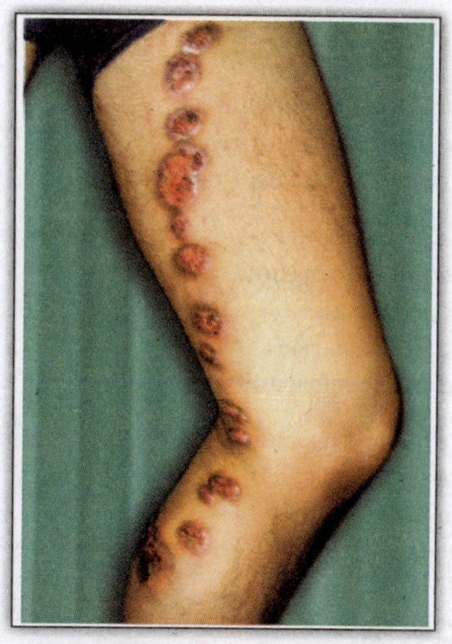

30. A female from Himachal pradesh presented with history of thorn prick a year back and now with verrucous lesion on leg. Biopsy image is shown below. What is most likely diagnosis?

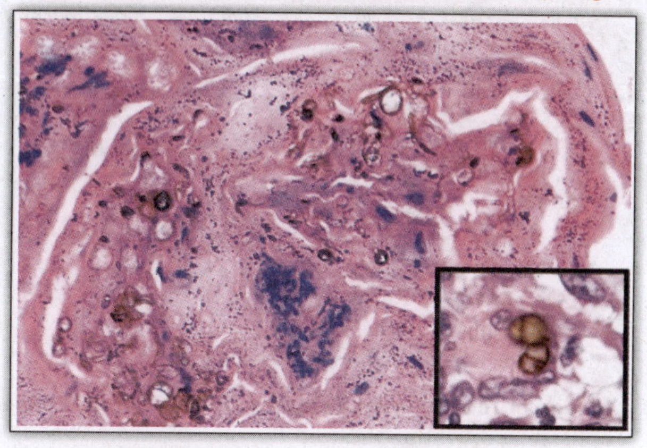

a. Sporotrichosis b. Chromoblastomycosis
c. Actinomycetoma d. Eumycetoma

31. An HIV positive patient develops diarrhea and faecal examination shows Cystoisospora belli. He was treated with cotrimoxazole. Diarrhea subsides but fever persists. Bone marrow examination was done and following picture was obtained. All are true about the organism EXCEPT:

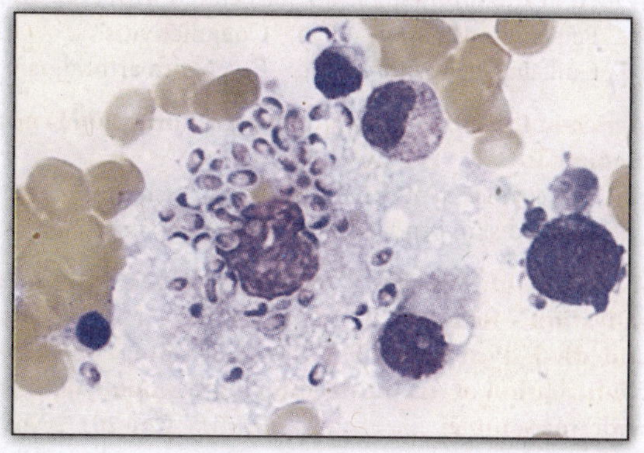

a. It is an intracellular yeast
b. It causes disseminated disease
c. It doesn't grow in SDA
d. Spores are highly infectious

32. **Beta (1-3)D glucan assay used for diagnosjs of?**
   a. Invasive candidiasis
   b. Cryotococcus encephalitis
   c. Rhino cerebral mucormycosis
   d. Pneumocystis jiroveci Pneumonia

33. **Which of the following types of malaria shows relapse?**
   a. Vivax and Falciparum
   b. Vivax and Ovale
   c. Vivax and Malariae
   d. Ovale and Falciparum

34. **In a case of Infective endocarditis the organism responsible is shown in the given picture. Identify the following organism.**

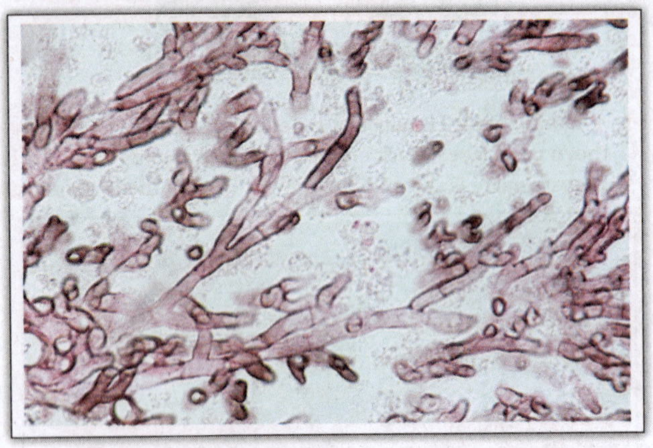

   a. Obtuse angled Mucor
   b. Obtuse angled Rhizopus
   c. Acute angled Penicillium
   d. Acute angled branching aspergillus

35. **Which of the following disinfectant is used to clean blood spillage in operation theatre?**
   a. Phenol based compound
   b. Alcohol based compound
   c. Chlorinated compounds
   d. Quaternary ammonium compounds

AIIMS MAY 2017

36. **Which of the following is not associated with zika virus?**
   a. Petechial rash b. Conjunctivitis
   c. Guillain barre syndrome d. Fever with arthralgia

37. **Which of the following staphylococcal infection is not toxin mediated?**
   a. Toxic shock syndrome b. Food poisoning
   c. Scalded skin syndrome d. Septic shock

38. **A child with history of dog bite comes with increased salivation, inability to drink water and hydrophobia and died. Post mortem Corneal scraping was taken for confirmation of diagnosis. Which test would you like to do with this sample?** ***(AIIMS May 2017, Nov 2016)***
   a. RT PCR
   b. Seller stain for negri bodies
   c. Indirect immunofluorescence
   d. Cell culture

39. **The following is a picture from scrapping of genital ulcer. Your diagnosis is?**
   a. Klebsiella granulomatis b. Hemophilus ducreyi
   c. Neisseria gonorrhoea d. Chlamydia trachomatis

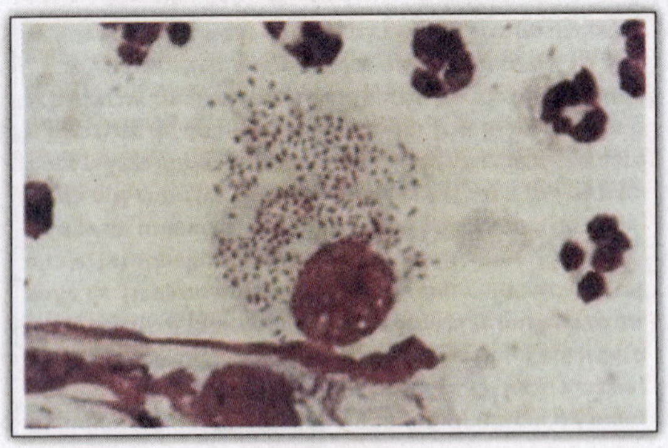

40. **Papain cleaves the immunoglobulin molecule into?** ***(AIIMS May 2017, AIPG 2014, DNB 2010)***
   a. 1 Fc and 1 Fab b. 1 Fc and 2 Fab
   c. 2 Fc and 1 Fab d. 2 Fc and 2 Fab

41. **Rhinosporidium seeberi belongs to?**
   a. Fungus
   b. Bacteria
   c. Aquatic protistan protozoa
   d. Virus

42. **Which of the following fits to the life cycle picture given below?**

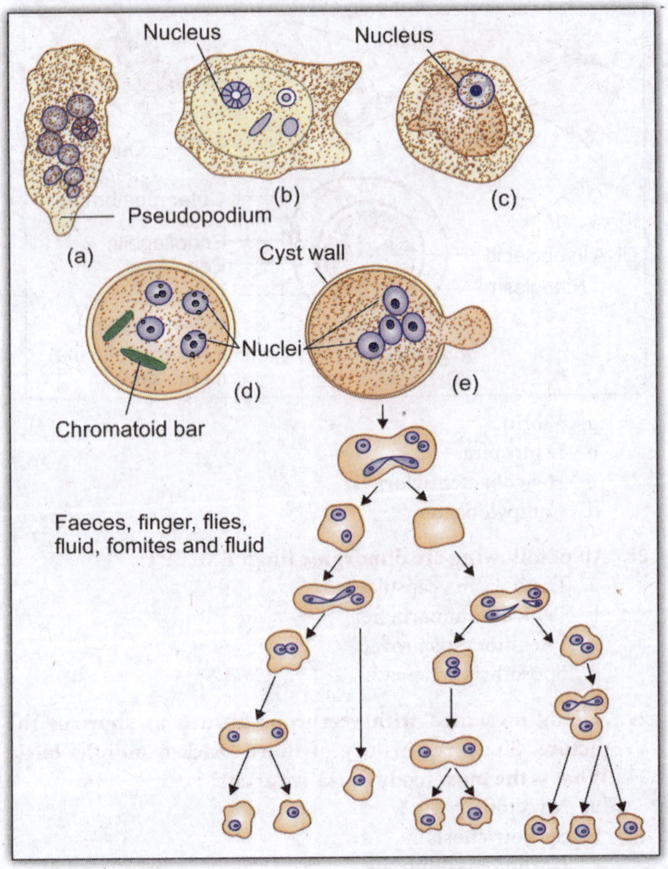

   a. B. coli b. E. histolytica
   c. A. duodenale d. E. vermicularis

43. Identify the organism from its egg in the picture?

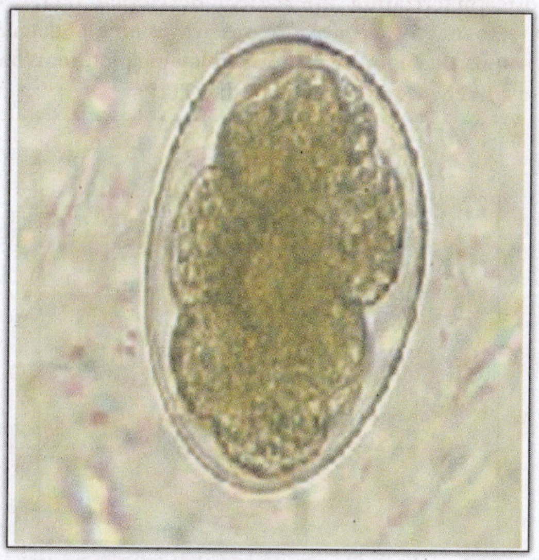

a. Enterobius vermicularis
b. Trichuris trichiura
c. Ascaris Lumbricoides
d. Necator americanus

44. Which of the following parasite's life cycle is shown below?

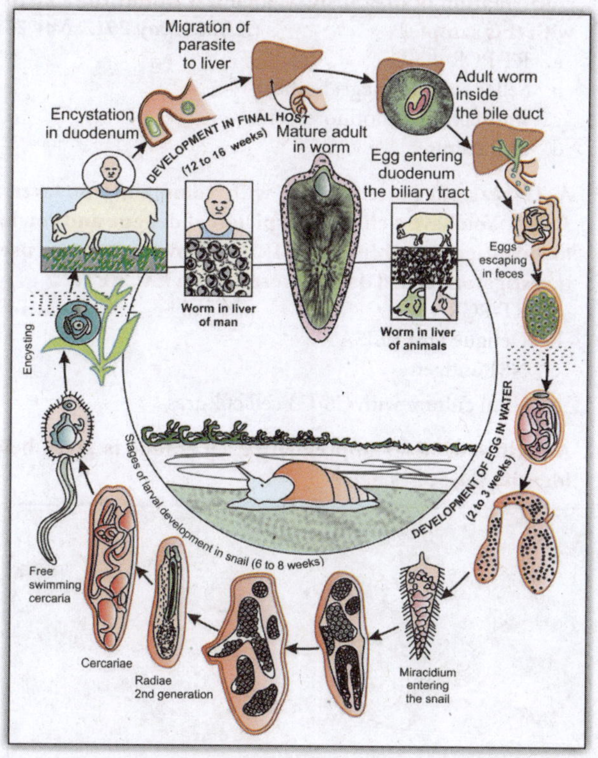

a. Fasciola buski
b. Fasciola hepatica
c. Paragonimus westermani
d. Clonorchis sinensis

45. Identify the organism in the slide?

a. Nocardia sp
b. Mycobacterium tuberculosis
c. Mycobacterium leprae
d. Actinomyces sp

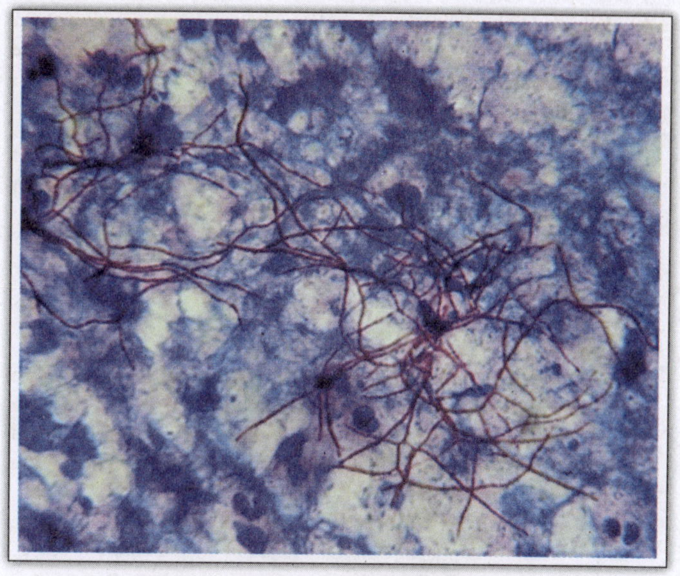

46. 1-3 β D glucan assay for fungi not used for?

a. Aspergillus
b. Pneumocystis
c. Cryptococcus
d. Pneumocystis jirovecii

47. A 20-year-old male with history of fever and enlarged lymph nodes and sore throat was suspected to have infectious mononucleosis and was ordered a Paul–Bunnell test. Which of the following is the principle of the test?

a. Heterophile antibody test
b. Neutralisation reaction
c. Complement mediated cell damage
d. Agglutination reaction

AIIMS NOVEMBER 2016

48. Which of the following statement regarding the intestinal nematode in the picture given below is correct?

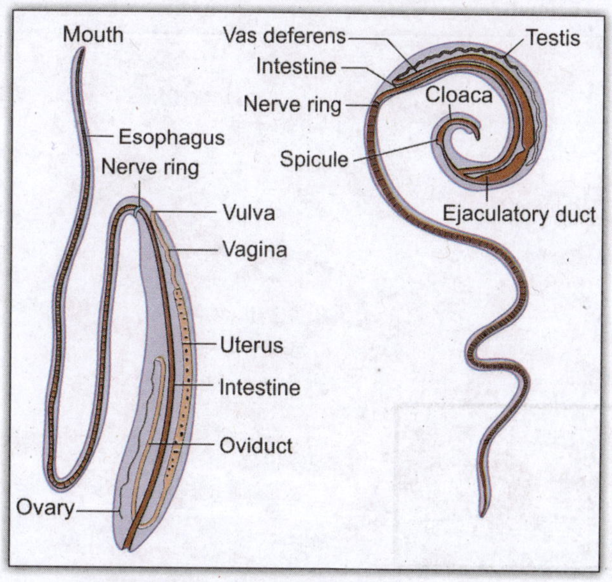

a. Drug of choice is triclabendazole
b. Site of attachment of adult worm is small intestine
c. Adult worm grows to 1–2 m in length
d. Eggs laid are infective in 10 days

49. Which of the following is most common systemic symptom during migration of larval phase of Helminths like Ancyclostoma, Strongyloides and Ascaris?

a. Eosinophilia
b. Pneumonitis
c. Liver failure
d. Larva migrans

50. Why schizonts of late trophozoite stage of plasmodium falciparum not seen in peripheral blood smear?

a. They are sequestrated in spleen
b. Adherence to capillary endothelium
c. Antigen antibody reaction
d. None

51. A 14-year-old presented with fever and chills for 3 days. On examination found to have signs of dehydration like positive skin pinch test and dry oral mucosa. Peripheral blood smear was done as shown in the picture below. Identify the organism?

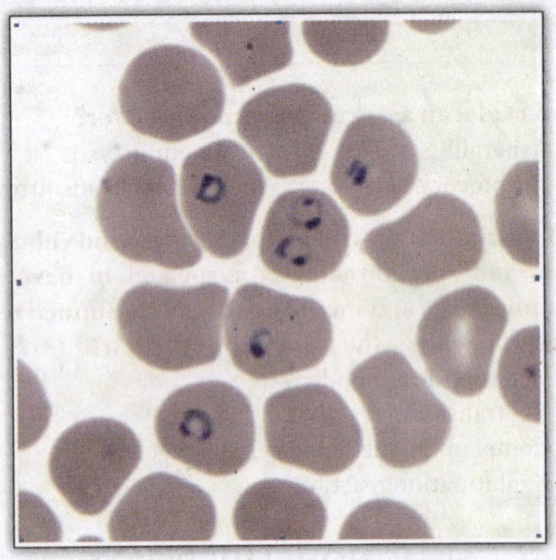

a. Plasmodium vivax
b. Plasmodium falciparum
c. Leishmania donovani
d. Salmonella typhi

52. Identify the given organism in the Gram staining slide given below?

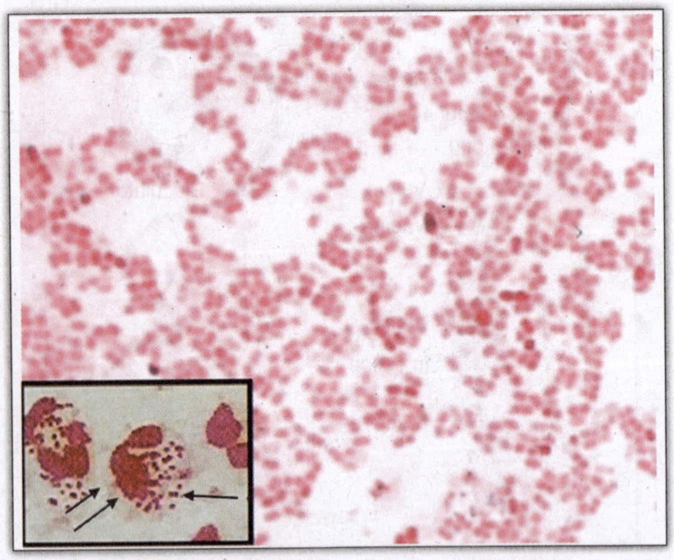

a. Staphylococcus aureus
b. Neisseria gonorrhoeae
c. Streptococcus pneumoniae
d. Haemophilus influenzae

53. A doctor does foleys catheterization for a ICU patient and postcatheterization the patient developed UTI. Catheter tip was sent for culture and was grown on blood agar. After 24 hours the blood agar shows following picture. What is the most likely causative agent of the UTI?

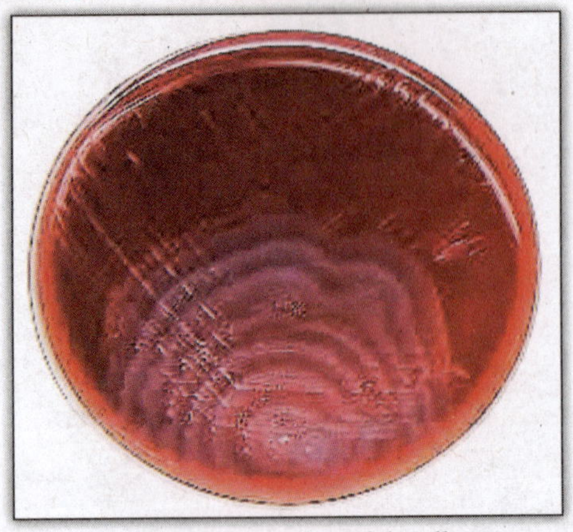

a. Escherichia coli
b. Klebsiella pneumoniae
c. Proteus mirabilis
d. Pseudomonas

54. A child with history of dog bite comes with increased salivation, inability to drink water and hydrophobia and died. Post mortem corneal scraping was taken for confirmation of diagnosis. Which test would you like to do with this sample? ***(AIIMS May 2017, Nov 2016)***

a. RT PCR
b. Seller stain for negri bodies
c. Indirect immunofluorescence
d. Cell culture

55. A 12-year-old patient came with complaints of fever for 3 days. You have a clinical suspicion of dengue and you have to investigate on him. All of the following test are useful investigation at 3rd day of presentation EXCEPT:

a. RT-PCR
b. Dengue IgM ELISA
c. NS1 antigen
d. Viral culture with C6/C3 cell cultures

56. A picture of silver impregnation technique is given below, identify the Spirochete?

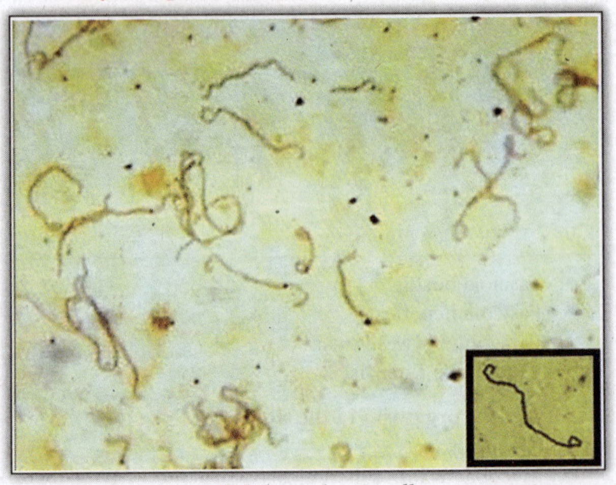

a. Treponema pallidium
b. Borellia recurrentis
c. Spirillum minus
d. Leptospira interrogans

57. **Which of the following is an obligate intracellular pathogen?**
   a. Coxiella burnetii b. Klebsiella
   c. Legionella d. Bartonella

AIIMS MAY 2016

58. **Which of the following bacteria is an obligate intercellular pathogen?**
   a. Coxiella brunettii b. Tropheryma whipplei
   c. Bartonella henselae d. Ehrlichia chaffeensis

59. **The complement complex that attacks bacterial membrane is?**
   a. C–12345 b. C–23456
   c. C–34567 d. C–56789

60. **A 27-year-old pregnant lady presented to AIIMS casualty with severe jaundice, altered sensorium, not responding to commands. Pelvic USG shows intrauterine fetal death. Liver function tests were done along with viral profile. The lab results are as tabulated below. The likely diagnosis is?**

Viral markers	Result
Anti IgM HAV	Nonreactive
Anti IgG HAV	Reactive
HbsAg	Nonreactive
Anti HbsAg	Nonreactive
Anti Hbc IgM	Nonreactive
Anti Hbc IgG	Reactive
Anti HCV IgG	Nonreactive
Anti HEV IgM	Reactive
Anti HEV IgG	Nonreactive

   a. Acute hepatitis E on chronic hepatitis A
   b. Acute hepatitis E on chronic hepatitis B
   c. Fulminant hepatitis due to chronic hepatitis B
   d. Fulminant hepatitis E infection

61. **The gram stained smear shown below is most consistent with?**

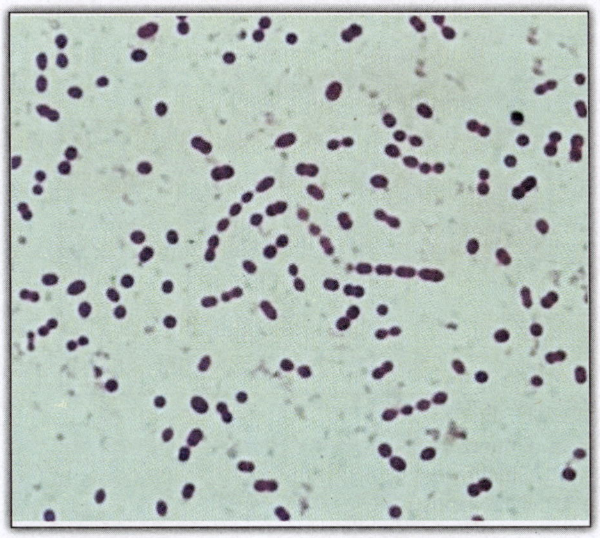

   a. S. pyogenes b. S. pneumonia
   c. S. aureus d. N. meningitides

62. **In patient with UTI; For urine culture, Cystiene Lactose Electrolyte Deficient (CLED) medium is preferred over McConkey agar because?** ***(AIIMS May 2016, Nov 2001)***
   a. Prevents growths of pseudomonas
   b. Differentiates lactose fermenters and non fermenters
   c. Promotes growths of Staph aureus and candida
   d. Inhibits the swarming growth of proteus spp

63. **Antigenic drift in influenza viruses?**
   a. Is exhibited only by influenza A viruses
   b. Affects predominantly the matrix protein
   c. Caused by frame shift mutation in the viral genome
   d. Responsible for seasonal epidemic of influenza

64. **A 23-year-old girl is brought to the emergency department with a two day history of fever, confusion with neck stiffness, hypotension and purpuric rash on her extremities as shown in the picture below. Her BP is 70/50 mm Hg. A lumbar puncture showed a cloudy CSF with total leukocyte count 4200 cells/cu mm, 91% neutrophils, protein – 198 mg/dl, glucose – 21 mg/dl. Correct description of organism causing this is?**

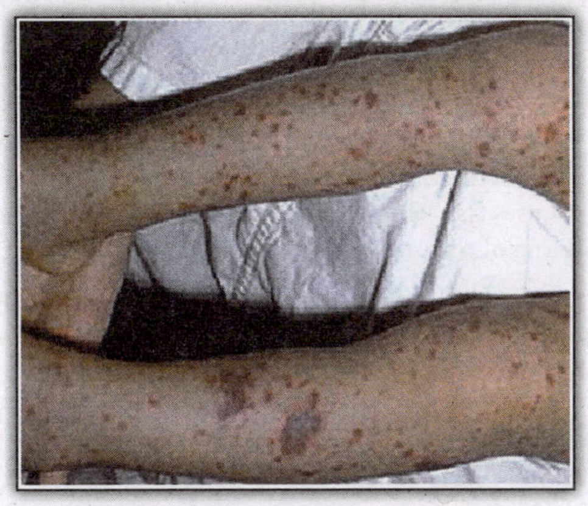

   a. Gram negative diplococcus, ferments glucose and maltose
   b. Gram positive diplococcic (lanceolate), catalase negative optochin sensitive
   c. Gram positive cocci in chains, catalyse negative and bacitracin sensitive
   d. Gram negative diplococcic (kidney bean shaped), oxidase positive

65. **A 47-year-old truck driver being investigated for odynophagia and watery diarrhea. Upper GI endoscopy showed gastric and esophageal candidiasis. A stool sample was sent to the parasitology laboratory. Microscopic wet mount of which is shown below. True statement regarding the helminth is?**

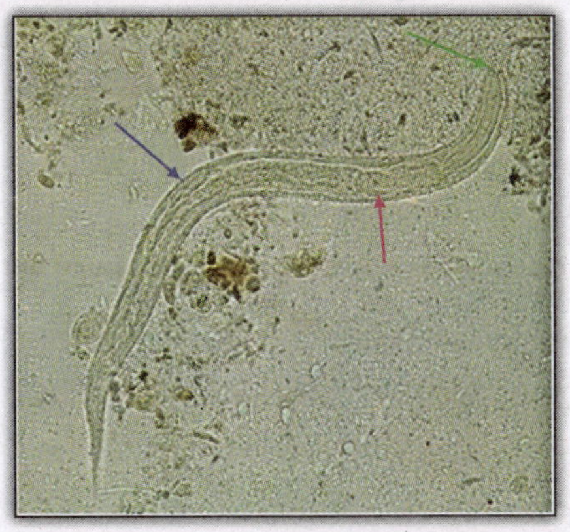

a. The infective stage of parasite shown is filariform larva
b. Adult female are capable of reproductive parthenogenesis
c. Transmitted through consumption of contaminated food and water
d. Drug of choice is thiabendazole

66. Egg of a helminth is shown below. Which of the following is true regarding the parasite?

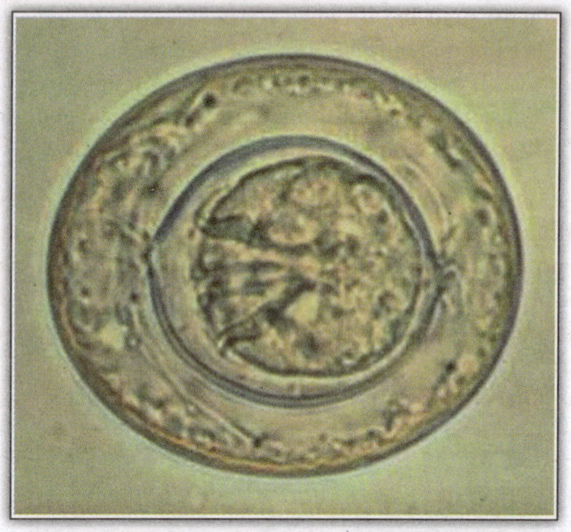

a. Both adult and larval stage of helminth can be seen in humans
b. It is acquired by consumption of improperly cooked pork
c. Causes transient self limiting infection in humans
d. Drug of choice is thiobendazole/albendazole

67. A 23-year-old patient presented to medicine OPD with history of abdominal pain and dysentery. Colonic biopsy sent for histopathology is as below. Most likely diagnosis is?

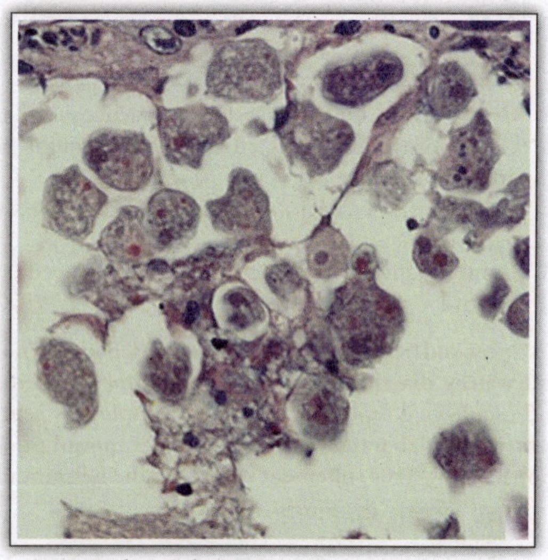

a. Intestinal amoebiasis
b. Enterobius vermicularis
c. Bacterial infectious diarrhea
d. Intertinal giardiasis

68. Parasite induced pernicious anemia is caused by?

a. Hymenolipis nana
b. Diphyllobothrium latum
c. Ankylostoma duodenale
d. Necator americanus

69. Autoinfection is characteristically seen all of the following infection EXCEPT:

a. H. nana
b. T. solium
c. E. vermicularis
d. Ascaris lumbricoides

70. Transfusion associated malaria has a shorter incubation period because the infection is caused by?

a. Sporozoites
b. Schizonts
c. Female gametocytes
d. Trophoziotes

AIIMS NOVEMBER 2015

71. A young lady presents with progressive dyspnea for 3 months. Lobectomy was done for cavitatory lesion in right lower lung. Histopathological appearence is seen in the picture. Most likely cause of disease and the number of layers that can be seen in the wall of parasite is?

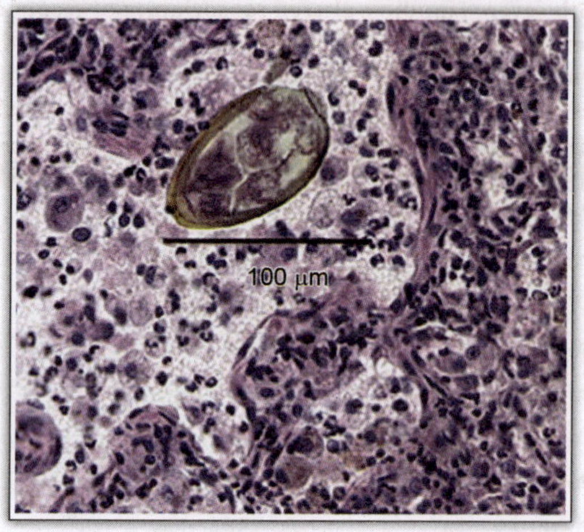

a. Echinococcus with 2 layers
b. Strongyloides with 2 layers
c. Paragonimus with 2 layers
d. Cysticercosis with 3 layers

72. Giemsa staining of a genital ulcer shows picture as shown. Identify the organism?

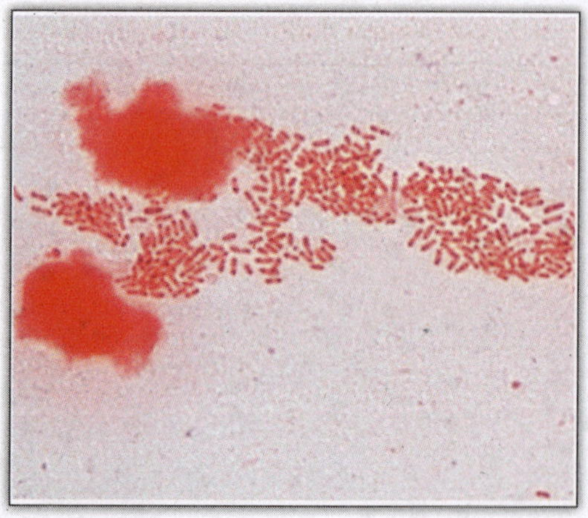

a. H. ducreyi
b. Gonorrhea
c. Chlamydia
d. Donovanosis

73. **For the life cycle shown in the picture below all are true except:**

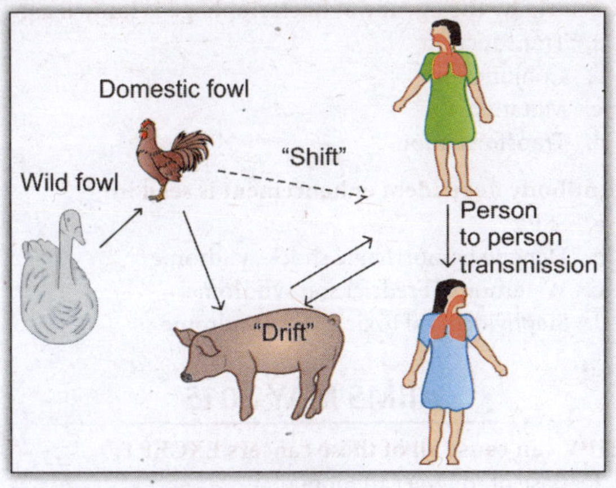

a. Pig acts as host
b. Segmented genome
c. Incubation period 4-5 days
d. Pandemic is caused by all serotypes

74. **All of the following are true about the disease shown in the life cycle given below EXCEPT:**

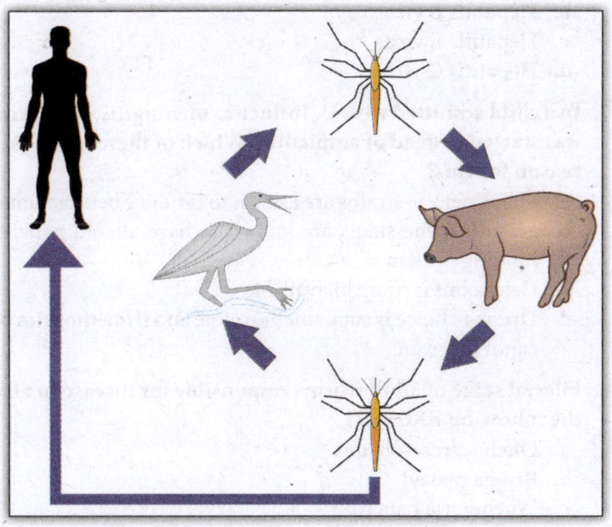

a. Pig is amplifier host
b. Paddy field
c. Nagayama strain
d. Caused by aedes

75. **Identify the parasite shown?**

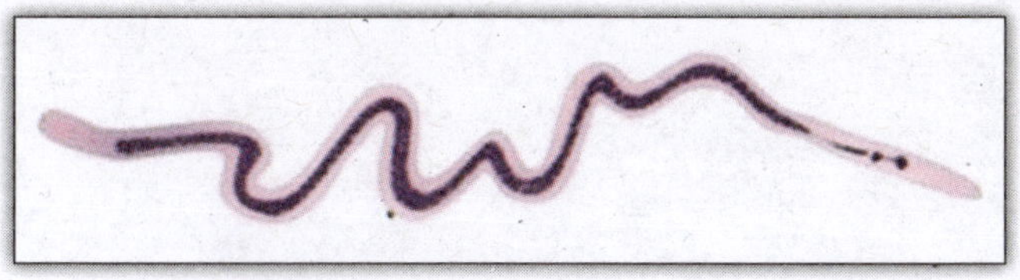

a. Loa Loa
b. Onchocerca volvulus
c. Brugia malayi
d. Wucheraria

76. **Trivalent influenza vaccine contains all EXCEPT:**

a. Influenza B
b. H1N1
c. H3N2
d. H2N1

77. **Stool sample from a patient is shown. How is this organism transmitted in humans?**

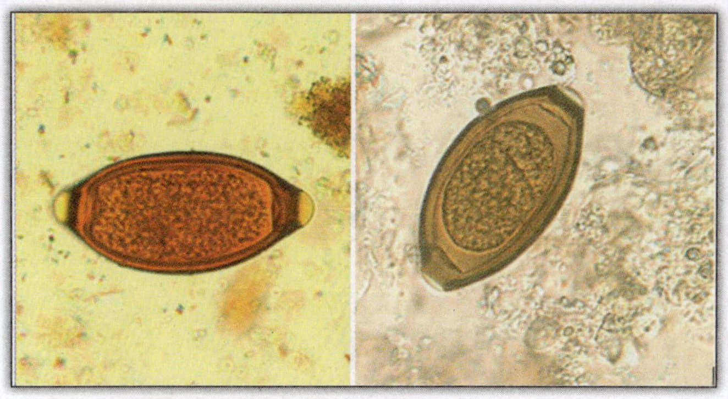

a. Ingestion of uncooked beef
b. Ingestion of egg contaminated in water
c. Penetration by filariform larva
d. Penetration by rhabditiform larva

78. **Serology profile of a patient is as follows. Anti HbS -, HBsAg -, HBV- DNA negative and Anti HBc IgM negative. Anti HbC IgG +ve. Most probable diagnosis is?**

a. Chronic hepatitis inactive state
b. Chronic hepatitis recovery state
c. Precore mutant infection
d. Window period

79. **A patient comes to clinic with a complaint of multiple episodes of loose watery stools for 3 days which starts after ingestion of shell fish at a local restaurant 3 days back. Other customers of restaurant had similar symptoms. The most common virus causing diarrhea in adults associated with shell fish ingestion is?**

a. Enterovirus 40, 41
b. Calcivirus
c. Rotavirus A
d. Norovirus

80. **Nasal biopsy of a patient with brain abscess is done. Identify the organism and stain used in the following picture?**

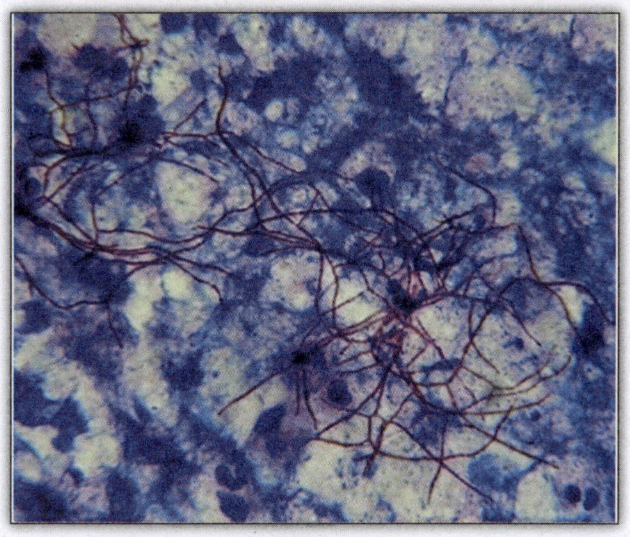

a. Streptococcus, Gram's stain
b. Staphylococcus, Gram's stain
c. Cryptococcus, India ink
d. Nocardia, Gram's stain

81. Various stages of which parasite is shown?

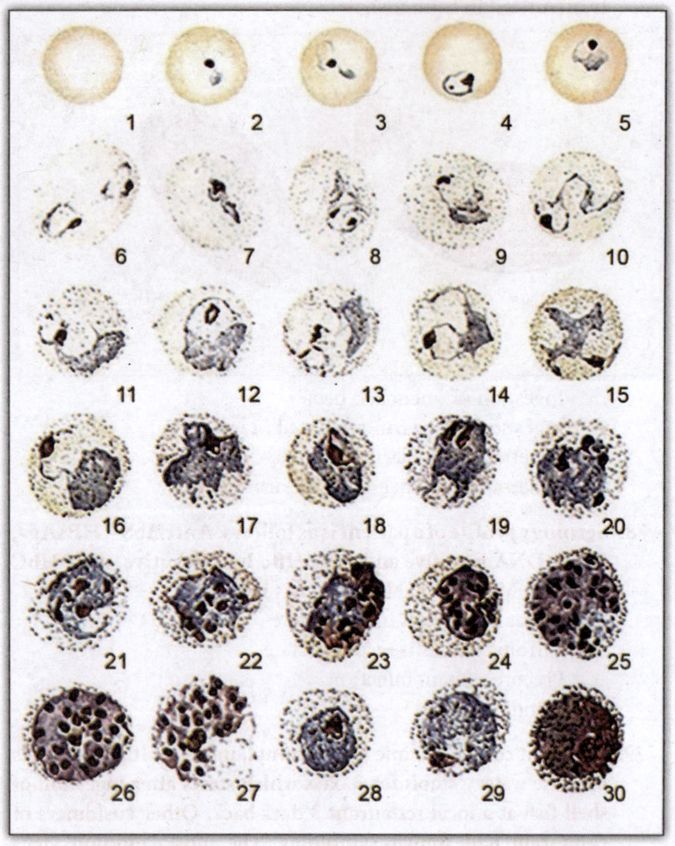

a. Plasmodium vivax b. Plasmodium malariae
c. Plasmodium falciparum d. Plasmodium ovale

82. A farmer presented with cervical lymphadenopathy with multiple discharging sinuses. HPE of the lymph node is shown. Which of the following stain is used for the diagnosis of the patient?

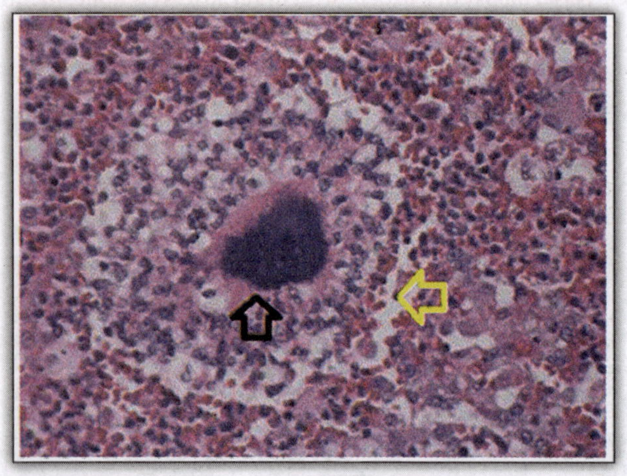

a. Grams stain b. AFB stain
c. PAS stain d. Methenamine silver

83. Transfer of DNA from a non-pathognomic to pathognomic bacteria by the agency of bacteriophage is known as?

a. Transduction
b. Conjunction
c. Mutation
d. Transformation

84. Antibody dependent enhancement is seen in?

a. SSPE
b. Dengue hemorrhagic shock syndrome
c. Waterhouse Fredrickson syndrome
d. Staphylococcal toxic shock syndrome

AIIMS MAY 2015

85. HPV can cause all of these cancers EXCEPT:

a. Base of tongue carcinoma
b. Tonsillar carcinoma
c. Nasopharyngeal carcinoma
d. Cancer carvix

86. Reverse transcriptase is a RNA dependent DNA polymerase. Which of these use in?

a. Hepatitis A virus
b. Hepatitis B virus
c. Hepatitis E virus
d. Hepatitis C virus

87. In a child admitted with H. Influenza meningitis, cefotaxime was started instead of ampicillin. Which of these is the likely reason for this?

a. H. influenzae strains are known to produce beta lactamase
b. H. influenzae stains are known to have altered pencillin binding protein
c. Cefotaxim is more bilavailable
d. Drug of choice is suphamethoxatole and trimethoprim but canot be given

88. Filarial stage of adult worms responsible for disease in all of the following EXCEPT:

a. Onchocerca volvulus
b. Brugia malayi
c. Wuchereria bancrofti
d. Mansonella ozzardi

89. Vibrio cholera acts by disrupting which of the following?

a. Hemidesmosome
b. Gap junctions
c. Zonula occludens
d. Zonula adherens

ANSWERS WITH EXPLANATIONS

AIIMS NOVEMBER 2018

1. Ans. (a) Pneumococcus

Ref: Bailey and Scott 13th ed page 407-408, Harrison 19th ed page 1011, Ananthanarayan 9th ed page 327

The most frequent pathogens of Bacterial meningitis according to age are as follows:

- **≥1 month and <3 months** – Group B streptococcus (39 percent), gram-negative bacilli (32 percent), Streptococcus pneumoniae (14 percent), Neisseria meningitidis (12 percent)
- **≥3 months and <3 years** – S. pneumoniae (45 percent), N. meningitidis (34 percent), group B streptococcus (11 percent), gram-negative bacilli (9 percent)
- **≥3 years and <10 years** – S. pneumoniae (47 percent), N. meningitidis (32 percent)
- **≥10 years and <19 years** – N. meningitidis (55 percent)
- **Adults > 20 years of age**- S. pneumoniae

Common Causes of Meningitis

Organism	Age group	Comment
Serogroup B streptococci *(Streptococcus agalactiae)*	Neonates to age 3 months	As many as 25% of mothers have vaginal carriage of serogroup B streptococci. Ampicillin prophylaxis during labor of women at high risk (prolonged rupture of membranes, fever, etc) or of known carriers reduces the incidence of infection in babies.
Escherichia coli	Neonates	Commonly have the K1 antigen.
Listeria monocytogenes	Neonates (< 1 month age); elderly (> 60 years), pregnant women and immunocompromised children and adults	Not unusual in patients with cell mediated immune deficiency
Haemophilus influenzae	Children 6 months to 5 years	Widespread use of vaccine greatly reduces the incidence of *H influenzae meningitis* in children.
Neisseria meningitidis	Most common pathogen in age group ≥10 years and <19 years 2nd most common pathogen in age group 3 months to 10 years	Polysaccharide vaccines against serogroups A, C, Y and W135 are used in epidemic areas and in association with outbreaks.
Streptococcus pneumoniae	**Most common cause in adults > 20 years of age** accounting to more than half cases. Most common pathogen from 3 month to 10 years of age. All age groups; highest incidence in the elderly	Often occurs with pneumonia; also with mastoiditis, sinusitis and basilar skull fractures.
Cryptococcus neoformans	AIDS patients	Frequent cause of meningitis

2. Ans. (a) Virus

Ref: Jawetz 26th Ed Pg 127

The interferons (IFNs) are critical cytokines that play a key role in defense against virus infections and other intracellular organisms, such as Toxoplasma gondii.

Protection of a cell from virus replication.

- The IFNs bind to their cellular receptor and activate the signal transducers, JAK and activators of transcription, STAT, signaling pathways.
- This process triggers activation of genes containing IFN-stimulated response elements or an IFN-γ–activated sequence.
- Some of these activated genes initiate production of selected proteins that inhibit virus replication.
- The different IFNs have overlapping biological activities such as antiviral actions antiproliferative actions and immunoregulatory actions.
- IFN-β has been used successfully to treat patients with multiple sclerosis, whereas IFN-γ has been shown to exacerbate this disease.
- They have also been used for the treatment of infections, malignancies, autoimmunity and immunodeficiency

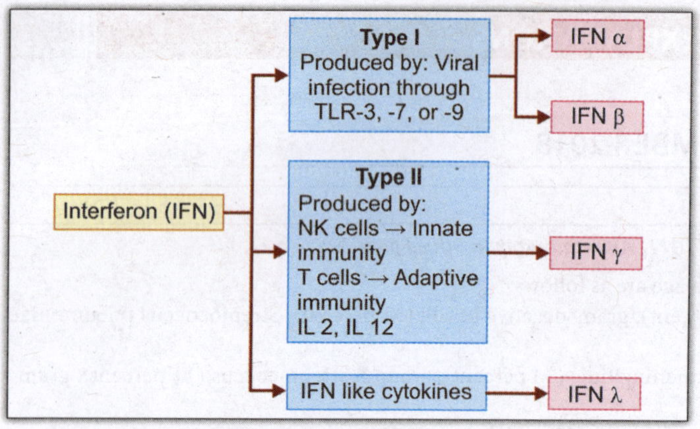

3. Ans. (c) Vibrio parahaemolyticus

Ref: Jawetz 24th ed ch 18, Harrison 19th Ed Pg 266,856

Vibrio parahaemolyticus is a halophilic bacterium that causes acute gastroenteritis following ingestion of contaminated seafood such as raw fish or shellfish. After an incubation period of 12–24 hours, nausea and vomiting, abdominal cramps, fever and watery to bloody diarrhea occur. Fecal leukocytes are often observed. (Jawetz)

Hints to Diagnosis

- **Calculation of food specific attack rate:**
  - As seen from the data, not all individuals have eaten all food items. It makes sense to calculate the food specific attack rate by calculating the percentage of people who have developed disease after eating the specific food item.
  - A **food-specific attack rate** is the number of persons who ate a specified food and became ill divided by the total number of persons who ate that food
  - **Overall attack rate** is the total number of new cases divided by the total population.

Analysis of Incidence of Food Poisoning

Food item	Total sick	Total number who consumed this food	Food specific attack rate (%)
Oyster	40	50	80
Hamburger	50	135	37
Salad	60	140	42.8
Ice cream	49	115	42.6

  - From the above table, we can see that most of the people who consumed oyster developed food poisoning.
  - Sewage, bacteria and viruses (e.g., the virus of hepatitis type A) may be 'concentrated in shellfish such as oysters and fish may carry **Vibrio parahaemolyticus, Salmonella spp.,** Clostridium botulinum type E and other organisms
  - However, Salmonella enteritidis is associated with chicken eggs.
- **Incubation period of 24 hours**

Staphylococcus aureus: Incubation period is 1–8 h
Yersinia enterocolitica: incubation period 5-10 days
Vibrio parahemolyticus; Incubation period 12-24 hours
Salmonella enteritidis: Incubation period 8–48 hour

Common Causative Organisms for Food Poisoning

Food item	Organism
Chicken	Shigella
Undercooked hamburger	E. coli (01 57:H7)
Fried rice or other reheated food	Bacillus cereus
Mayonnaise or creams	Staphylococcus aureus or Salmonella
Eggs	Salmonella
Uncooked foods or soft cheeses	Listeria
Seafood	Vibrio species, Salmonella, acute hepatitis A

4. Ans. (a) Nipah Virus

Ref: www.cdc.gov/vhf/nipah/transmission
https://www.cdc.gov/vhf/nipah/pdf/factsheet.pdf

The key points in the picture are pigs and bats. This directly points to agent the agent being Nipah virus.

Transmission

- Transmission of Nipah virus(NiV) to humans may occur after direct contact with infected bats, infected pigs, or from other NiV infected people.
- The NiV strain identified in the outbreak in Malaysia and Singapore (1999) appeared to have been transmitted initially from bats to pigs, with subsequent spread within pig populations. No occurrence of person-to-person transmission was reported.
- Conversely, person-to-person transmission of Nipah virus in Bangladesh and India is regularly reported. This is most commonly seen in the family and caregivers of Nipah virus-infected patients. Transmission also occurs from direct exposure to infected bats. A common example is consumption of raw date palm sap contaminated with infectious bat excretions.

5. Ans. (c) Organism is monoecious in nature so able to reproduce by using parthenogenesis

Ref: https://www.cdc.gov/dpdx/strongyloidiasis/index.html, Paniker's Medical Parasitology 8th Ed Pg 180

Hints to Diagnosis

- **Renal transplantation** - i.e. on Immunosuppressant therapy hence immunocompromised state.
- **3 months post transplant**
- **Diarrhea** i.e. Gastrointestinal symptoms.
- **Parasite** on the video which is larva of Strongyloides
- **Monoicous** are those species that bear both male and female reproductive organs on the same animal/plant. Strongyloides is a dioecious parasite with females greater in size than males.

The incidence of Strongyloides hyperinfection after renal transplantation is unknown and believed to be uncommon. Hyperinfection typically occurs during the first 3 months after transplantation with mortality rates reaching up to 50%.

Transmission of Strongyloides can occur from an infected renal allograft, most are the result of the uncontrolled proliferation of the nematode in an immunocompromised recipient with potential exposure before transplantation. The American Society of Transplantation recommends pretransplant screening with stool examination and Strongyloides stercoralis immunoglobulin G enzyme-linked immunosorbent assay (ELISA) antibody in recipients and donors from endemic areas or with eosinophilia

Strongyloides

Filariform larvae in contaminated soil penetrate the human skin and by various, often random routes, migrate into the small intestine. Historically it was believed that the L3 larvae migrate via the bloodstream to the lungs, where they are eventually coughed up and swallowed. However, there is also evidence that L3 larvae can migrate directly to the intestine via connective tissues. In the small intestine they molt twice and become adult female worms. The females live threaded in the epithelium of the small intestine and by parthenogenesis produce eggs , which yield rhabditiform larvae. The rhabditiform larvae can either be passed in the stool (see "Free-living cycle" above), or can cause autoinfection. In autoinfection, the rhabditiform larvae become infective filariform larvae, which can penetrate either the intestinal mucosa (internal autoinfection) or the skin of the perianal area (external autoinfection); in either case, the filariform larvae may disseminate throughout the body. To date, occurrence of autoinfection in humans with helminthic infections is recognized only in *Strongyloides stercoralis* and *Capillaria philippinensis* infections. In the case of *Strongyloides*, autoinfection may explain the possibility of persistent infections for many years in persons who have not been in an endemic area and of hyperinfections in immunosuppressed individuals

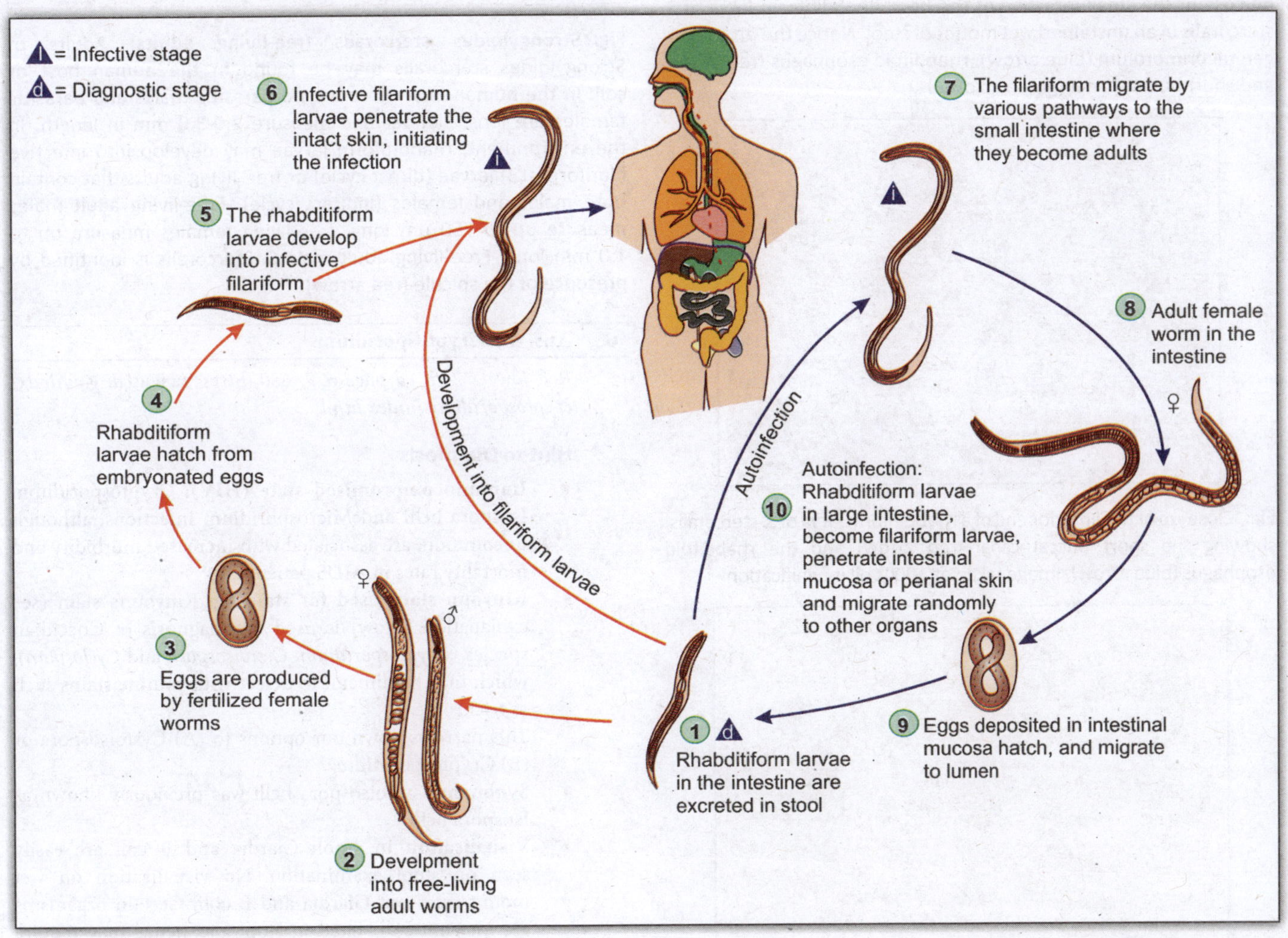

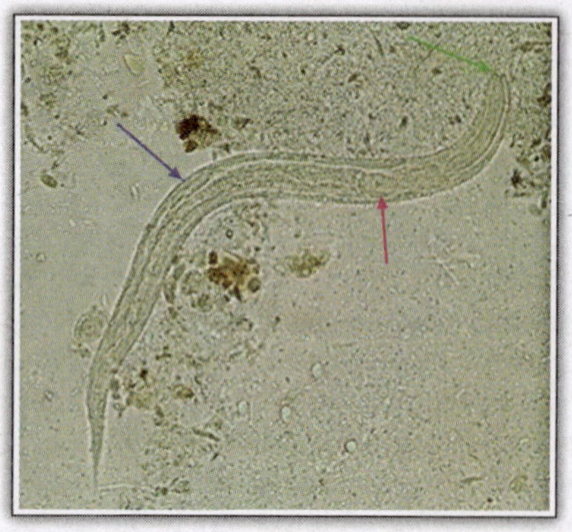

Fig: Strongyloides stercoralis first-stage rhabditiform (L1) larvae: The first-stage rhabditiform larvae (L1) of Strongyloides stercoralis are 180-380 µm long, with a short buccal canal, a rhabditoid esophagus and a prominent genital primordium. These L1 larvae are usually found in stool, as the eggs embryonate and hatch in the mucosa of the small intestine of the host. Rhabditiform larva of S. stercoralis in an unstained wet mount of stool. Notice the prominent genital primordium (blue arrow), rhabditoid esophagus (red arrow) and short buccal canal (green arrow)

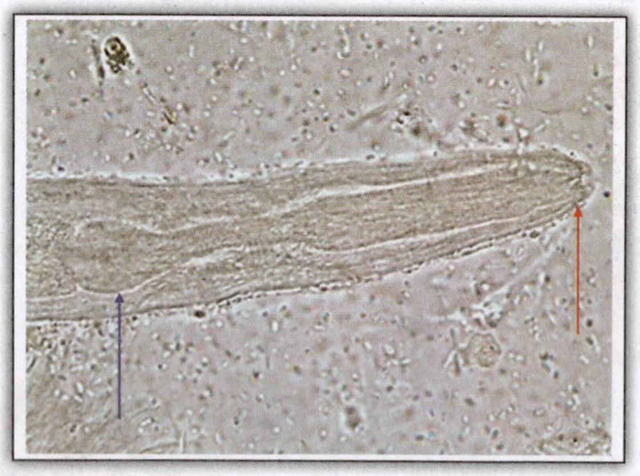

Fig: Close-up of the anterior end of a rhabditiform larva of S. stercoralis, showing the short buccal canal (red arrow) and the rhabditoid esophagus (blue arrow). Image taken at 1000x oil magnification

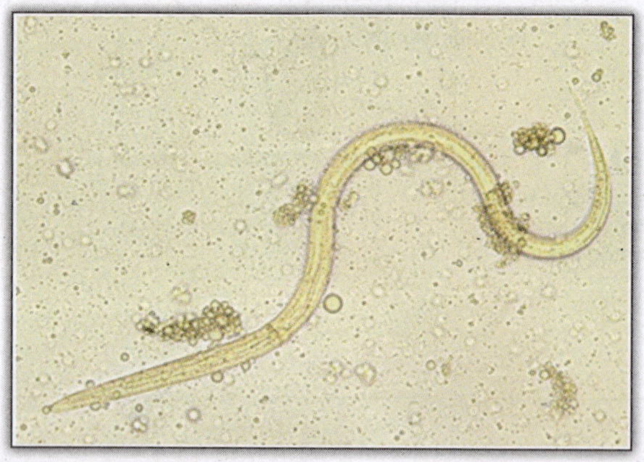

Fig: Strongyloides stercoralis third-stage filariform (L3) larvae: Infective, third-stage filariform larvae (L3) of Strongyloides stercoralis are up to 600 µm long. The tail is notched and the esophagus to intestine ratio is 1:1. Infective L3 larvae are found in soil and invade the human host by direct penetration of the skin. They may be found in respiratory specimens during cases of autoinfection.

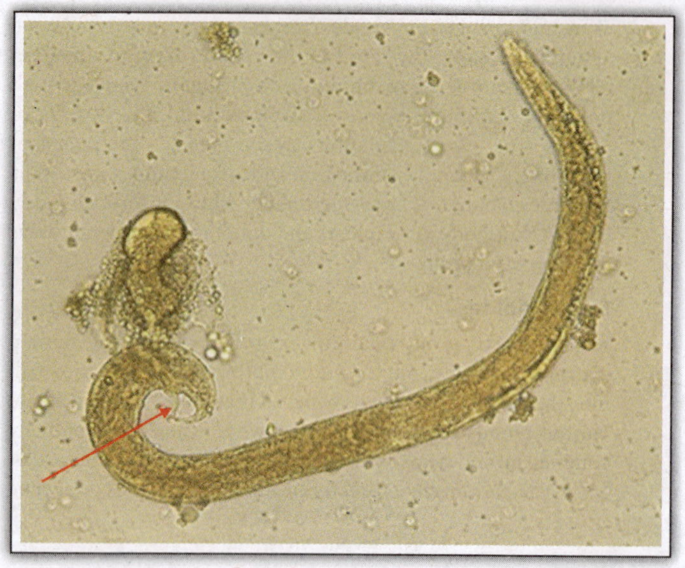

Fig: Strongyloides stercoralis free-living adults: Adults of Strongyloides stercoralis may be found in the human host or soil. In the human host there are no parasitic males and parasitic females are long, slender and measure 2.0-3.0 mm in length. In the environment, rhabditiform larvae may develop into infective filariform (L3) larvae (direct cycle) or free-living adults that contain both males and females (indirect cycle). Free-living adult males measure up to 750 µm long; free-living females measure up to 1.0 mm long. Free-living adult male S. Stercoralis is identified by presence of the spicule (red arrow)

6. **Ans. (b) Cryptosporidium**

Ref: Jawetz 24th ed page 679, 680, https://www.cdc.gov/dpdx/cryptosporidiosis/index.html

Hint to Diagnosis

- **Immunocompromised state (HIV):** Cryptosporidium, Isospora belli and Microsporidium infections, although uncommon, are associated with increased morbidity and mortality rates in AIDS patients.
- **Kinyoun stain used for staining:** Kinyoun's stain (see explanation below) is used for diagnosis of Coccidian species (*Cryptosporidium*, *Cystoisospora* and *Cyclospora*), which may be difficult to detect with routine stains such as trichrome.
  This narrows down our options to (A) Cystoisospora or (B) Cryptosporidium.
- **Synonym:** Cystoisospora belli was previously known as Isospora belli
- **Visualisation in stool:** Giardia and B coli are easily seen on stool examination. No visualization on wet mount rules out Giardia and B coli. Certain organisms are intermittently shed in stool and hence may require repeated sampling or concentration techniques.
- **Shape and size of the oocyst**: Cryptosporidium has round while Cystoisospora has oval oocysts. Also cryptosporidium is smallest in size amongst the provided options.

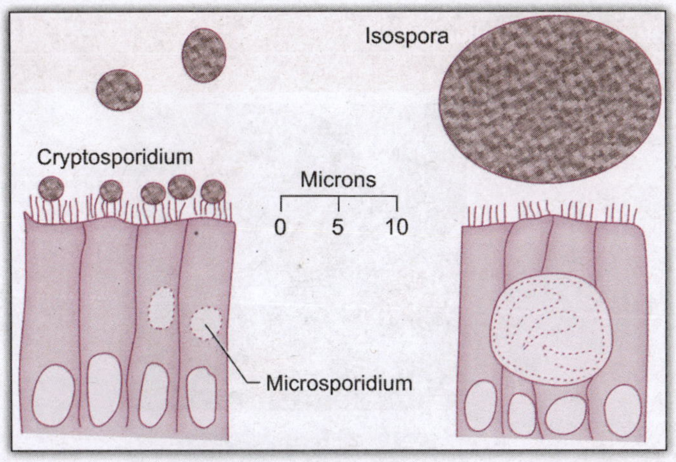

Fig: Diagram demonstrates the relative size and position of the trophozoites and cysts of Microsporidium, compared to Cryptosporidium and Isospora

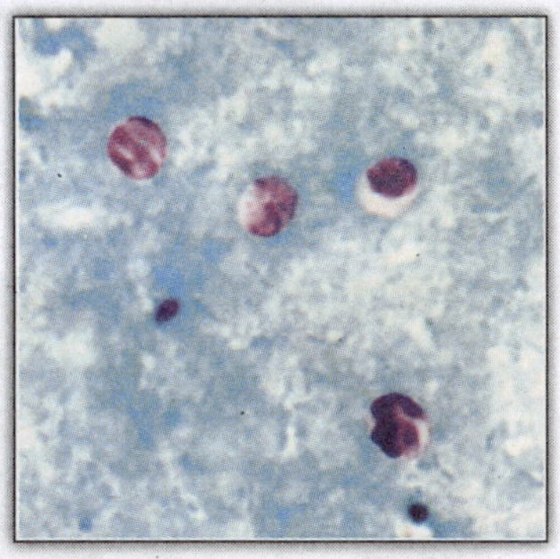

Fig: Cryptosporidium sp. oocysts stained with modified acid-fast. Oocysts are rounded and measure 4.2 to 5.4 µm in diameter. Sporozoites are sometimes visible inside the oocysts, indicating that sporulation has occurred. Staining of Cryptosporidium spp. oocysts can be variable. In particular, infections that are resolving can be accompanied by increasing numbers of non-acid-fast oocysts "ghosts."

Diagnosis of Intestinal Protozoal Infections			
Parasite	Stool ova & parasite	Fecal acid-fast stain	Stool antigen immunoassays
Giardia	+		+
Cryptosporidium	–	+	+
Isospora	–	+	
Cyclospora	–	+	
Microsporidia	–		

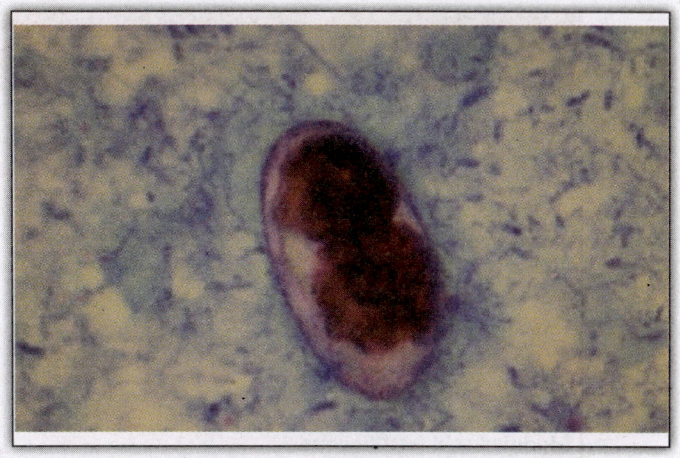

Fig: Mature Cystoisospora oocyst with two sporoblasts on modified acid-fast stain

The answer thus is (B) Cryptosporidium.

Cryptosporidium

- **Clinical features:**
- Immunocompetent: May be asymptomatic, or may cause febrile illness with diarrhea (watery), abdominal pain, nausea.
- **Immunocompromised:** Chronic persistent profuse diarrhea, weight loss, abdominal pain, sclerosing cholangitis.

Kinyoun's Carbol Fuschin

Modified Acid-Fast Staining Procedure

This technique is useful for the identification of oocysts of the coccidian species (*Cryptosporidium*, *Cystoisospora* and *Cyclospora*), which may be difficult to detect with routine stains such as trichrome. Unlike the Ziehl-Neelsen Modified Acid-Fast Stain, this stain does not require the heating of reagents for staining. There are four steps to this procedure requiring the following solutions:

- Absolute methanol
- **Acid alcohol:** 10 mL Sulfuric Acid + 90 mL Absolute ethanol. Store at room temperature.
- **Kinyoun's Carbol fuchsin:** May be purchased commercially.
- **3% Malachite green:** Dissolve 3 g of malachite green in 100 mL of distilled water. Store at room temperature.

Laboratory Diagnosis of Cryptosporidium

Stool examination

Wet mount:
Colorless spherical oocyst seen containing large and small granules (difficult to visualise in unstained preparation)
Fig: Cryptosporidium spp. oocysts (pink arrows) in wet mount. A budding yeast (brown arrow) is in the same field.

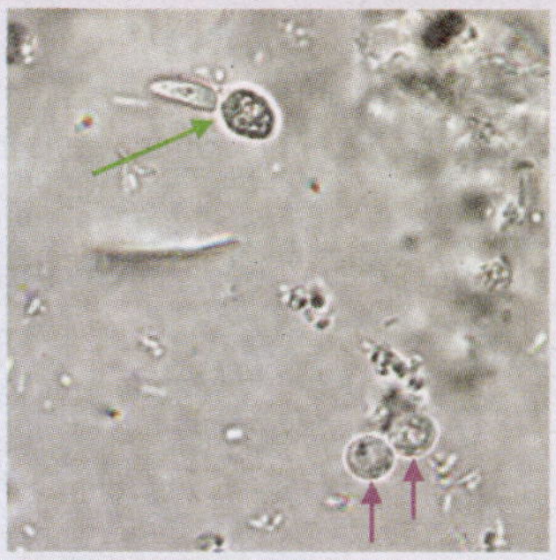

Laboratory Diagnosis of Cryptosporidium

Stool examination

ZN:
Red spheres against a blue background

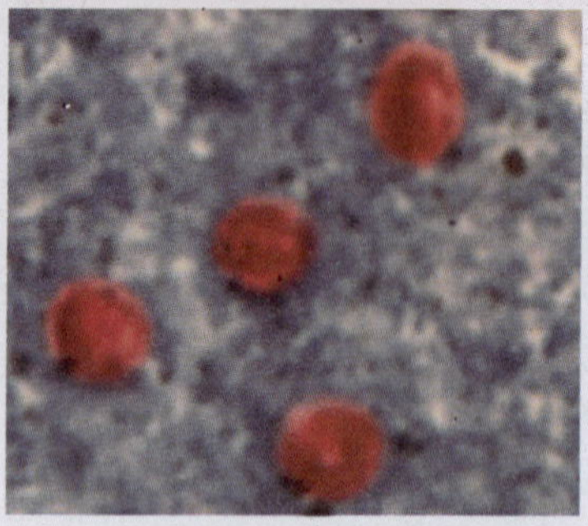

Modified acid fast/Kinyoun:
Oocysts are rounded and measure 4.2 to 5.4 µm in diameter. Sporozoites are sometimes visible inside the oocysts, indicating that sporulation has occurred.

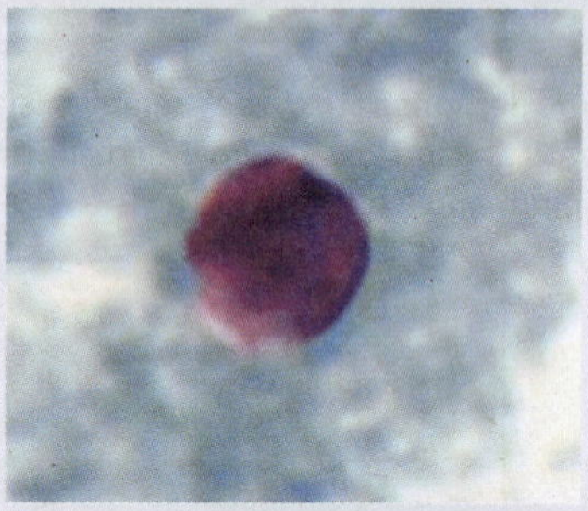

Fluorescent technique

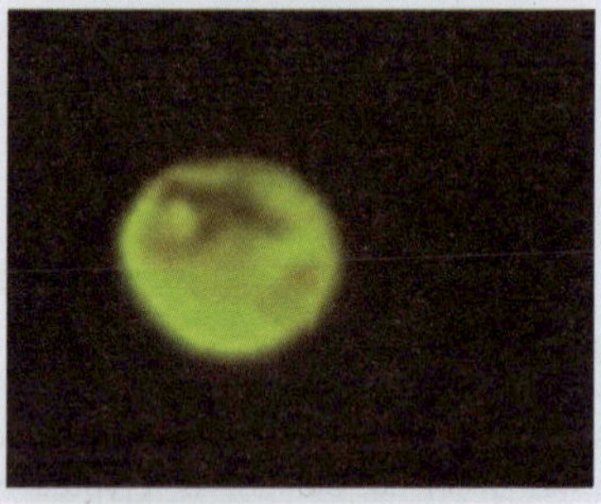

Indirect Immunofluorescence microscopy using monoclonal antibodies

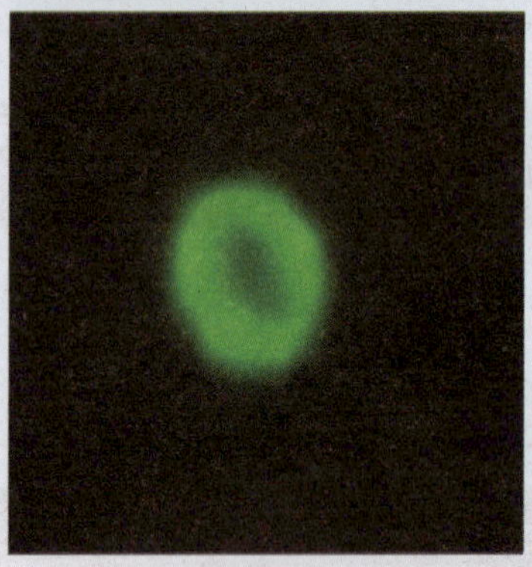

Serodiagnosis:

- Antibodies can be detected within 2 months of acute infection.
- Anti oocyst antibodies persist for 1 year and can be detected by ELISA and immunofluorescence.
- ELISA for detection of antigens in stools using monoclonal antibody → highly sensitive and specific

Histopathology

- Identification under light microscopy from apical surface of intestinal epithelium biopsy. Preferred site → Jejunum

7. **Ans. (c) Toluidine blue, glacial acetic acid and malachite green**

Ref: Manual of Microbiology 2nd ed by Kanika sharma page 121

- **Hint to diagnosis:** The clinical picture is highly suggestive of Diphtheria. Moreover, the slide shows a classical **"club shaped"** appearance which further supports the diagnosis. The stain typically used for such metachromatic granules is **Albert's stain.**
- **Pathogenesis:** Diphtheria toxin is absorbed into the mucous membranes and causes destruction of epithelium and a superficial inflammatory response. The necrotic epithelium becomes embedded in exuding fibrin and red and white cells, so that a grayish ***"pseudomembrane"*** is formed—commonly over the tonsils, pharynx, or larynx. Any attempt to remove the pseudomembrane exposes and tears the capillaries and thus results in bleeding.
- **Laboratory diagnosis:**
- Granules staining deeply with aniline dyes (metachromatic granules) are irregularly distributed within the rod (often near the poles) give the rod a beaded appearance
- Neisser and Albert's stain show bacilli with metachromatic granules and typical arrangement.
- Albert's stain contains Toluidine, glacial acetic acid, malachite green, ethyl alcohol, distilled water.

8. **Ans. (a) Pertussis (c) Faucial Diphtheria**

Ref: Jawetz 26th Ed Pg 269, Harrison's 19th Ed Pg 979
https://www.cdc.gov/infectioncontrol/pdf/guidelines/isolation-guidelines-H.pdf

NOTE

Most likely the question for wrongly framed and it should have been asked in "ALL EXCEPT" format. If its asked in the same format, Pertussis followed by Faucial Diphtheria will be the best answer

"Droplet nuclei" are tiny particles (1-10 microns range) that represent the dried residue of droplets. They may be formed by:

(a) Evaporation of droplets coughed or sneezed into the air or
(b) Generated purposefully by a variety of atomizing devices (aerosols).

- Particles in the 1-5 micron range are liable to be easily drawn into the alveoli of the lungs and may be retained there. (Not considered airborne are droplets and other large particles which promptly settle out)
- Amongst the given options, Pertussis and faucial diphtheria are transmitted by droplet infection. Atypical pneumonia is most commonly caused by mycoplasma, which also spreads by the same route. CDC guidelines suggest "Droplet" isolation for each of these.
- Pharyngeal (or faucial) diphtheria has always been the most virulent form of diphtheria.

Pertussis	
Causative organism	Bordetella pertussis

Contd...

Pertussis	
Pathogenesis	• Filamentous hemagglutinin and fimbriae mediate adhesion to ciliated epithelial cells and are essential for tracheal colonization. • The organism adheres to and multiplies rapidly on the epithelial surface of the trachea and bronchi and interferes with ciliary action. • The bacteria liberate the toxins and substances that irritate surface cells, causing coughing and marked lymphocytosis • Obstruction of the smaller bronchioles by mucous plugs results in atelectasis and diminished oxygenation of the blood. This probably contributes to the frequency of convulsions in infants with whooping cough
Mode of transmission	Droplet infection
Incubation period	2 weeks
Signs and symptoms	• **Stage I- Catarrhal stage:** mild coughing and sneezing. During this stage, large numbers of organisms are sprayed in droplets and the patient is highly infectious but not very ill • **Stage II - "Paroxysmal" stage**: the cough develops its explosive character and the characteristic "whoop" upon inhalation. This leads to rapid exhaustion and may be associated with vomiting, cyanosis and convulsions. The "whoop" and major complications occur predominantly in infants; paroxysmal coughing predominates in older children and adults. The white blood count is high (16,000–30,000/μL), with an absolute lymphocytosis • **Stage III - Convalescence - pertussis is a common cause of prolonged (4–6 weeks) cough in adults**
Laboratory Diagnosis	
Microscopy	• The organisms are minute gram-negative coccobacilli resembling • H influenzae. With toluidine blue stain, bipolar metachromatic granules can be demonstrated. A capsule is present.
Culture	• Bordet-Gengou medium (potato-blood-glycerol agar) • Charcoal-containing medium supplemented with horse blood (Regan lowe) is preferable because of the longer shelf life.
Other tests	Direct fluorescent antibody test, polymerase chain reaction
Treatment	Macrolides, Trimethoprim-sulfamethoxazole
Isolation	• 5 days after initiation of macrolide therapy • In untreated patients for 3-4 weeks
Prevention	Active immunization

9. **Ans. (a) Rk39 antigen based test is used for diagnosis**

Ref: Paniker's Medical parasitology 8th Ed Pg 54, Harrison's 19th Ed Pg 1390, CDC

This is a case of Visceral Leishmaniasis

(See details of Visceral Leishmaniasis in AIIMS May 2018 General Medicine) (see page no. 723)

Hints to Diagnosis

- Hepatosplenomegaly
- Fever
- Amastigote form of Leishmania donovani on Bone marrow aspirate

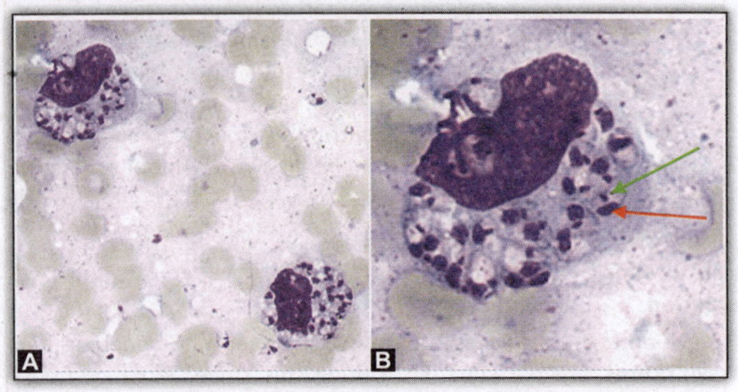

Figs A and B: Light-microscopic examination of a stained bone marrow specimen from a patient with visceral leishmaniasis— showing a macrophage containing multiple Leishmania amastigotes (the tissue stage of the parasite). Note that each amastigote has a nucleus (red arrow) and a rod-shaped kinetoplast (black arrow). Visualization of the kinetoplast is important for diagnostic purposes, to be confident the patient has leishmaniasis

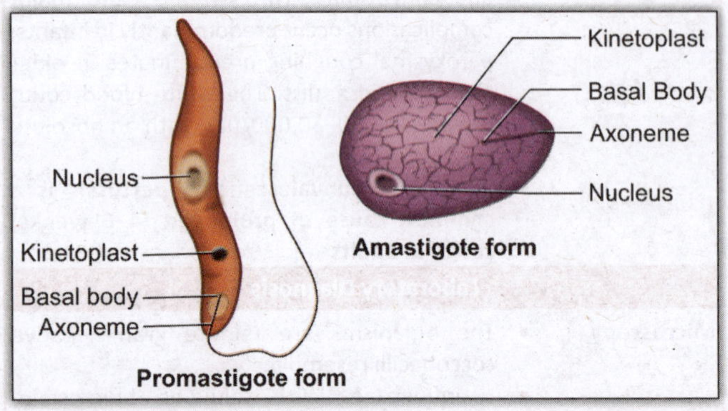

Fig: Morphological forms of Leishmania donovani

Let us Discuss the Options

Option (A) True

RK39 test is used for diagnosis of Leishmaniasis.

Option (B) False

- Organism is obligate intracellular organism hence can't be cultured
- Leishmania can be cultured on NNN medium (Novy, MacNeal and Nicolle → rabbit blood agar) and Schneider's Drosophila culture agar medium

Option (C) False

Buffy coat is used to diagnose the organism

Paniker's Medical parasitology 8th Ed Pg 58 states:

The number of amastigotes in peripheral blood is very scanty. Buffy coat is also most commonly found not positive. Bone marrow aspirate is the most common diagnostic specimen collected. Thus, buffy coat may be used, but it is most often not useful for diagnosis.

Option (D)

False: Leishmania is transmitted from sand fly not sheep.

10. Ans. (b) Entamoeba histolytica

Ref: Harrison's 19th Ed Pg 266, 852

- Grossly Mucoid stool suggests the presence of inflammatory diarrhea. Amongst the options, Entameba histolytica seems to be a more likely causative organism in this case. Giardia, C.perfringens and Staphylococcus, all cause non-inflammatory diarrhea
- A test for fecal leukocytes can suggest inflammatory disease in patients with diarrhea, although the predictive value of this test is still debated.
- Preparation is by a thin smear of stool on a glass slide, addition of a drop of methylene blue and examination of the wet mount
- A test for fecal lactoferrin, which is a marker of fecal leukocytes, is more sensitive and is available in latex agglutination and enzyme-linked immunosorbent assay formats.

Gastro Intestinal Pathogens Causing Acute Diarrhea

	Non inflammatory (enterotoxin)	Inflammatory (invasion or cytotoxin)	Penetrating
Location	Proximal small bowel	Colon or distal small bowel	Distal small bowel
Illness	Watery diarrhea	Dysentery or inflammatory diarrhea	Enteric fever
Stool findings	No fecal leukocytes; mild or no increase in fecal lactoferrin	Fecal polymorphonuclear leukocytes, increased fecal lactoferrin	Fecal mononuclear leukocytes
Causative organisms	Vibrio cholerae, enterotoxigenic Escherichia coli (LT and/or ST), entero aggregative E. coli, Clostridium perfringens, Bacillus cereus, Staphylococcus aureus, Aeromonas hydrophilia, Plesiomonas shigelloides, rotavirus, norovirus, enteric adenoviruses, Giardia lamblia, Cryptosporidium spp., Cyclospora	Shigella spp, Salmonella spp, Campylobacter jejuni, enterohemorrhagic E. coli, enteroinvasive E. coli, Yersinia enterocolitica, Listeria monocytogenes, Vibrio parahemolyticus, Clostridium difficile, A. hydrophila, P shigelloides, Entamoeba histolytica, Klebsiella oxytoca	Salmonella typhi, Y. enterocolitica

AIIMS MAY 2018

11. Ans: (a) Germ tube formation

Ref: Ananthnarayan 10th Ed Pg 616

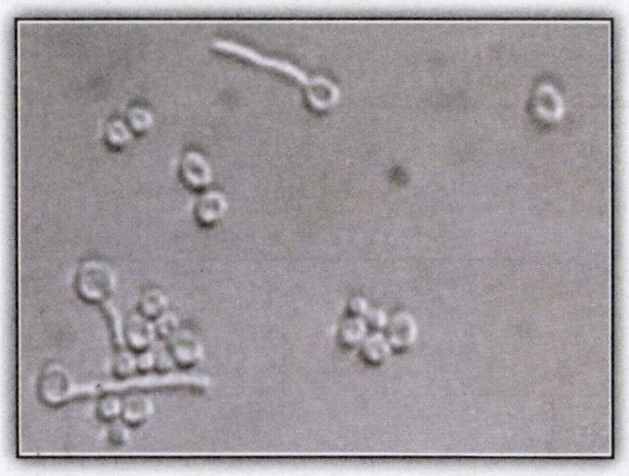

Fig: The picture shows formation of germ tube of Candida albicans

- Germ tube test **(Reynolds-Braude Phenomenon)** is the confirmatory test for Candida albicans
- When cells of Candida are incubated in serum at 370C for 2-4 hours Candida albicans produce short, slender, tube like structures called germ tubes.
- Germ tubes are short outgrowth, non-septate germinating hyphae.They are ½ the width and 3 – 4 times the length of the cell from which they arise. Buds and pseudo-hyphae can be distinguished from germ tubes by the constricted attachment at the point of origin. Germ tubes don't show constriction at the point of origin.
- Media used: Human pooled serum, bovine serum.

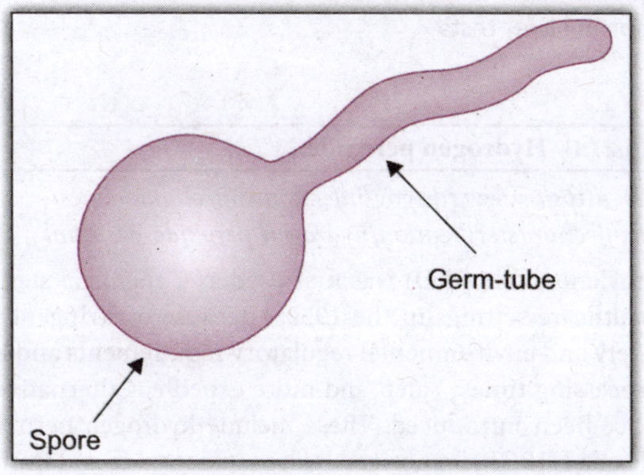

Fig: Germ tube- Candida albicans (Illustration)

12. Ans: (b) Cryptosporidium

Ref: Jawetz 24th ed page 679, 680, https://www.cdc.gov/dpdx/cryptosporidiosis/index.html

Repeat AIIMS Nov 2018 (See for explanation) (see page no. 248)

13. Ans: (a) IgM Anti HAV

Ref: Harrison's 19th Ed Pg 1994

NOTE

IgM is used for acute infection while IgG is used for chronic infection.

A typical battery of blood tests used for initial assessment of liver disease includes measuring levels of serum alanine and aspartate aminotransferases (ALT and AST), alkaline phosphatase (AlkP), direct and total serum bilirubin, and albumin and assessing prothrombin time. ***The most common causes of acute liver disease are viral hepatitis (particularly hepatitis A, B and C)***, drug-induced liver injury, cholangitis and alcoholic liver disease.

- Hepatocellular diseases that can cause jaundice include viral hepatitis, drug or environmental toxicity, alcohol and end-stage cirrhosis from any cause.
- Wilson's disease occurs primarily in young adults.
- Autoimmune hepatitis is typically seen in young to middle-aged women but may affect men and women of any age.
- Patients with alcoholic hepatitis typically have an AST-to-ALT ratio of at least 2:1 and the AST level rarely exceeds 300 U/L. Patients with acute viral hepatitis and toxin-related injury severe enough to produce jaundice typically have aminotransferase levels >500 U/L, with the ALT greater than or equal to the AST.
- While ALT and AST values <8 times normal may be seen in either hepatocellular or cholestatic liver disease, values 25 times normal or higher are seen primarily in acute hepatocellular diseases. Patients with jaundice from cirrhosis can have normal or only slightly elevated aminotransferase levels

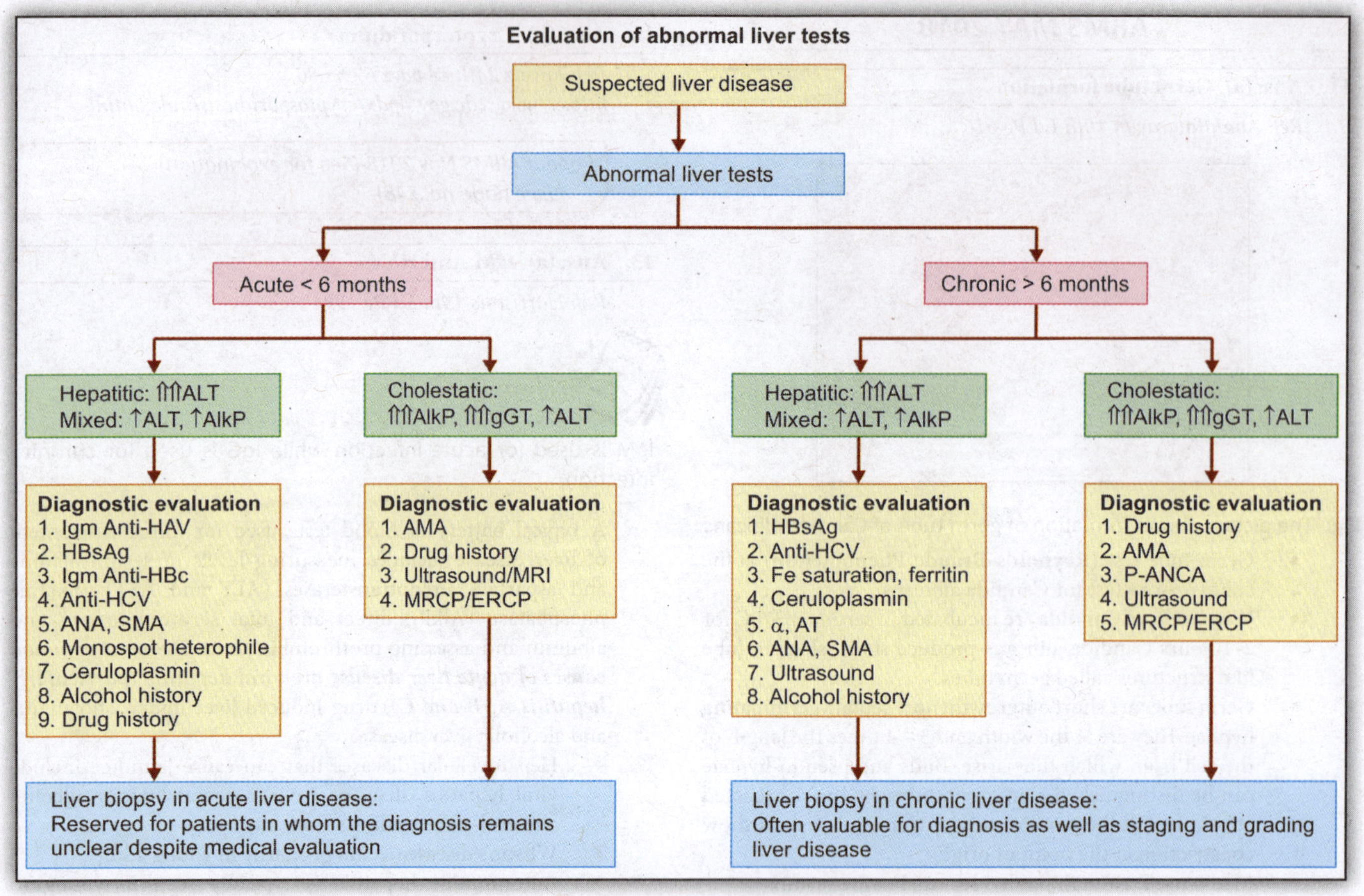

Fig: Algorithm for evaluation of abnormal liver tests

NOTE

- The presence of HBsAg, with or without IgM anti-HBc, represents HBV infection. If IgM anti-HBc is present, the HBV infection is considered acute; if IgM anti-HBc is absent, the HBV infection is considered chronic.
- Because it can take many weeks for hepatitis C antibody to become detectable, its assay is an unreliable test if acute hepatitis C is suspected.

14. Ans: (a) HAV

Ref: Jawetz 26th Ed page 507

(See table of "Clinical and Epidemiologic Features of Viral Hepatitis" in AIIMS May 2015) (see page no. 307-308)

Hepatitis A and E are two non-enveloped hepatitis virus. Thus, HAV infection is still possible with single donor plasma transfusion.

NOTE

They have given the clue in the question itself that Single donor plasma destroys enveloped viruses. Next time they might not give this information in the question.

15. Ans: (a) Hydrogen peroxide

Ref: https://www.cdc.gov/infectioncontrol/guidelines/disinfection/sterilization/hydrogen-peroxide-gas.html

Ethylene oxide (EtO) was first used as a chemical sterilant in healthcare settings in the 1950s. Because of stringent health, safety and environmental regulatory requirements and lengthy processing times, 'safer' and more expedient alternatives have since been introduced. These include hydrogen peroxide gas plasma (HPGP), vaporized hydrogen peroxide and immersion and vapor phase peracetic acid

16. Ans: (a) Dark field microscopy for T. Pallidum

Ref: Jawetz 27th Ed Pg 325

- Dark field microscopy for T.pallidum can be seen in the given image.
- The spirals of T. pallidum are so thin that they are not readily seen unless immunofluorescent stain or darkfield illumination is employed.
- A drop of tissue fluid or exudate is placed on a slide and a coverslip pressed over it to make a thin layer. The preparation is then examined under oil immersion with darkfield illumination for typical motile spirochetes.
- They can also be seen in tissues when stained by a silver impregnation method.

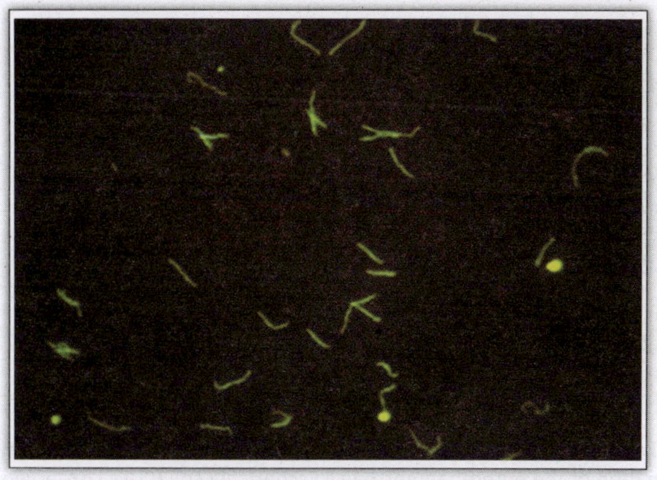

Fig: Treponema pallidum seen in Direct fluorescent antibody test

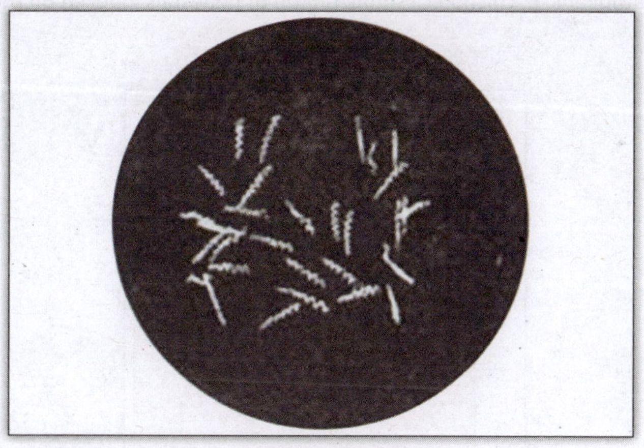

Fig: Treponema pallidum seen in dark field microscopy

17. Ans: (c) Complementation

Ref: Jawetz 24th ed ch 29

Complementation is the process by which two recessive mutations can supply each other's deficiency to produce a wild type phenotype. It is another method of genetic analysis used to determine whether two mutants, apparently defective in the same way, are defective in the same gene.

Complementation refers to the interaction of viral gene products in cells infected with two viruses, one or both of which may be defective. It results in the replication of one or both under conditions in which replication would not ordinarily occur. The basis for complementation is that one virus provides a gene product in which the second is defective, allowing the second virus to grow. The genotypes of the two viruses remain unchanged.

Phenotypic Mixing

A special case of complementation is phenotypic mixing, or the association of a genotype with a heterologous phenotype. This occurs when the genome of one virus becomes randomly incorporated within capsid proteins specified by a different virus or a capsid consisting of components of both viruses. If the genome is encased in a completely heterologous protein coat, this extreme example of phenotypic mixing may be called ***"phenotypic masking" or "transcapsidation."*** Such mixing is not a stable genetic change because, upon replication, the phenotypically mixed parent will yield progeny encased in capsids homologous to the genotype. The nucleocapsid of one virus becomes encased within an envelope specified by another, a phenomenon designated **"pseudotype formation."** There are many examples of pseudotype formation among the RNA tumor viruses.

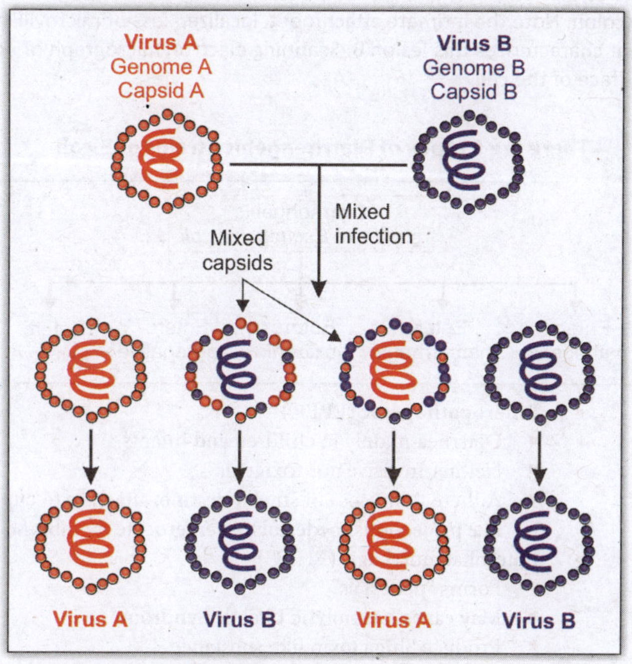

Fig: Phenotypic mixing produces pseudotypes: Progeny genomes with mixed capsid antigens

18. Ans: (c) Enteropathogenic E coli

Ref: Ananthanarayanan 7th Ed Pg 278

NOTE

The image shows pedestals of E coli. Both EHEC and EPEC form pedestals. But EHEC was not one of the options.

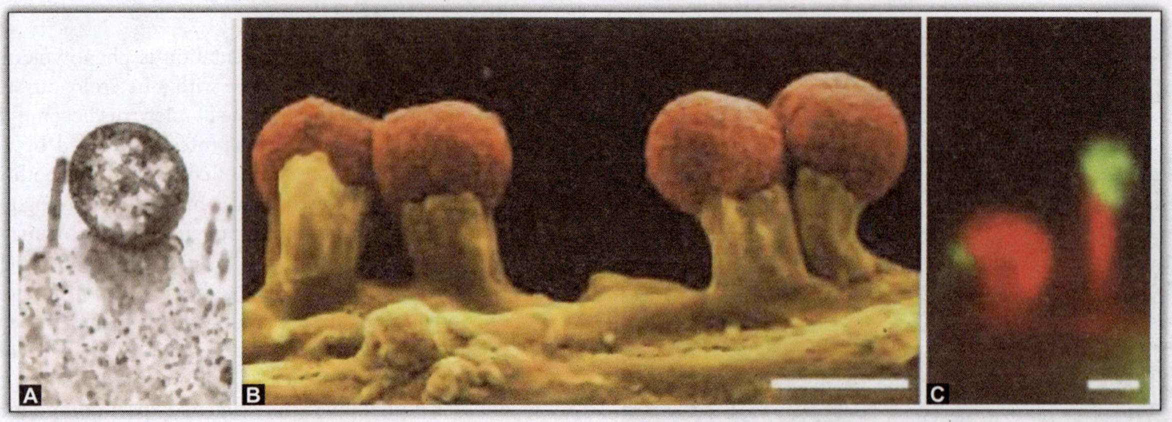

Figs A to C: Actin pedestal formation induced by EHEC and EPEC in vivo and on the surface of cultured cells. A. Transmission electron micrograph showing the characteristic attaching and effacing lesion formation of the enterohaemorrhagic Escherichia coli (EHEC) observed in colon. Note the intimate attachment, localized loss of microvilli and formation of a raised, pedestal-like structure beneath the bacterium that characterizes this lesion **B.** Scanning electron micrograph of enteropathogenic E. coli (EPEC) sitting on top of pedestals induced on the surface of the cell

There are 5 types of Diarrheagenic Strains of E.coli

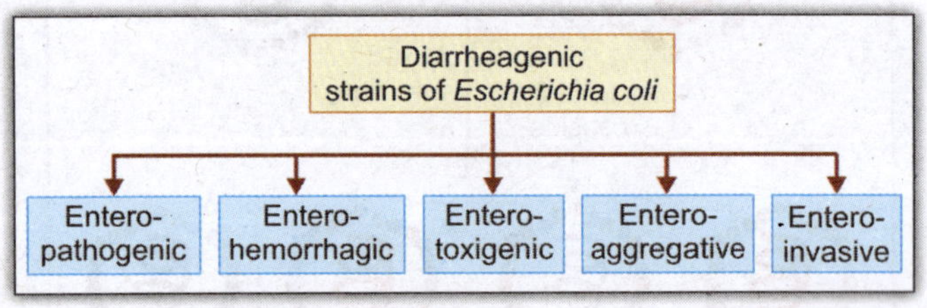

- **Enteropathogenic (EPEC)** -
  - Diarrhea mainly in children and infants.
  - Neither invasive nor toxigenic
  - Adhere to mucosa of small intestine, attach to to cup-like projections (pedestals) of enterocyte membrane
- Enterohaemorrhagic (EHEC) -
  - Forms "pedestals"
  - May cause haemolytic Uremic Syndrome
  - Produce Shiga toxin like substance

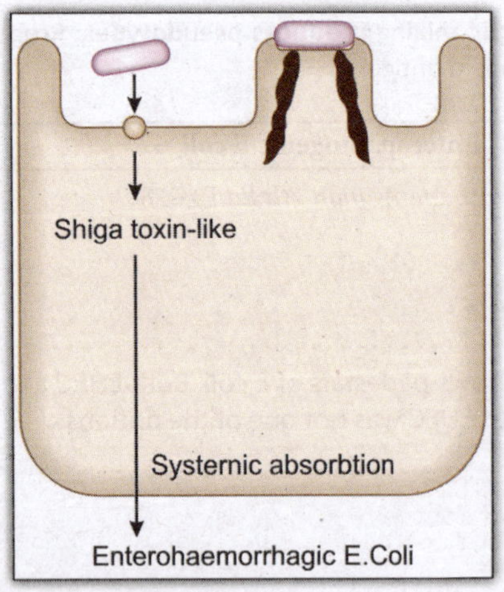

- **Enterotoxigenic (ETEC)** -
  - Causes Traveler's' diarrhea
  - First adhere to intestinal cells with fimbrial antigens and colonization factors (CFA) and then release toxins (Heat labile (LT) and heat stable toxins (ST))

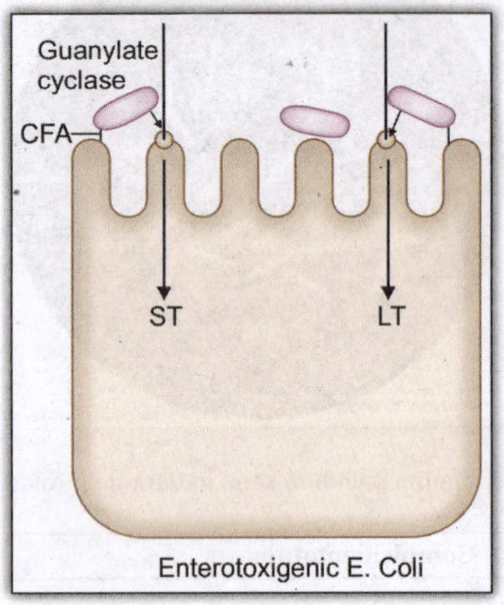

- **Enteroaggregative (EAEC):**
  - **Stacked brick appearance** in Hep 2 or glass with aggregative adhesive factor
  - Shortening of villi, haemorrhagic necrosis, edema, mononuclear infiltration of submucosa

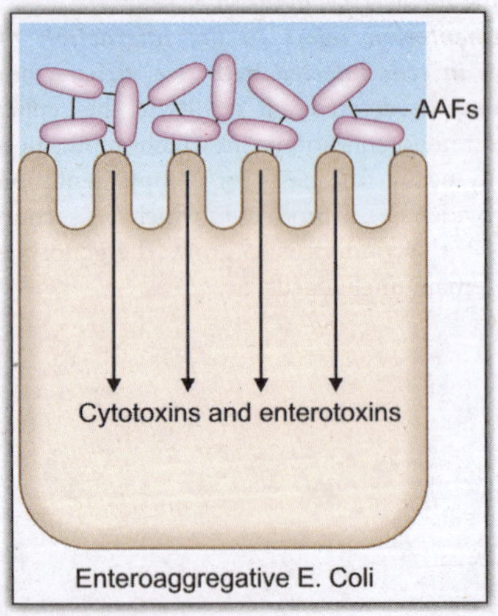

- **Enteroinvasive (EIEC):**
  - Invade intestinal epithelial cells in vivo with the help of a plasmid that codes for outer antigen (Virulence marker antigen-VMA).

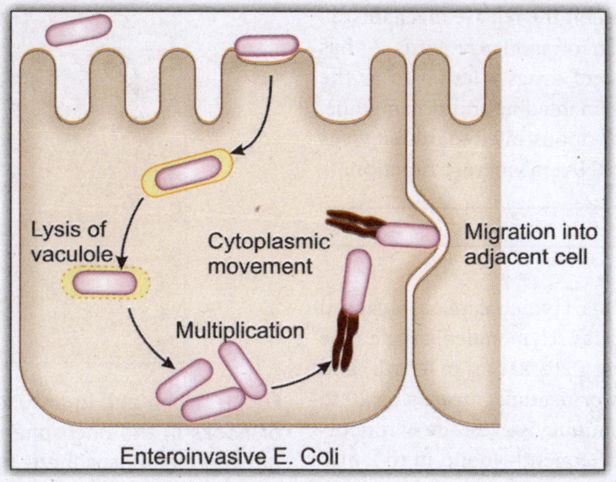

19. Ans: (b) Influenza A

Ref: Ananthanarayanan 7th Ed page 504

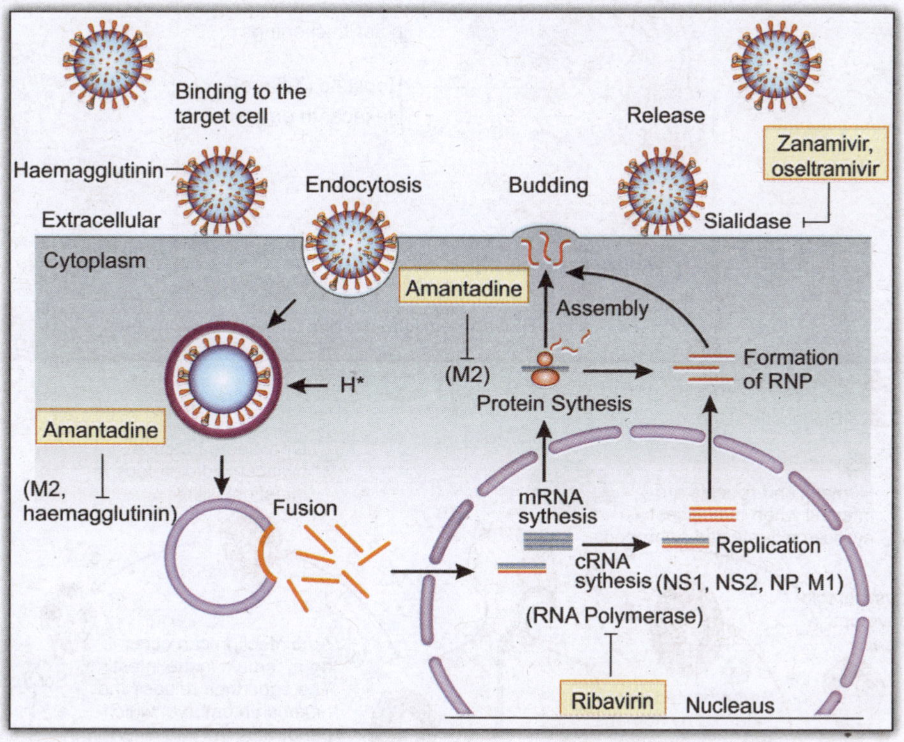

Fig: Life Cycle of Influenza virus with targets of therapeutic interventions

- **The surface of influenza virus A is decorated with three proteins: an M2 ion channel protein, the lectin haemagglutinin (H) and the enzyme sialidase (N).**
- Typically, the influenza virus adheres to the target host cell by using its surface glycoprotein haemagglutinin to recognize glycoconjugates such as GD1a that display terminal α-linked N-acetylneuraminic acid (α-Neu5Ac, compound 1a) residues.
- The virus is then endocytosed, fusion occurs and the host-cell machinery is engaged to produce the necessary viral components. Subsequent viral protein synthesis and particle assembly in the host cell prepares the virion progeny for the budding process to exit the host cell.
- The enzyme sialidase cleaves the terminal α-Neu5Ac residues from both the newly synthesized virion progeny glycoproteins as well as from the host-cell surface. The action of sialidase enables the host-cell-surface aggregated virion progeny to elute away from the infected cell and seek new host cells to infect.

- Both haemagglutinin and sialidase have been proposed as potential anti-influenza drug discovery targets.
- Zanamivir and oseltamivir efficiently block the action of sialidase and significantly inhibit the release mechanism.
- The M2 ion channel protein of influenza virus A has also been targeted by a class of drugs referred to as the adamantanes, which include amantadine and rimantadine.
- Last, ribavirin has also been demonstrated to inhibit virus replication by acting on the RNA polymerase function.

20. Ans: (a) Praziquantel

Ref: Jawetz 26th Ed Pg 736

The given picture is of Egg of H. nana. Hymenolepiasis is caused by two cestodes (tapeworm) species, Hymenolepis nana (the dwarf tapeworm, adults measuring 15 to 40 mm in length) and Hymenolepis diminuta (rat tapeworm, adults measuring 20 to 60 cm in length). Hymenolepis diminuta is a cestode of rodents infrequently seen in humans and frequently found in rodents.

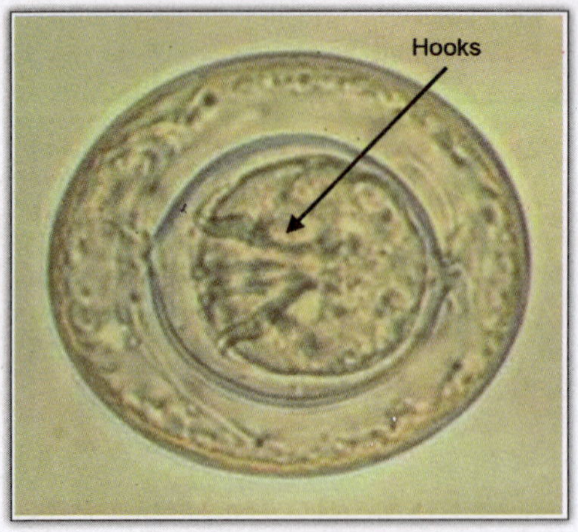

Fig: H. Nana egg in an unstained wet mount. Note the presence of hooks in the oncosphere and polar filaments within the space between the oncosphere and outer shell

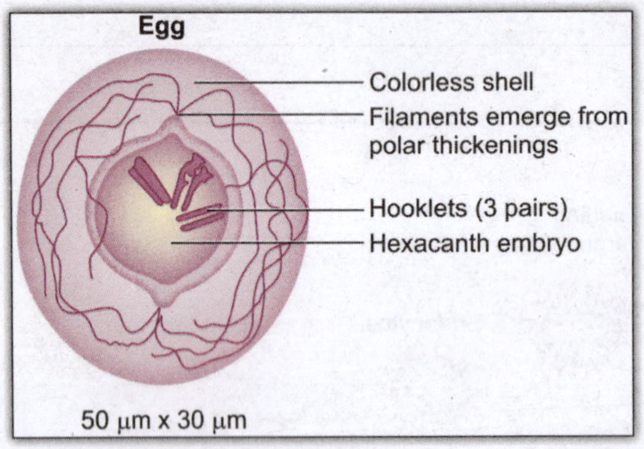

Fig: H. Nana egg-Illustrative

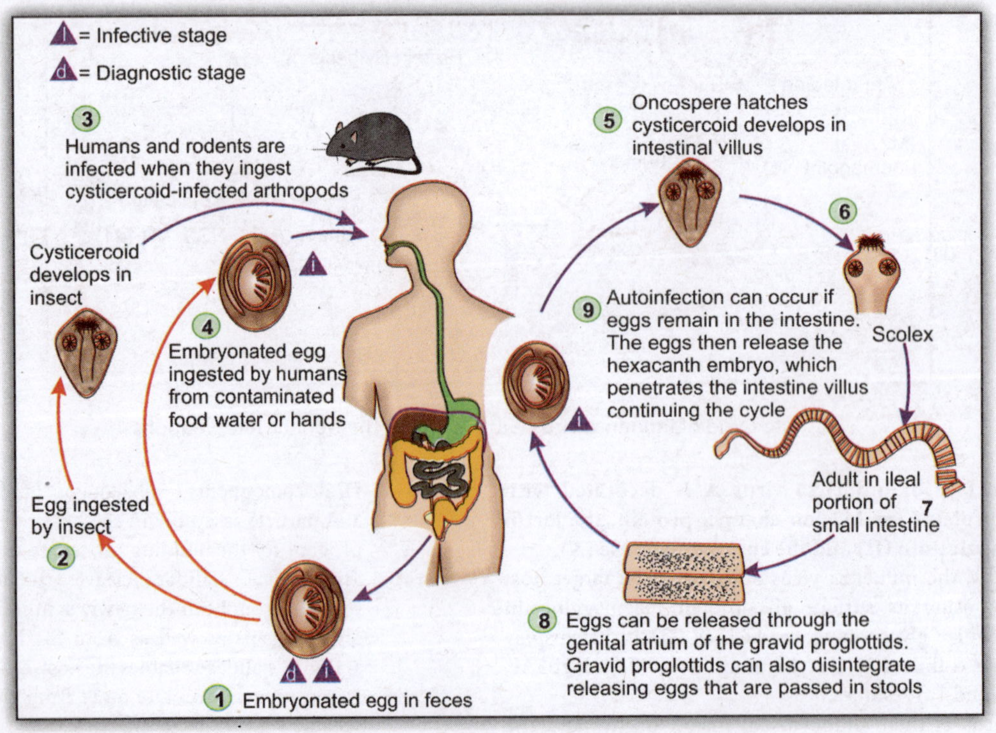

Fig: Life cycle of H Nana

Life cycle of H Nana: Eggs of *Hymenolepis nana* are immediately infective when passed with the stool and cannot survive more than 10 days in the external environment.. When eggs are ingested by an arthropod intermediate host (various species of beetles and fleas may serve as intermediate hosts), they develop into cysticercoids, which can infect humans or rodents upon ingestion and develop into adults in the small intestine. A morphologically identical variant, *H. nana* var. *fraterna*, infects rodents and uses arthropods as intermediate hosts. When eggs are ingested (in contaminated food or water or from hands contaminated with feces), the oncospheres contained in the eggs are released. The oncospheres (hexacanth larvae) penetrate the intestinal villus and develop into cysticercoid larvae. Upon rupture of the villus, the cysticercoids return to the intestinal lumen, evaginate their scoleces , attach to the intestinal mucosa and develop into adults that reside in the ileal portion of the small intestine producing gravid proglottids. Eggs are passed in the stool when released from proglottids through its genital atrium or when proglottids disintegrate in the small intestine. An alternate mode of infection consists of internal autoinfection, where the eggs release their hexacanth embryo, which penetrates the villus continuing the infective cycle without passage through the external environment. The life span of adult worms is 4 to 6 weeks, but internal autoinfection allows the infection to persist for years.

21. Ans: (b) Streptococcus pyogenes

Ref: Ananthnarayanan 7th Ed page 204, 210, KDT 7th Ed Pg 759

S. pyogenes is sensitive to Bacitracin.

- **Maxted's observation:** S. pyogenes is more sensitive to Bacitracin than any other streptococci.A solution of bacitracin is applied to inoculate blood agar to differentiate S. pyogenes from other streptococci. A wide zone of inhibition is seen.
- This is used for presumptive identification of S. pyogenes.
- Bacitracin is a polypeptide antibiotic and is active mainly against gram-positive organisms (both cocci and bacilli). Neisseria, H. influenzae, S. pyogenes, C.difficile.
- It acts by inhibiting cell wall synthesis at a step earlier than that inhibited by penicillin. Subsequently, it increases the efflux of ions by binding to cell membrane. It is bactericidal.
- Bacitracin is not absorbed orally. It is not given parenterally because of high toxicity, especially to the kidney.
- Use is restricted to topical application for infected wounds, ulcers, eye infections—generally in combination with neomycin, polymyxin, etc.
- It does not penetrate intact skin, therefore, is of little value in furunculosis, boils, carbuncles, etc.

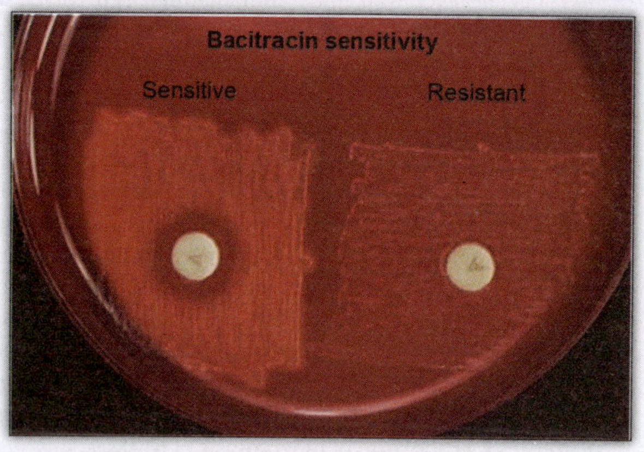

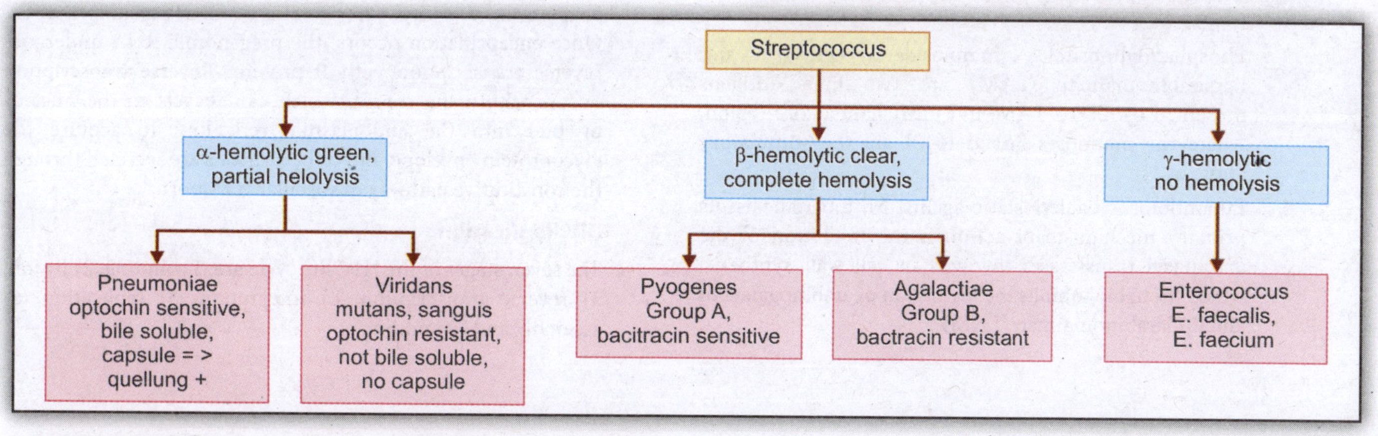

Basis of Typing/Sub-Classification of Bacteria	
Organism	**Basis of typing**
Streptococci	Carbohydrate -C (Lancefield classification)
Salmonella	O & H antigens (mainly O Ag)
Enterobacteria	Lactose fermentation
Shigella	*(Shigella dysentery Mannitol -Ve)*
Meningococci	Capsular polysaccharide Ag
Influenza virus	Ribonuclear protein Antigen (A,B,C)

22. Ans: (b) Till 24 hr after administration of antibiotic

Ref: Manual of Intensive Care Medicine By Richard S. Irwin and Rippe 5th Ed Pg 424; Ghai's 8th Ed Pg 565

Note

Irwin and Rippe's 5th Ed Pg 424 says; Respiratory isolation is indicated for upto 24 hours after starting antibiotic.
Park 24th Ed says; Isolation is recommended for 6 hours after effectively starting antibiotic. Since the latter is not in the options, we go with the first option.

- Meningococcal meningitis presents unique public health and infection control challenges. This diagnosis is suggested by the presence of a petechial or purpuric rash; however, this finding is neither sensitive nor specific.
- To prevent secondary cases of meningococcal meningitis among healthcare workers, all patients with presumed bacterial meningitis should initially be placed in respiratory isolation to prevent spread of infection by droplet infection.

AIIMS NOVEMBER 2017

23. Ans. (b) Tuberculosis

Ref: Prescott's Microbiology 9th ed page 744, Harrison 19th ed page 1103, http://www.who.int/tb/publications/use-of-lf-lam-tb-hiv/en/

Mycobacterial cell wall, lipoarabinomannan, is involved in the pathogen-host interaction and facilitates the survival of M. tuberculosis within macrophages. Tests based on the detection of mycobacterial lipoarabinomannan (LAM) antigen in urine have emerged as potential point-of-care tests for tuberculosis (TB). LAM antigen is a lipopolysaccharide present in mycobacterial cell walls, which is released from metabolically active or degenerating bacterial cells and appears to be present only in people with active TB disease. Urine-based testing would have advantages over sputum-based testing because urine is easy to collect and store and lacks the infection control risks associated with sputum collection. A low-cost point-of-care urine assay for lipoarabinomannan (LAM) used for screening patients prior to antiretroviral therapy (ART) rapidly diagnoses a proportion of tuberculosis (TB) cases.

Extra Edge

- Phosphatidylinositol mannoside (PIM) and lipoarabinomannan (LAM) are two lipid antigens presented by CD1b. LAM and PIM share a core region, where the mannoses linked to PI are the stimulatory antigens.
- Ethambutol is bacteriostatic against M. tuberculosis. Its primary mechanism of action is the inhibition of the arabinosyl transferases involved in cell wall synthesis, which probably inhibits the formation of arabinogalactan and lipoarabinomannan (LAM)
- LAM -B is a major antigen of M laprae which is distinct from LAM of M tuberculosis.

24. Ans. (b) HBV

Ref: Jawetz 24th ed page 496, 500

Two genera of viruses have Reverse transcriptase

1. Hepadna virus: Replicates through RNA intermediate. E.g. Hepatitis B virus
2. Retrovirus: Replicates through DNA intermediate. E.G. HIV virus

HBV Replication

The viral replication cycle are schematized. Blood borne virion circulating through the liver attach to the basolateral membranes through specific viral–host interactions. Pre-S1 protein on the envelope is believed to mediate viral attachment to as yet uncharacterized cellular membrane proteins. Once attached, the virus fuses with membrane protein in a slow temperature dependent reaction. Upon cellular entry, viral core is transported from the cytoplasm towards or into the nucleus while the DNA within the capsid undergoes maturation. ***The partially double stranded relaxed circular genome in the capsid is converted into a covalently closed; fully double stranded circular DNA (ccc DNA).*** The maturation of the genome is not dependent on any viral products but requires host machinery to remove covalently bound protein and RNA primers and complete double stranded synthesis. The ccc DNA amplifies viral infection, as it is the template for pregenomic RNA production. It also serves as the template for production of all the RNA species for the production of functional and structural viral protein.

Viral assembly is a complex multi-step reaction in which specific interactions between pregenomic RNA, P protein, host chaperonins and viral core proteins result in capsid formation. Once encapsidation occurs, the pregenomic RNA undergoes reverse transcription with P protein. Reverse transcription occurs within the capsid, which can recycle to the nucleus or bud into the endoplasmic reticulum to acquire the glycoprotein envelope. Enveloped virions are secreted through the constitutive pathway of vascular transport.

HIV Replication

The seven stages of the HIV life cycle are: 1) binding, 2) fusion, 3) reverse transcription, 4) integration, 5) replication, 6) assembly and 7) budding.

The Hiv Life Cycle

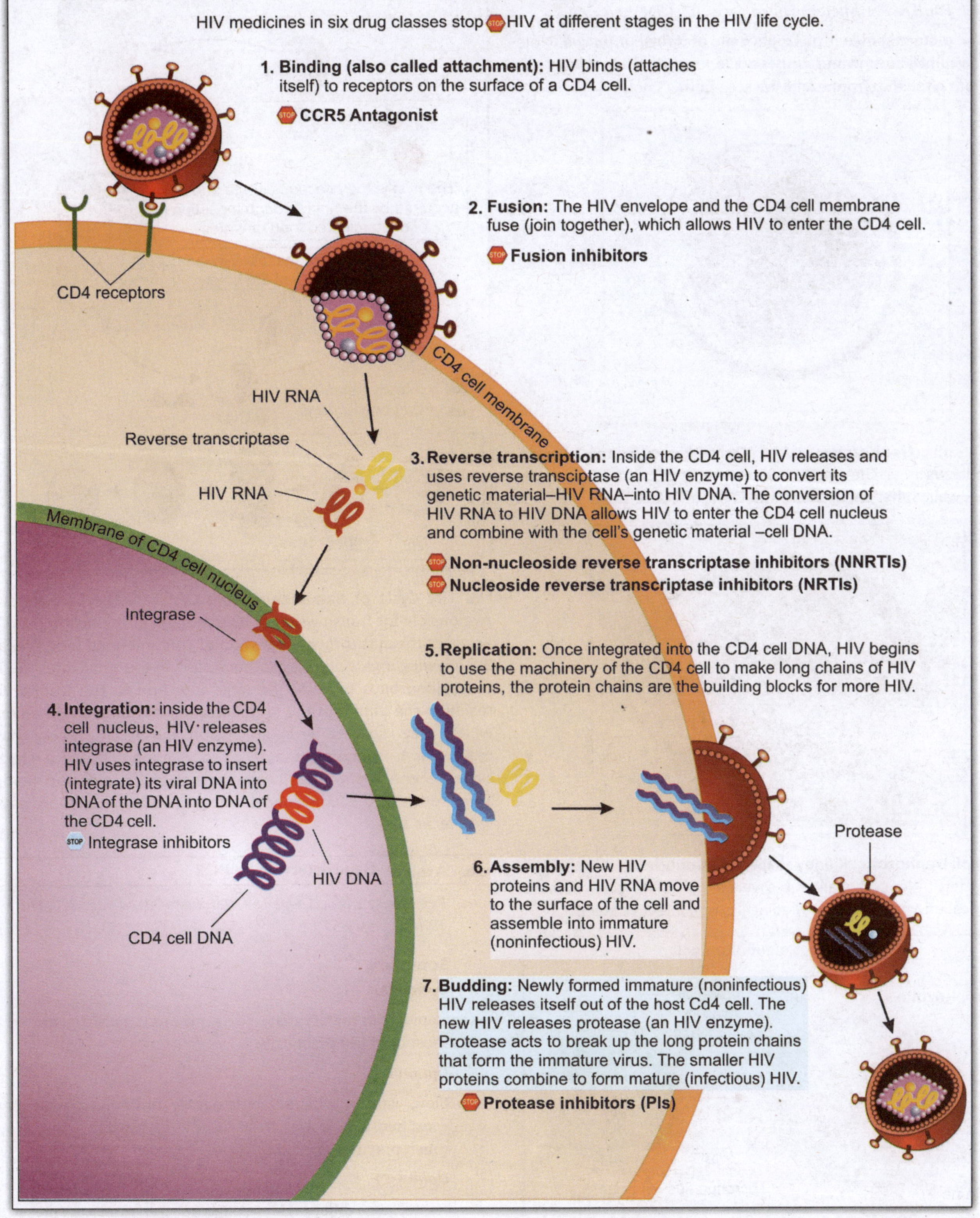

25. Ans. (b) Balantidium coli

Ref: Paniker Parasitology 7th ed page 107, CDC

The picture shown is of Trophozoite of *Balantidium coli*. Note the cilli all around and the Bean/Kidney shaped macronucleus. Both Cyst and Trophozoite are seen in the Stool

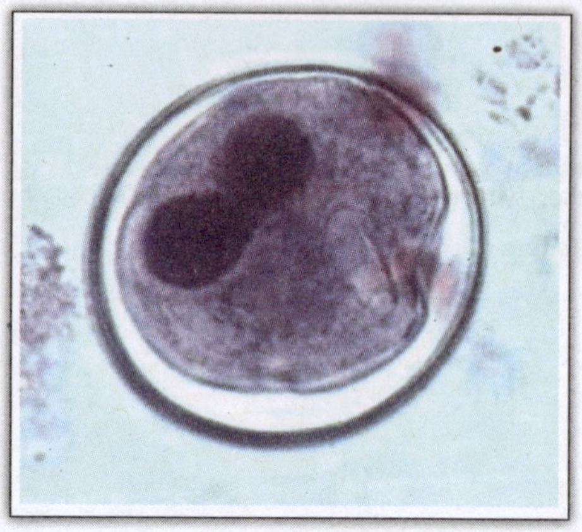

Fig: B. coli trophozoite cyst: Only kidney/bean shaped macronucleus is visible under microscope. It is covered by thick hard cyst wall. Spherical in shape and is the Infective stage.

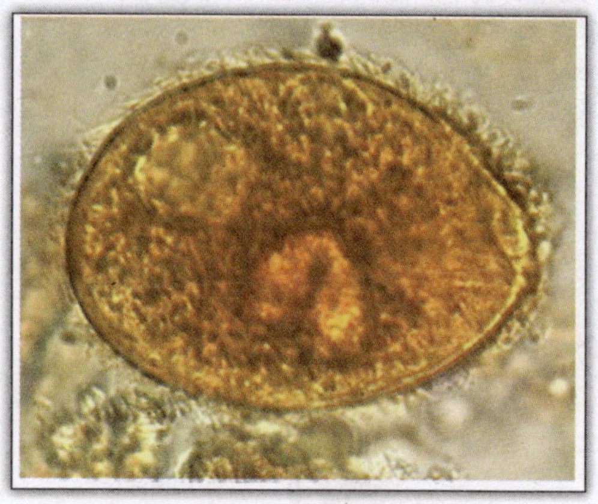

Fig: B. coli trophozoite: Kidney shaped Macronucleus and spherical micronucleus. No cyst wall but covered by visible cilia. Pointed anterior called Cystosome for feeding. Its non infective stage.

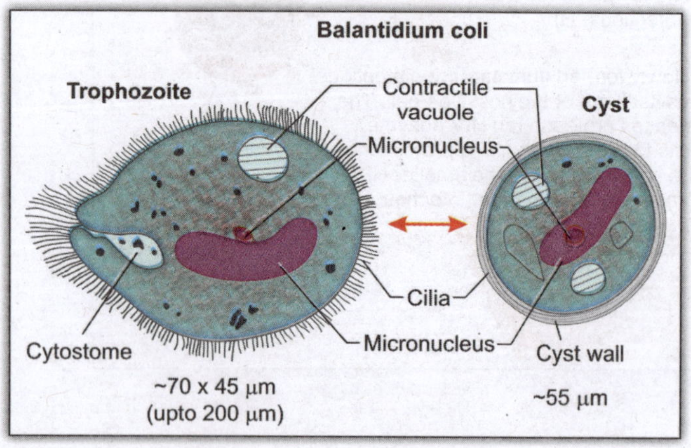

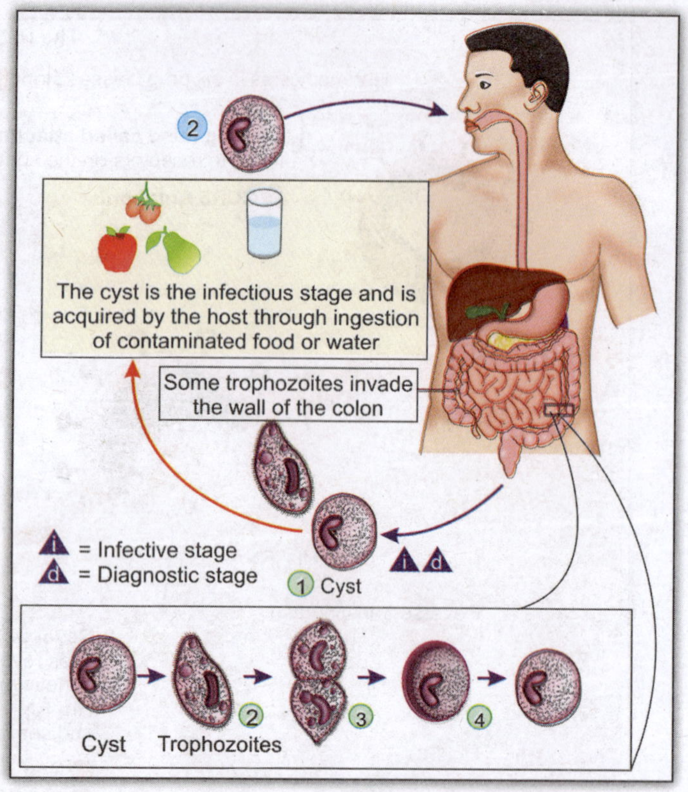

Fig: Life Cycle of Balantidium Coli: Cysts are the parasite stage responsible for transmission of balantidiasis **1**. The host most often acquires the cyst through ingestion of contaminated food or water **2**. Following ingestion, excystation occurs in the small intestine and the trophozoites colonize the large intestine **3**. The trophozoites reside in the lumen of the large intestine of humans and animals, where they replicate by binary fission, during which conjugation may occur **4**. Trophozoites undergo encystation to produce infective cysts **5**. Some trophozoites invade the wall of the colon and multiply. Some return to the lumen and disintegrate. Mature cysts are passed with feces **1**.

26. Ans. (c) Gene detection by PCR

Ref: Jawetz 24th ed page 187, Panikar 10th ed page 270, Harrison 19th ed page 857

Summary

Option (A)

Rapid, can differentiate toxigenic and nontoxigenic strain, most used test practically

Option(B)

Slow, can not differentiate toxigenic and nontoxigenic strain, most sensitive if we already know its a toxic strain. Not of much practical use

Option (C)

Rapid, can differentiate toxigenic and nontoxigenic strain. Newly approved for clinical testing, but appears to be more sensitive than enzyme immunoassay toxin testing and at least as specific

Option (D)

Colonoscopy is positive only when pseudomembrane develops, hence it is highly specific; but insensitive compared with other tests. Negative result does not rule out C. difficile

Administration of antibiotics results in proliferation of drug-resistant C difficile that produces two toxins. **Toxin A**, a potent enterotoxin that also has some cytotoxic activity, binds to the brush border membranes of the gut at receptor sites. **Toxin B** is a potent cytotoxin. Both toxins are found in the stools of patients with pseudomembranous colitis

The diagnosis of CDI is based on a combination of clinical criteria:

- Diarrhea (>3 unformed stools per 24 h for >2 days) with no other recognized cause plus
- Toxin A or B detected in the stool (by ELISA) or toxin producing C. difficile detected in the stool by PCR or culture or pseudomembranes seen in the colon.

Harrison's 19th Ed says

Despite the array of tests available for C. difficile and its toxins, no single traditional test has high sensitivity, high specificity and rapid turnaround. Most laboratory tests for toxins, including enzyme immunoassays, lack sensitivity. However, testing of multiple additional stool specimens is not recommended. ***Nucleic acid amplification tests, including PCR assays, have now been approved for diagnostic purposes and appear to be both rapid and sensitive while retaining high specificity***

Relative Sensitivity and Specificity of Diagnostic Tests for Clostridium Difficile Infection

Type of test	Relative sensitivitya	Relative specificitya	Comment
Stool culture for *C. difficile*	+ + + +	+ + +	Most sensitive test; specificity of + + + + if the *C. difficile* isolate tests positive for toxin; with clinical data, is diagnostic of CDI. Can not differentiate toxigenic from non toxigenic strain. **turn around time too slow for practical use**
Cell culture cytotoxin test on stool	+ + +	+ + + +	With clinical data, is diagnostic of CDI; highly specific but not as sensitive as stool culture; slow turnaround time
Enzyme immunoassay for toxin A or toxins A and B in stool	+ + to + + +	+ + +	With clinical data, is diagnostic of CDI; rapid results, but not as sensitive as stool culture or cell culture cytotoxin test. Can differentiate toxigenic vs nontoxigenic strain.
Enzyme immunoassay for *C. difficile* common antigen in stool	+ + + to + + + +	+ + +	Detects glutamate dehydrogenase found in toxigenic and nontoxigenic strains of *C. difficile* and other stool organisms; more sensitive and less specific than enzyme immunoassay for toxins; rapid results
PCR for *C. difficile* toxin B gene in stool	+ + + +	+ + + +	Detects toxigenic *C. difficile* in stool; newly approved for clinical testing, but appears to be more sensitive than enzyme immunoassay toxin testing and at least as specific
Colonoscopy or sigmoidoscopy	+	+ + + +	Highly specific if pseudomembranes are seen; insensitive compared with other tests

aAccording to both clinical and test-based criteria.

Note: + + + +, >90%; + + +, 71–90%; + +, 51–70%; +, 50%

27. Ans. (b) Leptospira

Ref: Anantnarayan 9th ed page 377, Jawetz 24th ed ch 25

The spirochetes (**Treponema, Borrelia, Leptospira**) are long, slender, helically coiled, spiral or corkscrew-shaped, gram-negative bacilli. They has an outer sheath or glycosaminoglycan coating. Inside the sheath is the outer membrane, which contains peptidoglycan and maintains the structural integrity of the organisms. **Endoflagella (axial filaments)** are the flagella-like organelles in the periplasmic space encased by the outer membrane. The endoflagella begin at each end of the organism and wind around it, extending to and overlapping at the midpoint. Inside the endoflagella is the inner membrane (cytoplasmic membrane) that provides osmotic stability and covers the protoplasmic cylinder.

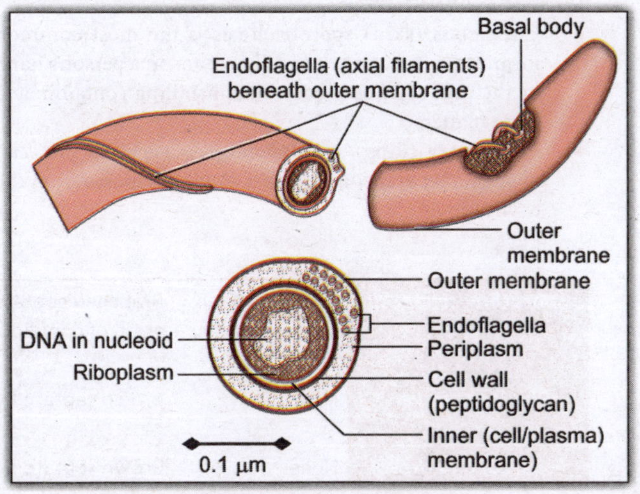

MICROBIOLOGY • Answers with Explanations

28. Ans. (c) Pneumocystis jiroveci

Ref: Ananthnarayan 9th Ed Page 593

Dimorphic fungi: Fungi that have two growth forms, such as a mold and a yeast. All dimorphic fungi are yeasts in humans (molds in dirt). Human infection is by spore inhalation, so no Person-Person transmission.

MNEMONIC for dimorphic fungi; **HB PSC** (use **HB** pencil in **PSC** exam)

- Histoplasma capsulatum
- Blastomycoses sermatidis
- Paracoccidiodes brasiliense
- Penicillium marneffei
- Sporothrix schenkii
- Coccidioides immitis
- Candida albicans

29. Ans. (b) Sporotrichosis

Ref: Jawetz 24th ed page 630-632, Ananthanarayanan 8th ed page 609

Similar Question was asked in AIIMS NOVEMBER 2012 Microbiology without Colour Plate

Sporothrix Schenckii

Sporothrix schenkii is a thermally dimorphic fungus that lives on vegetation. It is associated with a variety of plants—grasses, trees, sphagnum moss, rose bushes and other horticultural plants. Following traumatic introduction into the skin, S schenckii causes sporotrichosis, a chronic granulomatous infection. Multiple subcutaneous nodules and abscesses occur along the lymphatics. The incidence is higher among agricultural workers and sporotrichosis is considered an occupational risk for forest rangers, horticulturists and workers in similar occupations. Sporotrichosis (also known as **"rose gardener's disease"**) is a rare infection caused by Sporothrix. This fungus lives throughout the world in soil and on plant matter such as sphagnum moss, rose bushes and hay. People get sporotrichosis by coming in contact with the fungal spores in the environment.

Types of Sporotrichosis

- **Cutaneous (skin) sporotrichosis** is the most common form of the infection. It usually occurs on a person's hand or the arm after they have been handling contaminated plant matter.
- **Pulmonary (lung) sporotrichosis** is very rare but can happen after someone breathes in fungal spores from the environment.
- **Disseminated sporotrichosis** occurs when the infection spreads to another part of the body, such as the bones, joints, or the central nervous system. This form of sporotrichosis usually affects people who have weakened immune systems, such as people with HIV infection

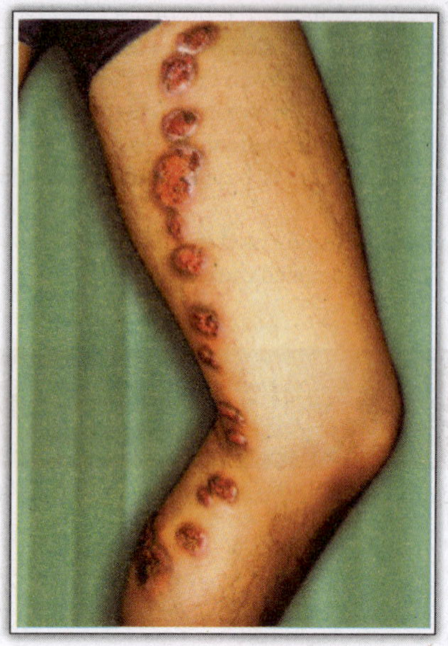

Fig: Noduloulcerative lesions **(sporotrichotic chancre)** appear along the lymphatics proximal to the initial inoculation injury site. It is the most common variety and accounts for 70–80% of the cases of cutaneous sporotrichosis. The extremities are affected most frequently. A noduloulcerative lesion at inoculation site and a string of similar nodules along the proximal lymphatics, with or without transient satellite adenopathy, characterizes this form.

30. Ans. (b) Chromoblastomycosis

Ref: Ananthanarayan Panikar 10th ed page 605

Hints in Question

- Thorn Prick signifies **"Traumatic inoculation"** of Fungus. The fungi that cause subcutaneous mycoses normally reside in soil or on vegetation. They enter the skin or subcutaneous tissue by traumatic inoculation with contaminated material. All 4 options are Subcutaneous mycosis and can enter through Traumatic Inoculation
- Superficial mycoses is frequently seen in Sub-Himalayan region including Himachal Pradesh.
- Out of all Subcutaneous mycoses, Verrucous lesion is typical of Chromoblastomycosis.

Chromoblastomycosis (chromomycosis) is a subcutaneous mycotic infection caused by traumatic inoculation by any of five recognized fungal agents that reside in soil and vegetation.

Sporothrix schenckii	Round or cigar shaped budding Yeast	Branched septate hyphae w/oval conidia at tip of conidiophores ("daisies")	Subcutaneous	*Sporotrichosis* (gardener's disease)
Phialophora verrucosa	None	Brown septate hyphae	Subcutaneous	*Chromoblastomycosis*
Fonsecaea pedrosoi	None	Brown septate hyphae and conidia	Subcutaneous	*Chromoblastomycosis*

Contd...

Pseudallescheria boydii	None	V-shaped septate hyphae with radiating chains of conidia	Subcutaneous	Mycetoma
Madurella mycetomatis	None	Brown septate branched hyphae	Subcutaneous	Mycetoma
Exophiala Bipolaris	None	Brown septate hyphae	Subcutaneous	Phaeohyphomycosis
Exserohilum	None	Brown septate hyphae	Subcutaneous	Phaeohyphomycosis

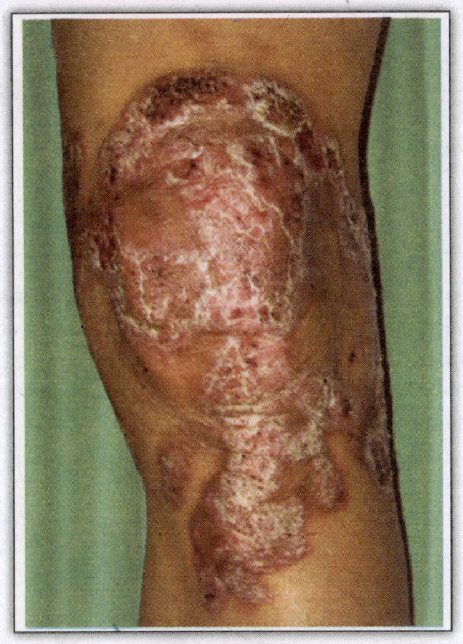

© Ran Yuping et al

Fig: Chromoblastomycosis Initial lesion: The initial erythematous papule grows slowly over months to years, the primary lesion becomes verrucous and wart-like with extension along the draining lymphatics

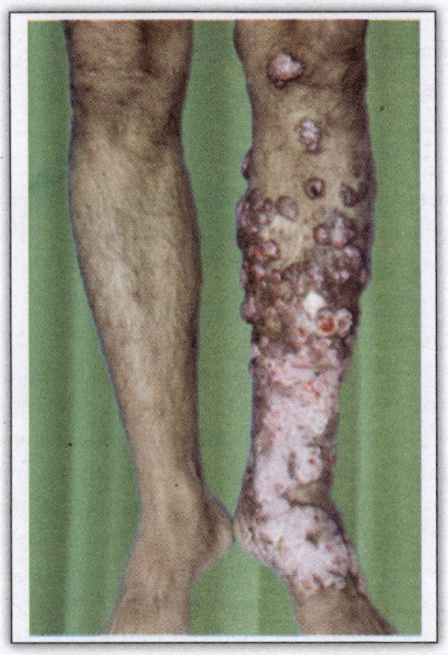

Fig: Chromoblastomycosis late lesion: Cauliflower-like nodules with crusting abscesses eventually cover the area. Small ulcerations or "black dots" of hemopurulent material are present on the warty surface. Rarely, elephantiasis may result from secondary infection, obstruction and fibrosis of lymph channels. Lymphedema is normally observed in the affected limb

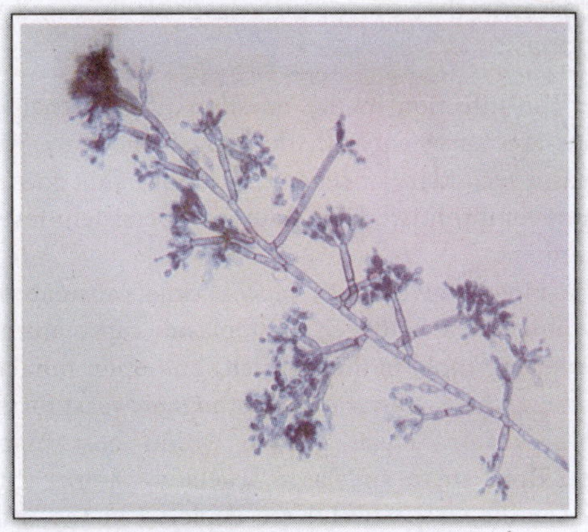

© CDC/Sherry Brinkman

Fig: Chromoblastomycosis Microscopy: Elliptical, brownish conidia from conidophore. The agents of chromoblastomycosis are identified by their modes of conidiation. The most frequent aetiological agents of CBM are- Fonsecaea pedrosoi, Phialophora verrucosa and Cladophialophora carrionii. Rhinocladiella aquaspersa

Light microscopy of lactophenol cotton blue preparation of colonies grown on Sabouraud's dextrose agar presenting with Conidiophores suberect, olivaceous brown, apically densely branched

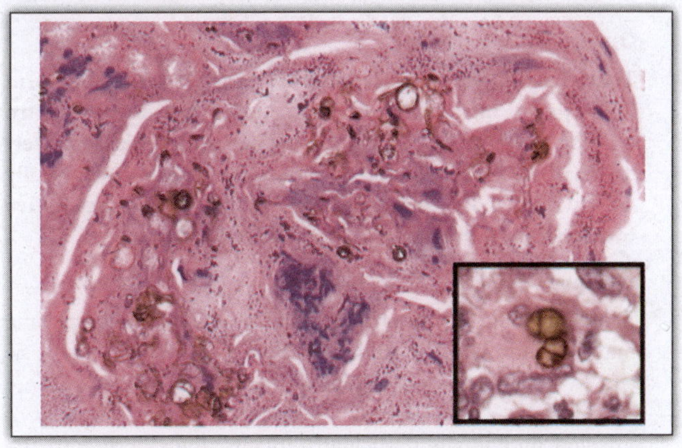

© Department of Pathology, Calicut Medical College

Fig: Chromoblastomycosis HPE: Histologic examination shows characteristic pseudoepitheliomatous hyperplasia in the epidermis and a mixed granulomatous inflammatory infiltrate with giant cells containing characteristic dark-brown, round sclerotic body resembling a **"copper penny"** i.e. Dark Brown Pigmented Yeast with reproduction by intracellular wall formation (septation) not budding. The agents of chromoblastomycosis are identified by their modes of conidiation. In tissue they appear the same, producing spherical brown cells (4–12 μm in diameter) termed muriform or sclerotic bodies that divide by transverse septation

31. Ans. (c) It doesn't grow in SDA

Ref: Jawetz 24th ed page 679, 680

NOTE

Cystoisospora belli, not Cryptosporidium was given in the exam. Cystoisospora belli, previously known as Isospora belli, is a parasite that causes an intestinal disease known as cystoisosporiasis

Clue: The infection in the question is protozoal while the options are consistent with the fungal infection. This points towards a secondary or second infection. This goes well with immunocompromised HIV status and persistent fever in spite of treatment.

The picture given is of Histoplasma capsulatum. It is a dimorphic fungal pathogen. Histoplasma capsulatum grows as a saprophytic mold in the soil (left) but, upon inhalation by a mammalian host, converts to a pathogenic yeast form (center) capable of intracellular growth within host macrophages (right). Both small and large vegetative spores (micro and macroconidia, respectively) are depicted in the mold form. Within the macrophage, yeast cells are shown within a membrane-bound phagosome and the macrophage nucleus is also depicted.

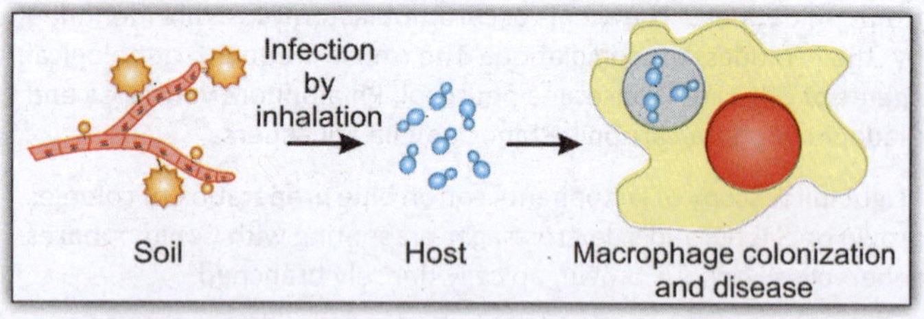

Option (A)

True; Histoplasma is a Dimorphic fungi. Oval yeasts form (2 × 4 μm) is intracellular in macrophages. In tissue or in vitro on rich medium at 37 °C, the hyphae and conidia convert to small, oval yeast cells. In tissue, the yeasts are typically seen within macrophages, as H capsulatum is a **facultative intracellular parasite**

Option (B)

True: Within macrophages, the yeasts of Histoplasma may disseminate to reticuloendothelial tissues such as the liver, spleen, bone marrow and lymph nodes. Severe disseminated histoplasmosis develops in a small minority of infected individuals particularly infants, the elderly and the immunosuppressed, including AIDS patients. In disseminated histoplasmosis, bone marrow cultures are often positive

Option (C)

False: Specimens are cultured in rich media, such as glucose-cysteine blood agar at 37 °C and on Sabouraud's agar or inhibitory mold agar at 25–30 °C. Cultures must be incubated for a minimum of 4 weeks.

Option (D)

True: Histoplasma spores circulate in the air after contaminated soil is disturbed. The spores are too small to see without a microscope. When people breathe in the spores, they are at risk for developing histoplasmosis. After the spores enter the lungs, the person's body temperature allows the spores to transform into yeast. The yeast can then travel to lymph nodes and can spread to other parts of the body through the bloodstream.

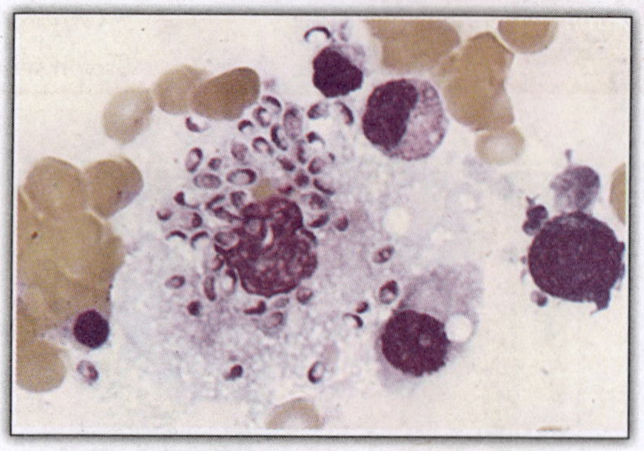

Fig: Histoplasma capsulatum: Wright stain of bone marrow aspirate revealed innumerable oval/crescent-shaped yeast cells in both intracellular and extracellular distribution, most prominently seen within marrow histiocytes. Also it is PAS positive and gave a positive Prussian blue reaction

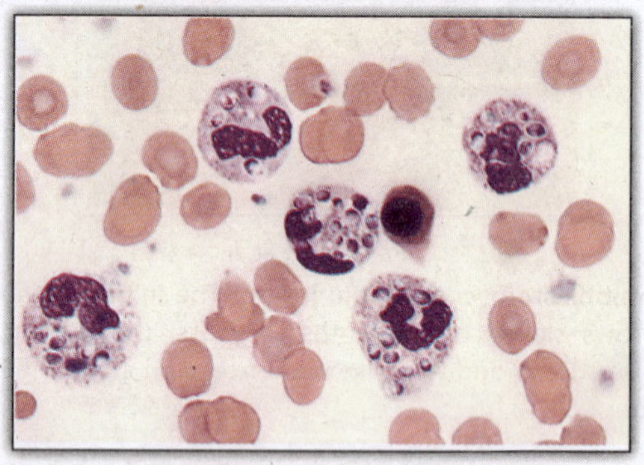

Fig: Histoplasma capsulatum inside neutrophils in a peripheral blood smear

32. Ans. (a) Invasive candidiasis

Ref: Toxicology of 1 - 3-Beta-Glucans: Glucans as a Marker for Fungal Exposure edited by Shih-Houng Young, Vincent Castranova page 203, 204, J. Clin. Microbiol. July 2014 vol. 52 no. 7 2328-2333

Similar Question was asked in AIIMS MAY 2017 Microbiology

(1–3)-β-D-glucan: A polysaccharide component of the cell wall of most fungi pyrogen test. A new fungal surrogate marker, (1–3)-β-D glucan, offers a noninvasive method for the potential surveillance and diagnosis of invasive fungal infections. Plasma β-glucan concentrations in normal subjects are less than 10 pg/ml. They increase in systemic fungal infections and have been shown to be high in deep mycoses, fungemias and antimycotic-responsive febrile episodes. Thus far, fungi reported to be involved in the elevation of β-glucan in blood include ***Aspergillus, Candida, Trichosporon, Cryptococcus, Saccharomyces, Fusarium, Acremonium and Ochroconis gallopavum***. *However, pulmonary cryptococcosis rarely seem to be associated with hyper-β-glucanemia unless it is invasive or extensive.* This may be due to a possible low content of β-glucan in the cell walls of Cryptococcus.

Consequently, to test for cryptococcosis, a latex agglutination test for glucronoxylomannan, abundant in the capsule should be employed. *For candidiasis, the β-glucan assay excels other Candida antigen tests, not only in that it is by far more sensitive, but also in that it covers all species of Candida, including C. glabraut and C. krusei, both of which often evade detection by the later on account of antigenic difference*

Extra Edge

- According to recent research published in the journal Molecular Microbiology, "The polysaccharide beta-1,6-glucan is a major component of the cell wall of Cryptococcus neoformans, but its function has not been investigated in this fungal pathogen.
- **KRE genes** are required for beta-1,6-glucan synthesis, maintenance of capsule architecture and cell wall protein anchoring in Cryptococcus neoformans
- The **Echinocandins** are a new class of antifungal agents that perturb the synthesis of the pervasive cell wall polysaccharide β-glucan by inhibiting 1,3-β-glucan synthase and disrupting cell wall integrity.

33. Ans. (b) Vivax and Ovale

Ref: Panikar 7th ed page 66

Hypnozoites (p.ovale and vivax) in liver are responsible for relapse when they reactivate. In Falciparum and Malariae Hypnozoites are not found hence relapse is not possible.

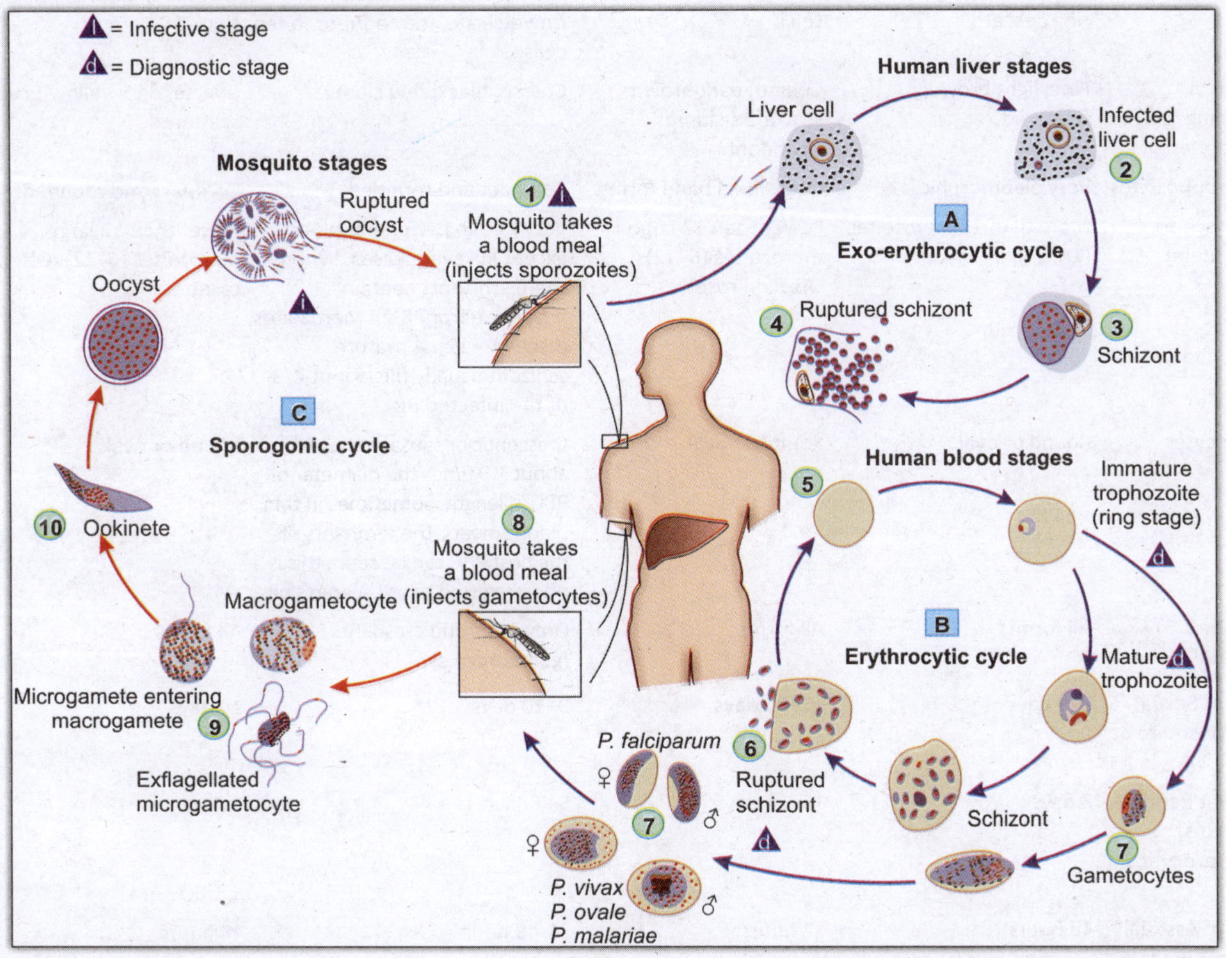

Source: CDC Illustrations

Fig: Life cycle of malaria parasite (Plasmodium): The malaria parasite life cycle involves two hosts. During a blood meal, a malaria-infected female Anopheles mosquito inoculates sporozoites into the human host **1**. Sporozoites infect liver cells **2** and mature into schizonts **3**, which rupture and release merozoites **4**. (Of note, in P. vivax and P. ovale a dormant stage [hypnozoites] can persist in the liver and cause relapses by invading the bloodstream weeks, or even years later.) After this initial replication in the liver (exo-erythrocytic schizogony **A**), the parasites undergo asexual multiplication in the erythrocytes (erythrocytic schizogony **B**). Merozoites infect red blood cells **5**. The ring stage trophozoites mature into schizonts, which rupture releasing merozoites. Some parasites differentiate into sexual erythrocytic stages (gametocytes) **7**. Blood stage parasites are responsible for the clinical manifestations of the disease. The gametocytes, male (microgametocytes) and female (macrogametocytes), are ingested by an Anopheles mosquito during a blood meal **8**. The parasites' multiplication in the mosquito is known as the sporogonic cycle **C**. While in the mosquito's stomach, the microgametes penetrate the macrogametes generating zygotes **9**. The zygotes in turn become motile and elongated (ookinetes) **10** which invade the midgut wall of the mosquito where they develop into oocysts **11**. The oocysts grow, rupture and release sporozoites **12**, which make their way to the mosquito's salivary glands. Inoculation of the sporozoites **1** into a new human host perpetuates the malaria life cycle.

Characteristic Features of the Malaria Parasite (Romanowsky-Stained Preparations)				
	P vivax (benign tertian malaria)	*P malariae* (quartan malaria)	*P falciparum* (malignant tertian malaria)	*P ovale* (ovale malaria)
Parasitized red cells	Enlarged, pale. Fine stippling (Schüffner's dots). Primarily invades reticulocytes, young red cells.	Not enlarged. No stippling (except with special stains). Primarily invades older red cells.	Not enlarged. Coarse stippling (Maurer's clefts). Invades all red cells regardless of age.	Enlarged, pale. Schüffner's dots conspicuous. Cells often oval, fimbriated, or crenated.
Level of usual maximum parasitemia	Up to 30,000/μL of blood.	Fewer than 10,000/μL.	May exceed 200,000/μL; commonly 50,000/μL.	Fewer than 10,000/μL.
Ring stage trophozoites	Large rings (1/3–1/2 red cell diameter). Usually one chromatin granule; ring delicate.	Large rings (1/3 red cell diameter). Usually one chromatin granule; ring thick.	Small rings (1/5 red cell diameter). Often two granules; multiple infections common; ring delicate, may adhere to red cells.	Large rings (1/3 red cell diameter). Usually one chromatin granule; ring thick.
Pigment in developing trophozoites	Fine; light brown; scattered.	Coarse; dark brown; scattered clumps; abundant.	Coarse; black; few clumps.	Coarse; dark yellow-brown; scattered.
Older trophozoites	Very pleomorphic.	Occasional band forms.	Compact and rounded.	Compact and rounded.
Mature schizonts (segmenters)	More than 12 merozoites (14–24).	Fewer than 12 large merozoites (6–12). Often in rosette.	Very rare in peripheral blood except in severe cases. When seen, schizonts contain anywhere from 8-24 merozoites (usually > 12). A mature schizont usually fills about 2/3 of the infected RBC.	Fewer than 12 large merozoites (6–12). Often in rosette.
Gametocytes	Round or oval.	Round or oval.	Crescentic or sausage shaped, about 1.5 times the diameter of RBC in length. Sometimes in thin blood smears, the remnants of the host RBC can be seen; this is often referred to as Laveran's bib.	Round or oval.
Distribution in peripheral blood	All forms.	All forms.	Only rings and crescents (gametocytes).	All forms.
Length of Sexual Cycle (Mosquito at 27 °C)	8–9 days	15–20 days	9–10 days	14 days
Prepatent Period (in Humans) (Preerythrocytic Cycle)	8 days	15–16 days	5–7 days	9 days
Length of Asexual Cycle (in Humans)	48 hours	72 hours	36-48 hours	48 hours

34. Ans. (d) Acute angled branching aspergillus

Ref: Paniker 9th ed page page 613

Candida species, Histoplasma and Aspergillus species are the most common of the many fungal organisms identified as causing Infective endocarditis **(Braunwald's Heart Disease 9th ed Page 1543)**

Option (A) and (B)

Zygomycetes (Mucor and Rhizopus): Irregular, broad, empty looking, non-septae hyphae branching at wide angles (Right angle). Also they are not well known to cause Infective endocarditis.

Option (C) and (D)

Penicillium and Aspergillus both have septate branched acute angled hyphae. Acute angle of Penicillium is 25°–45° while acute angle of Aspergillus is 45°. Secondly the characteristic helpful in distinguishing with Aspergillus is clear vacuoles alternating with basophilic zones. Thirdly Aspergillus is amongst the most common cause of fungal infective endocarditis while Penicillium endocarditis is rare.

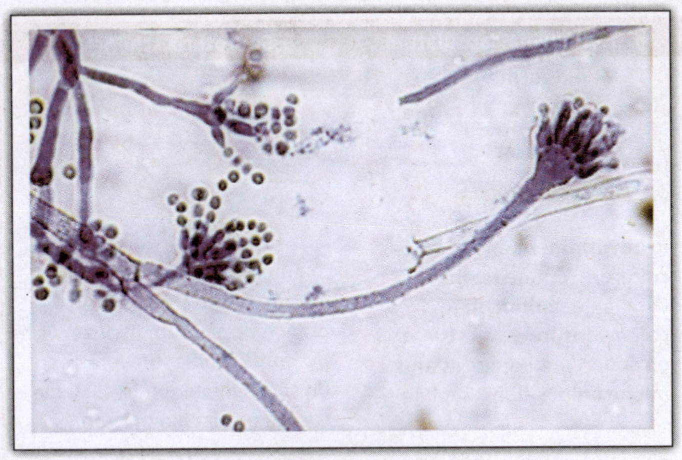

© Bouhaimed M

Fig: Aspergillus single hyphae in Grocott's methenamine silver (GMS) stain showing V-shaped/Acute angled, 45o septate, branched hyphae and radiating chains of conidia

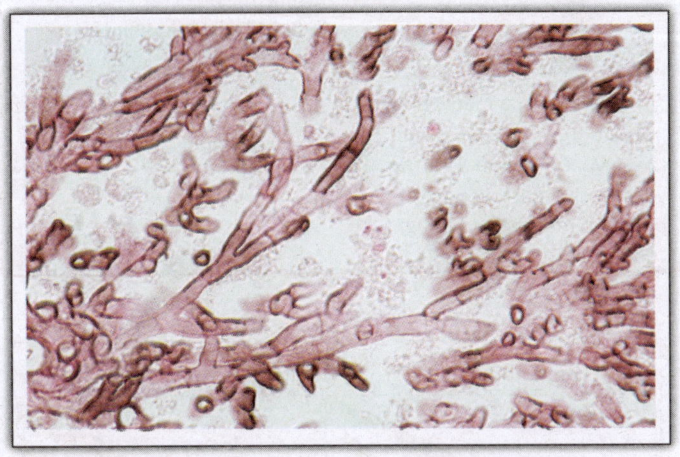

Fig: Aspergillus multiple hyphae in Grocott's methenamine silver (GMS) stained tissue section of lung showing narrow width, acute angled branched, septate hyphae

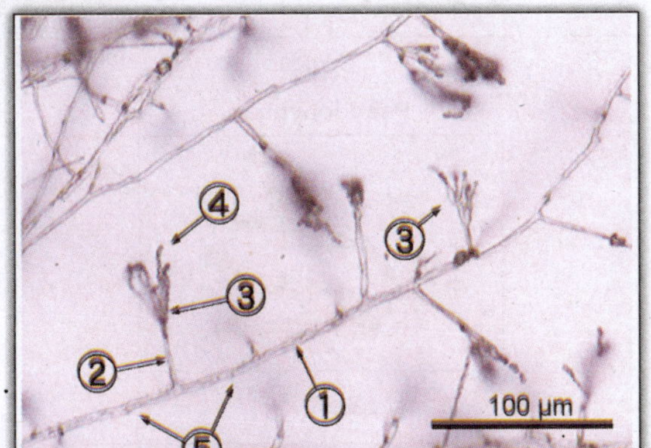

Fig: Penicillium single hyphae in Grocott's methenamine silver (GMS) stain showing Acute angled 25°–45° Septate, branched hyphae. Characteristic helpful in distinguishing with Aspergillus is clear vacuoles alternating with basophilic zones. Chains of conidia are produced by phialides, which are supported by branched conidiophores. Terminal conidium is oldest. 1. Hypha, 2. Conidiophore, 3. Phialide, 4. Conida, 5. Septa

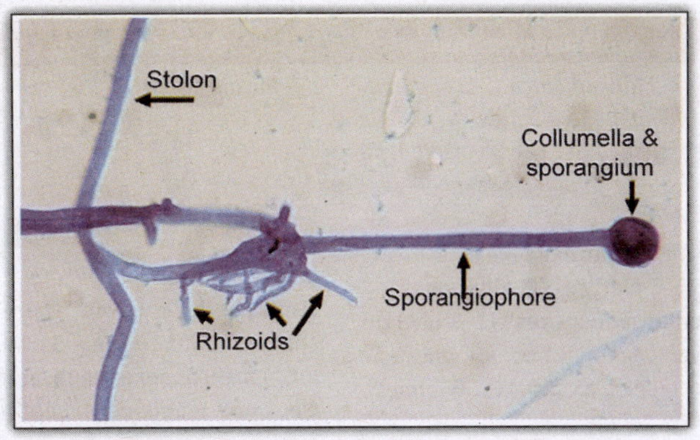

Fig: Zygomycetes- Rhizopus single hyphae- Pauciseptate/Aseptate Ribbon like, Right angled hyphae. Sporangiospores are produced inside a spherical structure, the sporangium. Sporangia are supported by a large apophysate columella atop a long stalk, the sporangiophore. Sporangiophores arise among distinctive, root-like rhizoids.

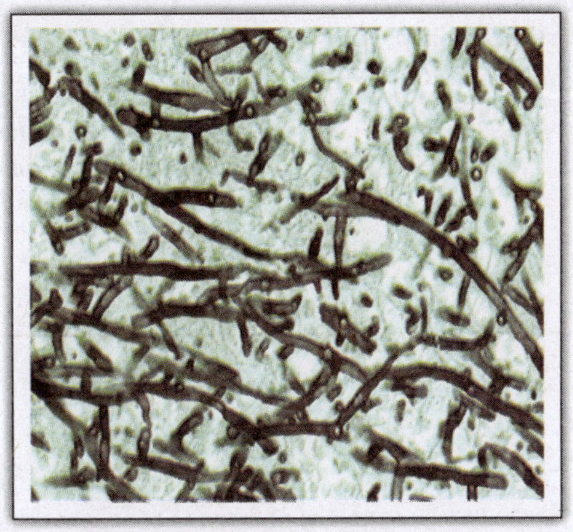

Fig: Zygomycetes- Rhizopus multiple hyphae- Pauciseptate/ Aseptate Ribbon like, Right angled hyphae.

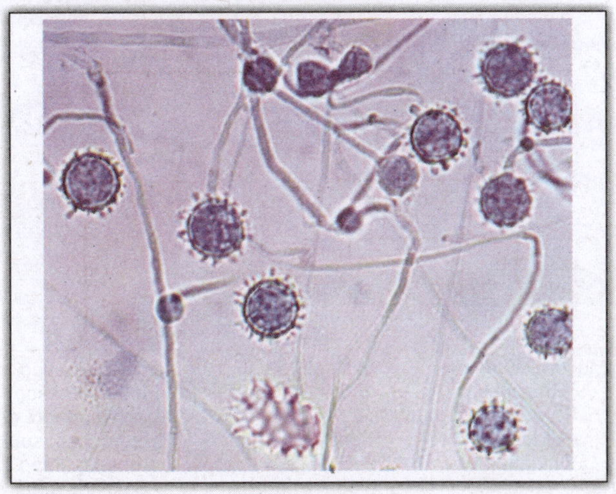

Fig: Histoplasma Hyaline septate hyphae. Large single celled Tuberculate macroconidium (with typical thick walls and radial, finger like projections) is a diagnostic structure of Histoplasma capsulatum. Histoplasma capsulatum exhibits thermal dimorphism growing in living tissue or in culture at 37C as a budding yeast-like fungus and in soil or culture at temperatures below 30C as a mould

Blastomyces spp.	Coccidioies spp.	Histoplasma capsulatum	Sporothrix schenckill
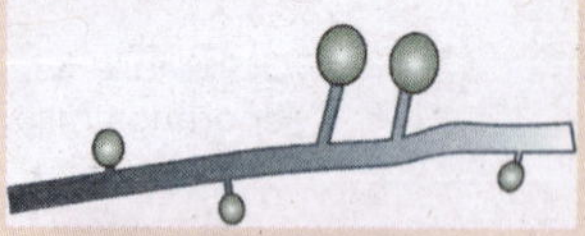 In **environment** and 25°C culture—**"Lolly-pop chlamydospores"** (2–3 uM) on varying lenght conidiophores attached to sepatate hyphae.	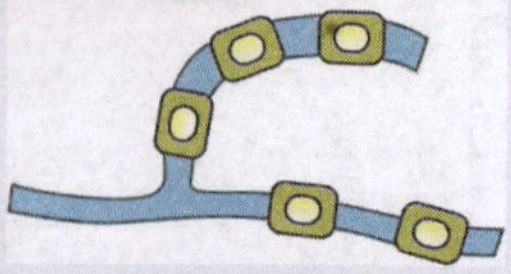 In **environment** and 25°C culture—thick walled "Barrel-shaped" (3 uM wide × 5 uM long) arthrospores separated by clear non-viable cells. Septate hyphae present	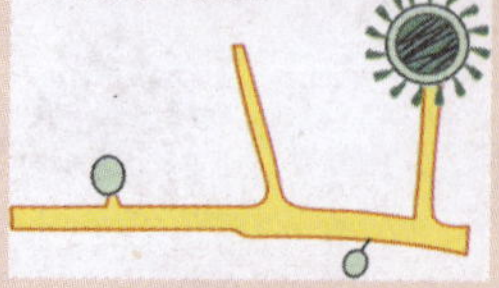 In **environment** and 25°C culture—septate hyphae with large **"tuberculate chlamydospores"** (8–104 uM) on short conidiophores and **microconidia** along hyphae	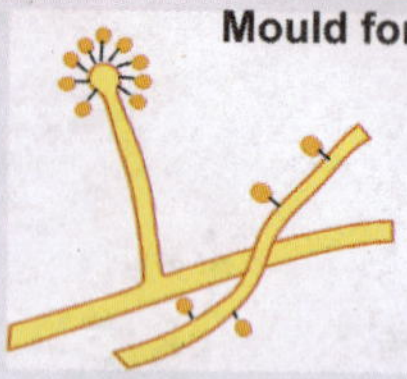 In **environment** and 25°C cyktyre—Fine (2uM wide) branching, septate hyphae with pyriform condia (flowerettes) on short conidiophores. Single condia occura along hyphae.
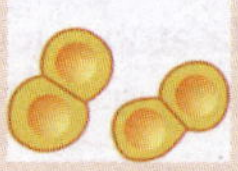 In **tissue** and fungal media at 37°C—**thick walled** yeast (5–20uM) with a **broad base** between monther adn daughter cells	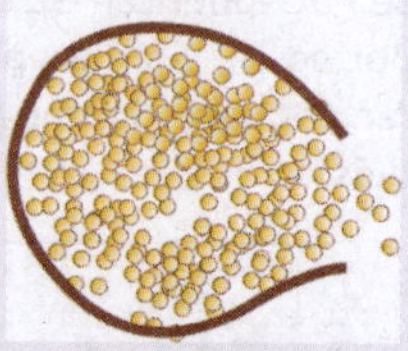 In **tissue** and speciallzed media at 37°C—immature (20–40uM) and mature **spherule** (50–250uM) containing infectious **endospores**	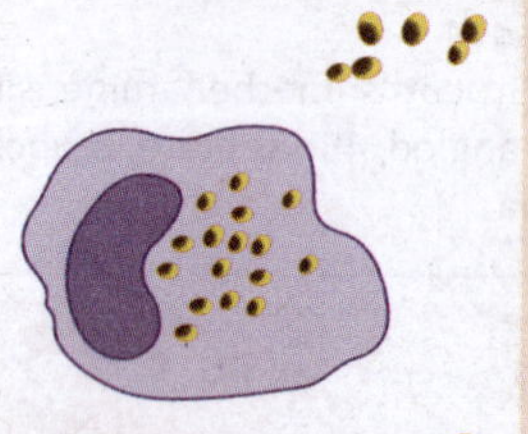 Yeast cells in a macrophage In **tissue**-intracellular, small (2–4uM). Culture at 37°C small yeast with a narrow base between mother and daughter cells	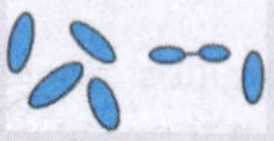 In **tissue** cigar-shaped (oval and fusiform), small (2uM wide × 3–8uM long) budding yeast. Culture at 37°C —small yeast similar to

NOTE

Grocott's silver. Both viable and dead hyphae are stained well with this method.

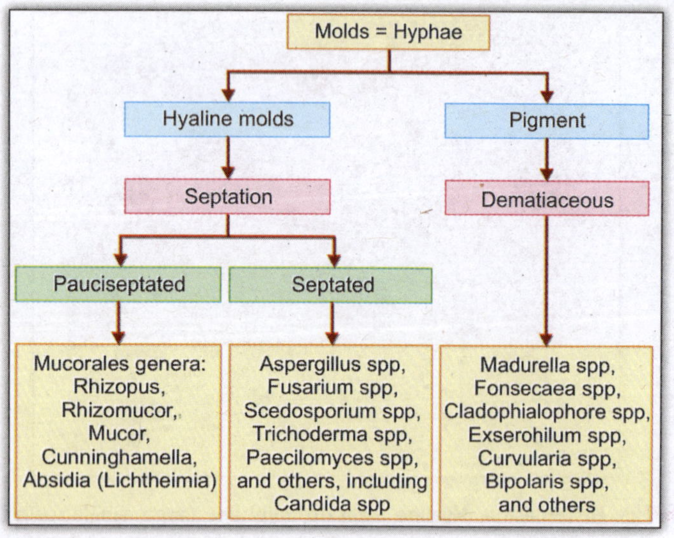

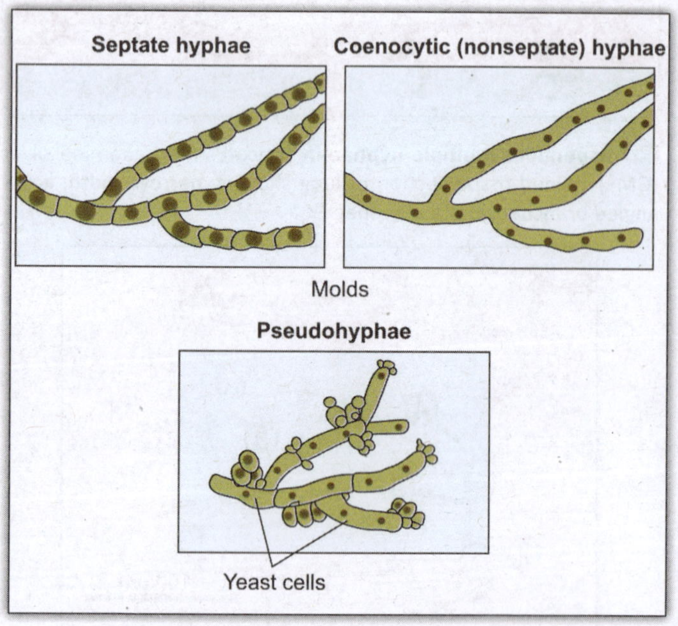

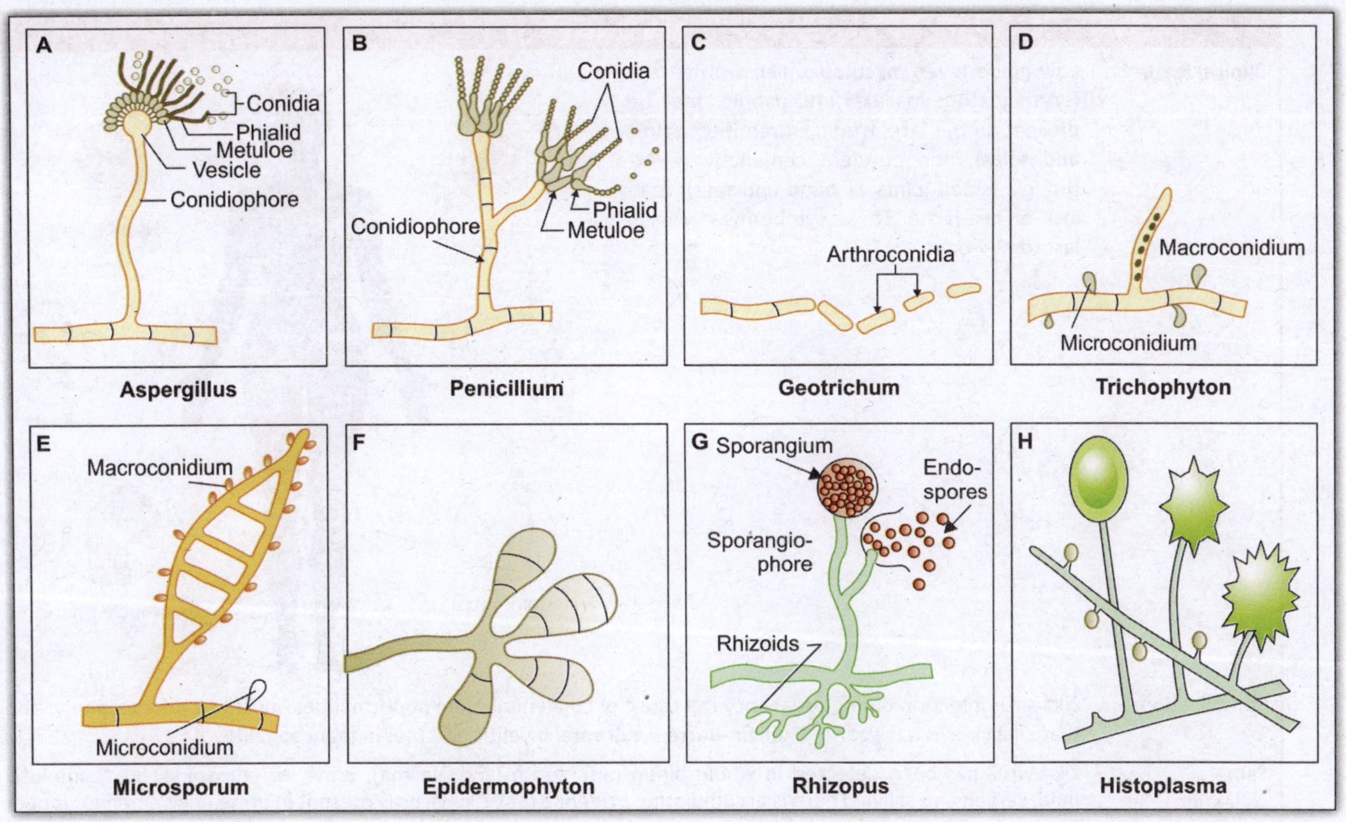

Fig: Legend—**A.** Aspergillus; **B.** Penicillium; **C.** Geotrichum; **D.** Trichophyton; **E.** Microsporum; **F.** Epidermophyton **G.** Rhizopus **H.** Histoplasma capsulatum

35. Ans. (c) Chlorinated compounds

Ref: Park 23rd ed page 129

Hypochlorites are the most widely used chlorine disinfectant, available as liquid (e.g. sodium hypochlorite) or solid (e.g. **calcium hypochlorite**). The most prevalent chlorine products are aqueous solutions of 5.25–6.15 percent of sodium hypochlorite, usually called household bleach. They have a broad spectrum of antimicrobial activity, do not leave toxic residues, are unaffected by water hardness, are inexpensive and fast acting, remove dried or fixed organisms and biofilms from surfaces

Work surfaces are to be decontaminated at least twice a day and after every spill of viable/infected material. Sodium hypochlorite available as 4% w/v solution is used as follows: Blood spillage is cleaned up using 1% hypochlorite solution. (Mix 1 part of ready made 4% w/v sodium hypochlorite solution with 3 parts of sterile water.) In general, a minimum concentration of 5,000 ppm (0.5%) hypochlorite is recommended to inactivate HIV present in a blood spill

AIIMS MAY 2017

36. Ans. (a) Petechial rash

Ref: Harrison 19th ed page 1314, http://www.who.int/mediacentre/factsheets/zika/en/, https://www.cdc.gov/zika/index.html

Rash of zika is maculopapular not petechial. Thrombocytopenia is reported only in few case reports and not common as in case of dengue.

Zika Virus	
Etiology	Zika virus is Ades mosquito-borne flavivirus
Transmission	Zika virus is primarily transmitted to people through the bite of an infected mosquito from the Aedes genus, mainly **Aedes aegypti** in tropical regions. ***Sexual transmission of Zika virus is also possible.*** Other modes of transmission such as blood transfusion are being investigated
Epidemiology	Zika virus was first identified in Uganda in 1947 in monkeys. It was later identified in humans in 1952 in Uganda and the United Republic of Tanzania. In July 2015 Brazil reported an association between Zika virus infection and Guillain-Barré syndrome. In October 2015 Brazil reported an association between Zika virus infection and microcephaly

Contd...

Zika Virus	
Clinical features	Low grade fever, maculopapular pruritic rash (erythematous macules and papules may be present on the face, trunk, extremities, palms and soles), non purulent conjunctivitis, Arthralgia (small joints of hand and feet), malaise or headache. These symptoms normally last for 2-7 days.
Complications	Zika virus infection during pregnancy is a cause of congenital brain abnormalities, including **microcephaly;** and that Zika virus is a trigger of **Guillain-Barré syndrome**, myelitis and meningoencephalitis
Sample collection	Zika virus has been detected in whole blood (also serum and plasma), urine, cerebrospinal fluid, amniotic fluid, semen and saliva. There is accumulating evidence that Zika virus is present in urine and semen for longer periods than in whole blood or saliva. **Specimens for nucleic acid testing (NAT) testing:** Whole blood, serum collected in a dry tube and/or urine collected from patients presenting with onset of symptoms ≤7 days **Serology (IgM detection):** Whole blood collected in a dry tube and serum collected from patients presenting with onset of symptoms ≥7 days

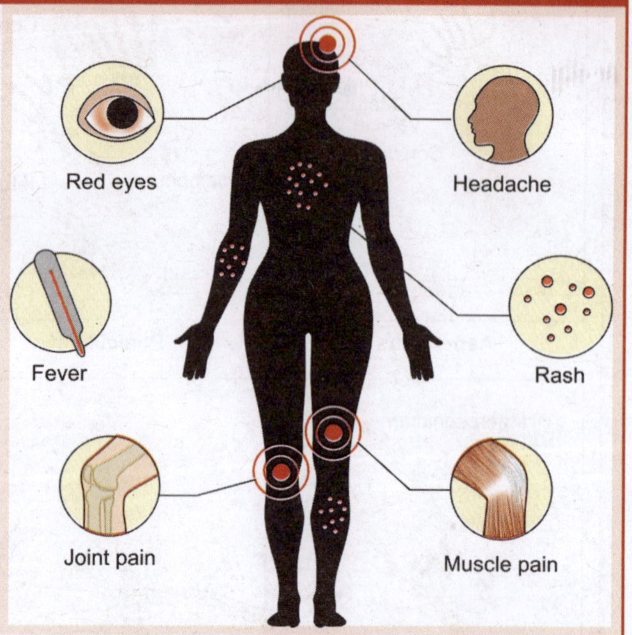

Algorithm of Diagnosis of Arbovirus Infection within 7 Days

Collect blood and urine
(keep a portion of blood as the first of a pair of serum samples)

↓

RT-PCRs for DENV, CHIK, ZIKV sequential or paralle testing

↓

Result for multiplex reactions	Interpretation
ZIKV pos, DENV neg, CHIK neg	ZIKV confirmed case
ZIKV neg, DENV neg, CHIK neg	DENV confirmed case
ZIKV neg, DENV neg, CHIK pos	CHIK confirmed case
ZIKV pos and/or DENV pos or CHIK pos	Co-detection and ZIKV confirmed case

Fig: A negative result for any PCR test does not conclusively rule out the infection

Zika Virus

Algorithm of Diagnosis of Arbovirus Infection after in 7 Days

Collect blood (serology and RT-PCR) and urine (RT-PCR where possible if more than one week after onset of symptoms (If collecting paired serum samples† allow 2–3 weeks between samples

- RT-PCR for ZIKV virus on urine and blood
  - Positive PCR: ZIKA confirmed case
  - Negative PCR: Zika virus infection not definitively ruled out → Test for IgM
- Test for IgM to DENV, CHIK and ZIKV, and other flaviviruses circulating where to exposure occurred

Result	Laboratory interpretation
ZIKV pos, DENV neg, CHIK neg	ZIKV probable case
ZIKV neg, DENV pos, CHIK neg	DENV probable case
ZIKV neg, DENV neg, CHIK pos	CHIK probable case
ZIKV pos, DENV neg, CHIK pos	ZIKV probable case + CHIK co-infection
ZIKV pos, DENV pos and/or CHIK pos	Probable flavivirus infection + CHIK co-infection

Final interpretation of result should be done in conjuction with clinical presentation

Other specimen types for RT PCR:
- Urine <30 days
- Semen <60 days

†For paired serum samples, a four-fold rise in IgM in the absence of a rise in antibody tites to other flaviviruses is further evidence of recent Zika virus infection

37. Ans. (d) Septic shock

Ref: Harrison 19th ed page 956, Prescott's 9th ed page 912

Staphylococcus aureus produces three types of toxin: cytotoxins, pyogenic toxin superantigens and exfoliative toxins.

Option (A) and (B)

The pyrogenic toxin superantigens are a family of small-molecular-size, structurally similar proteins that are responsible for two diseases: TSS and food poisoning. TSS results from the ability of enterotoxins and TSST -1 to function as T cell mitogens.

Option (C)

The exfoliative toxins are responsible for SSSS. The toxins that produce disease in humans are of two serotypes: ETA and ETB. These toxins are serine protease, which cleave desmosomal cadherins in the superficial layer of the skin, triggering exfoliation.

Option (D)

Septic shock/septicemia of *Staphylococcus* is not toxin mediated. Clinically, *S. aureus* sepsis presents in a manner similar to that documented for sepsis due to other bacteria.

38. Ans. (a) RT PCR

Ref: Anantnarayan 8th ed page 529

Repeat (See AIIMS Nov 2016 Microbiology for explanation) (see page no. 283)

39. Ans. (a) Klebsiella granulomatis

Ref: Jawetz 27th ed page 794

(See table of Sexually Transmitted Disease in Dermatology AIIMS May 2013) (see volume II)

Microscopy of STD's

Trick: in genital ulcer smear, Check if pathogen is intracellular or extracellular. If intracellular then check the lobes of the nucleus (Monocytes or Neutrophils)

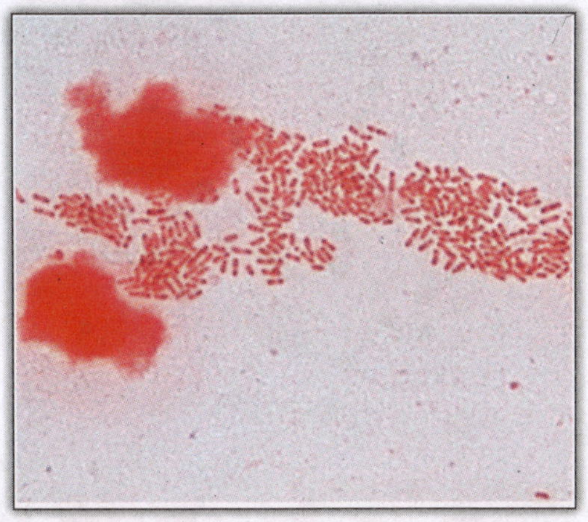

Fig: Haemophilus ducreyi on gram stain appearance of ulcer shows characteristic "Extracellular schools of fish" appearance. Haemophilus ducreyi causes chancroid **(soft chancre)**, a sexually transmitted disease. Chancroid consists of a ragged ulcer on the genitalia, with marked swelling and tenderness. The regional lymph nodes are enlarged and painful. The disease must be differentiated from syphilis, herpes simplex infection and lymphogranuloma venereum. **The small gram-negative rods** occur in strands in the lesions, usually in association with other pyogenic microorganisms. H ducreyi requires X factor but not V factor. It is grown best from scrapings of the ulcer base on chocolate agar containing 1% Iso Vitale X and vancomycin, 3 g/mL and incubated in 10% CO_2 at 33°C. There is no permanent immunity following chancroid infection. Treatment with intramuscular ceftriaxone, oral trimethoprim-sulfamethoxazole, or oral erythromycin often results in healing in 2 weeks

MNEMONIC = DUcreyi= Do You Cry= painful ulcer

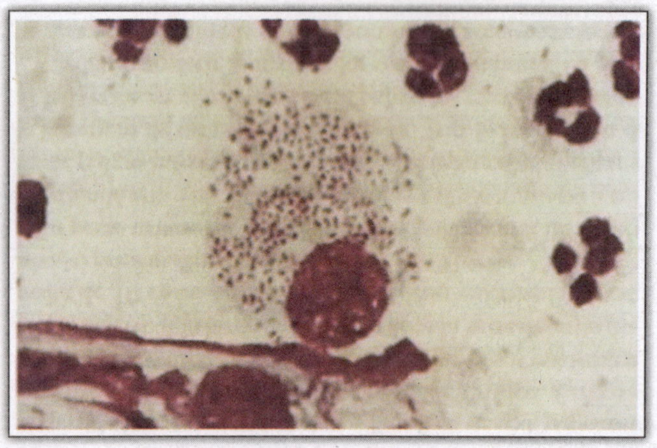

Fig: Donovanosis (granuloma inguinale) causes genital ulceration. The causative organism, Calymmatobacterium granulomatis reclassified as ***Klebsiella granulomatis. Donovan body*** (safety pin like inclusion bodies inside the monocyte

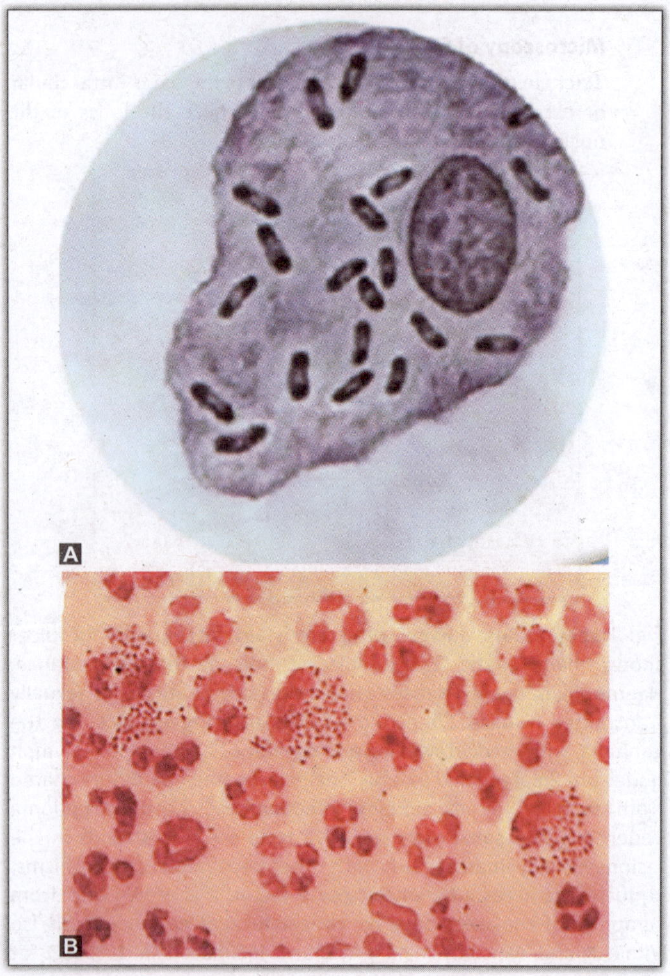

Fig: Neisseria is an intracellular Gram negative diplococci seen with polymorphonuclear leukocytes (see for multiple lobes of the nucleus) in urethral exudate

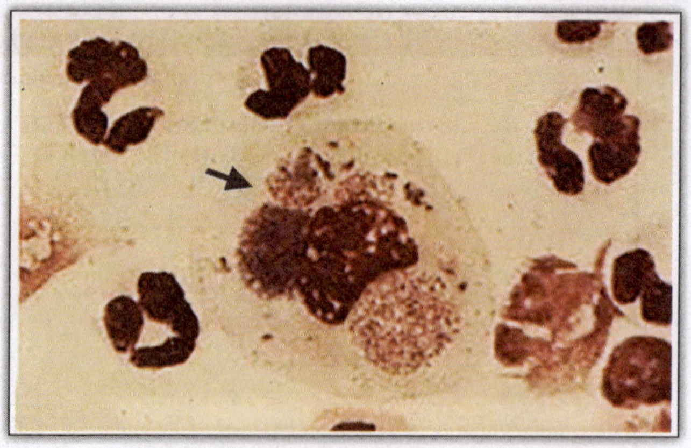

Fig: Chlamydia is gram-negative, obligate intracellular parasites. They must grow and reproduce within host cells. Intracytoplasmic Basophilic inclusion containing clamps of elementary bodies of Chlamydia -basophilic inclusions.

40. Ans. (b) 1Fc and 2 Fab

Ref: Jawetz 24th edition Chapter 44

Repeat AIPGMEE 2014, DNB December 2010

If an antibody molecule is treated with a proteolytic enzyme (e.g. Papain), peptide bonds in the hinge region are broken. This breakage produces two identical Fab fragments, which carry the antigen-binding sites and one Fc fragment, which is involved in placental transfer, complement fixation, attachment for various cells and other biologic activities.

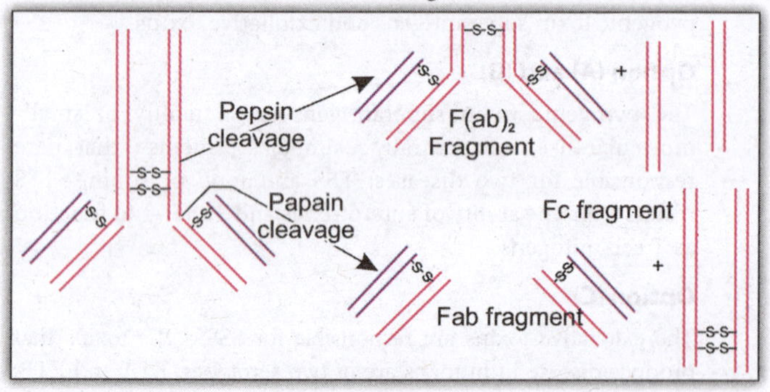

41. Ans. (c) Aquatic protistan protozoa

Ref: CDC, Dail and Hammar's Pulmonary Pathology: Non-neoplastic Lung Disease 3rd edition, page 404, Indian Journal of Medical Microbiology Year 2002 Volume 20 Issue 3 Page 119-131

"*R. seeberi* had first been regarded as a sporozoon by Malbran, its discoverer, in 1892, as a protozoan by Seeber who first published a description of the pathogen and then, as a phycomycete by Ashworth in 1923. Through molecular biological analysis of the organism's ribosomal DNA, Herr *et al.* classified the organism in a new clade which was named the ***Mesomycetozoa***, which includes fish and amphibian pathogens in the former ***DRIP clade (Dermocystidium, the rossette agent, Ichthyophonus and Psorospermium).*** It is of interest that the histopathology of these fish and amphibian diseases closely resembles that of rhinosporidiosis. In addition, morphological similarities were noted between *R. seeberi* and these pathogens. Indeed it was speculated by Herr *et al.* that some of these pathogens could be classified in the genus *Rhinosporidium* with the suggestion that *Rhinosporidium* is a monotypic genus. An independent group of workers supported this conclusion concerning taxonomy, in that their analysis of *R. seeberi* 18S rRNA from infected tissue showed that this organism is a protist "from a novel clade of parasites that infect fish and amphibians". These studies finally resolve the debate on the taxonomy of *R. seeberi*, particularly that it is not a classic fungus "but rather the first known human pathogen from the DRIPs clade, a novel clade of aquatic protistan parasites".

42. Ans. (b) E. histolytica

Ref: Paniker parasitology 6th ed page 24, Sternberg Pathology 5th ed page 1537

Entamoeba histolytica exists in three morphological forms Trophozoite, Precyst and Cyst. Tetranucleated cyst is the infective form and it divides into 8 uninucleated cysts as shown in the picture.

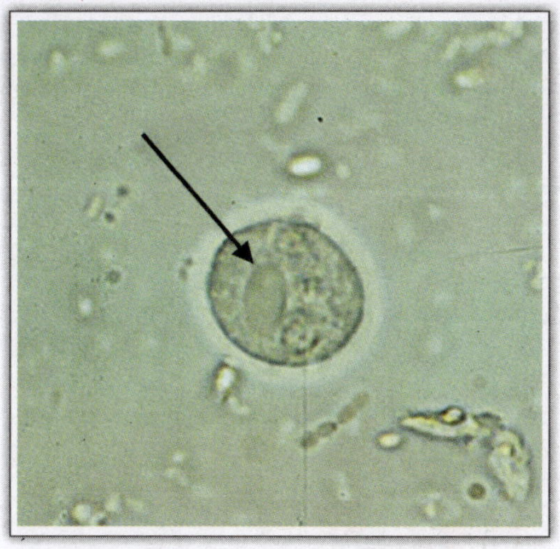

Fig: Cyst of E. histolytica/E. dispar in an unstained concentrated wet mount of stool. Notice the chromatoid bodies with blunt, rounded ends (arrow)

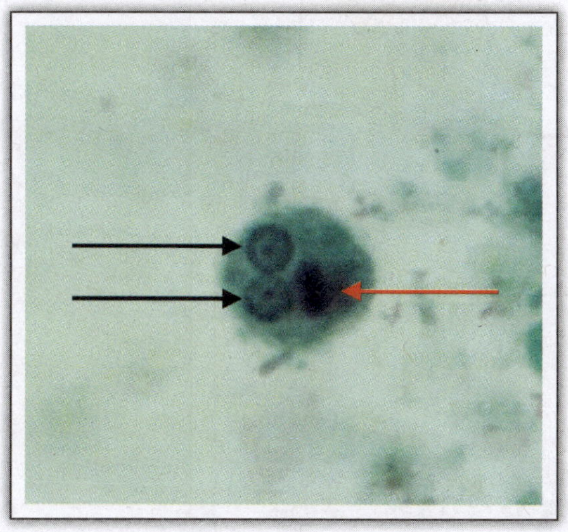

Fig: Cyst of E. histolytica/E. dispar stained with trichrome: Two nuclei are visible in the focal plane (black arrows) and the cyst contains a chromatoid body with typically blunted ends (red arrow)

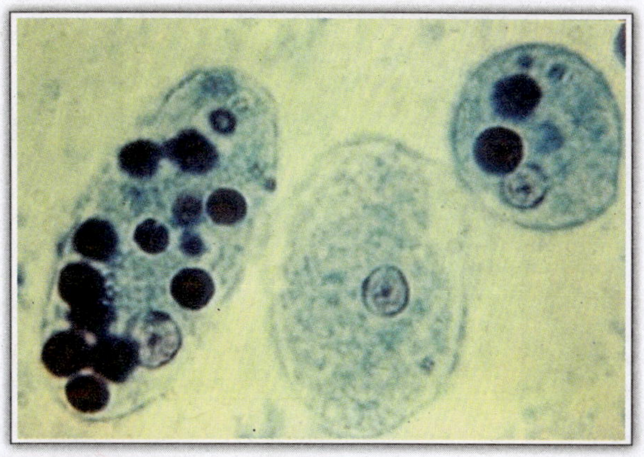

Fig: Trophozoites of E. histolytica with ingested erythrocytes stained with trichrome. The ingested erythrocytes appear as dark inclusions. The parasites above show nuclei that have the typical small, centrally located karyosome and thin, uniform peripheral chromatin

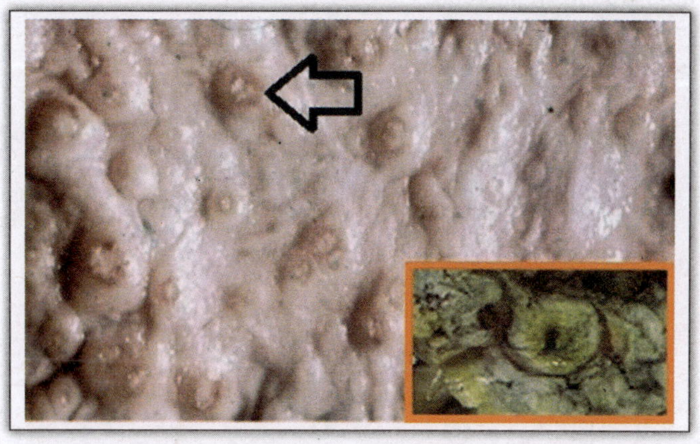

Fig: Gross intestinal specimen with Intestinal flask-shaped ulcers observed though rectosigmoidoscopy examination. Arrows indicate small colonic ulcers. Insat shows large flask shaped ulcer of later stages

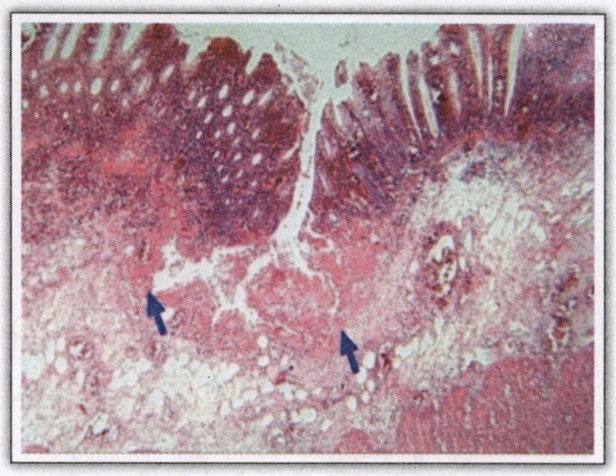

Fig: Colonic biopsy specimen in a patient with amoebiasis. A flask-shaped ulcer with a narrow opening and wide base (arrow) in the colon. Increased chronic inflammatory cells are seen within the lamina propria and an inflammatory exudate overlies the mucosa

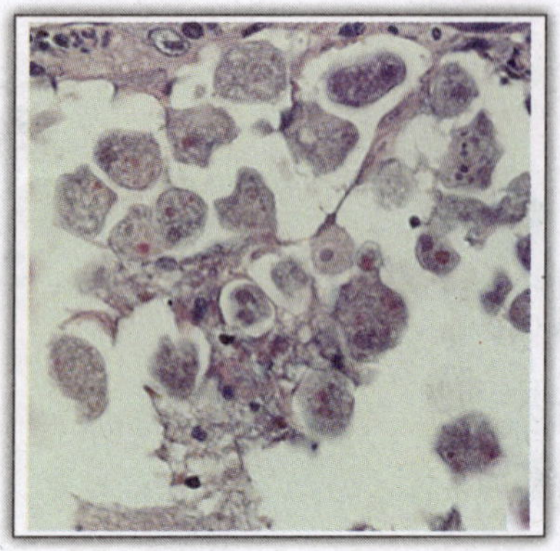

Source: CDC

Fig: Colonic biopsy High-magnification examination of the inflammatory exudate and ulcer base reveals typical trophozoites of Entamoeba histolytica. The sizes of trophozoites (arrow) are larger than those of macrophages. They have abundant amorphilic cytoplasm, small nuclei and erythrophagocytosis (phagocytosis of RBC) in some trophozoites

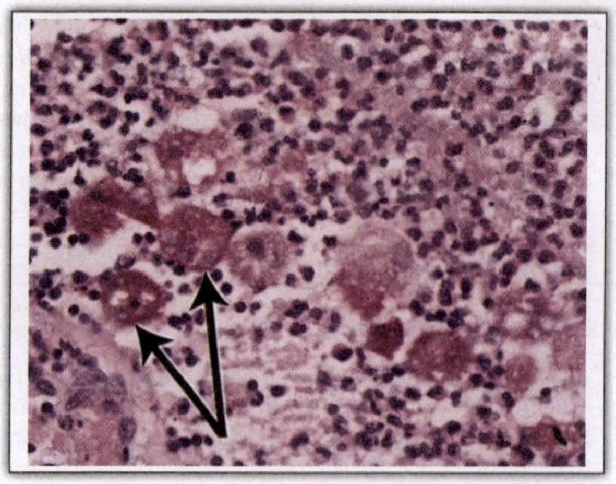

Fig: Liver biopsy: Biopsy obtained from the edge of amoebic liver abscess (HE and PAS stained, 20×). Notice the presence of trophozoites, hepatocytes and the large number of inflammatory cells

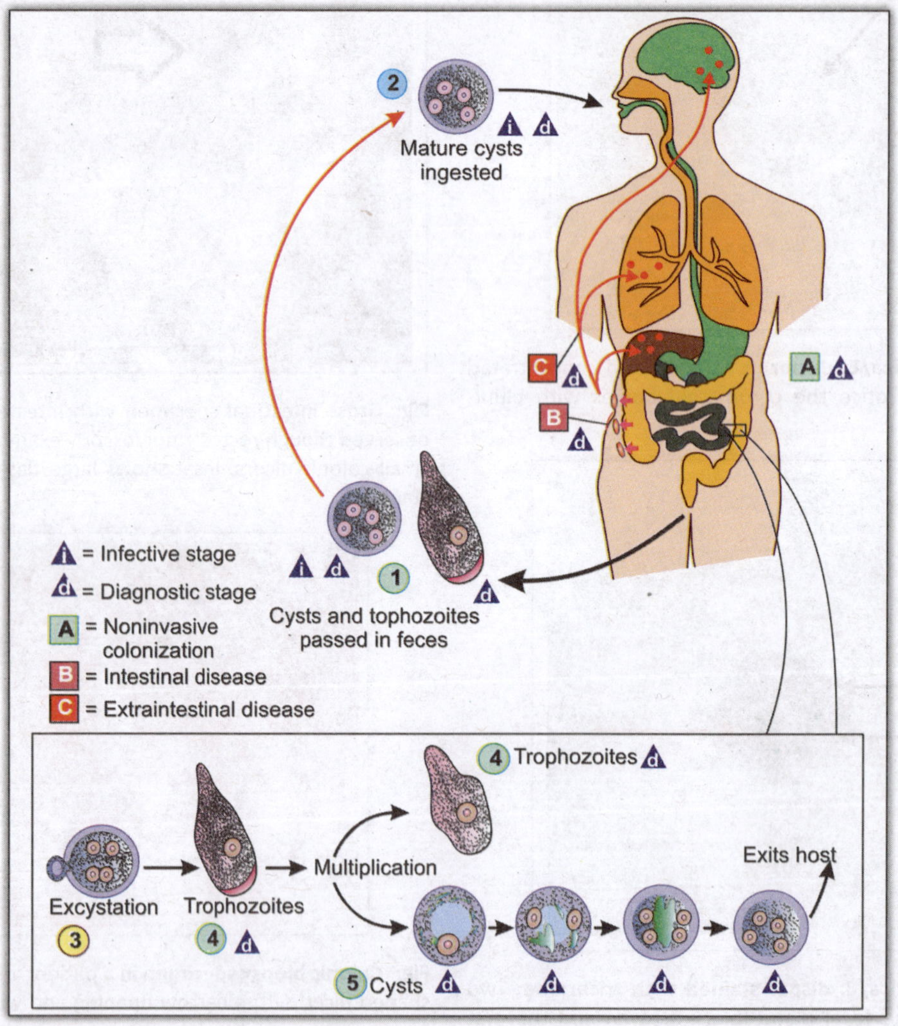

Source: CDC

FIG: Life cycle of E. Histolytica: Cysts and trophozoites are passed in feces **1**. Cysts are typically found in formed stool, whereas trophozoites are typically found in diarrheal stool. Infection by Entamoeba histolytica occurs by ingestion of mature cysts **2** in fecally contaminated food, water, or hands. **3** Excystation occurs in the small intestine and trophozoites **4** are released, which migrate to the large intestine.

The trophozoites multiply by binary fission and produce cysts **5** and both stages are passed in the feces **1**. Because of the protection conferred by their walls, the cysts can survive days to weeks in the external environment and are responsible for transmission. Trophozoites passed in the stool are rapidly destroyed once outside the body and if ingested would not survive exposure to the gastric environment. In many cases, the trophozoites remain confined to the intestinal lumen (**A**: noninvasive infection) of individuals who are asymptomatic carriers, passing cysts in their stool. In some patients the xtraintestinal sites such as the liver, brain and lungs (**C**: extraintestinal disease), with resultant pathologic manifestations. It has been established that the invasive and noninvasive forms represent two separate species, respectively E. histolytica and E. dispar. These two species are morphologically indistinguishable unless E. histolytica is observed with ingested red blood cells (erythrophagocystosis). Transmission can also occur through exposure to fecal mtrophozoites invade the intestinal mucosa (**B**: intestinal disease), or, through the bloodstream, eatter during sexual contact (in which case not only cysts, but also trophozoites could prove infective).

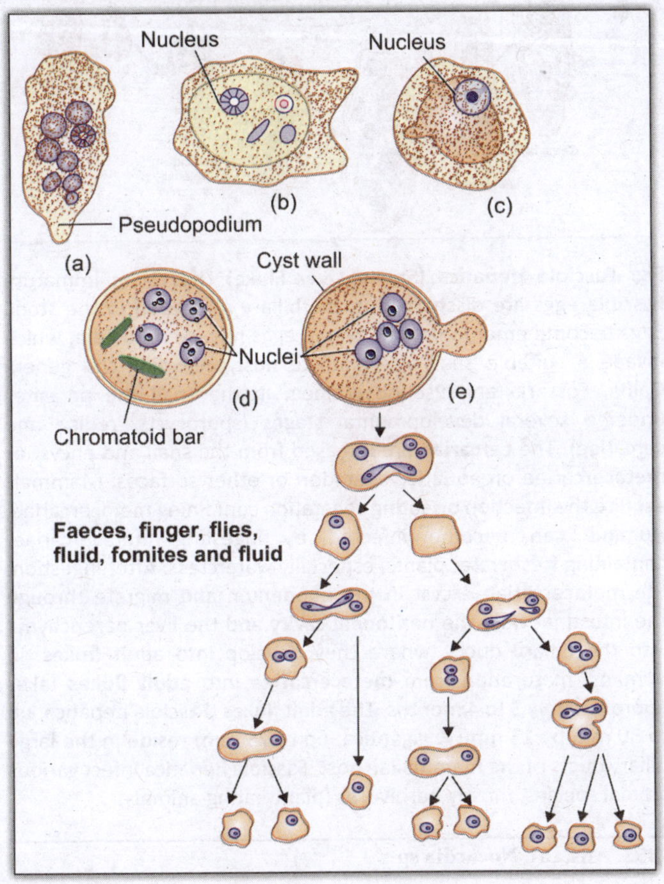

Fig Stages of Life cycle of E. Histolytica: a. Living trophozoite, b. Stained trophozoite, c. Precystic stage, d. Cystic stage: At the tetranucleate stage the cyst is infective to a new host. One tertanucleated cyst transforms to 8 uninucleated cyst, e. Encystment: The excystment is the process by which the cysts are transformed into the trophozoites.

43. Ans. (d) Necator americanus

Ref: Parasitology: A Conceptual Approach by Eric Loker, Bruce Hofkin- Page 48, CDC

Recall Bias

Two hookworms Nectar americanus and Ancylostoma duodenale eggs are similar and can not be differentiate. Ascaris Lumbricoides was the option not Ancylostoma duodenale. Hence the answer will be Necator Americanus

NOTE

Necator Americanus egg is non Bile stained. But the picture in the exam was yellowish due to iodine mount (in iodine wet mounts, both bile-stained and nonbile-stained helminthic ova are stained brown) and hence many students got confused and marked other options.

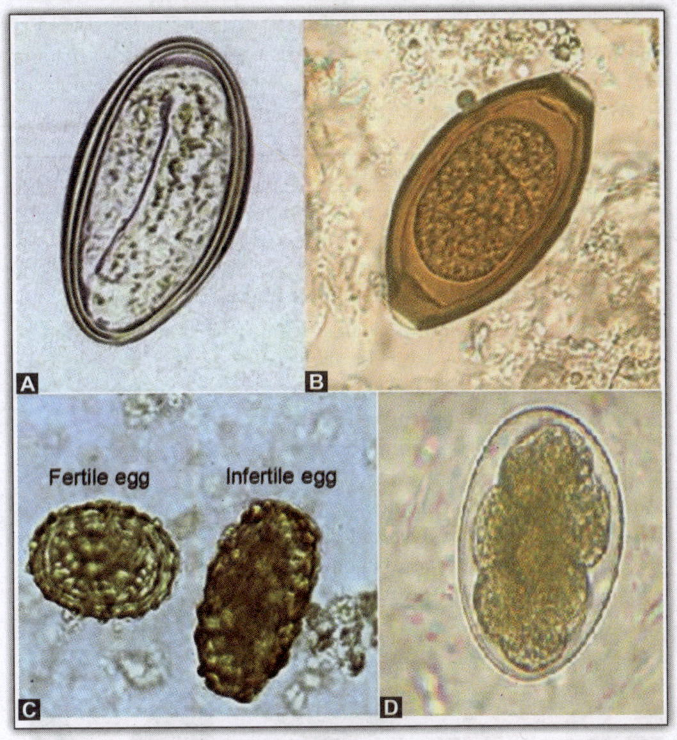

Figs A to D: Nematodes egg

A. **Enterobius vermicularis egg:** Elongate-oval and slightly flattened on one side. They are usually partially-embryonated when shed. Enterobiasis can be diagnosed by applying cellulose tape to the anus of a suspect patient, especially in the morning before the patient's first bowel movement. Eggs will adhere to the tape and can be seen microscopically.
B. **Trichuris trichiura egg (unstained wet mount):** Elongated barrel shaped with distinctive bipolar plugs, smooth outer shells. The eggs are unembryonated when passed in stool
C. **Ascaris lumbricoides egg:** Both fertilized and unfertilized Ascaris lumbricoides eggs are passed in the stool of the infected host.
   - **Fertilized eggs** are are rounded and have a thick shell with an external mammillated layer that is often stained brown by bile. Fertile eggs range from 45 to 75 µm in length.

- **Unfertilized eggs** are elongated and larger than fertile eggs (up to 90 μm in length). Their shell is thinner and their mammillated layer is more variable, either with large protuberances or practically none. Unfertile eggs contain mainly a mass of refractile granules.

D. **Ancylostoma duodenale or Necator americanus egg. (Circles represent RBC):** The eggs of Ancylostoma and Necator cannot be differentiated microscopically. The eggs are thin-shelled, colorless and measure 60-75 μm by 35-40 μm.

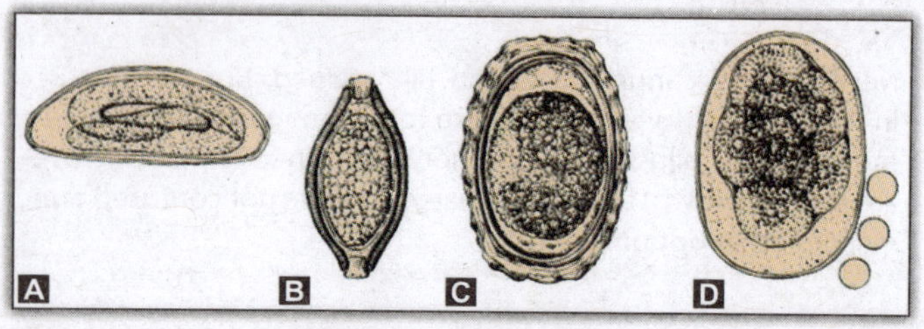

Figs A to D: A. Enterobius vermicularis egg; B. Trichuris trichiura egg; **C.** Ascaris lumbricoides egg; **D.** Ancylostoma duodenale or Necator americanus egg. (Circles represent RBC)

44. Ans. (b) Fasciola hepatica

Ref: BRS Microbiology and Immunology 4th ed page 208, Textbook of Parasitology by Chatterjee Page 187.

Fasciola Hepatica (Sheep Liver Fluke)

Disease: Fascioliasis is a parasitic infection typically caused by Fasciola hepatica, which is also known as "the common liver fluke" or "the sheep liver fluke."

Reservoir host: Sheep, cattle, humans

Mode of transmission: Ingestion of contaminated aquatic plants (watercress)

Progression in Humans: Cysts germinate in duodenum, exit through wall into liver and proceed to bile ducts, where they mature; eggs enter feces in bile

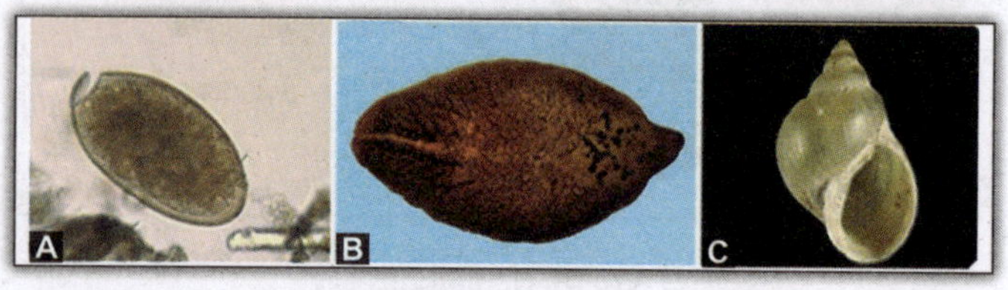

Credit: CDC

Figs A to C: Fasciola hepatica (Sheep liver fluke): A. Fasciola hepatica egg in an unstained wet mount (400 x magnification). F. Hepatica eggs are broadly ellipsoidal, operculated on one end and measure 130–150 μm by 60–90 μm; **B.** Adult Fasciola hepatica fluke stained with carmine (30 mm by 13 mm); **C.** Fossaria bulamoides, a snail host for F. hepatica

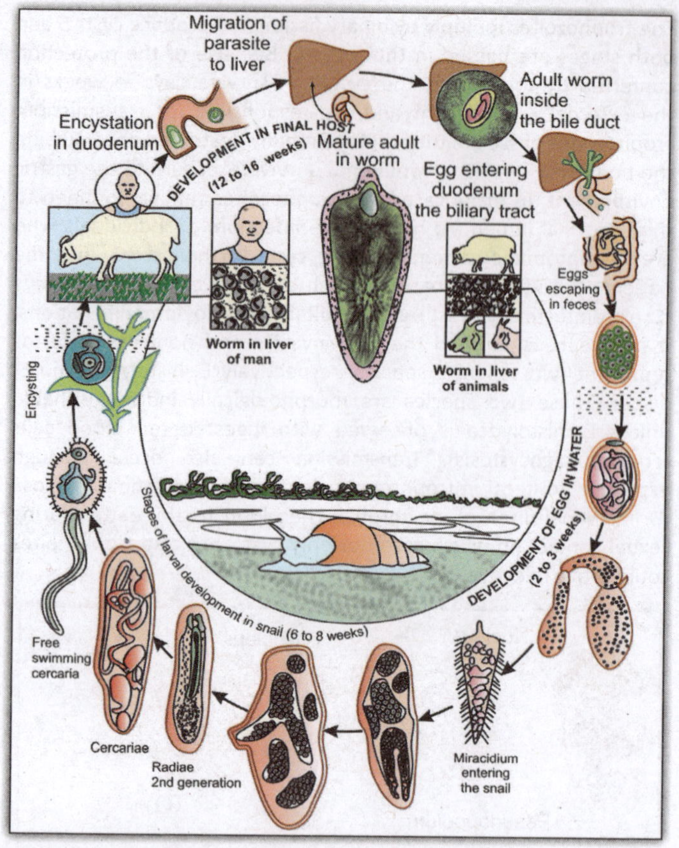

Fig: Fasciola Hepatica (Sheep Liver Fluke) Life cycle: Immature Fasciola eggs are discharged in the biliary ducts and in the stool. Eggs become embryonated in water, eggs release **miracidia,** which invade a suitable snail intermediate host, including the genera Galba, Fossaria and Pseudosuccinea. In the snail the parasites undergo several developmental stages (sporocysts, rediae and cercariae). The **cercariae** are released from the snail and encyst as **metacercariae** on aquatic vegetation or other surfaces. Mammals acquire the infection by eating vegetation containing metacercariae. Humans can become infected by ingesting metacercariae-containing freshwater plants, especially watercress. After ingestion, the metacercariae excyst in the duodenum and migrate through the intestinal wall, the peritoneal cavity and the liver parenchyma into the biliary ducts, where they develop into adult **flukes**. In humans, maturation from **metacercariae** into **adult flukes** takes approximately 3 to 4 months. The adult flukes (Fasciola hepatica: up to 30 mm by 13 mm; F. gigantica: up to 75 mm) reside in the large biliary ducts of the mammalian host. Fasciola hepatica infect various animal species, mostly herbivores (plant-eating animals).

45. Ans. (a) Nocardia sp

Ref: Jawetz 24th ed chapter 15, BRS Microbiology 4th ed page 39-41

Indirect repeat Microbiology AIIMS Nov 2016 (Different options, plus stain was also asked).

Nocardia

These bacteria are gram-positive, catalase-positive and partially acid-fast bacilli. Nocardiae form extensive branching substrates and aerial filaments that fragment after formation, breaking into coccobacillary cells. The cell walls contain mycolic acids that are shorter chained than those of Mycobacteria. They are considered to be weakly acid-fast, but if they are stained with the routine acid-fast reagent (carbol-fuchsin) but decolorized with 1–4% sulfuric acid instead of the stronger acid-alcohol decolorant, most isolates will stain acid-fast. Gram-stained smears reveal gram-positive bacilli, coccobacillary cells and branching filaments. With the modified acid-fast stain, most isolates will be acid-fast.

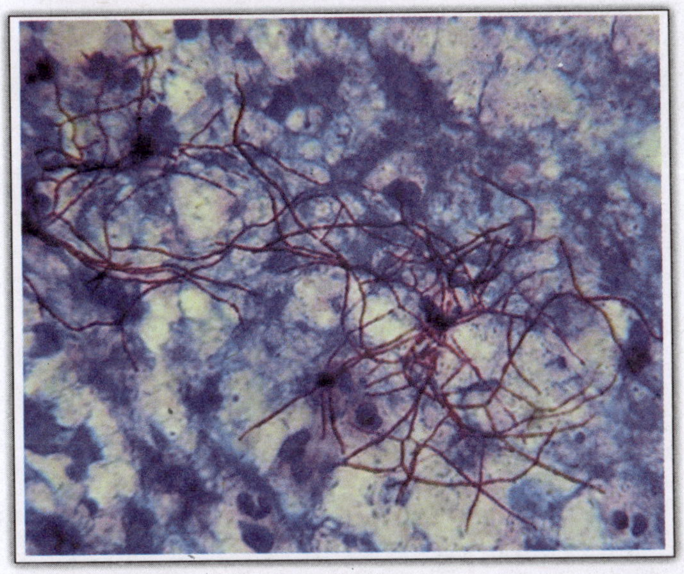

Fig: Nocardia, partially acid fast staining: (Pink in blue background). Partial Acid-Fast staining employed: Carbol fuscin stain (3 min), decolourize with 1% H2SO4 (until colour no longer comes off ~1 min) and counterstain with methyene blue (30 sec).

46. Ans. (c) Cryptococcus

Ref: Toxicology of 1 - 3-Beta-Glucans: Glucans as a Marker for Fungal Exposure edited by Shih-Houng Young, Vincent Castranova page 203, 204, J. Clin. Microbiol. July 2014 vol. 52 no. 7 2328-2333

Indirect repeat AIIMS NOV 2017 Microbiology (See for details of 1- 3 β D glucan)

47. Ans. (a) Heterophile antibody test

Ref: Ananthanarayan 9th ed 96-97, Textbook of Microbiology & Immunology By Subhash Chandra Parija 2nd ed page 483, Dorland's Medical Dictionary 32nd ed page 1896

Patient with primary EBV infection develops IgM antibodies that binds on antigen on RBC of other species particularly sheep and horse but not guinea pig kidney cells. Heterophile antibodies also occur in normal sera but these also binds to Guinea pig kidney cells. This forms the basis of Heterophile antibody test.

Paul–Bunnell test: Originally called as Heterophile Antibody test was first described by Paul and Bunnell for demonstration of heterophile antibodies in patients with infectious mononucleosis in 1932. It determined the highest dilution of the patient's serum that was capable of agglutinating sheep red blood cells by Hemagglutination. The Paul-Bunnell test is a useful test to screen for the presence of heterophile antibodies because it is simple and inexpensive.

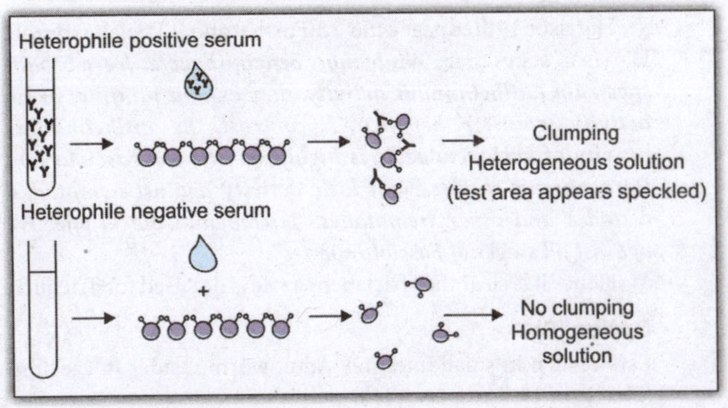

Paul-Bunnell-Davidsohn test AKA Davidson Differential Absorption Test

A type of heterophile antibody test for infectious mononucleosis, a modification of the Paul-Bunnell test that differentiates among three types of heterophile sheep erythrocyte agglutinins: those associated with infectious mononucleosis, those associated with serum sickness and natural antibodies against Forssman antigen. The patient's serum is absorbed with guinea pig kidney cells or with beef erythrocytes and centrifuged. Unabsorbed serum has an abnormally high heterophile antibody titer in infectious mononucleosis and serum sickness. Absorption with guinea pig kidney removes Forssman antibodies and serum sickness heterophile antibodies. Absorption with beef erythrocytes removes heterophile antibodies associated with infectious mononucleosis and serum sickness.

Note

Monospot test is a form of the heterophile antibody test which is used for the rapid screening of infectious mononucleosis

AIIMS NOVEMBER 2016

48. Ans. (d) Eggs laid are infective in 10 days

Ref: With text

The image is of Trichuris trichura

Recall Bias

Various versions of options were provided to us. We have sorted them on most commonly recalled options basis.

Option (A)

Ref: Medical Microbiology By Patrick R. Murray, Ken S. Rosenthal, Michael A. Pfaller 8th ed page 712; Benzimidazole is a broad spectrum anti helminthic agent that includes Mebendazole, Albendazole, Thiabendazole and Triclabendazole. Basic structure to all these agents are common; that is linked Benzene and Imidazole rings.

Ref: Jawetz 24th ed Table 46–4, Harrison 19th ed page 1416:

Triclabendazole is DOC for Fasciola hepatica. DOC for Trichuris is Albendazole 400 mg/day 1-3 days or Mebendazole 500 mg/day × 3 days or 100 mg BD × 3 days (Repeat in 2-3 weeks if necessary)

Harrison 19th ed page 246e-13; Further about Triclabendazole Harrison states that ***"While most benzimidazoles have broad-spectrum antihelminthic activity, they exhibit minimal or no activity against F. hepatica. In contrast, the antihelminthic ativity of triclabendazole is highly specific for Fasciola and Paragonimus species, with little activity against nematodes, cestodes and other trematodes. Triclabendazole is effective against all stages of Fasciola species"***

Hence it is clear that Triclabendazole is not used for Trichuris

Option (B)

Larva hatch in small intestine. Adult worm resides in caecum. (Harrison 19th ed page 1414)

Option (C)

Adult worm grows up to 3–5 cm (Harrison 19th ed page 1414)

Option (D)

Conventionally most microbiology textbooks gives 10 days. One such text is quoted here

Microbiology: A Clinical Approach-By Anthony Strelkauskas, Jennifer Strelkauskas, Danielle Moszyk-Strelkauskas Page 538; "Trichuris eggs are passed out of the body through the faeces and deposited in the soil. At this stage, the eggs are immature and not infective and they must incubate in the soil for 10 days before they embryonate and become infectious.

But CDC says it takes 15 to 30 days for the egg to mature and become infective. The confusion is cleared by the following reference.

Ref: Conns current therapy 2009: Medicine By CTI Reviews; *"Unembryonated egg passes to soil through feces of the previous host In the soil these eggs develop into segmented eggs (2 celled) and then into advanced cleavage stage. Once at this stage the eggs becomes embryonated (mature) and become infective. Immature eggs in soil takes 3 weeks to mature (Range = 15-30 days to mature, with minimum 10 days to mature)*

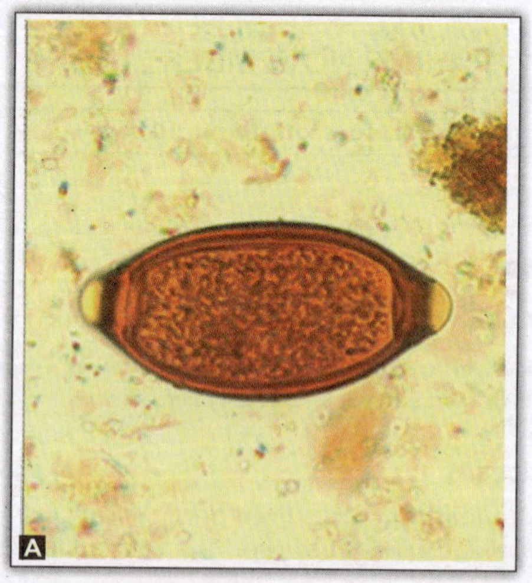

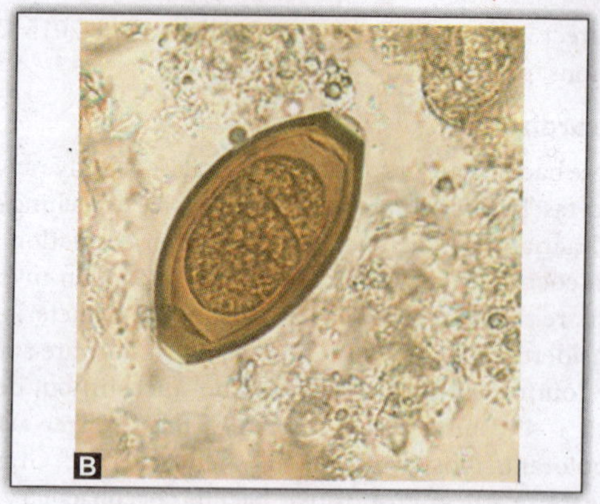

Figs A and B: A. Egg of Trichuris trichiura in an iodine-stained wet mount of stool. Elongated barrel shaped with distinctive bipolar plugs, smooth outer shells; **B.** Egg of T. trichiura in an unstained wet mount of stool

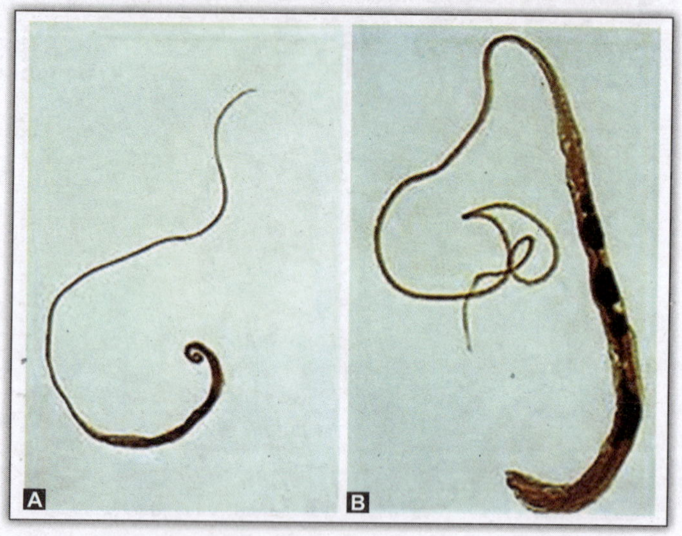

Figs A and B: A. Adult male trichuris (whipworm): 4 cm long, characteristic whiplike shape, posterior end is coiled with one protruding spicule; **B. Adult female trichuris:** 5 cm long, posterior end is not coiled, straight and blunt

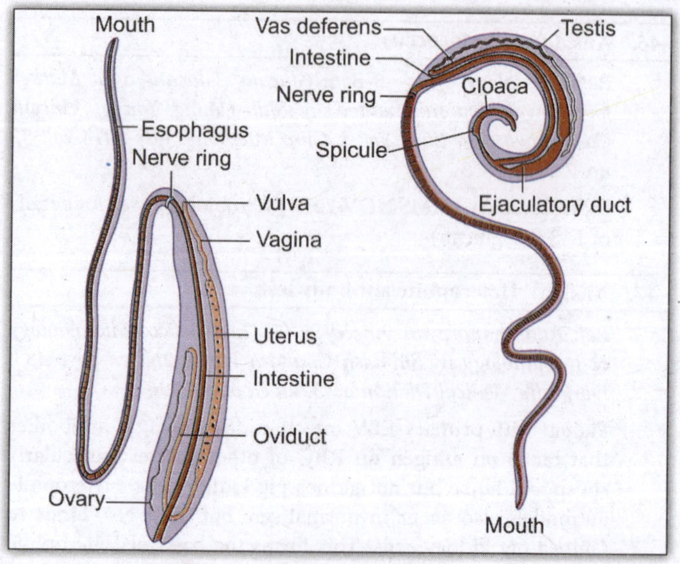

Fig: Adult Trichuris trichura male and female (Illustration)

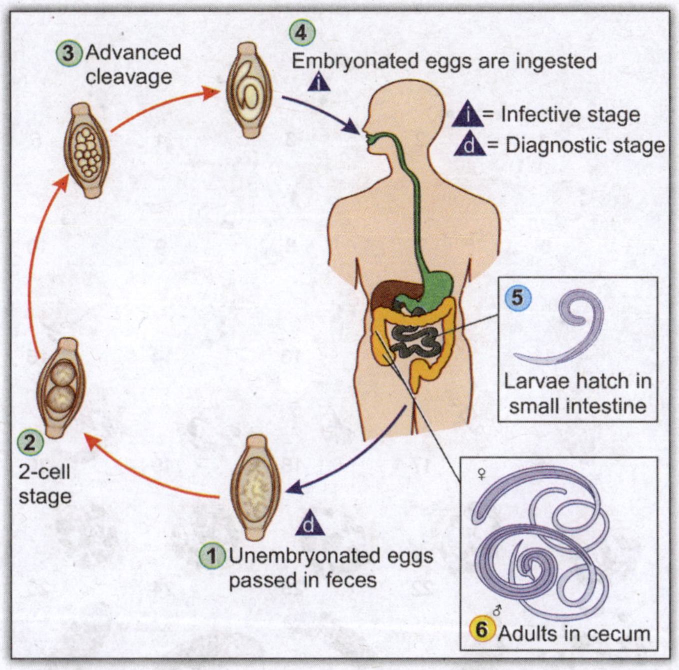

Fig: Life cycle of Trichuris trichura: (With permission from CDC) The unembryonated eggs are passed with the stool **1**. In the soil, the eggs develop into a 2-cell stage **2**, an advanced cleavage stage **3** and then they embryonate **4**; eggs become infective in 15 to 30 days (minimum 10 days). After ingestion (soil-contaminated hands or food), the eggs hatch in the small intestine and release larvae **5** that mature and establish themselves as adults in the colon **6**. The adult worms (approximately 4 cm in length) live in the cecum and ascending colon. The adult worms are fixed in that location, with the anterior portions threaded into the mucosa. The females begin to oviposit 60 to 70 days after infection. Female worms in the cecum shed between 3,000 and 20,000 eggs per day. The life span of the adults is about 1 year

49. Ans. (b) Pneumonitis

Ref: With text

Recall Bias

Many variants of recalls are were provided to us for this question. Some say that the common feature of the three helminths was asked. In that case except Liver failure all three are common to the three Helminths (Ancyclostoma, Strongyloides and Ascaris), hence its less likely to be asked in that format.

Larval ascariasis must be distinguished from toxocariasis, hookworm, Strongyloides stercomlis, schistosomiasis and TPE. **Ref: Manson's Tropical Diseases - Page 1522**

Option (A)

Eosinophilia is not a symptom

Ref: Community-Acquired Pneumonia -edited by Thomas J. Marrie Page 889

Migratory pulmonary infiltrates of varying sizes that are associated with eosinophilia are characteristic of the larval phase of ascariasis, hookworm and strongyloidiasis, tropical pulmonary eosinophilia caused by W. bancrofti or B. malayi, or Paragonimiasis

Ascaris, hookworm and Strongyloides are the most common causes of this syndrome among the intestinal helminths

Option (B)

Loeffler's syndrome—Nematode Pneumonitis: The phase of larval migration is a distinctive type of pneumonitis known as Loeffler's syndrome (simple pulmonary eosinophilia) characterised by mild group of symptoms, a scarcity of physical signs, a blood eosinophilia varying from less than 10% to 60% and transient pulmonary infiltration.

Loeffler syndrome has been more correctly termed pulmonary infiltrates with eosinophilia syndrome (Nelson 20th ed page 2079)

Ref: Nelson's 20th Ed page 1734

The most common symptoms due to these helminthes in patients with hookworms are due to pulmonary disease and obstruction of intestinal or biliary tract. LARVA migrating through these tissues cause allergic symptoms such as fever, cough, dyspnea, pulmonary infiltrates, dysnea. Vague abdominal pain may be seen. Ascaris worms may infiltrate biliary tract and block it. These worms may also infiltrate gut wall and may cause peritonitis.

Option (D)

Sometimes Larvae lose their way and wander around aimlessly in human body. This condition is known as Larva Migrans (Cutaneous and Visceral). The most common causative agent of Visceral Larva Migrans is Toxocara canis. Ferri's Clinical Advisor 2017 by Fred F. Ferri page 607

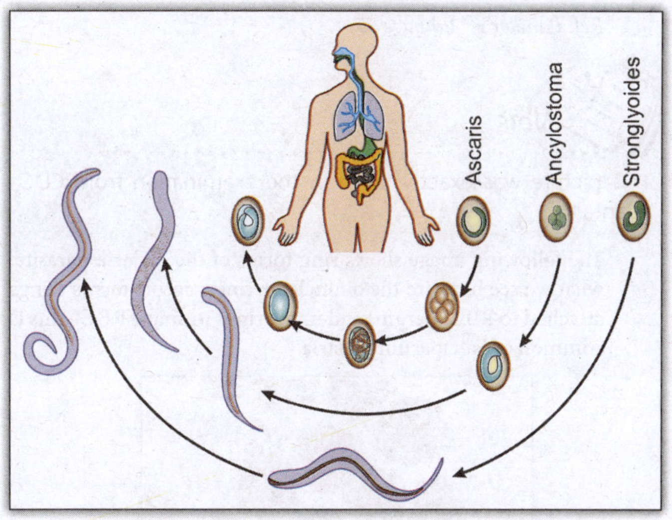

Life cycle of intestinal nematodes with a migratory phase through the langs. Eggs are passed in stool in Ascaris lumbricoides, Nectar americanus or Ancyclostoma duodenale or they hatch on their way out in Strongyloides. Ascaris eggs mature in soil and humans are infected upon ingestion of these eggs. With Hookworm and Strongyloides, humans are infected via skin penetration by Filariform Larva. *In all three infections, larvae pass through a migratory phase via the lungs before reaching maturity at their final habitat in the small intestine*

50. Ans. (b) Adherence to capillary endothelium

Ref: Paniker 6th ed page 80

In P. falciparum, stages of the asexual cycle; late trophozoite, early and mature schizonts are not ordinarily seen in peripheral blood, except in very severe or pernicious malaria.

The presence of P.falciparum schizonts in peripheral smears indicates a grave prognosis. The trophozoites usually disappear from peripheral circulation after about 24 hours. By then, a strain-specific high molecular weight antigen appears on the surface of the infected red cells, associated with knob-like projections on the erythrocyte membrane.

Such red cells disappear from peripheral circulation and adhere to the walls of venules and capillaries in internal organs—brain, heart, kidney, lungs, spleen, intestine, bone marrow, placenta. This cytoadherence causes sequestration of infected red cells in, these sites and is responsible for many of the serious complications of falciparum malaria, such as cerebral malaria.

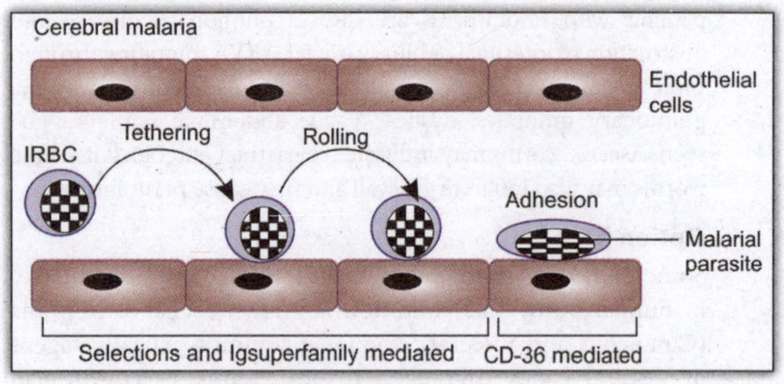

51. Ans. (b) Plasmodium falciparum

Ref: Paniker 6th Ed page 75

NOTE

This picture was exactly taken in the examination from CDC atlanta

The following image shows ring forms of the malaria parasite. what we see here are the bi nucleate rings, accole forms (rings attached to RBC margin) and many rings in single RBC. This is common of Falciparum malaria

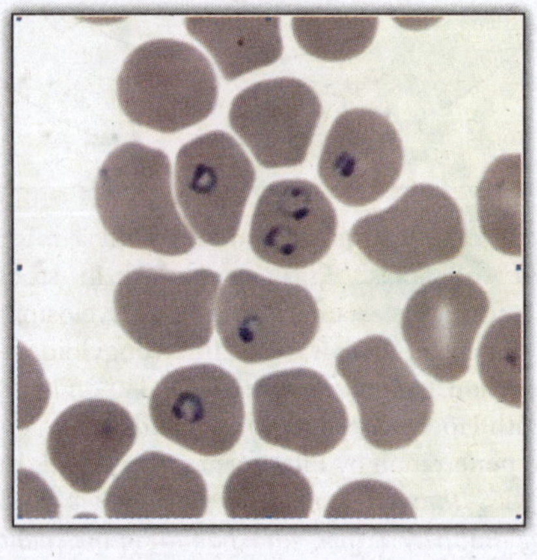

Source: CDC

Fig: Trophozoites ring stage of plasmodium falciparum

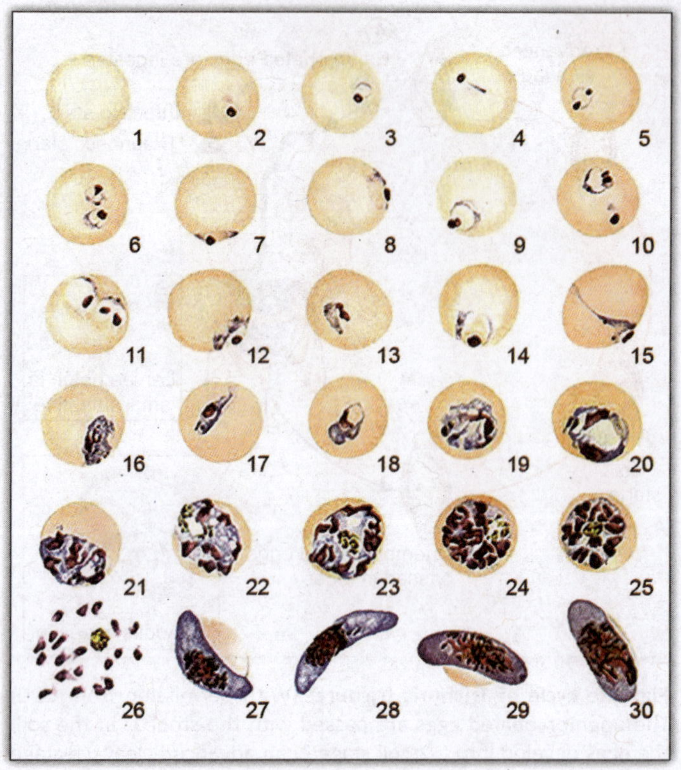

Fig: Plasmodium Falciparum: Blood Stage Parasites: Thin Blood Smears (Total 30)

Keys: 1. Normal red cell; **2–18.** Trophozoites (among these, Figs. 2-10 correspond to ring-stage trophozoite); **19–26.** Schizonts (Fig. 26 is a ruptured schizont); **27–28.** Mature macrogametocytes (female); Banana shaped; **29–30.** Mature microgametocytes (male); Banana shaped

52. Ans. (b) Neisseria gonorrhoeae

Ref: Anantnarayan 8th Ed page 224

NOTE

We have included the Insat for your better understanding. It was not provided in the exam.

First step: The organism is a gram negative organism. Therefore staphylococcus and streptococcus are ruled out. They are gram positive cocci.

Second step: The organism in question is a coccus. Niesseria species are gram negative diplococci. Hemophiluus species are gram negative coccobacillus or they have long bacillary forms. The organism in question is a diplococcus, most likely to be Neisseria Gonnorhea

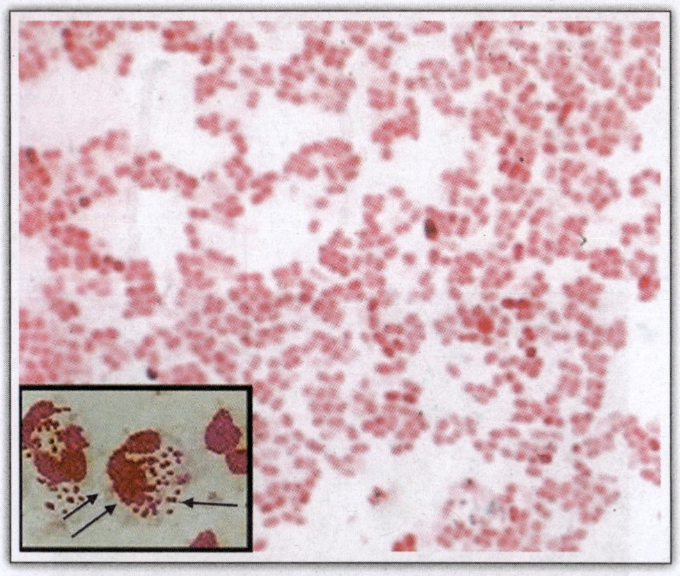

Fig: Gram negative cocci (Diplococci), insat shows intracellular Gram negative diplococci and polymorphonuclear leukocytes in urethral exudate; **Neisseria sp., Moraxella catarrhalis, Acinetobacter and Brucella**

53. Ans. (c) Proteus mirabilis

Ref: Anantnarayan 8th ed page 280

Swarming of Proteus on Blood agar: Proteus species move very actively by means of peritrichous flagella, resulting in "swarming" on solid media unless the swarming is inhibited by chemicals, such asphenylethyl alcohol or CLED (cystine lactose electrolyte deficient) medium. Swarming does not occur on MacConkey agar on which smooth , colorless colonies are formed.

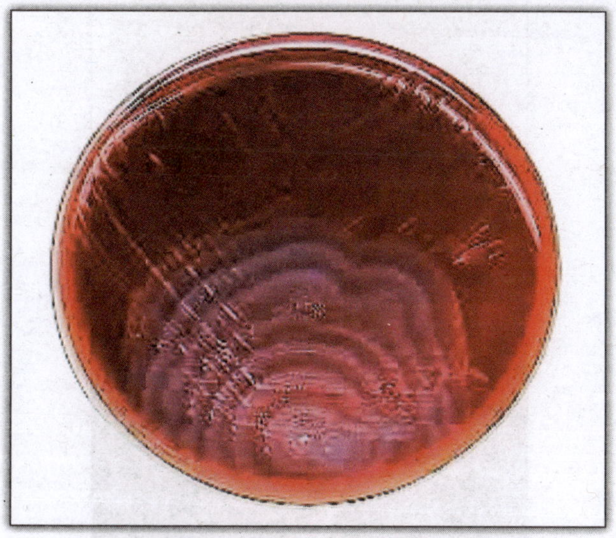

54. Ans. (a) RT PCR

Ref: Anantnarayan 8th ed page 529

Traditionally, rabies diagnosis is made by demonstration of rabies viral antigen by direct immunofluorescence (DIF) and mouse inoculation test (MIT). As per a ICMR funded project/ Study conducted by PGI chandigarh " 100 per cent sensitivity and specificity of RT-PCR as compared to 83.3 per cent of DIF and 66.7 per cent of Sellers stain for diagnosis of rabies. RTPCR also detected rabies viral infection earlier as compared to conventional tests and can also be used on ante-mortem samples" ***(Ref: Indian J Med Res 135, June 2012, pp 837-842)***

Harrison 19th ed page 1302: Once rabies is suspected, rabies-specific laboratory tests should be performed to confirm the diagnosis. Diagnostically useful specimens include serum, CSF, fresh saliva, skin biopsy samples from the neck and brain tissue (rarely obtained before death). Corneal impression smears are of low diagnostic yield and are generally not performed.

Harrison 19th ed page 896: Diagnosis can be made by finding rabies Virus antigen in brain tissue or in the neural innervation of hair follicles at the nape of the neck. PCR amplification of viral nucleic acid from CSF and saliva or tears may also enable diagnosis. Serology is frequently negative in both serum and CSF in the first week after onset of infection, which limits its acute diagnostic utility.

Postmortem Diagnosis of Rabies

- **Direct Immunofluorsce (DIF):** For post mortem diagnosis, the gold-standard diagnostic technique is to detect rabies virus antigen in infected tissues, preferably brain smears or touch impressions collected from a biopsy, by fluorescent antibody test (FAT). FAT is recommended by WHO and in 95–99% of cases, gives reliable results on fresh specimens within a few hours. FAT is direct immunofluorscence and relies on detection of antigens of rabies by antiserum. it uses specific monoclonal antibodies tagged with a dye.
- **Demonstration of Negri bodies:** Negri bodies are intracytoplasmic round oval purplish pink structures composed of fine fibrillar viral particles. They are demonstrated by histopathology from brain tissue especially hippocampus and cerebellum by ***Seller's technique***. The stain consists of methylene blue alcohol fixative and basic fuschin as staining agent.
- **Culture:** although culture of virus is ***most definitive*** way of detection of Rabies, but it is limited by high expertise required to perform the test. Virus can be cultured either directly into tissue culture cell lines (WI38, BHK21, CER) or direct intracerebral inoculation into mice. Though MIT has a sensitivity of more than 98.3 per cent and specificity of 100 per cent it is laborious, takes 2 to 3 week time and requires many experimental mice.
- **RT PCR:** It is a highly sensitive and specific test to detect rabies antigen.
- Serology of CSF

Coming to the options

Option (A)

RT PCR: In this question, it is the answer, because it has high specificity and sensitivity and relatively easier to perform and most importantly the sample is Corneal scraping which needs amplification.

Option (B)

Seller stain for negri bodies: Negri bodies are only demonstrated on neural tissue such as brain and not from corneal scrapings, skin and saliva

Option (C)

Indirect immunofluorescence: Direct immunofluorescence is used in diagnosis of rabies. Not indirect immunofluorescence

Option (D)

Cell culture: Although it is a definitive test, but it takes a long time and requires high skill plus the sample is Corneal scraping which needs amplification.

55. Ans. (b) Dengue IgM ELISA

Ref: Anantnarayan 8th ed page 519

Laboratory diagnosis methods for confirming dengue virus infection may involve detection of the virus, viral nucleic acid, antigens or antibodies, or a combination of these techniques. After the onset of illness, the virus can be detected in serum, plasma, circulating blood cells and other tissues for 4–5 days. During the early stages of the disease, virus isolation, nucleic acid or antigen detection can be used to diagnose the infection. At the end of the acute phase of infection, serology is the method of choice for diagnosis

Before day 5 of illness, during the febrile period, dengue infections may be diagnosed by virus isolation in cell culture, by detection of viral RNA by nucleic acid amplification tests (NAAT), or by detection of viral antigens by ELISA or rapid tests. Virus isolation in cell culture is usually performed only in laboratories with the necessary infrastructure and technical expertise. Viral antigen detectionby ELISA and dot blot assays directed against EM and NS1 can be used within 5-6 days of infection.

After day 5, dengue viruses and antigens disappear from the blood coincident with the appearance of specific antibodies. Serum IgM and IgG ELISA are therefore not used in early detection of dengue.

- **Viral isolation:** Isolation of virus can be done within 6 days of infection.
- RT-PCR viral nucleic acid detection are used for early detection of dengue.
- **Viral antigen detection:** ELISA and dot blot assays directed against EM and NS1. It can be within 6 days.
- **IgM ELISA:** IgM antibodies start forming 5 days after Infection. Antibody tests are not effective for diagnosing early infections.

56. Ans. (d) Leptospira interrogans

Ref: Ananthnarayan 8th ed page 372

Treponema Pallidum	Borrelia Burgdoferi	Leptospira
T pallidum are slender spirals measuring about 0.2 µm in width and 5–15 µm in length. The spiral coils are regularly spaced at a distance of 1 µm from one another. There are about 10 regular spirals. **Ends are smooth**	B burgdorferi is a spiral organism 20–30 µm long and 0.2–0.3 µm wide. **Large spirals;** The distance between turns varies from 2 to 4 µm. The organisms have variable numbers (7–11) of endoflagella and are highly motile. Both **ends are pointed**. Irregular spirals	Leptospirae are **tightly coiled (10-18 coils)**, thin, flexible spirochetes 5–15 µ m long, with very fine spirals 0.1–0.2 µ m wide; one end is often bent, forming a **hook or umbrella handle**. Secondary spirals give the leptospirae the appearance of brackets or the letter S

Contd...

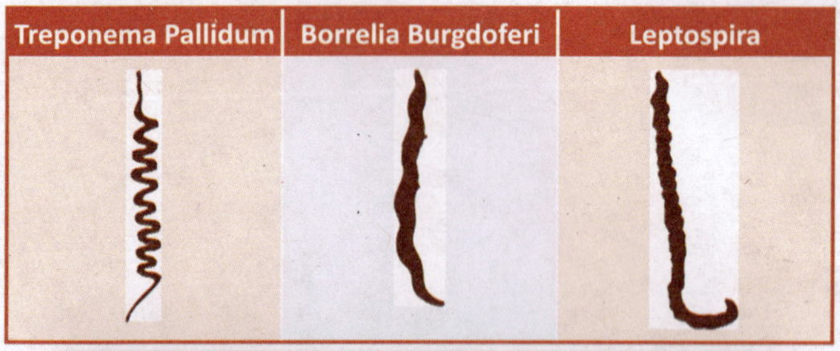

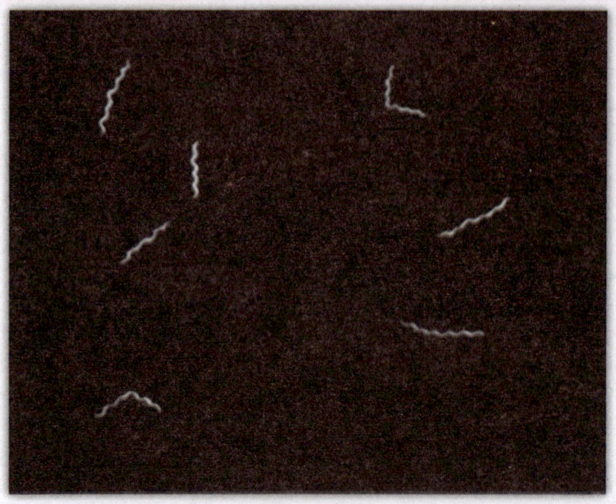

Fig: Treponema pallidum in dark field microscopy

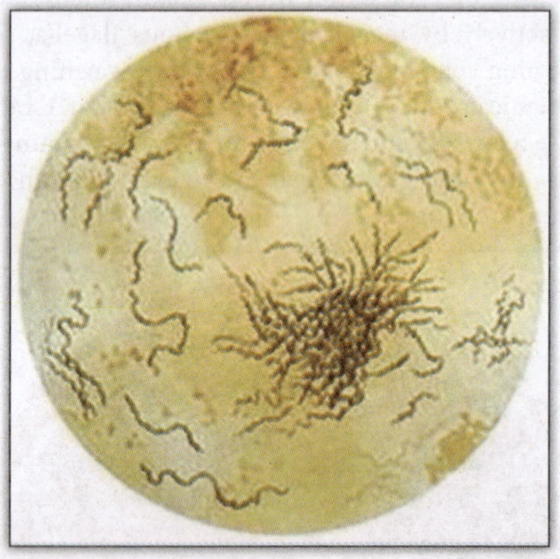

Fig: Treponema in silver impregnation

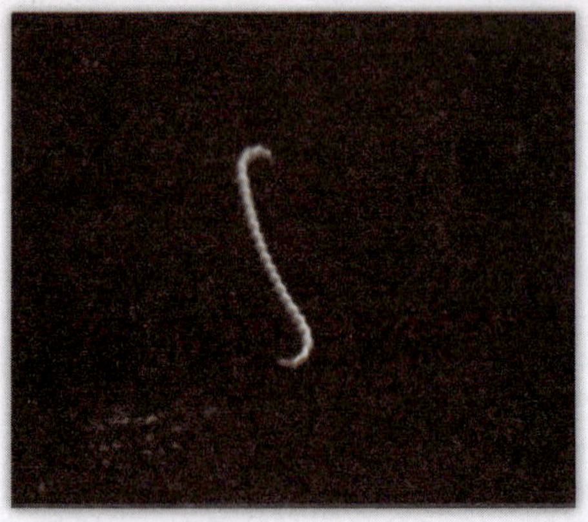

Fig: Leptospira in Dark field microscopy

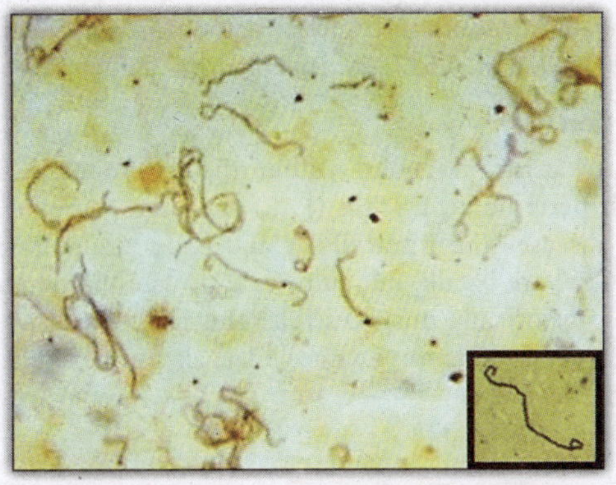

Fig: Leptospira in Silver impregnation

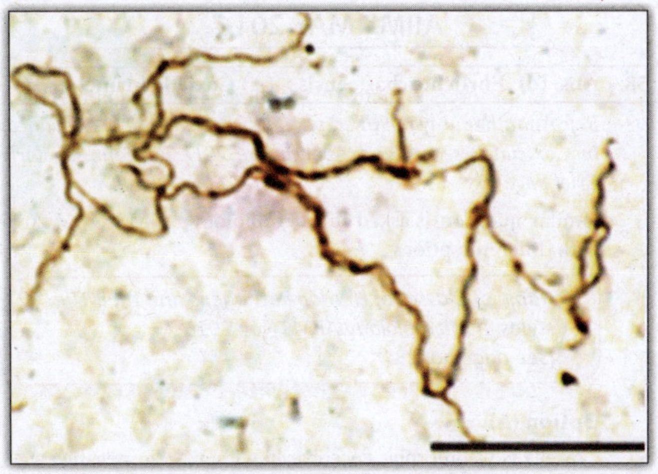

Fig: Borrelia Burgdorferi organisms shown by dark-filed microscopy; note the large and irregular spirals with pointed ends

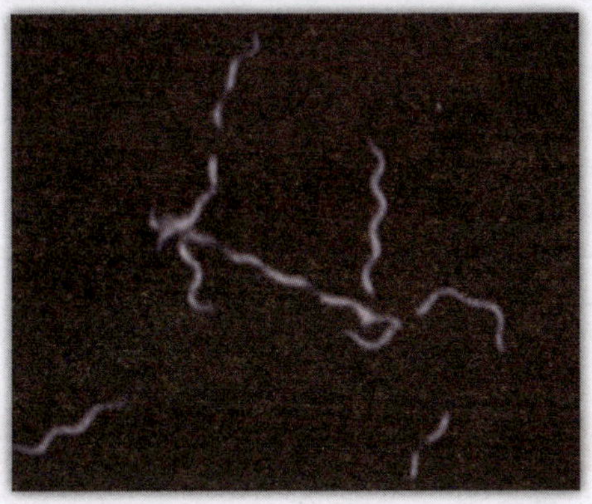

Fig: Borrelia Burgdorferi organisms shown by dark-filed microscopy

57. Ans. (a) Coxiella burnetii

Ref: Ananthanarayan 9th ed page 405, 409, 412, 411, Advances in Coxiella Research and Application: 2012 Edition: Scholarly Brief page 25

Similar question with different options was asked in Microbiology AIIMS MAY 2016 (see page no. 286)

Classes of Human Pathogens and Their Lifestyles

Taxonomic	Size	Site of Propagation	Examples
Prions	30–50 kD	Intracellular	Prion protein
Viruses	20–300 nm	Obligate intracellular	All viruses are obligate intracellular parasite
Bacteria	0.2–15 µm	Obligate intracellular	*Chlamydia trachomatis, Rickettsia,* Ehrlichia, ***Coxiella (recent host cell free growth shown in 2009)****, Mycobacterium laprae*
		Extracellular	Streptococcus pneumoniae, Staphylococcus aureus, Streptococcus pyogenes, Pseudomonas aeruginosa, Escherichia coli, etc.
		Facultative intracellular	*Mycobacterium tuberculosis, Non tuberculous mycobacteria, Nocardia, Brucella, Salmonella, Legionella,* Listeria, Diplococci (Neisseria), Legionella, Salmonella, Yersinia
Fungi	2–200 µm	Extracellular	Candida albicans
		Facultative intracellular	Histoplasma capsulatum, Cryptococcus neoformans
		Obligate intracellular	Pneumocystis jirovecii
Protozoa	1–50 µm	Extracellular	Trypanosoma gambiense
		Facultative intracellular	Trypanosoma cruzi
		Obligate intracellular	Leishmania donovani, Plasmodium, Toxoplasma gongii, Babesia,
Helminths	3 mm–10 m	Extracellular	Wuchereria bancrofti
		Intracellular	Trichinella spiralis

Mycobacterium tuberculosis is facultative intracellular while Mycobacterium laprae is obligate intracellular.
Obligate intracellular organisms can not be cultured on inert media while facultative intracellular organism can be cultured on inert media.
Intracellular organisms (both facultative and obligate) are protected from antibodies and complement.

AIIMS MAY 2016

58. Ans. (d) Ehrlichia chaffeensis > (A) Coxiella brunette

Ref: Ananthanarayan 9th ed page 405, 409, 412, 411, Advances in Coxiella Research and Application: 2012 Edition: Scholarly Brief page 25

Similar question is asked in Microbiology AIIMS NOV 2016 with different options

See table of Classes of Human Pathogens and their Life styles in Microbiology AIIMS Nov 2016 (see page no. 284)

Option (A)

Coxiella is pleomorphic coccobacilli with a Gram negative wall. It is an obligate intracellular pathogen infecting monocyte-macrophage cells. However Omsland et al. 2009 discovered the milestone advance of Coxiella host cell-free (axenic) growth. After Omsland many reserchers proved host free growth of Coxiella **However, C. burnetii was recently liberated from its host cell by a medium that supports axenic (host cell-free) growth.** Ref: Omsland A, Hackstadt T, Heinzen RA (2013) Bringing Culture to the Uncultured: Coxiella burnetii and Lessons for obligate intracellular bacterial pathogens. PLoS Pathog 9(9): e1003540. doi:10.1371/journal.ppat.1003540

Option (B)

Characteristic vacuoles within the macrophage that stain with periodic acid Schiff (PAS) stain are pathognomonic of the disease. The intracellular and extracellular PAS-positive material are bacilli, but cultures to isolate the organism have been historically unsuccessful. (This suggests that it is occur both intracellular and extracellular; also some studies in 2001 prove the same)

Ref: Jawetz 24E, 318

Option (C)

Bartonella are tiny Gram negative bacilli, which invade mammalian endothelial cells and blood cells. (Bartonella henselae is *Not obligate* but facultative Intracellular).

Option (D)

Ehrlichiae are small, Gram negative, obligate intracellular bacteria which have affinity towards blood cells.

59. Ans. (d) C -56789

Ref: Jawetz 24th ed page 139, Robbins 9th ed page 88-89

Complements System

Complements are acute phase proteins.

Liver synthesize central components. Spleen, macrophages. and intestinal mucosa can also synthesize.

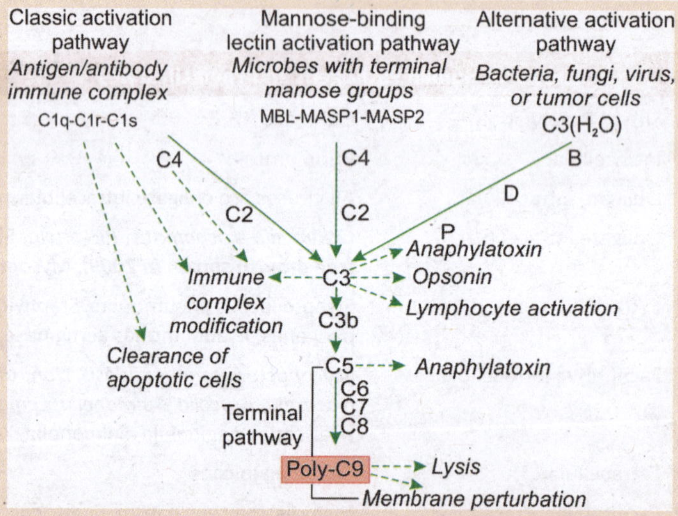

Classical pathway is activated by — IgM (most potent).

IgG (requires 2 molecules) and immune complexes (eg. in SLE).

In alternate C3 works on C3 convertase.

C3 convertase splits C3 into; **C_{3a} (Anaphylotoxin) + C3b (cell bound)**

Alternate pathway is activated by — Bacterial *endotoxin (mostpotent) and* zymogen, IgA & IgG_4, cobra venom

C3 is first common point between classical and alternate pathway. C3 is involved in both classical and alternate pathway.

Functions: Basic functions of complements are opsonization, chemotaxis, lysis of foreign cells and clumping of antigen bearing cells.

Role in innate immune response.

Biosynthesis of Complements

Complements	Site
C1	Intestinal epithelium

Contd...

C2, C4	Macrophages
C5, C8	Spleen
C3, C6, C9	Liver
C7	Not known
FAQ Complement, Leukotrienes, PGs	
• Most important opsonizing complement (major serum opsonin)	**C3b** (because of the presence of C3b receptors on the surface of many phagocytes)
• Most important chemotactin	C5a
• Anaphylotoxin	C5a (most potent), C3a, C4a
• MAC (membrane attack complex)	C5b-C6-C7-C8-C9
• SRS-A (slow reacting substances of anaphylaxis)	LT- C4, D4, E4
• Leukotriene which is chemotactic (promotes leucocyte adhesion)	LT-B4
• ↑Vascular permeability	LTC4, LTD4, LTE4
• Vasodilation	PGD2, PGE2, PGI2, PGF2α

60. Ans. (d) Fulminant hepatitis E infection

Ref: Jawetz 24th ed page 475-476, Harrison's 19th ed page 2009

Anti HEV IgM reactive status is characteristic of acute fulminant hepatitis E infection which is common in pregnancy.

Option (A)

There is no chronic state in hepatitis A

Option (B) and (C)

HbsAg +; Anti Hbs -/+; Anti Hbc + represents chronic state of Hepatitis B.

Interpretation of HAV, HCV and HDV Infections

Assay	Interpretation
Anti HAV IgM negative/ Anti HAV IgG negative	Most persons with these results have never contracted hepatitis A
Anti-HAV IgM-positive/ Anti HAV IgG negative	Acute infection with Hepatitis A
Anti HAV IgM positive/ Anti HAV IgG positive	Acute hepatitis A occurred within the last six months. By six months, the IgM reverts to negative
Anti HAV IgM negative/ Anti HAV IgG positive	Persons with this result are immune to hepatitis A. They have either been infected with the virus months or years in the past (with or without symptoms), or they have been vaccinated for hepatitis A. However, if they are currently ill, it is not likely to be due to hepatitis A
Anti HEV IgM negative/ Anti HEV IgG negative	Most persons with these results have never contracted hepatitis E
Anti-HEV IgM-positive/ Anti HEV IgG negative	Acute Fulminant Hepatitis E (Anti HEV IgM is detectable 2 to 9 weeks after exposure)
Anti HAV IgM positive/ Anti HAV IgG positive	Acute fulminant Hepatitis E (IgM is detected in both acute and chronic)

Contd...

Interpretation of HAV, HCV and HDV Infections

Anti HAV IgM negative/ Anti HAV IgG positive	Previously exposed or chronic hepatitis E (IgG is detected upto 12 years of infection)
Anti-HCV-positive	Current or past infection with HCV
Anti-HDV-positive, HBsAg- positive	Infection with HDV
Anti-HDV-positive, anti-HBc IgM-positive	Coinfection with HDV and HBV
Anti-HDV-positive, anti-HBc IgM-negative	Superinfection of chronic HBV infection with HDV

61. Ans. (b) S. pneumonia

Ref: Ananthnarayan 19th ed pages 200-221

The clinical picture is consistent with Gram positive cocci in pairs i.e. Diplococcus (Streptococcus pneumonae)

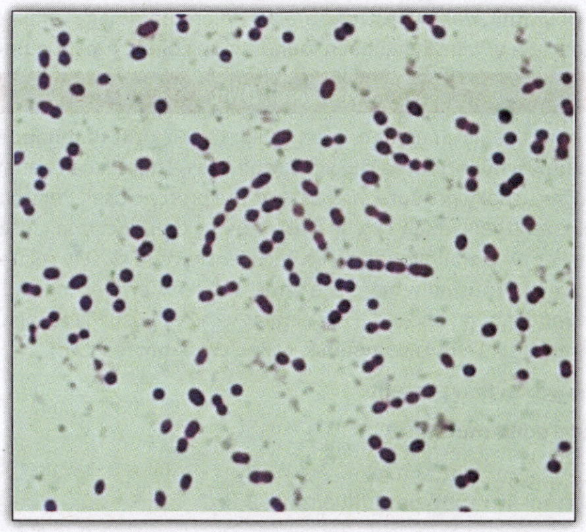

Fig: Gram positive cocci in group of two (diplococcus/Lancet shaped), although some very short chains may be seen: **Streptococcus Pneumoneae**

Option (A)

S. Pyogenes are Gram positive cocci in chains and pairs.

Option (B)

S. Pneumoniae are Gram positive cocci in pairs. Lanceolate shaped.

Option (C)

Staphylococci are Gram positive cocci in clusters

Option (D)

Neisseria are Gram negative cocci

62. Ans. (c) Promotes growths of Staph aureus and Candida

Ref: With text

Option (A)

CLED (cystine lactose electrolyte deficient), a non-inhibitory ideal medium for counting bacterial colonies. The medium supports growth of all urinary potential pathogens such as *E. coli*, Klebsiella, Pseudomonas, Streptococci, Staphylococci, Candida. P aeruginosa produces pale coloured colonies on MacConkey agar and green colonies on CLED medium. CLED supports the growth of wide range of pathogens but inhibits the swarming growth of proteus (Ref: Medical Microbiology Illustrated By S. H. Gillespie page 214)

Option (B)

Both CLED and MacConkey differentiate lactose fermenters with Non Fermenters. MacConkey agar, which is both a selective and differential medium, is a combination of bile salts, lactose and crystal violet (Koneman et al., 1997). Gram-negative bacteria are able to ferment lactose and produce pink-colored colonies distinguishing them from colorless bacteria that can not ferment the lactose. (Ref: Bailey & Scott's Diagnostic Microbiology 13th ed By Patricia Tille page 83).

Option (C)

CLED have advantages of distinguishing lactose from non-lactose fermenters (Similar to MacConkey agar) and inhibiting swarming of proteus and as CLED is less inhibitory to Staphylococcus, its use is strongly recommended. (Ref: Mackie & McCartne 14th Ed page 88)

Option (D)

Swarming does not occurs in MacConkey medium on which proteus produces colourless non lactose fermenting colonies. Bile salts present in MacConkey medium prevents swarming. (Ref: Textbook of Microbiology & Immunology By Subhash Chandra ParijaParija 2nd ed page 265)

Proteus species move very actively by means of peritrichous flagella, resulting in "swarming" on solid media unless the swarming is inhibited by chemicals, e.g. phenylethyl alcohol or CLED (cystine- lactose-electrolyte-deficient) medium. *(Ref: Jawetz 24th Ed page 251)*

63. Ans. (d) Responsible for seasonal epidemic of influenza

Ref: Ananthanarayan 9th ed page 499, Jawetz 24th ed page 542

Influenza Virus

- Family orthomyxoviridae
- ***Incubation period***: 18-72 hours
- ***Types***: A, B, C (No cross immunity and antigenically distinct)
- Both A and B have surface antigens, H (hemagglutinin), N (neuraminidase)
- **Major antigenic variations occur in A, some in B while C seems to be antigenically stable.**
- ***Rimantidine*** and ***Amantadine*** are used as prophylaxis for ***influenza A***

SUBTYPES: Influenza A viruses are divided into subtypes based on two proteins on the surface of the virus: the **hemagglutinin (H) and the neuraminidase (N).** There are 18 different hemagglutinin subtypes and 11 different neuraminidase subtypes. All known subtypes of influenza A viruses have been found among birds, except subtype H17N10 and H18N11 which have only been found in bats

Antigenic Drift	Antigenic Shift
Minor antigenic changes are termed antigenic drift that happen continually over time as the virus replicates. These small genetic changes usually produce viruses that are pretty closely related to one another, which can be illustrated by their location close together on a phylogenetic tree. Viruses that are closely related to each other usually share the same antigenic properties and an immune system exposed to an similar virus will usually recognize it and respond. (This is sometimes called **cross-protection**.)	Major antigenic changes in HA or NA, called antigenic shift. Shift results in a new influenza A subtype or a virus with a hemagglutinin or a hemagglutinin and neuraminidase combination that has emerged from an animal population that is so different from the same subtype in humans that most people do not have immunity to the new (e.g. novel) virus. Such a "shift" occurred in the spring of 2009, when an **H1N1 virus** with a new combination of genes emerged to infect people and quickly spread, causing a pandemic.
Cross protection present	Little or no cross protection
Due to **point mutation**	Due to **genetic reassortment** between human and avian influenza viruses.
Occurs in all 3 subtypes influenza A, B & C	Occurs only in Influenza A
Gradual change	Sudden change
Epidemics are rare	**Epidemics & Pandemics** are common

Contd...

Influenza Virus	
New subtypes are rare	Result in the appearance of a new subtype.

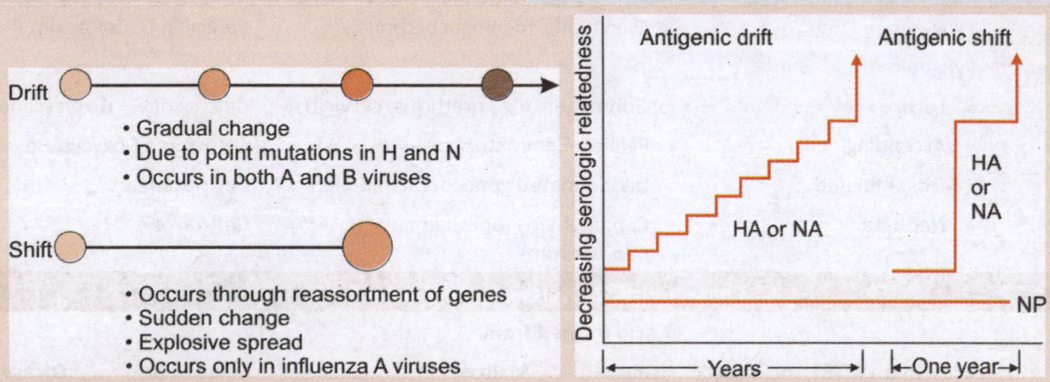

- In influenza virus antigen variation occurs mostly in Type A. (A>B>C). Influenza type C is antigenically stable or antigen variation does not occur.
- *Seasonal influenza is caused by H3N2 or HINI & Pandemic influenza is caused by Novel H1N1* **(Swine flu)**.
- *Highly pathogenic avian influenza is caused by H5N1 (Bird flu).*

Seasonal Influenza Vaccine	
Vaccination is currently the most effective measure for reducing the impact of influenza. Immunization is focused mainly on individuals at increased risk of complications of influenza infection and on individuals who might transmit influenza to such people. *A live attenuated, cold-adapted, temperature-sensitive, trivalent influenza virus vaccine administered by nasal spray was licensed in the United States in 2003.* It was the first live-virus influenza vaccine approved in the United States, as well as the first nasally administered vaccine in the United States	
Trivalent influenza vaccine	**Quadrivalent influenza vaccine**
World Health Organization make recommendations each year about which strains should be included in the vaccine. **Traditional flu vaccines (called "trivalent" vaccines) are made to protect against three flu viruses; an influenza A (H1N1) virus, an influenza A (H3N2) virus and an influenza B virus (Victoria or Yamagata lineages)**	**Quadrivalent vaccines:** Starting from the influenza season 2014–15 new quadrivalent combination vaccines containing four different influenza strains are gradually becoming available. These vaccines contain **two influenza A (H1N1 and H3N2 subtypes) and two influenza B (Victoria and Yamagata lineages) strains**

64. Ans. (a) Gram negative diplococcus, ferments glucose and maltose

Ref: Ananthanarayan 9th ed page 232

Its almost impossible to comment without a clinical history. Clinical history of Fever with rash and that of meningitis shall be given with or without the Lumbar puncture CSF analysis.

Option (A)

Gram negative diplococcus, ferments glucose and maltose—the organism is Neisseria Meningitidis—Causes Meninigits with CSF cloudy and with abundant cocci. Typical petechial rash occurs early in disease.

Option (B)

Gram positive diplococcic (lanceolate), catalase negative optochin sensitive—the organism is S. pneumoniae—Causes pneumonia, bronchitis, meningitis. Usually occur secondary to other pneumococcal infections.

Option (C)

Gram positive cocci in chains, catalyse negative and bacitracin sensitive—the organism is S. pyogenes—Causes respiratory infections, skin infections, genital onfections, abscesses.

Option (D)

Gram negative diplococcic (kidney bean shaped), oxidase positive—the organism is Neisseria gonorrhoeae—Causes Gonorrhoea, procitis, conjuctivits, arthritis, opthalmia neonatorum, bacteremia.

Important Clinical Features of Neisseriae			
Organism	Type of pathogenesis	Typical disease	Treatment
N. meningitides	Pyogenic	Meningitis, meningococcemia	Penicillin G, Cefotaxim & Ceftrioxone
N. gonorrhoeae	Pyogenic		
	• Local	Gonorrhea, e.g., urethritis, cervicitis	Ceftriaxone + Doxycycline
	• Ascending	Pelvic inflammatory disease	Cefoxitin + Doxycycline
	• Disseminated	Disseminated gonococcal infection	Ceftriaxone
	• Neonatal	Conjunctivitis (ophthalmia neonatorum)	Ceftriaxone

Characteristic of Neisseriae & M Catarrhalis						
		Acid formed from				
	Growth on MTM, mL, or NYC medium	Glucose	Maltose	Lactose	Sucrose or fructose	DNase
N gonorrhoeae	+	+	–	–	–	–
N meningitidis	+	+	+	–	–	–
M catarrhalis	-	-	–	–	–	+

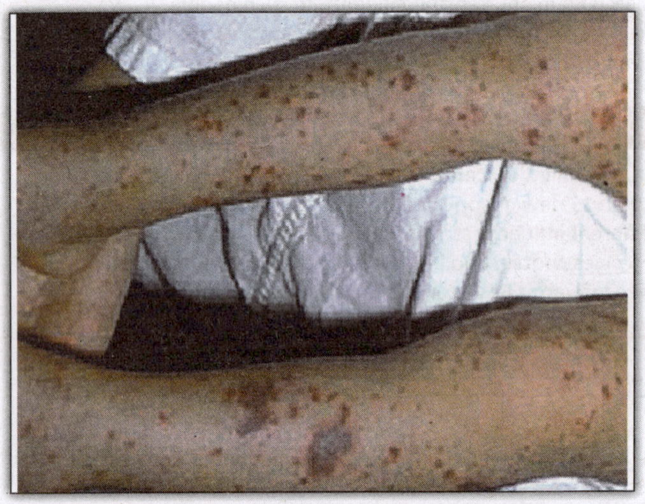

Fig: Nesseria meningitis: In meningococcal septicaemia, a rash is always a very important sign. The rash can appear anywhere on the body. Early skin rash looks like tiny pinpricks (pink, red, or purple). As the infection spreads through the system, the rash becomes more obvious. More bleeding under the skin may cause the spots to turn dark red or deep purple. The rash may resemble large bruises.

In infants and young children	In older children and adults
Fever	Fever
Disinterest in feeding	Vomiting and/or diarrhea
Irritability	Neck stiffness or aching
Extreme tiredness or floppiness	Backache
Dislike of being handled	Joint pains and sore muscles
Vomiting and/or diarrhea	General malaise, off food
Turning away from light	Drowsiness, confusion

Contd...

In infants and young children	In older children and adults
Drowsiness	Rash of red-purple pinprick spots or larger bruises.
Convulsions or twitching	Headache
Rash of red-purple pinprick spots or larger bruises	Photophobia (dislike of bright lights).

Glass test: One sign of meningococcal septicemia is that the rash doesn't fade when you apply pressure.

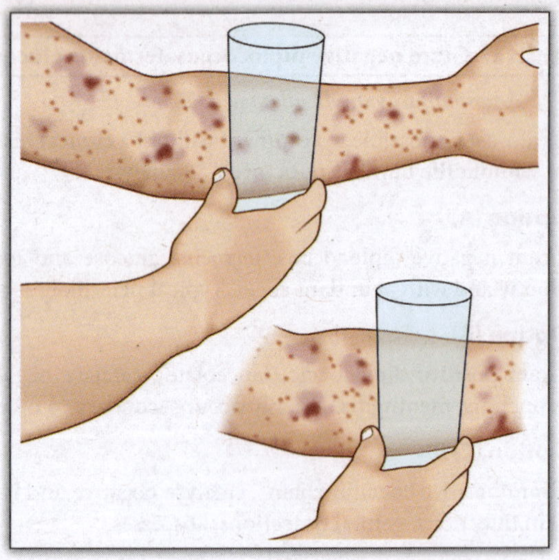

65. Ans. (b) Adult female are capable of reproductive parthenogenesis

Ref: Paniker`s Textbook of Medical Parasitology 7th ed page 178-181

The clinical pictures is consistent with immunocompromised state. However history of High Risk Behavious (Secual contact) can cause many other infections apart from HIV and that includes HTLV-1. The parasite colour plate is of Strongiloides. Now read following text

CDC says: Many studies have shown an association with strongyloides and infection with Human T-cell lymphotropic Virus-1 (HTLV-1). These studies have shown that people infected with HTLV-1 are more likely to become infected with Strongyloides and that once infected, are more likely to develop severe cases of strongyloidiasis. Of note, being infected with HIV/AIDS has not been shown to be a risk factor for developing Strongyloides or having a worse clinical course.

Further CDC says: Rarely, severe life-threatening forms of the disease called **hyperinfection syndrome** and disseminated strongyloidiasis can occur. These forms of the disease are more common in people who are on corticosteroids (prednisone for example) or other immunosuppressive therapies or who are infected with HTLV-1. In this situation, people become critically ill and should be taken to the hospital immediately.

Transmission of HTLV-I is believed to occur by sexual contact, from mother to child via breastfeeding and through exposure to contaminated blood just like HIV virus. Coinfection with HTLV-1 decreases IL-5 and IgE responses in patients with strongyloidiasis consistent with a relative switch from Th2 to Th1 response, Thus these patients lack a Th2 response. Steroid treatment acutely suppresses eosinophilia and T-cell activation.

Strongiloides infection can present as:

- **Acute infection:** Initial pruritic maculopapular rash or migrating linear urticaria (larva currans occurs on the trunk and buttocks). Intestinal infection at site of penetration; cough, SOB, wheezing, fever, Loffler's syndrome
- **Chronic infections (veterans 30 years later):** Intermittent cutaneous and enteric symptoms.
- **Hyperinfection Syndrome:** Seen in immunocompromised, uncontrolled, widespread dissemination of filariform larvae in blood stream, characterized by fever, vomiting, diarrhea, gram-negative sepsis/meningitis, pulmonary infiltrates, hypoxia, Periumbilical purpura.

Now coming to the options one by one:

Option (A)

It is smallest nematode known to cause human infections. Rhabditiform larvae is the most common form of parasite found in the feces. Whereas filariform larvae is the infective stage of parasite.

Option (B)

It was earlier believed that the female worms in the intestine are parthenogenetic and can produce offsprings without being fertilised by the male.

Option (C)

The infection is acquired by penetration of the skin by the filariform larvae when patient walks bare foot or by autoinfection.

Option (D)

Drug of choice of Strongyloids is Ivermectin. Thiobendazole is not been replaced by Ivermectin due to higher side effects.

	Parasitic Nematode				
Feature	*Ascaris lumbricoides* (Roundworm)	*Necator americanus, Ancylostoma duodenale* (Hookworm)	Strongyloides stercoralis	*Trichuris trichiura* (Whipworm)	*Enterobius vermicularis* (Pinworm)
Global prevalence in humans (millions)	807	576	100	604	209
Endemic areas	Worldwide	Hot, humid regions	Hot, humid regions	Worldwide	Worldwide
Infective stage	Egg	Filariform larva	Filariform larva	Egg	Egg
Route of infection	Oral	Percutaneous	Percutaneous or autoinfection	Oral	Oral
Gastrointestinal location of worms	Jejunal lumen	Jejunal mucosa	Small-bowel mucosa	Cecum, colonic mucosa	Cecum, appendix
Adult worm size	15–40 cm	7–12 mm	2 mm	30–50 mm	8–13 mm (female)
Pulmonary passage of larvae	Yes	Yes	Yes	No	No
Incubation period (days)	60–75	40–100	17–28	70–90	35–45
Longevity	1 y	*N. americanus*: 2–5 y *duodenale*: 6–8 y	Decades (owing to autoinfection)	5 y	2 months
Fecundity (eggs/day/worm)	240,000	*N. americanus*: 4000–10,000 *A. duodenale*: 10,000–25,000	5000–10,000	3000–7000	2000

Principal symptoms	Rarely gastrointestinal or biliary obstruction	Iron-deficiency anemia in heavy infection	Gastrointestinal symptoms; malabsorption or sepsis in hyperinfection	Gastrointestinal symptoms, anemia	Perianal pruritus
Diagnostic stage	Eggs in stool	Eggs in fresh stool, larvae in old stool	Larvae in stool or duodenal aspirate; sputum in hyperinfection	Eggs in stool	Eggs from perianal skin on cellulose acetate tape
Treatment	Mebendazole Albendazole Pyrantel pamoate Ivermectin Nitazoxanide	Mebendazole Pyrantel pamoate Albendazole	Ivermectin (DOC) Albendazole	Mebendazole Albendazole Ivermectin	Mebendazole Pyrantel pamoate Albendazole

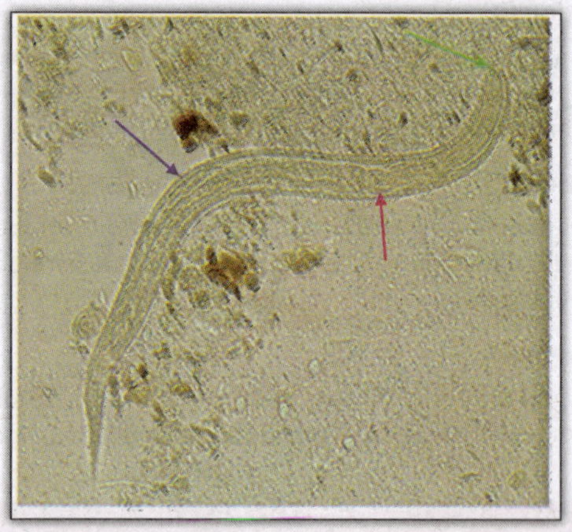

Source: CDC

Fig: Strongyloides stercoralis first-stage rhabditiform (L1) larvae: The first-stage rhabditiform larvae (L1) of Strongyloides stercoralis are 180–380 µm long, with a short buccal canal, a rhabditoid esophagus and a prominent genital primordium. These L1 larvae are usually found in stool, as the eggs embryonate and hatch in the mucosa of the small intestine of the host. Rhabditiform larva of S. stercoralis in an unstained wet mount of stool. Notice the prominent genital primordium (blue arrow), rhabditoid esophagus (red arrow) and short buccal canal (green arrow).

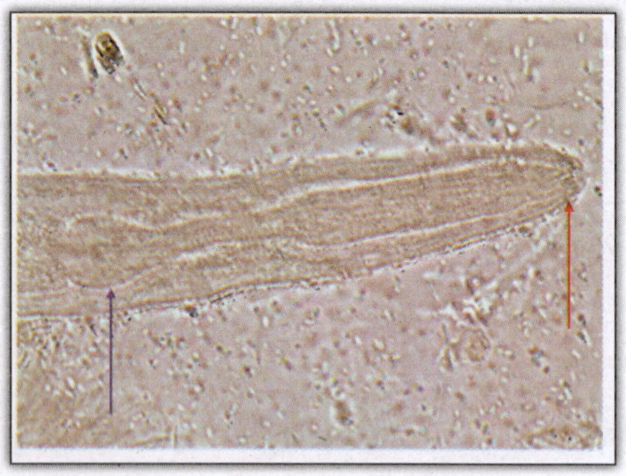

Source: CDC

Fig: Close-up of the anterior end of a rhabditiform larva of S. stercoralis, showing the short buccal canal (red arrow) and the rhabditoid esophagus (blue arrow). Image taken at 1000x oil magnification

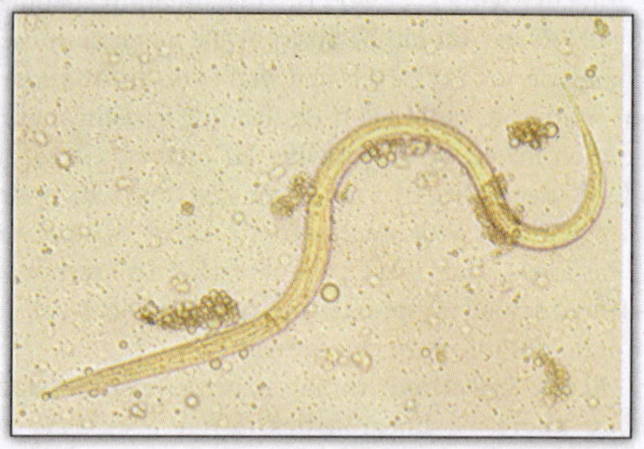

Source: CDC

Fig: Strongyloides stercoralis third-stage filariform (L3) larvae: Infective, third-stage filariform larvae (L3) of Strongyloides stercoralis are up to 600 µm long. The tail is notched and the esophagus to intestine ratio is 1:1. Infective L3 larvae are found in soil and invade the human host by direct penetration of the skin. They may be found in respiratory specimens during cases of autoinfection.

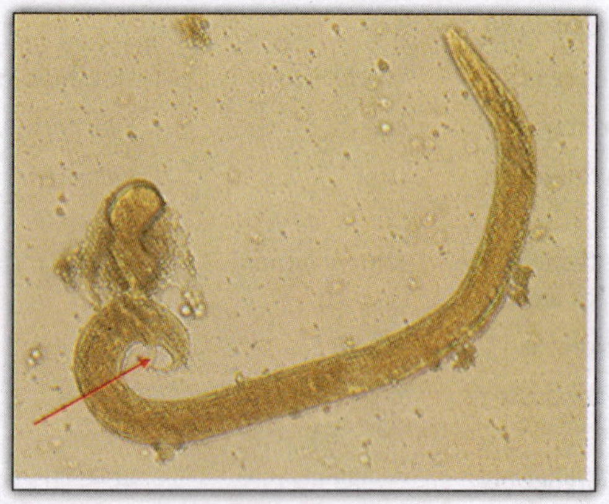

Source: CDC

Fig: Strongyloides stercoralis free-living adults: Adults of Strongyloides stercoralis may be found in the human host or soil. In the human host there are no parasitic males and parasitic females are long, slender and measure 2.0–3.0 mm in length. In the environment, rhabditiform larvae may develop into infective filariform (L3) larvae (direct cycle) or free-living adults that contain both males and females (indirect cycle). Free-living adult males measure up to 750 µm long; free-living females measure up to 1.0 mm long. Free-living adult male S. Stercoralis is identified by presence of the spicule (red arrow)

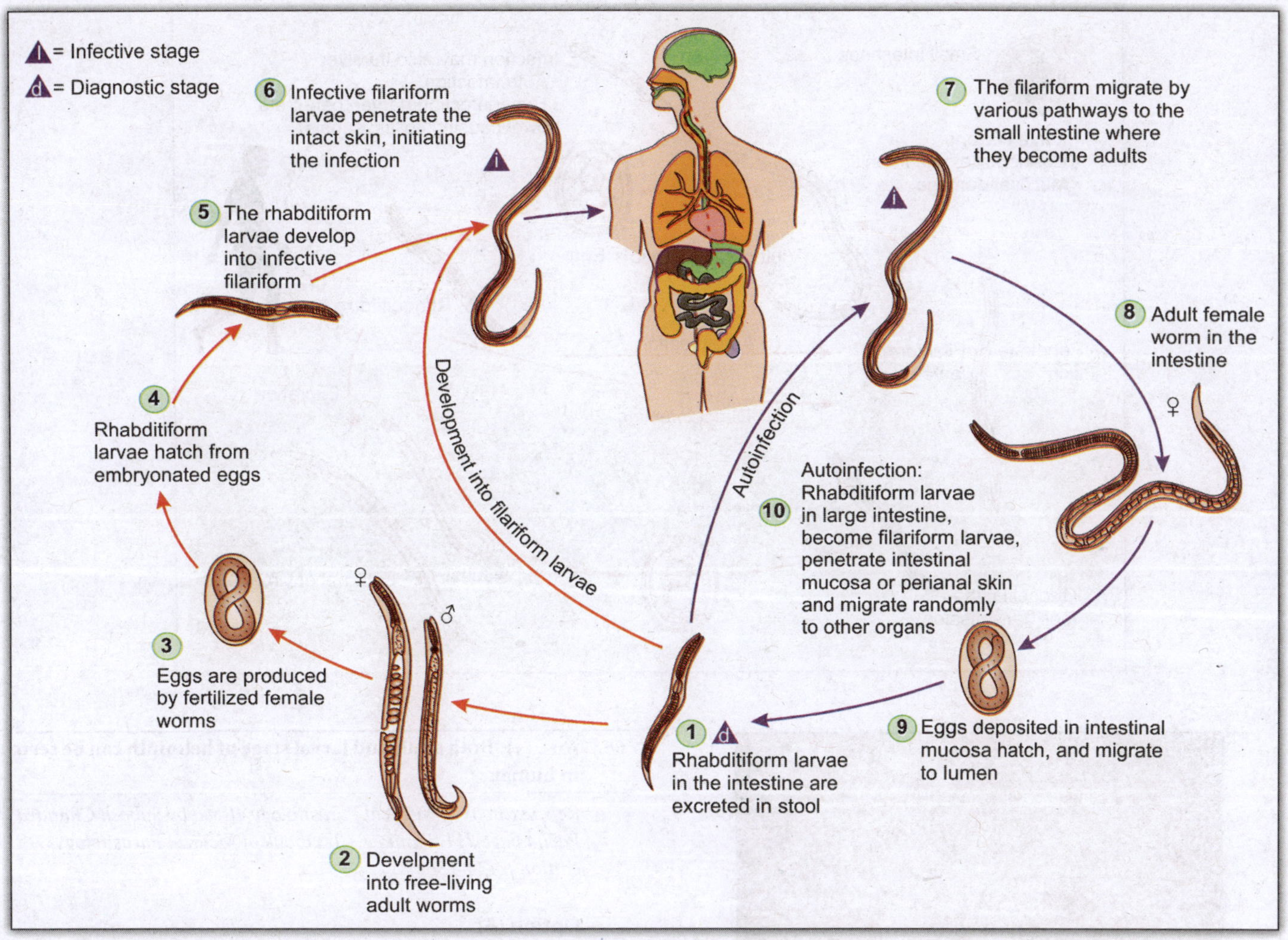

Source: CDC Illustrations

(A) **Life cycle of strongyloides:** The Strongyloides life cycle is more complex than that of most nematodes with its alternation between free-living and parasitic cycles and its potential for autoinfection and multiplication within the host. Two types of cycles exist:

Free-living cycle: The rhabditiform larvae passed in the stool **1** (see "Parasitic cycle" below) can either become infective filariform larvae (direct development) **6** or free living adult males and females **2** that mate and produce eggs **3** from which rhabditiform larvae hatch **4**. and eventually become infective filariform larvae **5**. The filariform larvae penetrate the human host skin to initiate the parasitic cycle (see below) **6**.

Parasitic cycle: Filariform larvae in contaminated soil penetrate the human skin **6** and by various, often random routes, migrate into the small intestine **7**. Historically it was believed that the L3 larvae migrate via the bloodstream to the lungs, where they are eventually coughed up and swallowed. However, there is also evidence that L3 larvae can migrate directly to the intestine via connective tissues. In the small intestine they molt twice and become adult female worms **8**. The females live threaded in the epithelium of the small intestine and by parthenogenesis produce eggs **9**, which yield rhabditiform larvae. The rhabditiform larvae can either be passed in the stool **1**(see "Free-living cycle" above), or can cause autoinfection **10**. In autoinfection, the rhabditiform larvae become infective filariform larvae, which can penetrate either the intestinal mucosa (internal autoinfection) or the skin of the perianal area (external autoinfection); in either case, the filariform larvae may disseminate throughout the body. To date, occurrence of autoinfection in humans with helminthic infections is recognized only in Strongyloides stercoralis and Capillaria philippinensis infections. In the case of Strongyloides, autoinfection may explain the possibility of persistent infections for many years in persons who have not been in an endemic area and of hyperinfections in immunosuppressed individuals

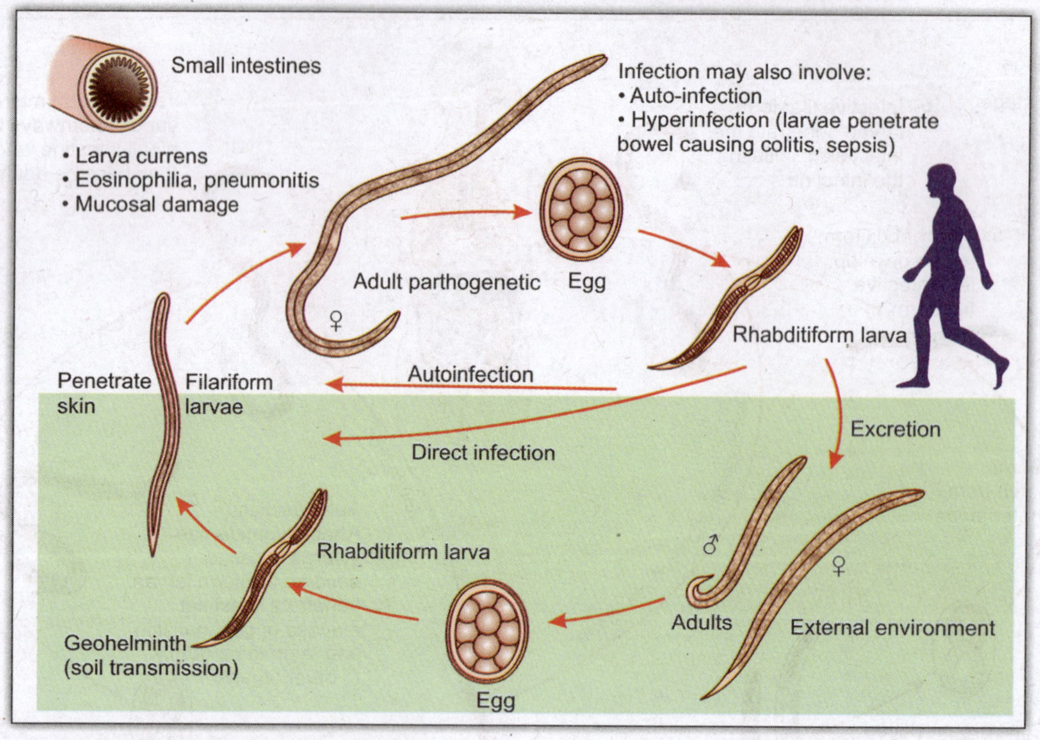

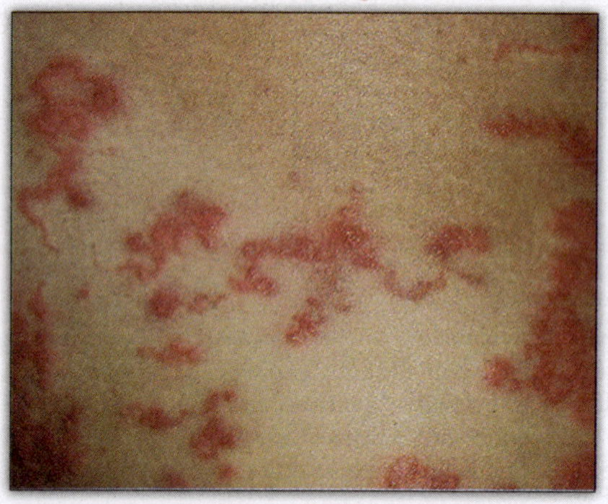

Fig: Strongyloides larva under the skin **(Cutaneous larva migrans)**

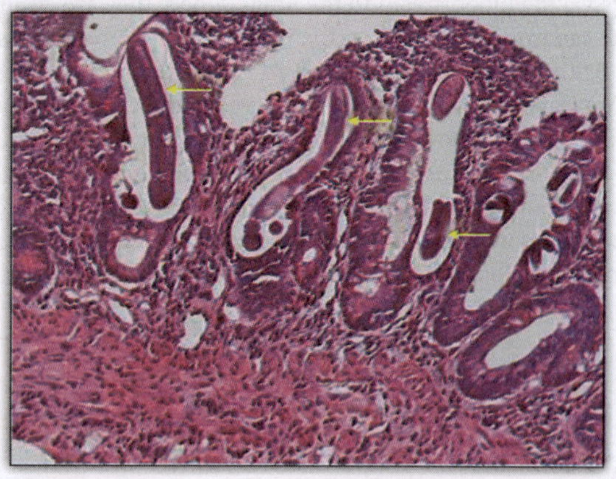

Fig: Duodenal biopsy showing Strongyloides stercoralis larval infection in the mucosal crypts (arrow) (HE).

66. Ans. (a) Both adult and larval stage of helminth can be seen in humans

Ref: Textbook of Medical Parasitology 4th ed by Subash Chandra Parija page 211, Paniker's Textbook of Medical Parasitology, 7th edition p.134-136

Option (A)

Hymenolepis nana does not necessarily need an intermediate host to complete its life cycle. Larvae can develop in spite of the high temperature of a human body. Adults live 4–6 weeks, but internal autoinfection allows hymenolepiasis to persist for years. Also see life cycle in color plates.

Option (B)

H. nana does not require an intermediate host and infection can occur directly from one infected person to another by fecal-oral transmission. Transmission is by contamination of food or water or from hands contaminated with feces. H. nana is the only cestode that parasitizes humans without requiring an intermediate host. It is possible for the worm's entire life cycle to be completed in the bowel, so infection can persist for years.

Option (C)

H. nana infection is either asymptomatic or severe, but not transient and self limiting. Hymenolepiasis is usually asymptomatic in adults. But prolonged infection or multiple Dwarf tapeworms especially in children can cause more severe symptoms due to inflammation of the intestinal mucosa. Heavy infections with H. nana can cause weakness, headaches, anorexia, abdominal pain and diarrhea.

Option (D)

Praziquantel is the drug or choice. Adults and children, 25 mg/kg in a single-dose therapy.

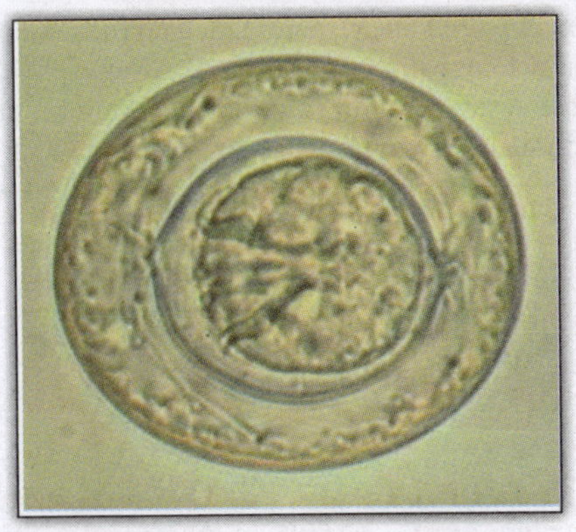

Fig: Egg of H. nana in an unstained wet mount. Note the presence of hooks in the oncosphere and polar filaments within the space between the oncosphere and outer shell

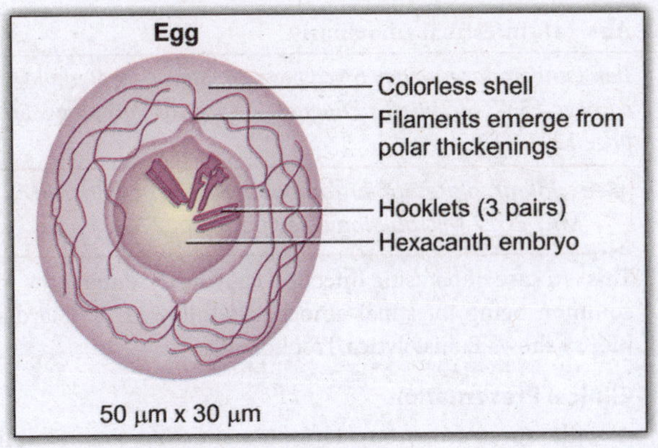

Fig: Egg of H Nana (Illustration)

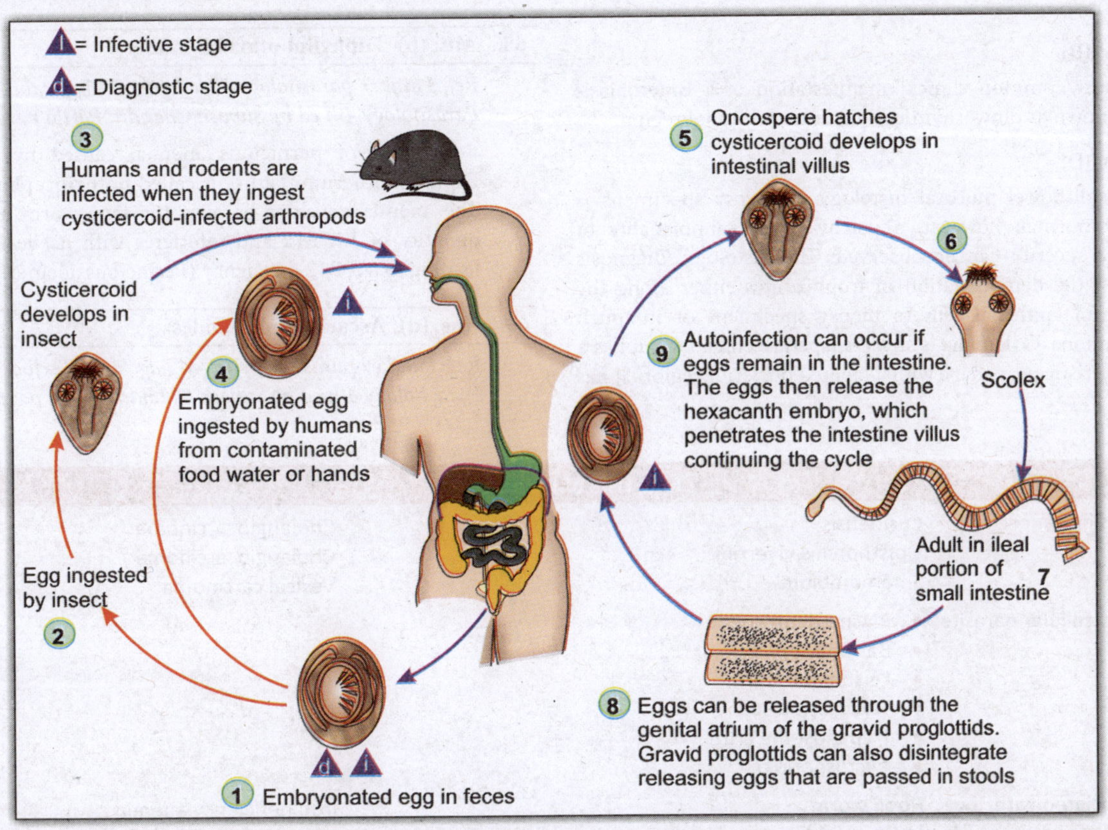

Fig: Fife cycle of h nana: Eggs of Hymenolepis nana are immediately infective when passed with the stool and cannot survive more than 10 days in the external environment **1**. When eggs are ingested by an arthropod intermediate host **2** (various species of beetles and fleas may serve as intermediate hosts), they develop into cysticercoids, which can infect humans or rodents upon ingestion **3** and develop into adults in the small intestine. A morphologically identical variant, H. nana var. fraterna, infects rodents and uses arthropods as intermediate hosts. When eggs are ingested **4** (in contaminated food or water or from hands contaminated with feces), the oncospheres contained in the eggs are released. The oncospheres (hexacanth larvae) penetrate the intestinal villus and develop into cysticercoid larvae **5**. Upon rupture of the villus, the cysticercoids return to the intestinal lumen, evaginate their scoleces **6**, attach to the intestinal mucosa and develop into adults that reside in the ileal portion of the small intestine producing gravid proglottids **7**. Eggs are passed in the stool when released from proglottids through its genital atrium or when proglottids disintegrate in the small intestine **8**. An alternate mode of infection consists of internal autoinfection, where the eggs release their hexacanth embryo, which penetrates the villus continuing the infective cycle without passage through the external environment **9**. The life span of adult worms is 4 to 6 weeks, but internal autoinfection allows the infection to persist for years.

Hymenolepiasis is caused by two cestodes (tapeworm) species, Hymenolepis nana (the dwarf tapeworm, adults measuring 15 to 40 mm in length) and Hymenolepis diminuta (rat tapeworm, adults measuring 20 to 60 cm in length). Hymenolepis diminuta is a cestode of rodents infrequently seen in humans and frequently found in rodents.

67. Ans. (a) Intestinal amoebiasis

Ref: Paniker parasitology 6th ed page 24, Sternberg Pathology 5th ed page 1537, Sternberg's Diagnostic Surgical Pathology, 5th Ed page 1321, CDC

See clolour plates of Entamoeba Histolytica in AIIMS MAY 2017 Microbiology (see page no. 276)

This is a case of parasitic infection causing dysentery, the most common being intestinal amoebiasis followed by Giardiasis. Biopsy shows E. histolytica Trophozoites

Clinical Presentation

A wide spectrum, from asymptomatic infection ("luminal amebiasis"), to invasive intestinal amebiasis (dysentery, colitis, appendicitis, toxic megacolon, amebomas), to invasive extraintestinal amebiasis (liver abscess, peritonitis, pleuropulmonary abscess, cutaneous and genital amebic lesions).

Option (B)

The most common clinical manifestation of a Enterobiasis (also known as pinworm infection) is an itchy anal region.

Option (D)

The small-bowel mucosal histology in biopsy specimens is usually normal; however, a patchy villous abnormality of variable severity can be observed. The histologic diagnosis rests on the demonstration of trophozoites either along the surface of epithelial cells in biopsy specimens or in touch preparations. G. lamblia is sickle-shaped; seen en face, it has a characteristic pear shape with a tapered posterior region. It has prominent paired nuclei, paired median rods, a curved median body and four pairs of flagellae. These morphologic features are most easily recognized on Giemsa-stained or trichrome-stained touch preparations

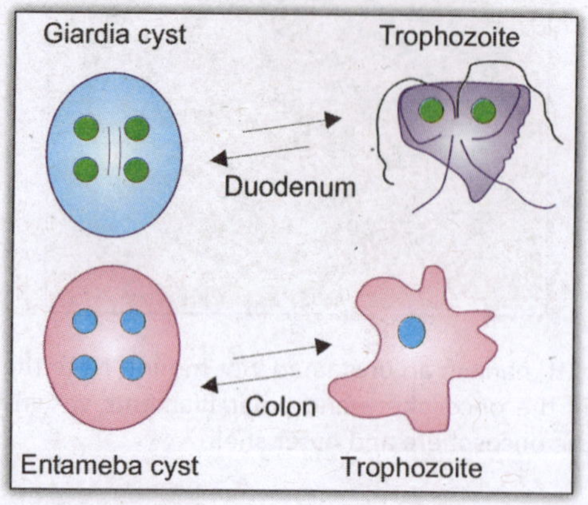

68. Ans. (b) Diphyllobothrium latum

Ref: Paniker parasitology 7th ed page 118, Textbook of Medical Parasitology 4th ed by Subash Chandra Parija page 184

A kind of pernicious anemia, caused by infection of Diphillobotherium latum, is called **bothriocephalus anemia.** The anemia develops because the tape worm absorbs large quantity of Vit B12 and interferes with its ileal absorption, leading to Vit B12 deficiency (Pernicious anemia)

69. Ans. (d) Ascaris lumbricoides

Ref: Paniker parasitology 6th ed page 169, Textbook of Medical Parasitology 4th ed by Subash Chandra Parija page 289

FAQ Lists of Parasitology

Parasite causing cancer	C. sinensis Opisthorchis viverrini S.hematobium	Cholangiocarcinoma Cholangiocarcinoma Vesical carcinoma
Obligate intracellular parasite	• Plasmodium spp • Babesia spp • Leishmania spp • Toxoplasma spp • Trypanosoma cruzi • Microsporidia	
Parasite associated with anemia	Hook worm (A.duodenal/N.americanus) Diphylobothrium latum Malaria Trichuris trichura Leishmania donovani	Iron deficiency anemia Megaloblastic anemia Hemolytic anemia Iron deficiency anemia Iron deficiency anemia
Charcoal Leyden crystals are seen in	• Entamoeba histolytica • Whipworm dysentry • Ascaris pneumonia • Bronchial asthma	
Protozoans cystic stage is not seen in	• Trichomonas vaginalis • Trichomonas intestinalis • Di-entamoeba fragilis • Entamoeba gingivalis	

FAQ Lists of Parasitology

No intermediate host	**Protozoa** • E. histolytica • Giardia lambdia • Chilomastix mesnili • Trichomonas vaginalis • Balantidium coli	**Helminths** • Enterobius vermicularis • Trichuris trichura • Ascaris lumbricoides • Ancylostoma duodenale • Necator americanus • H. nana
Two intermediate host	**Intermediate host** Snails & Crab Cyclops & Fis h Snail & Fish Snail & Plants	**Parasites** Paragonimus westermanii D. latum Clonorchis sinensis Fasciola spp.
Human is intermediate host in	• Man is definitive host for most parasites **except** the following, in which it is an intermediate host: ▪ **Plasmodium (malaria)** ▪ **Echinococcus granulosus (Hydatid worm)** ▪ **Toxoplasma** ▪ **Sarcocystis indonensis**	**MNEMONIC** = **P.E.T.S**
Epizootic (Amplifier or amplifying)	• *I*s a vertebrate host in which infectious agent multiply rapidly to high level and provide source of infection to blood feeding arthropode vector. Examples are: ▪ Arboviral encephalitis (Pigs in JE) ▪ House flea in plague ▪ Rodents in plague	
Autoinfection is seen in	• Capillariasis • **H.** nana • Enterobius Vermicularis • Strongyloides • Taenia solium	**MNEMONIC** = **C.H.E.S.T**
Non bile stained (colourless) egg in stool	• N. americana (Hook worm) • E.vermicularis • H.nana • A. duodanale (Hook worm)	**MNEMONIC** = **N.E.H.A**
Tests in parasitology	• **String test is positive with –** Giardia, Cryptosporidium, parahaemolyticus • **Skin snip is positive in –** Oncocercariasis • **Sabin Feldman dye test –** Toxoplasmosis • **Frenkel's skin test –** Toxoplasmosis • **Xenodiagnosis –** Chaga's disease • **Fairleys test –** Schistosomiasis • **Casoni's test –** Hydatid cyst • **Montegro test –** Leishmaniasis	

70. Ans. (d) Trophoziotes

Ref: Paniker's Textbook of Medical Parasitology 7th ed page 66-68

(See life cycle of Plasmodium in AIIMS Nov 2017 Microbiology) (see page no. 267)

Transfusion malaria: Blood transfusion can accidentally transmit malaria, if donor is infected with malaria. The parasites remain viable in blood bank for 1–2 weeks. As this condition is induced by direct infection of red cells by the merozoites, pre-erythrocytic schizogony and hypnozoites are absent. Relapse does not occur and incubation period is short.

NOTE

In the erythrocyte, the merozoites loses its internal organelles and appears as a rounded body with a vacoule in the centre. These parasites are called the ring forms or young trophozoites.

AIIMS NOVEMBER 2015

71. Ans. (c) Paragonimus with 2 layers

Ref: Paniker Parasitology 6th ed page 153, Topley Wilson 10th Edition

Recall Bias

None of the recaller confirmed any exactly same image for this question. There are two school of thoughts. Some recallers believe that it was Echinococcus, others think that it was Paragonimus. But most of the recallers confirmed that in options "Echinococcus with 2 layers" was mentioned. Now since the cyst wall of Echinococcus is 3 layered it is unlikely to be the answer.

Now coming to the image. Since sometimes it is very difficult to make out the number of layers of the cyst wall in the images. The better way is to check the corresponding number of layers in the options only and match them.

Three points to be considered in the question are:

- Incidence and prevalence of the parasite
- Prediliction to lung and other organs
- Number of cyst layers

Option (A)

Pulmonary Echinococcosis: The most common site for the primary Hydatid cyst is liver (63%) followed by lung (25%). The cyst wall consist of ***three layers:*** (1) The pericyst, of host origin and consisting of compressed lung tissue with an associated inflammatory host reaction evoked by the parasite and fibrosis; (2) The ectocyst (Acellular laminated hyaline material); and (3) The endocyst (cellular germinal layer). In the given diagram below; scheme of a hydatid cyst: (A) pericyst membrane (inflammatory host reaction); (B) laminated layer (parasite origin); (C) germinal layer; (D) Brood Capsule, (E). Daughter cyst.

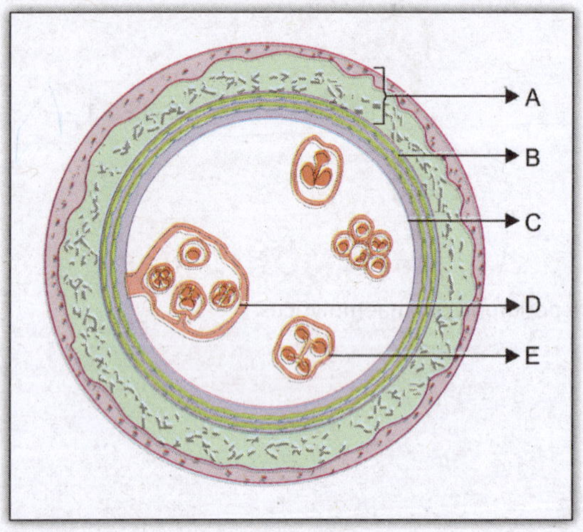

Option (B)

Strongyloides stercoralis may lead to cutaneous, pulmonary and intestinal manifestations along with hyperinfection. When larvae escape from the pulmonary capillaries into the alveoli, small hemorrhages may occur. Biopsy specimens containing these aberrantly migrating larvae may reveal a mild inflammatory response surrounding the parasite. Patchy infiltrates, diffuse interstitial pneumonitis and broncho-pneumonia may be detected. Larvae can be identified in sputum and bronchoalveolar lavage.

Option (D)

Histologically, the wall of a cysticercus cyst has **three distinct layers**; the outer cuticular layer, a middle cellular layer with pseudoepithelial structure and an inner reticular or fibrillary layer. The entire cyst is often surrounded by a pseudocapsule.

Option (C)

Paragonimus

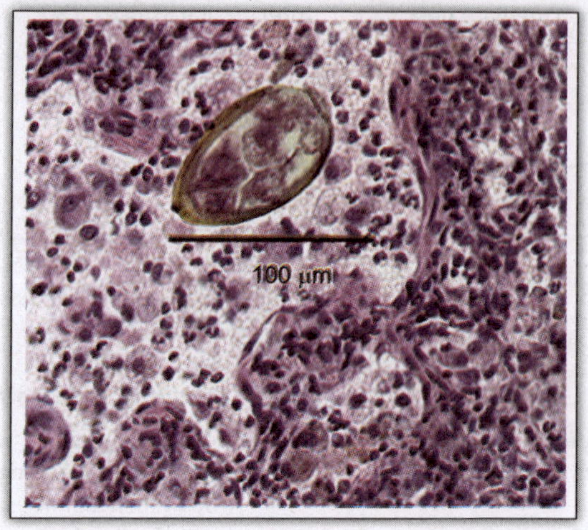

Source: CDC Atlanta

Fig: Paragonimus cyst: The pathologic lesions of paragonimiasis may be due to invasion and migration by the worms and host's immune responses to the invading parasites

- The basic pathology is the formation of a worm cyst primarily in the lungs. Usually located superficially, sometimes deep in the lung parenchyma contained dark red or rusty brown viscous fluid, red blood cells, inflammatory cells, eosinophils, necrotic tissue, Charcot-Leyden crystals and adult worms and ova.
- The adult worms are usually found at the periphery of the cyst, adhered to the cyst wall. Generally, a cyst contained paired worms, but single or more than two worms of the same or different species may be found.
- The cyst is communicated with bronchioles through which the cystic fluid, including the ova is discharged in the sputum to the exterior environment. If the sputum is swallowed as in case of young children, the ova can be detected in the faeces.
- Histopathologically, the worm cyst is composed of an outer fibro collagenous cyst wall with focal haemosiderinladen macrophages and an inner layer of congested blood vessels, inflammatory cells and normal or distorted ova.
- The size of the egg, approximately 85 micrometers, which was in the size range for Paragonimus spp. eggs.
- The presence of an operculum. This feature eliminates other helminth eggs in the same size range, Trichostrongylus, Ascaris (infertile) and Schistosoma japonicum.
- Location (lung tissue) where the eggs were found.

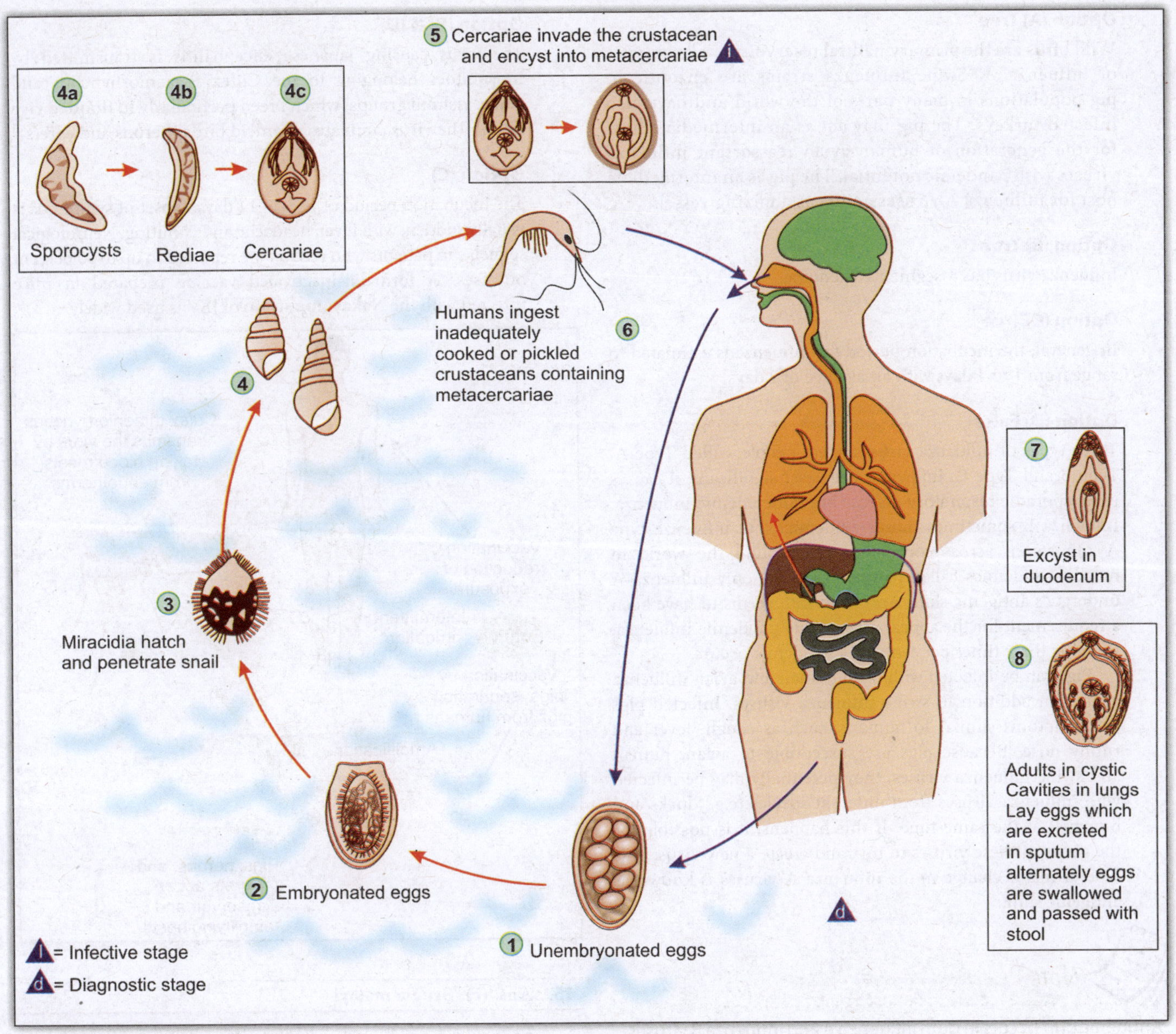

Source: CDC Illustrations

Fig: Life Cycle of Paragonimus: The eggs are excreted unembryonated in the sputum, or alternately they are swallowed and passed with stool ①. In the external environment, the eggs become embryonated ② and miracidia hatch and seek the first intermediate host, a snail and penetrate its soft tissues ③. Miracidia go through several developmental stages inside the snail ④: sporocysts ④a, rediae ④b, with the latter giving rise to many cercariae ④c, which emerge from the snail. The cercariae invade the second intermediate host, a crustacean such as a crab or crayfish, where they encyst and become metacercariae. This is the infective stage for the mammalian host ⑤. Human infection with P. westermani occurs by eating inadequately cooked or pickled crab or crayfish that harbor metacercariae of the parasite ⑥. The metacercariae excyst in the duodenum ⑦, penetrate through the intestinal wall into the peritoneal cavity, then through the abdominal wall and diaphragm into the lungs, where they become encapsulated and develop into adults ⑧ (7.5 to 12 mm by 4 to 6 mm). The worms can also reach other organs and tissues, such as the brain and striated muscles, respectively. However, when this takes place completion of the life cycles is not achieved, because the eggs laid cannot exit these sites. Time from infection to oviposition is 65 to 90 days.

72. Ans. (a) H. ducreyi

Ref: Jawetz 24th ed ch 19

See MICROSCOPY OF STD's (including H. Ducreyi) in AIIMS MAY 2017 Microbiology (see page no. 273)

73. Ans. (d) Pandemic is caused by all serotype

Ref: Jawetz and Topley Wilson 10th Ed

The picture above is of Influenza virus

See table of Influenza Virus in Microbiology AIIMS May 2016 (see page no. 474-475)

Option (A) True

Wild birds are the primary natural reservoir for all subtypes of influenza A. Swine influenza strains are enzootic in pig populations in many parts of the world and have also infected turkeys. The pig may act as an intermediate host for the generation of human avian reassortant influenza viruses with pandemic potential. The pig as an intermediate host for influenza A viruses acting as a mixing vessel.

Option (B) True

Influenza virus has 8-segmented genome.

Option (C) True

In general, the incubation period for influenza is estimated to range from 1 to 4 days with an average of 2 days.

Option (D) False

Three types of influenza viruses affect people, called Type A, Type B and Type C. Influenza C is least significant; it causes mild, sporadic respiratory disease but not epidemic influenza. Influenza B sometimes causes epidemics, but influenza type A can sweep across continents and around the world in massive epidemics called pandemics. Also, only influenza A undergoes antigenic shift. Antigenic shift seems to have been a requirement for the appearance of true pandemic influenza. Roughly three times per century, a pandemic occurs.

Pigs can be infected with both human and avian influenza viruses in addition to swine influenza viruses. Infected pigs get symptoms similar to humans, such as cough, fever and runny nose. Because pigs are susceptible to avian, human and swine influenza viruses, they potentially may be infected with influenza viruses from different species (e.g., ducks and humans) at the same time. If this happens, it is possible for the genes of these viruses to mix and create a new virus. This type of major change in the influenza A viruses is known as antigenic shift.

NOTE

Antigenic drift occurs in both influenza A and influenza B viruses, while antigenic shift is seen in Influenza A virus only.

74. Ans. (d) Caused by aedes

Ref: Jawetz 24th ed chapter 38, CDC Atlanta

Recall Bias

Some recalls said that the question was simply about identifying the disease i.e. Japanese encephalitis

Option (A)

Pigs are amplifying hosts, in that the virus reproduces in pigs and infects mosquitoes that take blood meals, but does not cause disease. The virus tends to spill over into human populations when infected mosquito populations build up explosively and the human biting rate increases (these culicines are normally zoophilic, i.e. they prefer to take blood meals from animals).

Option (B) & (D)

The virus causing Japanese encephalitis is transmitted by mosquitoes belonging to the **Culex** tritaeniorhynchus and Culex vishnui groups, which breed particularly in **flooded rice fields.** The virus circulates in ardeid birds (herons and egrets).

Option (C)

The incubation period of JE is 5–14 days. Onset of symptoms is usually sudden, with fever, headache and vomiting. Neurological sequelae in patients who recover are reported in up to 30 percent of cases. A formalin-inactivated vaccine prepared in mice infected with the **Nakayama strain** of JEV is used widely.

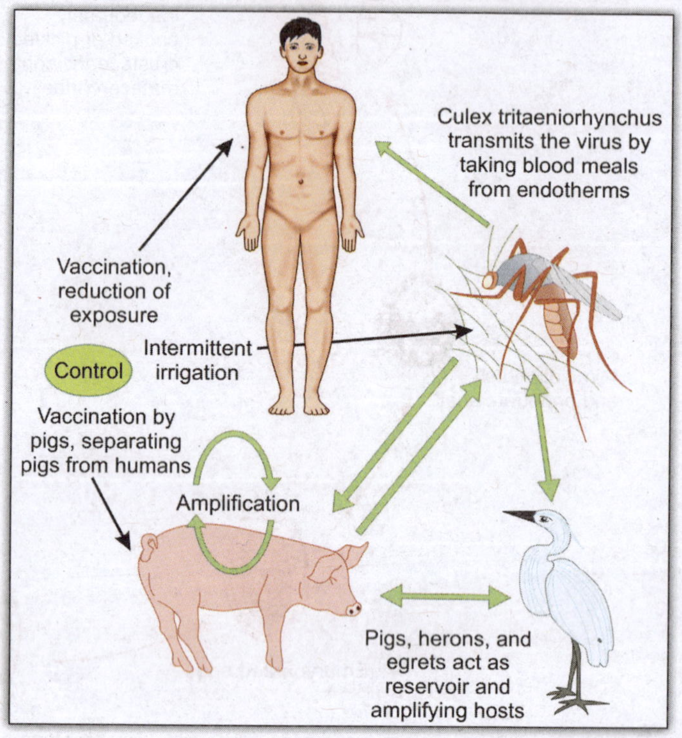

75. Ans. (c) Brugia malayi

Ref: Jawetz 24th ed chapter 46, Paniker Parasitology 6th ed page 203, CDC Atlanta, http://apps.who.int/iris bitstream/10665/37156/1/9241544899_eng.pdf

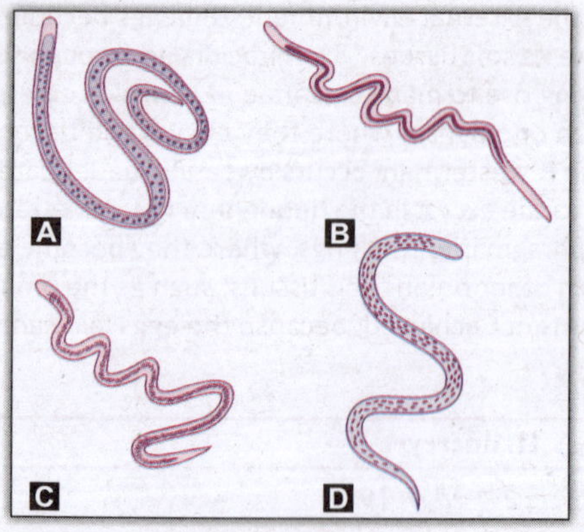

Figs A and B: The picture shows a schematic diagrams of Microfilarias of medical importance. **A.** Wuchereria bancrofti; **B.** Brugia malayi, **C.** Loa; **D.** Onchocerca volvulus

NOTE

Microfilariae are found in peripheral blood (in blood smear) only at night (nocturnal periodicity), largely at night or during crepuscular hours (subperiodicity), largely during daylight hours (diurnal periodicity), or without clear distinction (nonperiodic).

Microfilarias of Medical Importance

	(A) Wuchereria bancrofti	(B) Brugia malayi	(C) Loa Loa	(D) Onchocerca volvulus
Vector	Mosquito sp Depending on geographical distribution	Mansonia and Aedes	Deerflies (also known as mango flies or mangrove flies) of the genus Chrysops	Blackflies of the genus Simulium
Microfilaria found in	Blood (nocturnal periodicity)	Blood (nocturnal periodicity)	Blood (Diurnal)	Tissue (skin) (No periodicity, sample can be collected ay time)
Sheath	Present (unstained with haematoxylin, stains pale pink on giemsa)	Present (stains pink red on giemsa, unstained on haematoxylin), loose sheath with kinky curves	Present (stained pink with haematoxylin but unstained on giemsa)	**Absent**
Head space	Length= width (free of nuclei)	*Twice as long as width* (long head/cephalic space)	Short cephalic/head space	Long head space
Body	Smooth/Sweeping graceful curves	Folded in angular fashion	Irregular curves with **corkscrew appearance**	Long body with less curves
Body Nuclei	Well separated/dispersed yet numerous	Crowded and darkly stained	Coarse and crowded (**single row of nuclei** till the end of tail)	Well marked, moderately compact nuclei and elongated terminal nuclei
Interbody (amorphous mass seen in some sp)	**Stained pink with giemsa** but not satined with Haematoxylin	Not easily identified	Not easily identified	Not easily identified
Cytoplasm	Cytoplasm extends beyond the last nuclei	Terminal nuclei	Terminal nuclei (are irregularly spaced)	Cytoplasm extend beyond the last nuclei
Tail	Taper, Anucleate	Tapers, **Subterminal and terminal nuclei** (2 nuclei that appears connected by fine thread)	Taper, Nuclei irregularly spaced to extend to the tip of tail. Tails is sometimes flexed/coiled within the sheath.	Tapers to a sharp point, **typically flexed**, Anucleate

76. Ans. (d) H2N1

Ref: Jawetz 24th ed chapter 39, Topley & Wilson 10th Ed

See table of Influenza Virus in Microbiology AIIMS May 2016 (For season influenza vaccine (see page no. 274-275)

NOTE

Season flu vaccine is different from H1N1 vaccine. H1N1 vaccine does not provide protection against seasonal flu.

77. Ans. (b) Ingestion of egg contaminated in water

Ref: Jawetz 24th ed chapter 46, Paniker parasitology 6th ed page 166

Recall Bias

Some recalls says that in place of option (B) Feco oral route was given, which is also correct

See table of Parasitic Nematode in Microbiology AIIMS May 2016 (see page no. 291)

See Trichuris Trichura in AIIMS NOV 2016 Microbiology (see page no. 280)

Trichuris Trichiura (Whipworm)

Infection by T. trichiura occurs in humans when mature embryonated eggs containing the infective larvae are swallowed in contaminated food or water. The eggs are barrel shaped, brown in color, bile stained, triple shelled. It has colourless mucus plug at each pole and contain unsegmented ovum. Eggs float in saturated salt solution.

78. Ans. (b) Chronic hepatitis recovery state

Ref: Harrison 18th ed Table 304-5

Serologic Patterns of Hepatitis B Infection

HBsAg	HBeAg	Anti-HBc	Anti-HBs	Anti-HBe	Interpretation
+	+	IgM	–	–	Acute hepatitis B, high infectivity
+	+	IgG	–	–	Chronic hepatitis B, high infectivity
+	–	IgG	–	+	Late acute or chronic hepatitis B, low infectivity HBeAg–negative ("precore–mutant") hepatitis B (chronic or, rarely, acute)
+	+/–	+	+	+/–	HBsAg of one subtype and heterotypic anti–HBs (common) Process of seroconversion from HBsAg to anti– HBs (rare)
–	+/–	IgM	–	+/–	Acute hepatitis B Anti–HBc "window"
–	–	IgG	+	+	HBV infection in recent past, convalescence
–	–	IgG	+	–	HBV infection in distant past, recovery (Immune due to natural infection)
+	--	IgG	–	–	Simple carrier (Healthy carrier)
+	+	IgG	–	–	Super carrier (persistent carrier)
–	–	–	+	–	Immunization with HBsAg (after vaccination) Hepatitis B in the remote past (?) False–positive

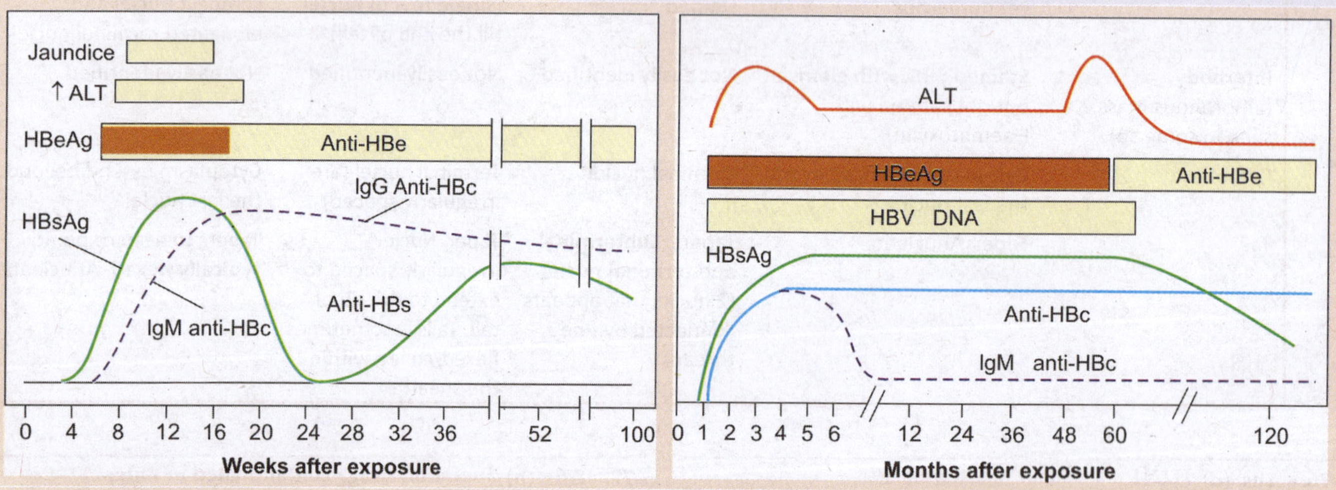

- **First virologic marker** detectable in serum within 1–12 weeks, usually between 8–12 weeks, is **HBsAg**
- **Anti-HBc is first antibody marker** to appear in HBV infection and is readily demonstrable in serum, beginning within the first 1–2 weeks after the appearance of HBsAg and preceding detectable levels of anti-HBs by weeks to months.
- After HBsAg disappears, antibody to HBsAg (anti-HBs) becomes detectable in serum and remains detectable indefinitely thereafter.
- The titer of HBsAg bears little relation to the severity of clinical disease. Indeed, an inverse correlation exists between the serum concentration of HBsAg and the degree of liver cell damage.
- Principal clinical usefulness of **HBeAg is as an indicator of relative infectivity**
- **Markers of replication:** HBeAg, HBV DNA (viral load): 2,000 IU/ml in his blood (= 10,000 copies/ml) HBeAg is a qualitative marker and HBV DNA a quantitative marker of this replicative phase, during which all three forms of HBV circulate, including intact virions.
- Pre-S1 and pre-S2 proteins are also expressed during periods of peak replication, but assays for these gene products are not routinely available

Contd...

- Because **HBcAg is intracellular** and, when in the serum, sequestered within an HBsAg coat, naked core particles do not circulate in serum and, therefore, HBcAg is not detectable routinely in the serum of patients with HBV infection.
- **Window period:** Time gap between disappearance of HBsAg and the appearance of anti-HBs. *During this "gap" or "window" period, anti-HBc may represent the only serologic evidence* of current or recent HBV infection
- Most instances of **isolated anti-HBc** represent hepatitis B infection in the remote past. Rarely, however, isolated anti-HBc represents low-level hepatitis B viremia, with HBsAg below the detection threshold; occasionally, isolated anti-HBc represents a cross-reacting or false-positive immunologic specificity
- Anti-HBc of the IgM class (IgM anti-HBc) predominates during the first six months after acute infection, whereas IgG anti-HBc is the predominant class of anti-HBc beyond six months.
- **After immunization** with hepatitis B vaccine, which consists of HBsAg alone, anti-HBs is the only serologic marker to appear
- Based on serological markers, hepatitis B carriers have classified into two types: super carriers and simple carriers. Super carriers have high titres of HBsAg and HBV DNA in their blood along with HBeAg.
- The **simple carrier** patient continues to shed HBsAg and the **super carrier** continues to shed HBsAg and HBeAg beyond the 24th week/6 months from the start of infection.

79. Ans. (d) Noro virus

Ref: Harrison 19th ed page 1285 Medical Microbiology By Patrick R. Murray, Ken S. Rosenthal, Michael A. Pfaller 8th ed Page 473, Bailey & Scott's Diagnostic Microbiology By Patricia Tille 13th ed Page 825, http://www.cdc.gov/norovirus/

- Norwalk virus belongs to the family of **Caliciviridae.** The genus name Norovirus is derived from Norwalk virus, the only species in the genus.
- **Norwalk virus**, the prototypical **norovirus**, was discovered during an epidemic of acute gastroenteritis in Norwalk, Ohio, in 1968.
- Norwalk virus belongs to the Norovirus is a non-enveloped, round, 27-nm particle with a 'ragged' outer edge but lacking a definite surface structure. It possesses a single capsid protein.
- **Noroviruses are the most important cause of epidemic non bacterial outbreaks of gastroenteritis worldwide.** The epidemiology of Norovirus infections include not only person-to-person spread but also mechanical transmission from hand to mouth. In addition to these modes of transmission, Noroviruses are often associated with outbreaks. Noroviruses are the major cause of viral gastroenteritis arising from eating **shellfish**
- Symptoms are sudden in onset and are accompanied by nausea and vomiting, which can be projectile and severe. Low-grade fever and diarrhea usually occur, the latter being relatively mild. In contrast to bacterial gastroenteritis, diarrheal stools do not contain blood, mucus, or white cells. In general, Norovirus infections are self-limiting and affected patients rarely need to be hospitalized

80. Ans. (d) Nocardia, Gram's stain

Ref: Jawetz 24th ed chapter 15, BRS Microbiology 4th ed page 39-41

Recall Bias

Some recallers believe that it was Streptococcus (you must know how to differentiate chains of streptococcus from filaments or nocardia; chains are more beaded and filaments are more branched). Some recallers think Cryptococcus in India ink was a separate question.

Nocardia

These bacteria are gram-positive, catalase-positive and partially acid-fast bacilli. Nocardiae form extensive branching substrates and aerial filaments that fragment after formation, breaking into coccobacillary cells. The cell walls contain mycolic acids that are shorter chained than those of Mycobacteria. They are considered to be **weakly acid-fast**, but if they are stained with the routine acid-fast reagent (carbol-fuchsin) but decolorized with 1–4% sulfuric acid instead of the stronger acid-alcohol decolorant, most isolates will stain acid-fast. **Gram-stained smears reveal gram-positive bacilli, coccobacillary cells and branching filaments.** With the modified acid-fast stain, most isolates will be acid-fast.

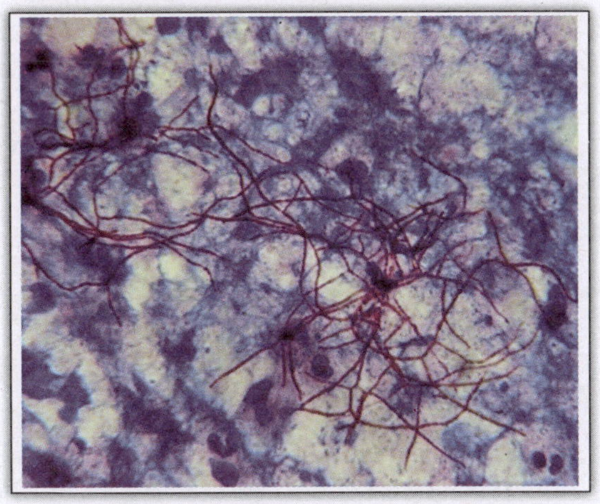

Fig: Nocardia, partially acid fast staining: (Pink in blue background). Partial Acid-Fast staining employed: Carbol fuscin stain (3 min), decolourize with 1% H_2SO_4 (until colour no longer comes off ~1 min) and counterstain with methyene blue (30 sec).

81. Ans. (a) Plasmodium vivax

Ref: Jawetz 24th ed Table 46-2 & 3, Paniker parasitology 6th ed page 79

This is a famous CDC illustration used commonly to demonstrate stages of different malaria parasite. The illustration has 30 sub numbered illustrations, hence Plasmodium Ovale and Plasmodium Malariae are ruled out (which have 25 sub illustrations each). The gametocytes in the illustration are round (not Banana shaped), hence Plasmodium falciparum is ruled out.

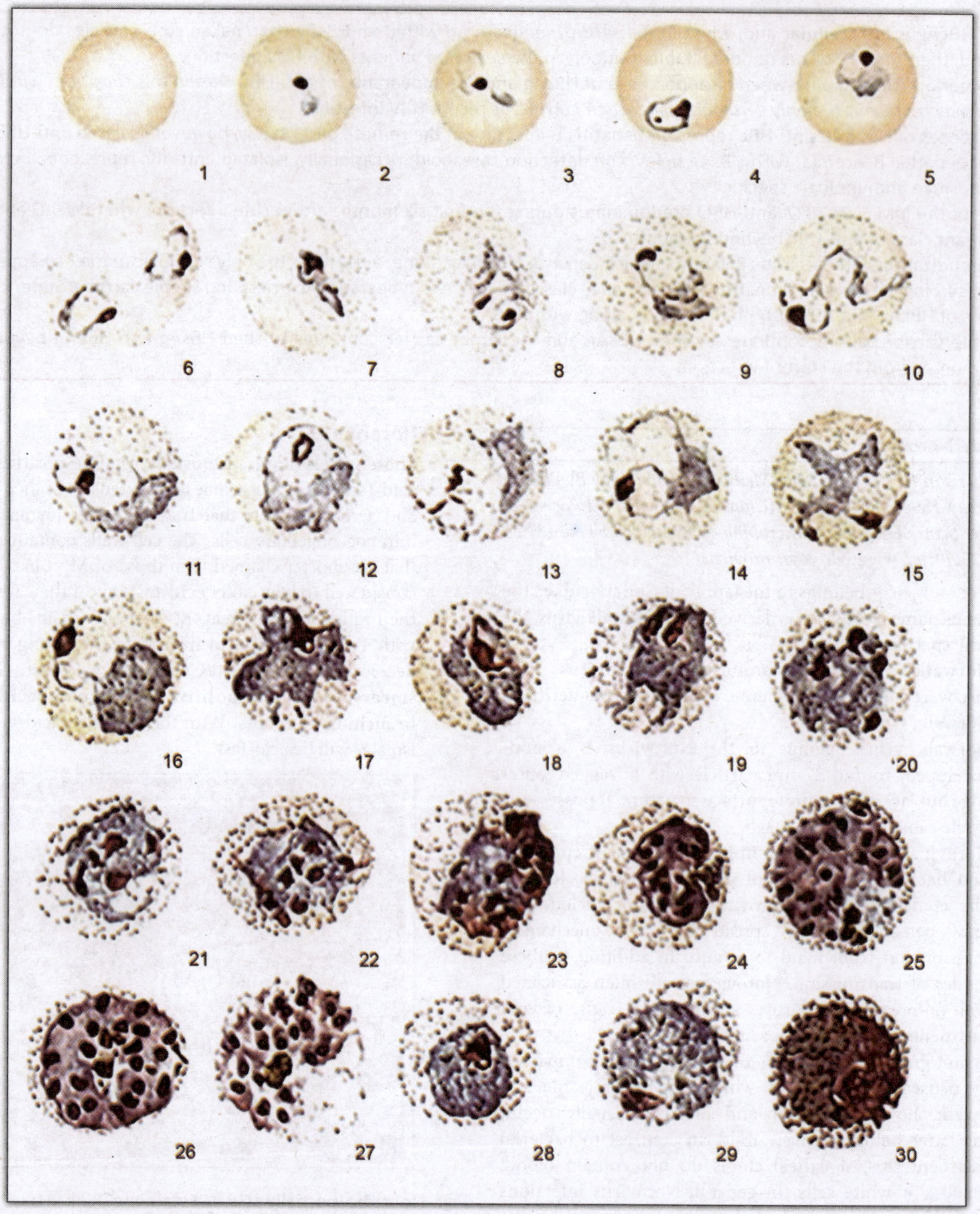

Fig: Plasmodium Vivax- Blood Stage Parasites: Thin Blood Smears

Keys: 1. Normal red cell; **2–6.** Young trophozoites (ring stage parasites); **7–18.** Trophozoites; **19–27.** Schizonts; **28–29.** Macrogametocytes (female)—Microgametocyte (male)

82. Ans. (a) Grams stain

Ref: BRS 4th ed page 103, Paniker 8th ed page 391-392

Actinomyces

General Characteristics

- Actinomyces is a filamentous, **non acid-fast, gram-positive bacilli**. Its filamentous growth and mycelialike colonies have a striking resemblance to fungi
- Is anaerobic, non spore forming, cast forming
- While individual bacteria are **rod-shaped**, Actinomyces colonies form **fungus-like branched** networks of hyphae
- Is found as a commensal organism in the gingival crevices and female genital tract.
- Causes chronic granulomatous infections, mainly of the soft tissues (although it also invades bone), with swelling and a tendency to form sinus tracts to the surface; exudate from these sinus tracts contains hard microcolonies called granules. Actinomyces has little respect for anatomic barriers.

Classification: The organism is related to the mycobacteria and belongs to the Actinomycetes.

· Attributes of pathogenicity. The organism grows contiguously in tissues with reduced oxygenation. Actinomycosis is most commonly caused by Actinomyces Israelii.

Clinical Disease

- Cervicofacial actinomycosis (**painless lumpy jaw**) most commonly begins after dental work is performed.
- Thoracic actinomycosis may involve the lungs and ribs.
- Abdominal actinomycosis starts in the ileocecal region and frequently produces sinus tracts to the skin surface.
- Mycetoma is an infection of the limb, with swelling, sinus tract formation and granules.

Laboratory diagnosis is by Gram stain of granules and anaerobic culture.

Treatment commonly involves penicillin and surgical drainage of necrotic tissues.

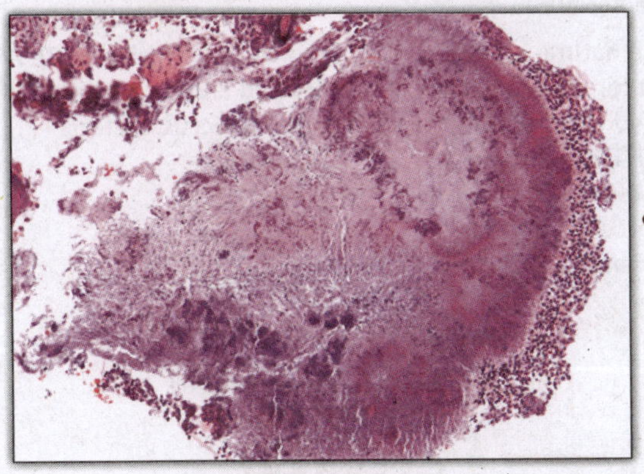

Fig: **Actinomyces H&E stain:** High magnification micrograph of a **sulfur granule** formed by actinomyces in the mandible. Histopathology - For most purposes, recognition is based on the appearances of sulphur granules using the ***hematoxylin and eosin (H&E) stain***. These granules actually represent colonies of A. israelii, a gram-positive, anaerobic filamentous bacteria

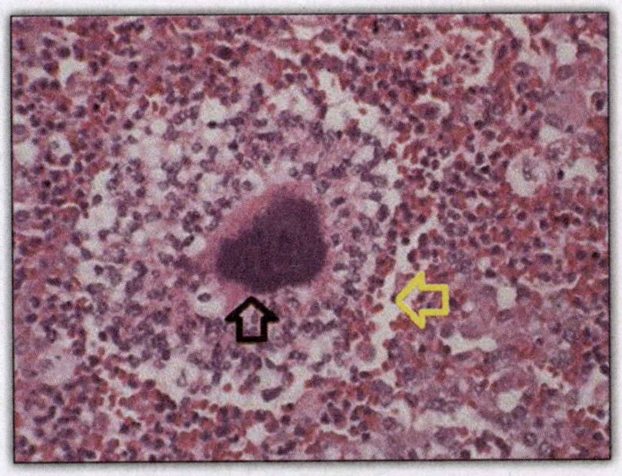

Fig: **Actinomyces grams stain:** Showing tangled mass of branching filaments (black arrow), surrounded by a hypocellular artifactual cleft (yellow arrow) surrounded by neutrophils and macrophages.

NOTE

Specific fungal stains such as the methenamine silver and periodic acid Schiff (PAS) stains are useful to ensure that fungi are present, but are seldom helpful for specific diagnosis. Actinomycete filaments also take up silver based stains

Actinomycosis Vs Nocardia

	Actinomycosis	Nocardia (Aerobic)
• Gram stain	Gram +ve filamentous branching	Gram +ve filamentous branching
• Acid fastness	Not	AFB +ve weak (but N. madurae AFB –ve)
• Morpho	• Non-motile • Non-sporing • Non-capsulated	• Non-motile • Non-sporing • Non-capsulated
• Infection in	In immunocompitant	In immunocompromised (HIV/AIDS)
• Clinical features	• Oro-cervicofacial (MC type)- woody/lump jaw • Appendix in GIT • PID in IUCD users (A. israelii)	• Airborn inhalation –thick sputum • CXR-Lt. lower lobe nodule with central cavitation
• Microscopy	Spidery colony & Sun-ray appearance: Ray fungus Sulphur granules	Paraffin bait technique
• Treatment	Penicillin	TMP-SMX/Sulfonamides

83. Ans. (a) Transduction

Ref: Ananthranayan 8th ed page 65-67, Jawetz 24th edition chapter 7

Bacterial Genetics		
Mechanism	**Comments**	**Study**
Conjugation	Transfer of genetic material between bacterial cells by direct cell to cell contact or by bridge like connections	Studied by **Lederburg and Tatum in Escherichia coli.**
Transduction	Donor DNA is carried in a virus phage coat (**Bacteriophage**) and is transferred into the recipient by the mechanism used for phage infection. Occasionally the DNA of bacteriophage combines with the DNA of bacterial cell.	Studied by **Lederburg and Zinder** in Salmonella.
Transformation	Direct uptake of donor DNA by the recipient cell, may be natural or forced. Relatively few bacterial species are naturally competent for transformation; these species assimilate donor DNA in linear form. Forced transformation is induced in the laboratory, where, after treatment with high salt and temperature shock, many bacteria are rendered competent for the assimilation of extracellular plasmids. The capacity to force bacteria to incorporate extracellular plasmids by transformation is fundamental to genetic engineering.	Studied by **Griffith (1928), Avery, McLeoid and McCarty (1944)** in **Pneumococcus** bacteria.

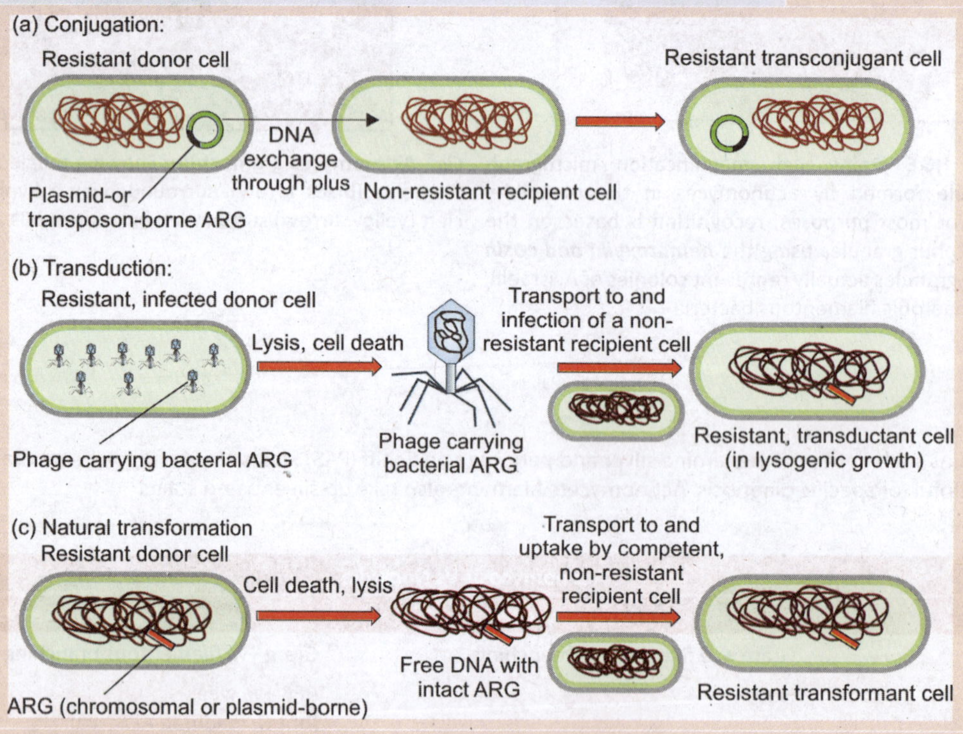

Footnote:
- Conjugation is mechanism of horizontal gene transfer as are transformation and transduction, although these two other mechanisms do not involve cell to cell conduct.
- Introduction of foreign DNA into eukaryotic cell is often called **transfection**

84. Ans. (b) Dengue hemorrhagic shock syndrome

Ref: Harrison 19th ed page 1322

Antibody-dependent enhancement (ADE) of virus infection is a process whereby virus-specific antibodies enhance the entry of virus into macrophages via interaction with Fc and/ or complement receptors. The phenomenon is observed with many diverse virus infections, for example, flaviviruses to poxviruses, with the common theme that they target macrophages as a site of infection.

The antiviral protein (i.e. The antibodies) bind to antibody Fc receptors. The most widely known example of ADE occurs in the setting of infection with dengue virus. In dengue virus infection, children aged <1 year are particularly susceptible, probably because of waning protective maternal antibody leading to infectious immune complexes resulting in exacerbation of infection. This enhancement of infectivity can **lead to dengue hemorrhagic fever or dengue shock syndrome.** ADE can also be seen in individuals subsequently infected with another dengue virus subtype to which there are cross-reactive antibodies. In such cases clinical course of the disease is more severe and those people have higher viremia.

This explains the observation that while primary (first) infection causes mostly minor disease (DF), secondary infection/reinfection is more likely to be associated with severe disease (DHF/DHS)

ADE of infection has also been reported in HIV.

AIIMS MAY 2015

85. Ans. (c) Nasopharyngeal carcinoma

Ref: Anantnarayan 9th ed page 553

Human Papilloma Virus	
Disease	**HPV TYPE**
Common warts (Verruca vulgaris)	2, 7
Plantar warts (verruca plantaris)	1, 2, 4, 63
Flat warts (Verruca plana)	3, 10
Anogenital warts (condyloma acuminatum)	6, 11, 42, 44 and others **(types 6 and 11 account for about 90% of all cases)** (75% by HPV-6)
Genital cancers	Highest risk: 16, 18, 31, 45 HPV types **(16 and 18 cause 70% of cervical cancer)** Other high-risk: 33, 35, 39, 51, 52, 56, 58, 59 Probably high-risk: 26, 53, 66, 68, 73, 82
Epidermodysplasia verruciformis	HPV types 5 and 8
Heck's disease- Focal epithelial hyperplasia (oral)	13, 32
Oral papillomas	6, 7, 11, 16, 32
HPV-positive oropharyngeal cancer	16
Laryngeal papillomatosis	6, 11

Virus Associated With Human Malignancy		
Virus Family	**Virus**	**Human cancer**
Papillomaviridae	Human papillomaviruses (HPV)	Genital tumors (Ca Cervix) Squamous cell carcinoma Oropharyngeal carcinoma (Tonsillar, Base of tongue, etc)
Herpesviridae	EB virus	Nasopharyngeal carcinoma Burkitt's lymphoma Hodgkin's disease B cell lymphoma
	Human herpesvirus 8	Kaposi's sarcoma
Hepadnaviridae	Hepatitis B virus	Hepatocellular carcinoma
Retroviridae	HTL virus	Adult T cell leukemia
	Human immunodeficiency virus	AIDS-related malignancies
Flaviviridae	Hepatitis C virus	Hepatocellular carcinoma

86. Ans. (b) Hepatitis B virus

Ref: Robbin's 9th ed page 615-16, Anantnarayan 9th ed page 540

HBV Structure and Genome

The HBV is a member of the Hepadnaviridae, a group of DNA-containing viruses that cause hepatitis in many animal species. HBV replication does not involve the integration of the virus in the DNA of the host cell, but integrated HBV frequently is found in cells. The integrated viruses generally have large deletions and rearrangements and usually become inactive. The genome of HBV is a partially double-stranded circular DNA molecule of 3200 nucleotides that encodes

- The precore/core region of a nucleocapsid "core" protein, the *hepatitis B core antigen (HBcAg)* and a precore protein designated hepatitis Be antigen (HBeAg). HBcAg is retained in the infected hepatocyte; HBeAg is secreted into blood and is essential for the establishment of persistent infection.
- Envelope glycoprotein, the *hepatitis B surface antigen (HBsAg)*, which may be produced and secreted into the blood in massive amounts. Blood HBsAg is immunogenic.
- A *DNA polymerase* with an error-prone reverse transcriptase activity that generates mutations in the genomes of replicating virus at a high rate.
- *HBV-X* protein, which acts as a transcriptional transactivator for many viral and host genes through interaction with various transcription factors. HBV-X is required for viral infectivity and may have a role in the development of hepatocellular carcinoma by regulating p53 degradation and expression.

Clinical and Epidemiologic Features of Viral Hepatitis					
Feature	**HAV**	**HBV**	**HCV**	**HDV**	**HEV**
Family	Picornaviridae	Hepadnaviridae	Flaviviridae	Unclassified	Unclassified
Genus	Hepatovirus	Orthohepadnavirus	Hepacivirus	Deltavirus	Hepevirus
Virion	27 nm, icosahedral	42 nm, spherical	60 nm, spherical	35 nm, spherical	30–32 nm, icosahedral
Envelope	No	Yes (HBsAg)	Yes	Yes (HBsAg)	No

Contd...

Clinical and Epidemiologic Features of Viral Hepatitis					
Feature	**HAV**	**HBV**	**HCV**	**HDV**	**HEV**
Genome	ssRNA	DsDNA	ssRNA	ssRNA	ssRNA
Stability	Heat & acid stable	Acid-sensitive	Ether-sensitive, acid-sensitive	Acid-sensitive	Heat-stable
Prevalence	High	High	Moderate	Low, regional	Regional
Incubation (days)	15–45, mean 30	30–180, mean 60–90	15–160, mean 50	30–180, mean 60–90	14–60, mean 40
Onset	Acute	Insidious or acute	Insidious	Insidious or acute	Acute
Age preference	Children, young adults	Young adults (sexual and percutaneous), babies, toddlers	Any age, but more common in adults	Any age (similar to HBV)	Young adults (20–40 years)
Transmission					
Fecal-oral	+++	–	–	–	+++
Percutaneous	Unusual	+++ (MC mode of transmission)	+++	+++	–
Perinatal	–	+++	±	+	–
Sexual	±	++	±	++	–
Clinical					
Severity	Mild	Occasionally severe	Moderate	Occasionally severe	Mild
Fulminant	0.1%	0.1–1% (most common, >50% of all cases of viral fulminant hepatitis)	0.1%	5–20% (highest chances of progression to fulminant hepatitis)	1–2%
Progression to chronicity	None (HAV remains self limited & does not progress to chronic liver disease	Occasional (1–10%) (90% of neonates)	Common (>50% – 85%)	Common (<5% coinfection, 80% upon super infection)	None
Carrier	None	0.1–30% 0.1-1% of blood donors in U.S & west	1.5–3.2% 0.2–1% of blood donors in US & west	Variable 1–10% in drug addicts & henophiliac	None
Hepatocellular carcinoma	No	Yes (neonatal infection)	Yes	No increase above HBV	None
Prognosis	Excellent	Worse with age, debility	Moderate	Acute → good, Chronic → poor	Good
Prophylaxis	IG Inactivated vaccine	HBIG Recombinant vaccine	None	HBV vaccine (none for HBV carriers)	Vaccine
Therapy	None	Interferon Lamivudine Adefovir Pegylated interferon Entecavir Telbivudine	Pegylated interferon plus ribavirin	Interferon ±	None

Footnote:
- Though prognosis of HDV with HBV is a bad prognosis, however prognosis of super infection is worse than coinfection.
- Likely hood of progression to chronic hepititis is maximum in HCV infection
- Likely hood of progression to fulminant hepatitis is maximum in HDV
- Most common viral cause of chronic hepatitis is HBV (because of its high incidence)
- Most common viral cause of fulminant hepatitis is HBV (because of its high incidence)

87. Ans. (a) H. influenzae strains are known to produce beta lactamase

Ref: Bailey and Scott 13th ed page 407-408, Harrison 19th ed page 1011, Ananthanarayan 9th ed page 327

Although widespread H. influenzae is capable of producing beta-lactamase (penicillin resistance), third-generation cephalosporins are not notably affected by the enzyme (i.e., ceftriaxone and cefotaxime) and may be effective therapeutic agents. β-Lactamase mediated resistance to ampicillin is common; β-lactam resistance by altered PBP (Penicillin binding protein) target is rare (≤1% of strains). Resistance to third- generation cephalosporins has not been documented.

88. Ans. (a) Onchocerca volvulus

Ref: Jawetz 24th page 691-698

Elephantiasis, a morbid gross enlargement of limbs, breasts and genitalia, is an immunopathologic response to long-continued filarial infection by Wuchereria or Brugia. Adult worms embedded in lymph tissues are the primary cause of these massive inflammatory and fibrotic reactions. **With *Onchocerca*, it is the microfilariae, actually elongated microscopic embryos, that cause the most severe damage.**

Many Authors argue for option D as it is non pathogenic. But it does cause few diseases and the adult worm is responsible for the same. Mansonella ozzardi is new world filarial, which is almost non-pathogenic but may cause **Ozzard's mansonelliasis (benign)** and occasionally hydrocele.

Similar question was asked in Jawet's Microbiology 24th ed page 698:

MCQ's. Pathologic effects of filariae in humans are caused by the adult worms in all but one species and in that case the principal damage is caused by the microfilariae. That species is (A) *Brugia malayi* (B) *Mansonella ozzardi* (C) *Dracunculus medinensis* (D) *Wuchereria bancrofti* (E) *Onchocerca volvulus* (F) *Loa loa Answer given is (E) Onchocerca – Jawetz 24/E, p698*

89. Ans. (c) Zonula occludens

Ref: Topley and Wilson, 10/E p, Chapter: Vibrio, p 11-12

Vibrio cholerae O1 causes diarrhea via the following five virulence factors: toxin coregulated pili, neuramidase, accessory cholera enterotoxin, zonula occludens toxin (ZOT) and cholera toxin (CT). **ZOT acts by loosening the tight junctions (zonnula occludens) of small-intestinal mucosa, thereby increasing intestinal permeability.**

Characteristic of Different Toxins

Toxins	Mechanism of action
Strychnine	• Post-synaptic inhibition of Neurotransmitter Glycine in spinal cord. • Acts on Antr.horn cell of spinal cord & inhibit post syneptic potential leading to release excitation.
Botulinum	• During the growth of *C botulinum* and during autolysis of the bacteria, toxin is liberated into the environment. • Seven antigenic varieties of toxin **(A to G)** are known. • Types **A, B and E (and occasionally F)** are the principal causes of human illness. Types A and B have been associated with a variety of foods and type E predominantly with fish products. Type C produces limberneck in birds; type D causes botulism in mammalsother than humans. • Botulinum toxin is absorbed from the gut and binds to receptors of presynaptic membranes of motor neurons of the peripheral nervous system and cranial nerves. • **Although all botulinum toxins have different molecular targets, they have same mechanism of action.** Proteolysis by the light chain of botulinum toxin of either **synaptobrevin, syntaxin, or SNAP-25** in the neurons **inhibits the release of acetylcholine at the synapse of peripheral nerves**, resulting in lack of muscle contraction and paralysis. • The SNARE proteins are synaptobrevin, SNAP 25 and syntaxin. The toxins of *C botulinum* types A and E cleave the 25,000-MW SNAP-25. Type B toxin cleaves synaptobrevin. • *C botulinum* toxins are among the most toxic substances known: The lethal dose for a human is probably about **1-2 µg**. The toxins are destroyed by heating for 20 minutes at 100°C.
Teatanus	• Tetanospasmin toxin inhibit presyneptic release of Neurotransmitter Glycin & GABA in CNS. • Toxins acts on Moter end plate, spinal cord, brain & sympathetic nervous system.
Cholera toxin	• Is a complex A-B toxin which is structurally and functionally similar to heat labile Enterotoxin of E. coli • Active **A subunit** regulates Adenylcyclase activity causing irreversible ADP ribosylation of GTP binding protein (cAMP acts as second messenger). • **B subunit is pentameric** binding subunit it binds GM gangliosides receptors in the intestinal epithelium
Zonula occludens toxin	Zonula occludens toxin. ZOT acts by loosening the **tight junctions** (zonnula occludens) of small-intestinal mucosa, thereby increasing intestinal permeability. Zonula occludens toxin modulates tight junctions through protein kinase C-dependent actin reorganization
Diphtheria toxin	• Produced by toxigenic or virulent strains **of *C. diphtheriae*.** • About 90-95% gravis and intermedius strains are toxigenic, while only 80-85% of mitis are so. • Diphtheria toxin is a protein and very potent exotoxin.Consist of **two functionally distinct polypeptide chains**.Both fragments are required for toxicity- • ***Fragment A***—N-terminal, It has enzymatic activity. It causes irreversible inhibition of protein synthesis by NAD^+ dependent ADP ribosylation of **EF-2** which results in cell death. • ***Fragment B***—C-terminal, responsible for Binding the toxin to the cells. The antibody to fragment B prevents the binding of toxin to the cells and is thus protective. • ***Pertussis toxin** also acts by ADP ribosylation*

Pathology

5

AIIMS NOVEMBER 2018

1. Which of the following is an immune privileged site? ***(AIIMS Nov 2018, 2015)***

a. Seminiferous tubule
b. Loop of henley
c. Area postrema
d. Optic disc

2. How will you differentiate a mediastinal mass due to thymoma from that due to acute lymphoblastic leukaemia (ALL)?

a. Tdt
b. CD 1a
c. CD3
d. Cytokeratin

3. Patient with retroperitoneal mass presents with intermittent fever, no history of weight loss or anorexia. After surgery mass was removed which showed a smooth fleshy mass and Histopathology showing small blue cells in a concentric fashion. What could be diagnosis?

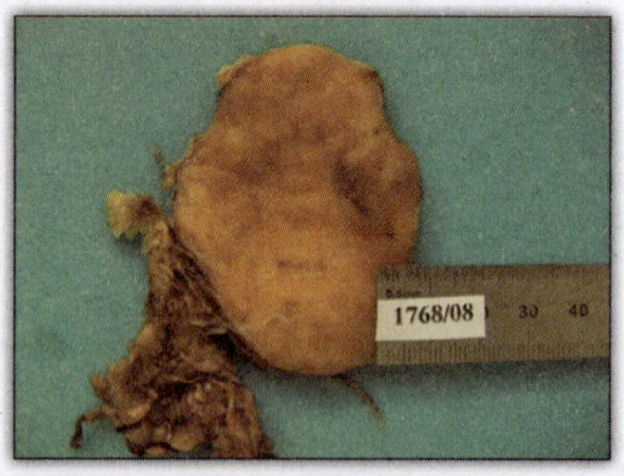

© Theodosopoulos T et al Case Rep Surg (2013)

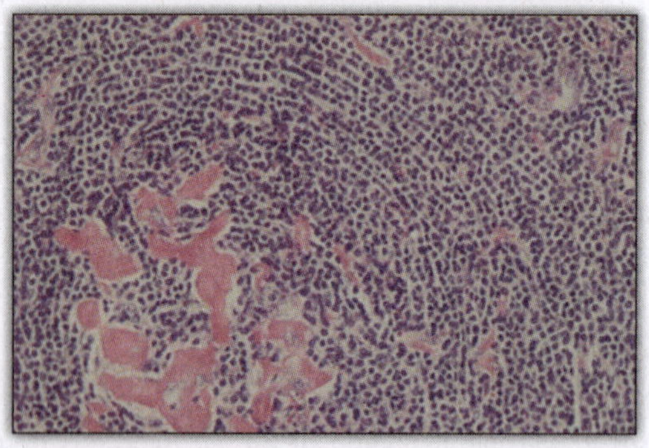

© Theodosopoulos T et al Case Rep Surg (2013)

a. Angiolymphoid hyperplasia
b. Non Hodgkin's lymphoma
c. IgG4 disease
d. Castleman's disease

4. Which of following Vacutainer tubes contains Sodium fluoride?

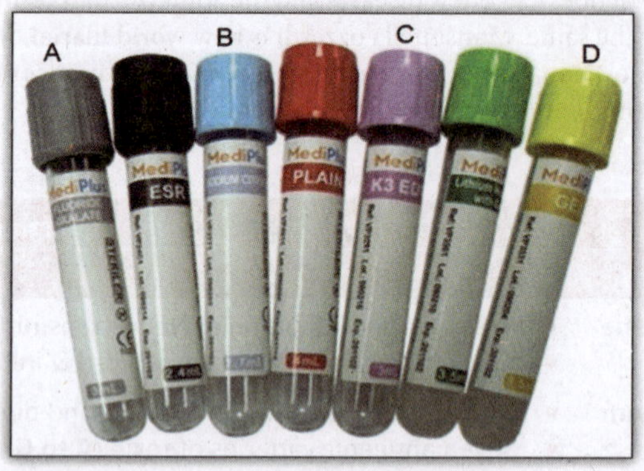

a. Tube A
b. Tube B
c. Tube C
d. Tube D

5. Which of following is not seen in apoptosis?

a. Swelling of cell organelles
b. Absence of inflammation
c. Gene mediated programmed cell death
d. Intact plasma membrane

6. Which of following help in recognition of necrotic cell debris produced as a result of inflammation ?

a. Toll like receptors
b. Neutrophil extracellular traps
c. Inflammasomes
d. P-selectin

7. Naive T cells gets activated by?

a. Dendritic cells
b. Macrophages
c. NK cells
d. B cells

8. Identify the inheritance pattern shown in pedigree diagram.

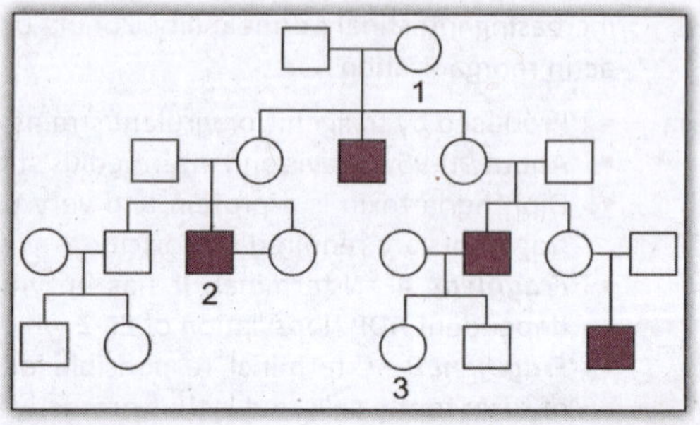

a. Autosomal recessive
b. X linked dominant
c. X linked recessive
d. Autosomal Dominant

9. What is the name of this process?

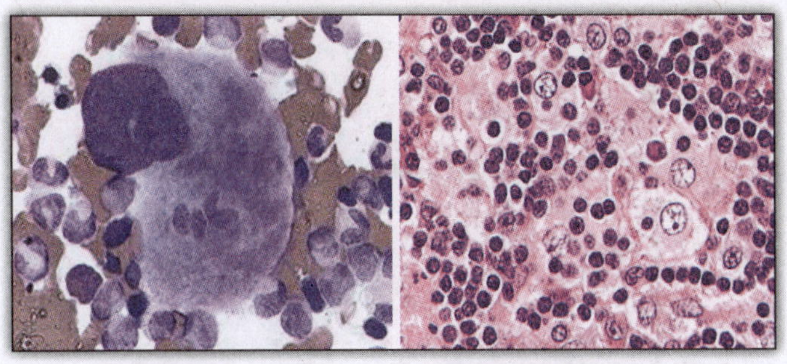

a. Necrosis
b. Phagocytosis
c. Emperipolesis
d. Autophagy

10. A patient comes with blunt road trauma. He is having severe bleeding. As a resident working there, you have asked for 2 Packed RBC and 4 platelet concentrates which have arrived from blood bank. Only one IV access is available for administering them. What should be done?

a. Transfuse platelet concentrates and keep packed RBCs at room temperature
b. Transfuse packed RBCs and keep platelet concentrates at room temperature
c. Transfuse platelet concentrates and keep packed RBCs at 2–6 degree C
d. Transfuse packed RBCs and keep platelet concentrates at 2–6 degree C

11. Tumour which causes phosphaturia and osteomalacia is?

a. Peripheral Nerve sheath tumour
b. Meningioma
c. Osteosarcoma
d. Fibrosarcoma

12. A patient presents with complaint of steatorrhoea. His Schilling test comes out to be abnormal while D-xylose test is normal. On duodenal biopsy normal villous are seen. Which of the following disease he would be suffering from?

a. Celiac disease
b. Ileal disease
c. Ulcerative colitis
d. Intestinal lymphangiectasia

13. A patient of road side blunt trauma presents to emergency. His blood group is not known and there is no time for cross matching. Which of the following FFP you would administer to him?

a. O Rh D +ve
b. O Rh D -ve
c. AB Rh D +ve
d. AB Rh D -ve

14. Antibody dependent cell cytotoxicity (ADCC) is shown by?

a. Only NK cells
b. NK cells and eosinophils
c. NK cells, neutrophils and macrophages
d. NK cells neutrophils and eosinophils

15. A 40 year old female comes with complaints of proteinuria. Immunofluorescence microscopy of renal pathology is shown in the image below. Which of the following could be diagnosis?

a. Lupus nephritis
b. Good pasture's Syndrome
c. FSGS
d. MPGN

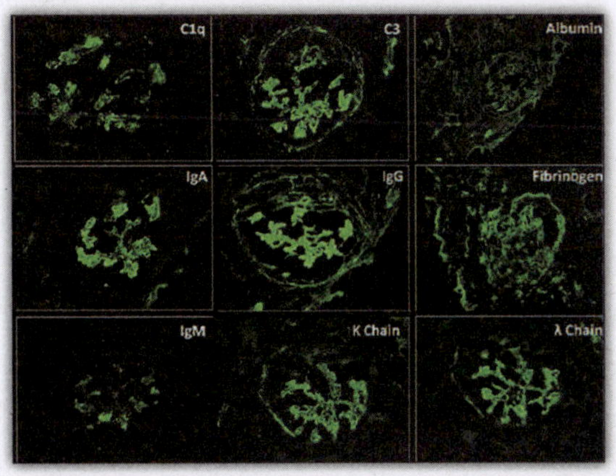

16. Which of following can't be diagnosed without positive anti-nuclear antibodies?

a. SLE
b. Sjogren's syndrome
c. Drug induced lupus
d. Scleroderma

17. A 14-year-old boy has major thalassemia and is on regular blood transfusion. Last time he presented with arrhythmia and iron overload was diagnosed and he is presently on chelators. This time when he approached for blood transfusion, while transfusing blood he felt anxious and felt back pain. What should the physician do?

a. Check urine for red colour
b. Stop blood transfusion and recheck clerical parameters
c. Continue Blood transfusion and do ECG
d. Monitor vitals and continue transfusion

18. A male diagnosed with Kartagener syndrome presents with complaints of infertility. Cause for infertility in this male is?

a. Epididymis obstruction
b. Oligospermia
c. Asthenospermia
d. Undescended testes

19. A young boy presents with pain in left ankle. On X-ray, lytic lesion is seen in calcaneus. Histopathological finding of lesion are shown. Most likely diagnosis is?

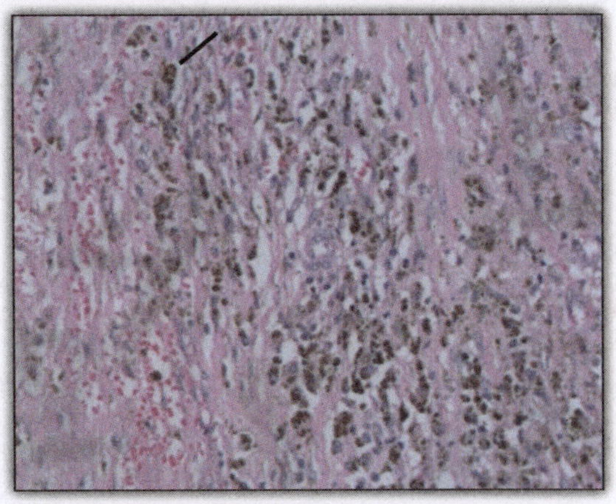

a. Ochronosis
b. Hemophilic pseudotumor
c. Pigmented villonodular Synovitis
d. Mycetoma

AIIMS MAY 2018

20. Which among the following is not seen in disorder or deficiency of elastin production?

a. Aortic dissection
b. Lens subluxation
c. Ligament hyperlaxity
d. Bone fracture

21. In Kartagener's syndrome cause of infertility is?

a. Oligospermia
b. Asthenospermia
c. Undescended testis
d. Epididymis obstruction

22. Best method to measure HbA1C is?

a. Affinity chromatography
b. Ion exchange Chromatography
c. Electrophoresis
d. Isoelectric focusing

23. Picture of light Microscope is shown below. Which of the marked labels is Condenser?

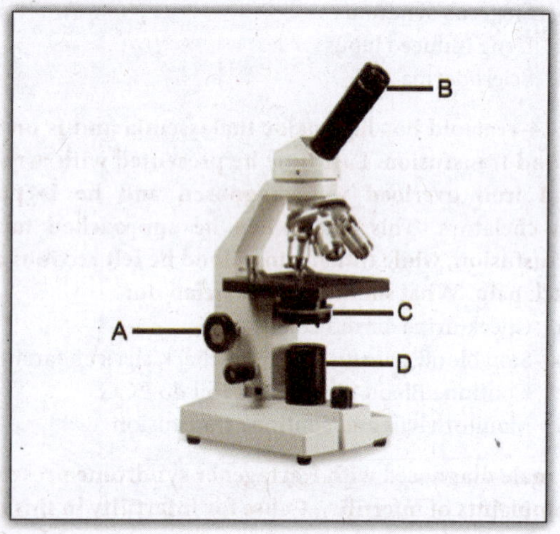

a. A
b. B
c. C
d. D

24. Which among the following laboratory investigation tells best about bleeding in DIC?

a. Decreased fibrinogen
b. Increased FDPs
c. Increased PT
d. Increased aPTT

25. Which of the following is not a provisional entity as per WHO 2016 classification of Acute leukemia?

a. AML with hyperploidy
b. B-ALL, BCR ABL1 like mutation
c. AML with BCR ABL1
d. Early T cell precursor leukemia/Lymphoma

26. Which of the following is the correct sequence of events in case of Leukocyte migration?

a. Stable adhesion– rolling- Activation of integrins– migration via endothelium
b. Activation of integrins– migration via endothelium– stable adhesion– rolling
c. Rolling- Activation of Integrins– Stable Adhesion– migration via endothelium
d. Rolling– Stable adhesion–Activation of integrins– migration via endothelium

27. Toluidine blue stain is used in the following picture for staining?

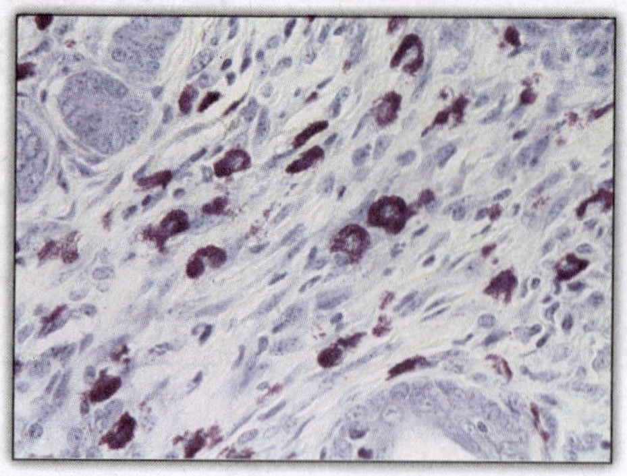

a. Mast cells
b. Melanocytes
c. Fibroblast
d. Perivascular macrophage

28. Which of the following stains is used for acid mucin?

a. PTAH
b. PAS
c. Alcian blue
d. Masson trichrome

29. A middle aged man comes with breathing difficulty. He gives history of working in a factory. Lung fibrosis and pleural thickening was observed and biopsy was taken. On histopathological examination following picture of lung parenchyma was seen. Most likely diagnosis is?

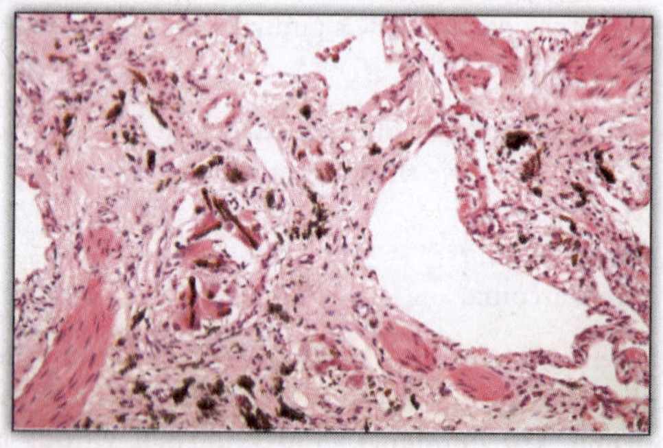

a. Silicosis
b. Coal workers pneumoconiosis
c. Asbestosis
d. Cotton fiber

30. A middle aged immunocompromised man came with fever and breathlessness. HRCT showed a middle lobe lesion with infiltration. Lung biopsy from the lesion is as below. Diagnosis is?

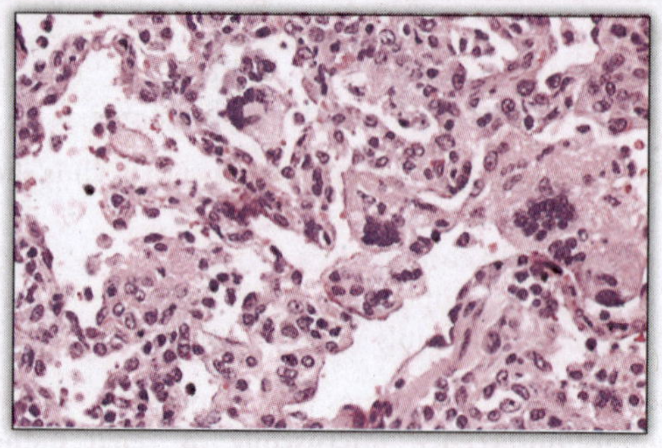

a. CMV organizing pneumonia
b. Cryptogenic organizing pneumonia
c. Small cell carcinoma lung
d. Organized Pneumonia with tuberculosis

31. Which of the following is correct about storage temperatures of blood components?
   a. RBC 20-24°C, Platelet -30°C, FFP 2-6°C
   b. RBC 2-6°C, Platelet 20-24°C, FFP -30°C
   c. RBC 2-6°C, Platelet -30°C, FFP 20-24°C
   d. RBC - 30°C, Platelet 2-6°C, FFP 20-24°C

32. Which of the following regarding blood transfusion is true?
   a. Started within 4 hours of receiving from blood bank
   b. Completed within 4 hours of receiving from blood bank
   c. Completed within 8 hours from the time of collection
   d. Wait till the patient is stable then transfuse, irrespective of time

33. A child with history of swelling in the leg, biopsy showing small round blue cells and diagnosed as Ewing's sarcoma on biopsy. What is the best method to detect t(11;22)?
   a. Conventional karyotyping
   b. FISH
   c. Next generation sequencing
   d. PCR

34. A 5-years-old child was presenting with proptosis. Microscopic examination has revealed round cell tumor positive for Desmin immunohistochemical marker. Most likely diagnosis is?
   a. Primitive Neuroectodermal Tumor (PNET)
   b. Embryonal rhabdomyosarcoma
   c. Lymphoma
   d. Leukemia

35. Following injury, a biopsy from the lesion on 4th day after the injury. Histopathology picture is shown below. This contains which type of collagen?

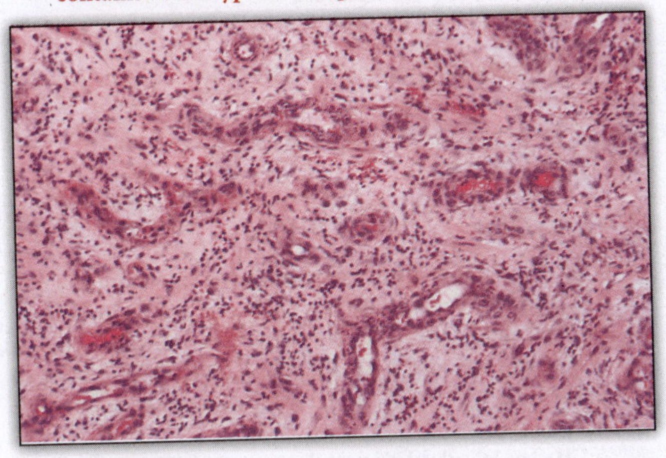

   a. Type I
   b. Type II
   c. Type III
   d. Type IV

36. Which is true about γδ T cells?
   a. A first line defense for bacterial peptide
   b. CD5
   c. CD4
   d. CD8

AIIMS NOVEMBER 2017

37. A 35-year-old depressed male comes with history of sudden difficulty in breathing since two days. His chest x ray showed bilateral diffuse infiltrate with prominent involvement of right middle and lower lobes. Patient could not be revived despite treatment. On autopsy the Lung gross specimen appears normal. Histopathological section of Lung biopsy is shown below. What is most likely diagnosis?

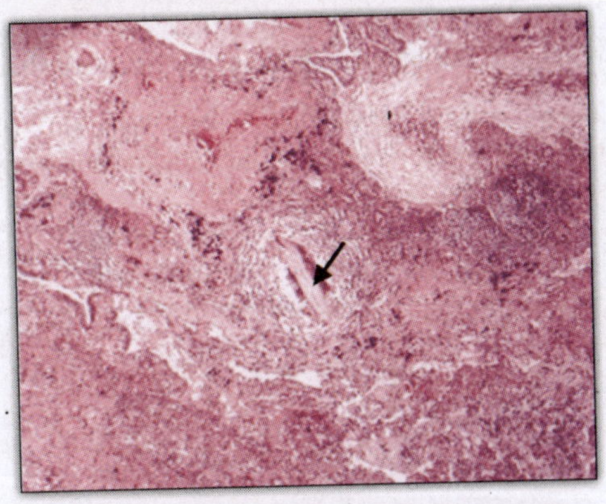

   a. Aspiration pneumonia with vegetative matter
   b. Necrotizing pneumonia
   c. Sarcoid granuloma
   d. Severe fungal pneumonia

38. In cases of Cancer breast based on which grade/stage of IHC staining, FISH for gene amplification would be done?
   a. HER 2 neu 1+   b. HER 2 neu 2+
   c. HER 2 neu 3+
   d. Done in all cases irrespective of IHC grade/stage

39. Fixative used for PAP smear is?
   a. 95% ethyl alcohol   b. 10% formalin
   c. Normal saline   d. Air drying

40. A patient presents with has 90% HbF and 3% HbA2. A peripheral blood smear was done. Which of the following picture/s will be seen?

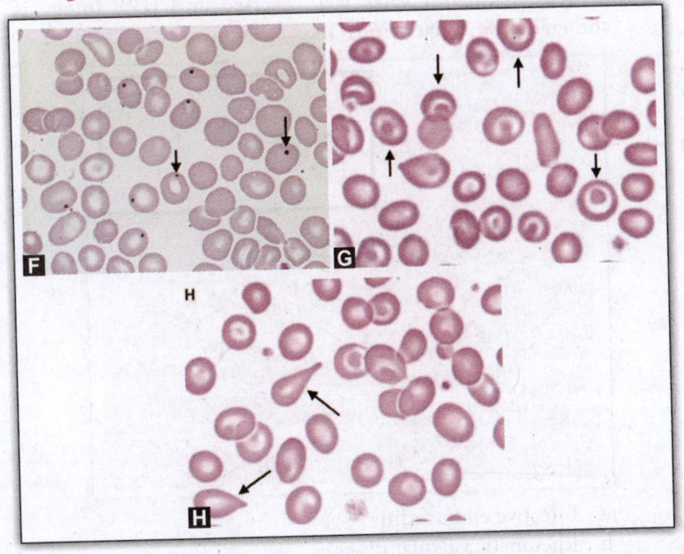

   a. F and G   b. F and H
   c. G and H   d. F, G and H

41. What is the sequence to be followed for blood sample collection for cross matching?

a. Ask patient to identify himself, Verification of patient details in file, blood collection, labeling at the nursing station
b. Ask the patient to identify himself, blood collection, cross check patient details, labelling at nursing station
c. Ask the patient to identify himself, labeling tibes bedside, blood collection, cross check patient details
d. Ask patient to identify himself, Verification of patient details in file, blood collection, labeling at the bedside

42. A male patient presented with bilateral proptosis. Histological specimen of the tumor shows following picture. Most likely diagnosis is?

a. Rhabdomyosarcoma b. Schwannoma
c. Leiomyoma d. Neurofibroma

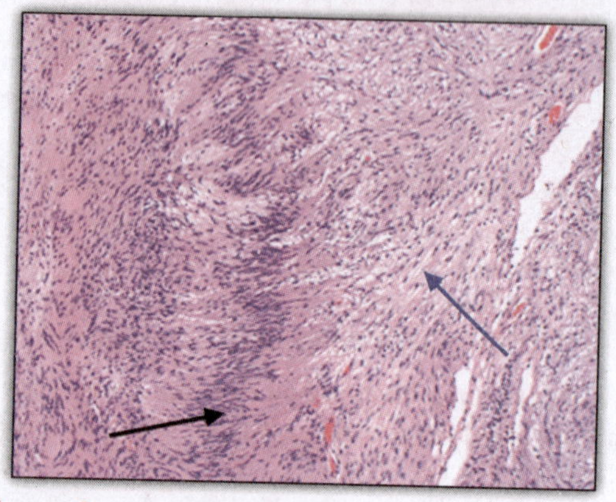

43. Chronic lymphocytic leukemia (CLL) and small lymphocytic lymphoma (SLL) cell of origin is?

a. Naive B cells in interfollicular zone
b. Lymphocytes in germinal center
c. Lymphocytes in peripheral zone
d. Bone marrow progenitors

44. A 30 year old male diagnosed with mitral stenosis with left atrial enlargement following severe dyspnea. Vegetations present on Mitral valve were excised and HPE image is shown below. What is most likely diagnosis?

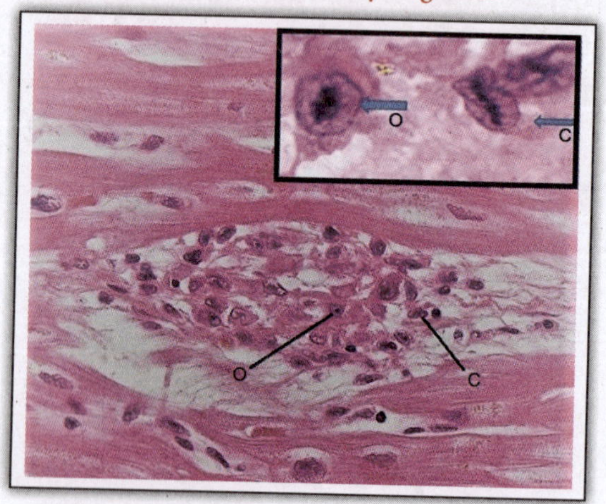

a. Infective endocarditis
b. Rheumatic valvular disease
c. Myxomatous degeneration
d. Sarcoidosis

45. A 43-year-old male comes with 6 month history of dysphagia. Barium swallow and endoscopy pictures are shown below. Biopsy of the growth most likely to show?

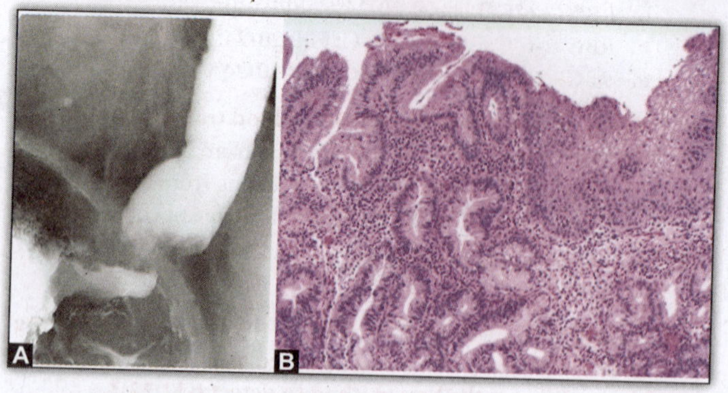

a. Squamous cell carcinoma
b. Adenocarcinoma
c. Large cell carcinoma
d. Barrett's esophagus

46. When you add Calcium and thromboplastin to PT which pathway gets activated?

a. Extrinsic pathway
b. Intrinsic pathway
c. Common pathway
d. Fibrinolysis

47. Blood is preserved in blood bank in which container which has shelf life of 35 days?

a. Citrate Phosphate Dextrose Adenine-1
b. Acid Citrate Dextrose
c. Citrate Phosphate Dextrose
d. Citrate Phosphate 2 Dextrose

48. For electrolyte estimation which of following anticoagulant is used?

a. Lithium heparin
b. Na fluoride
c. EDTA
d. Na citrate

49. A young donor came to the blood bank with platelet count 1.95 lac/mm3 is undergoing plasmapheresis for first time. He developed perioral numbness, tingling sensation during procedure. His vitals remain stable though. ECG showed tachycardia with ST-T changes. What is the reason for his symptoms?

a. He has low platelet count than required for procedure
b. Large infusion of ACD
c. 1st time donation
d. Low platelet index

50. A 5 year old child presents with bilateral proptosis. Which test is t be ordered to rule out Chloroma?

a. Peripheral Blood Smear b. WBC count
c. RBC count d. Platelet count

51. All of following are involved in Iron metabolism EXCEPT:

a. Ceruloplasmin b. Hepcidin
c. Transthyretin d. Ferritin

52. **Asymptomatic Hepatitis B is common in 2-3 % normal population, but there is increased risk of hepatocellular cancer due to?**
   a. Inability to produce inflammation against the organism
   b. High level of transaminases
   c. High rate of proliferation of hepatocytes
   d. Risk of integration of viral DNA with Host DNA

AIIMS MAY 2017

53. **A 35-year-old patient with history of high grade fever and Tonsillitis 2 months back now presents with cervical lymphadenopathy. His peripheral blood smear showed lymphocytosis with WBC count 22 × 109/L. Monospot test was negative. Tonsillectomy was done and it showed large cells mixed with lymphocytes. The cells were positive for CD20, EBV-LMP1, MUM1, CD 79a. Background cells were positive for CD3. The cells are negative for CD15. Your most probable diagnosis?**
   a. Infectious mononucleosis
   b. Hodgkin lymphoma
   c. EBV positive diffuse large B-cell lymphoma
   d. EBV positive mucocutaneous ulcer

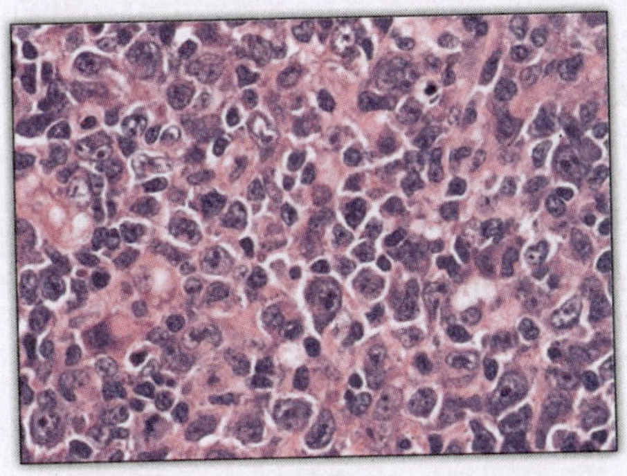

54. **A 20-year-old boy presented with persistent cervical lymphadenopathy for past 1 year. Histopathology of lymph node shows RS cell with focal nodularity and background T reactive lymphocytes. The cells were pósitive for CD20, LCA, EMA and negative for CD15 and CD30 and EBV negative. Diagnosis is?**
   a. Nodular lymphocyte predominant HL
   b. T cell rich B cell lymphoma
   c. Nodular sclerosis Hodgkin
   d. Lymphocytic rich HL

55. **MHC-2 seen in which cells?**
   a. Naive T cell
   b. Erythrocyte
   c. All nucleated cells
   d. B cells, dendritic cells and macrophages

56. **A 29-year-old female with history of polyarthalgia and back ache was investigated. She had nucleolar pattern of ANA in immunofluorescence. Which of the following is the best fit in her case?**
   a. Sclerodactyly, Raynaud's phenomenon, lung fibrosis
   b. Raynaud's phenomenon, parotid swelling, dry mouth
   c. Glomerulonephritis, malar rash, oral ulcer
   d. Genital ulcer, skin nodules, lung fibrosis

57. **A 30-year-old male presents with hypersalivation, dysphagia, sternal notch tenderness. On endoscopic biopsy histopathological picture is shown. Identify the lesion. What is most likely diagnosis?**

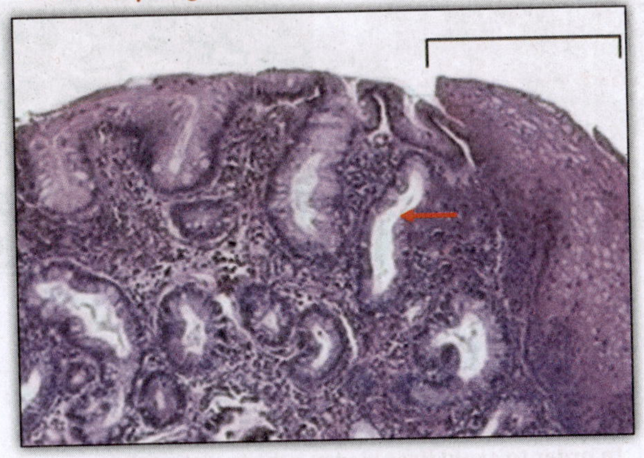

   a. Esophagitis
   b. Barrett's esophagus
   c. Squamous cell carcinoma
   d. Adenocarcinoma

58. **Which of the following is accurate regarding the intracellular iron metabolism in iron deficiency anemia?**
   a. Transferrin receptor 1—iron responsive elements (IRE) increases transferrin receptor mRNA concentration and synthesis.
   b. Transferrin receptor 1—iron responsive elements (IRE) decreases transferrin receptor mRNA concentration and increases synthesis
   c. Apoferritin mRNA—iron response element (IRE) decreases and ferritin synthesis decreases
   d. Apoferritin mRNA—iron response element decreases and ferritin synthesis increases

59. **A 50-year-old male diabetic presented with blurring of vision. Urine examination showed proteinuria. Fundus examination showed dot and blot haemorrhages, microaneurysm and cotton wool spots. Histopathology picture of kidney given shows?**

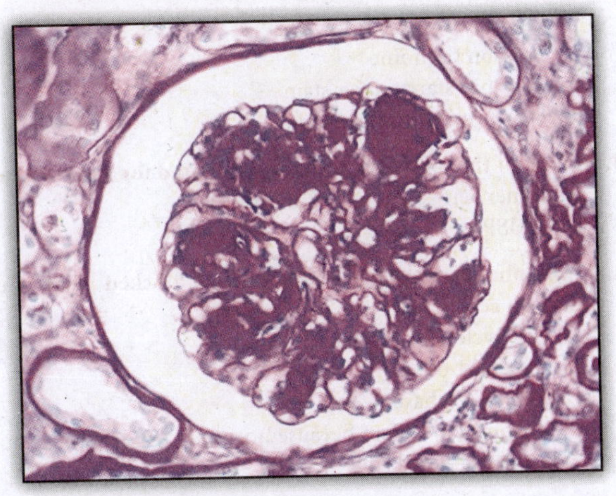

   a. Segmental sclerosis
   b. Kimmelstiel Wilson lesion
   c. Renal amyloidosis
   d. Crescents

60. **A 50-year-old male with frothy urine and periorbital edema proteinuria. The DIF and electron microscopic picture of the patient is given below. Diagnosis is?**

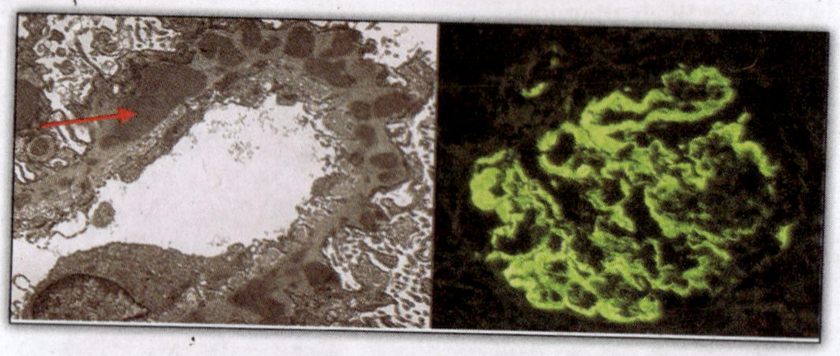

a. Crescentic glomerulonephritis
b. Minimal change disease
c. Membranoproliferative glomerulonephritis
d. Membranous glomerulonephritis

61. **In order to avoid liver biopsy, which of the following can be used as biochemical marker to diagnose liver fibrosis?**
a. Homocysteine and alkaline phosphatase
b. Transaminases
c. Serum laminin and hyaluronic acid
d. Unconjugated bilirubin and GGT

62. **Which stain is used in the staining of liver in the following diagram?**

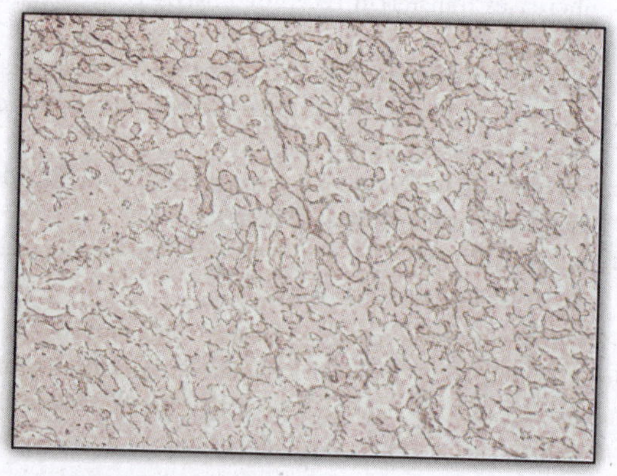

a. Grimelius' silver stain
b. Masson trichome
c. Warthin starry silver stain
d. Sweet reticulin silver stain

63. **Which of the following technology is used for gene editing?**
a. Genexpert
b. α PERT
c. CRISPR
d. Big Data

64. **If the phosphorylation of RB gene is blocked what is the effect on cell cycle?**
a. Cell cycle gets shorter
b. Affect G1 phase
c. Affect G2 phase
d. It would not affect because normally RB gene is in non-phosphorylated state

65. **Which gene is responsible for expression of self-antigen for deletion of immature T cell?**
a. NOTCH1
b. AIRE
c. RAG 1
d. RAG 2

66. **Which is the antigen that T cell never expresses throughout its development?**
a. PAX-5
b. Tdt
c. CD 34
d. CD 1a

67. **Which of the following can change the gene expression by methylation and acetylation without changing content of the gene**
a. Mutation
b. Inversion
c. Epigenetics
d. Amplification

68. **Acetone free methyl alcohol in Leishman's staining causes?**
a. Sterilizes the slide
b. Fixes the cells to the slide
c. Regulates the metabolism of the cells
d. Staining the cell

69. **A 26-year-old female with history of breathlessness comes with 5 g hemoglobin and normal WBC count, absolute reticulocyte count was 9. What will be the corrected reticulocyte count?**
a. 3
b. 4
c. 4.5
d. 5

70. **Red cell distribution width measures?**
a. Anisocytosis
b. Polychromasia
c. Poikilocytosis
d. Hypochromasia

71. **Latest marker on Mantle cell lymphoma is?**
a. SOX11
b. ITRA 1
c. MyD88
d. LMO2

72. **Which of the following is ALK positive cancer?**
a. Ewings sarcoma
b. Synovial sarcoma
c. Fibromatosis
d. Inflammatory myofibroblastic tumor

73. **A 70-year-old male presented with history of intractable diarrhea. His bone marrow and renal biopsy as shown below. Which of the following is the most appropriate diagnosis?**

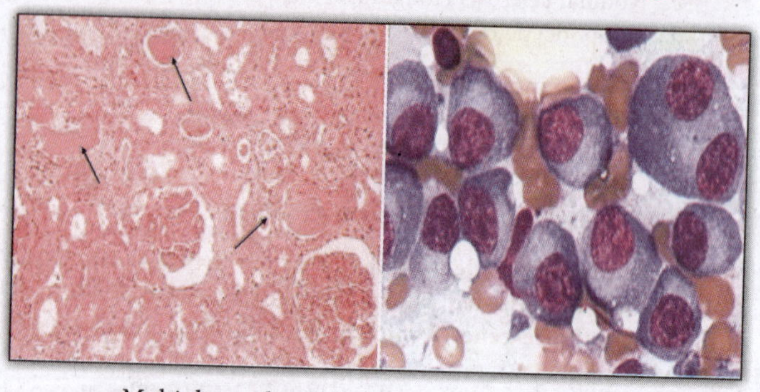

a. Multiple myeloma
b. Large cell lymphoma
c. Urate nephropathy
d. Visceral leishmaniasis

74. A 7-year-old patient presents with fever, weight loss. On examination with no organomegaly and no lymphadenopathy. Blood picture showed pancytopenia, bone marrow aspiration of the person is as given below. Your diagnosis is?

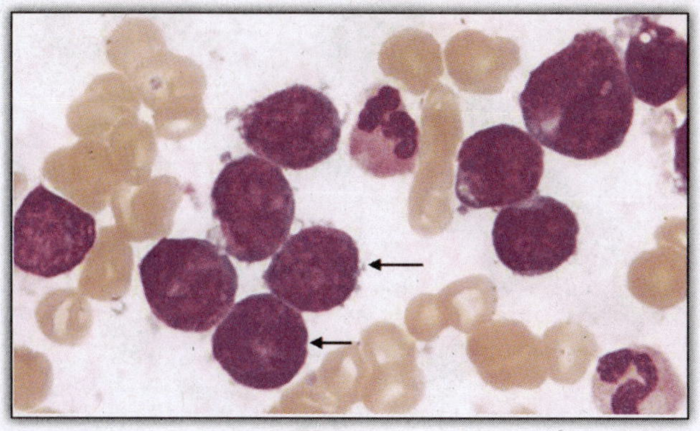

a. ALL
b. AML
c. Aplastic anaemia
d. Juvenile myelomonocytic leukemia

75. Which of the following is a negative acute phase reactant?

a. Ferritin b. CRP
c. Haptoglobin d. Albumin

AIIMS NOVEMBER 2016

76. Resolving power of light microscopy not affected by?

a. Sample thickness b. Focal length of eyepiece
c. Wavelength of light d. Aperture size

77. The following image is taken from a Neubauer chamber after charging of fluid. If the dilution factor is 20, what is the total cell count per cu mm?

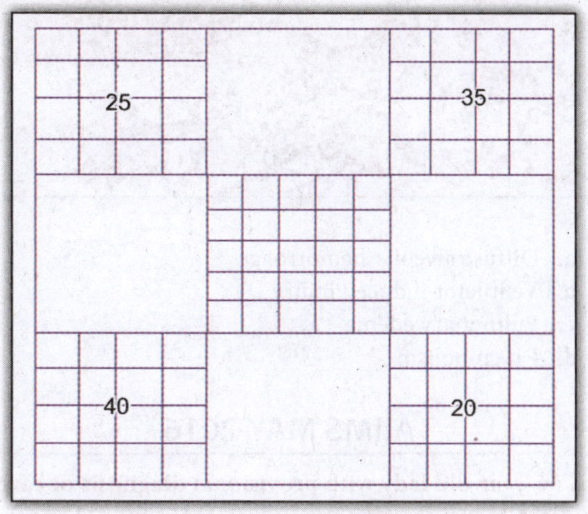

a. 3000 b. 6000
c. 7000 d. 11000

78. All are true about transfusion related acute lung injury (TRALI) EXCEPT:

a. Self Resolving in 2-3 weeks
b. Role of corticosteroids not clear
c. Morality < 10%
d. Supportive care is the mainstay of treatment

79. A person with HIV had neck pain, fever, vomiting, nausea and couldn't be survived. Autopsy specimen of brain and histopathological slide are provided. What is most likely diagnosis?

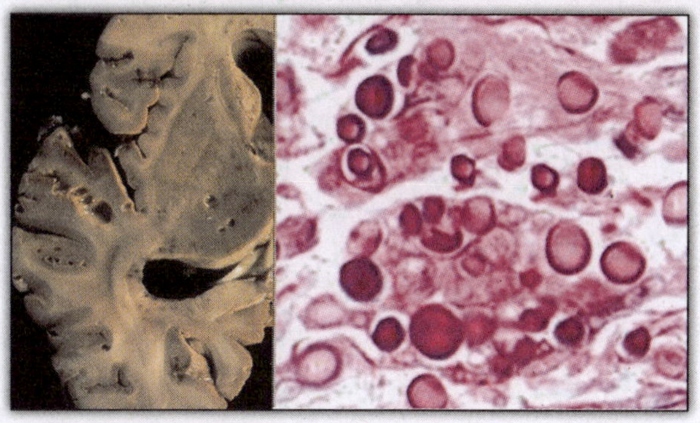

a. Herpes
b. *Toxoplasma gondii*
c. *Cryptococcus neoformans*
d. *Echinococcus multilocularis*

80. Which of the following cell marked in the following slide is increase in parasitic infection?

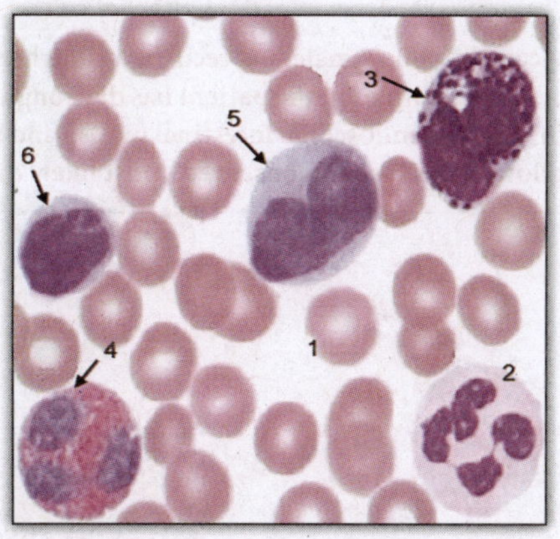

a. 1 b. 2
c. 3 d. 4

81. A patient was found to have splenomegaly, anemia and Jaundice. All of the following are true in this condition EXCEPT:

a. Increased urobilinogen b. Decreased haptoglobin
c. Increased LDH d. Low reticulocyte count

82. A 26-year-old female presents with pallor with hemoglobin 9.5%, PCV 30 and RBC count 2 million/mm^3. The most probable diagnosis is?

a. Sideroblastic anemia b. Iron deficiency anemia
c. Thalassemia d. Folic acid deficiency

83. Most common histopathological finding of rapidly progressing glomerulonephritis? ***(AIIMS Nov 2016, DNB 2006, 2002)***

a. Crescentic formation b. Mesangial proliferation
c. Loss of foot plate d. IgA deposition

84. Which of the following malignancy cannot be diagnosed on the basis of FNAC?

a. Adenocarcinoma of lung
b. Squamous cell carcinoma of lung
c. Follicular carcinoma of thyroid
d. Papillary carcinoma of thyroid

85. Given below is the histopathology of liver biopsy of a patient with hemochromatosis which of the following stain is used?

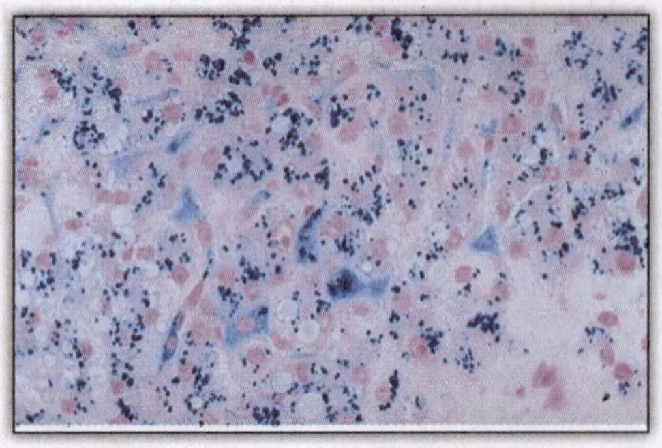

a. Prussian blue
b. Alcian blue
c. Von kossa
d. Crystal violet

86. Stain used to detect premalignant condition of Lip is?
(AIIMS Nov 2016, DNB June 2011)

a. Giemsa
b. Toluidine blue
c. Crystal violet
d. H and E

87. MHC antigen are absent in?

a. Neutrophil
b. Erythrocyte
c. Thrombocyte
d. Epithelial cell

88. A 24-year-old young male has recurrent diarrhea and loss of weight. On examination the patient has dry tongue and loss of skin turgor. On endoscopic intestinal biopsy and histopathology following picture was observed. Most likely diagnosis is?

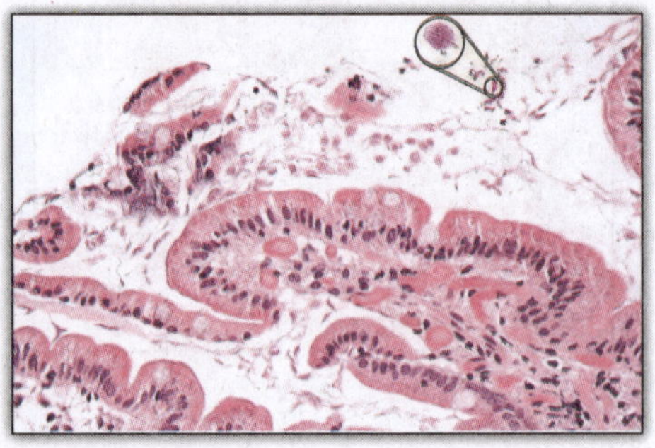

a. Whipple's disease
b. Giardiasis
c. *Entamoeba histolytica*
d. *H. pylori*

89. A 65-year-old female presents in december with history of chronic fatigue, cyanosis and pain in finger tips and cyanosis of the tip of nose along with dyspnoea. Peripheral blood picture is shown below. What is most likely finding?

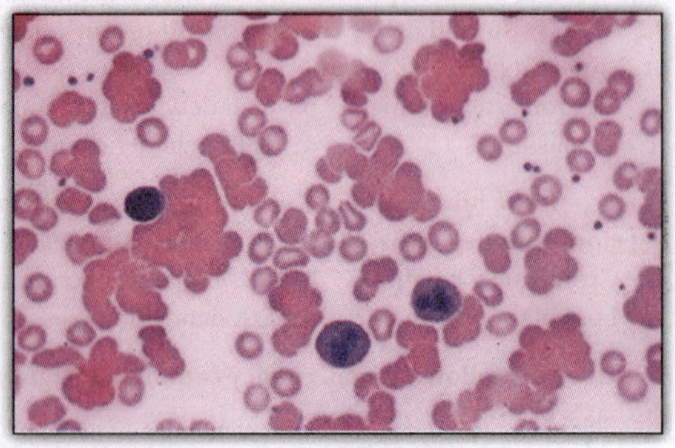

a. RBC clumps due to cold AIHA
b. RBC clumps due to warm AIHA
c. RBC clumps due to Hemoglobinopathy
d. RBC clumps due to G6PD deficiency

90. Urine cytology in a post renal transplant patient showed 2–3 pus cells and has raised serum creatinine. Marked structure in the image is?

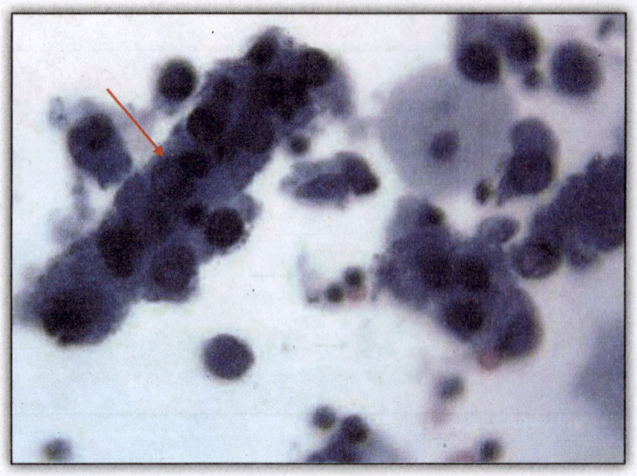

a. Hyaline cast
b. Decoy cells
c. Charcot leyden crystal
d. Tubular epithelial cells

91. A 25-year-old male with history of road traffic accident sustained fracture neck of femur and brought to the emergency. He was intubated for respiratory distress but dies in spite of ventilatory support. On autopsy the histopathological slide of lung is shown below. Most likely diagnosis is?

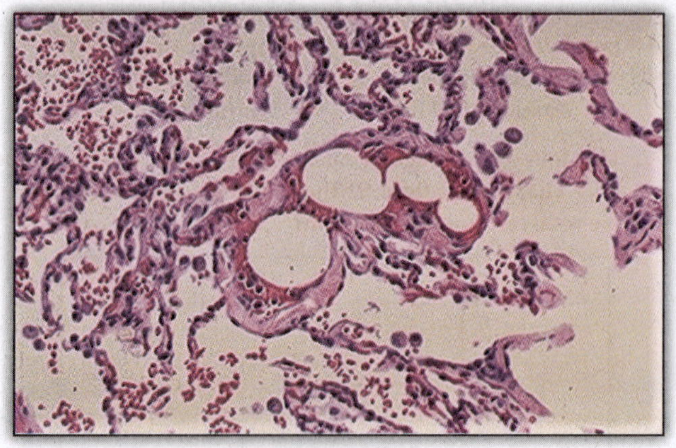

a. Diffuse alveolar hemorrhage
b. Ventilator induced injury
c. Pulmonary edema
d. Fat embolism

AIIMS MAY 2016

92. A 56-year-old lady with provisional diagnosis of carcinoma breast, biopsy was done and a series of immunohistochemical stains were done on breast biopsy specimen. Below are the photographs of ER, PR and HER2Neu. Which of the following best describes the prognosis of the patient representing - Column (A)?

a. Good prognosis
b. Poor prognosis
c. Good prognosis with transtuzumab
d. Good prognosis without transtuzumab

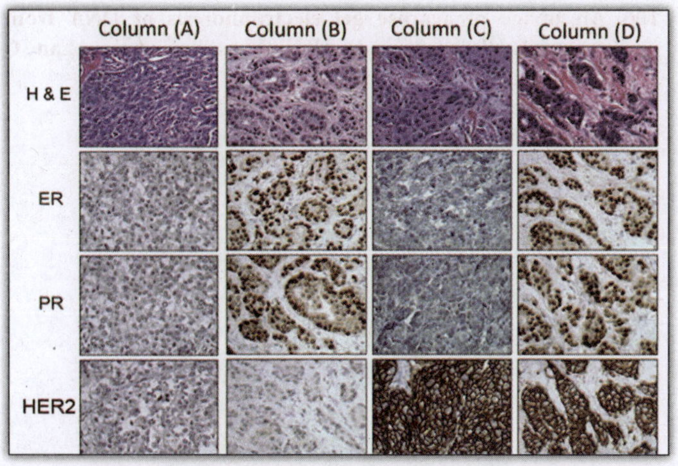

93. Direct immunofluorescence for IgG done on a kidney specimen as shown in the picture below. Most likely diagnosis is?

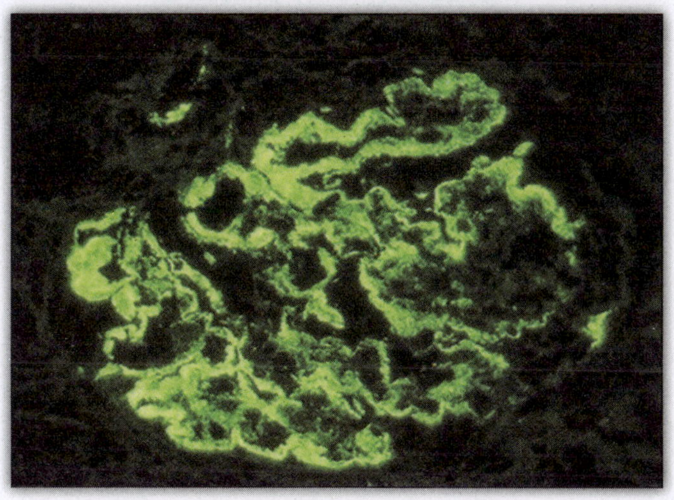

a. Membranous glomerulonephritis
b. Good pasture syndrome
c. Buerger's disease
d. Systemic lupus erythematosus

94. All are true regarding Giant cell tumor of bone EXCEPT:

a. Commonly seen in 20-40 years age group
b. Although benign it can metastasize to lung
c. Interspersed proliferating mononuclear cells are tumor cells
d. Multinucleated osteoclast like giant cells are the tumour cells

95. All are causes of a positive direct Coombs test EXCEPT:

a. Aplastic anemia
b. Hemolytic disease of newborn
c. Drug induced autoimmune haemolytic anemia
d. Haemolytic transfusion reaction

96. The following are antigen presenting cells EXCEPT:

a. M cell
b. Thymocyte
c. Macrophages
d. Langerhans cells

97. An image of Hematoxylin and Eosin stained section of patient with myocardial infraction shown below. Based on the findings, identify the age of infarct?

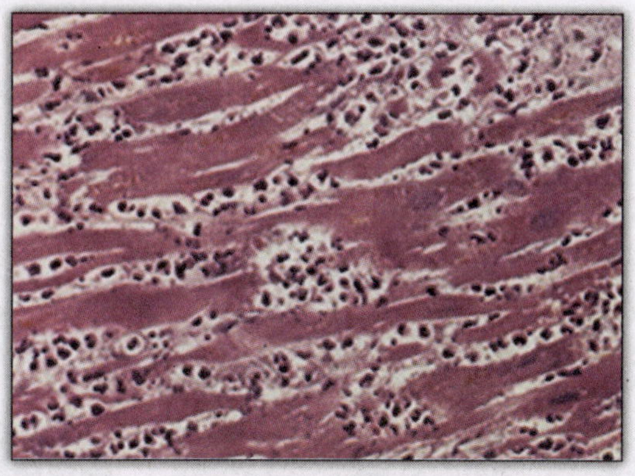

a. 6 hours
b. 1-2 days
c. 2 weeks
d. 3 weeks

98. Evaluate the specimen kidney shown below. Based on macroscopic examination the diagnosis is?

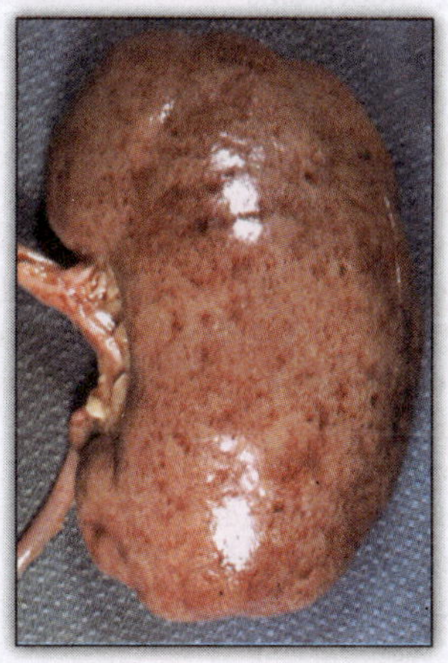

a. Amyloidosis
b. Flea bitten kidney due to malignant hypertension
c. Acute post streptococcal glomerulonephritis
d. Chronic glomerulonephritis

99. An image of H and E section of a tissue showing inflammation is shown below. Identify the marked cell?

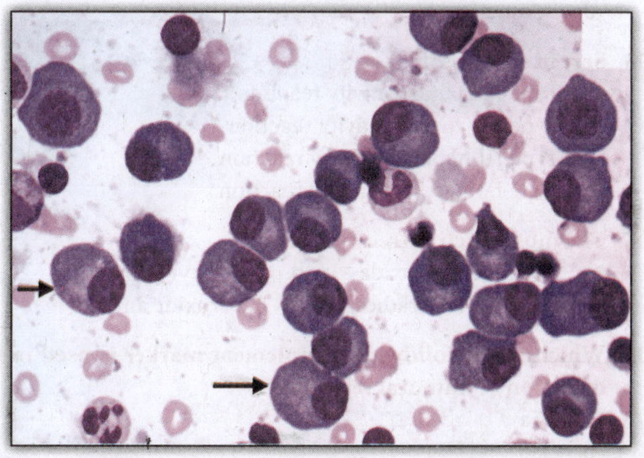

a. Plasma cell
b. Eosinophil
c. Lymphocyte
d. Macrophage

100. The image shown below is of mitral valve with presence of vegetations along the line of closure of valves. The most likely diagnosis based on the picture is?

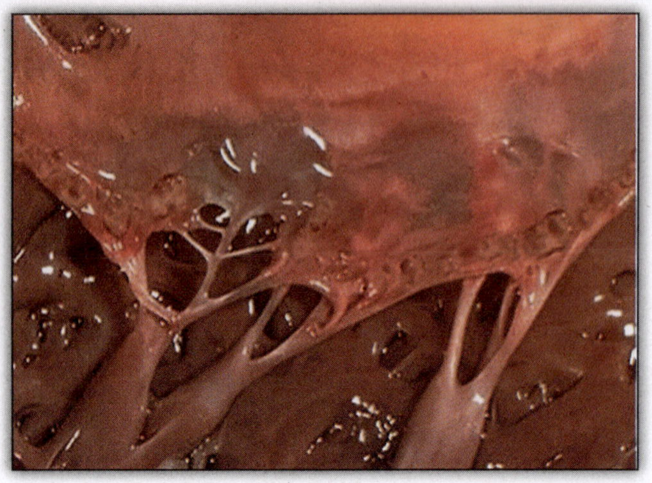

a. Rheumatic endocarditis
b. Infective endocarditis
c. Libman-sack endocarditis
d. NBTE

101. A 33-year-old female presented with 4 month history of persistent cough and hemoptysis. Bronchoscopic examination revealed a intrabronchial polyp. Biopsy shows small cell with salt and pepper chromatin, necrosis and mitotic figure of 5 per/10 HPF. On immunohistochemistry cells were intensely positive for synaptophysin/chromogranin. What is the diagnosis and grade of the tumour?

a. Carcinoid grade I
b. Atypical carcinoid grade II
c. Small cell carcinoid grade IV
d. Large cell neuroendocrine carcinoma stage IV

102. The surgical registrar has performed a testicular biopsy and has directed you to send it to histopathological examination. Operation theatre nurse asks you about the solution she should use to send the solution. You answer must be?

a. 10% neutral buffered formalin
b. Zenkers fixative
c. Gluteraldehyde
d. Bouin's fixative

103. Serum sickness is?

a. Type I hypersensitivity reaction
b. Type II hypersensitivity reaction
c. Type III hypersensitivity reaction
d. Type IV hypersensitivity reaction

104. The most reactive free radical is?

a. Hydrogen peroxide
b. Hydroxyl free radical
c. Peroxide free radical
d. Superoxide anion

105. Which of the following complement marker is used in the detection of humoral rejection?

a. C5a
b. C3d
c. C4d
d. C3b

106. An image of agarose gel electrophoresis of DNA from cultured cells is seen under UV light as shown below. Lane C in the picture represents?

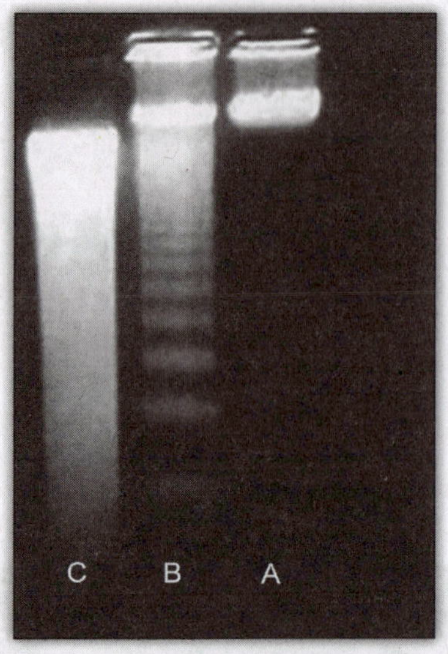

a. Majority of culture cells are apoptotic
b. Majority of cells with good DNA content
c. The cells in the culture are predominantly necrotic
d. Cells have mixture of normal and apoptotic cells

107. Packed red blood cells should be transfused?

a. Through 18 to 20 gauge IV catheter within 4 hours of receiving by patient side
b. Through 18 to 20 gauge IV catheter within 4 hours of issue from blood bank
c. Through 20 to 22 gauge IV catheter within 4 hours receiving by patient
d. Through 20 to 22 gauge IV catheter within 4 hours of issue from blood bank

108. The temperature at which RBC is stored in blood banks is?

a. –2° to –4°C
b. 2°–6°C
c. 20°–24°C
d. 37°C

109. All of the following are EBV positive lymphomas EXCEPT:

a. Lymphomatoid granulomatosis
b. Plasmablastic lymphoma
c. Nodular lymphocytic predominant Hodgkin's lymphoma
d. NK-T cell lymphoma

AIIMS NOVEMBER 2015

110. Which of the following is not specific but most important for regulation of iron metabolism?

a. Hepcidin
b. DMT-1
c. Ferroportin
d. Ferritin

111. Which of the following is an immune privileged site?
(AIIMS Nov 2018, 2015)

a. Seminiferous tubule
b. Loop of henle
c. Area postrema
d. Optic disc

112. There are different checkpoints in cell growth and regulations. Which is the primary checkpoint of cell growth and regulation?

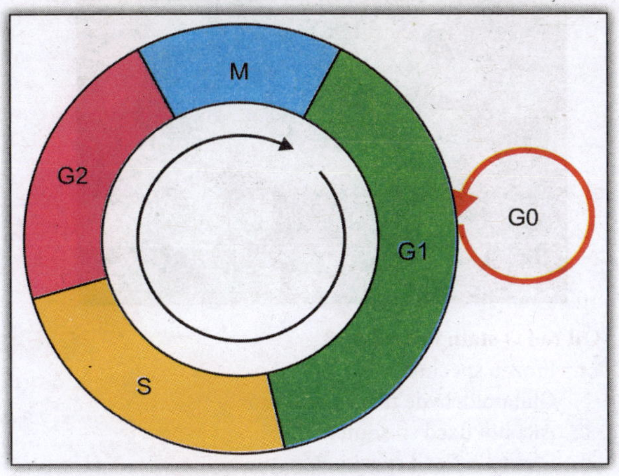

a. End of S phase
b. End of G1 phase
c. End of G2 Phase
d. End of M phase

113. Identify the urinary crystals shown?

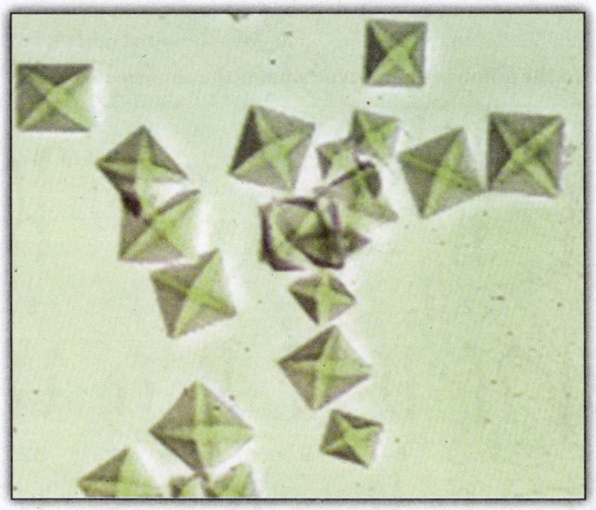

a. Calcium carbonate stone
b. Ammonium phosphate stone
c. Calcium oxalate stone
d. Uric acid

114. Which of the following statements about microalbuminuria is not true?

a. Cannot be detected by routine lab tests
b. Urine protein ranging from 20-200 mg/24 hours is called microalbuminuria
c. Microalbuminuria is an independent risk factor for CVS risk in diabetic patients
d. Microalbuminuria is earliest marker of diabetic nephropathy

115. About frozen section biopsy all are true EXCEPT:

a. Immediate definitive diagnosis of tumor
b. For detecting positive margins after resection
c. To confirm suspected metastasis
d. Sentinel lymph node biopsy in breast carcinoma

116. In the histopathology of schwannoma in picture below, the arrow marked area shows?

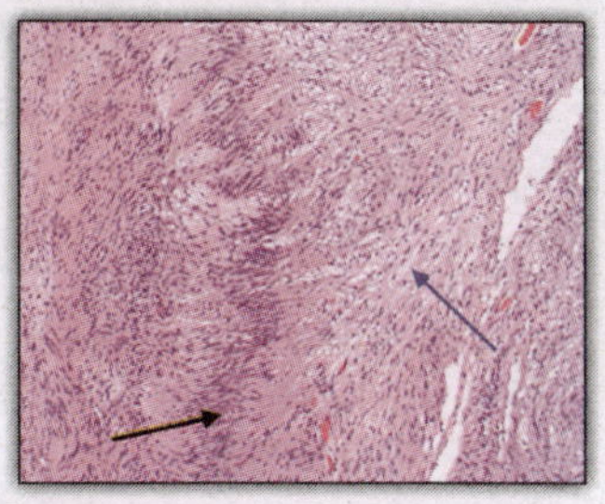

a. Myxoid tissue
b. Antony A pattern with verocay body
c. Antony B pattern with verucay cells
d. Antony C pattern - verucay cells

117. A 17-year-old patient presents with bleeding per rectum due to intussuception for which he was operated and histopathology was done for the resected segment as shown in the picture shown. Identify the pathology?

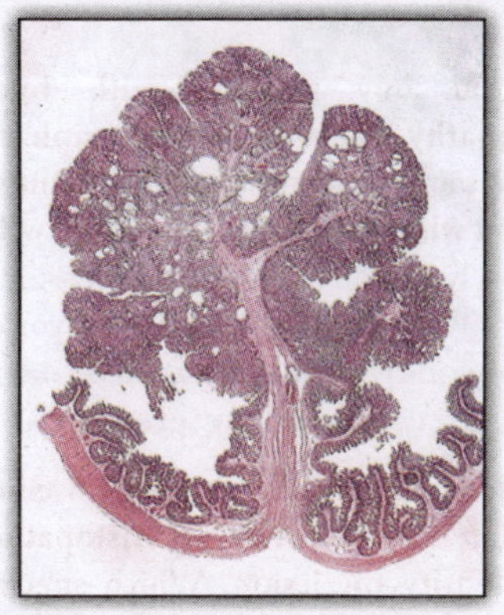

a. Tubulovillous adenoma b. Hamartomatous polyps
c. Juvenile polyposis syndrome
d. Adenocarcinoma

118. A 29-year-old athlete with family history of heart disease, suddenly collapsed and died during sport activity. Post mortem gross specimen of heart is shown below. Gross finding in figure shown below. Most likely diagnosis is?

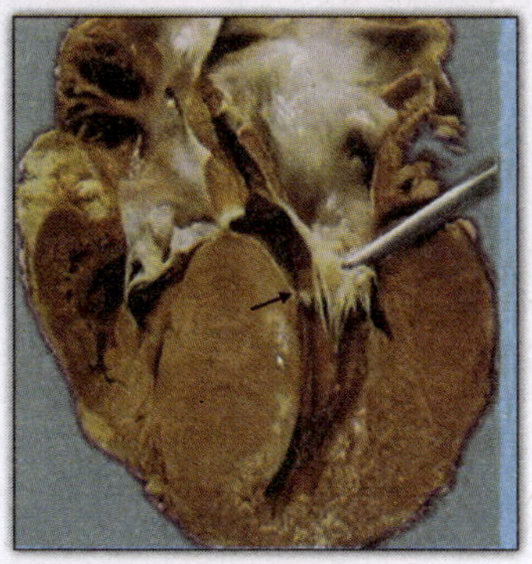

a. Hypertrophic cardiomyopathy
b. Rheumatic heart disease
c. Coronary heart disease
d. Arrhythmias

119. Most important prognostic factor in ALL is?

a. Hyperploidy b. TLC > 50,000
c. Organomegaly d. Response to therapy

120. Identify the gross cut section specimen of liver shown?

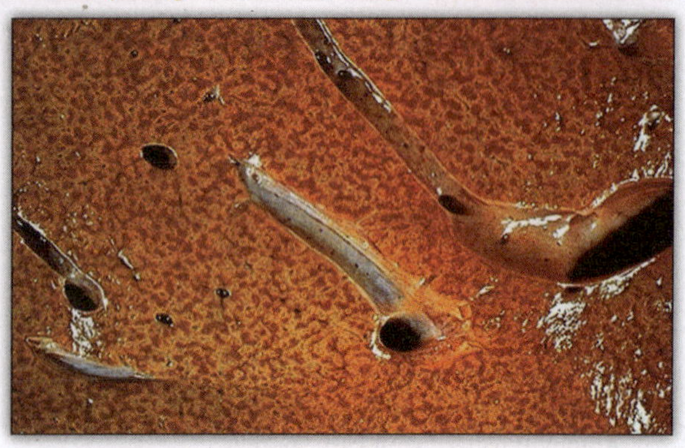

a. Nutmeg liver with dark areas of perivenular dead hepatocytes and gray areas of periportal viable hepatocytes
b. Nutmeg liver with dark areas of perivenular viable hepatocytes and gray periportal areas of dead hepatocytes
c. Amyloidosis with dark areas of perivenular dead hepatocytes and gray areas of periportal viable hepatocytes
d. Micronodular cirrhosis

121. A 17-year-old boy presents with bilateral cervical lymphadenopathy since 3 years. Lymph node biopsy is shown in the picture below. What is diagnosis? What is the etiology? And what characteristic feature will you look for?

a. Hodgkins lymphoma; EBV and Reed Sternberg cells
b. Hodgkins lymphoma; EBV and Embryo cell
c. Non Hodgkins lymphoma; HIV and Giant B cell
d. TB, Mycobacterium and tiny granuloma

122. A 30-year-old male engineer came with chief complaint of heart burn. On Endoscopic biopsy Histopathological picture is shown. Identify the lesion. Which special stain will be used? What additional feature is seen?

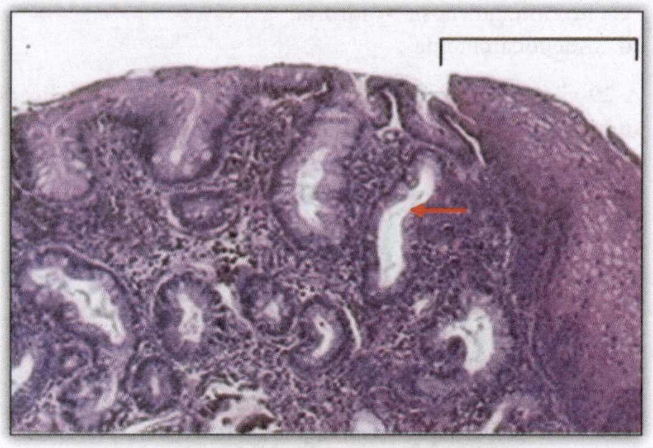

a. Esophagitis, mucin stain; erosions or ulceration
b. Barrett's esophagus, mucin stain, metaplasia
c. Squamous cell carcinoma, cytokeratin stain, keratin pearls
d. Adenocarcinoma, methylene blue, goblet cells

AIIMS MAY 2015

123. Following image was taken by attaching a camera to the microscope. The mechanism by which we view this image is?

a. By cathode ray tube
b. By dark field/phase condenser
c. Dichroic mirror
d. Phase plate

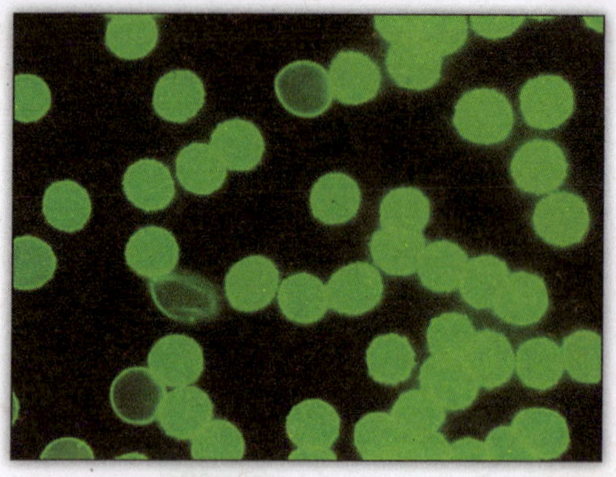

124. Oil red O stain is used for?

a. Frozen specimen
b. Glutaraldehyde fixed specimen
c. Alcohol fixed specimen
d. Formalin fixed specimen

125. The phenomenon where subsequent generations are at risk of earlier and more severe disease is known as?

a. Anticipation b. Mosaicism
c. Pleiotropy d. Dominance

126. ABO blood group is an example of?

a. Co dominance b. X linked inheritance
c. Autosomal recessive d. Mitochondrial inheritance

127. In the following karyotype what is the abnormality seen?

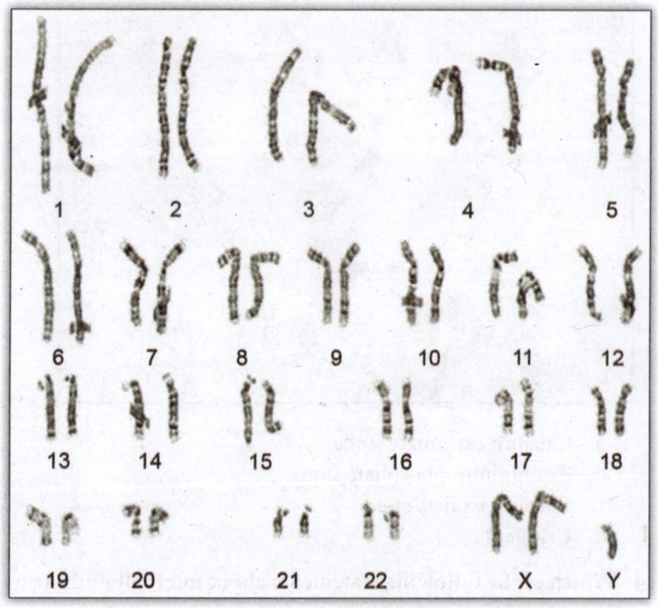

a. Gynecomastia with long thin limbs
b. Short stature with polydactyly
c. Webbed neck with widely spaced nipples
d. Rocker bottom feet

128. Platelet adhesion to collagen occurs via?

(AIIMS May 2015, Nov 2013)

a. Factor VIII b. Factor IX
c. Von-Willebrand factor d. Fibronectin

129. IgE receptor is present on?

a. Mast cell b. NK cell
c. B cell d. T cell

130. Best blood product to be given in a patient of multiple clotting factor deficiency with active bleeding?
a. Fresh frozen plasma
b. Whole blood
c. Packed BRCs
d. Cryoprecipitate

131. Which of the following is false about TRALI?
a. Develops within 24 hours
b. Mostly seen after sepsis and cardiac surgeries
c. It is a cause of non cardiogenic pulmonary edema
d. Plasma is more likely to cause it than whole blood

132. After and incised wound, new collagen fibrils are seen along with growing epithelium, the age of the wound is?
a. 4-5 days
b. About 1 week
c. 2-24 hours
d. 24-72 hours

133. Which collagen is typical of basement membrane?
a. Type I
b. Type II
c. Type III
d. Type IV

134. Most common nephropathy associated with malignancy?
a. Membranous glomerulonephritis
b. Minimal change disease
c. IgA nephropathy
d. Focal segmental glomerulosclerosis

135. A 45-year-old patient presents with fever, night sweats, weight loss. On X-ray a mass in apical lobe of lung is seen. On histopathology found to have caseous necrosis. This is because of?
a. Enzymatic degeneration
b. Hypersensitivity reaction with modified macrophages, lymphocytes and giant cells
c. Acute decease in blood supply
d. Decreased growth factors

136. Lymphatic spread is most commonly seen in which type of thyroid carcinoma?
a. Papillary
b. Medullary
c. Follicular
d. Lymphoma

137. A 48-year-old lady has hepatosplenomegaly with pancytopenia. On examination of the bone marrow, large cells are seen with crumpled paper appearance. Which of the following must have accumulated in these cells?
a. Sphingomyelins
b. Glucocerebrosides
c. Ceramides
d. Sulfatides

138. A 10-year-old boy presents with mass in the abdomen. On imaging the para-aortic Lymph node is enlarged. On biopsy starry sky appearance is seen. What is the underlying abnormality?
a. p53 gene mutation
b. RB gene mutation
c. Translocation involving BCR-ABL genes
d. Translocation involving MYC gene

139. In langerhans cell histiocytosis, the characteristic abnormality seen is?
a. Birbeck granules
b. Foamy macrophages
c. Plasma cell
d. Giant cell

AIIMS NOVEMBER 2018

1. Ans. (a) Seminiferous tubule

Ref: Robbin's 9th ed page 215, Gray's Anatomy 40th ed page 1263, Harrison 19th ed ch 318

Repeat Pathology AIIMS Nov 2015 (see page no. 393)

2. Ans. (d) Cytokeratin

REF: Harrison's 19th Ed Pg 120 e-2, Differential Diagnosis in Surgical Pathology By Paolo Gattuso Pg 295

Thymoma is an epithelial tumor and hence will be Cytokeratin positive whereas ALL will be positive for TdT, CD1a, and CD3 T-lymphoblastic lymphoma and thymoma are distinct primary mediastinal neoplasms that can have similar clinical presentations and overlapping histological features. Microscopic distinction is occasionally difficult because the immature lymphocytes associated with thymoma may resemble T-lymphoblastic leukaemia/lymphoma cells, morphologically and immunohistochemically.

3. Ans. (d) Castleman's disease

Ref: International, evidence-based consensus diagnostic criteria for HHV-8-negative/idiopathic multicentric Castleman disease.

Hint to Diagnosis

- Lack of constitutional symptoms like weight loss and anorexia essentially rules out NHL and favours Hyaline vascular histological subtype of Unicentric castleman's disease.
- Single retroperitoneal mass is more in favour of Unicentric Castleman's disease and rules out NHL and Multicentric Castleman's disease
- Concentrically arranged cells (onion peel fashion) is characteristic of Hyaline vascular subtype of Castleman's disease.
- **Option (A)** Patients with angiolymphoid hyperplasia with eosinophilia (ALHE) usually present with pink to red brown, dome shaped, dermal papules or nodules of the head or neck, especially around ears and over the scalp. ALHE is a vascular proliferation secondary to lymphoid and eosinophilic infiltration. Endothelial lining proliferation is characterised by eosinophilic vacuolated cytoplasm. Erroneously, the term Kimura's disease is sometimes used synonymously with angiolymphoid hyperplasia with eosinophilia. However, these diseases are nosologically and histologically totally unrelated.

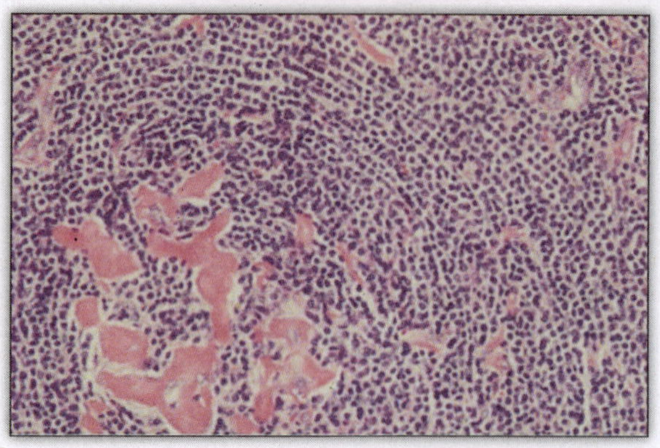

© Theodosopoulos T et al Case Rep Surg (2013)

Fig: Lymph node histopathology on Hematoxylin and eosin stain showing: Hyaline deposits are present within the germinal center. Hyaline vascular ("lollipop") lesion in which a follicle is radially penetrated by a sclerotic blood vessel. The follicle is surrounded by a broad mantle zone composed of concentric rings of small lymphocytes (so-called "onion skin").

Castleman disease is classified into following distinct disorders based on the number of regions of enlarged lymph nodes with characteristic histopathological features and the presence/absence of human herpesvirus 8 (HHV-8, also called Kaposi sarcoma associated herpesvirus [KSHV]) infection:

- **Unicentric Castleman disease (UCD)** involves one or more enlarged lymph node(s) in a single region of the body that demonstrates histopathological features that lie along a spectrum with hyaline vascular histopathological subtype on one end and plasma cell histopathologic subtype on the other. Constitutional symptoms are more commonly seen in patients with the plasma cell histopathological subtype of UCD. In contrast, signs and symptoms related to the hyaline vascular histopathological subtype are typically due to impingement and compression of neighboring structures (eg, airway, vessels) by the enlarging mass.
- **Multicentric Castleman disease** (MCD) involves multiple regions of lymph nodes that demonstrate CD histopathological features that lie along a spectrum with hypervascular histopathological subtype on one end and plasma cell histopathologic subtype on the other. These patients also have systemic inflammatory symptoms with generalized lymphadenopathy, hepatosplenomegaly, cytopenias, and organ dysfunction due to excessive proinflammatory cytokine increase (including interleukin IL-6). MCD is further subclassified according to the presence of HHV-8:

- **HHV-8-associated MCD:** Half of MCD cases are caused by HHV-8 infection in human immunodeficiency virus (HIV)-positive or otherwise immunocompromised individuals.
- **HHV-8-negative/idiopathic MCD (iMCD):** Another half of patients with MCD are HHV-8 negative. These cases are clinically and histopathologically identical to HHV-8-associated MCD, but the etiology is unknown.

Pathological Subtypes of UCD:

- **The hyaline vascular histopathologic subtype** of UCD is characterized by the following features:
  - **Small, regressed or atrophic germinal centers** which are often hyalinized, are depleted of lymphocytes.
  - **"Onion-skin appearance"** of the mantle zone around the germinal centers arranged in a concentric fashion.
  - **Germinal center "twinning" or "budding"** i.e. two or more closely adjacent atrophic germinal centers are encircled by a single mantle zone.
  - **"Lollipop appearance"** – Sclerotic blood vessels radially penetrate atrophic germinal centers.
  - **High endothelial venules in interfollicular zones** – The interfollicular lymphoid tissue contains numerous small blood vessels known as high endothelial venules that are lined by plump, activated endothelial cells.
  - **Tight aggregates of plasmacytoid dendritic cells** – These cells may also be appreciated in interfollicular regions, particularly with immunohistochemical stains for CD123
  - Obliterated sinuses and architectural disruption.
- **The plasma cell histopathologic subtype of UCD is characterized by the following features:**
  - **Interfollicular plasmacytosis** – The interfollicular region contains sheets of plasma cells.
  - **High endothelial venules in interfollicular zones** – The interfollicular lymphoid tissue contains numerous small blood vessels known as high endothelial venules that are lined by plump, activated endothelial cells.
  - **Large hyperplastic reactive germinal centers** – The germinal centers are often hyperplastic *(unlike the regressed germinal centers in hyaline vascular histopathologic subtype).*
  - **Follicle variability** – Abnormally enlarged or hyperplastic germinal centers are often present along with some regressed or "hyaline vascular"-like follicles in the same lymph node.
  - Patent sinuses with no architectural disruption.
- **Mixed histopathologic subtype of UCD** is characterized by a mix of hyaline vascular (predominantly regressed germinal centers) and plasma cell (interfollicular plasmacytosis) in the same lymph node.

4. Ans. (a) Tube A

Ref: Wintrobe's 12th ed page 1, Dacie and lewis practical hematology 10th ed page 7

Grey Vacutainer contains Sodium Fluoride + potassium oxalate which acts as antiglycolytic agent which preserves glucose up to 5 days, hence is used for glucose estimation.

Blood Collection System (Vacutainer System)

	Colour code	Additive	Blood draw	Mixing	Clinical use
Serum blos	Yellow/Golden (4)	Plain, No additive, Serum Separator Tube (SST) contains clot activator with gel separator at the bottom to separate blood from serum on centrifugation	4 mL 6 mL	5 times	Serum biochemistry, Dug monitoring, Serum immunology
	Red (3)	Plain, No additive, clot activator (Blood clots and serum is separated by centrifugation)	4 mL 4 mL 6 mL	5 times for plastic tubes, no mixing for glass tubes	Serum biochemistry, Dug monitoring, Serum immunology Blood bank profiles
Whole blood collection tubes	Lavender (6)	EDTA Liquid (Form calcium salts to remove calcium)	2 mL	8-10 times	Haematology (FBC), Blood Bank (Cross Match); gently invert bottle after filling to prevent clotting and platelet clumping
	Pink (7)	EDTA	2 mL	8-10 times	Blood grouping, cross matching, Direct coomb's test, Antenatal grouping
	Black (2)	Sodium citrate ESR	2 mL	8-10 times gently	Erythrocyte sedimentation rates

Contd...

Blood Collection System (Vacutainer System)					
	Colour code	**Additive**	**Blood draw**	**Mixing**	**Clinical use**
Plasma blood col	Grey (8)	Sodium Fluoride + potassium oxalate (Antiglycolytic agent preserves glucose up to 5 days)	2 mL	8- 10 times	For Glucose levels (Blood sugar)
	Light blue (1)	Buffered Sodium Citrate 3.2% (Form calcium salts to remove calcium) studies (9 volume of blood added to 1 volume of 109 mmol/L sodium citrate soL)	2 mL	3-4 times	Coagulation test (INR), Full draw required
	Green (5)	Plasma Separating Tube (PST) with Lithium Heparin (Anticoagulates with lithium heparin; Plasma is separated with PST gel at the bottom of the tube)	2 mL	8 10 times	Cytogenetics (chromosome studies), carboxy Hb, MethHb
Order of draw (Brackets): Blood culture packs (Read Sterile for Mnemonic), Followed by Light blue, Black, Red, Yellow, Green, Lavender, Pink, Grey (Stupid Boys bravely read, yet get low & poor Grades)					

Anticoagulants used for blood and their uses	
Sodium fluoride	Estimation of glucose since it inhibits enolase
Double oxalate	Used where vol of RBC is preserved like ESR , PCV
Sodium citrate	Coagulation studies and ESR by westergren's method
EDTA	EDTA is the preferred anticoagulant for blood counts because it produces complete anticoagulation with minimal morphologic and physical effects on cells
Heparin	Heparin is often used for red cell testing, osmotic fragility testing, and functional or immunologic analysis of leukocytes
ESR	All except coagulation studies

5. Ans. (a) Swelling of cell organelles

Ref: Robbin's 9th Ed Pg 7

Swelling of organelle is seen in Necrosis not Apoptosis.

See Table of NECROSIS VS APOPTOSIS in Pathology AIIMS MAY 2016 (see page no. 390)

6. Ans. (c) Inflammasomes

Ref: Robbin's 9th ed Pg 32

- Phagocytes, dendritic cells and many other cells, such as epithelial cells, express receptors that are designed to sense the presence of infectious pathogens and substances released from dead cells.
- These receptors have been called "**pattern recognition receptors"** because they recognize structures (i.e., molecular patterns) that are common to many microbes or to dead cells

Pattern Recognition Receptors

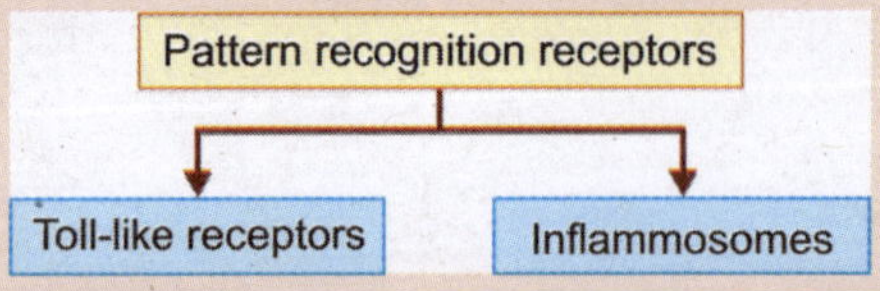

Toll-like receptors	Inflammasomes
Located in plasma membranes and endosomes, able to detect extracellular and ingested microbes provide defense against essentially all classes of infectious pathogens.	Multi-protein cytoplasmic complex that **recognizes products of dead cells**, like uric acid extracellular ATP, crystals and some microbial products
Recognition of microbes activates transcription factors that stimulate the production of a number of mediators of inflammation, antiviral cytokines (interferons)	Triggering of the inflammasome results in activation of caspase-1, which cleaves precursor forms of the inflammatory cytokine interleukin-1β (IL-1β) into its biologically active form

Contd...

Include mediators of inflammation, antiviral cytokines (interferons), and proteins that promote lymphocyte activation and even more potent immune responses.	IL-1 is an important mediator of leukocyte recruitment in the acute inflammatory response, and the leukocytes phagocytose and destroy dead cells.

About other options:

(B) Neutrophil extracellular traps (NETs)

These "traps" are extracellular fibrillar networks that are produced by neutrophils in response to infectious pathogens (mainly bacteria and fungi) and inflammatory mediators (such as chemokines, cytokines, complement proteins, and ROS). NETs contain a framework of nuclear chromatin with embedded granule proteins, such as antimicrobial peptides and enzymes. The traps provide a high concentration of antimicrobial substances at sites of infection, and prevent the spread of the microbes by trapping them in the fibrils. In the process, the nuclei of the neutrophils are lost, leading to death of the cells. The nuclear chromatin in the NETs, which includes histones and associated DNA, has been postulated to be a source of nuclear antigens in systemic autoimmune diseases, particularly lupus, in which affected persons react against their own DNA and Nucleoproteins

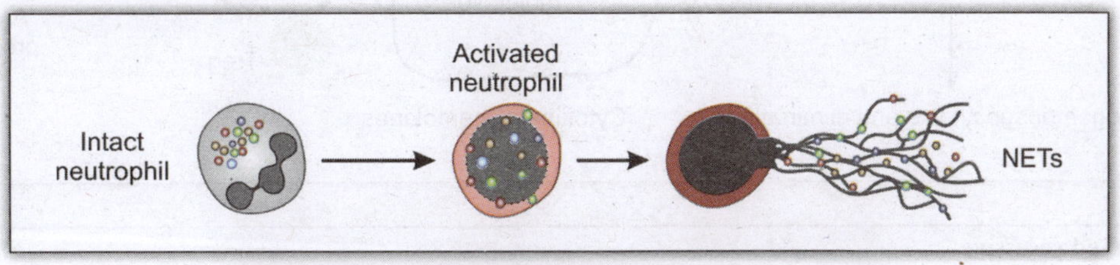

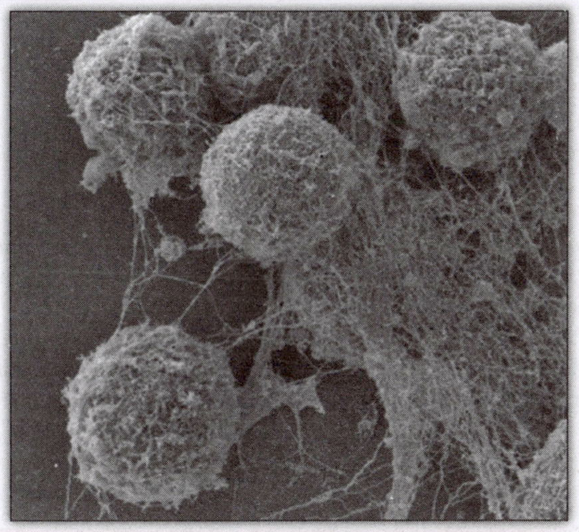

Fig: Scanning electron microscopy image of polymorphonuclear neutrophils undergoing NETosis

Option (D) P-selectin

P-selectin is an adhesion molecule which is distributed to the endothelial cell surface, where it can facilitate leukocyte binding.

7. Ans. (a) Dendritic cells; (b) Macrophages

Ref: Robbin's 9th Ed Pg 104,118

- The immune system contains several cell types that are specialized to capture microbial antigens and display these to lymphocytes.
- Foremost among these APCs are dendritic cells (DCs), **the major cells for displaying protein antigens to naive T cells to initiate immune responses**
- Dendritic cells (DCs), sometimes called interdigitating DCs, express high levels of class II MHC and T cell costimulatory molecules and function to capture and present antigens to T cells. DCs reside in and under epithelia, where they are strategically located to capture entering microbes; an example is the Langerhans cell of the epidermis.
- DCs also are present in the T cell zones of lymphoid tissues, where they present antigens to T cells circulating through these tissues, and in the interstitium of many nonlymphoid organs, such as the heart and lungs, where they are poised to capture the antigens of any invading microbes
- Naive CD4+ T lymphocytes recognize peptide antigens of self or microbial proteins in association with class II MHC molecules on the surface of DCs (or macrophages) that have processed the antigens

Also know:

Follicular variety of dendritic cells present antigens to B cells.

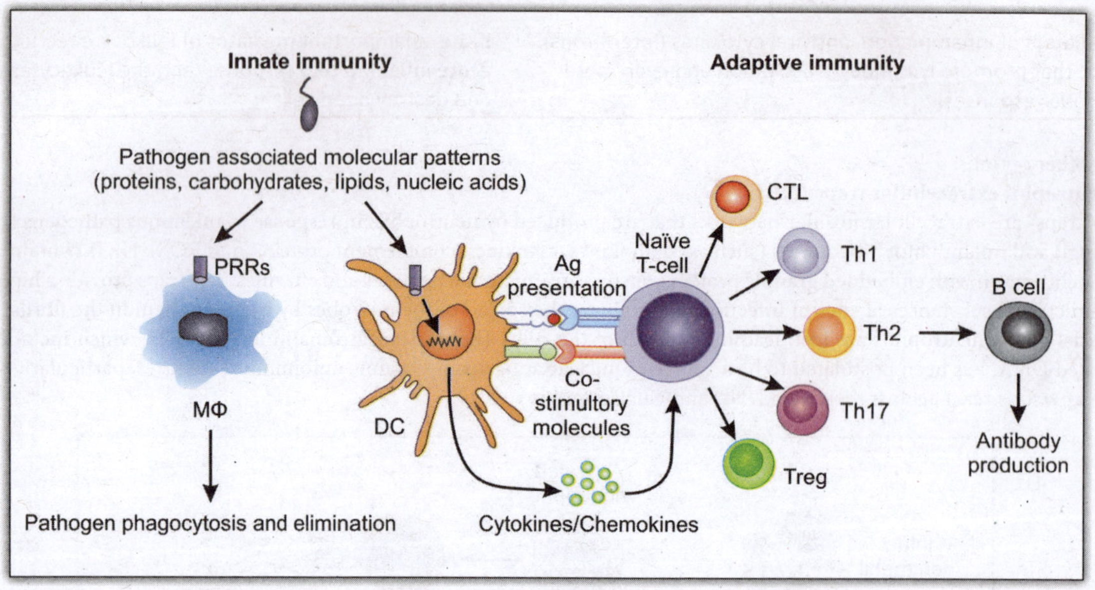

8. Ans. (c) X-linked recessive

Ref: Robbin's 9th Ed Pg 220

This pattern reflects an X-linked recessive inheritance

From the diagram, the following things are clear:

- Neither of the parents have the disease, so it is a recessive pattern.
- In the first generation, only the male child is affected. Both females are spared since they are heterozygous, however they serve as carriers.

  Thus, the inheritance is most likely X-linked.

  Heterozygous females rarely express the full phenotypic change, because they have the paired normal allele; although one of the X chromosomes in females is inactivated, this process of inactivation is random, which typically allows sufficient numbers of cells with the normal expressed allele to emerge.
- In the second generation (in the figure above), one male is affected while one daughter and one son have been spared. It is likely that the affected son inherited the disease-causing allele while the normal son has most likely inherited the normal allele from his mother. Both of them of course are homozygous for the X chromosome. Sons of heterozygous women have one chance in two of receiving the mutant gene.

X-linked recessive disorders are transmitted by heterozygous female carriers only to sons. An affected male does not transmit the disorder to sons, but all daughters are carriers.

Pedigree and Inheritance

How to read a pedigree chart?

However not a rule, but following scheme solves all the pedigree charts that use to come in PG entrance exams.

- **Check parents of the affected**
  - If both parents are normal (including carriers)- recessive
  - If any or both the parents are affected- dominant
- If dominant, check progeny/offspring of the affected male
  - If affected male affects females only- X-linked dominant
  - If affected male affects males only- Y-linked
  - If affected male affects both males and females- Autosomal dominant
  - If affected male do not transmit at all- Mitochondrial inheritance
- If recessive, check all affected
  - If both males and females are affected in the pedigree- Autosomal recessive
  - If only males are affected in the pedigree (female is affected only in the condition when father is affected and mother is carrier) - X-linked recessive
- For mitochondrial inheritance
  - Males are affected but do not transmit at all (0% transmission)
  - Females are affected and transmit to all the offsprings (100% transmission)

Contd...

Pedigree and Inheritance

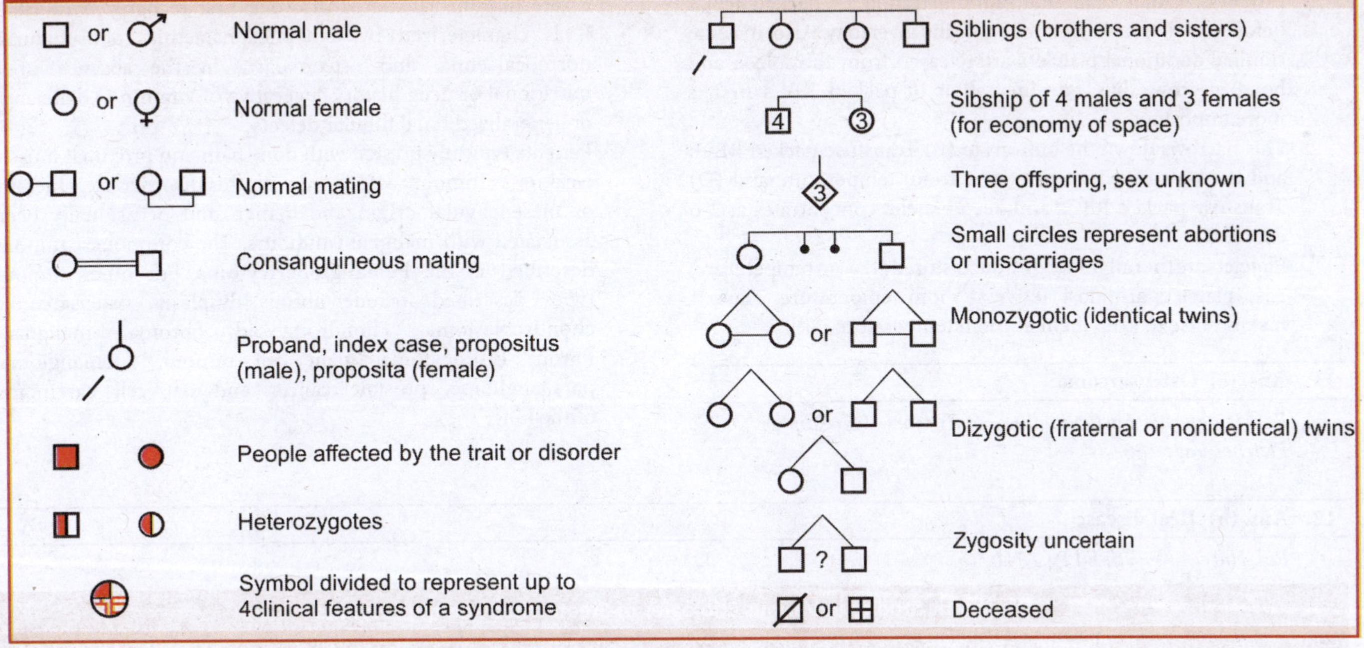

9. Ans. (c) Emperipolesis

Ref: Rosai and Ackerman's Surgical Pathology E-Book By Juan Rosai 10th Ed Pg 2327, 1801

Emperipolesis		
Description	Cells in living and intact state are seen in the cytoplasm of host cell without any damage.The host cells may be a megakaryocyte, monocyte, endothelial cell, fibroblast and a malignant cell.	
Physiological examples		
	Cell taken in	Host cell
Fetal liver	Erythroblast	Megakaryocyte
Circulation	Neutrophils, RBCs	Megakaryocyte
Brain	Lymphocytes	Glial cells
Pathological examples	Rosai Dorfman disease, autoimmune hemolytic anemia	

10. Ans. (b) Transfuse packed RBCs and keep platelet concentrates at room temperature

Ref: Miller's 8th ed Pg 1860

In this question, we need to weigh pros and cons of transfusion of both Packed RBCs and platelets and the sequence in which they are given, since we have just one intravenous access.

Scenario A: Transfusion of platelets followed by transfusion of packed RBCs:

Pros

- This will allow the packed RBCs to come back closer to room temperature. Transfusion of cold blood worsens hypothermia in a bleeding patient. Administration of unwarmed blood that has been stored at 4° C can decrease the recipient's temperature. This can worsen the pre existing coagulopathy. If the temperature decreases to less than 30° C, ventricular irritability and even cardiac arrest may occur.

Cons

- Transfusion of Platelet concentrate will not improve oxygen delivery to the tissues in this patient. Transfusion of RBCs (which contain haemoglobin) is essential for the same.
- Platelet concentrates do not aid volume status. They will not help improve haemodynamics much in this patient.

If care is taken to administer blood through a fluid warming device (warm water (37° to 38° C) bath or warming plates, one can avoid the complications of hypothermia due to cold blood products. Other than that, administration of packed RBCs before platelets is the better choice any given day. Also, in acute trauma, additional platelets are released from the spleen and bone marrow, thus, administration of packed RBCs first is more important.

This narrows down the options to (B) Transfuse packed RBCs and keep platelet concentrates at room temperature and (D) Transfuse packed RBCs and keep platelet concentrates at 2-6 degree C.

Platelets are the only blood products stored at room temperature. Also platelets are most active at room temperature. Thus, it makes sense to keep them at room temperature itself.

11. Ans. (c) Osteosarcoma

Ref: Diagnostic Histopathology of Tumors -Christopher D. M. Fletcher Page 1867

Acquired hypophosphataemic (oncogenic) osteomalacia is a rare tumour-associated disorder, first recognized in 1947. It is characterized by hypophosphataemia, phosphaturia, normocalcemia, and osteomalacia in the absence of a nutritional or drug history suggestive of vitamin D deficiency or generalized renal tubular defects

Patients typically present with bone pain and proximal muscle weakness. Tumours associated with this disorder are generally of mesenchymal origin and benign and occasionally been associated with malignant tumours. The commonest tumour described is the **hemangiopericytoma** but other tumour types described include fibrous dysplasia, osteosarcoma, chondroblastoma, chondromyxoid fibroma, malignant fibrous histiocytoma, giant cell tumour, haemangioma, paraganglioma, prostate cancer and oat cell carcinoma of the lung.

12. Ans. (b) Ileal disease

Ref: Harrison's 19th Ed Pg 1941

Diagnostic Studies in Various Etiologies of Steatorrhea and their Results

Test	Chronic pancreatitis	Ileal disease	Celiac disease	Bacterial overgrowth syndromes	Intestinal lymphangi ectasia
D-Xylose	Normal	Normal	Decreased	Normal or slightly abnormal	Normal
Schilling test	50% abnormal	Abnormal	Normal	Often abnormal	Normal
Duodenal mucosal biopsy	Normal	Normal	Abnormal (flat)	Normal	Abnormal : "dilated lymphatics"

Note:
- Abnormal Schilling test in chronic pancreatitis gives a normal result with pancreatic enzyme treatment
- Abnormal Schilling test in Bacterial overgrowth syndromes gives a normal result after antibiotic treatment.

13. Ans. (c) AB Rh D +ve

Ref: Wintrobe's 12th ed page 682, Miller's 8th Ed Pg 2441

- Patients with AB positive blood are universal plasma donors. Note that we are talking about plasma, which contains mainly antibodies, not packed RBCs which mainly contain antigens.
- Individuals with AB positive blood group contain all the antigens- A, B, Rh. Hence, the corresponding plasma will contain no antibody against these. Hence, it is the universal plasma donor.

Blood Group and Antibodies

Blood Group	Antigens	Antibodies
A positive	A, Rh	Anti-B
A negative	A	Anti-B, Anti-Rh (likely)
B positive	B, Rh	Anti-A
B negative	B	Anti-B, Anti-Rh (likely)
O positive	Rh	Anti-A, Anti-B
O negative	None	Anti-A, Anti-B, Anti-Rh (likely)
AB positive	A, B, Rh	None
AB negative	A,B	Anti-Rh (likely)

Note:
Anti-Rh antibodies do not form spontaneously in Rh negative individuals. They require a prior exposure.

14. Ans. (c) NK cells, neutrophils and macrophages

Ref: Robbin's 9th Ed Pg 108,114

- Antibodies cause disease in type II hypersensitivity by targeting cells for phagocytosis, by activating the complement system, and by interfering with normal cellular functions.
- The antibodies that are responsible typically are high-affinity antibodies capable of activating complement and binding to the Fc receptors of phagocytes.
- When circulating cells, such as erythrocytes or platelets, are coated (opsonized) with autoantibodies, with or without complement proteins, the cells become targets for phagocytosis by neutrophils and macrophages.
- These phagocytes express receptors for the Fc tails of IgG antibodies and for breakdown products of the C3 complement protein, and use these receptors to bind and ingest opsonized particles.

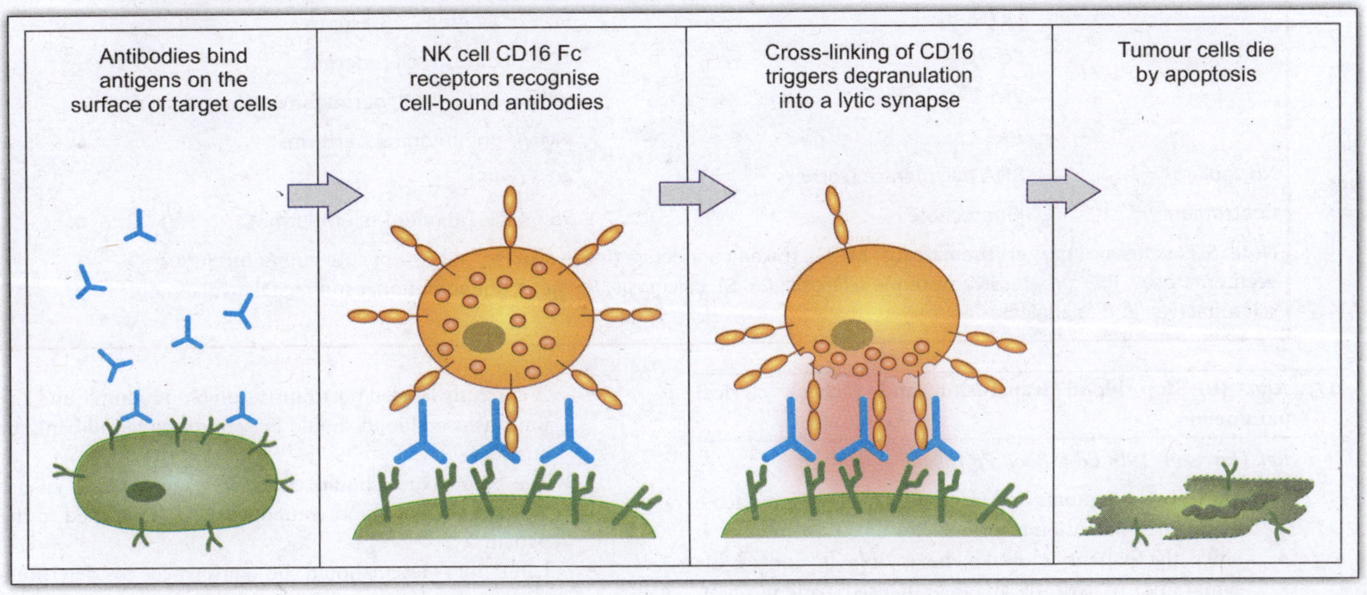

15. Ans. (a) Lupus nephritis

Ref: Rosai and Ackerman's Surgical Pathology 11th Ed Pg 971

- From the figure it is clear that antibodies are present against C1q, C3, Albumin, IgA, IgG, Fibrinogen, IgM, K chain and λ chain.
- Full range of antibodies under immunofluorescence, called **full house**, denotes severe antibody directed damage against kidney (called a full house immunofluorescence)
- In lupus nephritis, immunofluorescence studies reveal more than one class of immunoglobulin in a coarse granular pattern in the mesangium and peripheral capillary walls in all glomeruli.
- IgG is almost invariably present, but IgM and IgA are also frequently found.
- Both C3 and C1q are frequently found and the staining for Clq is particularly strong.
- **When all immunoglobulins and complement components are present, the pattern is often referred to as "full house," an immunofluorescent profile seen in all lupus classes and is considered characteristic of lupus nephritis.**
- Reactivity for fibrin and fibrinogen are commonly seen in crescentic and necrotizing lesions.
- Electron microscopy demonstrates large subendothelial electron-dense deposits usually accompanied by mesangial and sometimes subepithelial and/or intramembranous deposits

16. Ans. (d) Scleroderma

Ref: Harrison's 19th Ed Pg 379, 2134

Option (A) SLE

Antinuclear antibodies are present in over 95% of patients with SLE and are sensitive markers, but anti-dsDNA and anti-sm antibodies are more specific

Option (B)

Sjogren syndrome: Antinuclear antibodies are present in over 60% of patients. For diagnosis of this disease, the reaction of the patient's serum with Ro/SS-A and/or La/SS-B auto- antigens is one of the diagnostic criteria.

Option (C) Drug-induced lupus is a syndrome of positive Antinuclear antibodies

(Harrison). It is classically marked by antinuclear and antihistone antibodies and, in some cases, anti-double-stranded DNA (D -penicillamine, anti-TNF-α) or p-ANCA (minocycline) antibodies. Most people with drug-induced lupus develop antinuclear antibodies (80-95%), although people with drug-induced lupus caused by quinidine and minocycline often are ANA-negative.

Option (D) Scleroderma

Antinuclear autoantibodies are present in 95% patients with SSc and can be detected at disease onset.

Antinuclear Antibody (ANA) Patterns And Clinical Associations		
ANA Pattern	Antigen Identified	Clinical Correlate
Diffuse	Deoxyribonucleoprotein	Nonspecific
	Histones	Drug-induced lupus, lupus
Peripheral (rim)	ds-DNA	50% of SLE (specific)
Speckled	*U1-RNP*	*>90% of MCTD*
	Sm	30% of SLE (specific)
	Ro (SS-A)	Sjögrens 60%, SCLE, neonatal lupus, ANA(–) lupus
	La (SS-B)	50% of Sjögrens, 15% lupus
	Scl-70	40% of diffuse scleroderma
	PM-1	Polymyositis (PM), dermatomyositis
	Jo-1	PM w/ pneumonitis + arthritis
Nucleolar	RNA polymerase I, others	40% of PSS
Centromere	Kinetochore	75% CREST (limited scleroderma)

Note: SLE, systemic lupus erythematosus; MCTD, mixed connective tissue disease; SCLE, subacute cutaneous lupus erythematosus; PSS, progressive systemic sclerosis; CREST, *c*alcinosis, *R*aynaud phenomenon, *e*sophageal involvement; *s*clerodactyly; and *t*elangiectasia

17. Ans. (b) Stop blood transfusion and recheck clerical parameters

Ref: Harrison's 19th Ed E-Book Pg 138e-3

- The above symptoms and signs are suggestive an acute hemolytic transfusion reaction.
- Since the patient is awake, he is able to convey his symptoms. In case of an anaesthetised patient or an unconscious patient, checking for the color of urine can help in diagnosis of a reaction.
- Immune-mediated hemolysis occurs when the recipient has preformed antibodies that lyse donor erythrocytes.
- The patient above has been transfused multiple number of times. This places him at a risk of presence of preformed antibodies against antigens
- The ABO isoagglutinins are responsible for the majority of these reactions. However alloantibodies directed against other RBC antigens, i.e., Rh, Kell and Duffy, are responsible for more fatal hemolytic transfusion reactions.
- The most common cause of this reaction is human error.

Clinical Features

- **Fever, chest pain, nausea, flank pain, hypotension, nausea, flushing, dyspnea, anxiety.**
- Mainly the renal and coagulation systems are affected.
- The cause of acute renal failure from intravascular hemolysis is likely that Hb in the form of acid hematin precipitates in the distal tubule and causes mechanical tubular blockage.
- The magnitude of the precipitation probably is inversely related to the volume of urine flow and its pH.

Management

- When acute hemolysis is suspected the transfusion must be stopped immediately, intravenous access maintained and the reaction reported to the blood bank.
- A correctly labeled posttransfusion blood sample and any untransfused blood should be sent to the blood bank for analysis.
- The blood bank should check all paperwork to ensure that the correct blood component was transfused to the patient.
- Laboratory tests should be performed to determine the presence of hemoglobinemia: a direct antiglobulin test, repeat compatibility testing, repeat other serologic tests (i.e., ABO and Rh), and analysis of urine for hemoglobinuria.

Steps in the Treatment of a Hemolytic Transfusion Reaction

- Stop the transfusion.
- Maintain the urine output at a minimum of 75 to 100 mL/hr by the following methods:
  - Generously administer fluids intravenously and possibly mannitol 12.5 to 50 g, given over 5 to 15 minutes.
  - If intravenously administered fluids and mannitol are ineffective, administer furosemide (20 to 40 mg) intravenously.
- Alkalinize the urine; because bicarbonate is preferentially excreted in the urine, only 40 to 70 mEq of sodium bicarbonate per 70 kg of body weight is usually required to raise the urine pH to 8, whereupon repeat urine pH determinations indicate the need for additional bicarbonate.
- Assay urine and plasma hemoglobin concentrations.
- Determine platelet count, partial thromboplastin time, and serum fibrinogen level.
- Return unused blood to blood bank for repeat crossmatch.
- Send patient's blood and urine sample to blood bank for examination.
- Prevent hypotension to ensure adequate renal blood flow.

18. Ans. (c) Asthenospermia

Ref: Reproductive Endocrinology and Infertility edited by Douglas T. Carrell, C. Matthew Peterson page 375, Shaw's 15th Ed Pg 203

- ***Asthenospermia (Greek astheneia, weakness) is defined as <40% sperm motility or less than 32% with progressive motility.***
- Immotile cilia syndromes are a heterogeneous group of disorders in which sperm motility is reduced or absent.
- Kartagener syndrome is a subset of this disorder that presents with the triad of chronic sinusitis, bronchiectasis, and situs inversus. It is autosomal recessive disorder.
- Normally, 9 pairs of microtubules are organized around a central pair within the sperm tail and are connected by dynein arms (ATPase) that regulate microtubule and therefore sperm tail motion.
- Various defects in the dynein arms cause deficits in ciliary and sperm activity. Absence or defective action of dynein arms is present in Kartagener syndrome.
- This causes asthenospermia and hence infertility.

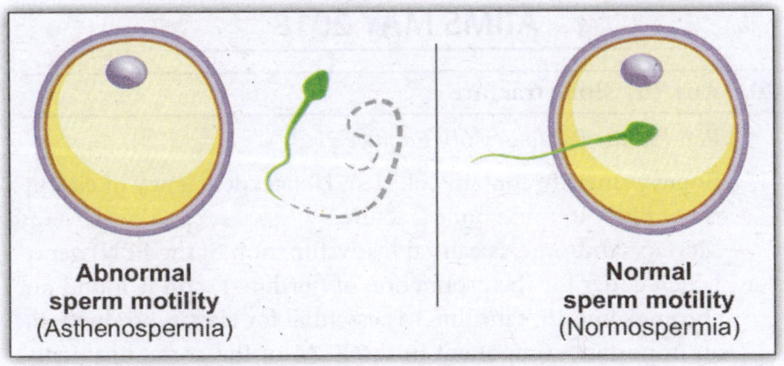

19. Ans. (b) Hemophilic pseudotumor

Ref: Orthopaedic Pathology by Vincent J. Vigorita 2nd ed page 586, Campbell 12th ed page 1166

Option (A)

Ochronosis is a syndrome caused by the accumulation of homogentisic acid in connective tissues. Ochronosis is predominantly a cutaneous disorder and does not show any lytic lesion of bone.

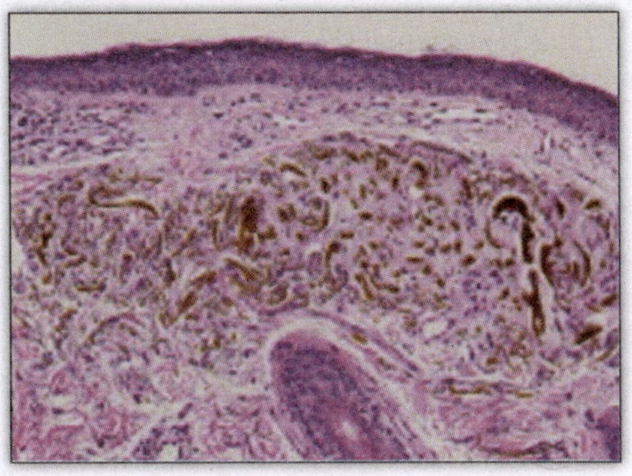

Fig: In the superficial dermis, there are sharply defined yellow-brown "banana" shaped deposits within homogenized elastotic fibers. There are scattered pigment-laden macrophages in the papillary dermis

Option (B)

Hemophilic pseudotumor is complication of Hemophilia. And since Hemophilia is a X-linked recessive disorder its exclusively seen in males. Radiograph reveals lytic lesion. Histologic examination confirmed that the masses represented a coagulum of blood products. The walls of the masses consisted of fibrous tissue with hemosiderin-laden macrophages

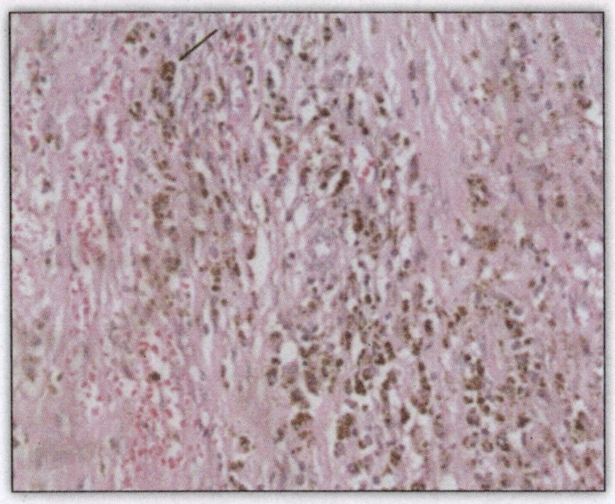

Fig: Inflammatory granulation tissue with hemosiderophages and evidence of old hemorrhages

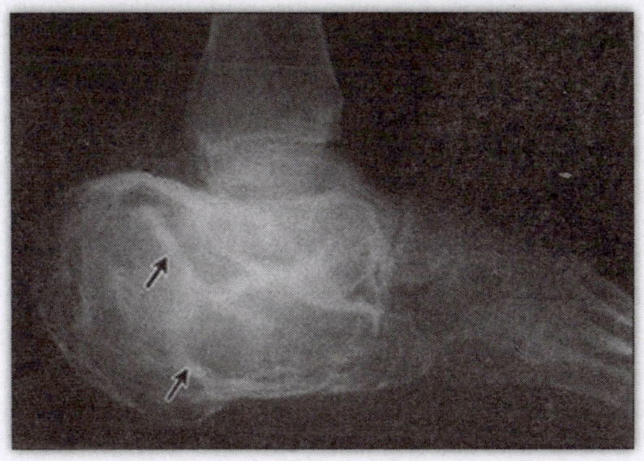

Fig: Patient of hemophilia with osseous pseudotumor of calcaneus. Radiograph of calcaneus shows well-defined, expansile, osteolytic lesion occupying entire calcaneus with scalloped appearance and contour deformity. Thick trabeculae (arrows) are also seen crossing osteolytic area. If chronic, cortical thickening is also noted as in this case

Option (C)

Pigmented villonodular Synovitis is a disease of synovium and a lytic lesion with in Calcaneum without any sign of involvement of synovium rules out Pigmented villonodular Synovitis.

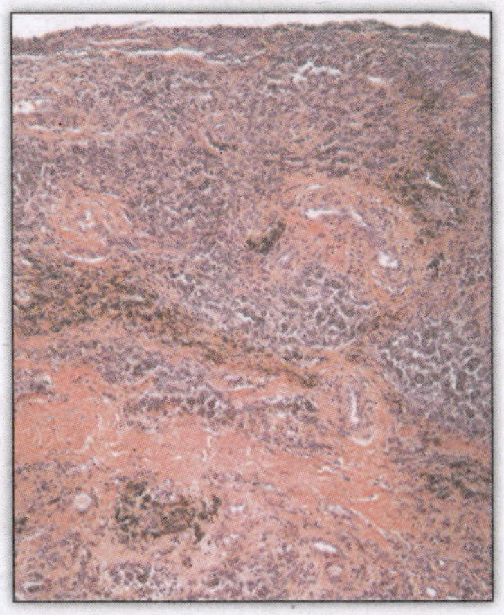

Fig: Micrograph of Pigmented villonodular Synovitis (PVNS) showing pigmented hemosiderin-laden macrophages (brown/red)

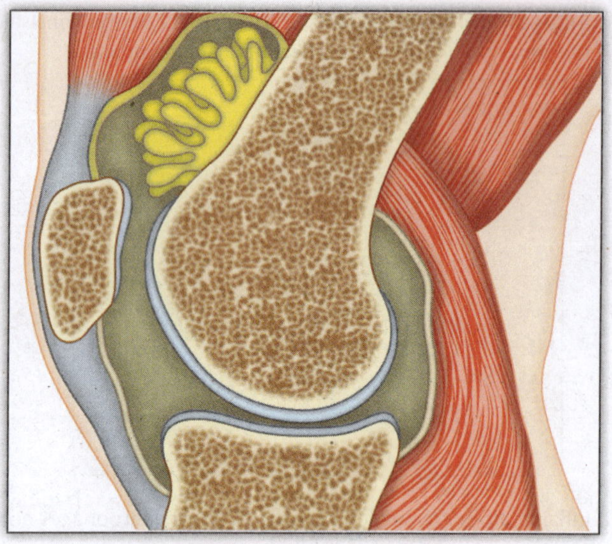

Fig: Pigmented villonodular Synovitis is a disease of abnormal growth of synovium. The additional tissue in the joint can cause pain, limit movements or cause the joint to lock, and in some cases, can destroy the normal joint structure. The knee is most commonly affected by this condition, though it can occur in other joints such as the hip, shoulder, elbow, ankle, or wrist

Option (D)

Mycetoma shows destructive lesions and sinuses of the bone not lytic lesions. **Mycetoma** is a chronic granulomatous disease with a progressive inflammatory reaction. Over the course of years, mycetoma progresses from small nodules to large, bone-invasive mutilating lesions. Mycetoma is usually caused when skin is repetitively broken and exposed to soil or water that contains the causal bacteria or fungi. Mycetoma presents as a triad of painless, firm subcutaneous masses, formation of multiple sinuses within the mass, and a purulent or seropurulent discharge containing sand-like particles called "grains," that can be white, yellow, red, brown, or black.

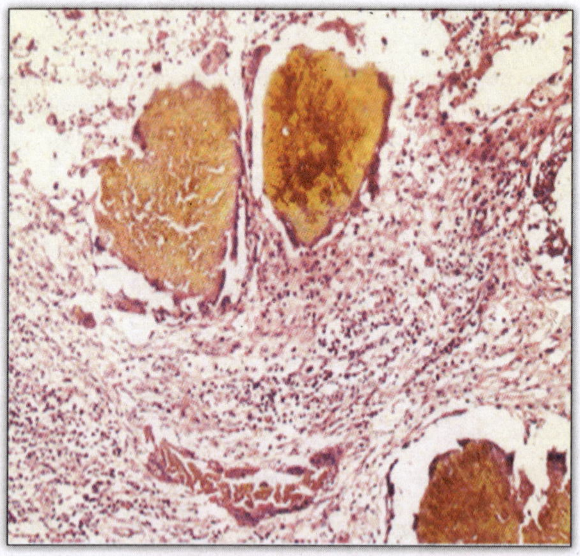

© Dr. Ahmed Fahal, Mycetoma Research Center, Khartoum, Sudan

Fig: Madurella mycetomi grains that tend to be large, light to dark brown in color, irregular outlines

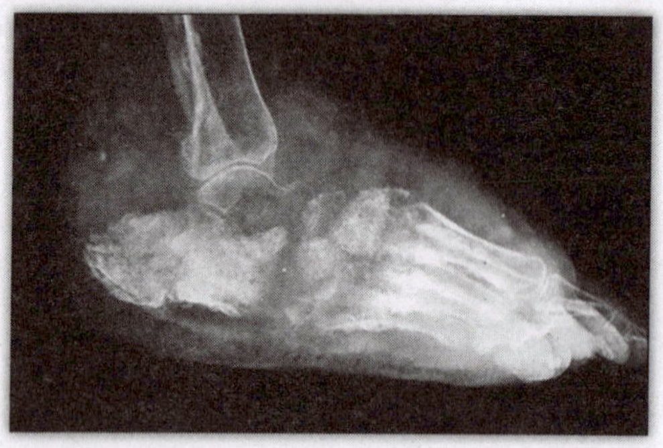

© Dr Ahmed Fahal, Mycetoma Research Center, Khartoum, Sudan

Fig: X-ray of foot eumycetoma showing massive soft tissue, periosteal reaction at the lower tibia, and multiple bone cavities involving most of the foot bones

AIIMS MAY 2018

20. Ans. (d) Bone fracture

Ref: Rubin's Pathology 6th Ed page 236

Bones primarily contain collagen. Hence, deficiency of elastin is not likely to cause bone fracture.

Marfan syndrome, is caused by dysfunction of the FBNI gene, which codes for the production of fibrillin-1, and is found on chromosome 15. Fibrillin-1 is essential for elastin production, an important component in the ECM of the aorta, ligaments and eyes **(Ref: Essential Human Development edited by Samuel Webster, Geraint Morris, Euan Kevelighan page 96)**

Diagnostic Criteria of Marfan Syndrome

Major criteria	Minor criteria
• Enlarged aorta • Tear in the aorta • Dislocation of the lens • Family history of the syndrome • At least four skeletal problems, such as flat feet or curved spine • Dural ectasia (enlargement of the lining that surrounds part of the spinal cord)	• Short sightedness (myopia) • Unexplained stretch marks • Loose joints

21. Ans. (b) Asthenospermia

Ref: Robbins 9th Edition, Page 283

Kartagener syndrome is seen in half of the patients with primary ciliary dyskinsia (autosomal recessive disorder caused by defects in ciliary motor proteins like dynein).

- Kartagener syndrome comprises of a triad of situs invertus, bronchiectasis and sinusitis
- It is also associated with male infertility due to sperm dysmotility (asthenospermia or asthenozoospermia).

22. Ans. (b) Ion exchange Chromatography

Ref: Clinical Chemistry, techniques, principles & correlations, Michael L. Bishop 6th Ed Pg 325,Tietz 5th Ed Pg 1443-1444

NOTE

If "High performance liquid chromatography" is provided in the options it will be the best answer

- There are a number of methods available for measurement of HbA1C. However, High performance liquid chromatography is used for standardisation of HbA1c assays. In the clinical laboratory, affinity chromatography is the preferred method of measurement.
- Standardization of glycosylated hemoglobin has been a continuing problem; there was no consensus on the reference method and no single standard is available to be used in the assays. Because of this, HbA1c values vary with the method and laboratory performing them.
- The International Federation of Clinical Chemistry and Laboratory Medicine (IFCC) developed a common definition for HbA1c and a reference method that specifically measures the concentration of only one molecular species of glycated A1c, the glycated N-terminal residue of the beta-chain of hemoglobin.
- This method, using either HPLC/electrospray mass spectrometry (HPLC-ESI/MS) or HPLC/capillary electrophoresis (HPLC-CE), is only used to standardize Atc assays and cannot be used for the clinical measurement of HbAlc.

Methods of Glycated Hemoglobin Measurement

Methods based on Structural Differences		
Immunoassays	Polyclonal or monoclonal antibodies toward the glycated N-terminal group of the β chain of hemoglobin	
Affinity chromatography	Separates based on chemical structure using borate to bind glycosylated proteins	Not temperature dependent Not affected by other hemoglobins
Methods based on Charge Differences		
Ion-exchange chromatography	Positive-charge resin bed	Highly temperature dependent Affected by hemoglobinopatheis
Electrophoresis	Separation is based on differences in charge	Hemoglobin F values >7% interferes
Isoelectric focusing	Type of electrophoresis using isoelectric point to separate	Pre-HbA$_1$c interferes
High-pressure liquid chromatography (HPLC)	A form on ion-exchange chromatography	Separates of all forms of glycosylated hemoglobin: A$_1$a, A$_1$b, A$_1$c

23. Ans. (c) Condenser

Ref: Essentials of Medical Microbiology by Apurba Sankar Sastry 2nd Ed Pg 10

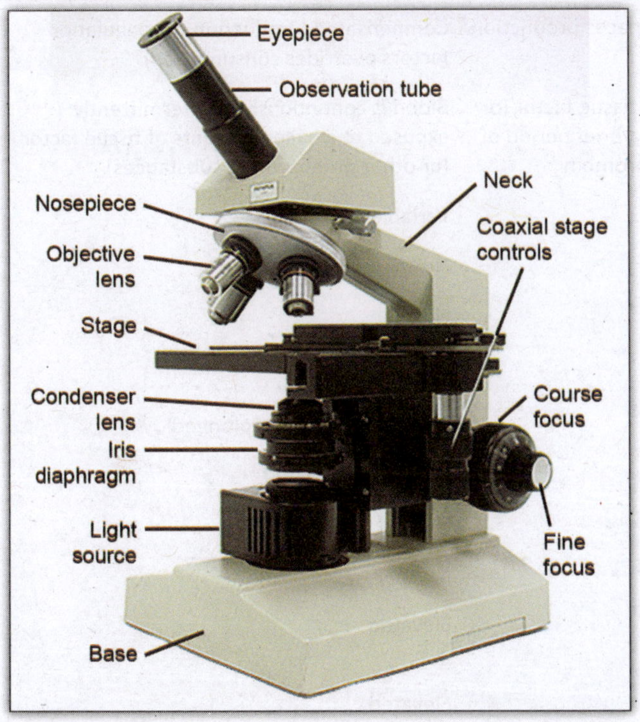

Fig: Parts and components of Light Microscope (Labeled)

Eyepieces: The eyepieces are the lenses at the top that the viewer looks through. To get the total magnification level, multiply the magnification of the objective used (ex: 10X eyepiece * 40X objective = 400X total magnification).

Tube: connects the eyepieces to the objective lenses.

Base: It is the bottom of the microscope, what the microscope stands on.

Arm: Structural element that connects the head of the microscope to the base.

Stage: The flat platform that supports the slides. Stage clips hold the slides in place.

Illuminator: A steady light source (110 volts) that shines up through the slide. Mirrors are sometimes used in lieu of a built-in light. If your microscope has a mirror, it is used to reflect light from an external light source up through the bottom of the stage.

Nose piece: Its a circular structure is where the different objective lenses are screwed in. To change the magnification power, simply rotate the turret.

Objective Lenses: Usually you will find 3 or 4 objective lenses on a microscope. The most common ones are 4X (shortest lens), 10X, 40X and 100X (longest lens). The higher power objectives (starting from 40x) are spring loaded. Spring loaded objective lenses will retract if the objective lens hits a slide, preventing damage to both the lens and the slide. All quality microscopes have achromatic, parcentered, parfocal lenses.

Rack Stop: This feature determines how far up the stage can go. Setting the rack stop is useful in preventing the slide from coming too far up and hitting the objective lens.

Condenser Lens: Condenser lenses focus the light, and are useful for attaining sharp images at magnifications of 400X and above. If the maximum power of microscope is 400X, a stage mounted 0.65 NA (or greater) condenser is ideal since it give you greater clarity without having to be focused separately. However, if microscope magnifying power is 1000X or above, focusable condenser lens with an N.A. of 1.25 or greater is needed.

Diaphragm or Iris: The diaphragm or iris is located under the stage and is an apparatus that can be adjusted to vary the intensity, and size, of the cone of light that is projected through the slide. As there is no set rule on which setting to use for a particular power, the setting depends on the transparency of the specimen and the degree of contrast you desire in your image.

24. Ans. (b) Increased FDPs

Ref: Harrison's 19th Ed Pg 737, Essentials of Haematology by Shirish Kawathalkar 2nd Ed Pg 442-447

NOTE

All the provided options parameters are deranged in acute DIC. However, since consumptive coagulopathy is the hallmark of DIC, FDP's are elevated in acute as well as chronic DIC.

"The most sensitive test for DIC is the FDP level. DIC is an unlikely diagnosis in the presence of normal levels of FDP." **(Ref: Harrison's 19th Ed Pg 737)**

"The fibrin degradation products (FDPs) that are generated in turn disrupt normal fibrin polymerization and fibrinogen binding to platelet surface αIIbβ3 (GPIIbIIIa), thus interfering with both fibrin clot formation and platelet aggregation, and effectively operating as pathological anticoagulant and antiplatelet agents. ***The consumptive coagulopathy, combined with the high concentration of FDPs, leads to the severe bleeding diathesis seen in decompensated DIC*** and accounts for the clinical observation that supportive therapy with Fresh Frozen Plasma (FFP) and platelet transfusions by themselves are generally insufficient to completely correct the bleeding diathesis. Clotting times become prolonged and the potential for clinically important bleeding increases"

As seen from above discussion, presence of high levels of FDP's worsens consumption coagulopathy and can cause severe bleeding. As a result, elevated FDP can act as an indicator of bleeding in DIC.

Disseminated Intravascular Coagulation

- DIC is a clinicopathologic syndrome characterized by widespread intravascular fibrin formation in response to excessive blood protease activity that overcomes the natural anticoagulant mechanisms.
- The most common causes are bacterial sepsis, malignant disorders such as solid tumors or acute promyelocytic leukemia, obstetric causes, trauma.
- The highlight of DIC is consumptive coagulopathy.

Acute Vs Chronic DIC

	Acute DIC	Chronic DIC
Status	Decompensated (Consumption overspaces production of coagulation factors)	Compensated (Production of coagulation factors overrides consumption)
Pathogenesis	Blood is exposed to large amounts of tissue factor (or other procoagulant substances) over a brief period of time, with significant generation of thrombin	Blood is continuously or intermittently exposed to smaller amounts of tissue factor (or other procoagulant substances)
Platelet count	Reduced	Variable
Prothrombin time (PT)	Prolonged	Normal
Activated partial thromboplastin time (aPTT)	Prolonged	Normal
Thrombin time	Prolonged	Normal to slightly prolonged
Plasma fibrinogen	Reduced	Normal to elevated
Plasma factor V	Reduced	Normal
Plasma factor VIII	Reduced	Normal
Fibrin degradation products (FDP)	Elevated	Elevated
D-dimer	Elevated	Elevated

25. Ans. (a) AML with hyperploidy

Ref: The 2016 revision to the World Health Organization classification of myeloid neoplasms and acute leukemia

AML with hyperploidy is not a provisional entity according to WHO 2016 classification.

Provisional Entities in WHO 2016 Classification	
Leukemia	**Myeloid origin**
AML with BCR-ABL *AML with mutated RUNX1* *B-lymphoblastic leukemia/ lymphoma, BCR-ABL1–like* *B-lymphoblastic leukemia/ lymphoma with iAMP21* *Early T-cell precursor lymphoblastic leukemia* *Natural killer (NK) cell lymphoblastic leukemia/ lymphoma*	Myeloid/lymphoid neoplasms with PCM1-JAK2 Provisional entity: Refractory cytopenia of childhood

26. Ans. (c) Rolling- Activation of Integrins– Stable Adhesion– migration via endothelium

Ref: Robin's 9th Ed Pg 35

The sequence of events in the recruitment of leukocytes from the vascular lumen to the extravascular space consists of

- **Margination and rolling along the vessel wall**: in postcapillary venules, circulating cells are swept by laminar flow against the vessel wall. Because the smaller red cells tend to move faster than the larger white cells, leukocytes are pushed out of the central axial column and thus have a better opportunity to interact with lining endothelial cells, especially as stasis sets in. If the endothelial cells are activated by cytokines and other mediators produced locally, they express adhesion molecules to which the leukocytes attach loosely. These cells bind and detach and thus begin to tumble on the endothelial surface, a process called rolling
- **Firm adhesion to the endothelium:** The rolling leukocytes are able to sense changes in the endothelium that initiate the next step in the reaction of leukocytes, which is firm adhesion to endothelial surfaces. This adhesion is mediated by integrins expressed on leukocyte cell surfaces interacting with their ligands on endothelial cells
- **Transmigration between endothelial cells:** After being arrested on the endothelial surface, leukocytes migrate through the vessel wall primarily by squeezing between cells at intercellular junctions. This extravasation of leukocytes, called diapedesis, occurs mainly in the venules of the systemic vasculature
- **Migration in interstitial tissues toward a chemotactic stimulus.**
After extravasating from the blood, leukocytes move toward sites of infection or injury along a chemical gradient by a process called chemotaxis. Both exogenous and endogenous substances can be chemotactic for leukocytes, including Bacterial products, Cytokines (especially those of the chemokine family), Components of the complement system, particularly C5, Products of the lipoxygenase pathway of arachidonic acid (AA) metabolism, particularly leukotriene B4 (LTB4). These mediators are produced in response to infections and tissue damage and during immunologic reactions.

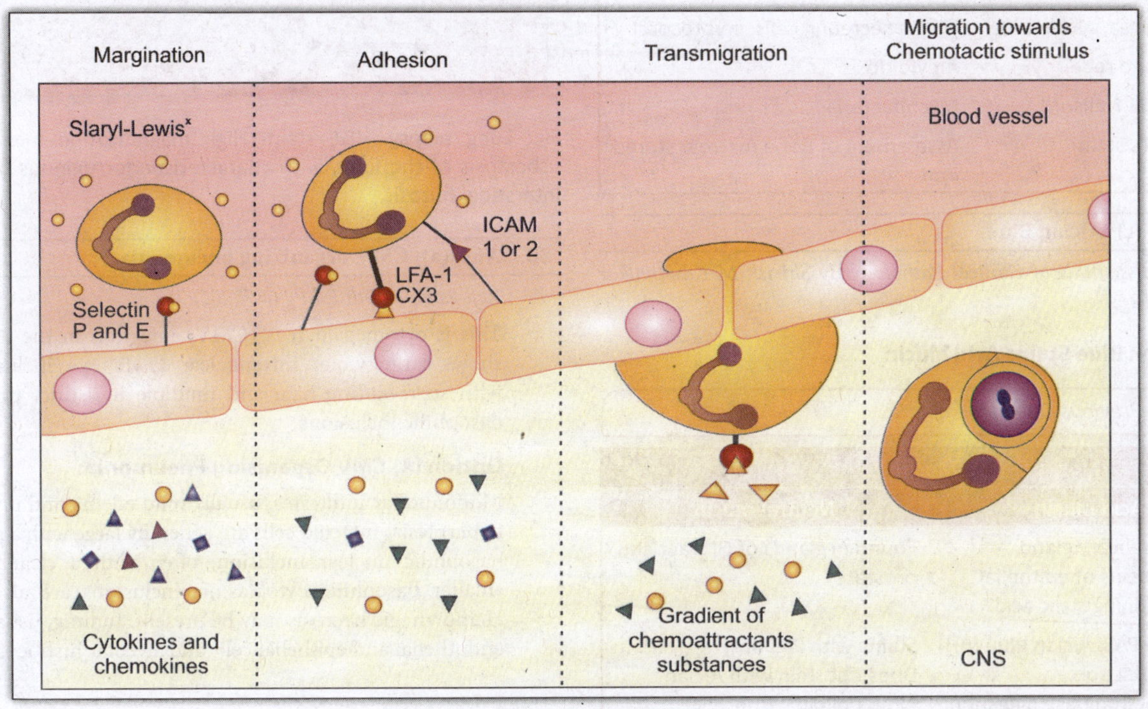

Leukocyte Migration

27. Ans. (a) Mast cells

Ref: Bancroft's histological techniques 7th Ed Pg 162, Essentials of Clinical Pathology by Shirish M Kawthalkar Pg 252

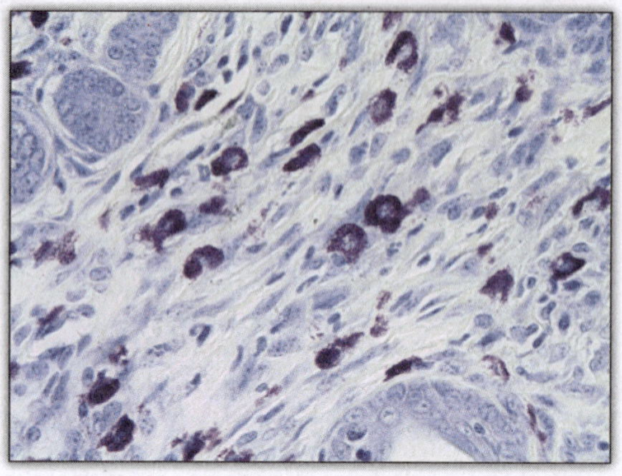

Fig: Mast cells are seen stained in Toluidine blue in the above figure

Toluidine blue (TB) is a **polychromatic dye** which can absorb different colours depending on how it binds chemically with various tissue. Mast cells are found in the connective tissue and their cytoplasm contains granules (metachromatic) composed of heparin and histamine. Toluidine blue should stain mast cells red-purple (**metachromatic staining**) and the background blue (**orthochromatic staining**)

Special Stains in Bone Marrow	
Stain	**Condition**
Reticulin stain	Marrow fibrosis
Periodic Acid Schiff	Complex Carbohydrates, fungi, tumor cells
Toluidine blue	Mast cells
Giemsa, Alcian blue	Mucin secreting cells, cryptococci
Congo red	Amyloidosis
Ziehl- Neilson	Mycobacteria
Perl's stain	Assessment of Bone marrow stored iron

28. Ans. (c) Alcian Blue

Ref: Essentials of Clinical Pathology By Shirish M Kawthalkar Pg 252

Alcian Blue Stains Acid Mucin

See Previous Question

Mucin	
Acid mucin	**Neutral mucin**
Found in salivary gland Typical mucins of epithelial cells containing sialic acid.	Found in glands of GI tract and prostate
Stain with PAS, Alcian blue (pH-2.5) colloidal iron. Resist hyaluronidase digestion	Stains with PAS only Does not stain with Alcian blue, Colloidal iron, Muscarmine,

Mucin	
Acid mucin	**Neutral mucin**
Note: **Acid mucin can also be of the sulfated mesenchymal type.** These contain hyaluronic acid and are found in tissue stroma. Stain with: Alcian blue (pH 2.5), colloidal iron, metachromatic dyes Do not stain with PAS. Digest Hyaluronic acid. Can be found in sarcomas.	

29. Ans. (c) Asbestosis

Ref: Robin's 9th Ed Pg 691-692

- Asbestos bodies, characteristic of asbestosis, are seen in the figure. Hence, asbestosis is the answer.
- Asbestos bodies are seen as golden brown, fusiform or beaded rods with a translucent center.
- They consist of asbestos fibers coated with an iron-containing proteinaceous material. Asbestos bodies apparently are formed when macrophages attempt to phagocytose asbestos fibers; the iron is derived from phagocyte ferritin.

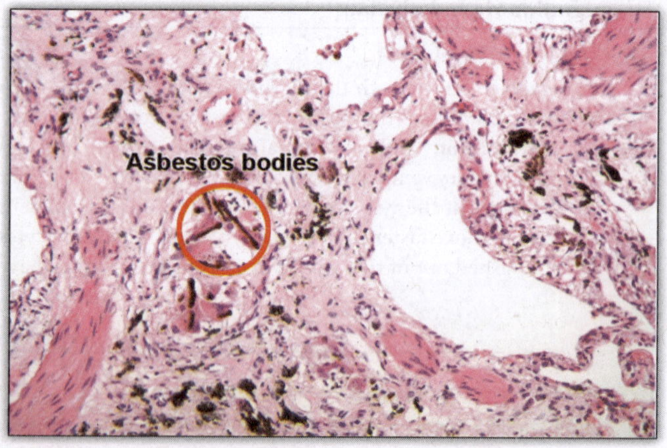

Fig: Lung biopsy. H&E stain- High magnification micrograph of asbestosis of the lung, with characteristic ferruginous bodies and interstitial fibrosis

30. Ans. (a) CMV organizing pneumonia

Ref: Robbin's 9th Ed Pg 687, 705, 717

This is cytomegalovirus (CMV) infection in the lung. CMV shows large violet intranuclear Owl's eye inclusion body with surrounding halo and multiple indistinct cytoplasmic, basophilic inclusions

Option (A) CMV Organising Pneumonia:

Mononuclear infiltrates, usually mild edema and pneumocyte hyperplasia. Infected cells are generally large with a prominent basophilic nuclear inclusion, often with a clear halo, and smaller basophilic cytoplasmic inclusions are also present. Hemorrhagic necrosis may be present. In lung, usually infects endothelial and epithelial cells and alveolar histiocytes.

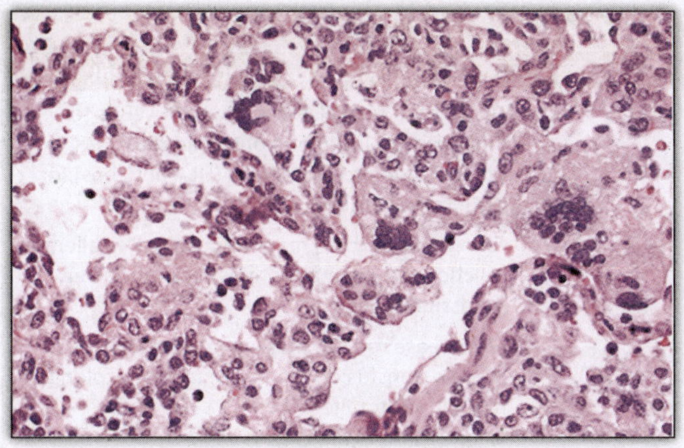

Fig: CMV organising pneumonia: Within consolidated areas, alveolar septa are expanded by hyperplastic type II pneumocytes, macrophages, edema, and alveoli contain numerous foamy macrophages, multinucleated viral syncytia, and fewer neutrophils. CMV shows large violet intranuclear Owl's eye inclusion body with surrounding halo and multiple indistinct cytoplasmic, basophilic inclusions

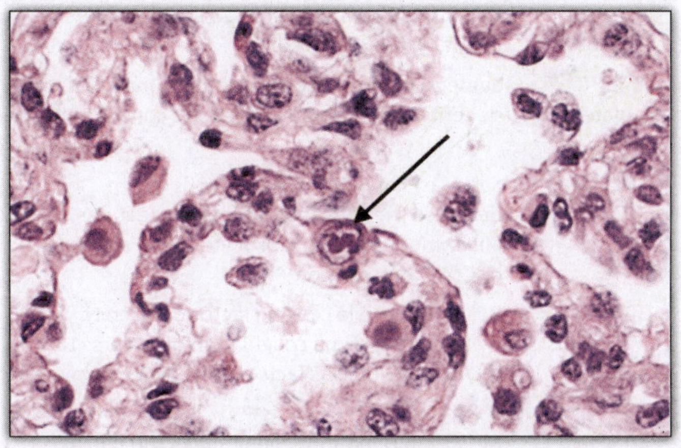

Fig: CMV organising pneumonia: Within consolidated areas, occasional pneumocytes are karyomegalic and the nucleus contains a single enlarged eosinophilic cytomegaloviral inclusion

Option (B)

Cryptogenic organizing pneumonia is a noninfectious inflammatory pulmonary process that leads to the formation of fibromyxoid connective tissue plugs in bronchioles and alveolar ducts (bronchiolitis obliterans) and organizing pneumonia within alveoli

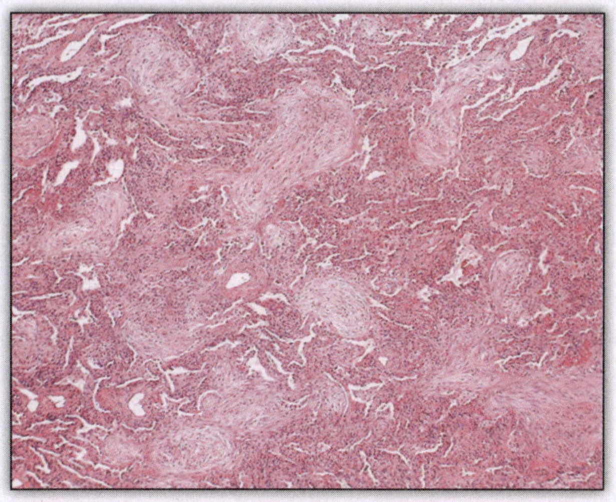

Fig: Cryptogenic organising pneumonia histopathology: This low magnification images shows numerous alveoli and alveolar ducts occupied by immature connective tissue and fibroblasts. This type of structure is sometimes referred to as a Masson body

Option (D)

Organized Pneumonia with tuberculosis will show Granuloma with central necrosis

31. Ans. (b) RBC 2–6°C, Platelet 20–24°C, FFP –30°C

Ref: Essentials of Haematology by Shirish Kawathalkar 2nd Ed Pg 396

RBC's: Whole blood is stored between 2–6 degree Celsius. Transfusion of whole blood must be started within 30 minutes of removal from refrigerator and completed within 4 hours.

Platelets: Platelets are stored at 20–24°C with continuous agitation in a device called platelet agitator. Maximum period of storage is 5 days. Units of platelets from different donors are pooled into one bag before transfusion. After pooling, the transfusion should be completed within 4 hours.

FFP: Collected → Frozen within 8 hours → rapidly frozen and stored at or below –18°C → thawed for 30–45 minutes at 30–37°C → then stored at 2–6°C to be used within 24 hours.

Blood Components and Indications For Use

Component	Composition	Volume	Storage	Indications and expected benefit
Whole blood	RBC and plasma (approx. Hct, 40%); WBCs; platelets	500 mL	2-6 °C	To increase red cell mass and plasma volume (plasma deficient in labile clotting factors V and VIII); for hypovolemic anemia, massive transfusion, or exchange transfusion in neonates
Packed RBCs	RBC and reduced plasma (approx. Hct, 75%); WBCs; platelets	250 mL	2-6 °C	To increase red cell mass in symptomatic anemia; 10 mL/kg raises Hct by 10%
RBCs, adenine-saline added	RBC and 100 mL of additive solution (approx. Hct, 60%); WBCs; platelets; little plasma	330 mL	2-6 °C	To increase red cell mass in symptomatic anemia; 10 mL/kg raises Hct by 8%

Contd...

Blood Components and Indications For Use				
Component	**Composition**	**Volume**	**Storage**	**Indications and expected benefit**
RBCs, leukocytes reduced (prepared by filtration)	>85% original volume of RBCs; <5 × 106 WBCs	>85% of original volume	2-6°C	To increase red cell mass; <5 × 10^6 WBCs to decrease the likelihood of febrile reactions, immunization to leukocytes (HLA antigens), or CMV transmission
RBCs, washed	RBCs (approx. Hct, 75%); reduced WBCs; no plasma	225 mL	2-6°C	To increase red cell mass; reduce risk of allergic reactions to plasma proteins; or reduce free potassium dose
RBCs, frozen	RBCs (approx. Hct, 75%);	225 mL	−80°C (−176°F)	To increase red cell mass; minimize febrile or allergic transfusion reactions; use for prolonged RBC blood storage
Granulocytes, pheresis	> 1 × 10^{10} granulocytes per unit 10–30 mL of RBC 1–6 × 10^6 platelet	220 mL	20-24°C	To provide granulocytes for selected patients with sepsis and severe neutropenia (Absolute neutrophil count <0.5 × 109/L i.e. <500/µl). Dose: Generally > 4 x 10^{10} once daily either until significant clinical improvement or ANC > 500/µl or 42 days, whichever comes earlier
RDP- Random donor platelet (Platelet concentrates)	Platelets (>5.5 × 10^{10}/unit); RBCs; WBCs; plasma	50 mL	20-24°C in platelet agitator	Bleeding due to thrombocytopenia or thrombocytopathy; 1 unit/10 kg raises platelet count by 17–50 × 10^9/L
SDP- Single donor platelet (Platelets pheresis)	Platelets (>3 × 1011/unit); RBCs; WBCs; plasma	300 mL	20-24°C in platelet agitator	Same as platelets; sometimes HLA matched; benefit is equivalent to 6 platelet concentrates
Platelets, leukocytes reduced	Platelets (as above); <5 × 10^6 WBCs/final dose of pooled or pheresis platelets	300 mL	20-24°C	Same as platelets; <5 × 10^6 WBCs to decrease the likelihood of febrile reactions, alloimmunization to leukocytes (HLA antigens), or CMV transmission
FFP; thawed plasma	FFP: All coagulation factors; thawed plasma: Reduced factors V and VIII	200 mL	-30°C thawed just before use	Best for multiple clotting factor deficiency. Treatment of some coagulation disorders; 10 mL/kg of FFP raises factor levels by a maximum of 25%
Cryoprecipitate (antihemophilic factor)	Fibrinogen; factors VIII and XIII; von Willebrand factor	15 mL	-30°C	MC use in Hypofibrinogenemia (<100 mg/dL) (1 unit/5 kg raises fibrinogen 70 mg/dL). Also used for factor XIII replacement (now not first-choice therapy for hemophilia A), von Willebrand disease, topical fibrin sealant

32. Ans. (b) Completed within 4 hours of receiving from blood bank

Ref: Essentials of Haematology by Shirish Kawathalkar 2nd Ed Pg 487-489

NOTE

Ideally it should be mentioned as removal from the refrigerator in the question. However for the sake of this question it can be taken equated to receiving from the blood bank.

Transfusion of whole blood must be started within 30 minutes of removal from refrigerator and completed within 4 hours of removal from refrigerator (i.e. receiving from the blood bank).

See Previous Question for Details

33. Ans. (b) FISH

Ref: Practical Soft Tissue Pathology by Jason L. Hornick 2nd Ed Pg 18

Cytogenetic and molecular genetic studies can be useful adjunctive tools in diagnosing Ewing sarcoma. The t(11;22)(q24;q12) chromosomal translocation or variants thereof are detectable in more than 95% of Ewing sarcomas and PNETs. The breakpoints of these translocations have indicated the involvement of the EWS gene on chromosome 22, the FL1-1 gene on chromosome 11, and the ERG gene on chromosome 21. This results in the production of the ***fusion genes EWS-FL1-1 for t(11;22) and EWS-ERG for t(21;22), which can be detected by reverse transcriptase polymerase chain reaction (RT-PCR) and fluorescence in situ hybridization (FISH) techniques.*** (Ref: Sternberg Surgical Pathology 5th ed page 242)

FISH studies may detect variant forms of the translocation that are negative by RT-PCR. Secondly, FISH methods detect proliferating cells that presumably are more likely to correlate with active disease, in contrast with RT-PCR, that can detect both proliferating and non proliferating cells. **(Ref: The Molecular Basis of Human Cancer edited by William B. Coleman, Gregory J. Tsongalis page 431)**

- Most cases of Ewing's sarcoma (85%) are the result of a translocation between chromosomes 11 and 22, which fuses the EWS gene of chromosome 22 to the FLI1 gene of chromosome 11.
- Ewing sarcoma/primitive neuroectodermal tumor (EWS/PNET) is a diagnostically challenging malignant round cell tumor with signature translocations involving the EWS gene.
- This translocation is detectable with both reverse transcriptase-polymerase chain reaction (RT-PCR) and fluorescence in situ hybridization (FISH) in formalin-fixed paraffin-embedded tissue. However, RT-PCR is less sensitive in formalin-fixed paraffin-embedded than frozen tissue. RT-PCR is suitable when frozen tissue is available.

Approach for Demonstration of Fusion Gene in Ewing's Sarcoma

Level	Technique	Comments
Chromosomal (metaphase)	Karyotyping	Requires fresh tissue
Chromosomal (interphase)	Fluorescent In Situ Hybridisation (FISH)	Best seen in formalin-fixed paraffin-embedded tissue. Specimen from Fine-needle aspirates, touch preparations, smears can also be used. Allows a more focused look on a specific genetic locus. Application of Centromere specific and sequence-specific probes
Fusion genes	Long range PCR	Difficult since introns can be large and breakpoints are not clustered Not robust for clinical applications
mRNA transcribed from fusion gene	RT-PCR	Suitable for frozen tissue, less sensitive for paraffin-embedded tissue. Fusion protein can be detected even if sample is not rich in tumor DNA, thus samples such as needle biopsies can be used. Detect more common fusions, rare fusions can be missed. Highly sensitive so contamination can be an issue.
Gene	Next Generation Sequencing	Allows sequencing examination of many genes in parallel. 25-500 genes are screened which are considered important for cancer. Comparatively less useful in sarcomas since panels are based on mutations in carcinoma and melanoma.
Fusion protein	Immunohistochemistry	Also detects wild-type protein and thus not specific.

34. Ans. (b) Embryonal rhabdomyosarcoma

Ref: Rosai and Ackerman's Surgical Pathology By John R. Goldblum 11th ed Pg 1872,

Clue to Diagnosis

- **Vimentin and Desmin** are positive for Mesenchymal tumors and soft tissue sarcomas. Embryonal Rhabdomyosarcoma is a Mesenchymal tumor hence Desmin is positive.
- **Age = 5 years** (Embryonal sarcoma; traditionally designated 'rhabdomyosarcoma is the most common primary orbital malignancy of childhood)
- **Proptosis:** Embryonal Rhabdomyosarcoma presents in the 1st decade (average 7 years) with rapidly progressive unilateral proptosis which may initially mimic an inflammatory process.
- **Round cells:** Rhabdomyosarcoma is histologically subclassified into embryonal, alveolar, and pleomorphic variants. The **rhabdomyoblast**—the diagnostic cell in all types contains eccentric eosinophilic granular cytoplasm rich in thick and thin filaments. ***Rhabdomyoblasts may be round or elongate; the latter are known as tadpole or strap cells***, and may contain cross-striations visible by light microscopy
- ***Embryonal sarcoma (traditionally designated 'rhabdomyosarcoma') is the most common primary orbital malignancy of childhood.*** The tumour is derived from undifferentiated mesenchymal cell rests, which have the potential to differentiate into striated muscle (Ref: Kanski 7th ed)
- Even in tumors with almost no discernible rhabdomyoblasts, desmin or muscle actin immunostains are positive in more than 95% of cases, and this is therefore the most reliable means of making the diagnosis in the routine setting.
- Desmin is an in intermediate filament that is a specific indicator for muscle differentiation, but it is present in both smooth and striated muscle. In general, only tumors with round rhabdomyoblasts or strap cells show positivity for this marker.
- Other markers for embryonal rhabdomyosarcoma: Sarcomeric Actin (one of the best markers), myoglobin, myosin, titin, Z-protein.

- Rhabdomyosarcomas are aggressive neoplasms that are usually treated with surgery and chemotherapy with or without radiation therapy.
- The histologic type and location of the tumor influence survival. ***The botryoid subtype has the best prognosis,*** while the anaplastic embryonal, pleomorphic, and alveolar variants are often fatal.

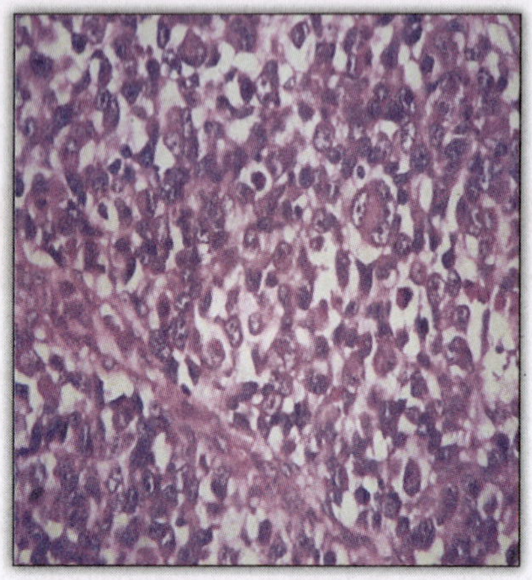

Fig: Histopathologic examination showed diffuse, Round to Spindle shaped tumor cells with abundant Red-Stained cytoplasm

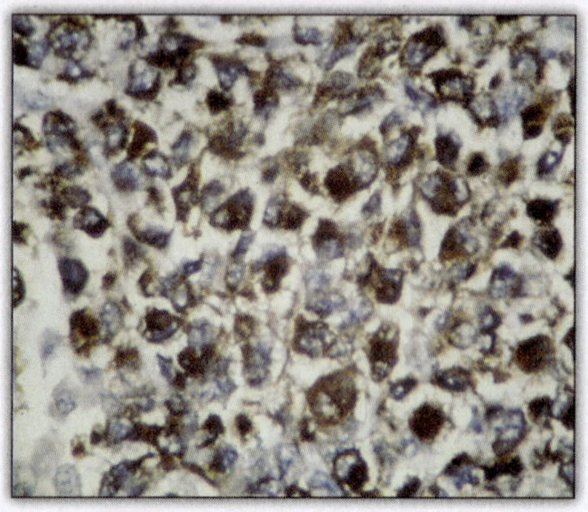

Fig: Embryonal rhabdomyosarcoma: desmin immunoreactivity in large eosinophilic cells (IHC ×40).

35. Ans. (c) Type III

Ref: Robin's 9th Ed Pg 23 and 108

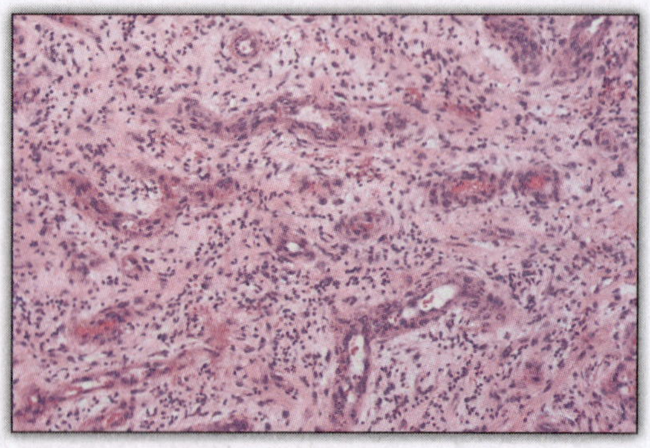

Fig: The picture is of Granulation tissue with proliferating capillaries and connective tissue with collagen producing fibroblasts and a mixed inflammatory infiltrate consisting of lymphocytes, plasma cells, eosinophilic and neutrophilic granulocytes and histiocytes

Fibroblasts and vascular endothelial cells proliferate in the first 24 to 72 hours (Day 1-3) of the repair process to form a specialized type of tissue called granulation tissue, which is a hallmark of tissue repair. The term derives from its pink, soft, granular appearance on the surface of wounds. Its characteristic histologic feature is the presence of new small blood vessels (angiogenesis) and the proliferation of fibroblasts. These new vessels are leaky, allowing the passage of plasma proteins and fluid into the extravascular space. Thus, new granulation tissue is often edematous. Granulation tissue progressively invades the incision space; the amount of granulation tissue that is formed depends on the size of the tissue deficit created by the wound and the intensity of inflammation. Hence, it is much more prominent in healing by secondary union. By 5 to 7 days, granulation tissue fills the wound area and neovascularization is maximal

At first a provisional matrix containing fibrin, plasma fibronectin, and type III collagen is formed, but this is replaced by a matrix composed primarily of type I collagen. (Robbins)

36. Ans. (a) A first line defense for bacterial peptide

Ref: Cell Signaling in Host–Pathogen Interactions by Diana Bahia 1st Ed Pg 113

- Gamma delta (γδ) T cells are the prototype of 'unconventional' T cells and represent a relatively small subset of T cells in peripheral blood.
- They are defined by expression of heterodimeric T-cell receptors (TCRs) composed of γ and δ chains. This sets them apart from the classical CD4+ helper T cells and CD8+ cytotoxic T cells that express αβ TCRs.
- Gamma-delta TCR binds directly to the antigens and does not require specialized antigen processing and presentation, as alpha-beta T cells do.
- These cells do not have a thymic differentiation phase and are derived directly from bone marrow precursors. They are positive for CD3, CD2, and CD7 but negative for CD4 and CD8, and they express cytotoxic granules in the cytoplasm.
- They are present primarily in mucocutaneous sites (skin, genital tract, GIT) where they serve as first responders to commonly encountered bacteria.
- Many antigens recognized by gamma delta T-cell are unconventional nonpeptide phosphoantigens, endogenous metabolites of cholesterol biosynthesis that are produced by bacteria.
- They participate in innate immune responses and also in tissue repair by expressing epithelial growth factors

AIIMS NOVEMBER 2017

37. Ans. (a) Aspiration pneumonia with vegetative matter

Ref: Robbin's 9th ed page 525

Chest X ray findings are suggestive of consolidation/ Pneumonia. Histopathological findings confirms aspiration pneumonia of vegetative matter.

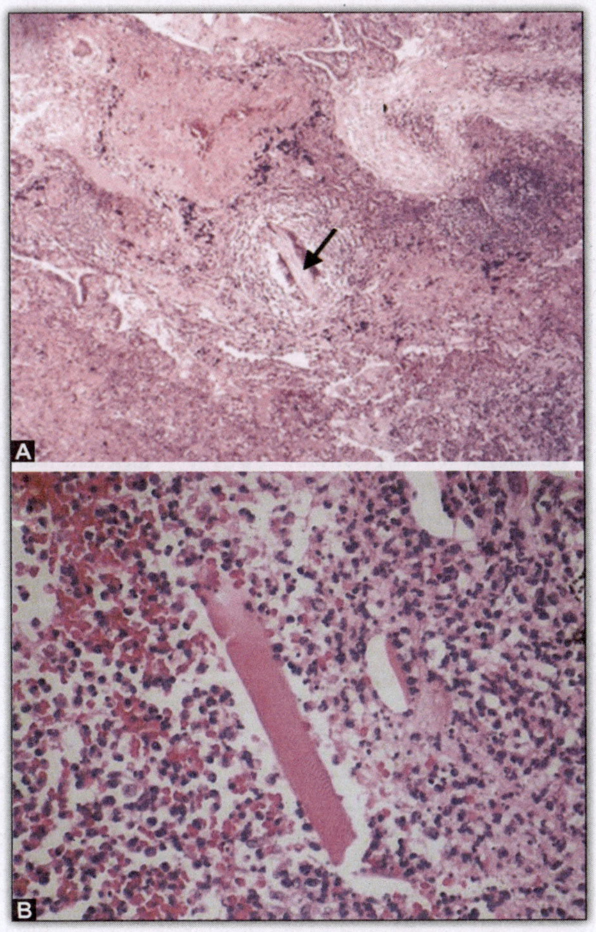

Figs A and B: (A) Aspiration Pneumonia due to Vegetative matter: Dense granulocytic infiltrate with Giant cells surround vegetable matter (arrow) in purulent exudates, organizing pneumonia (Top right corner) and Hyperemic capillaries; **(B)** Aspiration pneumonia showing skeletal muscle

Aspiration pneumonia: Most commonly food aspiration is due to vegetable matter (seeds), skeletal muscle, fat tissue, or fragments of bone. The most common vegetable matter seen in chronic aspiration is the starch grain or granule, found in legumes, including peas, beans, and lentils. The starch granule is about 100 μ in length, is eosinophilic and well demarcated and oval, and eventually degenerates as macrophages engulf the material. If foreign material is not present, a histologic diagnosis of aspiration pneumonia cannot be made. Acute exudative response in <24 h. Chronic changes include foreign body giant cell reaction and organizing pneumonia. Fibrosis and calcification can occur at later stages. Recurrent aspiration can lead to diffuse bronchiolitis in a miliary form.

38. Ans. (b) HER 2 neu 2+

Ref: Breast Cancer Management and Molecular Medicine edited by Martine J. Piccart, William C. Wood, Chie-Mien Hung, Lawrence J. Solin, Fatima Cardoso page 982

HER 2 NEU IHC INTERPRETATION

0 Negative

+1 Negative

+2 Equivocal (Requires FISH amplification to confirm)

+3 Positive

39. Ans. (a) 95% ethyl alcohol

Ref: With Text

Pap smears are wet-fixed (smears are immersed in fixative without allowing them to dry). Smears to be stained by Romanowsky stains are air-dried as fixation is affected during the staining procedure. Fixative used is either equal parts of ether and 95% ethanol, or 95% ethanol alone, 100% methanol, or 85% isopropyl alcohol. Fixation time of 10-15 minutes at room temperature is adequate. Smear may be left in fixative for 24 hour or more **(Ref: Pathology Practical Book by Harsh Mohan - 3rd ed Page 152)**

Ether is highly volatile and explosive, hence ether's use in alcohol as fixative was discontinued in late 1950s, leaving 95% ethyl alcohol alone as the standard fixative for PAP smear. **(Ref: Cytopreparation: Principles and Practice - By Gary Gill Springer Page 104)**

40. Ans. (d) F, G and H

Ref: Robbins 9th ed page 447, Wintrobe 12th ed page 1090

Presence of 90% HBF indicates Homozygous beta Thalassemia

(F) Howell-Jolly bodies

(G) Target cells

(H) Teardrop cells

All three are seen in Beta Thalassemia

The reference ranges are as follows:

- HbA_1: 95–98%
- HbA_2: 1.5–3.5% (usually<3.3%)
- HbF: < 2% (age-dependent)
- HbC: Absent
- HbS: Absent

Conditions Associated with Elevation of Hemoglobin F Levels

Condition	Percentage of hemoglobin F
beta-thalassemia triat	<10
Delta/beta-thalassemia triat	5–20
Deletional HPFH trait	20–40
Nondeletional HPFH trait	3–30
Homozygous delta/beta-thalassemia	100
Homozygous HPFH (deletional)	100
Homozygous beta-thalassemia	30–95
Homozygous hemoglobin S or hemoglobin S-beta-thalassemia	5–30
Hemoglobin S–HPFH	20–40
Hemoglobin E-beta thalassemia	10–50
Hemoglobin C-beta thalassemia	10–30

Fetal hemoglobin (HbF) has two alpha and two gamma chains (alpha2 gamma2). Adult hemoglobin A (HbA) has two alpha and two beta chains (alpha2 beta2), whereas hemoglobin A2 (HbA2) has two alpha and two delta chains (alpha2 delta2). Fetal hemoglobin (hemoglobin F, HbF) is the major hemoglobin present during gestation; it constitutes approximately 60 to 80 percent of total hemoglobin in the full-term newborn. It is almost completely replaced by adult hemoglobin (hemoglobin A, HbA) by approximately 6 to 12 months of age, and it amounts to less than 1 percent of total hemoglobin in the adult.

Among the inherited conditions associated with increased HbF levels in adults, some are primary and caused by mutation or genetic variation; these are termed hereditary persistence of HbF (HPFH). Others, such as those associated with sickle cell anemia and thalassemia, result from secondary responses to the dyserythropoiesis and hemolysis characteristic of these disorders, modulated by co-inherited genetic variation.

- **Hereditary Persistence of Fetal Hemoglobin:** HPFH is characterized by the presence of increased levels of HbF in adult life in the absence of relevant hematologic abnormalities. The amount of HbF is quite variable, ranging in the carriers from 2.0 to 30%, and this variability reflects a marked molecular heterogeneity.
- **Beta thalassemia:** HbF levels are normal or slightly elevated in beta thalassemia heterozygotes. Higher HbF (and HbA2) levels are found with mutations that involve promoter of the HBB gene, but variations in HbF levels also reflect the genetic background of the individual. In homozygous beta thalassemia, the proportion of HbF ranges from 10 percent in those with the milder alleles to almost 100 percent in homozygotes or compound heterozygotes with beta thalassemia.
- **Sickle cell anemia:** The predominant hemoglobin is S; Hb F is present in varying concentrations; and Hb A2 is normal. There is no Hb A.

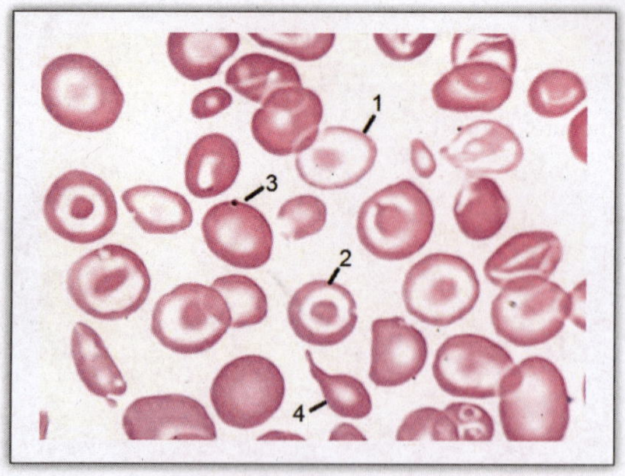

Fig: Blood picture of homozygous B thalassemia

Microcytic and hypochromic RBCs (1), Nucleated red cells, anisopoikilocytosis, target cells (2), Howell Jolly Bodies (3), Tear drop cells (4)

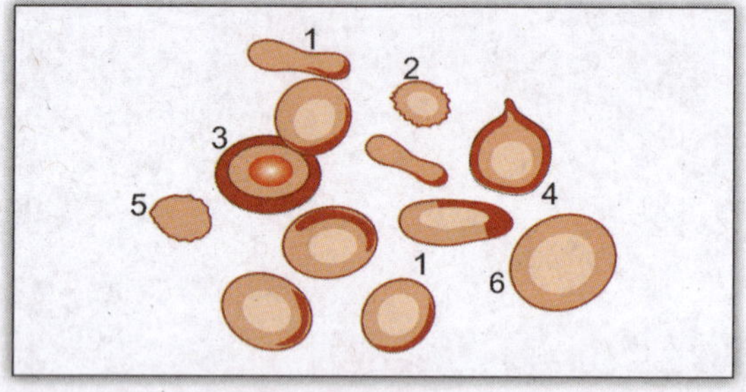

Poikilocytic red cells: (Elliptocytes (1), schistocytes (2), target cells (3), tear drop (4), spherocytes (5) and hypochromic (6) in Thalassemia major

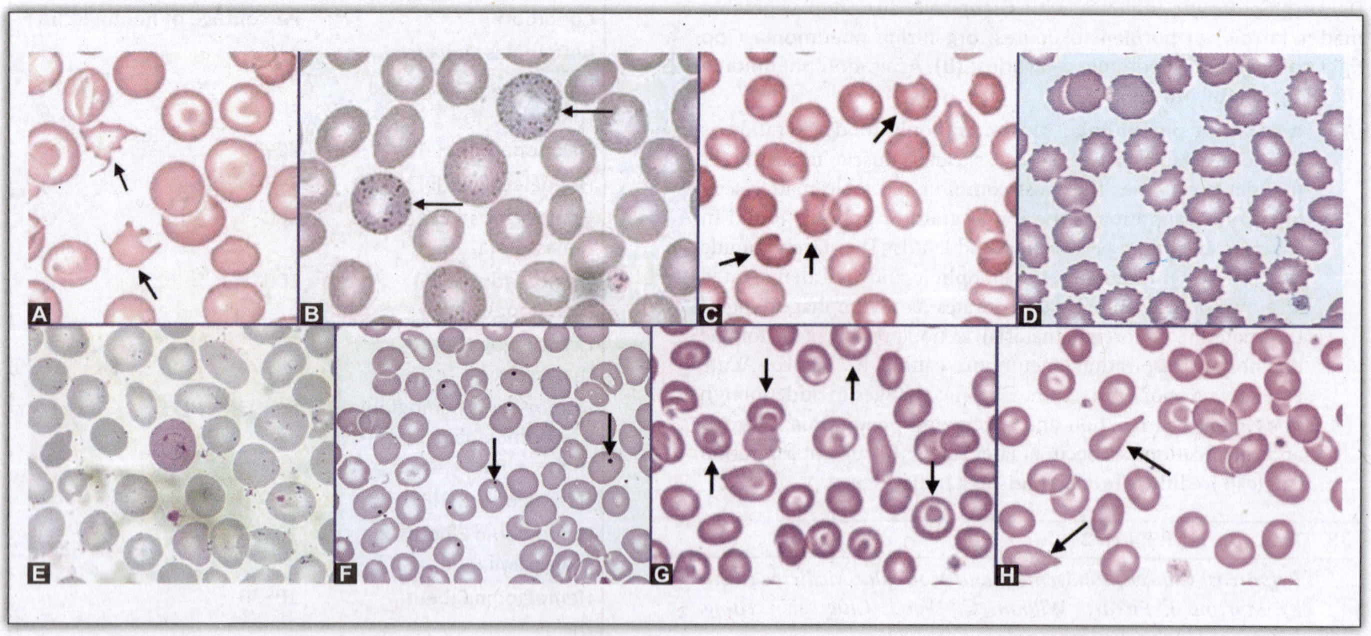

Figs A to H: **(A)** Acanthocytes; **(B)** Basophilic stippling; **(C)** Bite cells; **(D)** Burr cells; **(E)** Cabot Rings; **(F)** Howell-Jolly bodies; **(G)** Target cells and **(H)** Teardrop cells

Pathologic Red Cells in Blood Smears			
Red cell type	**Description**	**Underlying change**	**Disease state associations**
Acanthocyte (spur cell)	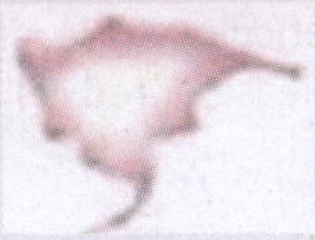 Irregularly spiculated red cells with projections of varying length and dense center	Altered cell membrane lipids	Abetalipoproteinemia, parenchymal liver disease, postsplenectomy
Basophilic stippling	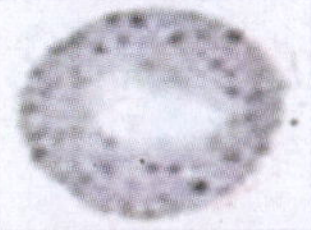 Punctuate basophilic inclusions	Precipitated ribosomes (RNA)	Coarse stippling: Lead intoxication, thalassemia Fine stippling: A variety of anemias
Bite cell (degmacyte)	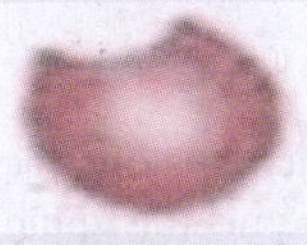 Smooth semicircle taken from one edge	Heinz body pitting by spleen	Glucose-6-phosphate dehydrogenase deficiency, drug-induced oxidant hemolysis
Burr cell (echinocyte) or crenated red cell	 Red cells with short, evenly spaced spicules and preserved central pallor	May be associated with altered membrane lipids	Usually artifactual; seen in uremia, bleeding ulcers, gastric carcinoma
Cabot rings	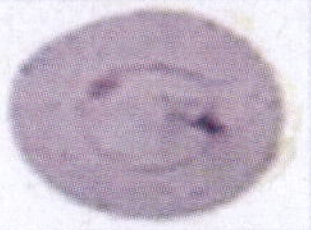 Circular, blue, threadlike inclusion with dots	Nuclear remnant	Postsplenectomy, hemolytic anemia, megaloblastic anemia
Ovalocyte (elliptocyte)	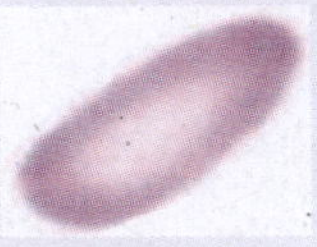 Elliptically shaped cell	Abnormal cytoskeletal proteins	Hereditary elliptocytosis
Howell-Jolly bodies	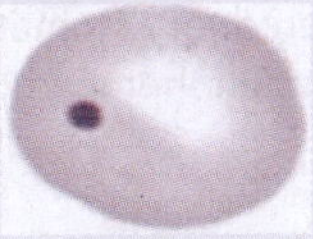 Small, discrete, basophilic, dense inclusions; usually single	Nuclear remnant (DNA)	Postsplenectomy, hemolytic anemia, megaloblastic anemia
Hypochromic red cell	Prominent central pallor	Diminished hemoglobin synthesis	Iron deficiency anemia, thalassemia, sideroblastic anemia
Macrocyte	Red cells larger than normal (>8.5 µm), well filled with hemoglobin	Young red cells, abnormal red cell maturation	Increased erythropoiesis; oval macrocytes in megaloblastic anemia; round macrocytes in liver disease
Microcyte	Red cells smaller than normal (<7.0 µm)	—	Hypochromic red cell
Pappenheimer bodies	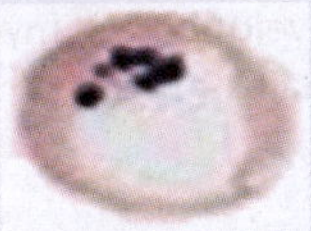 Small, dense, basophilic granules	Iron-containing siderosome or mitochondrial remnant	Sideroblastic anemia, postsplenectomy

Contd...

Pathologic Red Cells in Blood Smears			
Red cell type	**Description**	**Underlying change**	**Disease state associations**
Poly chromatophilia	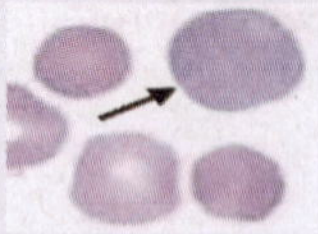 Grayish or blue hue often seen in macrocytic RBC lacking central pallor.	Ribosomal material 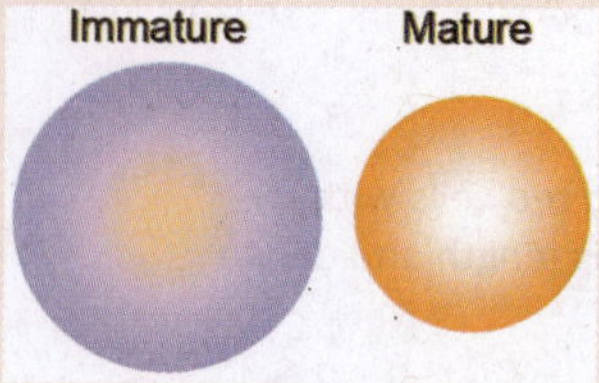	Reticulocytosis, premature marrow release of red cells
Rouleaux	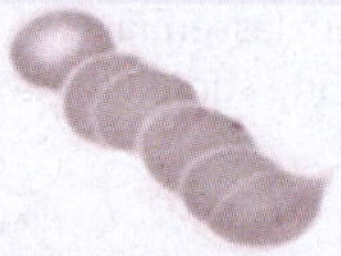 Red cell aggregates resembling stack of coins	Red cell clumping by circulating paraprotein	Paraproteinemia
Schistocyte (helmet cell)	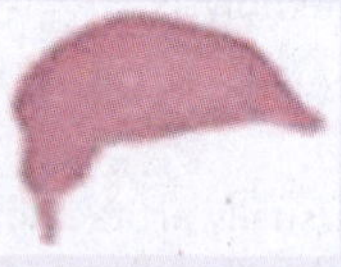 Distorted, fragmented cell; two or three pointed ends	Mechanical distortion in microvasculature by fibrin strands, disruption by prosthetic heart valve	Microangiopathic hemolytic anemia (disseminated intravascular coagulation, thrombotic thrombocytopenic purpura, prosthetic heart valves, severe burns)
Sickle cell (drepanocyte)	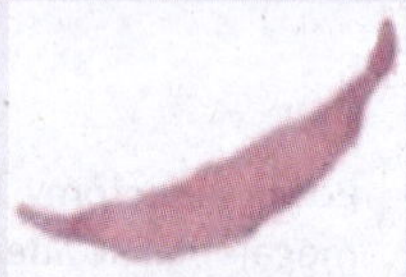 Bipolar, spiculated forms, sickle shaped, pointed at both ends	Molecular aggregation of HbS	Sickle cell disorders, not including S trait
Spherocyte	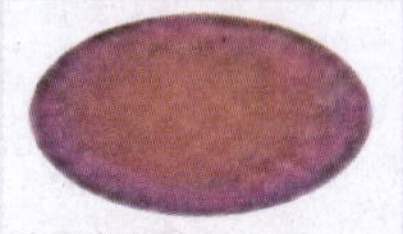 Spherical cell with dense appearance and absent central pallor, usually decreased diameter	Decreased membrane surface area	Hereditary spherocytosis, immunohemolytic anemia
Stomatocyte	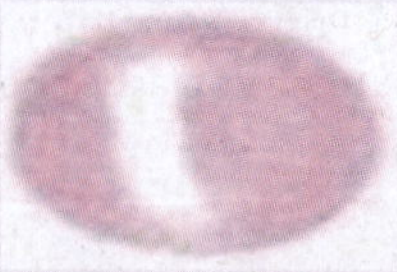 Mouth or cuplike deformity	Membrane defect with abnormal cation permeability	Hereditary stomatocytosis, Alcoholism, immunohemolytic anemia
Target cell (AKA-Mexican hat cells/ codocyte)	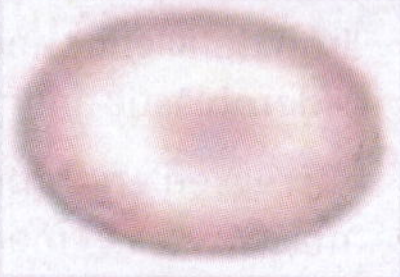 Target like appearance, often hypochromic	Increased redundancy of cell membrane	Liver disease, postsplenectomy, thalassemia, hemoglobin C disease
Teardrop cell (dacryocyte)	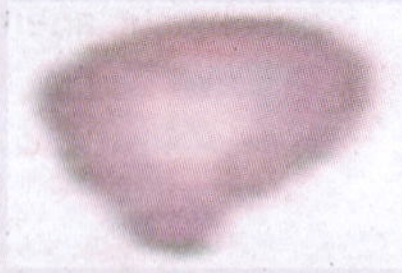 Distorted, drop-shaped cell	—	Myelofibrosis, myelophthisic anemia, Thalassemia

41. Ans. (d) Ask patient to identify himself, Verification of patient details in file, blood collection, labelling at the bedside

Ref: http://www.who.int/infection-prevention/publications/drawing_blood_best/en/

Recall Bias

There were many versions of options recalled. We have retained the best out of them. It is advised not to remember just answer but the complete steps.

Short Summary of method of collecting blood to be sent to blood bank for cross matching:

- Ask patient to identify themselves
- Cross check the patient's name against: File and blood request form
- Prepare patient and Take blood
- Label the test tube at patient's bedside only
- Crosscheck patient's details and ensure that name and CR No. is matching on both the tubes and form.

WHO Guidelines on Drawing Blood Best Practice in Phlebotomy		
Step 1	Assemble equipment	Laboratory sample tubes, vacuum-extraction blood tubes, blood-sampling devices (safety-engineered devices or needles and syringes, tourniquet, alcohol hand rub, 70% alcohol swabs, gauze or cotton-wool, laboratory specimen labels, writing equipment, laboratory forms, leak-proof transportation bags and containers, Puncture-resistant sharps container
Step 2	Identify and prepare the patient	Introduce yourself to the patient, and ask the patient to state their full name. Match the patient's details with the laboratory form, to ensure accurate identification. Discuss the test to be performed and obtain verbal consent
Step 3	Select the site	Extend the patient's arm and inspect the antecubital fossa or forearm. Locate a vein of a good size that is visible, straight and clear. The vein should be visible without applying the tourniquet. Apply the tourniquet about 4–5 finger widths above the venepuncture site and re-examine the vein.
Step 4	Perform hand hygiene and put on gloves	Wash hands with soap and water, and dry with single use towels or if hands are not visibly contaminated, clean with alcohol rub – use 3 mL of alcohol rub on the palm of the hand, and rub it into fingertips, back of hands and all over the hands until dry. After performing hand hygiene, put on well-fitting, non-sterile gloves
Step 5	Disinfect the entry site	Clean the site with a 70% alcohol swab for 30 seconds and allow to dry completely
Step 6	Take blood	Anchor the vein by holding the patient's arm and placing a thumb BELOW the venepuncture site. Ask the patient to form a fist so the veins are more prominent. Enter the vein swiftly at a 30 degree angle or less. Once sufficient blood has been collected, release the tourniquet BEFORE withdrawing the needle. Withdraw the needle gently and apply gentle pressure to the site with a clean gauze or dry cotton
Step 7	Fill the laboratory sample tubes	Use evacuated tubes with a needle and tube holder. If a syringe or winged needle set is used, best practice is to place the tube into a rack before filling the tube. Before dispatch, invert the tubes containing additives for the required number of times
Step 8	Draw samples in the correct order	Draw blood collection tubes in the correct order, to avoid cross-contamination of additives between tubes.
Step 9	Clean contaminated surfaces and complete patient procedure	Discard the used needle and syringe or blood sampling device into a puncture resistant sharps container. Bedside labeling, which is typically the patient's first and last names, file number, date of birth, and the date and time when the blood was taken. ***Check the label and forms for accuracy***. Discard used items into the appropriate category of waste. Perform hand hygiene again. ***Recheck the labels on the tubes and the forms before dispatch.***
Step 10	Prepare samples for transportation	Pack laboratory samples safely in a plastic leak-proof bag with an outside compartment for the laboratory request form.
Step 11	Clean up spills of blood or body fluids	If blood spillage has occurred clean it up

42. Ans. (b) Schwannoma

Ref: Robbins 9th ed page 1314

Histopathological features of Schwannoma is a hot favorite topic of AIIMS exam now a days. Asked in different forms in AIIMS NOV 2017, NOV 2015, NOV 2014, MAY 2014

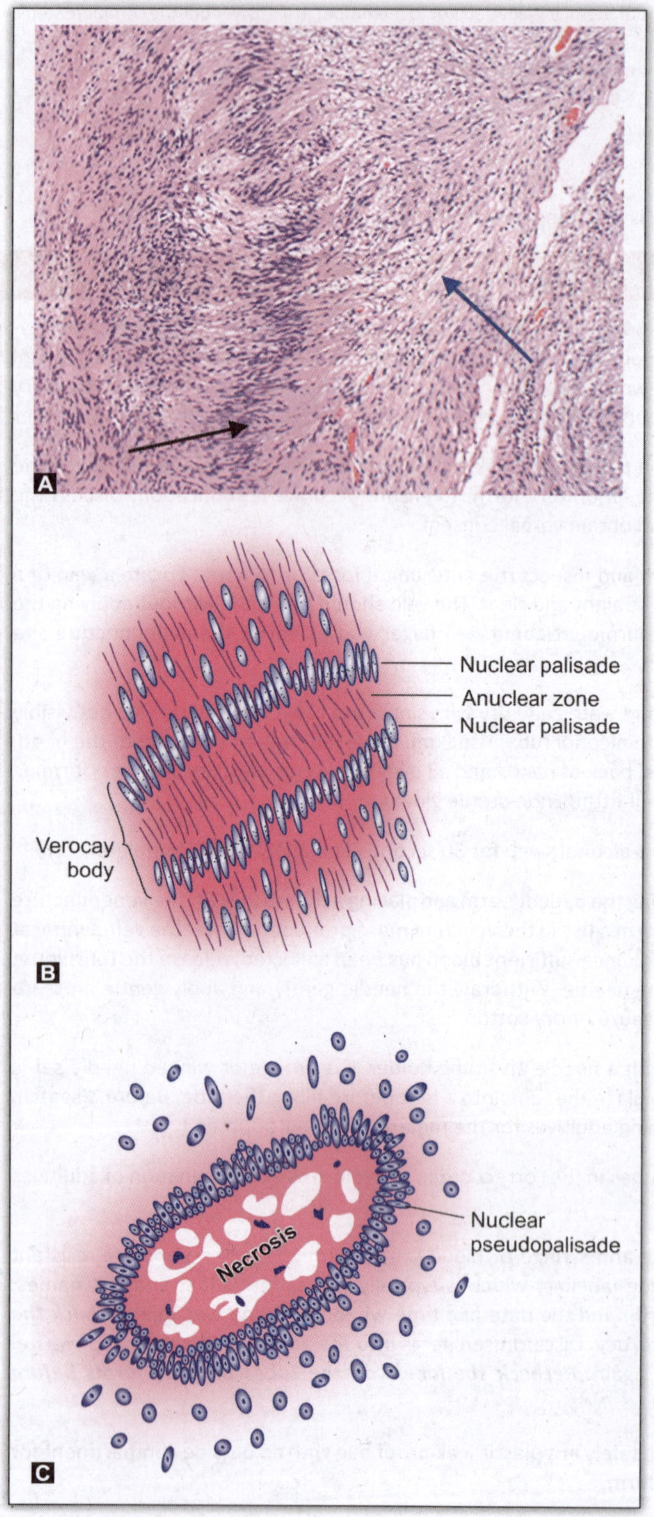

Figs A to C: The black arrow represents nuclear Palisading called verocay Bodies in Antomi A patter of Schwannoma

Schwannoma

Schwannomas are well-circumscribed, encapsulated masses that are attached to the nerve but can be separated from it. Tumors form firm, gray masses that may have areas of cystic and xanthomatous change. The defining histomorphologic features of schwannomas are eponymously named after the individuals who described them during the process of classification: in 1910 the Uruguayan neuropathologist Jose Verocay described the phenomenon of opposing rows of palisaded nuclei separated by eosinophilc, anuclear fibrillary processes now known as **"Verocay bodies,"** and a decade later in 1920 the Swedish neurologist Nils Antoni described the characteristic mixed architectural pattern of schwannomas, with

- In the **Antoni A pattern** of growth, elongated cells with cytoplasmic processes are arranged in fascicles in areas of moderate to high cellularity and scant stromal matrix; the **"nuclear-free zones"** of processes that lie between the regions of nuclear palisading are termed Verocay bodies.
- In the **Antoni B pattern** of growth, the tumor is hypocellular and consists of a loose meshwork of cells, microçysts and myxoid stroma.

In both areas the individual cells have an elongated shape and regular oval nuclei. Electron microscopy shows basement membrane deposits encasing single cells and collagen fibers. Because the lesion displaces the nerve of origin as it grows, silver stains or immunostains for neurofilament proteins demonstrate that axons are largely excluded from the tumor, although they may become entrapped in the capsule. The Schwann cell origin of these tumors is borne out by their **S-100 immunoreactivity**. A variety of degenerative changes may be found in schwannomas, including nuclear pleomorphism, xanthomatous change, and vascular hyalinization. Malignant change is extremely rare, but local recurrence can follow incomplete resection.

What Are Palisades and Pseudopalisades?

A palisade is a strong fence or protective perimeter made of a row of wooden poles or stakes driven into the ground. Pathologists examining the microscopic appearance of certain tumors noted arrangements of elongated nuclei stacked in neat rows and attached the descriptive term ***"palisades"*** on the basis of their resemblance to the forts. Nuclear palisades may be considered ***"primary"*** when they reflect a natural tendency of the nuclei to develop this distinctive pattern of growth or ***"secondary"*** when the alignment forms as a response to external influences such as necrosis. The latter have been termed ***"pseudopalisades"*** to distinguish them from primary palisades. Although not pathognomonic, palisades are most often seen in schwannomas, whereas pseudopalisades are typical of glioblastomas.

43. Ans. (a) Naive B cells in interfollicular zone

REF: Robbins Basic pathology 10th ed page 467

CLL/ SLL - B cells originate from Pre/Post Germinal center memory B cell or Naive B cell. Chronic Lymphocytic Leukemia (CLL) and Small Lymphocytic Lymphoma (SLL) disorders differ only in the degree of peripheral blood lymphocytosis.

Types of lymphoid leukemias and non-hodgkin lymphomas		
Diagnosis	**Cell of origin**	**Salient clinical features**
Neoplasms of immature B and T cells		
B-cell acute lymphoblastic leukemia/ lymphoma	Bone marrow precursor B cell	Predominantly children; symptoms relating to marrow replacement and pancytopenia; aggressive
T-cell acute lymphoblastic leukemia/lymphoma	Precursor T cell (often of thymic origin)	Predominantly adolescent males; thymic masses and variable bone marrow involvement; aggressive
Neoplasms of mature B cells		
Burkitt lymphoma	Germinal-center B cell	Adolescents or young adults with extranodal masses; uncommonly presents as "leukemia"; aggressive
Diffuse large B-cell lymphoma	Germinal-center or post germinal center B cell	All ages, but most common in adults; often appears as a rapidly growing mass; 30% extranodal; aggressive
Extranodal marginal zone lymphoma	Memory B cell	Arises at extranodal sites in adults with chronic inflammatory diseases; may remain localized; indolent
Follicular lymphoma	Germinal-center B cell	Older adults with generalized lymphadenopathy and marrow involvement; indolent
Hairy cell leukemia	Memory B cell	Older males with pancytopenia and splenomegaly; indolent
Mantle cell lymphoma	Naive B cell	Older males with disseminated disease; moderately aggressive
Multiple myeloma/solitary plasmacytoma	Post germinal center bone marrow homing plasma cell	Myeloma: older adults with lytic bone lesions, pathologic fractures, hypercalcemia, and renal failure; moderately aggressive Plasmacytoma: isolated plasma cell masses in bone or soft tissue; indolent
Small lymphocytic lymphoma/ chronic lymphocytic leukemia	Naive B cell or memory B cell	Older adults with bone marrow, lymph node, spleen, and liver disease; autoimmune hemolysis and thrombocytopenia in a minority; indolent
Neoplasms of mature T cells or NK cells		
Adult T-cell leukemia/lymphoma	Helper T cell	Adults with cutaneous lesions, marrow involvement, and hypercalcemia; occurs mainly in Japan, West Africa, and the Caribbean; aggressive
Peripheral T-cell lymphoma, unspecified	Helper or cytotoxic T cell	Mainly older adults; usually presents with lymphadenopathy; aggressive
Anaplastic large-cell lymphoma	Cytotoxic T cell	Children and young adults, usually with lymph node and soft-tissue disease; aggressive
Extranodal NK/T-cell lymphoma	NK-cell (common) or cytotoxic T cell (rare)	Adults with destructive extranodal masses, most commonly sinonasal; aggressive
Mycosis fungoides/Sézary syndrome	Helper T cell	Adult patients with cutaneous patches, plaques, nodules, or generalized erythema; indolent
Large granular lymphocytic leukemia	Two types: cytotoxic T cell and NK cell	Adult patients with splenomegaly, neutropenia, and anemia, sometimes

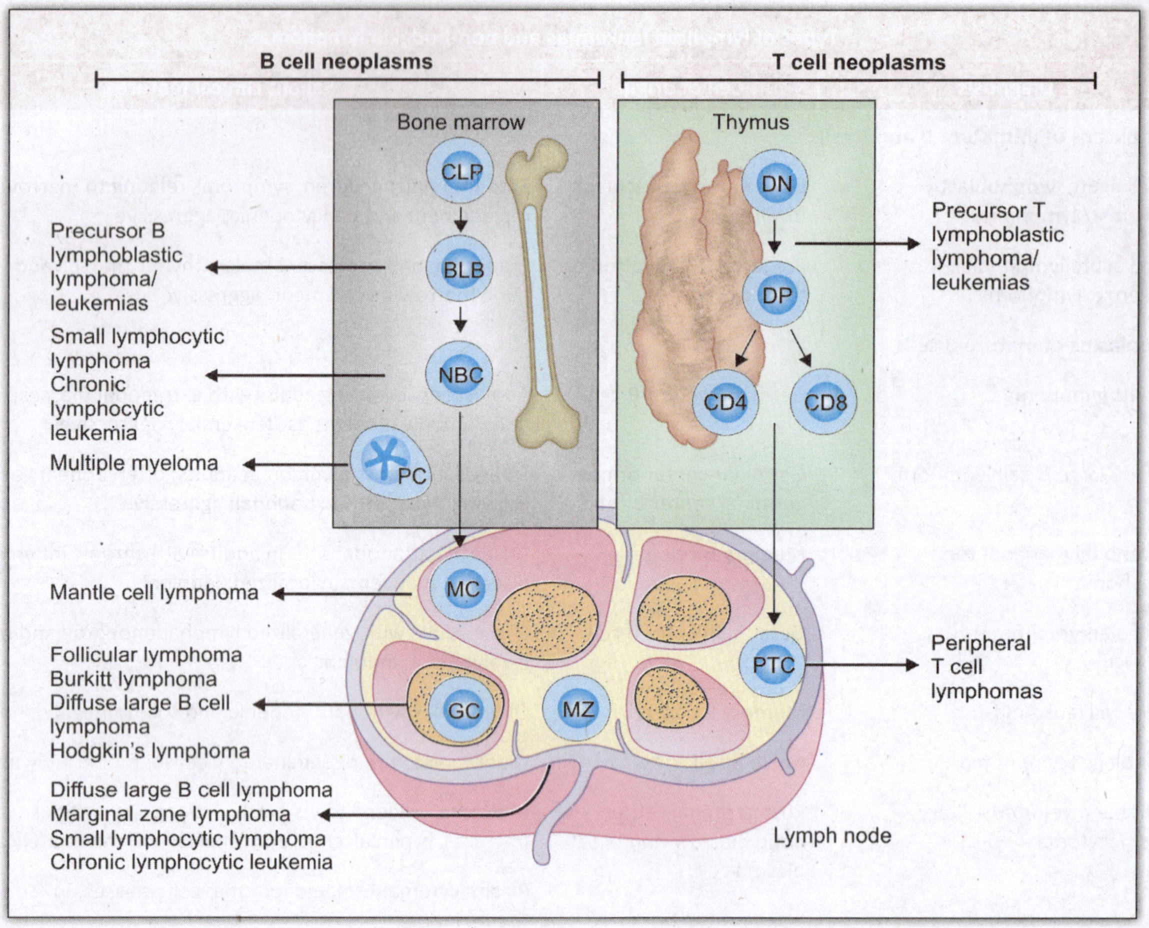

44. Ans. (b) Rheumatic valvular disease

Ref: Harrison 19th ed page 2152, Robbins 9th ed page 425

WHO diagnostic criteria of diagnosis of Rheumatic heart disease is described in Medicine AIIMS MAY 2015 (see page no. 791-792)

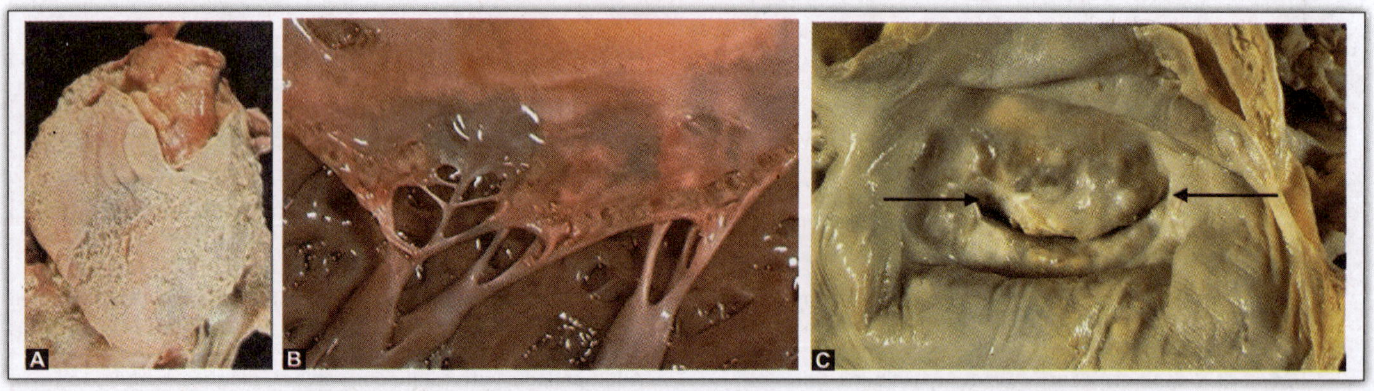

Figs A to C: **(A)** Rheumatic Heart disease Gross: Bread and Butter pericarditis; **(B)** Rheumatic Heart disease Gross: Valvular vegetation-Irregular, warty, firm, along the line of closure of valves and **(C)** Rheumatic Heart disease Gross: Fibrous bridging across the valves and calcification causes "Fishmouth" or "Buttonhole" stenosis

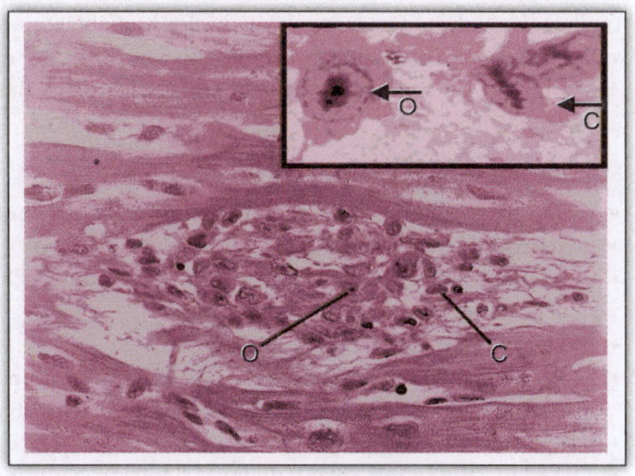

Fig: Rheumatic Heart disease HPE: Aschoff bodies or Rheumatic granuloma demarcated by

1. Anitschkow cells (Specialized Histiocytes which appears caterpillar like in cross section-marked as C and owl's eye in longitudinal section- marked as O) associated with fibrinoid necrosis
2. Scattered Plasma cells and T lymphocytes
3. Aschoff cells (Inflammatory Giant cells)

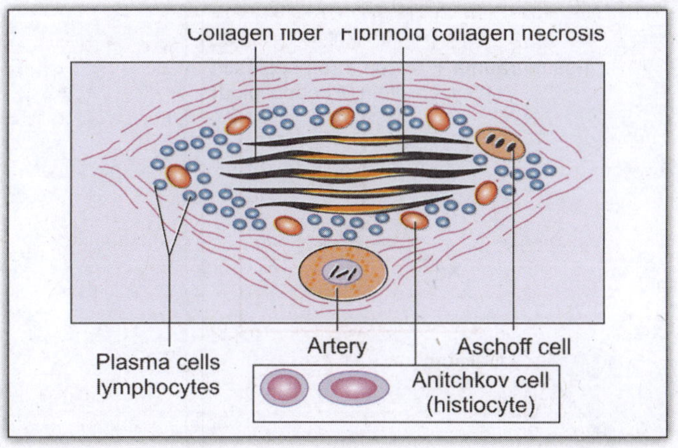

45. Ans. (b) Adenocarcinoma

Ref: Robbins Basic pathology 10th ed page 596, Schwartz's 9th ed chapter 25

It is not possible to determine the histology of esophageal tumors by their radiographic appearance, however some findings may improve specificity. The vast majority of adenocarcinomas arise from Barrett's esophagus and typically occur in the distal (Lower ⅓) esophagus. These tumors have a propensity to invade the gastric cardia and fundus. On the other hand Squamous cell carcinoma is commonly seen in upper and Middle third of esophagus.

Clue to Diagnosis:

- Barium swallow picture shows Apple core deformity of the lower end of esophagus typical of adenocarcinoma
- Microscopically, Barrett esophagus is frequently present adjacent to the tumor. Right half of this slide is Barrett esophagus and left half is Adenocarcinoma.

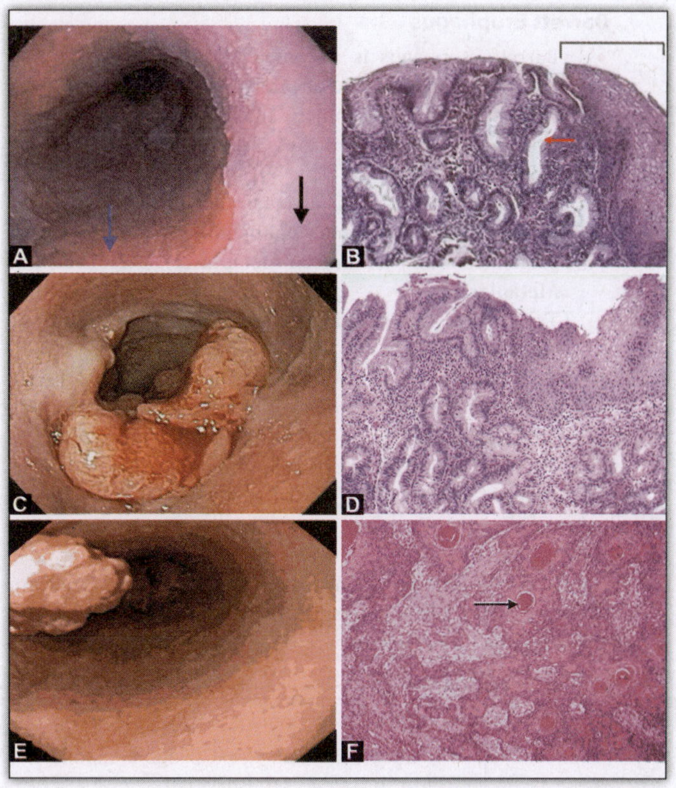

Figs A to F: (A) Barrett esophagus endoscopy: Esophageal squamous epithelium (Black arrow) is replaced by metaplastic columnar epithelium (Blue arrow- Salmon coloured mucosa in Endoscopy); **(B) Barrett esophagus histopathology:** Esophageal squamous epithelium is replaced by metaplastic columnar epithelium containing intestinal goblet cells (Red arrow). Note the squamous epithelium on the right side and columnar epithelium on the left side; **(C) Adenocarcinoma Esophageal endoscopy:** Upper-gastrointestinal endoscopy showing lower-esophageal ulceroproliferative tumor measuring 2.5 cm × 2.5 cm. Lower third esophageal cancers are mostly adenocarcinoma; **(D) Adenocarcinoma of Esophagus Histopathology:** Microscopically, Barrett esophagus is frequently present adjacent to the tumor. Right half of this slide is Barrett esophagus and left half is Adenocarcinoma. Tumors most commonly produce mucin and form glands, often with intestinal-type morphology; less frequently tumors are composed of diffusely infiltrative signet-ring cells (similar to those seen in diffuse gastric cancer); **(E) Squamous cell carcinoma esophagus endoscopy:** In contrast to adenocarcinoma, half of squamous cell carcinomas occur in the middle third of the esophagus. Early lesions appear as small, gray-white, plaque-like thickenings. It is polypoid or exophytic and protrude into and obstruct the lumen. Or it can either ulcerated or diffusely infiltrate. These may invade surrounding structures including the respiratory tree, causing pneumonia; the aorta, causing catastrophic exsanguination; or the mediastinum and pericardium and **(F) Squamous cell carcinoma esophagus Histopathology:** Typical keratinizing conventional, well differentiated squamous cell carcinoma with keratin pearls (arrow). Most squamous cell carcinomas are moderately to well-differentiated. Squamous cell carcinoma begins as an in situ lesion termed **squamous dysplasia**

Barrett Esophagus

- Barrett esophagus is a complication of long standing gastroesophageal reflux, occurring over time in up to 10% of patients with symptomatic GERD.
- It is single most important risk factor of esophageal adenocarcinoma
- In Barrett esophagus distal squamous mucosa is replaced by metaplastic columnar epithelium as a response to prolonged injury **(columnar metaplasia; AKA Intestinal Metaplasia)**
- Two criteria are required for the diagnosis of Barrett esophagus:
  1. Endoscopic evidence of columnar epithelium lining above the gastroesophageal junction
  2. Histological evidence of intestinal metaplasia in biopsy specimen from columnar epithelium

Locations of Goblet cells: Goblet cells are glandular simple columnar epithelial cells whose sole function is to secrete mucin, which dissolves in water to form mucus. They use both apocrine and merocrine methods for secretion. They are found scattered among the epithelial lining of organs, such as the intestinal and respiratory tracts. They are found inside the trachea, bronchus, and larger bronchioles in respiratory tract, small intestines, the colon, and conjunctiva in the upper eyelid. They may be an indication of metaplasia, such as in Barrett's esophagus.

Staining of Goblet Cell-Alcian Blue

- Common "routine" stain (not an immunohistochemical stain) to detect mucins
- At pH 2.5, detects acidic mucins, At pH 1.0, detects highly acidic mucins
- Stained parts are blue to bluish-green
- PAS-Alcian blue may be best pan mucin combination; PAS also stains glycogen, but predigestion with diastase will remove the glycogen
- Alcian blue-high iron diamine detects sulfomucins (brown) and sialomucins (blue)

46. Ans. (a) Extrinsic Pathway

Ref: Robbins Basic pathology 10th ed page 104

Adding Thromboplastin and calcium will activate Extrinsic pathway.

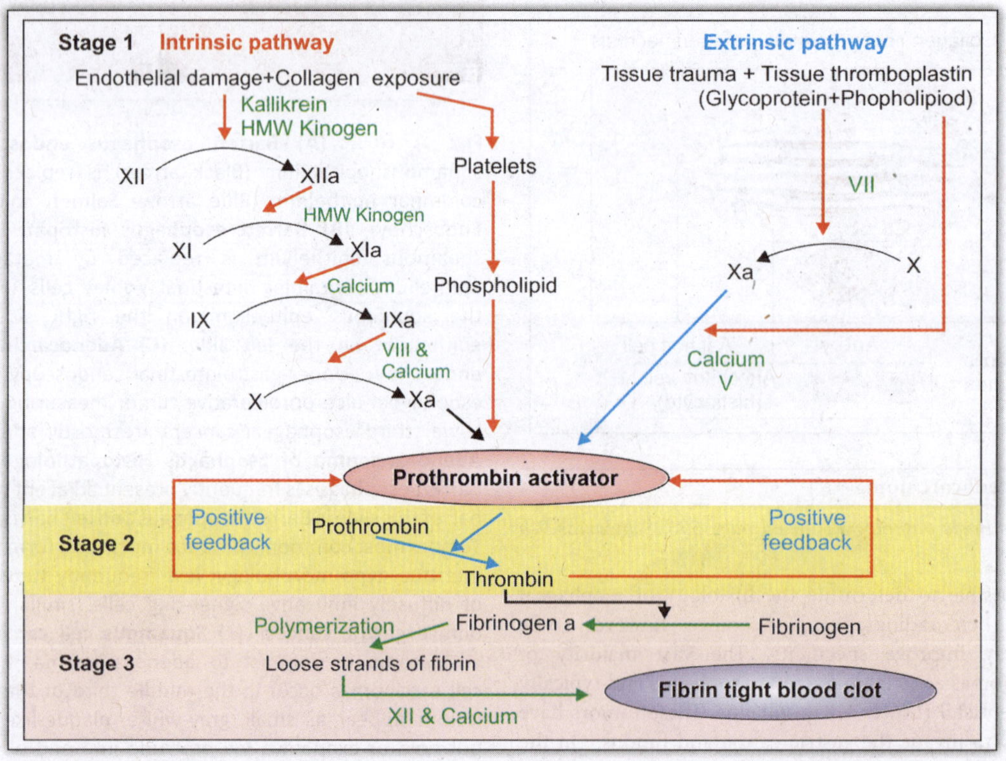

47. Ans. (a) Citrate Phosphate Dextrose Adenine-1

Ref: Wintrobe's clinical hematology 12th ed page 675

Shelf life of Blood Components	
Component	**Period of storage /life**
RBC (ACD- acid citrate dextrose, CPD-Citrate Phosphate dextrose, CP2D- Citrate Phosphate Double Dextrose)	21 days
RBC (CPDA 1- Citrate phosphate dextrose Adenine 1)	35 days

Contd...

Shelf life of Blood Components	
Component	**Period of storage /life**
RBC (Adsol)	42 days
Platelets	5 days
Granulocytes	24 hours
Factor VIII	2 days
Factor V	4-5 days
Factor XI	6-7 days

48. Ans. (a) Lithium heparin

Ref: Essentials in Hematology and Clinical Pathology By Ramadas Nayak 1st Ed Pg 337

- For electrolyte estimation we need to get serum first and for getting serum coagulation is required and hence anticoagulants are not added. It's done in Red coloured vacutainer system which contains no anticoagulant. If we still have a select a best answer then Heparin will be the best answer.
- Heparin can be added for instantaneous anticoagulation and to prevent haemolysis after the blood is drawn. Haemolysis may cause spurious elevation in serum potassium report. Minimal heparin is added, just to wet inner surface of syringe.
- Heparin is also used in osmotic fragility test (for spherocytosis), Red cell enzyme studies (G6PD and PK studies), Arterial blood gas analysis.
- Sodium fluoride is an antiglycolytic agent which inhibits use of glucose by blood cells.Used for estimation of blood glucose
- EDTA (Ethyl Diamine Tetra Acectic acid) chelates calcium and is used for CBC, HbF estimation and Hb electrophoresis.
- Sodium citrate chelates calcium and is used in anticoagulation studies and estimation of ESR

49. Ans. (b) Large infusion of ACD

Ref: Wintrobe's Clinical Hematology 12th Ed page 674

Perioral numbness with tingling sensation points towards Hypocalcemia. ECG changes are also consistent with Hypocalcemia. Now we need to look into options to check which one causes hypocalcemia.

The anticoagulant used for essentially all transfusable blood components today is citrate, which chelates ionized calcium in donor blood, making it unavailable to the calcium-dependent stages of coagulation. After transfusion, citrate is readily metabolized into bicarbonate by the liver of the recipient. Apheresis donors face the additional potential complication of transient hypocalcemia from the citrate infused when anticoagulated blood components are returned to them from the apheresis device. Symptoms consist of tingling or muscle cramps. Citrate symptoms are treated by slowing the flow of the device or giving the donor oral calcium supplements. Intravenous calcium infusions are needed only during prolonged apheresis procedures such as those for HPC collection

ECG Changes in Hypocalcemia
(2.1 mmol/L or 9 mg/dL)

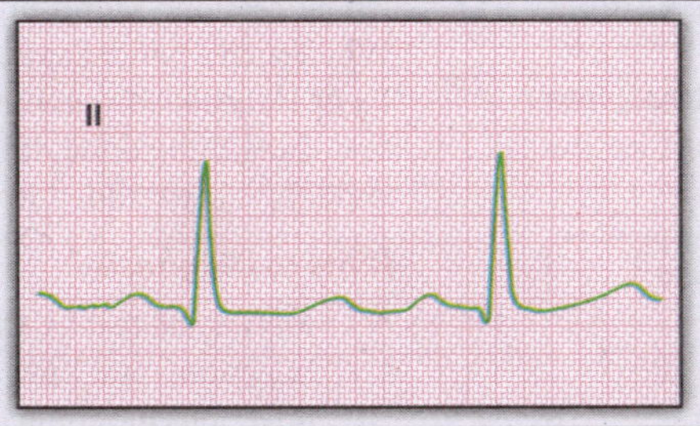

Main ECG change is **prolonged QT** interval mainly due to prolonged ST
Narrow QRS complex
Reduced PR interval
T wave flattening and inversion
Prominent U-wave

50. Ans. (a) Peripheral Blood smear

Ref: Robbins basic pathology 10th ed page 480

AML occasionally presents as a localized soft-tissue mass known variously as a myeloblastoma, granulocytic sarcoma, or chloroma. AML can usually be diagnosed from the peripheral smear, but bone marrow aspirate and biopsy should always be performed to determine proper classification

51. Ans. (c) Transthyretin

Ref: Wintrobe 11th ed page 811, Robbin's 9th ed page 649

Option (A)

Ceruloplasmin is copper containing enzyme with ferroxidase activity

Option (B)

Hepcidin is produced in the liver, present in the plasma and excreted through the kidneys. Hepcidin expression is increased with iron overload induced by carbonyl iron, suggesting that its production might be part of a compensatory response to limit iron absorption expression of hepcidin is decreased in the setting of iron deficiency anemia, hypoxia, or inflammation.

Finally, patients with inappropriate expression of hepcidin develop an iron-restricted anemia.
It is structurally similar to antimicrobial peptides involved in innate immunity, and it has been shown to have antimicrobial properties.

Option (C)

Transthyretin (TTR) is a transport protein in the serum and cerebrospinal fluid that carries the thyroid hormone thyroxine (T4) and retinol-binding protein bound to retinol. This is how transthyretin gained its name: transports thyroxine and retinol.

Option (D)

Once in the cytosol, iron enters a chelatable pool from which it is used by several enzymes or is stored in ferritin.

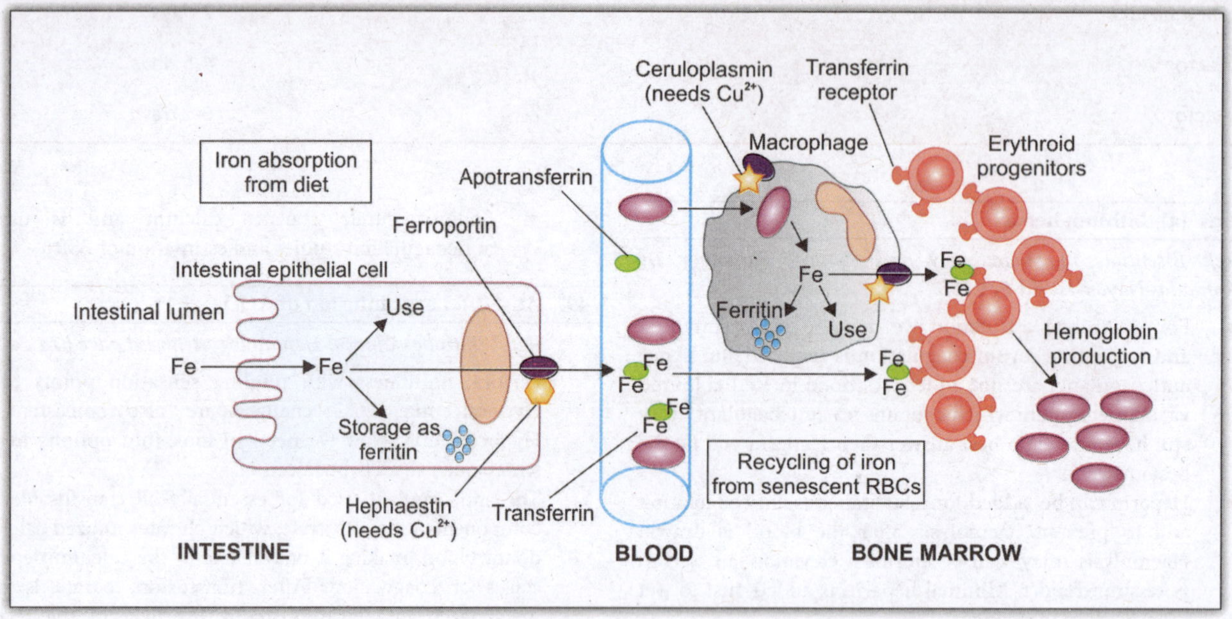

52. Ans. (d) Risk of integration of viral DNA with Host DNA

Ref: Int J Exp Pathol. 2001 Apr; 82(2): 77–100.

Chronic hepatitis B virus (HBV) infection is a major global cause of hepatocellular carcinoma (HCC). There are two explanations for the development of HCC in patients who have apparently recovered from chronic HBV infection.

1. HBV DNA may persist in low concentration in the serum and liver tissue after the disappearance of HBsAg from the serum.
2. Alternatively, HBV DNA may become integrated into host DNA during an early stage of infection before the elimination of the virions

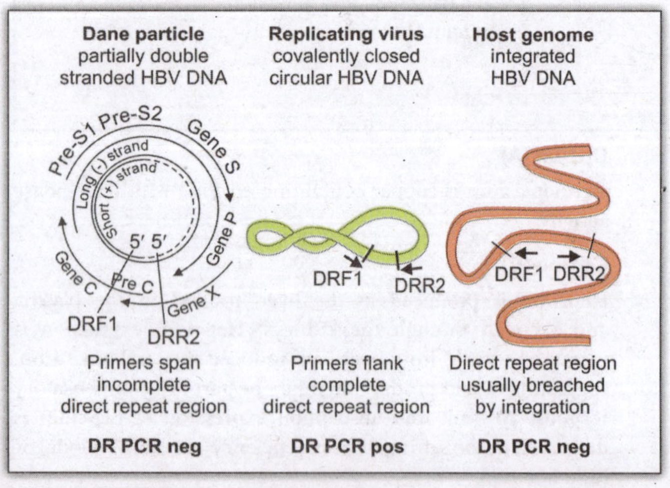

AIIMS MAY 2017

53. Ans. (a) Infectious mononucleosis

Ref: Robbins 9th ed page 436, Devita 8th ed page 2423, Harrison 19th ed page 1168, Modern Pathology (2012) 25, 1149–1159 doi:10.1038/modpathol.2012.70; published online 25 May 2012

This is the most controversial and difficult question of the whole session. Monospot negative is given to confuse you. When such a patient appears to OPD and a provisional diagnosis of Infectious mononucleosis is made, monospot test is the first thing to be done. If monospot comes negative, Hodgkins and DLBCL are added in the list of differentials.

Hints to Diagnosis

- Monospot test is the screening method of active EBV infection and negative monospot cannot rule out infectious mononucleosis. Tests for heterophile antibodies are positive in 40% of patients with 1M during the first week of illness and in 80-90% during the third week. Test is positive up to 3 months. If monospot test is negative other confirmatory serological tests are done which is positive in this case.
- The latent membrane protein 1 (LMP-1) is one of the EBV-encoded proteins believed to have an important role in B-cell immortalization by inducing the expression of bcl-2, which inhibits programmed death of the infected cells. LMP-1 is also considered to be an oncogene, and deletions near the 3 end of the LMP-1 gene, in a region that affects the half-life of the LMP-1 protein, have been

reported in some lymphoproliferative disorders. (Devita 8th ed page 2423)

- The monospot test is not recommended for general use. The antibodies detected by monospot can be caused by conditions other than infectious mononucleosis. Moreover, studies have shown that the monospot produces both false positive and false negative results. For example, the heterophile antibodies detected by monospot are often not present in children with infectious mononucleosis. At best, the monospot test may indicate that a person has a typical case of infectious mononucleosis, but does not confirm the presence of EBV infection.
- Lymphocytosis is characteristic of IM and not seen in DLBCL
- Lage cells in the background points to IM, DLBCL will show sheets of large cells only
- IHC profile of both IM and DLBCL are not exactly same but matching and cannot be differentiated on the basis of markers provided in the question, except CD3 positive cells in the background seen in IM but not seen in DLBCL
- CD 15 negative rules out Classical Hodgkins.

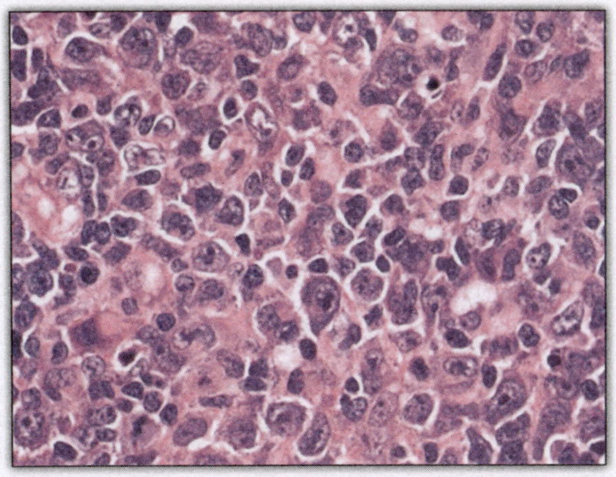

Fig: Characteristic morphological features of infectious mononucleosis cases. Ulceration of tonsillar mucosa and geographic ulcer. Focal distortion of normal tissue architecture. Polymorphous infiltrates consisting of scattered immunoblasts in a background of numerous small mature lymphocytes and plasma cells

Features	Infectious Mononucleosis	EBV Positive Diffuse Large B-cell Lymphoma
Age group	Adolescent/Young adults	Most common in older age groups (Most common lymphoma of adult group)
Fever, tonsillitis, lymphadenopathy	Present	Present
Peripheral leucocytosis	Present with large atypical cells (10000–20000/µL). Lymphocytosis is usually demonstrable, with >10% atypical lymphocytes (Downey cells)	No
Monospot test (Heterophile reaction)	Positive. (Note: Monospot negative infectious mononucleosis is known, although uncommon. In such cases, serological tests and titres need to be seen)	May be positive
Histology	Large cells on background of lymphocytes	Large cells in sheets only, hardly any background cells
Markers	Both B cells and T cell markers CD20+, CD 30+, MUM1/IRF4+, occasional CD3+ immunoblast-like cells, CD10- (Germinal center marker), CD15-, BCL-6, BCL2 weekly +,	B Cell markers (CD 19, CD20, CD3, CD5, CD10, CD45, CD 79a, Bcl-2, Bcl-6, Ki-67, IRF-4/MUM-1, MYC
Splenomegaly	Almost in all cases	May be present

About Option (B) Hodgkin's Lymphoma:

CD 15 negative rules out classical Hodgkin's. Both Hodgkins and RS cells are CD 15 positive.

Option (C) EBV Positive Diffuse Large B Cell Lymphoma:

- Diffuse large B cell lymphoma is the most common type of lymphoma in adults, accounting for approximately 50% of adult NHLs.
- It includes several subtypes that share an aggressive natural history.
- The majority of patients (57%) presented with cervical lymphadenopathy.
- The other common presenting symptoms were growth or ulcer on the tonsil (38%), dysphagia or foreign-body sensation (36%), odynophagia or otalgia (20%), change in voice (5.8%)
- Although the median age at presentation is about 60 years, diffuse large B cell lymphomas can occur at any age; they constitute about 15% of childhood lymphomas.
- Patients typically present with a rapidly enlarging, often symptomatic mass at one or several sites.
- Extranodal presentations are common. Although the gastrointestinal tract and the brain are among the more frequent extranodal sites, tumors can appear in virtually any organ or tissue.
- The neoplastic B cells are large (at least three to four times the size of resting lymphocytes) and vary in appearance from tumor to tumor.
- In many tumors, cells with round or oval nuclear contours, dispersed chromatin, several distinct nucleoli, and modest amounts of pale cytoplasm predominate.

- These mature B cell tumors express pan-B cell antigens, such as CD19 and CD20.
- Many also express surface IgM and/or IgG. Other antigens (e.g., CD10, BCL2) are variably expressed.
- EBV-associated diffuse large B cell lymphomas arise in the setting of the acquired immunodeficiency syndrome (AIDS), iatrogenic immunosuppression (e.g., in transplant recipients), and the elderly.
- In the post-transplantation setting, these tumors often begin as EBV-driven polyclonal B cell proliferations that may regress if immune function is restored.

Option (D) EBV Positive Mucocutaneous Ulcer:

Generally seen in immunocompromised patients. Also, large cells show CD30 strong positive and CD20 reduced expression.

54. Ans. (a) Nodular lymphocyte predominant HL

Ref: Robbins's 9th ed page 441

Read this question in connection and continuation to previous question. CD15-points towards Hodgkins Lymphoma. Then see other features to find out Subtype

Hodgkins Lymphoma

- **Essential for the diagnosis of Hodgkin lymphoma is the Reed-Sternberg (RS) cell**, a very large cell (15 to 45 µm in diameter) with an enormous multilobate nucleus, exceptionally prominent nucleoli and abundant, usually slightly eosinophilic cytoplasm. Particularly characteristic are cells with two mirror-image nuclei or nuclear lobes, each containing a large (inclusion-like) acidophilic nucleolus surrounded by a clear zone, features that impart an **owl-eye appearance**. The nuclear membrane is distinct.
- Typical RS cells and variants have a characteristic immunophenotype, as they ***express CD15 and CD30 and fail to express CD45*** (common leukocyte antigen), B cell antigens, and T cell antigens. As we shall see, "classic" RS cells are common in the mixed-cellularity subtype, uncommon in the nodular sclerosis subtype, and rare in the lymphocyte predominance subtype; in these latter two subtypes, other characteristic RS cell variants predominate.
- The events that transform Reed Sternberg cells and alter their appearance and gene expression programs are still unclear. One clue stems from the involvement of EBV. **EBV is present in the RS cells in as many as 70% of cases of the mixed-cellularity subtype and a smaller fraction of other "classical" forms of Hodgkin lymphoma.** More important, the integration of the EBV genome is identical in all RS cells in a given case, indicating that infection precedes (and therefore may be related to) transformation and clonal expansion.
- Thus, as in Burkitt lymphoma and B cell lymphomas in immunodeficient patients, EBV infection probably is one of several steps contributing to tumor development, particularly of the mixed-cellularity subtype.

Reed-Sternberg cells (and variants) are large cells with very striking "Inclusion-like" eosinophilic nucleoli. Try and identify them using the following diagram:

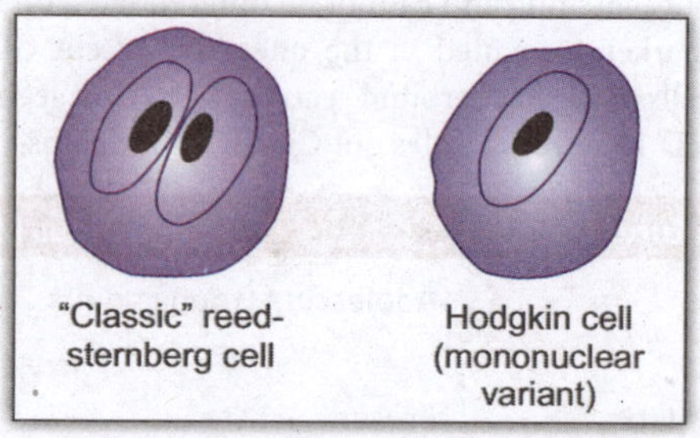

The lacunar cell variant has a folded or multilobulated nucleus lying within a clear space with fine pink bands radiating outwards from the nucleus; the latter are artifacts caused by shrinkage of the cell during processing in the laboratory.

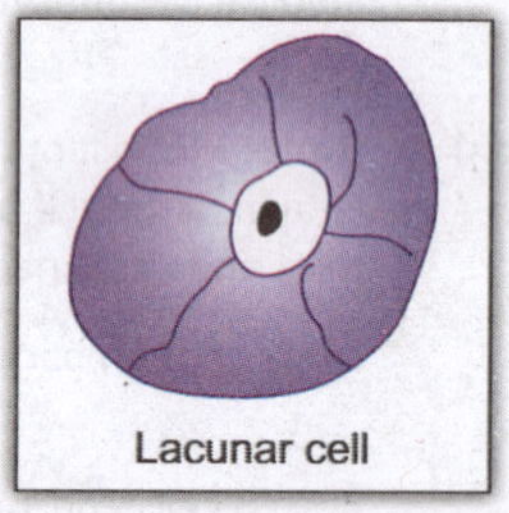

Fig: Reed Sternberg cells and its variants

Subtypes of Hodgkin's Lymphoma

Subtype	Morphology and immunophenotype	Typical clinical features
Nodular sclerosis	Frequent **lacunar cells** and occasional diagnostic **RS cells**; background infiltrate composed of T lymphocytes, eosinophils, macrophages, and plasma cells; fibrous bands dividing cellular areas into nodules. RS cells CD15+, CD30+; usually EBV-	**Most common subtype**; usually stage I or II disease; frequent mediastinal involvement; equal occurrence in males and females (F = M), most patients are young adults
Mixed cellularity	Frequent mononuclear and diagnostic RS cells; background infiltrate rich in T lymphocytes, eosinophils, macrophages, plasma cells; RS cells CD15+, CD30+; 70% EBV+	More than 50% present as stage III or IV disease; M greater than F; biphasic incidence, peaking in young adults and again in adults older than 55
Lymphocyte predominance	Frequent mononuclear and diagnostic RS cells; background infiltrate rich in T lymphocytes; RS cells CD15+, CD30+; 40% EBV+	Uncommon; M greater than F; tends to be seen in older adults
Lymphocyte depletion	Reticular variant: Frequent diagnostic RS cells and variants and a paucity of background reactive cells; RS cells CD15+, CD30+; most EBV+	Uncommon; more common in older males, HIV-infected individuals, and in developing countries; often presents with advanced disease
Lymphocyte predominance	Frequent L & H (popcorn cell) variants in a background of follicular dendritic cells and reactive B cells; RS cells CD20+, CD15-, C30-; EBV-	Uncommon; young males with cervical or axillary lymphadenopathy; mediastinal

55. Ans. (d) B cells, dendritic cells and macrophages

Ref: Robbins 9th ed page 102

Indirect repeat Pathology AIIMS NOV 2016 (All except was asked, See for explanation) (see page no. 375)

MHC-2 is seen in all antigen presenting cell including B cell, macrophages and dendritic cells.

56. Ans. (a) Sclerodactyly, Raynaud's phenomenon, lung fibrosis

Ref: Robbins 9th ed page 125

This is a case of systemic sclerosis or scleroderma sclerodactyly, Raynauds and lung fibrosis are all seen in scleroderma

- Antinuclear antibodies (ANAs) are directed against nuclear antigens and can be grouped into four categories:
  - Antibodies to DNA
  - Antibodies to histones
  - Antibodies to nonhistone proteins bound to RNA
  - Antibodies to nucleolar antigens.
- The most widely used method for detecting ANAs is ***indirect immunofluorescence.***
- The pattern of nuclear fluorescence suggests the type of antibody present in the patient's serum. Four basic patterns are recognized:
  - **Homogeneous or diffuse nuclear staining:** Usually reflects antibodies to chromatin, histones, and occasionally, double-stranded DNA.
  - **Rim or peripheral staining patterns:** Most often indicative of antibodies to double-stranded DNA.
  - **Speckled pattern:** Refers to the presence of uniform or variable-sized speckles. This is one of the most commonly observed patterns of fluorescence and therefore the least specific. It reflects the presence of antibodies to non-DNA nuclear constituents. Examples include Sm antigen, ribonucleoprotein, and SS-A and SS-B reactive antigens.
  - **Nucleolar pattern:** Presence of a few discrete spots of fluorescence within the nucleus and represents antibodies to RNA. This pattern is reported most often in patients with systemic sclerosis.

Scleroderma/Systemic Sclerosis (SS)

- An immunologic disorder characterized by excessive fibrosis in multiple tissues, obliterative vascular disease, and evidence of autoimmunity, mainly the production of multiple autoantibodies.
- It is commonly called scleroderma because the skin is a major target, but this disorder is better labeled "systemic" because lesions are present throughout the body.
- Cutaneous involvement is the usual presenting manifestation and eventually appears in approximately 95% of cases, but it is the visceral involvement—of the gastrointestinal tract, lungs, kidneys, heart, and skeletal muscles—that is responsible for most of the related morbidity and mortality.
- SS can be classified into two groups on the basis of its clinical course:
  - **Diffuse scleroderma**, characterized by initial widespread skin involvement, with rapid progression and early visceral involvement.
  - **Limited scleroderma**, with relatively mild skin involvement, often confined to the fingers and face. Involvement of the viscera occurs late, so the disease in these patients generally has a fairly benign course. This clinical presentation is also called the CREST syndrome because of its frequent features of calcinosis, Raynaud phenomenon, esophageal dysmotility, sclerodactyly, and telangiectasia.
- SS affects women three times more often than men, with a peak incidence in the 50- to 60-year age group.
- There is a substantial overlap in presentation between SS and RA, SLE, and dermatomyositis.
- The distinctive feature of SS is the striking cutaneous involvement. Almost all patients exhibit Raynaud phenomenon, a vascular disorder characterized by reversible vasospasm of the arteries.
- Typically the hands turn white on exposure to cold, reflecting vasospasm, followed by change to blue as ischemia and cyanosis supervene. Finally, the color changes to red as reactive vasodilation occurs.
- Progressive collagen deposition in the skin leads to atrophy of the hands, with increasing stiffness and eventually complete immobilization of the joints.
- Difficulty in swallowing results from esophageal fibrosis and resultant hypomotility. Eventually, destruction of the esophageal wall leads to atony and dilation.
- Malabsorption may appear if the submucosal and muscular atrophy and fibrosis involve the small intestine.
- Dyspnea and chronic cough reflect the pulmonary changes; with advanced lung involvement, secondary pulmonary hypertension may develop, leading to right-sided cardiac failure.
- Renal functional impairment secondary to both the advance of SS and the concomitant malignant hypertension is frequently marked.
- Virtually all patients of systemic sclerosis have ANAs that react with a variety of nuclear antigens.
- Two ANAs strongly associated with systemic sclerosis have been described.
- DNA topoisomerase I (anti-Scl 70), is highly specific. Depending on the ethnic group and the assay, it is present in 10% to 20% of patients with diffuse systemic sclerosis. Patients who have this antibody are more likely to have pulmonary fibrosis and peripheral vascular disease.
- Anticentromere antibody, is found in 20% to 30% of patients, who tend to have the CREST syndrome or limited cutaneous systemic sclerosis. Only rarely does the same patient have both antibodies.

57. Ans. (b) Barrett's esophagus

Ref: Robbin's 9th ed page 757, Basic histology Text and Atlas by Luiz Carlos Junqueira 11th ed chapter 4, Text Book of Histology Krishna Garg 4th Edn Page 93, 94

Repeat Pathology AIIMS NOV 2015 (see page no. 405) (Same slide was given, also stain and additional feature was asked) (See for details)

See Details of Barrett's Esophagus in AIIMS NOV 2017 Pathology (see page no. 352)

58. Ans. (a) Transferrin receptor 1—iron responsive elements (IRE) increases transferrin receptor mRNA concentration and synthesis.

Ref: Williams Hematology 8th ed Chapter 42

- The regulation of iron metabolism at the cytoplasmic mRNA level by interaction of iron-regulatory protein (IRP-1) and the iron-responsive elements (IREs) to **apoferritin mRNA (Mechanism 1) and transferrin receptor (TfR) mRNA (Mechanism 2).**
- When the cytoplasmic iron concentration is low, IRP-1 binds to the IREs of both mRNAs. ***This represses the translation of apoferritin mRNA***, where the IRE is at the 5′ end of the mRNA, thereby reducing the amount of apoferritin formed.
- It stabilizes ***and increases the translation of TfR mRNA*** where the IRE is at the 3′ end of the mRNA, thereby increasing the amount of TfR formed.
- Conversely, when there is an abundance of iron in the cytoplasm, IRP-1 is displaced from both species of mRNA. This results in derepression of apoferritin synthesis and destabilization and degradation of TfR mRNA.

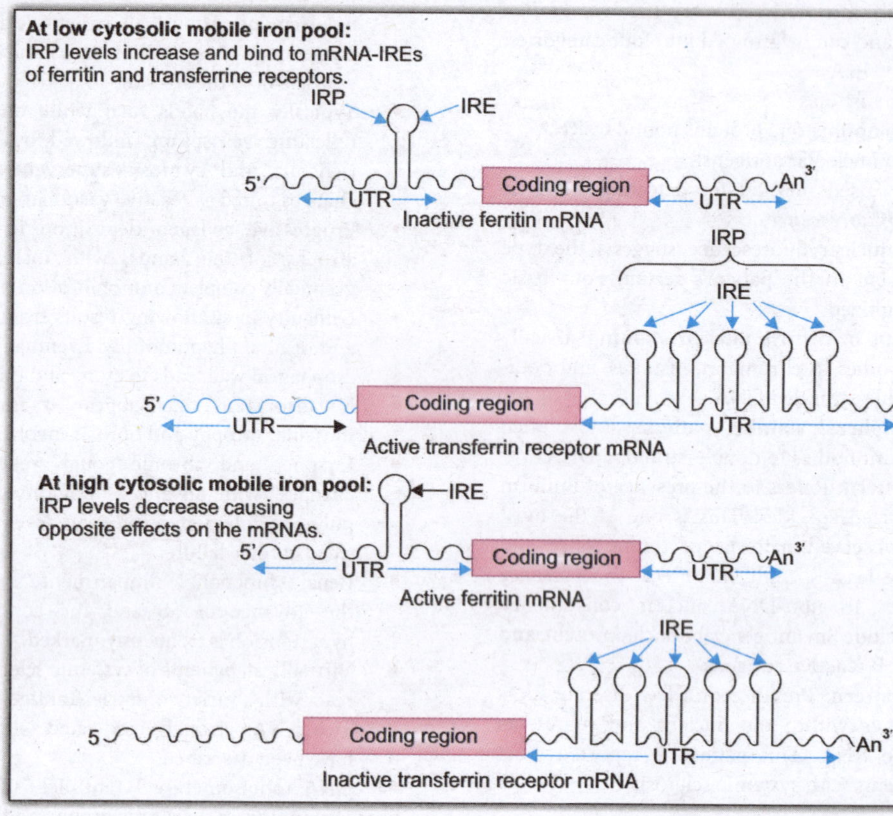

59. Ans. (b) Kimmelstiel Wilson lesion

Ref: Robbin's Basic Pathology 10th edition. Pg 781-783

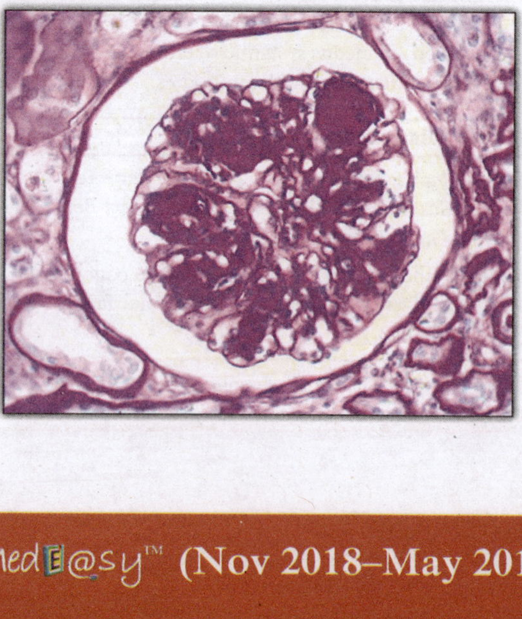

Kimmelstiel Wilson Lesion in Diabetic Nephropathy

- Nodular glomerulosclerosis describes a glomerular lesion made distinctive by ball-like deposits of a laminated matrix situated in the periphery of the glomerulus.
- These nodules are PAS-positive and usually contain trapped mesangial cells. This distinctive change has been called the Kimmelstiel-Wilson lesion, after the two pathologists who first described it.
- Nodular glomerulosclerosis is encountered in approximately 15% to 30% of persons with long-term diabetes and is a major contributor to morbidity and mortality.
- Diffuse mesangial sclerosis also may be seen in association with old age and hypertension; by contrast, the nodular form of glomerulosclerosis, once certain unusual forms of nephropathies have been excluded, is essentially pathognomonic of diabetes.

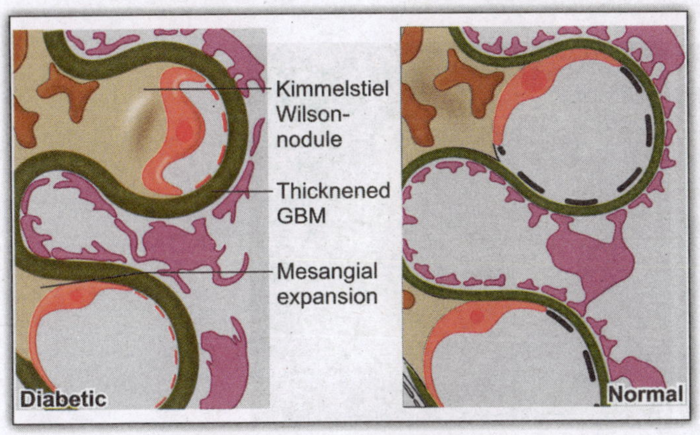

60. Ans. (d) Membranous glomerulonephritis

Ref: Robbin's 9th ed ch 20,

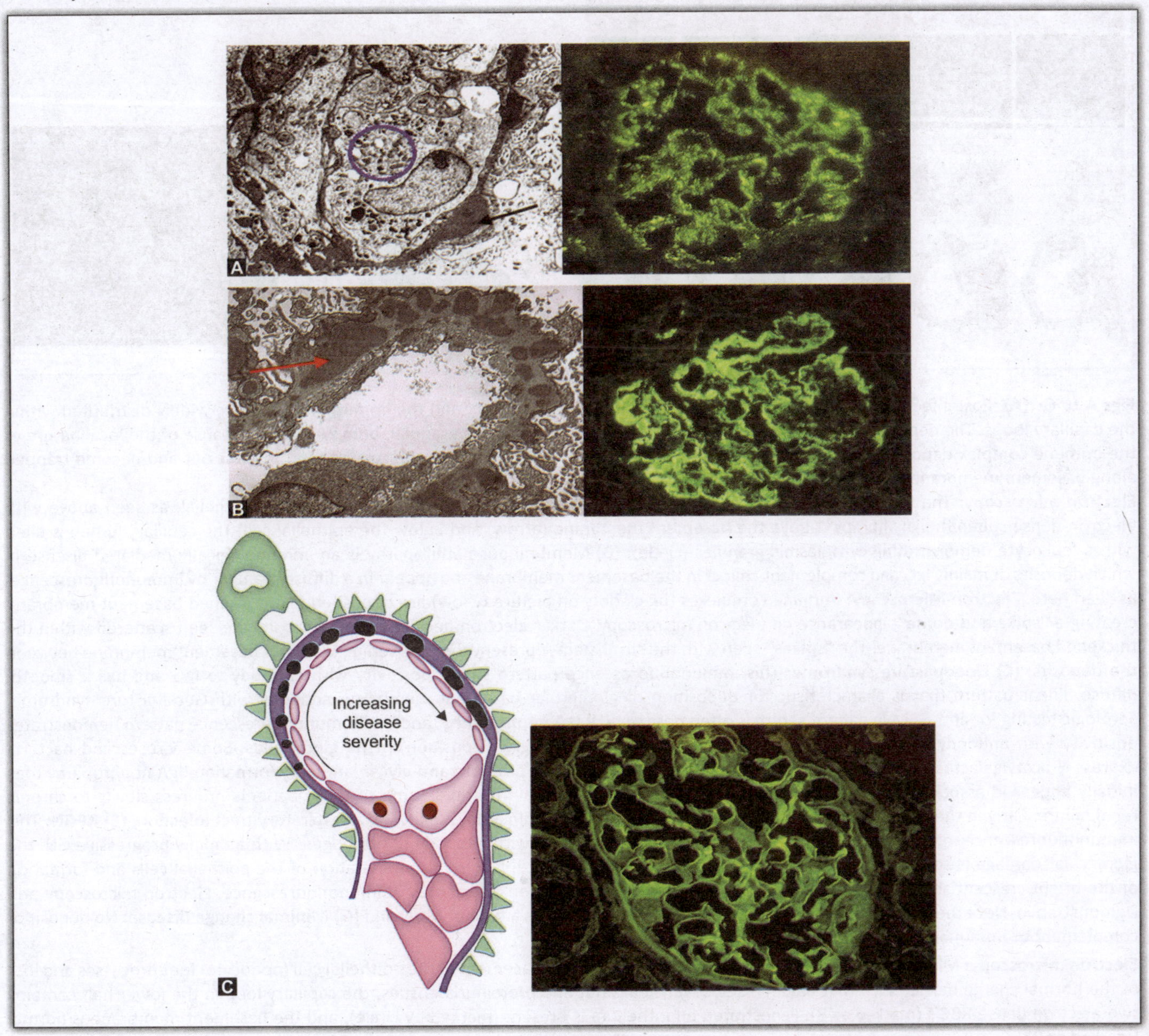

Figs A to G:

http://unckidneycenter.org/kidneyhealthlibrary/glomerular-disease/membranous-nephropathy

See table of Major Primary Glomerulonephritis in PATHOLOGY AIIMS NOV 2016 (see page no. 373 and 381)

Immunofluorescence picture of membranous glomerulonephritis was asked in Pathology AIIMS MAY 2016, now they have added electron microscopy picture in the same question. Two patterns of deposition of immune complexes as seen by immunofluorescence microscopy:

1. Granular, characteristic of circulating and in situ immune complex nephritis
2. Linear, characteristic of classic anti-GBM disease

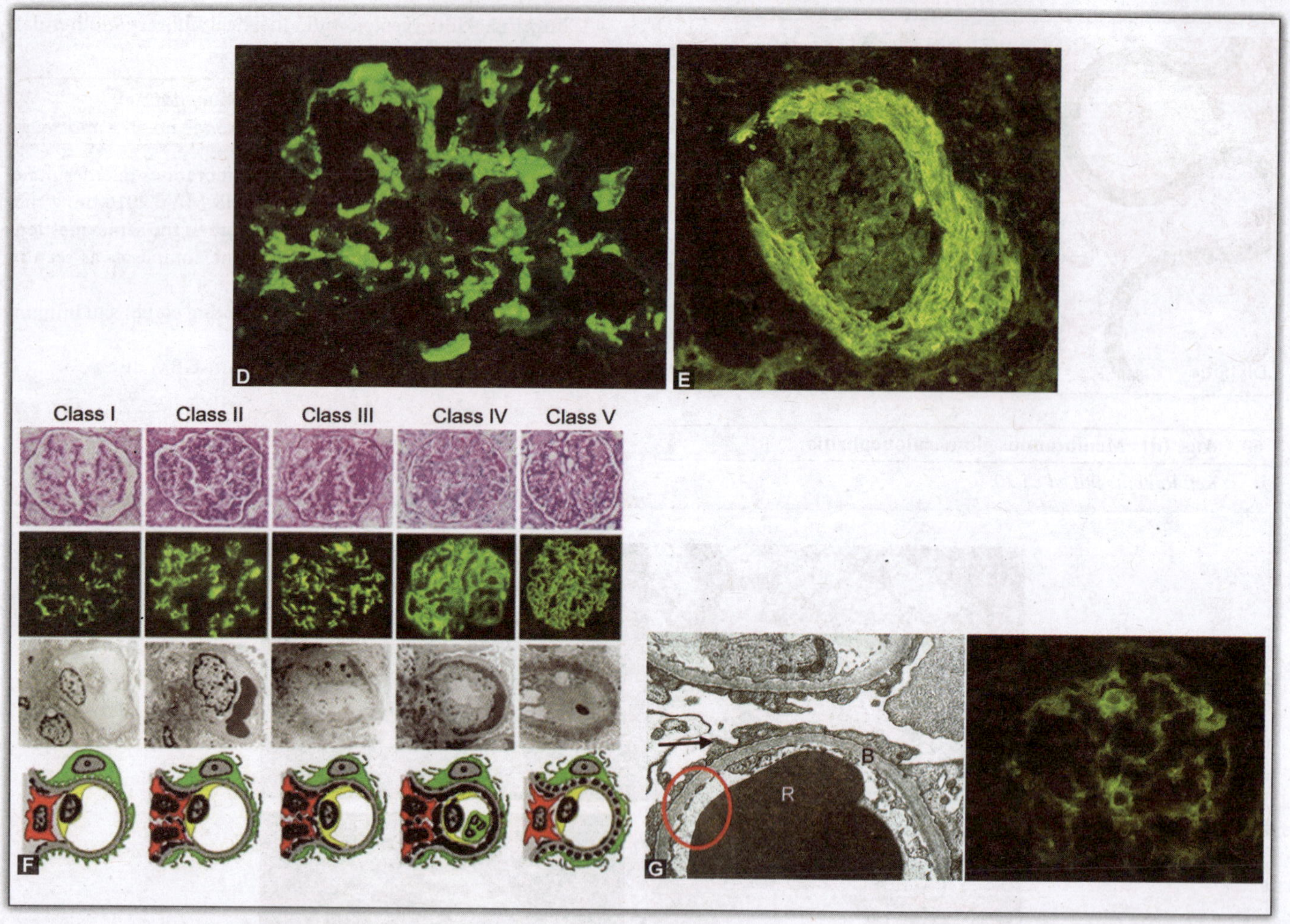

Figs A to G: (A) Post-infectious glomerulonephritis is immunologically mediated, and the immune deposits are widely distributed within the capillary loops. The deposits are seen here with bright green fluorescence in a granular, bumpy pattern because of the focal nature of the immune complex deposition process. In type III hypersensitivity, antigen-antibody complexes tend to filter out and become trapped along basement membranes, such as those in glomerular capillaries.

Electron microscopy: The immune deposits of post-infectious glomerulonephritis are predominantly subepithelial, as seen above with electron dense subepithelial "humps" above the basement membrane (arrow) and below the epithelial cell. The capillary lumen is filled with a leukocyte demonstrating cytoplasmic granules (circle); **(B)** Membranous nephropathy is an immunologically mediated disease in which deposits of mainly IgG and complement collect in the basement membrane and appear in a diffuse granular by immunofluorescence, as seen here. **Electron Microscopy:** Immune complexes (black dots on picture below) are deposited in a thickened basement membrane creating a **"spike and dome"** appearance on electron microscopy. Darker electron dense immune deposits are seen scattered within the thickened basement membrane. The **"spikes"** seen with the silver stain represent the intervening matrix of basement membrane between the deposits; **(C) Goodpasture syndrome:** This immunofluorescence pattern shows positivity with antibody to IgG and has a smooth, diffuse, linear pattern that is characteristic for deposition of glomerular basement membrane antibody with Goodpasture syndrome. Serologic testing for anti-GBM in patient serum is often positive; **(D) IgA nephropathy**, and the immunofluorescence pattern demonstrates positivity with antibody to IgA. Note that the pattern is that of mesangial deposition in the glomerulus. Some viruses and bacteria express N-acetylgalactosamine on their cell surfaces so that infection may promote anti-glycan antibody formation. IgA nephropathy may initially appear in association with an upper respiratory or gastrointestinal infection. Some of these patients progress slowly to chronic renal failure. Early in the course, there may be gross hematuria, often within 3 days following a respiratory tract infection; **(E) RPGN:** This immunofluorescence micrograph of a glomerulus demonstrates positivity with antibody to fibrinogen. With a rapidly progressive GN, the glomerular damage is so severe that fibrinogen leaks into Bowman's space, leading to proliferation of the epithelial cells and formation of the bright crescent shown here; **(F) Lupus** glomerulonephritis classes: on microscopy, Immunofluorescence, Electron microscopy and Demonstrative. Note the increasing granularity on immunofluorescence. Its a type of MGN and **(G) Minimal change disease:** No deposit of complement or immunoglobulins are recognized (nil deposit disease)

Electron microscopy: Minimal change disease (MCD) is characterized by effacement of the epithelial cell (podocyte) foot processes and loss of the normal charge barrier such that albumin selectively leaks out and proteinuria ensues. the capillary loop in the lower half contains two electron dense RBC's (marked as R). Fenestrated endothelium is present (marked by circle), and the basement membrane is normal (marked as B).

61. Ans. (c) Serum laminin and hyaluronic acid

Ref: Zakim and Boyer's Hepatology: A Textbook of Liver Disease E-Book By Thomas D. Boyer, Arun J. Sanyal, Norah A Terrault, Keith D Lindor page 119, Complications of Cirrhosis: Evaluation and Management edited by Andrew Keaveny, Andrés Cárdenas page-39

Non-invasive methods have been proposed as surrogate markers for liver biopsy. It was shown that serum hyaluronic acid (HA) and laminin (LN) levels increase with the development of liver fibrosis and has been proved its utility.

Simplest non-invasive index of liver fibrosis is AST/ALT ratio.

Non-invasive biomarkers of liver fibrosis are direct (Class 1) and indirect (Class 2).

- **Non-specific markers:** Includes age, gender, laboratory markers of liver injury or dysfunction including aspartate transaminase (AST), alanine transaminase (ALT), gamma glutamyl transferase (GGT), bilirubin, heptoglobin, platelet count, prothrombin time, cholesterol, apoprotein A1 and alpha 2 macroglobulin (A2M).
- **Specific markers:** Includes extracellular matrix proteins like hyaluronic acid (HA), serum laminin, matrix metaloproteinase-2, tissue inhibitor of metaloproteinase-1, amino-terminal peptide of type III procollagen.

Biomarkers of Liver Fibrosis

Test	Components	Pitfalls
AST/ALT ratio	AST, ALT	Alcohol, muscle breakdown
AST/platelet ratio index	AST, platelet count	Alcohol, muscle breakdown, extrahepatic cause of thrombocytopenia
FIB-4	Age, AST, ALT, platelet count	Alcohol, muscle breakdown, extrahepatic cause of thrombocytopenia
NAFLD fibrosis score	Age, BMI, diabetes (the presence of), AST, ALT, albumin, platelet count	Alcohol, muscle breakdown, extrahepatic causes of thrombocytopenia malnutrition
FibroSure/Fibro test	Age, sex, bilirubin, GGT, apoliprotein A1, haptoglobin, and α_2-macroglobulin	Alcohol, Gilbert syndrome, renal disease, hemolysis, statin, use, inherited dyslipidemia
HepaScore/FibroScore	α_2-Macroglobulin, bilirubin, GGT, hyaluronic acid	Alcohol, Gilbert syndrome, renal disease, extrahepatic fibrosis
FibroMeter	Age, sex, platelet count, α_2-macroglobulin, ALT, AST GCT, INR, blood urea nitrogen	Alcohol, Gilbert syndrome, renal disease, anticoagulation
FibroSpect	α_2-Macroglobulin, hyaluronic acid, tissue inhibitor of metalloproteinase	Renal disease, extrahepatic fibrosis, chronic inflammatory diseases
Enhanced liver fibrosis score	Hyaluronic acid, tissue inhibitor of metalloproteinase, N-terminal propeptide of type III procollagen	Renal disease, extrahepatic fibrosis, chronic inflammatory diseases

62. Ans. (d) Sweet reticulin silver stain

Ref: Bancroft's Theory and Practice of Histological Techniques pg-334, http://library.med.utah.edu/WebPath/HISTHTML/MANUALS/RETIC.PDF

In pathology, the reticulin stain, is a popular staining method in histology. It is used to visualize reticular fiber and used extensively in liver histopathology. Gordon & Sweet's Staining Protocol for Reticulin is commonly used.

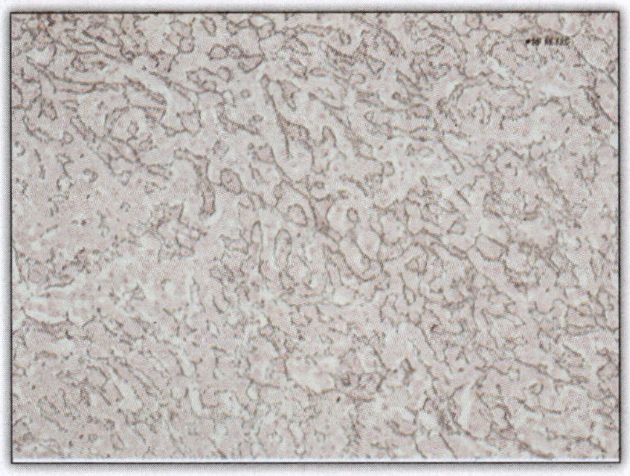

Fig: Gordon & Sweet's Staining Protocol for Reticulin staining in Liver histology

- A silver impregnation technique that demonstrates reticular fibers. Reticulum is a support function of the body and is abundant in liver, spleen, and kidney. In a normal liver the fibers are will defined strands, but necrotic and cirrhotic liver show discontinuous patterns. Reticulum also forms characteristic patterns in relationship to certain tumor cells.
- **Principle:** The tissue is oxidized, then sensitized with the iron alum, which is replaced with silver. The silver is reduced with formalin to its visible metallic state.
- Reticulin fibers have little natural affinity for silver solutions so, they must be treated with potassium permanganate to produce sensitised sites on the fibers where silver deposition can be initiated.
- The silver is in a form readily able to precipitate as metallic silver (diamine silver solution) The Optimal pH for maximum uptake of silver ions is pH 9.0.
- A reducing agent, formalin, causes deposition of silver in the form of metal. Any excess silver in the unprecipitated state is removed by treating with hypo.
- Gold chloride treatment renders the preparation permanent and produces a neutral black colour of high intensity.

63. Ans. (c) CRISPR

Ref: Genome Editing by Kursad Turksen page 3

CRISPR: Clustered Regularly Interspaced Palindromic Repeats are segments of prokaryotic DNA containing short, repetitive base sequences.

- Editing genes can mean removing or replacing an existing gene, switching a gene on or off, or inserting a new gene altogether.
- Whatever the aim, the first step is always to find the stretch of DNA that codes for the gene and grab hold of it, so a cut can be made.
- CRISPR not only finds the target gene and locks on, it also delivers an enzyme that cuts the DNA with unprecedented accuracy.
- The reason it is able to manage this precision double act is because CRISPR is made of ribonucleic acid (RNA)—a molecule that can be tailor-made to perfectly match a sequence of DNA or to bind to a protein.
- CRISPR RNA does both jobs—one end is custom-made to match the target gene's DNA sequence, and the other end binds to a DNA-cutting enzyme, or nuclease.
- The **CRISPR-Cas9 system** for genome editing consists of a small RNA molecule, called single guide RNA (sgRNA), and a nonspecific endonuclease, Cas9.
- The small RNA molecule forms a complex with Cas9 and provides sequence specificity to the system by interacting with its genomic target according to the Watson-Crick base-pairing rules.
- In contrast to ZFNs and TALENs, which require complete reengineering of the enzymes for reprogramming, the simple modification of the sgRNA is sufficient to reprogram Cas9 to target any sequence of interest. The simplicity of CRISPR-Cas9 reprogramming, its high efficacy, and its multiplexing capability have propelled this technology to forefronts of genome editing.
- Each repetition is followed by short segments of spacer DNA from previous exposures to foreign DNA (e.g., a virus or plasmid).

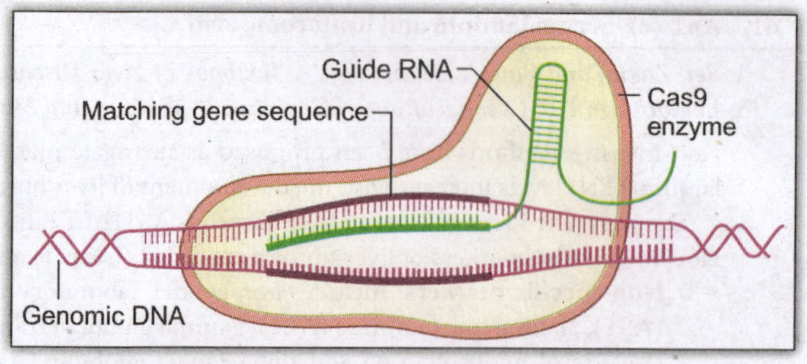

Fig: CRISPR

Also Know

GeneXpert- used in Nucleic Acid Amplification Tests, e.g. identification of Mycobacterium tuberculosis and rifampicin resistance by polymerase chain reaction—The Xpert MTB/RIF detects DNA

64. Ans. (b) Affect G1 phase

Ref: Robbins 9th ed page -184

- As development proceeds, however, two gaps are incorporated into the cell cycle: gap 1 (G1) between mitosis (M) and DNA replication (S), and gap 2 (G2) between DNA replication (S) and mitosis (M).
- Although each phase of the cell cycle circuitry is monitored carefully, the transition from G1 to S is believed to be an extremely important checkpoint in the cell cycle "clock."
- Once cells cross the G1 checkpoint they can pause the cell cycle for a time, but they are obligated to complete mitosis.
- In G1, however, cells can remove themselves entirely from the cell cycle, either temporarily (quiescence, or G0) or permanently (senescence).
- Indeed, during development, as cells become terminally differentiated, they exit the cell cycle and enter G0. Cells in G0 remain there until external cues, such as mitogenic signaling, push them back into the cell cycle.
- In G1, therefore, diverse signals are integrated to determine whether the cell should progress through the cell cycle, or exit the cell cycle and differentiate, and Rb is a key hub integrating external mitogenic and differentiation signals to make this decision.

The cyclins and CDKs promote cell cycle progression, while the CDK inhibitors stop it. The balance between the two groups of molecules determines whether the cell proliferates or is quiescent.

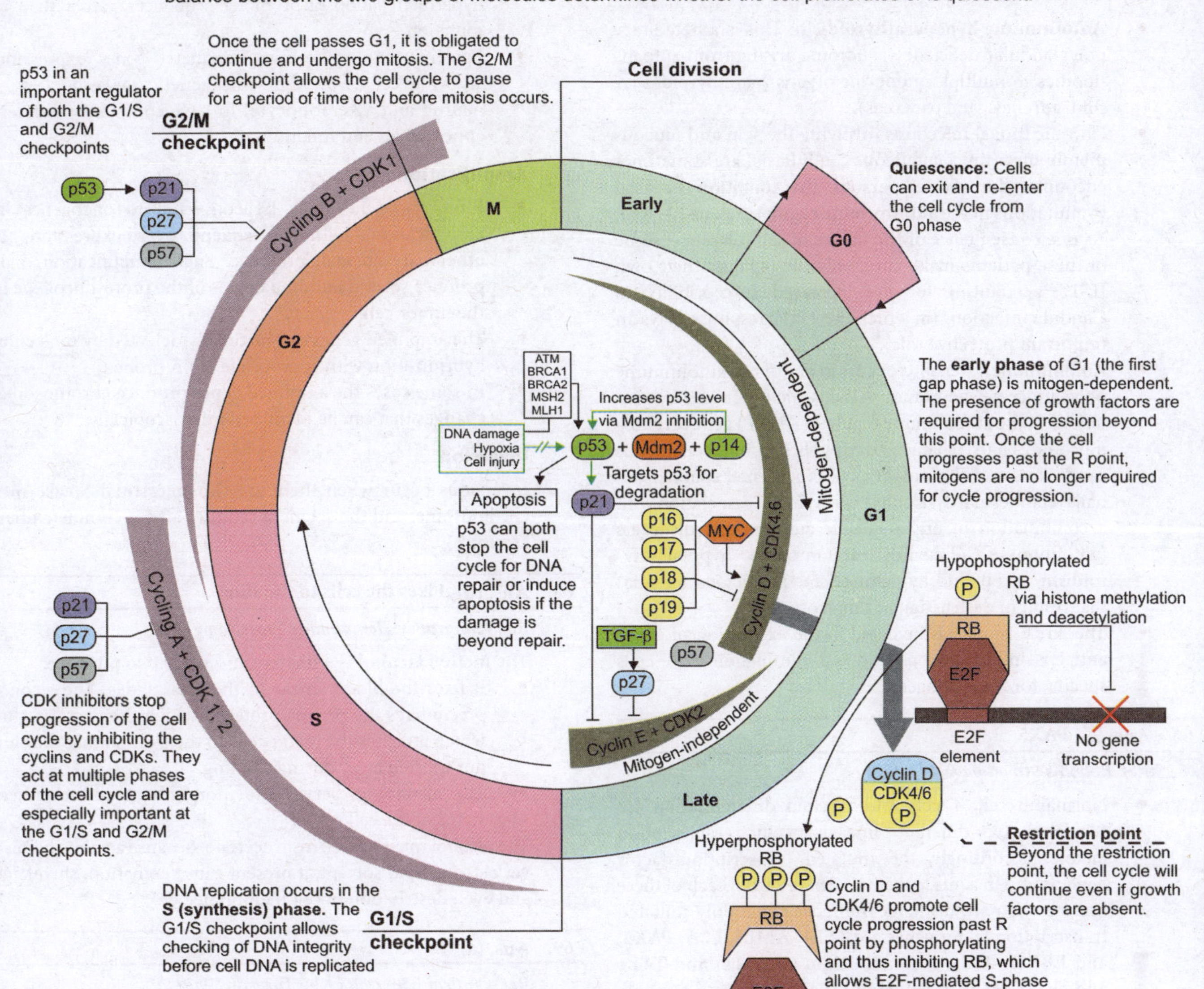

AB — autosomal dominant inheritance

Germline mutation of *RB1* gene cause **retinoblastoma**, an embryonic cancer of the retina. Since RB inhibits cell cycle progression, it is protective against uncontrolled cell proliferation and thus is a **tumour suppressor (ts).** According to the **Knudson two-hit hypothesis** for recessive ts genes, both alleles of the *RB1* gene must be lost for cancer to develop.
In the **hereditary form**, one allele of the *RB1* gene is mutated or deleted in the germ cells. The other allele is lost via a somatic mutation later on. The hereditary form features bilateral, multifocal retinal involvement and typically manifests early, before the age of 1.
Sporadic retinoblastoma is more common and is often unilateral and unifocal in origin. The age of onset is usually later, between the ages of 1 and 2.

p53 — autosomal dominant inheritance

Germline mutations of *p53* gene causes **Li-Fraumeni syndrome**, in which multiple cancers develop at a relatively young age (<45). Breast cancer, osteosarcoma, leukemia, lymphoma, and adrenocortical carcinomas are the most common cancers found in *Li-Fraumeni syndrome*.
Similar to retinoblastoma, the two-hit hypothesis applies to Li-fraumeni syndrome as well. One allele of *p53* is lost in the germline and the second allele is lost somatically. The risk of cancer is dominantly inherited.
p53 is called the "guardian of the genome". It is lost in almost every type of cancer because its loss confers a significant survival advantage, leading to rapid, unchecked proliferation and evasion of apoptosis.

Oncogenes	Tumour suppressors
The lack of inhibition or gain of function of which will lead to cancer.	The increased inhibition or loss of function of which will lead to cancer.
Cyclins	RB
Cyclins-dependent kinases (CDKs)	p53
E2F	p21, p27, p57 (CIP/KIP/WAF)
MYC	p14/ARF
Mdm2	p16/INK4a, p17, p18, p19
	TGF-β receptor
	BRCA1, BRCA2
	ATM

65. Ans. (b) AIRE

Ref: Robbins Basic Pathology 9th ed Page 145

- **Autoimmune hypoparathyroidism:** This is a hereditary polyglandular deficiency syndrome arising from autoantibodies to multiple endocrine organs (parathyroid, thyroid, adrenals, and pancreas).
- Chronic fungal infections involving the skin and mucous membranes (mucocutaneous candidiasis) are sometimes encountered in affected persons. This condition is caused by mutations in the **autoimmune regulator gene (AIRE).** As one consequence of the failure of self tolerance, some of these patients make autoantibodies against their own IL-17, accounting for the increased susceptibility to Candida infections (in which the TH17 response plays an important protective role).
- Autoimmune adrenalitis occurs in one of two autoimmune polyendocrine syndromes: APS1, which is caused by mutations in the autoimmune regulator (AIRE) gene on chromosome 21 and is characterized by chronic mucocutaneous candidiasis and abnormalities of skin, dental enamel, and nails (ectodermal dystrophy) occurring in association with a combination of organ-specific autoimmune disorders (autoimmune adrenalitis, autoimmune hypoparathyroidism, idiopathic hypogonadism, pernicious anemia) that result in destruction of target organs.
- The AIRE protein is involved in the expression of tissue antigens in the thymus and the elimination of T cells specific for these antigens.

66. Ans. (a) PAX5

Ref. Robbins 9th ed page 431-433

- Normal B cell, T cell, and myeloid differentiation are regulated by different lineage-specific transcription factors; accordingly, the mutated transcription factor genes found in acute leukemias derived from each of these lineages also are distinct. The most commonly mutated transcription factor genes are **TEL1, AML1, E2A, PAX5, and EBF in ALLs of B cell origin (B-ALLs) and TAL1 and NOTCH1 in T cell ALLs (T-ALLs).**
- CD34- Hemopoeitic progenitor cell antigen.
- CD1a+ T cells are normal component of T cell repertoire
- Terminal deoxynucleotidyl transferase (TdT), an enzyme specifically expressed in pre-B and pre-T cells, is present in more than 95% of cases of ALL.

67. Ans. (c) Epigenetics

Ref: Robbin's 9th ed page 176

Epigenetics

- Epigenetics refers to reversible, heritable changes in gene expression that occur without mutation. Such changes involve post-translational modifications of histones and DNA methylation, both of which affect gene expression.
- In normal, differentiated cells, the major portion of the genome is not expressed. These regions of the genome are silenced by DNA methylation and histone modifications.
- On the other hand, cancer cells are characterized by a global DNA hypomethylation and selective promoter localized hypermethylation.
- Indeed, it has become evident during the past several years that tumor suppressor genes are sometimes silenced by hypermethylation of promoter sequences, rather than by mutation.
- Epigenetic modifications regulate gene expression, allowing cells with the same genetic make-up (e.g., a neuron and a keratinocyte) to have completely different appearances and functions.

Amplification

- Proto-oncogenes may be converted to oncogenes by amplification, with consequent over expression, of otherwise normal proteins. Such amplification may produce several hundred copies of the proto-oncogene in the tumor cell.
- The amplified genes can be readily detected by molecular hybridization with appropriate DNA probes.
- In some cases the amplified genes produce chromosomal changes that can be identified microscopically.

Inversion

Inversions occur when there are two interstitial breaks in a chromosome, and the segment reunites after a complete turnaround.

68. Ans. (b) Fixes the cells to the slide

Ref: Laboratory Hematology Practice pg-285

The methyl alcohol is a fixative and solve two purpose:

- It fixes the blood smear to the glass slides. The alcohol precipitates the plasma proteins, which then acts as glue which attaches the blood cells to the slide so that they are not washed away during staining.
- The alcohol preserves the morphology and chemical status of the cell.

The alcohol must be free from acetone, because acetone being a very strong lipid solvent, if present cause crenation, shrinkage and even destruction of cell membrane.

69. Ans. (a) 3

Ref: Clinical hematology by Turgeon. Page 77

Corrected reticulocyte count = Reticulocyte % × Hematocrit/ Expected Hematocrit

Or

Corrected Reticulocyte Count = Recticulocyte % × Hemoglobin/Expected Hemoglobin = $9 \times 5/15 = 3$

70. Ans. (a) Anisocytosis

Ref: Wintrobe's Clinical Hematology, 12th ed page 4

Red Cell Distribution Width (RDW)

- The red cell distribution width (RDW) is a red cell measurement that quantitates cellular volume heterogeneity reflecting the range of red cell sizes within a sample.
- RDW is particularly useful in characterizing microcytic anemia, allowing to distinguish between uncomplicated iron deficiency anemia (high RDW, normal to low MCV) and uncomplicated heterozygous thalassemia (normal RDW, low MCV), although other tests are usually required to confirm the diagnosis.

- RDW is also useful in identifying red cell fragmentation, agglutination, or dimorphic cell populations (including patients who have had transfusions, have sideroblastic anemias, or have been recently treated for a nutritional deficiency).
- The red cell indices represent mean values and do not reveal any variation that may exist within a population of cells. Also, the indices do not detect two or more populations differing in size or other characteristics.
- The MCV can be normal if there are combined abnormalities, such as when iron deficiency (decreased MCV) is accompanied by a megaloblastic anemia (increased MCV). For these purposes, it is important to examine the peripheral blood smear.
- Also, the electronically derived RDW allows for recognition of these phenomena because it quantifies the degree of heterogeneity of RBC size (i.e., **Anisocytosis**) in a population of cells, and this has proven to be of value. The upper limit of normal values for RDW is 14.6%.
- An increased RDW value is an early and pronounced finding in iron deficiency and most megaloblastic anemias; no differences from normal are seen in heterozygous thalassemia. In iron deficiency, the RDW value may become abnormal even before the MCV falls below the lower limits of normal.
- **Poikilocytosis:** Variation in shape of cells e.g. Sickle cell, Burr cell, schistocytes, ovalocytes, etc.
- **Polychromasia:** (also known as Polychromatophilia) is a disorder where there is an abnormally high number of immature red blood cells found in the bloodstream as a result of being prematurely released from the bone marrow during blood formation. (Poly- refers to many, and -chromasia means color.)
- **Hypochromasia**: Hypochromia is characterized by an increase in central pallor. It is said to be present when greater than 1/2 of the cell diameter has central pallor. Hypochromia is caused by a deficiency in the production of hemoglobin, which is usually the result of iron deficiency caused by chronic hemorrhage.

71. Ans. (a) SOX11

Ref: Robbin's 9th Ed. Pg- 435

Mantle Cell Lymphoma

Mantle cell lymphoma is composed of cells resembling the naive B cells found in the mantle zones of normal lymphoid follicles. It constitutes approximately 4% of all NHLs and occurs mainly in men older than 50 years of age.

Immunophenotypic and Genetic Features

- Almost all tumors have an (11;14) translocation that fuses the cyclin D1 gene to the IgH locus. This translocation dysregulates the expression of cyclin D1, a cell cycle regulator, and is believed to be an important mediator of uncontrolled tumor cell growth. The tumor cells usually coexpress surface IgM and IgD, pan-B cell antigens (CD19 and CD20), and CD5. Mantle cell lymphoma is most readily distinguished from CLL/SLL by the absence of proliferation centers and the presence of cyclin D1 protein.
- The constant expression of SOX11 in most MCL including cases negative for CCND1 & CCND2 translocations, and its virtually absence in subtypes of tumors with a very indolent behaviour suggest that SOX11 contribute to the pathogenesis of this lymphoma and it's aggressive clinical behaviour

72. Ans. (d) Inflammatory myofibroblastic tumor

Ref: Diagnostic Histopathology of Tumors By Christopher D. M. Fletcher 4th ed page 810

Anaplastic Lymphoma Kinase (ALK)

Anaplastic lymphoma kinase (ALK) also known as ALK tyrosine kinase receptor or CD246 (cluster of differentiation 246) is an enzyme that in humans is encoded by the *ALK* gene.

ALK positive neoplasms are:

- Anaplastic large cell lymphoma
- Adenocarcinoma of lung
- Familial neuroblastoma
- Inflammatory myofibroblastic tumor: 50% of inflammatory myofibroblastic tumors have rearrangements involving the ALK gene on chromosome 2p23
- Adult and pediatric renal cell carcinomas
- Esophageal squamous cell carcinoma
- Breast cancer notably the inflammatory subtype
- Colonic adenocarcinoma
- Glioblastoma multiforme
- Anaplastic thyroid cancer

73. Ans. (a) Multiple Myeloma

Ref: Wintrobe's clinical hematology 12th ed page 2378

One of the most common and inadequately managed symptoms that patients with multiple myeloma (MM) experience as a result of cancer treatment is diarrhea. Diarrhea in patients with MM often is severe enough to warrant dose reduction, delays, or discontinuation of chemotherapy.

Multiple myeloma is a neoplastic plasma cell dyscrasia (PCD) characterized by a clinical pentad: (a) anemia (most common clinical feature-normochromic, normocytic in most patients, but macrocytosis may be observed as well) (b) a monoclonal protein in the serum or urine or both. M protein (M component, myeloma protein, or M spike) is a hallmark of the disease (c) abnormal bone radiographs and bone pain, (d) hypercalcemia: Calcium can precipitate in the kidneys and aggravate renal insufficiency and (e) renal insufficiency or failure: The pathologic lesion of myeloma kidney consists of monoclonal light chains in the tubules in the form of dense, often laminated, tubular casts. These casts contain albumin and Tamm-Horsfall protein. An important feature of myeloma kidney is that it is primarily a tubular rather than a glomerular disease.

Plasma Cell Neoplasms

These B-cell proliferations contain neoplastic plasma cells that virtually always secrete a monoclonal Ig or Ig fragment. Collectively, the plasma cell neoplasms (often referred to as dyscrasias) account for about 15% of the deaths caused by lymphoid neoplasms. The most common and deadly of these neoplasms is multiple myeloma. Multiple myeloma (plasma cell myeloma), the most important monoclonal gammopathy, usually presents as tumorous masses scattered throughout the skeletal system. Solitary myeloma (plasmacytoma) is an infrequent variant that presents as a single mass in bone or soft tissue.

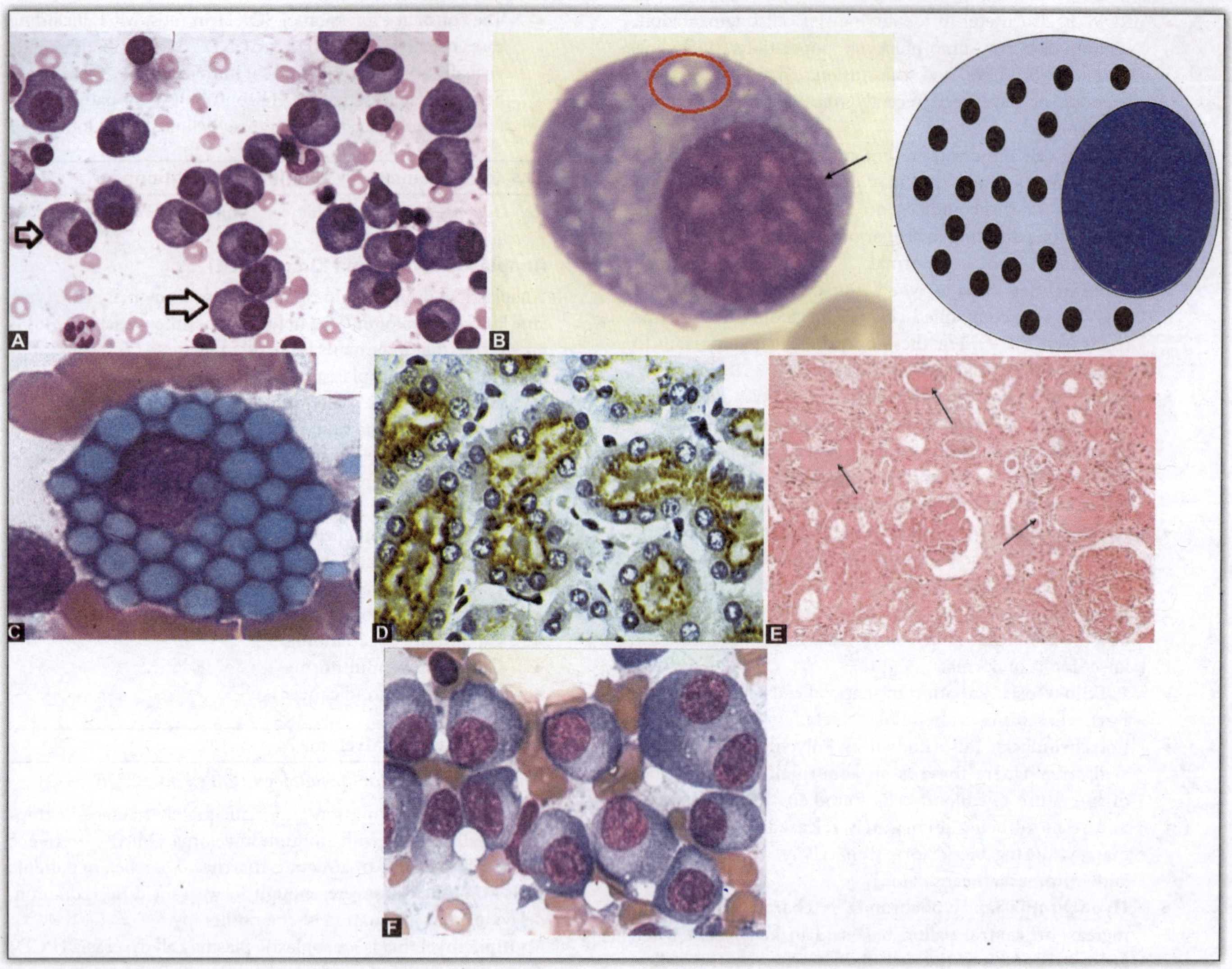

Figs A to F: (A) Plasma cell have basophilic cytoplasm containing pale zones of extensive golgi apparatus and an eccentric nucleus with heterochromatin in a characteristic cartwheel or clock face arrangement. The plasma cells are well differentiated morphologically. The more mature cells have clumped nuclear chromatin, abundant cytoplasm, low nuclear-cytoplasmic ratio; **(B) Plasma cell high definition (classical):** Basophilic (blue) cytoplasm, Cartwheel eccentric nucleus (arrow), and pale golgi apparatus in cytoplasm (red circle); **(C)** Plasma cell myeloma, morphologic variants based on cytoplasmic features. So-called **Mott cell with abundant "grape-like"** cytoplasmic inclusions of immunoglobulin; Fig: **(D) Plasma cell myeloma:** Section of kidney showing renal tubular lambda deposition with casts reflecting renal tubular Bence Jones protein reabsorption **(Immunoperoxidase, anti-lambda light chain)**. Immunohistochemical stains on marrow biopsy sections are often valuable to essential in the diagnosis of plasma cell neoplasms. They may be used to: 1. Assess the quantity of plasma cells in marrow biopsies; 2. Identify monoclonal plasma cell proliferations; 3. Distinguish myeloma from other neoplasms; **(E) Bence Jones cast nephropathy** in multiple myeloma is associated with glassy, fracturing casts occluding the tubular lumina (arrows). Multinucleated giant cells surround some casts and **(F) Bone marrow biopsy in multiple myeloma:** Plasma cells with basophilic cytoplasm, eccentric nuclei, and "clock face" chromatin

74. Ans. (a) ALL

Ref: Wintrobe's clinical hematology 12th ed page 1892-1908

Features	ALL	AML	Juvenile myelomonocytic leukemia
Age group:	Mostly children	Mostly adults	70% are children less than 1 year old.
Lymphadenopathy	More common	Less common	Less common
Bone marrow			Myelocytic and Monocytic Differentiation (5-30%-Monocyte), decreased megakaryocytes, Blast+ promonocyte less than 20%

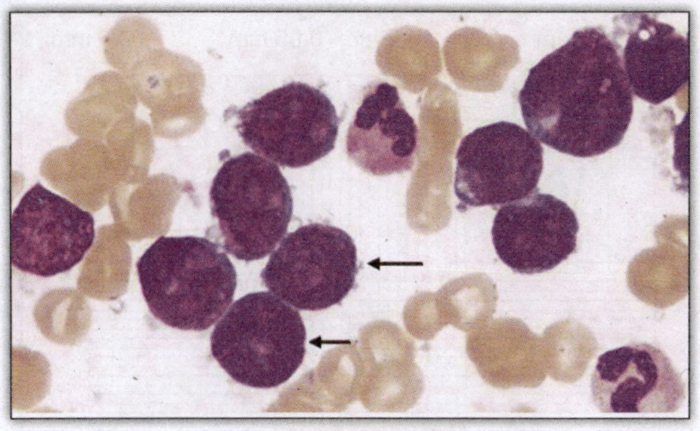

Fig: Acute Lymphoid Leukemia (ALL)

Acute Lymphoid Leukemia (ALL):

- These are neoplasms of immature B cells or T cells which are referred to as lymphoblasts (long arrows)
- 85% of all cases are B-ALLs which manifest typically as childhood acute leaukemias while rest are T-ALLs which manifest as thymic 'lymphomas' in adolescents specially males.
- Marrow is hypercellular, packed with lymphoblasts which replace the normal marrow elements.
- Blasts are larger, with scanty cytoplasm as compared to small lymphocytes.
- As compared to myeloid blasts, lymphoblasts have more condensed chromatin, less conspicuous or absent nucleoli and lesser cytoplasm without granules.
- However morphological differentiation is not absolute and definitive diagnosis is based on immunohistochemistry.
- Histochemical stains are also helpful as lymphoblasts are **MPO negative** and show **PAS positive** cytoplasmic granules.
- ALL is the commonest cancer in children but it has about 95% remission rate with aggressive chemotherapy and 75–85% complete cure rates.
- Yet it is the leading cause of cancer deaths in children.

75. Ans. (d) Albumin

Ref: Robbins Pathology 10th ed page 86, Bailey 26th ed page 9, Clinical Laboratory Medicine 2nd edited by Kenneth D. McClatchey Page 265

Acute-phase proteins are defined as those proteins whose plasma concentrations increase (positive acute phase proteins) or decrease (negative acute-phase proteins) by at least 25% during inflammatory states.

Negative phase proteins are consumed for the production of positive phase proteins during inflammatory reactions.

Acute Phase Reactant	
Positive acute phase reactant	**Negative acute phase reactant**
• CRP (C- Reactive protein) • Alpha-1 Antitrypsin • Ceruloplasmin • Fibrinogen • IL-1, IL-6, TNF-α • Haptoglobulin	• Albumin and Prealbumin • Transferrin • Retinol binding protein • Transthyretin

76. Ans. (a) Sample thickness

Ref: Harsh Mohan, Pathology Practical Book 3rd ed page 5, Microbiology: A Laboratory Manual, 5th edition, Cappuccino, J.S. and Sherman, N., Benjamin/Cummings Science Publishing

Resolving power, also called spatial resolution or horizontal resolution represents the capacity of the optical system or a lens to produce seprate images of object very close to each other. When a lens cannot discriminate, that is, when the two objects appear as one, it has lost resolution.

The resolving power of a lens is dependent on the wavelength of light used and the numerical aperture, which is a characteristic of each lens and imprinted on each objective. The **numerical aperture is defined as a function of the diameter of the objective lens in relation to its focal length.** It is doubled by use of the substage condenser; which illuminates the object with rays of light that pass through the specimen obliquely as well as directly.

Resolving Power (R) = 0.61 **λ/NA**

Where

λ – Wavelength of incident light

NA – Numerical aperture of the lens system.

Resolving power of standard microscope is 200 nm.

Numerical aperture has the property that it is constant for a beam as it goes from one material to another, provided there is no optical power at the interface.

The relationship between wavelength and numerical aperture is valid only for increased resolving power when light rays are parallel. **Therefore, the resolving power is dependent on another factor, the refractive index.**

$$NA = n \sin \theta \approx \sim n \frac{D}{2f}$$

Where n = Refractive index, D = Diameter of lens, f = Focal length of lens

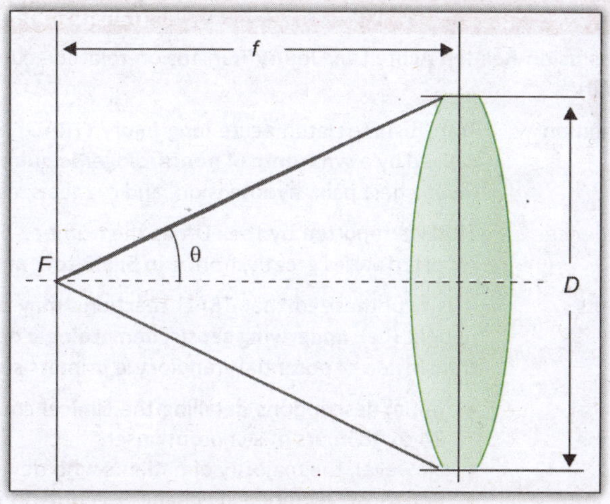

Depth of field: This is the longitudinal resolving power of the microscope. It is the distance between the nearest object plane that is in focus and the farthest object plane that is also in focus. When considering resolution in optical microscopy, a majority of the emphasis is placed on point-to-point lateral resolution in the plane perpendicular to the optical axis. Another important aspect to resolution is the axial (or longitudinal) resolving power of an objective, which is measured parallel to the optical axis and is most often referred to as depth of field.

77. Ans. (b) 6000

Ref: Textbook Of Practical Physiology By G K Pal 2nd ed page 57, District Laboratory Practice in Tropical Countries, Monica Cheesbrough, 2nd ed, pg 119-120

Large Square Area = 1 mm × 1mm = 1 mm^2

The depth of the chamber is 0.100 mm (space between the glass slide and cover slip)

Leukocytes/ WBC are counted in the 4 large squares with normally 1:20 dilution and RBC are counted in 80 small squares with normally 1:200 dilution

Volume of large square = 1 mm^2 × 0.1 mm = 0.1 mm^3 = 0.1μL = 1 × 10^{-4} mL

Volume of small square = 0.05 mm × 0.05 mm × 0.1 mm = 0.00025 mm^3 = 0.00025μL

$$\text{RBC concentration} = \frac{\text{Number of counted erythrocytes} \times \text{Dilution}}{\text{Number of counted squares} \times \text{Volume above one large square}}$$

$$\text{WBC concentration} = \frac{\text{Number of counted Leukocytes} \times \text{Dilution}}{\text{Number of counted squares} \times \text{Volume above one large square}}$$

Hence WBC concentration = 120 × 20/4 × 0.1 = 2400/0.4 = 6000

Alternatively

Cells counted in 4 squares = n = (25+35+40+20) = 120

Total volume of 4 square = 4 × 0.1cu.mm=0.4 cu.mm

So, 0.4 cu.mm volume contains 120 cell.

Therefore, 1 cu.mm or, per dL = (120 × 2.5) = 300

If 20 times diluted fluid contains 300 cells,

Undiluted concentration will be 300 x 20 = 6000

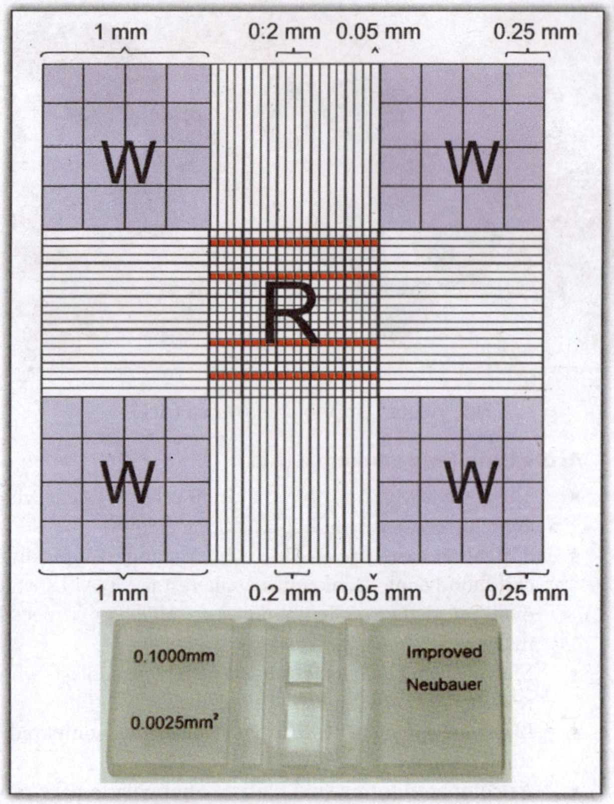

78. Ans. (a) Self Resolving in 2–3 weeks

Ref: Wintrobe's 12th ed page 699, Harrison 19th ed page 138 e5

TRALI is the new love of AIIMS exams.

TRALI is also asked in Pathology AIIMS MAY 2015 (With different options)

Transfusion-Related Acute Lung Injury	
Transfusion-Related Acute Lung Injury Transfusion-related acute lung injury (TRALI) is the most common cause of transfusion related fatalities	
Definition	Transfusion-related acute lung injury (TRALI) most commonly presents as severe respiratory distress of sudden onset, caused by a **syndrome of noncardiogenic pulmonary edema resembling the adult respiratory distress syndrome.** Chills, fever, chest pain, hypotension, and cyanosis, as well as the usual manifestations of pulmonary edema, may be seen.
Incidence	TRALI is reported by the FDA as the number-one cause of transfusion-associated fatality. The incidence of TRALI being reported varies greatly, from **1 in 5,000 to 1 in 13,000**
Events	It is hypothesized that TRALI reactions may be the result of two cumulative events: the first event is linked to the patient (i.e., **underlying sepsis, hematologic disease, and/or postsurgical status**), and the second event is related to the transfusion of potential granulocyte primers such as inflammatory cytokines, active lipids, and/or alloantibodies.
Clinical course	• Initial descriptions detailing the clinical course for TRALI suggested quick resolution of hypoxemia, generally within **24 to 48 hours** of symptom onset. • However, the majority of patients who develop TRALI will require ICU admission and ventilator support. • For those requiring mechanical ventilation, these early reports described a mean duration of ventilator support lasting approximately 40 hours. • In contrast, subsequent evidence suggests that most cases will require respiratory support for a longer period (e.g. approximately 3 to 10 days). • These more contemporary data frequently report composite outcomes from cases of TRALI and possible TRALI/ transfused ARDS and limit the study population to the critically ill. • Such cases are likely to represent the more severe end of the clinical spectrum. In contrast, milder cases of TRALI and/ or possible TRALI/transfused ARDS may go undiagnosed or unreported.

Contd...

Transfusion-Related Acute Lung Injury	
Mortality	5–10% in general 40–50% in critically ill patients
Risk factors	• Testing the donor's plasma for anti-HLA antibodies can support this diagnosis. • The implicated donors are frequently **multiparous women.** • The transfusion of plasma from male and nulliparous women donors reduces the risk of TRALI. • Recipient factors that are associated with increased risk of TRALI include smoking, chronic alcohol use, shock, liver surgery (transplantation), mechanical ventilation with >30 cm H_2O pressure support and positive fluid balance treatment is supportive, and patients usually recover without sequelae If TRALI or possible TRALI/transfused ARDS are suspected, the transfusion should be discontinued immediately.
Diagnosis	The diagnosis of a TRALI reaction is based on the onset of acute lung injury (ALI) **within/up to 6 hours of transfusion.** ALI is characterized by an acute onset of hypoxemia (oxygen saturation <90% by pulse oximetry for a patient breathing room air or a $PaO_2/FiO_2 \leq 300$ mm Hg), bilateral infiltrates on frontal chest radiograph, and no evidence of circulatory overload. Based on studies of adult respiratory distress syndrome, which has similar pulmonary manifestations, it has been suggested that agglutination of granulocytes and complement activation occur in the pulmonary vascular bed, leading to capillary endothelial damage with consequent fluid leak into the alveoli.
Prevention	The AABB requires evaluation of donors implicated in TRALI. Donors whose plasma is implicated in such reactions should be examined for the presence of granulocyte specific and HLA antibodies that react with recipient leukocytes. It is recommended to avoid further transfusion of plasma-containing products from implicated donors found to have anti-HLA or antigranulocyte antibodies. **Recently, the AABB recommended that blood banks minimize the production of high-plasma-content components** (such as FFP and apheresis platelets) from donors at risk for alloimmunization (e.g., women with a history of pregnancy). Ultimately, criteria for TRALI susceptibility will have to be clarified in order to prevent it effectively.
Management	**Management** of the patient with either TRALI or possible TRALI/transfused ARDS is supportive, with oxygen supplementation for the correction of hypoxemia being the cornerstone of treatment. Hemodynamic monitoring may be required to determine whether fluid overload is a factor; if not, diuretics are of no proven value. Very high doses of corticosteroids may be of benefit in transfusion-related acute lung injury, probably by blocking granulocyte aggregation and consequent vascular damage. Non-invasive respiratory support with continuous positive airway pressure (CPAP) or bilevel positive airway pressure (BiPAP) may be sufficient in less severe cases, but endotracheal intubation with invasive mechanical ventilation is often required. The available evidence suggests that most patients who develop either TRALI or possible TRALI/transfused ARDS will require ventilatory support (approximately 70 to 80 percent). **Steroids**—the routine use of corticosteroids when TRALI is suspected is not recommended.

79. Ans. (c) ***Cryptococcus neoformans***

Ref: Sternberg's Diagnostic Surgical Pathology 5th Ed page 377, Harrison 19th ed page 1263, HIV disorders of the brain; pathology and pathogenesis Frontiers in Bioscience 11, 718-732, January 1, 2006

Harrison 19th ed page 1263: Opportunistic infections causing neurologic Diseases in Patients with HIV Infection are: Toxoplasmosis, Cryptococcosis, Cytomegalovirus, Syphilis, Mycobacterium tuberculosis, HTLV-I infection, Amebiasis

About Option (D)

Brain involvement only occurs in <2% of patients infected with *E. granulosus*

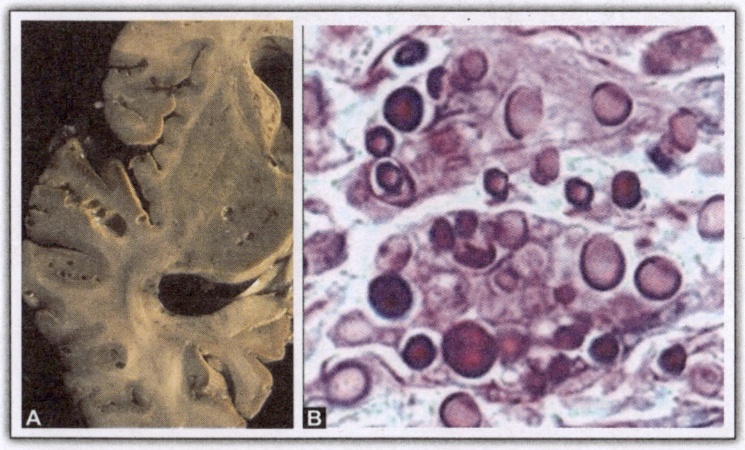

Figs A and B: (A) Cryptococcus infection of Brain Gross: Multiple small cystic lesion of brain giving a Swiss cheese appearance; **(B) Cryptococcus infection of Brain Histopathology:** Cryptococcus (an encapsulated yiest) appears as a spherical, encapsulated structure, which is surrounded by large empty spaces. Confirmed on India ink preparation

	Herpes	Toxoplasma gondii	Cryptococcus Neoformans
Gross (Brain)	Advanced HSV encephalitis shows diffuse softening and edema, accentuated by **hemorrhagic necrosis of the inferior frontal and temporal lobes.**	Multiple foci of **Hemorrhagic necrosis** with 3-5 nm tachyzoites (cysts). Focal, variable in size but generally large, of irregular borders and can affect any part of the brain, with strong predilection to basal ganglia and brainstem.	Gelatinous grayish material within the subarachnoid space and multiple small cysts within the parenchyma giving a **Swiss cheese appearance**, especially prominent at basal ganglia. As the infection spreads the perivascular space **(Virchow Robin)** may become distended & filled with same mucoid, gelatinous material originated from the cryptococcal capsule
Histopathology	**Cowdry A amphophilic intranuclear inclusions of 90 nm to 100 nm "target" capsids.** Without treatment, extensive necrosis, macrophage reaction and neovascularization develop. The degree of necrosis (especially in the frontal & temporal lobes, frequently bilateral) & inflammatory & reactive changes are more severe than any other viral encephalitis and can be detected by imaging.	Histologically, acute lesions differ from chronic abscesses. **1. Acute lesions**: Poorly circumscribed, contain necrotic & hemorrhagic areas with scanted inflammatory cells & abundant intracellular tachyzoites & parenchymal oocysts. **2. Chronic lesions** develope after treatment, well demarcated cysts with microglial nodules and macrophages in the adjacent brain parenchyma, where parasites are difficult to find.	Cystic lesions in the basal ganglia consist of aggregates of organisms confined to the **Virchow-Robin spaces**, which are enlarged. In tissue sections, the Cryptococcus appears as a **spherical, encapsulated structure**, which is surrounded by large empty spaces result of the abundant mucoid material secreted by the yeasts. The **capsule of Cryptococcus** can be visualized more clearly with special staining methods and silver impregnations, such as Gomori methenamine and Grocott, PAS and mucicarmine.

80. Ans. (d) 4

Ref: Atlas and Text of Hematology, Tejender Singh, Chapter 1

The question has 2 components. One is the basic microbiology knowledge that Eosinophils are increased in Parasitic infections, and second is the identification of eosinophils in the peripheral smear.

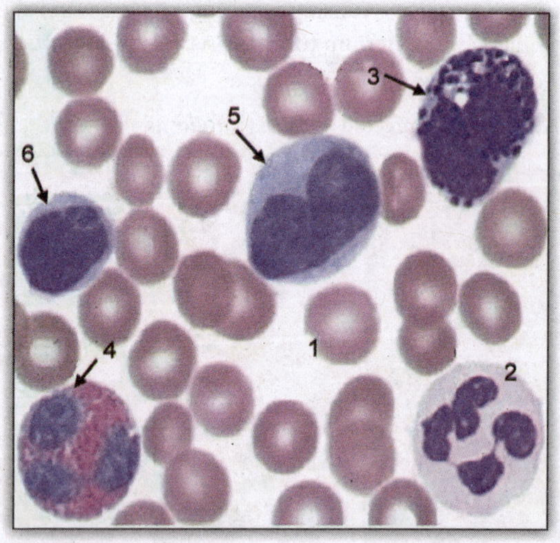

Fig: Peripheral smear: 1= RBC, 2= Neutrophil, 3= Basophil, 4= Eosinophil, 5= Monocytes, 6= Lymphocytes

Cells of Peripheral Smear				
Cells	**Description**	**Cells/mm³ of blood**	**Duration of development and life span**	**Function**
Erythrocytes (RBC) (Marked as 1)	Biconcave, anucleate disc, salmon coloured, diameter 7-8μm	4-6 million	D-15 days LS-100-120 days	Transport oxygen and CO_2
Leukocytes (WBC)	Spherical nucleated cell	4000-11000		
Granulocytes				
• Neutrophil (Marked as 2)	Multilobed nucleus, inconspicuous cytoplasmic granules, diameter 10-12 μm	3000-7000	D-14 days LS-14 hours to few days	Phagocytize bacteria
• Eosinophil (cell 4)	Bilobed nucleus, red cytoplasmic granules, diameter 10-14 μm	100-400	D-about 14 days LS-about 5 days	Kills parasitic worms, complex role in allergy and asthma
• Basophil (Marked as 3)	Bilobed nucleus, large purplish-black cytoplasmic granules, diameter 10-14 μm	20-50	D-about 1-7 days LS-a few hours to few days	Release histamine and other mediators of inflammation; contain heparin and anticoagulant
Agranulocytes				
• Lymphocyte (Marked as 6)	Spherical or indented nucleus, pale blue cytoplasm, diameter 5-17 μm	1500-3000	D-days to weeks LS-hours to years	Mount immune response by direct cell attack or via antibodies
• Monocyte (Marked as 5)	U or kidney shaped nucleus, grey -blue cytoplasm, diameter 14-24 μm	100-700	D-about 2-3 days LS-months	Phagocytosis; develop into macrophages in the tissue
Platelets	Discoid cytoplasmic fragments containing granules, stain deep purple, diameter 2-4 μm	150,000- 400,000	D-4-5 days LS-5-10 days	Seal small tears in blood vessels, instrumental in blood clotting

81. Ans. (d) Low reticulocyte count

Ref: Robbins 9th ed page 409

Recall Bias

The term Hemolytic anemia was not mentioned in the Question. It was a case based question.

This is a case of Hemolytic anemia

Features shared by all uncomplicated hemolytic anemias include

- Decreased red cell life span,
- Compensatory increase in erythropoiesis (Reticulocytosis)
- Retention of the products of degraded red cells (including iron) by the body. Urobilinogen, Bilirubin and LDH are all breakdown products of RBC and hence are increased in Hemolytic anemia.
- Because the recovered iron is efficiently recycled, red cell regeneration may almost keep pace with the hemolysis. Consequently, *hemolytic anemias are associated with erythroid hyperplasia in the marrow and increased numbers of reticulocytes in the peripheral blood.*
- Regardless of cause, intravascular hemolysis leads to hemoglobinemia, hemoglobinuria, and hemosiderinuria. The conversion of heme to bilirubin can result in unconjugated hyperbilirubinemia and jaundice.
- Massive intravascular hemolysis sometimes leads to acute tubular necrosis. *Haptoglobin*, a circulating protein that binds and clears free hemoglobin, is completely depleted from the plasma, which also usually contains high levels of *lactate dehydrogenase* (LDH) as a consequence of its release from hemolyzed red cells.

82. Ans. (d) Folic acid deficiency

Ref: Robbins 9th ed page 422

MCV (Mean Corpuscular Volume in fL) = PCV (Hematocrit in %)/RBC (mil/mm³) × 10

= 30/2 × 10

= 150 fL (Which is >100, hence macrocytic anemia)

NOTE

Even without doing any calculations the answer is very evident as folic acid deficiency is the only option causing Macrocytic anemia in the options provided (The odd one out rule)

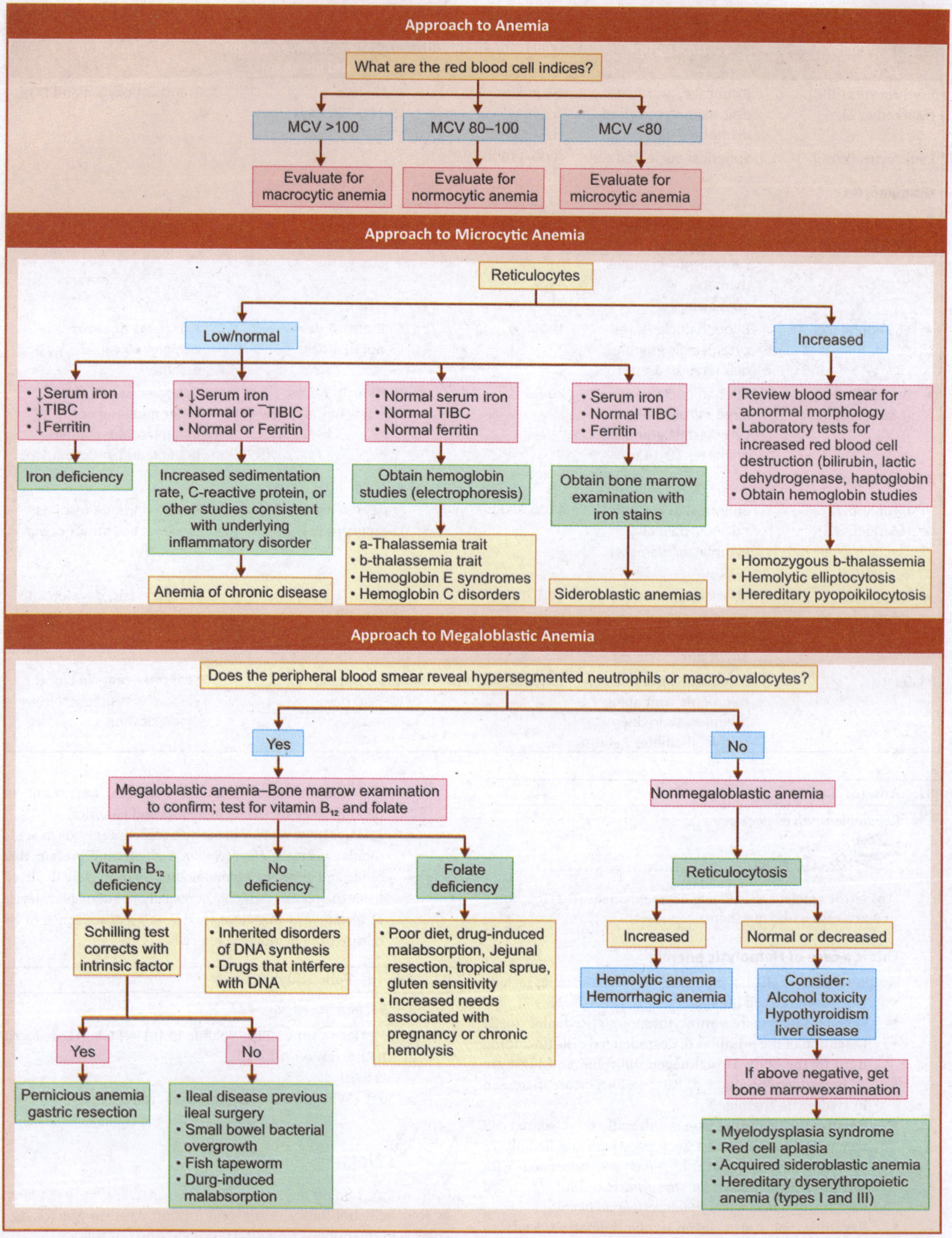
Approach to Anemia
What are the red blood cell indices?
MCV >100
MCV 80–100
MCV <80
Evaluate for macrocytic anemia
Evaluate for normocytic anemia
Evaluate for microcytic anemia
Approach to Microcytic Anemia
Reticulocytes
Low/normal
Increased
• ↓Serum iron • ↓TIBC • ↓Ferritin
Iron deficiency
• ↓Serum iron • Normal or ¯TIBIC • Normal or Ferritin
Increased sedimentation rate, C-reactive protein, or other studies consistent with underlying inflammatory disorder
Anemia of chronic disease
• Normal serum iron • Normal TIBC • Normal ferritin
Obtain hemoglobin studies (electrophoresis)
• a-Thalassemia trait • b-thalassemia trait • Hemoglobin E syndromes • Hemoglobin C disorders
• Serum iron • Normal TIBC • Ferritin
Obtain bone marrow examination with iron stains
Sideroblastic anemias
• Review blood smear for abnormal morphology • Laboratory tests for increased red blood cell destruction (bilirubin, lactic dehydrogenase, haptoglobin • Obtain hemoglobin studies
• Homozygous b-thalassemia • Hemolytic elliptocytosis • Hereditary pyopoikilocytosis
Approach to Megaloblastic Anemia
Does the peripheral blood smear reveal hypersegmented neutrophils or macro-ovalocytes?
Yes
No
Megaloblastic anemia–Bone marrow examination to confirm; test for vitamin B12 and folate
Vitamin B12 deficiency
No deficiency
Folate deficiency
Schilling test corrects with intrinsic factor
Yes
No
Pernicious anemia gastric resection
• Ileal disease previous ileal surgery • Small bowel bacterial overgrowth • Fish tapeworm • Durg-induced malabsorption
• Inherited disorders of DNA synthesis • Drugs that intèrfere with DNA
• Poor diet, drug-induced malabsorption, Jejunal resection, tropical sprue, gluten sensitivity • Increased needs associated with pregnancy or chronic hemolysis
Nonmegaloblastic anemia
Reticulocytosis
Increased
Normal or decreased
Hemolytic anemia Hemorrhagic anemia
Consider: Alcohol toxicity Hypothyroidism liver disease
If above negative, get bone marrowexamination
• Myelodysplasia syndrome • Red cell aplasia • Acquired sideroblastic anemia • Hereditary dyserythropoietic anemia (types I and III)

83. Ans. (a) Crescentic formation

Ref: Robbins 9th ed page 532

The characteristic and most common histologic finding associated with RPGN is the presence of crescents **(crescentic GN).** The diseases causing crescentic GN may be associated with a known disorder or it may be idiopathic. When the cause can be identified, about 12% of the patients have anti-GBM antibody–mediated crescentic GN with or without lung involvement; 44% have immune complex GN with crescents; and the remaining 44% have pauciimmune crescentic GN. All have severe glomerular injury.

Major Primary Glomerulonephritis						
Disease	Most frequent clinical presentation	Pathogenesis	Light microscopy	Fluorescence microscopy	Electron microscopy	Comments
Post streptococcal glomerulonephritis (PSGN)	Acute nephritis	Antibody mediated: circulating or planted antigen	Enlarged hypercellular glomeruli, **Diffuse proliferation,** leukocytic infiltration (both neutrophil and monocytes), Crescent form in severe disease	Granular IgG, IgM and C3 in GBM and mesangium	Subepithelial Humps	Develops 1-3 weeks after acute infection with nephritogenic strains Complement level returns to normal in 6-8 weeks
Goodpasture syndrome	Rapidly progressive glomerulonephritis	Anti GBM antibodies (α-3 chain of Type IV collagen) COL4 A3 antigen	Diffuse proliferative RPGN, Focal necrotizing lesion and crescents in >50% of glomeruli	**Linear IgG** and C3; fibrin in crescents	No deposits; GBM disruption; fibrin	Type II hypersensitivity
Idiopathic RPGN	Rapidly progressive glomerulonephritis	Anti GBM antibody Immune complex ANCA-associated	**Proliferation**, focal necrosis, **crescents**	Linear IgG and C3 (Type I) Granular IgG or IgA or IgM (Type II) Negative or equivocal (Type III)	No deposits Deposits may be present No deposits	There may occur rapidly progressive renal failure **Fibrin** leakage more strongly contributes to crescent formation Parietal epithelial cells, monocytes, macrophages undergo proliferation
Membranous glomerulopathy	Nephrotic syndrome **(MC cause of nephrotic syndrome in adults)**	In situ antibody-mediated antigen unknown	Diffuse capillary wall thickening	Granular IgG and C3 diffuse	Subepithelial deposits	Affects patients between 30-50 years age. **MC Nephropathy of malignancy Lung > Breast/ Stomach)**
Minimal change Disease	Nephrotic syndrome (m.c cause of nephrotic syndrome in children)	Unknown, loss of glomerular polyanion: podocyte injury	Normal, lipids in proximal tubular cells	Negative	Loss of foot processes, no deposits, fusion of foot processes with normal appearing glomeruli is characteristic	Serum Complement level is normal Excellent prognosis with steroid treatment

Contd...

Major Primary Glomerulonephritis						
Disease	**Most frequent clinical presentation**	**Pathogenesis**	**Light microscopy**	**Fluorescence microscopy**	**Electron microscopy**	**Comments**
Focal segmental glomerulosclerosis	Nephrotic syndrome, non nephritic proteinuria	Unknown, ablation nephropathy Plasma factor: Podocyte injury	Focal and segmental sclerosis and hyalinosis, collapse of GBM, lipid droplets, foam cells	Focal; IgM and C3	Loss of foot processes, focal detachment of epithelial cells with denudation	Collapsing glomerulopathy (typical in HIV) is a variant with characteristic of proliferation and hypertrophy of podocytes. Other variants are Glomerular tip lesion variant, cellular variant, Perihilar variant and NOS (Not otherwise specified- m.c) variant
Membranoproliferative glomerulonephritis (MPGN) Type 1	Nephrotic syndrome	Immune complex	Mesangial proliferation, basement membrane thickening, splitting, glomerular cell proliferation, leukocytic infiltration, **double contour or tram track appearance,** proliferation of mesangial cells	IgG + C3 : Clq +C4	Subendothelial deposits	
Dense deposit disease (MPGN Type II)	Hematuria Chronic Renal Failure	Autoantibody alternative complement pathway		C3+/- IgG, no Clq or C4	Dense deposits Intra membranous deposits	Positive for C3 NeF or C3 nephritic factors
Henoch-Schönlein purpura (IgA nephropathy/ Berger's disease)	Recurrent hematuria or proteinuria		Focal and segmental proliferative GN, mesangial widening	IgA +/- IgG. IgM and C3 in mesangium, Properdin deposition	Mesangial and paramesangial dense deposits	Most common cause of GN worldwide Follows 1-2 days after Respiratory or G.I tract infection Serum C3 normal Recurrence common
Chronic Glomerulonephritis	Chronic renal failure	Variable	Hyalinised Glomeruli	Granular and negative		

Footnote

Whereas IgA nephropathy is typically an isolated renal disease, similar IgA deposits are present in a systemic disorder of children, Henoch-Schönlein purpura

M.C cause of Nephritic syndrome is Rapidly Progressive Glomerulonephritis (RPGN) (Post Streptococcal and Non Streptococcal)

GN without proliferative changes are: Minimal Change Disease, Membranous GN, Diabetic nephropathy, Amyloidosis

84. Ans. (c) Follicular carcinoma of thyroid

Ref: Robbins 9th ed page 1097, Bailey 26th ed page 765, Schwartz 9th ed page 1364

Repeat Pathology AIIMS NOV 2014 (With different options)

The diagnosis of "follicular lesion" is the most common diagnosis of thyroid FNA specimens. The cytological differential diagnosis includes nodular hyperplasia, follicular adenoma, follicular carcinoma, and follicular variant of papillary carcinoma. **An inherent limitation of thyroid FNA is its inability to distinguish follicular adenoma from follicular carcinoma.** The reason for this limitation is that the diagnostic distinction between follicular adenoma and carcinoma is based on capsular and/or vascular invasion by the neoplastic cells.

The hallmark of all follicular adenomas is the presence of an intact, well-formed capsule encircling the tumor. Careful evaluation of the integrity of the capsule is therefore critical in distinguishing follicular adenomas from follicular carcinomas, which demonstrate capsular and/or vascular invasion. Thyroid FNA is considered only a screening test to identify a patients with high risk of follicular carcinoma.

(Ref: The Washington Manual of Surgical Pathology edited by Peter A. Humphrey, Louis P. Dehner, John D. Pfeifer page 338)

85. Ans. (a) Prussian blue

Ref: Robbins 9th ed page 532

NOTE

Golden-yellow hemosiderin is stained blue with the Prussian blue stain

Hemochromatosis

The morphologic changes in hereditary hemochromatosis are all responses to the deposition of hemosiderin in the following organs (in decreasing order of severity): liver, pancreas, myocardium, pituitary, adrenal, thyroid and parathyroid glands, joints, and skin.

The term **"hemosiderosis"** is used to denote a relatively benign accumulation of iron. The term **"hemochromatosis"** is used when organ dysfunction occurs. Hemochromatosis can be primary (the cause is probably an autosomal recessive genetic disease) or secondary (excess iron intake or absorption, liver disease, or numerous transfusions). Hemochromatosis leads to bronze pigmentation of skin, diabetes mellitus (from pancreatic involvement), and cardiac arrhythmias (from myocardial involvement).

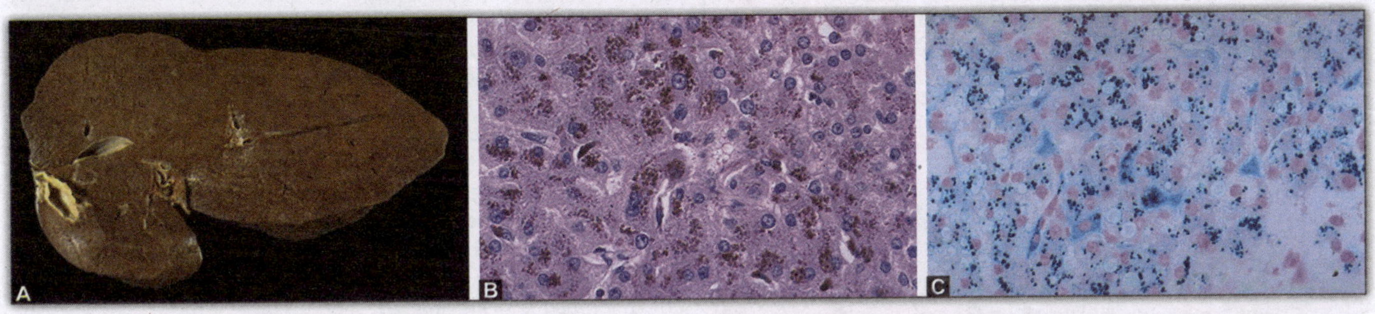

Figs A to C: (A) Hemochromatosis Liver Gross: The dark brown color of the liver on sectioning is due to extensive iron deposition in hereditary hemochromatosis (HHC). HHC results from a mutation involving the hemochromatosis gene (HFE) that leads to increased iron absorption from the gut; **(B) Hemochromatosis Liver Histopathology H and E staining:** The hepatocytes and Kupffer cells here are full of granular brown deposits of hemosiderin from accumulation of excess iron in the liver. The iron accumulation may lead to a micronodular cirrhosis (so called "pigment" cirrhosis) and **(C) Hemochromatosis Liver Histopathology Prussian Blue staining:** A Prussian blue iron stain demonstrates the blue granules of hemosiderin in hepatocytes and Kupffer cells. In the liver, iron becomes evident first as golden-yellow hemosiderin granules in the cytoplasm of periportal hepatocytes, which stain blue with the Prussian blue stain

86. Ans. (b) Toluidine blue

Ref: Oral and Maxillofacial Surgery, Lars Anderssons, Karl-Erik Kahnberg, M page 604, Indian journal of dental research 2007 Volume: 18 Issue: 3 Page: 101-105, Mehrotra et al. Molecular Cancer 2006 5:11.

Toluidine blue has been demonstrated as to be an effective tool for screening of premalignant leisons or oral cancers reoccurance in high risk populations. Mitotic index is a clinically important parameter in cancer pathology. **Toluidine Blue detect efficiently and rapidly mitotic figures in sections of formalin-fixed paraffin-embedded human tissues especially in oral cavity**

87. Ans. (b) Erythrocyte

Ref: Robbins 9th ed page 102

RBCs are neither nucleated nor Antigen presenting cells hence does not have MHC on it.

The MHC gene products are classified into 3 categories. Class I and II encode cell surface glycoproteins involved in antigen presentation. Class III genes encode components of the complement system.

Human MHC Gene Products

Major histocompatibility complex (MHC): A cluster of genes located in close proximity, e.g. on **human chromosome 6,** that encode the histocompatibility antigens (MHC molecules).

	Class I	Class II
Genetic loci (partial list)	HLA-A, -B, and -C	HLA-DP, -DQ, and -DR
Polypeptide composition	MW 45,000 + β_2 M (MW 12,000)	α chain (MW 33,000), β chain (MW 29,000), Ii chain (MW 30,000)
Cell distribution	All nucleated somatic cells	Antigen-presenting cells (macrophages, B cells, Dendritic cells etc), activated human T cells
Present peptide antigens to	CD8 T cells	CD4 T cells
Size of peptide bound	8–11 residues	10–30 or more residues

88. Ans. (b) Giardiasis

Ref: Sternburg's Diagnostic Surgical Pathology 5th ed page 1313

This is a case of infectious diarrhea due to *Giardia lamblia* infection of the small intestine.

Option (A)

Whipple disease, a chronic systemic illness with numerous gastrointestinal features such as diarrhea and malabsorption, is caused by *Tropheryma whippleii*, a rod-shaped microorganism. The diagnosis of Whipple disease is usually based on the identification of **PAS-positive**, diastase-resistant inclusions in small-intestinal biopsy specimens. Positive gut mucosal biopsy specimens demonstrate infiltration of the lamina propria; muscularis mucosae; and, in some cases, submucosa by macrophages with a ***foamy gray-blue*** cytoplasm. The number of intraepithelial lymphocytes is not increased.

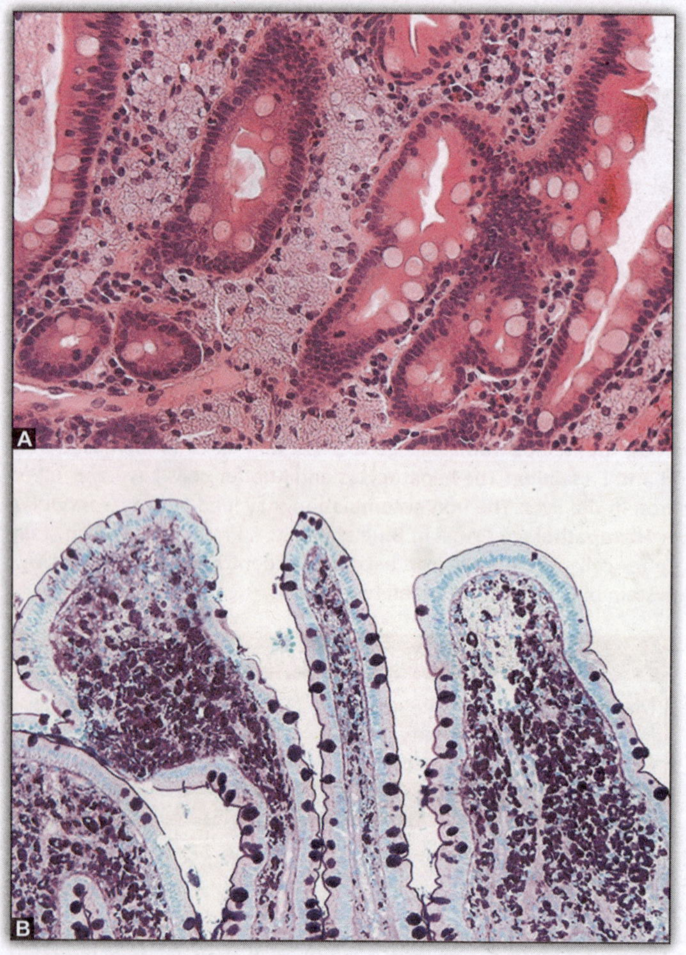

Figs A and B: (A) Whipple's disease high magnification H&E stain, Duodenal biopsy: The images show the characteristic foamy macrophages are present in the lamina propria; **(B) Whipple's disease PAS stain, Duodenal biopsy:** Duodenum villi of Whipples disease with Foamy infiltrate in lamina propria on a PAS stain

Option (B)

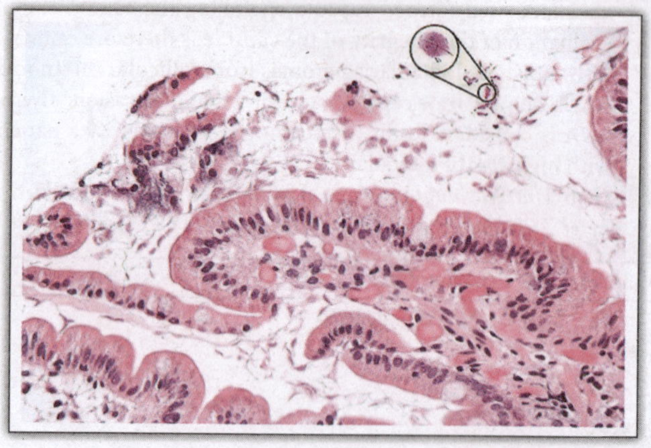

Fig: Intestinal biopsy showing Giardia: The small pear-shaped trophozoites live in the duodenum and become infective cysts that are excreted. They produce a watery diarrhea. A useful test for diagnosis of infectious diarrheas is stool examination for ova and parasites. Although pathologists usually encounter Giardia in duodenal biopsy specimens, the organism has been found in the gastric antrum, ileal specimens, and even colonic biopsy specimens. The small-bowel mucosal histology in biopsy specimens is usually normal; however, a patchy villous abnormality of variable severity can be observed. The histologic diagnosis rests on the demonstration of trophozoites either along the surface of epithelial cells in biopsy specimens or in touch preparations. The organism is approximately the same size as the enterocyte nucleus. In profile, the trophozoite of *G. lamblia* is sickle-shaped; seen en face, it has a characteristic pear shape with a tapered posterior region. It has prominent paired nuclei, paired median rods, a curved median body, and four pairs of flagellae. These morphologic features are most easily recognized on Giemsa-stained or trichrome-stained touch preparations

Option (C)

Increased chronic inflammatory cells are seen within the lamina propria, and an inflammatory exudate overlies the mucosa. High-magnification examination of the inflammatory exudate reveals typical trophozoites of *Entamoeba histolytica*.

Option (D)

A close association exists between peptic ulcer disease and gastric infection with Helicobacter pylori. Some authors think gastric heterotopia or metaplasia is an important predisposing factor for the effect of H. pylori because the organism is found in these ectopic gastric tissues by H and E, silver, or modified Giemsa stain techniques.

The organism is not usually found on normal small-intestinal epithelium or on gastric mucosa in which intestinal metaplasia has occurred.

89. Ans. (a) RBC clumps due to cold AIHA

Ref: Wintrobe's Clinical Hematology, 12th Ed page 964

Hints to Diagnosis

- High age ruled out hemoglobinopathies
- Spherocyte is visible on the Peripheral smear which is seen in Hereditary spherocytosis and Autoimmune hemolytic anemia
- RBC clamps in the peripheral smear indicates AIHA
- History of cell lysis in Winter is typical of cold AIHA

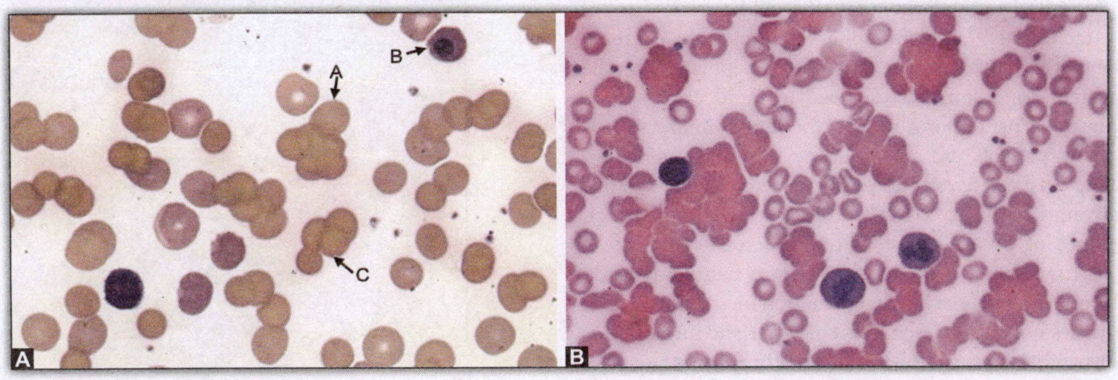

Cold Agglutination Disease (CAD)

- Mild, chronic hemolytic anemia with exacerbations in the winter is the general rule for CAD. Rarely does the hemoglobin drop below 7 g/dL.
- Acrocyanosis can occur from agglutination of RBCs in the cooler vessels of the hands, ears, nose, and feet. Digits may become cold, stiff, painful, or numb and may turn purplish. Limbs may manifest livedo reticularis, a mottled appearance that is readily reversible upon warming of the affected area.
- The self-limited, postinfectious CAD tends to affect younger patients, whereas the chronic idiopathic form is a disease of the elderly, with peak incidence at ~age 70 years.

Serologic Overview of Hemolytic Anemias

	Cold agglutinin disease (CAD)	Paroxysmal cold hemoglobinuria (PCH)	Mixed warm and cold autoimmune hemolytic anemia	Warm autoimmune hemolytic anemia	Drug-induced hemolytic anemia
Percentage of cases	16–32%	32% (children); rare in adults	7–8%	40–70%	12–18%
Direct antiglobulin test	C3	C3	IgG ± complement	IgG ± C3; rarely C3 alone	IgG or C3; occasionally IgG ± C3
Ig	IgM	IgG	IgG, IgM	IgG, occasionally with IgA or IgM	IgG
RBC eluate	Nonreactive	Nonreactive	IgG	IgG	IgG or nonreactive
Antibody specificity	I > i >> *Pr*	P	Panreactive	Panagglutinin	Rh-related
			Unclear > *I* > others	Rarely Rh	Drug-dependent

90. Ans. (b) Decoy cell

Ref: With text

Eyes can see what we already know. And since Decoy cell was most possibly new to the examinee, it was missed by most and marked as Hyaline cast.

A renal transplant patient with raised serum creatinine is indicative of Renal failure post transplant. Pus cells are in normal range (0-4 p.v.f.) indicative of non infectious pathology or Viral pathology. For Hyaline cast they could have asked without putting this particular case scenario. Also note that Urine casts are best seen in Urine microscopy routine without adding any stain and the slide provided is a stained slide. Now read following text.

Harrison 19th ed page 490, 923: Certain viruses are typically seen only in immunosuppressed patients. BK virus (polyomavirus hominis 1) has been documented in the urine of bone marrow transplant recipients and, like adenovirus, may be associated with hemorrhagic cystitis.

Harrison 19th ed page 925: The papovaviruses BK virus and JC virus (polyomavirus hominis types 1 and 2) have been cultured from the urine of **kidney transplant recipients** (as they have from that of HSC transplant recipients) in the setting of profound immunosuppression. High levels of BK virus replication detected by PCR in urine and blood are predictive of pathology, especially in the setting of renal transplantation. Urinary excretion of BK virus and BK viremia are associated with the development of ureteral strictures, polyomavirus-associated nephropathy (1-10% of renal transplant recipients), and (less commonly) generalized vasculopathy

Brenner and Rector's The Kidney, 8th ed ch 65: Replication of BK virus, with shedding of infected uroepithelial cells **(decoy**

cells) into the urine occurs in more than one third of renal transplant recipients. The clinical features associated with such replication include none (most common), acute and chronic allograft dysfunction, and hemorrhagic cystitis.

Sternburg Diagnostic Surgical Pathology, 5th Ed page 1747: Recently, particularly after the widespread use of FK506 (tacrolimus) and mycophenolate mofetil in renal transplantation, polyomavirus interstitial nephritis became an important condition that can lead to rapid graft failure. The polyomavirus responsible for the renal injury is BK virus. Many patients are under heavy immunosuppression because of suspected rejection. Urine cytology is positive for polyomavirus-infected cells **(decoy cells);** however, the presence of decoy cells does not necessarily indicate a polyomavirus interstitial nephritis. BK virus can be detected in the blood with polymerase chain reaction in active case. The diagnostic lesion is the presence of characteristic intranuclear inclusions with a dense peripheral chromatin ring in the nuclei of tubular epithelial cells. Sometimes the infected cells contain large "smudgy" nuclei or large vacuolated nuclei.

Diagnosis of BK Virus Infection

- Nucleic acid amplification test (NAAT) like DNA PCR and RNA PCR of Blood
- NAAT of Urine
- Biopsy (core biopsy from medulla)
- Urine Decoy cell

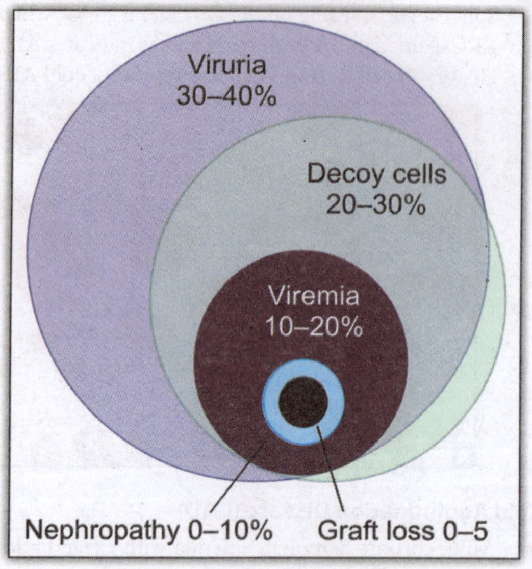

Fig: Type and prevalence of BK virus (BKV) infections in kidney transplant recipients

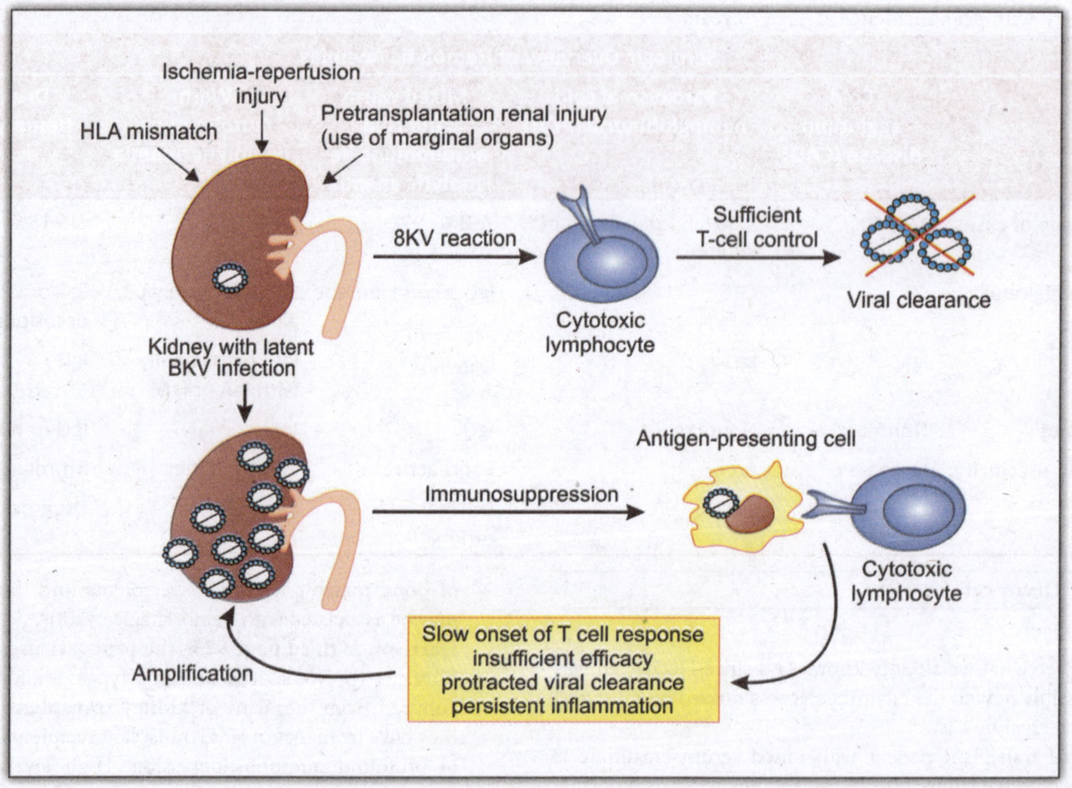

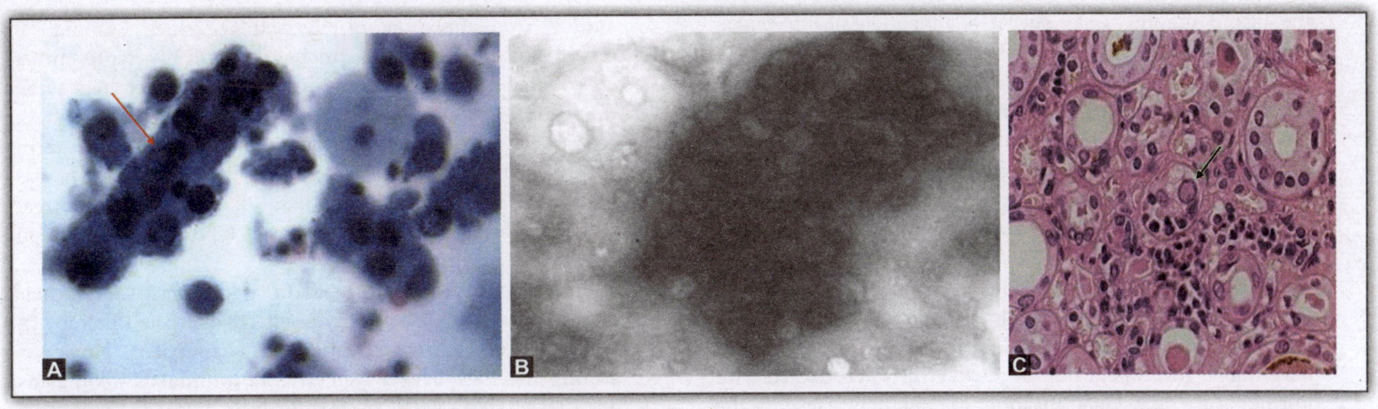

Figs A to C: (A) Decoy cell in Urine Papanicolaou stain: Disperse decoy cells and cellular cylinders containing compacted decoy cells. When they appear, these cylinders are pathognomic of kidney damage. Decoy cells are renal tubular or uroepithelial cells with intranuclear BK Virus inclusion bodies. Note that the Decoy cell aggregates in the form of cylinders looks like Hyaline cast. Decoy cells are seen by three methods, 1. Electon microscopy, 2. Phase contrast microscopy and 3. Papanicolaou stain; **(B) Urine Electron Microscopy with Haufen:** There are no accurate, noninvasive tests to diagnose BK polyomavirus nephropathy, But recently Electron microscopic qualitative detection of cast-like, three-dimensional polyomavirus aggregates **("Haufen" German = heap, hive, pile)** in the urine accurately predicts BK polyomavirus nephropathy. Haufen detection was correlated with pathology in concomitant renal biopsies and BK viruria (decoy cell shedding and viral load assessments by PCR) and BK viremia (viral load assessments by PCR). Haufen originated from renal tubules containing virally lysed cells, and the detection of Haufen in the urine correlated tightly with biopsy confirmed BK polyomavirus nephropathy (concordance rate 99%); **(C) BK Virus Nephropathy:** Amphophilic large intranuclear inclusions with a dense peripheral chromatin ring in the nuclei of tubular epithelial cells. Variable degree of interstitial inflammation, fibrosis and atrophy. Similar appearance to cellular rejection

91. Ans. (d) Fat embolism

Ref: Robbins, 9th ed page 91

History of trauma and fracture of lower limb are risk factors of Fat embolism. Histopathological slide also suggest fat embolism. It can also be seen with extensive soft tissue trauma, burn injuries, severe fatty liver, and very rarely with orthopedic procedures

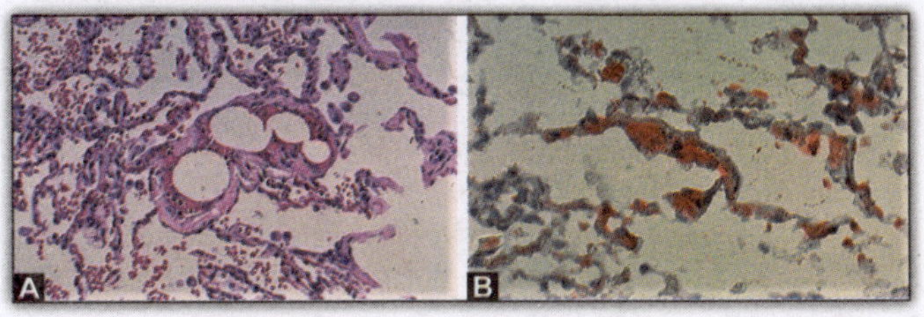

Figs A and B: (A) Fat embolism Histopathology: The clear rounded holes in the small pulmonary arterial branch in this section of lung are characteristic for fat embolism. Fat embolism syndrome is most often a consequence of trauma with long bone fractures; **(B) Fat embolism- An Oil Red O stain demonstrates the fat globules within the pulmonary arterioles.** The globules stain reddish-orange. The cumulative effect of many of these gobules throughout the lungs is similar to a large pulmonary embolus, but the onset of dyspnea is usually 2 to 3 days following the initiating event, such as blunt trauma with bone fractures

AIIMS MAY 2016

92. Ans. (b) Poor prognosis

Ref: Sternberg Pathology 5th ed Page 321, Devita 10th ed page 1243

NOTE

Only Column (A) was given in the exam. We have included the other columns for better understanding of the concept

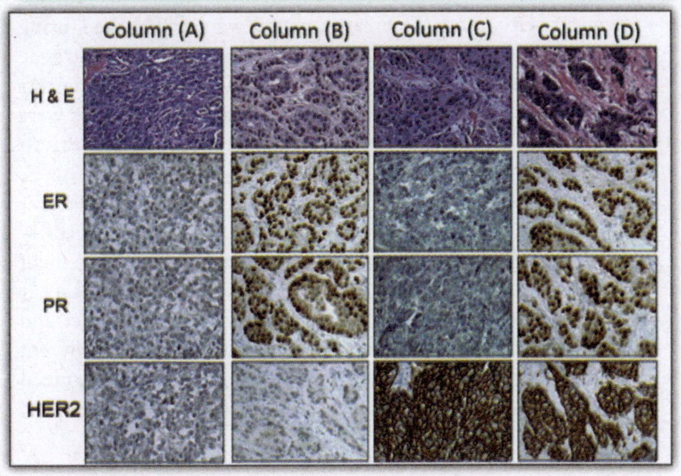

Fig: Breast tissue biopsy

ER and PR (on any tissue of the body) are stained brown in the "nucleus" on the other hand HER2 is stained brown in the membrane (peripheries)

Column (A): ER (-), PR (-), HER2 (-) [TRIPLE NEGATIVE]
Column (B): ER (+), PR (+), HER2 (-)
Column (C): ER (-), PR (-), HER2 (+)
Column (D): ER (+), PR (+), HER2 (+)

Reporting guidelines: ASCO and the CAP have issued recommendations for reporting the results of immunohistochemical assays for ER and PR. Studies using both IHC and the ligand binding assay suggest that patients with higher hormone receptor levels have a higher probability of response to hormonal therapy, but expression as low as 1% positive staining has been associated with clinical response. As a result, the guidelines recommend classifying all cases with at least 1% positive cells as receptor positive. For patients with low ER expression (1% to 10% weakly positive cells), the decision on endocrine therapy should be based on an analysis of its risks and potential benefits.

Quantification of ER and PR: There is a wide range of receptor levels in cancers as shown by the biochemical ligand binding assay and as observed with IHC. Patients whose carcinomas have higher levels have improved survival when treated with hormonal therapy. Quantification systems may use only the proportion of positive cells or may include the intensity of immunoreactivity:

- **Number of positive cells:** The number of positive cells can be reported as a percentage or within discrete categories.

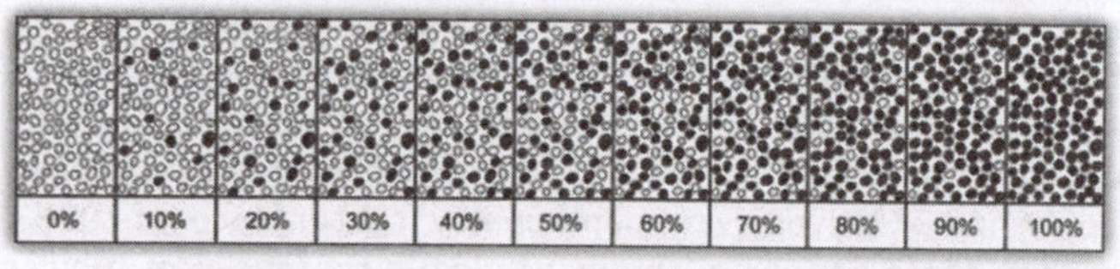

- **Intensity:** Refers to degree of nuclear positivity (i.e., pale to dark). The intensity can be affected by the amount of protein present, as well as the antibody used and the antigen retrieval system. In most cancers, there is heterogeneous immunoreactivity with pale to darkly positive cells present.

Molecular Classification of Breast Cancer

Early studies of transcription profiles using DNA microarrays identified several molecular subtypes of breast cancer. Groupings of breast cancers were established using computational methods that evaluated similarities in the gene expression profiles generated for individual breast cancers among large cohorts of breast cancer samples. Clusters were identified based on common gene expression patterns driven by overexpressed genes.

The first study of this type identified four major molecular subtypes of breast cancer: i) ER+/luminal, ii) HER2+ (HER2-enriched), iii) basal-like, and iv) normal-like. Subsequent transcription profiling studies of invasive breast cancer demonstrated that these molecular subtypes are distinct and reproducible between breast cancer cohorts and using different gene sets for cluster analysis. The currently recognized molecular subtypes of breast cancer are

- Luminal A (ER+)
- Luminal B (ER+/HER2-enriched)
- HER2+ (HER2-enriched)
- Basal-like
- Claudin-low, and
- Normal-like

Luminal A and Luminal B Breast Cancers

ER+ breast cancers occur most frequently and comprise two major molecular classifications: luminal A and luminal B. ***Luminal A breast cancers are the most common, with a frequency of 28% to 31%.*** Luminal B breast cancers are characterized by ER positivity accompanied by amplification and/or overexpression of the HER2 gene. Luminal B breast cancers occur less frequently, typically representing approximately 20% of patients in any given data set. In general, the two ER+ breast cancer subtypes, luminal A and luminal B, are associated with a **good prognosis** and excellent long-term survival (approximately 80% to 85% 5-year survival), whereas the ER– subtypes (HER2+ and basal-like) are difficult to treat and are associated with poor prognosis (approximately 50% to 60% 5-year survival).

The ability of patients with ER+ breast cancers to survive their disease reflects the availability of effective targeted therapy in the form of anti-estrogen treatment (e.g. tamoxifen). **However, among the ER+ breast cancers, the luminal B neoplasms are associated with a significantly worse prognosis, compared with the luminal A subtype.** The differences in patient outcomes are due in part to variations in response of luminal A and luminal B breast cancers to anti-estrogen treatment. Therapy targeted to HER2-overexpressing breast cancers (including the luminal B subtype) with trastuzumab (Herceptin; Genentech), either concurrent or sequential with adjuvant chemotherapy, has improved survival for these breast cancer subtypes.

HER2 + Breast Cancers

HER2 is a member of the human epidermal growth factor receptor family, which also includes EGFR (alias HER1), HER3, and HER4. In breast cancer and some other cancers, HER2 behaves as an oncogene, exerting its oncogenic effects through overexpression, either via the normal gene or secondary to gene amplification. HER2+ breast cancers represent approximately **17% of all breast cancers,** with a frequency of 12% to 21% across different data sets. HER2 overexpression (HER2+) in breast cancer is associated with **poor clinical outcomes,** but is also predictive of positive therapeutic responses to anti-HER2 drugs (e.g. trastuzumab). **HER2+ breast cancers are typically ER–, so treatment for these cancers does not include anti-estrogenic hormonal therapies.** Rather, therapies for the HER2+ breast cancers are based on combinations of targeted drugs (e.g. trastuzumab) and cytotoxic chemotherapy. **Since the introduction of targeted therapy for HER2+ breast cancers, the long-term outcomes for these patients have improved dramatically.**

Basal-Like and Claudin-Low Breast Cancers

Together, the basal-like and Claudin-low molecular subtypes represent subsets of **triple-negative breast** cancers (as classified by immunohistochemistry), lacking expression of ER and PR (ER–/PR–) and also lacking amplification of ERBB2 (HER2–). **Basal-like breast cancers represent approximately 15% of all breast cancers.** The basal-like breast cancers have high rates of cell proliferation and **extremely poor clinical outcomes.** *These cancers are associated with distinct risk factors, including early-onset menarche, younger age at first full-term pregnancy, high parity combined with lack of breast feeding, and abdominal adiposity.* Basal-like breast cancers respond to preoperative chemotherapy. Despite the observation of pathological complete response in some patients with basal-like breast cancers, overall these patients have a very poor prognosis, perhaps related to a higher likelihood of relapse in those patients in whom pathological complete response was not achieved.

Claudin-low breast cancers represent approximately 10% of all breast cancers. These breast cancers are enriched for markers of epithelial-to-mesenchymal transition and stem cell-like and/or tumor-initiating cell features. Similar to the basal-like cancers, claudin-low breast cancers respond to some chemotherapeutic agents, but patients have **poor recurrence-free and overall survival outcomes.**

Normal-like breast cancers: The normal-like breast cancers are so designated because they tend to cluster closely with normal breast epithelium in microarray studies. It is not yet clear whether this is a distinct molecular subtype of breast cancer or simply a grouping of breast cancers that are not otherwise classifiable because of contaminating normal epithelium. Nevertheless, this subset of breast cancer is routinely reported in gene expression studies.

93. Ans. (a) Membranous glomerulonephritis

Ref: Robbin's 9th ed ch 20, http://unckidneycenter.org/kidneyhealthlibrary/glomerular-disease/membranous-nephropathy

See Details of Membranous Glomerulonephritis in AIIMS MAY 2017 PATHOLOGY (see page no. 359)

Robbins

Two patterns of deposition of immune complexes as seen by immunofluorescence microscopy:

- Granular, characteristic of circulating and in situ immune complex nephritis
- Linear, characteristic of classic anti-GBM disease

Out of the options provided only Membranous Glomerulonephritis and SLE shows granular pattern. Most students think the image was a midway between linear and granular, hence some of them got confused and marked Goodpasture syndrome (Linear IgG deposits). Less granularity does not rules out MGN. Students also recalled that IgG was written on the right corner of the image. Membranous Glomerulonephritis is a slowly progressive disease and hence the quantification of the granularity depends on the stage of the MGN. The same can be easily understood by the stages of LUPUS nephritis which is a secondary form of MGN, But we are not considering it as answer because its far less common compared to MGN. **85% of MGN cases are classified as primary membranous glomerulonephritis—that is to say, the cause of the disease is idiopathic (of unknown origin or cause). SLE is amongst the secondary cause (rest of 15%).**

94. Ans. (d) Multinucleated osteoclast like giant cells are the tumour cells

Ref: Robbins 9th ed ch 26, Robbins 8th ed page 1233, Sternberg pathology 5th ed page 271-273, Apley 9th ed page 202

We have included this question in pathology as it includes some important Histopathological points

Option (A)

It usually arises in individuals in their 20s to 40s, Hence correct

Option (B)

Giant-cell tumors are locally invasive benign tumor, in adults involve both the epiphyses and the metaphysis, but in adolescents they are confined proximally by the growth plate and are limited to the metaphysis. The majority arise around the knee (distal femur and proximal tibia), but virtually any bone can be involved. Occasionally, they present with pathologic fractures. Most are solitary; however, multiple or multicentric tumors do occur, especially in the distal extremities. Giant-cell tumors often erode into the subchondral bone plate and destroy the overlying cortex, producing a bulging soft-tissue mass delineated by a thin shell of reactive bone. The margins with the adjacent bone are fairly circumscribed but seldom sclerotic. The biologic unpredictability of these neoplasms complicates their management. Conservative surgery such as curettage is associated with a 40% to 60% recurrence rate, and up to **4% metastasize to the lungs**

Option (C) and (D)

They are **mostly composed of uniform oval mononuclear cells that constitute the proliferating component of the tumor.** Scattered within this background are numerous osteoclast-type giant cells having 100 or more nuclei that resemble those of the mononuclear cells. Necrosis, hemorrhage, hemosiderin deposition, and reactive bone formation are common secondary features.

95. Ans. (a) Aplastic anemia

Ref: Wintrobe 12th ed page 960-961, Robbin's 9th ed ch 14, Robbins 8th ed page 653

The diagnosis of immunohemolytic anemia requires the detection of antibodies and/or complement on red cells from the patient. This is done using the **direct Coombs antiglobulin test,** in which the patient's red cells are mixed with sera containing antibodies that are specific for human immunoglobulin or complement. If either immunoglobulin or complement is present on the surface of the red cells, the multivalent antibodies cause agglutination, which is easily appreciated visually as clumping. In the **indirect Coombs antiglobulin test,** the patient's serum is tested for its ability to agglutinate commercially available red cells bearing particular defined antigens.

Direct Antiglobulin Test (Dat, Direct Coombs Test)

In 1908, Moreschi described antiglobulin reactions as an aid to RBC agglutination. This work went largely unnoticed until 1945, when the investigation of anti-RBC antibodies was revolutionized with the development of the antiglobulin test by Coombs, Mourant, and Race and its application to identifying IgG-coated RBCs in **hemolytic disease of the newborn (HDN)** in 1946. The principle of the DAT (direct Coombs test) is quite simple. To ascertain if patient RBCs are coated with immunoglobulin, complement, or both, antisera with reactivity to human immunoglobulin and/or complement molecules is added to a suspension of the RBCs in question, providing the necessary cross-link to elicit agglutination. The test is performed by first washing the RBCs to remove nonspecifically attached proteins. Following the addition of antiserum (antihuman globulin, AHG), the mixture is centrifuged to enhance agglutination. The result is interpreted by resuspending the RBCs gently and observing carefully for clumps. Negative reactions are further incubated at room temperature, centrifuged, and read again, as this additional incubation promotes positive reactions in the presence of complement. Initial testing is done with polyspecific

AHG (antisera), which contain anti-IgG, anti-C3d, and, occasionally, some anti–light-chain activity. Monospecific reagents differentiate between IgG and C3d to further define the specificity.

Outside of Autoimmune Hemolytic Anemia, a Positive DAT may also be seen with (Wintrobes 12th ed page 961)

- Alloantibodies in a recipient of RBC or plasma transfusion
- Antibodies from maternal circulation that cross the placenta and coat the fetal RBCs
- Antibodies directed against certain drugs that bind to the RBC membrane (e.g., penicillin)
- Nonspecifically adsorbed proteins including immunoglobulins and Wharton's jelly
- RBC-bound complement
- Antibodies produced by passenger lymphocytes in transplanted organs or hematopoietic components

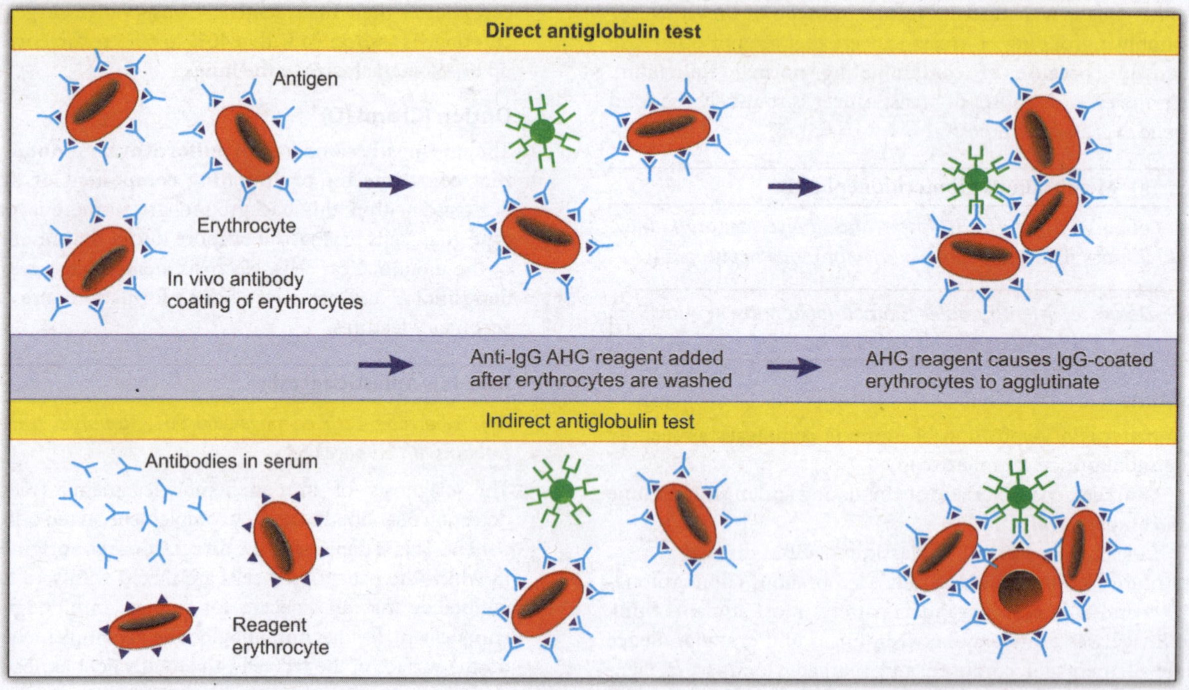

Indirect Antiglobulin Test (Iat, Indirect Coombs Test)

Approximately 80% of patients with AIHA have autoantibodies in their serum as well as on their RBCs. The antibodies in their serum or plasma and the antibodies eluted from their RBCs are detected by the indirect antiglobulin test (IAT; more commonly known as the antibody screen). Unlike the DAT, which uses patient RBCs with reagent serum, the IAT tests patient serum against reagent RBCs. Immunoglobulin from the patient serum attaches to the reagent RBCs and is detected with antiglobulin sera, which cross-link the RBCs together and produce agglutination, as in the DAT.

96. Ans. (b) Thymocyte

Ref: Wintrobe's 12th ed 408-409, Robbins 8th ed page 187

Antigen-Presenting Cells

The development of humoral and cell-mediated immunity depends on complex cellular interactions that involve lymphocytes and nonlymphoid cells. Activation of lymphocytes by antigen requires its processing and presentation by another cell that is commonly known as an antigen-presenting cell (APC). Antigen-presenting cells fall into two categories: professional and non-professional.

- **Professional APC:** Those that express MHC class II molecules along with co-stimulatory molecules and pattern recognition receptors are often called professional antigen-presenting cells. All professional APCs also express MHC class I molecules as well. Macrophages promptly capture foreign substances, and antigen processing and presentation was first demonstrated there. Other professional APCs are the DCs (Dendritic Cells) and B lymphocytes. Langerhans cells are one of the most well studied types of immature dendritic cell
- **The nonprofessional APCs** express MHC class I molecules. Nonprofessional antigen presenting cells include Fibroblast, glial cell, renal tubular epithelial cells, pancreatic beta islet cells, Thymic epithelial cells (not thymocytes)

Option (A)

Specialized cells, called M cells or microfold cells, are overlaying lymphoid tissue in the Peyer's patches. In face, M cells overlay GALT and have a highly invaginated basolateral membrane in which antigen-presenting cells (APCs), such as macrophages and dendritic cells resides. Structurally and functionally M cells are antigen transporting but not antigen presenting cells. *(Ref: Principles of Mucosal Immunology By Society for Mucosal Immunology edited by Philip D Smith page 294, Mucosal Immunology by Jiri Mestecky, Warren Strober, Michael W. Russell, Hilde Cheroutre, Bart N. Lambrecht, Brian L Kelsall 4th ed page 46)*

However there are conflicting evidence suggesting that M cells can act as APC by itself. According to one reference **"The evidence presented thus far suggests that M cells serve primarily in antigen transport and, to a lesser extent, in antigen processing"**

Hence for the purpose of this question we suggest M cells to be APC because Thymocytes are clearly not APC.

Professional Antigen Presenting Cells	B cell	Macrophage	Dendritic cell
Antigen uptake	+++ Surface immunoglobulin (antigen-specific)	+++ Phagocytosis	+++
Major histocompatibility	Constitutive	Inducible	Constitutive
Complex expression	+++ to ++++	– to +++	++++
Co-stimulatory activity	Inducible	Inducible	Constitutive
	– to +++	– to +++	++++
Antigen presented	Toxins Viruses Bacteria	Extracellular and Vesicular bacteria	Viruses Allergens?
Location	Lymphoid tissues Peripheral blood	Wide body distribution	Wide body distribution Epithelia
Indications: +++, strong; ++++, very strong; –, negative			

97. Ans. (b) 1-2 days

Ref: Robbins 9th ed page 542

The picture shows coagulative necrosis with dense neutrophilic infiltration consistent with 1-3 days old myocardial infarction, hence option B is best available answer

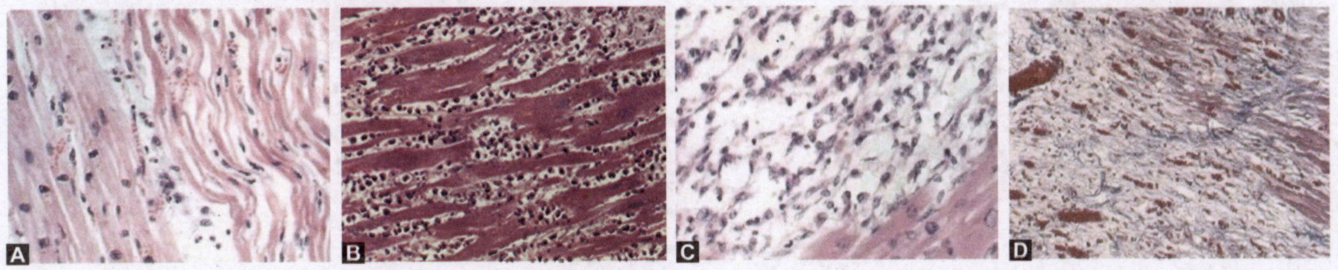

Figs A to D: (A) < 24 hour old infarct: Showing coagulative necrosis along with wavy fibers (elongated and narrow). compared with adjacent normal fibers (at left). Widened spaces between the dead fibers contain edema fluid and scattered neutrophils; **(B) 1–3 days old infarct:** Reperfusion contraction band/coagulative necrosis with Dense polymorphonuclear leukocytic infiltrate in area of acute myocardial infarction; **(C) 3 to 7 days old infarct:** Dead myocytes begin to disintegrate and are removed by macrophages and enzyme proteolysis. There is proliferation of fibroblasts with formation of granulation tissue, which progressively replaces necrotic tissue. Nearly complete removal of necrotic myocytes by phagocytosis (approximately 7 to 10 days); **(D) > 2 Weeks old infarct:** Granulation tissue characterized by loose collagen and abundant capillaries

Evolution of Morphologic Changes in Myocardial Infarction

Time	Gross features	Light microscope	Electron microscope
Reversible injury			
0–½ hour	None	None	Ralaxation of myofibrils; glycogen loss; mitochondrial swelling
Irreversible injury			
½–4 hours	None	Usually none; variable **waviness of fibers** at border may be present	Sarcolemmal disruption; mitochondrial amorphous densities
4–12 hours	Dark mottling (occasional)	**Early coagulation necrosis (loss of nuclei) with wavy fibers**; edema; hemorrhage	

Contd...

12–24 hours	Dark mottling	Ongoing **coagulation necrosis with wavy fibers**; pyknosis of nuclei; myocyte hypereosinophilia; marginal **contraction band necrosis**; early neutrophilic infiltrate
1–3 days	Mottling with yellow-tan infarct center	Coagulation necrosis, with loss of nuclei and striations; **brisk interstitial infiltrate of neutrophils**
3–7 days	Hyperemic border; central yellow-tan softening	Beginning disintegration of dead myofibers, with dying neutrophils; early phagocytosis of dead cells by macrophages at infarct border
7–10 days	Maximally yellow-tan and soft, with depressed red-tan margins	Well-developed phagocytosis of dead cells; early formation of fibrovascular granulation tissue at margins
10–14 days	Red-gray depressed infarct borders	Well-established granulation tissue with new blood vessels and collagen deposition
2–8 weeks	Gray-white scar, progressive from border toward core of infarct	Increased collagen deposition, with decreased cellularity
>2 months	Scarring complete	Dense collagenous scar

98. Ans. (b) Flea bitten kidney due to malignant hypertension

Ref: Sternberg Pathology 5th ed page 1733-1735, Robbins 9th ed ch 20

The given specimen of Kidney shows characteristic Flea Bitten Appearance of Malignant Hypertension.

Malignant Hypertension and Accelerated Nephrosclerosis

Malignant nephrosclerosis is the form of renal disease associated with the malignant or accelerated phase of hypertension

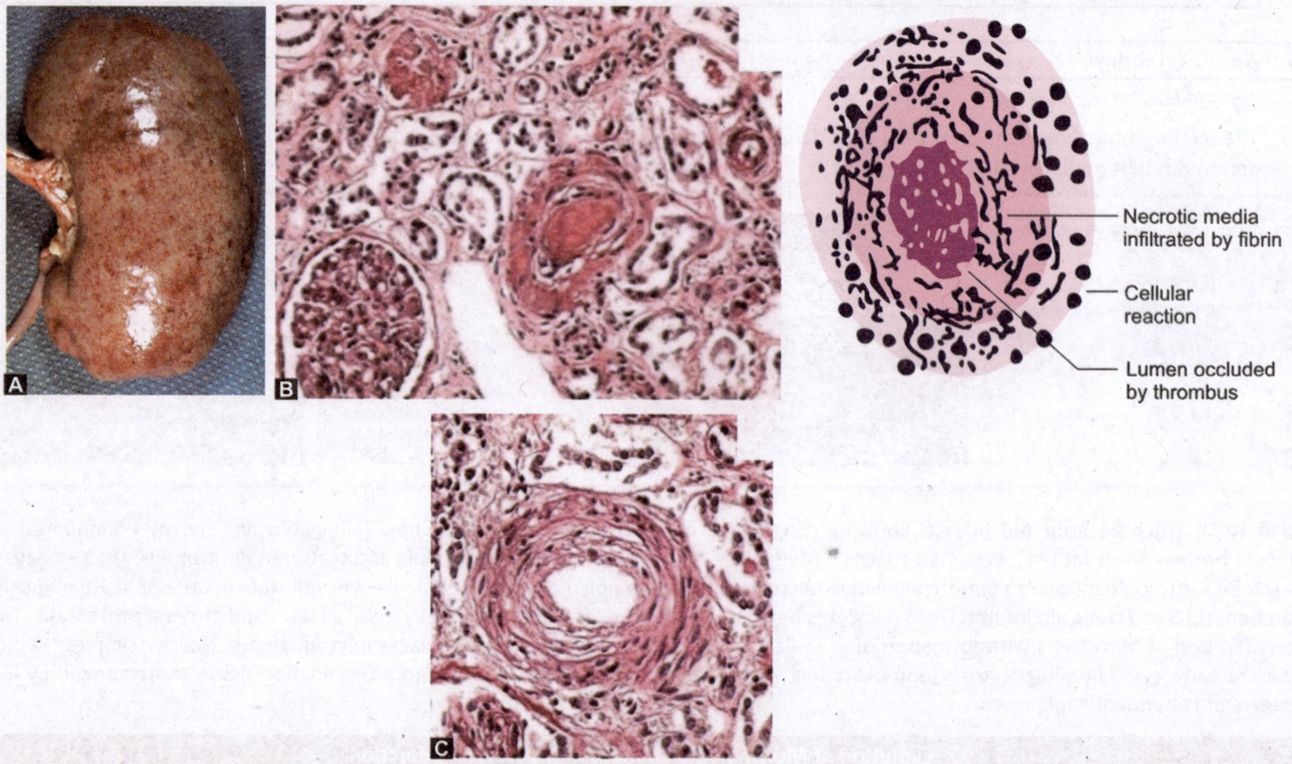

Figs A to C: (A) On gross inspection the kidney size depends on the duration and severity of the hypertensive disease. Small, pinpoint petechial hemorrhages may appear on the cortical surface from rupture of arterioles or glomerular capillaries, giving the kidney a peculiar "flea-bitten" appearance Two histologic alterations characterize blood vessels in malignant hypertension; **(B) Fibrinoid necrosis of arterioles.** This appears as an eosinophilic granular change in the blood vessel wall, which stains positively for fibrin by histochemical or immunofluorescence techniques. This change represents an acute event; it may be accompanied by limited inflammatory infiltrate within the wall, but prominent inflammation is not seen. Sometimes the glomeruli become necrotic and infiltrated with neutrophils, and the glomerular capillaries may thrombose; **(C) Hyperplastic arteriolitis (onion-skin lesion):** In the interlobular arteries and arterioles, there is intimal thickening caused by a proliferation of elongated, **concentrically arranged smooth muscle cells**, together with fine concentric layering of collagen and accumulation of pale-staining material that probably represents accumulations of proteoglycans and plasma proteins. This alteration has been referred to as onion-skinning because of its concentric appearance. The lesion, also called hyperplastic arteriolitis, correlates well with renal failure in malignant hypertension. There may be superimposed intraluminal thrombosis. The arteriolar and arterial lesions result in considerable narrowing of all vascular lumens, ischemic atrophy and, at times, infarction distal to the abnormal vessels.

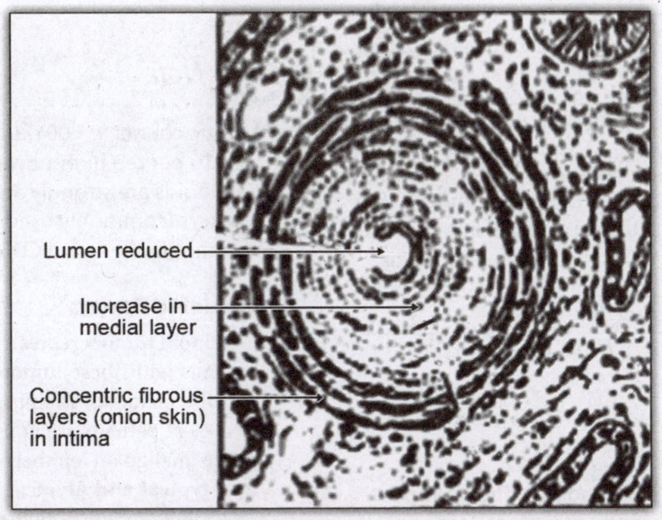

Vascular Pathology of Hypertension	Hyaline arteriosclerosis	Hyperplastic arteriosclerosis
Renal condition	In kidney it is called is **benign nephrosclerosis**	In kidney it is called as **malignant nephrosclerosis**
Etiology	Characteristic of **benign hypertension**. May also occur in diabetes and ageing	Characteristic of **malignant hypertension**
Pathogenesis	Two processes participate in the arterial lesions: 1. Medial and intimal thickening, as a response to hemodynamic changes, aging, genetic defects, or some combination of these 2. Hyaline deposition in arterioles, caused partly by extravasation of plasma proteins through injured endothelium and partly by increased deposition of basement membrane matrix in response to chronic hemodynamic stress. In diabetic microangiography the underlying etiology is hyperglycemia-induced endothelial cell dysfunction	Result from long standing benign hypertension, with eventual injury to arteriolar walls, or the initiating injury may spring de novo from arteritis, a coagulopathy, or some injury causing acute exacerbation of the hypertension. In any case, the result is increased permeability of the small vessels to fibrinogen and other plasma proteins, endothelial injury, focal death of cells of the vascular wall, and platelet deposition. This leads to the appearance of **fibrinoid necrosis** of arterioles and small arteries, swelling of the vascular intima, and intravascular thrombosis. Mitogenic factors from platelets (e.g., PDGF), plasma, and other cells cause hyperplasia of intimal smooth muscle of vessels, resulting in the **hyperplastic arteriolosclerosis** that is typical of malignant hypertension and further narrowing of the lumens.
Gross	Either normal or moderately reduced in size. Fine, leathery granularity of the surface	Kidney size depends on the duration and severity of hypertensive disease. Small, pinpoint petechial hemorrhages may appear on the cortical surface from rupture of arterioles or glomerular capillaries, giving the kidney a peculiar **"flea-bitten" appearance.**
Microscopy	Homogenous pink, hyaline thickening of arteriolar wall with luminal narrowing. Medial hypertrophy, reduplication of the elastic lamina, and increased myofibroblastic tissue in the intima, which combine to narrow the lumen. This change, called fibroelastic hyperplasia, often accompanies hyaline arteriolosclerosis	Two histologic alterations characterize blood vessels in malignant hypertension: • **Fibrinoid necrosis of arterioles.** This appears as an eosinophilic granular change in the blood vessel wall, which stains positively for fibrin by histochemical or immunofluorescence techniques. • **Concentric, laminated, onion skinned** thickening of arteriolar wall with luminal narrowing. The laminations consist of smooth muscle cells with thickened, reduplicated basement membranes The lesion, also called hyperplastic arteriolitis, correlates well with renal failure in malignant hypertension. There may be superimposed intraluminal thrombosis. The arteriolar and arterial lesions result in considerable narrowing of all vascular lumens, ischemic atrophy and, at times, infarction distal to the abnormal vessels.

99. Ans. (a) Plasma cell

Ref: Robbins 9th ed page 97

The findings of the arrow marked cell are consistent with Plasma cell.

See Details of PLASMA CELL NEOPLASMS in AIIMS MAY 2017 PATHOLOGY (see page no. 365-366)

100. Ans. (a) Rheumatic endocarditis

Ref: Robbins 8th ed page 567

See Details of RHEUMATIC ENDOCARDITIS in AIIMS NOV 2017 PATHOLOGY (see page no. 351-352)

One do not need to see the picture to arrive at a diagnosis as it is clearly mentioned that the vegetations are along the line of closure on the mitral valves, pointing towards rheumatic endocarditis.

101. Ans. (b) Atypical carcinoid grade II

Ref: Robbin's 8th ed page 729, Devita 8th ed page 1724

NOTE

Earlier NET was excluded by TNM staging. The European Neuroendocrine Tumor Society and the American Joint Committee on Cancer classify, or stage, NET by primary tumor (T), lymph node involvement (N), and distant metastasis (M). TNM staging represents a new system of NET classification. But in the question there is no mention of Tumor size, Nodal status or metastasis. The examiner is mostly talking about grade not stage. There are chances of recall bias also.

Devita States

The classification of bronchial carcinoid tumors has been a subject of debate. The 2004 World Health Organization (WHO) classification recognizes 4 major types of lung neuroendocrine tumors (NETs):

- Typical carcinoid (also called bronchial carcinoid, Kulchitsky cell carcinoma-I [KCC-I])
- Atypical carcinoid (also called well-differentiated neuroendocrine carcinoma and KCC-II)
- Large cell/Intermediate small cell neuroendocrine carcinoma
- Small cell neuroendocrine carcinoma (also called KCC-III)

These tumors are further grouped in a 3-tiered grading system as low grade (TC), intermediate grade (AC), and high grade (LCNEC and SCLC) NETs

In 2010, the World Health Organization (WHO) updated its classification of NET based on tumor site of origin, clinical syndrome, and differentiation

Summary of Diagnostic Criteria and Grading of Lung Neuroendocrine Tumors Based on the 2004 World Health Organization Classification

	Typical carcinoid	Atypical carcinoid	Large cell NET	Small cell lung carcinoma
Grade	Low	Intermediate	High	High
Morphology	Well differentiated	Well differentiated	Poorly differentiated	Poorly differentiated
Mitosis per 10 HPF	<2	2-10	>10 (median 70)	>10 (median 80)
Necrosis	None	Present (focal punctate)	Present (extensive)	Present (extensive)

NOTE

- Mitotic counts (P <001) (<10 per ten high-power fields vs. >10 per ten high-power fields) is related to prognosis
- Carcinoids are strongly and diffusely positive for NE markers (commonly used markers include synaptophysin, chromogranin A, and CD56/NCAM).

Carcinoid Tumors

Carcinoid tumors represent 1% to 5% of all lung tumors. Most patients with these tumors are younger than 40 years of age, and the incidence is equal for both sexes. Approximately 20% to 40% of patients are nonsmokers. Carcinoid tumors are low-grade malignant epithelial neoplasms that are subclassified into **typical and atypical carcinoids.** *Typical carcinoids have no p53 mutations or abnormalities of BCL2 and BAX expression, while atypical carcinoids show these changes in 20% to 40% and 10% to 20% of tumors, respectively.*

Clinical Features

The clinical manifestations of bronchial carcinoids emanate from their intraluminal growth, their capacity to metastasize, and the ability of some of the lesions to elaborate vasoactive amines. Persistent *cough, hemoptysis, impairment of drainage of respiratory passages with secondary infections, bronchiectasis, emphysema, and atelectasis* are all by-products of the intraluminal growth of these lesions.

Most interesting, albeit rare, are functioning lesions capable of producing the classic carcinoid syndrome, that is, intermittent attacks of diarrhea, flushing, and cyanosis. Overall, most bronchial carcinoids do not have secretory activity and do not metastasize to distant sites but follow a relatively benign course for long periods and are therefore amenable to resection. The reported 5- to 10-year survival rates are 87% and 87% for typical carcinoids, 56% and 35% for atypical carcinoids, 27% and 9% for large cell neuroendocrine carcinoma, and 9% and 5% for small cell carcinoma, respectively.

(Devita) **Bronchial carcinoid tumors are frequently discovered on chest radiograph. The most common symptoms are pneumonia, hemoptysis, and cough.**

102. Ans. (d) Bouin's fixative

Ref: With Text

Sternberg's Diagnostic Surgical Pathology, 5th Edition page 1930: The quality of the preparation is one of the major problems in evaluating testis biopsies in infertility. Unfortunately, 10% formalin introduces significant artifact in testicular specimens. Nuclei tend to shrink and appear denser; tubular margins have a somewhat undulating appearance; and tubules shrink slightly, creating a larger interstitial space. Nevertheless, diagnoses can be made on formalinized, albeit suboptimal, tissue. **Optimal fixation is rendered with Bouin and Hollande solutions (both containing picric acid)**, which eliminate artifacts introduced by formalin. Nuclear detail is superior, aiding in identification of cell types and in ascertaining whether enlarged germinal cells along the tubular basement membrane are giant spermatogonia or malignant germ cells. Urologists should have Bouin or Hollande solutions available before the biopsy.

	Fixatives Used in Pathology				
	Fixative	**Method of fixation**	**Contents**	**Advantages**	**Disadvantages**
ALCOHOL	Ethanol	Denaturing by removal of water causing coagulation and cell shrinkage	95% ethyl alcohol	Quick and give good nuclear details hence used in enzyme histochemistry, molecular analysis, impression smears, blood smears. Preserves glycogen and crystals	Not used in routine because causes excessive hardening. Dissolves lipid
	Carnoy's	—	60% ethanol, 30% chloroform, 10% glacial acetic acid	Cytological fixative, Rapid penetration, Nuclear details, Fixes RNA, preserves glycogen	Hemolyse RBC, dissolves cytoplasmic elements
	Methacarn	—	60% methanol, 30% chloroform, 10% glacial acetic acid		
ALDEHYDE S	Neutral buffered formalin (NBF)	Cross-linking by adding side chains of basic amino acids (especially Lysine). Active ingredient **methylene glycol**, the hydrated form of formaldehyde and the two coexist in an equilibrium	10% of 37% formaldehyde solution, in a neutral pH. It is 4% aqueous solution of formaldehyde often called 10% formalin because it is made by 10 fold dilution of formalin.	Most commonly used fixative, routine fixative, can be used in IHC and molecular analysis, Long term storage. Neutral pH and osmotic pressure equals to ECF.	Paradox between the rate of penetration of formaldehyde and its rate of fixation may be due to the fast penetration of methylene glycol and slow fixation rate of formaldehyde
	Glutaraldehyde	Cross-linking	Generally, 2% v/v of glutaraldehyde to water/PBS	Fixes quickly hence used in **electron microscopy,** preservation of collagen	Causes deformation of α helix structure of protein, hence not good for IHC. Slow penetration, must be refrigerated
	Paraformaldehyde (PFA)	Cross-linking	Generally, 4% w/v of paraformaldehyde to Water/PBS		
PICRIC ACID BASED	Bouin's	**Both denaturing and cross linking** (picric acid penetrates slow and coagulates proteins with out chemical interaction, acetic acid penetrates quickly and opposes the tissue shrinkage caused by picric acid)	25% of 37% formaldehyde solution, 70% picric acid, 5% acetic acid	Routine fixative, Penetrates well, Fixative of choice for **Testicular Biopsies.** Gives nuclear details. Not causes much hardness of tissue	Picric acid stains bellow. Picric acid causes cell shrinkage, Picric acid causes DNA methylation hence PCR molecular diagnosis cannot be done, cannot be used for IHC, Lysis of RBC, dissolves some proteins.
MERCURIC CHLORIDE	Zenker's	Denaturing by binding to sulphydryl and amino groups. Mercury based fixatives provide excellent nuclear details and are used in evaluating lymphoma	5% mercuric chloride (w/v), 2.5% potassium dichromate (w/v), 5% glacial acetic acid (v/v), water	Routine fixative, preserves mitochondria, excellent nuclear details. Specially used for hematopoietic and reticuloendothelial tissue	Causes some tissue hardness. Not used in IHC, not used with metal instruments, Must be washed overnight to remove chromate, Must be prepared fresh, Require Iodine treatment to remove Mercury before staining. potentially toxic hence difficult to dispose.

Contd...

	Fixatives Used in Pathology				
	Fixative	**Method of fixation**	**Contents**	**Advantages**	**Disadvantages**
	B5	—	5.4% mercuric chloride (w/v), 1.1% Sodium acetate (w/v), 4% formaldehyde (v/v), Water	Cytoplasmic - nuclear staining. For LN, Spleen, bone marrow	Must be prepared fresh, timed exposure required as overexposure causes hardening, Require Iodine treatment to remove Mercury before staining
OXIDISING AGENT	Osmium tetraoxide	Denaturation	Osmium tetraoxide	Preserves micostructure hence used in **electron microscopy**	Interferes with staining. low penetration limits role in light microscopy

Footnote

- Fixatives can be placed into two categories; denaturing fixatives and cross-linking (or addition) fixatives
- In most tissue a volume of fixative 15 times the volume of tissue is required to fix the tissue adequately within 12 to 18 hours.
- NBF is most commonly used fixative for routine histopathology
- Glutaraldehyde and osmium tetroxide are recommended for fixation of tissues for electron microscopy.

103. Ans. (c) Type III hypersensitivity reaction

Ref: Robbins 9th ed page 207-208

Acute serum sickness is the prototype of a systemic immune complex disease; it was once a frequent sequel to the administration of large amounts of foreign serum (e.g., serum from immunized horses used for protection against diphtheria). In modern times the disease is infrequent, but it is an informative model that has taught us a great deal about systemic immune complex disorders

Hypersensitivity Reactions			
TYPE 1: Allergy/ Atopy/Anaphylaxis	**True Anaphylaxis** Free Ag → fixed IgE (on mast cell)		Wheal and Flare reaction, Casoni's test, anaphylaxis, Praunitz Kustner reaction, Theobald smith phenomenon, Schultz dale phenomenon, Atopic dermatitis,
	Pseudoanaphylaxis (Anaphylactoid reaction) Free Ag → direct degranulation of mast cell (not IgE mediated)		Iodine-containing radio contrast (mc), aspirin and muscle relaxants, morphine
TYPE 2: Antibody dependent cytotoxic hypersensitivity	Free Ab → fixed Ag	IgM IgG/complement mediated	Autoimmune hemolytic anemia Hemolytic disease of the newborn (erythroblastosis fetalis) Autoimmune thrombocytopenic purpura Goodpasture's syndrome Pemphigus vulgaris Bullous pemphigoid Acute rheumatic fever Pernicious anemia Myasthenia gravis Graves' disease Hyperacute graft rejection
		ADCC- antibody-dependent cell mediated cytotoxicity	Acute transplant rejection (Vascular)
TYPE 3: Immune complex	Free Ag + Free Ab → **Immune complex**		Serum sickness Arthus reaction Systemic lupus erythematosus (SLE) Immunoglobulin therapy Acute necrotizing vasculitis Polyarthritis nodosa Post streptococcal glomerulonephritis Shick's test

Contd...

Hypersensitivity Reactions			
TYPE 4: Delayed hypersensitivity, cell-mediated, antibody-independent	Ag +T cell mediated (CD4/CD8)	**Delayed:** CD4 mediated (contact and tuberculin types within 72 hours, Granulomatous type; 21-28 days)	Contact dermatitis Mantoux (tuberculin) test Lepromin test Multiple sclerosis Phlyctenular keratoconjunctivitis Jones mote reaction (cutaneous basophilic hypersensitivity) Chronic transplant rejection
		Direct cell toxicity:Cytotoxic CD8 T cell mediated	Perforin dependent killing Fas-FasL dependent killing Graft vs Host disease Acute transplant rejection (Cellular)

Graft Rejection	
Hyperacute	Type 2
Acute	Type 4 >2 (both if provided) Acute cellular rejection = type 4 (better prognosis) Acute vascular rejection = type 2
Chronic	Type 4
# Graft rejection is type 4 hypersensitivity unless type is provided	

104. Ans. (b) Hydroxyl free radical

Ref: Robbins 9th ed page 47

Free radicals are chemical species that have a single unpaired electron in an outer orbit. Energy created by this unstable configuration is released through reactions with adjacent molecules, such as inorganic or organic chemicals—proteins, lipids, carbohydrates, nucleic acids—many of which are key components of cell membranes and nuclei. Reactive oxygen species (ROS) are a type of oxygen-derived free radical whose role in cell injury is well established. ROS are produced normally in cells during mitochondrial respiration and energy generation, but they are degraded and removed by cellular defense systems.

Properties of The Principal Free Radicals Involved in Cell Injury				
Properties	$O_2^{\bar{\cdot}}$ Superoxide ion	H_2O_2 hydrogen peroxide	$^{\cdot}OH$ hydroxyl radical	$ONOO^-$
Mechanisms of production	Incomplete reduction of O_2 during oxidative phosphorylation; by phagocyte oxidase in leukocytes	Generated by SOD from O_2- and by oxidases in peroxisomes	Generated from H_2O by hydrolysis, e.g., by radiation; from H_2O_2 by Fenton reaction; from $O_2^{\bar{\cdot}}$	Produced by interaction of $O_2^{\bar{\cdot}}$ and NO generated by NO synthase in many cell types (endothelial cells, leukocytes, neurons, others)
Mechanisms of inactivation	Conversion to H_2O_2 and O_2 by SOD	Conversion to H_2O and O_2 by catalase (peroxisomes), glutathione peroxidase (cytosol, mitochondria)	Conversion to H_2O by glutathione peroxidase	Conversion to HNO_2 by peroxiredoxins (cytosol, mitochondria)
Pathologic effects	Stimulates production of degradative enzymes in leukocytes and other cells; may directly damage lipids, proteins, DNA; acts close to site of production	Can be converted to $^{\cdot}OH$ and OCl-, which destroy microbes and cells; can act distant from site of production	**Most reactive oxygen-derived free radical**; principal ROS responsible for damaging lipids, proteins, and DNA	Damages lipids, proteins, DNA
Free radicals are chemical species that have a single unpaired electron in an outer orbit				

105. Ans. (c) C4d

Ref: Robbins 9th ed ch 6

Deposition of the complement breakdown product C4d in allografts is a strong indicator of humoral rejection, because C4d is produced during activation of the complement system by the antibody-dependent classical pathway. The importance of making this diagnosis is that it provides a rationale for treating affected patients with B cell–depleting agents.

106. Ans. (c) The cells in the culture are predominantly necrotic

Ref: Robbin's 9th ed ch 5, Robbins 8th ed page 27

The picture is exact replica of Robbins 9th ed Figure 1-23.

Agarose gel electrophoresis of DNA extracted from culture cells. Ethidium bromide stain; photographed under ultraviolet illumination.

Lane A, Viable cells in culture.

Lane B, Culture of cells exposed to heat showing extensive apoptosis; note ladder pattern of DNA fragments, which represent multiples of oligonucleosomes.

Lane C, Culture showing cell necrosis; note diffuse smearing of DNA.

Robbin's states: Apoptotic cells exhibit a characteristic breakdown of DNA into large 50- to 300-kilobase pieces. Subsequently, there is cleavage of DNA by Ca2+- and Mg2+-dependent endonucleases into fragments whose sizes are multiples of 180 to 200 base pairs, reflecting cleavage between nucleosomal subunits. The fragments may be visualized by electrophoresis as DNA "ladders"

Necrosis versus Apoptosis		
Morphological Features		
	Apoptosis	**Necrosis**
Outset	Shrinking of cytoplasm, condensation of nucleus	Swelling of cytoplasm and mitochondria
Plasma membrane	**Blebbing** of plasma membrane without loss of integrity	Loss of membrane integrity
Chromatin	Aggregation of chromatin at the nuclear membrane.	
Organelles	Mitochondria become leaky due to pore formation involving proteins of the bcl-2 family.	Disintegration (swelling) of organelles
Vesicles	Formation of membrane bound vesicles (**Apoptotic bodies:** Cytoplasm and tightly packed organelles, with or without pyknotic nuclear fragments)	No vesicle formation, complete lysis
Terminal	Fragmentation of cell into smaller bodies	Total cell lysis
Inflammation	Absent	Present
Physiological Features		
	Apoptosis	**Necrosis**
Extent	Localized effect that destroys individual cells	Affects groups of contiguous cells
Induction	Self-Induced by physiological stimuli (lack of growth factors, changes in hormonal environment)	Evoked by non-physiological/external disturbances (complement attack, lytic viruses, hypothermia, hypoxia, ischemica, metabolic poisons)
Phagocytosis	Phagocytosis by adjacent cells or macrophages	Phagocytosis by macrophages
Immune system	No inflammatory response	Significant inflammatory response
Biochemical Features		
	Apoptosis	**Necrosis**
Regulation	Tightly regulated process involving activation and enzymatic steps	Loss of regulation of ion homeostasis
Energy input	Energy (ATP)-dependent (active process, does not occur at 4°C)	No energy requirement (passive process, also occurs at 4°C)
DNA	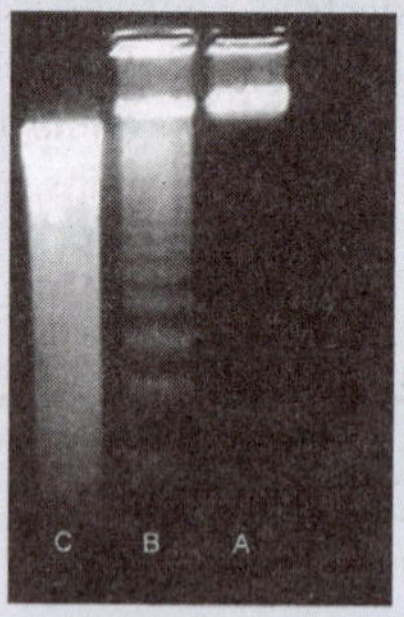 Non-random mono- and oligonucleosomal length fragmentation of DNA (Lane B: **Ladder pattern after agarose gel electrophoresis**)	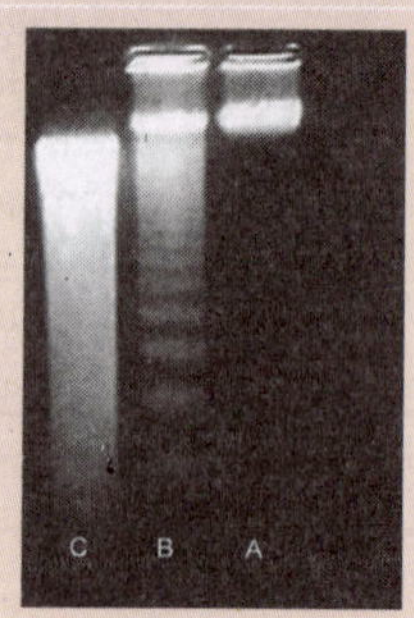 Random digestion of DNA (Lane C: **smear of DNA after agarose gel electrophoresis**)

Contd...

Timing	Prelytic DNA fragmentation	Postlytic DNA fragmentation (= late event in cell death)
Biochemical events	Release of various factors (cytochrome C, AIF) into cytoplasm by mitochondria. Activation of caspase cascade. Alterations in membrane asymmetry (translocation of phosphatidylserine from the cytoplasmic to the extracellular side of the membrane)	

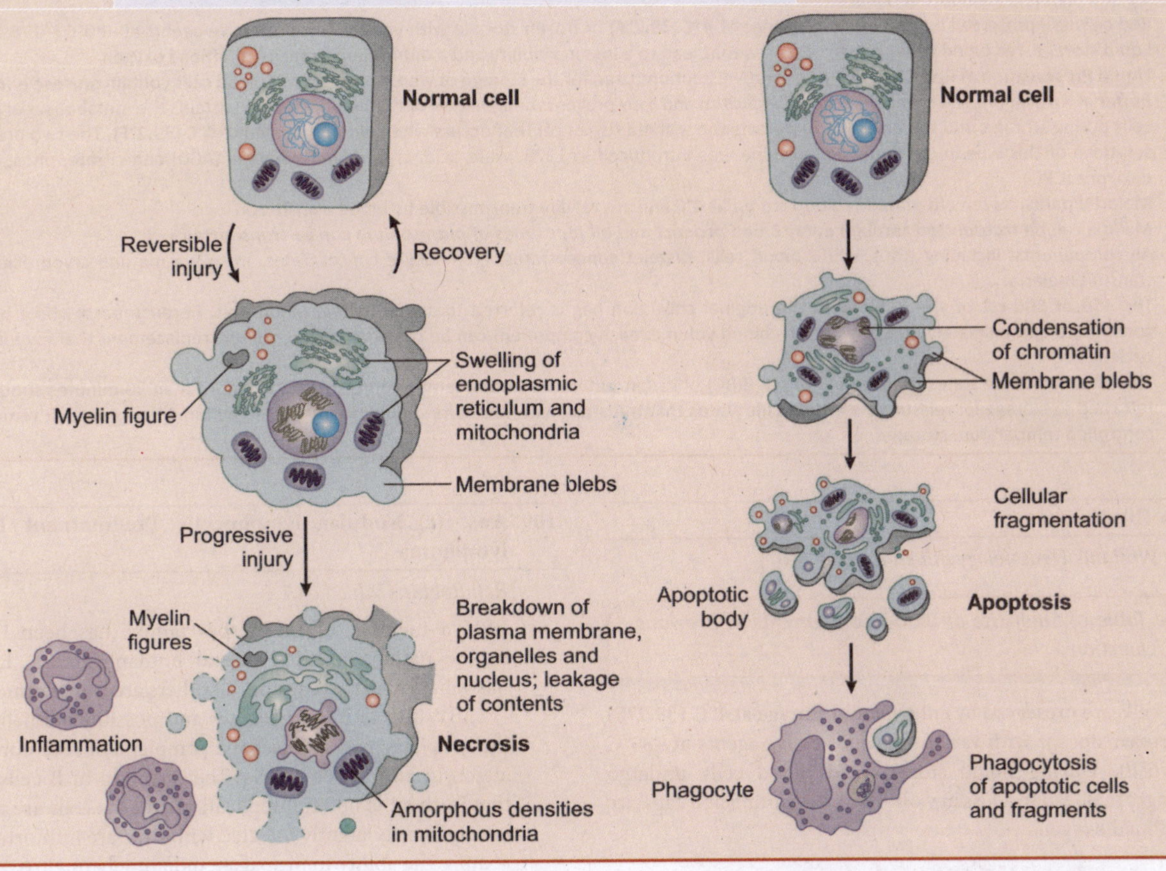

107. Ans. (b) Through 18 to 20 gauge IV catheter within 4 hours of issue from blood bank

Ref: Wintrobe 12th ed page 675, WHO Clinical Transfusion Practice Guidelines, American Society of Hematology 2012 Clinical Practice Guide on Red Blood Cell Transfusion

There are three components of the answers:

- **Time limit from the issue from the blood bank:** For whole blood and Packed RBC are to be transfused with in 4 hours of issue from the blood bank The 30-minute rule states that red blood cell (RBC) units left out of controlled temperature storage for more than 30 minutes should not be returned to storage for reissue; the 4-hour rule states that transfusion of RBC units should be completed within 4 hours of their removal from controlled temperature storage.
- **Time limit from the receiving by the patient side:** No such guidelines available as the time of transfusion is not related to the receiving end but the issuing end.
- **Size of the IV cannula used for transfusion:** In adults, 18 to 20-gauge catheter is recommended to provide good flow rate without too much discomfort for the patient. In neonates and pediatric patients RBCs can be safely administered through 22, 24 or 26-gauge needle.

Shelf Life of Blood Components

Component	Period of storage/life
RBC (CPD-A1)	35 days
RBC (Adsol)	42 days
Platelets	5 days
Granulocytes	24 hours

Contd...

Shelf Life of Blood Components	
Component	**Period of storage/life**
Factor VIII	2 days
Factor V	4-5 days
Factor XI	6-7 days

Footnote

[a]WBCs and platelets are nonfunctional

- Red cells are preserved by either liquid storage at **4°C (39.2°F)** or frozen storage with various cryoprotective agents at –80°C (–176°F). During liquid storage, red blood cells undergo changes that lead to a loss in viability and a diminished capacity to offload oxygen
- **Liquid Preservation of Red Cells:** The preservative solutions used for the storage of whole blood or red blood cells contain ***glucose and a citrate buffer*** at an acid pH. The citrate ion chelates calcium and thus prevents coagulation of the blood, glucose sustains the metabolism of red blood cells during storage, and the acid pH counteracts the marked rise of pH that occurs when blood is cooled to **4°C (39.2°F).** The two preservative solutions of this type in use until CPD-adenine was introduced in 1978, were acid, citrate, and dextrose (ACD) and citrate, phosphate, and dextrose (CPD)
- **Malarial parasites remain viable** in blood stored at 4°C and are readily transmissible by blood transfusion
- Malaria can be ***transmitted through every blood product and all four types of plasmodium can be transmitted***"
- All components, including RBCs, white blood cells, platelet concentrates, granulocyte concentrates, fresh plasma and cryoprecipitate can transmit malaria
- The **450 or 500 mL** of whole blood in the original collection bag is referred to as one whole blood unit. Because each whole blood unit constituted approximately 10% of a donor's blood volume, each component can be considered roughly **10%** replacement therapy for an adult patient.
- The **30-minute rule** states that red blood cell (RBC) units left out of controlled temperature storage for more than 30 minutes should not be returned to storage for reissue; the **4-hour rule** states that transfusion of RBC units should be completed within 4 hours of their removal from controlled temperature storage.

108. Ans. (b) 2°–6°C

Ref: William's Hematology 8th ed chapter 140

See Table of Shelf Life of Blood Components In Previous Question

Red cells are preserved by either liquid storage at **4°C (39.2°F)** or frozen storage with various cryoprotective agents at –80°C (–176°F). During liquid storage, red blood cells undergo changes that lead to a loss in viability and a diminished capacity to offload oxygen

109. Ans. (c) Nodular lymphocytic Predominant Hodgkin's lymphoma

Ref: Robbin's 9th ed ch 7

EBV, a member of the herpes family, has been implicated in the pathogenesis of several human tumors. Except for nasopharyngeal carcinoma, all others are B-cell tumors.

EBV infects B lymphocytes and possibly epithelial cells of the oropharynx. EBV uses the complement receptor **CD21** to attach to and infect B cells. The infection of B cells is latent; that is, there is no viral replication and the cells are not killed, but the B cells latently infected with EBV are immortalized and acquire the ability to propagate indefinitely in vitro.

Oncogenic Viruses		
Oncogenic DNA Viruses		
Virus	**Disease**	**Cancer**
Papova viridae Papilloma virus (some)	Warts, including STD genital warts	Uterine (cervical) cancer
Epstein-Barr virus	Infectious mononucleosis	African form of Burkitt lymphoma B-cell lymphomas in immuno suppressed individuals (particularly in HIV infection or undergoing immuno suppressive therapy after organ transplantation) A subset of Hodgkin lymphoma Nasopharyngeal and some gastric carcinomas and rare forms of T cell lymphomas and natural killer (NK) cell lymphomas.
Hepadna virus Hepatitis B virus (HBV)	Hepatitis B (infectious hepatitis)	Liver cancer
Adenoviridae	Acute respiratory disease; Common cold	Adenocarcinomas (cancer of glandular epithelial tissues)

Contd...

Poxviridae	Smallpox; Cowpox	Miscellaneous
Oncogenic RNA Viruses of the Family Retroviridae		
Virus	Cancer	
Human T-cell leukemia virus (HTLV-1; HTLV-2)	Adult T-cell leukemia, Lymphoma	
Sarcoma viruses of cats, chickens, rodents	Sarcomas (cancer of connective tissues)	
Mammary tumor virus of mice	Mammary gland tumors	
Feline leukemia virus (FeLV)	Feline leukemia	

AIIMS NOVEMBER 2015

110. Ans. (a) Hepcidin

Ref: Wintrobe 11th ed page 811, Robbin's 9th ed page 649

Hepcidin is a protein that is known to play a central role in iron homeostasis in the body. Iron absorption is regulated by hepcidin, a small circulating peptide that is synthesized and released from the liver in response to increases in intrahepatic iron levels. Hepcidin inhibits iron transfer from the enterocyte to plasma by binding to ferroportin and causing it to be endocytosed and degraded. As a result, as hepcidin levels rise, iron becomes trapped within duodenal cells in the form of mucosal ferritin and is lost as these cells are sloughed. Thus, when the body is replete with iron, high hepcidin levels inhibit its absorption into the blood. Conversely, with low body stores of iron, hepcidin synthesis falls and this in turn facilitates iron absorption. By inhibiting ferroportin, hepcidin not only reduces iron uptake from enetrocytes but also suppresses iron release from macrophages, which are an important source of the iron that is used by erythroid precursors to make hemoglobin. This, as we shall see, is important in the pathogenesis of anemia of chronic diseases.

But Hepcidin is not specific for iron metabolism. Hepcidin is induced by

- Inflammation
- Interleukin–6 (IL-6), an inflammatory cytokine, signals through the JAK-STAT (Janus Kinase—Signal Transducer and Activator of Transcription) pathway to mediate this effect
- Anemia that is associated with chronic inflammation (anemia of inflammation or AI) is probably due to inflammation mediated upregulation of hepcidin. AI manifests as a microcytic, hypochromic anemia that is refractory to iron supplementation.
- In addition to the above-mentioned factors, hypoxia is also known to induce hepcidin and this effect is mediated by stabilization of the hypoxia-inducible factors 1 and 2 (HIF-1 and HI

111. Ans. (a) Seminiferous tubule

Ref: Robbin's 9th ed page 215, Gray's Anatomy 40th ed page 1263, Harrison 19th ed ch 318

(Robbins says) Some antigens are hidden (sequestered) from the immune system, because the tissues in which these antigens are located do not communicate with the blood and lymph. Thus, self-antigens in these tissues do not induce tolerance but fail to elicit immune responses and are essentially ignored by the immune system. This is believed to the case for the **testis, eye, and brain**, all of which are called *immune privileged sites* because it is difficult to induce immune responses to antigens introduced into these sites. If the antigens of these tissues are released, for example, as a consequence of trauma or infection, the result may be an immune response that lead to prolonged tissue inflammation and injury. This is the postulated mechanism for post-traumatic orchitis and uveitis.

The above statement Robbins only talks about the Immune privileged organs not tissue. Only option (B) Loop of Henle can be ruled out from the above text. Now read following texts from Harrison and Gray's

(Harrison says) Some autoantigens reside in immunologically privileged sites, such as the brain or the **anterior chamber of the eye**. If the privileged site is damaged by trauma or inflammation, or if T cells are activated elsewhere, proteins expressed at this site can become the targets of immunologic assault. Such an event may occur in multiple sclerosis and sympathetic ophthalmia, in which antigens uniquely expressed in the brain and eye, respectively, become the target of activated T cells.

(Gray's says) Although the CNS has long been considered to be an immunologically privileged site, lymphocyte surveillance of the brain may be a normal, low-grade activity that is enhanced in disease.

Now come to the conclusion:

Gynecology by 10 teachers 19th ed page 88: Sertoli cells are highly specialized cells that maintain the integrity of seminiferous epithelium (so that spermatogenesis can occur in an immune privileged area) as well as nourish the developing sperm. This complex blood-testis barrier provides an immunologically privileged site.

112. Ans. (b) End of G1 phase

Ref: Robbin's 9th ed page 25

Cells in G1 progress through the cycle and reach the critical stage at the G1/S transition, known as restriction point, rate limiting step for replication. Upon passing this restriction point, normal cells become irreversibly committed to DNA replication.

Cell Cycle

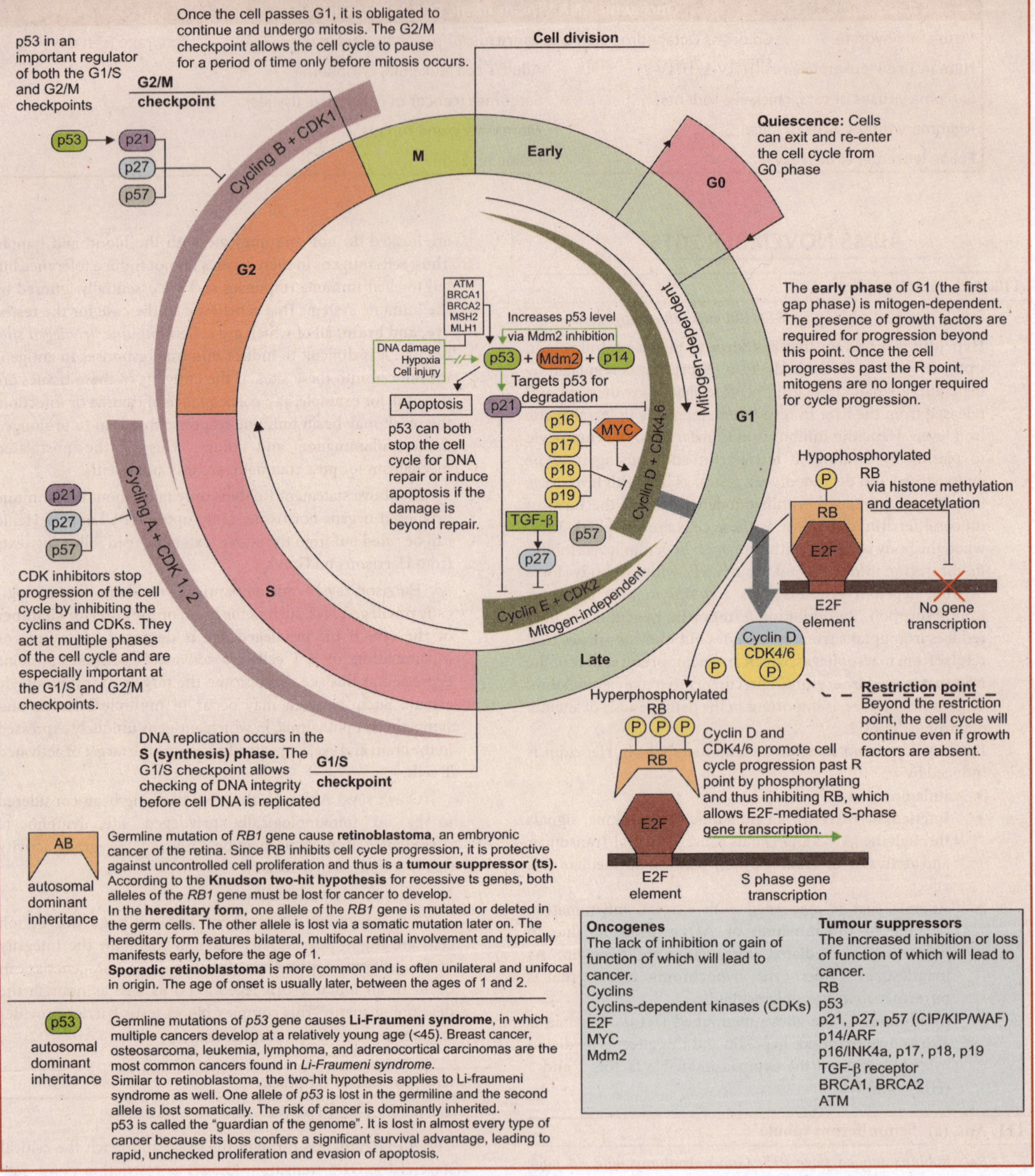

AB

autosomal dominant inheritance

Germline mutation of *RB1* gene cause **retinoblastoma**, an embryonic cancer of the retina. Since RB inhibits cell cycle progression, it is protective against uncontrolled cell proliferation and thus is a **tumour suppressor (ts)**.
According to the **Knudson two-hit hypothesis** for recessive ts genes, both alleles of the *RB1* gene must be lost for cancer to develop.
In the **hereditary form**, one allele of the *RB1* gene is mutated or deleted in the germ cells. The other allele is lost via a somatic mutation later on. The hereditary form features bilateral, multifocal retinal involvement and typically manifests early, before the age of 1.
Sporadic retinoblastoma is more common and is often unilateral and unifocal in origin. The age of onset is usually later, between the ages of 1 and 2.

p53

autosomal dominant inheritance

Germline mutations of *p53* gene causes **Li-Fraumeni syndrome**, in which multiple cancers develop at a relatively young age (<45). Breast cancer, osteosarcoma, leukemia, lymphoma, and adrenocortical carcinomas are the most common cancers found in *Li-Fraumeni syndrome.*
Similar to retinoblastoma, the two-hit hypothesis applies to Li-fraumeni syndrome as well. One allele of *p53* is lost in the germiline and the second allele is lost somatically. The risk of cancer is dominantly inherited.
p53 is called the "guardian of the genome". It is lost in almost every type of cancer because its loss confers a significant survival advantage, leading to rapid, unchecked proliferation and evasion of apoptosis.

Oncogenes	**Tumour suppressors**
The lack of inhibition or gain of function of which will lead to cancer.	The increased inhibition or loss of function of which will lead to cancer.
Cyclins	RB
Cyclins-dependent kinases (CDKs)	p53
E2F	p21, p27, p57 (CIP/KIP/WAF)
MYC	p14/ARF
Mdm2	p16/INK4a, p17, p18, p19
	TGF-β receptor
	BRCA1, BRCA2
	ATM

113. Ans. (c) Calcium oxalate stone

Ref: Henry's Clinical diagnosis and management 22 ed page 469

The crystals shown is typical Envelope shaped Calcium Oxalate dihydrate crystal

Urinary Crystals			
Crystal	**Shape**	**Favorable pH**	**Comments**
Calcium oxalate dihydrate 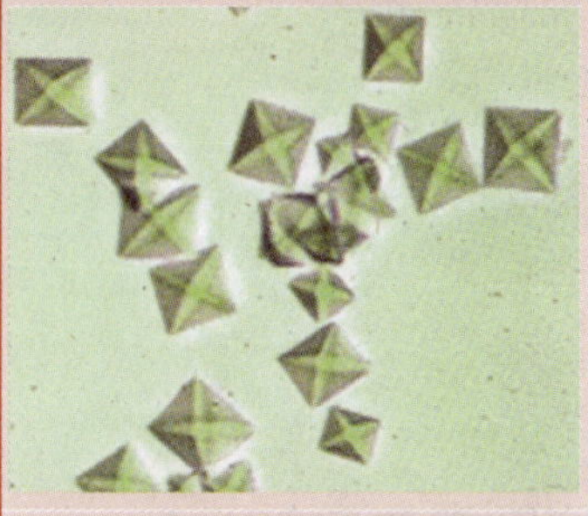	Colorless Octahedron (**Envelope shaped**), diamond shape	Acidic or pH insensitive in the physiologic pH range of 5 to 8	Artifact of storage (can develop in stored urine). Associated with food high in oxalate (tomatoes, asparagus, ascorbic acid
Calcium oxalate monohydrate 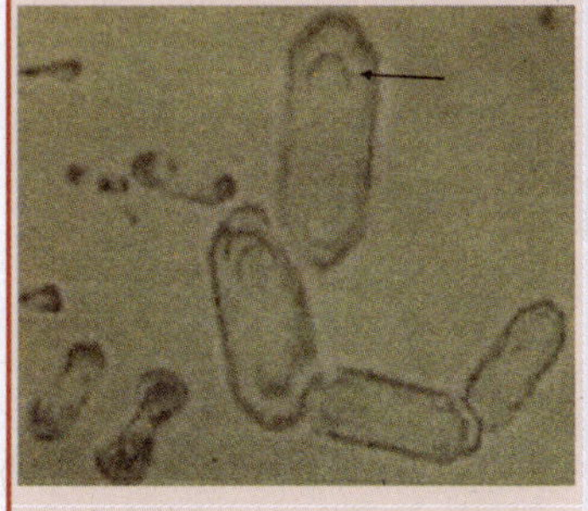	Colorless, Spindle (arrow), oval (**Hemp seed)**, or dumbbell shape,	Acidic or pH insensitive in the physiologic pH range of 5 to 8	Associated with food high in oxalate (tomatoes, asparagus, ascorbic acid
Calcium oxalate monohydrate (picket fence) 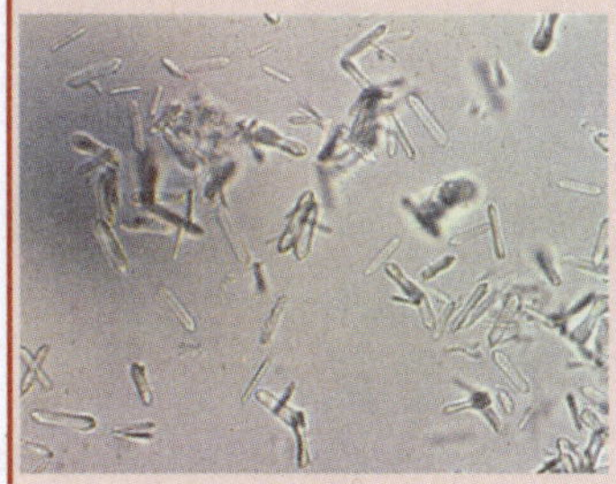	A particular form of calcium oxalate monohydrate are flat, elongated, six-sided crystals ("**picket fences**") which are the larger crystals	Acidic or pH insensitive in the physiologic pH range of 5 to 8	Seen in ethylene glycol toxicosis
Calcium carbonate 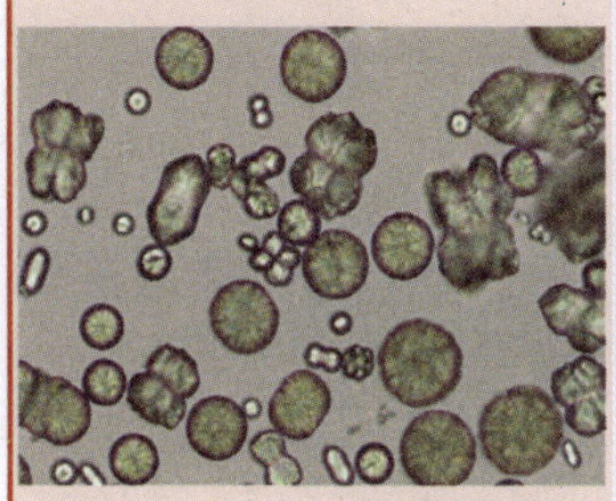	Yellow to colorless **dumbells or spheres with radial striations**	Alkaline urine	Usually large crystals and can be readily observed at low magnification.
Uric acid 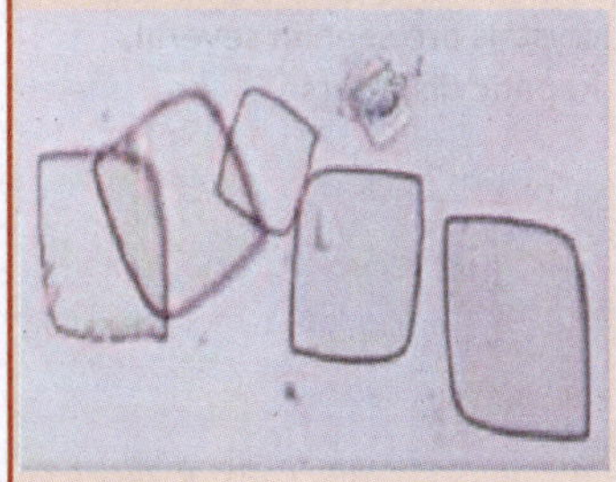	Amber in color, Rhomboic, 4 sided plates, prism, oval with pointed ended	5-5.5 (Acidic Urine)	

Contd...

Urinary Crystals			
Crystal	**Shape**	**Favorable pH**	**Comments**
Ammonium biurate 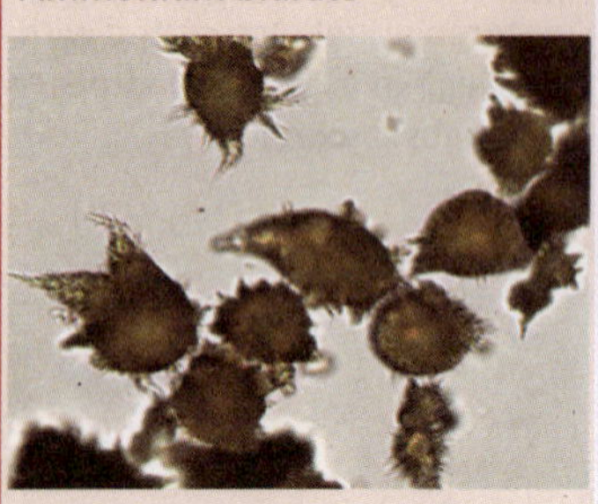	Brown or yellow-brown spherical bodies with irregular protrusions **("thorn-apples")**	Alkaline pH	Can be observed under low magnification
Struvite crystals (magnesium ammonium phosphate, triple phosphate) 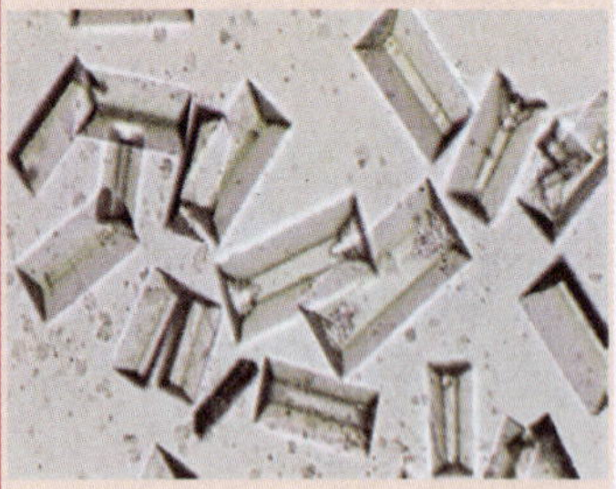	Colorless, three-dimensional, prism-like crystals (**"coffin lids"**)	Neutral and Alkaline pH is favourable.	UTI with urease positive bacteria promote struvite crystalluria
Calcium phosphate 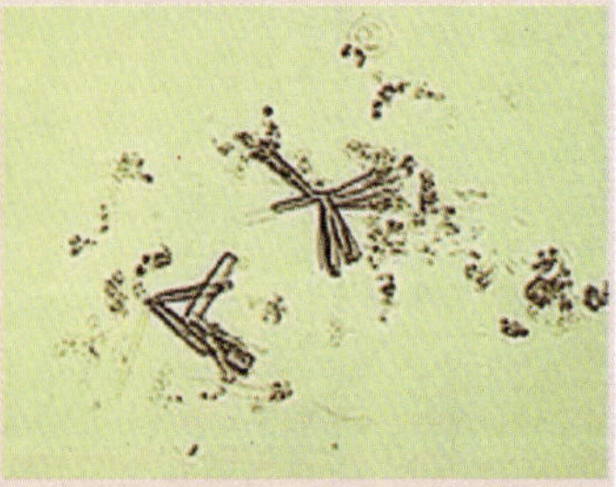	Large flat-shaped plates or wedge-shaped prisms in rosettes. Single prisms are usually blunt on one end and pointed on the other end.	Alkaline urine	
Hippuric acid 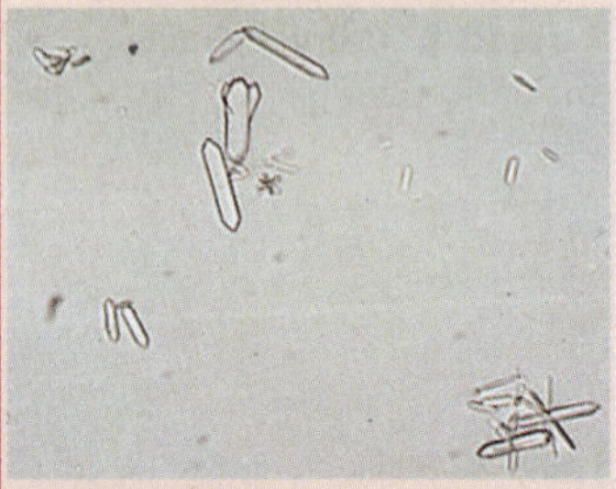	Colorless prisms, plates, or needle-like often conglomerated into masses		
Bilirubin crystals 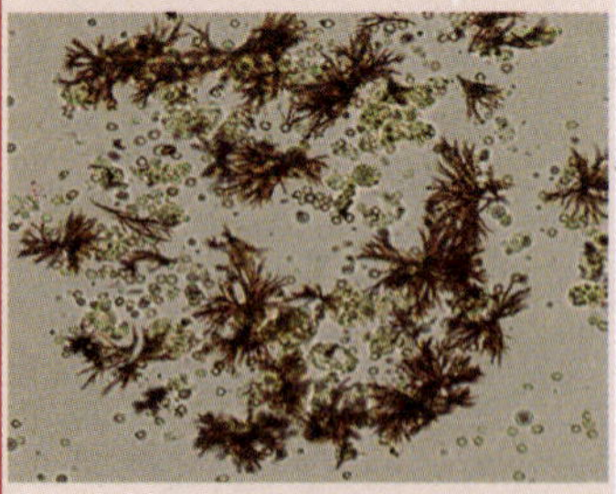	Yellow-brown **needles or granules**. Form from conjugated bilirubin.		They are frequently attached to the surface of cells. Bilirubin crystals are seen in several hepatic disorders

Contd...

Urinary Crystals			
Crystal	Shape	Favorable pH	Comments
Cystine crystals 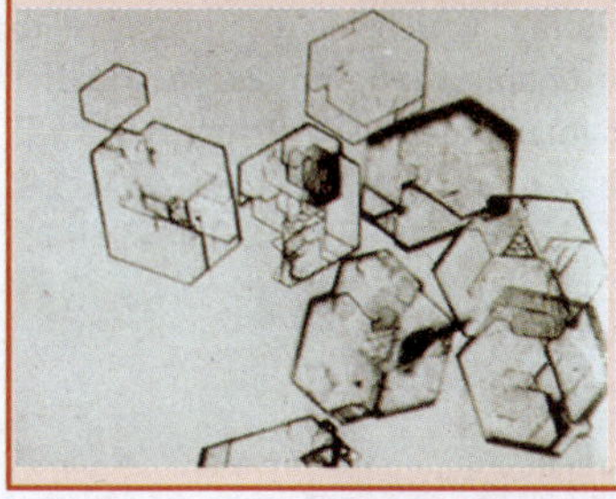	Flat colorless, thin, **hexagonal** plates with equal or unequal sides	Acidic urine	Cystine crystals are found in the inherited condition, **cystinuria.** Cystine crystals are the most frequent cause of kidney stones in children.

114. Ans. (b) Urine protein ranging from 20-200 mg/24 hours is called microalbuminuria

Ref: With Text

Option (A)

Robbin's 8th ed pg 1145: Microalbuminuria is the presence of albumin in urine above the normal level but below the detectable range of conventional urine dipstick methods.

Option (B)

Harrison 18th ed ch 344: Microalbuminuria is defined as **30–299 mg/d** in a 24-h collection or 30–299 μg/mg creatinine in a spot collection (preferred method).

Option (C)

Harrison 18th ed ch 344: Both microalbuminuria and macroalbuminuria in individuals with DM are associated with increased risk of cardiovascular disease.

Henry's clinical diagnosis and management 22 ed page 452: In diabetic patients, microalbuminuria is associated with a 4 to 6 fold increase in cardiovascular mortality and independent risk factor for renal mortality.

Option (D)

The earliest manifestation of diabetic nephropathy is appearance of low amount of albumin in urine (>30 mg/day, but <300 mg/day) that is microalbuminuria.

115. Ans. (a) Immediate definitive diagnosis of tumor

Ref: Introduction to Biopsy Interpretation and Surgical Pathology By J.C.E. Underwood page 100

Indications for Frozen Sections

- Provide a diagnosis that will allow the surgeon to make an intraoperative decision regarding further surgery during that operative event.
- Assess margins when additional excision to attain a negative margin is an option.
- Assess adequacy of diagnostic tissue in a biopsy specimen from an open or a complicated procedure. For example, a bone biopsy in the operating room may yield only reactive bone, and a second biopsy procedure may be avoided with frozen section.
- Plan the workup of the specimen. The need for cytogenetics, flow cytometry, and other special studies should reasonably be evaluated prior to fixation. Tissue for protocols or banking may need to be sampled.
- Plan for resources. Scheduling of operating room time for definitive procedure pending permanents may be require faster diagnosis.

From above list of indications option (D) is not clear, now read following text.

Option (D)

Ref: Breast Cancer Research Protocols By Susan A. Brooks, Adrian Harris 2006 Humana press page 104: Some authors advocate frozen section of the sentinel lymph nodes, whereas others institutions never use frozen section because of sampling errors in their settings. The decision to incorporate frozen section evaluation into one's program depends on the comfort level of the pathologist and surgeon.

Ref: Eur J Surg Oncol. 2009 Mar; 35(3):276-80: Intraoperative frozen section examination of the sentinel node is a useful predictor of axillary lymph node status in breast cancer patients. Seventy-two percent of the patients with metastatic disease were correctly diagnosed and spared a second surgical procedure.

Ref: Histopathology. 1999 Jul; 35(1):14-8. In up to 10% of cases, the final paraffin sections will reveal micrometastases that were not detected by the frozen section, and in these patients axillary lymph node dissection will have to be performed in a second session.

116. Ans. (b) Antony A pattern with verocay body

Ref: Robbins 9th ed page 1314

Histopathological features of Schwannoma is a hot favorite topic of AIIMS exam now a days. Asked in different forms in AIIMS NOV 2017, NOV 2015, NOV 2014, MAY 2014

See Details of Schwannoma in AIIMS NOV 2017 Pathology (see page no. 348)

117. Ans. (b) Hamartomatous polyps

Ref: Robbin's 9th ed page 809

This is a case of Peutz Jegher's syndrome which in which multiple Hamartomatous polyps are found.

Hamartomatous polyps occur sporadically and in the context of various genetically determined or acquired syndromes (Peutz-Jeghers syndrome, Cowden syndrome, Bannayan-Ruvalcaba-Riley syndrome, Cronkhite-Canada syndrome, Tuberous sclerosis)

Because the morphology of Peutz-Jeghers polyps can overlap with that of sporadic hamartomatous polyps, the presence of multiple polyps in the small intestine, mucocutaneous hyperpigmentation, and a positive family history are key to the diagnosis.

Peutz-Jeghers syndrome is a rare autosomal dominant syndrome presents at a median age of 11 years with multiple GI hamartomatous polyps and mucocutaneous hyperpigmentation. The latter takes the form of dark blue to brown macules around the mouth, eyes, nostrils, buccal mucosa, palmar surfaces of the hands, genitalia, and perianal region. These lesions are similar to freckles but are distinguished by their presence in the buccal mucosa. Peutz-Jeghers polyps can initiate **intussusception**, which is occasionally fatal.

Intestinal Polyps

Definition: A polyp is an abnormal growth of tissue projecting from a mucous membrane. If it is attached to the surface by a narrow elongated stalk, it is said to be pedunculated. If no stalk is present, it is said to be sessile. Polyps are most common in the colon but may occur in the esophagus, stomach, or small intestine.

Classification: In general, intestinal polyps can be classified as non-neoplastic or neoplastic in nature. The most common neoplastic polyp is the adenoma, which has the potential to progress to cancer. The non-neoplastic polyps can be further classified as inflammatory, hamartomatous, or hyperplastic.

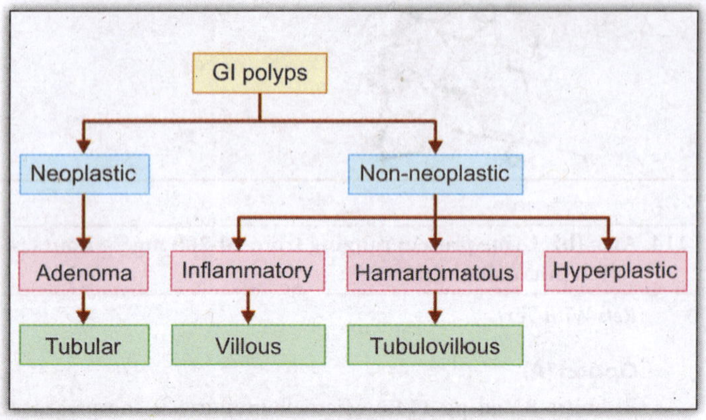

Intestinal Polyps			
Polyp	**Histologic appearance**	**Risk of malignancy**	**Comments**
Adenoma	0.3 to 10 cm in diameter often pedunculated or large sessile, with the surface of both types having a texture resembling velvet or a raspberry, due to the abnormal epithelial growth pattern	Characterized by the presence of epithelial dysplasia, precursors to colorectal cancer	Sub classified as **A-1: tubular (**small, pedunculated, small rounded, or tubular, glands), <20% villous element **A-2: tubulovillous** (mixture of tubular and villous elements) **A-3: villous** (larger sessile covered by slender villi) based on their architecture. >80% villous element
Serrated adenoma (Serrated = **Saw tooth)**	**Serrated architecture** throughout the full length of the glands, ***including the crypt base***, *Overlap histologically with hyperplastic polyps* (see Footnote), but are more commonly found in the right/ proximal colon. Horizontalization of the crypts, **L shaped** (red arrow) **or inverted T shaped** (green arrow) base branching of the crypt	Malignant potential but lack typical cytologic features of dysplasia that are present in other adenomas	Subtypes are: **(B-1) Sessile serrated adenoma/polyp,** showing asymmetrical serrated crypts and dilated crypts. **(B-2) Traditional serrated adenoma**, with prominent complex serration and hypereosinophilic cells. Mostly found at rectosigmoid junction.
Inflammatory **(C)**	Dilated glands, epithelial hyperplasia, superficial erosions, inflammatory infiltrate and lamina propria fibromuscular hyperplasia	No malignant potential	Forms as part of the solitary rectal ulcer syndrome
Hamartomatous polyp	Can present in different forms depending on the syndrome they are seen in (i.e. Juvenile polyp/Peutz Jeghers). Sporadic hamartomatous polyp has overlapping histology with Peutz Jeghers type Hamartomatous polyp	No malignant potential	Peutz-Jeghers syndrome, Cowden syndrome, Bannayan Ruvalcaba Riley syndrome, Cronkhite-Canada syndrome are syndromic Hamartomatous polyps

Contd...

Intestinal Polyps			
Polyp	**Histologic appearance**	**Risk of malignancy**	**Comments**
Hyperplastic polyp	Subtytes are: **(D-1) Microvesicular:** Serrations are limited to 1/2 to 2/3 of crypts (base is spared), mostly found in left/distal colon and rectum. Cells have microvesicular mucin droplets **(D-2) Goblet cell rich Hyperplastic polyp:** Typically less than 5 mm.. . Delayed shedding and crowding of goblet cells. Mucosal thickening	No malignant potential	Hyperplastic polyposis syndrome. They must be distinguished from sessile serrated adenomas, a histologically similar lesions that have malignant potential (see footnote)
Peutz-Jeghers type Hamartomatous polyp **(E)**	Multiple GI **hamartomatous polyps**. Large and pedunculated with a lobulated contour. Characteristic **arborizing network** of connective tissue, smooth muscle, lamina propria, and glands lined by normal-appearing intestinal epithelium. The arborization **(Christmas tree appearance)** and presence of smooth muscle intermixed with lamina propria are helpful in distinguishing polyps of Peutz-Jeghers syndrome from juvenile polyps.	Increased risk	Peutz-Jeghers syndrome
Juvenile polyp (Juvenile type Hamartomatous polyp) (F)	Sporadic are solitary, <3 cm in diameter, typically pedunculated, smooth surfaced, reddish lesions. A typical juvenile polyp demonstrate multiple mucus retention cysts/gland dilatation (blue arrow), inflammatory cell infiltrate and ***unlike PJS absence of smooth-muscle proliferation***.	Dysplasia may develop. Juvenile polyposis syndrome is associated with increased risk of colonic adenocarcinoma	Autosomal dominant **Juvenile polyposis syndrome (JPS);** >3 hamartomatous polyps in colorectum or polyps throughout GIT or any number of polyp with family history of JPS

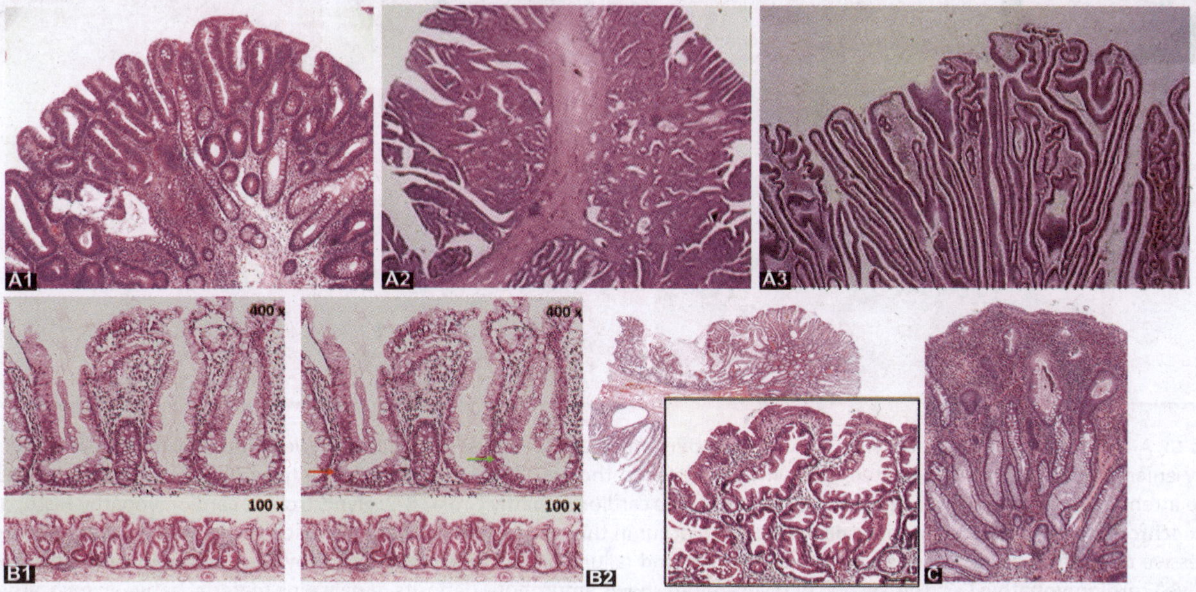

Figs A to F:

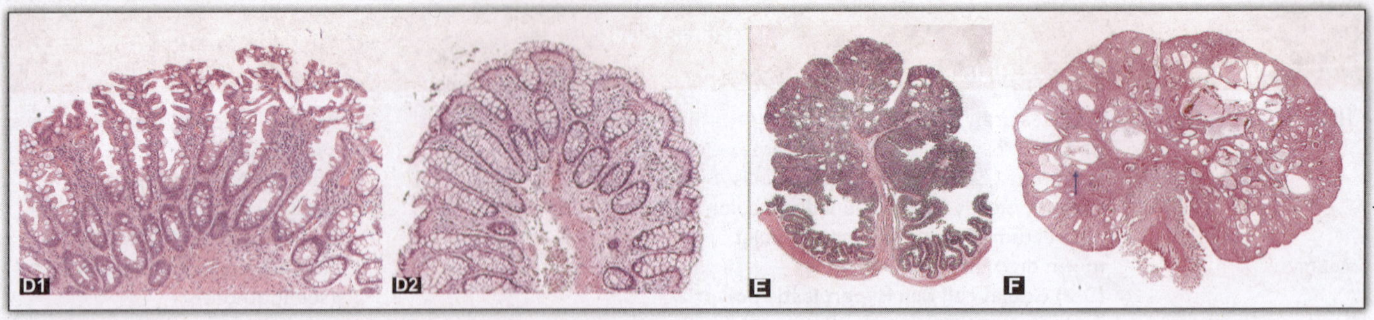

Figs A to F: A-1: Tubular Adenoma; A-2: Tubulovillous Adenoma; A-3: Villous Adenoma; B-1- Sessile serrated adenoma/polyp; B-2- Traditional serrated adenoma; **(C)** Inflammatory Polyp; D-1 : Microvesicular hyperplastic polyp; D-2: Goblet cell rich Hyperplastic polyp; **(E)** Peutz-Jeghers type Hamartomatous Polyp; **(F)** Juvenile Polyp (Juvenile type Hamartomatous polyp)

118. Ans. (a) Hypertrophic cardiomyopathy

Ref: Robbins 9th ed page 569, Harrison 19th ed page 1569

The history is self explanatory and one need not even see the Gross picture given, to come to a diagnosis. Read Following lines of Harrison

"Hypertrophic cardiomyopathy usually presents between the ages of 20 and 40 years. Dyspnea on exertion is the most common presenting symptom, reflecting elevated intracardiac filling pressures. Chest pain with either an atypical or typical exertional pattern occurs in more than half of symptomatic patients and is attributed to myocardial ischemia from high demand and abnormal intramural coronary arteries in the hypertrophied myocardium. Palpitations may result from atrial fibrillation or ventricular arrhythmias. Much less common are episodes of presyncope or syncope, often related to heavy exertion. Of grave concern is the possibility that the first manifestation of disease may be sudden death from ventricular tachycardia or fibrillation. ***Hypertrophic cardiomyopathy is the most common lesion found at autopsy of young athletes dying suddenly***"

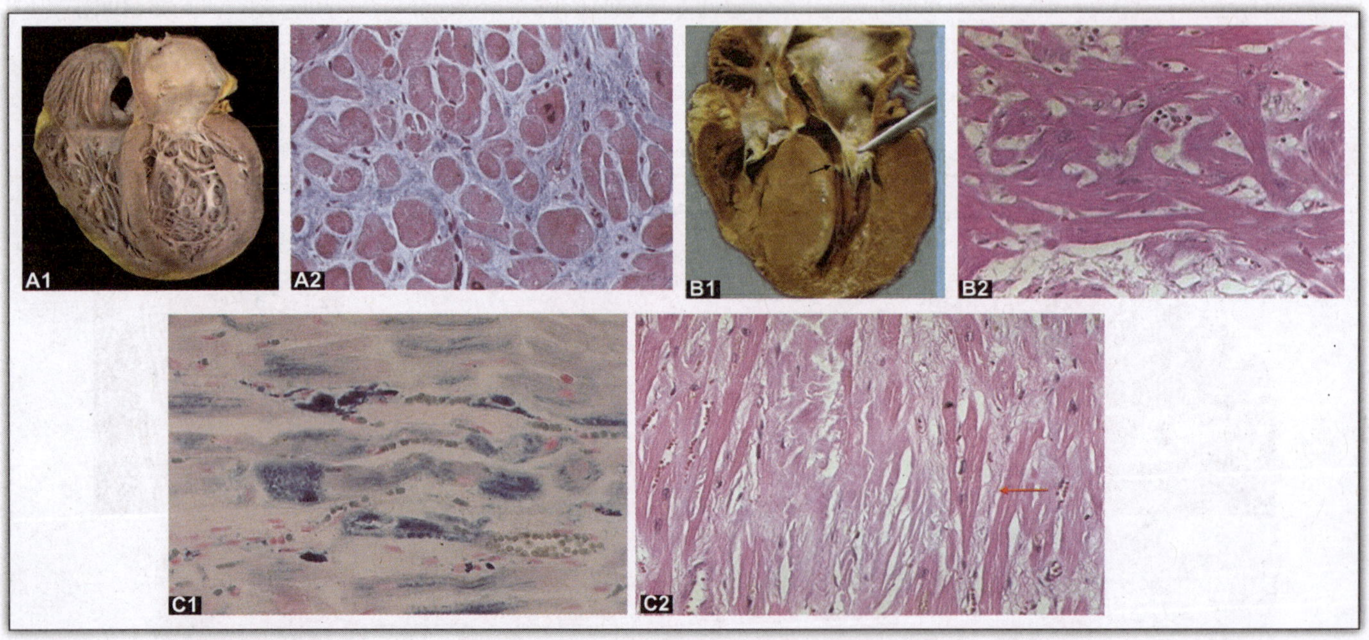

Figs A to C: A-1: Dilated cardiomyopathy gross: All 4 chambers are dilated, most severe in the left ventricle which appears globular. Heart is usually enlarged and flabby; A-2: Dilated Cardiomyopathy Histpathology: Most muscle cells are hypertrophic with enlarged nuclei but some are attenuated, stretched and irregular; B-1: Hypertrophic cardiomyopathy Gross; B-2: Hypertrophic cardiomyopathy Histopathology; C-1: **Hemochromatosis,** with excessive iron deposition, can occur in the heart as shown here microscopically with Prussian blue iron stain. The excessive deposition of iron leads to heart enlargement and failure similar to a cardiomyopathy, making hemochromatosis a form of **"restrictive" cardiomyopathy**; C-2: This section of myocardium shows amorphous deposits of pale pink material between myocardial fibers. This is characteristic for amyloid. Amyloidosis is a cause for an **"infiltrative"** or **"restrictive" form of cardiomyopathy**. It is a nightmare for anesthesiologists when intractable arrhythmias occur during surgery on such patients.

Types of Cardiomyopathy			
	Dilated	Restrictive	Hypertrophic
Ejection fraction (normal >55%)	Usually <30% when symptoms severe	25-50%	>60%
Left ventricular diastolic dimension (normal <55 mm)	>60 mm	>60 mm (may be decreased)	Often decreased
Left ventricular wall thickness	Decreased	Normal or increased	Markedly increased
Atrial size	Increased	Increased; may be massive	Increased; related to abnormal
Valvular regurgitation	Related to annular dilation; mitral appears earlier, during decompensation; tricuspid regurgitation in late stages	Related to endocardial involvement; frequent mitral and tricuspid regurgitation, rarely severe	Related to valve-septum interaction; mitral regurgitation
Common first symptoms	Exertional intolerance	Exertional intolerance, fluid retention early	Exertional intolerance; may have chest pain
Congestive symptoms*	Left before right, except right prominent in young adults	Right often dominates	Left-sided congestion may develop late
Physical examination	Moderate to severe cardiomegaly; S3, S4, Atrioventricular valve regurgitation, especially mitral	Mild to moderate cardiomegaly; S3 or S4, Atrioventricular valve regurgitation; inspiratory increase in venous pressure **(Kussmaul sign)**	Mild cardiomegaly Apical systolic thrill and heave; brisk carotid upstroke, S4 common, Systolic murmur that increases with Valsalva maneuver
Chest radiograph	Moderate to marked cardiac enlargement, especially left ventricular Pulmonary venous hypertension	Mild cardiac enlargement Pulmonary venous hypertension	Mild to moderate cardiac enlargement Left atrial enlargement
Electrocardiograph (ECG)	Sinus tachycardia Atrial and ventricular arrhythmias ST-segment and T wave abnormalities Intraventricular conduction defects	Low voltage Intraventricular conduction defects Atrioventricular conduction defects	Left ventricular hypertrophy ST-segment and T wave abnormalities Abnormal Q waves Atrial and ventricular arrhythmias
Arrhythmia	Ventricular tachyarrhythmia; conduction block in Chagas' disease, and some families. Atrial fibrillation.	Ventricular uncommon except in sarcoidosis conduction block in sarcoidosis and amyloidosis. Atrial fibrillation.	Ventricular tachyarrhythmias; atrial fibrillation
Echocardiography	Left ventricular dilation and dysfunction Abnormal diastolic mitral valve motion secondary to abnormal compliance and filling pressures	Increased left ventricular wall thickness and mass Small or normal-size left ventricular cavity Normal systolic function Pericardial effusion	Asymmetric septal hypertrophy Narrow left ventricular outflow tract Systolic anterior motion of the mitral valve Small or normal-sized left ventricle
Radionucleotide studies	Left ventricular dilation and dysfunction (RVG)	Infiltration of myocardium (^{201}Tl) Small or normal-sized left ventricle (RVG) Normal systolic function (RVG)	Small or normal-sized left ventricle (RVG) Vigorous systolic function (RVG) Asymmetric septal hypertrophy (RVG or ^{201}Ti)

Contd...

Types of Cardiomyopathy			
	Dilated	**Restrictive**	**Hypertrophic**
Cardiac catheterization	Left ventricular enlargement and dysfunction Mitral and/or tricuspid regurgitation Elevated left- and often right-sided filling pressures Diminished cardiac output	Diminished left ventricular compliance "Square root" sign in ventricular pressure recordings Preserved systolic function Elevated left- and right-sided filling pressures	Diminished left ventricular compliance Mitral regurgitation Vigorous systolic function Dynamic left ventricular outflow gradient
Valvular regurgitation	Related to annular dilation; mitral appears earlier, during decompensation; tricuspid regurgitation in late stages	Related to endocardial involvement; frequent mitral and tricuspid regurgitation, rarely severe	Related to valve-septum interaction; mitral regurgitation
Mechanism of heart failure	Impairment of contractility (**Systolic Dysfunction**)	Impairment of compliance (**Diastolic Dysfunction**)	Impairment of compliance (**Diastolic Dysfunction**)
Gross changes	**A-1:** All 4 chambers are dilated, most severe in the left ventricle which appears globular. Heart is usually enlarged and flabby (weighing approx 2-3 times from normal heart). The wall thickness may be normal as the hypertrophy is masked by the dilatation.	Ventricles are of approximately normal size or slightly enlarged, cavities are not dilated, myocardium is firm and non compliant.	**B-1:** Marked left ventricular hypertrophy, with asymmetric bulging of a very large interventricular septum into the left ventricular chamber (aka asymmetric septal hypertrophy)
Microscopic changes	**A-2:** Most muscle cells are hypertrophic with enlarged nuclei but some are attenuated, stretched and irregular. Interstitial and endocardial fibrosis of variable degree- blue on Trichome stain	There may be only patchy or diffuse interstitial fibrosis. Etiology specific findings can be seen.	**B-2:** Most important histologic features of myocardium in HCM are: • Extensive **myocyte hypertrophy** to a degree unusual in other conditions. • **Haphazard disarray** of bundles of myocyte, individual monocyte and sarcomere within cells (termed myofiber disarray) • **Interstitial fibrosis.**
Etiology	**Most common:** Alcoholic or Idiopathic **Infective:** Viral (Coxsackie, adenovirus, HIV, hepatitis C) Parasitic (T. Cruzi- Chagas' disease, toxoplasmosis) Bacterial (diphtheria), Spirochetal (Borellia burgdorferi- Lyme disease) Rickettsial- (Q fever), Fungal (with systemic infection) **Noninfective:** Granulomatous inflammatory disease (Sarcoidosis, Giant cell myocarditis) Hypersensitivity myocarditis, Polymyositis, dermatomyositis, Collagen vascular disease Peripartum cardiomyopathy, Transplant rejection	**Most common:** Amyloidosis **Infiltrative (Between Myocytes):** Amyloidosis (Primary-light chain amyloid, Familial-abnormal transthyretin, Senile-normal transthyretin or atrial peptides), Inherited metabolic defects **Storage (Within Myocytes):** Hemochromatosis (iron), *Inherited metabolic defects* (Pompe's, Forbes, Carnitine transport defect, Fabry's disease, Gaucher disease, Danon's disease (lysosome associated membrane protein, LAMP2), Hemochromatosis, Familial amyloidosis, Barth syndrome, Friedreich's ataxia)	**Most common:** Idiopathis Hypertrophic subaortic stinosis (IHSS) **Genetic:** This is the best characterized genetic cardiomyopathy, for which more than 400 individual mutations have been identified in 11 sarcomere genes. More than 80% of the mutations are in the beta-myosin heavy chain, the cardiac myosin-binding protein C, or cardiac troponin T **Pseudohypertrophic:** Inherited metabolic diseases **Secondary hypertrophy:** Cardiovascular causes

Contd...

Types of Cardiomyopathy			
	Dilated	Restrictive	Hypertrophic
	Toxic: Alcohol, Catecholamines: amphetamines, cocaine, Chemotherapeutic agents: (anthracyclines, trastuzumab), Interferon Other therapeutic agents (hydroxychloroquine, chloroquine), Drugs of misuse (emetine, anabolic steroids), Heavy metals: lead, mercury, Occupational exposure: hydrocarbons, arsenicals **Metabolic:** Nutritional deficiencies (thiamine, selenium, carnitine), Electrolyte deficiencies (calcium, phosphate, magnesium) Endocrinopathy (Thyroid disease Pheochromocytoma, Diabetes), Obesity, Hemochromatosis **Inherited Metabolic Pathway Defects:** (few) **Familial:** Skeletal and cardiac myopathy Dystrophin-related dystrophy (Duchenne's, Becker's), Mitochondrial myopathies (e.g., Kearns-Sayre syndrome), Arrhythmogenic ventricular dysplasia, Hemochromatosis **Overlap with Restrictive Cardiomyopathy :** Minimally dilated cardiomyopathy", Hemochromatosis, Amyloidosis, Hypertrophic cardiomyopathy ("burned-out") **Idiopathic:** **Miscellaneous:** Arrhythmogenic right ventricular dysplasia (may also affect left ventricle), Left ventricular noncompactiona, Peripartum cardiomyopathy **Tako-Tsubo Cardiomyopathy**	**Fibrotic:** Radiation, Scleroderma Endomyocardial: Tropical endomyocardial fibrosis Hypereosinophilic syndrome (Löffler's endocarditis), Carcinoid syndrome, Radiation, Drugs: e.g., serotonin, ergotamine **Overlap with Other Cardiomyopathies:** Hypertrophic cardio myopathy/"pseudohypertroph ic, Minimally dilated" cardiomyopathy (Early stage dilated cardiomyopathy, Partial recovery from dilated cardiomyopathy), Sarcoidosis **Idiopathic**	
Note: Restrictive cardiomyopathy is not a pathological entity but rather a description of hemodynamic condition due to stiffness of ventricles. Heart size and walls are essentially normal on gross.			

119. Ans. (d) Response to therapy

Ref: Robbin's 9th ed page 590, Devita's 6th ed p-2240, Nelson 17th ed p- 1695, Wintrobe's Clinical Hematology 11th ed Table 80.2, William's Haematology 8th ed

Wintrobes states: Many clinical and biologic characteristics previously identified as prognostic factors for adult patients with ALL have lost predictive value as therapy has evolved and become more intensive. In contrast, **age, WBC count at presentation, and initial response to therapy have remained strong predictors of outcome,** as have immunophenotypic and cytogenetic features

Three of the most important predictive factors are:
- Age of the patient at the time of diagnosis
- Initial leukocyte count
- Speed of response to treatment

Among these, response to the treatment with steroid is the most consistent prognostic marker.

Prognostic Factors of ALL		
Determinants	**Favourable**	**Unfavourable**
WBC count/µL	Low (<50000)	High (>100000)
Age	2-10 years	<1 and >10 years
Sex	Female	Male
Race	White	Black
Hepatosplenomegaly and lymphadenopathy	Absent	Present
Testicular involvement	Absent	Present
CNS	Absent	Overt
FAB classification	L1	L2
PLOIDY	Hyperdiploidy (>50 chromosomes)	Hypodiploidy (<45 chromosomes)
Cytogenetic markers	Trisomy 4, 10, 17 t(12:21) (TEL:AML1)	t(9:22) (BCR:ABL) t(4:11) (MLL AF4) t(1:19)
Time of remission	<14 days	>28 days
Minimal residual disease	$<10^{-4}$	$>10^{-3}$
Immunophenotype	Early pre B cell	T cell, pre B cell

- Failure to achieve Complete Remission within 4 weeks of starting treatment or after one course of induction chemotherapy has been considered an independent unfavorable prognostic factor
- Early pre-B cell ALL comprises approximately two-thirds of cases of childhood ALL and is associated with a favorable prognosis. Although most early pre-B lymphoblasts are CALLA positive, CALLA expression does not appear to have independent prognostic significance.
- Pre-B cell ALL accounts for approximately 20% of childhood ALL and has been associated with a poorer outcome compared to early pre-B cell ALL.

120. Ans. (b) Nutmeg liver with dark areas of perivenular viable hepatocytes and gray periportal areas of dead hepatocytes

Ref: Robbin's 9th ed page 129

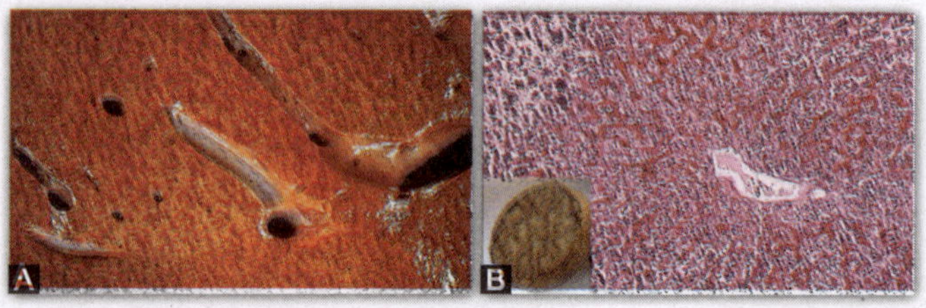

Figs A and B: (A) Chronic passive congestion gross; **(B)** Chronic passive congestion Histology

Nutmeg Liver; Liver with Chronic Passive Congestion and Hemorrhagic Necrosis

Morphology. The cut surfaces of congested tissues are often discolored due to the presence of high levels of poorly oxygenated blood. Microscopically, acute pulmonary congestion exhibits engorged alveolar capillaries often with alveolar septal edema and focal intra-alveolar hemorrhage. In chronic pulmonary congestion the septa are thickened and fibrotic, and the alveoli often contain numerous hemosiderin-laden macrophages called **heart failure cells.** In **acute hepatic congestion**, the central vein and sinusoids are distended; centrilobular hepatocytes can be frankly ischemic while the periportal hepatocytes—better oxygenated because of proximity to hepatic arterioles—may only develop fatty change. In **chronic passive hepatic congestion** the centrilobular regions are grossly red-brown and slightly depressed (because of cell death) and are accentuated against the surrounding zones of uncongested tan liver (nutmeg liver- so-called because it resembles the cut surface of a nutmeg). Microscopically, there is centrilobular hemorrhage, hemosiderin-laden macrophages, and degeneration of hepatocytes. Because the centrilobular area is at the distal end of the blood supply to the liver, it is prone to undergo necrosis whenever the blood supply is compromised.

NOTE

- Conditions associated with hepatic venous congestion causing nutmeg liver include:
  - Hepatic veno-occlusive disease
  - Budd-Chiari syndrome
  - Congestive hepatopathy - Right-sided cardiac decompensation (Right heart failure) constrictive pericarditis
- Nutmeg is the seed of the tree in genus Myristica, roughly egg-shaped

121. Ans. (a) Hodgkins lymphoma; EBV and Reed Sternberg cells

Ref: Robbin's 9th ed page 608-611, Wintrobe's Clinical Hematology 12th Ed Table 96.3 page 2155, William's Hematology 8th ed ch: 99, Nelson 19th ed page 1739

See Details of Hodgkin's Lymphoma in MAY 2017 PATHOLOGY (see page no. 356)

Clues from the History are

- **Age:** Lymphoma is the third most common cancer in pediatric age group. It is the most common cancer in adolescence accounting for > 25% of newly diagnosed cancers in persons **15 to 19** years old. Hodgkin's lymphoma is the most common malignancy in adolescence. It is uncommon less than 14 years of age.
- **Bilateral Lymphadenopathy:** Detection of an unusual mass or swelling in the superficial, supradiaphragmatic lymph nodes **(60–70% cervical and supraclavicular, 15–20% axillary) is the most common presentation of Hodgkin lymphoma**. Only 15 to 20 percent of patients have subdiaphragmatic disease at presentation.

Lymphadenopathy is usually **nontender** and has a "**rubbery**" consistency. Although any lymph node group can be involved, cervical and supraclavicular adenopathy are the most common physical findings in Hodgkin's lymphoma

122. Ans. (b) Barrett's esophagus, mucin stain, metaplasia

Ref: Robbin's 9th ed page 757, Basic histology Text and Atlas by Luiz Carlos Junqueira 11th ed chapter 4, Text Book of Histology Krishna Garg 4th Edn Page 93, 94

See Details of Barrett's Esophagus in AIIMS NOV 2017 PATHOLOGY (see page no. 352)

NOTE

In option (B) it was metaplasia not dysplasia. Metaplasia is mandatory for diagnosis of Barrett, however different grades of dysplasia may or may not be seen with Barrett

Metaplasia, Dysplasia and Neoplasia

	Metaplasia	Dysplasia	Neoplasia
Definition	One differentiated cell type is replaced by another cell type	Loss in uniformity of the individual cells as well as loss in their architectural orientation	Abnormal mass of tissue, the growth of which exceeds and is un-coordinated and persist in the same excessive manner after cessation of the stimuli.
Reversibility	Reversible	May or may not be reversible	Non reversible
Tissue of occurrence	Occurs in both epithelial (squamous, columnar) and mesenchymal/ connective tissue (osseous, cartilaginous)	Occurs only in epithelium.	Occurs in almost all types of tissue of the body.
Cellular changes	Normal differentiation maintained, only cell type changes.	**Distorted cellular development i.e. Pleomorphism**, nuclear hypercromatia with a high nuclear to-cytoplasmic ratio, mitosis, loss of polarity, ***loss in the uniformity*** *of the individual cells as well as a* ***loss in their architectural orientation***	**Benign:** Well differentiated single cell proliferation with or without atypia. **Malignant:** Variable degree of differentiation and pleomorphism (Well differentiated to anaplastic), high Nucleo Cytoplasmic ratio, hyperchromatic nuclei, irregular nuclear membrane, prominent nucleoli.
Mitosis	Normal in number, location and configuration	Increase in number, normal configuration, confined within epithelium.	Increase in number, abnormal configuration and bizzare mitotic figure (malignant tumors), spread in adjacent structures.
Mechanism	Reprogramming of stem cells through cytokines, growth factors.	When chronic irritation continues in metaplastic or hyperplastic tissue.	Genetic changes due to external stimuli allow excessive and unregulated proliferation that becomes autonomous
Natural history	Reversible on withdrawal of stimuli	May regress on removal stimulus or may progress to higher grade of dysplasia or carcinoma in situ	Not reversible

Contd...

Metaplasia, Dysplasia and Neoplasia			
	Metaplasia	**Dysplasia**	**Neoplasia**
Example	• **Columnar to squamous-** Respiratory epithelium in chronic smoker and vitamin A deficiency, excretory duct epithelium of salivary gland pancreas or bile duct due to stones • **Squamous to columnar** – Barrett's esophagus Bone formation in muscles: Myositis ossificans	• Cervix – Carcinoma in situ • Bronchial mucosa • Barrett's oesophagus	• Benign: Lipoma, Fibroma, Chondroma, Adenoma, Papilloma, Cystadenoma etc • Malignant: Carcinoma- Squamous cell carcinoma, Melanoma, Adenocarcinoma etc • Sarcoma- Fibrosarcoma, Chondrosarcoma, Rhabdomyosarcoma, Leiomyosarcoma, Liposarcoma etc

Footnote
- **Anaplasia: Lack of differentiation, mostly seen in malignant neoplasia**
- **When dysplastic changes are marked and involved the entire thickness of epithelium but the lesion remain confined by the basement membrane, it is considered as preinvasive neoplasm and referred to as *carcinoma in situ***

AIIMS MAY 2015

123. Ans. (c) Dichroic mirror

Ref: Bailey and Scott 13th ed page 76-79

This topic was asked because of the latest Nobel Prize. On October 8, 2014, the Nobel Prize in Chemistry was awarded to **Eric Betzig, William Moerner and Stefan Hell** for development of super-resolved fluorescence microscopy.

A **fluorescence microscope** is an optical microscope that uses fluorescence and phosphorescence instead of, or in addition to, reflection and absorption. Typical components of a fluorescence microscope are a **light source** (xenon arc lamp or mercury-vapor lamp are common; more advanced forms are high-power LEDs and lasers), the **excitation filter**, the **dichroic mirror** (or dichroic beamsplitter), and the **emission filter**.

Principle: Certain dyes, called fluors or fluorochromes, can be raised to a higher energy level after absorbing ultraviolet (excitation) light. When the dye molecules return to their normal, lower energy state, they release excess energy in the form of visible (fluorescent) light. This process is called fluorescence.

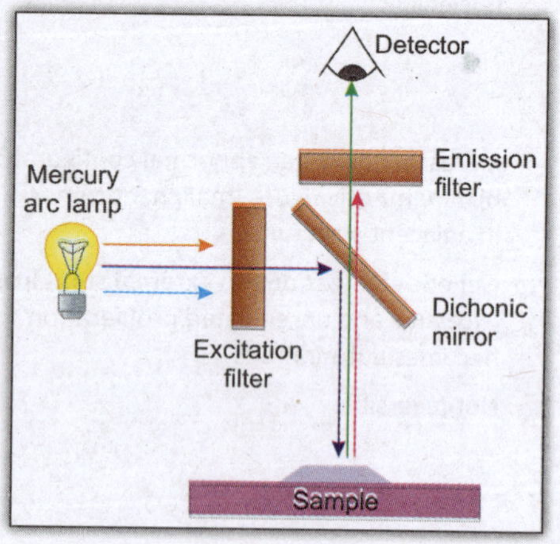

An excitation filter passes light of the desired wavelength to excite the fluorochrome that has been used to stain the specimen. A barrier filter in the objective lens prevents the excitation wavelengths from damaging the eyes of the observer. When observed through the ocular lens, fluorescing objects appear brightly lit against a dark background. The color of the fluorescent light depends on the dye and light filters used.

Fluorescent dye	Acridine orange	Auramine	Calcoflour White
Excitation light	Blue	Blue	Violet
Exciter filter Wavelength	450-490 λ	450-490 λ	355-425 λ
Barrier filter Wavelength	515 λ	515 λ	460 λ
Use	It stains all nucleic acids, so it is non-specific. All microorganisms and host cells will stain and give a bright orange fluorescence	For mycobacteria. They appear bright yellow or orange against a greenish background	For detection of fungi and some parasites such as microsporidia

124. Ans. (a) Frozen specimen

Ref: Sternberg's Diagnostic Surgical Pathology 5th ed page 980

Oil red O is physical method of staining that relies on the affinity for solubility of dye in lipid than the dye solvent. Alcoholic fixatives should be avoided because they act as lipid solvents. A positive control is usually not needed as most of the tissue contains some fat. Oil red O staining must be performed on cryostat sectioned frozen tissue. Lipids are solubilized by organic solvents used in traditional paraffin embedding.

Lipid Stains	Sudan stains (Sudan III, IV, Sudan Back-B, Oil Red O)	Oil Red O (AKA Sudan Red) largely replaced Sudan III and Sudan IV. Used for staining neutral triglycerides and lipids on frozen sections and some lipoproteins on paraffin sections. Oil Red O is also used in a technique for staining latent fingerprints
	Osmium tetra oxide	As a lipid stain, it is useful in scanning electron microscopy (SEM)

125. Ans. (a) Anticipation

Ref: Robbin's pathology 9th ed page 242, 804

Anticipation: This term refers to the phenomenon whereby clinical features of genetic syndrome worsen with each successive generation, as if the mutation becomes increasingly deleterious as it is transmitted from a man to his grandsons and great-grandsons. Anticipation is common in trinucleotide repeat disorders, such as Huntington's disease and myotonic dystrophy, where a dynamic mutation in DNA occurs.

Examples of Diseases Showing Anticipation	
Autosomal dominant	Several spinocerebellar ataxias Huntington's disease – CAG Myotonic dystrophy – CTG Dyskeratosis congenita – TTAGGG (telomere repeat sequence)
Autosomal recessive	Friedreich ataxia (GAA triplet repeat) (Note: Friedreich ataxia does not usually exhibit anticipation because it is an autosomal recessive disorder.
X linked	Fragile X syndrome – CGG
Without expression type	Crohn's disease Behçet's disease

Terms used in Genetics and Inheritance	
Anticipation	This term refers to the phenomenon whereby clinical features of genetic syndrome worsen with each successive generation, as if the mutation becomes increasingly deleterious as it is transmitted from a man to his grandsons and great-grandsons. Anticipation is common in trinucleotide repeat disorders, such as **Huntington's disease** and **myotonic dystrophy**, where a dynamic mutation in DNA occurs
Dominance	Dominance in genetics is a relationship between alleles of one gene, in which the effect on phenotype of one allele masks the contribution of a second allele at the same locus. The first allele is dominant and the second allele is recessive. The first allele is dominant and the second allele is recessive. For genes on an autosome (any chromosome other than a sex chromosome), the alleles and their associated traits are autosomal dominant or autosomal recessive. Dominance is a key concept in **Mendelian inheritance** and classical genetics.
Codominance	Although gene expression and Mendelian traits are usually described as dominant or recessive, in some cases both of the alleles of gene pair contribute to the phenotype a condition called co-dominance. **Histocompatibility and blood group** antigens are good example of condominant inheritance.
Epistasis	Epistasis is the phenomenon of the effect of one gene being dependent on the presence of one or more 'modifier genes', the genetic background. Thus, epistatic mutations have different effects in combination than individually. if genes A and B are mutated, and each mutation by itself produces a unique phenotype but the two mutations together show the same phenotype as the gene A mutation, then gene A is epistatic and gene B is hypostatic. For example, the **gene for male pattern baldness is epistatic to the gene for red hair**
Pleiotropism	In pleiotropism, a single gene affects a number of phenotypic traits in the same organism. These pleiotropic effects often seem to be unrelated to each other. Consequently, a mutation in a pleiotropic gene may have an effect on some or all traits simultaneously. An example is **phenylketonuria**, a human disease that affects multiple systems but is caused by one gene defect
Mosaicism	Mosaicism denotes the presence of two or more populations of cells with different genotypes in one individual who has developed from a single fertilized egg. Mosaicism can result from various mechanisms including chromosome non-disjunction, anaphase lag and endoreplication. The most common form of mosaicism found through prenatal diagnosis involves **trisomies.** In rare cases, **intersex** conditions can be caused by mosaicism where some cells in the body have XX and others XY chromosomes (46, XX/XY)
Genetic Heterogeneity	Genetic heterogeneity is a phenomenon in which a single phenotype or genetic disorder may be caused by any one of a multiple number of alleles or non-allele (locus) mutations. **Mental Illnesses, Autism, Cystic fibrosis, Retinitis Pigmentosa**

126. Ans. (a) Co dominance

Ref: Robbin's pathology 9th ed page 140

See Table of Terms Used in Genetics and Inheritance in Previous Question

127. Ans. (a) Gynecomastia with long thin limbs

Ref: Robbin's 9th ed page 166-167, Nelson 18th ed ch 81 and 56, Harrison's 18th ed table 349-2

Karyotype is 47 XXY which is of Klinefelter's syndrome

Klinefelter's Syndrome	
Genetics	The chromosomal aberration most often results from meiotic nondisjunction of an X chromosome during parental gametogenesis; the extra **X chromosome is maternal in origin in 54% and paternal in origin in 46% of patients.** Increased maternal age predisposes to meiotic nondisjunction and to this syndrome, but in most instances maternal age is not advanced. The ***47,XXY complement is the most common chromosomal pattern in persons with Klinefelter syndrome (80%);*** some have mosaic patterns
Incidence	Approximately 1/500 newborn males has a 47,XXY chromosome complement, representing the most common sex chromosomal aneuploidy in males
Clinical Features	
Psychiatric behaviour	Because behavioral or psychiatric disorders may often be apparent long before defects in sexual development, the condition should be considered in all boys with mental retardation and in children with psychosocial, learning, or school adjustment problems. Affected children may be *anxious, immature, excessively shy, or aggressive, and they may engage in antisocial acts.* **Fire-setting behavior** has been observed in some of these children
IQ and Learning	Full-scale IQ scores may be normal, with verbal IQ being somewhat decreased. Verbal cognitive defects and underachievement in reading, spelling, and mathematics are common. By late adolescence, most boys with Klinefelter syndrome have generalized learning disabilities, most of which are language based, and are 4 to 5 grade levels behind.
Physical characteristic	The height of patients with Klinefelter's syndrome tends to be increased. The patients tend to be **tall, slim, and underweight** and to have **relatively long legs,** but body habitus can vary markedly.
Sexual characteristic	The **testes tend to be small for age**, but this sign may become apparent only after puberty, when normal testicular growth fails to occur. The phallus tends to be smaller than average, and **cryptorchidism or hypospadias** may occur in a few patients. About 80% of adults have **gynecomastia;** they have sparser facial hair, most shaving less often than daily. The most common testicular lesions are spermatogenic arrest and Sertoli cell predominance. **Azoospermia and infertility** are usual, although rare instances of fertility are known. Antisperm antibodies have been detected in one quarter of tested specimens. Decreased libido
Other	Increased risk of breast tumors, thromboembolic disease, obesity, diabetes mellitus, varicose veins

128. Ans. (c) Von-Willebrand factor

Ref: Robbin's 9th ed page 80, 117, Dacie and Lewis Practical Haematology 11th Ed page 395-396

Activation of Platelets

The main step in platelet function are adhesion, activation with shape change and aggregation. When the vessel wall is damaged, the subendothelial structures, including basement membrane, collagen and microfibrils, are exposed. Platelet adhesion to the subendothelium of an injured vessel wall is a complex process that requires the contributions of several adhesive proteins.

Endothelial injury brings platelets into contact with the subendothelial ECM, which includes among its constituents *Von-Willebrand factor (vWF),* a large multimeric protein that is synthesized by EC. vWF is held fast to the ECM through interactions with collagen and also binds tightly to Gp1b, a glycoprotein found on the surface of platelets. These interactions allow vWF to act as a sort of molecular glue that binds platelets tightly to denuded vessel walls.

vWF binds to collagen and microfibrils and then captures platelet via initial binding to GPIb. Resulting in initial monolayer of adhering platelets. Fibronectin is an essential adhesive substrate in many fundamental biological processes. Platelets possess 2 main receptors for this protein, α5β1 and αIIbβ3. Platelet adhesion to purified fibronectin has been shown to depend on both glycoprotein (GP) IIb/IIIa and very late antigen (VLA)-5 under both static and flow conditions.

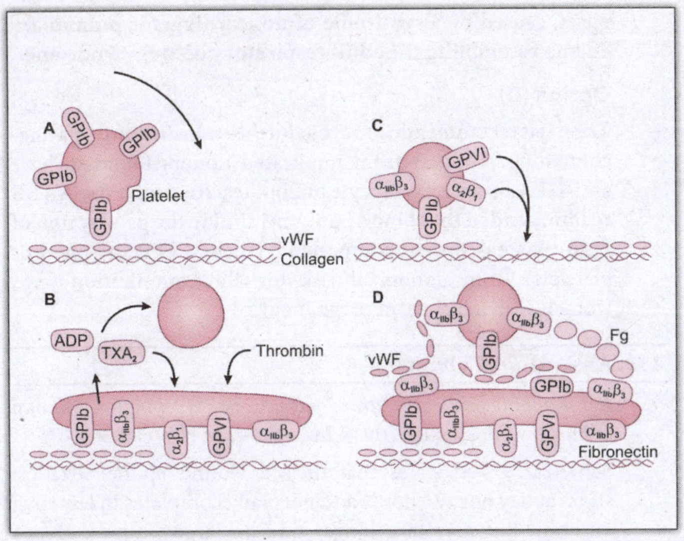

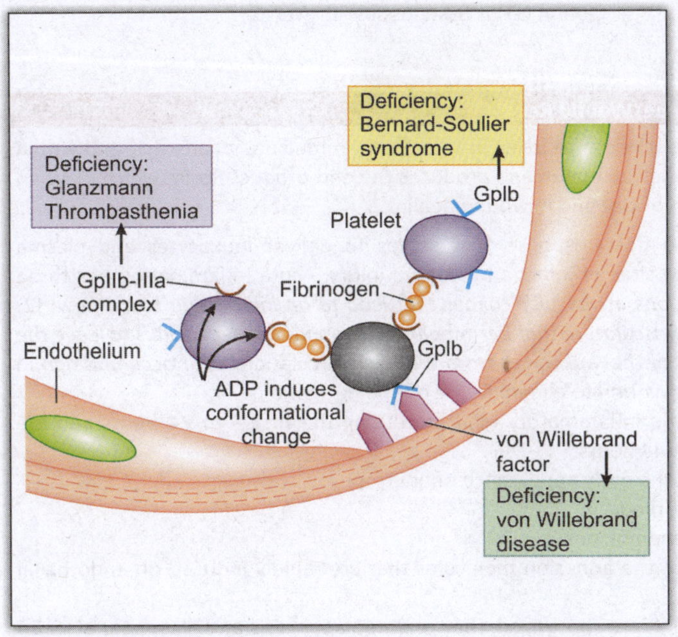

129. Ans. (a) Mast cell

Ref: Robbin's 9th ed page 111

Immediate hypersensitivity is a tissue reaction that occurs rapidly (typically within minutes) after the interaction of antigen with IgE antibody that is bound to the surface of mast cells in a sensitized host. The reaction is initiated by entry of an antigen, which is called an allergen because it triggers allergy. Many allergens are environmental substances that are harmless for most persons on exposure. Some people apparently inherit genes that make them susceptible to allergies. This susceptibility is manifested by the propensity of such persons to mount strong TH2 responses and, subsequently, to produce IgE antibody against the allergens. The IgE is central to the activation of the mast cells and release of mediators that are responsible for the clinical and pathologic manifestations of the reaction. Immediate hypersensitivity may occur as a local reaction that is merely annoying (e.g., seasonal rhinitis, or hay fever), severely debilitating (asthma), or even fatal (anaphylaxis).

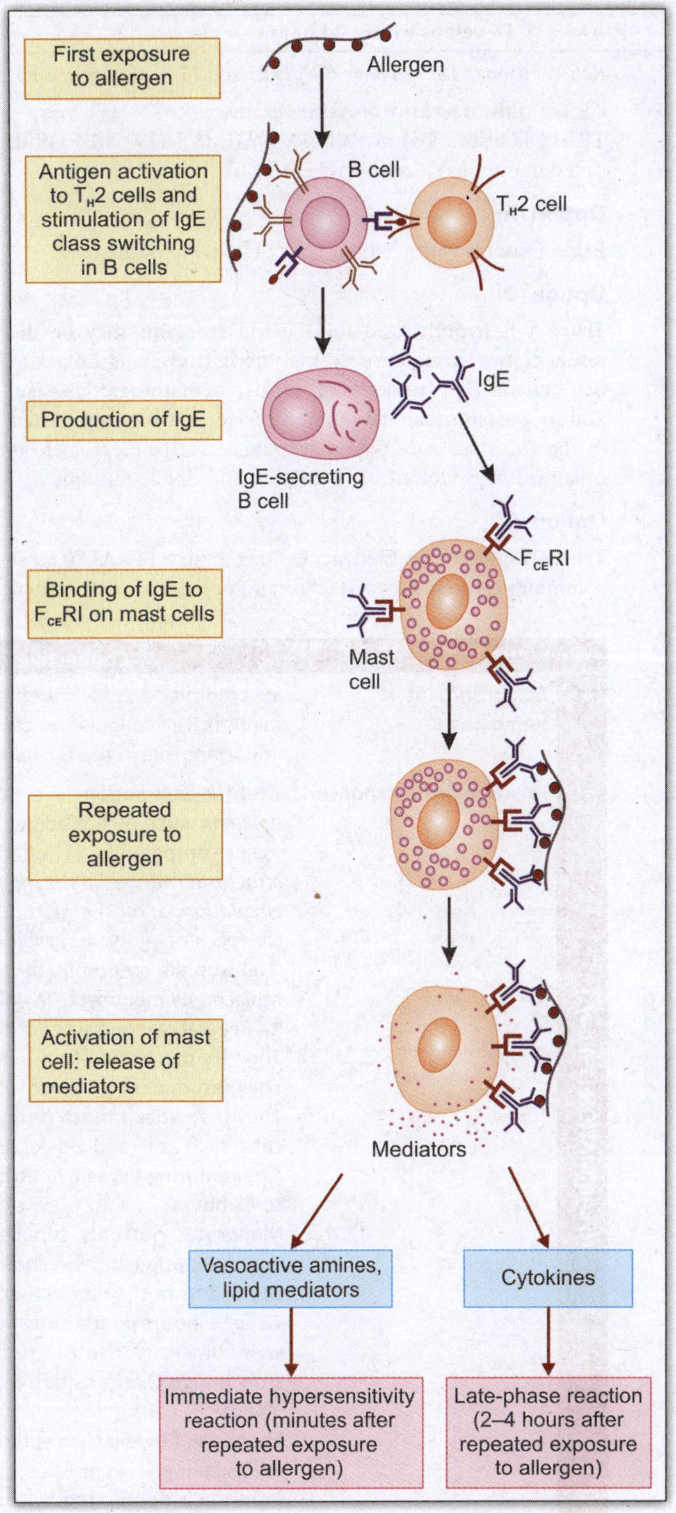

130. Ans. (a) Fresh frozen plasma

Ref: Wintrobe 12th ed page 677, Harrison 19th ed page 138 e3

See Table of " Blood Components and Indications for Use" in AIIMS MAY 2018 PATHOLOGY (see page no. 339)

Frozen blood products (plasma, cryoprecipitate) take 10 to 30 minutes to thaw. It may take the same amount of time to perform an uncomplicated cross match.

131. Ans. (a) Develops within 24 hours

Ref: Wintrobe's 12th ed page 699, Harrison 19th ed page 138 e5

TRALI is the new Love of AIIMS exams

TRALI is also asked in Pathology AIIMS NOV 2016 (With different options) (See for table of TRALI)

Option (A)

False: Onset is within 6 hour (not 24 hour) of transfusion

Option (B)

True: It is hypothesized that TRALI reactions may be the result of two cumulative events: the first event is linked to the patient (i.e., **underlying sepsis, hematologic disease, and/or postsurgical status**), and the second event is related to the transfusion of potential granulocyte primers such as inflammatory cytokines, active lipids, and/or alloantibodies.

Option (C)

True: Transfusion-related acute lung injury (TRALI) most commonly presents as severe respiratory distress of sudden onset, caused by a **syndrome of noncardiogenic pulmonary edema resembling the adult respiratory distress syndrome.**

Option (D)

True: It is recommended to avoid further transfusion of plasma-containing products from implicated donors found to have anti-HLA or antigranulocyte antibodies. **Recently, the AABB recommended that blood banks minimize the production of high-plasma-content components** (such as FFP and pheresis platelets) from donors at risk for alloimmunization (e.g., women with a history of pregnancy)

132. Ans. (d) 24-72 hours

Ref: Robbin's pathology 9th ed page 65-66, Washington Manual of Surgery 5th ed page 109, Schwartz 9th ed ch 9

Schwartz 9th ed states that incised wound epithelialization starts at day one (24 hour) and normally completes in less than 48 hour, But may take longer time in large wounds. Hence Option (D) is best possible answer

Connective Tissue/Wound Repair		
INFLAMMATION (1-4 days)	**Establishment of hemostasis**	Severed blood vessels with any smooth muscles in their walls immediately constrict, and within minutes, the coagulation cascade is initiated and produces the end-product fibrin, which plays an important role in the formation of clot and in wound healing.
	Inflammatory response	*Acute inflammation* is a rapid host response that serves to deliver leukocytes and plasma proteins, such as antibodies, to sites of infection or tissue injury. Acute inflammation has three major components: (1) *alterations in vascular caliber that lead to an increase in blood flow*, (2) *structural changes in the microvasculature that permit plasma proteins and leukocytes to leave the circulation*, and (3) *emigration of the leukocytes* from the microcirculation, *their accumulation* in the focus of injury, and *their activation* to eliminate the offending agent Neutrophils predominate in the inflammatory infiltrate during the **first 6 to 24 hours** and are replaced by monocytes in 24 to 48 hours. • Several reasons account for the early appearance of neutrophils: They are more numerous in the blood They respond more rapidly to chemokines They may attach more firmly to the adhesion molecules that are rapidly induced on endothelial cells, such as P- and E-selectins. After entering tissues, neutrophils are short-lived; they **undergo apoptosis and disappear after 24 to 48 hours.** Monocytes not only survive longer but may proliferate in the tissues, and thus become the dominant population in chronic inflammatory reactions. Derived from circulating monocytes, **macrophages achieve significant numbers in the wound by 48 to 96 hours postinjury** and remain present until wound healing is complete (Schwartz 9th ed) Less numerous than macrophages, T-lymphocyte numbers peak at about 1 week postinjury and truly bridge the transition from the inflammatory to the proliferative phase of healing (Schwartz 9th ed) There are, however, exceptions to this pattern of cellular infiltration. In certain infections—for example, those produced by **Pseudomonas bacteria—the cellular infiltrate is dominated by continuously recruited neutrophils for several days; in viral infections, lymphocytes may be the first cells to arrive; in some hypersensitivity reactions, eosinophils may be the main cell type.**

Contd...

PROLIFERATION (4 -12 days)	**Epithelialization and angiogenesis**	Endothelial cells also proliferate extensively during this phase of healing. These cells participate in the formation of new capillaries (angiogenesis), a process essential to successful wound healing. Epithelialization is the critical aspect of wound-healing events. It restores the barrier between the wound and the external environment. **The process begins within 1 day of injury and is seen as thickening of the epidermis at the wound edge. Re-epithelialization is complete in less than 48 hours in the case of approximated incised wounds, but may take substantially longer in the case of larger wounds, in which there is a significant epidermal/dermal defect** (Schwartz 9th ed). Epithelialization of wounds occurs via the migration of epithelial cells from the edges of the wound and from remaining epidermal skin appendages. Migration of epithelial cells occurs at the rate of **1 mm/day** in clean, open wounds. Primarily closed wounds have a contiguous epithelial layer at **24 to 48 hours.** (Washington Manual of surgery 5th ed)
	Migration and proliferation of fibroblasts/Granulation	Migration and proliferation of fibroblasts and deposition of connective tissue, which, together with abundant vessels and interspersed leukocytes, has a pink, granular appearance and hence is called *granulation tissue.* **By 3 to 5 days, the specialized granulation tissue that is characteristic of healing is apparent**. Collagen is the main protein secreted by fibroblasts. It provides strength and structure and facilitates cell motility in the wound. **Collagen is synthesized at an accelerated rate for 2 to 4 weeks**, greatly contributing to the tensile strength of the wound. Oxygen, vitamin C, α-ketoglutarate, and iron are important cofactors for the cross-linkage of collagen fibers. If these are not present, wound healing may be poor. **Wound contraction begins 4 to 5 days after wounding and continues for 12 to 15 days** or longer if the wound remains open.
MATURATION	**Scar formation** **Connective tissue remodeling**	The deposition of matrix at the wound site follows a characteristic pattern: *Fibronectin and collagen type III constitute the early matrix scaffolding, glycosaminoglycans and proteoglycans represent the next significant matrix components, and collagen type I is the final matrix* (Schwartz 9th ed) Maturation and reorganization of the fibrous tissue (remodeling) to produce the stable fibrous scar. It begins at approximately **21 days after wounding**. At the outset of scar remodeling, collagen synthesis is downregulated, and the cellularity of the wound decreases. During scar remodeling, collagen is broken down and replaced by new collagen that is denser and organized along the lines of stress.

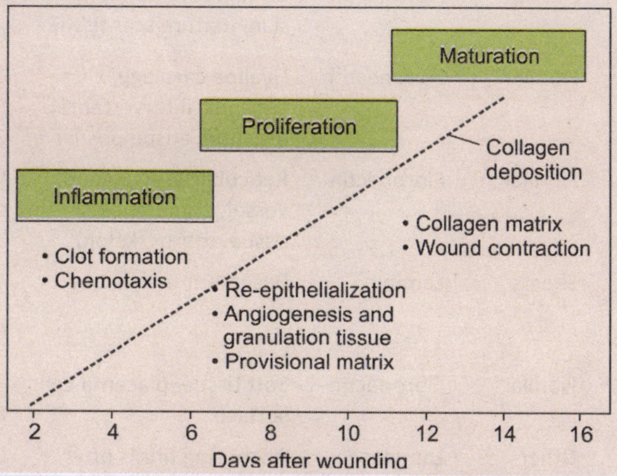

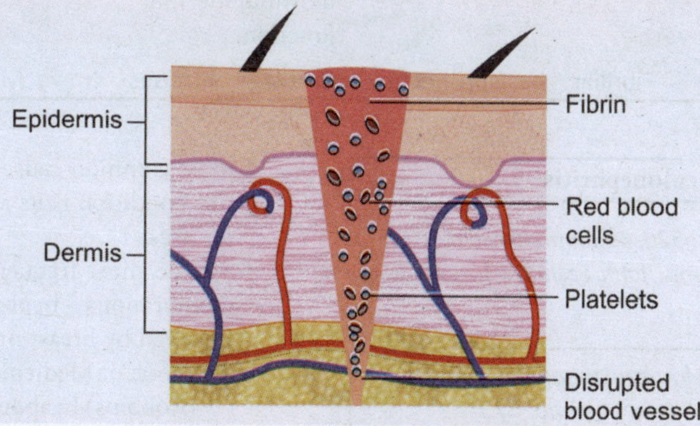

Contd...

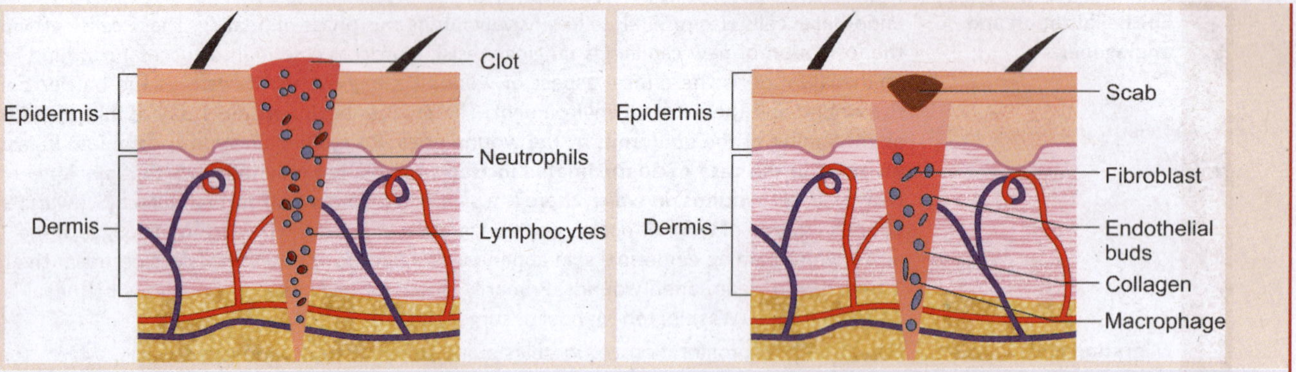

Wound Strength:

- Carefully sutured wound have tensile strength of 70% of unwounded skin largely because of placement of sutures
- When sutures are removed, usually at the end of first week the wound strength is approximately 10%
- **Then there is rapid gain of strength for next 4 weeks**
- **By 6 months, the wound reaches 80% of the bursting strength of unwounded tissue.** It is important to note that a well-healed wound never achieves the strength of unwounded tissue. This process reaches a plateau at 12 to 18 months, but it may last indefinitely. (Washington Manual of Surgery)

133. Ans. (d) Type IV

Ref: Robbin's 9th ed page 63

Types of Collagen and Associated Diseases

	Chains	Structure	Anchor	Tissue	Disease
TYPE 1 (MC=90%)	2(a1)+(a2)	Fibrillar	Fibronectin	Bone, teeth, tendon, skin, mature scar tissue	Arthrochalasis EDS-type 7 Osteogenesis imperfecta
TYPE 2	3 (a1)	Fibrillar	Fibronectin	Hyaline cartilage, vitreous, intervertebral disc (nucleuspulposus)	Collaginopathies type 2 and 11e.g. Stickler syndrome Achondrogenesis type 2
TYPE 3	3 (a1)	Fibrillar	Fibronectin	Reticular fibers, blood vessel, granulation tissue, uterus, keloid	Vascular Ehlers-Danlossyndrome (EDS)-type-3, Hypermobility EDS-type-4
TYPE 4	2(a1)+(a2) all BM or (a3-6) GBM	Sheets	Laminin	Basement membrane	Alport syndrome Goodpasture's syndrome
TYPE 5	(a1)+(a2)+(a3)	Fibrillar	Fibronectin	Soft tissue, placenta,cell surface	Ehlers-Danlos syndrome (EDS), classical-type 1 and 2
TYPE 7	3(a1)	Other	Laminin	Anchoring fibrils of dermoepidermal junction	Dystrophic epidermolysis bullosa
TYPE 9	(a1)+(a2)+(a3)	Fibrillar	Fibronectin	Cartilage, vitreous	Multiple epiphyseal dysplasia

134. Ans. (a) Membranous glomerulonephritis

Ref: Robbin's 9th ed page 526, Comprehensive Clinical Nephrology By Richard J. Johnson, John Feehally, Jurgen Floege 5th ed page 335

See Table of Major Primary Glomerulonephritis in Pathology AIIMS Nov 2016 (see page no. 373)

Membranous nephropathy is the most common nephropathy associated with malignancy. Membranous nephropathy is the most common cause of NS in the elderly. A unique feature of this condition is its association with malignancy in up to 20% of cases.

The most frequently reported carcinoma associated with membranous nephropathy is bronchogenic carcinoma, followed by breast or gastric and colon adenocarcinoma (API Textbook of Medicine 9th ed Page 1625)

(Robbins) In about 85% of cases, membranous nephropathy is caused by autoantibodies that cross-react with antigens expressed by podocytes. In the remainder (secondary membranous nephropathy), it occurs secondary to other disorders, including

- Infections (chronic hepatitis B, syphilis, schistosomiasis, malaria)
- Malignant tumors, particularly carcinoma of the lung and colon and melanoma
- Systemic lupus erythematosus and other autoimmune conditions
- Exposure to inorganic salts (gold, mercury)
- Drugs (penicillamine, captopril, nonsteroidal antiinflammatory agents)

135. Ans. (b) Hypersensitivity reaction with modified macrophages, lymphocytes and giant cells

Ref: Robbin's 9 th ed page 480

The clinical picture is of Tuberculosis.

Microscopically, the inflammation produced with TB infection is **granulomatous**, with epithelioid macrophages and Langhans giant cells along with lymphocytes, plasma cells, maybe a few PMN's, fibroblasts with collagen, and characteristic **caseous necrosis** in the center. The inflammatory response is mediated by a **type IV hypersensitivity** reaction. This can be utilized as a basis for diagnosis by a TB skin test.

Caseous necrosis is encountered most often in foci of **tuberculous infection.** The term **"caseous" (cheeselike)** is derived from the friable white appearance of the area of necrosis. On microscopic examination, the necrotic area appears as a collection of fragmented or lysed cells and amorphous granular debris enclosed within a distinctive inflammatory border; this appearance is characteristic of a focus of inflammation known as a granuloma.

A granuloma is a focus of chronic inflammation consisting of a microscopic aggregation of macrophages that are transformed into epithelium-like cells, surrounded by a collar of mononuclear leukocytes, principally lymphocytes and occasionally plasma cells. Frequently, epithelioid cells fuse to form giant cells in the periphery or sometimes in the center of granulomas. These giant cells may attain diameters of 40 to 50 μm. They have a large mass of cytoplasm containing 20 or more small nuclei arranged either peripherally **(Langhans-type giant cell)** or haphazardly **(foreign body–type giant cell).** There is no known functional difference between these two types of giant cells, yet some pathologists persist in describing them—perhaps because they make nice exam questions!

Immune granulomas are caused by a variety of agents that are capable of inducing a cell-mediated immune response. This type of immune response produces granulomas usually when the inciting agent is poorly degradable or particulate. In such responses macrophages engulf foreign protein antigen, process it, and present peptides to antigen-specific T lymphocytes, causing their activation. The responding T cells produce cytokines, such as IL-2, which activates other T cells, perpetuating the response, and IFN-γ, which is important in activating macrophages and transforming them into epithelioid cells and multinucleate giant cells.

The prototype of the immune granuloma is that caused by infection with ***Mycobacterium tuberculosis.*** In this disease the granuloma is referred to as a tubercle. It is often characterized by the presence of central caseous necrosis. In contrast, caseous necrosis is rare in other granulomatous diseases. The morphologic patterns in the various granulomatous diseases may be sufficiently different to allow reasonably accurate diagnosis by an experienced pathologist.

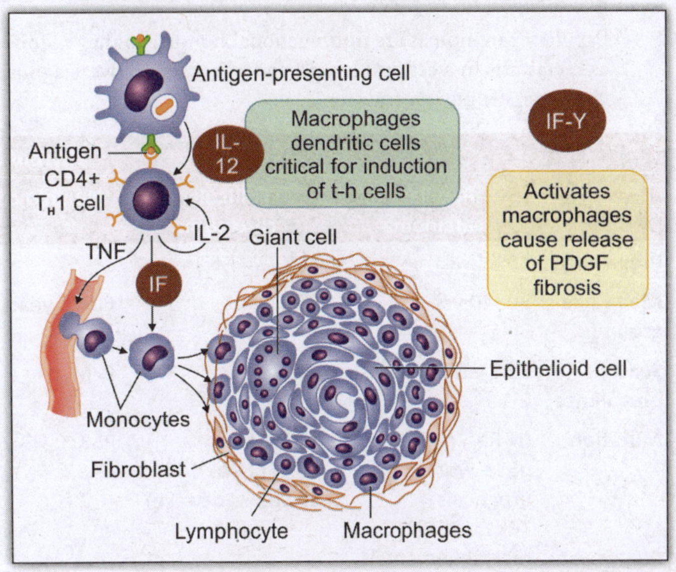

Fig: Mechanism of type IV hypersensitivity in formation of granuloma

Diseases with Granulomatous Inflammation		
Disease	**Cause**	**Tissue reaction**
Tuberculosis	*Mycobacterium tuberculosis*	**Caseating granuloma** (tubercle): focus of activated macrophages (epithelioid cells), rimmed by fibroblasts, lymphocytes, histiocytes, occasional Langhans giant cells; central necrosis with amorphous granular debris; acid-fast bacilli
Leprosy	*Mycobacterium leprae*	Acid-fast bacilli in macrophages; **noncaseating granulomas**
Syphilis	*Treponema pallidum*	Gumma: microscopic to grossly visible lesion, enclosing wall of histiocytes; plasma cell infiltrate; central cells necrotic without loss of cellular outline
Cat-scratch disease	Gram-negative bacillus	Rounded or stellate granuloma containing central granular debris and recognizable neutrophils; giant cells uncommon
Sarcoidosis	Unknown etiology	**Noncaseating granulomas** with abundant activated macrophages
Crohn disease (inflammatory bowel disease)	Immune reaction against intestinal bacteria, self-antigens	Occasional **noncaseating granulomas** in the wall of the intestine, with dense chronic inflammatory infiltrate

136. Ans. (a) Papillary

Ref: Robbin's 9th ed page 733

Papillary carcinomas are nonfunctional tumors, so they manifest most often as a painless mass in the neck, either within the thyroid or as metastasis in a cervical lymph node. A preoperative diagnosis usually can be established by fine-needle aspiration on the basis of the characteristic nuclear features.

Thyroid Carcinoma						
	Papillary carcinoma	Follicular carcinoma	Hurthle cell Ca	Anaplastic carcinoma	Medullary carcinoma	Lymphoma
Prevalence	80% (MC)	10% (2nd MC)	3%	1%	5%	<1%
Mean Age group	30- 40 yrs	> 50 years	60-75 years	Elderly (7th to 8th decade)	Familial c- young age, Sporadic- 50-60 years	Older pts (Late 60's)
Sex prevalence	F:M ratio 2:1	F:M 3:1	F>M	F>M	F:M ratio 1.5:1	F:M ratio 2:1
Mutation	(N-Ras, gsp, c-myc, p53)- worse prognosis. TRK1, (RET/PTC rearrangements) MET PTEN (rare)	MET, RAS PTEN (asso. With Cowden's disease)	P53 RAS	P53 P21/WAF LOH	RET protooncogene (sporadic & familial) APC	
Risk factors	**External radiation** especially <5 years of age (usually 5 years after exposure)	Geographical distribution with **Iodine deficiency** causing long standing goitre	Radiation to neck, Iodide deficiency	Dedifferentiation in setting of previous thyroid pathology **(preexisting goiter**, FTC, PTC)	**Familial MEN 2A or 2B**, C cell hyperplasia may be premalignant	**Hashimoto's disease**
Cell type	Follicular	Follicular	Follicular, oxyphilic cells	wide variety of cell types	Parathyroid C cells	Non Hodgkin's B cell type
Pathology	Very seldom encapsulated, well-defined follicles with only minimal papillary architecture, **Orphan Annie eye nuclei, Psammoma bodies**	Majority are encapsulated Follicles containing colloid are present	Variant of Follicular, Abundant, granular, eosinophilic cytoplasm due to abundant mitochondria **(Hurthle/ Askanazy cells),** vascular or capsular invasion	Regions of spontaneous necrosis and hemorrhage. **Angioinvasion**, Spindle cell, giant cell (osteoclast like) with intranuclear cytoplasmic invaginations	Neuroendocrine neoplasms, Presence of **amyloid stroma,** MCT is associated with the secretion of **calcitonin** (but not associated with hypocalcemia)	
Origin	Solitary or multifocal	Solitary mostly	Often multifocal & bilateral (about 30%)		Familial cases are multicentric	
Clinical features	Slow growing painless thyroid mass, cervical lymphadenopathy is a common initial presentation	Painless thyroid mass, 1% cases maybe associated with hyperthyroidism, cervical lymphadenopathy is an uncommon initial presentation (about 5%)	Painful palpable thyroid mass (MC clinical sign). Symptoms more suggestive of malignancy (dysphagia, dyspnea, coughing, choking spells, hoarseness)	Dysphonia, Dysphagia, Dyspnea, cervical tenderness, and a painful, rapidly enlarging neck mass. Early fixity to adjacent structures is characteristic. SVC syndrome can also be part of the findings	The presence of both neck mass and an elevated calcitonin level is virtually diagnostic of MCT, Unilateral (80%) in sporadic disease, bilateral in 90% of familial patients. Palpable cervical lymphadenopathy (15 to 20%). Diarrhoea may be seen in some cases (due to secretion of 5HT)	Rapidly growing painless mass (Goitre) in a short period Respiratory distress, hoarseness, fever, dysphagia

Contd...

Thyroid Carcinoma						
	Papillary carcinoma	Follicular carcinoma	Hurthle cell Ca	Anaplastic carcinoma	Medullary carcinoma	Lymphoma
Metastasis	Lymph node (**Lateral aberrant thyroid**) Blood borne (less common, occur esp. If extra thyroidal, i.e infiltrated capsule) to lungs	Lymph node involvement is unusual & occurs in <10% of cases. Blood borne distant spread is more common (**Osteolytic bone mets**, lung, liver)	Unlike PTC & FTC, spread to lymph nodes is a poor prognosis (70% mortality), More invasive than FTC, metastasize more frequently to bones	Direct spread	Early spread to lymphatics, Later **Osteoblastic** to bones	Lymphatic
Investigations	FNAC of mass or lymph node, Tumour marker: **Thyroglobulin** (no prognostic value pre surgical)	In 1% cases, warm nodule may be seen on scintiscan FNAC does not differentiate between follicular ca & adenoma (Hence frozen section may be required) **Thyroglobulin** positive	a. Do not take up RAI b. Vascular or capsular invasion and can, therefore, not be diagnosed by FNAB **thyroglobulin** positive	FNAC Positive for epithelial markers like cytokeratin but negative for thyroglobulin	a. FNAC b. Tumour markers: Calcitonin b. Do not take up RAI c. Serum calcium: hyperparathyroidism d. Urinary catecholamines-pheochromocytoma e. CEA & calcitonin gene related peptide	a. FNAC, Large needle (Trucut) biopsy, b. USG-classic pseudocystic pattern
Recurrence	Less thyroglobulin levels used for monitoring recurrence	More common. Serum thyroglobulin levels used for monitoring recurrence	Presently Recurrent tumours are incurable	Lethal hence patients do not survive in the first place		
Prognosis	Excellent (93% 10 years survival rate for most favourable stages) Thyroglobulin is used as prognostic indicator for recurrence post surgically	Poorer than papillary better than Hurthle cell, although this disparity is more prominent after 10-15 years, (Poorly differentiated FTC and well-differentiated FTC have 60% & 85% 10-year survival rates)	Poor	Very poor	MEN 2A usually has a more favorable long-term outcome than MEN 2B or sporadic MCT	Good
Comments	Least malignant, associated with dystrophic calcification	Pulsatile secondaries are seen	Highest incidence of metastasis amongst differentiated thyroid cancers	Most malignant, Radiotherapy reqd along with surgery	Rule out pheochromocytoma & hyperparathyroidism	May be asso. With generalized Non-Hodgkin's lymphoma

137. Ans. (b) Glucocerebrosides

Ref: Nelson 20th ed page 710, Robbin's 9th ed page 153

Repeat AIIMS Pediatrics May 2013 (except that in May 2013 it was asked in a 3 year old child)

Gaucher's disease should be considered in the differential diagnosis of patients with unexplained organomegaly, who bruise easily, have bone pain, or have a combination of these conditions. Bone marrow examination usually reveals the presence of Gaucher cells (large cells with **crumbled paper appearance**). All suspected diagnoses should be confirmed by determination of the acid β-glucosidase (Glucocerebrosidases) activity in isolated leukocytes or cultured fibroblasts, and by identification of their specific acid β-glucosidase gene mutations.

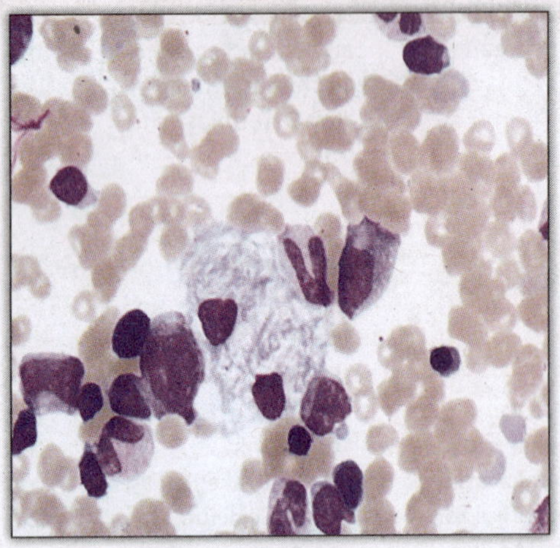

In **Gaucher disease**, the degradation stops at the level of **glucocerebrosides**, which accumulate in the phagocytes. These phagocytes—the Gaucher cells— become enlarged, with some reaching a diameter as great as 100 μm, because of the accumulation of distended lysosomes, and acquire a pathognomonic cytoplasmic appearance characterized as **"wrinkled tissue paper"**. No distinct vacuolation is present .

138. Ans. (d) Translocation involving MYC gene

Ref: Robbin's 9th ed page 436

The clinical picture is of Burkitt Lymphoma with characteristic histopathological Starry Sky appearance and c-MYC gene translocations on chromosome 8

Burkitt's Lymphoma:

- Classified into- Endemic (African) type, Non endemic (sporadic) type, HIV associated aggressive type
- BL tumor cells are intermediate in size (Medium size) and typically have round or oval nuclei and two to five distinct nucleoli. There is a moderate amount of basophilic or amphophilic cytoplasm that often contains small, lipid-filled vacuoles (a feature appreciated only on smears).
- Medium-sized lymphoma cells (Burkitt cells) have a very high proliferative rate and frequent mitotic figures. The rate of proliferation, as determined with Ki-67 staining, is at or above 95 percent
- These cells are characterized by a high rate of spontaneous apoptosis with interspersed macrophages engorged with cellular debris as a result of the high cell turnover rate (high rate of apoptosis and cell proliferation) leading to the characteristic "starry sky" pattern in marrow and lymph nodes
- Nuclear contours are round to oval without cleaves or folds, a key feature in the distinction from diffuse large cell lymphoma
- Nuclear remnants are phagocytosed by benign macrophages (tangible body macrophages)
- BL cells are mature B cells, positive for CD19, CD20, CD22, and CD79a, and have monotypic surface IgM; they lack CD5 and CD23.
- BL cells also show immunologic similarity to germinal center cells of B-cell follicles rather than activated B cells, being positive for BCL6, CD10, Tcl1, and CD38, and negative for Mum-1, CD44, CD138, and Bcl-2.
- All forms are associated with c-MYC gene translocations on chromosome 8. Most translocations fuse MYC with the IgH gene on chromosome 14, but variant translocations involving the κ and λ light chain loci on chromosomes 2 and 22, respectively, are also observed. The net result of each is the same—the dysregulation and overexpression of MYC protein.
- Essentially all endemic type and about 20% of sporadic cases tumors are latently infected by EBV. It was the first tumor to be etiologically associated with a virus
- Most tumors occur at extra nodal sites- commonest presentation for endemic type is a mass involving mandible and for sporadic type, mass involving the ileocaecum and peritoneum.
- Very aggressive tumor but responds well to intensive chemotherapy.
- Most children and young adults have very high rates of complete cure but prognosis is guarded in adults.

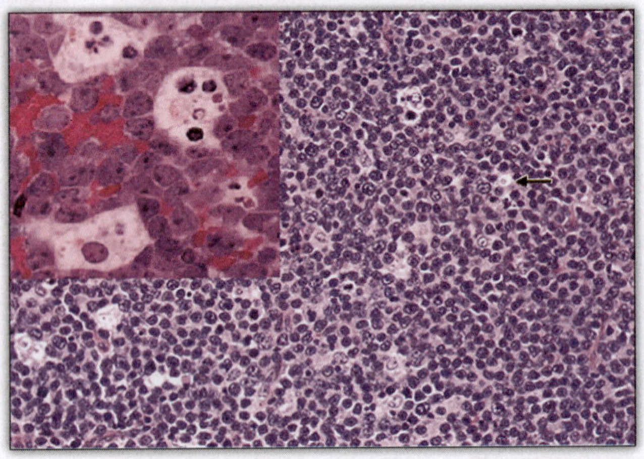

139. Ans. (a) Birbeck granules

Ref: Robbin's 8th ed chapter 13, Handbook of Practical Immunohistochemistry edited by Fan Lin, Jeffrey Prichard page 487, Rook's 8th ed p- 55.9

Langerhans Cell Histiocytosis

- The term *histiocytosis* is an "umbrella" designation for a variety of proliferative disorders of dendritic cells or macrophages.
- Langerhans cell histiocytoses, a spectrum of proliferations of a special type of immature dendritic cell called the **Langerhans cell**. In most instances, these proliferations are monoclonal and therefore likely to be neoplastic in origin.
- Langerhans cells have abundant, often vacuolated cytoplasm and vesicular nuclei containing linear grooves or folds. *The presence of **Birbeck granules** in the cytoplasm is characteristic.* Birbeck granules are pentalaminar tubules, often with a dilated terminal end producing a **tennis racket–like appearance**, which contain the protein **langerin**. In addition, the tumor cells also typically express **HLA-DR, S-100, and CD1a.**

- LCH can now be identified on the basis of immunoreactivity to cell surface markers such as CD-ia and more specifically **CD-207 (Langerin),** which differentiates it from other dendritic disorders

Langerhans Cell Histiocytosis Presents as Several Clinicopathologic Entities

There are three types of LCH, one localised type involving bones and lungs (Eosinophilic granuloma) and two systemic types.

1. **Multifocal multisystem Langerhans cell histiocytosis (Letterer-Siwe disease)**
   - Occurs most frequently **before 2 years** of age but occasionally affects adults.
   - A dominant clinical feature is the development of cutaneous lesions resembling a seborrheic eruption, which is caused by infiltrates of Langerhans cells over the front and back of the trunk and on the scalp.
   - Most of those affected have concurrent **hepatosplenomegaly, lymphadenopathy, pulmonary lesions,** and (eventually) **destructive osteolytic bone lesions.**
   - Extensive infiltration of the marrow often leads to **anemia, thrombocytopenia,** and a predisposition to recurrent infections, such as otitis media and mastoiditis.
   - In some instances the tumor cells are quite anaplastic; such tumors are sometimes referred to as Langerhans cell sarcoma. The course of untreated disease is rapidly fatal. With intensive chemotherapy, 50% of patients survive 5 years.
2. **Unifocal and multifocal unisystem Langerhans cell histiocytosis (eosinophilic granuloma)**
   - **Eosinophilic granuloma**, the **localized form** of LCH described in 1940, occurs in children and young adults with **predilection to head and neck especially temporal and frontal bones**
   - Characterized by proliferations of Langerhans cells admixed with variable numbers of eosinophils, lymphocytes, plasma cells, and neutrophils. Eosinophils are usually, but not always, a prominent component of the infiltrate.
   - Involvement of the posterior pituitary stalk of the hypothalamus leads to diabetes insipidus in about 50% of patients. The combination of calvarial bone defects, diabetes insipidus, and exophthalmos is referred to as the **Hand-Schuller-Christian triad**. Many patients experience spontaneous regression; others can be treated successfully with chemotherapy.
3. **Pulmonary Langerhans cell histiocytosis** represents a special category of disease, most often seen in adult smokers, which may regress spontaneously upon cessation of smoking. It usually comprises a polyclonal population of Langerhans cells, suggesting that it is a reactive hyperplasia rather than a true neoplasm.

Pharmacology

6

AIIMS NOVEMBER 2018

1. Morphine should never be given in:
a. Ischemic pain b. Biliary colic
c. Cancer pain d. Post operative pain

2. A drug which is sold only at prescription of registered medical practitioner is under which schedule?
a. Schedule X b. Schedule H
c. Schedule P d. Schedule G

3. An infant presents to pediatrician with jaundice. His serum unconjugated bilirubin levels are 33 mg/dl. Which of the following drug mother would have taken in 3rd trimester of pregnancy?
a. Chloroquine b. Ampicillin
c. Cotrimoxazole d. Azithromycin

4. Which antimalarial drug is gametocidal for all species of Plasmodia?
a. Quinine b. Chloroquine
c. Primaquine d. None of the above

5. Dapsone which is used as antibacterial, antifungal and immunomodulator. Which of following describes its mechanism of action?
a. By inhibiting cell wall synthesis
b. By inhibiting protein synthesis in ribosomes
c. By inhibiting sterol in cell wall
d. By competing with PABA in folic acid synthesis

6. All of the following drugs require dose reduction in renal failure EXCEPT:
a. Amphotericin B b. Doxycycline
c. Gentamicin d. Vancomycin

7. Low volume of distribution indicates:
(AIIMS Nov 2018, 2015)
a. Low efficacy
b. Decreased distribution in tissues and organ
c. Short biological life
d. Poor bioavailability

8. Loading dose of a drug depends upon:
(AIIMS Nov 2018, May 2018)
a. Volume of distribution
b. Clearance
c. Half-life
d. Route of administration

9. Phase I trial is done for which of the following?
a. Dose b. Pharmacokinetics
c. Efficacy d. Safety

10. All are side effects of Salbutamol EXCEPT:
(AIIMS Nov 2018, May 2018)
a. Tremors b. Hypoglycemia
c. Hypokalemia d. Tachycardia

11. Store in a cool place as referred over medicines is:
(AIIMS Nov 2018, 2015)
a. Freezing point of water
b. Zero °C
c. 2-4°C
d. 8 to 15°C

12. Active metabolite of Nitroprusside acts by/through:
a. Phospholipase A2 b. Guanylyl Cyclase
c. Phosphokinase 1,2 d. Through IP3

13. Primary action of nitrates in a patient of angina is:
a. By reduction of preload
b. By reduction of afterload
c. Coronary vasodilation
d. Decrease Heart rate

14. A hypertensive patient was on Beta blocker with his blood pressure poorly controlled. He was prescribed verapamil. This would result in:
a. Atrial fibrillation
b. Torsades de pointes
c. Bradycardia with AV block
d. Tachycardia

15. Mechanism by which Ach decreases Heart rate is:
a. Delayed diastolic depolarisation
b. Increase in plateau
c. Decrease Preload
d. Slows AV conduction

16. Lithium use in pregnancy leads to which of the following defects?
a. Neural tube defects
b. Cardiac defects
c. Urogenital defects
d. Facial defects

17. Antitubercular drug which causes ophthalmic toxicity is:
a. Ethambutol
b. Isoniazid
c. Rifampicin
d. None of the above

18. Which drug is used to prevent acute mountain sickness?
a. Digoxin b. Dexamethasone
c. Diltiazem d. Acetazolamide

19. A patient was on Indinavir, lamivudine, zidovudine and ketoconazole. He develops breast hypertrophy, nephrolithiasis, hyperlipidemia and central obesity. Which out of four drug could be cause of all side effects?

a. Indinavir b. Lamivudine
c. Zidovudine d. Ketoconazole

20. A patient is on sodium valproate. Carbamazepine is added to his prescription. Which of the following side effect increases?

a. Hyperammonemia b. Hepatotoxicity
c. Pancreatitis d. Thrombocytopenia

21. The technique given in the picture is used for:

a. Preparing monoclonal antibodies
b. Preparing cell line for virus culture
c. Process of genetic engineering
d. Synthesis of vaccine

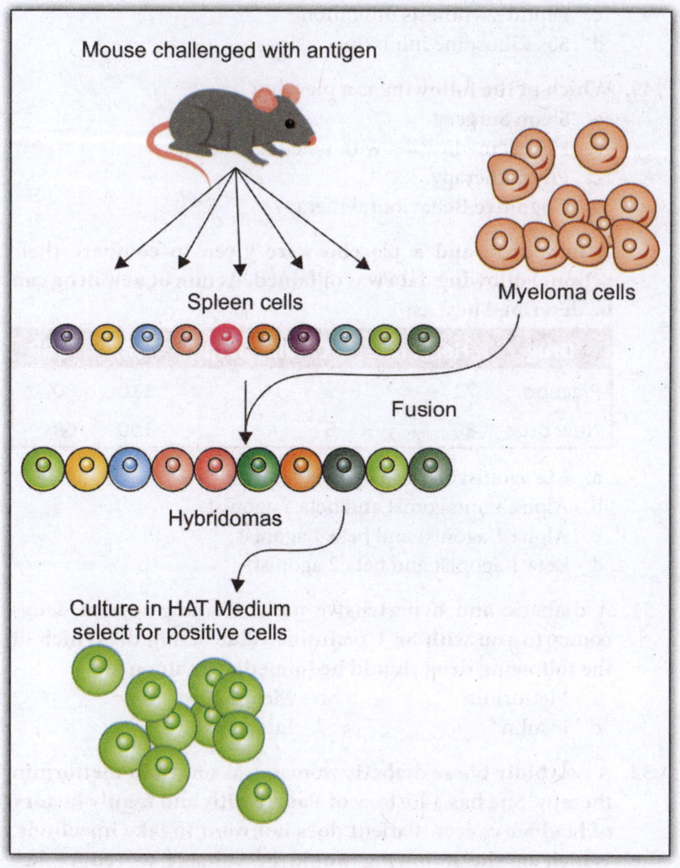

22. All of the following drug increase bleeding when patient is on warfarin EXCEPT:

a. Isoniazid b. Carbamazepine
c. Cimetidine d. Amiodarone

AIIMS MAY 2018

23. All of the following are used in the treatment of Typhoid fever EXCEPT: ***(AIIMS May 2018, AI PG 2008)***

a. Azithromycin
b. Amikacin
c. Ceftriaxone
d. Ciprofloxacin

24. Therapeutic index is a measure of:

a. Safety b. Efficacy
c. Potency d. Dose variability

25. Loading dose of a drug depends upon:
(AIIMS Nov 2018, May 2018)

a. Volume of distribution b. Clearance
c. Half-life d. Route of administration

26. Which of the following parameter is used to assess the rate of drug absorption:

a. Tmax b. Cmax
c. Half-life d. Area under the curve

27. From which of the following routes, bioavailability of the drug is likely to be 100 percent?

a. Intramuscular b. Intravenous
c. Subcutaneous d. Intradermal

28. First pass metabolism is bypassed by all EXCEPT:

a. Oral b. Intravenous
c. Sublingual d. Subcutaneous

29. Effect of Potassium ionophore valinomycin on beta cells of pancreas is:

a. Decrease secretion of insulin
b. Increase secretion of Insulin
c. Increase secretion of C-peptide secretion increases
d. No change in Insulin secretion

30. A patient require ceftriaxone 180 mg. You have a 2 mL syringe with 10 divisions per mL. The vial contains 500 mg/5mL of ceftriaxone. How many divisions in the 2 mL syringe will you fill to give 180 mg ceftriaxone?
(AIIMS May 2018, Nov 2017)

a. 1.8 b. 18
c. 20 d. 9

31. Which of the following is not an adverse effect of salbutamol?

a. Hypoglycemia b. Hypokalemia
c. Tremors d. Tachycardia

32. Treatment of choice for late cardiovascular syphilis is:

a. Benzathine penicillin 7.2 million units in three divided doses
b. Benzathine penicillin 2.4 million units single dose
c. Benzyl penicillin 12–24 million units for 21 days
d. Tetracycline 2 g daily

33. Manufacturer of a drug company labels the drug contains 500 mg paracetamol. On govt. analysis, it was found to contain only 200 mg of drug. Which type of drug it is known as?

a. Counterfeit drug b. Spurious drug
c. Adulterant drug d. Misbranded drug

34. Sudden discontinuation of which of the following drugs can result in agitation, anxiety and insomnia:

a. Venlafaxine b. Imipramine
c. Valproate d. Olanzapine

35. Heparin acts via which of the following adjuvants?

a. Antithrombin III
b. Protein C
c. Protein S
d. Thrombomodulin

36. **A 21-year-old medical student comes to emergency after experiencing repeated vomiting. Resident gives him an antiemetic drug which leads to abnormal posturing. Which of following drug he was administered?**
   a. Metoclopramide b. Ondansetron
   c. Domperidone d. Dexamethasone

37. **Which drug is likely to cause flagellated pigmentation of skin?**
   a. Bleomycin b. Minocycline
   c. Vincristine d. Daunorubicin

38. **New drug recently approved for Amyotrophic Lateral Sclerosis is:**
   a. Edaravone b. Piracetam
   c. Ceftriaxone d. Doxycycline

39. **Which of the following drugs is not used in Rheumatoid arthritis?**
   a. Febuxostat b. Leflunomide
   c. Etanercept d. Methotrexate

40. **Which of the following drugs is commonly used in cancer associated thromboembolism?**
   a. Low molecular weight heparin
   b. Unfractionated heparin
   c. Direct thrombin inhibitors
   d. Warfarin

41. **A drug which is sold only at prescription of registered medical practitioner is under which schedule?**
   (AIIMS Nov 2018, May 2018)
   a. Schedule X b. Schedule H
   c. Schedule P d. Schedule G

42. **Which of the following is wrongly matched regarding mechanism of action of anti-fungal drugs?**
   a. Azoles: Inhibit lanosterol alpha demethylase thereby preventing ergosterol synthesis
   b. Flucytosine: Inhibit microtubule thereby preventing mitosis
   c. Echinocandins: Inhibit glycan synthesis by inhibiting beta 1,3 glycan synthase
   d. Amphotericin B: Impair barrier mechanism in cell membrane

43. **Which of the following drugs is correctly matched with its mechanism of action?**
   a. Tenofovir—Inhibits assembly of proviral components into viral proteins
   b. Enfuvirtide—An entry inhibitor- Inhibits viral entry by binding to CCR5 receptor
   c. Ritonavir—A nucleoside reverse transcriptase inhibitor
   d. Dolutegravir—inhibits integration of viral DNA into host

AIIMS NOVEMBER 2017

44. **Drug of choice for Insomnia in blind people is:**
   a. Latanoprostene b. Zerviate
   c. Tasimelteon d. Ramelteon

45. **A patient in labour ward was given opioid analgesic. Which drug should be kept ready for emergency?**
   a. Atropine b. Naloxone
   c. Lignocaine d. Fentanyl

46. **The most important mechanism of antibiotic resistance in biofilms is:**
   a. Increased adhesion
   b. Increased efflux of antibiotic
   c. Low mitotic rate
   d. Decreased diffusion of antibiotic

47. **What instructions you would give to a lactating mother regarding drug usage?**
   a. Breastfed child just before taking next dose, when plasma concentration of drug is least
   b. Give longer half lives drug to her
   c. No advice as most of drugs are excreted negligibly in breast milk
   d. Tell the mother to breastfeed when the drug is least efficacious

48. **Mechanism of action of Vancomycin is:**
   a. Cell membrane inhibition
   b. Cell wall synthesis inhibition
   c. Peptide synthesis inhibition
   d. 50s Ribosome inhibition

49. **Which of the following is a placebo?**
   a. Sham Surgery
   b. Herbal medication with no effect known
   c. Physiotherapy
   d. Cognitive Behavioural therapy

50. **A new drug and a placebo were given to compare their action. Following data was obtained. Action of new drug can be described best as:**

Drug	Heart rate	Cardiac output	SBP	DBP
Placebo	72	5	110	80
New drug	86	6	150	68

   a. M2 agonist and M3 agonist
   b. Alpha 1 antagonist and beta 1 agonist
   c. Alpha 1 agonist and beta 1 agonist
   d. Beta 1 agonist and beta 2 agonist

51. **A diabetic and hypertensive patient taking several drugs comes to you with Sr. Creatinine value 5.7mg/dl. Which of the following drug should be immediately stopped?**
   a. Metformin b. Metoprolol
   c. Insulin d. Linagliptin

52. **A morbidly obese diabetic woman was on failed metformin therapy. She has a history of Pancreatitis and family history of bladder cancer. Patient does not want to take injections. Which of the following would be suitable to reduce her glucose levels?**
   a. Sitagliptin b. Pioglitazone
   c. Canagliflozin d. Liraglutide

53. **A person on antitubercular treatment taking following drugs develops tingling sensation. Which of the following is added to the regimen?**
   - Rifampicin: 15 mg/kg/day (10 to 20 mg/kg/day)
   - Isoniazid: 10 mg/kg/day (10 to 15 mg/kg/day)
   - Pyrazinamide: 35 mg/kg/day (30 to 40 mg/kg/day)
   - Ethambutol 20 mg/kg/d (15 mg to 25 mg/kg/day)

   a. Folic acid b. Cobalamine
   c. Pyridoxine d. Thiamine

54. A patient requires ceftriaxone 180 mg. You have a 2 mL syringe with 10 divisions per mL. The vial contains 500 mg/5mL of ceftriaxone. How many divisions in the 2 mL syringe will you fill to give 180 mg ceftriaxone?

(AIIMS May 2018, Nov 2017)

a. 1.8 b. 18
c. 20 d. 9

55. Drug that decrease size of prostate is:

a. Flutamide b. Tamsulosin
c. Finasteride d. Sildenafil

56. A friend of yours is going on a hill station trip next morning and he had history of motion sickness. He asked you for prescribing some drug. What would you prescribe?

a. Dimenhydrinate 1 hour before journey
b. Ranitidine one night before and 1 hour before trip
c. Omeprazole one hour before trip
d. Scopolamine transdermal patch a night before

57. A patient presented with pain in the right lower quadrant of abdomen. He has history of renal stones in right kidney. He was prescribed an opioid which is partial agonist at mu receptors and antagonist at kappa receptors. The likely drug given was:

a. Pentazocin b. Tramadol
c. Buprenorphine d. Fentanyl

58. A patient comes with acute exacerbation of bronchial asthma. Salbutamol inhalation was given and no improvement was noticed. Hence, Intravenous corticosteroids and Aminophylline was added and condition improved. What is the mechanism of action of corticosteroids in this condition?

a. They increase bronchial responsiveness to salbutamol
b. They cause direct bronchodilation when used with xanthenes
c. They increase mucociliary clearance
d. They indirectly increases effectivity of xanthines on adenosine receptors

AIIMS MAY 2017

59. Drug of choice for prophylaxis of Pneumocystis jirovecii in an immunocompromised patient is:

a. Cotrimoxazole b. Amoxycillin
c. Dexamethasone d. Cephalosporin

60. Mechanism of action of protease inhibitors is:

a. It inhibits translation
b. It inhibits assembly of virus protein
c. It inhibits proviral RNA synthesis
d. Inhibits conversion of RNA to DNA

61. A 40-year-old patient came with complaints of spikes of fever and difficulty in breathing. Transesophageal echo found out vegetations in the heart. The culture showed positive for Burkholderia cepacia. Which of the following is the first line management? Drug of choice for Burkholderia cepacia pneumonia is:

a. Aminoglycosides and colistin
b. Carbapenems and 3rd generation cephalosporins
c. Tigecycline and cefepime
d. Cotrimoxazole with 3rd generation cephalosporin

62. Storage of drug in the tissues is suggested by:

a. Small volume of distribution
b. Large volume of distribution
c. Excretion in urine
d. Excretion in saliva

63. A patient came with complaints of high grade fever and altered sensorium. He was diagnosed to be suffering from meningococcal meningitis. Which of the following is the most appropriate empirical treatment option? Empirical drug of choice for treatment of meningococcal meningitis:

a. Ceftriaxone b. Gentamycin
c. Cefepime d. Cefoxitin

64. An epileptic adult man is on levetiracetam therapy 1 g BD. He is seizure free for 2 years. Now, he started developing irritability and lability of mood that is affecting his daily life. What should the doctor do?

a. Stop levetiracetam therapy suddenly
b. Taper the drug over 6 months
c. Continue the medication for another 3 years
d. Stop levetiracetam and start another antiepileptic

65. A 70-year-old patient has diabetes mellitus and hypertension. He presents with renal failure and does not want to take insulin. Which antidiabetic drug will you prefer in this patient that does not require dose modification in renal disease?

a. Linagliptin b. Vildagliptin
c. Exenatide d. Repaglinide

66. All are idiosyncratic reactions to Carbamazepine EXCEPT:

a. Rash b. Steven Johnson syndrome
c. Blurred vision d. Agranulocytosis

67. Components of lente insulin are:

a. 30% amorphous + 70% crystalline
b. 30% crystalline + 70% amorphous
c. Same as NPH insulin
d. Only 70% amorphous

68. Mechanism of action of Oseltamivir is:

a. Neuraminidase inhibitor
b. Blocks viral M2 protein
c. Fusion inhibitor
d. RNA dependent DNA polymerase inhibitor

69. Antidote for overdose of fibrinolytic therapy is?

(AIIMS May 2017, Nov 2015)

a. Heparin b. Epsilon amino caproic acid
c. Protamine d. rTPA

70. A drug X was administered by continuous IV infusion at the rate of 1.6 mg/min. Clearance of drug X is 640 ml/min. If the t1/2 of the drug is 1.8 hours, what would be the plasma concentration of drug after achieving steady state?

a. 2.5 mg/L b. 5 mg/L
c. 7.5 mg/L d. 10 mg/L

71. A patient was administered 200 mg of a drug. 75 mg of the drug is eliminated from the body in 90 minutes. If the drug follows first order kinetics, how much drug will remain after 6 hours?

a. 12.5 mg b. 25 mg
c. 30 mg d. 50 mg

72. A 60-year-old patient who had myocardial infarction 2 weeks back with TG- 262 mg/dl, LDL- 124 mg/dl, HDL - 32 mg/dL. Which of the following will you use?
a. Atorvastatin 80 mg
b. Rosuvastatin 10 mg
c. Rosuvastatin + Fenofibrate
d. Fenofibrate

73. Which of the following is a bactericidal drug for *Mycobacterium leprae*?
a. Ofloxacin
b. Ciprofloxacin
c. Amoxicillin
d. Erythromycin

74. Which of the following disease modifying anti-rheumatoid drugs acts by increasing extracellular adenosine?
a. Methotrexate
b. Leflunomide
c. Sulfasalazine
d. Chloroquine

75. Which of the following is a P glycoproteins inducer?
a. Ketoconazole
b. Rifampicin
c. Erythromycin
d. Itraconazole

76. In an animal model how will you show vasomotor reversal of Dale?
a. Block of α1 followed by stimulation of β1
b. Block of α1 followed by stimulation of β2
c. Block of β1 followed by block of α1
d. Block of β1 followed by block of β2

AIIMS NOVEMBER 2016

77. Which of the following is not used in osteoporosis?
a. PTH
b. Denosumab
c. Milnacipran
d. Strontium ranelate

78. A patient is started on Thioamide. Which of the following is not a life threatening/ serious side effect of Thioamide?
a. Agranulocytosis
b. Aplastic anemia
c. Liver toxicity
d. Lung fibrosis

79. All of the following are included in a Drug literature EXCEPT:
a. Expiry date
b. Common Side effects
c. Rare side effects
d. Common drug interaction

80. Which of the following is not true for rifabutin when compared to rifampicin?
a. Rifabutin has a longer half-life than rifampicin
b. Rifabutin has lesser incidence of drug interactions
c. Rifabutin is more efficacious against MAC as compared to Rifampicin
d. Rifabutin is more efficacious for pulmonary TB than rifampicin

81. Antidote of benzodiazepine overdose is:
a. Naloxone
b. Naltrexone
c. Flumazenil
d. Acamprosate

82. Which of the following is the least commonly preferred site of insulin injection?
a. Dorsal aspect of arm
b. Periumbilical
c. Lateral aspect of thigh
d. Anterior aspect of thigh

83. Drug used safely in renal failure is:
a. Linagtiptin
b. Sitagliptin
c. Vildagliptin
d. Saxagliptin

84. Digoxin is obtained from a plant source and has a half-life of 40 hours. How does this information helps in formulating the prescription?
a. Loading dose is required to achieve immediate effect
b. Regimen for smooth discontinuation
c. To adjust maintenance dosing for achieving therapeutic blood levels
d. Long half-life allows alternate day dosing

85. Which of the following correctly represents the sequence of rate of topical drug absorption?
a. Posterior auricular > Scalp > Scrotum > Dorsal aspect of hand > Sole
b. Posterior auricular > Scrotum > Scalp> Dorsal aspect of hand > Sole
c. Scalp> Scrotum> Posterior auricular> Dorsum of hand> Sole
d. Scrotum > Scalp> Posterior auricular > Dorsal aspect of hand > Sole

86. A patient on MDI (Metered dose Inhaler) has been advised to take 2 puff twice a day. Which of the following instruction for reusing the MDI is not correct?
a. 2 puffs must be 1 minute apart
b. Patient must rinse the mouth between the puff
c. Shake the inhaler before each dose
d. Cleaning the inhaler after every use

87. The following graph shows effect of three drugs on BP and Heart rate. Which of the following statement is correct about this graph?

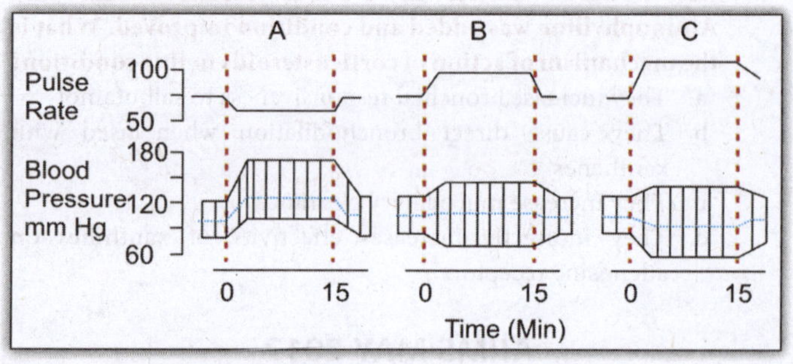

a. Drug A is isoprenaline
b. Fall in HR of Drug A could be prevented by Muscarinic antagonist
c. Drug B is Epinephrine
d. Drug C is Norepinephrine

88. Which of the following statement regarding following graph is correct?

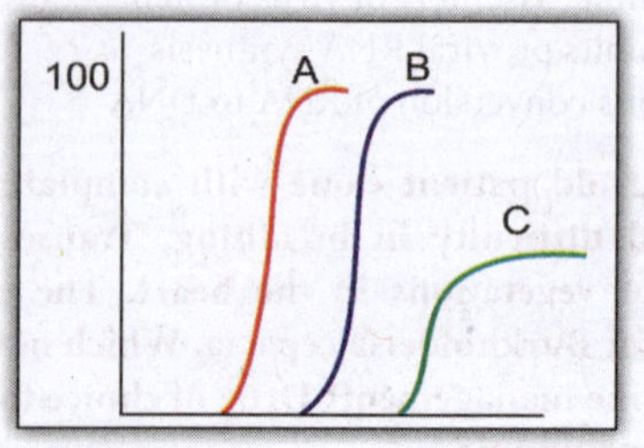

a. Both A and B are full agonists
b. B is more Potent than A
c. C produces antagonism which is non-competitive
d. A is more efficacious than B, but potency is same

89. **Increased bleeding time is found in a health care provider. He was enquired about NSAID use but denied. Bleeding time is prolonged in all of the following drugs EXCEPT:**
   a. Vitamin K b. Antidepressant
   c. Theophylline d. Cephalosporin

AIIMS MAY 2016

90. **Nimodipine is approved for use in:**
   a. Subarachnoid hemorrhage
   b. Subdural hemorrhage
   c. Extradural hemorrhage
   d. Intracerebral hemorrhage

91. **The drug that produces least inhibition of CYP450 is:**
   a. Omeprazole b. Rabeprazole
   c. Lansoprazole d. Pantoprazole

92. **The treatment of choice for erythrodermic psoriasis is?**
   a. Topical steroid b. Corticosteroid
   c. Methotrexate d. Topical Coal tar

93. **Post marketing surveillance is part of which of the following phase of clinical trials?**
   a. Phase 0 b. Phase 1
   c. Phase 2 d. Phase 4

94. **The anti-emetic activity of metoclopramide is mainly because of?**
   a. D2 antagonism b. 5-HT4 antagonism
   c. 5-HT4 agonism d. 5-HT3 antagonism

95. **ARB inhibitor with additional PPAR-γ agonist activity is?**
   a. Losartan b. Candesartan
   c. Telmisartan d. Eprosartan

96. **All of the following are G2 phase inhibitors EXCEPT:**
   a. Paclitaxel b. Etoposide
   c. Topotecan d. Daunorubicin

97. **All of the following are GpIIb/IIIa receptor inhibitor EXCEPT:**
   a. Abciximab b. Prasugrel
   c. Eptifibatide d. Tirofiban

98. **Vasomotor reversal of dale is demonstrated by?**
   a. Fall in blood pressure by high dose intravenous Ach
   b. Increase in blood pressure following administration of IV propranolol
   c. Fall in blood pressure by ganglionic blocker
   d. Fall in blood pressure by adrenaline pretreated with phentolamine

99. **One of the following is pharmacological effects of adrenaline which does not play a role in its management of anaphylaxis?**
   a. Stimulation of vascular alpha receptors
   b. Stimulation of pre-synaptic alpha receptors
   c. Bronchodilatation by stimulation of beta 1 receptors
   d. Stimulation of beta two receptors on heart

100. **Which of the following does not contribute to the therapeutic levels of IV dopamine for the purpose of acute shock?**
   a. Stimulation of cardiac beta 1 receptor
   b. Release of Noradrenaline to cause positive ionotropic effect
   c. Stimulation of renal dopimergic receptor to increase renal perfusion
   d. Stimulation of vasomotor alpha 1 receptor

AIIMS NOVEMBER 2015

101. **Dopamine in dose concentration at 3-5 mcg/kg/min acts predominantly on:**
   a. α1- Blood vessels b. β1- Heart
   c. D1- Renal vessels d. D2- Striatum

102. **Low volume of distribution indicates:**
   a. Low efficacy *(AIIMS Nov 2018, 2015)*
   b. Decreased distribution in tissues and organ
   c. Short biological life
   d. Poor bioavailability

103. **Low dose aspirin act as anti-platelet drug by inhibiting:**
   a. TXA2 synthesis b. TXB2 synthesis
   c. Endothelin d. Lipoxygenase

104. **Which of the following is a gender specific side effect caused by valproate?**
   a. Tremor b. Alopecia
   c. Weight gain d. PCOD

105. **Drug of choice for bird flu is:**
   a. Oseltamivir b. Ribavirin
   c. Zanamivir d. Peramivir

106. **Penicillinase acts on which bond of penicillin G, numbered in the figure below?**

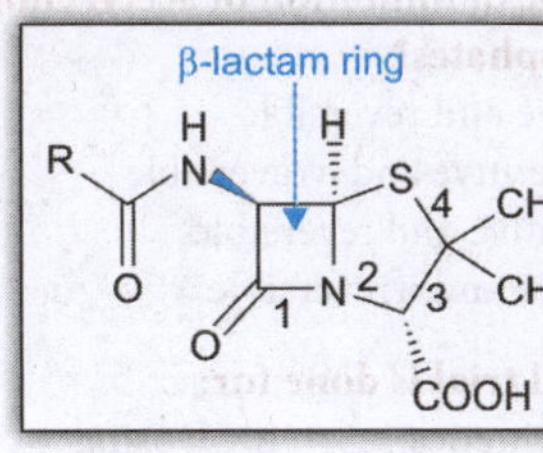

   a. 1 b. 2
   c. 3 d. 4

107. **Anti-epileptic drug which can cause progressive visual field defect is:**
   a. Phenobarbitone b. Vigabatrin
   c. Ethosuximide d. Valproate

108. **Which is an oral drug for hepatitis-C treatment?**
   a. Lamivudine b. Ribamivir
   c. Ledipasvir d. Peg IFN α

109. **Etanerecept mechanism of action is by:**
   a. TNF alpha inhibitor b. Selective COX inhibitor
   c. IL-1 inhibition d. IL-6 inhibition

110. **Which of the following is a calcineurin inhibitor?**
   a. Cyclosporine b. Methotrexate
   c. Leflunomide d. Mycophenolate Mofetil

111. **Which of the following is a latest drug approved for MDR TB?**
   a. Bedaquiline b. Tipranavir
   c. Levofloxacin d. Linezolid

112. **What will be advice given to a bisphosphonate taking patient?**
   a. Take tab before meals with full glass of water
   b. Take tab after meals with full glass of water
   c. Discontinue if gastroesophageal discomfort persists
   d. Discontinue if bone pain persists

113. Drug which doesn't inhibit nucleic acid synthesis?

a. Rifampicin b. Fluoroquinolones
c. Nitrofurantoin d. Linezolid

114. Drug whose absorption is increased after fatty meal:

a. Griseofulvin b. Amphotericin-B
c. Nimesulide d. Ampicillin

115. Antidote for overdose of fibrinolytic therapy is:

a. Heparin b. Epsilon amino caproic acid
c. Protamine d. rTPA

116. Store in a cool place as referred over medicines is: *(AIIMS Nov 2018, 2015)*

a. Freezing point of water b. 0°C
c. 2-4°C d. 8 to 15°C

117. Schedule of drug to be sold only on prescription are:

a. Schedule H b. Schedule P
c. Schedule S d. Schedule X

118. What is the rationale behind xenobiotic metabolism by CYP enzymes?

a. Increase in water solubility
b. Increase in lipid solubility
c. Conversion to an active metabolite
d. Makes it suitable to evaporate through skin surface

119. What is the type of inhibition of acetyl cholinesterase caused by organophosphates?

a. Competitive and reversible
b. Non competitive and irreversible
c. Uncompetitive and reversible
d. Competitive and irreversible

120. Phase 1 clinical trial is done for:

a. Pharmacokinetics b. Dosing
c. Drug Safety d. Drug Efficacy

AIIMS MAY 2015

121. All of these drugs can cause hearing loss EXCEPT:

a. Metronidazole b. Vancomycin
c. Kanamycin d. Quinine

122. Methacholine acts at which of the following receptors? *(AIIMS May 2015, May 2014)*

a. M1 b. M2
c. M3 d. M4

123. Which of the following is a protease inhibitor?

a. Saquinavir b. Nevirapine
c. Abacavir d. Enfuvirtide

124. Diuretic which can be given in mild to moderate hypertension is?

a. Loop diuretic
b. Thiazide
c. Osmotic diuretic
d. Potassium sparing diuretic

125. Best anti-hypertensive drug in pulmonary hypertension:

a. Bosentan b. Amlodipine
c. Frusemide d. Digoxin

126. Which of the following does not act by increasing insulin secretion?

a. Exenatide b. Sitagliptin
c. Rasiglitazone d. Repaglinide

127. Nitroglycerine is used sublingual because:

a. Non ionic, more lipid soluble
b. Ionic but still more lipid soluble
c. Ionic and less lipid soluble
d. Non-ionic less lipid soluble

ANSWERS WITH EXPLANATIONS

AIIMS NOVEMBER 2018

1. Ans. (b) Biliary colic

Ref: KDT 7th ed page 474, Miller's 8th Ed page 2257

- In patients with cholelithiasis and biliary tract obstruction, the use of opiates should be limited preoperatively because these drugs can cause spasm of the choledochoduodenal sphincter (sphincter of Oddi) and a subsequent increase in intra biliary tract pressure.
- These effects appear to be more pronounced for *fentanyl, morphine, and meperidine* and less severe for opiate agonist-antagonists.
- Intraoperatively, opiates may be used with the recognition that the possible development of sphincter of Oddi spasm can be treated directly with naloxone or by relaxing smooth muscle tone with either glucagon or nitroglycerin(which induces release of nitric oxide).
- Biliary colic due to disease or morphine responds to sublingual GTN or isosorbide dinitrate.

Precautions with Morphine

Condition	Comment
Infants and the elderly	More susceptible to the respiratory depressant action
Respiratory insufficiency (emphysema, pulmonary fibrosis, cor pulmonale), sleep apnea	Precaution must be exercised. May abolish the respiratory drive
Bronchial asthma	Can precipitate an attack by its histamine releasing action.
Head injury	• Raised Intracranial pressure (ICP) caused by CO2 retention, especially dangerous in patients with head injury, since they already have raised ICP. • Even therapeutic doses can cause marked respiratory depression in these patients. • Vomiting, miosis and altered mentation produced by morphine interfere with assessment of progress in head injury cases.
Hypotensive states and hypovolaemia	May cause exaggerated hypotension
Undiagnosed acute abdominal pain	Can aggravate certain conditions, e.g. diverticulitis, biliary colic, pancreatitis. Inflamed appendix may rupture.
Elderly male	May cause acute urinary retention

2. Ans. (b) Schedule H

Ref: KDT 7th Ed page 4,5

As per drug rules, majority of drugs including all antibiotics must be sold in retail only against a prescription issued to a patient by a registered medical practitioner. These are called 'prescription drugs', and in India they have been placed in the schedule H of the Drugs and Cosmetic Rules (1945) as amended from time to time.

Drugs and Cosmetic Rules of 1945

It contains 168 rules from 1 to 168 and 25 Schedules from Schedule A to Schedule Y. Different type of forms are also given for different type of approvals from drug authorities.

Schedule A	Forms and applications
Schedule B	Fees for test or analysis by the Central Drugs Laboratories or State Drugs Laboratories
Schedule C	Biological and Special Products
Schedule D	Class of Drugs: Extent and conditions of exemption
Schedule E	List of Poisonous Substances under the Ayurvedic (including Siddha) and Unani Systems of Medicine
Schedule F	Requirements for the functioning and operation of a Blood Bank and/or for preparation of Blood Components. Vaccines, Antisera, Diagnostic Antigens
Schedule G	Hormonal preparations
Schedule H	Prescription Drugs
Schedule I	Omitted
Schedule J	Disease and ailment (by whatever name described) which a drug not purport to prevent or cure.
Schedule K	Class of drug: Extent and conditions of exemption

Contd...

Drugs and Cosmetic Rules of 1945	
Schedule L	Good Laboratory Practice
Schedule M	Good manufacturing practices and requirements of premises, plant and equipment for Pharmaceutical product.
Schedule N	List of Minimum Equipment for the Efficient Running of a Pharmacy
Schedule O	Standard for Disinfectant Fluids
Schedule P	Life Period and Pack size of Drugs
Schedule Q	List of Dyes, colours and Pigments permitted to be used in Cosmetics and Soaps
Schedule R	Standards for condoms made of rubber latex intended for single use and other mechanical contraceptives
Schedule S	Standard for cosmetics
Schedule T	Good manufacturing practices for Ayurvedic, Siddha and all Unani medicines
Schedule U	I – Particulars to be shown in the manufacturing records. II – Records of Raw Materials III – Particulars to be recorded in the analytical records
Schedule V	Standards for patent or proprietary medicines.
Schedule Y	Requirements and guidelines for permission to import and/or manufacture of New Drug for sale or to undertake clinical Trials.

3. Ans. (c) Cotrimoxazole

Ref: KDT 7th Ed page 707

- Co-trimoxazole is a 5:1 mixture of two antibiotics, sulfamethoxazole (SMX) and trimethoprim (TMP).
- SMX-TMP is believed to cause kernicterus in neonates by displacing bilirubin from plasma albumin, and hence it is not to be used in last trimester of pregnancy or in neonates. Sulfonamide competes with bilirubin binding sites on albumin.
- Also, Neonatal haemolysis and methemoglobinaemia can occur if it is given near term, the former can cause raised bilirubin.
- Trimethoprim being an antifolate, there is theoretical teratogenic risk.

4. Ans. (c) Primaquine

Ref: KDT 7th Ed page 821

- Gametocidal refers to elimination of the male and female gametes of Plasmodia formed in the patient's blood. Gametocidal action is of no benefit to the patient being treated, but will reduce the transmission to mosquito.
- Primaquine is gametocidal to all species of Plasmodia, while artemisinins have weak lethal action on early-stage but not mature gametes.
- Gametes exposed to proguanil or pyrimethamine may fail to carry on the life cycle normally in the mosquito.

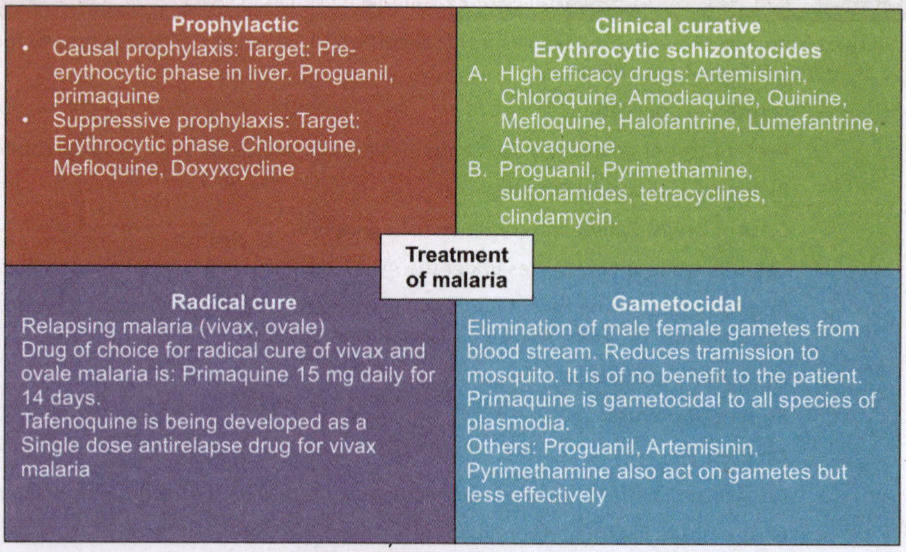

5. Ans. (d) By competing with PABA in folic acid synthesis

Ref: KDT 7th ed page 780, Goodman Gilman 12th ed page 1089

- Dapsone is chemically related to sulfonamides and has the same mechanism of action, i.e. **inhibition of PABA incorporation into folic acid by folate synthase.** The antibacterial action of dapsone is antagonized by PABA. It is effective in leprosy at doses lower than that in
- Dapsone is active against certain protozoa as well. Combined with pyrimethamine, it is an alternative to sulfadoxine-pyrimethamine for *P. falciparum* and *Toxoplasma gondii infections*, as well as for the fungus *Pneumocystis jirovecii*.
- Anti-inflammatory property has been detected in dapsone. It is used in dermatology for its anti-inflammatory properties, particularly in sterile (noninfectious) pustular diseases of the skin.
- Dapsone prevents the respiratory burst from myeloperoxidase, suppresses neutrophil migration by blocking integrin mediated adherence, inhibits adherence of antibodies to neutrophils, and decreases the release of eicosanoids and blocks their inflammatory effects; all these actions are likely to be important in autoimmune skin diseases.
- Dapsone is approved for use in dermatitis herpetiformis and leprosy. It is particularly useful in the treatment of linear immunoglobulin A (IgA) dermatosis, bullous systemic lupus erythematosus, erythema elevatum diutinum, and subcorneal pustular dermatosis.

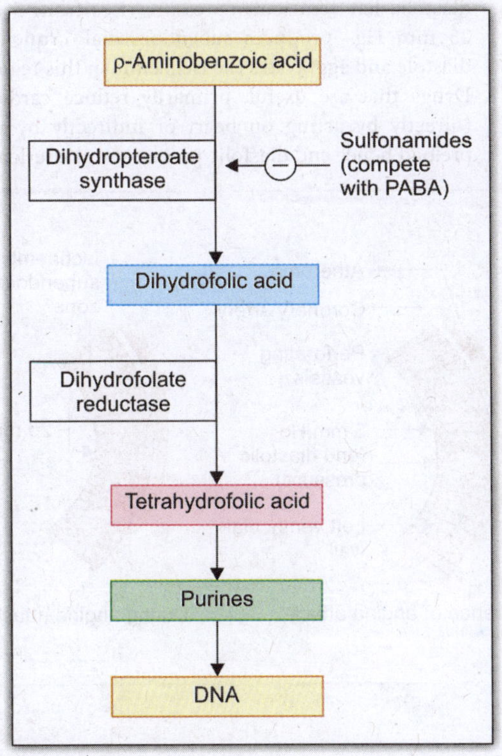

6. Ans. (b) Doxycycline

Ref: KDT 7th Ed page 68,69

Tetracyclines (except Doxycycline) have an anti-anabolic effect and accentuate uraemia.

Antimicrobial Requiring Dose Reduction/Avoidance in Renal Failure

Reduce dose even in mild failure	Reduce dose only in moderate/severe failure	Drugs to be avoided
Aminoglycosides	Metronidazole	Nitrofurantoin
Cephalosporins	Fluoroquinolones	Nalidixic acid
Amphotericin B	Cotrimoxazole	Talampicillin
Vancomycin	Clarithromycin	Tetracycline
Ethambutol	Meropenem	(Except
Flucytosine	Imipenem	Doxycycline)
	Carbenicillin	

7. Ans. (b) Decreased distribution in tissues and organ

Ref: KDT 7th ed page 18, Katzung 8th ed page 38

Repeat AIIMS Nov 2015 Pharmacology (See for explanation) (see page no. 472)

8. Ans. (a) Volume of distribution > (d) Route of administration

Ref: KDT 7th Ed page 33

- **Loading dose** is a single or few quickly repeated doses given in the beginning to attain target concentration rapidly. It may be calculated as—

Loading dose = Target Plasma Concentration X Volume of Distribution/Bioavailability

- Thus, loading dose is governed only by Volume of distribution and not by Clearance or t1/2.
- Bioavailability is also an important determinant of loading dose.
- It is a measure of the fraction (F) of administered dose of a drug that reaches the systemic circulation in the unchanged form.
- Route of administration is an important determinant of bioavailability. For example, IV route gives almost 100% bioavailability, while those given by G.I route are subjected to First pass metabolism and so on.

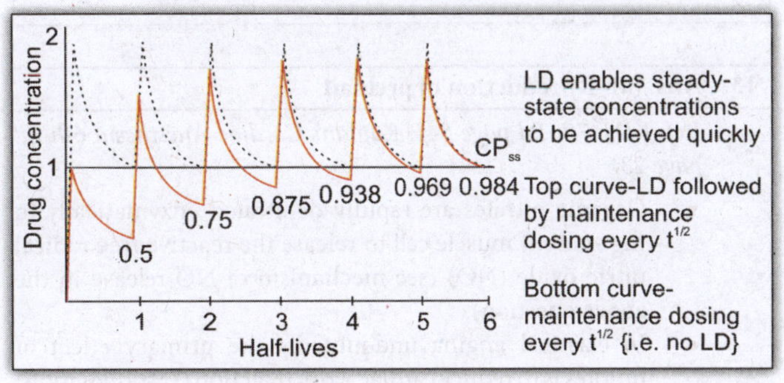

9. Ans. (D) Safety

Ref: KDT 7th ed page 63-64, Katzung 12th ed page 75, Goodman's Gillman 12th Ed page 79

Although Phase I trial is the beginning of Pharmacokinetic study of the drug it is done primarily for safety profile of the drug.

See table of "Clinical Trial and Preclinical Testing" in AIIMS May 2016 Pharmacology (see page no. 463)

10. Ans. (b) Hypoglycemia

Ref: KDT 7th Ed page 223

Repeat (AIIMS May 2018 Pharmacology) (see page no. 435)

11. Ans. (d) 8 to 15 C

Ref: Park 23nd ed page 100; http://apps.who.int/medicinedocs/en/d/Js4885e/6.5.html

Repeat (AIIMS Nov 2015 Pharmacology) (see page no. 484)

12. Ans. (b) Guanylyl cyclase

Ref: KDT 7th Ed page 303

Inhibition of PDE-5, the cGMP degrading isoenzyme in cavernosal and vascular smooth muscle, results in accumulation of cGMP and marked potentiation of NO action.

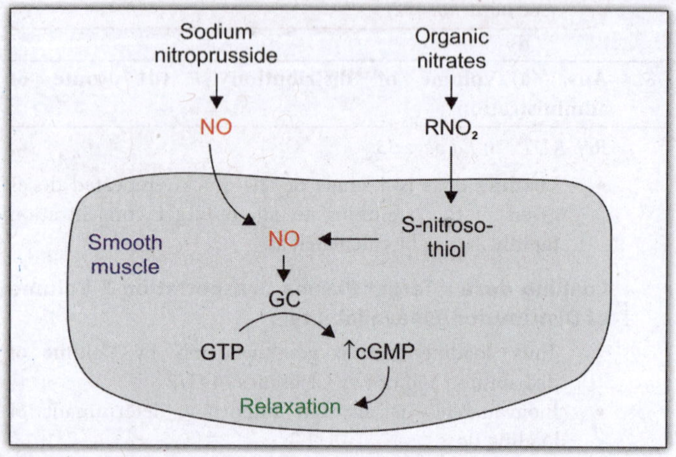

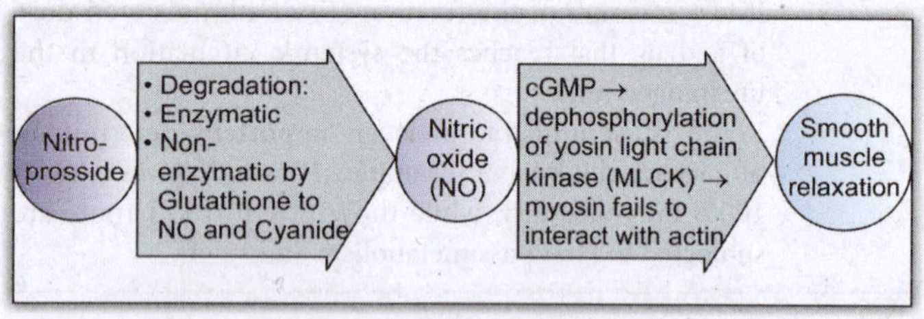

13. Ans. (a) By reduction of preload

Ref: KDT 7th Ed page 541, Kaplan's Cardiac Anesthesia 6th Ed page 236

- Organic nitrates are rapidly denitrated enzymatically in the smooth muscle cell to release the reactive free radical nitric oxide (NO) (see mechanism of NO release in the above question).
- In classical angina undoubtedly the primary effect of nitrates is to reduce cardiac work by action (vasodilatation) on peripheral vasculature, though increased blood supply to ischaemic area may contribute.

Angina

It is precipitated by a mismatch in Oxygen demand-supply ratio to the heart.

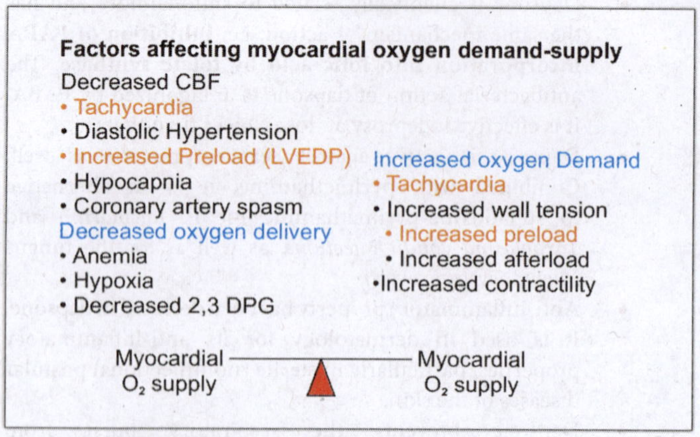

- Blood vessels supplying the deeper tissues are perforating branches of larger coronary arteries which run epicardially. The blood flow to deeper cardiac tissues occurs during diastole.
- Patients having angina often have severe arteriosclerotic affliction of these coronary arteries
- The coronary obstruction is 'fixed'; blood flow fails to increase during increased demand despite local factors mediated dilatation of resistance vessels and this causes ischaemic pain.
- Due to inadequacy of ischaemic left ventricle, the end diastolic left ventricular pressure rises from 5 to about 25 mm Hg—produces subendocardial 'crunch' during diastole and aggravates the ischaemia in this region.
- Drugs that are useful, primarily reduce cardiac work (directly by acting on heart or indirectly by reducing preload hence end diastolic pressure, and afterload).

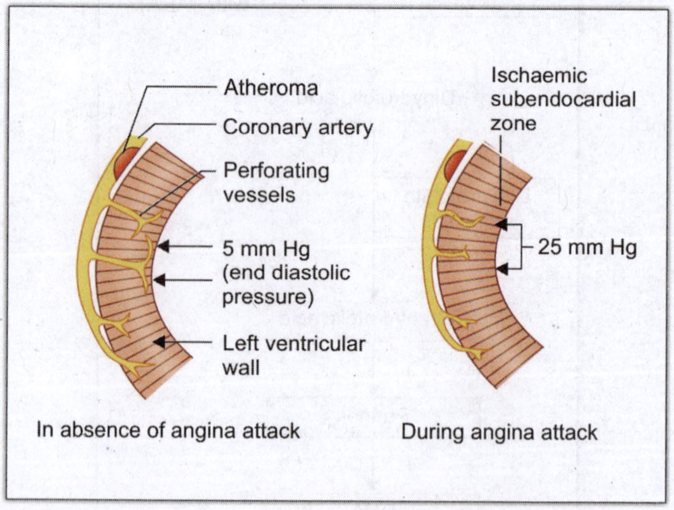

Effect of Nitrates		
Preload	**Intracardiac**	**Afterload**
• Preferential action at comparatively lower doses • **Main mechanism of action** Venodilation → peripheral pooling of blood → decreased venous return → preload on heart is reduced → end diastolic size and pressure are reduced → decreased cardiac work according to Laplace's law → reduction in ventricular radius decreases the tension that must be generated in the ventricular Wall → decreased O2 consumption. Decrease in end diastolic pressure abolishes the subendocardial crunch by restoring the pressure gradient across ventricular wall due to which subendocardial perfusion occurs during diastole.	Main mechanism of relief **in Prinzmetal angina**. Preferentially relaxation of bigger conducting coronary arteries than arterioles or resistance vessels → Favourable redistribution of blood flow to ischaemic areas	At slightly higher doses: arteriolar dilatation → slight decrease in total peripheral resistance (t.p.r.) or afterload on heart → BP falls → contributes to the reduction in cardiac work which is directly proportional to aortic impedance
Note: In ischemic zones, dilatation of autoregulatory resistance vessels increases blood flow, while in the non-ischaemic zones, resistance vessels maintain their tone → flow does not increase, or may decrease to compensate for increased flow to ischaemic zone.		

14. Ans. (c) Bradycardia with AV block

Ref: KDT 7th Ed page 535

Effect of Beta Blocker and Calcium Channel Blockers on The Heart			
Site	**Beta blocker**	**Verapamil**	**Effect**
SA node	Decreased slope of phase 4 depolarization	Decreased slope of phase 4 depolarization	Bradycardia
AV node	Prolongation of AV nodal effective refractory period (ERP)	Prolongation of AV nodal effective refractory period (ERP)	AV Nodal Block
Mechanism	Antiarrhythmic action is exerted primarily because of cardiac adrenergic blockade	Depresses Ca2+ mediated depolarization thus suppresses automaticity and reentry dependent on slow channel response	

As seen, these drugs have an additive effect and will cause bradycardia and AV block.

15. Ans. (a) Delayed diastolic depolarisation

Ref: KDT 7th Ed page 103

- The cardiac muscarinic receptors are of the M2 subtype.
- **ACh hyperpolarizes the SA nodal cells and decreases their rate of diastolic depolarization.**
- As a result, rate of impulse generation is reduced—bradycardia or even cardiac arrest may occur.
- At the A-V node and His-Purkinje fibers refractory period (RP) is increased and conduction is slowed: P-R interval increases and partial to complete A-V block may be produced. However, this is not a direct cause of fall in heart rate.
- The force of atrial contraction is markedly reduced and RP of atrial fibers is abbreviated.
- Due to nonuniform vagal innervation, the intensity of effect on RP and conduction of different atrial fibers varies— inducing inhomogeneity and predisposing to atrial fibrillation or flutter.
- Ventricular contractility is also decreased but the effect is not marked.

16. Ans. (b) Cardiac defects

Ref: KDT 7th Ed page 449

Lithium causes foetal goiter, cardiac and other abnormalities, especially in the period of growth and development, i.e, after day 56 of fetus.

Teratogenic Effects of Common Anticonvulsant Medications		
Drug	**Abnormalities described**	**Pregnancy category**
Valproate	Neural-tube defects, clefts, skeletal abnormalities, developmental delay	D
Phenytoin	Fetal hydantoin syndrome: craniofacial anomalies, fingernail hypoplasia, growth deficiency, developmental delay, cardiac defects, clefts	D
Lithium	Ebstein anomaly (mc), Fetal goitre, cleft palate in experimental animals	D

Contd...

Teratogenic Effects of Common Anticonvulsant Medications		
Drug	**Abnormalities described**	**Pregnancy category**
Carbamazepine	Fetal hydantoin syndrome, spina bifida	D
Phenobarbital	Clefts, cardiac anomalies, urinary tract malformations	D
Lamotrigine	Inhibits dihydrofolate reductase, lowering fetal folate levels. Registry data suggest increased risk for clefts	C
Topiramate	Registry data suggest increased risk for clefts	C
Levetiracetam	Theoretical—skeletal abnormalities and impaired growth in animals at doses similar to or greater than human therapeutic doses	C

17. Ans. (a) Ethambutol

Ref: KDT 7th Ed page 769

(See table of "Antitubercular Drug" in AIIMS May 2014 Pharmacology) (see Volume II)

- Loss of visual acuity/colour vision, field defects due to optic neuritis is the most important dose and duration of Ethambutol therapy dependent toxicity.
- Patients should be instructed to stop the drug at the first indication of visual impairment.
- Earlier it was contraindicated in children because young children may be unable to report early visual impairment, but it is now allowed with due precaution.
- With early recognition and stoppage of the drug, visual toxicity is reversible.
- Ethambutol is contraindicated in patients with optic neuritis.

18. Ans. (d) Acetazolamide

Ref: KDT 7th Ed page 587

- When they first arrive at a high altitude, many individuals develop transient "mountain sickness." This syndrome develops 8–24 h after arrival at altitude and lasts 4–8 days.
- It is characterized by headache, irritability, insomnia, breathlessness, and nausea and vomiting. It appears to be associated with cerebral edema. The low PO2 at high altitude causes arteriolar dilation, and if cerebral auto regulation does not compensate, there is an increase in capillary pressure that causes increased transudation of fluid into brain tissue.
- All forms of high-altitude illness are benefited by descent to lower altitude and by treatment with the diuretic acetazolamide.
- Acetazolamide is a carbonic anhydrase inhibitor, and results in stimulated respiration, increased PaCO2, lowering of CSF and brain pH, and reduced formation of CSF.
- When cerebral edema is marked, large doses of glucocorticoids are often administered as well. Their mechanism of action is unsettled.

19. Ans. (a) Indinavir

Ref: KDT 7th ed page 805, Harrison 19th ed page 1274

Nephrolithiasis and crystalluria are a unique toxicity caused by Indinavir amongst anti retroviral drugs.

See table of "Antiretroviral Drugs used in the Treatment of HIV Infection" in AIIMS MAY 2015 Pharmacology (see page no. 487)

20. Ans. (b) Hepatotoxicity

Ref: KDT 7th Ed page 417

A rare but serious adverse effect of valproate is fulminant hepatitis; occurs only in children (especially below 3 years). Those with hepatic disease or who receive other anticonvulsant or hepatotoxic drug are at greater risk.

21. Ans. (a) Preparing monoclonal antibodies

Ref: KDT 7th ed page 871-72, 884, Jawetz 26th ed page 133

- In the given figure, we can see myeloma cells to the right, and a single cell to the left, which then forms a homogenous clone of cells after combining with myeloma cells.
- Immunoglobulins that arise from a single clone of cells, e.g., in a plasma cell tumor (myeloma), are homogeneous and are referred to as monoclonal. Monoclonal antibodies can be produced by fusing a myeloma cell with an antibody-producing lymphocyte.
- Such hybridomas can produce unlimited quantities of monoclonal antibodies in vitro.
- **Polyclonal antibodies:**
- Antibodies that arise in an animal in response to a single complex antigen are heterogeneous because they are formed by many different clones of cells, each expressing an antibody capable of reacting with a different antigenic determinant on the complex antigen.
- These antibodies are said to be polyclonal.

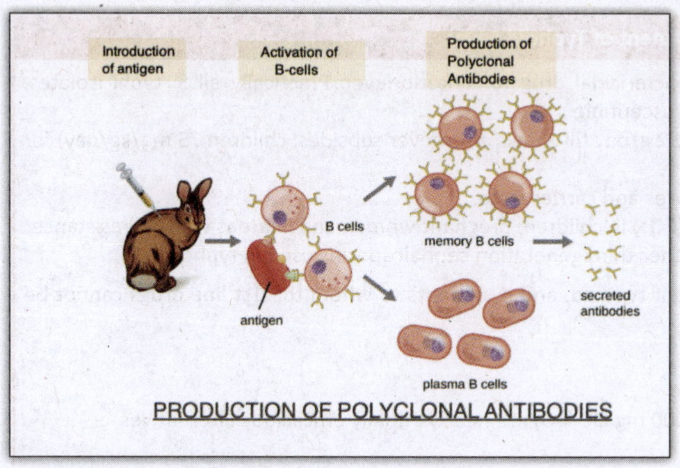

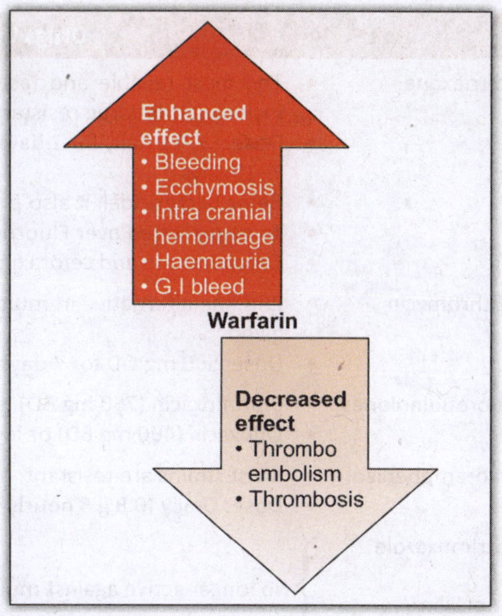

22. Ans. (b) Carbamazepine

Ref: KDT 7th Ed page 26,767

Warfarin is an anticoagulant drug that acts by interfering with synthesis of Vitamin K dependent clotting factors.

Conditions Affecting the Action of Warfarin

Condition	Mechanism
Conditions Enhancing the Action of Warfarin	
Debility, malnutrition, malabsorption, prolonged antibiotic therapy	Decreased supply of Vitamin K to liver
Newborns	Low level of Vitamin K and clotting factors
Liquid paraffin (habitual use)	Reduced vitamin K absorption
Broad-spectrum antibiotics	Inhibit gut flora and reduce Vitamin K production
Liver disease, chronic alcoholism	Liver disease, chronic alcoholism
Newer cephalosporins (ceftriaxone, cefoperazone)	Same mechanism as Warfarin-additive action
Long acting sulfonamides, Indomethacin, phenytoin and probenecid	Displace warfarin from plasma protein binding
Chloramphenicol, erythromycin, celecoxib, isoniazid, cimetidine, allopurinol, amiodarone, metronidazole. (Tolbutamide, phenytoin inhibit warfarin metabolism and vice versa)	Inhibition of warfarin metabolism
Hyperthyroidism	Faster degradation of clotting factors
Conditions Reducing the Action of Warfarin	
Barbiturates (except benzodiazepines), carbamazepine, rifampin and griseofulvin	Induction of metabolism of oral anticoagulants.
Oral contraceptives	Increase blood levels of clotting factors

Note:
The dose of anticoagulant determined during therapy with enzyme inducer drugs would be higher, If the same is continued after withdrawing the inducer-marked hypoprothrombinemia can occur, and fatal bleeding has been reported.

AIIMS MAY 2018

23. Ans. (b) Amikacin

Ref: KDT 7th Ed page 712, Jawetz 26th Ed page 376

- Aminoglycosides are not effective in treating Salmonella enteric fevers because the Salmonellae are **intracellular** and the aminoglycosides do not enter the cells.
- Cefepime being a 4th generation cephalosporin, can be used against Salmonella, though not routinely used.

Drugs Used for Treatment of Typhoid Fever	
Ceftriaxone	• The most reliable and fastest acting bactericidal drug for enteric fever. Practically all S. typhi isolates, including multidrug resistant ones, are susceptible. • Dose: i.v. 4 g daily for 2 days followed by 2 g/day till 2 days after fever subsides; children 75 mg/kg/day) for 7–10 days • Being bactericidal, it also prevents relapses and carrier state. • To be preferred over Fluoroquinolones (FQs) in children, pregnant women and in areas with FQ resistance. • Cefoperazone and cefotaxime are the other third generation cephalosporins used in typhoid.
Azithromycin	• 2nd line alternative in multidrug resistant typhoid, and in patients to whom the 1st line drugs cannot be given • Dose: 500 mg OD for 7 days
Fluoroquinolones	• Ciprofloxacin (750 mg BD) is mostly used. • Ofloxacin (400 mg BD) or levofloxacin (500 mg OD/BD) are nearly equally efficacious alternatives
Chloramphenicol	• Most strains are resistant • Dose: Orally (0.5 g 6 hourly till fever subsides, then 0.25 g 6 hourly for 5–7 days).
Cotrimoxazole	No longer active against multi drug resistant thyroid
Ampicillin/ Amoxicillin	

24. Ans. (a) Safety

Ref: KDT 7th Ed page 55, Lippincott 6th Ed page 35

"The gap between the therapeutic effect dose response curve (DRC) and the adverse effect DRC defines the safety margin or the therapeutic index of a drug."

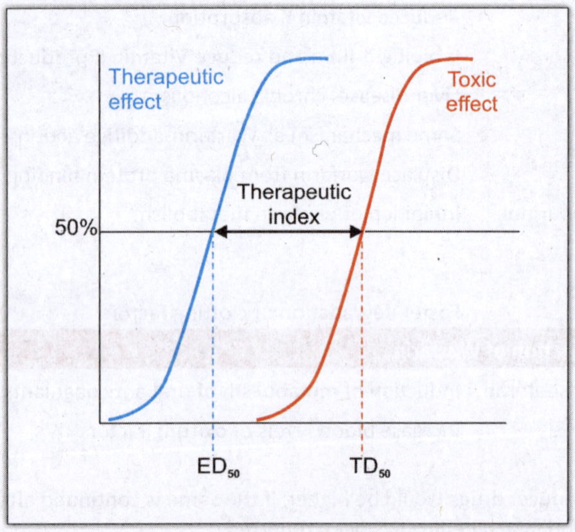

Fig: Therapeutic index

$$\text{Therapeutic index} = \frac{\text{Median Lethal Dose}}{\text{Median Effective Dose}}$$

Or LD_{50}/ED_{50}

Where: Median effective dose (ED_{50}) is the dose which produces the specified effect in 50% individuals and median lethal dose (LD_{50}) is the dose which kills 50% of the recipients.

More about the Dose Response Curve

Simple dose response curve hyperbolic in shape while log DRC is sigmoid in shape. There are three important parameters- potency, efficacy and slope	
Potency	It is the measure of the amount of drug needed to produce the response. Drug producing same response at lower dose is more potent (in DRC more the dose response curve towards left, greater is the potency i.e. A > B > C > D) 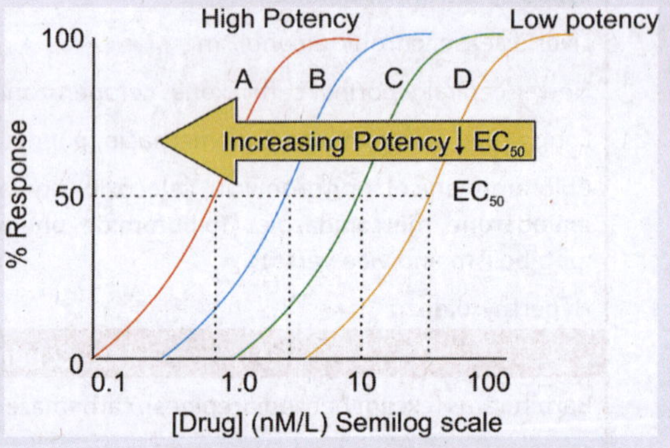
Efficacy	It is the maximum effect produced by a drug. It is clinically more important than potency. (On DRC- More is the peak of curve greater is its efficacy i.e. A>B>C>D) 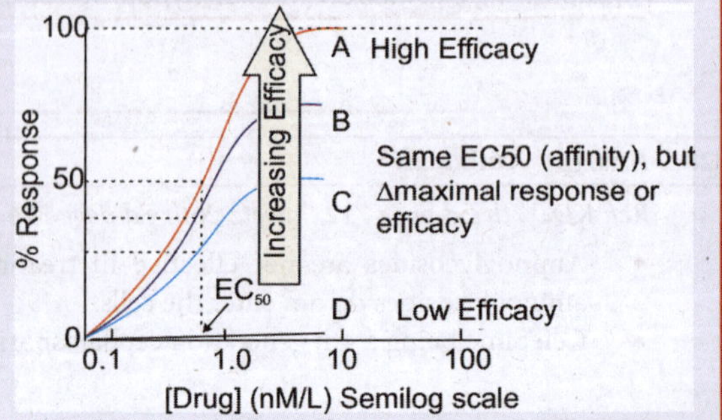

Contd...

Slope	Steeper is the slope more are the chances of getting the response drastically with increase in dose. I.e. steep DRC means narrow therapeutic index

25. Ans. (a) Volume of distribution > (D) Route of administration

Ref: KDT 7th Ed page 33

Repeat AIIMS NOV 2018 Pharmacology (see page no. 427)

26. Ans. (a) Tmax

Ref: Basic Pharmacokinetics and Pharmacodynamics by Sara E. Rosenbaum Ch 9; Pharmacology: Principles and Practice By Miles Hacker page 256

The three important pharmacokinetic parameters that describe the plasma level-time curve and useful in assessing the bioavailability of a drug are

- **Peak Plasma concentration (Cmax):** The point of maximum concentration of drug in plasma is called as the peak and the concentration of drug at peak is known as peak plasma concentration. It is also called as peak height concentration and maximum drug concentration. Cmax is expressed in mcg/mL. The peak level depends upon
  - Dose administered
  - Rate of absorption, and
  - Rate of elimination.

  The peak represents the point of time when absorption rate equals elimination rate of drug. The portion of curve to the left of peak represents **absorption phase** i.e. when the rate of absorption is greater than the rate of elimination. The section of curve to the right of peak generally represents **elimination phase** i.e. when the rate of elimination exceeds rate of absorption
- **Time of peak concentration (tmax):** The time for drug to reach peak concentration in plasma (after extravascular administration) is called as the time of peak concentration. Tmax is the time at which absorption rate and elimination rate are equal. ***It is expressed in hours and is useful in estimating the rate of absorption***. Onset time and onset of action are dependent upon tmax.
- **Area under the curve (AUC):** It represents the total integrated area under the plasma level-time profile and expresses the total amount of drug that comes into the systemic circulation after its administration. AUC is expressed in mcg/mL/hours. It is the most important parameter in evaluating the bioavailability of a drug from its dosage form as it represents the extent of absorption.

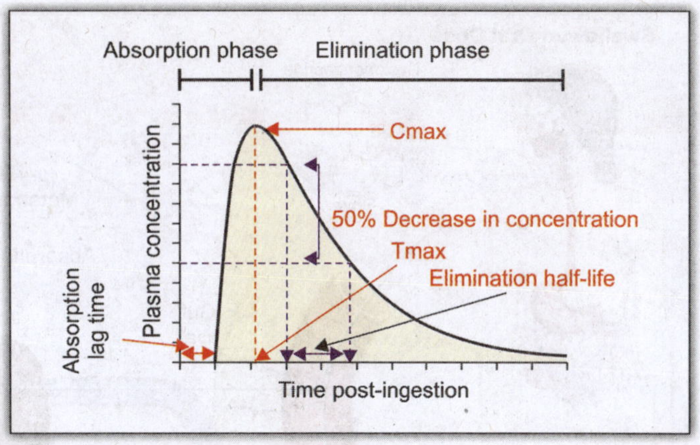

27. Ans. (b) Intravenous

Ref: KDT 7th Ed page 9, 16

- Bioavailability refers to the rate and extent of absorption of a drug from a dosage form as determined by its concentration-time curve in blood or by its excretion in urine.
- It is a measure of the fraction (F) of administered dose of a drug that reaches the systemic circulation in the unchanged form.
- Different routes of administration affect the drug's bioavailability.
- ***Bioavailability of drug injected i.v. is around 100%***, but is frequently lower after oral ingestion because— (a) the drug may be incompletely absorbed. (b) the absorbed drug may undergo first pass metabolism in the intestinal wall/liver or be excreted in bile.
- Incomplete bioavailability after s.c. or i.m. injection is less common, but may occur due to local binding of the drug.

28. Ans. (a) Oral

Ref: KDT 7th Ed page 6, 8, 16, 27

First Pass Metabolism

- This refers to metabolism of a drug during its passage from the site of absorption into the systemic circulation. The major site for first pass metabolism is the liver and intestine.
- Drugs entering through oral route undergo first pass metabolism to a great extent.
- Sublingual administration of a drug bypasses the liver (enters venous system) and drugs with high first pass metabolism can be absorbed directly into systemic circulation.
- Parenteral routes bypass the liver and intestines as a site of first pass metabolism.

Note

Limited presystemic metabolism can occur in the skin (transdermally administered drug) and in lungs (for drug reaching venous blood through any route). Drug entering from any systemic route is exposed to first pass metabolism in lungs, but its extent is minor for most drugs.

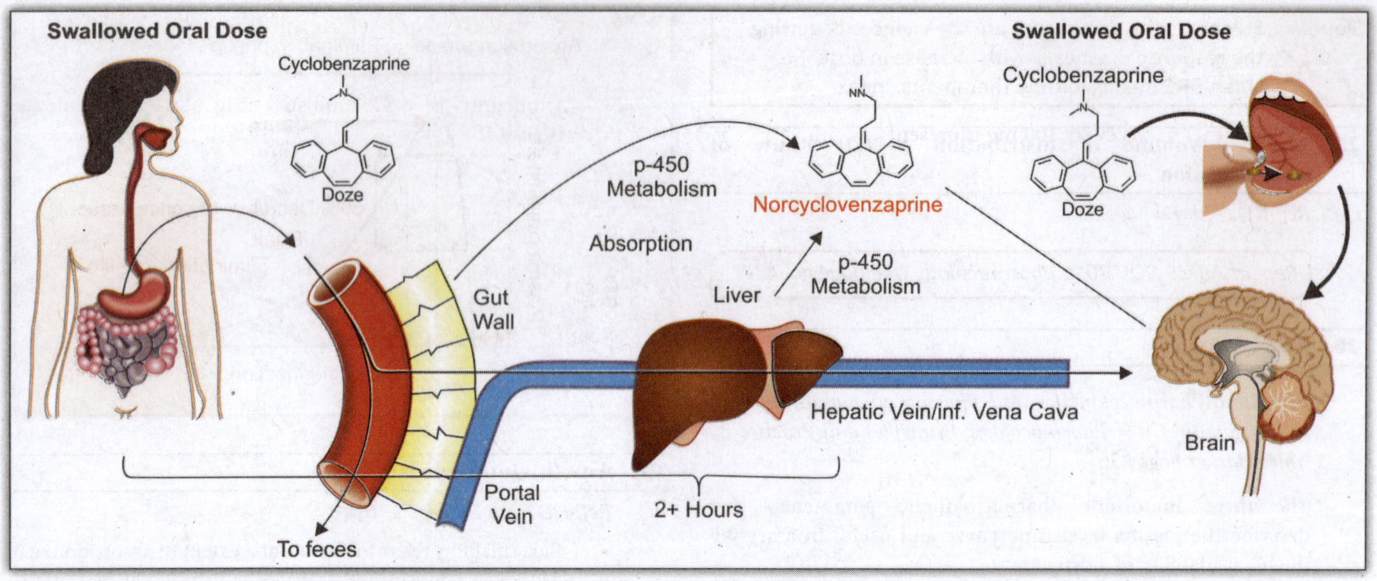

29. Ans. (a) Decreased secretion of insulin

Ref: KDT 7th Ed page 259, Treatment of EARLY DIABETES R. Camerini-Davalos page 85

- The inflow of potassium in islet cells is mediated, in part, by an oubain-sensitive ATPase.
- The outflow of potassium is by passive movement driven by electrochemical gradient of potassium across plasma membrane
- The Beta cells of islets of Langerhans have a glucose sensing mechanism dependent on entry of glucose into β cells (through GLUT1) and its phosphorylation by glucokinase.
- Normally, glucose entry and metabolism leads to activation of the glucosensor which indirectly inhibits the ATP-sensitive K^+ channel (K^+ ATP) resulting in **partial depolarization of the β cells.**
- This increases intracellular calcium availability and causes release of insulin.
- Valinomycin allows potassium to permeate inside mitochondria and dissipate proton gradient.
- Thus, there is increased inflow of potassium into cells, thereby causing a state of hyperpolarization and decreasing the release of insulin.

Secretagogues-Mechanism of Action

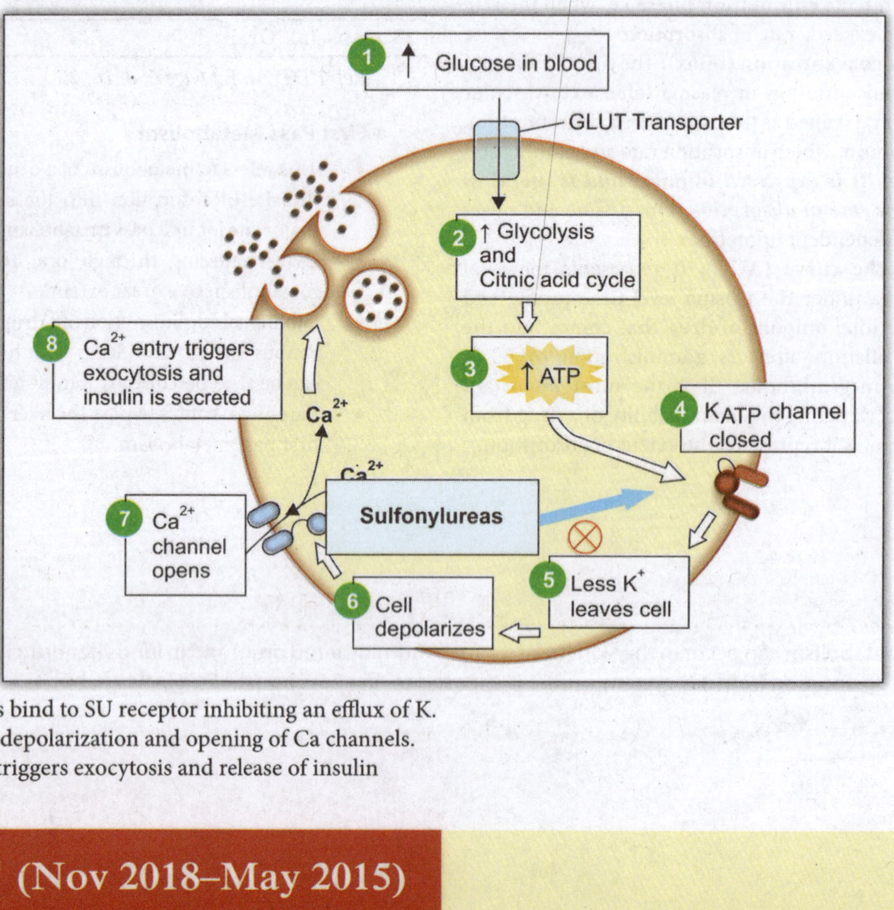

- Sulfonylureas bind to SU receptor inhibiting an efflux of K.
- This leads to depolarization and opening of Ca channels.
- Influx of Ca triggers exocytosis and release of insulin

30. Ans. (b) 18

Ref: Pharmaceutical Calculations By Howard C. Ansel 14th ed page 428

500 mg/5mL means every 100 mg is present in 1 mL,
So, 180 mg will be present in 1.8 mL
10 divisions per mL means 0.1 mL per division
So, 1.8 mL will be present in 18 divisions

NOTE

Please read the question carefully. *Number of* ***divisions*** in 2 mL syringe has been asked, not amount of drug in mL.

31. Ans. (a) Hypoglycemia

Ref: KDT 7th Ed page 223

- Salbutamol is a β2 agonistic drug used to terminate attacks of asthma.
- Its β2:β1 selectivity ratio is 10

Side effects:

- Muscle tremors are the dose related side effect.
- Palpitations, restlessness, nervousness, throat irritation and ankle edema can also occur. Hypokalaemia is a possible complication.

32. Ans. (a) Benzathine penicillin 7.2 million units in three divided doses

Ref: KDT 7th Ed Page 720,763; Harrison's 19th Ed page 1136

For late syphilis including cardiovascular syphilis, benzathine penicillin 2.4 MU weekly for 3 weeks is recommended.

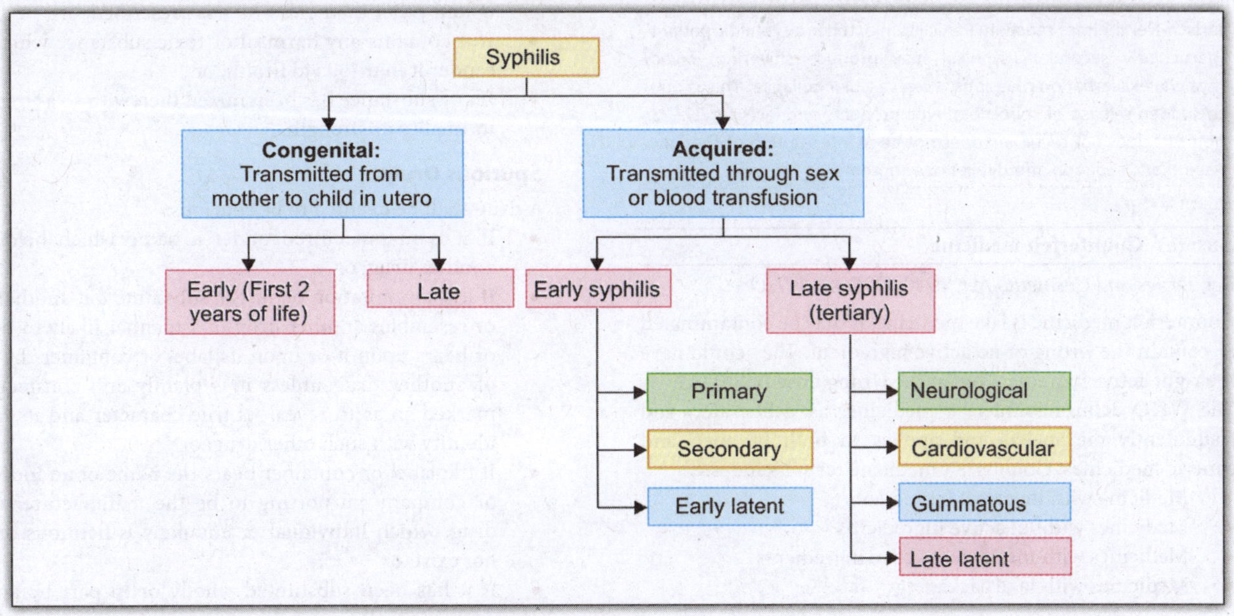

Fig: WHO classification of syphilis

- Cardiovascular manifestations of syphilis, usually appearing 10–40 years after infection, are attributable to endarteritis obliterans of the vasa vasorum which provide the blood supply to large vessels.
- Cardiovascular involvement results in uncomplicated aortitis, aortic regurgitation, saccular aneurysm (usually of the ascending aorta) or coronary ostial stenosis.
- Linear calcification of the ascending aorta on chest x-ray films suggests asymptomatic syphilitic aortitis, as arteriosclerosis seldom produces this sign.
- *T. pallidum* has not shown any resistance and PnG is the drug of choice.

Treatment of Syphilis		
Stage of syphilis	**Patients without penicillin allergy**	**Patients with penicillin allergy**
Primary, secondary, or early latent	Penicillin G benzathine (single dose of 2.4 mU IM)	Tetracycline HCl (500 mg PO qid) or doxycycline (100 mg PO bid) for 2 weeks
Late latent (or latent of uncertain duration), cardiovascular, or benign tertiary	Penicillin G benzathine (2.4 mU IM weekly for 3 weeks)	Tetracycline HCl (500 mg PO qid) or doxycycline (100 mg PO bid) for 4 weeks

Contd...

Treatment of Syphilis		
Stage of syphilis	**Patients without penicillin allergy**	**Patients with penicillin allergy**
Neurosyphilis (asymptomatic or symptomatic)	Aqueous crystalline penicillin G (18–24 mU/d IV, given as 3–4 mU q4h or continuous infusion) for 10–14 days *Or* Aqueous procaine penicillin G (2.4 mU/d IM) plus oral probenecid (500 mg qid), both for 10–14 days	Desensitization and treatment with penicillin. Ceftriaxone (2 g/d either IM or IV for 10–14 days) can be used; however, cross-reactivity between penicillin and ceftriaxone is possible
Syphilis in pregnancy	According to stage	Desensitization and treatment with penicillin

Footnote:
- If CSF examination is abnormal, treat as Neurosyphilis

Also Know

Jarisch-Herxheimer reaction: Penicillin injected in a syphilitic patient (particularly secondary syphilis) may produce shivering, fever, myalgia, exacerbation of lesions, even vascular collapse. This is due to sudden release of spirochetal lytic products and lasts for 12–72 hours. It does not recur and does not need interruption of therapy. Aspirin and sedation afford relief of symptoms

33. Ans. (a) Counterfeit medicine

Ref: Drugs and Cosmetics Act, 1940, USFDA, WHO

Counterfeit medicine is fake medicine. It may be contaminated or contain the wrong or no active ingredient. They could have the right active ingredient but at the wrong dose (USFDA).

The WHO defines counterfeit medicines as 'deliberately and fraudulently mislabeled' and applies to both branded and generic medicines. Counterfeit medicine term includes:
- Medicine with incorrect ingredients
- Medicines without active ingredients
- Medicines with insufficient active ingredients
- Medicines with fake packaging

Misbranded Drugs

A drug shall be deemed to be misbranded:
- If it is so colored, coated, powdered or polished that damage is concealed or if it is made to appear of better or greater therapeutic value than it really is; or
- If it is not labeled in the prescribed manner; or
- If its label or container or anything accompanying the drug bears any statement, design or device which makes any false claim for the drug or which is false or misleading in any particulars

Adulterated Drugs

A drug shall be deemed to be adulterated:
- If it consists in whole or in part, of any filthy, putrid or decomposed substance; or
- If it has been prepared, packed or stored under insanitary conditions where by it may have been contaminated with filth or whereby it may have been rendered injurious to health; or
- If its container is composed, in whole or in part, of any poisonous or deleterious substance which may render the contents injurious to health; or
- If it bears or contains, for purposes of colouring only, a colour other than one which is prescribed; or
- If it contains any harmful or toxic substance which may render it injurious to health; or
- If any substance has been mixed therewith so as to reduce its quality or strength.

Spurious Drugs

A drug shall be deemed to be spurious:
- If it is manufactured under a name which belongs to another drug; or
- If it is an imitation of, or is a substitute for, another drug or resembles another drug in a manner likely to deceive or bears upon it or upon its label or container the name of another drug unless it is plainly and conspicuously marked so as to reveal its true character and its lack of identity with such other drug; or
- If the label or container bears the name of an individual or company purporting to be the manufacturer of the drug, which individual or company is fictitious or does not exist; or
- If it has been substituted wholly or in part by another drug or substance; or
- If it purports to be the product of a manufacturer of whom it is not truly a product.

34. Ans. (a) Venlafaxine

Ref: Katzung 13th Ed page 524-525, Goodman Gilman 13th Ed page 273

- Agitation, anxiety and insomnia are associated with withdrawal of antidepressants. Other symptoms include flu-like symptoms, insomnia, nausea, imbalance, sensory disturbances, and hyperarousal.
- Amongst the options, Venlafaxine is an SNRI, while Imipramine is a TCA. Both are antidepressants.
- There are 2 points in favor of Venlafaxine in this question-
  - Imipramine withdrawal usually manifests 48 hours after withdrawal due to its longer t1/2 as compared to Venlafaxine.
  - There are no cholinergic symptoms like sweating, piloerection which are present with Imipramine withdrawal.
- **Antidepressant withdrawal syndrome:**

- **SSRI/SNRI withdrawal:** A temporary deficiency of synaptic serotonin occurs with abrupt withdrawal of an SSRI. This deficiency is compounded by the fact that down-regulated receptors will remain in their relatively hypoactive state for days to weeks. This is believed to result in antidepressant discontinuation syndrome directly or indirectly via downstream effects on other neurotransmitter systems (e.g., norepinephrine, dopamine, and γ-amino-butyric acid) implicated in depressive and anxiety disorders.
- **TCA withdrawal:** Because tricyclic antidepressants and MAOIs also are serotonergically active, the same mechanism is implicated for their respective antidepressant discontinuation syndromes; however, tricyclic antidepressants also affect the **cholinergic system**, so rapid discontinuation may cause signs of **parkinsonism and problems with balance.**
- **MAO inhibitor withdrawal:** Because MAOIs cause changes in the alpha2-adrenergic and dopaminergic receptors, their discontinuation may cause agitation and **psychosis.**

35. Ans. (a) Antithrombin III

Ref: KDT 7th Ed page 617

- Heparin acts indirectly by activating plasma antithrombin III (AT III, a serine proteinase inhibitor).
- The heparin-AT III complex then binds to clotting factors of the intrinsic and common pathways (Xa, IIa, IXa, XIa, XIIa and XIIIa) and inactivates them but not factor VIIa operative in the extrinsic pathway. At low concentrations of heparin, factor Xa mediated conversion of prothrombin to thrombin is selectively affected.
- The anticoagulant action is exerted mainly by inhibition of factor Xa as well as thrombin (IIa) mediated conversion of fibrinogen to fibrin.
- Antithrombin III is itself a substrate for the protease clotting factors; binds with the protease to form a stable complex (suicide inhibitor). However, in the absence of heparin, the two interact very slowly. **Heparin enhances the action of AT III** in two ways:
  - Long heparin molecule provides scaffolding for the clotting factors (mainly Xa and IIa) as well as AT III to get bound and interact with each other.
  - Heparin induces conformational change in AT III to expose its interactive sites.

    A specific pentasaccharide sequence, which is present in only some of the heparin molecules, binds to AT III with high affinity to induce the conformational change needed for rapid interaction with clotting factors.
- Inhibition of IIa requires both the mechanisms, but Xa inhibition can occur by mechanism 'b' alone
- Low concentrations of heparin prolong aPTT without significantly prolonging PT. High concentrations prolong both. Thus, low concentrations interfere selectively with the intrinsic pathway, affecting amplification and continuation of clotting, while high concentrations affect the common pathway as well.

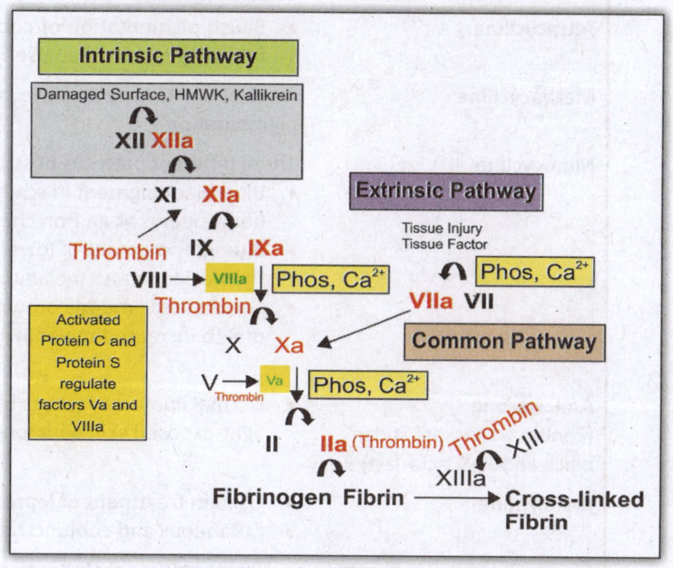

36. Ans. (a) Metoclopramide

Ref: KDT 7th Ed page 665, Katzung 13th Ed page 1070

- Metoclopramide is a D2 antagonist,5-HT3 antagonist and 5-HT4 agonist.
- The central antidopaminergic (D2) action of metoclopramide on CTZ is clearly responsible for its antiemetic property. However, D2 antagonism can result in extrapyramidal side effects.
- Sedation, dizziness, loose stools, muscle dystonia (especially in children) are the main side effects of Metoclopramide.
- Ondansetron is a 5HT antagonist. It does not act on Dopamine receptors.
- Domperidone acts only on D2 receptors in the g.i.t, with minimal central activity. Hence extrapyramidal effects are rare.

37. Ans. (a) Bleomycin

Ref: Weedon's Skin Pathology Essentials by Ronald. B. Johnston 2nd ed page 296, Goodman Gilman 13th ed page 1193

Name	Predilection and clinical key features	Histopathology
Drug deposits and pigmentation		
Antimalarial drugs	• Various pigmentations possible: ▪ Ochronosis-like deposits ▪ Pretibial pigment with slate-gray to blue-black	
Phenothiazines	• Progressive gray-blue pigment in sun-exposed areas • Stain with Fontana–Masson (melanina) but not Perls' (hemosiderin)	
Tetracyclline	• Bluish pigmentation of cutaneous osteomas and bluish-green pigmentation in areas of trauma following tetracycline use	
Methacyclline	Antibiotic with may produce gray-black pigmentation in light-exposed areas and conjunctival pigmentation	
Minocycline	Three different patterns possible: • Blue-black pigment in scars, related to hemosiderin or an iron chelate of minocycline • Blue-gray pigment of lower legs and arms (hemosiderin and melanin) • Generalized "muddy brown" pigmentation due to increased melanin in basal layer	• Pigment in macrophages, dermal dendrocytes and eccrine myoepithelial cells (localized patterns) • Extremity pigmenation stains with Perls' (hemosiderin) and Fontana—Masson (melanin), not PAS • Scar pigmentation stains with Perls' only and not Fontana
Amlodarone (Fontana–Masson, sudan black and PAS, acid-fast)	• Dermal lipofuscin causes blue-gray pigment in light-exposed skin with long-term use	• Yellow-brown granules of lipofuscin found in macrophages (around vessels at papillary and reticular junction)
Clofazimine	• Used in treatment of leprosy, DLE • Cutaneous and conjunctival pigmentation with reddish-blue hue	
Chemotherapeutic agents	• Pigmentation of skin may occur following bleomycin, busulfan, doxorubicin, etc. ▪ Bleomycin (cytotoxic antibiotic used in Hodgkin's disease and testicular cancer) may cause "flagellate pigmentation" (linear hyperpigmented streaks often on chest and back) ▪ Similar pigmentation ("flagellate mushroom dermatitis") may be seen with ingestion of raw shiitake mushrooms	

38. Ans. (a) Edaravone

Ref: Lange clinical neurology 10th Ed page vii, 251

- ***Edaravone is a drug newly approved for the treatment of Amyotrophic lateral sclerosis.***
- It is the first drug introduced for the treatment of Amyotrophic Lateral Sclerosis after around 20 yrs.
- Edaravone has anti-oxidant properties.
- Oxidative stress caused by free radicals is believed to be one of the causes of nerve cell death in ALS.
- It has a neuroprotective effect and slows the progression of ALS by removing free radicals in the nervous system.
- It is administered 60 mg intravenously (into the bloodstream) in 28-day cycles. The treatment starts with a patient receiving the therapy for 14 consecutive days, followed by a two-week drug-free period. Patients then receive an infusion during 10 of the next 14 days, followed by a two-week drug-free period.

39. Ans. (a) Febuxostat

Ref: KDT 7th Ed page 217

Febuxostat is a recently introduced nonpurine xanthine oxidase inhibitor, equally or more effective than allopurinol in lowering blood uric acid level in patients with hyperuricaemia and gout.

Anti Rheumatoid Drugs	
Disease modifying antirheumatic drugs (DMARDs)	• **Non biological drugs:** ▪ **Immunosuppressants:** Methotrexate, Azathioprine, Cyclosporine ▪ Sulfasalazine ▪ Chloroquine or Hydroxychloroquine ▪ Leflunomide **(Gold and penicillamine are obsolete DMARDs.)** • **Biological agents** ▪ **TNFα inhibitors:** Etanercept, Infliximab, Adalimumab ▪ IL-1 antagonist: Anakinra
Adjuvant drugs	**Corticosteroids:** Prednisolone and others

Drugs used in Gout
Acute gout
NSAIDs Colchicine Corticosteroids

Contd...

Chronic Gout	
Uricosurics	**Synthesis inhibitors**
Probenecid Sulfinpyrazone	Allopurinol Febuxostat

40. Ans. (a) Low molecular weight heparin

Ref: "Optimal Treatment Approaches of Cancer-Induced Thrombosis" American College of Cardiology 2017 guidelines

- Current guideline-endorsed therapy options for cancer-associated thrombosis include **low molecular weight heparin (LMWH), unfractionated heparin (UFH), warfarin, and fondaparinux.**
- **All current guidelines recommend LMWH for at least 3-6 months in cancer-associated VTE**, with the potential to treat indefinitely in patients with active malignancy and ongoing treatment.
- UFH can be considered for patients with renal insufficiency, and fondaparinux can be considered for patients with heparin-induced thrombocytopenia (HIT).

Cancer and Thromboembolism

- Venous thromboembolism (VTE) is a highly prevalent and significant cause of both morbidity and mortality in patients with cancer.
- Virchow's triad summarizes the multi-factorial risks associated with VTE development, cancer-induced hypercoagulability(pro-coagulant and inflammatory cytokines), endothelial and vessel wall damage (chemotherapy-induced interleukin and tumor necrosis factor release as well as indwelling catheters needed for medication administration), and venous stasis (immobility and venous external compression).
- Risk for VTE and recurrent VTE is highest among patients with hematologic malignancies, lung cancer, gastrointestinal cancer (stomach/colon), pancreatic cancer, kidney cancer, and bone cancer, patients with myelodysplastic disorder, and in patients with distant metastases
- VTE management in patients with cancer requires a complicated balance between high recurrence risk and concerns for significant hemorrhagic complications.
- Additionally, patients with cancer frequently have comorbid conditions (e.g., renal failure, thrombocytopenia) or use of medications that interact with and limit the safe use of many anticoagulant medications.
- Finally, these patients require frequent interruptions in therapy for invasive procedures; have medication-induced dietary changes affecting vitamin K intake, and potential intolerance for oral administration due to GI adverse effects associated with chemotherapy.

41. Ans. (b) Schedule H

Ref: KDT 7th Ed page 4,5

Repeat AIIMS NOV 2018 (See for explanation)

As per drug rules, majority of drugs including all antibiotics must be sold in retail only against a prescription issued to a patient by a registered medical practitioner. These are called 'prescription drugs', and in India they have been placed in the schedule H of the Drugs and Cosmetic Rules (1945) as amended from time to time.

42. Ans. (b) Flucytosine: Inhibit microtubule thereby preventing mitosis

Ref: KDT 7th Ed page 790

Option(A) True

Imidazoles and triazoles acts by inhibiting the fungal cytochrome P450 enzyme *'lanosterol 14-demethylase'* and thus impair ergosterol synthesis leading to a cascade of membrane abnormalities in the fungus.

Option(B) False

Flucytosine is a *pyrimidine antimetabolite* which is inactive as such i.e. it is a Prodrug. After uptake into fungal cells, it is converted into 5-fluorouracil and then to 5-fluorodeoxyuridylic acid which is an inhibitor of thymidylate synthesis. Thymidylic acid is a component of DNA.

Option (C) True

Echinocandins (e.g. Caspofungin, Micafungin, Anidulafungin) a new class of potent semisynthetic antifungal antibiotics with a complex cyclic lipopeptide structure. it *inhibits the synthesis of β-1, 3-glucan,* which is a unique component of the fungal cell wall.

Option (D) True

Amphotericin B: Impair barrier mechanism in cell membrane. The polyenes (name polyene is derived from their highly double bonded structure for which Amphotericin B is a prototype) have high affinity for ergosterol present in fungal cell membrane. Polyenes combine with fungal cell wall and get inserted into the membrane and orient themselves to form a ***'micropore'*** with interior hydrophilic side and outer lipophilic side, thus cell permeability is markedly increased.

Mechanism of Action of Anti Fungals

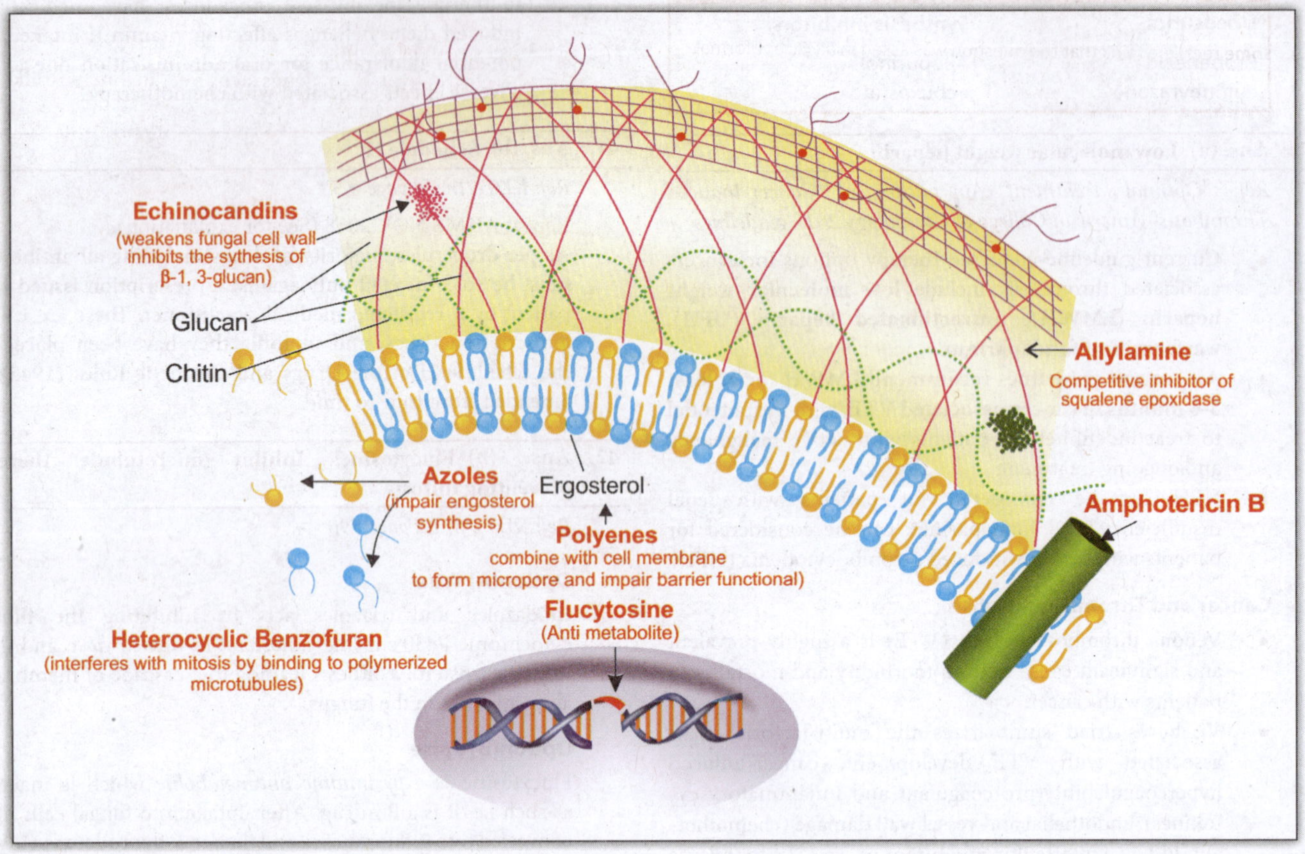

43. Ans. (d) Dolutegravir—inhibits integration of viral DNA into host

Ref: KDT 7th ed page 805, Harrison 19th ed page 1277, Lippincott 6th Ed page 579-583

See table of "Targets and Mechanism of Antiretroviral Drugs" in AIIMS MAY 2017 (see page no. 446)

Dolutegravir is an HIV-1 antiviral agent. It inhibits HIV integrase by binding to the active site and blocking the strand transfer step of retroviral DNA integration in the host cell.

AIIMS NOVEMBER 2017

44. Ans. (c) Tasimelton

Ref: Sleep Medicine by Nick Antic 1st Ed Ch 35; Manual of Clinical Psychopharmacology

By Alan F. Schatzberg 8th Ed

- Given the inability of light to treat insomnia in the blind, an alternative therapy is required that will entrain the circadian clock, and therefore the sleep/wake cycle.
- Both melatonin and a melatonin agonist have been shown to reset the circadian clock in the totally blind.
- Tasimelteon is a melatonin MT1/MT2 agonist and is safe and effective.
- Ramelteon (Rozerem) is a specific melatonin MT1/MT2 receptor agonist that was approved in 2005 as the first FDA-approved hypnotic that is not a controlled substance.
- **In 2014, a second MT1/MT2 agonist, tasimelteon, was approved for the treatment of non-24-hour sleep-wake disorder in totally blind individuals. While not approved for other forms of insomnia, tasimelton has a clinical profile similar to that of ramelteon.**

45. Ans. (b) Naloxone

Ref: K.D Tripathi 7th Ed page 472, 483

- Apnoea of the newborn may occur when morphine is given to the mother during labour.
- The blood-brain barrier of the foetus is undeveloped; morphine attains higher concentration in foetal brain than in that of mother.
- Naloxone 10 µg/kg injected in the umbilical cord is the treatment of choice. Naloxone is the drug of choice for morphine poisoning (0.4–0.8 mg i.v. every 2– 3 min: max 10 mg) and for reversing neonatal asphyxia due to opioid use during labour (10 µg/kg in the cord).
- It is also used to treat overdose with other opioids and agonist-antagonists (except buprenorphine).
- Naloxone (high dose) can prevent buprenorphine effect, but does not reverse it when given afterwards; does not precipitate buprenorphine withdrawal; probably because of more tight binding of buprenorphine to opioid receptors.

46. Ans. (d) Decrease diffusion of antibiotic

Ref: Goodman and Gilman's 12th ed, page 1367; HPIM 19th ed page 145 e4 and 161 e1

Recall Bias

Some recallers think that the question was asked in all Except format

Biofilm mechanism of resistance of antibiotics includes all EXCEPT:

A. Increased excretion of antibiotics (Answer)
B. Mechanical barrier
C. Decreased diffusion of antibiotic
D. Adherence

"Bacterial and fungal biofilms are colonies of slowly growing cells that are enclosed within an exopolymer matrix. The exopolysaccharide is negatively charged, which restricts positively charged antibiotics from reaching their target. This physical barrier restricts the diffusion of antimicrobial molecules and sometimes binds them. To be effective against infections in these compartments, antibiotics have to be able to penetrate the biofilm and endothelial barriers." ***Ref: Goodman and Gilman***

From the above explanation it is clear that resistance is because of restriction of antibiotics to reach target site and sometimes biofilm adheres the antibiotics, for sure it is not the increased efflux or excretion of antibiotics. ***Ref: Harrison's 19th ed 145 e 4 and 161 e1:***

- Biofilms are surface associated communities of bacteria, often embedded in a matrix, that allow the microbes to persist and to resist the effects of host immunity and antimicrobial agents.
- Growth in biofilms leads to altered microbial metabolism, production of extracellular virulence factors, and decreased susceptibility to biocides, antimicrobial agents, and host defense molecules and cells.
- Examples of microbial biofilm growth associated with human disease are:
  - *P. aeruginosa* growing on the bronchial mucosa during chronic infection
  - Staphylococci and other pathogens growing on implanted medical devices
  - Dental pathogens growing on tooth surfaces to form plaque

47. Ans. (a) Breastfed child just before taking next dose, when plasma concentration of drug is least

Ref: Katzung's 13th ed page 1020

This line from Katzung gives you the answer: *"If the nursing mother must take medications and the drug is a relatively safe one, she should optimally take it 30–60 minutes after nursing and 3–4 hours before the next feeding. In some cases this may allow time for drugs to be partially cleared from the mother's blood, and the concentrations in breast milk will be relatively low."*

Readers please be careful if 'option a' was not as given in question then the answer would be 'option c', see the following line, from Katzung:

"Despite the fact that most drugs are excreted into breast milk in amounts too small to adversely affect neonatal health, thousands of women taking medications do not breast-feed because of misperception of risk. Unfortunately, physicians contribute heavily to this bias. It is important to remember that formula feeding is associated with higher morbidity and mortality in all socioeconomic groups."

Important points regarding drug use during lactation:

- Most drugs are excreted into breast milk and are detectable also, but the amount is too small to adversely affect neonatal health
- The concentration of drugs achieved in breast milk is usually low. Therefore, the total amount the infant would receive in a day is substantially less than what would be considered a "therapeutic dose."
- Most antibiotics taken by nursing mothers can be detected in breast milk.
  - Tetracycline concentrations in breast milk are approximately 70% of maternal serum concentrations and present a risk of permanent tooth staining in the infant.
  - Isoniazid rapidly reaches equilibrium between breast milk and maternal blood. The concentrations achieved in breast milk are high enough so that signs of pyridoxine deficiency may occur in the infant if the mother is not given pyridoxine supplements.
- Most sedatives and hypnotics achieve concentrations in breast milk sufficient to produce a pharmacologic effect in some infants.
  - Barbiturates taken in hypnotic doses by the mother can produce lethargy, sedation, and poor suck reflexes in the infant.
  - Chloral hydrate can produce sedation if the infant is fed at peak milk concentrations.
  - Diazepam can have a sedative effect on the nursing infant, but, most importantly, its long half-life can result in significant drug accumulation.
- Opioids such as heroin, methadone, and morphine enter breast milk in quantities potentially sufficient to prolong the state of neonatal narcotic dependence if the drug was taken chronically by the mother during pregnancy.
  - If conditions are well controlled and there is a good relationship between the mother and the physician, an infant could be breast-fed while the mother is taking methadone. She should not, however, stop taking the drug abruptly; the infant can be tapered off the methadone as the mother's dose is tapered. The infant should be watched for signs of narcotic withdrawal.
  - Although codeine has been believed to be safe, a recent case of neonatal death from opioid toxicity revealed that the mother was an ultra rapid metabolizer of cytochrome 2D6 substrates, producing substantially higher amounts of morphine. Hence, polymorphism in maternal drug metabolism may affect neonatal exposure and safety. A subsequent case control study has shown that this situation is not rare. The FDA has published a warning to lactating mothers to exert extra caution while using painkillers containing codeine.
- Minimal use of alcohol by the mother has not been reported to harm nursing infants. Excessive amounts of alcohol, however, can produce alcohol effects in the infant. Nicotine concentrations in the breast milk of smoking mothers are low and do not produce effects in the infant.
- Lithium enters breast milk in concentrations equal to those in maternal serum. Clearance of this drug is almost

completely dependent upon renal elimination, and women who are receiving lithium may expose the infant to relatively large amounts of the drug.

- Radioactive substances such as iodinated 125I albumin and radioiodine can cause thyroid suppression in infants and may increase the risk of subsequent thyroid cancer as much as tenfold. Breast feeding is contraindicated after large doses and should be withheld for days to weeks after small doses. Similarly, breast-feeding should be avoided in mothers receiving cancer chemotherapy or being treated with cytotoxic or immunomodulating agents for collagen diseases such as lupus erythematosus or after organ transplantation.

48. Ans. (b) Cell wall synthesis Inhibition

Ref: Katzung 13th ed 773

- Vancomycin inhibits cell wall synthesis by binding firmly to the D-Ala-D-Ala terminus of nascent peptidoglycan pentapeptide. This inhibits the transglycosylase, preventing further elongation of peptidoglycan and crosslinking.
- Beta-lactam antibiotics, structural analogs of the natural D-Ala-D-Ala substrate, covalently bind to the active site of PBPs. This binding inhibits the transpeptidation reaction and halts peptidoglycan synthesis, and the cell dies. Beta-lactam antibiotics kill bacterial cells only when they are actively growing and synthesizing cell wall.

Classification of Antibiotics

Mechanism of action	Examples
Inhibit cell wall synthesis	• Fosfomycin • Cycloserine • Bacitracin • Vancomycin • β lactam antibiotics (includes penicillins, cephalosporins, monobactams, carbapenems, and β lactamase inhibitors)
Cause leakage from cell membranes	Polypeptides- Polymyxins, Colistin, Bacitracin. Polyenes-Amphotericin B, Nystatin, Hamycin.
Inhibit protein synthesis	Tetracyclines, Chloramphenicol, Erythromycin, Clindamycin, Linezolid.
Cause misreading of m-RNA code and affect permeability	Aminoglycosides-Streptomycin,Gentamicin,
Inhibit DNA gyrase	Fluoroquinolones-Ciprofloxacin and others.
Interfere with DNA function	Rifampin, Metronidazole.
Interfere with DNA synthesis	Acyclovir,Zidovudine.
Interfere with intermediary metabolism	Sulfonamides, Sulfones, PAS, Trimethoprim, Pyrimethamine, Ethambutol.

49. Ans. (a) Sham Surgery

Ref: Principles and Practice of Surgery By O James Garden 7th ed page 139

The confusion is between (A) Sham surgery and (B) Herbal medication with no effect known. Option (C) Physiotherapy and Option (D) CBT are known therapies with known effects and hence can not be used as Placebo.

Placebo (Latin- I shall please) is a substance or treatment with no active therapeutic effect. A placebo may be given to a person in order to deceive the recipient into thinking that it is an active treatment.

To establish whether or not the benefit of a particular surgical intervention is due to the 'placebo effect', the intervention must be investigated using a placebo-controlled RCT. In surgery, these placebo-controls are referred to as 'sham procedures/ surgeries'. One placebo controlled, randomized blinded trial of arthroscopic lavage versus arthroscopic debridement versus sham knee surgery in patients with osteoarthritis demonstrated no benefit to either arthroscopic lavage or debridement when compared to sham surgery (Moseley et al., 2002)

If the herbal medicine cannot be administered in a predetermined standardized formulation, it will be impossible to keep the treatment blinded. Otherwise also use of herbal medicines as placebo may not be always possible because of ethical and technical issues. For example, Herbal medicines have strong and prominent smell and taste. (***Ref: Drug Discovery and Clinical Research By S K Gupta page 435***)

A single herb can contain hundreds of natural constituent and most of herbal medicines contains mixture of herbs. It becomes almost impossible to ascertain the effect. Clinical effects of herbal medicines are often related to traditional knowledge, experience of Individual practitioners, theory and concepts of traditional medicine. (***Ref: The Problem of Herbal Medicines Legal Status By JL Valverde page 12***). Hence herbal medicines are not ideal for placebo effect.

NOTE

Nocebo is the opposite of placebo, and refers to negative psychodynamic effect evoked by the pessimistic attitude of the patient, or by loss of faith in the medication and/or the physician. Nocebo effect can oppose the therapeutic effect of active medication.

50. Ans. (d) Beta 1 agonist and beta 2 agonist

Ref: KDT 7th ed page 101, 127,130

The new drug increases heart rate, cardiac output, systolic blood pressure but decreases diastolic blood pressure.

Let us review actions at various receptors:

M_1			M_2	M_3
• Location and function subserved	Authonomic ganglia: Gastric glands: CNS	Depolarization (late EPSP) Hist. release, action secretion learning, memory motor functions	*SA node:* Hyperpolarization, ↓ rate of impulse generation *AV node*: α velocity of conduction *Atrium:* shortening of APD, ↓ contractility *Ventricle:* ↓ contractility (slight) (receptors sparse) Cholinergic nerve endings: ↓ ACh release *CNS:* tremor, analgesia *Visceral smooth muscle*: contraction	Visceral smooth muscle: contraction Iris: Constriction of pupil Ciliary muscle: Contraction Exocrine glands: secretion Vascular endothelium: release of NO→ vasodilatation

α actions	β actions
• Constriciton of arterioles and veins → rise in BP ($\alpha_1 + \alpha_2$) • Heart—little action, arrhythmia at high dose (α_1)	Dilatation of arterioles and veins → fall in BP (α_2) Cardiac stimulation (α_1), ↑ rate, force and conduction velocity

Now let us discuss the options:

Option (A)

M2 agonist and M3 agonist

M2 agonism will decrease heart rate, and hence cardiac output will decrease (C.O = heart rate X Stroke Volume).

Option (B)

Alpha 1 antagonist and beta 1 agonist

Alpha 1 antagonism will decrease SBP and Beta 1 agonism will increase heart rate and cardiac output may increase.

Option (C)

Alpha 1 agonist and beta 1 agonist

Alpha 1 agonism will increase SBP. However, DBP will increase due to vasoconstriction due to alpha 1 action. Beta 1 agonism will increase heart rate. Cardiac output will increase.

Option (D)

Beta 1 agonist and beta 2 agonist

Beta 1 agonism will increase heart rate. Beta 2 agonism will cause vasodilatation thus causing fall in DBP. Cardiac output will increase. This drug seems to have isoprenaline-like action on the body. SBP may increase. Also, it matches the parameters in the question and hence is the answer.

Adr: $\alpha_1 + \alpha_2 + b_1 + \beta_2$ and weak β_3 action

NA: $\alpha_1 + \alpha_2 + \beta_1 + \beta_2$ but no β_3 action

Iso: $\beta_1 + \beta_2 + \beta_3$ nut no a action

51. Ans. (a) Metformin

Ref: KDT 7th ed page 276, Harrison 19th ed page 2413

In addition to general restrictions for use of oral hypoglycaemics, metformin is contraindicated in hypotensive states, heart failure, severe respiratory, hepatic and renal disease, as well as in alcoholics because of increased risk of lactic acidosis (KDT)

Metformin should not be used in patients with renal insufficiency (glomerular filtration rate [GFR] <60 mL/min any form of acidosis, unstable congestive heart failure (CHF), liver disease, or severe hypoxemia. Some feel that these guidelines are too restrictive. The National Institute for Health and Clinical Excellence in the United Kingdom suggests that metformin be used at a GFR >30 mL/min, with a reduced dose when the GFR is <45 mL/min. (Harrison)

52. Ans. (c) Canagliflozin

Ref: Harrison 19th ed page 2414, Lippincott's 4th Ed page 295, KDT 7th Ed page 274, 277, 278

See table of Glucose-Lowering Therapies for type 2 Diabetes AIIMS MAY 2015 Pharmacology

Clue:

There are 4 prerequisites given in this question.

1. There is history of pancreatitis so the replacement drug should not have pancreatitis in its side effects.
2. Family history of Bladder cancer, hence the replacement drug should not have side effect of Bladder cancer risk.
3. Patient does not want to take injections so the drug needs to be given orally.
4. Patient is Obese hence preferred drug should have characteristic of weight loss

Option (A)

Sitagliptin is given orally and does not causes bladder cancer but it is known to cause pancreatitis. Sitagliptin has no effect on body weight. There are postmarketing reports of acute pancreatitis (fatal and nonfatal) and severe allergic and hypersensitivity reactions. Sitagliptin should be immediately discontinued if pancreatitis or allergic and hypersensitivity reactions occur. Hence should be avoided in this case.

Option (B)

Pioglitazone is given orally, does not cause pancreatitis but it is known to increase the risk of Bladder cancer. Side effects include weight gain. Hence can not be given in this case

Option (C)

Canagliflozin is in a class of medications called sodium-glucose co-transporter 2 (SGLT2) inhibitors. It is given orally.

Acute pancreatitis is a very rare side effect with an incidence <1%. Harrison 19th ed says "As part of the FDA approval of canagliflozin in 2013 postmarketing studies for cardiovascular outcomes and for monitoring bladder and urinary cancer risk are underway. Apart from this it also causes weight loss hence is ideal in the given patient.

Option (D)

Liraglutide is recently developed long-acting GLP-1 agonist. It does not cause Bladder cancer. It also causes weight loss. But It's known to cause pancreatitis and is given as subcutaneous injection once daily. Liraglutide is contraindicated in individuals with a history of pancreatitis and should be permanently discontinued if pancreatitis develops. Hence, it can not be given in this case.

53. Ans. (c) Pyridoxine

Ref: K.D Tripathi 7th Ed page 916, Harrison 19th ed page 1116

- The symptoms of the patient are related to the deficiency of pyridoxine caused by isoniazid.
- Isoniazid reacts with pyridoxal to form a hydrazone, and thus inhibits generation of pyridoxal phosphate. Isoniazid also combines with pyridoxal phosphate to interfere with its coenzyme function. Due to formation of hydrazones, the renal excretion of pyridoxine compounds is increased. Thus, isoniazid therapy produces a pyridoxine deficiency state.
- Pyridoxine is used to prevent and treat (10–50 mg/day) isoniazid induced neurological disturbances.
- Acute isoniazid poisoning has been successfully treated with massive doses (in grams) of pyridoxine.

54. Ans. (b) 18

Ref: Pharmaceutical Calculations By Howard C. Ansel 14th ed page 428

500 mg/5mL means every 100 mg is present in 1 mL,
So 180 mg will be present in 1.8 mL
10 divisions per mL means 0.1 mL per division
So, 1.8 mL will be present in 18 divisions

55. Ans. (c) Finasteride

Ref: KDT 7th Ed Page 302

Finasteride is a competitive 5 alpha reductase inhibitor and is used in benign hypertrophy of prostate along with alpha 1 blockers like tamsulosin.

The α1 blockers afford faster (within 2 weeks) and greater symptomatic relief than **finasteride which primarily affects static component of obstruction** and has a delayed onset (around six months) for clinical improvement. The α1 blockers do not affect prostate size, but are more commonly used. Concurrent treatment with both produces greater symptomatic relief.

Some details about Finasteride:

- Competitive inhibitor
- Relatively selective for 5 α-reductase ***type 2 isoenzyme*** (predominates in male urogenital tract.)
- Patients with large prostate (volume > 40 ml) obtain greater relief than those with smaller gland.
- Up to 20% reduction in prostate size may be obtained.
- Withdrawal of the drug results in regrowth of prostate, but with continued therapy benefit is maintained for ***3 years or more.***
- **Other uses: Finasteride has also been found effective in male pattern baldness** (promotes hair growth and prevents further hair loss), **although hair follicles have primarily type 1 enzyme.** Onset- 3 months, effective till 1 year after cessation.
- **Side effects:** decreased libido, impotence and decreased volume of ejaculate (each in 3–4% patients). Gynaecomastia, skin rashes, swelling of lips are rare.

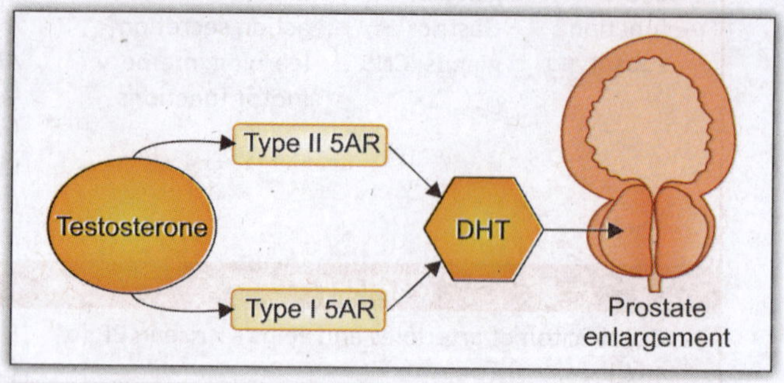

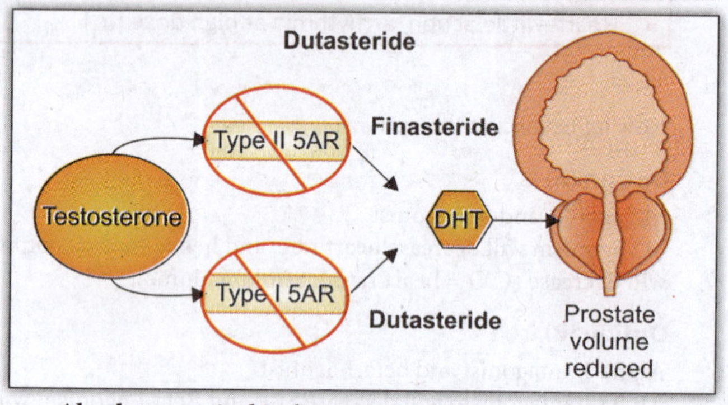

Absolute surgical indications include

a. Refractory urinary retention (failing at least one attempt at catheter removal),
b. Recurrent urinary tract infection from BPH
c. Recurrent gross hematuria from BPH,
d. Bladder stones from BPH
e. Renal insufficiency from BPH
f. Large bladder diverticula

56. Ans. (d) Scopolamine transdermal patch a night before

Ref: KDT 7th Ed page 168, 664, Harrison 19th ed page 260

- Antiemetics with anticholinergic- antihistaminic property are the first choice drugs for motion sickness. Antidopaminergic and anti-HT3 drugs are less effective.
- All anti-motion sickness drugs act better when taken 1/2–1 hour before commencing journey. Once sickness has started, it is more difficult to control; higher doses/ parenteral administration may be needed.
- Dimenhydrinate (anti histaminic with anticholinergic activity) should be taken 1 hour before the journey. It affords protection from motion sickness for 4–6 hours, but produces sedation and dryness of mouth

Scopolamine: A transdermal patch can be applied behind the pinna containing 1.5 mg of hyoscine (scopolamine), to be given at least 4 hours before journey and to be replaced after 72 hours (3 days) if needed. Oral dose 0.4–0.6 mg one hour before travel and then TID may be recommended. Scopolamine is the most effective drug for motion sickness. With the advantage of it having mild side effects, scopolamine seems to be the drug of choice.

57. Ans. (c) Buprenorphine

Ref: K.D Tripathi 7th Ed page 479

Opioid drugs and their actions on opioid receptors		
Strong opioid agonist	Morphine, Methadone, Heroin, Fentanyl	
Moderate opioid agonist	Codeine, Dihydrocodeine, Dextropropoxyphene	
Mixed agonist/antagonist	Buprenorphine	Partial/weak μ agonist + kappa antagonist
	Pentazocine	Partial μ agonist with agonist activity at κ receptors too
	Levallorphan	Antagonist on μ-opioid receptor and agonist on kappa receptors
Weak opioid agonist	Tramadol **(Atypical opioid)**	Weak μ opioid receptor agonist Very low affinity for κ and δ opioid receptor. Inhibits reuptake of Noradrenaline and 5-HT, increases 5-HT release, activates monoaminergic spinal inhibition of pain.
Pure antagonist	Naloxone, Naltrexone, Nalmefene	

58. Ans. (a) They increase bronchial responsiveness to salbutamol

Ref: K.D.Tripathi 7th Ed page 229

KDT 7th Ed says: "Corticosteroids afford more complete and sustained symptomatic relief than bronchodilators or cromoglycate; improve airflow, reduce asthma exacerbations and may influence airway remodeling, retarding disease progression. They also increase airway smooth muscle responsiveness to β agonists and reverse refractoriness to these drugs. Inhaled corticosteroids have thus markedly changed the outlook on asthma therapy"

Asthma attack not responding to intensive bronchodilator therapy: start with high dose of a rapidly acting i.v. glucocorticoid which generally acts in 6–24 hours—shift to oral therapy for 5–7 days and then discontinue abruptly or taper rapidly.

AIIMS MAY 2017

59. Ans. (a) Cotrimoxazole

Ref: KDT 7th edition page 706 to 708

- ***Cotrimoxazole is drug of choice for both treatment and prophylaxis of P. jirovecii (Previously known as P. carinii) infection.***
- Cotrimoxazole is a fixed dose combination of trimethoprim and sulfamethoxazole.
- The required plasma concentration ratio of sulfamethoxazole: trimethoprim is 20:1, which shows synergistic activity against most organisms. This is achieved by dose ratio of 5:1, because trimethoprim has high tissue distribution. For example, 1 Double Strength (DS) tablet = sulfamethoxazole 800 mg + trimethoprim 160 mg.
- For curative treatment of PCP = High dose cotrimoxazole (4-6 DS tablets per day) + prednisone or methylprednisolone as adjunctive
- For prophylaxis of PCP low dose is used (1 DS tablet daily).

Drugs of Choice for Infectious Disease Prophylaxis	
Disease	**Drug of choice**
Anthrax	Ciprofloxacin/Doxycycline
Cholera	Doxycycline
Diphtheria	Penicillin/Erythromycin
Endocarditis	Amoxycillin/Clindamycin
Gonorrhoea/Syphilis	Procaine penicillin
Group B Streptococcal infection	Ampicillin
Influenza A and B	Oseltamivir
H. influenzae Type B	Rifampicin
Herpes simplex	Acyclovir
Malaria	Chloroquine (for susceptible)/Mefloquine/ Doxycycline (endemic area or chloroquine resistant)
Meningococcal meningitis	Rifampicin
Mycobacterium Avium Complex (MAC)	Azithromycin/Clarithromycin
Otitis media	Amoxicillin
Pertussis (Whooping cough)	Azithromycin/Erythromycin
Plague	Tetracycline
Pneumocystis jirovecii	Cotrimoxazole/Atovaquone/ Dapsone
Rheumatic fever	Benzathine penicillin
Rickettsial infections	Tetracyclines
Surgical prophylaxis	Cefazolin
TB	INH with/without Rifampicin
Toxoplasmosis	Cotrimoxazole
Urinary tract infections	Cotrimoxazole

60. Ans. (b) Inhibits assembly of virus protein

Ref: Goodman & Gilman's 12th ed page 1628 to 1659; KDT 7th ed page 805, Harrison's 19th Ed page 1274

Let us go through individual options:

Option (A)

It inhibits translation and **Option (C)** It inhibits proviral RNA synthesis.

Translation and transcription of HIV viral DNA is by using host (human) enzymes so as of now no drugs target this system.

Option (D)

Inhibits conversion of RNA to DNA

NRTI & NNRTI inhibit reverse transcriptase thereby inhibiting conversion of RNA to DNA.

Option (B)

It is correct mechanism of protease inhibitors. Function of HIV protease is cleavage of gag and pol precursor polypeptides and other precursor proteins to final structural proteins of mature virion.

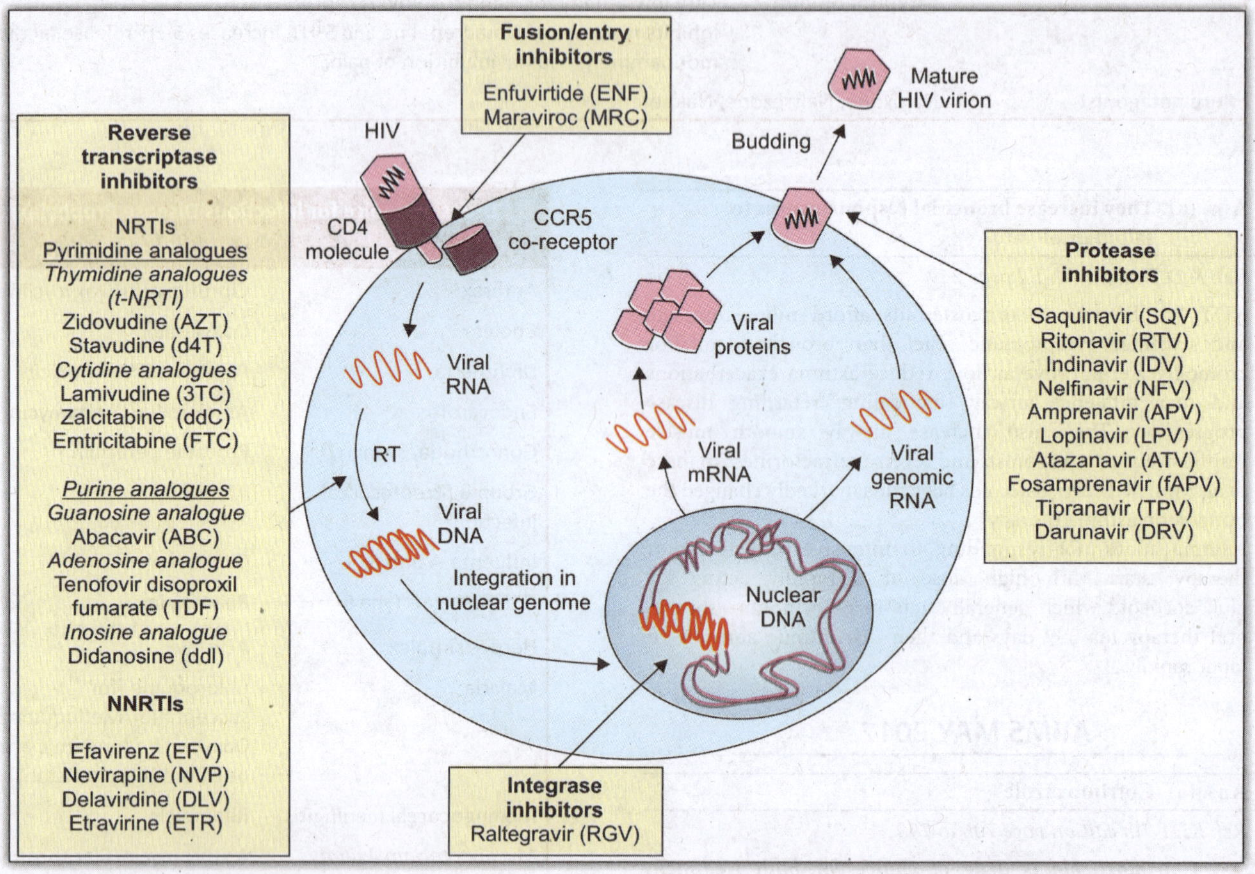

Fig: Pathogenesis and targets of antiretroviral drugs (trends in pharmacological sciences)

Targets and Mechanism of Antiretroviral Drugs

Target	Normal function in virus	Drug class	Mechanism of action
gp41	HIV attaches through gp 160 (which includes gp120 & gp41) → gp 41 fuses viral envelop to host membrane → entry of virus	Enfuvirtide (Entry inhibitor)	Binds to gp41 → does not allow conformational changes that allow fusion of virusè blocks entry of virus into host cell.
CCR5		Maraviroc (Entry inhibitor)	Binds specifically to host protein ccr5 → blocks entry
RT (Reverse transcriptase)	RT then converts viral RNA to DNA	NRTI [Nucleoside/ Nucleotide (tenofovir)] e.g. zidovudine, lamivudine, etc.	These drugs are purine or pyrimidine analogues that enter cells get phosphorylated and then blocks replication by 2 ways: (1) Competitively inhibits incorporation of native nucleotides. (2) once incorporated terminates elongation of nascent DNA because NRTI lack 3' hydroxyl group

Contd...

Targets and Mechanism of Antiretroviral Drugs			
Target	**Normal function in virus**	**Drug class**	**Mechanism of action**
		NNRTI (Nonnucleoside) e.g. nevirapine	Bind to NNRTI binding pocket in enzyme RT which is separate from catalytic site and cause change in 3D structure of the enzymeè reducing its activity.
Integrase	Incorporates viral DNA into host DNA.	Integrase inhibitor e.g. Raltegravir	These drugs bind to integrase enzyme and prevent viral DNA strand transfer to host DNA
Protease	Proteolytic cleavage of gag and pol precursor polypeptides and other precursor proteins to final structural proteins of mature virion	Protease inhibitors e.g. ritonavir, saquinavir, etc.	HIV protease inhibitors are peptide-like chemicals that competitively inhibit the action of the viral protease thereby blocking formation of mature virions.

61. Ans. (d) Cotrimoxazole with 3rd generation cephalosporin

Ref: Katzung 13th ed page 802, 904, Harrison's 19th ed page 1048

NOTE

Trimethoprim-sulfamethoxazole (TMP-SMX), also known as co-trimoxazole

- **What Harrison's 19th Ed page 1048 says:**
  - B cepacia is intrinsically resistant to most antimicrobials.
  - TMP-SMX, meropenem, and doxycycline are most effective drugs.
  - Empirical treatment of choice is TMP-SMX or meropenem
  - Some strains are susceptible to third-generation cephalosporins and fluoroquinolones
  - When serious pulmonary infection is there, e.g. cystic fibrosis then combination therapy is suggested, but combination of meropenem and TMP-SMX is antagonistic.
  - Resistance to all agents has been reported.
- **What Katzung page 904 says**

  DOC for B. Cepacia is TMP-SMX and alternative agents are Ceftazidime, chloramphenicol.

62. Ans. (b) Large volume of distribution

Ref: KDT 7th ed page 21, Katzung 8th ed page 38

Indirect repeat Pharmacology AIIMS Nov 2015 (was asked in reverse form i.e. What happen in Low volume of distribution)

- **The extent and pattern of distribution of a drug depends on its:**
  - Lipid solubility
  - Ionization at physiological pH (a function of its pKa)
  - **Extent of binding to plasma and tissue proteins:** Drugs extensively bound to plasma proteins are largely restricted to the vascular compartment and have low volume of distribution, e.g. diclofenac and warfarin
  - Presence of tissue-specific transporters
  - Differences in regional blood flow
- Volume of distribution is the apparent volume required to contain the amount of drug homogeneously at the concentration found in the plasma
- Drugs having high volume of distribution get sequestrated in various tissues and are unequally distributed and tend to have longer duration of action.
- Due to sequestration may exert local toxicity, e.g. tetracyclines on bone and teeth, chloroquine on retina, streptomycin on vestibular apparatus, emetine on heart and skeletal muscle.
- Large volume of distribution indicates good drug storage. Small volume of distribution means drug stays in vascular compartment either due to high plasma protein binding or due to less lipid solubility, therefore less drug is distributed to tissues. Lesser the distribution lesser will be the storage.

63. Ans. (a) Ceftriaxone

Ref: Harrison's 19th ed table 147-1 page 780, 889.

Meningitis can be broadly classified into community acquired (usual case) or hospital acquired. The empirical therapy for both of these is discussed in the table below.

Type of Meningitis	MC Cause	Empirical Treatment	Addition to Empirical R_x	Rationale
Community acquired meningitis	*S. pheumoniae* (50%) and N. *meningitidis* (25%)	3rd/4th gen cephalosporin (ceftriaxone, cefotaxime, cefepime) + vancomycin + acyclovir + dexamethasone	+ Ampicillin	3 months of age, those >55, or immunocompromised (to cover *Listeria monocytogens*)
			+ Metronidazole	In patients with otitis, sinusitis, or mastoiditis (to cover gram-negative anaerobes)
			+ Doxycycline	In tick season (tick-borne bacterial infections)

Contd...

Type of Meningitis	MC Cause	Empirical Treatment	Addition to Empirical R_x	Rationale
Hospital acquired meningitis	Staphylococci and gram -ve organisms *(P. aeruginosa)*	Vancomycin + ceftazidime or cefepime or meropenem		Ceftriaxone and cefotaxime do not provide activity against CNS infection with pseudomonas therefore replaced by active agents

Meningococcal Meningitis				
Empirical Rx	**DOC if suceptible**	**DOC if resistance to Pencillin G**	**Chemoprophylaxis for adults and children >1 year**	**Alternate chemoprophylaxis for adults**
Ceftriaxone or cefotaxime	Penicillin G	Ceftriaxone or cefotaxime	2-day regimen of rifampin (not recommended in pregnancy)	One dose of azithromycin (500 mg) or one im dose of ceftriaxone (250 mg)

64. Ans. (b) Taper the drug over 6 months

Ref: Katzung 13th ed page 414, Harrison's 19th ed page 2556

This question is about whether to stop levetiracetam or to switch to different antiepileptic due to adverse effects of levetiracetam. Levetiracetam is a well tolerated antiepileptic with very few adverse effects.

- The usual adverse effects include: somnolence, asthenia, ataxia, and dizziness.
- Less common but important: mood and behavioral changes.
- Rare: Psychotic reaction

Stopping an Antiepileptic

Stopping or switching an antiepileptic is mandated based on 2 parameters

- Seizure free period and
- Compliance or adverse effect of the drug
  - The appropriate seizure free interval is unknown and undoubtedly varies for different forms of epilepsy. It is reasonable to attempt withdrawal of antiepileptic after 2 years seizure free period if the patient meets the following criteria:

  a. Complete medical control of seizures for 1–5 years;
  b. Single seizure type, either focal or generalized;
  c. Normal neurologic examination, including intelligence; and
  d. Normal EEG.

Withdrawal of therapy should be gradual over a period of 2 to 3 months.

Switching to Different Antiepileptic

- If seizure free period is not sufficient to withdraw or seizures are not controlled by the drug or if there is significant toxicity then switching to another antiepileptic may be considered.
- "This is usually done by maintaining the patient on the first drug while a second drug is added. The dose of the second drug should be adjusted to decrease seizure frequency without causing toxicity. Once this is achieved, the first drug can be gradually withdrawn (usually over weeks unless there is significant toxicity). The dose of the second drug is then further optimized based on seizure response and side effects. Monotherapy should be the goal whenever possible".

Based on above explanation ***option A*** and ***option C*** are wrong.

Option (B)

Tapering is usually 2 to 3 months but may vary with different drugs and different scenarios. Therefore over 6 months can be regarded as true.

Option (D)

The patient is seizure free for 2 years, but other criteria like type of seizure, neurologic examination and EEG has not been mentioned in question. Remember that all the criteria need to be met to stop the drug. This could have been the answer if tapering of levetiracetam over a period and then gradually shifting to other antiepileptic would have been mentioned.

65. Ans. (a) Linagliptin

Ref: KDT 7th ed page 275, Katzung 13th ed page 1090 & 1091

Indirect Repeat (Different case description and options) Pharmacology AIIMS NOV 2016

Dipeptidyl Peptidase-4 (DPP-4) Inhibitors

- Sitagliptin, Vildagliptin, Saxagliptin, Alogliptin, Linagliptin.
- The dose of Sitagliptin, Vildagliptin and saxagliptin should be reduced if GFR falls below 50-60 ml/min.
- Linagliptin is safe in renal failure or hepatic impairment. There is no dose adjustment required for linagliptin in renal failure patients (which is the only oral drug currently licensed for this use)

66. Ans. (c) Blurred vision

Ref: Katzung 13th ed page 410, Harrison's 19th ed page 383

Diplopia (not blurred vision) is a adverse effect of carbamazepine not an idiosyncratic reaction

- MC drugs causing Steven Johnson syndrome are (Harrison's 19th *page* 383): Sulfonamides, nevirapine, allopurinol, lamotrigine, aromatic anticonvulsants (including phenytoin, carbamazepine, and barbiturates), and NSAIDs, specifically oxicam.

- Unpredictable reactions or type B or Bizarre reactions varies from patient to patient and are not due to drug as such. These include idiosyncratic reactions (IR) and allergy.
- Unpredictable reactions are rare. Carbamazepine is known for unpredictable reactions.
- Adverse drug effects are due to drug's off target actions and on contrary reason for IRs is unpredictable and is considered to be related to patient.

Idiosyncratic Reactions due to Carbamazepine are	Adverse Effects of Carbamazepine are
• **MC IR is:** Erythematous skin rash (SJS)	• **MC dose-related adverse effects of carbamazepine** are diplopia and ataxia.
• **Dangerous IRs** but rare include: Aplastic anemia and agranulocytosis.	• Other dose-related complaints include mild gastrointestinal upsets, unsteadiness, and, at much higher doses, drowsiness.
• **Other IRs** leukopenia (common idiosyncratic blood dyscrasia) and hepatic dysfunction (rare)	• Hyponatremia and water intoxication are rare and may be dose related.

67. Ans. (a) 30% amorphous + 70% crystalline

Ref: KDT 7th ed page 264

Lente insulin is a combination of 30% semilente (amorphous) and 70% ultralente (crystalline) insulin zinc suspension

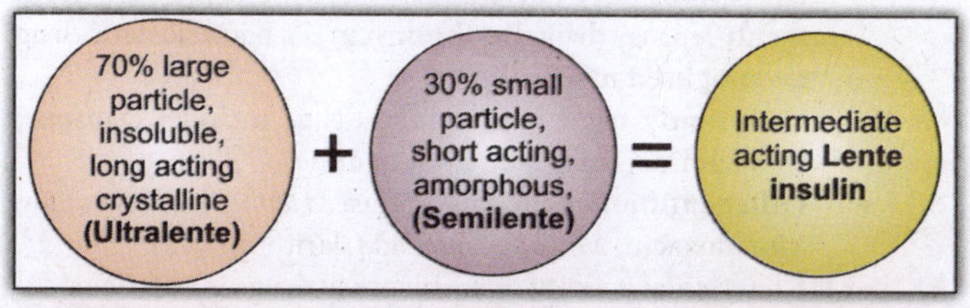

Insulins		
Highly purified mono-component insulin	Porcine Actrapid-Regular	Short acting
	Porcine Monotard-Lente	Intermediate acting
	Porcine Insulatard- NPH	
	Porcine Mixtard	30% regular, 70% Isophane
Human insulin	Human Actrapid-Regular	Short acting
	Human Monotard-Lente	**Intermediate acting**
	Human Insulatard- NPH	
	Human Mixtard	30% regular, 70% Isophane
Insulin analogues	Insulin lispro Insulin aspart Insulin glulisine	Ultra short acting
	Insulin glargine	Long acting

Contd...

Insulins

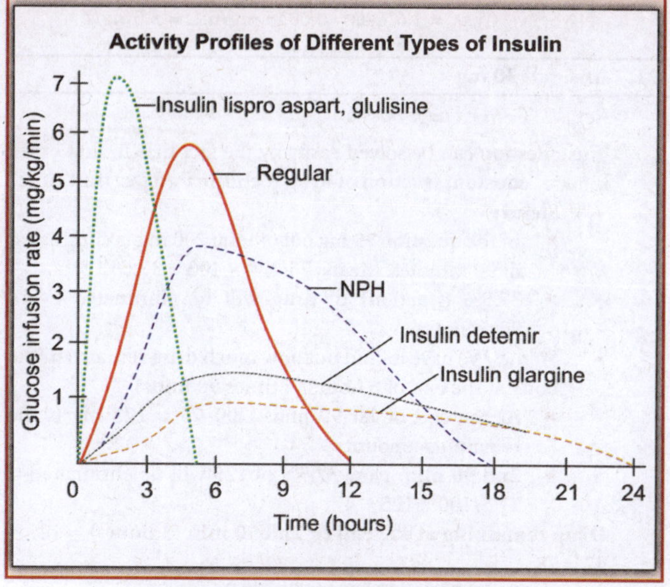

68. Ans. (a) Neuraminidase inhibitor

Ref: Harrison's 19th Ed page 21 5e-l, Katzung 13th ed page 886

- Oseltamivir and zanamivir are anti influenza agents
- Influenza A is divided into various subtypes based on H (haemagglutinin) and N (Neuraminidase) into various subtypes. Important being H5N1 (avian), H1N1 (swine), H1N2 and H3N2.
- Neuraminidase inhibitors: **Oseltamivir** and **Zanamivir**
  - Influenza virus requires neuraminidase to sialic acid residues in host membrane to get released from the cell
  - Neuraminidase inhibitors interfere with release of progeny influenza virus from infected host cells, thus halting the spread of infection within the respiratory tract.
  - Inhibition of viral neuraminidase results in clumping of newly released influenza virions to each other and to the membrane of the infected cell.
  - Active against both influenza A and B
- **Amantadine** and its α-methyl derivative **rimantadine**, block the M2 proton ion channel (*Option B*) of the virus particle and inhibit uncoating of the viral RNA within infected host cells, thus preventing its replication
  - Active against influenza A only

69. Ans. (b) Epsilon amino caproic acid

Ref: Goodman 12th ed page 867, Katzung 12th page 616

Repeat Pharmacology AIIMS NOV 2015 (See for explanation)

70. Ans. (a) 2.5 mg/L

Ref: KDT 7th ed page 32

- Plasma steady state concentration (Cpss) is achieved after repeated administration of drug leading to a balance between drug input and elimination.
- Cpss is directly proportional to the dose rate and inversely to the clearance of the drug and the relation is as follows:

Cpss = Dose rate/Clearance

Dose rate = 1.6 mg/mL, Clearance = 640 mL/min

Cpss = 1.6/640 = 0.0025 mg/mL = 2.5mg/L

71. Ans. (c) 30 mg

Ref: KDT 7th ed page 30

This question can be solved easily by the fact that in first order kinetic **"constant fraction of drug is eliminated per unit time"**

- ***Step 1:***
  - In the question 75 mg out of total 200 mg is eliminated in 90 minutes. Means 75/200 × 100 = 37.5%
  - 37.5% (fraction) of drug will be eliminated every 90 minutes
- ***Step 2:*** We have to find out how much drug remains in the body at the end of 6 hours (4 times 90 mins)
  - At the end of 1st 90 mins: 200–75 = 125 mg is the remaining amount
  - **2nd 90 min:** Now 37.5% of 125 will be eliminated = 37.5/100 × 125 = 47

Drug remaining at the end of 2nd 90 min (3 hours) = 125 – 47 = 78

- **3rd 90 min:** 37.5% of 78 = 29.25

Drug remaining at the end of 3rd 90 min (4½ hours) = 78–29.25 = 48.75

- **4th 90 min:** 37.5% of 48.75 = 18.3

Drug remaining at the end of 4th 90 min (6 hours) = 48.7–18.3 = 30.4 = 30 mg

Thus the answer

72. Ans. (a) Atorvastatin 80 mg

Ref: CMDT 2017 page 1263-64

- When lipid lowering agents are indicated the treatment is started with HMG Co-A reductase inhibitors (statins)

Option (C) Rosuvastatin + Fenofibrate

Combination therapy is rarely indicated. Only ezetimibe plus simvastatin has shown benefit in trials even though very small. Gemfibrozil and HMG-CoA reductase inhibitors increases the risk muscle and liver disease more than either drug alone.

Option (D) Fenofibrate

Fibrates are used to reduce triglycerides and increase HDL levels, which is not the case here and also first line therapy is always statins.

This table shown below serves as a guide to type of therapy to be used under specific conditions.

Indications	Treatment recommendation
Presence of clinical atherosclerotic cardiovascular disease	High intensity statin or moderate intensity statin if over age 75
Primary elevation of LDL cholesterol ≥190 mg/dL (4.91 mmol/L)	High intensity statin
Age 40–75 Presence of diabetes LDL ≥70 mg/dL (1.81 mmol/L)	Moderate intensity statin Or high intensity statin if 10-year CVD risk 7.5% or higher
Aged 40–75 No clinical atherosclerotic cardiovascular disease or diabetes LDL 70–189 mg/dL (1.81–4.91 mmol/L) Estimated 10-year CVD risk 7.5% or higher	Treat with moderate-to-high intensity statin

As per the table above patient comes under 1st category (presence of clinical cardiovascular disease). It is also important to point out that even if the patient is not having deranged lipid profile he may be started with statin therapy.

- **High intensity statin therapy:** lowers LDL cholesterol by approximately 50%.
  - Atorvastatin 40–80 mg ***(Option A)*** and rosuvastatin 20–40 mg/day
- **Moderate intensity statins** lower LDL cholesterol by approximately 30–50%.
  - Atorvastatin 10–20 mg, rosuvastatin 5–10 mg ***(Option B)***, simvastatin 20–40 mg, pravastatin 40–80 mg, and lovastatin 40 mg.

73. Ans. (a) Ofloxacin

Ref: KDT 7th ed page 782, 783

- Among the given options ofloxacin, ciprofloxacin and amoxicillin have bactericidal activity, but only ofloxacin is anti-leprosy drug. Erythromycin is a bacteriostatic drug and not used in leprosy.
- **Commonly used** anti-leprosy drugs include: Dapsone, Clofazimine, Rifampin, Ethionamide.
- **Other antibiotics** effective against *M leprae* are: Ofloxacin, Moxifloxacin, Minocycline and Clarithromycin
- Bactericidal activity of anti-leprosy drugs is as follows
  - **Rifampicin:** Up to 99.99% *M.leprae* are killed in 3–7 days by 600 mg/day dose.
  - **Ofloxacin:** Over 99.9% bacilli were found to be killed by 22 daily doses of ofloxacin monotherapy.
  - **Clarithromycin:** Monotherapy with 500 mg daily caused 99.9% bacterial killing in 8 weeks.

74. Ans. (a) Methotrexate

Ref: Harrison's 19th ed page 2145

This is a direct line from Harrison's ***"At the dosages used for the treatment of RA, methotrexate has been shown to stimulate adenosine release from cells, producing an anti-inflammatory effect."***

Other salient points from the above text are as follows:

- Conventional DMARDs include ⇒ hydroxychloroquine, sulfasalazine, methotrexate, and leflunomide
- Onset of action is delayed by ⇒ 6 to 12 weeks
- **DMARD of choice for rheumatoid arthritis is** ⇒ Methotrexate
- **Methotrexate** ⇒ stimulates adenosine release ⇒ anti-inflammatory effect

- **Leflunomide** ⇒ inhibitor of pyrimidine synthesis ⇒ equally effective as methotrexate as both monotherapy and combination therapy
- **Hydroxychloroquine** ⇒ does not delay radiographic; therefore not a true DMARD. (Disease modifying anti-rheumatic drugs DMARDs by definition reduce the disease activity and retard the progression)
- **Sulfasalazine** ⇒ delays radiographic progression of disease
- Other drugs that are rarely used include: Minocycline, gold salts, penicillamine, azathioprine, and cyclosporine

75. Ans. (b) Rifampicin

Ref: KDT 7th ed page 13-15

- Transport of drugs across membranes can occur through various pathways, one of them being primary active transport which involves transport of solutes against electrochemical gradient. P-glycoprotein is most well known primary active transporter
- **Location:** Intestinal mucosa, renal tubules, bile canaliculi, choroidal epithelium, astrocyte foot processes around brain capillaries (the blood-brain barrier), testicular and placental microvessels.
- P-gp is a non-selective transporter developed by body to deal with xenobiotics.
- **Function:** Pumps out many drugs/metabolites and thus limits their intestinal absorption, penetration into brain, testes and foetal tissues as well as promotes biliary and renal elimination.
- **For example,** Digoxin and cyclosporine have low oral bioavailability in spite of good oral absorption because of P-gp. P-gp pumps out the drug from epithelium back into the lumen.
- **Inducers and inhibitors:** It acts in synergy with CYP3A4, Usually the xenobiotics inducing and inhibiting CYPs also induce and inhibit P-gp.
- **Inhibitors** of p-gp quinidine, verapamil, erythromycin, etc., enhance oral bioavailability.
- **Inducers** of p-gp like rifampin and phenobarbitone reduce the oral bioavailability of these drugs.

Remaining **options (A), (C), (D)** are p-gp inhibitors.

76. Ans. (b) Block of α1 followed by stimulation of β2

Ref: KDT 7th ed page 131, 140

Recall Bias

Many variants of different permutation and combination of alpha and beta receptors were recalled. Not going into the confusion of recalls just remember the correct answer

Indirect repeat Pharmacology AIIMS MAY 2016 (See for explanation)

AIIMS NOVEMBER 2016

77. Ans. (c) Milnacipran

Ref: Harrison's 18th Ed, Ch: 353; KDT 7th ed page 340

Option (B): Denosumab

It is a human monoclonal antibody which inhibits osteoclast differentiation and function as well as promotes their apoptosis. It is a treatment option for postmenopausal osteoporosis when no other drug is appropriate. Ref: KDT 7th ed page 346

Option (C)

Another SNRI (Selective serotonin-norepinephrine reuptake inhibitors), milnacipran, has been studied extensively as an antidepressant. In addition to their use in major depression, other applications of the SNRIs include the treatment of pain disorders including neuropathies and fibromyalgia. Ref: Katjung 12th ed page 525

Option (D)

Strontium ranelate is composed of two atoms of strontium bound to an organic ion, ranelic acid. Although not yet approved for use in the USA, this drug is used in Europe for the treatment of osteoporosis. Ref Katzung 12th ed page 778

Drugs Used in Osteoporosis

Drug	Mode of action	Remarks
Parathormone (PTH)	PTH stimulates the production of the active metabolite of vitamin D. PTH receptor is a G protein coupled receptor. (PTH) acts on PTH-receptor located on the osteoblast membrane and induces RANKL production—indirectly activating osteoclast differentiation and function. PTH promotes both bone formation and resorption in part by stimulating the proliferation and differentiation of osteoblasts and osteoclasts	**Teriparatide** is a recombinant preparation of 1–34 residues of amino terminal of human PTH has been recently introduced for the treatment of severe osteoporosis. It duplicates all the actions of long (1–84) PTH. Injected s.c. 20 µg once daily, it acts only for 2–3 hours, and has been found to increase bone mineral density in osteoporotic women
Estrogen	Majority of estrogen (and androgen) effects on bone resorption are mediated indirectly through paracrine factors produced by osteoblasts. These actions include (1) increasing IGF-I and TGF and (2) suppressing IL-1, IL-6, TNF, and osteocalcin synthesis. The indirect estrogen actions primarily decrease bone resorption. Estrogens reduce bone turnover, prevent bone loss, and induce small increases in bone mass of the spine, hip, and total body. E	Both oral and transdermal routes are available. For oral estrogens, the standard recommended doses have been 0.3 mg/d for esterified estrogens, 0.625 mg/d for conjugated equine estrogens, and 5 mg/d for ethinyl estradiol. For transdermal estrogen, the commonly used dose supplies 50 mg estradiol per day. pidemiologic databases indicate that women who take epidemiologic replacement have a 50% reduction, on average, of osteoporotic fractures, including hip fractures.

Contd...

Drugs Used in Osteoporosis		
Drug	**Mode of action**	**Remarks**
Progestins	Neither medroxyprogesterone acetate nor micronized progesterone appears to have an independent effect on bone; at lower doses of estrogen, norethindrone acetate may have an additive benefit	In women with a uterus, daily progestin or cyclical progestins at least 12 days per month are prescribed in combination with estrogens to reduce the risk of uterine cancer. Medroxyprogesterone acetate and norethindrone acetate blunt the high-density lipoprotein response to estrogen, but micronized progesterone does not.
SERM (Selective estrogen receptor modulator)	Competitive partial agonist inhibitor of estradiol at the estrogen receptor	Two SERMs are used currently in postmenopausal women: **Raloxifene,** which is approved for the prevention and treatment of osteoporosis, and **Tamoxifen**, which is approved for the prevention and treatment of breast cancer. In contrast to tamoxifen, raloxifene is not associated with an increase in the risk of uterine cancer or benign uterine disease. Raloxifene increases the occurrence of hot flashes but reduces serum total and low-density lipoprotein cholesterol, lipoprotein (a), and fibrinogen.
Bisphosphonates	Bisphosphonates are structurally related to pyrophosphates, compounds that are incorporated into bone matrix. BPN specifically impair osteoclast function and reduce osteoclast number, in part by inducing apoptosis. Recent evidence suggests that the nitrogen-containing BPN also inhibit protein prenylation, one of the end products in the mevalonic acid pathway, by inhibiting the enzyme farnesyl pyrophosphate synthase.	Postmenopausal osteoporosis and Steroid induced osteoporosis **Bisphosphonate — Relative Potency** **1st generation BPN** Etidronate — 1 Tiludronate — 10 **2nd generation BPN** Pamidronate — 100 Alendronate — 100–500 Ibandronate — 500–1000 **3rd generation BPN** Risedronate — 1000 Zoledronate — 5000
Calcitonin	The principal effects of calcitonin are to lower serum calcium and phosphate by actions on bone and kidney. Calcitonin suppresses osteoclast activity by direct action on the osteoclast calcitonin receptor. Calcitonin inhibits osteoclastic bone resorption. Although bone formation is not impaired at first after calcitonin administration, with time both formation and resorption of bone are reduced. Human calcitonin monomer has a half-life of about 10 minutes. Salmon calcitonin has a longer half-life	Calcitonin preparations are approved by the FDA for Paget's disease, hypercalcemia, and osteoporosis in women >5 years past menopause. A **nasal spray** containing calcitonin (200 IU/d) is available for treatment of osteoporosis in postmenopausal women. Calcitonin is not indicated for prevention of osteoporosis and is not sufficiently potent to prevent bone loss in early postmenopausal women.
Denosumab	Denosumab is a fully human monoclonal antibody to RANKL, the final common effector of osteoclast formation, activity, and survival. Denosumab binds to RANKL, inhibiting its ability to initiate formation of mature osteoclasts from osteoclast precursors and to bring mature osteoclasts to the bone surface and initiate bone resorption. Denosumab also plays a role in reducing the survival of the osteoclast.	A novel agent that was given twice yearly by SC administration in a randomized controlled trial in postmenopausal women with osteoporosis has been shown to increase BMD. **It is a treatment option for postmenopausal osteoporosis when no other drug is appropriate.**
Fluoride	Fluoride accumulates in bones and teeth, where it may stabilize the hydroxyapatite crystal. Such a mechanism may explain the effectiveness of fluoride in increasing the resistance of teeth to dental caries, but it does not explain its ability to promote new bone growth.	At present, fluoride is not approved by the FDA for treatment or prevention of osteoporosis, and it is unlikely to be. Fluoride remains an experimental agent despite its long history and multiple studies.

Contd...

Drugs Used in Osteoporosis		
Drug	**Mode of action**	**Remarks**
Strontium ranelate	It suppresses bone resorption (block differentiation of osteoclasts while promoting their apoptosis) well as stimulates bone formation. Unlike bisphosphonates, denosumab, or teriparatide, this drug increases bone formation markers while inhibiting bone resorption markers.	Reserve drug for elderly women >75 years age who have already suffered osteoporotic fracture and are unable to tolerate BPNs. Although not yet approved for use in the USA, this drug is used in Europe for the treatment of osteoporosis.
Thiazide diuretics	The principal application of thiazides in the treatment of bone mineral disorders is in reducing renal calcium excretion.	Thiazides may increase the effectiveness of PTH in stimulating reabsorption of calcium by the renal tubules or may act on calcium reabsorption secondarily by increasing sodium reabsorption in the proximal tubule.

78. Ans. (d) Lung fibrosis

Ref: KDT 7th ed page 252, Goodman Gilman 10th Ed page 990

Option (A)

The most dangerous complication is **agranulocytosis,** an infrequent but potentially fatal adverse reaction

Option (B)

Aplastic anemia is rare but irreversible and potentially life threatening

Option (C)

Both Propylthiourcila and Metrimazole (PTU> Metrimazole) can cause fatal liver failure, hence PTU is reserved to the patient allergic to Metrimazole.

Antithyroid Drugs (Thioamides)

This term has also been applied to all thyroid inhibitors. The thioamides methimazole and propylthiouracil are major drugs for treatment of thyrotoxicosis. The thiocarbamide group is essential for antithyroid activity.

Pharmacokinetics

The short plasma half-life of these agents (1.5 hours for propylthiouracil and 6 hours for methimazole) has little influence on the duration of the antithyroid action or the dosing interval because both agents are accumulated by the thyroid gland. For propylthiouracil, giving the drug every 6–8 hours is reasonable since a single 100 mg dose can inhibit 60% of iodine organification for 7 hours. Since a single 30 mg dose of methimazole exerts an antithyroid effect for longer than 24 hours, a single daily dose is effective in the management of mild to moderate hyperthyroidism.

Both thioamides cross the placental barrier and are concentrated by the fetal thyroid, so that caution must be employed when using these drugs in pregnancy. Of the two, propylthiouracil is preferable in pregnancy because it is more strongly protein-bound and therefore crosses the placenta less readily. In addition, it is not secreted in sufficient quantity in breast milk to preclude breast-feeding.

Mechanism of Action

Inhibiting the thyroid peroxidase-catalyzed reactions and blocking iodine organification. In addition, they block coupling of the iodotyrosines. They do not block uptake of iodide by the gland. Propylthiouracil and (to a much lesser extent) methimazole inhibit the peripheral deiodination of T4 and T3. Since the synthesis rather than the release of hormones is affected, the onset of these agents is slow, often requiring 3–4 weeks before stores of T4 are depleted

Toxicity

- Adverse reactions to the thioamides occur in 3–12% of treated patients.
- Most reactions occur early. The most common adverse effect is a **maculopapular pruritic rash,** at times accompanied by systemic signs such as fever. Rare adverse effects include an urticarial rash, vasculitis, arthralgia, a lupus-like reaction, cholestatic jaundice, hepatitis, lymphadenopathy, hypoprothrombinemia, exfoliative dermatitis, polyserositis, and acute arthralgia.
- The most dangerous complication is **agranulocytosis,** an infrequent but potentially fatal adverse reaction. It occurs in 0.3–0.6% of patients taking thioamides, but the risk may be increased in older patients and in those receiving high-dose methimazole therapy (over 40 mg/d). The reaction is usually rapidly reversible when the drug is discontinued, but antibiotic therapy may be necessary for complicating infections. Colony-stimulating factors Agents Used in Anemias; Hematopoietic Growth Factors) may hasten recovery of the granulocytes.

Contraindications

Metrimazole is associated with birth defects hence Propylthiouracil is Drug of choice during pregnancy

79. Ans. (a) Expiry date

Ref: Ethical criteria for medicinal drug promotion. World Health Organization [Online]. 1988 May 13;[8 screens] Available from: http://www.who.int/medicinedocs/collect/edmweb/pdf/whozip08e/whozip08e.pdf

It is a legal requirement that all pharmaceutical products must carry the date of manufacture and date of expiry on their label. *(Ref KDT 7th ed page 73)*. Here 'Label' means the packaging cover not the drug literature leaflet provided inside the cover box.

WHO criteria for ethical medicinal drug promotion dictate that promotional literature should contain following information:

The name(s) of the active ingredient(s) using either international nonproprietary names (INN) or the approved generic name of the drug.

- The brand name
- Amount of active ingredient(s) per dose
- Other ingredients known to cause problems, i.e. adjuvant
- Approved therapeutic uses
- Dosage form or dosage schedule
- Safety information including side effects and major adverse drug reactions, precautions, contraindications and warnings, and major drug interactions
- Name and address of manufacturer or distributor
- Reference to scientific literature as appropriate

80. Ans: (d Rifabutin is more efficacious for pulmonary TB than rifampicin

Ref: KDT 7th ed page 771, Goodman 10th Ed page 805

Rifabutin has better activity against MAC organisms than rifampin and is active in vitro against

The1 rifamycins (rifampin, rifabutin, rifapentine) are related macrocyclic antibiotics produced by Amycolatopsis mediterrane; rifampin is a semisynthetic derivative of rifamycin B.

Rifabutin (Ansamycin)

General Pharmacology And Antibacterial Spectrum

Rifabutin is derived from rifamycin and is related to rifampin. It has significant activity against M tuberculosis, M avium-intracellulare, and M fortuitum. Rifabutin shares a common mechanism of action with rifampin (inhibition of mycobacterial RNA polymerase) but is more active in vitro. ***Rifabutin s less active against M.tuberculosis, and more active against MAC than rifampin. Majority of M.tuberculosis isolates resistant to R are cross resistant to rifabutin. Thus, it is not an option for treatment of MDR-TB.*** It is active in vitro against MAC bacteria isolated from HIV-infected (typically *M. avium*) and non–HIV-infected individuals (~40% *M. intracellulare*). Rifabutin also inhibits the growth of many strains of *M. tuberculosis*. Cross-resistance between rifampin and rifabutin is common in *M. tuberculosis*, although some strains are resistant to rifampin yet sensitive to rifabutin. Most *M. avium* strains resistant to rifampin are still sensitive to rifabutin. Some rifampin-resistant strains may appear susceptible to rifabutin in vitro, but a clinical response is unlikely because the molecular basis of resistance, rpoB mutation, is the same.

Pharmacokinetics

Rifabutin is both substrate and inducer of cytochrome P450 enzymes. Rifabutin is given orally, usually at 300 mg/day. Following GI absorption, it is metabolized by hepatic CYPs and eliminated in a biphasic manner with a mean terminal t1/2 of ~45 hours, predominantly in urine and bile. Dosage adjustment is not necessary in patients with impaired renal function. Because it is a less potent inducer, rifabutin is indicated in place of rifampin for treatment of tuberculosis in HIV-infected patients who are receiving concurrent antiretroviral therapy with a protease inhibitor or nonnucleoside reverse transcriptase inhibitor.

Oral bioavailability of rifabutin is low (~20%), but t½ is much longer (>30 hours). Rifampicin is well absorbed orally, (bioavailability is ~ 70%), but food decreases absorption; rifampin is to be taken in empty stomach. The t½ of rifampin is variable (2–5 hours).

Dose

300 mg (5 mg/kg) OD oral; RIBUTIN 150 mg tab.

Therapeutic uses

Rifabutin is effective for the prevention of MAC infection in HIV infected individuals and can decrease the frequency of MAC bacteremia. Azithromycin or clarithromycin is more effective and less likely to interact with HAART drugs. Rifabutin also is commonly substituted for rifampin in the treatment of tuberculosis in HIV-infected patients, as it has a less profound CYP-dependent drug interaction. Rifabutin also is used in combination with clarithromycin and ethambutol for the therapy of MAC disease. The primary indication of rifabutin is for prophylaxis and treatment of MAC infection in HIV-AIDS patients. For prophylaxis of MAC, rifabutin alone 300 mg/day is an alternative to azithromycin/clarithromycin, while for treatment of MAC infection, it is combined with 2–3 other anti-MAC drugs.

Side Effect Profile

Rifabutin generally is well tolerated in persons with HIV infection; primary reasons for discontinuation of therapy include rash (4%), GI intolerance (3%), and neutropenia (2%). Overall, neutropenia occurred in 25% of patients with severe HIV infection who received rifabutin. Uveitis and arthralgia have occurred in patients receiving rifabutin doses > 450 mg daily in combination with clarithromycin or fluconazole. Patients should be cautioned to discontinue the drug if visual symptoms occur. Like rifampin, the drug causes an orange-tan discoloration. Rarely, thrombocytopenia, a flu-like syndrome, hemolysis, myositis, chest pain, and hepatitis have occurred. Although less potent than rifampin, rifabutin does induce hepatic CYPs and can decrease the t1/2 of a number of drugs, including zidovudine, prednisone, digitoxin, quinidine, ketoconazole, propranolol, phenytoin, sulfonylureas, and warfarin.

Also know about Rifapentin

Rifapentine is an analog of rifampin. It is active against both *M tuberculosis* and *M avium*. As with all rifamycins, it is a bacterial RNA polymerase inhibitor, and cross-resistance between rifampin and rifapentine is complete. Like rifampin, rifapentine is a potent inducer of cytochrome P450 enzymes, and it has the same drug interaction profile. Toxicity is similar to that of rifampin.

Rifapentine and its microbiologically active metabolite, 25-desacetylrifapentine, have an elimination half-life of 13 hours. Rifapentine 600 mg (10 mg/kg) once weekly is indicated for treatment of tuberculosis caused by rifampin-susceptible strains during the continuation phase only (ie, after the first 2 months of therapy and ideally after conversion of sputum cultures to negative). Rifapentine should not be used to treat HIV-infected patients because of an unacceptably high relapse rate with rifampin-resistant organisms.

Rifapentine (PRIFTIN) has a longer t1/2 than rifampin and rifabutin, which allows once-weekly dosing. It has an intermediate capacity to induce CYPs, between rifabutin and rifampin. In HIV-infected patients, rifapentine may select for rifamycin resistance; rifabutin is therefore preferred in this situation

81. Ans. (c) Flumazenil

Ref: KDT 7th ed page 401, Katzung 11th Ed page 421

Flumazenil is one of several 1,4-benzodiazepine derivatives with a high affinity for the benzodiazepine binding site on the GABAA receptor that act as competitive antagonists. It blocks many of the actions of benzodiazepines, zolpidem, zaleplon, and eszopiclone, but does not antagonize the central nervous system effects of other sedative-hypnotics, ethanol, opioids, or general anesthetics.

Flumazenil is approved for use in reversing the central nervous system depressant effects of benzodiazepine overdose and to hasten recovery following use of these drugs in anesthetic and diagnostic procedures. Although the drug reverses the sedative effects of benzodiazepines, antagonism of benzodiazepine-induced respiratory depression is less predictable.

When given intravenously, flumazenil acts rapidly but has a short half-life (0.7 - 1.3 hours) due to rapid hepatic clearance. Because all benzodiazepines have a longer duration of action than flumazenil, sedation commonly recurs, requiring repeated administration of the antagonist.

Adverse effects of flumazenil include agitation, confusion, dizziness, and nausea. Flumazenil may cause a severe precipitated abstinence syndrome in patients who have developed physiologic benzodiazepine dependence. In patients who have ingested benzodiazepines with tricyclic antidepressants, seizures and cardiac arrhythmias may follow flumazenil administration.

82. Ans. (c) Lateral aspect of thigh

Ref: Goodman 11th Ed page 1059, KDT 7th ed page 259

- Insulin usually is injected subcutaneously in the abdomen (below costal margins to illiac crest and and 2 inches away from umblicus), buttock, anterior thigh, or dorsal arm.
- Factors that determine the rate of absorption of insulin after subcutaneous administration include the site of injection, the type of insulin, subcutaneous blood flow, smoking, regional muscular activity at the site of the injection, and the volume and concentration of the injected insulin.
- Rotation of insulin injection sites traditionally has been advocated to avoid lipohypertrophy or lipoatrophy. The abdomen is the preferred site of injection in the morning because insulin is absorbed more rapidly from that site than from the arm. If the patient refuses to inject into the abdomen, it is preferable to select a consistent injection site for each component of insulin treatment (e.g., prebreakfast dose into the thigh, evening dose into the arm).
- Increased subcutaneous blood flow (brought about by hot baths or exercise) increases the rate of insulin absorption. In the upright posture, subcutaneous blood flow diminishes considerably in the legs and to a lesser extent in the abdominal wall. An altered volume or concentration of injected insulin affects the rate of absorption and the duration of action. When regular insulin is mixed with lente or ultralente insulin, some of the regular insulin becomes modified, causing a partial loss of the short-acting component. Injections of mixtures of insulin preparations thus should be made without delay. There is less delay in absorption of regular insulin when it is mixed with NPH insulin.
- Subcutaneous insulin administration may result in anti-insulin IgG antibody formation. In most patients, circulating anti-insulin antibodies do not alter the pharmacokinetics of the injected hormone. Rarely, the pharmacokinetics of the insulin preparations can be altered, potentially leading to increased postprandial hyperglycemia (owing to decreased action of regular insulin) but nighttime hypoglycemia (owing to the prolonged action of intermediate insulin). Because of concerns that IgG anti-insulin antibodies could cross the placenta and cause fetal hyperglycemia by neutralizing fetal insulin or cause fetal or neonatal hypoglycemia due to unpredictable release of insulin from antigen-antibody complexes, it is recommended that only human insulin be used during pregnancy.

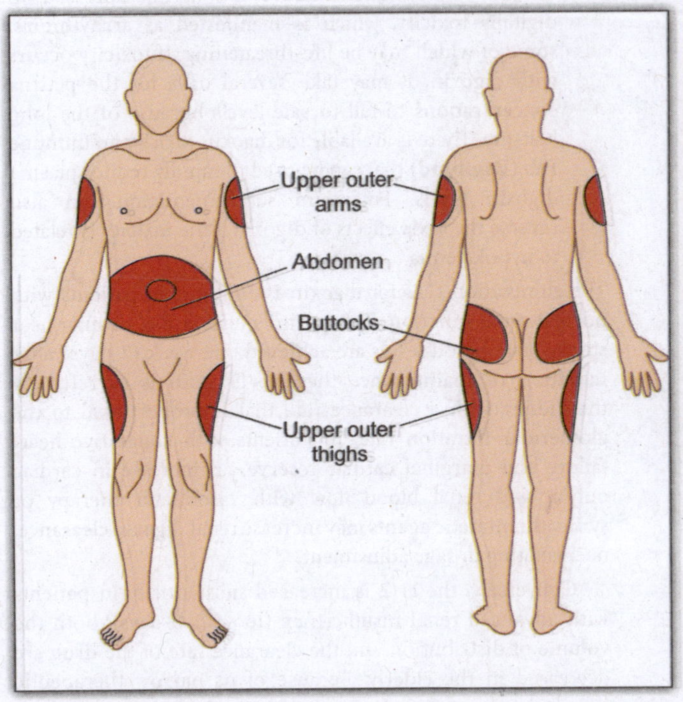

83. Ans. (a) Linagliptin

Ref: KDT 7th ed page 275, ABC of Diabetes by Tim Holdt 7th ed page 37

Dipeptidyl peptidase-4 (DPP-4) inhibitors

- Sitagliptin, vildagliptin, saxagliptin, alogliptin, Linagliptin.
- The dose of sitagliptin, vildagliptin and saxagliptin should be reduced if GFR falls below 50–60 ml/min.
- Linagliptin is safe in renal failure or hepatic impairment. There is no dose adjustment required for linagliptin in renal failure patients (which is the only oral drug currently licensed for this use)

84. **Ans. (c) To adjust maintenance dosing for achieving therapeutic blood levels**

Ref: Lippincott 4th Ed page 307

Pharmacokinetics of Digoxin

The long half-life of digitalis compounds necessitates special considerations when dosing.

- With a half-life of 40 hours. This permits once-a-day dosing; near steady-state blood levels are achieved one week after initiation of maintenance therapy. Digoxin would require several days of constant dosing to reach steady-state, therapeutic plasma levels. Therefore, when initiating treatment, a special dosing regimen involving "loading doses" is used to rapidly increase digoxin plasma levels. This process is termed "digitalization."
- For digoxin, the therapeutic plasma concentration range is 0.5 - 1.5 ng/ml. It is very important that therapeutic plasma levels are not exceeded because digitalis compounds have a relatively narrow therapeutic safety window.
- Plasma concentrations above 2.0 ng/ml can lead to digitalis toxicity, which is manifested as arrhythmias, some of which may be life-threatening. If toxicity occurs with digoxin, it may take several days for the plasma concentrations to fall to safe levels because of the long half-life. There is available for digoxin toxicity an immune Fab (**Digibind**) that can be used to rapidly reduce plasma digoxin levels. Potassium supplementation can also reverse the toxic effects of digoxin if the toxicity is related to hypokalemia

The elimination t1/2 for digoxin is 36 hours in patients with normal renal function. This permits once-a-day dosing; near steady-state blood levels are achieved one week (7 days) after initiation of maintenance therapy. Digoxin is excreted by the kidney with a clearance rate that is proportional to the glomerular filtration rate. In patients with congestive heart failure and marginal cardiac reserve, an increase in cardiac output and renal blood flow with vasodilator therapy or sympathomimetic agents may increase renal digoxin clearance, necessitating dosage adjustment.

Conversely, the t1/2 is increased substantially in patients with advanced renal insufficiency (to ~3.5–5 days); both the volume of distribution and the clearance rate of the drug are decreased in the elderly. Because of its narrow therapeutic index, the drug must be used with caution in patients with renal insufficiency and in the elderly.

Calculation of Loading Dose

It follows from the above, that to achieve a target Cp, the Vd of the drug must be known.

LD = Vd × target Cp (Plasma concentration)

e.g. to achieve a target Cp of 1.5 μg/L for digoxin (Vd - 500 L)

LD (μg) = 500 (L) × 1.5 (μg/L) = 750 μg D

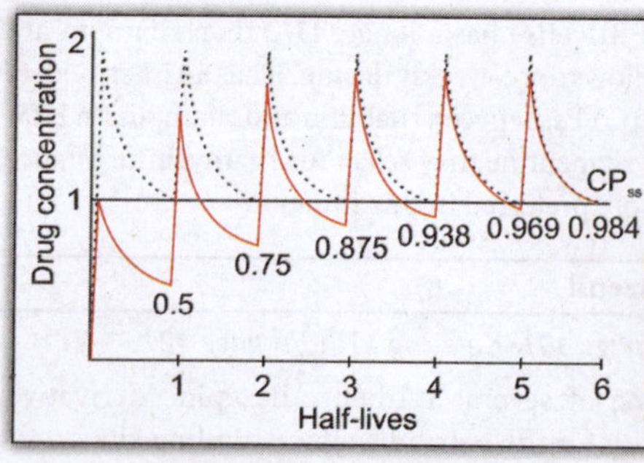

The t½ provides an index of:

- The time-course of drug elimination
- The time-course of drug accumulation
- Choice of dose interval

85. **Ans. (b) Posterior auricular > Scrotum > Scalp> Dorsal aspect of hand > Sole**

Ref: With text

Ref: Encyclopedia of Controlled Drug Delivery - Volume 2 - By Edith Mathiowitz Page 979; Numerous studies have been performed on this topic giving different results with main controversy regarding highest absorption from Scrotum of Postauricular region. Old books and Earlier studies quotes scrotum with highest rate of absorption while latest books and later further studies found that Posterior auricular area shows better absorption. Anatomic sites may be ranked in the following order of decreasing permeability: **Postauricular region > Scrotum> Abdomen > Scalp> Forearm > Foot > Sole**

The stratum corneum differs in thickness, with the palm and sole being the thickest (400-600 μm) followed by the general body stratum corneum (10-16 μm), and the scrotum (5 μm). Facial and post-auricular regions have the thinnest stratum corneum. Permeability generally is inversely proportional to the thickness of the stratum corneum but thickness is only one variable in determining regional differences in drug penetration. **Ref: Goodman Gilman 12th ed page 1803**

Passage through the outermost layer is the rate-limiting step for percutaneous absorption. A hydrated stratum corneum allows more percutaneous absorption. Transport of most drugs is a passive thermodynamic process, and heat generally increases penetration. **Ref: Goodman Gilman 12th ed page 1803**

86. **Ans. (d) Cleaning the inhaler after every use**

Ref: OP Ghai 7th ed page 363, Rau's Respiratory Care Pharmacology by Douglas S. Gardenhire page 50

Metered Dose Inhaler (MDI)

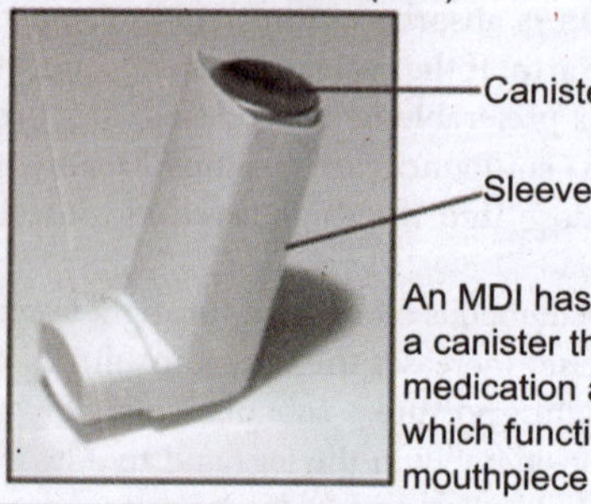

An MDI has two parts: a canister that contains medication and a sleeve which functions as a mouthpiece

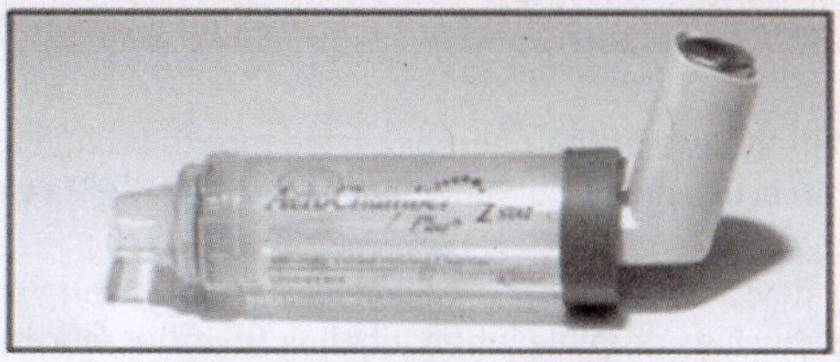

MDI Inserted into a Spacer

Use of Metered Dose Inhaler

Generic Recommendations That Apply All pMDI

- Remove mouthpiece cover of pMDI from boot
- Prime pMDI as directed in package insert
- Clean and dry boot of pMDI based on manufacturer's guidelines
- Track remaining doses after each use

Critical Steps in Use of the Open Mouth Technique With pMDIs'

- Remove cap, inspect for foreign matter, and push canister into nozzle receptacle of mouthpiece actuator
- Hold MDI in vertical position, shake inhaler, and, if not used recently, discharge priming dose
- Exhale to functional residual capacity (easier for subject) or to residual volume
- Hold MDI about 1 inch in front of open mouth or, alternatively, place in mouth with teeth apart and with tongue flat
- Begin to breathe in slowly through mouth while actuating inhaler by pressing down on canister. Inspiration should take about 3-4 seconds
- Continue inhaling to total lung capacity and hold breath for up to 10 seconds (only one puff for inhalation)
- Exhale normally, shake canister, wait 20-30 seconds to allow valve to refill, and repeat dose if prescribed
- Keep a diary of number of uses or use a counting device to keep track of number of actuations used Note: If you have trouble aiming the MDI at your open mouth, you can place the mouthpiece directly in your mouth and rest it on the lower front teeth without sealing your lips around it.

Critical Steps in Use of the Closed Mouth Technique With pMDI

- Remove mouthpiece cover and check for foreign objects
- Shake inhaler thoroughly
- Prime pMDI into air if it is new or has not been used for several days
- Sit up straight or stand up
- Exhale all the way out
- Place pMDI between teeth
- Ensure that tongue does not block pMD1 by keeping it flat under mouthpiece
- Seal lips
- Actuate pMDI as you begin to inhale slowly
- Hold breath for 10 seconds or as long as possible
- **Wait 1 minute before administering another puff of medicine**
- Repeat steps 2 through 10 until dosage prescribed by physician is reached
- After using a corticosteroid, rinse mouth after last puff of medicine
- Spit water out and do not swallow any
- Replace mouthpiece cover on pMDI after each use

Critical Steps in Soft Mist inhaler (Respimat) Use

- Close mouthpiece cap; press safety catch while pulling off clear base
- On label of inhaler, write discard date- 3 mnths from date cartridge is inserted into device
- Remove medication cartridge from box
- Push narrow end of cartridge into inhaler
- Return clear base to mouthpiece assembly
- Hold inhaler upright, with cap closed, to avoid accidental release of dose
- Turn clear base one-half turn
- Point inhaler toward ground and press dose release button
- Continue steps 6 through 8 until mist of medication is seen
- Once mist is visible, repeat steps 6 through 8 three times
- Once primed, turn clear base one-half turn and open mouthpiece cap
- Breathe out, slowly emptying lungs; close lips around mouthpiece without covering air vents 13. Point inhaler to back of throat, keeping inhaler parallel to ground
- While inhaling slowly and deeply, press dose release button; continue to breathe in slowly for as long as possible
- Hold breath for 10 seconds or as long as possible
- Repeat steps 12 through 15 until prescribed dose has been completed
- When complete, replace mouthpiece cover on inhaler

Contd...

Use of Metered Dose Inhaler

To Inhale a Corticosteroid

Use the same procedure as described in the use of the open or closed mouth technique with these exceptions:

- If you use a bronchodilator and a corticosteroid, inhale the bronchodilator first and wait 1-2 minutes before inhaling the corticosterold
- Always use an extension or spacer device when inhaling a corticosteroid. If you do not have such a device, try to hyperextend (straighten) your head and neck as much as possible when inhaling (in other words, look at the ceiling)
- Rinse your mouth and throat with water after finishing

Common Errors in Use

The number of patients using pMDIs incorrectly ranges from 12% to 89%, according to available studies." • Failure to coordinate actuation with inhalation (27%) • Too short a period of breath-hold after inhalation (26%) • Too rapid an inspiratory flow rate (19%) • Inadequate shaking and mixing of contents before use (13%) • Abrupt cessation of inspiration as aerosol strikes throat (6%) • Actuation at total lung capacity (4%) • Firing actuation into mouth but inhaling through 0880 (2%) • Exhaling during actuation • Placing wrong end of inhaler in mouth, or holding in wrong (nonvertical) position • Failure to take cap off before use • Firing of MDI multiple times during a single inhalation • Covering air vents on specific inhalers ResPimat)

Cleaning pMDI Frequency of cleaning:

Once a week and as needed Look at hole where drug sprays out from inhaler

Clean inhaler if you see powder in or around hole

Remove pMDI canister from plastic container so that it does not get wet

Rinse plastic container with warm water and shake out to remove excess water

Dry overnight

Replace canister inside mouthpiece and recap mouthpiece

Cleaning Respimat Frequency of cleaning:

Once a week and as needed Remove mouthpiece cover Wipe outside of mouthpiece with damp cloth

Wipe metal piece inside mouthpiece with damp cloth Clean outside of inhaler with damp cloth when needed

Recap mouthpiece Store in cool, dry place

Check Canister Fullness

The best approach is to keep a patient log of use, showing date of initial use and subsequent numbers of actuations each day.

If a pMDI is used regularly (e.g., two actuations four times daily), the projected date of depletion can be calculated.

For occasional use, tallies at the end of the day on a self-stick note kept in a convenient place, such as the bathroom, can be useful.

Counting devices can be purchased that count the no. of actuations during use.

Some manufacturers have a built-in counter on the actuator (e.g., ProAir, Ventolin, and Flovent). Canister flotation in water is no longer recommended; it is imprecise, varies with different drugs, and can clog pMDI nozzles.

87. Ans. (c) Drug B is Epinephrine

Ref: KDT 7th ed page 133

NOTE

- The original graph has a third parameter of Peripheral resistance along with Heart rate and BP. In examination however only Heart rate and BP was provided in the graph.
- Isoproterenol is better known as Isoprenaline

This question is based upon knowledge of action of direct sympathomimetics.

Direct Sympathomimetics

They act directly as agonists on alpha and beta adrenoceptors -Adrenaline, Nor-adrenaline, isoprenaline (isoproterenol), phenylephrine, methox, xylomctazoline, salbutamol and many others

Aid to Diagnosis

Out of three curves only Drug A shows decrease heart rate. Out of Epinephrine, Norepinephrine and Isoprenaline only Norepinephrine will show decreased HR (See table below)

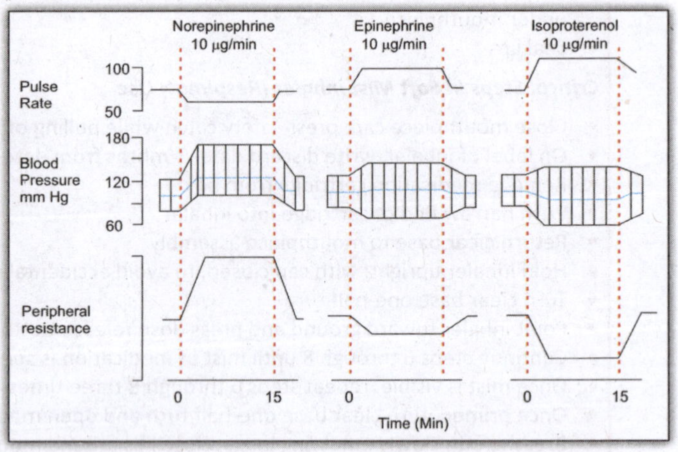

Thus according to the figure

Drug A (Norepinephrine) showed increase in systolic, diastolic and mean pressure with constant pulse pressure and falling HR.

Drug B (Epinephrine) showed increase in systolic, steady mean pressure, fall in diastolic and rise in HR.

Drug C (Isopretrenol) showed first increase then decrease and steady state of systolic with increasing HR

Regarding Option (B); The effects of Drug A (Fall in heart rate), that is Noradrenaline is blocked/ antagonised by beta blockers like propanolol not Muscarinics.

Drug	Action of Receptors
Adrenaline	α1, α 2, β1, β2 and weak β3
Nor-adrenaline	α 1, α 2, α 1, α 3, No β2 action
Isopreternol	β1, β2, β3, No α action

	Adrenaline	Nor-adrenaline	Isopreternol
Heart Rate	↑	↓	↑↑
Cardiac Output	↑↑	–	↑↑
Systolic BP	↑↑	↑↑	↑
Diastolic BP	↑↓	↑↑	↑↑
Mean Bp	↑	↑↑	↓
Bronchial Muscle	↓↓	–	↓↓
Interstitial Muscle	↓↓	↓	↓
Blood Sugar	↑	↑–	↑
Blood Flow To Skin	↓	↓	–
Blood To Skeletol Muscle	↑↑	↓	↓
Kidney Blood Flow	↓	↓	–
Liver Blood Flow	↑↑	–	↑↑
Coronary	↑	↑	↑

88. Ans. (a) Both A and B are full agonists

Ref: Karzung 12th ed page 7, 30, KDT 7th ed page 53

Option (A): A and B are full Agonist having maximum possible efficacy, hence correct statement

Option (B): Is false because potency of A > B > C

Option (D): Efficacy of A = B > C, hence this statement is also false

Option (C): C is not a non competitive antagonist as the starting point is different, C is hence partial agonist

Dose Response Curve	
Simple dose response curve hyperbolic in shape while log DRC is sigmoid in shape. There are three important parameters- potency, efficacy and slope	
Potency	It is the measure of the amount of drug needed to produce the response. Drug producing same response at lower dose is more potent (in DRC more the dose response curve towards left, greater is the potency i.e. A > B > C > D) 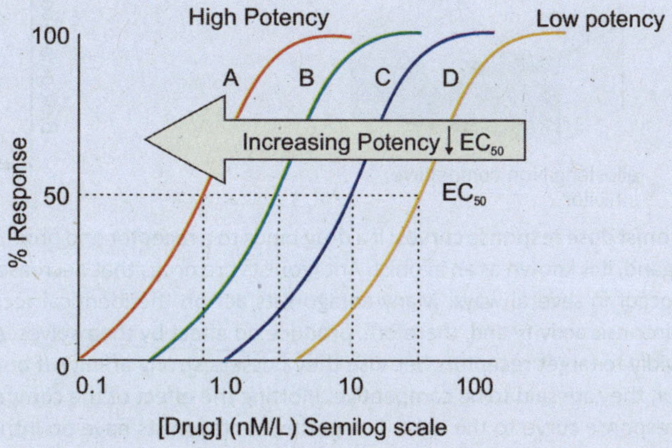

Contd...

Dose Response Curve	
Efficacy	It is the maximum effect produced by a drug. It is clinically more important than potency. (On DRC- More is the peak of curve greater is its efficacy i.e. A>B>C>D)
Slope	Steeper is the slope more are the chances of getting the response drastically with increase in dose. I.e. steep DRC means narrow therapeutic index

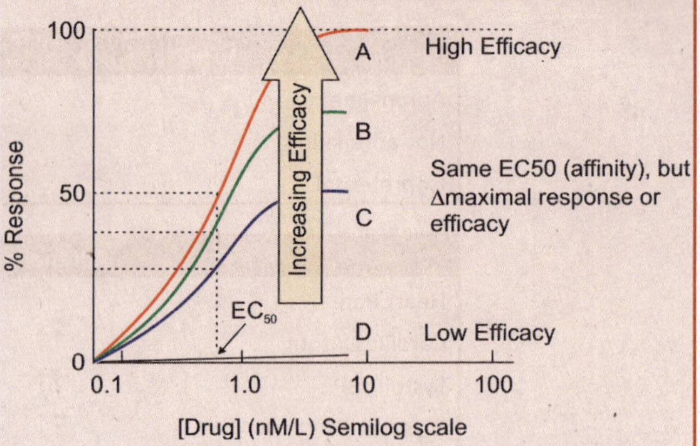

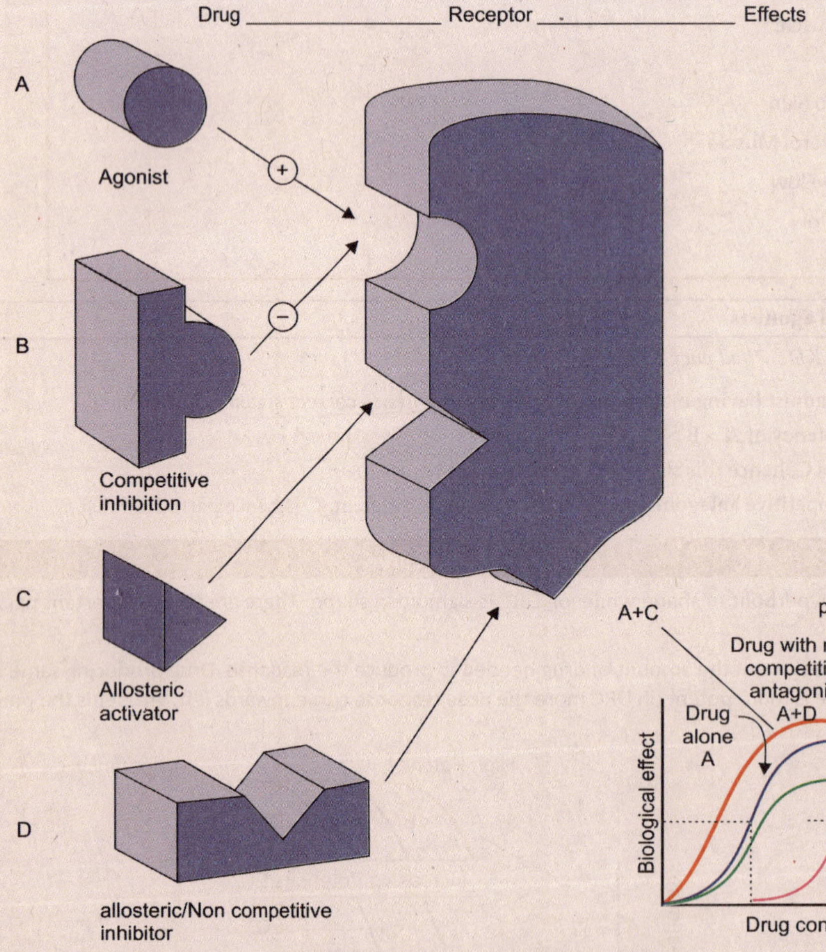

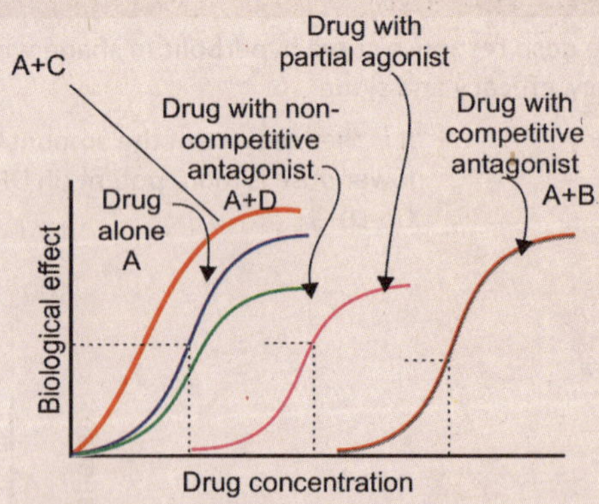

Agonist and anatgonist dose response curves: If a drug binds to a receptor and produces a biologic response that mimics the response to the endogenous ligand, it is known as an agonist. Antagonists are drugs that decrease the actions of another drug or endogenous ligand. Antagonism may occur in several ways. Many antagonists act on the identical receptor macromolecule as the agonist. Antagonists, however, have no intrinsic activity and, therefore, produce no effect by themselves. Although antagonists have no intrinsic activity, they are able to bind avidly to target receptors because they possess strong affinity. If both the antagonist and the agonist bind to the same site on the receptor, they are said to be competitive. Plotting the effect of the competitive antagonist characteristically causes a shift of the agonist dose-response curve to the right. Competitive antagonists have no intrinsic activity. If the antagonist binds to a site other than where the agonist binds, the interaction is noncompetitiveâ€ or allosteric. It decreases the efficacy of a drug.

Contd...

Dose Response Curve

Examples of Competitive and Noncompetitive Antagonism.

A. Competitive Antagonism, where both the agonist (Isoproterenol) and the antagonist (Propranolol) bind reversibly to the same receptor subtype (β-adrenoceptor). In the presence of the competitive antagonist, the dose-response curve is shifted to the right in a parallel manner

B. Non-competitive antagonism. Phenoxybenzamine binds irreversibly (with covalent bonds) to α-adrenergic receptors. This reduces the fraction of available receptors, and reduces the maximal effect that can be produced by the agonist.

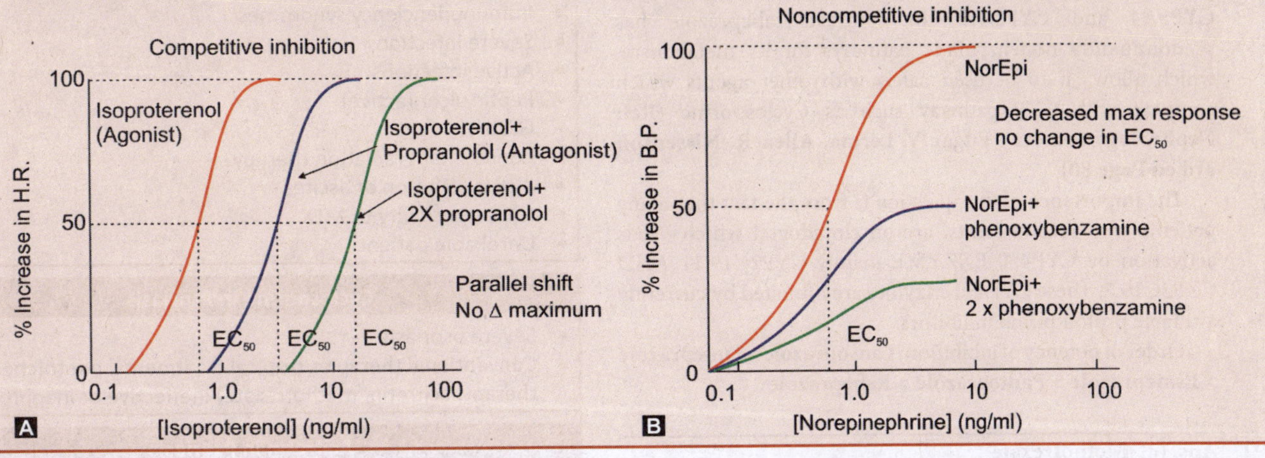

89. Ans. (a) Vitamin K

Ref: KDT 7th ed page 616, Goodman Gillman 11th ed page 954

Vitamin K is procoagulant not anticoagulant.

Drugs Affecting Platelet Function and Mechanism of Action

Interfering with platelet membrane	Inhibition of prostaglandin pathways	Inhibition of platelet phosphodiesterase	Unknown mechanism of action
Tricyclic antidepressant Amitriptyline, Imipramine	Antiplatelet: Aspirin, clopidogrel	Caffeine	Acetazolamide
SSRI; citalopram, Escitalopram, fluoxetine Fluvoxamine, paroxetine Sertraline	NSAID (Indomethacin, ibuprofen, naproxen, diclofenac, ketorolac)	Dipyridamole Cilostazol	Ethacrynic acid
Antipsychotic; Chlorpromazine	Furosemide	Aminophylline	Hydroxychloroquine
Anesthetic; Cocaine, Lidocaine	Calcium channel blockers; Verapamil	Theophylline	Nitroprusside
Antihistamine; Promethazine, Diphenhydramine	Hydralazine	Vinblastine	Cyproheptadine
Isoproterenol	Cyclosporine	Vincristine	Nitroglycerin
Beta blockers; Propranolol	Hydrocortisone	Colchicine	Famotidine
Antibiotics: Penicillin Ampicillin, Cephalothin, Carbenicillin		Papaverine	Cimetidine

AIIMS MAY 2016

90. Ans. (a) Subarachnoid hemorrhage

Ref: KDT 7th ed page 540, 550

Nimodipine, a member of the dihydropyridine group of calcium channel blockers, has a high affinity for cerebral blood vessels and appears to reduce morbidity after a subarachnoid hemorrhage. nimodipine is claimed to be particularly selective for cerebral blood vessels. Splice variants in the structure of the α1 channel subunit appear to account for these differences.

91. Ans. (b) **Rabeprazole**

Ref: Goodman Gilman 12th Ed page 1312, Clinical Pharmacy and Therapeutics by Roger Walker P- 17

Out of the given options drug that causes least inhibition of CYP450 is Rabeprazole

All of the PPIs, except rabeprazole, are metabolized predominantly by hepatic CYP450 enzymes, in particular CYP3A4 and CYP2C19. In contrast, rabeprazole has predominantly nonenzymatic pathways for its metabolism, which allows it to be used safely with other agents which compete with CYP pathway such as Cyclosporine **(Ref: Nephrology Secrets - Edgar V. Lerma, Allen R. Nissenson 3rd ed Page 80)**

The importance of this question is from the fact that many patients who receive stents, are on clopidogrel which needs activation by CYP450 ENZYME mainly CYP2C19.11 AND CYP2C19.7. These CYP450 enzymes are inhibited by currently available proton pump inhibitors.

Order of potency of inhibition: **Lansoprazole > Omeprazole > Esmeprazole > Pantoprazole > Rabeprazole**

92. Ans. (c) **Methotrexate**

Ref: Goodman Gilman 12th Ed page 1820, 1809, KDT 7th ed page 882

Treatment of erythrodermic psoriasis is

- Methotrexate
- Cyclosporine
- Acitretin

Quick review of some therapies in psoriasis

Methotrexate In Psoriasis

Indications

- Severe psoriasis
  - Chronic plaque psoriasis (>10–15% BSA or interference with employment or social functioning)
  - Pustular psoriasis (generalized or localized)
  - Erythrodermic psoriasis
  - Psoriatic arthritis (moderate to severe)
  - Severe nail psoriasis
- Psoriasis not responding to topical treatments, photo(chemo) therapy and/or systemic retinoids

Contraindications (Absolute or Relative)

- Impaired kidney function (creatinine clearance <60 ml/min)
- Severe anemia, leukopenia and/or thrombocytopenia
- Significant liver function abnormalities, hepatitis (active and/or recent), severe fibrosis, cirrhosis, excessive alcohol intake
- Concomitant hepatotoxic medications

Contd...

Methotrexate In Psoriasis

- Concomitant medications that increase MTX levels, e.g. trimethoprim–
- Sulfamethoxazole
- Significantly reduced pulmonary function
- Pregnancy or lactation
- Currently planning to have children (male and female patients)‡
- Immunodeficiency syndromes
- Severe infections
- Active infections
- Peptic ulcer (active)
- Gastritis
- Concomitant radiation therapy
- Pleural effusion or ascites
- Hypersensitivity to MTX
- Unreliable patient

Cyclosporine in Psoriasis

- Severe psoriasis
- Conventional therapies (topical treatments, photo(chemo) therapy, acitretin, methotrexate) ineffective or inappropriate

Acitretin in Psoriasis

Indications	Contraindications
• Severe psoriasis that cannot be managed by topical treatments or photo(chemo)therapy • Monotherapy is indicated for erythrodermic or pustular psoriasis • Combination therapy is indicated for chronic plaque psoriasis	• Severe liver dysfunction • Severe kidney dysfunction (elimination reduced) • Pregnancy or lactation • Women of childbearing potential who cannot guarantee adequate contraception during and up to 3 years following discontinuation of acitretin • Hyperlipidemia, especially hypertriglyceridemia, that cannot be controlled • Concomitant medications that interfere with retinoid bioavailability or whose • Metabolism is altered† • Concomitant hepatotoxic drugs, e.g. methotrexate • Poorly controlled diabetes mellitus • History of pancreatitis • Excessive alcohol intake • Use of contact lenses • Unreliable patient

93. Ans. (d) **Phase 4**

Ref: KDT 7th ed page 63-64, Katzung 12th ed page 75, Goodman's and Gilman 12th Ed page 79

Clinical Trial and Preclinical Testing

Preclinical Phase

- Before starting the clinical trials on a drug, the pharmaceutical companies would conduct pre-clinical studies which involve; ***In vitro* experiments, *In vivo* experiments**
- As such, these studies would use wide range of doses of the study drug in order to obtain the following preliminary data: **Efficacy, Toxicity, Pharmacokinetics**
- These data would assist the companies in deciding whether the particular drug candidate possesses the scientific merit for developing as **'Investigational New Drug** (IND).

Clinical Trials

	Designation	Study	Population	Sample size	End point/specific end point
Phase 0	Human **microdosing studies**	*Pharmacodynamics and pharmacokinetics* (no data on safety or efficacy, being by definition a single **sub-therapeutic dose**)	Healthy volunteers	10 to 15	*Pharmacodynamics and pharmacokinetics*
Phase 1	First stage of testing in human subjects	***Safety*** (AKA- pharmacovigilance is most important), dose-ranging tolerability, pharmacokinetics, and pharmacodynamics. 70% of new drugs pass this phase. **Phase 1A** (Single Ascending Dose), **Phase 1A** (Multiple Ascending Dose):	Healthy volunteers or individuals with target disease	20-100	Safety
Phase 2	Phase 2B: **Pivotal studies**	**Phase 2A:** *Dosing requirements* (how much drug should be given), **Phase 2 B:** *Efficacy* (how well the drug works), toxicity and continue Phase I safety assessments. Phase 2 trials have the **highest rate of drug failures**, and only 25% of innovative drugs move on to phase 3.	Individuals with target disease	100-300	Efficacy (specific end point= Cardiac output)
Phase 3	Randomized controlled multicenter trials, **"pre-marketing phase"**	How *effective* the drug is, in comparison with current 'gold standard' treatment (most expensive, time-consuming and difficult trials). **Phase 3A**: conducted after efficacy of the study drug but before the regulatory submission of New Drug Application. **Phase 3B:** conducted after regulatory submission of New Drug Application but before the approval and launch of the study drug. If phase 3 results meet expectations, application is made for permission to market the new agent. Marketing approval requires submission of a **New Drug Application (NDA)**—or for biologicals, a Biological License Application—to the FDA.	Individuals with target disease	300–3,000 or more	Efficacy (specific end point= Reduction in mortality rate)

Contd...

Phase 4	Postmarketing surveillance Trial	Safety surveillance (pharmacovigilance, designed to detect any rare or long-term adverse effects)	Individuals with target disease as well as new age groups, genders, etc.	Thousands	Efficacy (specific end point = Reduction in mortality rate)

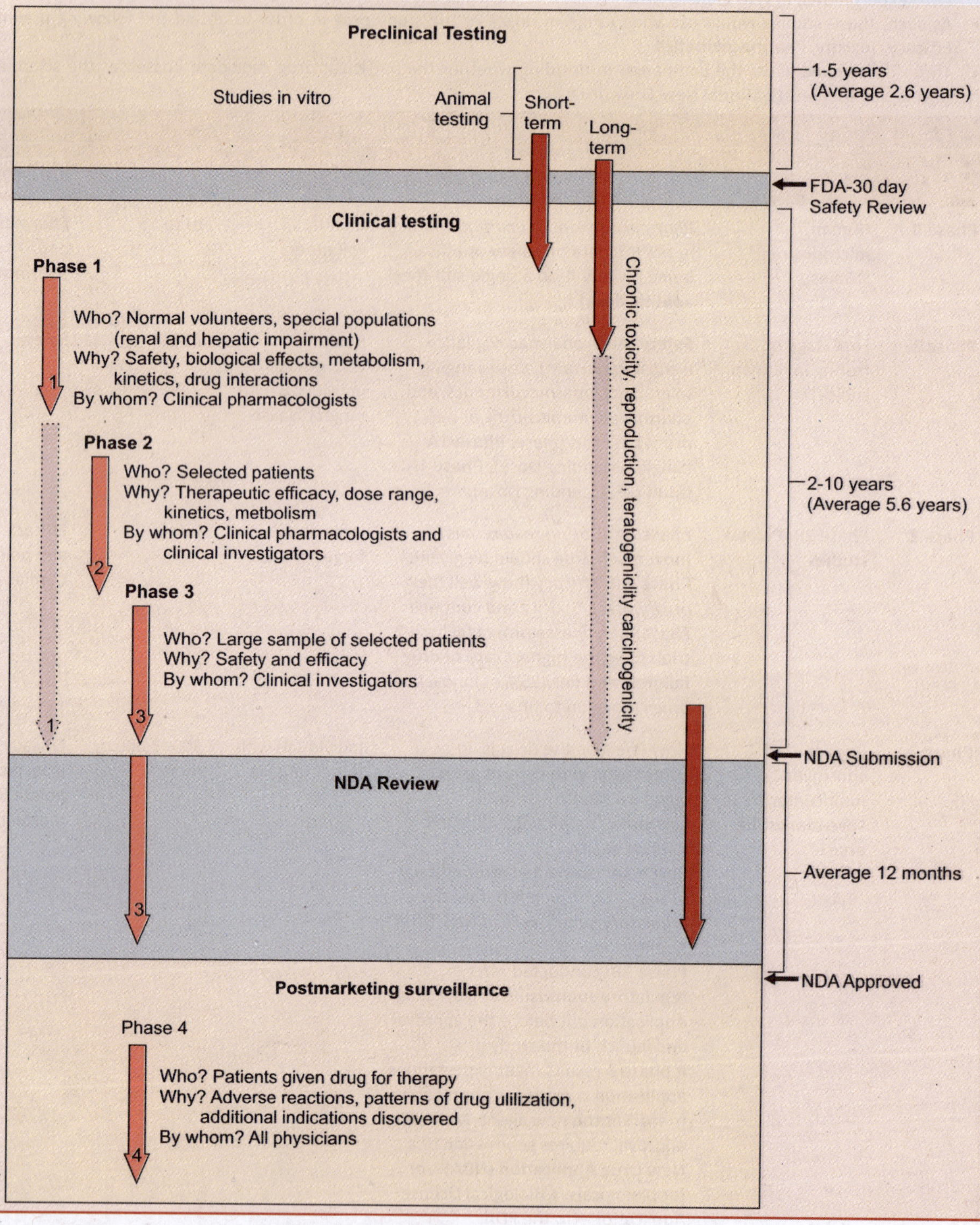

94. Ans. (a) D2 antagonism

Ref: Goodman Gilman 12th Ed page 1788, KDT 7th ed page 664

Anti-emetics with D2 blocking action are chlorpromazine and related neuroleptics like triflupromazine, prochlorperazine, etc. and prokinetic drug metoclopramide. (KDT 7th ed page 951)

Metoclopramide acts through **both dopaminergic and serotonergic receptors** (KDT 7th ed page 665)

Metoclopramide

Mechanism of action: Metoclopramide, one of the oldest true prokinetic agents, stimulates coordinated contractions that enhance transit.

Mechanism of Action of Metaclopramide	
D2 Antagonism	The central antidopaminergic (D2) action of metoclopramide on CTZ is clearly responsible for its **antiemetic property.** Hastening gastric emptying and enhancing LES tone by augmenting ACh release. However, clinically this action is secondary to that exerted through 5HT4 receptors.
5-HT_4 agonism	Metoclopramide acts in the g.i.t. to enhance ACh release from myenteric motor neurons. **The gastric hurrying and LES tonic effects are mainly due to this action**
5-HT_3 antagonism	The central anti 5-HT3 action appears to be significant only when large doses are used to control CINV

Therapeutic use:

- Therapeutic Use and Pharmacokinetics Metoclopramide is indicated in symptomatic patients with gastroparesis, in whom it may modestly improve gastric emptying.
- Metoclopramide injection is used as an adjunctive measure in medical or diagnostic procedures such as intestinal intubation or contrast radiography of the GI tract.
- In general, its greatest utility lies in its ability to ameliorate the nausea and vomiting that often accompany GI dysmotility syndromes.
- It is used to ameliorate nausea and vomiting after chemotherapy.

Dosage

Metoclopramide is available for oral and parenteral use. The usual initial oral dose range is 10 mg, 30 minutes before each meal and at bedtime. The onset of action is within 30–60 minutes after an oral dose. In patients with severe nausea, an initial dose of 10 mg can be given intramuscularly (onset of action 10–15 minutes) or intravenously (onset of action 1–3 minutes). For prevention of chemotherapy-induced emesis, metoclopramide can be infused at 1–2 mg/kg of body weight, administered over at least 15 minutes, beginning 30 minutes before the chemotherapy is begun and repeated as needed every 2–3 hours. Alternatively, a continuous intravenous infusion may be given (3 mg/kg of body weight before chemotherapy, followed by 0.5 mg/kg of body weight per hour for 8 hours). The usual pediatric dose for gastroparesis is 0.1–0.2 mg/kg of body weight per dose, given 30 minutes before meals and at bedtime.

Adverse Effects

- The major side effects of metoclopramide include extrapyramidal effects. Dystonias, usually occurring acutely after intravenous administration, and parkinsonian symptoms that may occur several weeks after initiation of therapy generally respond to treatment with anticholinergic or antihistaminic drugs and are reversible upon metoclopramide discontinuation.
- Tardive dyskinesia also can occur with chronic treatment (months to years) and may be irreversible.
- Metoclopramide can elevate prolactin levels by blocking the inhibitory effect of dopamine on pituitary lactotropes.
- Methemoglobinemia has been reported in premature and full-term neonates receiving metoclopramide.

95. Ans. (c) Telmisartan

Ref: Goyal S, Arora S, Bhatt TK, Das P, Sharma A, Kumari S, Arya DS. Modulation of PPAR-gamma by telmisartan protects the heart against myocardial infarction in experimental diabetes. ***Chemico Biological Interaction. 2010 May 14;185(3):271-80.***

PPAR is one of the favourite research topic in AIIMS Pharmacology department. AIIMS website's pharmacology page ennumerates around 37 research articles, 8 involving PPAR, 4 involving Telmisartan and 3 involving both PPAR and Telmisartan

Telmisartan, a unique ARB, improves left ventricular remodeling of infarcted heart by activating PPAR gamma. Telmisartan prevents unfavorable cardiac remodeling through a reduction of cardiac hypertrophy and fibrosis. An anti-inflammatory effect and PPAR-gamma activation were suggested to be important in addition to suppression of Ang II activity.

A novel action of several AT1 antagonists is partial agonist activity at the peroxisome proliferator-activated receptor γ (PPAR-γ) — a nuclear receptor expressed primarily in adipose tissue. PPAR-γ regulates the gene expression of proteins involved in the differentiation of adipocytes from precursor fibroblast-like cells and the storage of fatty acids.

96. Ans. (a) Paclitaxel

Ref: Goodman Gilman 12th Ed page 1672, 1708-1711, KDT 7th ed page 866, 875

Phase specificity of anticancer drugs:

- **G1:** Vinblastine.
- **S:** Mtx, cytarabine, fludarabine, 6-TG, 6-MP, 5-FU, hydroxyurea, mitomycin C, doxorubicin, daunorubicin.
- **G2:** Daunorubicin, bleomycin, etoposide, topotecan.
- **M:** Vinca alkaloids and Taxans are M phase specific

Classification of Cancer Chemotherapy Agents

Group	Subgroups and agents	Acute toxicity	Delayed toxicity	Uses
Alkylating Agents • Alkylation of DNA at N7 and O6 position of Guanine→DNA crosslinking b/n 2 strands→ prevents duplication • AA are commonly used in chronic leukemia • AA are **non-phase specific** • AA causes secondary leukemia in 4-5 years	**Nitrogen Mustard**			
	1. Mechlorethamine (First anticancer drug)	CINV-chemo induced nausea vomiting (4hr-48hrs) Myelosuppression	Myelosuppression (delayed type-onset=7d, Nadir=10-14d, recovery = 21-28d) Alopecia	MOPP-Hodgkin's lymphoma
	2. Cyclophosphamide [CP → 4hydroxyCP ↔ aldophosphamide → Acrolein (toxic) and **phosphamide mustard** (Therapeutic active metabolite)]	CINV Myelosuppression (CP>Ifo)	Myelosuppression (CP>Ifo) Alopecia, SIADH Hemorrhagic cystitis (Ifo>CP) Sec cancer-transitional cell cancer of bladder	Wagner's granulomatosis DOC CMF-Breast, small cell lung ca Broad spectrum
	3. Ifosfamide → 4-hydroxy ifosfamide → **Ifosfamide mustard** (Therapeutic active metabolite), by product **Chloroacetaldehyde** (Neurotoxic)	CINV Myelosuppression (CP>Ifo) Neurotoxicity (Ifo>CP)	Myelosuppression (CP>Ifo) Alopecia Hemorrhagic cystitis (Ifo>CP)	Broad spectrum Lung, breast, ovary, sarcoma, testis, germ cell tumor
	4. Melphalan amino acid derivative of mechlorethamine	CINV Myelosuppression	Myelosuppression No alopecia	Multiple myeloma DOC Can replace C in CMF
	5. Chlorambucil	Myelosuppression CINV is rare	Myelosuppression No alopecia	CLL, Hodgkin's
	Nitrosoureas (lipophilic-crosses BBB)		Nitrosoureas causes delayed Myelosuppression (onset-15d, Nadir-4 wks, recovery-6wks)	
	1. Carmustine (BCNU-bis chloro nitroso urea)	CINV (severe-2 hrs)	Myelosuppression, male infertility, Pulmonary fibrosis	Brain tumors DOC (Glioblastoma multi-forme, Astrocytoma, Medulloblastoma)
	2. Lomustine (CCNU)	CINV (severe-2 hrs)	Myelosuppression Interstitial lung disease	Do
	3. Semustine (methyl CCNU)	CINV (severe-2 hrs)	Myelosuppression	Do
	4. Streptozocin (methyl-ation of protein and nucleic acid)	CINV (severe-2 hrs)	No Myelosuppression	Pancreatic islet cell tumor Carcinoid tumor
	Alkyl Sulfonates (Intra strand cross linking of DNA by 2 N7 Guanine)			
	Busulfan (Dealkylating agent)	Hyperuricemia (MC)	Sterility, gynecomastia, seizures, Skin pigmentation, Adrenal insufficiency Pulmonary fibrosis (specific)	CML-DOC until imatinib Conditioning of BM transplant
	Ethyl enamines			
	Thiotepa (Organophosphorous)	CINV	Myelosuppression	Seldom used now

Contd...

Classification of Cancer Chemotherapy Agents				
Group	**Subgroups and agents**	**Acute toxicity**	**Delayed toxicity**	**Uses**
Non Classical Alkylating Agents • Acts on RNA and Protein synthesis not/ mild DNA	**Triazenes**			
	Dacarbazine (Active-methyl carbonium ion)	CINV-severe	Permanent sterility Myelosuppression (early/classical)	MAID-sarcoma, ABVD-Hodgkin's Malignant melanoma (most active agent)
	Procarbazine (autoxidize spontaneously, Active-Azoprocarbazine, crosses BBB)	CINV, MAO inhibitor Disulfiram like reaction	Myelosuppression, Dermatitis Leukemogenic, teratogenic	MOPP-Hodgkin's PCV-Glioblastoma
	Altretamine	CINV-severe Hypotension	Neurotoxic Nephrotoxic	Refractory ovarian cancer
Alkylating Like Agents	**Platinum Compounds**			
1st gen platinum Inactivated by aluminum	Cisplatin	CINV (most emetogenic) Hypo Mg, K, Ca sec to hypo Mg)	Myelosuppression Ototoxicity, Secondary leukemia, sensory ataxia, Predominant large fiber sensory neuronopathy	CMF-Solid malignancies
2nd generation platinum, Cross resistance-cisplatin	Carboplatin	CINV (cis>carbo)	Myelosuppression (carbo>cis) No nephrotoxicity	Less potent than cisplatin (1:4) GemCarco-lung cancer
3rd generation platinum No cross resistance	Oxaliplatin	PSN pathy (reversible hand and foot, temp loss)	Neurotoxicity (dose limiting) No nephrotoxicity PSN pathy (irreversible, hand, foot, leg, arm, temp loss, propio loss)	FOLFOX- colon cancer Cis/carboplatin resistance
Antimetabolites • S phase specific • Inhibits DNA synthesis • No acute toxicities • Commonly used in acute leukemias	Folate Antagonists			
	Methotrexate		Hepatotoxicity (portal/ periportal/ bridging fibrosis and cirrhosis) Myelosuppression Mucositis and thrombocytopenia (Leucovorin does not reverse neurotoxicity)	Choriocarcinoma DOC ALL, Osteosarcoma, RA, ectopic Myasthenia, psoriasis, meningeal leukemia (intrathecal route), Ankylosing spondylitis
	Pemetrexed; newer congener of Mtx primarily targets the enzyme thymidylate synthase		Mucositis, diarrhoea, myelosuppression are similar to Mtx, but a painful, itching erythematous rash, mostly involving the hands and feet, 'handfoot syndrome' is quite common.	Mesothelioma, non-small cell lung
	Purine Analogue			
	6 Thioguanine		Myelosuppression Hepatotoxicity	Adult acute leukemia
	6 Mercaptopurime		Myelosuppression, hepatotoxicity	Childhood acute leukemia

Contd...

Classification of Cancer Chemotherapy Agents

Group	Subgroups and agents	Acute toxicity	Delayed toxicity	Uses
	Fludarabine		Myelosuppression, Flu like symptoms (fever, myalgia, arthralgia)	
	Cladribine		Myelosuppression, Nephrotoxic, CINV	Hairy cell leukemia
	Pentostatin		Nephrotoxic	Hairy cell leukemia
	Pyrimidine Analogue			
	5 Fluorouracil (5-FU)		GI upset-diarrhea (MC) Hand foot syndrome, CINV Myelosuppression, neurotoxicity Cerebellar ataxia	
	Cytarabine		Stomatitis, CINV, Cerebellar ataxia Myelosuppression	AML
	Capecitabine		CINV, Diarrhea, Hand foot syndrome Myelosuppression (<5FU)	Metastatic breast cancer Metastatic colorectal cancer
	Gemcitabine		CINV, Myelosuppression (dose limiting)	Pancreatic cancer DOC Bladder and Non-small cell lung Ca
Antibiotics	**Anthracyclins**	Topoisomerase 2 inhibitor (mc),	Quinone Free radical injury and intercalation b/n DNA strands	Membrane binding (responsible for cardiotoxicity)
	Doxorubicin (Adriamycin)	CINV, Alopecia	Myelosuppression (dose limiting, neutropenia > thrombocytopenia) Cardiotoxicity (cardiomyopathy, CHF) Radiation recall Hand foot syndrome	Broad spectrum Solid tumors and sarcomas (rhabdo/leiomyosarcoma, Kaposi sarcoma)
	Daunorubicin	CINV, Alopecia	Myelosuppression, cardiotoxicity, radiation recall	Narrow spectrum AML
	Idarubicin (synthetic Daunorubicin analogue)	CINV, Alopecia, Red urine (not hematuria)	Myelosuppression, cardiotoxicity, radiation recall	AML (more efficacious than daunorubicin)
	Mitoxantrone	CINV, Bluish discoloration of nails	Myelosuppression (dose limiting) Lower cardiotoxicity	
	Other Antibiotics			
	Bleomycin (Glyco peptide Antibiotic) Free radical injury→ds-ss DNA breaks, have both DNA and Fe binding domain	Allergic reaction Hypotension	Pulmonary fibrosis (dose limiting) Mucocutaneous toxicity Marrow sparing	HL, NHL, SCC Malignant pleural effusion Ascitis (sclerosing agent)
	Mitomycin- C Acts as alkylating agent	CINV	Hemolytic uremic syndrome Pulmonary fibrosis 8th nerve damage	Radiosensitizer-DOC SCC

Contd...

Classification of Cancer Chemotherapy Agents				
Group	**Subgroups and agents**	**Acute toxicity**	**Delayed toxicity**	**Uses**
	Dactinomycin Inhibits all forms of DNA dependent RNA synthesis, r-RNA most sensitive	CINV	Myelosuppression Alopecia Radiation recall	Pediatric tumors (Ewing's, wilm's, Rhabdomyosarcoma) Radiosensitizer
	Actinomycin	CINV Desquamation	Myelosuppression Alopecia	Pediatric tumors (Ewing's, wilm's, Rhabdomyosarcoma) Radiosensitizer
	Plicamycin	CINV		
Enzyme	L-Asparaginase (inhibits protein synthesis of tumor cell by depletion of L-Asparagine)	Anaphylaxis/ hypersensitivity-fever, chills, rash, urticaria (bronchochospasm, hypotension if severe)	Hypercoagulable state Pancreatitis, Hepatotoxicity Marrow sparing, no alopecia	ALL Ineffective in solid tumors (normal cells spared)
Plant Derived	**Vinca Alkaloids**	**M phase specific**	Inhibits tubulin polymerization	Mitotic inhibitors
	Vincristine	Alopecia	Symmetric, sensory motor large/small fiber PSNpathy SIADH, Marrow sparing	Lymphosarcoma, Wilm's, Ewing's Remission of childhood acute leukemia.
	Vinblastine	Alopecia (Vc>Vb)	Symmetric, sensory motor large/small fiber PSNpathy (Vc>Vb) Myelosuppression	Hodgkin's, testicular carcinoma
	Epipodophyllotoxins	Topoisomerase 2 inhibitor	***G2 phase***	
	Etoposide (VP-16)	CINV, Hypotension	Myelosuppression, early onset secondary leukemia (1-3 years) alopecia, Length-dependent sensory predominant PSNpathy, autonomic neuropathy	
	Teniposide (VP-26)			
	Taxans	***M phase specific***	Enhance tubulin polymerization	Spindle poison
	Paclitaxel	Hypersensitivity	Symmetric, predominantly sensory large-fiber > small-fiber PSNpathy (stocking glove type) Myelosuppression	Cisplatin resistance Relapse and resistant breast/ovary ca
	Docetaxel (more potent)	Hypersensitivity	Myelosuppression, Symmetric, predominantly sensory large-fiber > small-fiber PSNpathy (is less frequent)	Cisplatin resistance, Relapse-resistant br/ ovary ca
	Camptothecin	Topoisomerase 1 inhibitor	ss DNA breaks	**G2 phase**

Contd...

Classification of Cancer Chemotherapy Agents				
Group	**Subgroups and agents**	**Acute toxicity**	**Delayed toxicity**	**Uses**
	Topothecan	CINV	Myelosuppression (dose limiting)	
	Irinothecan (active = SN-38)	CINV, Cholinergic syndrome (SLUDGE) including early diarrhea-24hrs	Myelosuppression, cholinergic syndrome (SLUDGE) including late diarrhea 3-10d (dose limiting)	Advanced colorectal ca- DOC
Miscellaneous	Arsenic Trioxide (degradation of PMLI and RARα protein)	Headache, light headedness CINV	Cardiotoxicity (QT prolongation, arrhythmias), Myelosuppression Syndrome-fever, fluid retention, wt gain, rash	APL-induction in tretinoin relapse and refractory
	Hydroxyurea (inhibits ribonucleotide reductase→inhibits DNA synthesis) Hydroxyurea has 100% oral bioavailability	CINV	Myelosuppression (dose limiting) Hyperpigmentation	CML AML-blast crisis
	Imatinib (Bcr-Abl Tyrosine kinase inhibitor)	CINV	Fluid retention, Ankle and perioral edema	CML-chronic phase GIST with Ckit tyrosine kinase
	Dasatinib and Nilotinib (novel agents-TK inhibitors)			CML- imatinib resistance/intolerance

97. Ans. (b) Prasugrel

Ref: Goodman's and Gilman 12th Ed page 870

Prasugrel is a thienopyridine. The thienopyridine include ticlopidine, clopidogrel, and prasugrel, drugs that target $P2Y_{12}$, a key ADP receptor on platelets.

Features of GPIIB/IIIA Antagonists			
Feature	**Abciximab**	**Eptifibatide**	**Tirofiban**
Description	Fab fragment of humanized mouse monoclonal antibody	Cyclical KGD-containing heptapeptide	Nonpeptidic RGD mimetic
Specific for GPIIb/IIIa	No	Yes	Yes
Plasma half-life	Short (min)	Long (2.5 h)	Long (2.0 h)
Platelet-bound half-life	Long (days)	Short (s)	Short (s)
Renal clearance	No	Yes	Yes

GPIIb/IIIA Receptor Antagonists

As a class, parenteral GPIIb/IIIa receptor antagonists have an established niche in patients with acute coronary syndromes. The three agents in this class are abciximab, eptifibatide, and tirofiban.

Mechanism of Action

A member of the integrin family of adhesion receptors, GPIIb/IIIa is found on the surface of platelets and megakaryocytes. GPIIb/IIIa is the most abundant receptor. GPIIb/IIIa is inactive on resting platelets. When platelets are activated, inside-outside signal transduction pathways trigger a conformational activation of the receptor. Once activated, GPIIb/IIIa binds adhesive molecules, such as fibrinogen and, under high shear conditions, vWF. Once bound, fibrinogen and/or vWF bridge adjacent platelets together to induce platelet aggregation.

Although abciximab, eptifibatide, and tirofiban all target the GPIIb/IIIa receptor, they are structurally and pharmacologically distinct. Abciximab is a Fab fragment of a humanized murine monoclonal antibody directed against the activated form of GPIIb/IIIa. Abciximab binds to the activated receptor with high affinity and blocks the binding of adhesive molecules. In contrast to abciximab, eptifibatide and tirofiban are synthetic small molecules. Eptifibatide is a cyclic heptapeptide that binds GPIIb/IIIa because it incorporates the KGD motif, whereas tirofiban is a nonpeptidic tyrosine derivative that acts as an RGD mimetic. Abciximab has a long half-life and can be detected on the surface of platelets for up to 2 weeks. Eptifibatide and tirofiban have shorter half-lives.

Dosing

All of the GPIIb/IIIa antagonists are given as an IV bolus followed by an infusion. Because they are cleared by the kidneys, the doses of eptifibatide and tirofiban must be reduced in patients with renal insufficiency.

Side Effects

In addition to bleeding, thrombocytopenia is the most serious complication. Thrombocytopenia is immune-mediated and is caused by antibodies directed against neoantigens on GPIIb/IIIa that are exposed upon antagonist binding. With abciximab, thrombocytopenia occurs in up to 5% of patients. Thrombocytopenia is severe in 1% of these individuals. Thrombocytopenia is less common with the other two agents, occurring in 1% of patients.

Indications

Abciximab and eptifibatide are used in patients undergoing percutaneous coronary interventions, particularly those with acute MI. Tirofiban is used in high-risk patients with unstable angina. Eptifibatide also can be used for this indication

98. Ans. (d) Fall in blood pressure by adrenaline pretreated with phentolamine

Ref: KDT 7th ed page 131, 140

The α blockers abolish the pressor action of Adr (injected i.v. in animals), which then produces only fall in BP due to β2 mediated vasodilatation. This was first demonstrated by Sir HH Dale (1913) and is called vasomotor reversal of Dale. Ergot alkaloids are the adrenergic antagonists with which Dale demonstrated the vasomotor reversal phenomenon.

Propranolol blocks vasodilatation and fall in BP evoked by isoprenaline and enhances the rise in BP caused by Adr. There is re-reversal of vasomotor reversal that is seen after a blockade

Drug	Action of Receptors
Adrenaline	α1, α2, β1, β2 and weak β3
Nor-adrenaline	α1, α2, α1, α3, No β2 action
Isoproternol	β1, β2, β3, No α action

Note:
- α_1 presents in blood vessels–causes vasoconstrictions, increases blood pressure
- β_2 – presents in blood vessels, causes vasodilatation – decrease in blood pressure
- At lower concentration of adrenaline β2 – receptors are more sensitive
- At higher concentration adrenaline acts on all receptors

Effects of Adrenaline on Blood Pressure

To observe effects of adrenaline on blood pressure, we have to give adrenaline intravenous rapidly (In dog)

Step 1: When we give adrenaline intravenously, initially the concentration of adrenaline is high.
- So it will act on α_1, β_2.
- But actions of α_1 (vasoconstriction), will predominate over actions of β_2 (vasodilatation)
- So there will be rise in blood pressure

Step 2: Within few second level of adrenaline will decrease due to its rapid metabolism and neuronal re- uptake
- At lower concentration only action of β_2 will predominate
- So only fall in Blood pressure seen

Step 3: So at this level you can observe initially rise in blood pressure and then after fall in blood pressure. This is called biphasic response (It is not vasomotor reversal of dale)

Step 4: After biphasic response if we administer non-selective alpha blocker
- It blocks the alpha receptors, hence α_1 mediated vasoconstriction Now, if you give Adrenaline again what will happen?
- Only β_2 mediated action occur (why?- because α_1 receptors are blocked by alpha blocker)
- So only fall in blood presser is seen, rather than biphasic response
- This phenomenon is called Vasomotor reversal of Dale

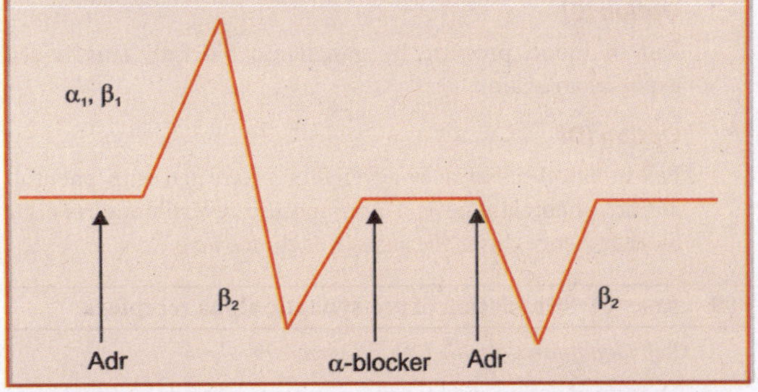

What is Re-reversal

As name suggests re-reversal, we have to reverse the action which happened in Vasomotor reversal of Dale. For this

Step 1. First we give adrenaline intravenously and observe **biphasic response**

Step 2. Now, second step, we give non Selective Beta Blocker (instead of non selective alpha blocker). It blocks the β_2 receptors, hence β_2 mediated vasodilatation will be blocked

Step 3. Now, if you give Adrenaline again what will happen?
- Only α_1 **mediated action occur-vasoconstriction-rise in blood pressure** (why? because β_2 receptors are blocked by beta blocker)
- So only rise in blood presser is seen, rather than biphasic response

This phenomenon is called Re-reversal of Vasomotor reversal of Dale

Contd...

What is Re-reversal

Re-reversal of vasomotor reversal

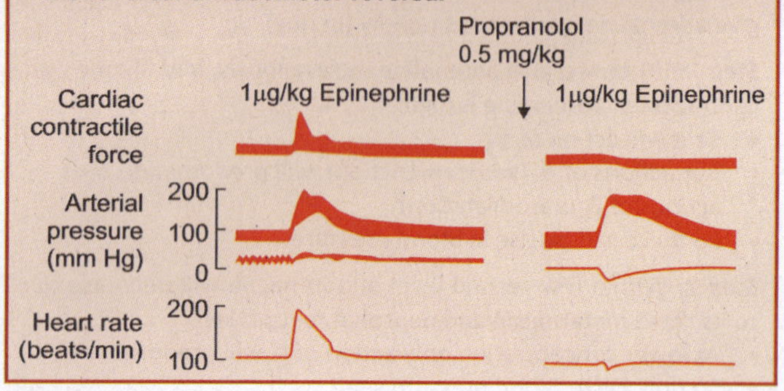

So

1. If only fall in BP- Vasomotor reversal of Dale
2. Only Rise in BP - Re-reversal of Vasomotor reversal of Dale.

Lets Now Check the Options

Option (A)

Fall in blood pressure by high dose intravenous Ach : Ach is not an alpha blocker, hence it cant be an answer.

Option (B)

Increase in blood pressure following administration of IV propranolol : in vasomotor reversal of Dale, only fall in pressure happens, this therefore can also not be an answer.

Option (C)

Fall in blood pressure by ganglionic blocker: This is self explanatory again.

Option (D)

Fall in blood pressure by adrenaline pretreated with phentolamine: phentolamine is a non specific reversible adrenergic blocker, hence this is the answer of choice here.

99. Ans. (b) Stimulation of pre-synaptic alpha receptors

Ref: Goodman Gilman 12th Ed page 199

The role of prejunctional alpha receptors is to inhibit the release of nor epinephrine, therefore this action doesn't play any role in management of anaphylaxis. The α 2A and α 2C adrenergic receptors are the principal prejunctional receptors that inhibit sympathetic neurotransmitter release; the a2B adrenergic receptors also may inhibit transmitter release at selected sites. Clinical uses of epinephrine are based on its actions on blood vessels, heart, and bronchial muscle.

A major use is to provide rapid relief of hypersensitivity reactions, including anaphylaxis, to drugs and other allergens. Other effects mentioned in the options are required for mitigation of anaphylaxis.

- Stimulation of vascular alpha receptors caused constrictions of veins and therefore keeps blood in arterial circulation. It also causes vasoconstriction of splanchnic circulation to divert blood to important organs such as brain.
- Bronchodilation of beta 2 receptors help to breathe.
- Stimulation of beta-1 causes heart to contract.

100. Ans. (c) Stimulation of renal dopaminergic receptor to increase renal perfusion

Ref: KDT 7th ed page 507, Goodman Gilman 12th Ed page 355

Dopamine at a dose of 1 to 3 μg/kg/min has been termed **"renal-dose dopamine"** and has traditionally been used to provide selective renal vasodilation in patients at risk for renal dysfunction. However, it is now clear that although low-dose dopamine may increase blood flow to the renal cortex, blood flow to the renal medulla may actually decrease.

Given the relatively hypoxic environment of the renal medulla under normal circumstances, this effect is potentially harmful.

Furthermore, the increase in urine output that occurs with low-dose dopamine is due primarily to a direct tubular natriuretic effect rather than to renal vasodilation.

In a well-conducted, large, randomized trial, low-dose dopamine did not reduce the incidence of acute renal failure in patients with early renal dysfunction.

Dopamine has a number of other potentially detrimental effects, including inhibition of hypoxic ventilatory drive, impairment of ventilation-perfusion matching in the lung, and suppression of the secretion of some anterior pituitary hormones, such as prolactin, growth hormone, and thyrotropin.

AIIMS NOVEMBER 2015

101. Ans. (b) β1- Heart

Ref: KDT 7th ed page 507, Goodman Gilman 12th Ed page 355

The effects of dopamine are dose-dependent.

- Low doses of dopamine (<3 g/kg per min) stimulate the DA1 and DA2 receptors and cause vasodilation of the splanchnic vasculature.
- Moderate doses (3–5 g/kg per min) stimulate the beta1 receptors and cause an increase in cardiac output with little or no change in heart rate or SVR.
- At higher doses (5 g/kg per min) the effects of dopamine on the alpha 1 receptors overwhelm the dopaminergic receptors, and vasoconstriction ensues, leading to an increase in SVR, LV filling pressures, and heart rate.

102. Ans. (b) Decreased distribution in tissues and organ

Ref: KDT 7th ed page 18, Katzung 8tt ed page 38

The **volume of distribution** is a hypothetical volume of fluid into which a drug is dispersed.

Once a drug enters the body, from whatever route of administration, it has the potential to distribute into any one of three functionally distinct compartments of body water or to become sequestered in a cellular site.

- **Plasma compartment**: If a drug has a very large molecular weight or binds extensively to plasma proteins, it is too large to move out through the endothelial slit junctions of the capillaries and, thus, is effectively trapped within the plasma (vascular) compartment. As a consequence, the drug distributes in a volume (the plasma) that is about six percent of the body weight or, in a 70-kg individual, about 4 L of body fluid, e.g. heparin

- **Extracellular fluid**: If a drug has a low molecular weight but is hydrophilic, it can move through the endothelial slit junctions of the capillaries into the interstitial fluid. However, hydrophilic drugs cannot move across the lipid membranes of cells to enter the water phase inside the cell. Therefore, these drugs distribute into a volume that is the sum of the plasma water and the interstitial fluid, which together constitute the extracellular fluid. This is about twenty percent of the body weight, or about 14 L in a 70-kg individual, e.g. aminoglycoside.
- **Total body water**: If a drug has a low molecular weight and is hydrophobic, not only can it move into the interstitium through the slit junctions, but it can also move through the cell membranes into the intracellular fluid. The drug, therefore, distributes into a volume of about sixty percent of body weight, or about 42 L in a 70-kg individual, e.g. ethanol.
- In pregnancy, the fetus may take up drugs and thus increase the volume of distribution. Drugs that are extremely lipid-soluble, such as thiopental may also have unusually high volumes of distribution.

Apparent Volume of Distribution

The volume into which drugs distribute is called the apparent volume of distribution, or Vd. Another useful way to think of this constant is as the partition coefficient of a drug between the plasma and the rest of the body. Presuming that the body behaves as a single homogeneous compartment with volume V into which drug gets immediately and uniformly distributed

V = dose administered i.v/Plasma concentration

Apparent volume of distribution can be defined as "the volume that would accommodate all the drug in the body, if the concentration throughout was the same as in plasma". Thus, it describes the amount of drug present in the body as a multiple of that contained in a unit volume of plasma.

- **Lipid-insoluble drugs do not enter cells**- V approximates extracellular fluid volume, e.g. streptomycin, gentamicin 0.25 L/kg.
- **Distribution is not only a matter of dilution, but also binding and sequestration.** Drugs extensively bound to plasma proteins are largely restricted to the vascular compartment and have low values, e.g. diclofenac and warfarin (99% bound) V = 0.15L/kg.
- **Drugs sequestrated in other tissues** may have, V much more than total body water or even body mass, e.g. digoxin 6 L/kg, propranolol 4 L/kg, morphine 3.5 L/kg, because most of the drug is present in other tissues, and plasma concentration is low. Therefore, in case of poisoning, drugs with large volumes of distribution are not easily removed by haemodialysis.

A large Vd has an important influence on the half-life of a drug, because drug elimination depends on the amount of drug delivered to the liver or kidney (or other organs where metabolism occurs) per unit of time. Delivery of drug to the organs of elimination depends not only on blood flow, but also on the fraction of the drug in the plasma. **If the Vd for a drug is large, most of the drug is in the extraplasmic space and is unavailable to the excretory organs. Therefore, any factor that increases the volume of distribution can lead to an increase in the half-life and extend the duration of action of the drug.** An exceptionally large Vd indicates considerable sequestration of the drug in some organ or compartment.

103. Ans. (a) TXA2 synthesis

Ref: KDT 7th ed page 609, Katzung 12th ed page 638

Aspirin alters the balance between TXA_2, which promotes aggregation, and PGI_2, which inhibits it. Aspirin inactivates cyclo-oxygenase (COX)-acting mainly on the constitutive form COX-1-by irreversibly acetylating a serine residue in its active site. This reduces both TXA_2 synthesis in platelets and PGI_2 synthesis in endothelium. Oral administration is relatively selective for platelets because of presystemic elimination. Furthermore, vascular endothelial cells can synthesise new enzyme via regeneration of COX-1 and via COX-2, whereas platelets (which contain only COX-1 and have no nuclei) cannot. After administration of aspirin, TXA_2 synthesis does not recover until the affected cohort of platelets is replaced in 7-10 days. Consequently, low doses of aspirin given once every 24 or 48 hours decrease the synthesis of TXA_2 without drastically reducing PGI_2 synthesis.

Clinical trials have demonstrated the efficacy of aspirin in several clinical settings with similar efficacy over a dose range of 50-1500 mg per day, all of which doses nearly completely abolish platelet thromboxane biosynthesis. Adverse effects of aspirin, mainly on the gastrointestinal tract, are, **however, clearly dose-related, so a low dose (often 75 mg once daily)** is usually recommended for thromboprophylaxis.

Goodman and Gilman States

In platelets, the major cyclooxygenase product is thromboxane A_2, a labile inducer of platelet aggregation and a potent vasoconstrictor. **Aspirin blocks production of thromboxane A_2 by acetylating a serine residue near the active site of platelet cyclooxygenase (COX-1), the enzyme that produces the cyclic endoperoxide precursor of thromboxane A_2.** Since platelets do not synthesize new proteins, the action of aspirin on platelet cyclooxygenase is permanent, lasting for the life of the platelet (7 to 10 days). Thus, repeated doses of aspirin produce a cumulative effect on platelet function. Complete inactivation of platelet COX-1 is achieved when 160 mg of aspirin is taken daily. Therefore, aspirin is maximally effective as an antithrombotic agent at doses much lower than those required for other actions of the drug. Numerous trials indicate that aspirin, when used as an antithrombotic drug, is maximally effective at doses of 50 to 320 mg per day. Higher doses do not improve efficacy; moreover, they potentially are less efficacious because of inhibition of prostacyclin production, which can be largely spared by using lower doses of aspirin. Higher doses also increase toxicity, especially bleeding.

104. Ans. (d) PCOD

Ref: KDT 7th ed page 407, Goodman Gillman 12th ed page 5 97

The question is straight forward in the present form. Whether or not its a side effect of Valproate, PCOD is the only Gender specific option provided.

There has been increasing concern about sodium valproate being an iatrogenic cause of polycystic ovary syndrome (PCOS). Polycystic ovary syndrome represents a complex neuroendocrine disorder with multiple determinants; menstrual irregularities may be a frequently seen phenomenon in women with bipolar illness, at least partially independent of psychotropic drug therapy.

105. Ans. (a) Oseltamivir

Ref: Harrison's 19th Ed page 21 5e-l

Recall Bias

Some students think that the question was asked as " All of the following can be used in Bird flu EXCEPT:" Answer in that case will be Ribavirin as it is inconsistent on clinical trials.

Influenza A Virus Including Subtype H1N1

Influenza A (H1N1) virus is a subtype of influenza A virus and was the most common cause of human influenza (flu) in 2009. Some strains of H1N1 are endemic in humans and cause a small fraction of all influenza-like illness and a small fraction of all seasonal influenza. Other strains of H1N1 are endemic in pigs (swine influenza) and in birds (avian influenza).

The virus isolated from patients in the United States was found to be made up of genetic elements from four different flu viruses:
- North American swine influenza
- North American avian influenza
- Human influenza
- Swine influenza virus.

Pandemic	On June 11, 2009, the WHO declared an H1N1 pandemic, moving the alert level tophase 6, marking the first global pandemic since the 1968 Hong Kong flu.
Cause of death	A study conducted in coordination with the University of Michigan Health Service published in the December 2009 American Journal of Roentgenology warning that H1N1 flu can cause **pulmonary embolism**, surmised as a leading cause of death in this current pandemic.
Pregnancy	The research team of Andrew Miller MD showed pregnant patients are at increased risk.
Virulence	The virulence of swine flu virus is mild and the mortality rates are very low.
Outbreak	H5N1; Hong kong H9N2; China H9N2; Hong kong H7N7; Netherlands 2004/05 H5N1; H7N3; Canada, H10N7; Egypt H5N1 in 13 new countries including India H5N1 in China, Egypt, Indonesia, Nigeria
Drug categories	Two groups of drugs are currently available for the treatment or prophylaxis of influenza infections: • **Adamantanes:** The adamantanes (amantadine and rimantadine) are effective only against influenza A and are associated with several toxic effects and with rapid emergence of drug-resistant variants. *This potential for the development of resistance especially limits the use of the adamantanes for the treatment of influenza, although the drugs still have a place in planning for prophylaxis during an epidemic.* • **Newer class of neuraminidase inhibitors:** The neuraminidase inhibitors (zanamivir and oseltamivir) interfere with the release of progeny influenza virus from infected host cells, a process that prevents infection of new host cells and thereby halts the spread of infection in the respiratory tract. These have activity against both influenza A and B viruses. *A key advantage of the neuraminidase inhibitors, and a major difference from the adamantanes, is that development of resistance is very rare* ▪ **Zanamivir** is approved for treatment of influenza among children aged ≥7 years. ▪ **Oseltamivir** is approved for treatment and chemoprophylaxis among persons aged ≥1 year. Recommended treatment and chemoprophylaxis dosages of oseltamivir for children vary by the weight of the child ▪ **Peramivir,** a newer agent in clinical trials, has also been shown to be a potent and selective inhibitor of influenza A and B neuraminidases. ▪ **Ribavirin**, a nucleoside analogue has been used in the treatment of human influenza A virus infections, usually administered orally or by aerosolization, and occasionally by the IV route for severe infections or in immunocompromised hosts. A consistent benefit has not been observed in clinical studies, and **currently ribavirin is not considered to be a drug of choice for influenza A infection**

Contd...

Influenza A Virus Including Subtype H1N1	
Drug therapy	• **Oseltamivir**, sold under the trade name Tamiflu and is taken orally in capsules or as a suspension, used to treat and prevent both Influenza virus A and Influenza virus B. • Oseltamivir is a prodrug (active metabolite, the free carboxylate of oseltamivir) and is the first orally active ***neuraminidase inhibitor*** serving as a competitive inhibitor towards sialic acid. • Oseltamivir is approved for use in persons age 1 and over. There is also currently an FDA Emergency Use authorization temporarily allowing the use of Tamiflu in children less than one year old. • **Treatment dosage:** The usual adult dosage for treatment of influenza is 75 mg twice daily for 5 days, beginning within 2 days of the appearance of symptoms and with decreased doses for children and patients with renal impairment. • **Prophylaxis dosage**: Standard prophylactic dosage is 75 mg once daily for patients aged 13 and older, which has been shown to be safe and effective for up to six weeks. • **Co-administration with probenecid:** It has been suggested that co-administration of oseltamivir with probenecid could extend a limited supply of oseltamivir. Probenecid reduces renal excretion of the active metabolite of oseltamivir.

106. Ans. (a) 1

Ref: KDT 7th ed page 716, Goodman 12th ed page 1478

Bacteria also can destroy b-lactam antibiotics enzymatically via the actions of b-lactamases. The substrate specificities of some of these enzymes are relatively narrow; such enzymes are sometimes referred to as penicillinases or cephalosporinases. Beta lactam antibiotics act on the lactam ring internal amide bond. Penicillinase acts on the same internal amide bond before beta lactam antibiotics can act on it.

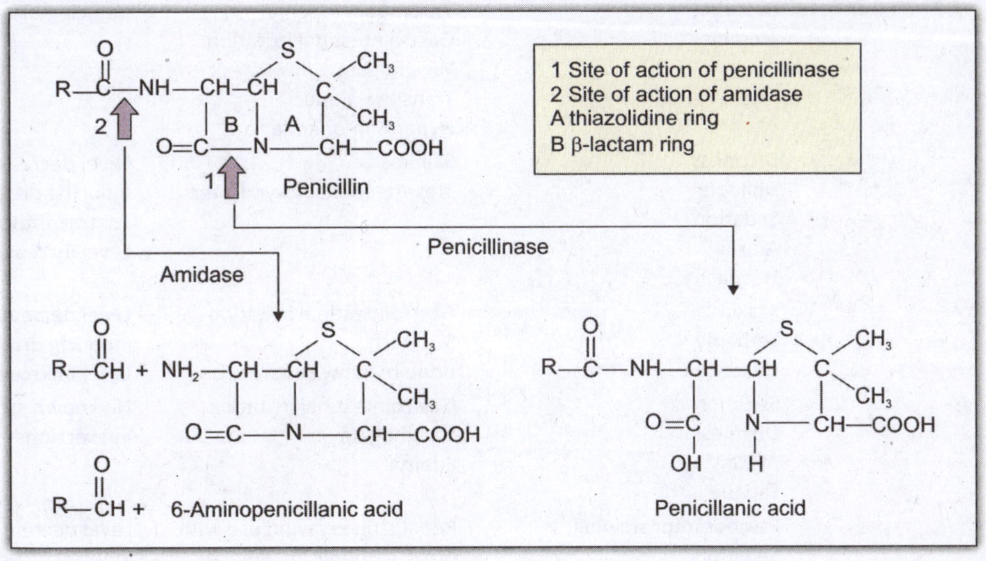

In general, gram-positive bacteria produce and secrete large amounts of b-lactamase. Most of these enzymes are penicillinases. The staphylococcal penicillinase is encoded in a plasmid that may be transferred to other bacteria and is inducible by substrate.

In gram-negative bacteria, b-lactamases are strategically located in the periplasmic space between the inner and outer cell membranes for maximal protection of the microbe. b-lactamases of gram-negative bacteria are encoded either in chromosomes or plasmids, and may be constitutive or inducible.

107. Ans. (b) Vigabatrin

Ref: Katzung 9th Ed page 561

Vigabatrin

Mechanism of Action

Vigabatrin is an **irreversible inhibitor of GABA aminotransferase (GABA-T)**, the enzyme responsible for the degradation of GABA. It apparently acts by increasing the amount of GABA released at synaptic sites, thereby enhancing inhibitory effects. Vigabatrin may also potentiate GABA by inhibiting the GABA transporter.

Clinical use

Vigabatrin is useful in the **treatment of partial seizures and West's syndrome**.

Side Effect Profile

- Typical toxicities include **drowsiness, dizziness, and weight gain.**
- Less common but more troublesome adverse reactions are **agitation, confusion, and psychosis; preexisting mental illness is a relative contraindication.**
- The drug was delayed in its worldwide introduction by the appearance in rats and dogs of a reversible **intramyelinic edema**; this phenomenon has not been observed in any patient to date.

- More recently, unfortunately, long-term therapy with vigabatrin has been associated with development of **visual field defects** in up to one third of patients. This adverse effect may not be reversible, and vigabatrin may therefore be relegated to use in patients—such as those with infantile spasms—who are refractory to other treatments.

Side Effects of Common Anti Epileptics

Generic Name	Adverse Effects: Neurologic	Adverse Effects: Systemic	Drug Interactions
Phenytoin (diphenyl-hydantoin	Dizziness Diplopia Ataxia Incoordination Confusion	Gum hyperplasia Lymphadenopathy Hirsutism Osteomalacia Facial coarsening Skin rash	Level increased by isoniazid, sulfonamides, fluoxetine Level decreased by enzyme-inducing drugs[a] Altered folate metabolism
Carbamazepine	Ataxia Dizziness Diplopia Vertigo	Aplastic anemia Leukopenia Gastrointestinal irritation Hepatotoxicity Hyponatremia	Level decreased by enzyme-inducing drugsa Level increased by erythromycin, propoxyphene, isoniazid, cimetidine, fluoxetine
Valproic acid	Ataxia Sedation Tremor	Hepatotoxicity Thrombocytopenia Gastrointestinal irritation Weight gain Transient alopecia Hyperammonemia	Level decreased by enzyme-inducing drugs[a]
Lamotrigine	Dizziness Diplopia Sedation Ataxia Headache	Skin rash Stevens-Johnson syndrome	Level decreased by enzyme-inducing drugsa and oral contraceptives Level increased by valproic acid
Ethosuximide	Ataxia Lethargy Headache	Gastrointestinal irritation Skin rash Bone marrow suppression	Level decreased by enzyme-inducing drugs[a] Level increased by valproic acid
Gabapentin	Sedation Dizziness Ataxia Fatigue	Gastrointestinal irritation Weight gain Edema	No known significant interactions
Topiramate	Psychomotor slowing Sedation Speech or language problems Fatigue Paresthesias	Renal stones (avoid use with other carbonic anhydrase inhibitors) Glaucoma Weight loss Hypohidrosis	Level decreased by enzyme-inducing drugs[a]
Tiagabine	Confusion Sedation Depression Dizziness Speech or language problems Paresthesias Psychosis	Gastrointestinal irritation	Level decreased by enzyme-inducing drugs[a]
Phenobarbital	Sedation Ataxia Confusion Dizziness Decreased libido Depression	Skin rash	Level increased by valproic acid, phenytoin
Primidone	Same as phenobarbital		Level increased by valproic acid, phenytoin

Contd...

Side Effects of Common Anti Epileptics			
	Adverse Effects		
Generic Name	Neurologic	Systemic	Drug Interactions
Clonazepam	Ataxia Sedation Lethargy	Anorexia	Level decreased by enzyme-inducing drugs[a]
Felbamate	Insomnia Dizziness Sedation Headache	Aplastic anemia Hepatic failure Weight loss Gastrointestinal irritation	Increases phenytoin, valproic acid, active carbamazepine metabolite
Levetiracetam	Sedation Fatigue Incoordination Mood changes	Anemia Leukopenia	No known significant interactions
Zonisamide	Sedation Dizziness Confusion Headache Psychosis	Anorexia Renal stones Hypohidrosis	Level decreased by enzyme-inducing drugs[a]
Oxcarbazepine	Fatigue Ataxia Dizziness Diplopia Vertigo Headache	See carbamazepine	Level decreased by enzyme-inducing drugs[a] May increase phenytoin
Lacosamide	Dizziness Ataxia Diplopia Vertigo	GI irritation Cardiac conduction (PR interval prolongation)	Level decreased by enzyme-inducing drugs[a]
Rufinamide	Sedation Fatigue Dizziness Ataxia Headache Diplopia	GI irritation Leukopenia Cardiac conduction (QT interval prolongation)	Level decreased by enzyme-inducing drugs[a] Level increased by valproic acid May increase phenytoin

108. Ans. (c) Ledipasvir

Ref: Harrison 19th ed page 2049

Simeprevir, boceprevir, sofosbuvir, ledipasvir: All are oral agents for chronic hepatitis C. None is used as single agent. Sofosbuvir and Ledipasvir need not be combined with interferon.

Ledipasvir is a HCV NS5A inhibitor with potent antiviral activity against HCV genotypes 1a and 1b. In the non-transplant setting, the combination therapy (SOF + ledipasvir ± RBV) has shown higher than 95% cure rates of genotype 1

Latest Guidelines for Treatment of Hepatitis C	
Screening	• Screening for HCV infection must be recommended in targeted populations defined according to the local epidemiology of HCV infection, ideally within the framework of national plans. • Screening for HCV infection must be based on the detection of anti-HCV antibodies. • Rapid diagnostic tests (RDT) can be used instead of classical enzyme immunoassays to facilitate anti-HCV antibody screening and improve access to care. • If anti-HCV antibodies are detected, HCV RNA should be determined by a sensitive molecular method to identify patients with on-going infection. • RDTs use various matrices, including serum, plasma, but also fingerstick capillary whole blood or, for some of them, oral (crevicular) fluid, facilitating screening without the need for venous puncture, tube centrifugation, freezing and skilled labour. RDTs are simple to perform at room temperature without specific instrumentation or extensive training.

Contd...

Latest Guidelines for Treatment of Hepatitis C	
Diagnosis	• The diagnosis of acute and chronic HCV infection is based on the detection of HCV RNA by a sensitive molecular method (lower limit of detection <15 IU /ml) • Anti-HCV antibodies are detectable by enzyme immunoassay (EIA) in the vast majority of patients with HCV infection, but EIA results may be negative in early acute hepatitis C and in profoundly immunosuppressed patients • Anti-HCV antibodies are the first-line diagnostic test for HCV infection • In the case of suspected acute hepatitis C or in immunocompromised patients, HCV RNA testing should be part of the initial evaluation • If anti-HCV antibodies are detected, HCV RNA should be determined by a sensitive molecular method • Anti-HCV-positive, HCV RNA negative individuals should be retested for HCV RNA three months later to confirm true convalescence
Pretreatment Assessment	• The causal relationship between HCV infection and liver disease should be established • The contribution of comorbid conditions to the progression of liver disease must be evaluated and appropriate corrective measures implemented • Liver disease severity should be assessed prior to therapy. Identifying patients with cirrhosis is of particular importance, as their prognosis is altered and their treatment regimen may be adapted • Fibrosis stage can be assessed by non-invasive methods initially, with liver biopsy reserved for cases where there is uncertainty or potential additional aetiologies • HCV RNA detection and quantification should be made by a sensitive assay with a lower limit of detection of ≤15 IU/ml • The HCV genotype and genotype 1 subtype (1a/1b) must be assessed prior to treatment initiation and will determine the choice of therapy • IL28B genotyping has no role in the indication for treating hepatitis C with the new DAAs (Directly acting agents) • HCV resistance testing should not be performed prior to therapy, because the SVR rates are very high both in patients without and with detectable amounts of resistance-associated variants by means of population sequencing at baseline (with the exception of patients infected with subtype 1a who receive the combination of PegIFN-α, ribavirin and simeprevir)
Goal of therapy in hepatitis C	• The goal of therapy is to cure HCV infection to prevent hepatic cirrhosis, decompensation of cirrhosis, HCC, severe extra-hepatic manifestations and death • The endpoint of therapy is undetectable HCV RNA in a sensitive assay (≤15 IU/ml) 12 weeks (SVR12) and 24 weeks (SVR24) after the end of treatment • In patients with advanced fibrosis and cirrhosis, HCV eradication reduces the rate of decompensation and will reduce, albeit not abolish, the risk of HCC. In these patients surveillance for HCC should be continued • In patients with decompensated cirrhosis, HCV eradication reduces the need for liver transplantation. Whether HCV eradication impacts mid- to long-term survival in these patients is unknown
Various drugs for Hepatitis C	• PegIFN-α2a Once weekly subcutaneous injection of 180 μg (or less if dose reduction needed) • PegIFN-α2b Once weekly subcutaneous injection of 1.5 μg/ kg (or less if dose reduction needed) • Ribavirin Two capsules in the morning and 3 in the evening if body weight < 75kg, or Three capsules in the morning and 3 in the evening if body weight ≥75 kg • Sofosbuvir One tablet once daily (morning • Simeprevir One capsule once daily (morning) • Daclatasvir One tablet once daily (morning) • Sofosbuvir/ledipasvir: Tablets containing 400 mg of sofosbuvir and 90 mg of ledipasvir. One tablet once daily (morning) • Paritaprevir/ombitasvir/ritonavir Two tablets once daily (morning) • Dasabuvir, Tablets containing 250 mg of dasabuvir One tablet twice daily (morning and evening)
Treatment	Combination therapy with pegylated **interferon alfa (PEG-IFN alfa)** and the nucleoside analogue **ribavirin** is the current standard of care in patients infected with hepatitis C virus (HCV). Patients with HCV genotype 1 have a much less favorable response to therapy and are treated for 12 months, compared with patients infected with genotypes 2 and 3, in whom a 6-month course of therapy is sufficient. If viremia is present after 6 months, additional therapy has a negligible benefit, and treatment should be stopped in all patients regardless of the viral genotype. With HIV coinfection, all patients with a response to therapy at the end of 6 months should receive an additional 6 months of combination therapy regardless of the genotype. Patients with acute HCV infection should be treated for 6 months. The addition of protease inhibitors to the combination of PEG-IFN alfa and ribavirin is becoming the new standard of care for the treatment of chronic HCV infection. Regimens that include a protease inhibitor significantly improve sustained virological response rates in patients with genotype 1 HCV infection.

109. Ans. (a) TNF alpha inhibitor

Ref: Katzung 12th Ed page 648, Goodman Gilman 12th ed page 1826

Cytokines play a central role in the immune response and in autoimmune conditions like rheumatoid arthritis. Although a wide range of cytokines are expressed in the joints of rheumatoid arthritis patients, TNF-α appears to be particularly important in the inflammatory process.

TNF-α affects cellular function via activation of specific membrane-bound TNF receptors (TNFR1, TNFR2). Three drugs interfering with TNF have been approved for the treatment of rheumatoid arthritis and other rheumatic diseases

	Adalimumab	Infliximab	Etanercept
Mechanism of action	Fully human IgG1 anti-TNF monoclonal antibody. This compound complexes with soluble TNF- and prevents its interaction with p55 and p75 cell surface receptors. This results in down-regulation of macrophage and T cell function	Chimeric (25% mouse, 75% human) IgG1 monoclonal antibody that binds with high affinity to soluble and possibly membrane-bound TNF-	Recombinant fusion protein consisting of two soluble TNF p75 receptor moieties linked to the Fc portion of human IgG1, it binds TNF- molecules and also inhibits lymphotoxin-.
Pharmacokinetics	Half-life of 20 days	The terminal half-life is 12 days without accumulation after repeated dosing at the recommended interval of 8 weeks. After intermittent therapy, infliximab elicits human antichimeric antibodies in up to 62% of patients	The drug is slowly absorbed, with peak concentration 72 hours after drug administration. Etanercept has a mean serum elimination half-life of 4.5 days
Route of administration	Subcutaneous	Intravenous infusion	Subcutaneous
Dose	The usual dose in rheumatoid arthritis is 40 mg every other week, although increased responses may be evident at higher dosages. In psoriasis, 80 mg is given at week 0, 40 mg at week 1, and then 40 mg every other week thereafter	Infliximab is given as an intravenous infusion at doses of 10 mg/kg, although the usual dose is 5 mg/kg every 8 weeks.	Etanercept is given subcutaneously in a dosage of 25 mg twice weekly or 50 mg weekly. In psoriasis, 50 mg is given twice weekly for 12 weeks followed by 50 mg weekly
Indications	Approved for the treatment of rheumatoid arthritis, ankylosing spondylitis, psoriatic arthritis, juvenile idiopathic arthritis, plaque psoriasis and Crohn's disease. It decreases the rate of formation of new erosions. It is effective both as monotherapy and in combination with methotrexate and other DMARDs	Infliximab is approved for use in rheumatoid arthritis, ankylosing spondylitis, psoriatic arthritis, and Crohn's disease. It is being used in other diseases, including psoriasis, ulcerative colitis, juvenile chronic arthritis, Wegener's granulomatosis, giant cell arteritis, and sarcoidosis	Etanercept is approved for the treatment of rheumatoid arthritis, juvenile chronic arthritis, psoriasis, psoriatic arthritis, and ankylosing spondylitis. It can be used as monotherapy although over 70% of patients taking etanercept are also using methotrexate.
Side effects	In common with the other TNF-α "blocking agents, the risk of bacterial infections and macrophage-dependent infection (including tuberculosis and other opportunistic infections) is increased,	↑ incidence of bacterial infections, including URTI. As a Potent macrophage inhibitor (activation of latent tuberculosis). Rare cases of leukopenia, hepatitis, activation of hepatitis B, and vasculitis have been documented.	↑ bacterial infections especially soft tissue infections and septic arthritis. Activation of latent tuberculosis is Lower with etanercept than with other TNF-α blocking agents.

Contd...

	Adalimumab	Infliximab	Etanercept
	although it remains very low. A low incidence of newly formed double-stranded DNA (dsDNA) antibodies and antinuclear antibodies (ANAs) has been documented when using adalimumab, but clinical lupus is extremely rare. Rare leukopenias and vasculitis, apparently associated with adalimumab, have been documented.	The incidence of positive ANA and dsDNA antibodies is increased, although clinical lupus erythematosus remains an extremely rare occurrence and the presence of ANA and dsDNA does not contraindicate the use of infliximab. **Infusion site reactions correlate with anti-infliximab antibodies. These reactions occur in approximately 11%** of patients, and the combined use of antihistamines and H2 blocking agents apparently prevents some of these reactions.	Opportunistic infections can rarely occur when using etanercept. The incidence of solid malignancies is not increased, but as with other TNF-α blocking agents one must be alert for lymphomas While positive ANAs and dsDNAs may be found in patients receiving this drug, these findings do not contraindicate continued use if clinical lupus symptoms do not occur. Injection site reactions occur in 40% of patients. Anti-etanercept antibodies are present in up to 16% of treated patients

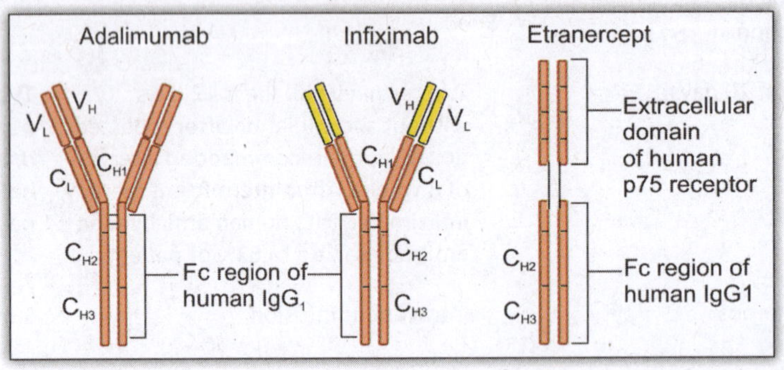

110. Ans. (a) Cyclosporine

Ref: KDT 7th ed page 838, Katzung 12th ed page 986

Calcineurin Inhibitors		
Mechanism of action	These drugs bind to an immunophilin (cyclophilin for cyclosporine or FKBP-12 for tacrolimus), resulting in subsequent interaction with calcineurin to block its phosphatase activity. Calcineurin is required for movement of a component of the nuclear factor of activated T lymphocytes (NFAT) into the nucleus NFAT, in turn, is required to induce a number of cytokine genes, including that for interleukin-2 (IL-2), a prototypic T-cell growth and differentiation factor.	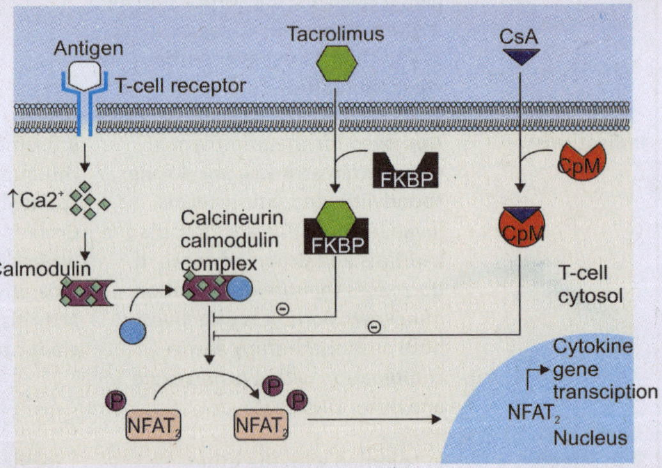
Classification	**Systemic**	**Topical**
	Cyclosporine Tacrolimus	Tacrolimus Pimecrolimus
Cyclosporine	• Produced by the fungus species *Beauveria nivea* • Can be administered intravenously or orally **Pharmacokinetics:** Cyclosporine is extensively metabolized in the liver by CYP3A and to a lesser degree by the gastrointestinal (GI) tract and kidneys. Cyclosporine and its metabolites are excreted principally through the bile into the feces. Cyclosporine also is excreted in human milk. In the presence of hepatic dysfunction, dosage adjustments are required. **No adjustments generally are necessary for dialysis or renal failure patients.**	

Contd...

Calcineurin Inhibitors	
	Indications: • Cyclosporine is FDA-approved for the treatment of psoriasis. Other cutaneous disorders that typically respond well to cyclosporine are atopic dermatitis, alopecia areata, epidermolysis bullosa acquisita, pemphigus vulgaris, bullous pemphigoid, lichen planus, and pyoderma gangrenosum. • Clinical indications for cyclosporine are kidney, liver, heart, and other organ transplantation; rheumatoid arthritis. **Side effects** • The principal adverse reactions to cyclosporine therapy are renal dysfunction, tremor, hirsutism, hypertension, hyperlipidemia, and gum hyperplasia • Hyperuricemia may lead to worsening of gout, increased P-glycoprotein activity, and hypercholesterolemia. • Nephrotoxicity occurs in the majority of patients treated and is the major indication for cessation or modification of therapy. • Hypertension occurs in ~50% of renal transplant and almost all cardiac transplant patients. • Combined use of calcineurin inhibitors and glucocorticoids is particularly diabetogenic, **although this apparently is more problematic in patients treated with tacrolimus.** • Cyclosporine, as opposed to tacrolimus, is more likely to produce elevations in low-density lipoprotein (LDL) cholesterol. • Hepatotoxicity can also occur; therefore, liver function should be periodically assessed. • Infections in patients taking CsA are common and may be life-threatening. Viral infections due to herpes group and cytomegalovirus (CMV) are prevalent. • Lymphoma may occur in all transplanted patients due to the net level of immunosuppression and has not been linked to any one particular agent. • Anaphylactic reactions can occur on parenteral administration.
Tacrolimus	• Tacrolimus is a macrolide antibiotic produced by ***Streptomyces tsukubaensis.*** • Like cyclosporine, tacrolimus inhibits T-cell activation by inhibiting calcineurin. Tacrolimus binds to an intracellular protein, **FK506-binding protein-12 (FKBP-12)**, an immunophilin structurally related to cyclophilin. • Tacrolimus is available for oral administration as capsules (0.5, 1, and 5 mg), as a sterile solution for injection (5 mg/mL) and topically for cutaneous application. **Topical uses:** • In commercially available topical formulations (0.03% and 0.1%), tacrolimus ointment is effective in and approved for the treatment of **atopic dermatitis** in adults (0.03% and 0.1%) and children (0.03%). • Other uses in dermatology include intertriginous psoriasis, vitiligo, mucosal lichen planus, graft-versus-host disease, allergic contact dermatitis, and rosacea. It is applied to the affected area twice a day and generally is well tolerated. • A major benefit of topical tacrolimus compared with topical glucocorticoids is that tacrolimus does not cause skin atrophy and therefore can be used safely in locations such as the face and intertriginous areas. • Common side effects at the site of application are transient erythema, burning, and pruritus, which tend to improve with continued treatment. However, topical tacrolimus should be used with extreme caution in patients with Netherton's syndrome because these patients have been shown to develop elevated blood levels of the drug after topical application. **It is recommended that patients using tacrolimus use sunscreen and avoid excessive UV exposure** **Systemic uses** Tacrolimus is indicated for the prophylaxis of solid-organ allograft rejection in a manner akin to cyclosporine and as rescue therapy in patients with rejection despite "therapeutic" levels of cyclosporine. Dosages are intended to achieve blood trough levels of 5–15-ng/mL. Pediatric patients generally require higher doses than do adults.
Tacrolimus	**Side effects:** • Nephrotoxicity, neurotoxicity (tremor, headache, motor disturbances, seizures), GI complaints, hypertension, hyperkalemia, hyperglycemia, and diabetes are all associated with tacrolimus use. • **As with cyclosporine, nephrotoxicity is limiting.** • Tacrolimus has a negative effect on pancreatic b cells, and **glucose intolerance and diabetes mellitus are well-recognized complications of tacrolimus-based immunosuppression.**
	• As with other immunosuppressive agents, there is an increased risk of secondary tumors and opportunistic infections. **Notably, tacrolimus does not adversely affect uric acid or LDL cholesterol**
Sirolimus	• Does not affect calcineurin. • Blocks m TOR *mammalian target of rapamycin*, Inhibition of mTOR blocks cell-cycle progression at the $G_1 \rightarrow S$ phase transition
Everolimus	• Everolimus (40-0-[2-hydroxy] ethyl-rapamycin) is closely related chemically and clinically to sirolimus but has distinct pharmacokinetics. The main difference is a shorter half-life and thus a shorter time to achieve steady-state concentrations of the drug

111. Ans. (a) Bedaquiline

Ref: Mandell, Douglas, and Bennett's Principles and Practice of Infectious Diseases 8th ed page 474, FDA news release. 2012. Dec 31, [Last accessed on 2013Feb 15]. Available from: http://www.fda.gov/NewsEvents/Newsroom/PressAnnouncements/ucm333695.htm.

The Food and Drug Administration (FDA), on 28 December 2012, granted accelerated approval to SIRTURO™ (bedaquiline) Tablets as a part of combination therapy in adults with multi-drug-resistant TB (MDR-TB). [It is the first new anti-TB drug to be approved after 1998 (rifapentine was approved in 1998) and the first anti-TB drug with a novel mechanism of action to be approved after 40 years (rifampicin was approved in 1974). It is also the first to be introduced specifically for the treatment of MDR-TB in combination with other drugs.

Mechanism of Action

Bedaquiline, a diarylquinoline, binds to subunit c of mycobacterial ATP synthase (an enzyme essential for the energy production in *M. tuberculosis*) and inhibits its activity. It is highly selective for mycobacterial ATP synthase enzyme compared to homologous eukaryotic enzyme (Selectivity Index >20 000).

Dose

Bedaquiline is available as 100 mg tablet for oral administration. Its bioavailability is enhanced in presence of food. It is eliminated mainly in feces. Bedaquiline should be administered as directly observed therapy (DOT) along with standard MDR-TB regimen. Recommended dose is 400 mg once daily for 2 weeks followed by 200 mg thrice weekly for 22 weeks. After 24 weeks of bedaquiline therapy, MDR-TB regimen should be continued as per national TB treatment guidelines.

Side Effects

The most common side-effects reported with bedaquiline therapy are nausea (30%), arthralgia (26%), headache (22%), hemoptysis (14%), chest pain (9%), anorexia (7%), and rash (6%). **Important cardiovascular adverse effect is QT prolongation. Concurrent use of other QT-prolonging drugs causes additive QT prolongation.** Other important adverse effect is elevation of hepatic transaminases, which is moderate and reversible on discontinuation of therapy. There are no clinical data in pediatric patients, adolescents (<18 yrs), and pregnant and lactating women. **The safety and efficacy of bedaquiline for treatment of drug-sensitive TB, extra-pulmonary TB, and HIV-infected patients is not established. Therefore, use of bedaquiline is not recommended in these settings.**

112. Ans. (a) Take tab before meals with full glass of water

Ref: KDT 7th ed page 333

See table of "Drugs used in Osteoporosis" in Pharmacology AIIMS Nov 2016 (see page no. 451 to 453)

<table>
<tr><th colspan="2">Bisphosphonates</th></tr>
<tr><td>Mechanism of action</td><td>They have a strong affinity for bone, especially areas undergoing remodeling. The bisphosphonates decrease osteoclastic bone resorption via several mechanisms, including 1) inhibition of the osteoclastic proton pump necessary for dissolution of hydroxyapatite, 2) decrease in osteoclastic formation/activation, 3) increase in osteoclastic apoptosis (programmed cell death), and 4) inhibition of the cholesterol biosynthetic pathway important for osteoclast function.</td></tr>
<tr><td>Classification</td><td>Based on their side chains, the bisphosphonates are grouped into first-, second-, and third generation drugs.
<ul>
<li>First-generation drugs (e.g., medronate, clodronate, and etidronate) contain minimally modified side-chains or a chlorophenyl group (e.g., tiludronate) and are the least potent agents.</li>
<li>Second-generation aminobisphosphonates (e.g., pamidronate, alendronate, and ibandronate) contain an N-atom in the side chain and are 10–100 times more potent than the first-generation drugs.</li>
<li>Third-generation drugs (e.g., risedronate and zoledronate) contain an N-atom within a heterocyclic ring and are up to 10,000 times more potent than first-generation drugs.</li>
</ul>
<table>
<tr><th>Bishosphonate</th><th>Relative potency</th></tr>
<tr><td>First generation BPNs</td><td></td></tr>
<tr><td>Etidronate</td><td>1</td></tr>
<tr><td>*Tiludronate</td><td>10</td></tr>
<tr><td>Second generation BPNs</td><td></td></tr>
<tr><td>Pamidronate</td><td>100</td></tr>
<tr><td>Alendronate</td><td>100–500</td></tr>
<tr><td>*Ibandronate</td><td>500–1000</td></tr>
<tr><td>Third generation BPNs</td><td></td></tr>
<tr><td>Risedronate</td><td>1000</td></tr>
<tr><td>Zolendronate</td><td>5000</td></tr>
</table></td></tr>
<tr><td>Indications</td><td><ul>
<li>Etidronate, risedronate, alendronate, ibandronate, pamidronate, tiludronate, and zoledronic acid, comprise an important drug group used for the treatment of disorders of bone remodeling, such as osteoporosis and Paget's disease, as well as for treatment of bone metastases and hypercalcemia of malignancy</li>
<li>Alendronate, risedronate, and ibandronate have been approved for the prevention and treatment of osteoporosis.</li>
</ul></td></tr>
</table>

Contd...

Bisphosphonates	
	• Zoledronic acid is also approved for the treatment of postmenopausal osteoporosis. • Second- and third-generation bisphosphonates also may act as anticancer drugs by inhibiting the activation of cancer-associated proteins, such as Ras, through suppression of geranylgeranylation and farnesylation
Adverse reactions	• These include diarrhea, abdominal pain, and musculoskeletal pain. • Alendronate, risedronate, and ibandronate are associated with esophagitis and esophageal ulcers. To minimize the risk of esophageal irritation, patients should remain upright for at least 30 minutes (60 minutes for ibandronate) after taking a bisphosphonate. Symptoms often abate with fastidious adherence to recommendations for taking these drugs. **If symptoms persist, a proton pump inhibitor at bedtime may be helpful.** The oral drugs may be better tolerated when taken once weekly or monthly, with no reduction in efficacy. **Patients with active upper GI disease should not be given oral bisphosphonates.** • Osteonecrosis of the jaw has been reported with bisphosphonates. Etidronate is the only member of the class that causes osteomalacia following long-term, continuous administration.
Pharmacokinetics	All oral bisphosphonates have very limited bioavailability. **They should be administered with a full glass of water following an overnight fast and at least 30 minutes before breakfast.** They are excreted primarily by the kidneys and are not recommended for patients with a creatinine clearance of less than 30 mL/min. • Alendronate, risedronate, and ibandronate are orally active agents for osteoporosis, although less than one percent of the administered dose is absorbed. • Alendronate and risedronate may be dosed once daily or once weekly, whereas ibandronate is administered once monthly • Food significantly interferes with absorption. Bisphosphonates should be administered with 6 to 8 ounces of plain water at least 30 minutes (60 minutes for ibandronate) before eating breakfast or taking other medications. • The bisphosphonates are rapidly cleared from the plasma, primarily because they avidly bind to the hydroxyapatite mineral of bone. • Once bound to bone, they are cleared over a period of hours to years. Elimination from the body is primarily through renal clearance, and the bisphosphonates should not be given to individuals with severe renal impairment. • For patients unable to tolerate oral bisphosphonates, intravenous ibandronate and zoledronic acid are alternative treatments for osteoporosis. Intravenous ibandronate is administered once every 3 months, and zoledronic acid is administered once yearly.

113. Ans. (d) Linezolid

Ref: KDT 7th ed page 668, Goodman Gilman 12th ed page 1535

Classification of antibiotics based upon mechanism of Action and examples

Classification of Antibiotics	
Mechanism of action	**Examples**
Inhibit cell wall synthesis	• Fosfomycin • Cycloserine • Bacitracin • Vancomycin • β lactam antibiotics (includes penicillins, cephalosporins, monobactams, carbapenems, and β lactamase inhibitors)
Cause leakage from cell membranes	Polypeptides- Polymyxins, Colistin, Bacitracin. Polyenes-Amphotericin B, Nystatin, Hamycin.
Inhibit protein synthesis	Tetracyclines, Chloramphenicol, Erythromycin, Clindamycin, Linezolid
Cause misreading of m-RNA code and affect permeability	Aminoglycosides-Streptomycin, Gentamicin
Inhibit DNA gyrase	Fluoroquinolones-Ciprofloxacin and others
Interfere with DNA function	Rifampin, Metronidazole
Interfere with DNA synthesis	Acyclovir, Zidovudine
Interfere with intermediary metabolism	Sulfonamides, Sulfones, PAS, Trimethoprim, Pyrimethamine, Ethambutol

114. Ans. (a) Griseofulvin

Ref: Katzung 12th ed page 855, Goodman Gilman 12th ed page 1585, KDT 7th ed page 15

Griseofulvin is best absorbed when taken with a fatty meal. Presence of food dilutes the drug and retards absorption. Further, certain drugs form poorly absorbed complexes with food constituents, e.g. tetracyclines with calcium present in milk; moreover food delays gastric emptying. Thus, most drugs are absorbed better if taken in empty stomach. However, there are some exceptions, e.g. fatty food greatly enhances lumefantrine absorption.

Increased absorption of drugs with fatty food is seen in: Albendazole, praziquantel, Itroconazole, Mebendazole, Griseofulvin, Posaconazole, Artemether-lumefantrine

NOTE

Carbohydrates reduces the absorption of Isoniazid

115. Ans. (b) Epsilon amino caproic acid

Ref: Goodman 12th ed page 867, Katzung 12th page 616

Aminocaproic Acid

Aminocaproic acid (AMICAR) is a Lys analog that competes for Lys binding sites on plasminogen and plasmin, thus blocking the interaction of plasmin with fibrin. ***Aminocaproic acid is thereby a potent inhibitor of fibrinolysis and can reverse states that are associated with excessive fibrinolysis.***

The main problem with its use is that thrombi that form during treatment with the drug are not lysed. For example, in patients with hematuria, ureteral obstruction by clots may lead to renal failure after treatment with aminocaproic acid. Aminocaproic acid has been used to reduce bleeding after prostatic surgery or after tooth extractions in hemophiliacs. Aminocaproic acid is absorbed rapidly after oral administration, and 50% is excreted unchanged in the urine within 12 hours.

For intravenous use, a loading dose of 4–5 g is given over 1 hour, followed by an infusion of 1 g/h until bleeding is controlled. No more than 30 g should be given in a 24-hour period. Rarely, the drug causes myopathy and muscle necrosis.

116. Ans. (d) 8 to 15°C

REF: Park 23nd ed page 100; http://apps.who.int/medicinedocs/en/d/Js4885e/6.5.html

The following terms relate to temperature and medical supplies. It is important to follow the manufacturer's recommended storage conditions for all products.

Drug Storage Instructions	
Store frozen	Some products, such as certain vaccines, need to be transported within a cold chain and stored at -20°C (4°F). Frozen storage is normally for longer-term storage at higher-level facilities.
Store at 2°-8°C (36°-46°F)	Some products are very heat sensitive but must not be frozen. These are usually kept in the first and second part of the refrigerator (never the freezer). This temperature is appropriate for storing vaccines for a short period of time.
Keep cool	Store between 8°-15°C (45°-59°F)
Store at room temperature:	Store at 15°-25°C (59°-77°F)
Store at ambient temperature	Store at the surrounding temperature. This term is not widely used due to significant variation in ambient temperatures. It means "room temperature" or normal storage conditions, which means storage in a dry, clean, well ventilated area at room temperatures between 15° to 25°C (59°-77°F) or up to 30°C, depending on climatic conditions

117. Ans. (a) Schedule H

Ref: KDT 7th ed page 5, http://cdsco.nic.in/html/copy%20of%201.%20d and cact121.pdf, http://www.mohfw.nic.in/showfile.php?lid=3036

As per drug rules, majority of drugs including all antibiotics must be sold in retail only against a prescription issued to a patient by a registered medical practitioner. These are called 'Prescription Drugs', and in India they have been placed in the schedule H of the Drugs and Cosmetic Rules.

Drugs and Cosmetic Rules of 1945	
It contains 168 rules from 1 to 168 and 25 Schedules from Schedule A to Schedule Y. Different type of forms are also given for different type of approvals from drug authorities.	
Schedule A	Forms and applications
Schedule B	Fees for test or analysis by the Central Drugs Laboratories or State Drugs Laboratories
Schedule C	Biological and Special Products
Schedule D	Class of Drugs: Extent and conditions of exemption
Schedule E	List of Poisonous Substances under the Ayurvedic (including Siddha) and Unani Systems of Medicine
Schedule F	Requirements for the functioning and operation of a Blood Bank and / or for preparation of Blood Components. Vaccines, Antisera, Diagnostic Antigens
Schedule G	Hormonal preperations

Contd...

Drugs and Cosmetic Rules of 1945	
Schedule H	Prescription Drugs
Schedule I	Omitted
Schedule J	Disease and ailment (by whatever name described) which a drug not purport to prevent or cure.
Schedule K	Class of drug: Extent and conditions of exemption
Schedule L	Good Laboratory Practice
Schedule M	Good manufacturing practices and requirements of premises, plant and equipment for Pharmaceutical product.
Schedule N	List of Minimum Equipment for the Efficient Running of a Pharmacy
Schedule O	Standard for Disinfectant Fluids
Schedule P	Life Period and Pask size of Drugs
Schedule Q	List of Dyes, colours and Pigments permitted to be used in Cosmetics and Soaps
Schedule R	Standards for condoms made of rubber latex intended for single use and other mechanical contraceptives
Schedule S	Standard for cosmetics
Schedule T	Good manufacturing practices for Ayurvedic, Siddha and all Unani medicines
Schedule U	• Particulars to be shown in the manufacturing records. • Records of Raw Materials • III – Particulars to be recorded in the analytical records
Schedule V	Standards for patent or proprietary medicines.
Schedule Y	Requirements and guidelines for permission to import and/or manufacture of New Drug for sale or to undertake clinical Trials.

118. Ans. (a) Increase in water solubility

Ref: Goodman Gillman 12th Ed page 124, 125, KDT 7th ed page 14

Substances foreign to the body, or xenobiotics, are metabolized by the same enzymatic pathways and transport systems that are utilized for dietary constituents. Xenobiotics to which humans are exposed include environmental pollutants, food additives, cosmetic products, agrochemicals, processed foods, and drugs. Many xenobiotics are lipophilic chemicals that, in the absence of metabolism, would not be efficiently eliminated and would accumulate in the body, possibly causing toxicity. Most xenobiotics are subjected to metabolic pathways that convert these hydrophobic chemicals into more hydrophilic derivatives that are readily eliminated in urine or bile. Many xenobiotics which induce or inhibit P-gp also have a similar effect on the drug metabolizing isoenzyme CYP3A4, indicating their synergistic role in detoxification of xenobiotics.

119. Ans. (d) Competitive and irreversible

Ref: Goodman Gillman 12th ed page 242, Katzung 12th Ed page 106, KDT 7th ed page 99

Organophosphates and carbamates are insecticides that are usually used in rural areas. These products are readily absorbed through the skin, lungs, mucous membranes and gastrointestinal tract. **Organophosphates induce a competitive and irreversible inhibition of pseudocholinesterase and acetylcholinesterase (AChE) whereas carbamates have competitive but reversible inhibition (transient) as they spontaneously hydrolyze within 48 h.**

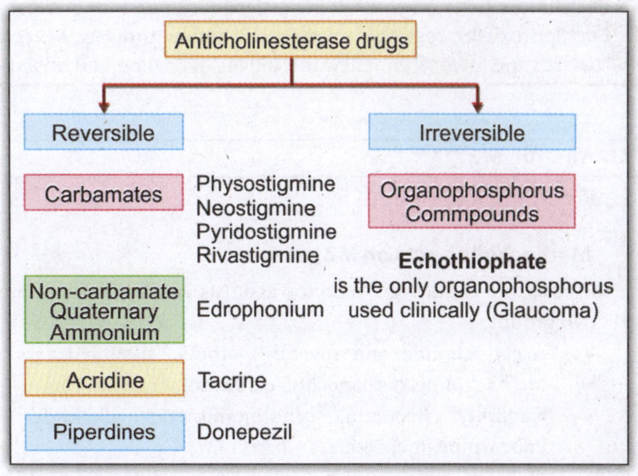

120. Ans. (c) Drug safety

Ref: KDT 7th ed page 63-64, Katzung 12th ed page 75, Goodman's and Gilman 12th Ed page 79

See table of "Clinical Trial and Preclinical Testing" in Pharmacology AIIMS May 2016 (see page no. 463)

AIIMS MAY 2015

121. Ans. (a) Metronidazole

Ref: KDT 7th ed page 586, 742, 744

Ototoxic Drugs		
	Predominantly cochleotoxic	Predominantly vestibulotoxic
Aminoglycosides (Most common)	*Exclusively **outer hair cells**; particularly of the basal* coil of the cochlea Kanamycin, Neomycin, Amikacin, Sisomycin, dihydrostreptomycin	Streptomycin, gentamycin, tobramycin
Diuretics	Furosemide and ethacrynic acid: (inhibits Na+ K+ ATPase of stria vascularis) Reversible damage to cochlea, may cause irreversible damage too	
Salicylates	Reversible damage to cochlea (Possibly they interferes at enzymatic level)	
Antimalarials	Mostly reversible damage; Quinine, Chloroquinine (Vasoconstriction of striae and cochlea)	
Cytotoxic drugs	*Major effect on **outer hair cells;*** Nitrogen mustard, Platinum compounds (cisplatin and carboplatin) Vincristine/Vinblastine	
Desferrioxamine	Mostly permanent cochlear damage	
Analgesics	Indomethacin, ibuprofen, phenyl butazone	
Chemicals	Tobacco, marijuana, carbon monoxide	
Miscellaneous	Erythromycin, ampicillin, propylthiouracil, propanolol	

Footnote:
- Although most ototoxic drugs are both cochleotoxic and vestibulotoxic however they are either predominantly cochleotoxic or vestibulotoxic
- Neomycin is most ototoxic Aminoglycoside
- Netilmicin is least ototoxic Aminoglycoside
- Streptomycin and gentamicin are the most vestibulotoxic aminoglycosides
- Loop diuretics such as ethacrynic acid and furosemide may potentiate the ototoxic effects of the aminoglycosides and should be avoided when possible.
- **Vestibulotoxicity**; may result in vertigo, oscillopsia, and impairment of balance particularly in the dark.
- **Cochleotoxicity**; results in hearing loss and/or tinnitus. AG cochleotoxicity typically affects ***first the high frequency*** and then extends towards the lower frequency and ranges over time in a dose-dependent manner

122. Ans. (b) M2

Ref: KDT 7th ed page 101

Methacholine acts on M2 receptor

Muscarinic cholinergic receptor agonists can be divided into two groups:
- Acetyl choline and several synthetic choline esters : Methacholine, bethanochol, carbachol
- Naturally occurring cholinomimetic alkaloids : Pilocarpine, muscarine, and arecoline
- Methacholine (acetyl-b-methylcholine) differs from ACh chiefly in its greater duration and selectivity of action. Its action is more prolonged because the added methyl group increases its resistance to hydrolysis by cholinesterases.
- Carbachol and bethanochol, unsubstituted carbamoyl esters, are completely resistant to hydrolysis by cholinesterases and thus survive long enough to be distributed to areas of low blood flow.
- Carbachol retains substantial nicotinic activity, particularly on autonomic ganglia; both its peripheral and its ganglionic actions are probably due, in part, to the release of endogenous ACh from the terminals of cholinergic fibers.
- Of the three major natural plant alkaloids, muscarine acts almost exclusively at muscarinic receptor sites, arecoline also acts at nicotinic receptors, and pilocarpine has a dominant muscarinic action but causes anomalous cardiovascular responses (the sweat glands are particularly sensitive to this drug).

Muscarinic Activity (Some Choline Esters)							
Muscarinic Agonist	Susceptibility to Cholinesterases (I)	Cardiovascular	Gastrointestinal	Urinary Bladder	Eye Topica	Antagonism by Atropine	Nicotinic Activity
Acetylcholine	+++	++	++	++	+	+++	++
Methacholine	+	+++	++	++	+	+++	+
Carbachol	–	+	+++	+++	++	+	+++
Bethanechol	-	+	+++	+++	++	+++	–

Remember that methacholine acts on M2 and Bethanochol acts on M3 Receptors

123. Ans. (a) **Saquanivir**

Ref: KDT 7th ed page 805, Harrison 19th ed page 1274

Antiretroviral Drugs Used in the Treatment of HIV Infection			
Drug	**Indication**	**Dose in Combination**	**Toxicity**
NRTI			
Zidovudine (AZT, azidothymidine, Retrovir, 3'azido-3'-deoxythymidine)	Treatment of HIV infection in combination with other antiretroviral agents	200 mg q8h or 300 mg bid	Anemia, granulocytopenia, myopathy, *lactic acidosis, hepatomegaly with steatosis,*
	Prevention of maternal-fetal HIV transmission		
Didanosine (Videx, Videx EC, ddI, dideoxyinosine, 2',3'-dideoxyinosine)	For treatment of HIV infection in combination with other antiretroviral agents	Should be administered on an empty stomach 60 kg: 200 mg bid <60 kg: 125 mg bid Enteric coated: 60 kg: 400 mg qd < 60 kg: 250 mg qd	Pancreatitis, peripheral neuropathy, *lactic acidosis, hepatomegaly with steatosis*
Zalcitabine (ddC, HIVID, 2'3'-dideoxycytidine)	In combination with other antiretroviral agents for the treatment of HIV infection	0.75 mg tid	Peripheral neuropathy, *pancreatitis, lactic acidosis, hepatomegaly with steatosis, oral ulcer,* **One toxicity unique to zalcitabine is oral ulceration and stomatitis**
Stavudine (d4T, Zerit, 2'3'-didehydro-3'-dideoxythymidine)	Treatment of HIV-infected patients in combination with other antiretroviral agents	60 kg: 40 mg bid <60 kg: 30 mg bid	Peripheral neuropathy, *pancreatitis, lactic acidosis, hepatomegaly with steatosis, lipodystrophy*
Lamivudine (Epivir, 2'3'-dideoxy-3'-thiacytidine, 3TC)	In combination with other antiretroviral agents for the treatment of HIV infection	300 mg qd	**Least toxic antiretroviral** *Neutropenia, pancreatitis in pediatric, exacerbation of hepatitis*
Emtricitabine (FTC, Emtriva)	In combination with other antiretroviral agents for the treatment of HIV infection	200 mg qd	**Chemically related to lamivudine; hence one of the least toxic ART.** Hyperpigmentation in sun exposed areas, *exacerbation of hepatitis*
Abacavir (Ziagen)	For treatment of HIV infection in combination with other antiretroviral agents	300 mg bid	**Unique and potentially fatal hypersensitivity syndrome** (fever, rash, nausea, vomiting, malaise or fatigue, and loss of appetite)
Tenofovir (Viread)	For use in combination with other antiretroviral agents when treatment is indicated	300 mg qd	Well tolerated except flatulence, *Potential for renal toxicity (not proved)*
NNRTI			**MC toxicity is rash**
Delavirdine (Rescriptor)	For use in combination with appropriate antiretrovirals when treatment is warranted	400 mg tid	Skin rash, abnormal LFT, *erythema multiforme, Stevens-Johnson syndrome*
Nevirapine (Viramune)	In combination with other antiretroviral agents for treatment of progressive HIV infection	200 mg/day × 14 days then 200 mg bid	Skin rash, Hepatotoxicity, *Stevens-Johnson syndrome*

Contd...

Antiretroviral Drugs Used in the Treatment of HIV Infection			
Drug	**Indication**	**Dose in Combination**	**Toxicity**
Efavirenz (Sustiva)	For treatment of HIV infection in combination with other antiretroviral agents	600 mg qhs	Neuropsychiatric symptoms (Vivid dreams, depression) Rash, *Abnormal LFT, **potentially teratogenic**, Stevens-Johnson syndrome*
Etravirine	Pending	Pending	Rash, headache, dizziness, nausea, diarrhea
PROTEASE INHIBITORS			PI can cause lipodystrophy, hyperlipidaemia, Type- 2 DM
Saquinavir mesylate (Invirase—hard gel capsule)	In combination with other antiretroviral agents when therapy is warranted	1000 mg + 100 mg ritonavir bid	GI symptoms (Diarrhea, vomiting, abdominal discomfort), *hyperglycemia, lipodystrophy*
(Fortovase—soft gel capsule)	For use in combination with other antiretroviral agents when treatment is warranted	1200 mg tid	Diarrhea, nausea, abdominal pain, headaches, hyperglycemia, fat redistribution, lipid abnormalities
Ritonavir (Norvir)	In combination with other antiretroviral agents for treatment of HIV infection when treatment is warranted (may alter levels of many other drugs, including saquinavir)	600 mg bid	GI symptoms (Diarrhea, vomiting, abdominal discomfort), Peripheral and perioral paresthesias, *hyperglycemia, lipodystrophy*
Indinavir sulfate (Crixivan)	For treatment of HIV infection in combination with other antiretroviral agents when antiretroviral treatment is warranted	800 mg q8h or 800 mg + 100 mg ritonavir bid or 1000 mg q8h when used with efavirenz or nevirapine	**Unique toxicity is crystalluria and nephrolithiasis,** unconjugated hyperbilirubinemia, *hyperglycemia, lipodystrophy*
Nelfinavir mesylate (Viracept)	For treatment of HIV infection in combination with other antiretroviral agents when antiretroviral therapy is warranted	1250 mg bid	Secretory diarrhoea, *hyperglycemia, lipodystrophy, May contain traces of the potential carcinogen/teratogen (ethyl methane sulfonate)*
Amprenavir (Agenerase) Fosamprenavir (Lexiva)	In combination with other antiretroviral agents for treatment of HIV infection	1200 mg bid or 600 mg + 100 mg ritonavir bid or 1200 mg + 200 mg ritonavir qd 1400 mg bid or 700 mg + 100 mg ritonavir bid	GI symptoms (Diarrhea, vomiting, abdominal discomfort), Skin rash, *oral paresthesias, abnormal LFT, hyperglycemia, lipodystrophy*
Lopinavir/ritonavir (Kaletra)	For treatment of HIV infection in combination with other antiretroviral agents	400 mg/100 mg bid	GI symptoms (Diarrhea, vomiting, abdominal discomfort), *Hypercholesterolemia, hyperglycemia, lipodystrophy*
Atazanavir (Reyataz)	For treatment of HIV infection in combination with other antiretroviral agents	300 mg qd +Ritonavir 100 mg qd when given with efavirenz	Unconjugated hyperbilirubinemia, *PR prolongation, hyperglycemia, fat maldistribution*
Tipranavir (Aptivus)	In combination with 200 mg ritonavir for combination therapy in treatment-experienced adults	500 mg + 200 mg ritonavir twice daily	Diarrhea, nausea, fatigue, headache, skin rash, hepatotoxicity, intracranial hemorrhage

Contd...

Antiretroviral Drugs Used in the Treatment of HIV Infection			
Drug	**Indication**	**Dose in Combination**	**Toxicity**
Darunavir (Prezista)	In combination with 100 mg ritonavir for combination therapy in treatment-experienced adults	600 mg + 100 mg ritonavir twice daily with food	Diarrhea, nausea, headache
FUSION INHIBITORS			
Enfuvirtide (Fuzeon)	In combination with other agents in treatment-experienced patients with evidence of HIV-1 replication despite ongoing antiretroviral therapy	90 mg SC bid	<u>Injection site reactions, hypersensitivity reactions,</u> *lymphadenopathy, Pneumonia*
Maraviroc (Selzentry)	In combination with other antiretroviral agents in treatment experienced adults infected with only CCR5-tropic HIV-1 that is resistant to multiple antiretroviral agents	150–600 mg bid depending upon concomitant medications	Hepatotoxicity, nasopharyngitis, fever, cough, rash, abdominal pain, dizziness, fever, musculoskeletal symptoms
Raltegravir (Isentress)	In combination with other antiretroviral agents in treatment experienced patients with evidence of ongoing HIV-1 replication	400 mg bid	Nausea, rash

Note: Most prominent toxicities in underlines, Rare toxicities in italics

124. Ans. (b) Thiazide

Ref: Harrison 19th ed page 1623

KDT 7th ed page 561: Though not as effective as ACE inhibitors in reversing left ventricular hypertrophy, some recent trials in mild to moderate hypertension have found thiazides to reduce left ventricular mass. The JNC 7 recommends instituting low-dose (12.5–25 mg) thiazide therapy, preferably with added K+ sparing diuretic, as a first choice treatment of essential hypertension, especially in the elderly. Higher doses are neither more effective nor safe. If the low dose (25 mg/day) fails to reduce BP to desired level, another antihypertensive should be added, rather than increasing dose.

- **Thiazides: Low-dose thiazide diuretics often are used as first-line agents alone or in combination with other antihypertensive drugs.** Thiazides inhibit the Na^+/Cl pump in the distal convoluted tubule and hence increase sodium excretion. In the long term, they also may act as vasodilators. Thiazides are safe, efficacious, inexpensive, and reduce clinical events. They provide additive blood pressure lowering effects when combined with beta blockers, angiotensin-converting enzyme inhibitors (ACEIs), or angiotensin receptor blockers (ARBs). Owing to an increased incidence of metabolic side effects (hypokalemia, insulin resistance, increased cholesterol), higher doses generally are not recommended.
- Potassium-sparing diuretics, amiloride and triamterene, act by inhibiting epithelial sodium channels in the distal nephron. These agents are weak antihypertensive agents but may be used in combination with a thiazide to protect against hypokalemia.
- **Loop diuretics:** The main pharmacologic target for loop diuretics is the Na^+-K^+-$2Cl^{âe}$ cotransporter in the thick ascending limb of the loop of Henle. Loop diuretics generally are reserved for hypertensive patients with reduced glomerular filtration rates [reflected in serum creatinine >220 μmol/L (>2.5 mg/dL), CHF, or sodium retention and edema for some other reason, such as treatment with a potent vasodilator, e.g., minoxidil.

125. Ans. (a) Bosentan

Ref: Harrison 19th ed page 1660

Harrison 18th ed Table 250–2. Principles of Drug Treatment of Pulmonary Arterial Hypertension has been removed from the 19th edition of Harrison. This table recommends to Test vasoreactivity, if vasoreactive calcium blockers in high doses are the drugs of choice. Typically, these patients require high doses (e.g., nifedipine, 240 mg/d, or amlodipine, 20 mg/d).

19th ed Harrison gives a table of FDA approved therapies of PAH which does not mention calcium Channel Blockers.

Harison 19th ed states; There are several approved agents for PAH including prostacyclin and prostacyclin analogues, phosphodiesterase-5 inhibitors, a soluble guanylyl cyclase stimulator and endothelin receptor antagonists, that have improved the outlook dramatically. Although there is no cure for PAH, current pharmacologic therapies improve morbidity and, in some cases, mortality too.

Approved Therapies for the Treatment of Pah			
Generic name	**Route of administration**	**Drug class**	**Indication**
Epoprostenol	IV	Prostacyclin derivative	Treatment of PAH to improve exercise capacity
Iloprost	Inhaled	Prostacyclin derivative	Treatment of PAH to improve a composite endpoint consisting of exercise tolerance, symptoms (NYHA Class), and lack of deterioration
Treprostinil	IV or SC	prostacyclin derivative	Treatment of PAH to diminish symptoms associated with exercise
Treprostinil	Inhaled	prostacyclin derivative	Treatment of PAH to improve exercise ability
Treprostinil	Oral	prostacyclin derivatives	Treatment of PAH to improve exercise ability
Bosentan	Oral	Non-selective endothelin receptor antagonist	Treatment of PAH to improve exercise capacity and to decrease clinical worsening
Ambrisentan	Oral	Endothelin receptor antagonist	Treatment of PAH to Improve exercise capacity and delay clinical worsening
Macitentan	Oral	Non-selective endothelin antagonist	Treatment of PAH to improve exercise capacity and delay clinical worsening
Sildenafil	Oral	PDE5 inhibitor	Treatment of PAH to improve exercise capacity and delay clinical worsening
Tadalafil	Oral	PDE5 inhibitor	Treatment of PAH to improve exercise ability
Riociguat	Oral	Soluble guanylyl cyclase stimulator	Treatment of PAH to improve exercise capacity and delay clinical worsening

126. Ans. (c) Rosiglitazone

Ref: Harrison 19th ed page 2414, Lippincott's 4th Ed page 295

Following glucose lowering agents don't work by increasing insulin secretion

- **Biguanides (metformin):** The main mechanism of action of metformin is reduction of hepatic glucose output, largely by inhibiting hepatic gluconeogenesis. Metformin also slows intestinal absorption of sugars and improves peripheral glucose uptake and utilization.
- **Thiozolidinediones or glitazones (Rosiglitazone, pioglitazone)**: Although the exact mechanism by which the TZDs lower insulin resistance remains to be elucidated, they are known to target the peroxisome proliferator activated receptor (PPAR) a nuclear hormone receptor. Ligands for PPAR regulate adipocyte production and secretion of fatty acids as well as glucose metabolism, resulting in increased insulin sensitivity in adipose tissue, liver, and skeletal muscle.
- **Alpha glucosidase inhibitors (Acarbose and miglitol):** These drugs are taken at the beginning of meals. They act by delaying the digestion of carbohydrates, thereby resulting in lower postprandial glucose levels. Both drugs exert their effects by reversibly inhibiting membrane-bound glucosidase in the intestinal brush border.

Glucose-Lowering Therapies for type 2 Diabetes						
	Mechanism of action	**Examples**	**A1C reduction (%)[a]**	**Agent-specific advantages**	**Agent-specific disadvantages**	**Contraindications**
Oral						
Biguanides	↓Hepatic glucose production, weight loss, glucose, utilization, insulin resistance	Metformin	1–2	Weight loss	Lactic acidosis, diarrhea, nausea	Serum creatinine >1.5 mg/dL (men) >1.4 mg/dL (women), CHF, radiographic contrast studies, seriously ill patients, acidosis
α–Glucosidase inhibitors	↓Glucose absorption	Acarbose, Miglitol	0.5–0.8	Reduce postprandial glycemia	GI flatulence, liver function tests	Renal/liver disease
Dipeptidyl peptidase IV inhibitors (Insulin secretagogues)	Prolong endogenous GLP-1 action	Saxagliptin, Sitagliptin, Vildagliptin	0.5–1.0	Does not cause hypoglycemia		Reduce dose with renal disease

Contd...

Glucose-Lowering Therapies for type 2 Diabetes						
	Mechanism of action	Examples	A1C reduction (%)[a]	Agent-specific advantages	Agent-specific disadvantages	Contraindications
Sulfonylureas (Insulin secretagogues)	↑Insulin secretion.	**1st generation** Chlorpropamide Tolazamide Tolbutamide **2nd generation** Glimepiride Glipizide Glipizide (extended release) Glyburide	1–2	Lower fasting blood glucose	Hypoglycemia, weight gain	Renal/liver disease
Meglititinides (Insuli secretagogues—nonsulfonylureas)	↑Insulin secretion	Repaglinide Nateglinide	1–2	Short onset of action, lowers postprandial glucose	Hypoglycemia	Renal/liver disease
Thiazolidinedi-ones	↓Insulin resistance, ↑glucose utilization	Rosiglitazone, Pioglitazone	0 5–1.4	Lower insulin requirements	Peripheral edema, CHF, weight gain, fractures, macular edema; rosiglitazone may increase risk of MI	Congestive heart failure, liver disease
Parenteral						
Insulin	↑Glucose utilization and other anabolic actions	Porcine insulin, Human insulin, Insulin analogue	No limit	Known safety profile	Injection, weight gain, hypoglycemia	
GLP-1 agonist (Insulin secretagogues)	↑Insulin, ↓Glucagon, slow gastric emptying	Exenatide, liraglutide	0.5–1.0	Weight loss	Injection, nausea, ↑risk of hypoglycemia with insulin secretagogues	Renal disease, agents that also slow GI motility
Amylin agonist[b]	Slow gastric emptying, ↓Glucagon	Pramlintide	0.25–0.5	Reduce postprandial glycemia, weight loss, Used in both Type 1 and Type 2 DM	Injection, nausea, ↑risk of hypoglycemia with insulin	Agents that also slow GI motility
Medical nutrition therapy and physical activity	↓Insulin, resistance, ↑insulin secretion	Low-calorie, low-fat diet, exercise	1–2	Other health benefits	Compliance difficult, long term success low	

127. Ans. (a) Non ionic, more lipid soluble

Ref: Foye's principle of medicinal chemistry Page 505

Nitroglycerin is an organic ester or nitric acid. The nitro group makes it non polar and soluble through lipid bio membranes. Hence it is used in emergency medicine sublingually because of its faster absorption, and given sublingually, liver is bypassed and its metabolism is liver is avoided. In humans, peak concentrations of nitroglycerin are found in plasma within 4 minutes of sublingual administration; the drug has a t1/2 of 1–3 minutes.

Sublingual organic nitrates should be taken at the time of an anginal attack or in anticipation of exercise or stress. Such intermittent treatment provides reproducible cardiovascular effects. However, frequently repeated or continuous exposure to high doses of organic nitrates leads to a marked attenuation in the magnitude of most of their effects. The magnitude of tolerance is a function of dosage and frequency of use.

Tolerance may result from a reduced capacity of the vascular smooth muscle to convert nitroglycerin to NO (i.e., true vascular tolerance), or to the activation of mechanisms extraneous to the vessel wall (i.e., pseudo tolerance).

Forensic Medicine

7

AIIMS NOVEMBER 2018

1. A person was brought dead to the casualty and autopsy was performed to find the cause of death. On external examination only finding found was a mark on the chin as in first pic. And on internal examination of neck there was the finding on the anterior surface of neck as shown below. Your possible diagnosis is:

(AIIMS Nov 2018, 2017, May 2017)

a. Throttling
b. Smoothering
c. Hanging
d. Ligature strangulation

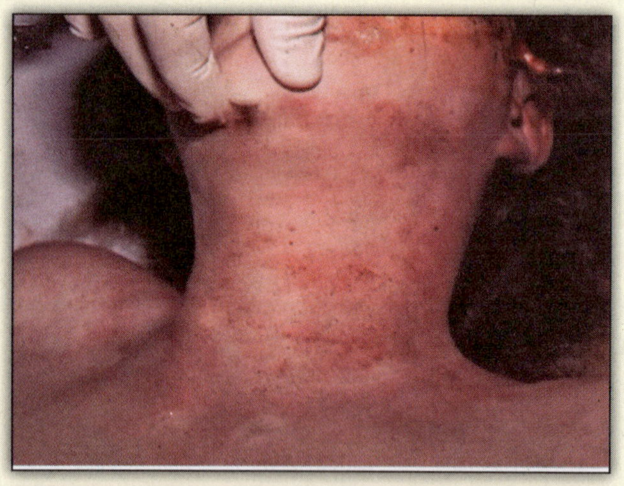

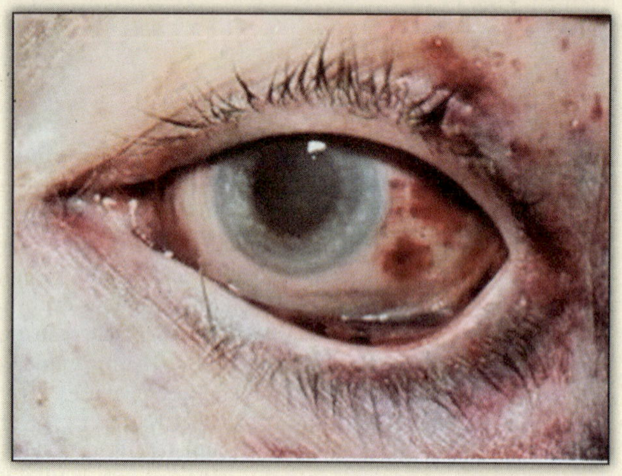

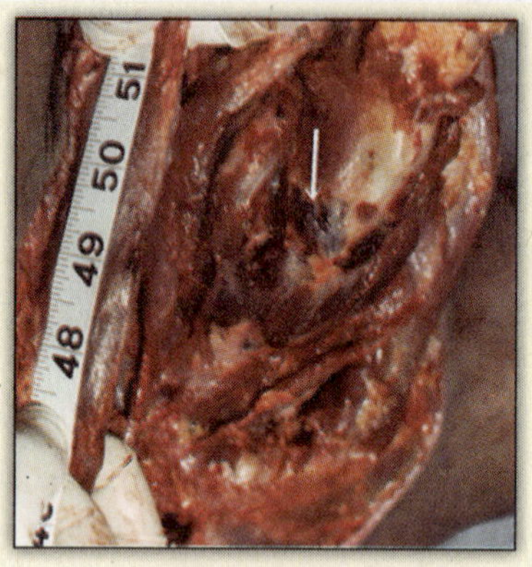

2. Bullet fingerprinting refers to:

a. Primary markings of bullet
b. Secondary markings of bullet
c. Fingerprints of human on bullet
d. Artifacts produced on bullet as a result of handling

3. Identify the fracture in the given image:

a. Hinge fracture
b. Ring fracture
c. Gutter fracture
d. Pond fracture

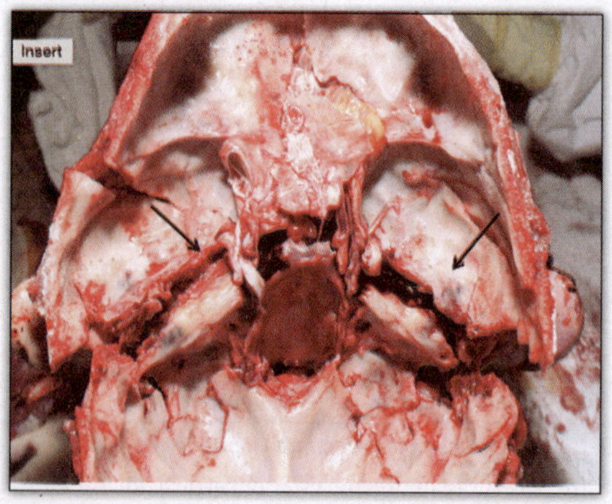

4. A 18-year-old girl was brought to OPD. On examination labia majora separated, labia minora is flabby, fourchette tear present and vagina is roomy but Hymen is intact. What could be possible?

a. True virgin
b. Pseudo virgin
c. Premenstrual stage
d. Molestation

5. Cause of decreased tissue perfusion in case of smoke filled room is:
a. Hypoxic hypoxia
b. Stagnant hypoxia
c. Anemic hypoxia
d. Histotoxic hypoxia

6. As per Govt of India Ministry of Health and family welfare, victim of sexual assault can be examined till:
a. 4 days b. 5 days
c. 7 days d. 10 days

7. On request of patient, a hospital have to give medical records within:
a. 48 hours b. 72 hours
c. 120 hours d. 7 days

8. Hyperpigmentation of hands as given in the image below is due to which poisoning?
a. Arsenic
b. Mercury
c. Lead
d. Chromium

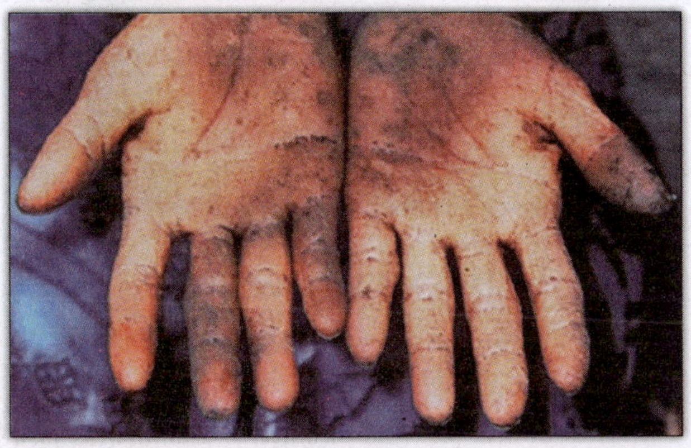

©Jaishankar M, Tseten T, Anbalagan N, Mathew BB, Beeregowda KN - Interdiscip Toxicol (2014)

9. Aggravated sexual act as per POCSO Act includes all EXCEPT:
a. By threatening
b. By group or gang of people
c. In sectarian or communal violence
d. By police officers

AIIMS MAY 2018

10. Which of the following is a difference between female and male skull?
a. Frontal and parietal eminence prominent in female skull
b. Teeth are comparatively larger in female
c. Frontal and parietal eminence are more prominent in females
d. Supra tympanic crest is present in females

11. Which of the following is true about Borrowed Servant Doctrine?
a. Hospital administration is responsible for the actions of interns and trainees
b. A nurse assisting a surgery is the borrowed servant of the hospital
c. Doctor assisting a surgeon in operation theatre is borrowed servant of surgeon
d. Anaesthetist coming for surgery when asked by Surgeon is borrowed servant of surgeon

12. First-hand knowledge rule is applicable on:
a. Handwriting expert
b. Doctor as witness
c. Bomb expert
d. Common witness

13. A 14-year-old girl comes with left humerus fracture and cigar burn marks on general examination. What would you do?
a. Tell to your colleague
b. Report it to authority as you feel it is case of physical abuse
c. Call social worker
d. Give the treatment & send back the patient

14. Match the following correctly:

1	Abrus precatorius	a	Blue rocket
2	Spanish fly	b	Brown sugar
3	Aconite	c	Blister beetle
4	Heroin	d	Gunchi

a. 1-b 2-c 3-a 4-d b. 1-c 2-a 3-d 4-b
c. 1-d 2-c 3-a 4-b d. 1-d 2-c 3-b 4-a

15. Calculate the age of a fetus having CRL 21 cm, while the total length of the fetus is 31 cm, Testis at the superficial inguinal ring and talus is present.
a. 4-5 months
b. 5-6 months
c. 6-7 months
d. 7-8 months

16. True statement about plant given in picture is:
a. It causes AV block
b. Root is the poisonous part of plant
c. Physostigmine is used to treat its toxicity
d. Atropine is antidote

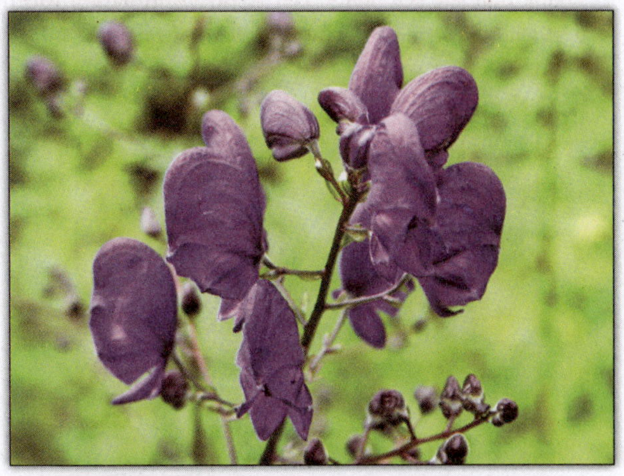

17. Match the following:
a. 1-a 2-b 3-c 4-d
b. 1-d 2-a 3-b 4-c
c. 1-b 2-a 3-b 4-c
d. 1-a 2-b 3-d 4-c

1	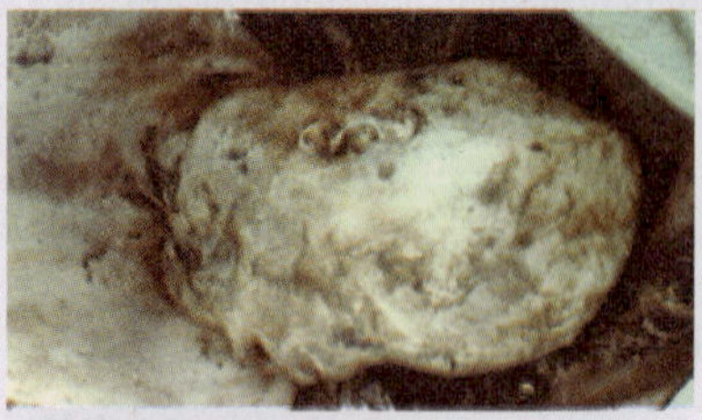	a	Marbling
2	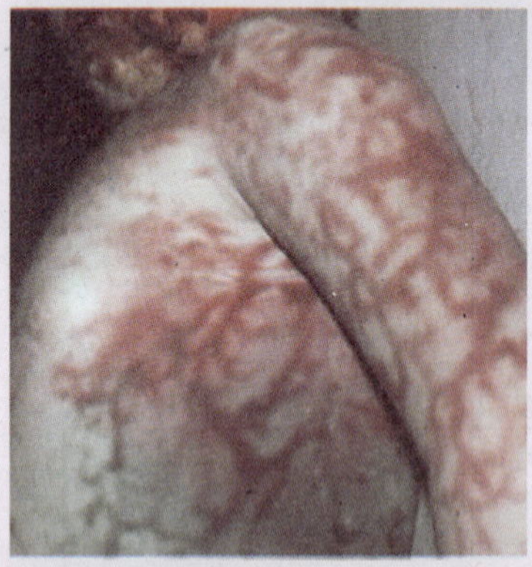	b	Mummification
3	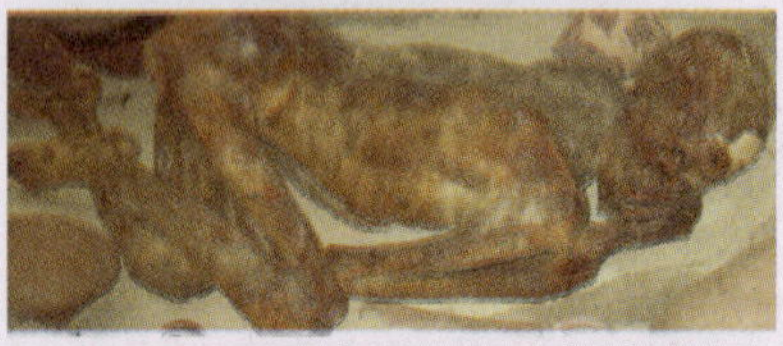	c	Postmortem Lividity
4	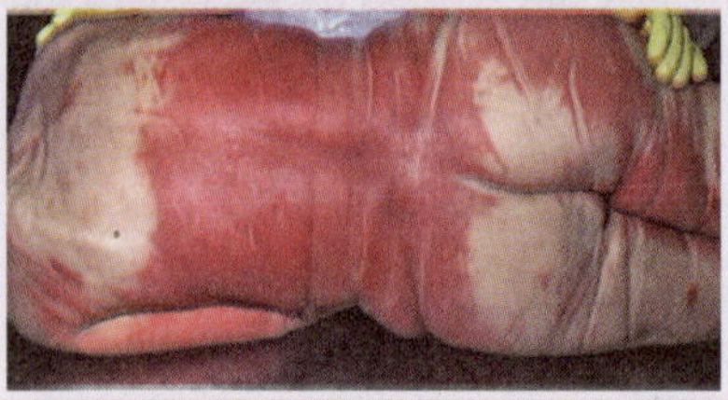	d	Adipocere

18. An allegedly 14-year-old girl ran away with an adult male for which he is booked for kidnapping. However, the girl is saying that she is a major. Her X-ray examination was then performed. Estimate her radiological age from the following X-rays?

a. 13 -14 years
b. 16-17 years
c. 17-19 years
d. 19-21 years

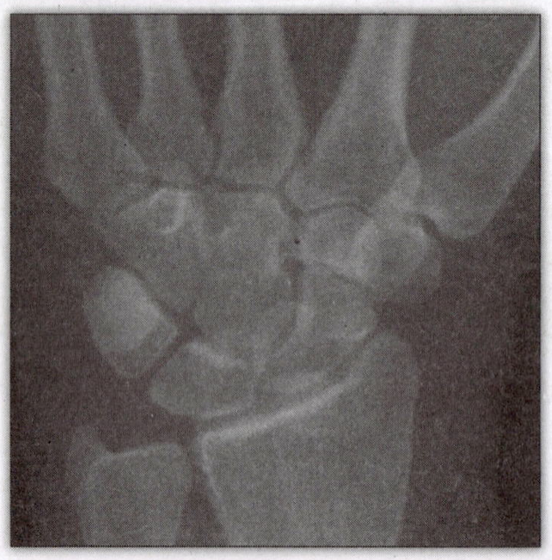

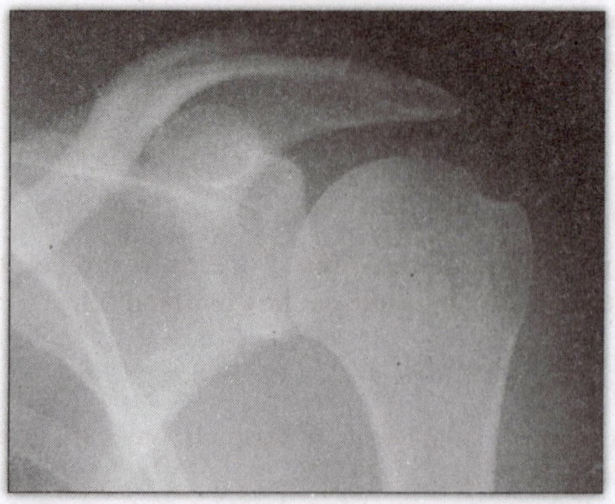

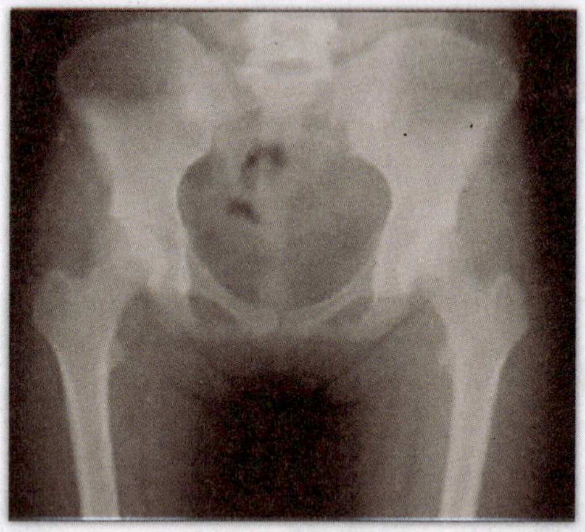

AIIMS NOVEMBER 2017

19. A person was brought to the casualty brought dead and autopsy was performed to find the cause of death. On external examination only finding found was a mark on the chin as in first pic. And on internal examination of neck there was the finding on the anterior surface of neck as shown below. Your possible diagnosis is:

(AIIMS Nov 2018, 2017, May 2017)

a. Throttling
b. Smothering
c. Hanging
d. Ligature strangulation

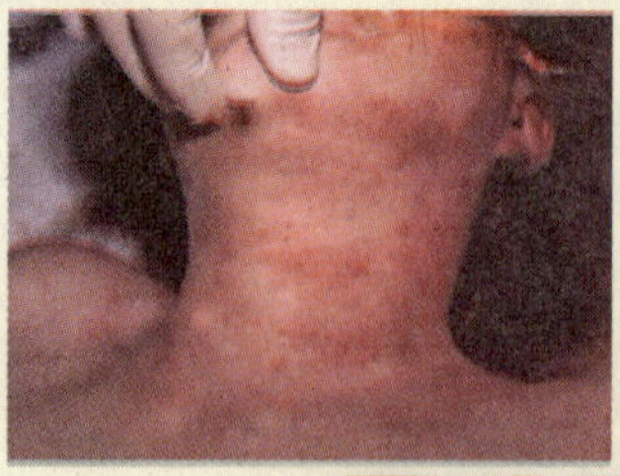

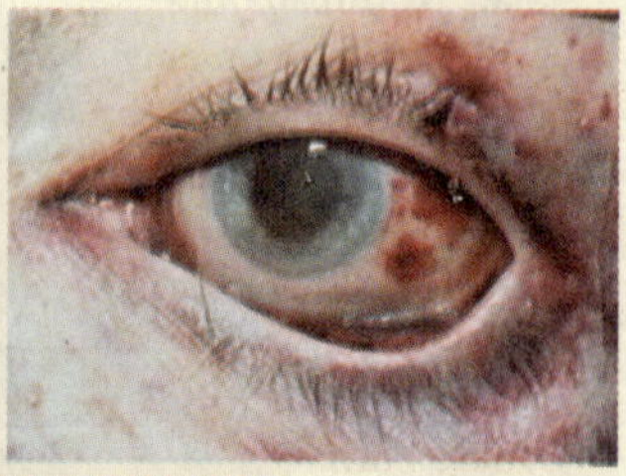

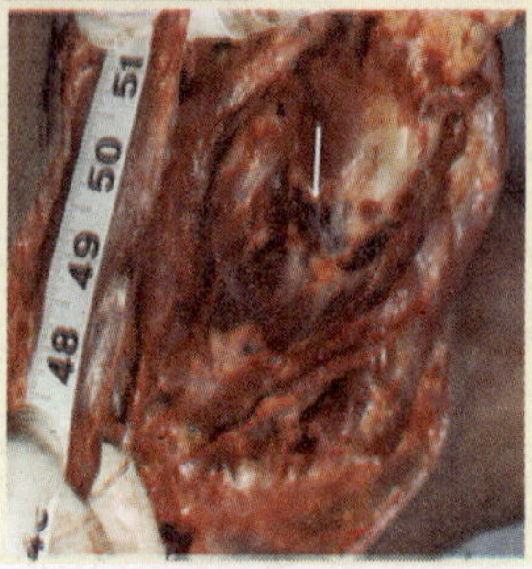

20. Black foot disease is caused by: *(AIIMS Nov 2017, AI PG 2014)*

a. Arsenic
b. Mercury
c. Cadmium
d. Lead

21. Atropine can be used in all EXCEPT:

a. Endrin
b. Baygon
c. Parathion
d. Tik20

22. A 14-year-old rape victim with 22 weeks pregnancy came for examination. All can be done EXCEPT:

a. Male doctor can perform physical examination in presence of female attendant
b. Urine Pregnancy test is not required
c. Vaginal swab is not necessary
d. A gynecologist can do termination of pregnancy with her consent

23. According to Nysten's rule order of appearance of rigor mortis is:

a. Orbicularis oculi, Facial muscles, Upper limb, Thorax
b. Orbicularis oculi, Neck, Thorax, Upper limb
c. Neck, Muscles of eyelid, Upper limb, Thorax
d. Facial muscles, Muscles of eyelid, Thorax, Upper limb

24. Match the following:

A	Cocaine	i	Purple haze
B	LSD	ii	White lady
C	Capsicum	iii	Gunchi
D	Abrus Precatorius	iv	Hunan hand

a. A-i B-ii C-iii D-iv
b. A-ii B-i C-iv D-iii
c. A-iii B-i C-ii D-iv
d. A-i B-iii C-iv D-ii

25. Match the following: *(AIIMS Nov 2017, 2016)*

Ethical duties of doctors	a	Declaration of Oslo	1
Therapeutic abortion	b	Declaration Geneva	2
Human experimentation	c	Declaration of Tokyo	3
Torture	d	Declaration of Helsinki	4

a. 1 b, 2 a, 3 d, 4 c
b. 1 b, 2 c, 3 a, 4 d
c. 1 a, 2 c, 3 b, 4 d
d. 1 a, 2 d, 3 b, 4 c

26. In a case of a gunshot injury to skull with entry wound surrounded by abrasion collar and tattooing and an exit wound along with metal fragments of bullet inside the bullet track, what will be preserved for calculating the range of firing:

a. Hair
b. Bullet pieces
c. Blood
d. Clothes

27. Criminal responsibility of insane is defined as?

a. Curren's rule
b. Durham's rule
c. McNaughten's rule
d. American law institute test

AIIMS MAY 2017

28. Which of the following is correct regarding corporo-basal index of sacrum?

a. Breadth of first sacral vertebra × 100/breadth of fifth lumbar vertebra
b. Breadth of fifth lumbar vertebra × 100/breadth of all sacral vertebra
c. Breadth of first sacral vertebra × 100/breadth of base of sacrum
d. Breadth of fifth lumbar vertebra × 100/breadth of base of sacrum

29. Which of the following is false regarding teeth features and ethnicity?

a. In Negroes the teeth are broad and extra cusps
b. Caucasians have carabelli cusp on labial surface of mandibular molar
c. Shovel shaped incisors in Mongoloids
d. Absent upper 3rd molar in Mongoloids

30. An adult came to casualty with complaints of rapid heart rate and angina like pain. On examination everything else was normal except for episodic tachycardia with occasional extrasystole and amblyopia. Most likely cause is:

a. Chronic nicotine poisoning
b. Cannabis intoxication
c. Arsenophagia
d. Cocainism

31. A young adult came with casualty with history of some substance abuse. His pulse was 130 beats/minute, respiratory rate 30/min, blood gas analysis revealed metabolic acidosis, hypocalcemia and electrolyte imbalance. Blood urea – 100 mg/dL, creatinine – 4 mg/dL. Urine analysis showed calcium oxalate crystals. He improved on gastric lavage, ethanol, sodium bicarbonate, calcium gluconate and 4-methyl pyrazole. What is the substance he consumed?

a. Ethylene glycol
b. Methyl alcohol
c. Formaldehyde
d. Paraldehyde

32. Death in jackknife position is due to:

a. Burking
b. Positional asphyxia
c. Traumatic asphyxia
d. Wedging

33. A person was brought to the casualty brought dead and autopsy was performed to find the cause of death. On external examination only finding found was a mark on the chin as in first pic. And on internal examination of neck there was the finding on the anterior surface of neck as shown below. Your possible diagnosis is: *(AIIMS Nov 2018, 2017, May 2017)*

a. Throttling
b. Hanging
c. Smothering
d. Ligature strangulation

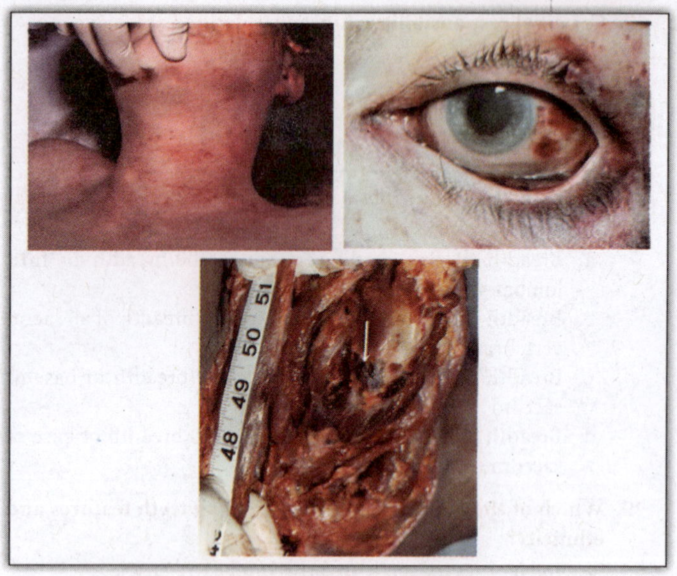

34. **While performing Autopsy of a patient who died of Myocardial infarction. On triphenyl tetrazolium stain, color of normal viable part of heart will be:**

(AIIMS May 2017, Nov 2016)

a. White
b. Red
c. Blue
d. Dark brown

AIIMS NOVEMBER 2016

35. **A dead male fetus was bought by police for autopsy. The weight of fetus is 1000-gram, crown rump length of 23 cm. Intestine is full of meconium, Pupillary membrane absent, nails appeared and testes is at Superficial inguinal ring. What is the estimated age of the fetus?**

a. 6 months
b. 7 months
c. 8 months
d. 9 months

36. **Which of the following is not used for Tattooing?**

a. Osmium blue
b. Vermilion
c. India Ink
d. Prussian blue

37. **Saint Anthony fire is seen in:**

a. Alcoholism
b. Ergotism
c. Cocaine
d. Datura

38. **Patient was brought to emergency with head trauma, with no attendant available. Neurosurgeon want to perform Surgery but no one is available to give consent. Under which section of IPC the doctor can proceed with surgery?**

a. 90
b. 91
c. 92
d. 93

39. **While performing Autopsy of a patient who died of Myocardial infarction. On triphenyl tetrazolium stain, color of normal viable part of heart will be:**

(AIIMS May 2017, Nov 2016)

a. White
b. Red
c. Blue
d. Dark Brown

40. **A farmer in a village of Central India consumes lot of cereals, suddenly developed symptoms of dizziness, spasticity. What is most likely diagnosis?**

a. Lathyrus sativus
b. Papaver somniferum
c. Cannabis sativus
d. Argemone

41. **Which of the following about the MTP Act is correct?**

a. There is no need to remove the IUD in case of an abortion
b. USG is mandatory for all patients undergoing MTP
c. Can be done up to 72 days
d. Can be done by only RMP registered for abortion under MTP Act

42. **A 24-year-old male with unknown history, presented in Emergency with altered sensorium and Pinpoint pupils. His Blood pressure was 140/90 mm Hg and respiratory rate of 8/min. Most likely diagnosis is:**

a. Pontine Hemorrhage
b. Opioid intoxication
c. Alcohol intoxication
d. Benzodiazepam

43. **Match the following:W** *(AIIMS Nov 2017, 2016)*

Ethical duties of doctors	a	Declaration of Oslo	1
Therapeutic abortion	b	Declaration Geneva	2
Human experimentation	c	Declaration of Tokyo	3
Torture	d	Declaration of Helsinki	4

a. 1 b, 2 a, 3 d, 4 c
b. 1 b, 2 c, 3 a, 4 d
c. 1 a, 2 c, 3 b, 4 d
d. 1 a, 2 d, 3 b, 4 c

44. **A patient comes with nausea vomiting and ascending paralysis. Most likely cause of poisoning is:**

a. Datura
b. Strychnos nux-vomica
c. Conium maculatum
d. Opium

45. **Which of the following is not a radiological signs of child abuse?**

a. Metaphyseal fracture
b. Corner fracture pattern
c. Bucket handle fracture
d. Sub epiphyseal microfracture

46. **A doctor who is transmitted HIV infection to an otherwise HIV negative patient, due to use of infected needles comes under which section of IPC?**

a. 166
b. 202
c. 203
d. 269

47. **A married village lady with comes with history of intake of unknown substance and kerosene like smell from mouth and SpO_2 was around 80, BP 80/60 mm Hg and pulse 50/min. Which of the following is not done in emergency?**

a. Atropine
b. Vasopressors
c. Gastric lavage
d. Maintain airway

48. The color seen in the lesion in the picture below is due to:

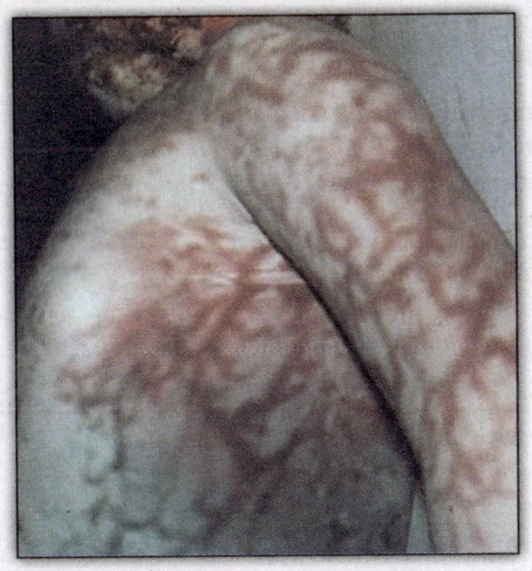

a. Reduced hemoglobin
b. Methemoglobin
c. Sulphmethemoglobin
d. Hematoma

49. In burns, all are signs inhalational injury EXCEPT:

a. Singeing of hairs, lashes, eyebrows
b. Yellow sputum
c. Improper exchange of gases
d. Hoarseness of voice

AIIMS MAY 2016

50. According to Transplantation of Humans Organs Act, all of the following specialist are authorised for pronouncing brain death EXCEPT:

a. Neurosurgeon
b. Surgeon performing the liver transplant
c. Patient's attending doctor
d. RMP in charge of the hospital

51. Biomedical research involving humans' subjects is guided by code of ethics formed by:

a. International code of medical ethics
b. Hippocratic oath
c. Declaration of Geneva
d. Declaration of Helsinki

52. In cases of examination of victims of sexual offence, toluidine blue test is used to identify:

a. Clotted blood on injuries
b. Healed micro injuries
c. Dried seminal stains
d. Recent micro injuries

53. In fingerprint reader, the prints of eight fingers are recorded including all EXCEPT:

a. Thumb
b. Middle finger
c. Ring finger
d. Little finger

54. In the skeletal remains of a suspected male in a building collapse, the length of humerus is 24.5 cm. The predicted height of the person will be:

a. 93 cm
b. 110 cm
c. 130 cm
d. 143 cm

55. Estimate the bone age from the X-ray film of the wrist joint shown below:

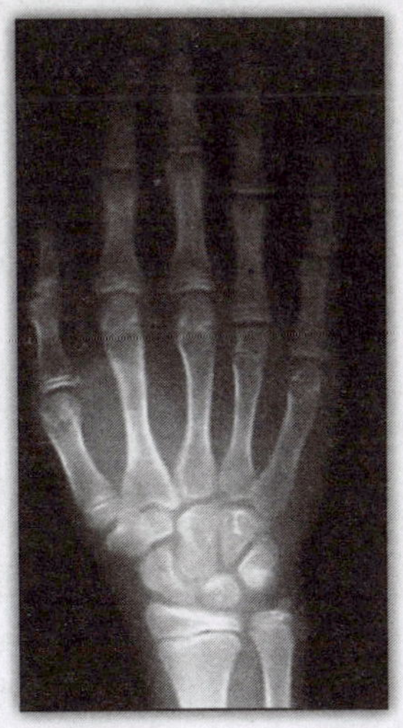

a. Less than 15 years
b. Less than 17.5 years
c. Between 18–19 years
d. Between 20–22 years

56. The posture of body as seen in the picture given below is due to:

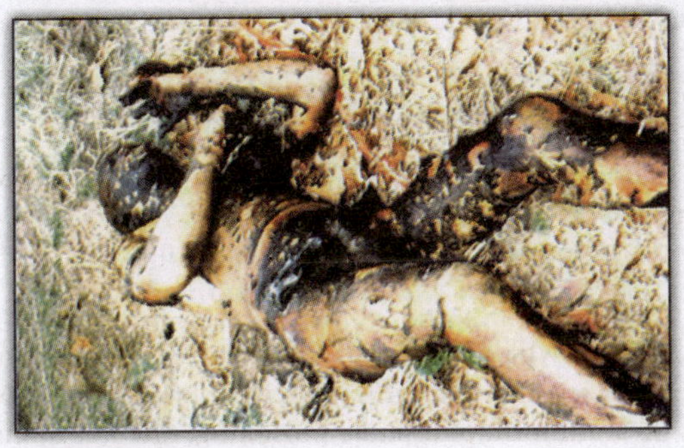

a. Rigor mortis
b. Cadaveric spasm
c. Pugilistic attitude
d. Postmortem caloricity

57. The type of injury shown in the given picture is:

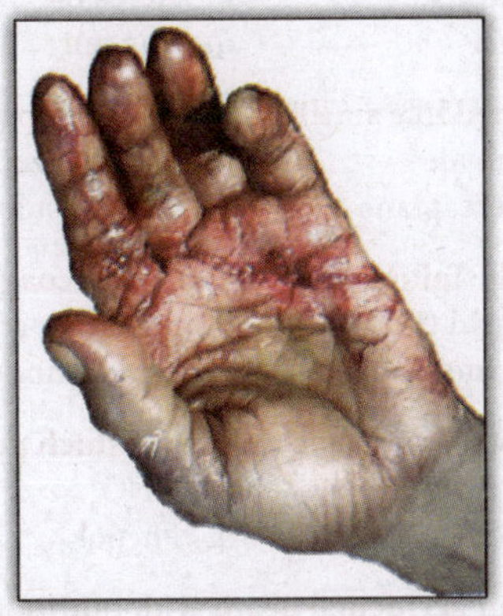

a. Abrasion
b. Lacerated wound
c. Chop wound
d. Incised wound

58. Based on the firearm injury in the given image, the range of firearm is:

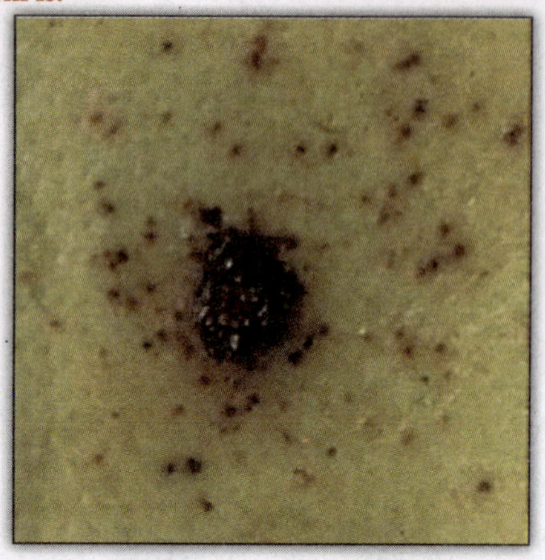

a. Point blank range b. Close range
c. Distant range d. Intermediate range

59. In case of infant deaths, Ploucquets test is carried out at autopsy suggest live birth by:

a. Increase in weight of lungs in relation to body weight following respiration
b. Presence of air in middle ear
c. Presence of air in stomach and duodenum
d. Change in shape of chest

AIIMS NOVEMBER 2015

60. Which of the following is not used in detoxification of chronic alcohol dependence?

a. Acamprosate b. Flumazenil
c. Naltrexone d. Disulfiram

61. A doctor who performed the autopsy on a 26-year-old married women committing suicide found the cause of death to be aluminum phosphide poisoning. She was summoned in a court of law where he willingly hid this information. This is punishable under which section?

a. IPC 193 b. CrPC 175
c. CrPC 69 d. IPC 189

62. In bomb blast all injuries are seen EXCEPT:

a. Lacerations b. Abrasion
c. Fracture d. Puncture

63. Shoe polished like smell is seen in which poisoning?

a. Paraldehyde b. Nitrobenzene
c. Thiomercaptane d. Copper sulphate

64. Which of the following does not cause coagulative necrosis?

a. Nitric acid (HNO_3) b. Sulphuric acid (H_2SO_4)
c. Hydrochloric acid(HCl) d. Hydrofluoric acid (HF)

65. Boiled lobster syndrome is seen in which poisoning?

a. Boric acid b. HNO_3
c. H_2SO_4 d. Phenol

66. In case of an accidental death with multiple skull fractures, Which of the following rule is used to determine 1st, 2nd and consecutive fractures?

a. Durham's rule b. Puppe's rule
c. Ashley rule d. McNaughten's rule

67. Ashley's rule is used for the determination of:

a. Age b. Sex
c. Race d. Stature

68. Ewing postulate deals with relationship between:

a. Trauma and tumor b. Trauma and MI
c. Trauma and SAH d. Trauma and poisoning

69. As per National Crime Bureau most common mode of suicide in India is:

a. Drowning b. Poisoning
c. Fall from height d. Hanging

70. Which of these statements is false about snake bite:

a. Antivenom is not effective in Humpnosed Pit Viper bite
b. Cobra venom is neurotoxic
c. Atropine premedication should be used before administering Neostigmine
d. Neostigmine has a role in krait bite

71. A man throws sulphuric acid on his wife's face due to some delusion. Which of the following is incorrect about the chemical burn of the face?

a. Blistering vesicles
b. Red line of demarcation absent
c. Ulcerated patch present
d. Absence of Singeing of hair

AIIMS MAY 2015

72. Sweating is absent in:

a. Heat syncope b. Miner' s cramps
c. Heat stroke d. Heat exhaustion

73. Segmentation of blood in blood vessel in Retina after death is called as:

a. Kennedy phenomenon b. Taches noire
c. Rokitansky sign d. Kevorkian sign

74. Legal age of sexual consent is:

a. 18 years b. 20 years
c. 16 years d. 15 years

75. Lower two parts of sternal body fuses by what age:

a. 8 years
b. 10 years
c. 12 years
d. 14 years

76. A bomb blast took place in Delhi following which 2 persons died. All of the following are true about these types of injuries EXCEPT:

a. Force of explosion is mostly directional
b. Force of explosion decreases rapidly
c. Injuries occur due to burns or air blast
d. Bruise, laceration and fractures are triad of main injuries seen

77. The high court has the power to stay the execution of a pregnant woman according to which section of criminal procedure code?

a. 416 CrPC
b. 417 CrPC
c. 418 CrPC
d. 419 CrPC

78. Mr. X fired his gun at Mr. Y who moved and escaped with the bullet only grazed his thigh. There was only a little bleeding and no other significant injury. Mr. Y registered a FIR against Mr. X. Mr. X is liable for arrest under which section of the Indian Penal Code?

a. 302
b. 304
c. 324
d. 326

79. The knot in judicial hanging is placed at:

a. Below the chin
b. The back of the neck
c. Choice of hangman
d. The angle of jaw

80. Acrid (pear like) smell is seen with:

a. Nitrobenzene
b. Ether
c. Paraldehyde
d. Phenol

81. A person was advised by his orthopedician to get regular dressing of his wound done, but the patient did not give much care. The patient visited after sometime at which time the orthopedician again advised regular dressing but did not do the dressing himself as he was busy. Finally, the wound enlarged involving the underlying bone and the patient developed osteomyelitis. Which of the following is a true statement?

a. Doctor is guilty under avoidable negligence
b. Doctor guilty under last clear chance doctrine
c. The doctor is not guilty because of contributory negligence
d. The doctor is guilty because of prescribing wrong medicines

82. In car accident, two dead bodies were found from the front seats of the car. Which of the following in postmortem examination will help to identify driver from front passenger EXCEPT:

a. Seat belt abrasion over left shoulder
b. Steering wheel imprint
c. Sparrow foot marks
d. Whiplash injury

83. A man fell from 35 feet height. Eyewitnesses say that he landed directly on his feet. Which of the following injuries will confirm this fact?

a. Ring fracture of foramen magnum + lumbar spine injury
b. Gutter fracture skull + cervical spine injury
c. Pond fracture skull + cervical spine injury
d. Depressed fracture skull + cervical spine injury

84. Rat hole injury is associated with:

a. Postmortem artifact
b. Animal bite
c. Firearm injury
d. Razor blade

AIIMS NOVEMBER 2018

1. Ans. (a) Throttling

Ref: Reddy 33rd ed page 352, Knight's Forensic Pathology 4th ed page 374

NOTE

The pictures are representative pictures, not the exact pictures that were given in the exam. Although any number of variants and permutation combination of Asphyxial injuries are possible, it is beyond the scope of this book and we will be concentrated on the Hallmark findings.

Option (A)

External bruising of the neck in Manual strangulation/ Throttling can be very minimal as in this case. But internal findings of multiple hematomas are consistent with manual strangulation.

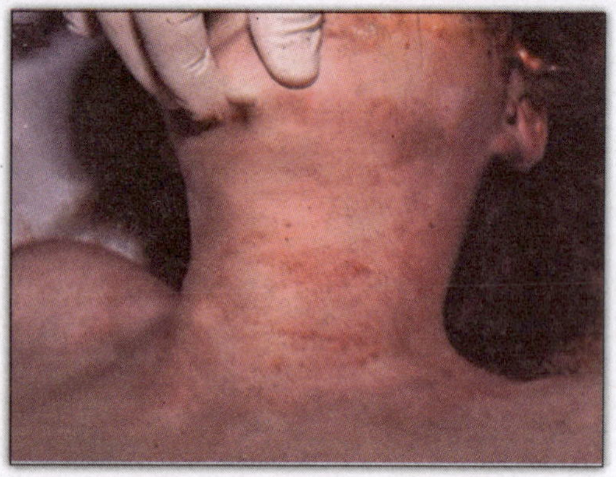

Fig: Manual strangulation/Throttling external: Injuries to the neck in homicidal manual strangulation deaths may be quite subtle. A mark semilunar mark of thumb or nail is often visible below the chin or high in the neck. Fingerprint abrasions are visible on the neck

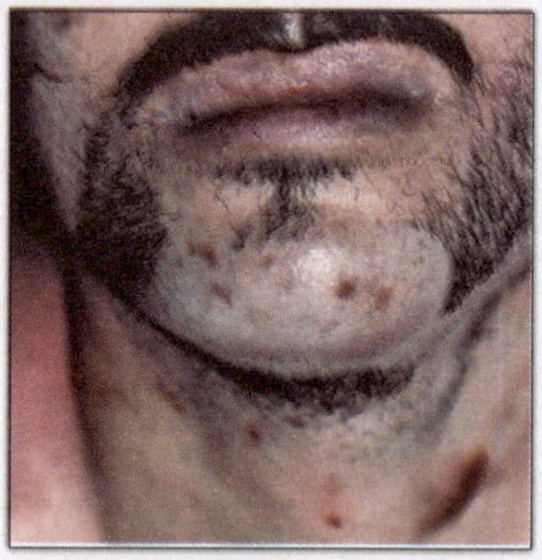

Fig: Manual strangulation/Throttling: This is a case of manual strangulation. One cannotice semilunar finger nail abrasions on the chin and a contusion on the left and right angle of the lower lip together with multiple nail abrasions on the right side of the neck and a big abraded contusion over the left clavicle. Such lesions indicate attempted smothering while manually strangulating the victim.

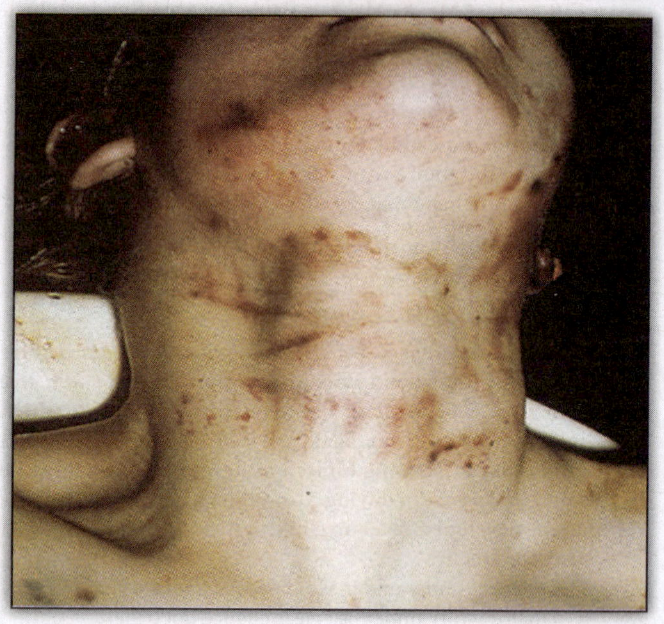

Fig: Multiple irregular unpatterned abrasions on the neck in case of Throttling

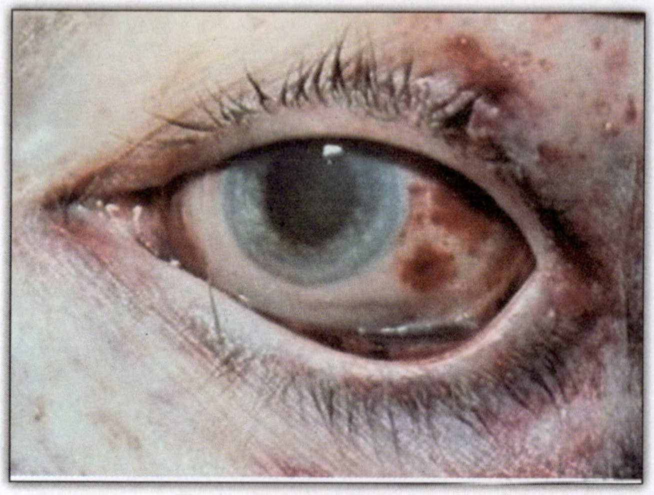

Fig: Conjunctival haemorrhages/petechiae in manual strangulation

NOTE

Tardieu spots were first described by French police surgeon Ambroise Auguste Tardieu as minute hemorrhages on the surfaces of the lungs, heart, conjunctiva and other body parts. Its pathognomonic sign of asphyxial deaths.

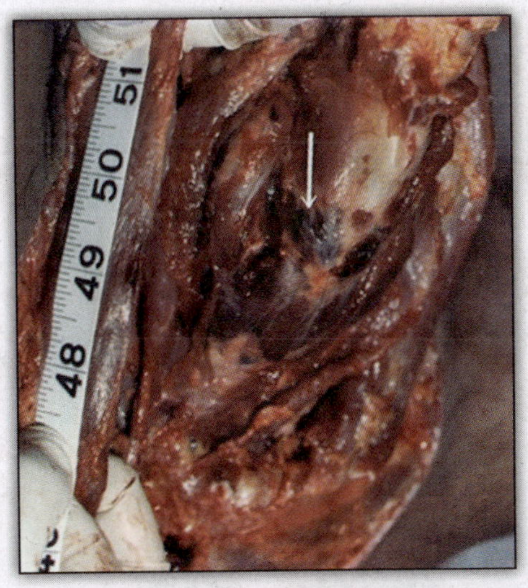

Fig: Manual strangulation/Throttling internal:
Arrow pointing hematoma

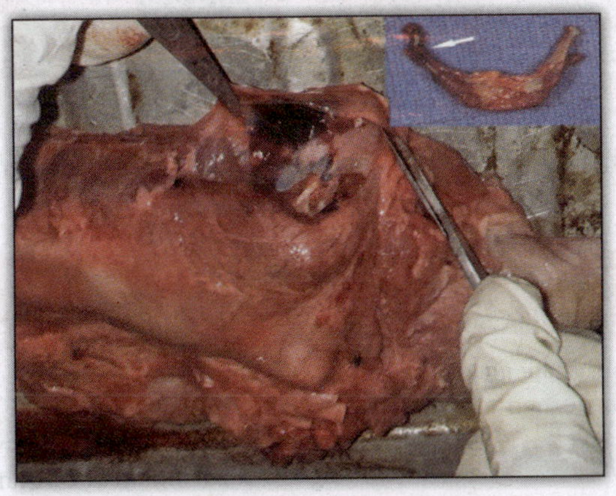

Fig: Manual strangulation/Throttling internal: Forceps pointing hematoma and Hyoid bone fracture in Insat ©Medeasy, Dr Shashank Sharma

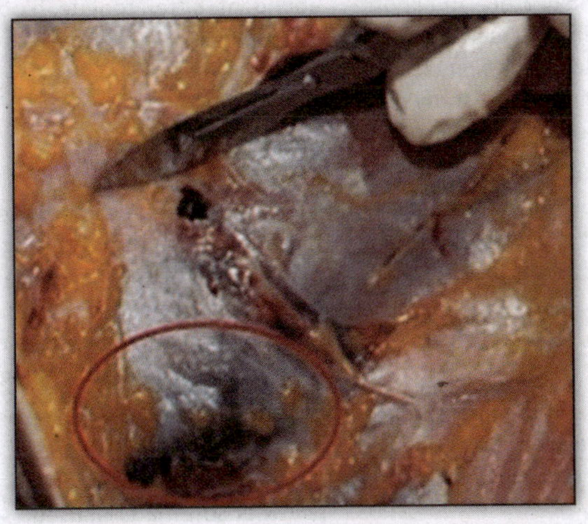

Fig: Manual strangulation/Throttling internal:
Hematoma visible without deep dissection © Nouma Youssef

Option (B)

Smothering is characterized by Facial and gum injury. Also, there won't be any internal findings in neck dissection normally.

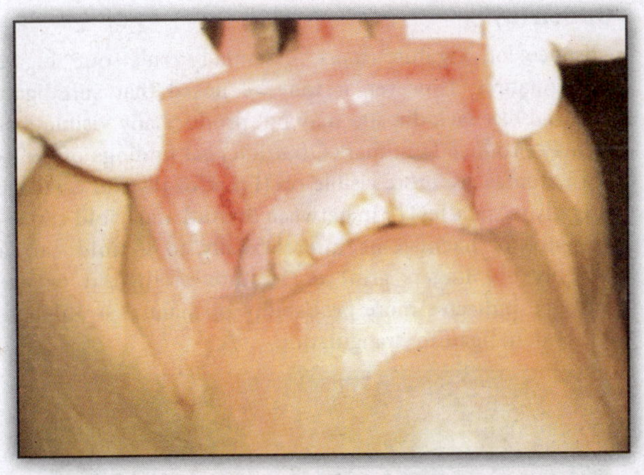

Fig: Smothering external: Bruising of inside of mouth. Note that the Bruising and/or laceration of Oral mucosa in Smothering needs to be differentiated from the Petechial hemorrhage which is seen in all cases of Asphyxia death

Option (C)

Hanging can be ruled out in absence of any ligature mark or know mark.

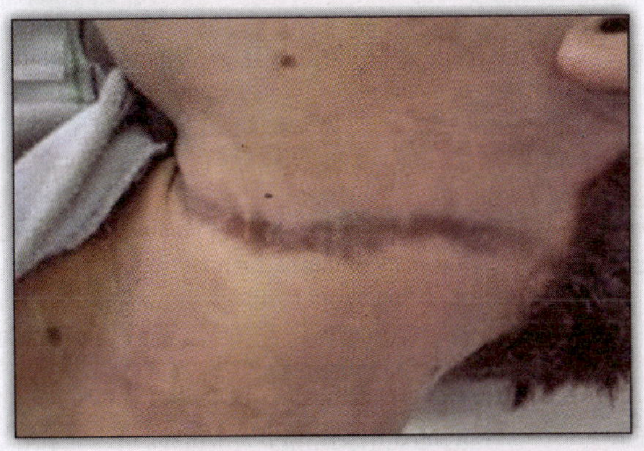

Fig: Hanging External: Ligature mark is oblique, incomplete and high in neck

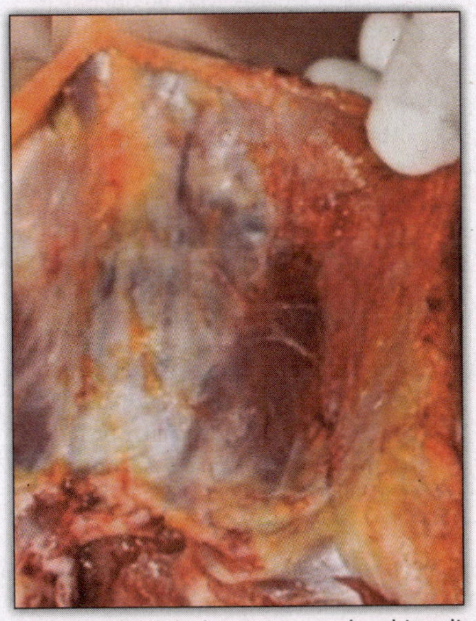

Fig: Hanging Internal: Underlying tissue pale white glistening, no bruising, hemorrhage/hematoma of underlying structures

Option (D)

Absence of Ligature mark essentially rule out Ligature strangulation. However, it may be noted that soft ligature material like sari, dupatta may not produce any visible marks or may produce faint marks, but internal findings of bruises/ haematomas are more visible on (Front of thyroid cartilage + laterally in muscles) or in between thyroid and hyoid cartilage. Presence of haematoma inferolaterally to thyroid cartilage (thumb and fingers grip) or fracture of thyroid or hyoid cartilage indicates more probability of manual strangulation rather than ligature strangulation.

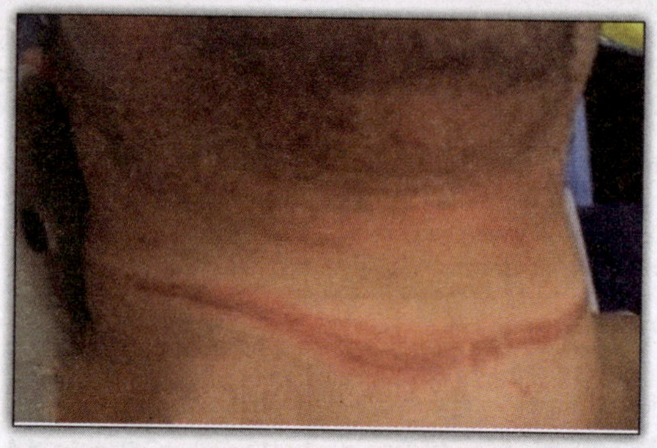

Fig: Ligature strangulation external: Ligature mark which is transverse, circular, complete, in lower neck

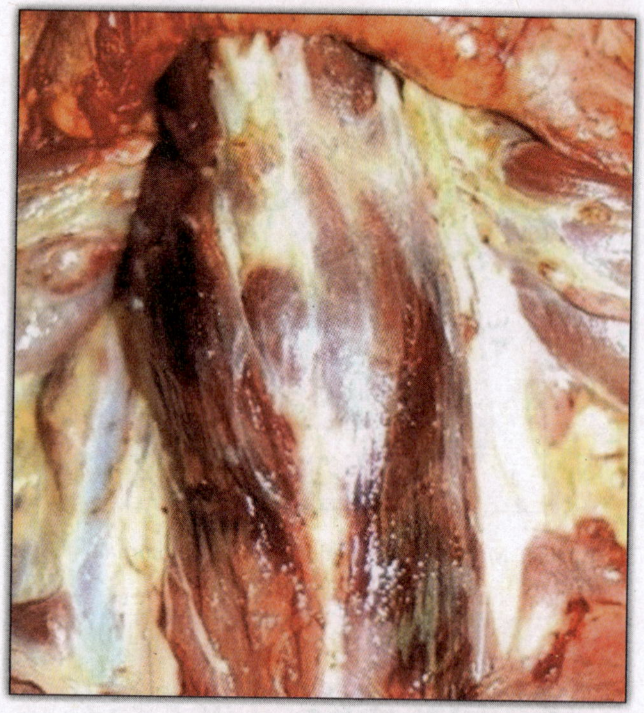

Fig: Ligature strangulation internal: Anterior neck "strap" muscle hemorrhage in a strangulation case

Signs of Asphyxial Death

Condition	External finding/ligature mark	Autopsy/internal finding	Other significant findings
Hanging	Oblique, incomplete, high-between thyroid and hyoid cartilage or above hyoid **Note:** Running noose may cause horizontal ligature mark.	Underlying tissue pale white glistening, no bruising, hemorrhage/hematoma of underlying structures.	Swollen cyanosed face Dribbling of saliva, semen at meatus, suicide note, **Amussat sign** (tears in intima of carotids).
Ligature strangulation	Transverse/Horizontal, circular, complete, across the middle or lower part of neck, at or below the level of thyroid cartilage. May be oblique if person is strangled or dragged.	Bruising, hemorrhage of the subcutaneous tissue and muscles of neck, especially underneath the ligature and knot. There may be bruising or laceration of the sheath of carotid arteries. Fracture thyroid cartilage. (Picture will show distinctly visible red bleeding point).	Face is congested, swollen and cyanosed. **Tardieu's spots** more abundant, bitten tongue, blood stained froth.
Manual strangulation, throttling	Abrasions and bruises on the front and sides of the neck.	Bruise: Oval or round and 1.5–2 cm in size. Bruises made by tips of thumbs are more prominent than with other fingers. Multiple abrasions present due to struggle.	Extravasation of blood in subcutaneous tissues underneath the external marks of bruising and abrasions is the most significant internal sign. Inward compression **fracture of hyoid bone** is the most diagnostic finding of throttling.
Smothering	Abrasions and bruises around the mouth, inner side of mouth, gums, tongue, lips, nostrils, chin, border of mandible. Fracture nasal none/ cartilage.	Injuries on the inside of the lips from pressure of teeth are seen. Bruising of gums or sometimes tears of delicate tissues are seen.	Most common mode is by plastic bag in suicidal and Pillow in homicidal. Minimal facial injury if pillow or soft material used.

Summary:

- Ligature mark + underlying hematoma with or without Thyroid fracture = **Ligature strangulation**
- Ligature mark without underlying hematoma with or without hyoid fracture = **Hanging**
- Nail marks/no marks, no ligature with underlying hematoma of neck muscles = **Throttling**
- Signs of asphyxia + facial injury/fracture nasal bone/cartilage along with injury inner side of lips = **Smothering**

2. **Ans. (b) Secondary markings of bullet**

Ref: APC Essentials of Forensic Medicine and Toxicology By Anil Aggrawal 1st ed page 191

In all rifled firearms, the bullet is slightly larger than the barrel (so that it can provide perfect obturation). Thus, as it passes through the barrel, not only do the lands and grooves leave their mirror image on it (**primary markings**), but also the unique linear markings which are specific to each gun (**secondary markings**). Because of the infinite possible variations, each gun leaves its own characteristic secondary markings on the bullet, which are often called the **"fingerprint of the gun/ bullet/ ballistic"**. The phrase is however not entirely correct; while fingerprints do not change during the life an individual, markings made by guns change gradually over the life of a gun — as it wears out more and more. They can also altered by the gun owner very easily by cleaning it repeatedly. They are synonymous with individual or accidental characteristics of a fired bullet.

Primary and Secondary Markings of Bullet

	Primary markings	Secondary markings
Visibility	Visible through naked eye	Often not visible through naked eye
Information	Gives information of manufacturer	Gives information of Individual gun
Due to	Each company has different number of rulings, their widths and depths, the direction of their rotation and twist etc	Individual variations in each gun like • Variations in minor details of rifling at the time of manufacturing itself • Repeated wear and tear of each gun • Gun cleaning activities • Metallic fouling, each time a shot is fired

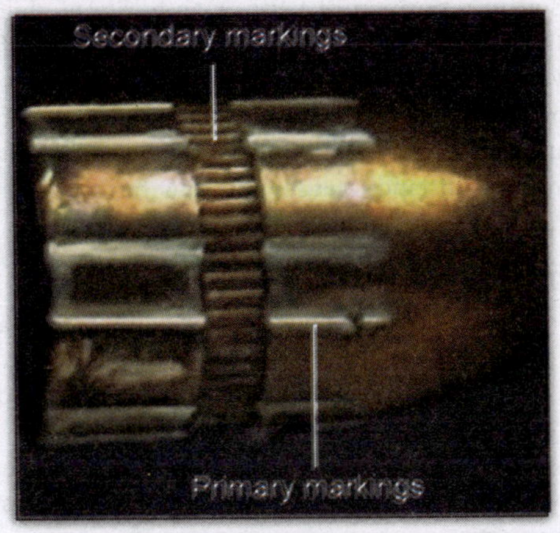

Fig: Primary and secondary markings of the bullet

3. **Ans. (a) Hinge fracture**

Ref: Parikh's 6th ed page 4.9, Gautam Biswas 3rd ed page 293, Reddy 33rd ed page 247

(See table of "Important Fractures in Forensic Medicine" in AIIMS May 2015 Forensic Medicine)

Transverse Hinge Fracture AKA- Motorcyclist's fracture: It is name given to a fracture of base of skull in which the skull base is broken down into two separate anterior and posterior halves and they move independently of each other. It is a type of hinge fracture. The fracture line runs on the base of middle cranial fossa following the petrous temporal bone.

4. **Ans. (b) Pseudo virgin**

Ref: Concise Textbook of Forensic Medicine & Toxicology By Sharma 2nd ed page 119

This question is basically to test your knowledge of True vs False (Pseudo) virgin. Rest of the options are fillers

True Versus False Virgin

	True virgin	False virgin
Hymen	Intact	Intact but elastic type
Labia majora	Firm and lie in apposition	Separated and flabby
Labia minora	Soft and sensitive, Pink	Brownish separate and elongated
Fourchette and posterior commissure	Intact	Torn
Vestibule	Narrow	Wide
Vaginal orifice	Orifice does not allow penetration of more than one finger	Admits 2 or more fingers
Vaginal cavity	Narrow with rugose on wall	Enlarged and roomy. Rugose on wall may be absent

5. **Ans. (c) Anemic hypoxia**

Ref: Gautam Biswas 3rd ed page 586

Asphyxiant gas is a non-toxic or toxic gas which causes respiratory embarrassment leading to unconsciousness or death by asphyxiation. Smoke filled room will most likely cause Carbon monoxide poisoning. CO combines reversibly with hemoglobin to form carboxyhemoglobin (COHb) producing **anemic hypoxia** (blood O_2-carrying capacity is reduced). It has a high affinity for Hb (about 250 times more than O_2).

Types of Hypoxia

Type of hypoxia	Pathophysiology	Arterial pO_2	O_2 content of arterial blood	Examples
Anemic hypoxia	Due to reduced O_2 carrying capacity	Normal	Reduced	Anemia (Reduced RBC, Reduced Hb) CO poisoning
Hypoxic hypoxia	Inadequate gas exchange	Reduced	Reduced	High altitude Respiratory disease
Histotoxic hypoxia	Inability of cells to utilize available O_2	Normal	Normal	Cyanide poisoning
Stagnant hypoxia	Due to slow circulation	Normal	Normal	Circulatory shock Congestive heart failure

6. Ans. (a) 4 days

Ref: Ministry of Health and Family Welfare Guidelines & Protocols: Medico-legal care for survivors/victims of Sexual Violence https://mohfw.gov.in/sites/default/files/953522324.pdf

- If a woman reports within 96 hours (4 days) of the assault, all evidence including swabs must be collected, based on the nature of assault that has occurred.
- The likelihood of finding evidence after 72 hours (3 days) is greatly reduced; however, it is better to collect evidence up to 96 hours in case the survivor may be unsure of the number of hours lapsed since the assault.
- The spermatozoa can be identified only for 72 hours after assault. So, if a survivor has suffered the assault more than three days ago, taking swabs for spermatozoa are to be refrained from. In such cases swabs should only be sent for tests for identifying semen. Evidence on the outside of the body and on materials such as clothing can be collected even after 96 hours.
- Blood must be collected within 3 days and urine within 4 days in drug facilitated sexual assaults.

7. Ans. (b) 72 hours

Ref: A Review of Forensic Medicine & Toxicology by Gautam Biswas 3rd Ed Pg 7

On request for medical records, either by the patients or legal authorities, the same should be issued within the period of 72 hour. This applies to a doctor in his private capacity, in case of indoor patients whom he/she might have treated/operated in hospital/nursing home.

8. Ans. (a) Arsenic

Ref: Gautam Biswas 3rd Ed Pg 492

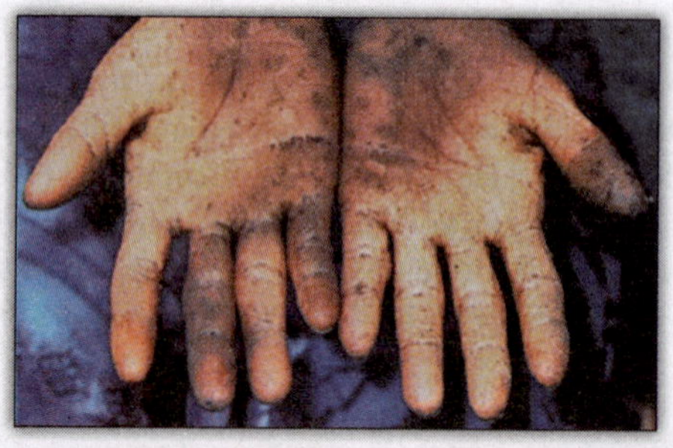

Fig: Arsenic keratosis, so called "raindrops on a dusty road"

- The common appearance of the dark brown patches with scattered pale spots is sometimes described as "raindrops on a dusty road".
- In severe cases, the pigmentation extends broadly over the chest, back, and abdomen. Pigment changes have been observed in populations chronically consuming drinking water containing 400 ppb or more arsenic.
- Arsenical hyperkeratosis occurs most frequently on the palms and soles.
- Keratoses usually appear as small corn-like elevations, 0.4 to 1 centimeter (cm) in diameter.
- In most cases, arsenical keratoses show little cellular atypia and may remain morphologically benign for decades. In other cases, cells develop marked atypia (precancerous) and appear indistinguishable from Bowen's disease, which is an in situ squamous cell carcinoma.
- Basal cell carcinomas have also been reported. Confounding factors for arsenic-induced skin cancer may include exposure to sunlight, chronic liver disease, and nutritional status.

9. Ans. (a) By threatening

Ref: Protection of Children from Sexual Offences Act, 2012

An offence is treated as "aggravated" when committed by a person in a position of trust or authority of child such as a member of armed forces or security forces, police officer, public servant; management staff of jail, remand home government or private hospital, educational and religious institution; gang sexual assault; commission of sexual assault using weapons or corrosive substance; causes grievous hurt. Further details of the definition are outlined below.

Aggravated Sexual Assault:

- Whoever, being a police officer, commits sexual assault on a child:
  - Within the limits of the police station or premises where he is appointed; or
  - In the premises of any station house whether or not situated in the police station to which he is appointed; or
  - In the course of his duties or otherwise; or
  - Where he is known as, or identified as a police officer; or
- Whoever, being a member of the armed forces or security forces, commits sexual assault on a child:

- Within the limits of the area to which the person is deployed; or
  - In any areas under the command of the security or armed forces; or
  - In the course of his duties or otherwise; or
  - Where he is known or identified as a member of the security or armed forces; or
- Whoever being a public servant commits sexual assault on a child; or
- Whoever being on the management or on the staff of a jail, or remand home or protection home or observation home, or other place of custody or care and protection established by or under any law for the time being in force commits sexual assault on a child being inmate of such jail or remand home or protection home or observation home or other place of custody or care and protection; or
- Whoever being on the management or staff of a hospital, whether Government or private, commits sexual assault on a child in that hospital; or
- Whoever being on the management or staff of an educational institution or religious institution, commits sexual assault on a child in that institution; or
- Whoever commits gang sexual assault on a child.
  Explanation: When a child is subjected to sexual assault by one or more persons of a group in furtherance of their common intention, each of such persons shall be deemed to have committed gang sexual assault within the meaning of this clause and each of such person shall be liable for that act in the same manner as if it were done by him alone; or
- Whoever commits sexual assault on a child using deadly weapons, fire, heated substance or corrosive substance; or
- Whoever commits sexual assault causing grievous hurt or causing bodily harm and injury or injury to the sexual organs of the child; or
- Whoever commits sexual assault on a child, which:
  - Physically incapacitates the child or causes the child to become mentally ill as defined under clause (l) of section 2 of the Mental Health Act, 1987 or causes impairment of any kind so as to render the child unable to perform regular tasks, temporarily or permanently; or
  - Inflicts the child with human immunodeficiency virus or any other life-threatening disease or infection which may either temporarily or permanently impair the child by rendering him physically incapacitated, or mentally ill to perform regular tasks; or
- Whoever, taking advantage of a child's mental or physical disability, commits sexual assault on the child; or
- Whoever commits sexual assault on the child more than once or repeatedly; or
- Whoever commits sexual assault on a child below twelve years; or
- Whoever, being a relative of the child through blood or adoption or marriage or guardianship or in foster care, or having domestic relationship with a parent of the child, or who is living in the same or shared household with the child, commits sexual assault on such child; or
- Whoever, being in the ownership or management or staff, of any institution providing services to the child, commits sexual assault on the child in such institution; or
- Whoever, being in a position of trust or authority of a child, commits sexual assault on the child in an institution or home of the child or anywhere else; or
- Whoever commits sexual assault on a child knowing the child is pregnant; or
- Whoever commits sexual assault on a child and attempts to murder the child; or
- Whoever commits sexual assault on a child in the course of communal or sectarian violence; or
- Whoever commits sexual assault on a child and who has been previously convicted of having committed any offence under this Act or any sexual offence punishable under any other law for the time being in force; or
- Whoever commits sexual assault on a child and makes the child to strip or parade naked in public, is said to commit aggravated sexual assault.

Salient Features of POCSO Act 2018

- Minimum punishment for rape made 10 years
- Minimum punishment of twenty years to a person committing rape on a woman aged below 16.
- Minimum punishment of 20 years rigorous imprisonment and maximum Death penalty/Life imprisonment for committing rape on a girl aged below 12.
- Fine imposed shall be just and reasonable to meet the medical expenses and rehabilitation of the victim
- Police officer committing rape anywhere shall be awarded rigorous imprisonment of minimum ten years.
- Investigation in rape cases to be completed within two months.
- No anticipatory bail can be granted to a person accused of rape of girls of age less than sixteen years.
- Appeals in rape cases to be disposed within six months.

AIIMS MAY 2018

10. Ans. (a) Frontal and parietal eminence prominent in female skull

Ref: Gautam Biswas 3rd Ed page 24

Male Versus Female Skull		
General	Larger, heavier, thick walled, prominent muscular ridge	Smaller, lighter, thin walled, smooth muscular ridge
Cranial capacity	Larger (1450–1550 cc)	Smaller (1300–1350 cc)
Glabella	More prominent	Less prominent
Supraorbital/ supraciliary ridge	More prominent	Less prominent
Frontal and Parietal eminence	Less prominent	More prominent
Zygomatic arch	More prominent	Less prominent
Occipital protuberance	More prominent	Less prominent

Contd...

Male Versus Female Skull		
Orbits	Square, rounded margins, small	Rounded, sharp margins, large
External Auditory meatus	Bony ridge along upper border (Supra tympanic crest) is prominent	Supra tympanic crest often absent
Mastoid process	Large, round, blunt	Small, smooth, pointed
Digastric groove	Deep	Shallow
Condylar facet	Long, narrow	Short, broad
Palate	Large, U-shaped, broad	Small, parabolic
Teeth	Larger (100 mm)	Smaller (95 mm)
Foramen magnum	Relatively large, long	Small, round

11. Ans. (c) Doctor assisting a surgeon in operation theatre is borrowed servant of surgeon

Ref: Gautam Biswas 3rd ed page 21

'Borrowed servant doctrine': An employee may serve more than one employer, e.g. the nurse employed by a hospital to assist in operations will be the 'borrowed servant' of the operating surgeon during the operation, and the servant of the hospital for all other purposes. *A physician may be liable for the negligence of a nurse employed by the hospital under the borrowed servant doctrine depending upon the factual context.*

Working Example: The classical example occurs in the operating room. Although the scrub nurse or operating room technician is an employee of the hospital, he/she is paid and controlled by the administration of the hospital for the purpose of a specific operation. But that same employee is directed or controlled by the surgeon during the operation, therefore, depending on the facts of the case, the negligent liability of the scrub technician may vicariously involve the surgeon performing the operation rather than the hospital that employs the technician.

Option (A)

The statement is true but not related to Borrowed Servant Doctrine. Interns and Residents are employee of the Hospital and they are Borrowed servant for the Physician or surgeon giving orders to them.

Option (B)

A nurse assisting a surgery is the borrowed servant of the Operating surgeon not the hospital.

Option (C)

Doctor assisting a surgeon in operation theatre is borrowed servant of surgeon. In fact, all the OT staff or any assistant of the Surgeon are borrowed servant of the operating surgeon for the time of surgery.

Option (D)

Anaesthetist coming for surgery from outside hospital/ freelance on request of the surgeon is not the employee of the Hospital. Hence Anesthetist and Surgeon do not have a common employer. Plus Anesthesia is independent domain and both Surgeon and Anesthetist are independently liable for their actions without being in a Servant relationship to each other.

12. Ans. (d) Common witness

Ref: Gautam Biswas 3rd ed Pg 50

- A witness is a person who gives sworn testimony (evidence) in a court of law as regards facts and/or inferences that can be drawn from these.
- There are 2 type of witnesses—Common and expert.
- A common witness gives evidence about the facts observed or perceived by him. No special knowledge is required for tendering the evidence by him.

Common Versus Expert Witness		
	Common witness	Expert Witness
Definition	**118 IEA-** Gives evidence about the fact observed or perceived by him	**45 IEA-** person skilled in Arts, Medicine, Science etc
Drawing inference	Not allowed	Allowed
Opinion on other witness	Not allowed	Allowed
Volunteering a statement	Not allowed	Allowed
Responsibility	Less responsibility	More responsibility
Punishment on false evidence	Less punishment	More punishment
Conduct money	Cannot claim	Can claim
Example	Any common person	Handwriting expert, forensic expert, doctor, chemist etc.

13. Ans. (b) Report it to authority as you feel it is case of physical abuse

Ref: Gautam Biswas 3rd ed page 331

This is a case of Battered Baby syndrome, which is a criminal offence and hence a medicolegal matter.

Option (A)

Telling a colleague will be breach of privacy of the patient and it's also not a privileged communication. It can only help you to make a diagnosis if not already made.

Option (B) and (C)

Since it is a Medical Legal matter the Authorities (Police in this case) needs to be informed. A social worker is generally called by the police if required, however a doctor can also call a social worker but not before informing the police.

Option (D)

There is no question of sending back the patient in a Medicolegal case. Battered Baby syndrome is a serious offence.

Battered Baby Syndrome

Definition: A battered child is one who has received repetitive physical injuries as a result of nonaccidental violence produced by a parent or a guardian. It is also called Caffey syndrome, Caffey-Kempe syndrome, maltreatment syndrome or parent-infant traumatic stress syndrome.

Characteristic injuries of Battered baby syndrome are:

- Laceration of the oral mucosa along with labial frenulum of the lower lip is a characteristic lesion.
- Slap marks, lash mark, knuckle punches, pinch mark [**butterfly-shaped bruise** with one wing (caused by thumb) larger than other
- **Intracranial Hemorrhage-(shaken baby syndrome or infantile whiplash syndrome):** Due to striking the child with fist or object or against a wall, dropping the child or vigorous shaking of the infant.
- **Eyes:** Retinal hemorrhages and lens displacement may be seen.
- **Cigarette burns:** Small circular pitted burns indicate deliberate stubbing of cigarette ends.
- **Skeletal injuries:** Bony injuries include transverse fractures, impacted fractures, spiral fractures, metaphyseal chip fractures, subperiosteal hematoma, and multiple deformities of the long bones and rib cage of the body due to multiple healed fractures and callus formation.

14. Ans. (c) 1-d 2-c 3-a 4-b

Ref: Review of Forensic Medicine and Toxicology by Gautam Biswas 3rd ed Pg 519

The table indicates the local vernacular names of certain poisons:

Scientific and Vernacular Names of Certain Poisons		
Poison	**Name**	**Image**
Abrus precatorius	Rati, Gunchi, Jequirity	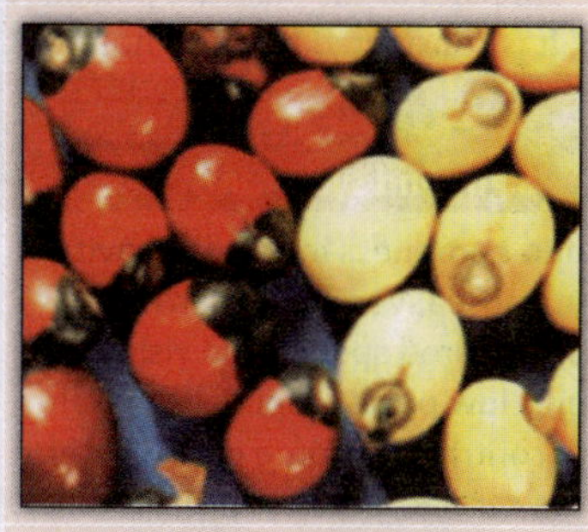
Spanish fly	Blister beetle	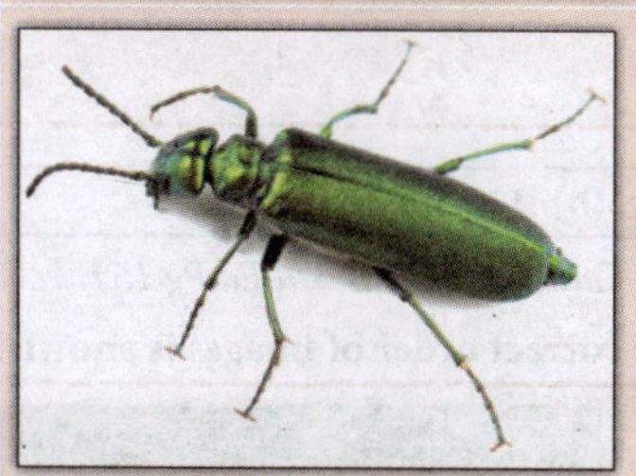
Aconite	Monk's hood, mitha zaher, bish, wolf's bane, women's bane, devil's helmet or blue rocket	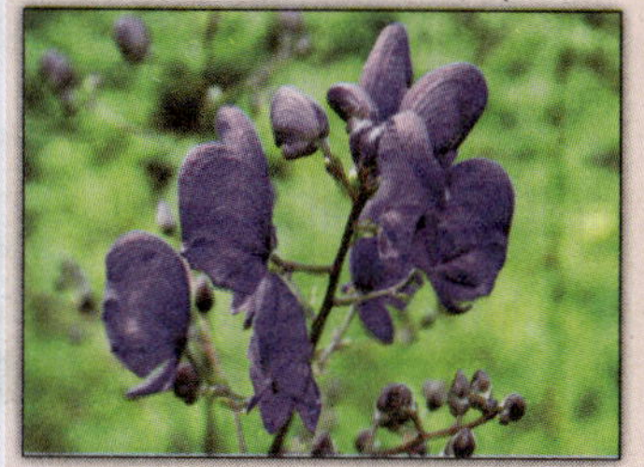
Heroin (derived from Papaver somniferum)	Brown sugar, smack	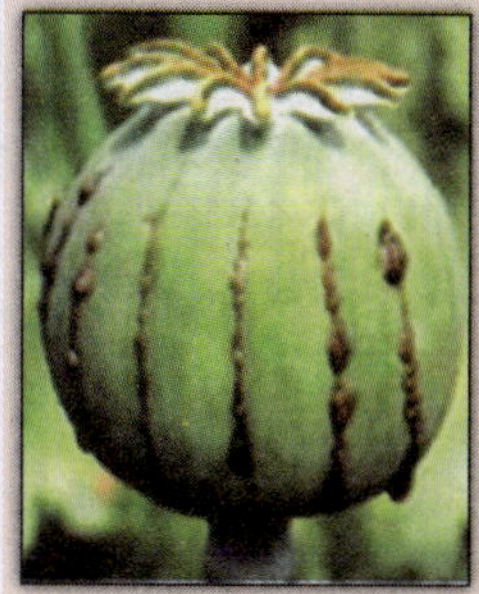 Papaver somniferum

15. Ans.(c) 6- 7 months

Ref: Forensic Medicine and Toxicology By Rabindra Nath Karmakar 5th Ed Pg 259

The presence of testis at superficial inguinal ring indicates that the gestational age is 7 months. Based on length of the fetus, the gestational age can be calculated as follows:

Calculation of Gestational Age	
For the first 5 months	After 5 months
Hasse's rule: Square root of the length (in cm) of the fetus is the age in months.	**Morison's rule:** Age in lunar months multiplied by 5 is the length (in cm) of the fetus.

By Morison's rule:

Length of fetus = Gestational age × 5
Hence Gestational age = Length of fetus/5 = 31/5 = 6 months
Hence the answer is (C) 6–7 months

16. Ans. (b) Root is the poisonous part of the plant

Ref: Gautam Biswas 3rd Ed page 576

- The image shows flowers of Aconite.
- All parts of the plant are poisonous but the root and root tubers are the most potent.
- It is considered the ideal homicidal poison. Aconite has no antidote, and its treatment is mainly supportive.

Aconite/Mitha Bish/Mitha Zahar			
Signs and symptoms	Fatal dose and period	Specific treatment	Comments
Tingling and numbness in the oral cavity, salivation, nausea, vomiting, diarrhoea, giddiness, impaired speech and vision, convulsions, low pulse, pupils alternately dilate and contract, become dilated later. Death from cardiac arrest or resp. paralysis	1 g root, 250 mg extract, 25 drops tincture, 4 mg alkaloid. Average fatal period 6 hours	No antidote. Supportive management. Gastric lavage with tannic acid/ $KMnO_4$, Atropine/ Novocaine Artificial resp. with O_2	• All plant parts are poisonous. Root is most poisonous. **Sweet taste (Mitha zahar)** • Destroyed in the body hence difficult to detect after death • Accidental/Homicidal poisoning • Arrow poison, Cattle poison, Abortifacient

17. Ans. (b) 1-d 2-a 3-b 4-c

Ref: Gautam Biswas 3rd Ed Pg 151

The correct order of images is shown below:

1	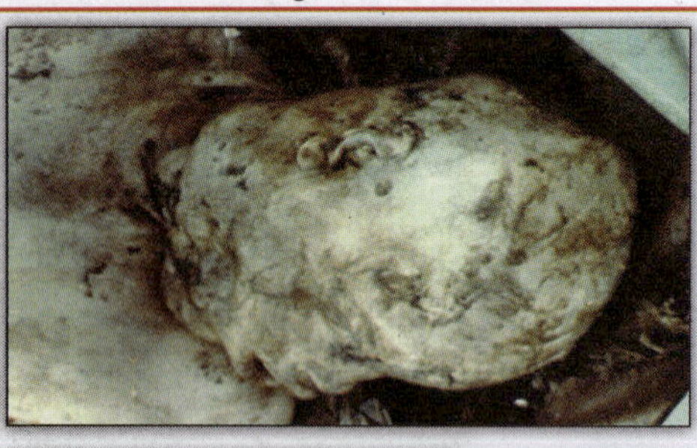	d	**Adipocere:** Conversion of fatty tissues into fatty acids. Rancid smell. Gains moisture and undergo hydrolysis. Ideal conditions are warm temperature, moisture, (hot and humid) less air, bacteria, and fat splitting enzymes. Time required = 1 week (5–15 days)
2	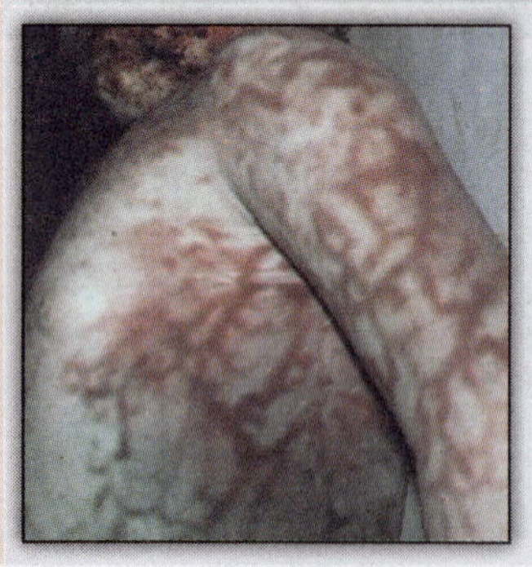	a	**Marbling:** Decomposition of hemoglobin to sulphmethemoglobin in the blood vessels causes a greenish or reddish-brown staining of the inner walls of the superficial vessels. This is seen as linear branching patterns, which gives a **'marbled' ('road map')** appearance of the skin. Marbling commences after 24 hours. In summers, 'marbling' is seen in 36–48 hours after death.

Contd...

3	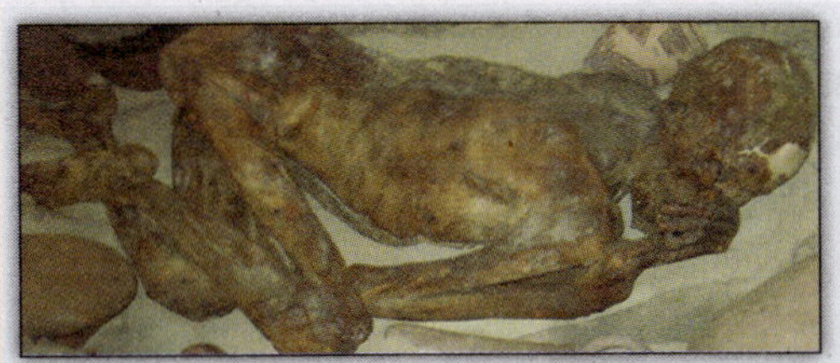	b	**Mummification:** Dehydration or desiccation. Odorless. Ideal condition are High temperature, dry condition, and free circulation of air 3–12 months.
4	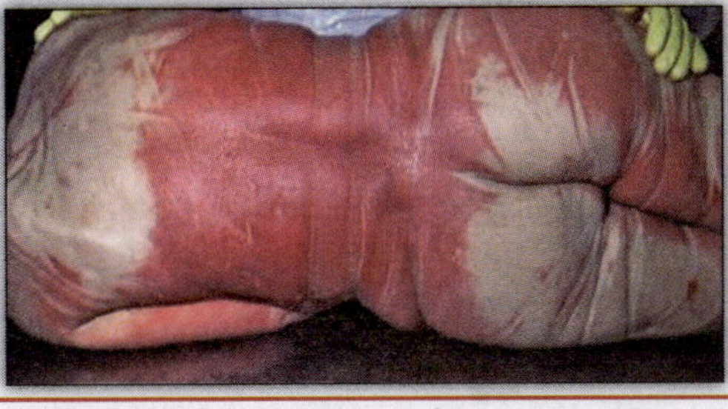	c	**Postmortem Lividity**: Livor mortis has been variously named as postmortem hypostasis, postmortem lividity, postmortem staining, suggillations, vibices, and so on.

18. Ans. (d) 19-21 years

Ref: Gautam Biswas 3rd Ed Pg 72

Let us discuss the findings of each X-ray:

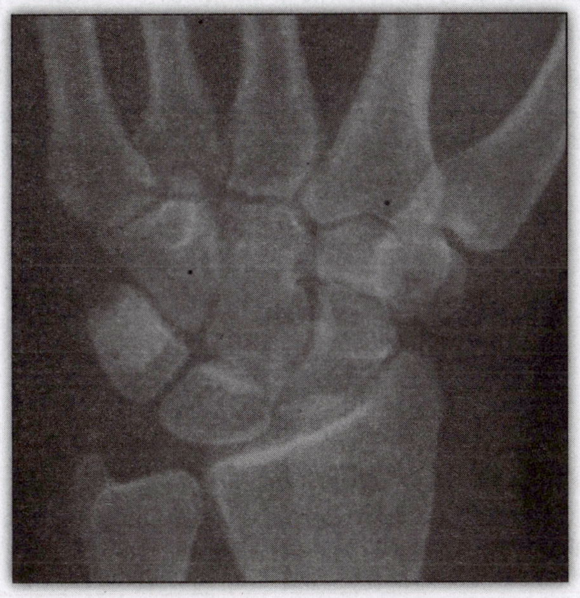

- **X-ray wrist:**
  Pisciform has appeared → Age > 12–17 years
  Lower end of both, radius and ulna have fused → Age > 17 years

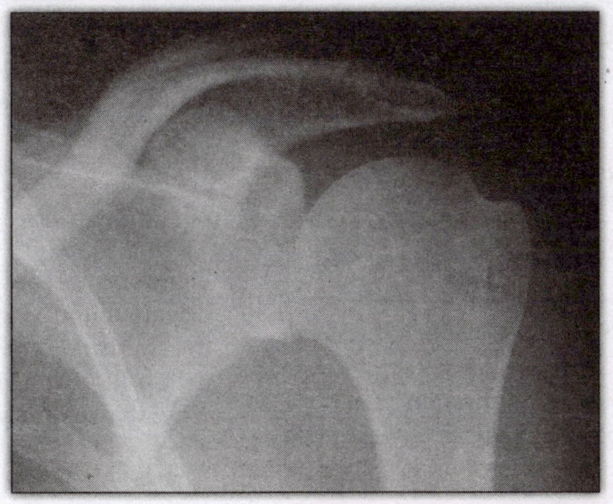

- X-ray Shoulder → Greater tubercle, lesser tubercle, head of humerus have fused with the shaft → Age > 18 years

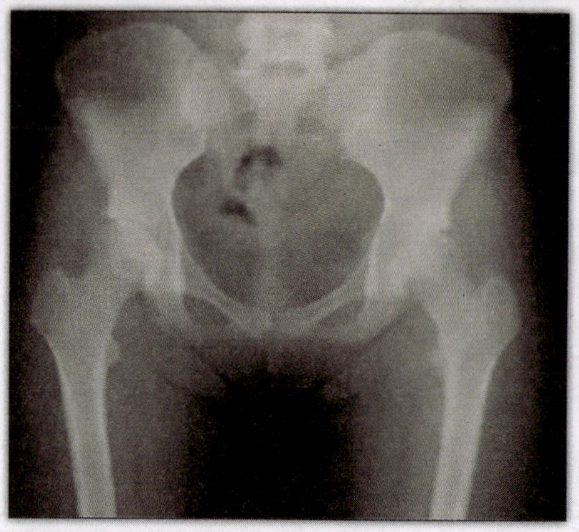

- X-ray Pelvis → Iliac crest, ischial tuberosity have fused → Age >20 years

Hence, the answer is (D) 19-21 years

Identification of Age		
Identification of age by Galstaun chart (most accepted) age in years		
Ossification center	**Girls (years)**	**Boys (years)**
Elbow	13-15 (Head of radius-14, Olecranon -15)	15-17 (Head of radius-16, Olecranon -17)
Wrist	16-17 (Lower end of radius-16.5, lower end of ulna-17) (Pisciform- last bone in the wrist- 12-17)	18-19 (Lower end of radius-16-17, lower end of ulna-18) (Pisiform- last bone in the wrist- 9-12)
Shoulder	17-18	19-20
Iliac crest	17-19	19-20
Ischial tuberosity	20	20
Inner end of clavicle	20	22
Lower end of femur	14-17	14-17
Lower end of tibia	14-15	15-17
Identification of age by Carpal bones		
There are 8 carpal bones and Pisiform is last to appear. Approximate age before appearance of Pisiform can be given from the number of carpal bones. i.e. **Total number of carpal bones = Age in years** At 9th year all 8 carpal bones are present.		

AIIMS NOVEMBER 2017

19. Ans. (a) Throttling

Ref: Reddy 33rd ed page 352, Knight's Forensic Pathology 4th ed page 374

Repeat (See AIIMS Nov 2018 Forensic Medicine for explanation) (see page no. 500)

20. Ans. (a) Arsenic

Ref: Nageshkumar G Rao 2nd ed page 465, Gautam Biswas 3rd ed page 492

Blackfoot disease due to platelet activation and hypercoagulability of blood in peripheral arteries is observed in endemic areas of arsenicism. Chronic exposure also causes diabetes, vasospasm and peripheral vascular insufficiency (blackfoot disease—peripheral vascular disease characterized by systemic arteriosclerosis resulting in dry gangrene and spontaneous amputations of affected extremities)

NOTE

Blackfoot disease is an endemic peripheral vascular disease found among the inhabitants of a limited area on the southwest coast of Taiwan, where artesian well water with a high concentration of arsenic has been used for more than eighty years.

	Clinical features	Fatal dose	Management	Comments
Arsenic	Burning pain, severe vomiting, tenesmus, bloody diarrhoea with mucus shreds, cramps. **Red velvet gastric mucosa. Rain drop pigmentation. Mee's lines. Blackfoot disease**	120-200 mg 24 hours	Demulcents and Lavage, Fresh hydrated **ferric oxide (Antidote)** Chelation-BAL	Rigor mortis lasts longer. **Mimics cholera.** Arsenic neuritis resembles chronic alcoholism

21. Ans. (a) Endrin

Ref: Gautam Biswas 3rd ed page 601, KDT 7th ed page 111

Endrin is an Organochlorine Pesticide with no antidote available. Treatment is symptomatic. Parathion and TIK20 are Organophosphates. Baygon is a Carbamate. For both Organophosphate and Carbamates Atropine is the Antidote.

Pesticides Classification

Insecticides are classified into three groups: Contact poisons, stomach poisons and fumigants.

- **Contact poisons** are those which kill insects primarily by contact, e.g., pyrethrum, DDT, HCH, dieldrin.
- **Stomach poisons** are those which when ingested cause the death of the insects, e.g., paris green, sodium fluoride.
- **Fumigants** are those which give off vapours which have a lethal effect on the insects, e.g., sulfur dioxide. This classification is by no means a rigid one, because a contact poison can also be a stomach poison.

Most of the present-day insecticides available for vector control (excluding inorganic chemicals and larvicidal oils) may be classified conveniently into 3 groups based on their chemical composition

- **Group I:** Organochlorine compounds
- **Group II:** Organophosphorus compounds
- **Group III:** Carbamates

Organophosphorus	Alkyl phosphates	TEPP: Tetraethyl pyrophosphate HETP: Hexaethyl tetraphosphate OMPA: Octa methyl pyrophoramide Malathion: Killbug, Bugsoline Dimefox Isopestox
	Aryl phosphates	Parathion: Follidol, Killphos, Ekato Methylparathion: Metacide Chlorthion Diazion: **Tik 20** Chlorpyriphos
Carbamates	Aldicarb: Temik Aminocarb: Matacil Approcarb: **Baygon** Carbaryl: Sevin Carbofuran: Furaxdan	
Organochlorides	DDT	
	BHC	GBH: Gamma benzene hexachloride Lindane: Gamma hexachloro cyclohexane
	Cyclodienes	Aldrin Dieldrin Endosulfan: Thiodan
	Endrin **(most toxic organochloride)** Heptachlor: Isobenzan: Chlordane: Chlordecone: Kepone Dechlorane: Mirex	
	Toxaphene	
Pyrethroids	Allethrin: Active ingredient of Raid Imiprothrin: Active ingredient of Raid Ant and Roach Killer Bifenthrin: Active ingredient of *Talstar, Capture, Ortho Home Defense Max* Beta-Cyfluthrin: Active ingredient in Baygon Transfluthrin: Active ingredient in Baygon Cyphenothrin: Active ingredient of K2000 Insect spray sold in Israel	

22. Ans. (d) A gynecologist can do termination of pregnancy with her consent

Ref: Forensic Medicine and Toxicology Rabindra Nath Karmakar 5th ed page 357, Review of Forensic Medicine and Toxicology By Gautam Biswas 2nd ed page 19

Option (A)

True: Male doctor can perform physical examination in presence of female attendant. This is a universal truth for all physical examinations of a female patient by a male doctor irrespective of age and complaints.

Option (B)

True: Since patient is already 22 weeks pregnant, urine pregnancy test is neither required nor productive. USG can be done straight away

Option (C)

True: Since the rape occurred 22 weeks ago there is no point in taking Vaginal swab now. Hence, vaginal swab is not taken at this point

Option (D)

False: According to MTP Act, pregnancy above 20 weeks cannot be terminated

As per consent rules, child below 18 years cannot give consent to suffer harm like MTP (Sec 87 IPC). Hence, there are two falsehood in this statement.

23. Ans. (b) Orbicularis oculi, Neck, Thorax, Upper limb

Ref: Gautam Biswas 3rd ed page 143, APC Essentials of Forensic Medicine and Toxicology

By Anil Aggrawal 1st ed page 124

Recall Bias...

Lot of permutation combination of the sequences were recalled. Its advised students must not remember the answer but the correct sequence of the Rigor mortis.

Nysten's law: After French Pathologist Pierre-Hubert Nysten who proposed the law in 1811. is applicable to voluntary muscles only. It states that the muscles closest to the brain goes into Rigor mortis first and those which are farthest goes into Rigor mortis last. Hence, it is also known as *Proximodistal progression of Rigor Mortis.* This it appears in the order of (**Mnemonic**- in the multiples of 3)

- Eyelids (orbicularis oculi) [2 hrs]
- *Jaw first and then facial muscles* [3 hrs] (since temporalis and masseter are placed high on face but effect is seen on jaw so jaw shows RM first and then facial muscles)
- Neck, Thorax [4-5 hrs]
- Upper limb (from shoulder to the hand) [6 hrs]
- Abdomen, lower limb (from the hip to the foot) [9 hrs]
- Small muscles of fingers and toes [12 hrs]

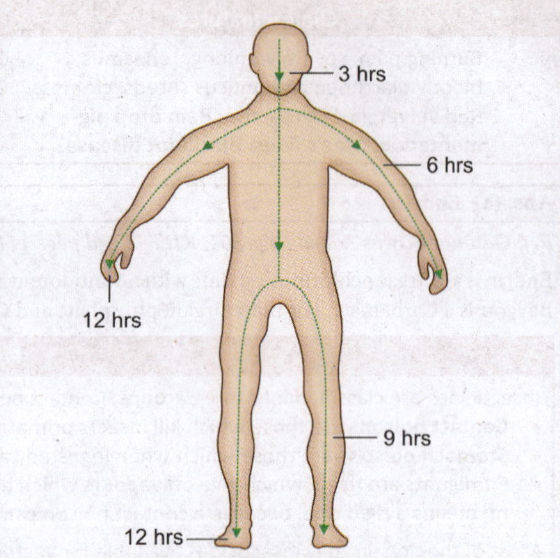

Nysten's rule: Proximo-distal progression of Rigor Mortis

24. Ans. (b) A-ii B-i C-iv D-iii

Ref: Gautam Biswas 3rd ed page 519, 521, 622

'Hunan hand' ('Chilli Willy') is a painful contact dermatitis seen in people with continuous and prolonged exposure to chilli peppers containing capsaicin

Abrus Precatorius is also known as Rati, Gunchi, Jequirity

Story of Purple Haze: Jimi Hendrix is world's greatest electric guitar player, had a short career. Hendrix's first big success was "Purple Haze,". The moment that turned Hendrix into a star in his homeland was his incendiary performance (literally—he closed his set by lighting his guitar on fire) at the Monterey International Pop Festival. After Monterey, the Jimi Hendrix Experience became one of the hottest rock bands anywhere. And Jimi Hendrix became a guitar god. With fame came drugs—most notably LSD, the "Purple Haze" variety, which was known as "Monterey Purple" before the festival and took on the name of Hendrix's famous song ever after.

Street Names of Common Psychotropic Drugs

Amphetamine	Black beauty, Hearts, Speed, LA, Truck driver
Methamphetamine (Methyl homolog of amphetamine)	Ice, Speed, Chalk, Crystal, Crank, Glass, Fire, Meth, yabba
Cocaine	Coke, Crack, Candy, Pasta, Bazooka, Rock, Snuff, Snow or white lady
Flunitrazepam	Roofies, R2, roofenol, roche, rope, forget pill
GHB	Grievous bodily harm, Georgia home boy, Liquid G, Liquid ecstasy, Scoop

Contd...

Street Names of Common Psychotropic Drugs	
Ketamine	K, Ket, Cat Vitamins, Special K, Vitamin K, Super acid, smack K, kit-kat
Liquid gold	Slang for urine of amphetamine addicts sold on the streets
LSD	Acid, Blotters, Boomer, Cubes, Dots, Microdot, Red/Green Dragon, Yellow sunshine, Purple Haze, Monterey Purple
MDMA	Ecstasy, XTC, Molly, Combining 'ecstasy' with psilocybin mushrooms is called 'hippy flipping'.
Morphine	Miss Emma, Monkey, White stuff
Opium	Big O, Black stuff, Gum, Hop
Phencyclidine (PCP)	Angel dust, super kools, dips, wack, rocket fuel, crystal, tic-tac, purple rain, zombie

25. Ans. (a) 1 b, 2 a, 3 d, 4 c

Ref: Gautam Biswas 3rd ed page 6, Reddy 33rd ed page 26, 400, 647

Repeat (See AIIMS Nov 2016 FMT for explanation) (see page no. 523)

26. Ans. (a) Hair

Ref: Reddy 33rd ed page 216, Nageshwar Rao 2nd ed page 279-285

See table of "Shotgun Firearm Injuries" in AIIMS May 2015 FMT (see page no. 547-548)

The aim of any Ballistic study is to identify the range, direction and weapon. Firearm injuries are broadly classified into Entry wound and Exit wound.

Option (A)

Range of gunshot injury can be determined by Tattooing, Blackening, Abrasion collar/Grease collar, Singeing of Hairs, Grease collar. All of them are seen at entry wound. Singeing and Abrasion collar are seen in Contact-range and Close range gunshot injury. Blackening will be seen till Short range and Tattooing will be seen till intermediate range gunshot injury.

Option (B)

Bullet pieces might or might not be found in the gunshot injury irrespective of the range of gunshot.

Option (C)

Blood cannot determine the range of gunshot, in fact it has nothing to do with the gunshot injury.

Option (D)

Since the injury is at the Skull, there is no point preserving the cloths.

27. Ans. (c) Mc Naughten's rule

Ref: Parikh Forensic 6th Edn Page 6.29, Gautam Biswas 3rd ed page 416

McNaughten rule: *Nothing is an offence which is done by a person who, at the time of doing it, by reason of unsoundness of mind, is incapable of knowing the nature of the act, or what he is doing is either wrong or contrary to the law". Note:* **Voluntary drunkenness/intoxication is not a defence u/s 84 IPC.** "McNaughten was an accused in a criminal case. He, while laboring under the delusion of persecution, shot Mr. Drummond, the private secretary of the Prime Minister Sir Robert Peel, at London, in mistake of the latter."

To assess the criminal responsibility of insane persons, certain other rules have come into use in subsequent periods in different countries at different times.

- **Durham's rule (1954):** An accused person is not criminally responsible, if his unlawful act is the product of mental disease
- **Curren's rule (1964):** An accused person is not criminally responsible, if at the time of committing the act, he did not have the capacity to regulate his conduct to the requirements of the law as a result of mental disease
- **American Law Institute test (1970):** A person is not responsible for criminal conduct, if at the time of such conduct as a result of mental disease, the person lacked adequate capacity either to appreciate the wrongfulness of his conduct or to conform his conduct to the requirements of law.
- **The Brawner rule (1972)** argues that insanity should be decided by a Jury. Under this proposal, Juries are allowed to decide the 'insanity question' as they see fit.

AIIMS MAY 2017

28. Ans. (c) Breadth of first sacral vertebra × 100/breadth of base of sacrum

Ref: Reddy 33rd Ed page 64

Identification of Sex	
According to Krogman, the degree of accuracy in sexing adult skeletal remains is as follows:	
Entire skeleton	100%
Pelvis and skull	98%
Pelvis alone	95%
Skull alone	90%
Long bones only	80%

Contd...

Identification of Sex by Pelvis and Sacrum	Male	Female
Pelvic inlet	Deep and narrow	Shallow and wide
Ilium	Less expanded	More expanded, splayed walls
Iliac fossa	Shallow	Deep
Suprapubic arch	Narrow, V-shaped, angle <70°	Wide, U-shaped, >90°
Ischial tuberosity	Inverted	Everted
Obturator foramen	Ovoid	Triangular
Greater sciatic notch	Narrow, deep, <90°	Wide, shallow, >90°
Preauricular sulcus	Narrow, shallow and without marked edges	Broad and deep in parous women
Ischiopubic (Washburn) index $\frac{\text{Pubic length (in mm)}}{\text{Ischial length (in mm)}} \times 100$	73-94	91-150
Sciatic notch Index (Best criteria) $\frac{\text{Width of sciatic notch}}{\text{Depth of sciatic notch}} \times 100$	4-5	5-6
Corporo-Basal Index $\frac{\text{Breadth of body of 1st sacral vertebra}}{\text{Breadth of base of sacrum}} \times 100$	>42	<42
Sacral Index $\frac{\text{Transverse diameter of base of sacrum}}{\text{Anterior length of sacrum}} \times 100$	<114	>114
Subpubic angle	V-shaped angle 70°-75°	Rounded, U-shaped, broader (90-100°) angle

Identification of Sex by Human Sternum	Male	Female
Ashley rule (AKA 149 Rule)	Sternal length >149 mm	Sternal length <149 mm
Hyrtl's rule	Body is longer and more than twice the length of manubrium	Body is shorter and less than twice the length of manubrium
Breadth	More	Less
Length of mesosternum (Body of sternum)	>95 mm	<80 mm
Level of upper margin	Lower part of body of T2	Lower part of body of T3
Sternal index = $\frac{\text{Length of manubrium}}{\text{Length of body}} \times 100$	46.2	54.3
Sternal foramen	Twice as common as in females	Less common

Footnote:
- **Rule of 149:** Ashley (1956) proposed this rule for European population
- **Rule of 136:** This rule was given by Ashley (1956) for the population of East Africa.
- For Indian population rule of 136 is better applied (Jit et al. 1980, Ankit et al. 2013)
- Ashley's rules are predictive but not conclusive. Jit et al. applied "Rule of 136" by which they determined the sex of 86% male and 78% female, but individually he cannot say if any particular sternum given is definitely male of female

29. Ans. (b) Caucasians have carabelli cusp on labial surface of mandibular molar

Ref: Knight's Forensic Pathology 4th Ed page 559, Gautam Biswas 3rd ed page 71

Option (A) True

In Negroes the teeth are broad and extra cusps

Option (B) False

Caucasians have carabelli cusp on mesial/palatal surface (not labial surface) of upper/maxillary molar (not mandibular molar)

> **NOTE**
> Caucasians is an umbrella taxon (term) for Europeans/whites/Americans.

A cusp is an occlusal or incisal eminence on a tooth. Canine teeth, otherwise known as cuspids, each possess a single cusp, while premolars, otherwise known as bicuspids, possess two each. Molars normally possess either four or five cusps. For roots, term used is trifurcated, bifurcated etc. carabelli cusp is an additional cusp.

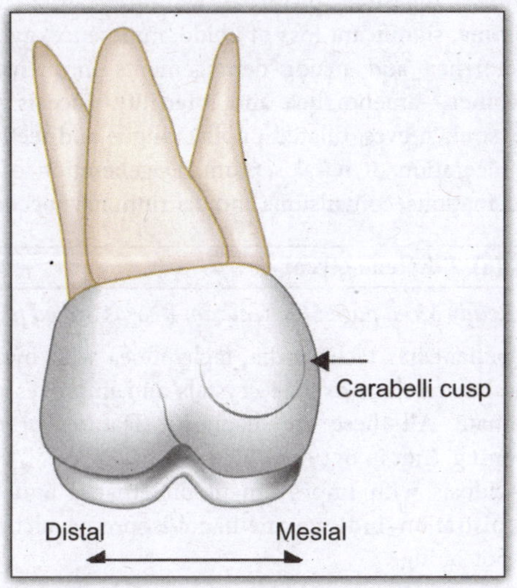

Option (C) True

Incisors of Mongoloids are shovel shaped

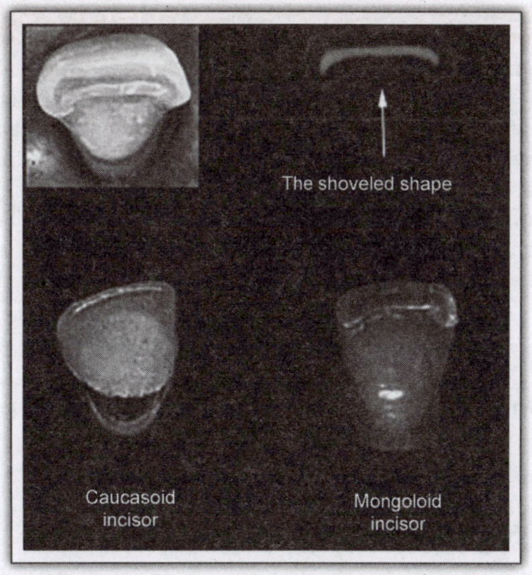

Option (D) True

Taurodontism, especially in maxillary molars, enamel pearls on premolars and congenital lack of upper 3rd molars are commonly seen in Mongoloids.

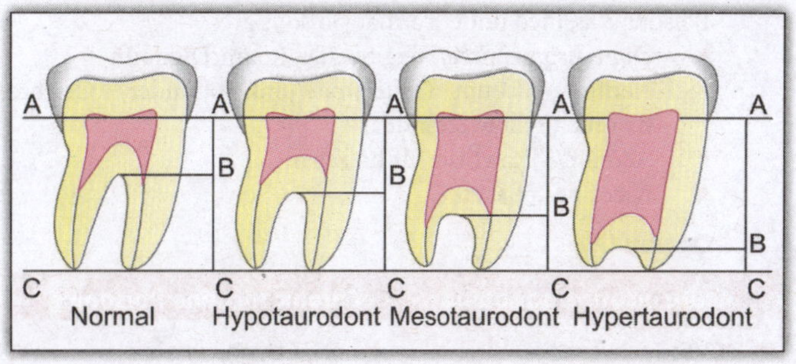

Identification of Race			
	Negro/Black, Aryan, Indian	European/Caucasians	Mongols
Skull type	Dolichocephalic (long headed)	Mesaticephalic (moderate headed)	Brachycephalic (broad headed)
Cephalic index	70-74.9	75-79.9	80 and above
Height index	72	71	75
Nasal index	55	46	50
Dental features	Two lingual cusps on mandibular first premolars	Long pointed canine roots. Lateral incisor in upper jaw is smaller than the central, especially in females. Carabelli's tubercle/cusp is an anomalous cusp on the mesial palatal surface of the upper 1st permanent molars, most commonly seen among Europeans (75–85%) (50% of American whites and 34% of Afro-Americans).	Bull-tooth or 'taurodontism' especially in maxillary molars, Enamel pearls (small nodules of enamel on tooth surface of premolars) and congenital lack of upper 3rd molars are commonly seen in Mongoloids. Shovel-shaped uppercentral incisors

Contd...

Cross section of hair	Kidney shaped	Oval	Round

Footnote:
- Race of a dead remains can be determined by cephalic index, height index and nasal index.
- Cephalic index also known as breadth index is obtained by multiplying maximum transverse breadth by 100 and dividing it by maximum anteroposterior diameter. The breadth is the greatest diameter across the skull above the mastoid process. The length is measured between the glabella and the external occipital protuberance.
- Taurodontism is an aberration of teeth that lacks the constriction at the level of the cemento-enamel junction characterized by elongated pulp chambers and apical displacement of bifurcation or trifurcation of the roots, giving it a rectangular shape. The term means 'bull like' teeth, and derived from similarity of these teeth to those of cud chewing animals.

30. Ans. (a) Chronic nicotine poisoning

Ref: Reddy 33rd ed page 615, Krishan Vij 5th ed page 526, Gautam Biswas 3e/p-577

NOTE

Best answer for the question specifically is Digitalis purpurea (foxglove) as the term Extrasystole is classically described with Digitalis. But since it was not provided in the options the next best answer will nicotine as it is a cardiac poison

Poisons classified under cardiac poisons are:
- Digitalis purpurea/Foxglove/Digitoxin/Digitalin
- Nerium odorum (True/white/pink oleander) Cerebra thevetia (Yellow oleander)
- Aconite/Mitha bish/Mitha zahar
- Nicotine/tobacco

Option (A)

Acute nicotine poisoning	Chronic nicotine Poisoning
• **CVS:** Tachycardia followed by bradycardia, hypotension, arrhythmia, tachypnea followed by respiratory depression and collapse. • **GIT:** Burning acid sensation, nausea, vomiting, abdominal pain, salivation and odor of tobacco. • **CNS:** Headache, restlessness, confusion, vertigo, sweating, convulsions and coma.	• **RS:** Cough, wheeze, dyspnea, chronic bronchitis and lung cancer may develop. • **CVS:** Anemia, palpitations, irregularity of heart beats, angina pectoris and Berger's disease. • **GIT:** Anorexia, vomiting and diarrhea. • **CNS and others:** Impaired memory, amblyopia, blindness, tremors, insomnia, anxiety and headache.

Option (B)

Cannabis intoxication presents as stage of excitement followed by stage of narcosis (respiratory and CVS depression)

Option (C)

Acute arsenic poisoning features: Hypotension, pulmonary edema, ARDS, circulatory collapse, ventricular tachycardia and fibrillation.

Chronic arsenic poisoning features: CVS: Chronic nephritis and cardiac failure causing dependent edema Plus 4 stages 1. GIT disturbances 2. Catarrhal changes 3. Skin rashes 4. Nervous disturbances.

Option (D)

Cocainism/chronic cocaine poisoning manifests as emaciation, anorexia, digestive disturbances, tachycardia tachypnoea, insomnia, significant loss of libido, impotence, gynecomastia, galactorrhea and major derangements in menstrual cycle in women—amenorrhea and infertility. Face is pale, shifty gaze, sunken eyes, dilated pupils, tongue and teeth are black, and ulceration of nasal septum. Degeneration of CNS with hallucinations, convulsions and delirium may occur.

31. Ans. (a) Ethylene glycol

Ref: Reddy 33 ed page 583, Gautam Biswas 3rd ed page 555, 556

The patient has tachycardia, tachypnoea with hypocalcemia, urine has calcium oxalate crystals and improves on calcium gluconate. All these are diagnostic features or oxalic acid poisoning. (not in options)

Acidosis with improvement on ethanol and fomepizole administration indicate methanol/isopropyl alcohol/glycolic acid poisoning.

Ethylene glycol when consumed, is metabolized into:
- **Glycolic acid** (methanol like kinetics i.e. ethanol has a much higher affinity for alcohol dehydrogenase than methanol and ethylene glycol. Presence of ethanol will therefore, inhibit formation of toxic metabolites from methanol and ethylene glycol.
- **Oxalic acid**

Oxalic Acid Poisoning			
Clinical features	Lethal dose	Management	Comments
Sour taste, burning pain, bloody mucus, vomiting, albuminuria, oxaluria, shock, cramps, convulsions, coma, coffee ground vomitus, hypocalcemia	15–20 g 1–2 hours	Specific antidotecalcium (Chalk) Lavage with lime water (not warm water), 10 mL 10% Ca. Gluconate	Used in bleaching, calico prints, erase forgery attempts. Present in Rhubarb, Tomato, Spinach

32. Ans. (b) Positional asphyxia

Ref: Gautam Biswas 3rd ed page 161, Oxford Handbook of Forensic Medicine

By Jonathan P. Wyatt, Tim Squires, Guy Norfolk page 108, Bernard Knight 4th ed page 365

Note: Some books intermix Traumatic asphyxia with Positional asphyxia. Following are the views of eminent forensic experts of country including chief editors of JIAFM.

Jackknife is the specific position used for surgical procedure where person is on prone position with high abdomen head and legs are at lower level. It is purely due the specific position of the subject. So, it is positional asphyxia.

If the position of body is unyielding for normal respiration to occur then it must be positional or postural asphyxia, while in traumatic asphyxia it is the external force which plays the major role. And if we consider jackknife position to be traumatic asphyxia then there is no place for positional asphyxia to be defined as an entity.

Examples of positional asphyxia:

- Positional/restraint asphyxia may occur in hogtying (individual is placed in a prone position, their hands are cuffed together behind their back, and their ankles are bound and tied to their wrists).
- **Jackknife:** It includes positional asphyxia due to head and chest lying below the level of waist such that the abdominal contents press the diaphragm to further restrict respiratory movements of lungs. Accidentally while climbing a window, the waist is on the window, legs lying outside, and head and chest suspended inside. As a method of torture—person may be suspended head down from a horizontal pole placed under the knees with the wrists bound to the ankles ('parrot's perch', 'jack' or 'Pau de Arara').

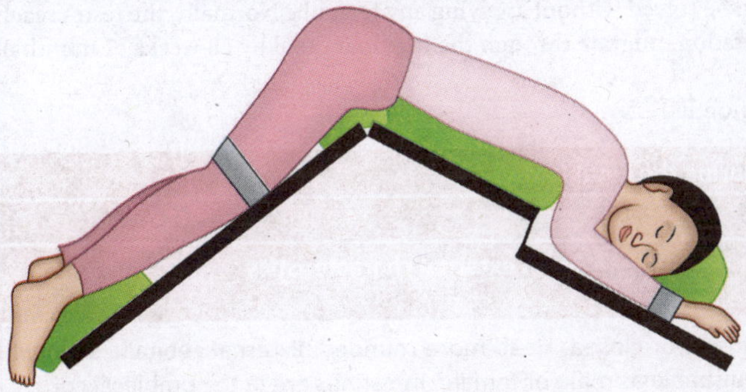

"Patient's abdomen lies flat on the bed. The bed is scissored so the hip is lifted and the legs and head are low. Similar to the **jackknife** except the legs are bent at the knee at a 90°. Also called the side-lying position, it is like the **jackknife** except the patient is on his or her side."

33. Ans. (a) Throttling

Ref: Reddy 33rd ed page 352, Knight's Forensic Pathology 4th ed page 374

Repeat AIIMS NOV 2018 Forensic Medicine (See for explanation) (see page no. 500)

34. Ans. (b) Red

Ref: Gautam Biswas 3rd ed page 133, Reddy 33rd ed page 146, Robbin's 9th ed ch, J Punjab Acad Forensic Med Toxicol 2012;12(1):60

Immersion of tissue slices in a solution of triphenyl tetrazolium chloride (TTC) gives red color (Brick red in Robbins) to the healthy area (where lactate dehydrogenase activity is preserved), but infarcted area appears pale if seen in about 4 hours the results are, however, inconsistent.

In the table on same page however, Gautam Biswas states "at 0–6 hours—No change" triphenyltetrazolium chloride (TTC) test negative.

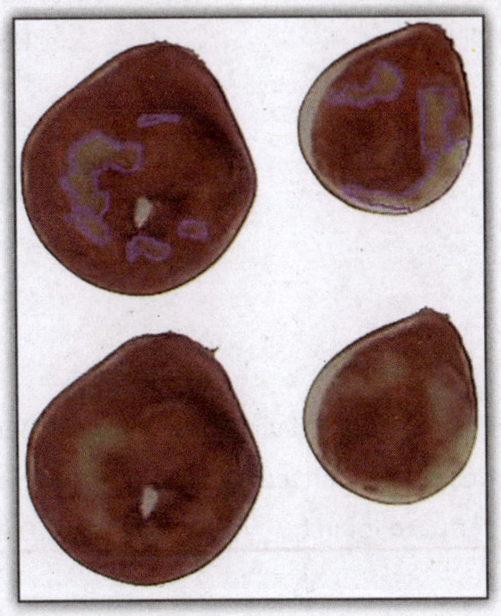

Fig: Staining of Sliced myocardium by Triphenyltetrazolium chloride (TTC) stain on autopsy. The infarct is unstained/ pale below and is being measured by perimetric software above (blue perimetry). Normal myocardium is red stained.

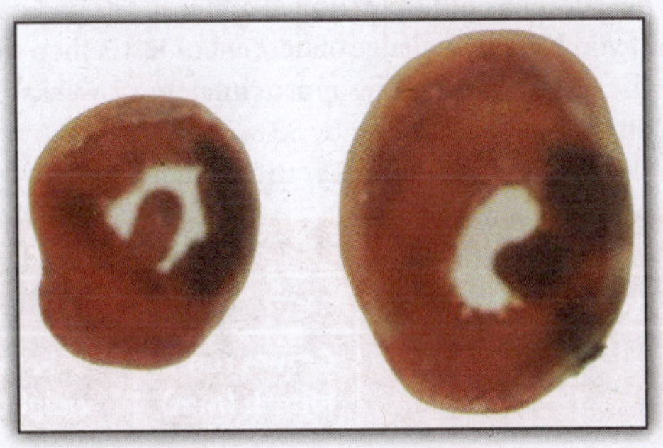

Fig: Blood perfused myocardium slice soaked with 10% formalin after tetrazolium staining which turns the blood a dark brown color.

There are two forms of tetrazolium:

1. Nitro blue Tetrazolium (NBT)
2. Triphenylte trazolium chloride (TTC)

Myocardial infarction can be demonstrated by triphenyl tetrazolium chloride or by nitro bluete trazolium dye test in an unfixed and fresh heart by immersing the slices of heart from suspected area or different areas of heart in these chemical dyes. The color of infracted area remains pale yellow (unstained) and the normal heart with intact dehydronases stains red with TTC and Blue with NBT dye.

Immersion of tissue slices in a solution of triphenyl tetrazolium chloride (TTC) gives red color (Brick red in Robbins) to the healthy area (where Lactate dehydrogenase activity is preserved), but infarcted area appears pale if seen in about 4 hours the results are, however, inconsistent.

In blood-perfused hearts the infarct is often hemorrhagic. The extravasated blood is often a dark red color and difficult to differentiate from tetrazolium stain. For that reason, heart slices are soaked in 10% formalin after tetrazolium staining which turns the blood a dark brown color.

Autopsy Staining of Myocardium	Nitro blue tetrazolium chloride (NBT)	Triphenyl tetrazolium chloride (TTC)
Cost of chemical	100 dollars/gm	4 dollars/gm
Characteristic	Cannot cross cell membrane	Can cross cell membrane
Clinical use	Not cross membranes and therefore can only be used with sliced tissue. The slicing disrupts enough cells that the nitro blue will react with the exposed cytosol	Can cross cell membrane, hence it can be used to both stain slices as well as perfusate. TTC is quite toxic and will cause the heart to stop beating instantly. Therefore, the heart must be in a Langendorff apparatus where coronary perfusion will persist even if the heart stops beating. It cannot be used in the in situ heart
Normal myocardium	Blue	Brick red
Necrosed/infarcted myocardium	Pale yellow (unstained)	Pale yellow (unstained)
Perfused Infarct	Dark brown on adding formalin	Dark Brown on adding formalin

AIIMS NOVEMBER 2016

35. Ans. (b) 7 months

Ref: Parikh 6th ed page 5.67, Forensic Medicine By Rabindra Nath Karmakar 5th ed page 259

This question has multiple clinical applications and can be solved by applying any of them if not all of them simultaneously.

- If you have knowledge of descent of testis then this question can be solved without applying any formula. Normally, the testes reach the inguinal region by approximately 12 weeks' (4 months) gestation, migrate through the inguinal canal by 28 weeks (7 months), and reach the scrotum by 33 weeks
- Fetal weight is 1000 gm at the Intrauterine age of 28 weeks (7 months)

Criteria for Estimating Age during the Fetal Period

Age (weeks) Menstrual	Age (weeks) Fertilization	Crown rump length (mm)	Fetal weight (g)	Main external characteristics
11	9	50	8	Eyes closing or closed. Head more rounded. External genitalia still not distinguishable as male or female. Intestines are in the umbilical cord.
12	10	61	14	Intestines in abdomen. Early fingernail development.
14	12	87	45	Sex distinguishable externally. Well-defined neck.
16	14	120	110	Head erect. Lower limbs well developed.
18	16	140	200	Ears stand out from head.
20	18	160	320	Vernix caseosa present. Early toenail development.
22	20	190	460	Head and body (lanugo) hair visible.
24	22	210	630	Skin wrinkled and red.
26	24	230	820	Fingernails present. Lean body.
28	26	250	1000	Eyes partially open. Eyelashes present.
30	28	270	1300	Eyes open. Good head of hair. Skin slightly wrinkled.
32	30	280	1700	Toenails present. Body filling out. Testes descending.
34	32	300	2100	Fingernails reach fingertips. Skin pink and smooth.
38	36	340	2900	Body usually plump. Lanugo hairs almost absent. Toenails reach toe tips.
40	38	360	3400	Prominent chest; breasts protrude. Testes in scrotum or palpable in inguinal canals. Fingernails extend beyond fingertips.

(Ref: William's 24th ed table 7.1)

- Lastly by calculating Crown Heel length (CHL) and applying it to Hasse's formula. Note that CRL not CHL is given in the question. Hence, we need to calculate the CHL first.

  CRL = 2/3 Crown Heel length. Hence, Crown Heel length CHL = 3/2 CRL

CHL = 3/2 × 23 = 34.5

Applying Hasse's rule Age = CHL/5 = 34.5/5 = 6.9 = 7 months

Identification of Intrauterine Age	
Hasse's rule	Up to 5 months, square root of length of fetus in cm is the age of fetus
	After 5 months, age in lunar months mustiplied by 5 is the Crown heel length of the fetus, i.e. 1/5th of the Crown heel length of the fetus in cm gives the age in lunar months. Sometimes separately referred to as **Morison's rule**

36. Ans. (a) Osmium blue

Ref: Reddy 33rd ed page 92, Textbook of Forensic Medicine and Toxicology Nagesh Kumar G Rao Page 105-106

Tattoo marks are fairly good identification marks for both living and dead.

Pigments Used

Carbon dust, Indian Ink, Indigo, Chinese black, Prussian blue, Cinnabar, Vermilion, Cobalt

Tattoo Removal

- Surgically by skin grafting
- Electrolysis
- Corrosives (chemical)
- Burning
- Laser removal

NOTE

A tattoo removed by electrolysis or laser removal (to hide their criminal identity) can be identified by tattoo pigments in sentinel lymph nodes. Tattoo pigments found in draining lymph nodes are often mistaken for malignant metastasis

37. Ans. (b) Ergotism

Ref: Reddy 33rd ed page 556, Gautam Biswas 3rd ed page 522

	Signs and symptoms	Fatal dose	Management	Comments
ergot (Claviceps purpurea) (Ergotism AKA: St. Anthony's Fire, St. Vitus's Dance)	Acute: GI symptoms, colicky pain, tingling, cramps, hypoglycaemia and anuria. Chronic Ergotism has two forms: gangrenous (St. Anthony's Fire) or convulsive (St. Vitus' Dance).	Uncertain dose and period	Lavage-tannic acid. Amyl nitrate inhalation. Vasodilators	• Active principle: **Ergotoxin, Ergotamine, Ergometrine** • **Gangrenous ergotism resembles Raynaud's**

Ergotamine was the first alkaloid derived, from fungus **Claviceps. purpurea,** for medicinal use. It was first isolated and structurally characterized, in 1918, by Arthur Stoll of the Chemical Company Kern and Sandoz (now Novartis International AG), in Switzerland.

Poisoning due to consumption of ergot infected rye by humans as well as other mammals is referred to as ergotism. Although other grasses may also become infected with C. purpurea, it most commonly occurs on rye.

There are two sets of symptoms that are recognized in cases of ergot poisoning: **convulsive and gangrenous ergotism**. In gangrenous ergotism, the victim may lose parts of their extremities, such as toes, fingers, ear lobes, arms and legs may be lost accompanied by burning pain. This type of ergotism causes gangrene due to constriction of blood vessels.

The first major outbreak occurred in the **Rhine Valley,** in 857 AD and in 944 AD, 40, 000 deaths were recorded as a result of gangrenous ergotism. It was at this time that the symptoms (but not the etiology) from consumption of ergot was called **Holy Fire**. "Fire" because of the burning, prickling sensations, in the extremities, that were experienced by the victims of gangrenous ergotism, and "Holy" because of the belief that this was a punishment from God.

In 1039, another outbreak occurred in France during which a series of hospitals dedicated to St Anthony were built in order to care for the victims of ergotism, and hence the name **St. Anthony's Fire**. Patients often find relief from ergotism probably due to the absence of rye bread from the victims' diet during their care in the hospital.

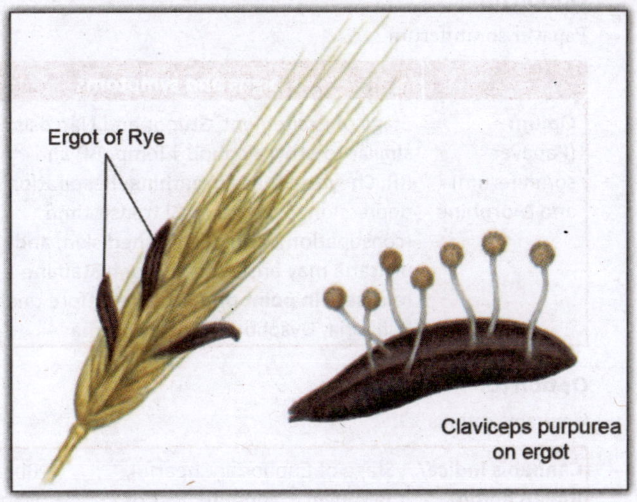

38. Ans. (c) 92

Ref: Reddy 33rd ed page 53, Gautam Biswas 3rd ed page 23

Emergency Cases

If a patient is unconscious and there is an imminent danger to the life of the patient and there is no designated surrogate or the surrogate is unavailable, then the law presumes that consent has been deemed to be given (implied consent, Sec. 92 IPC). For implied consent to apply, the injured must require emergency treatment to save life or limb and the treatment rendered must be so limited. Once the emergency treatment is no longer required, the doctrine of implied consent does not govern.

IPC 90	Consent known to be given under fear or misconception
IPC 91	Exclusion of acts which are offences independently of harm caused
IPC 92	***Act done in good faith for benefit of a person without consent;*** Nothing is an offence by reason of any harm which it may cause to a person for whose benefit it is done in good faith, even without that person's consent, if the circumstances are such that it is impossible for that person to signify consent, or if that person is incapable of giving consent, and has no guardian or other person in lawful charge of him from whom it is possible to obtain consent in time for the thing to be done with benefit
IPC 93	***Communication made in good faith:*** No communication made in good faith is an offence by reason of any harm to the person to whom it is made, if it is made for the benefit of that person. E.g. A surgeon, in good faith, communicates to a patient his opinion that he might not live. The patient dies in consequence of the shock. The surgeon has committed no offence, though he knew it to be likely that the communication might cause the patient's death.

39. Ans. (b) Red

Ref: Gautam Biswas 3rd ed page 133, Reddy 33rd ed page 146, Robbin's 9th ed ch, J Punjab Acad Forensic Med Toxicol 2012;12(1):60

Repeat AIIMS MAY 2017 FMT (See for explanation) *(see page no. 517)*

Immersion of tissue slices in a solution of **triphenyl tetrazolium chloride (TTC)** gives red color (Brick red in Robbins) to the healthy area (where Lactate dehydrogenase activity is preserved), but infarcted area appears pale if seen in about 4 hours the results are, however, inconsistent.

In the table on same page however, Gautam Biswas states "at 0–6 h - No change; triphenyl tetrazolium chloride (TTC) test negative.

40. Ans. (a) Lathyrus sativus

Ref: Reddy 33rd ed page 628, Gautam Biswas 3rd ed page 631

Option (A)

Lathyrus Sativus: This is a variety of pulse and is the staple food for the low-income groups in some areas of Central India known to cause paralysis. **Active Principle** b-N-oxalyl amino-alanine (BOAA), a neurotoxic amino acid present in the seed cotyledon.

Signs and Symptoms

Neurolathyrism, progressive spastic paraplegia A spastic gait develops characterized by 'walking on tiptoes' with the legs crossing scissor-wise. Later, complete paraplegia occurs. The knee jerks are increased, ankle clonus is marked and Babinski's sign is present.

Option (B)

Papaver somniferum

	Signs and symptoms	Fatal dose	Management	Comments
Opium (Papaver somniferum) and **Morphine**	Stage of Excitement, Stupor and Narcosis, similar to ethyl alcohol. ↓Temp, BP and RR. **Cheyne-Stokes breathing**, Respiration depression, Cyanosis, ↓GI transit time (constipation), Pruritus, flushed skin, and urticaria may arise because of histamine release, **Pin point pupils** dilate before death, Euphoria, Dysphoria, Seizure, coma	200 mg morphine, 2 mg opium 9–12 hours	Gastric Lavage, Naloxone 0.4-0.8 mg IV/IM every 10-15 min till pupil dilates. Artificial respiration, O_2	• **Raw flesh like smell** • **Poison of choice for suicide** • **High physical dependence**

Option (C)

Cannabis sativus

Cannabis Indica/ Indian hemp/ Hashish in Egypt/ Marijuana in America/Dagga in Africa	Stage of Euphoria: Chearful, Talkative, ↑ appetite, loss of perception, visual hallucinations Stage of Narcosis: drowsiness, confusion, ataxia, deep sleep. (used as **stupefying poison** before rape and robbery) **Run amok, Sexual Jealousy crimes**	Bhang- 10 g/kg, Ganja- 8 g/kg Charas- 2 g/kg 12 hours	Gastric lavage, Saline purgation, IV fluids, O_2, Artificial respiration, Tranquilizers	• Active principle = **Delta-9** THC (Tetrahydrocannabinol) • Preparations: **Charas-** resinous exudates of leaves and stem- 25 to 40% THC, **Hashish**-Concentrated charas, **Ganja** – flowering top- 25% THC, **Bhang-** Dried leaves- 15% THC, **Majun-** sweetmeat made of bhang- 15% THC

Option (D)

Argemone Mexicana (Prickly Poppy): It grows wild all over India in the cold season. The argemone or *katkar* oil causes **epidemic dropsy**. The oil from the seeds is sometimes used as an adulterant of mustard oil or other edible oil, i.e. the consumption is in mistake with the **OIL and not CEREALS. Active Principles** The plant contains two alkaloids—berberine and protopine. The oil contains two alkaloids, sanguinarine and dihydrosanguinarine. They cause abnormal permeability of blood vessels. Marked edema of the legs, and sometimes **generalized anasarca.** PNS Tingling and hyperesthesia of skin and tenderness of the calf muscles. The jerks are feeble or absent. Ocular Dimness of vision.

Food Adulterants				
Disease	**Toxin**	**Adulterant**	**Added to**	**Effects**
Endemic ascitis Pictow Disease in Canada Winton Disease in New Zealand	Pyrrolizidine alkaloids	ragwort (S. jacobea) rattleweed (Crotalaria retusa) Jhunjhunia in India	Millet seeds (Panicum miliare)- GONDHI in India Accidently by milk from cows feeding on these plants	Hepatotoxic, hepatic veno-occlusive disease and liver cancer
Neurolathyrism or Lathyrism	β-oxalyl-amino-alanine (BOAA) structural analogue of the neurotransmitter glutamate	Lathyrus sativus (also known as Grass pea, Khesari Dal or Almorta)	Bengal gram and Red gram	lack of strength in or inability to move the lower limbs, emaciation of gluteal muscles (buttocks)-characteristic
Osteolathyrism or odoratism	β-aminopropionitrile (BAPN) (antirheumatic agent in veterinary medicine)	Lathyrus odoratus seeds (sweet peas)	Bengal gram and Red gram	collagen cross-linking deficiency- weakness and fragility of connective tissue (i.e., skin, bones, and blood vessels (angiolathyrism)
Epidemic dropsy	Benzophenanthridine alkaloids, sanguinarine and dihydro-sanguinarine	Argemone mexicana (Mexican prickly poppy)- "PivlaDatura" or "Satyanashi" in India	Mustard oil	inhibition of Na+-K+-ATPase activity of heart - Proteinuria, edema, nephrotic syndrome, headache, nausea, loose bowels, erythema and breathlessness

41. Ans. (d) Can be done by only RMP registered for abortion under MTP Act

Ref: Gautam Biswas 3rd ed page 34

Option (A)

There is no mention of IUD in the MTP Act, however in gynecological practice if IUD fails and conception occurs then IUD needs to be removed before MTP

Option (C) and (D)

Section 1: Short title, extent and commencement	This Act may be called the Medical Termination of Pregnancy Act, 1971. It extends to the whole of India except the State of Jammu and Kashmir. Adopted by Kashmir and Mizoram in 1980
Section 2: Definition	"Guardian" means a person having the care of the person of a minor or a lunatic; "Lunatic" has the meaning assigned to it in Sec. 3 of the Indian Lunacy Act, 1912 (4 of 1912) "Minor" means a person who, under the provisions of the Indian Majority Act, 1875 (9 of 1875), is to be deemed not to have attained his majority, **"Registered medical practitioner"** shall have one or more of the following experience or training in gynecology and obstetrics, namely; In the case of a medical practitioner, who was registered in a State Medical Register immediately before the commencement of the Act, experience in the practice of gynecology and obstetrics for a period of not less than **three years;** In the case of a medical practitioner, who is registered in a State Medical Register: (i) if he has completed **six months** of house surgency in gynecology and obstetrics; or (ii) unless the following facilities are provided therein, if he had experience at any hospital for a period of **not less than one year** in the practice of obstetrics and gynecology or

Contd...

	If he has assisted a registered medical practitioner in the performance of **twenty-five cases** of medical termination of pregnancy of which **at least five have been performed independently**, in a hospital established or maintained or a training institute approved for this purpose by the government. This training would enable the Registered Medical Practitioner (RMP) to do only 1st Trimester terminations (up to 12 weeks of gestation). For terminations up to twenty weeks the experience or training as prescribed under sub rules (1), (2) and (4) shall apply. In case of a medical practitioner who has been registered in a State Medical Register and who holds a post-graduate degree or diploma in gynecology and obstetrics, the experience or training gained during the course of such degree or diploma.
Section 3: When Pregnancies may be terminated by RMP	A RMP shall not be guilty of any offence under that Code if any pregnancy is terminated by him in accordance with the provisions of this Act. Under MTP Act, pregnancy cannot be terminated after 20 weeks of pregnancy. Where the length of the pregnancy does not exceed twelve weeks if such medical practitioner is, or Where the length of the pregnancy exceeds twelve weeks but does not exceed twenty weeks, if not less than two registered medical practitioners are. Above 20 weeks, the pregnancy can be terminated only on therapeutic considerations, i.e. to save the life of the mother. In such cases, decision can be taken by a single doctor. The consent referred to in sub-section (4) of section 3 shall be given in Form C
Section 4: Place where pregnancy may be terminated	No place shall be approved under **clause (b) of section 4,** In case of first trimester, that is, up to 12 weeks of pregnancy:- A gynecology examination/labor table, resuscitation and sterilization equipment, drugs and parental fluid, back up facilities for treatment of shock and facilities for transportation; and **In case of second trimester, that is, up to 20 weeks of pregnancy:** An operation table and instruments for performing abdominal or gynecological surgery; Anaesthetic equipment, resuscitation equipment and sterilization equipment; Drugs and parental fluids for emergency use, notified by Government of India from time to time.
Section 5: Exceptions of Sections 3 and 4	The provisions of Sec.4 and so much of the provisions of sub-section (2 of Sec. 3 as relate to the length of the pregnancy and the opinion of not less than two registered medical practitioner, shall not apply to the termination of a pregnancy by the registered medical practitioner in case where he is of opinion, formed in **good faith,** that the termination of such pregnancy is **immediately necessary (Emergency)** to save the life of the pregnant woman. Notwithstanding anything contained in the Indian Penal Code (45 of 1860), the termination of a pregnancy by a person who is not a registered medical practitioner shall be an offence punishable under that Code, and that Code shall, to this extent, stand modified.
Section 6: Power to make rules	Lies with the central government
Section 7: Power to make regulations	Lies with the state government
Section 8: Protection of action taken in good faith	No suit for other legal proceedings shall lie against any registered medical practitioner for any damage caused likely to be caused by anything which is in good faith done or intended to be done under this Act
Amendment	Amendment on 18th December 2002, shall come into effect from 18th June, 2003 Word Lunatic was replaced by Mentally Ill In section 5 of the principal Act, for sub-section (2) and the Explanation thereto, the following shall be substituted, namely: Notwithstanding anything contained in the Indian Penal Code, the termination of pregnancy by a person who is not a registered medical practitioner shall be an offence punishable with rigorous imprisonment for a term which shall not be less than two years but which may extend to seven years under that Code, and that Code shall, to this extent, stand modified. Whoever terminates any pregnancy in a place other than that mentioned in section 4, shall be punishable with rigorous imprisonment for a term which shall not be less than two years but which may extend to seven years. Any person being owner of a place which is not approved under clause (b) of section 4 shall be punishable with rigorous imprisonment for a term which shall not be less than two years but which may extend to seven years.

42. Ans. (b) Opioid intoxication

Ref: Gautam Biswas 3rd ed page 537

	Benzodiazepine Poisoning	Alcohol Intoxication	Opioid Intoxication	Pontine Hemorrhage
Pupil	Contracted	Dilated in intoxication/contracted in comatose (macevans sign)	Classical pin point pupil	Contracted > Pin point
Respiratory rate	Normal vitals		Hypoventilation	Hyperventilation
Blood pressure	Normal vitals		Hypotension	Uncontrolled hypertension

43. Ans. (a) 1 b, 2 a, 3 d, 4 c

Ref: Gautam Biswas 3rd ed page 6, Reddy 33rd ed page 26, 400, 647

Various Declarations Adopted by WMA in Chronological Order		
Declaration of Geneva (revised form of Hippocrates's oath)	Ethical duties of doctors, humanitarian goal of medicine	Geneva, Switzerland 1948
Declaration of **H**elsinki (adopted with Nuremberg code-1947)	**H**uman experimentation and research ethics	Helsinki, Finland 1964
Declaration of Sydney	Organ transplantation	Sydney, Australia 1968
Declaration of Oslo	Therapeutic abortion	Oslo, Norway, 1970
Declaration of **T**okyo	**T**orture is contrary to laws of humanity	Tokyo, Japan 1975
Declaration of Lisbon	The rights of the patients	Lisbon, Portugal 1981 (amended in 1995 and 2005)
Declaration of Madrid	Euthanasia is unethical	Madrid, Spain 1987
Declaration of Malta	**Hunger strikers** (urges physicians to resuscitate them, but restrains physicians from intervening when a valid and informed refusal has been made)	St. Julians, Malta 1991 (revised in 1992 and 2006)
Declaration of Ottawa	Right of the child for health care	Ottawa, Canada 1998 (amended in 2009)
Declaration of Delhi	Health effects of climate changes	New Delhi 2009

44. Ans. (c) Conium maculatum

Ref: Gautam Biswas 3rd ed page 575, Reddy 33rd ed page 614

Conium or Hemlock causes ascending paralysis, Datura and opium causes descending paralysis while strychnine causes medullary paralysis.

	Signs and symptoms	Fatal dose	Management	Comments
Conium/hemlock	Nausea, vomiting, diarrhea, mousy odor in breath, Ingestion causes burning in the mouth and throat, gastric inflammation, slow respiration and pulse, mental confusion, tremors and blindness, dilated pupils. This is followed by ***progressive ascending paralysis*** of limbs, and the patient dies of asphyxia due to respiratory paralysis	1 cm of plant few hours (60 mg coniine)	Gastric lavage with 5% tannic acid artificial resp, O_2	• **Mousy odor** • Hemlock was administered to ***Socrates,*** the Greek Philosopher in 399 BC for execution.

45. Ans. (d) Subepiphyseal Microfracture

Ref: Gautam Biswas 3rd ed page 333, Reddy 33rd ed page 445, Grainger and Allison's Diagnostic Radiology 5th ed ch 68

Summary

Multiple collective microfractures are the cause of other radiological signs of Nonaccidental injury/child abuse and per se Microfracture is not visible radiologically.

Oski's Pediatrics

Principles and Practice edited by Julia A. McMillan, Ralph D. Feigin, Catherine DeAngelis, M. Douglas Jones 4th ed page 154: (CML) Classic metaphyseal fracture of long bones is the most specific fracture of inflicted injuries, considered pathognomonic for abuse. This so, called Corner fracture, Bucket Handle fracture, Metaphyseal flag or Metaphyseal fragment fracture has been studied and shown to be a series of planar microfracture through the most immature portion of long bones. This fragmented portion of the bone depending on the projection of the X-ray will appear as a fragment (Corner fracture) or semilunar loop (Bucket handle fracture)

Pediatric Radiology

The Requisites By Johan G. Blickman, Bruce R. Parker, Patrick D. Barnes 3rd ed page 202: Periosteal avulsion with microfractures of the growing bone at its metaphyseal insertion is considered to be the causative mechanism. It is most likely caused by the force generated in the shaking of the child.

The following circumstances should alert the physician to the possibility of NAI (Non accidental injury)/Child abuse:

- The presence of an inappropriate, inconsistent, or conflicting history.
- The presence of unexplained soft tissue injury.
- The presence of a healing fracture or the presentation of the child in a shocked or dehydrated state resulting from a delay in seeking medical help.
- Radiological evidence of trauma exceeds that expected from the clinical history.
- The presence of skeletal injuries with a high specificity for abuse.

Signs of Child Abuse	
Skeletal injuries	**Surface injuries**
Bony injuries include transverse fractures, impacted fractures, spiral fractures, metaphyseal chip fractures, subperiosteal hematoma, and multiple deformities of the long bones and rib cage of the body due to multiple healed fractures and callus formation. Multiple rib fractures also occur along posterior angle of ribs on side-to-side squeezing. The fractured ribs heal by callus formation in 1–2 weeks, giving characteristic appearance of a knob (knob fractures), and on X-ray 'string of beads' appearance is seen in paravertebral gutter. In whiplash movement of arms and legs, typical ***'corner' or 'bucket-handle' fractures*** in the metaphyseal region may be seen.	Butterfly-shaped bruise with one wing (caused by thumb) larger than other. CNS: Injuries are inflicted by throwing the child, striking the child with fist or object or against a wall, dropping the child or vigorous shaking of the infant (shaken baby syndrome or infantile whiplash syndrome) leading to intracranial hemorrhage. The triad of injuries includes encephalopathy, retinal hemorrhages and SDH. SDH is the most consistent component of the triad and may be the first clinical sign identified on CT scan.

The following fractures, which occur infrequently, are considered to have a high specificity for abuse:

- Metaphyseal, rib and scapular fractures
- Fractures of the outer third of the clavicle
- Sternal fractures
- Spinous process fractures

Fractures that occur frequently but have a low specificity for abuse are:

- Midclavicular fractures
- Simple linear skull fractures of the parietal bone
- Single diaphyseal fractures, with the exception of spiral fractures of the humerus
- Greenstick fractures

Radiology of Nonaccidental Injury

The spectrum of injuries encompassed by the terms nonaccidental injury (NAI) or child abuse range from the well documented physical and sexual abuse to the less frequently publicized emotional abuse, neglect, deprivation and abandonment. The radiologist's role is to provide an objective assessment of the radiology and this is best carried out in the absence of any contact with the patient or his/her family.

Metaphyseal Fractures

Also known as corner or bucket handle fractures, metaphyseal fractures are highly characteristic of and specific for NAI with an incidence of between 11% and 28%. They are most commonly seen in nonmobile abused infants under 18 months of age, and are most frequent around the knees and ankles but also occur at the shoulder, elbow, wrists and hips. They may be bilateral. Metaphyseal fractures do not usually occur in children over 2 years of age.

Diaphyseal Fractures

Are the most common fracture in child abuse and are said to occur four times more frequently in NAI than metaphyseal fractures. The femur, humerus and tibia are the most frequently injured bones. No one pattern or type of diaphyseal fracture is specific to NAI.

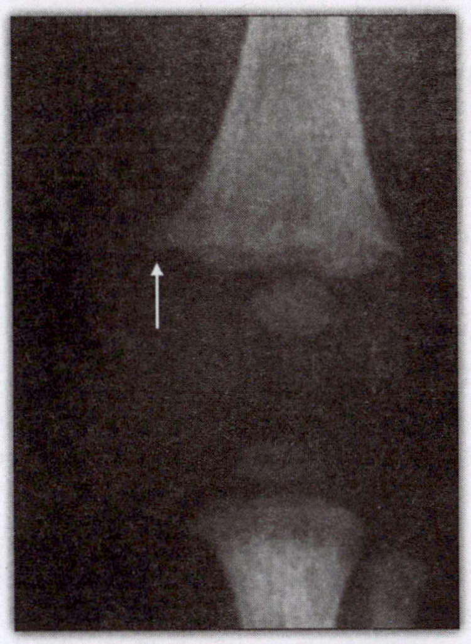

Fig: (A) Anteroposterior radiograph of the knees in a child having undergone NAI reveals "corner" fracture (arrows) on the medial aspect of the distal femur

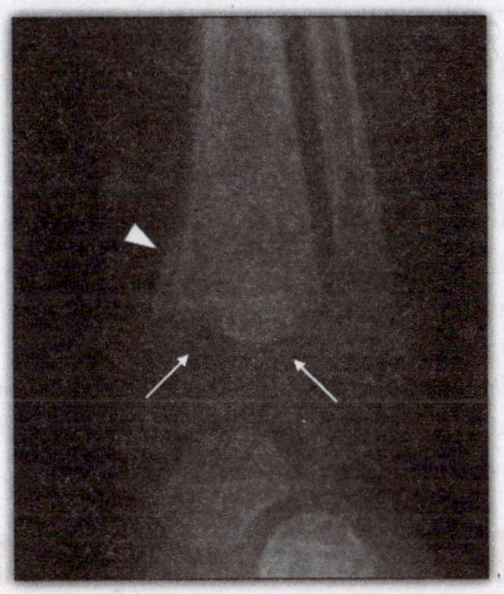

Fig: (B) Anteroposterior radiograph of the ankle in a child having undergone NAI evidences a "bucket-handle" fracture (arrows) of the distal tibia. Since the lesion is extensive, an associated periosteal reaction is seen (arrowhead)

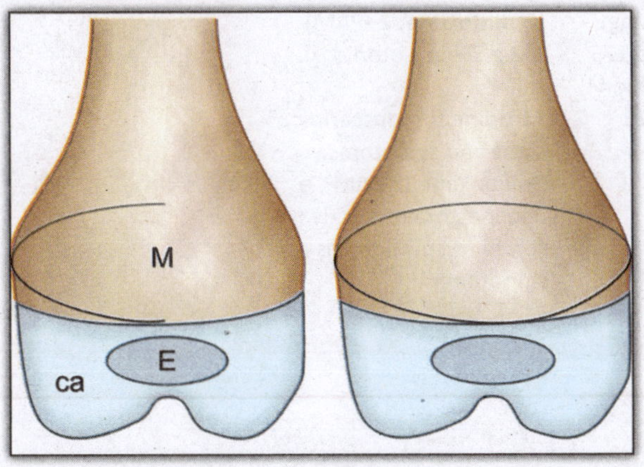

Fig: (C) Diagram of a classic metaphyseal lesion depicts a "corner" incomplete fracture (left) and a "bucket-handle" complete fracture (right). M = metaphysis; E = osseous portion of the epiphysis; ca = cartilaginous portion of the epiphysis. The black line corresponds to the fracture line

46. Ans. (d) 269

Ref: Reddy 33rd ed page 55

Option (A) IPC 166

Public servant disobeying law, with intent to cause injury to any person.

Option (B) IPC 202

Intentional omission to give information of offence by person bound to inform shall be punished with imprisonment of either description for a term which may extend to six months, or with fine, or with both.

Option (C) IPC 203

Giving false information respecting an offence committed.—Whoever knowing or having reason to believe that an offence has been committed, gives any information respecting that offence which he knows or believes to be false, shall be punished with imprisonment of either description for a term which may extend to two years, or with fine, or with both.

Option (D) IPC 269

Negligent act likely to spread infection of disease dangerous to life: Whoever unlawfully or negligently does any act which is, and which he knows or has reason to believe to be, likely to spread the infection of any disease dangerous to life, shall be punished with imprisonment of either description for a term which may extend to six months, or with fine, or with both.

47. Ans. (b) Vasopressor

Ref: Gautam Biswas 3rd ed page 627

Specific Odors of Poisons	
Acetone smell	Aspirin (salicylic acid), Alcohol, Chloroform
Aromatic smell	Chloral hydrate
Burnt rope like smell	Marijuana (Cannabis)
Bitter almond	Cyanide, Hydrocyanic acid
Coal gas like smell	Carbon monoxide
Garlic smell	Arsenic, **Phosphorous**, Thallium, Tellurium, Selenium
Fishy/Garlic odor of phosphine	**Zinc phosphide**, Aluminum phosphide
Kerosene like smell	Kerosene, Organophosphates, Organochlorides
Mousy odor	Conium/hemlock
Moth ball like smell	Naphthalene, Camphor
Phenolic/hospital like smell	Carbolic acid
Pear (Acrid) like smell	**Chloral hydrate, Paraldehyde**
Raw flesh like smell	Opium
Rotten egg like smell	Hydrogen sulfide (H_2S), carbon disulfide, **Disulfiram**, Mercaptans, N acetylcysteine
Shoe polish like smell	Nitrobenzene
Sweet	Aconite
Vinegar	Acetic acid, Hydrofluoric acid

Kerosene like smell is seen in Kerosene, OPC poisoning. Point in favor of OPC poisoning are:

- OPC poisoning is much more common than Hydrocarbon (Kerosene) poisoning.
- Bradycardia with Hypotension
- Suicide with Kerosene is rare while suicide with OPC is very common
- Kerosene poisoning is mostly accidental in children

Option (A)

Atropine is considered as clinical antidote of OPC poisoning. Atropine has no role to play in Kerosene poisoning except that few authors have written about Atropine challenge test in case of query of OPC poisoning. A number of authors have recommended the "atropine challenge" as an aid to diagnosis. When given to a normal person who has not been exposed to cholinesterase inhibitors, a 2 mg dose of atropine (0.025-0. 050/kg in pediatric cases) causes:

- A dry mouth.
- An increase in heart rate of about 35 beats/minute (max 35-45 beats/min) within 3-5 minutes of an IV dose and 35-45 minutes of IM dose
- Blurred near-vision.
- Dry, hot skin
- Mydriasis (pupillary dilation)

Most of these effects will dissipate within 4–6 hours, except blurred near-vision which may persist for 24 hours. (Sidell 1997). It has been suggested that when these physiological changes do not occur with this dose (sometimes referred to as an atropine challenge), this is indicative of cholinesterase inhibitor toxicity. (Clark 2002; Erdman 2004)

Hydrocarbons may be used as diluents in liquid formulations of cholinesterase inhibitors. In cases of ingestion, aspiration pneumonitis with acute respiratory distress syndrome may add to the muscarinic respiratory effects of the poison, but is unresponsive to atropine. (Reigart and Roberts 1999)

Option (B)

Vasopressors have no role in either Hydrocarbon (Kerosene) or OPC poisoning. Hence, it is the most likely answer.

Option (C)

Gastric lavage is a part of treatment in OPC poisoning while is contraindicated in Kerosene poisoning (with certain exceptions)

Gastric lavage in Kerosene poisoning should never be done without intubation, as there is a risk of aspiration. Gastric lavage and emesis are contraindicated in Kerosene poisoning except:

- When the patient presents within 1 hour of ingestion or large amount of ingestion (>4 mL/kg). Gastric lavage with warm water containing 5 percent sodium bicarbonate administered with extreme care to prevent entry into respiratory tract is beneficial with large amount of kerosene consumption (more than 4 mL/kg weight)
- When the patient is in coma.
- When kerosene is mixed with pesticides, heavy metals and other toxin

The following measures, performed before nasogastric lavage, may minimize the risk of aspiration:

- Endotracheal intubation with a balloon-cuffed endotracheal tube
- Left lateral decubitus with mild Trendelenburg positioning
- Pinching off the nasogastric tube and withdrawing it quickly after the procedure is complete

	Signs and symptoms	Fatal dose	Management	Comment
Organophosphous compounds (Malathion, Diazinon, Tik-20)	Muscarinic: **Mnemonic = SLUDGE -BBB;** Salivation, Lacrimation/ **chromodacryorrhea** (shedding of red tears due to accumulation of porphyrin in lacrimal glands), Urination, Defecation, GI upset, Emesis, Bronchospasm, Blurred vision (Miosis), Bradycardia Nicotinic: Fatigue, weakness, cramps, dyspnea, cyanosis CNS: Confusion, Stupor, Coma, convulsions, Contracted pupils Organophosphorus-induced *delayed-onset polyneuropathy* (**OPIDP**): after **2 to 4 weeks** central peripheral-distal axonopathy type with secondary demyelination.	IV/IM Fatal dose is half the oral fatal dose Orally: HETP-350 mg, OMPA-175 mg, TEPP- 100 mg, parathione 175 mg, malathion and TIK-20 1 g	Decontaminate, Gastric lavage, **Clinical Antidote: Atropine** 2 mg IV/IM every 15-30 minutes, **specific antidote: Oxime (Pralidoxime; 2 -PAM)** 1-2 g 5% in isotonic saline. Atropine for muscarinic signs and symptoms. Pralidoxime (2-PAM), a cholinesterase reactivator, for nicotinic signs and symptoms	• **Kerosene/Garlic smell** • **Resists putrefaction**

NOTE

- Avoid intravenous fluid overload, as it may precipitate pulmonary edema.
- For patients who have ingested large quantities of hydrocarbons with significant systemic toxicity and who presented within 60 minutes of ingestion, gastric emptying using nasogastric lavage is suggested.

MNEMONIC = CHAMP

- **C** : Camphor
- **H** : Halogenated hydrocarbons (e.g. trichloroethane, trichloroethylene)
- **A** : Aromatic hydrocarbons (e.g., benzene, toluene, xylene)
- **M** : Metal additives (e.g. arsenic, mercury) in hydrocarbon base
- **P** : Pesticide additives (e.g. organophosphates) in hydrocarbon base

- Activated charcoal (AC) should NOT be administered to patients with a single agent ingestion of a hydrocarbon without systemic toxicity for the following reasons:
  - AC administration increases the risk of spontaneous vomiting and additional pulmonary aspiration.
  - AC does not bind well to hydrocarbons.

48. Ans. (c) Sulphmethemoglobin

Ref: Gautam Biswas 3rd ed page 147, Reddy 33rd ed page 166

Marbling of Skin

The blood vessels provide an important route through which the bacteria can spread with ease throughout the body. Their passage is marked by the decomposition of hemoglobin to sulphmethemoglobin in the blood vessels, which causes a greenish or reddish-brown staining of the inner walls of the superficial vessels. This is seen as linear branching patterns, which gives a 'marbled' ('road map') appearance of the skin. Areas where visible: It appears first in the shoulder, roots of the limbs, thighs, sides of abdomen, chest and neck. Onset: In summers, 'marbling' is seen in 36–48 hours after death.

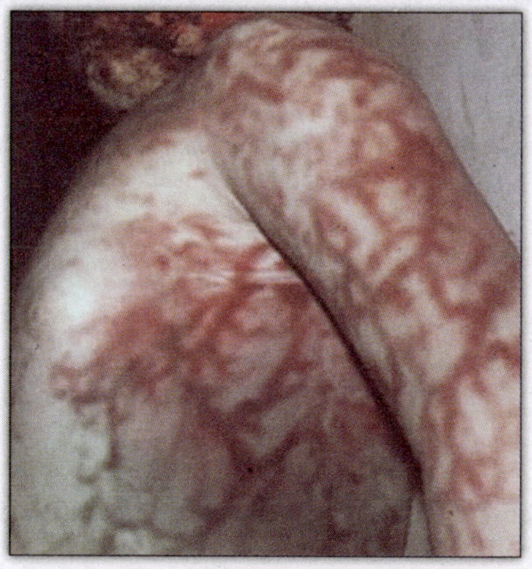

49. Ans. (a) Singeing of hairs, lashes, eyebrows

Ref: Gautam Biswas 3rd ed page 274, www.up todate.com

Inhalation injury is a nonspecific term that refers to damage to the respiratory tract or lung tissue from heat, smoke, or chemical irritants carried into the airway during inspiration. The term is often used synonymously with smoke inhalation injury. It is rare to find isolated inhalational burn injury and signs of Flame burn like Singeing of hairs, lashes, eyebrows are often seen.

Singeing of facial hairs however can be seen in inhalational injury, they cannot specifically tell us airway involvement as they are due to Flame burns. Now the dispute arises about the Yellow sputum. We talked to many FMT faculty and Professors and they all provided us one dictum and one opinion:

- **Dictum:** Singeing of hairs, lashes, eyebrows is a sign of Flame burn (also it is no specific sign of airway involvement)
- **Opinion:** Inhalational injury invariably leads to secondary infection of airway and hence Yellow sputum, hence a tell-tale sign of airway involvement (the initial finding however might be the sooty carbonaceous sputum).

Physical findings that are specific to Airway involvement/ Inhalational injury are:

- Singed nasal vibrissae
- Soot in the oropharynx, nasal passages, proximal airways
- **Sooty carbonaceous sputum**
- **Brassy cough**
- Hoarseness, and stridor, which increase the work of breathing and may lead to respiratory fatigue with sub- and suprasternal retractions.

Signs of lower respiratory tract injury may include any or all of the following:

- Tachypnea
- Decreased breath sounds
- Wheezing
- Rales and Rhonchi
- Use of accessory respiratory muscles

With inhalation, there is laryngeal, tracheal and respiratory burns that may progress to adult respiratory distress syndrome

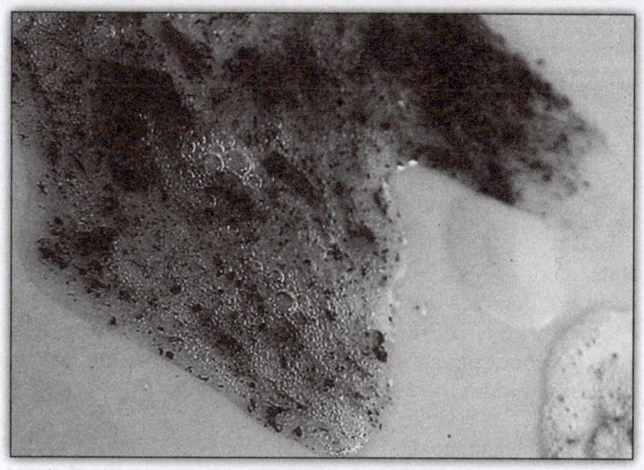

Fig: Sooty Carbonaceous Sputum

FORENSIC MEDICINE • Answers with Explanations

50. Ans. (b) Surgeon performing the liver transplant

Ref: Gautam Biswas 3rd ed page 30, Reddy 33rd ed page 651

Transplantation of Human Organ Act 1994	
Section 1	Human organ was replaced by **"HUMAN ORGAN AND TISSUE"** (Tissue except blood) in 2011 Amendment
Section 2 (i)	2011 Amendment clarified Near relative as; spouse, son, daughter, father, mother, brother, sister, grandfather, grandmother, grandson, granddaughter
Section 2 (f)	Section 2 (f) of The Transplantation of Human Organs Act 1994 states that, a "donor" means any person not less than 18 years of age, who voluntarily authorizes the removal any of his/her organ removal for therapeutic purposes.
Section 2 (q)	Introduced in 2011 Amendment; TRANSPLANT COORDINATOR; a person appointed by the hospital for coordinating all matters related to transplantation.
	Aims at regularization and monitoring of organ donation, harvesting and transplantation in its various aspects A person declared brain dead is legally and clinically dead **Aims:** • Put an end to money making/commercial transplant • Brain dead patients as suitable donors for organ transplantation (valid only when declared dead by brain death certification committee) • Allows cadaveric donation to those in need • Allows live donor to donate its organs to close relatives only (up to uncle and aunts) • Allows mutual swapping of organs between two families in need (recent amendment) • Exceptional cases of live donors are transferred to AUTHORIZATION COMMITTEE for prior approval
Section 3 (6)	Where any human organ is to be removed from the body of a person in the event of his brain-stem death, no such removal shall be undertaken unless such death is certified, in such form and in such manner and on satisfaction of such conditions and requirements as may be prescribed, by a **Board of medical experts** consisting of the following namely: • The registered medical practitioner in charge of the hospital in which brain-stem death has occurred • An independent registered medical practitioner, being a specialist, to be nominated by the registered medical practitioner specified in cause (i), from the panel of names approved by the Appropriate authority • A neurologist or a neurosurgeon to be nominated by the registered medical practitioner specified in clause (i), from the panel of names approved by the Appropriate Authority • The registered medical practitioner treating the person whose brain-stem death has occurred
Section 9 (1A)	When donor or recipient being near relative is a foreign national, prior approval of Authorization committee is required (2011 Amendment)
Section 9 (1B)	No organ or tissue shall be removed from a Minor for the purpose of transplantation before his/her death (2011 Amendment)
Section 9 (1C)	No organ or tissue shall be removed from a Mentally challenged for the purpose of transplantation before his/her death (2011 Amendment)
Section 18 (a)	Punishment for members of medical profession is Previously: Imprisonment up to 5 years and fine of ₹ 10, 000 (Original) **After 2011 Amendment:** Imprisonment up to 10 years and fine up to rs 20 lakh (2011 Amendment) Removal of name from medical register for 2 years for 1st offence and permanently for subsequent offence **Punishment for commercial dealings in human organs**: Punishable with imprisonment for a term from 5 to 10 years and fine of 25 lakh to 1 crore

Note:

Cadaveric donation of organs can be done to anyone in need but only after the consent of the close relatives or person in possession of dead body even if dead person has declared his body to be donated in his will

- Live donor can only donate to close relatives (mother father sister brother son daughter, grandparents, uncle aunt).
- Cases in which live donor wants to donate to
  - Not close relative
  - Foreign nationals
  - To a person to whom he is emotionally attached or stayed together for a long time

Such cases are transferred to AUTHORIZATION COMMITTEE which investigates the cases and enquire about the background of such cases by looking at various documents and proof. It may grant permission or dismiss the case as it may deem fit.

- Dead Bodies in which the medicolegal investigations are pending cannot be used for transplantation activities in any case. However, if police officer/medicolegal officer is satisfied that organ removal will not hamper criminal inquest/enquiry, he can allow for the same.
- In unclaimed bodies, after 48 hours, consent for transplant can be given by hospital authority/employer/head of institution

51. Ans. (d) Declaration of Helsinki

Ref: Nageshwar Rao 2nd ed page 24, Gautam Biswas 3rd ed page 6

See Table of "Various Declarations Adopted by WMA in Chronological Order" In FMT AIIMS Nov 2016 (see page no. 523)

52. Ans. (d) Recent micro injuries

Ref: J Forensic Sci. 1997 Mar;42(2):316-9, McCauley J, Guzinski G, Welch R, Gorman R, Osmers F (1987) Toluidine blue in the corroboration of rape in adult victim. Am J Emerg Med 5:105–108 152.

All forensic medicine textbooks give reference of either of these two articles in bibliography.

"Application of toluidine blue dye increased the detection rate of posterior fourchette lacerations". Toluidine blue is an important tool to detect and document genital and perianal injuries following sexual assault. Application of toluidine blue dye and its subsequent removal from unstained areas by means of a destaining reagent, such as diluted acetic acid or a lubricant has been shown to increase the detection rate of **recent posterior fourchette lacerations** from 16% to 40% in adult rape victims.

53. Ans. (d) Little finger

Ref: Handbook of Fingerprint recognition by David Maltoni page 163, Forensic Science: The Basics, Second Edition Kathy Mirakovits Page 158

The little fingers are never recorded because they are not particularly well suited for fingerprint comparison.

Dactylography

AKA: Dactuloscopy, Dermatographics, Galton systen, Fingerprint study

Sir Henry Galton (1892) depending on the arrangements of papillary ridges classified the finger prints into 4 major o primary types.

Arch = 7% (Plain and Tented)

Loop = 65% (Most common, Ulnar loop and Radial loop)

Whorl = 25% (Circular, Spiral clockwise, Spiral Counterclockwise)

Composite: Mixed of all three patterns above (2-3%)

Whole pattern Loop pattern Arch pattern

There exist four types of fingerprint readers:

Optical readers take a visual image of the fingerprint using a digital camera. Cheap and used in mobiles

Capacitive or **CMOS readers** use capacitors and thus electrical current to form an image of the fingerprint

Ultrasound fingerprint readers costly

Thermal

Note:

The little fingers are never recorded because they are not particularly well suited for fingerprint comparison

Most suitable fingerprints in fingerprint scanners : **Index finger > Thumb > Middle finger > Ring finger**.

Most suitable for ink impression fingerprints on papers/documents: **Thumb > Index finger > Middle finger > Ring finger**

- Fingerprints are formed during **Intrauterine life.**
- Fingerprints are 100% accurate method of identification
- In practice minimum **12 points matching** is considered as proof of identity (In India), however traditionally **16 points matching** is considered by most foreign Authors. Question can be asked in two forms. Minimum matching and normally considered
- No two person can have same Finger prints, not even identical twins
- Chances of two person having identical fingerprints is **1 in 64000 million**
- Faint and invisible finger prints (**Latent Fingerprints**) can be made visible by special techniques like **Aluminum hydroxide.**
- Finger prints can be taken from dead bodies and even putrified bodies.
- The first Finger print Bureau in world was established at **Kolkata** on 12th June 1897 at Writer's building.

54. Ans. (d) 143 cm

Ref: Nageshwar Rao 2nd ed page 105, Reddy 33 ed page 85

Length of long bones is calculated by Hepburn osteometric board and Total stature is calculated by Karl Pearson formula. Total Length = 70. 64 + (2.9 × Length of humerus) = 70.64 + (2.9 × 24.5) = 70.64 + 71.05 = 141.69 (closest is 143)

Identification of Race			
	Negro/Black, Aryan, Indian	**European/Caucasians**	**Mongols**
Skull type	Dolichocephaly (long headed)	Mesaticephaly (moderate headed)	Brachycephaly (broad headed)
Cephalic index	70-74.9	75-79.9	80 and above
Height index	72	71	75
Nasal index	55	46	50
Dental features	Two lingual cusps on mandibular first premolars	Long pointed canine roots. Lateral incisor in upper jaw is smaller than the central, especially in females. **Carabelli's tubercle/cusp** is an anomalous cusp on the mesial palatal surface of the upper 1st permanent molars, most commonly seen among Europeans (75–85%) (50% of American whites and 34% of Afro-Americans).	**Bull-tooth or 'taurodontism'** especially in maxillary molars, **Enamel pearls** (small nodules of enamel on tooth surface of premolars) and ***congenital lack of upper 3rd molars*** are commonly seen in Mongoloids. **Shovel-shaped** uppercentral incisors
Cross section of hair	Kidney shaped	Oval	Round

* Race of a dead remains can be determined by Cephalic index, Height index and Nasal index

\# Cephalic index also known as Breadth index is obtained by multiplying maximum transverse breadth by 100 and dividing it by maximum anteroposterior diameter. The breadth is the greatest diameter across the skull above the mastoid process. The length is measured between the glabella and the external occipital protuberance.

% **Taurodontism** is an aberration of teeth that lacks the constriction at the level of the cemento-enamel junction characterized by elongated pulp chambers and apical displacement of bifurcation or trifurcation of the roots, giving it a rectangular shape. The term means **'bull like' teeth,** and derived from similarity of these teeth to those of cud chewing animals.

** Maximum length of long bones are measured with osteometric board (**Hepburn osteometric board** modified by Trevor), not tapes or calipers as it is not accurate. If incomplete skeleton is found, but individual bones not fragmented individual bones are measured by osteometric board and multiplication factors applied to obtain the stature according to **Karl Pearson's formula**

To calculate stature by length of long bones

Trotter and Glaister formulae/Karl Pearson formulae > Multiplication factor > Thumb rules

Karl pearson formulae for males: Humerus 70.64 + (2.9 x humerus length)

Femur 81.3 + (1.88 x femur length)

Multiplication factors for male: Humerus 7.08

Femur 3.60

Tibia 4.20

Note: Both Karl Pearson formula and Multiplication factors are different for males and females. Mostly male formula is asked. Very slight difference in female formula and also practically it does not makes much difference. Hence, we have mentioned only male's formula.

Thumb rule

- Humerus is 20%, tibia is 22%, femur is 27%, and vertebral column is 34% of total skeleton. 2-4 cm is added for soft tissue to get total height
- In fully extended both arms, measurement from tip of right middle finger tip to left gives the total height of body
- (Length of one arm × 2) + 30 cm for both clavicles + 4 cm for sternum id equal to stature
- Vertex to symphysis pubis = half of stature
- Sternal notch to symphysis pubis × 3.3 = stature
- Height of a person is max in the morning after sleep due to muscles relaxed and diurnal variation is 1 to 5 cm

55. Ans. (b) Less than 17.5 years

Ref: Reddy 33 rd ed fig 4.27, 4.28

In the given picture plate: All the 8 carpals bone have appeared i.e. age is more than 9–12 years (pisiform is last to appear) lower end of radius fusion occur at 18–19 years and lower end of ulna fusion occur at 17–18 years. In the above picture lower end of radius and ulna have not ossified (epiphyseal plate is visible. Hence the age of the child is between 12 and 17–18 years. Hence, less than 17.5 years is most correct answer.

In human anatomy, there are 8 carpal bones which can be classified as either belonging to two transverse rows, or three longitudinal columns.

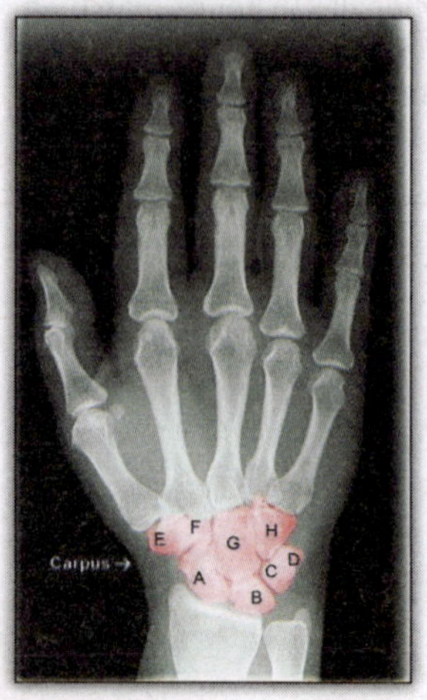

Original photo is by Dr. Jochen Lengerke at de. wikipedia
A = Scaphoid B = Lunate
C = Triquetrum D = Pisiform
E = Trapezium F = Trapezoid
G = Capitate H = Hamate
1 = Radius 2 = Ulna 3 = Metacarpus

Identification of Age		
Identification of Age by Galstaun Chart (Most Accepted) Age in Years		
Ossification Center	**Girls (Years)**	**Boys (Years)**
Elbow	13-15 (Head of radius-14, Olecranon -15)	15-17 (Head of radius-16, Olecranon -17)
Wrist	16-17 (Lower end of radius-16.5, lower end of ulna-17) (Pisiform- last bone in the wrist- 12-17)	18-19 (Lower end of radius-16-17, lower end of ulna-18) (Pisiform- last bone in the wrist- 9-12)
Shoulder	17-18	19-20
Iliac crest	17-19	19-20
Ischial tuberosity	20	20
Inner end of clavicle	20	22
Lower end of femur	14-17	14-17
Lower end of tibia	14-15	15-17

Identification of Age by Carpal Bones

There are 8 carpal bones and Pisiform is last to appear. Approximate age before appearance of Pisiform can be given from the number of carpal bones. i.e. **Total number of carpal bones = Age in years**
At 9th year all 8 carpal bones are present.

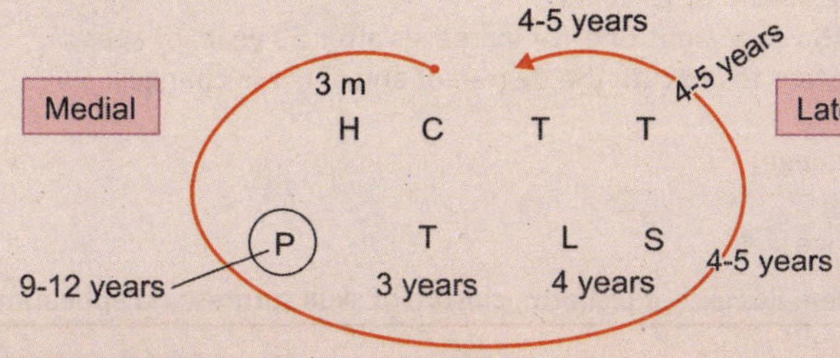

Identification of Age by Sternum

	Appearance	Fusion	
Manubrium	5-6 months intra uterine	60 years with body	
Body 1st segment	5-6 months intra uterine	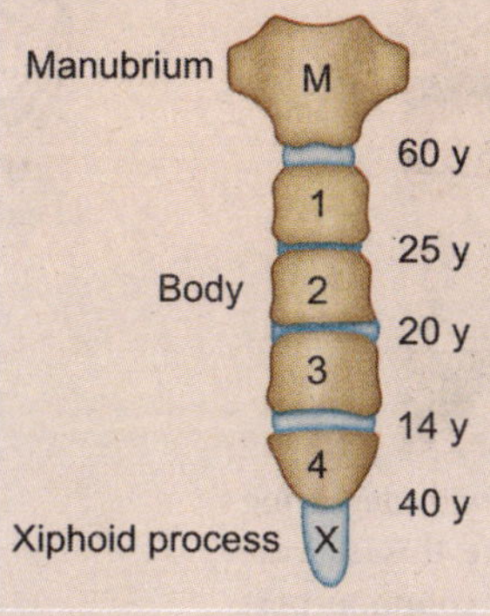	14-25 years from below upwards
Body 2nd segment	7 months intra uterine		
Body 3rd segment	7 months intra uterine		
Body 4th segment	10 months intra uterine		
Xiphoid	3 years	40 years with body of sternum	

Identification of Age by Dental Pattern

Stack's method	Stack evolved a method to estimate the age from the weight of the erupting teeth of fetus and infant. He provided a regression line of weight of growing dental tissues against age **(from 5 months in utero to postnatal age of 7 months)**
Boyde's method	This method, applicable mainly to estimate age of dead infants, is based on counting the number of cross striations in the enamel of teeth (incremental lines) from *neonatal line* onwards. Neonatal line is formed soon after birth and can be seen in about 3 weeks, or by electron microscopy 1–2 days after birth

Contd...

Miles' method	The amount of wear on all three permanent molars occurs at comparable rates which can be assessed, and age estimation made on the basis of comparison to the baseline. Miles also developed a method to determine age at death by measuring the thickness of enamel and dentin from neonatal line and divided it by appropriate daily rate of formation
Gustafson's method	Age estimation consists of microscopic examination of longitudinal section of central part of the tooth to assess changes in teeth as a result of wear and tear with advancing age. Estimate age between **25–60 years.** Useful only while examining a dead body or skeletal remains, as teeth need to be extracted for examination. It is based on criteria given 6 criteria • **Attrition:** Wearing down of occlusal surface due to mastication, first involving enamel, then dentin and lastly pulp. • **Periodontosis:** Retraction of gum margin and loosening of tooth exposing the neck and adjacent parts of roots. • **Secondary dentin:** Progressive infilling of the dental pulp cavity, decreases the size of cavity and may completely obliterate it. • **Cementum apposition:** Cementum increase in thickness around the root due to changes in tooth position, continuously deposited throughout life and forms incremental lines. • **Root resorption:** Involves both cementum and dentin. Starts at apex and extends upwards. • **Root transparency:** Occurs in root from below upwards in lower jaw and above downwards in upper jaw due to rarefaction of the dentin tissue. ***Most reliable of all criteria.*** **NOTE:** • Periodontosis is estimated before tooth is extraction • Tooth is ground down on glass slabs from both sides to about 1 mm, which allows estimation of transparency, then it is further ground to about ¼ mm for microscopic examination. • Anterior teeth are more suitable than posterior teeth. Merit decreases from incisors to premolars, molars are quite unsuitable. • All changes are absent at 15 years. • Error is ± 10–15 years. Limit of error increases after 50 years of age. 0-3 points are allotted to indicate the degree of any of these changes: 0–No change 1–Beginning of change 2–Obvious change 3–Maximum change
Note: Fusion of epiphysis occurs earlier in females except pisiform, closure of skull sutures and appearance of third molar (controversial)	

56. Ans. (c) Pugilistic attitude

Ref: Reddy 33rd ed page 322, Gautam biswas 3rd ed page 270

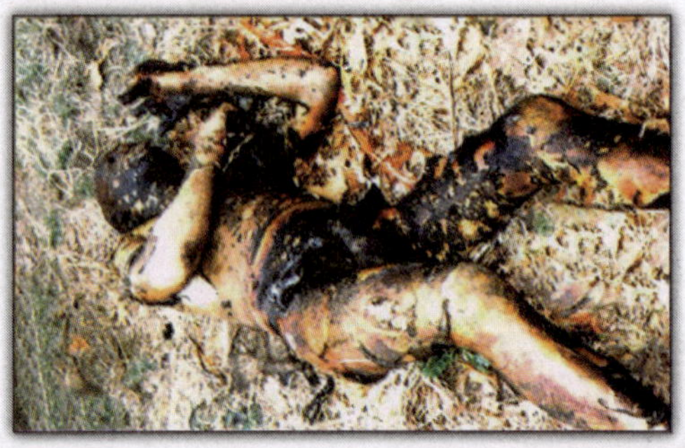

Given photograph shows a charred/burnt body with degloving (peeling off) of skin at hands and various parts, i.e. this is a case of thermal death by dry heat/flame burn. Most common post mortem muscle change in such cases is **Pugilistic attitude/ Boxers/Defense/Fencing attitude.** It is due to heat stiffening which causes coagulation of muscle proteins and dehydration. Legs are flexed at hips and knees. Arms are flexed at elbows and held out in front of the body and fingers are hooked as claws. Flexor muscles being bulkier contract more and causes an attitude of generalized flexion. Can occur in both antemortem and postmortem burns. Dead bodies while being cremated attains a posture of ***"sit up and beg"*** due to this phenomenon. Rigor mortis spreads uniformly and sequentially in nonthermal deaths. Cadaveric spasm takes place in a single group of muscles. Postmortem caloricity cannot be shown in the picture.

57. Ans. (b) Lacerated wound

Ref: Principles of Forensic Medicine and Toxicology by Rajesh Bardale page 186

NOTE

In the Examination Lacerated wound of the chest was given.

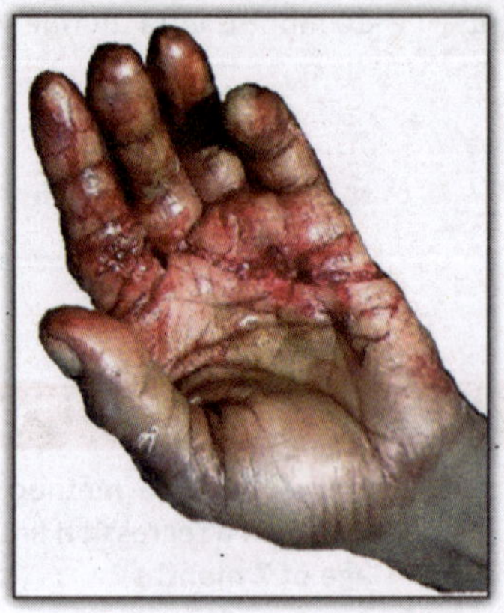

Copyright: Dr Vaibhav Bharat

Fig: Lacerated wound of Hand: With irregular shape and margins (contrary to incised wound), Length greater than depth (contrary to chop wound).

Difference Between Incised, Lacerated and Stab Wounds			
Trait	**Incised wound**	**Lacerated wound**	**Stab wound**
Manner of production	By sharp objects or weapons	By blunt objects or weapons	By pointed, sharp or pointed blunt weapon
Site	Anywhere	Usually over bony prominences	Anywhere, usually chest and abdomen
Margins	Smooth, even, clean-cut and everted	Irregular and often undermined, serrated, minute tears in margins	Clean- cut parallel edges, smooth → pointed sharp Lacerated → pointed blunt
Abrasions on edges	Absent	Usually present	Negative Present with Handle bruise
Bruising	No adjacent bruising of soft tissues	Bruising of surrounding and underlying	Rare
Shape	Linear or spindle shaped; tail and head present	Varies: Usually irregular, shallow tail	Linear or irregular; fish tail may be present
Dimensions	Usually longer than deep; often after gaping	Usually longer than deep	Depth greater than length and breadth
Depth of wound	Structures deeply cut to the depth of the wound	Small strands of tissue at the bottom bridge across margins	Structures cleanly cut
Haemorrhage	Usually profuse and external spurting of blood may be seen	Slight except scalp and external	Varies, usually internal
Hair bulbs	Cleanly cut	Crushed or torn	Usually clean cut
Bones	May be cut	May be fractured	May be punctured
Foreign bodies	Absent	Usually present	Usually absent
Clothes	May be cut	May be torn	May be cut
Note: A thick glass produces atypical incised wound which might look like a Lacerated wound			

58. Ans. (d) Intermediate range

Ref: Reddy 33rd ed page 219

See table of "Shotgun Firearm Injuries" in AIIMS May 2015 FMT (see page no. 547-548)

59. Ans. (a) Increase in weight of lungs in relation to body weight following respiration

Ref: Reddy 33rd ed page 439, Gautam Biswas 3rd ed page 324

Signs/Tests for Live Birth	
Signs of live birth as Recognized by the Civil law	• Cry of the baby- Vagitus vaginalis and Vagitus uterinu • Movement of any part of body • Sneezing and yawning • Heartbeat

Sign of Live Birth as Recognized by Criminal Law	**External signs:**
	• Shape of chest and its measurements: increase AP diameter and circumference
	• Changes in skin
	  ▪ Color -bright red at birth
	Brick red- 2nd to 3rd day
	Yellowish -3rd to 6th day
	Normal-7th to 10th day
	  ▪ Desquamation of skin -begins over abdomen by 2nd day and is completed by 3rd to 4th day
	  ▪ Vernix caseosa
	• Caput succedaneum
	• Cephalohaematoma
	• Change in the umbilical cord
	  ▪ Cut margin dries up by about 2 hours

	▪ The cord dries up about 24 hours. ▪ Red ring appears around umbilicus on the 2nd day. ▪ Cord falls off by 4th-5th day and complete healing of the surface occurs.

Contd...

Signs/Tests for Live Birth

Internal signs/tests

- Position of highest point of diaphragm goes down from 3rd- 4th ribs to 6th/7th ribs.
- Examination of lungs
- **Ploucquet test:** Weight of lungs is 1/70 of total body weight before respiration and becomes 1/35 (increases) after respiration
- **Fodere (static) test:** weight of unrespired lungs is 30 to 40 g and becomes 60 to 70 gm after respiration
- **Hydrostatic test/Rayget test/floatation test:** Unrespired lungs sink in water while respired lungs float in water If there is milk in stomach, it points to live birth. According to this test, non respired lungs sink in water and respired lungs hydrostatic test is not necessary if milk is present in stomach.
- Histological examination of the lungs: Cuboidal/columnar epithelium before respiration and flat squamous epithelium after respiration
- Consistency: Changes from dense firm (liver like) to soft and spongy

- Findings in the stomach and intestine-
  - **Breslau's second life test:** Live born infant swallows air into the stomach during respiration, and if present in small intestine it further confirms live birth. Both ends of stomach and intestine are tied with a knot and air bubbles are seen under water when incision is given on stomach and intestine.
  - Demonstration of air in X-ray.
  - Presence of milk/honey in stomach.
- Meconium - large intestine is completely free of meconium within 24 hours after birth.
- Change in the heart- closure of foramen ovale occurs within 3 months after birth.
- Change in blood vessels-
  - Umbilical arteries (medial umbilical ligament) – start contracting within 10 hours after birth and obliteration completed by 3rd day.
  - Umbilical vein (ligamentum teres) -start contracting by 2nd to 3rd day after birth and completely obliterate by 4th to 6th day.
  - Ductus arteriosus (ligamentum arteriosum) starts to obliterate by 2nd to 3rd day after birth and completed by 7 to 10 days.
  - Ductus venosus(ligamentum venosum) starts to obliterate by 3rd to 4th day after birth and completed by 10 days.
- Incremental line in the enamel of the teeth-one of the surest signs of live birth.
- **Wredin's test:** Test of air in middle ear. The middle ear at birth is filled with gelatinous substance, and at varying interval, it is replaced by air which enters through the Eustachian canal. The time at which this takes place is variable, and therefore the test is of no value
- Presence of some ossification centers e.g. at the lower end of radius, heads of humerus and femur and capitulum of humerus.
- Changes in the blood-
  - Nucleated RBC is absent in peripheral circulation within 24 hours.
  - Fetal haemoglobin 55% to 60% at birth.
- Closure of fontanelle.

AIIMS NOVEMBER 2015

60. Ans. (b) Flumazenil

Ref: Gautam Biswas 3rd ed page 620

Flumazenil is an antidote of Benzodiazepine, and is not used in Alcohol dependence.

Treatment and Prophylaxis of Opium and Alcohol Dependence Syndrome

	Acute withdrawal	Prophylaxis of Withdrawal and Maintenance	Craving	Relapse	Treatment
alcohol	Benzodiazepines Chlordiazepoxide	Acamprosate Naltrexone	Acamprosate Naltrexone	Naltrexone Disulfiram (antabuse)	**Acute**: IV glucose, insulin, benzodizepines, Thiamine **Chronic**: Disulfiram, Citrated calcium carbimide (temposil) Chlorpromazine, Clonidine
Opium	Beta blocker, clonidine Needed short term	Methadone > Buprrnorphine > Codeine	Propranolol relieves anxiety and craving	Naltrexone	IV/IM Naloxone (nalmefen) followed by oral naltrexone for maintenance.

61. Ans. (a) IPC 193

Ref: Gautam Biswas 3rd ed page 471, Parikh 6th ed page 1.10, http://bombayhighcourt.nic.in/libweb/oldlegislation/ipc1860/index.html

The case in question is of Suicide not attempted suicide plus the autopsy is performed hence we can presume that the doctor in question is a government doctor. In both the cases the doctor is bound to inform the police (Section 202 IPC). However, it is point worthy to note that a medicolegal autopsy is not performed without informing the police. Hence, we can presume that the doctor had already informed the police and section 202 IPC is not applicable.

191	**Perjury definition**: A witness who after taking oath or making a solemn affirmation, willfully makes a false statement which he knows or believes to be the false
192	Fabricating false evidence (definition)
193	**Punishment for Perjury/false evidence:** Whoever intentionally gives false evidence in any stage of a judicial proceeding, or fabricates false evidence for the purpose of being used in any stage of a judicial proceeding, shall be punished with imprisonment of either description for a term which may extend to seven years, and shall also be liable to fine

NOTE

- Both 192 and 193 IPC were given in the option, since IPC 192 talks about the definition of giving false evidence and section 193 talks about the punishment of giving false evidence, option (B) 193 IPC is the better answer.
- Don't get confused by Section 202 IPC (If given in option). Section 201, 202 IPC is applicable if a doctor fails to Inform the police about the cases which he is bound to inform even if not asked, like Poisoning, Rape. On the other hand, Section 193 IPC is applicable when doctor gives false evidence/Conceals evidence in the court of law or the investigating officer.
- **Government doctor**: Bound to report all cases of poisoning whether suicidal or accidental or homicidal Sec. 39 CrPC, bound to report all cases of unnatural deaths Sec. 40 CrPC
- **Private practitioner**: Bound to report all unnatural deaths, bound to report only homicidal poisoning CrPC: 39 and not accidental/suicidal

62. Ans. (c) Fracture

Ref: Reddy 33rd ed page 240, Gautam Biswas 3rd ed page 290, Parikh 6th ed page 4.183, APC Essentials of Forensic Medicine and Toxicology By Anil Aggrawal 1st ed page 235, Sabiston 19th ed page 612, Bailey 26th ed page 430

Fracture is seen in tertiary blast injury but is not a component of Marshall's triad.

Types of Blast Injuries				
	Primary	Secondary	Tertiary	Quaternary
Mechanism	Effect of pressure differential (waves) on victim	Due to primary and secondary projectiles/ fragments/flying debris. Most common blast injuries	Due to individual being thrown by blast wind, i.e. Victim's body becomes a projectile	Not due to primary, secondary and tertiary injury. E.g. Inhalation/ absorption of toxins/ infections of blast
Organs affected	Gas filled organs like; Ear drum> Lungs (Blast Lung = Butterfly pattern on CXR) > GIT	Any body part may be affected. Injuries consist of typical **Marshalls triad**: Puncture **Laceration, Abrasions, Bruises *(Mnemonic LAB)*** with tattoing of body (Although fractures do occur in blast injuries, they are non specific and are not a part of Classic Marshall's triad)	Any body part may be affected. Fracture and traumatic amputation	Any body part may be affected. Burns, crush injury,
Underwater blast	Increased Primary blast injury	Decreased secondary blast injury	Decreased tertiary blast injury	Decreased quaternary blast injury

Contd...

Types of Blast Injuries				
	Primary	Secondary	Tertiary	Quaternary
Force of Explosion	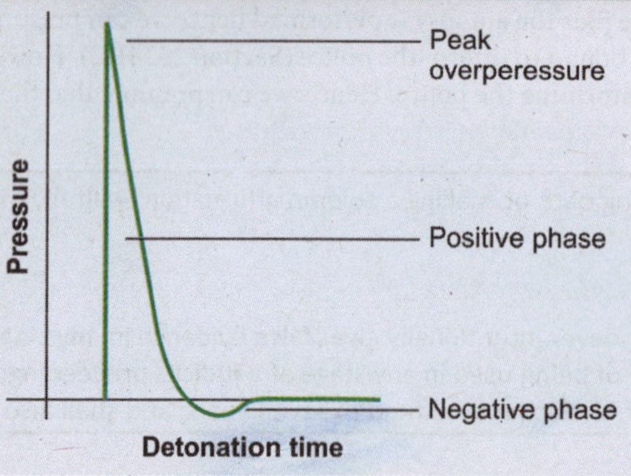		Force of explosion is directional as it travels from source of detonation to the surrounding in positive part of dynamic over compression wave and from surrounding to center of source during negative part of dynamic over compression wave. Force of explosion decreases rapidly as it lasts for few milliseconds only	

Footnote:

- Gas- or air- containing structures (**Hollow organs like lungs, Bowel, ear drums**) within the body are most affected by primary blast injury, because a pressure difference develops between the body surface and internal organ.
- Most common affected organ in Air blast: TM > LUNG > GIT
- Most common affected organ in Underwater blast with head inside: TM> GIT
- Most common affected organ in Air Blast with body underwater: TM> LUNG> GIT
- Most common affected organ in Underwater blast with body inside but head outside: GIT
- Most severely affected organ in Air Blast: LUNGS
- Most severely affected organ in Underwater blast: GIT
- Pulmonary barotrauma is the **most common cause of death** and morbidity in blast injury.
- Colon is the most common site of hemorrhage and perforation in GIT
- Risk factors: Close to detonation, closed room, against the wall
- All types of blast injury are usually evident if an individual is very close to the epicenter of the explosion
- When a high explosive is detonated, it produces shock wave which spreads concentrically from the explosion site at the speed of sound, causing a tremendous blast effect.
- **Intracranial hemorrhage** occurs with considerable frequency
- Blast effect is easily transmitted in water. The **hollow viscera are mainly prone to underwater explosions** and since there are no injuries due to secondary impact, the victim presents very little external but massive internal damage

63. Ans. (b) Nitrobenzene

Ref: Forensic Medicine and Toxicology By R. N. Karmaka 3rd ed page 70

See Table of Specific Odor of Poisons in ENT November 2016 (see page no. 525)

Nitrobenzene is an organic compound with the chemical formula $C_6H_5NO_2$. It is a water-insoluble pale, yellow oil with shoe polish-like odor. Approximately 97% of nitrobenzene is consumed in the production of aniline, which is a precursor to rubber chemicals, pesticides, dyes (particularly azo dyes), explosives, and pharmaceuticals.

64. Ans. (d) Hydrofluoric acid (HF)

Ref: Reddy 33rd ed page 530, Gautam Biswas 3rd ed page 482, APC Essentials of Forensic Medicine and Toxicology by Anil Aggrawal 1st ed page 458

Corrosive mineral acid produces coagulative necrosis on contact due to exothermic reaction

Corrosive alkali cause liquefaction necrosis on contact and causes more severe injury due to their hygroscopic action.

Hydrofluoric acid is the only acid that produces liquefactive necrosis

Acids are hydrogen containing substances that on dissolution in water produces hydronium ions. They produce coagulative necrosis of tissue on contact. Hydrofluoric acid is a prominent exception, since it produces liquefactive necrosis.

Sabiston 18th ed chapter 22; Hydrofluoric acid is a toxic substance used widely in both industrial and domestic settings and is the ***strongest inorganic acid*** known. Such burns are managed differently from other acid burns in general. Hydrofluoric acid produces dehydration and corrosion of tissue by free hydrogen ions. In addition, the fluoride ion complexes with bivalent cations such as calcium and magnesium to form insoluble salts. Systemic absorption of the fluoride ion can then induce intravascular calcium chelation and hypocalcemia, which causes ***life threatening arrhythmias.*** All patients with hydrofluoric acid burns are admitted for cardiac monitoring, with particular attention paid to ***prolongation of the QT interval.***

Bailey 26th ed page 400: It is best not to split-skin graft these hydrofluoric acid wounds initially, but to do this at a delayed stage.

Corrosive Injury		
	Acid injury	**Alkali injury**
Incidence	Less common	More common
Severity	Less severe	More severe
Ingestion- Most common site in GIT	Stomach (Antrum and pylorus) > Esophagus (because squamous epithelium of Esophagus is resistant to acid)	Esophagus > Stomach (Columnar epithelium of stomach is more resistant to alkali)
Type of injury	Coagulative necrosis (Except Hydrofluoric acid)	Liquefactive necrosis
Eschar formation	Common	Less common

65. Ans. (a) Boric acid

Ref: Gautam biswas 3rd ed page 485, Principles of Clinical Toxicology 3rd ed page 221

Boric Acid

Used as antiseptic, insecticide (cockroach), flame retardant and neutron absorber. Previously used for the treatment of napkin dermatitis. Ingestion causes generalized erythema creating a **boiled lobster appearance** with extensive areas of desquamation (d/d toxic epidermal necrolysis/staph scalded skin syndrome). Death is due to circulatory collapse. Activated charcoal is not used.

66. Ans. (b) Puppe's rule

Ref: Reddy 33rd ed page 225, APC Textbook of Forensic Medicine and Toxicology By Anil Aggrawal page 282

Bullet Kinetics and Injury

Size and configuration of damage caused by bullet depends on:
- Kinetic energy lost by bullet
- Type of tissue along the tract (elastic versus non elastic e.g. bone)

Caliber	Caliber technically means diameter of the inside of the bore (**land to land**) in 1/100th of an inch. Distance between two diametrically opposite lands. Thus, caliber 22 means 22/100 inch = 0.22	X = Bore diameter 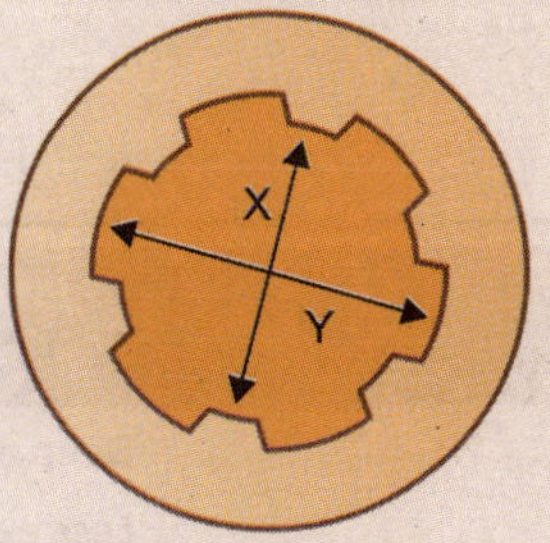 Y = Groove diameter
Stability of bullet	A bullet while passing through a rifled barrel rotates or spins on its longer axis. The spin • Imparts gyroscopic stability • In view of its stability, it increases the accuracy with which a target can be hit • Prevents the bullet from wobbling as it travels in the air	
Energy	Amount of energy transferred is given by the formula **KE = 1/2 MV2** It shows that velocity rather than weight plays a greater role in determining the kinetic energy possessed by the bullet.	

As a bullet projectile moves through a body, it creates because of its intrinsic energy a temporary (cylindrical) cavity along its tract that quickly collapse upon itself within milliseconds of its formation. The cavity created is many times larger than the diameter of the bullet with maximum point of expansion occurring at the point where the bullet is traveling sideways (greatest degree of jaw).

- Bullets fired from handguns are propelled by **low velocity, have low energy** (50-100 J) and result in low energy transfer wounds characterized by injuries confined to wound tract
- Rifle bullets are **high velocity, high energy** (2000–3000 J) have potential to cause high energy transfer wounds producing temporary cavity

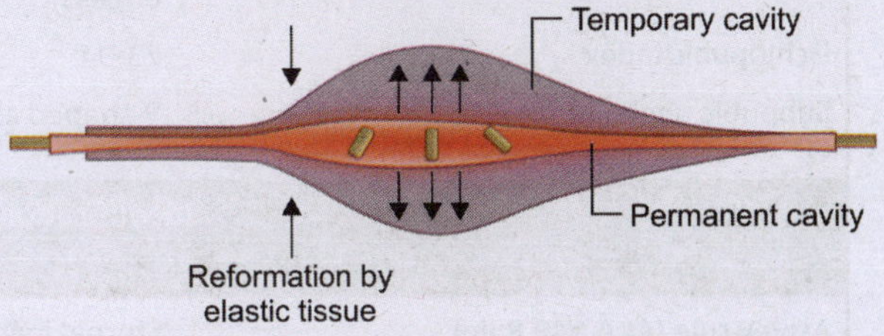

Cavitation due to shock waves of gun shot

Contd...

Bullet Kinetics and Injury	
Puppe's rule is used to determine sequence of shots when more than one shot have been fired at the cranium. First enunciated by Georg Puppe (1867-1925) of Germany. The rule states that when two fracture line intersects each other, the second fracture line never crosses the first one. **Principle:** First bullet will cause certain fracture lines to radiate from the hole it causes. The fracture lines emaciating from the second bullet hole will stop at the lines caused by first hole. The fracture lines emaciated from the third bullet hole will stop at the lines caused by both 1st and 2nd hole and so on.	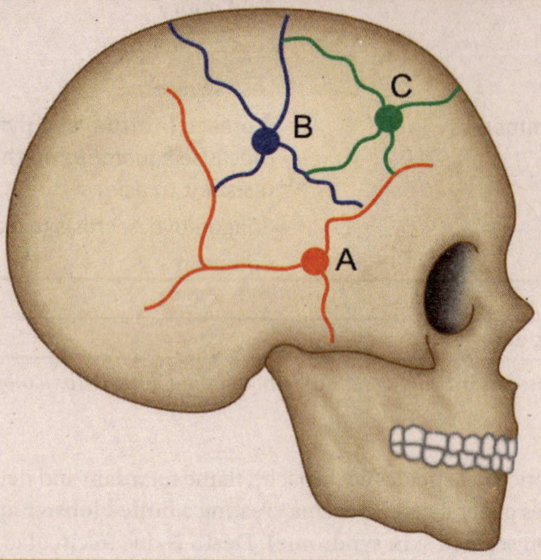

67. Ans. (b) Sex

Ref: APC Essentials of Forensic Medicine and Toxicology By Anil Aggrawal 1st ed page 50, J Punjab Acad Forensic Med Toxicol 2009; 9(1):12-5

Identification of Sex	
According to **Krogman**, the degree of accuracy in sexing adult skeletal remains is as follows	
Entire skeleton	100%
Pelvis and skull	98%
Pelvis alone	95%
Skull alone	90%

Identification of Sex by Pelvis		
	Male	Female
Pelvic inlet	Deep and narrow	Shallow and wide
Ilium	Less expanded	More expanded, splayed walls
Iliac fossa	Shallow	Deep
Suprapubic arch	Narrow, V-shaped, angle <70°	Wide, U-shaped, >90°
Ischial tuberosity	Inverted	Everted
Obturator foramen	Ovoid	Triangular
Greater sciatic notch	Narrow, deep, <90°	Wide, shallow, >90°
Preauricular sulcus	Narrow, shallow and without marked edges	Broad and deep in parous women
Ischiopubic index	73-94	91-150
Subpubic angle	V-shaped angle 70°-75°	Rounded, U-shaped, broader (90-100°) angle
Identification of Sex By Human Sternum		
	Male	Female
Ashley rule (AKA 149 Rule)	Sternal length > 149 mm	Sternal length < 149 mm
Hyrtl's rule	Body is longer and more than twice the length of Manubrium	Body is shorter and less than twice the length of Manubrium
Breadth	More	Less

Contd...

Length of Mesosternum (Body of sternum)	>95 mm	<80 mm
Level of upper margin	Lower part of body of T2	Lower part of Body of T3
Sternal index = $\frac{\text{Length of Manubrium}}{\text{Length of body}} \times 100$	46.2	54.3
Sternal foramen	Twice as common as in females	Less common

Footnote:
- **Rule of 149:** Ashley (1956) proposed this rule for European population
- **Rule of 136:** This rule was given by Ashley (1956) for the population of East Africa.
- For Indian population rule of 136 is better applied (Jit et al 1980, Ankit et al 2013)
- Ashley's rules are predictive but not conclusive. Jit et al applied "Rule of 136" by which they determined the sex of 86% male and 78% female, but individually he can't say if any particular sternum given is definitely male of female

68. Ans. (a) Trauma and tumor

Ref: Parikh 6th ed page 4.89

Ewing's postulate showing relationship between trauma and new growth consists of:
- Evidence of **previous integrity** of the part affected
- Undeniable and **adequate trauma** must be proven
- A **reasonable interval** (neither too short not too long) must elapse between the time of trauma and appearance of tumor
- The disease/tumor must arise exactly at the site of injury
- The tumor must be **confirmed pathologically**

69. Ans. (d) Hanging

Ref: www. ncrb. nic. in

On an average, more than one lakh persons commit suicides every year in the country during the decadal period from 2004 to 2014

The highest incidents of 16,307 suicides were reported in Maharashtra followed by 16,122 suicides in Tamil Nadu and 14,310 suicides in West Bengal accounting for 12.4%, 12.2% and 10.9% respectively of total suicides. The means adopted for committing suicide varied from the easily available means such as consumption of poison, jumping into the well etc. to more painful means such as self-inflicted injuries, hanging, shooting, etc. Like previous year, **'Hanging' (41.8%), Consuming 'Poison' (26.0%), 'Self-immolation' (6.9%) and 'Drowning'** (5.6%) were the prominent means of committing suicides.

70. Ans. (d) Neostigmine has a role in krait bite

Ref: Reddy 33rd ed page 565, Parikh 6th ed page 9.47, Harrison 19th ed page 2736, Snake Bite: Indian Guidelines and Protocol page 425, http://www. Apiindia. org/medicine_update_2013/chap94.pdf

Government of India, Health and Family Welfare Department has prepared a National Snakebite Management Protocol. The question is most probable based on it.

Recall Bias

Some of the students recalled a different set of options. In both the cases the answer would be same.
E. Hump-nosed Pit viper does not respond to ASV
F. ASV is the routine treatment of all the snake bites
G. Supportive measure like ventilation useful with ASV
H. Neostigmine is given in krait bite

Option (A) and (E)

India is estimated to have the highest snakebite mortality in the world. The Big Four" namely common cobra (Naja naja), Russell's viper (Dabiola russelii), saw-scaled viper (Echis carinatus) and common krait (Bungarus caeruleus) are highly venomous and believed to be responsible for most of the poisonous bites in India. However, this assumption of great four, has led to nonidentification of other poisonous species which are going unnoticed and leading to deaths. The recent discovery of the hump-nosed pit viper, capable of causing life threatening symptoms has demonstrated this. This non recognition has led the ASV manufacturers to produce antivenom only against these four species only.

Option (B)

Cobra

Neurotoxic (neuro paralysis + convulsions because effects CNS), Krait : neurotoxic (neuroparalysis only. no convulsions), Vipers: vasculotoxic, Sea snake: myotoxic.

In cobra and krait bites neuroparalysis is a prominent feature.

	Signs and symptoms	Fatal dose	Management	Comments
Elapids **(Cobra, Krait) -neurotoxic**	Local burning, bite marks, muscle weakness, cramps, ptosis, paralysis, dysphagia, convulsions	Cobra-15 mg Krait-6 mg Few hours	Clean and torniquete, Specific/polyvalent antivenin (20 mL around bite, 20 mL IM, 20 mL IV) Elapids specific-Atropine 0.6 mg + Neostigmine 0.5 mg (for Cobra only)	Fangs long, canalised so can give lethal dose through the cloths. Neurotoxins and cholinesterases are predominant in Elapid venom

Contd...

	Signs and symptoms	Fatal dose	Management	Comments
Vipers **(Russell's, Saw scaled)-vasculotoxic**	Vomiting, hemolysis, haemorrhages, pupils dilated, renal tubular necrosis, collapse	Viper-40 mg Few days	General treatment same. Viper specific: heparin and fibrinogen	Fangs short, fixed, grooved so cannot bite effectively through clothes. Hemolysin and thromboplastin are predominant in viper venom
***Sea Snakes*-myotoxic**	Generalized muscle pain, myoglobinuria, hyperkalemia	Uncertain. Not fatal.	General treatment same	

Option (C)

To counteract the neuroparalytic symptoms, neostigmine is the drug of choice but unfortunately it works well in postsynaptic poison like that of cobra only. in case of presynaptic poisons like krait, it is of no use. Atropine is always administered before neostigmine to block the anticipated muscarinic side effects of neostigmine in a dose of 0.5 mg.

Option (D) and (H)

Neostigmine is an anticholinesterase, which is particularly effective in postsynaptic neurotoxins such as those of cobra and is not useful against presynaptic neurotoxin i. e. common Krait and the Russell's viper

Option (F) and (G)

See national snake bite management protocol below:

National Snake Bite Treatment Protocol (India)

Patient Assessment phase: On arrival

- Deal with any life-threatening symptoms on presentation, i.e. **Airway, Breathing and Circulation.**
- If there is evidence of a bite where the skin has been broken, give **Tetanus Toxoid**
- Routine use of antibiotic is not necessary, although it should be considered if there is evidence of cellulitis or necrosis.

Diagnosis Phase: General Principles

- Wherever possible, identify the snake responsible for the bite
- Determine if any traditional medicines have been used, they can sometimes cause confusing symptoms.
- Determine the exact time of the bite. This can give indications as to the progression of any symptoms
- All patients will be kept under observation for a minimum of **24 hours**
- Many species, particularly the Krait and the Hump-nosed pit viper are known for the length of time it can take for symptoms to manifest. Often this can take between 6 to 12 hours

Diagnosis Phase: Symptoms

	Cobra	Krait	Russell's Viper	Saw Scaled Viper	Humpnosed Pit Viper
Local pain tissue damage	Yes	No	Yes	Yes	Yes
Ptosis/Neurological signs	Yes	Yes	Yes	No	No
Haemostatic abnormalities	No	No	Yes	Yes	Yes
Renal complications	No	No	Yes	No	Yes
Response to neostigmine	Yes	No	No	No	No
Response to ASV	Yes	Yes	Yes	Yes	No

Diagnosis Phase: Investigations

- **20 Minute Whole Blood Clotting Test (2OWBCT)** considered the most reliable test of coagulation and can be carried out without specialist training
- Other Useful Tests (depending on availability)
  - Haemoglobin/PCV/Platelet count/PT/APTT/FDP/D-Dimer
  - Peripheral Smear
  - Urine Tests for Proteinuria/RBC/Haemoglobinuria/Myoglobinuria
  - Biochemistry for Serum creatinine/urea/Potassium
  - Oxygen saturation/PR/BPi RR/Postural Blood Pressure
  - ECG/X-ray/CT/Ultrasound (The use of X-Ray and ultrasound are of unproven benefit, apart from identification of bleeding in Viperine bites)
  - ABG (if facilities available)

Contd...

Treatment phase: Pain Management

- Pain can be relieved with oral paracetamol (Adult dose of 500-1000m9 4-6 hourly. Paediakic dose 10mg/kg every 4-6 hourly orally) or Mild opiates such as Tramadol, 50 mg can be used orally
- Aspirin should not be used due to its adverse impact on coagulation.
- Do not use nonsteroidal anti-inflammatory drugs (NSAIDs) as they can cause bleeding.

Treatment Phase: Anti Snake Venom (ASV)

- Anti-snake venom (ASV) is the **mainstay of treatment**. In India, polyvalent ASV, i.e. effective against all the four common species; Russell's viper, common cobra, common Krait and saw-scaled viper and no monovalent ASVs are available.
- The polyvalent Anti snake venom used in India is found ineffective for bites from **Humpnose pit viper** and less effective against Sochurek's saw scaled viper'
- ASV is produced both in **liquid and lyophilized forms.** There is no evidence to suggest which form is more effective.
- Liquid ASV requires a reliable cold chain and has 2-year shelf life. Lyophilized ASV, in powder form, has 5-year shelf life and requires only to be kept cool.
- Each vial is 10 mL of reconstituted ASV.
- ASV is recommended to be administered in the initial dose of **8-10 Vials**
- Children should receive the same ASV dosage as adults.
- All ASV to be administered over **1 hour** at constant speed.
- Local administration of ASV near or at the bite site should not be done. It is ineffective, painful and can raise the intracompartmental pressure.
- After initial ASV dose, no additional ASV should be given until the next clotting test at **6 hours.** This is due to the inability of the liver to replace clotting factors in less than 6 hours.
- Purely local swelling, even if accompanied by a bite mark from an apparently venomous snake, is not ground for administering ASV
- No test dose of ASV is required

Treatment Phase: Repeat ASV

- After **6 hours** a further coagulation test should be performed and a further dose should be administered in the event of continued coagulation disturbance.
- This dose should also be over 1 hour. CT tests and repeat doses of ASV should continue on a 6 hourly pattern until coagulation is restored, unless a species is identified as one against which polyvalent ASV is not effective.
- The repeat dose should be **5 - 10 vials** of ASV i.e. half to one full dose of the original amount
- 20 vials (10 + 10) is the maximum dose of ASV that should be given to a neurotoxically envenomed patient.

Prevention of ASV Reactions - Prophylactic Regimes

Two regimens are normally recommended:

- 100 mg of Hydrocortisone and HI antihistamine (10 mg Chlorpheniramine Maleate; 22.5 mg IV pheniramine maleate IV or 25 mg Promethazine HCL I.M.) 5 minutes before ASV administration. The dose for children is 0.I–0.3 mg/kg of antihistamine IV and 2 mg/kg of Hydrocortisone IV Antihistamine should be used with caution in pediatric patients.
- 0.25–0.3 mg adrenaline 1:1000 given subcutaneously

Treatment phase: Treating Complications/Supportive Measures

ARF: Peritoneal dialysis

For hypotension: Usually crystalloids are used for volume expansion. Dopamine can be used dose being is 5-10 μg/kg/minute in normal saline or glucose solutions as IV Drip

Persistent bleeding: Adding clotting factors, fresh frozen plasma (FFP)

Neurological sequelae: Early referral to well-equipped center for management of respiratory failure with Mechanical Ventilation. Elective Endotracheal Intubation and Ventilation while transferring the patient to higher center.

71. Ans. (a) Blistering vesicles

Ref: Parikh 6th ed page 4.168, Gautam Biswas 3rd ed page 484, APC Essentials of Forensic Medicine and Toxicology By Anil Aggrawal 1st ed page 233 table 6

Recall Bias

Some recallers believe that there was another set of options

A. Absence of signing of hair
B. Presence of red line of demarcation
C. Burn at lower level to where acid falls
D. Presence of ulcerated patch

In these options, (B) is incorrect

In chemical burns characteristically, there are ulcerated patches, no blisters, hair is not singed and the red line of demarcation is absent.

Types of Burn Injuries			
	Dry heat burns	Scald (moist heat burns)	Chemical burns
Cause	Flame or heated solid or radiant heat	Steam or liquid near boiling point > 60°C	Corrosive acid, alkali
Site	At or above the site of contact (as flames tends to rise up)	At or below the site of contact (as liquid tends to flow down). More severe at the point of contact	At or below the site of contact
Edge	Deep burns may fade into more superficial burns, so sharply defined edges may not be present	Sharply defined edges usually present	Sharply defined edges usually present
Skin	Dry, shriveled, charred (if deep)	Sodden (saturated with water) and bleached	Destroyed/Corroded and stained
Blisters/vesicles	At the circumference of the burnt area	Most marked over burnt area	Absent with corrosives. Seen with specific chemicals only, called as Vesicants
Red line of demarcation	Present	Present	Absent
Charring (soot)	Present	Absent	May be present, in case of mineral acids
Singeing of hairs	Present	Absent	Absent
Ulcerated patch	Absent	Absent	Present
Trickle marks	Absent	Present	Present
Scar	Thick and cause disfigurement	Thin and less disfigurement	Thick, Keloid scar, much disfigurement

AIIMS MAY 2015

72. Ans. (c) Heat stroke

Ref: Reddy 33rd ed page 319; Gautam biswas 3rd ed page 264

Clinical Effects of Hyperthermia on Body				
	Heat stroke Heat hyperpyrexia	Heat exhaustion	Heat cramps Miners/strokers/fireman cramps	Heat syncope/heat prostration
Etiology	Impaired thermoregulation impaired sweating	Profuse sweating, Excessive salt and water loss	Profuse sweating, Excessive salt and water loss	Profuse sweating, Excessive salt and water loss + cutaneous vasodilatation
Mechanism	Impaired sweating leading to hyperthermia	Systemic loss of salt and water and inadequately replaced	Local loss in a strenuously working group of muscle, replaced by plain water only leads to dilutional hyponatremia and muscle cramp	Systemic loss followed by systemic and cerebral hypotension l/t sudden collapse
Features	• Rapid onset • Raised body temperature 40 C or more • Delirium convulsion electrolyte imbalance • Dilated pupil followed by pin point pupil • Hot dry skin • Impaired sweating • Tachycardia hypotension	• Insidious onset • Low fever • Dilated pupil • Sweating present • Cool clammy skin • Tachycardia hypotension	Muscle cramps in a localized group of muscles only.	No rise in temperature Seen in tropics and deserts Systolic BP<100

73. Ans. (d) Kevorkian sign

Option (A) Kennedy Phenomenon

Surgical alteration of firearm wounds makes it difficult to interpret whether it was an entry wound or exit wound.

Option (B) Tache Noir

Triangular (base at limbus) discoloration of sclera seen after 3-4 hours of death.

Option (C) Rokitansky sign

There is no such sign in Forensic medicine or otherwise. In forensic medicine Rokitansky method is used in autopsy.

Option (D)

Kevorkian sign is a postmortem change that occurs in the retinal vessels.

- It is characterized by fragmentation of blood column in the retinal vessels.
- It appears **within minutes** after death and lasts for about **1 hour**.
- It can be visualized by using an **ophthalmoscope**.

74. Ans. (a) 18 years

Ref: Gautam Biswas 3rd ed page 367

- When the female is wife of male, age for sexual consent is 15 years
- When the female is not wife of male, age for sexual consent: 18 years

NOTE

consent may be a valid defense if the girl is between 16-18 years and the male is not more than 5 year older than the female

75. Ans. (d) 14 years

Ref: Gautam Biswas 3rd ed table 4.9, Parikh's 6th ed page 2.9

See Table of Identification of Age in FMT AIIMS May 2016

76. Ans. (d) Bruise, laceration and fractures are triad of main injuries seen

Ref: Reddy 33rd ed page 240, Gautam Biswas 3rd ed page 290, Parikh 6th ed page 4.183, APC Essentials of Forensic Medicine and Toxicology By Anil Aggrawal 1st ed page 235, Sabiston 19th ed page 612, Bailey 26th ed page 430

See Table of Types of Blast Injuries in FMT AIIMS NOV 2015 (see page no. 535-3536)

77. Ans. (a) 416 CrPC

Ref: Principles of Forensic Medicine and Toxicology by Rajesh Bardale Page 334

Criminal Procedure Code 1973	
2 (c) CrPC	Defines cognizable offences i.e. arrest without warrant (rape, murder, dacoity)
26 CrPC	Division of offences
39 CrPC	Inform police about every illegal event (**A government doctor is bound to report all cases of poisoning whether suicidal or accidental or homicidal to police**) (A private practitioner is bound to inform only homicidal poisoning) Noncompliance/ not reporting in above matters is punishable under section 176 IPC, Giving false information on such matters is punishable under section 177 IPC
40 CrPC	Inform police about every death (**A government doctor is bound to inform all unnatural deaths to police**)
53 CrPC	Procedure of examination of accused (can be done w/o consent if on request of SI)
53 (a) CrPC	Procedure of examination of RAPE accused
54 CrPC	Accused himself can ask court to get him medically examined to prove his innocence
61-69 CrPC	Summons
160 CrPC	Police IO has the power to summon any witness (except female, male <15 years)
161 CrPC	Police recording of statement in cases
164 (a) CrPC	Procedure of examination of RAPE VICTIM
164 CrPC	MAGISTRATE recording of statement in cases
174 CrPC	Police inquest
174 (3) CrPC	Procedure in dowry death
175 CrPC	Power to summon persons (Medical practitioner can be summoned by IO and he is bound to attend)
176 CrPC	Magistrate inquest (custodial death, dowry death, death in mental asylum)
291 CrPC	This is accepted as evidence in a higher court when it has been recorded and attested by a magistrate in the presence of the accused who had an opportunity of cross examining the witness
357 (c) CrPC	Free treatment by all medical institution to rape/acid attack victims
409 CrPC	Withdrawl of cases by session judge
410 CrPC	Withdrawl of cases by judicial magistrate
411 CrPC	Withdrawl of cases executive magistrate
412 CrPC	Reasons to be recorded for withdrawal of cases
416 CrPC	Postponement of execution of a pregnant woman (up to 6 months after delivery) or change it to life imprisonment by high court

78. Ans. (c) 324

This is a case of simple injury by dangerous weapon

Section 324 IPC is Voluntarily causing Hurt by Dangerous Weapons
Section 326 IPC is Voluntarily causing Grievous injury by Dangerous Weapons

Dangerous Weapon

Any instrument for **shooting** stabbing or cutting, or any instrument which, used as a weapon of offence, is likely to cause death, or by means of fire or any heated substance, or by means of any poison or any corrosive substance, or by means of any explosive substance, or by means of any substance which it is deleterious to the human body to inhale, to swallow, or to receive into the blood, or by means of any animal.

IPC 302	Punishment for murder
IPC 303	Punishment for murder by life-convict
IPC 304	Punishment for culpable homicide not amounting to murder
IPC 304A	**Causing death by gross negligence**—Whoever causes the death of any person by doing any rash or negligent act not amounting to culpable homicide, shall be punished with imprisonment of either description for a term which may extend to **two years**, or with fine, or with both
IPC 304B	Dowry death Where the death of a woman is caused by any burns or bodily injury or occurs otherwise than under normal circumstances *within seven years of her marriage* and it is shown that soon before her death she was subjected to cruelty or harassment by her husband or any relative of her husband for, or in connection with, any demand for dowry, such death shall be called "dowry death" and such husband or relative shall be deemed to have caused her death. Whoever commits dowry death shall be punished with imprisonment for *a term which shall not be less than seven years but which may extend to imprisonment for life.*

79. Ans. (d) The angle of jaw

Ref: Reddy 33ed page 303

Hanging		
Cause of death	In Judicial hanging death takes place due to fracture dislocation at the level of **2nd and 3rd cervical vertebra** which is caused by sudden drop. Fracture dislocation of 1st and 2nd vertebra is less common. The most frequent cause of death by hanging is **obstruction of the cervical blood vessels**. Fracture of the spine and the base of the skull are rarely observed in cases of death by hanging and if so, generally only in cases of a fall from a certain height ("drop") as in judicial hanging	
	Judicial Hanging	**Non-Judicial Hanging**
Manner of death	Legally as punishment	Homicidal, suicidal
Cause of death	Fracture dislocation of c2-c3 > c3 c4 due to drop by 5 to 7 meters/15 to 20 feet approx	Due to compression by ligature asphyxia -15 kg, Compression of carotids-3 to 5 kg, Compression of jugulars-2 kg
Knot	Atypical hanging–below right jaw most commonly (below chin most effective)	Typical or Atypical
Pathophysiology	Rupture of brain stem between pons and medulla leading to immediate unconsciousness. No or minimal signs of asphyxia	Asphyxia
	Typical Hanging When the knot ligature is present at nape of neck i.e. Centrally over the occiput	**Atypical Hanging** When the knot ligature is present at site other than nape of neck. Commonest location of the knot is near the mastoid process or angle of mandible. Occasionally it may be under the chin
	Antemortem Hanging	**Postmortem Hanging**
Motive	Usually suicidal (Homicidal only in Lynching)	Homicidal
Ligature mark	Well developed with parchment like base and is yellow or brown	Not well developed
Saliva	Dribbling of saliva present	Absent

Contd...

Injuries	No other injuries seen	Other injuries causing death seen
Signs of asphyxia	Present	Absent
Circumstantial evidence	Closed room No signs of struggle	Signs of struggle present
Drag marks on body	May be seen	Not seen
Suicide note	May or may not be present	Never present
Rope fibers	May be seen in the hands	Not seen

80. Ans. (c) Paraldehyde

Ref: With text

See table of Specific Odor of Poisons in ENT Nov 2016 (see page no. 525)

Recall Bias

Some people think Chloral Hydrate was option (A) in place of Nitrobenzene. In that case Chloral Hydrate will be marginally a better answer than Paraldehyde.

Forensic medicine books give both Chloral hydrate and Paraldehyde as Acrid/Pear Like smell but some Pharmacology books mentions Chloral hydrate only.

Forensic medicine textbooks place both Chloral hydrate and Paraldehyde on the same spectrum to causes Acrid (Pear) like smell, but pharmacology books specifies that "Pear like smell is of Chloral hydrate, while Paraldehyde smells chemical like" **(Ref: Pharmacology By Gary C. Rosenfeld, David S. Loose Board review series 4th ed page 321, Current Diagnosis and Treatment Emergency Medicine 7th ed ch 47)**

Modern Medical Toxicology By Pillay 4th ed page 204: Paraldehyde poisoning shows pungent odor. In the table Pillay gives Paraldehyde with Chloral Hydrate in Acrid/Pear like smell.

81. Ans. (b) Doctor guilty under last clear chance doctrine

Ref: RN Karmakar FMT 4th ed page 375

It is that chance that the physician gets to take precautionary measures against the damages resulted from the negligent act of the patient. If the physician fails to prevent such damages of the patient even after getting clear time (last chance to clear the potential harm) he cannot bring forward the plea of contributory negligence.

Scenario 1

If the orthopedician advised to take care of the wound by so and so means, and the patient did not take care, and did not come to the OPD when complaint started, and then resulted in osteomyelitis – No Negligence

Scenario 2

Orthopedician applied too tight bandage/plaster/(or orthopaedician missed a fracture scaphoid, one of MC fractures missed) and advised the patient to return to OPD if numbness, pain, swelling etc. happen or progress. The patient does not pay attention to warning symptoms and does not seek medical attention further. Consequently gangrenous necrosis occur. Doctor can plea Doctrine of Avoidable Consequence Rule to reduce the amount of damages to be paid significantly.

Scenario 3

Orthopedician did an undercorrected closed reduction (wrong by Dr). Patient continued to take the limb in use despite instructions of doctor (wrong by patient). Deformity/malunion resulted. Contributory negligence: Wrong by doctor + wrong by patient. Doctrine of Avoidable Consequence Rule: Wrong by doctor + patient avoids reasonable steps to avoid consequence.

Scenario 4

Orthopaedician performs surgery on wrong limb – res ipsa loquitur- criminal negligence.

Defence/Doctrine in Favor and Against a Doctor

Defense for Doctors against Negligence	Doctrine in Favor of Patient for Negligent Doctor
No duty owed to plaintiff Duty discharged according to prevailing standards Informed consent (civil cases only)	**Res ipsa loquitur:** Means 'the thing or fact speaks for itself". Applies to both civil and criminal negligence. Error is so self-evident that the patient's lawyer need not prove the doctor's guilt with medical evidence. The doctor has to prove his innocence ex: wrong limb surgery
Contributory negligence Composite negligence Corporate negligence Vicarious liability Borrowed servant doctrine Product liability by manufacturer	**Doctrine of common knowledge:** In an act involving omission or commission in application of common knowledge. It is a variant of res ipsa loquitur. Here, the patient must prove the act of commission or omission, but he need not produce evidence to establish the standard of care.
Therapeutic misadventure Medical maloccurrence Error of judgement Calculated risk doctrine	**Novus actus interveniens:** New act intervened to break the chain of causation A was suffering from injury after assault by B and admitted in hospital. Negligence of Dr C (say leaving swab after laparotomy) breaks the chain of blame from assailant B to Dr C
Res judicata Res indicate Good samaritan doctrine Doctrine of avoidable consequence rule	**Last clear chance doctrine:** Negligence after negligence of patient despite getting a last chance to avoid the damage

82. Ans. (c) Sparrow foot marks

Ref: Parikh's 6th ed p 4.134-136, Reddy 33rd ed page 281, Gautam Biswas 3rd ed page 285

Recall Bias

Some students feel that the question was not to differentiate between Driver and passenger but just the Identification of Driver.
In car accident, driver and front passenger both died. Which of the following in post mortem examination will help to identify driver EXCEPT: **(a) Seat belt over left shoulder (ans)** (b) Sparrow footmark on the head (c) Whiplash injury to spinal cord (d) Steering wheel impact
The answer will change if only identification of driver is asked. In case of point of differentiation of Driver and passenger is asked, both peculiar points of identification of Driver and Front seat passenger will help to differentiate.

Injuries Sustained by Vehicle Occupants

	Driver	Front seat passenger	Rear seat Passenger
Incidence	Highest	In between	Lowest
Warning of collusion	Yes	No	No
Windscreen injury (Sparrow foot mark)	Yes	Yes	No
Steering wheel injury	Yes	No	No
Dashboard injuries	Yes	Yes	No
Whiplash Injury	Less common because driver is mostly warned and gets time to embrace the steering	Yes. More common than driver	Possible but not common
Seat belt abrasions	On right shoulder in India, On left shoulder in west	On left shoulder in India, On right shoulder in west	No

Note:
- Frequency of injuries of road traffic accident: **Pedestrians injury > Driver injury > Front seat passenger > Rear seat passengers**
- There may be peculiar facial lacerations due to contact with the shattered windscreen known as **'sparrow foot marks'**
- **In Whiplash Injury** there is usually a history of a low velocity rear-end collision in which the occupant's body is forced against the car seat while his or her head flips backwards and then recoils in flexion.

83. Ans. (a) Ring fracture of foramen magnum + lumbar spine injury

Ref: Parikh's 6th ed page 4.9, Gautam Biswas 3rd ed page 293, Reddy 33rd ed page 247

Fall from height causes following spinal- cranial injuries:
- Burst fracture of cervical spine
- Lumbar vertebra fracture
- Ring fracture of foramen magnum
- Ring of the atlas (Jefferson's fracture)

Important Fractures in Forensic

Ring fracture	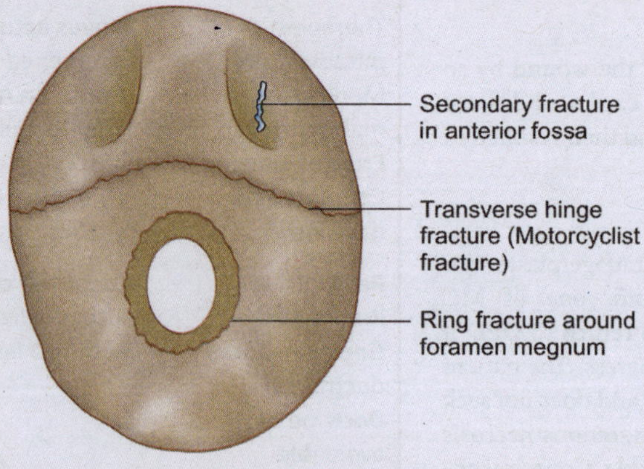	This is a type of fissure fracture that encircles the base of skull around the **foramen magnum,** running from the sella turcica, partly through petrous ridges and then going posteriorly and medially, joining in the posterior fossa. In the front, the fracture may pass through the middle ear and roof of the nose. As a result, the skull gets separated from the spine. In **feet-first impact,** forces transferred upward can result in significant pelvic trauma, as well as a 'ring fracture' of the skull, as forces drive the spinal column upward into the cranial cavity

Contd...

Motorcyclist's fracture	It is name given to a fracture of base of skull in which the skull base is broken down into two separate anterior and posterior halves and they move independently of each other. It is a type of **hinge fracture**. The fracture line runs on the base of middle cranial fossa following the petrous temporal bone.
Depressed fracture/ Fracture *a la signature*	When a portion of fractured bone is driven inwards it is known as depressed fracture. It is also called *'fracture-a-la-signature'* (**signature fracture**), as the shape often points towards the shape of the offending weapon. They are caused by blows with a heavy weapon having small striking surface, such as hammer, axe, brick or chopper.
Pond/Indented/Ping pong ball fracture	This is a smooth concave depression without a fracture line resulting from in buckling of skull, occurring only in the elastic skull of **infants and children** (prior to 4 years of age). A dent is produced instead of cracking. May occur due to obstetric forceps
Comminuted/spider-web/mosaic fracture	Two or more intersecting lines of fracture divide the bone into three or more fragments. It is caused by blows with weapons having large striking surface, such as heavy iron bar, or from a bullet.
Blow out fracture	This is due to blunt trauma to the eye wherein the forces are transmitted via the globe to the bony orbit, causing disruption of the orbital walls. ***Teardrop sign***: The fracture is most commonly involves the thin medial wall and/or orbital floor that results in radiographically, a soft tissue 'teardrop' or polypoid mass in the roof of the maxillary antrum.
Gutter fracture	Part of the thickness of the bone is removed so as to form a gutter, e.g. oblique bullet wounds. It is usually accompanied by comminuted depressed fracture of the inner table of skull
Countercoup injury	Occurs on the opposite side of impact
Fissured fracture	Caused by heavy weapon striking broad surface
Diastatic fracture	Separation of skull sutures
Undertaker's fracture	Rough handling of dead bodies by undertaker leads to fracture dislocation of C6-C7. This fracture dislocation is called as **undertaker's fracture** and may resembles antemortem injury.

84. Ans. (c) Firearm injury

Ref: Reddy 33rd ed page 218

Shotgun Firearm Injuries

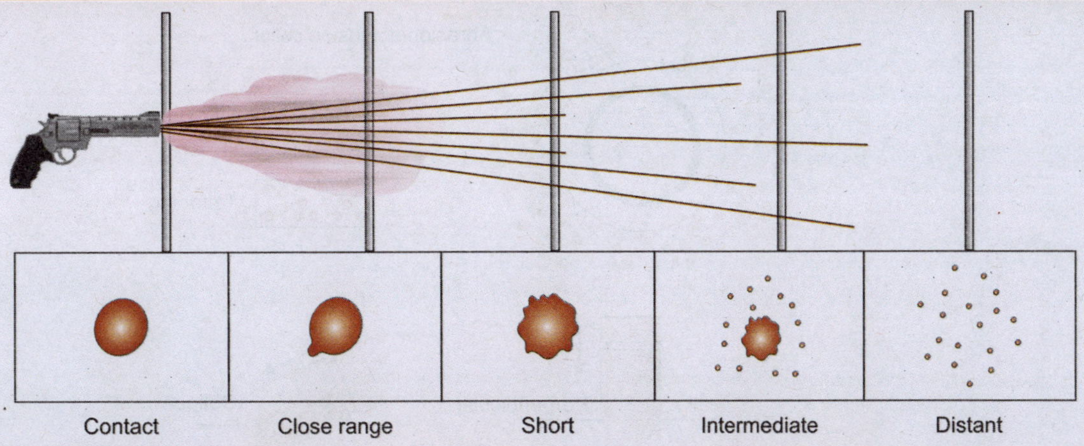

	Contact/Point Blank range	Close range	Short range	Intermediate range	Long/Distant shot
Distance	Contact	Up to 1 meter	1-2 meters	2-4 meters	>4 meters
Size	Large lacerated with cavitation due to gases.	Bullet size entry wound	Single circular aperture 4-5 cm in diameter.	Central hole with small peripheral Satellite holes	Central hole absent . Small individual

Contd...

Shotgun Firearm Injuries

Shape	Shotgun entry wound is round, elliptical, cruciate, triangular, and single up to 30 cm. Edges are normally inverted (may be everted due to bone underneath or gases coming out)	Between 30 cm to 1 m, the rim of the wound is irregular and often called a **'Rat-hole'** in the USA because of the nibbled edges, the same appearance is called **'scalloping'** in the UK. There may be annular abrasion and bruising/ "rat nibbling"	Irregular margins of central entry wound without any satellite wounds	Irregular margins of a central entry wound with few satellite independent entry wounds are seen from 2 meters and above	Widespread pattern of pellet wounds as all pellets show independent entry wound from 4 meters onwards.
Abrasion ring/ Grease collar	Present	Present	Absent	Absent	Absent
Burning and Singeing of hair	Present	Present	Absent	Absent	Absent
Soot Blackening/Smudging	Present	Present	Present	Absent	Absent
Tattooing/stippling	Independent tattoo marks absent	Independent tattoo marks absent	Independent tattoo marks absent	Independent tattoo marks seen (Reddish brown in antemortem gunshot, while Pale/yellow/ greyish brown in postmortem gunshot)	Absent
Muzzle imprint	Present in tight contact, Incomplete in loose contact	Absent	Absent	Absent	Absent

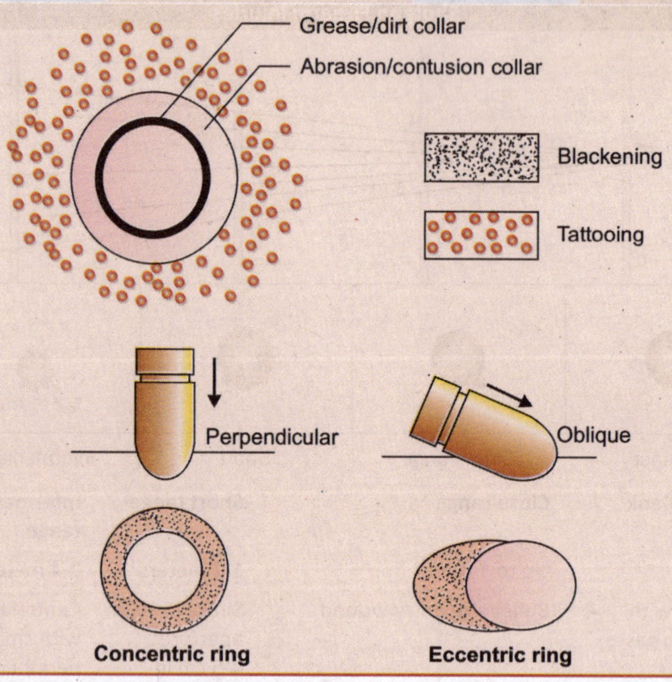

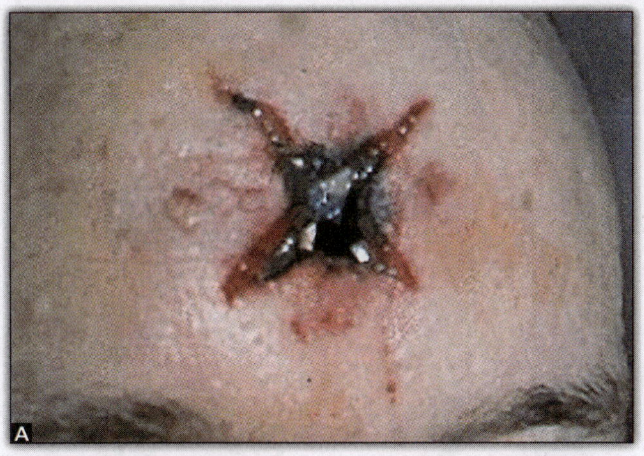

Fig: Contact Shotgun bullet entry wound: Since the barrel contacts the skin, the gases released by the fired round go into the subcutaneous tissue and caused the star shaped laceration. Note the grey black soot and faint abrasion ring

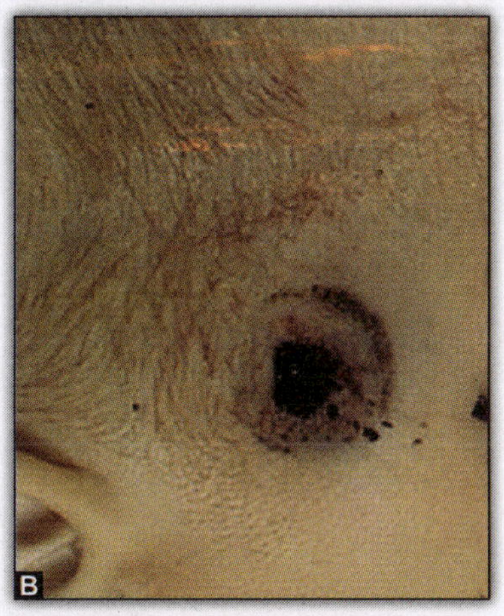

Fig: Contact Shotgun bullet entry wound: An abrasion ring, formed when the force of the gases entering below the skin blow the skin surface back against the muzzle of the gun, is seen here in this contact range gunshot wound to the right temple

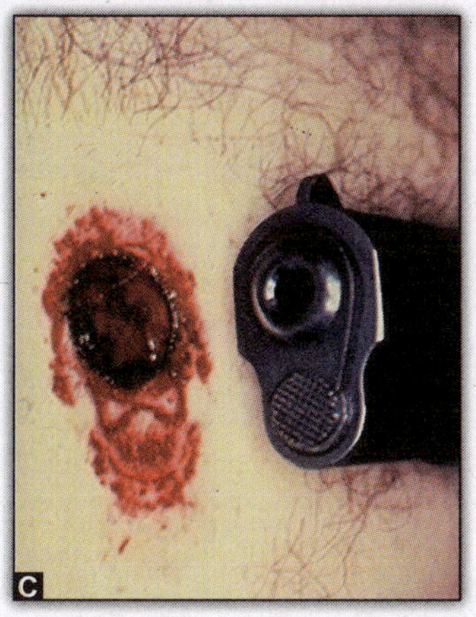

Source: Todd C. Grey University of Utah

Fig: Contact Shotgun bullet entry wound: The abrasion ring, and a very clear muzzle imprint, are seen in this contact range gunshot wound.

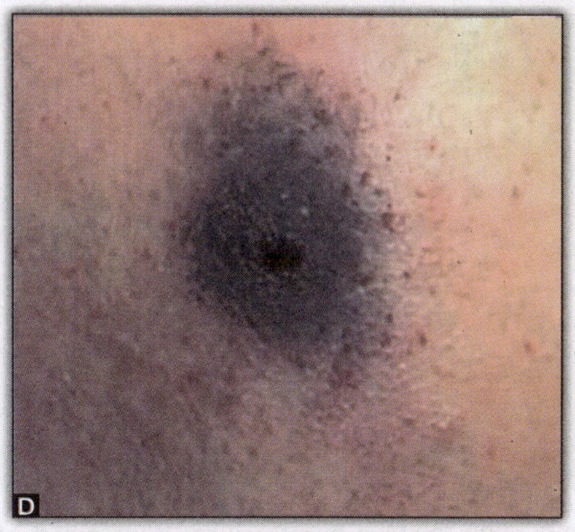

Fig: Close range Shotgun bullet entry wound: With dark circular soot deposition and minor stippling after that, but no independent Tattooing

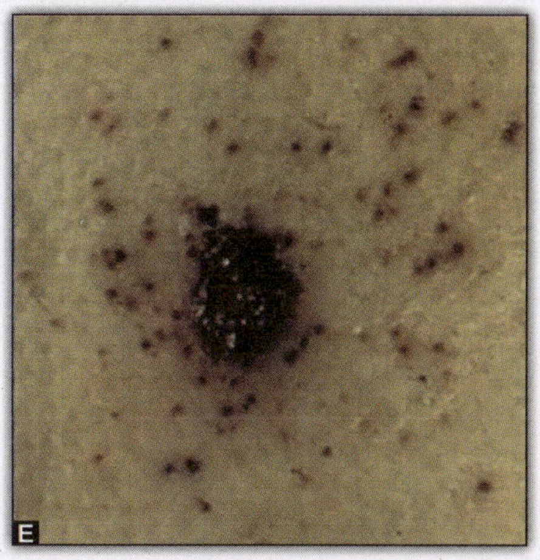

Fig: Intermediate range Shotgun bullet wound which is not angled, with powder tattooing but no soot/blackening

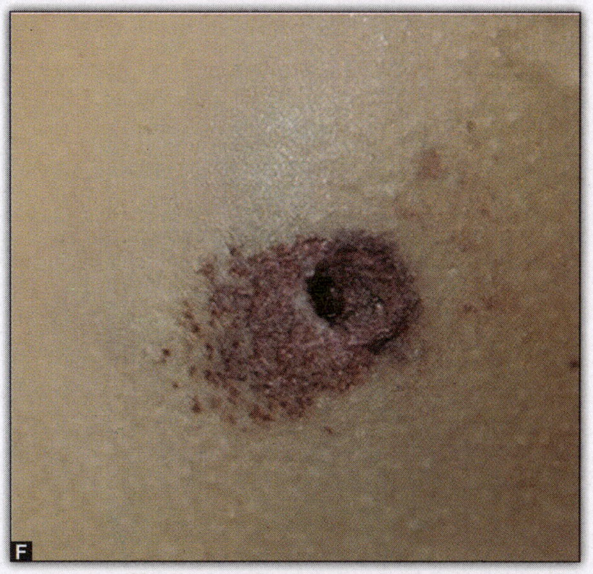

Fig: Intermediate range Shotgun bullet wound which is angled, with powder tattooing but no soot/blackening

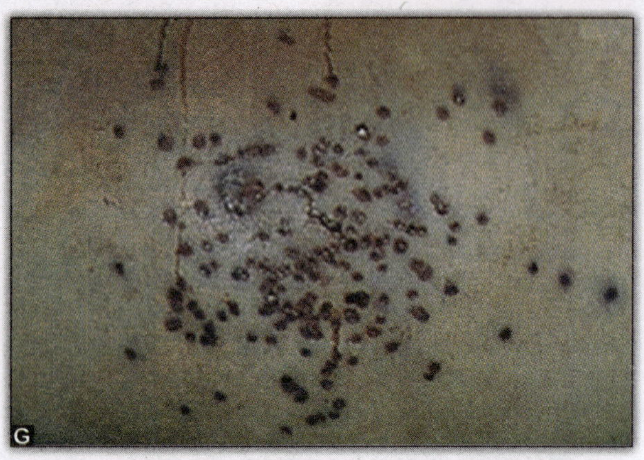

Fig: Distant range shotgun bullet wound: Widespread pattern of pellet wounds as all pellets show independent entry wound from 4 meters onwards. Both soot and tattooing is absent

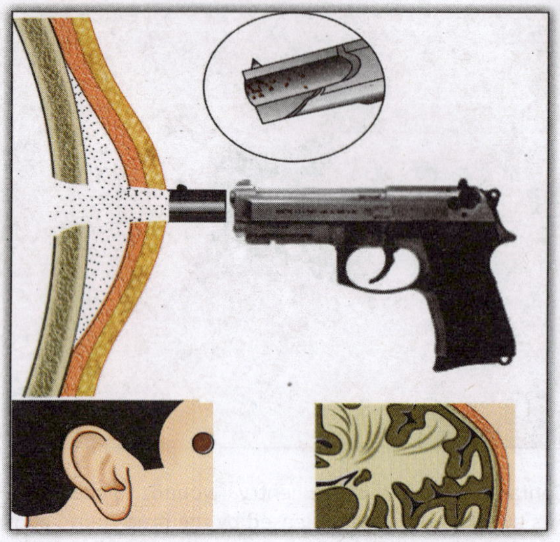

8

Preventive & Social Medicine

AIIMS NOVEMBER 2018

1. An intern spilled blood on the floor, what should be done next?

a. Mop the floor
b. Cover the floor with absorbent material
c. Clean with 0.5% Sodium hypochlorite
d. Inform the infection control board of the hospital

2. A known case of Tuberculosis is now resistant to isoniazid and rifampicin. Which of the following regimen should be prescribed to him?

a. 6 drugs for 6 months followed by 4 drugs for 18 months
b. 6 drugs for 6 months followed by 4 drugs for 12 months
c. 5 drugs for 4 month followed by 4 drugs for 1 month & 3 drugs for 5 months
d. 4 drugs for 4 months followed by 6 drugs for 12 months

3. In a trial involving 200 people, Blood pressure was measured before and after giving a drug. Test of significance to be used for this is?

a. Unpaired t-test b. Paired t-test
c. Chi-square test d. ANOVA

4. In a trial on ischemic cerebral infarct and ischemic cerebral stroke mean and Standard deviation were calculated. Test of significance to be used to compare data?

a. Paired t-test b. Unpaired t-test
c. Chi-square test d. ANOVA

5. Period of isolation recommended for Measles is?

a. From onset of catarrhal stage to rash
b. From onset of fever to rash
c. From onset of symptoms to 3 days
d. 3 days before and 4 days after rash

6. Which of the following vaccine is not included in Universal Immunization Programme?

a. Influenza
b. Rota virus
c. Measles & Rubella
d. Adult Japanese encephalitis

7. Maternal mortality rate is defined as?

a. Maternal deaths per 1000 live births
b. Maternal deaths per 100000 live births
c. Maternal deaths per 1000 births
d. Maternal deaths per 100 live births

8. True about screening tests done in series is?

a. Sensitivity increases specificity decreases
b. Sensitivity decreases specificity increases
c. Sensitivity and specificity increases
d. Sensitivity and specificity decreases

9. The symbol shown below represents?

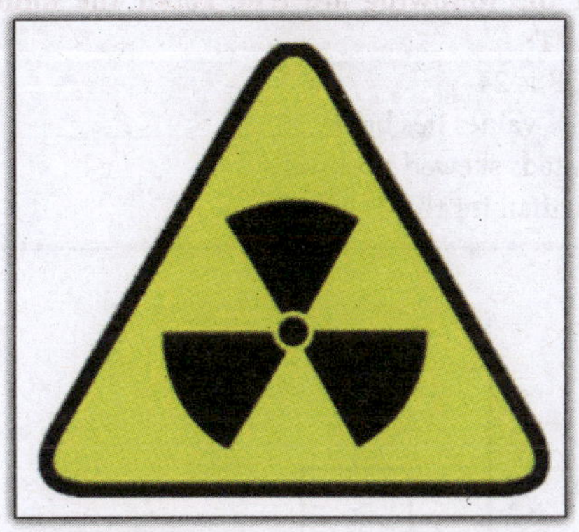

a. Cytotoxic waste
b. Radiation hazard
c. Biomedical waste management
d. Bioterrorism

10. BCG vaccine has been shown to be most effective against?

a. Pulmonary tuberculosis
b. Extrapulmonary tuberculosis
c. CNS and disseminated tuberculosis
d. Childhood tuberculosis

11. The drug kit in the picture is used for treatment of?
(AIIMS Nov 2018, 2015)

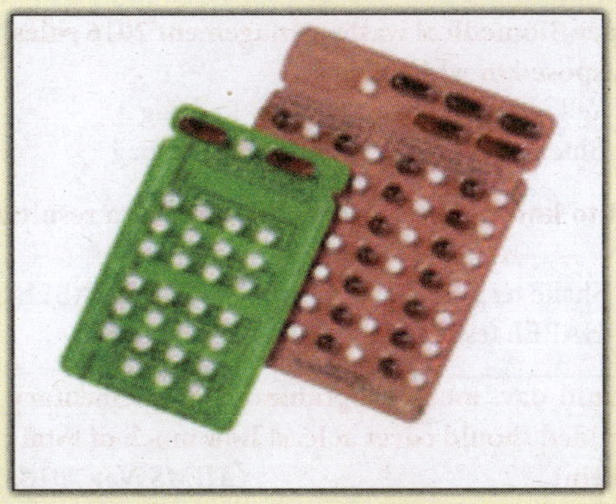

a. HIV b. Leprosy
c. Tuberculosis d. Urethral discharge

12. Which of the following is true for following graph?
a. Mean = Median = Mode
b. Mean = Median ≠ Mode
c. Mean = Mode ≠ Median
d. Mean ≠ Median ≠ mode

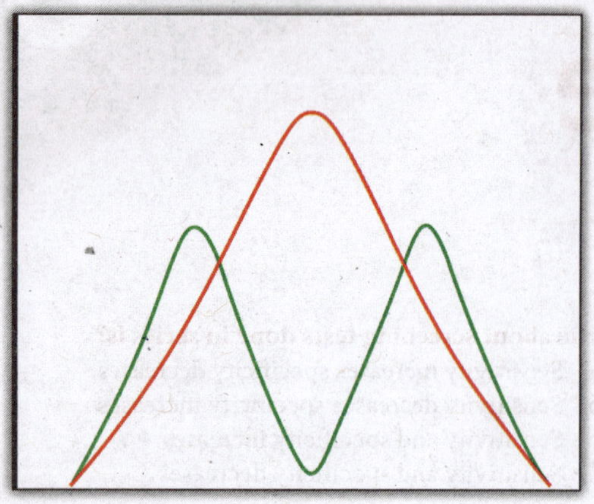

13. All of the following are true about the following image EXCEPT:
a. IQR is 24
b. 75% values lies below 36
c. Data is skewed positively
d. Median for this is 24

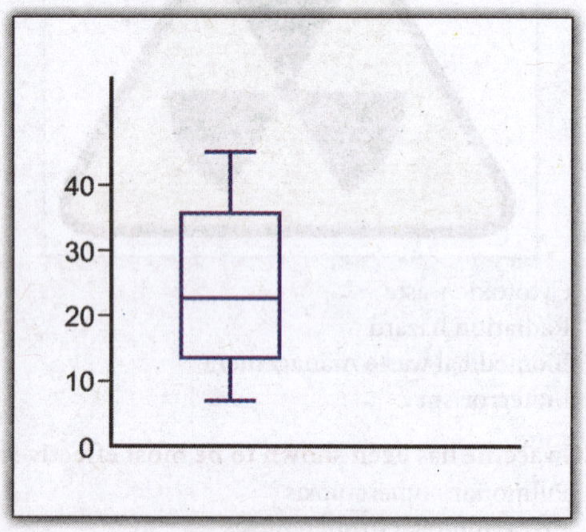

14. A community reports around 40-50 cases of dengue per week. This week 48 cases are reported. This is termed as?
a. Endemic
b. Outbreak
c. Epidemic
d. Sporadic

15. As per Biomedical waste management 2016 rules, blood bag is disposed in which bag ?
a. Yellow bag
b. Red bag
c. Blue box
d. White bag

16. Test to know about vaccine damaged as a result of freezing is?
a. Shake test
b. Modified HABEL test
c. HABEL test
d. Schick test

17. In mid-day meal programme, Supplementary nutrition provided should cover at least how much of total calorie and protein? ***(AIIMS Nov 2018, Nov 2017)***
a. ⅓ calorie, ½ protein
b. ½ calorie, ⅓ protein
c. ½ calorie,⅔ protein
d. ⅔ calorie, ½ protein

AIIMS MAY 2018

18. LaQshya initiative is for?
a. Improvement in labor room services
b. Providing ANC care on 9th of every month
c. Cash Benefits on delivery in Govt. hospitals
d. Providing IFA tablets to pregnant women to correct anemia

19. Incubation period for LGV is?
a. 3–5 days
b. 7–10 days
c. 3–30 days
d. 9–90 days

20. At sub center, number of infants to be registered is approximately?
a. 50
b. 100
c. 150
d. 200

21. Drug of choice for scrub typhus is? ***(AIIMS May 2018, Nov 2017)***
a. Doxycycline
b. Azithromycin
c. Ciprofloxacin
d. Chloramphenicol

22. Chi square test is not applicable for which of the following?
a. Resting heart rate (beats/min) and age in years
b. Tumor (benign or malignant) and type of surgery
c. Age group and cancer stage
d. Sex and stage of cancer

23. Which of the following parameters is used to determine the sensitivity of vaccine due to heat?
a. VVM
b. VCM
c. VMV
d. VMM

24. Which is the correct order of margin of error in the following diagram?

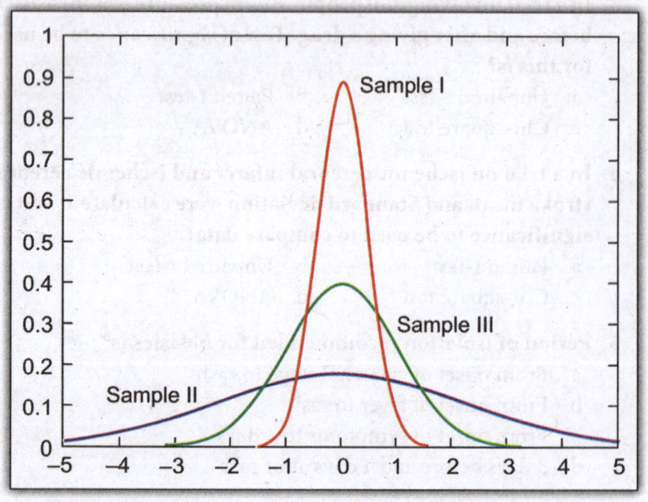

a. I > II > III
b. III > II > I
c. III < I > II
d. III < II > I

25. Under NHM, which committee makes plan for village health?
a. Village health sanitation and nutrition committee (VHNSC)
b. Rogi Kalyan Samiti (RKS)
c. Panchayat Health Committee
d. Village health planning committee (VHPC)

26. Blinded staggers and alkali disease in livestock is due to?
a. Selenium
b. Manganese
c. Magnesium
d. Chromium

AIIMS NOVEMBER 2017

27. Which of the following OPV vaccine vials is/are usable based on the Vaccine Vial Monitor (VVM) color change?

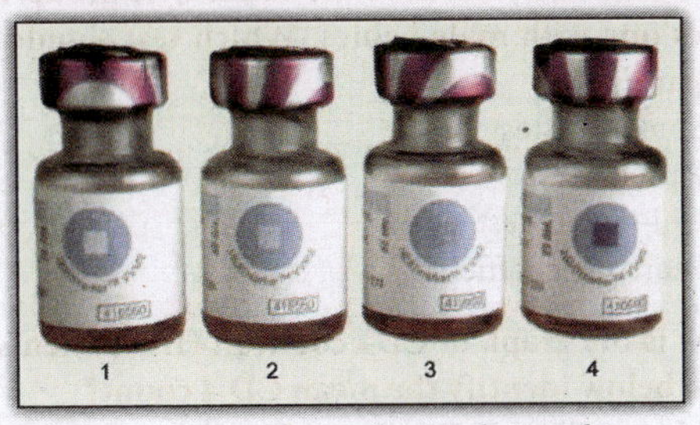

a. Only 1 b. Both 1 and 2
c. Both 3 and 4 d. 1, 2, and 3

28. A doctor uses a highly sensitive test on a patient and the result is positive. What does this mean?
a. Highly likely that patient has the disease
b. Highly unlikely that patient has the disease
c. If the prevalence is high, then the patient is likely to have the disease
d. If it is a rare disease, then the patient is likely to have the disease

29. Chronic liver disease is classified using Child–Pugh class A to C, employing the added score from above. Class A = 5–6, Class B = 7–9 and Class C = 10–15. What is the type of data in this scoring system?
a. Ordinal b. Qualitative
c. Nominal d. Continuous

30. In a subcenter with a Crude birth rate of 20, what will be the expected number of Antenatal care (ANC) registrations in a year?
a. 60 b. 80
c. 100 d. 120

31. While testing the health hazards on a group of people after giving a new drug and or placebo. The following results were obtained. Based on these results what is the absolute risk reduction and relative risk reduction in %?

	Total subjects	People affected
New drug	15230	1600
Placebo	15229	1830

a. 10% and 0.9% b. 0.1% and 0.9%
c. 1% and 10% d. 1% and 9%

32. Prevalence of Leprosy in India, as of 31st march 2016 is?
a. 0.66/10000 population b. 0.66/ 1 lakh population
c. 9.7/ 10000 population d. 9.7/ 1 lakh population

33. A randomized control trial comparing efficacy of two drugs found to have significant difference in activity ($p < 0.01$), however in reality there was no difference between two drugs. This is called?
a. Alpha error b. Beta error
c. 1-Alpha d. 1-Beta

34. Viral Hemorrhagic fever reported in India is?
a. Crimean Congo Hemorrhagic fever
b. Yellow fever
c. Ebola
d. Marburg

35. Drug of choice for scrub typhus is?
(AIIMS May 2018, Nov 2017)
a. Doxycycline b. Azithromycin
c. Ciprofloxacin d. Chloramphenicol

36. A 18 year male comes with pruritus over hand as shown in the picture. Causative organism shown in the picture is?

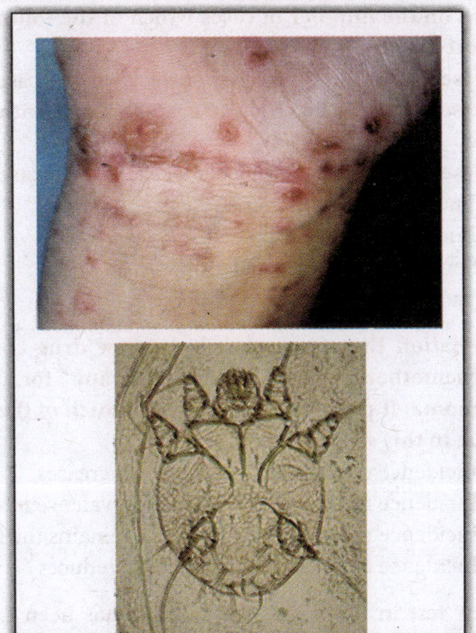

a. Sarcoptes scabiei b. Pediculus capitis
c. Ixodid Tick d. Xenopsylla cheopis

37. In mid-day meal programme, Supplementary nutrition provided should cover at least how much of total calorie and protein?
(AIIMS Nov 2018, 2017)
a. ⅓ calorie, ½ protein b. ½ calorie, ⅓ protein
c. ½ calorie,⅔ protein d. ⅔ calorie, ½ protein

AIIMS MAY 2017

38. A researcher said he has discovered a new drug which is effective in chronic hypertensives with a *P* value of <0.10. Which of the following is true regarding the same?
a. The test is 90% reproducible
b. 90% of test results could have occurred by chance
c. Not more than 10% of the people benefitted by the drug could be due to chance
d. 90% of patients will be benefitted by giving the drug

39. Which point in the below natural history of disease marks the onset of symptoms?

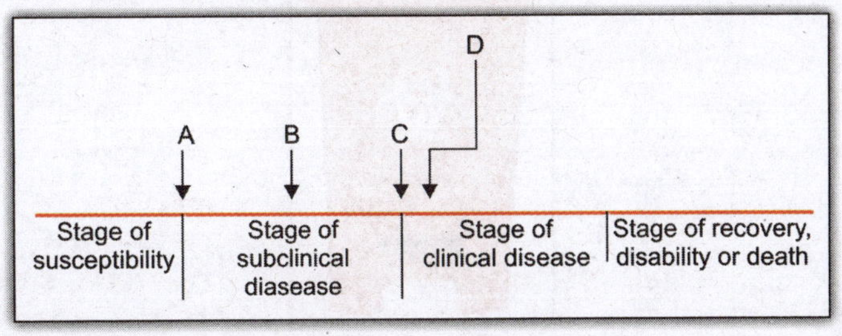

a. A b. B
c. C d. D

40. A child with sputum negative and chest X-ray suggestive of tuberculosis. Next step to do according to revised RNTCP criteria?

a. NAAT b. Culture
c. Line probe assay d. Tuberculin test

41. The following are the disease frequencies in a population. Based on the number of cases which of the following is the correct match

Disease 1-Usually 40-50 case per week with 48 cases last week

Disease 2-Usually less than 10 cases in a year with 1 case last week

Disease 3-Usually 2-3 cases per week, with 13 cases last week

a. Endemic, epidemic, sporadic
b. Endemic, sporadic, epidemic
c. Sporadic, endemic, epidemic
d. Pandemic, endemic, sporadic

42. A radiation therapist prescribes a new drug combination of chemotherapy and immunotherapy for metastatic melanoma. It prolongs the survival. Which of the following is true in this situation?

a. Incidence reduces and prevalence increases
b. Incidence remains the same and prevalence increases
c. Incidence reduces and prevalence remains the same
d. Incidence increases and prevalence reduces

43. A new test in black line (below line) has been designed to diagnose a disease condition. The test is being applied to both normal and diseased population. The graph of which is given below. Which of the following is correct regarding the test?

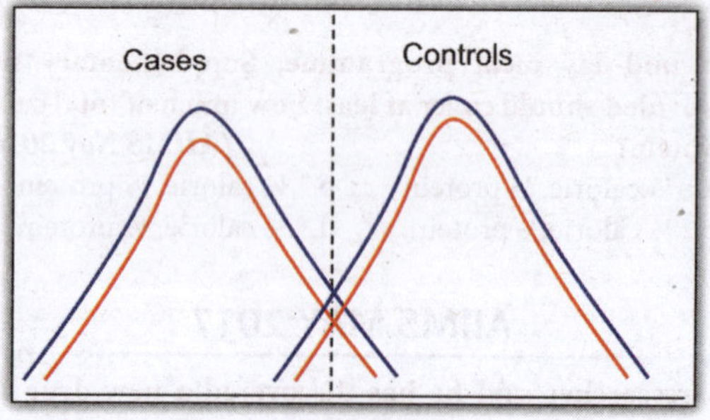

a. High sensitivity high specificity
b. Low sensitivity low specificity
c. Low sensitivity high specificity
d. High sensitivity low specificity

44. Which biomedical waste is disposed in the bag shown below?

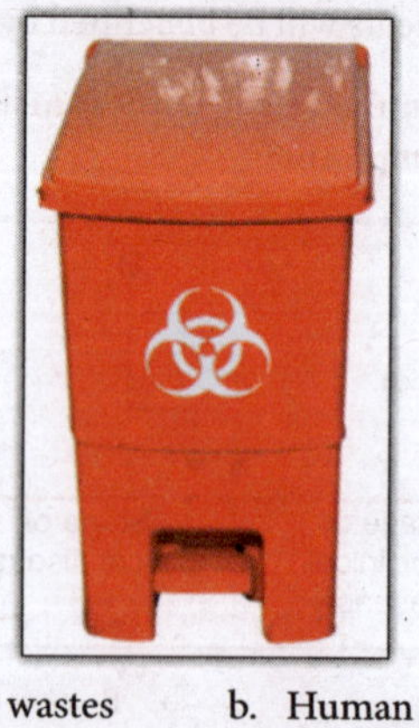

a. Laboratory wastes b. Human anatomical waste
c. Sharp waste d. Soiled plastic waste

45. A study was conducted with the objective to compare the incidence of postpartum depression using depression score (Edinburgh depression scale) depression in mother as compared to the sex of the child. One group with female babies one with male babies. Which test should be used to compare?

a. Student's t test
b. Paired t test
c. Chi-square test
d. Pearson's coefficient

46. Below is the graph of CD4 count in HIV patients. From the graph below identify the mean CD 4 count?

a. Mean will be 300
b. Mean more than 350
c. Mean anywhere between 300 to 400
d. Mean less than 300

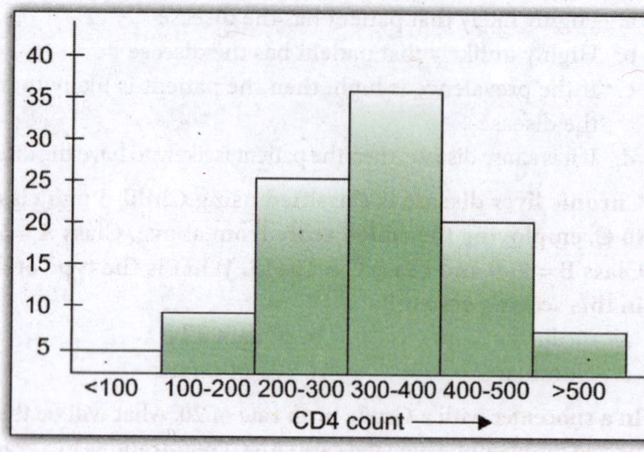

AIIMS NOVEMBER 2016

47. A study was conducted to see the effect of pulse oximeter readings in neonates with and without micropore. A plot between the two values was drawn as shown in the figure. Which of the following conclusion of the figure is correct?

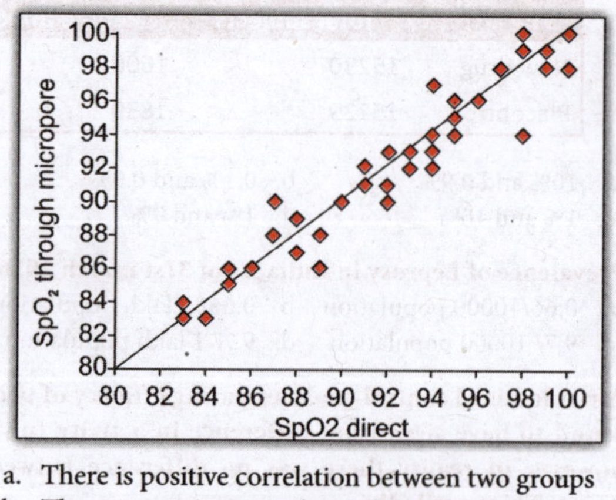

a. There is positive correlation between two groups
b. There is negative correlation between two groups
c. There is no correlation between two groups
d. The data is insufficient to comment

48. A study was conducted in three villages with three different water sources. Prevalence of Typhoid carrier was studied in three villages. What type of study is this?

a. Cross sectional study b. Cohort study
c. Field trial d. Case control study

49. **Histopathological confirmation of ovarian cancer was done in a cohort of patients screened with CA 125 testing. 60/100 women who were tested positive with this test actually had ovarian cancer. 20/100 women who tested negative with this test had ovarian cancer. What is the negative predictive value of this test?**
   a. 20/100 b. 40/100
   c. 60/100 d. 80/100

50. **The intraocular pressure (IOP) was measured in a population of 400 people above the age of 65. The mean IOP was 25 mm Hg and standard deviation was 10 mm Hg. What is the range that would contain the IOP of 95% of the population?**
   a. 22- 24 b. 24-26
   c. 26-28 d. 28-30

51. **In a study was conducted to know the number of positive axillary lymph nodes in 20 MRM surgeries in carcinoma of breast patients. A graph is plotted and there are three marking on the curve below. Based on the distribution type of curve which of the following is correct?**

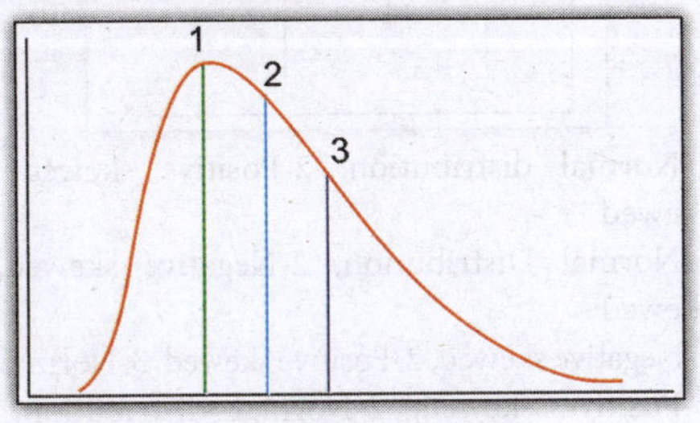

   a. 1 = Mean, 2 = Median, 3 = Mode
   b. 1 = Median, 2 = Mean, 3 = Mode
   c. 1 = Mode, 2 = Mean, 3 = Median
   d. 1 = Mode, 2 = Median, 3 = Mean

52. **Which of the following is best for determining the threshold for diagnosis of a positive test?**
   a. Chi square test b. Pearson coefficient
   c. Analysis of variance d. Receptor operator curve

53. **If the relative risk is 1, then which of the following statement is correct?**
   a. There is a positive association between the effect and cause
   b. There is a negative association between the effect and cause
   c. There is no increase in risk because for the occurrence of the effect
   d. Cannot be commented upon because of inadequate data

54. **According to new RNTCP guidelines, Suspected case of pulmonary TB are all EXCEPT:**
   a. Confirmed case of extrapulmonary tuberculosis with cough of any duration
   b. Diabetic patient with any duration of cough
   c. HIV patient with any duration of cough
   d. History of contact with sputum positive TB patient with any duration of cough

55. **Ponderal index is?**
   a. Head circumference to abdominal circumference ratio
   b. Mid upper arm circumference to Head circumference ratio
   c. Height in cm to cube of weight in Kg
   d. Square root of height in feet by weight in grams

AIIMS MAY 2016

56. **What will be the 95% confidence interval in a study estimated prevalence of 10% and sample size of 100?**
   a. 4–16
   b. 2–18
   c. Inadequate information to calculate 95% CI
   d. 7–13

57. **An obstetrician used APGAR score to assess health of 30 newborn infants. The result showed most of them with score >7. The data distribution is?**
   a. Normal distribution b. Negatively skewed
   c. Positively skewed d. Symmetrically skewed

58. **To design a study for a disease whose prevalence in community is 10%. Alpha error has to be kept at 5% with a relative precision of 20% and power of study 80%. What will be the sample size of the study?**
   a. 3600 b. 1800
   c. 900 d. 600

59. **The best study design to access the association between smoking and lung cancer in a relatively quick time, Which of the study design is preferred?**
   a. Case control study
   b. Cohort study
   c. Randomized controlled trial
   d. Cross sectional study

60. **If study subjects are selected according to the potential factor that will influence the outcome of the study, then the sampling is?**
   a. Systemic random sampling
   b. Stratified random sampling
   c. Simple random sampling
   d. Clustered random sampling

61. **If we say that there is no significant association between two variables and if truly an association exists. Then it is called?**
   a. Type I error b. Type II error
   c. Systematic error d. Random error

62. **All of the following are continuous variable EXCEPT:**
   a. Weight in Kgs
   b. Blood group (A, B, AB, O)
   c. Age in years and months
   d. Height in cms

63. **In primary health care, ABC and VED are related to?**
   a. National program evaluation
   b. Drug inventory
   c. Staff management
   d. Vaccination coverage assessment

64. **ASHA worker duty includes all of the following EXCEPT:**
   a. Give immunization to all eligible children in the village
   b. Escort all pregnant mothers to hospitals for delivery
   c. Screen village population for noncommunicable disease
   d. Ensure success of all program under ANM

65. **Which of the following indicator is used for growth monitoring at anganwadi center?**
   a. Height for age b. Mid arm circumference
   c. Weight for age d. Height for weight

66. In India, psychiatrists are not posted at?
a. District hospitals
b. Military hospitals
c. Primary health centers
d. Hospitals attached to medical colleges

67. As per RNTCP, the sputum samples collected in a suspected TB patient are labelled as?
a. A, B
b. α, β
c. 1, 2
d. Y, Z

68. True regarding survey conducted for Total goiter rate is?
a. Goiter are classified into three grades not visible, palpable, visible
b. Goiter is classified as endemic if TGR ≥ 10%
c. Indicator of Iron deficiency anemia in the population
d. Field survey of TGR does not require doctors

69. Which of the following is true for iron prophylaxis as per National iron plus program for Iron deficiency anemia?
a. 20 mg of elemental iron and 100 microgram of folic acid to 2-5 year old children weekly for a year
b. 45 mg of elemental iron and 400 microgram of folic acid to 2-5 year old children biweekly for a year
c. 100 mg of elemental iron and 500 microgram of folic acid to pregnant women biweekly for a year
d. 100 mg of elemental iron and 500 microgram of folic acid to pregnant women weekly for a year

70. All the statements are true about the disease EXCEPT:
a. Incidence is a probability that a healthy individual will develop the disease during specified period
b. Incidence will decrease if a new drug is effective in reducing mortality from the disease
c. Incidence measures the absolute risk of developing the disease
d. Incidence decreases if a particular prevention program is effective

AIIMS NOVEMBER 2015

71. Identify the vector and disease transmitted by the vector shown in the following picture?

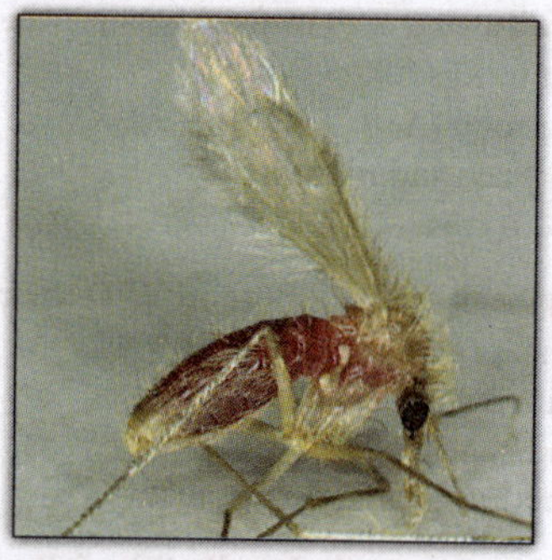

a. Anopheles, Malaria
b. Culex, Japanese encephalitis
c. Sand fly, Visceral leishmaniasis
d. Tsetse fly, sleeping sickness

72. Data description given below is called as?
a. Box whiskers plot
b. Stem and leaf plot
c. Forest plot
d. Funnel plot

0	9
1	2, 8, 3, 9, 5
2	0, 3, 9, 2
3	9, 8, 2, 5, 7, 8, 8
4	9, 3, 2, 6
5	8, 9, 0, 3, 5
6	6, 7, 5
7	1

73. The following box plot shows the distribution of three sets of data around the mean. What is the correct sequence of inference from this box plot?

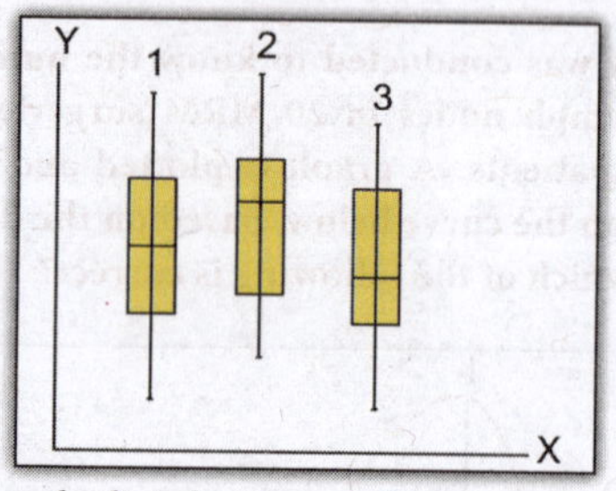

a. 1-Normal distribution, 2-Positive skewed, 3-Negative skewed
b. 1-Normal Distribution, 2-Negative skewed, 3-Positive skewed
c. 1-Negative skewed, 2-Positive skewed, 3-Normal distribution
d. 1-Positive skewed, 2-Normal distribution, 3-Negative skewed

74. A 28-year-old female had delivered a baby 15 days back. The baby has now fallen sick and the woman does not have resources to take the baby to the hospital. Under which scheme can the mother avail free transport to hospital?
a. JSSY
b. JSSK
c. Indira Gandhi matritva yojana
d. ICDS

75. Which of the following is true about Rashtriya swasthya bima yojana?
a. Valid for 4 members i.e. BPL couple and 2 dependents
b. Valid in government hospitals only
c. Valid only within the particular district in which they are enrolled
d. Can get cashless benefit in all enlisted hospitals showing smart card and fingerprints

76. What will be the result if mortality of a disease is decreased but not cured?
a. Prevalence increase
b. Prevalence decrease
c. Incidence increase
d. Incidence decrease

77. In a study 125 females of 16-25 years with mean diastolic blood pressure of 70 mm Hg and standard deviation of 10 mm Hg. The value of lower 5th percentile will be?
a. 50.4 b. 60
c. 67.5 d. 89.6

78. A researcher selected all possible samples from a population and derived and plotted the mean and standard deviation of each sample on linear graph. This can be done by using?

a. Population distribution b. Sampling distribution
c. Sample distribution d. Continuous distribution

79. A doctor record Blood sugar levels of Diabetic patients and then History was taken regarding risk factors and comorbidities. To find the probabilities the plot used is?

a. Venn diagram b. Pie diagram
c. Histogram d. Tree diagram

80. Breast milk is deficient in?

a. Iron and vitamin A
b. Iron and vitamin C
c. Phosphorous and vitamin C
d. Phosphorous and vitamin A

81. The following scatter plot of four different samples shows the correlation between weight and height in the samples. The coefficient of correlation of all the 4 samples taken together is 0.60. What will be the net correlation coefficient?

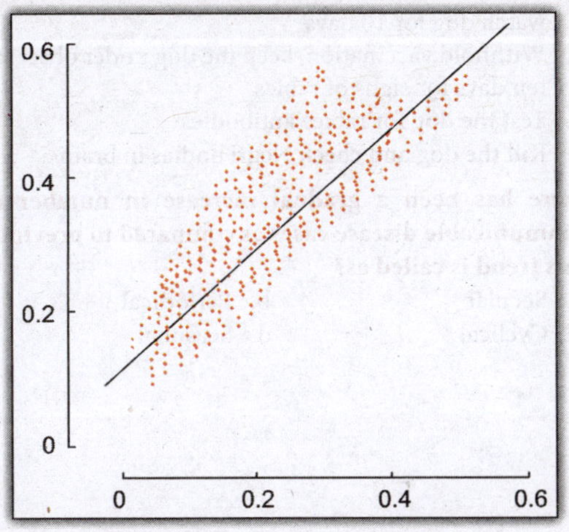

a. More than 0.60 b. Less than 0.60
c. 0.60 d. Cannot be calculated

82. Method of assessment of best correlation between exposure and outcome is?

a. Cross sectional study b. Case control study
c. Cohort study d. RCT

83. The drug kit in the picture is used for treatment of? *(AIIMS Nov 2018, 2015)*

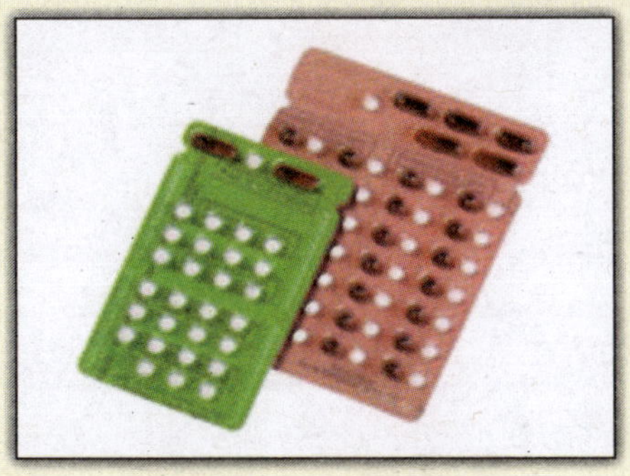

a. HIV b. Leprosy
c. Tuberculosis d. Urethral discharge

84. All are true about Randomization in clinical trial EXCEPT:

a. Reduces confounding
b. Decreases selection bias
c. Ensure comparability of two groups
d. Increase external validity of the trial

85. A latex agglutination test for diagnosis of meningitis was approved. Calculate the sensitivity and specificity of the test based on the data given below?

	Test positive	Test negative
Diseased	27	3
Non diseased	5	95

a. Sensitivity 90%, Specificity 95%
b. Sensitivity 95%, Specificity 90%
c. Sensitivity 80%, Specificity 90%
d. Sensitivity 75% Specificity 95%

86. Which is true regarding Malaria as per revised National drug policy 2013?

a. Primaquine is contraindicated in pregnancy and infants
b. Presumptive treatment with chloroquine is recommended
c. P. falciparum is treated with ACTs and Primaquine is not given with ACTs
d. P. vivax is treated with chloroquine for 3 days and Primaquine for 7 days

AIIMS MAY 2015

87. In a study, two groups of newborns are checked for their weights based on whether their mothers received food supplements or not. The appropriate test which can be used for comparing the data is?

a. Paired T-test b. Chi square test
c. Fischer exact test d. Student's T-test

88. Human developmental index is a composite measure which used?

a. Life expectancy at age one, literacy and infant mortality
b. Freedom, spice and right to express oneself
c. Life expectancy at birth, knowledge and decent standard of living
d. Life expectancy at birth, infant mortality and quality of life

89. In a group of 100 people, the average GFR is 85 ml/min with a standard deviation of 2.5. What is the range for 90% confidence interval?

a. 81-89 b. 80-90
c. 70-100 d. 75-95

90. Food safety and standards authority of india comes under which ministry?

a. Ministry of consumer affairs food and public distribution
b. Minister of agriculture
c. Rural statistics
d. Ministry of health and family welfare

91. A researcher wants to do a study of blood levels of lipids among people who smoke and those who do not. But he is now concerned that the smokers might differ from non-smokers in their diet, exercise, etc as well. This concern is known as?

a. Recall bias b. Interviewer bias
c. Information bias d. Selection bias

92. Tuberculin test is a cheap and easily available test. In which of the following situation there is high failure in the interpretation of the test?

a. Environmental mycobacterium infections are less
b. High prevalence of disease
c. High percentage of immunized people
d. HIV cases are less

93. In a survey of sleep apnea scores among 10 people, the highest sample of 58 was entered by mistake as 85. This will affect the result as?

a. No change in mean, increased median
b. Increased mean, no change in median
c. Increased mean, increased median
d. Increased mean, decreased median

94. Haddon matrix is related to?

a. Hypertensive disorders
b. Communicable diseases
c. Maternal and child mortality
d. Injury prevention

95. The blood pressure data of 200 persons were collected. The first quartile BP of the data was 94 mm Hg and third quartile was 100 mm Hg. How many patients have blood pressures between the 3rd and 4th quartile is?

a. 200
b. 100
c. 50
d. 25

96. Data about recent trends of immunization in the community can be found by?

a. District level health survey
b. Rural survey
c. Sample registration system
d. Census data

97. Window period is defined as the time taken from?

a. Entry in cell to expulsion of first viral particle
b. Entry of pathogen to appearance of first clinical symptoms
c. Exposure to laboratory detection of disease
d. Entry to maximum communicability

98. 'Nikshay' is newly launched central government software. It is used for tracking?

a. High-risk newborns
b. Malaria
c. Tuberculosis
d. High-risk pregnancies

99. Sensitivity measures?

a. True positive
b. False positive
c. True negative
d. False negative

100. Screening is not useful in which carcinoma?

a. Testicular carcinoma
b. Carcinoma Colon
c. Carcinoma Breast
d. Carcinoma Prostate

101. A boy complained of unprovoked bite by a local dog in the community. The dog was later caught by the local animal authorities and appeared to be healthy. The most appropriate course of action wound be? ***(AIIMS May 2015, 2014)***

a. Give post-exposure prophylaxis to the bitten person and watch dog for 10 days
b. Withhold vaccination, keep the dog under observation for ten days for signs of rabies
c. Test the dog for rabies antibodies
d. Kill the dog and check Negri bodies in brain

102. There has been a gradual increase in number of non-communicable disease cases as compared to previous years. This trend is called as?

a. Secular
b. Periodical
c. Cyclical
d. Seasonal

AIIMS NOVEMBER 2018

1. Ans. (b) Cover the floor with absorbent material

Ref: Park 23rd ed page 129, WHO Guidelines on Drawing Blood: Best Practices in Phlebotomy.

NOTE

Next step is asked. Hence before chemically treating the floor it is necessary to dispose off the broken glass and excess blood on floor.

Blood spillage may occur because a laboratory sample breaks in the phlebotomy area or during transportation, or because there is excessive bleeding during the procedure. In this situation, clean up the spillage and record the incident, using the following procedure.

- Wear a pair of non-sterile gloves.
- Use tongs or a pan and brush to sweep up as much of the broken glass (or container) as possible. Do not pick up pieces with your hands.
- Discard the broken glass in a sharps container. If this is not possible due to the size of the broken glass, wrap the glass or container in several layers of paper and discard it carefully in a separate container. Do not place it in the regular waste container.
- ***Use disposable paper towels to absorb as much of the body fluids as possible.***
- Wipe the area with water and detergent until it is visibly clean.
- Saturate the area again with **sodium hypochlorite 0.5%** (10 000 ppm available chlorine). This is a 1:10 dilution of 5.25% sodium hypochlorite bleach, which should be prepared daily.
- Rinse off the tongs, brush and pan, under running water and place to dry.
- Remove gloves and discard them.
- Wash hands carefully with soap and water, and dry thoroughly with single-use towels.
- Record the incident in the incident book if a specimen was lost, or persons were exposed to blood and body fluids.

Hypochlorites are the most widely used chlorine disinfectant, available as liquid (e.g. sodium hypochlorite) or solid (e.g. **calcium hypochlorite**). The most prevalent chlorine products are aqueous solutions of 5.25–6.15 percent of sodium hypochlorite, usually called household bleach. They have a broad spectrum of antimicrobial activity, do not leave toxic residues, are unaffected by water hardness, are inexpensive and fast acting, remove dried or fixed organisms and biofilms from surfaces

Work surfaces are to be decontaminated at least twice a day and after every spill of viable/infected material. Sodium hypochlorite available as 4% w/v solution is used as follows: Blood spillage is cleaned up using 1% hypochlorite solution. (Mix 1 part of readymade 4% w/v sodium hypochlorite solution with 3 parts of sterile water.) In general, a minimum concentration of 5,000 ppm (0.5%) hypochlorite is recommended to inactivate HIV present in a blood spill

2. Ans. (a) 6 drugs for 6 months followed by 4 drugs for 18 months

Ref: Park 23rd ed page 191

NOTE

In India we still use conventional regimen no the Shortened regimen for MDR TB

Multidrug-resistant TB (MDR-TB) is caused by TB bacteria that are resistant to at least isoniazid and rifampicin, the two most effective anti-TB drugs. These patients need second-line treatment.

Options for treatment of MDR-TB include the conventional MDR treatment regimen (total duration of therapy generally 20 to 26 months) or a shortened regimen (total duration of therapy 9 to 12 months)

- **Conventional regimen** (total duration 20 to 26 months) for treatment of MDR-TB consists of an intensive phase (administration of at least ***five effective drugs for at least 6 months*** after sputum culture conversion), followed by a continuation phase administration of at least **four effective drugs given for 18 to 24 months** beyond sputum culture conversion (performed monthly until negative)
- **Shortened regimen commonly known as the Bangladesh regime**— The shortened MDR-TB regimen for pulmonary tuberculosis (9 to 11 months) was described by the WHO in 2016; it is appropriate for nonpregnant patients with MDR-TB. The shortened regimen consists of the following components: **Intensive phase** – Four months (daily) of seven drugs: high-dose isoniazid (15 to 20 mg/kg/day), ethambutol, pyrazinamide, moxifloxacin, kanamycin, prothionamide, and clofazimine. There has not been substantial experience with substitution of the injectable agent for bedaquiline in the shortened regimen. **Continuation phase** – Five months (daily) of four drugs: ethambutol, pyrazinamide, moxifloxacin, and clofazimine.

Conventional Regimen for MDR TB	
Duration	20 to 26 months
DRUGS	
Intensive phase	Administration of at least **five effective drugs for at least 6 months** after sputum culture conversion): **First line** :Susceptible first-line drugs if any (including pyrazinamide and/or ethambutol), a fluoroquinolone, and bedaquiline (if available) **or** an injectable agent (amikacin, kanamycin, or capreomycin). **Other alternative agents** include linezolid, clofazimine, and cycloserine. **If there are not at least five active drugs available** in these categories, other add-on agents include ethionamide, high-dose isoniazid, para-aminosalicylic acid, delamanid, and a carbapenem (meropenem or imipenem) plus clavulanate.
Continuation phase	**At least four effective drugs** given for 18 to 24 months beyond sputum culture conversion (performed monthly until negative).

Shortened Regimen for MDR TB	
Duration	9-12 months
Criteria	Nonpregnant patients with MDR-TB who meet the following criteria: • Absence of extrapulmonary disease • Access to all component antituberculous drugs in the regimen: moxifloxacin, kanamycin, prothionamide, clofazimine, high-dose isoniazid, pyrazinamide, ethambutol • No resistance to the drugs in the regimen (except isoniazid resistance) • No previous exposure to drugs in the regimen for more than one month
DRUGS	
Intensive phase	**Four months (daily) of seven drugs**: High-dose Isoniazid (15 To 20 Mg/Kg/Day), Ethambutol, Pyrazinamide, Moxifloxacin, Kanamycin, Prothionamide, And Clofazimine.
Continuation phase	**Five months (daily) of four drugs:** ethambutol, pyrazinamide, moxifloxacin, and clofazimine.

3. Ans. (b) Paired t-test

Ref: Biostatistics BY Mahajan 7th ed page 134, Park 22nd ed page 795

Blood pressure is a quantitative data and measuring BP in same individual before and after medication will require Paired t-test.

Statistical Tests					
Qualitative data		**Quantitative data**			
Fischer's test Small sample size >20% of cells have expected values <5	**Chi Square Test** Large sample size <20% of cells have expected values <5	**Z-test** (2 sample groups) Sample is large (n>100)	**Student 't' Test** (2 sample groups) Sample is small		**ANOVA** More than 2 sample groups
			Paired 't' test Same Sample (e.g :Before & After)	**Unpaired 't' test** 2 independent samples	

4. Ans. (b) Unpaired t-test

Ref: Biostatistics BY Mahajan 7th ed page 134, Park 22nd ed pg 795

(See table of "Statistical Tests" in previous question)
(see page no. 560 and 610)

Mean and standard deviation calculation is possible in Quantitative data only. Also there are 2 independent sample groups of ischemic cerebral infarct and ischemic cerebral stroke. Hence Unpaired t test is to be applied.

5. (c) From onset of symptoms to 3 days

Ref: Park 23rd Ed Pg 120, 126, 150

Isolation period of Measles is controversial because park mentioned different figures at different places 3 days after rash (page 126) and 7 days after rash (page 150). CDC says 4 days after onset of rash. Going by CDC and park both combined 3 days after rash is the correct answer. Also 7 days after rash is not provided in the options.

Period of Isolation	
Chicken pox	Until all lesions crusted, usually 6 days after onset of rash
Measles	From onset of catarrhal stage to 3rd day of rash
German measles	None (except that Women in 1st trimester or sexually active, non immune women in childbearing years not using contraceptive measures should not be exposed)
Cholera, diphtheria	3 days after tetracycline started, until 48 hours of antibiotics (or negative cultures after treatment)
Shigellosis, salmonellosis	Until 3 consecutive negative stool culture
Hepatitis A	3 weeks
Influenza	3 days after onset
Polio	2 weeks in adults, 6 weeks in pediatrics
Sputum positive Tuberculosis	Until 3 weeks of effective chemotherapy
Herpes zoster	6 days after onset of rash
Mumps	Until swelling subsides (now changed from 9 days to 5 days)
Pertussis	4 weeks or until paroxysms cease
Meningococcal meningitis/ streptococcal pharyngitis	Until first 6 hours of effective antibiotic therapy

6. Ans. (a) Influenza

Ref: Pak 23rd ed page 122, ***https://mohfw.gov.in/sites/default/files/5628564789562315.pdf***

NOTE

JE vaccination is provided as part of Routine Immunization programme in 154 districts in 15 states. (Mainly UP, West Bengal, Assam, Bihar).

Schedule:

1st dose: 9-12 months
2nd dose- 16-24 months
Dose: 0.5 ml S/C left upper arm
DIluent- phosphate buffer
Maximum age- 15 years

Under UIP, following Vaccines are Provided:

- BCG (Bacillus Calmette Guerin)
- DPT (Diphtheria, Pertussis and Tetanus Toxoid)
- OPV (Oral Polio Vaccine)
- Measles
- Hepatitis B
- TT (Tetanus Toxoid)
- Japanese Encephalitis vaccination (in selected high disease burden districts)
- Hib containing Pentavalent vaccine (DPT+HepB+Hib) (In selected States)

Diseases Protected by Vaccination under UIP:

- Diphtheria
- Pertussis
- Tetanus
- Polio
- Tuberculosis
- Measles
- Hepatitis B
- Japanese Encephalitis (commonly known as brain fever)
- Meningitis and Pneumonia caused by Haemophilus Influenzae type b

7. Ans. (b) Maternal deaths per 100000 live birth

Ref: Park 24th Ed page 593, 484

Maternal mortality ratio: Number of maternal deaths during a given time period per 100,000 live births during the same time-period.

Total no. of female deaths due to complications of pregnancy, childbirth or within 42 days of delivery from "puerperal causes" in an area during a given year)	x 1000 (or 100,000)
Total no. of live births in the same area and year	

The Value of MMR is 130/ 100000 (2014-16)

Maternal mortality rate: Number of maternal deaths in a given period per 100,000 women of reproductive age during the same time-period.

8. Ans. (b) Sensitivity decreases specificity increases

Ref: Park 24th ed page 149, Lecture Notes on Epidemiology By Professor Dr Abdul Rashid Khan, Professor K.A. Narayan 2nd ed page 149

Two screening tests done in series increase specificity and decrease sensitivity

Two screening tests done in parallel increase sensitivity and decrease specificity

9. Ans. (b) Radiation hazard

Ref: ***https://aerb.gov.in/index.php/english/radiation-symbol***

The "Trefoil" is a radiation symbol for radiation hazards.

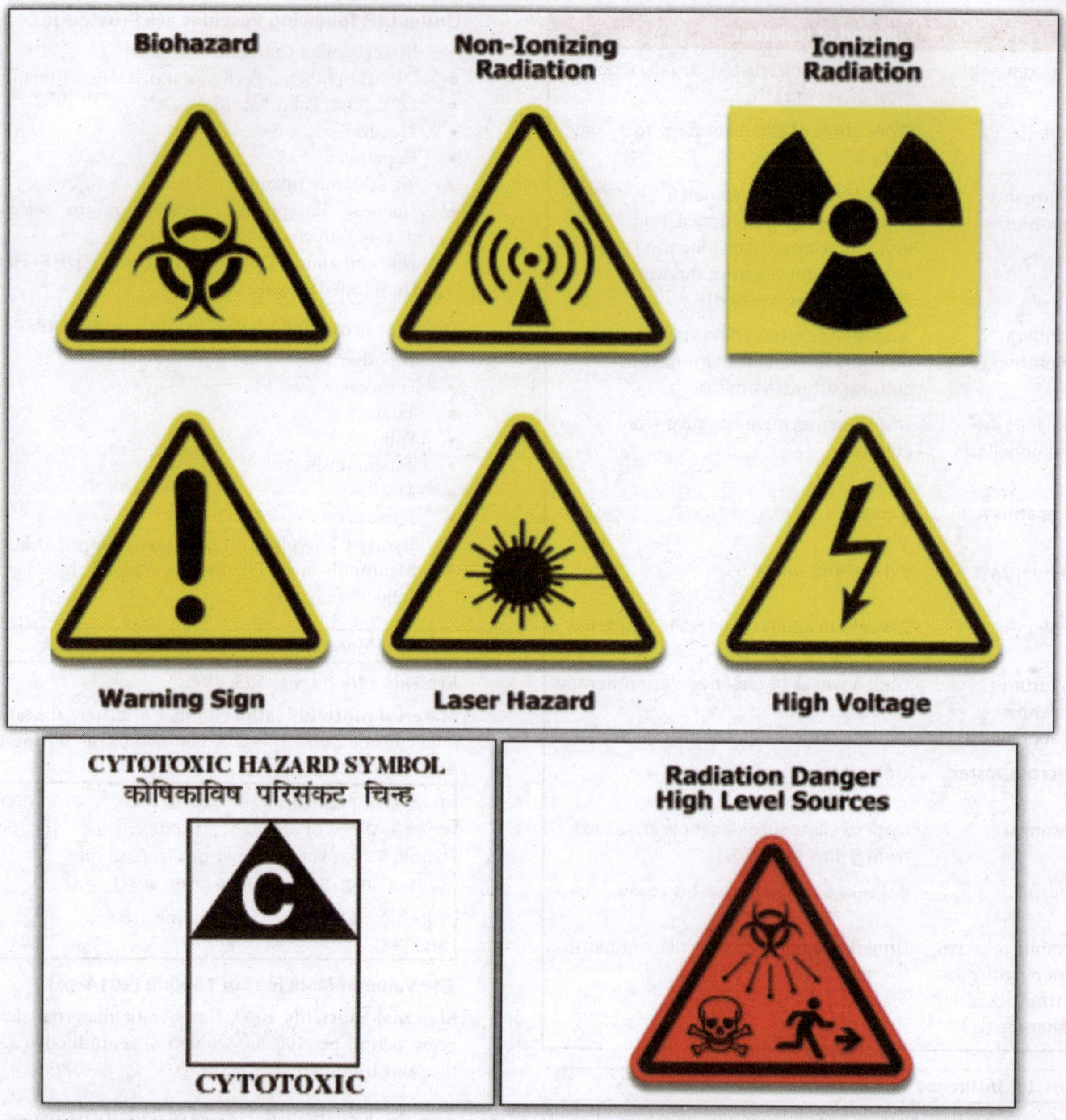

Fig: This symbol is also being promoted by International Atomic Energy Agency as Radiation symbol for sealed sources

10. Ans. (c) CNS and Disseminated Tuberculosis

Ref: Park 24th Ed Pg 210

There is evidence that BCG plays a valuable role in preventing severe forms of childhood tuberculosis viz meningitis and miliary tuberculosis.

11. Ans. (b) Leprosy

Ref: Park 23rd ed page 322, http://www.searo.who.int/entity/leprosy

- The red capsules contain Rifampicin which is to be taken once a month (300 mg X 2 on the first day of the month), while white tablets contain Dapsone. The green strip is for PauciBacillary while red one is for Multibacillary Leprosy.
- In the Multibacillary strip, the 3 additional dark colored capsules contain Clofazimine (100 mg X3).
- The Capsules and the single Dapsone tablet segregated at the top are to be taken on the first day of each month of treatment.

Blister Packs of MDT of Leprosy

The treatment of leprosy is in the form of Multi Drug Therapy (MDT), which is the combination of two or three of the following drugs:

1. Cap. Rifampicin
2. Tab. Dapsone
3. Cap. Clofazimine

Four types of standard regimens are available in blister packs for treatment of leprosy; MDT is provided in convenient-to-use blister calendar packs (BCPs) with medicine for four weeks or 28 days, which is loosely referred to as one month. BCPs for PB leprosy contain two medicines and that for MB leprosy contain three medicines. BCPs for children contain the same medicines as the BCPs for adults but in smaller doses.

Leprosy Regimen			
Adult MB leprosy	Rifampicin: 600 mg once a month supervised Clofazimine 300 mg once monthly supervised and 100 mg on alternate days or 50 mg daily self-administered Dapsone 100 mg once monthly supervised with 100 mg daily self-administered	Duration: 12 months (12 blister packs)	Follow up: once a year for 5 years
Child (ages 10 – 14) MB leprosy	Rifampicin: 450 mg once a month supervised Clofazimine 150 mg once monthly supervised and 50 mg on alternate days Dapsone 50 mg once monthly supervised with 50 mg daily self-administered	Duration: 12 months (12 blister packs)	Follow up: once a year for 5 years
Child (ages 6 – 9) MB leprosy	Rifampicin 300 mg once monthly + Clofazimine 100 mg once monthly supervised and 50 mg twice weekly + Dapsone 25 mg once monthly supervised with 50 mg daily self-administered	Duration: 12 months (12 blister packs)	Follow up: once a year for 5 years
Adult PB leprosy	Rifampicin: 600 mg once a month supervised Dapsone: 100 mg daily self-administered (For adults with body weight below 45 kg the dose of rifampicin should be 450 mg once monthly and dapsone 50 mg daily)	Duration: six months (six blister packs)	Follow up: once a year for 2 years
Child PB leprosy	Rifampicin 300 mg (0–5 years) or 450 mg (6–14 years) once monthly supervised Dapsone 25 mg (0–5 years) or 50 mg (6–14 years) daily	Duration: six months (six blister packs)	Follow up: once a year for 5 years

The appropriate dose for children under 10 years of age can be decided on the basis of body weight. [Rifampicin: 10 mg per kilogram body weight, clofazimine: 1 mg per kilogram per body weight daily and 6 mg per kilogram monthly, dapsone: 2 mg per kilogram body weight daily. The standard child blister pack may be broken up so that the appropriate dose is given to children under 10 years of age. Clofazimine can be spaced out as required.

**Rarely, it may be considered advisable to treat a patient with a high bacillary index (BI) for more than 12 months. This decision may only be taken by specialists at referral units after careful consideration of the clinical and bacteriological evidence

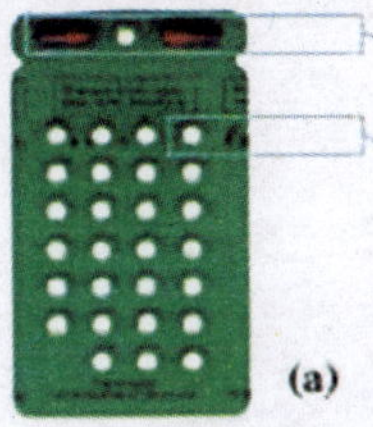

(a)

PB adult blister pack

PB adult treatment:

Once a month: Day 1
- 2 capsules of rifampicin (300 mg X 2)
- 1 tablet of dapsone (100 mg)

Once a day: Days 2–28
- 1 tablet of dapsone (100 mg)

Full course: 6 blister packs

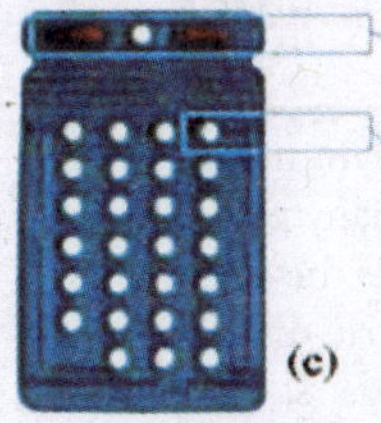

(c)

PB child blister pack

PB child treatment (10–14 years):

Once a month: Day 1
- 2 capsules of rifampicin (300 mg+150 mg)
- 1 tablet of dapsone (50 mg)

Once a day: Days 2–28
- 1 tablet of dapsone (50 mg)

Full course: 6 blister packs

For children younger than 10, the dose must be adjusted according to body weight.

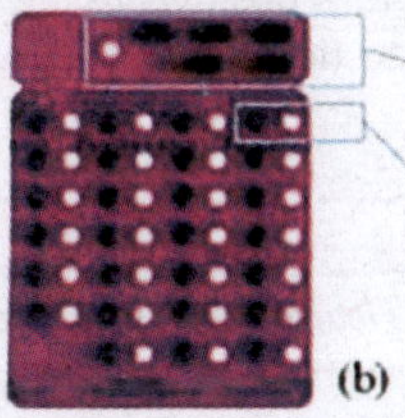

(b)

MB adult blister pack

MB adult treatment:

Once a month: Day 1
- 2 capsules of rifampicin (300 mg X 2)
- 3 capsules of clofazimine (100mg X 3)
- 1 tablet of dapsone (100 mg)

Once a day: Days 2–28
- 1 capsule of clofazimine (50 mg)
- 1 tablet of dapsone (100 mg)

Full course: 12 blister packs

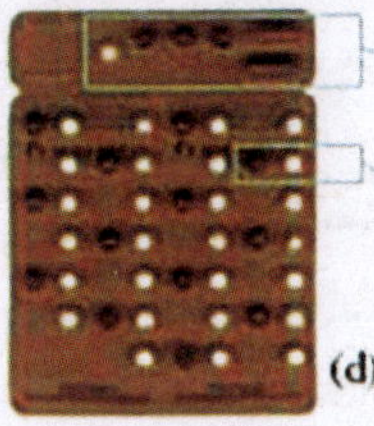

(d)

MB child blister pack

MB child treatment (10–14 years):

Once a month: Day 1
- 2 capsules of rifampicin (300 mg+150 mg)
- 3 capsules of clofazimine (50 mg X 3)
- 1 tablet of dapsone (50 mg)

Once a day: Days 2–28
- 1 capsule of clofazimine every other day (50 mg)
- 1 tablet of dapsone (50 mg)

Full course: 12 blister packs

For children younger than 10, the dose must be adjusted according to body weight.

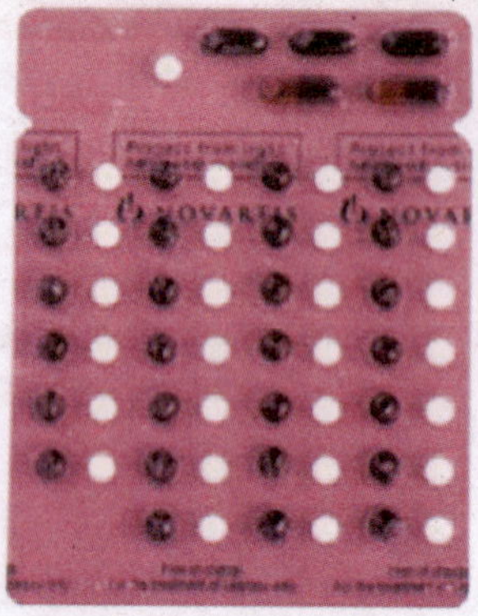

Top 2 lines break off: detachable):
Clofazimine 300 mg (three capsules of 100 mg), Rifampcin 600 mg (two capsules of 300 mg) and Dapsone 100 mg (one tablet of 100 mg)

Unsupervised Daily treatment (Day S2-28): Clofazimine 50 mg (one capsule of 50mg) Every day and dapsone 100 mg (one tablet of 100 mg) Every day
Duration of treatment: 12 blister packs to be taken within 12-18 months

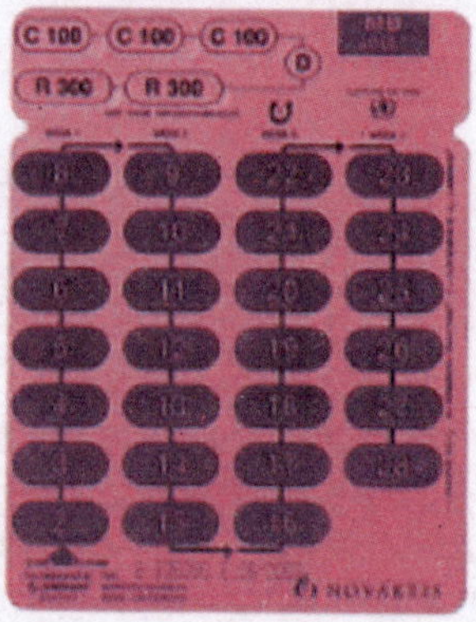

Back view of the MB Adult MDT blister pack
R = Rifampicin: monthly supervised dose is 600 mg (2 capsules, each of 300 mg).
C = Clofazimine 100 mg: monthly supervised dose is 300 mg (3 Capsules).
D = Dapsone: monthly supervised dose is 100 mg (1 tablet).
The figures 2-28 represent 4 weeks of unsupervised clofazimine (50 mg) every day and Dapsone (100 mg) daily.
Actual size of blister pack: 106 mm x 140 mm

12. Ans. (b) Mean = Median ≠ Mode

Ref: Oxford Handbook of Medical statistics page 182, Park 23rd ed page 847

(See table of "Measure of Central Tendency" in AIIMS Nov 2016 PSM) (see page no. 584)

Distributions don't have to be unimodal to be symmetric. They can be bimodal (two peaks) or multimodal (many peaks). The following bimodal distribution is symmetric, as the two halves are mirror images of each other. In a symmetric distribution, the mean, mode and median all fall at the same point. **In bimodal distribution the mean and median are still in the center, but there are two modes: one on each peak**

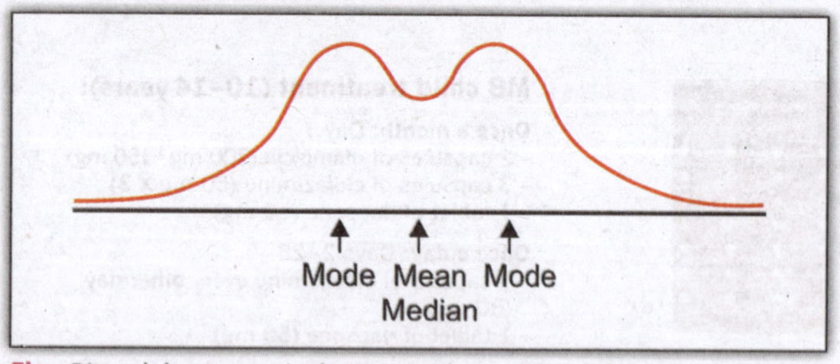

Fig: Bimodal symmetrical curve with 2 modes and Mean = Median

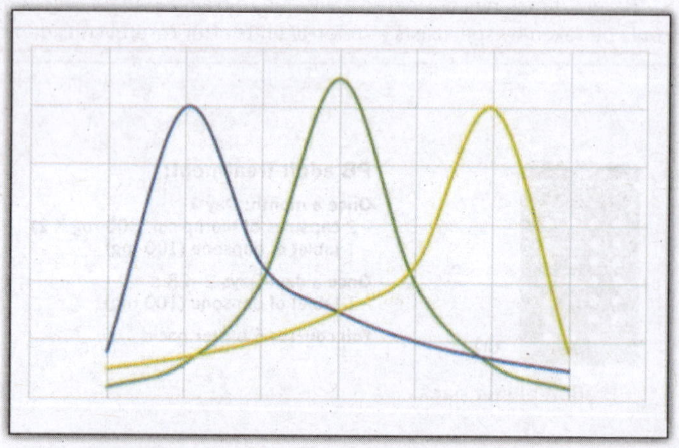

Fig: The bell curve is shown in comparison to a positively-skewed (right skewed) curve and a negatively-skewed (left-skewed) curve. Don't get confused with this graph

13. Ans. (c) Data is skewed positively

Ref: Statistics: An Interactive Text for the Health and Life Sciences by Goteti Bala Krishnamurty, Patricia Kasovia-Schmitt, David J. Ostroff Page 117, Essentials of Inferential Statistics - By Malcolm O. Asadoorian, Demetrius Kantarelis Page 49

In the given picture of Box whiskers plot, the 1st Quartile Q_1 is at 12, Q_2 is at 24 and Q_3 is at 36

Option (A) True:

IQR (Inter Quartile range) is $Q_3 - Q_1 = 36–12 = 24$

Option (B) True:

75% data lies below Q_3 or third quartile

Option (C) False:

Skewness is reflected if the median (Q_2) is closer to one end of the box.

- If Q_2 is closer to Q_3 = Positive or Right skew
- If Q_2 is closer to Q_1 = Negative or Left Skew

In the given Box whiskers plot Q_2 is closer to Q_1 hence its a Negative skew.

Option (D) True:

Median = Q_2 = 24 in the given plot

Box whiskers plot: A box-and-whiskers plot or box plot is a virtual representation of the distribution of data set. It displays a five—number summary for a variable (minimum, maximum, first and third quartiles, and median). It consists of a rectangle (the box) with one end at the lower (or first) quartile Q_1 and the other end at the upper (or third) quartile Q_3. Usually, the lower quartile is calculated as the median of the lower half of the ordered data list and is referred to as the lower hinge. The upper quartile is calculated as the median of the upper half of the ordered data list and is referred to as the upper hinge. The line parallel to the ends cut the box at the median.

Q_1: The first quartile is the middle (the median) of the lower half of the data set. One-fourth (25%) of the data lies below the first quartile, and three-fourths (75%) lies above.	Q_2: The second quartile is another name for the median of the entire set. One-half (50%) of the data lies below the second quartile, and one-half (50%) lies above.	Q_3: The third quartile is the middle (the median) of the upper half of the data set. Three-fourths (75%) of the data lies below the third quartile and one-fourth (25%) lies above.

Construction of the Box and Whiskers Plot Requires that a Box is drawn such that

- Ends of the box are at Q_1 and Q_3
- A vertical line is drawn within the box which indicated median which is measure of center
- Lines drawn from left end of box to minimum value and from right end of box to maximum value, these lines are called Whiskers
- Symmetry is reflected if the median is at the middle of the box.
- Skewness is reflected if the median is closer to one end of the box.
  - If Q_2 is closer to Q_3 = Positive or Right skew
  - If Q_2 is closer to Q_1 = Negative or Left Skew
- Length of the box = Interquartile range (IQR) = $Q_3 - Q_1$

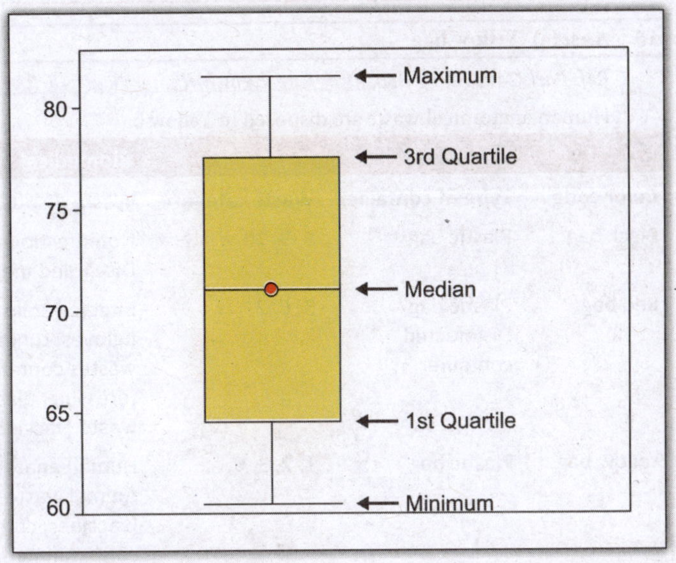

14. Ans. (a) Endemic

Ref: Park 24th Ed Pg 98

Some Important Definitions		
Term	**Description**	**Example**
Epidemic	The "unusual" occurrence in a community or region of disease, specific health-related behavior or other health- related events clearly in excess of "expected occurrence". The amount of disease occurring in the past, in the absence of an epidemic, defines the "expected" frequency.	Cholera, chickenpox. Modern "slow" epidemics- Coronary disease
Endemic	It refers to the constant presence of a disease or infectious agent within a given geographic area or population group, without importation from outside; may also refer to the "usual" or expected frequency of the disease within such area or population group.	Common cold
Hyperendemic	The disease is constantly present at a high incidence and/or prevalence rate and affects all age groups equally	

Contd...

Some Important Definitions		
Holoendemic	"Holoendemic" a high level of infection beginning early in life and affecting most of the child population, leading to a state of equilibrium such that the adult population shows evidence of the disease much less commonly than do the children	Malaria
Sporadic	The cases occur irregularly, haphazardly from time to time, and generally infrequently. The cases are so few and separated widely in space and time that they show little or no connection with each other, nor a recognizable common source of infection. A sporadic disease may be the starting point of an epidemic when conditions are favorable for its spread.	Polio, tetanus, herpes-zoster and meningococcal meningitis.
Pandemic	An epidemic usually affecting a large proportion of the population, occurring over a wide geographic area such as a section of a nation, the entire nation, a continent or the world	Influenza pandemics of 1918 and 1957, cholera El Tor in 1962 (still continuing) & acute hemorrhagic conjunctivitis in 1971 and 1981.

15. Ans. (a) Yellow bag

Ref: Park 24th Ed Pg 830, http://mpcb.gov.in/biomedical/pdf/BMW_Rules_2016.pdf

Human anatomical waste are disposed in Yellow bag

Biomedical Waste Disposal

Color code	Type of container	Waste category	Waste disposed	Treatment options
Black bag	Plastic bag	5, 9, 10	Noninfectious waste (papers, plastic covers), Discarded medicines & cytotoxic drugs	Disposal in secure land fills
Red bag	Plastic bag/ Disinfected container	3, 6, 7	Infected solid disposable wastes other than sharps (gloves, tunings, catheters, iv sets), Infected solid wastes contaminated with blood and body fluids (dressing, plaster, linen), Microbiology/ Biotech waste (vaccines, cultures)	Autoclave, Microwave, chemical treatment
Yellow bag	Plastic bag	1, 2, 3, 6	Human anatomical waste Animal waste, Microbiology/ Biotech waste (vaccines, cultures), Infected solid wastes contaminated with blood and body fluids (dressing, plaster, linen)	Incineration
Blue bag	Plastic bag/ Puncture proof container	4, 7	Solid sharps (needles, syringes, scalpels, blades), Infected solid disposable wastes other than sharps (gloves, tunings, catheters, iv sets)	Autoclave, Microwave, chemical treatment, destruction and shredding

16. Ans. (a) Shake Test

Ref: Park 24th Ed Pg 118, 119

Freeze Damage To Vaccine : The vaccines that are freeze sensitive will get spoiled if they get frozen. Causes of Vaccine freezing are:

- Improper storage in ILR
- Cold climates and ambient temperature is less than 0C
- Storage and transport with non-conditioned frozen ice-packs
- Defective ILR
- Incorrect thermostat adjustment
- Untrained or improperly trained staff handling vaccine/ cold chain

The ***"Shake Test"*** is used to check whether freeze sensitive vaccines have been damaged by exposure to temperature below 0 C. After it has thawed, a vial of vaccine that has been frozen no longer has the appearance of a cloudy liquid but tends to form flakes that settle down at the bottom of the vial. There is only one way to conduct a Shake test. The protocol must not be altered.

Procedure:

Test Vial: Take a vaccine vial you suspect that may have been frozen - This is "Test Vial"

Frozen Control Vial: Take a vaccine vial of the same antigen, same manufacturer, and same batch number as the suspect vaccine vial you want to test.

- Freeze solid this vial at -20 C overnight in deep freezer and this is "frozen control" vial and label it accordingly to avoid its usage.
- Let it Thaw. Do NOT HEAT it.
- Hold the control and the test vials together between thumb and the forefinger and vigorously shake the vials for 10–15 seconds.
- Place both vials to rest on a flat surface, side by side observe them for 30 minutes.
- Compare for rate of sedimentation. If the sedimentation in the "Test Vial" is slower than the "Frozen Control Vial" the vaccine has not been damaged. It passed the shake test. Use the vaccine batch - it is not damaged.

- If the sedimentation is similar in both vials or if sedimentation is faster in "Test Vial" than in the "Frozen vial" the vaccine is damaged. It failed in the shake test. Do NOT use. Notify your supervisor.

17. Ans. (a) ⅓ calorie, ½ protein

Ref: Park 24th Ed Pg 616, 698

Repeat (See AIIMS Nov 2017 PSM for explanation) (see page no. 575)

AIIMS MAY 2018

18. Ans. (a) Improvement in labor room services

Ref: http://pib.nic.in/newsite/PrintRelease.aspx?relid=177532

LaQshya- Labor Room Quality Improvement Initiative has been launched by Ministry of Health and Family Welfare under National Health Mission in 2017.

LaQshya- Labor Room Quality Improvement Initiative	
Goal	Reduce preventable maternal and newborn mortality, morbidity and stillbirths associated with the care around delivery in Labor room and Maternity OT and ensure respectful maternity care.
Objectives	• To reduce maternal and newborn mortality & morbidity due to APH, PPH, retained placenta, preterm, preeclampsia & eclampsia, obstructed labor, puerperal sepsis, newborn asphyxia, and sepsis, etc. • To improve Quality of care during the delivery and immediate post-partum care, stabilization of complications and ensure timely referrals, and enable an effective two-way follow-up system. • To enhance satisfaction of beneficiaries visiting the health facilities and provide Respectful Maternity Care (RMC) to all pregnant women attending the public health facility
Scope	Following facilities would be taken under LaQshya initiative on priority: • All government medical college hospitals. • All District Hospitals & equivalent health facilities. • All designated FRUs and high case load CHCs with over 100 deliveries/60 (per month) in hills and desert areas.
Strategies	• Reorganizing/aligning Labor room & Maternity Operation Theater layout and workflow as per 'Labor Room Standardization Guidelines' and 'Maternal & Newborn Health Toolkit' issued by the Ministry of Health & Family Welfare, Government of India. • Ensuring that at least all government medical college hospitals and high caseload district hospitals have dedicated obstetric HDUs as per GoI MOHFW Guidelines, for managing complicated pregnancies that require life-saving critical care. • Ensuring strict adherence to clinical protocols for management and stabilization of the complications before referral to higher centers.
Interventions	• Ensuring availability of optimal and skilled human resources as per case-load and prevalent norms through rational deployment and skill upgradation. • Ensuring skill assessment of all staff of LR & Maternal OT through OSCE (Objective Structured Clinical Examination) testing as per Dakshata guidelines for delivery of 'zero-defect' quality obstetric and newborn care. Enhance proficiency of labor room and operation theater staff for management of the complications through skill-lab training, simulations and drills. Ensuring that staff working in the labor room and maternity OT are not shifted from maternity duty to other departments/wards frequently. • Sensitizing care-providers for delivery of respectful maternity care and close monitoring of language, behavior and conduct of the labor room, OT & HDU Staff. 4. Creating an enabling environment for natural birthing process. • Implementation of Clinical Guidelines, Labor Room Clinical Pathways, Referral Protocols, safe birth checklist (in labor room and Obstetric OT) and surgical safety check-list. • Ensuring round the clock availability of Blood transfusion services, diagnostic services, drugs & consumables. • Ensuring availability of triage area and functional newborn care area. • Ensuring systematic facility-level audit of all cases of maternal/neonatal deaths, stillbirth, and maternal near

19. Ans. (c) 3–30 days

Ref: Park 23rd ed page 332, Harrison's 19th Ed page 2404

Option (A)

3-5 days is typical of Chancroid

Option (B)

9-90 days is typical of syphilis

NOTE

Harrison's 19th Ed states incubation period of LGV to be 3 days - 6 weeks which is not provided in the options and is best fitting with 3–30 days. Also Park categorically mentions 3–30 days and most likely the question is taken from Park directly

Lymphogranuloma Venereum: It commonly presents with swelling of lymph nodes in the groin. Although initially there is a small, painless ulcer of the genitalia **3–30 days** after exposure it may pass unrecognized and resolve spontaneously. Untreated, the disease may cause extensive lymphatic damage resulting in elephantiasis of the genitalia. The antibiotics used are doxycycline, erythromycin and tetracycline. Benefit in late cases, e.g. with rectal stricture is slight. Surgical operation may be of benefit in cases with extensive elephantiasis or deformity.

20. Ans. (b) 100

Ref: Park 23rd Ed Pg 524, 567, http://nhsrcindia.org/sites/default/files/Better_Planning_of_Work_at_Sub_Center_Level.pdf

NOTE

If not provided otherwise we must consider Non high focus states

At Subcenter level, a population of approximately 5000, ***we expect 100 infants in non-high focus states*** and 150-200 in high-focus states, with an equal number of pregnancies. This translates to 60 children per month for immunization and 15 children per immunization session in non-high focus states. In high focus states, there would be around 100 children per month and 25 children per immunization session.

21. Ans. (a) Doxycycline

Ref: Park 23rd ed page 300, Harrison 19th ed page 152e-3

Tetracycline (Doxycycline) is the drug of choice for the treatment of epidemic louse-borne typhus, murine typhus, scrub typhus, tick typhus, Rocky Mountain spotted fever, and Mediterranean spotted fever

Typhus group

Rickettsia prowazekii	Epidemic typhus (louse-borne typhus), Brill-Zinsser disease	Louse (Human body louse)	Humans	Fever, chills, myalgia, rash (no eschar), headache severe illness if untreated	Central Africa, Asia, Central, North, and South America
Rickettsia typhi	Murine typhus, endemic typhus (flea-borne typhus)	Flea	Rodents	Fever, headache, myalgia, rash (no eschar); milder illness than epidemic typhus	Tropical and subtropical areas worldwide
Orientia (formerly Rickettsia) tsutsugamushi	Scrub typhus	Larval trombiculid mites (chigger) (True reservoir)	Rodents	Fever, headache, rash (50% have eschar), lymphadenopathy, atypical lymphocytes	Asia-Pacific region from maritime Russia and China to Indonesia and North Australia to Afghanistan

22. Ans. (a) Resting heart rate (beats/min) and age in years

Ref: Park 23rd Ed page 73, Biostatistics BY Mahajan 7th ed pg 134

(See table of "Statistical Tests" in AIIMS May 2018 PSM) (see page no. 560 and 610)

Chi square test is done for Qualitative data. Heart rate is a Quantitative data hence ruled out

23. Ans. (a) VVM

Ref: Park 23rd Ed page 110

Vaccine Vial Monitor

A vaccine vial monitor (VVM) is a label containing a heat sensitive material which is placed on a vaccine vial to register cumulative heat exposure over time. The combined effects of time and temperature cause the inner square of the VVM to darken, gradually and irreversibly.

A direct relationship exists between the rate of color change and temperature:

- The lower the temperature, the slower the color change.
- The higher the temperature, the faster the color change.

The VVM is a circle with a small square inside it. It can be printed on a product label, attached to the cap of a vaccine vial or tube, or attached to the neck of an ampoule. The inner square of the VVM is made of heat sensitive material that is light at the starting point and becomes darker with exposure to heat. At the starting point, the inner square is a lighter color than the outer circle. From then on, until the temperature and/or duration of heat reaches a level known to degrade the vaccine beyond acceptable limits, the inner square remains lighter than the outer circle.

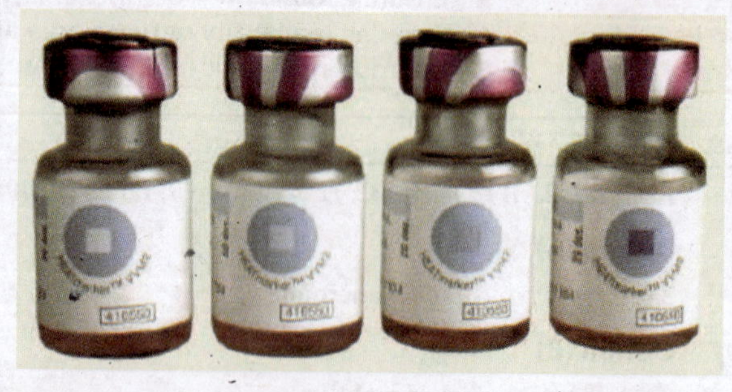

At the discard point, the inner square is the same color as the outer circle. This reflects that the vial has been exposed to an unacceptable level of heat and the vaccine degraded beyond acceptable limits. The inner square will continue to darken with heat exposure until it is much darker than the outer circle. Whenever the inner square matches or is darker than the outer circle, the vial must be discarded. VVMs are located either on the label or on the top of the cap or on the neck of the ampoule depending on the type of vaccine (liquid or freeze-dried). VVM for liquid type vaccines are placed on custom labels to allow reference to VVM readings even though those vials have been opened and intended to be used in subsequent sessions according to multi-dose vial policy (MDVP). VVM for freeze dried vaccines are placed either on top of the cap (vials) or on the neck of the ampoule so it is discarded by the time of reconstitution. Since freeze-dried vaccines must be discarded within six hours or at the end of the session whichever comes first, VVM can only be referred until the time of reconstitution.

Rule 1: If the inner square is lighter than the outer circle, the vaccine can be used provided that the expiry date has not passed.

Rule 2: If the inner square is the same color or darker than the outer circle, the vaccine must not be used.

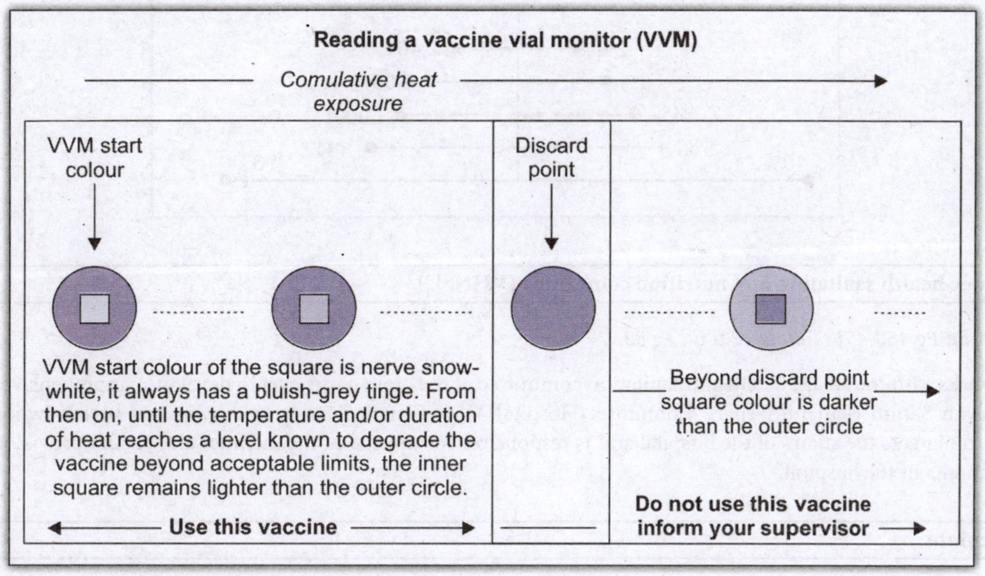

24. Ans. (c) III < I > II

Ref: Park 23rd Ed Pg 850

Recall Bias

We are not sure about the labeling used in the graph so read the question carefully in the exam and then mark the answer accordingly based on the concept.

Margin of error is inversely proportional to the sample size. Larger the sample size lower will be the margin of error. Hence in the given diagram Sample II will have largest margin of error.

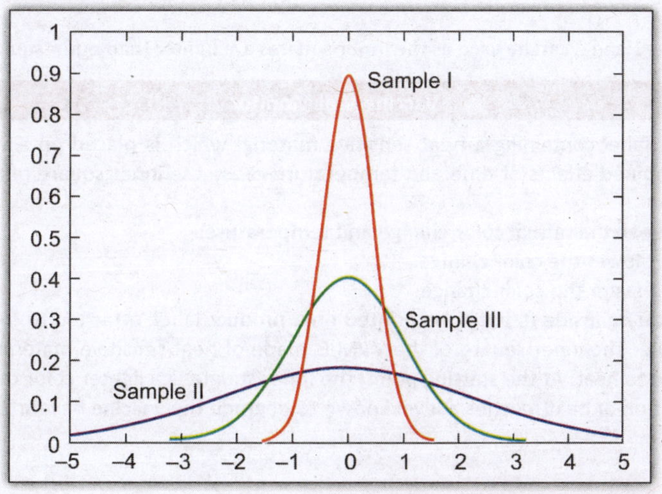

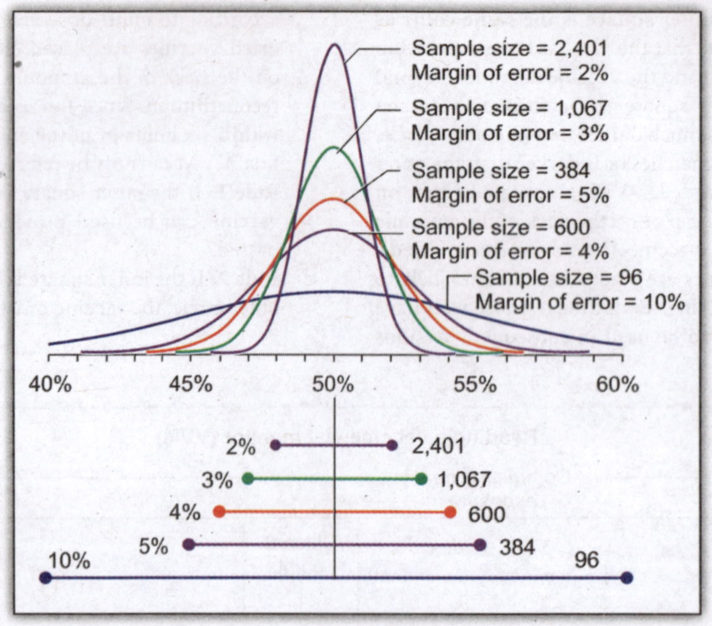

25. Ans. (a) Village health sanitation and nutrition committee (VHNSC)

Ref: Park 23rd Ed Pg 450-451, Taneja 12th Ed Pg 82

- ASHA works with the village health and sanitation committee of the gram panchayat to develop comprehensive village health plan.
- Rogi Kalyan Samiti (Patient Welfare Committee/Hospital Management Society is a registered society whose members act as trustees to manage the affairs of the hospital and is responsible for upkeep of the facilities and ensure provision of better facilities to the patients in the hospital.

26. Ans. (a) Selenium

Ref: Trace Elements in Human and Animal Nutrition By E Underwood 2nd Ed Pg 344

- Blind staggers is an acute syndrome in cattle and sheep characterized by wandering and stumbling of animals with impaired vision.
- Alkali disease is a chronic form of selenosis of animals characterized by emaciation.
- Selenium toxicity is caused by consumption of seleniferous plants.

AIIMS NOVEMBER 2017

27. Ans. (b) Both 1 and 2

Ref: Park 24th ed page 118

From the above image only vial 1 and 2 can be used as the inner squares are lighter than outer squares.

Vaccine Vial Monitor

A vaccine vial monitor (VVM) is a label containing a heat sensitive material which is placed on a vaccine vial to register cumulative heat exposure over time. The combined effects of time and temperature cause the inner square of the VVM to darken, gradually and irreversibly.

- A direct relationship exists between the rate of color change and temperature:
- The lower the temperature, the slower the color change.
- The higher the temperature, the faster the color change.

The VVM is a circle with a small square inside it. It can be printed on a product label, attached to the cap of a vaccine vial or tube, or attached to the neck of an ampoule. The inner square of the VVM is made of heat sensitive material that is light at the starting point and becomes darker with exposure to heat. At the starting point, the inner square is a lighter color than the outer circle. From then on, until the temperature and/or duration of heat reaches a level known to degrade the vaccine beyond acceptable limits, the inner square remains lighter than the outer circle.

Contd...

Vaccine Vial Monitor

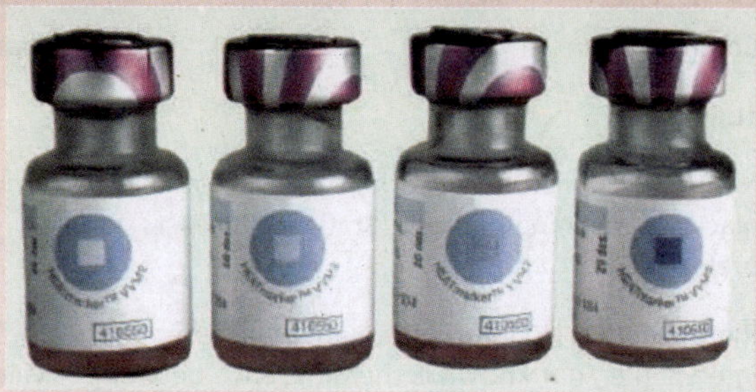

At the discard point, the inner square is the same color as the outer circle. This reflects that the vial has been exposed to an unacceptable level of heat and the vaccine degraded beyond acceptable limits. The inner square will continue to darken with heat exposure until it is much darker than the outer circle.

Whenever the inner square matches or is darker than the outer circle, the vial must be discarded. VVMs are located either on the label or on the top of the cap or on the neck of the ampoule depending on the type of vaccine (liquid or freeze-dried). VVM for liquid type vaccines are placed on custom labels to allow reference to VVM readings even though those vials have been opened and intended to be used in subsequent sessions according to multi-dose vial policy (MDVP). VVM for freeze dried vaccines are placed either on top of the cap (vials) or on the neck of the ampoule so it is discarded by the time of reconstitution. Since freeze-dried vaccines must be discarded within six hours or at the end of the session whichever comes first, VVM can only be referred until the time of reconstitution.

Rule 1: If the inner square is lighter than the outer circle, the vaccine can be used provided that the expiry date has not passed.

Rule 2: If the inner square is the same color or darker than the outer circle, the vaccine must not be used.

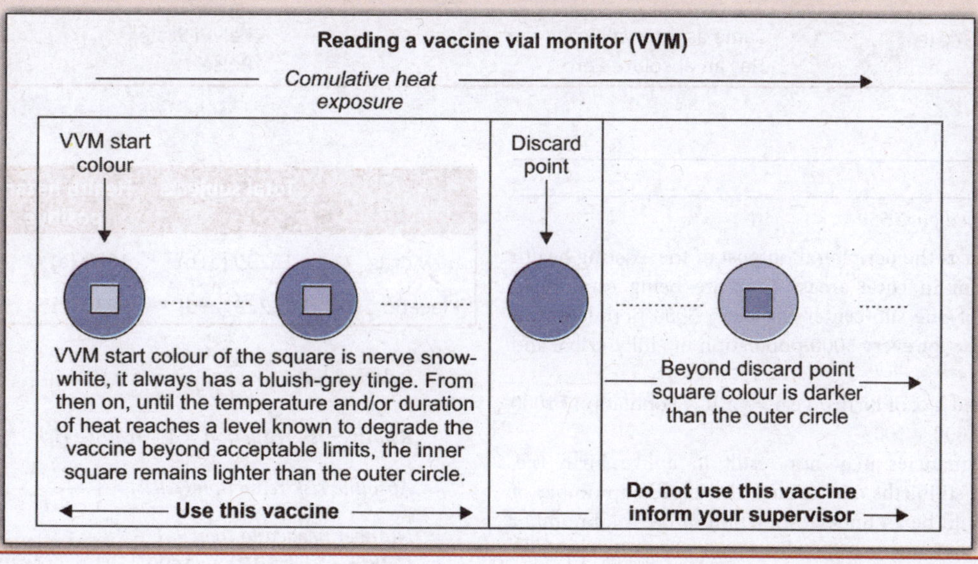

28. Ans. (c) If the prevalence is high, then the patient is likely to have the disease

Ref: Park 24th ed page 149

Sensitivity of a screening test is its ability to detect correctly those who have the disease. Sensitivity and specificity can be considered fixed properties of a diagnostic test unaffected by the prevalence (Common or rare) of the disease. On the other hand Predictive value depends on the prevalence of the disease. **Positive predictive value:** The PPV of a test is a proportion that is useful to clinicians since it answers the question: 'How likely is it that this patient has the disease given that the test result is positive? Predictive value" reflects the **diagnostic power of the test.** The predictive accuracy depends upon sensitivity, specificity and disease prevalence. The "predictive value of a positive test" indicates the probability that a patient with a positive test result has, in fact, the disease in question. *The more prevalent a disease is in a given population, the more accurate will be the predictive value of a positive screening test.* The predictive value of a positive result falls as disease prevalence declines.

$$\text{Positive predictive value} = \frac{\text{True positives}}{\text{True positives} + \text{False positives}}$$

29. Ans. (a) Ordinal

Ref: High Yield Biostatistics 4th ed page 2-3

Child Pugh is an Ordinal scale as there is Rank order with Class A = 5–6, Class B = 7–9 and Class C = 10–15

Statistical Scales		
Name	**Comments**	**Examples**
Categorical scale (For Qualitative data)		
Nominal scale	No implication of order/ ratio, Data cannot be placed in meaningful order (Statistically least preferable)	Hindus, Muslims, Christians
Ordinal scale	Rank ordered. No information about size of interval (i.e., not known is the difference between the 1st and 2nd rank is the same as between 2nd and 3rd)	1st, 2nd, 3rd Mild, moderate, severe TNM staging Child Pugh Class A = 5–6, Class B = 7–9 and Class C = 10–15
Dichotomous scale	Data fall into 2 groups only	Died/ Alive
Metric scale (for quantitative data)		
Interval Scale	Meaningful Intervals between items Do not have an absolute zero Do not have meaningful ratios	Difference between 50°C and 60°C is the same as that between 30°C and 40°C But 60°C is not twice as hot as 30°C because 0°C does not mean complete absence of heat
Ratio Scale	Same as Interval Scale Has an absolute Zero	Kelvin Scale Pulse

30. Ans. (a) 60

Ref: Park 24th ed page 559

The sub-center is the peripheral outpost of the existing health delivery system in rural areas. They are being established on the basis of one sub-center for every 5000 population in general and one for every 3000 population in . hilly, tribal and backward areas.

Hence Expected No. of Births/ year = CBR X Population / 1000 = 20 × 5000/ 1000 = 100

As some pregnancies may not result in a live birth (i.e. abortions and stillbirths may occur), the expected number of live births would be an under-estimation of the total number of pregnancies. Hence, a correction factor of 10% is required, i.e. add 10% to the figure obtained above. So, the total number of expected pregnancies **(Z) = Y + 10% of Y = 100 + 10 = 110**

As a thumb rule, in any given month, approximately half the number of pregnancies estimated above should be in records. I.e. ANC registrations should be minimum 110/ 2 = 55 which is approximately 60

To ensure complete registration, it is essential that the ANM should know the estimated number of pregnancies to be registered annually in her area. Calculating the expected number of annual pregnancies in the area will help her judge how good her pregnancy registration is and help her judge whether she has an adequate stock of the supplies required to provide routine ANC

31. Ans. (c) 1% and 10%

Ref: High Yield Biostatistics 4th ed page 92-93

Lets first redraw the table

	Total subjects	Health hazard positive	Health hazard negative
new drug	15230 (a+b)	1600 (a)	13400 (b)
Placebo	15229 (c+d)	1830 (c)	13620 (d)

Relative risk = $\left(\frac{a}{a+b}\right)-\left(\frac{c}{c+d}\right)$

Relative risk reduction = 1 – relative risk

Absolute risk reduction (ARR) = $\left(\frac{c}{c+d}\right)-\left(\frac{a}{a+b}\right)$

Number needed to treat = 1/ARR

Relative Risk (RR) = (1600/15230) / (1830/15229) = 0.87 (0.9 Rounded off)

Relative risk reduction (RRR) = 1- Relative Risk = 1- 0.9 = 0.1 or 10%

Absolute Risk Reduction (ARR) = (1830/15229) - 1600/ 15230 = 0.01 = 1%

32. Ans. (a) 0.66/10000 population

Ref: NLEP Annual Report http://nlep.nic.in/pdf/revised%20annual%20report%2031st%20March%202015-16.pdf

Recall Bias

Some recallers think that Annual new case detection rate (ANCDR) was asked

If prevalence was asked then 0.66/10000 population

If Annual New case detection rate was asked then it is 9.71/ lakh population or 0.97/10000 population.

During the year 2015–16, Annual New Case Detection Rate (ANCDR) of 9.71 per 1 lakh population Prevalence Rate (PR) of 0.66 per 10,000 population

It has been observed that trend of two important indicators of National Leprosy Eradication Program, India i.e. Annual New Case Detection Rate (ANCDR) and Prevalence Rate (PR) are almost static since 2006–2007.

In addition, the percentage of grade II disability amongst new cases detected has been increased from 3.10% (2010–2011) to 4.61% (2014–2015), which indicates that the cases are being detected late in the community and there may be several cases which are lying undetected or hidden

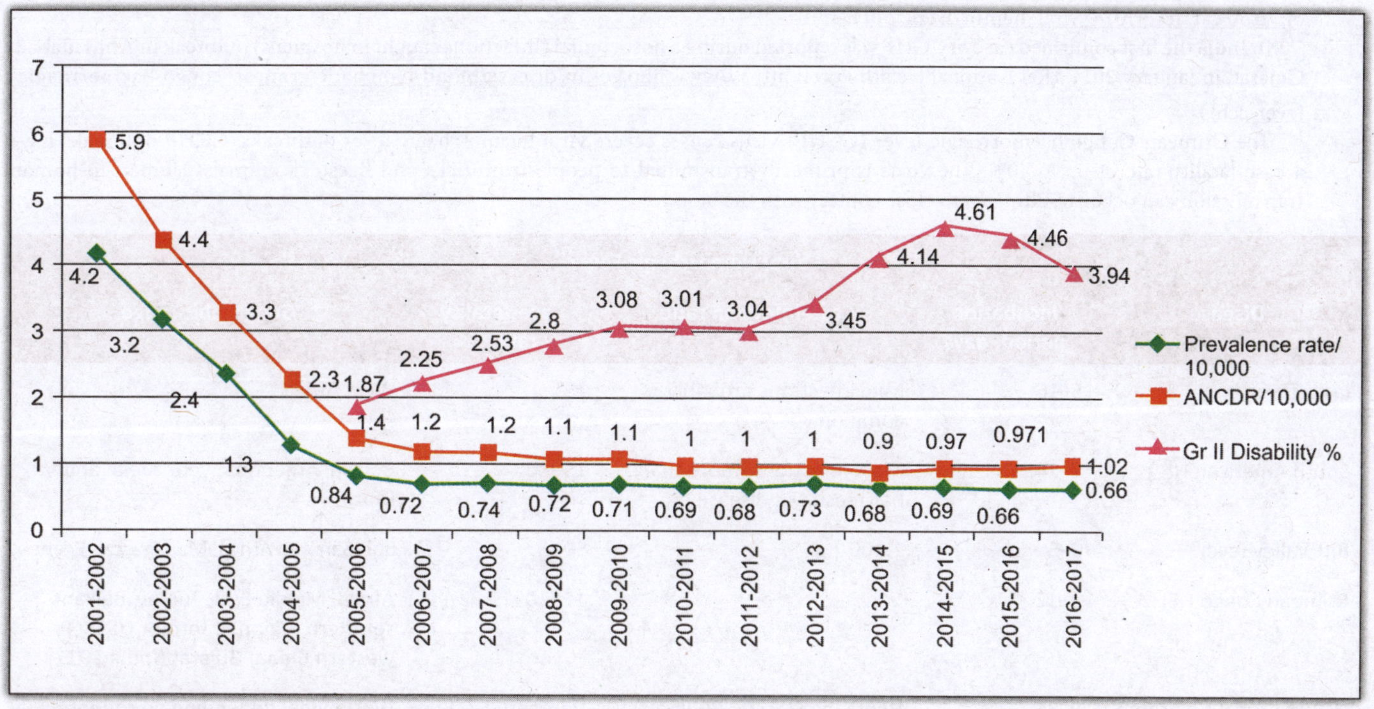

33. Ans. (a) Alpha error

Ref: High Yield Biostatistics 4th ed page 28, 29

Types of Error	
Type 1 error	**Type II error**
Alpha error	*Beta error*
False negative	*False positive*
Rejecting null hypothesis when its true	*Accenting null hypothesis when its false*
• There is no real difference however we find a difference • An example of this would be if a test shows that a woman is pregnant (H0: she is not) when in reality she is not, or telling a patient he is sick (H0: he is not), when in fact he is not	• We fail to observe a difference when in reality there is a difference • An example of this would be if a test shows that a woman is not pregnant (H0: she is not), when in reality, she is

Tabulated relations between truth/falseness of the null hypothesis and outcomes

	Null hypothesis (H_0) is true	Null hypothesis (H_0) is false
Reject null hypothesis	Type I error False positive	Correct outcome True Positive
Fail to reject null hypothesis	Correct outcome True Negative	Type II error False negative

34. Ans. (a) Crimean Congo Hemorrhagic fever

Ref: With Text

Agents causing VHFs are distributed worldwide. Although there are 12 viruses that are capable of causing hemorrhagic fevers, only 2 are consistently seen in India. In the Indian scenario, however, Dengue and Dengue hemorrhagic fever, and Kyasanur Forest Disease (KFD) infection are seen and are endemic (even hyperendemic). There is also an increasing recent interest in the Ebola virus as the current 2014 epidemic in the African subcontinent may soon spread beyond its boundaries and indeed some cases have already been reported from outside of the main affected region. (Ref: Update on Tropical Fever page 153 http://www.apiindia.org/pdf/monograph_2015_update_on_tropical_fever/014_viral_hemorrhagic.pdf)

In India the first confirmed case of CCHF was reported during a nosocomial (Infections caught in hospitals) outbreak in Ahmadabad, Gujarat, in January 2011. (Ref National Health Portal https://www.nhp.gov.in/disease/blood-lymphatic/crimean-congo-haemorrhagic-fever-cchf)

The Crimean-Congo haemorrhagic fever (CCHF) virus causes severe viral haemorrhagic fever outbreaks. CCHF outbreaks have a case fatality rate of up to 40%. The virus is primarily transmitted to people from ticks and livestock animals. Human-to-human transmission can occur resulting from close contact with the blood

Viral Hemorrhagic Fever

Disease	Incubation period, days	Case-infection ratio	Case-fatality rate, %	Geographic range
lassa fever	5–16	Mild infections probably common	15	West Africa
South American HF	7–14	Most infections (more than half) result in disease	15–30	Bolivia, Argentina, Venezuela, and Brazil
Rift Valley fever	2–5	1:100	50	Sub-Saharan Africa, Madagascar, Egypt
Crimean Congo HF	3–12	1:5	15–30	Africa, Middle East, Turkey, Balkans, southern region of former USSR, western China, Gujarat (India 2011)
HF with renal syndrome	9–35	Hantaan, >1:1.25; Puumala, 1:20	Hantaan, 5–15; Puumala, <1	Worldwide, depending on rodent reservoir
Hantavirus pulmonary syndrome	7–28	Very high	40–50	America
Marburg or Ebola HF	3–16	High	25–90	Sub-Saharan Africa
Yellow fever	3–6	1:2–1:20	20	Africa, South America
Dengue HF/dengue shock syndrome	2–7	Nonimmune, 1:10,000; heterologous immune, 1:100	<1 with supportive treatment	Tropics and subtropics worldwide
Kyasanur Forest/Omsk HF	3–8	Variable	0.5–10	Mysore (India)/ western Siberia

35. Ans. (a) Doxycycline

Ref: Park 23rd ed page 300, Harrison 19th ed page 152e-3

Repeat AIIMS MAY 2018 (See for explanation) (see page no. 568)

Tetracycline (Doxycycline) is the drug of choice for the treatment of epidemic louse-borne typhus, murine typhus, scrub typhus, tick typhus, Rocky Mountain spotted fever, and Mediterranean spotted fever

36. Ans. (a) Sarcoptes scabiei

Ref: Rook's 8th Ed page 38.36, Park 23rd ed page 782

The image in the question shows four pairs of legs, two anterior and two posterior. The legs don't have claws. There is no siphon mechanism on the head. The legs aren't attached to the thorax alone. Thus it is a case of sarcoptes scabies. Scabies is an infestation of the skin by the mite Sarcoptes scabiei.

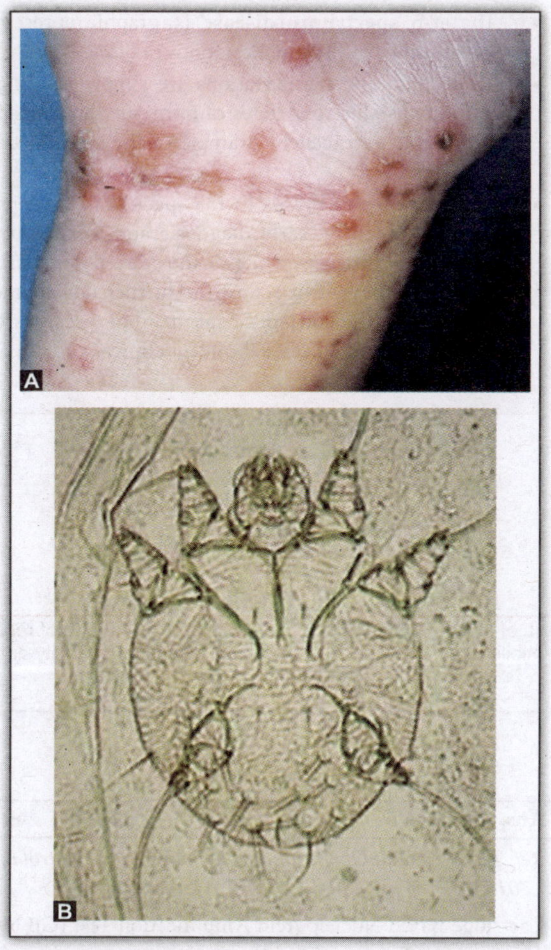

Figs A and B: **(A) Classic scabies** typically manifests as an intensely pruritic eruption with a distribution on sides and webs of the fingers, wrists, axillae, areolae, and genitalia are among the common sites of involvement. Crusted scabies, a less common variant that primarily occurs in the setting of reduced cellular immunity and is associated with a heavy mite burden, is characterized by thick scale, crusts, and fissures. Pruritus is the most prominent and common clinical feature of scabies. Host type I and IV hypersensitivity reactions involving multiple cell lines underline the pathophysiology of the scabietic rash and pruritus. The itch is characteristically described as intense, intractable and generalized pruritus that usually spares the scalp. It is worse at night and after a hot shower, but occasionally patients are asymptomatic. The diagnosis of scabies is confirmed through the detection of scabies mites, eggs, or feces with microscopic examination; **(B) Sarcoptes scabiei var. hominis:** Mite identified by light microscopy (100x amplification) in skin scrapings of a burrow (after 10% KOH). It has an ovoid body, flattened dorsoventrally. The adult female = 0.4 x 0.3 mm and Adult male = 0.2 x 0.15 mm. The body is creamy white and is marked by transverse corrugations, and on its dorsal surface by bristles and spines (denticles). There are four pairs of short legs; the anterior two pairs end in elongated peduncles tipped with small suckers. In the female, the rear two pairs of legs end in long bristles (setae), whereas in the male bristles are present on the third pair and peduncles with suckers on the fourth. The mites burrow into the upper layer of the skin but never below the stratum corneum. The burrows appear as tiny raised serpentine lines that are grayish or skin-colored and can be a centimeter or more in length

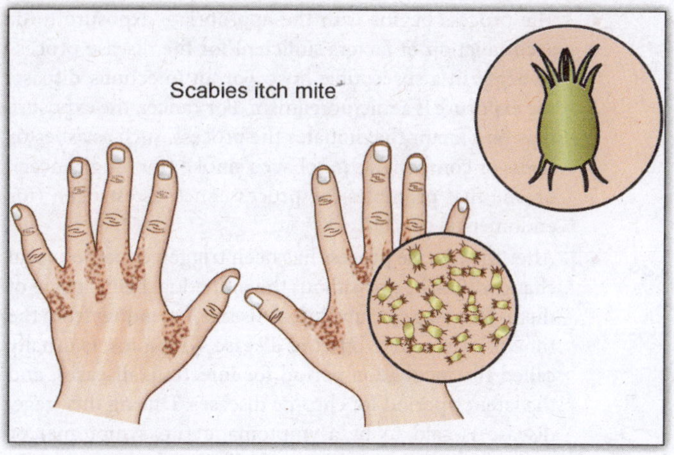

37. Ans. (a) ⅓ calorie, ½ protein

Ref: Park 24th Ed Pg 616, 698

Principles of Mid-day Meal

- The meal should be a supplement and not a substitute to the home diet
- The meal should supply at least 1/3 of the total calories and 1/2 of the total protein need
- The cost of the meal should be reasonably low
- The meal should be such that it can be prepared easily in schools; no complicated cooking process should be involved
- As far as possible, locally available foods should be used; this will reduce the cost of the meal, and
- The menu should be frequently changed to avoid monotony

AIIMS MAY 2017

38. Ans. (c) Not more than 10% of the people benefitted by the drug could be due to chance

Ref: Oxford Handbook of Medical Statistics Page 248

- This question is based on basic biostatistics.
- The *P* (probability) value is used when we wish to see how likely it is that a hypothesis is true. The hypothesis is usually that there is *no* difference between two treatments, known as the "null hypothesis".
- The *P* value gives the probability of any observed difference having happened by chance.
- $P = 0.5$ means that the probability of the difference having happened by chance is 0.5 in 1, or 50:50.
- Similarly, a *P* value of less than 0.10 means that the probability of it happening by chance is 10%.
- Thus, according to our question, the probability that the drug affected the chronic hypertensives by chance is less than 10%. Hence, 90% of the subjects were benefitted by the drug.

39. Ans. (c) C

Ref: Park 24th ed page 40, CDC

- Natural history of disease refers to the progression of a disease process in an individual over time, in the absence of treatment.

- The process begins with the appropriate exposure to or accumulation of factors sufficient for the disease process to begin in a susceptible host. For an infectious disease, the exposure is a microorganism. For cancer, the exposure may be a factor that initiates the process, such as asbestos fibers or components in tobacco smoke (for lung cancer), or one that promotes the process, such as estrogen (for endometrial cancer).
- After the disease process has been triggered, pathological changes then occur without the individual being aware of them. This stage of subclinical disease, extending from the time of exposure to onset of disease symptoms, is usually called the incubation period for infectious diseases, and the latency period for chronic diseases. During this stage, disease is said to be asymptomatic (no symptoms) or inapparent. This period may be as brief as seconds for hypersensitivity and toxic reactions to as long as decades for certain chronic diseases.
- Although disease is not apparent during the incubation period, some pathologic changes may be detectable with laboratory, radiographic, or other screening methods. Most screening programs attempt to identify the disease process during this phase of its natural history, since intervention at this early stage is likely to be more effective than treatment given after the disease has progressed and become symptomatic.
- The **onset of symptoms** marks the transition from subclinical to clinical disease. Most diagnoses are made during the stage of clinical disease. In some people, however, the disease process may never progress to clinically apparent illness. In others, the disease process may result in illness that ranges from mild to severe or fatal. Ultimately, the disease process ends either in recovery, disability or death.
- The term **"spectrum of disease"** is a graphic representation of variations in the manifestations of disease.
- These different manifestations are simply reflections of individuals' different states of immunity and receptivity. Leprosy is an excellent example of the spectral concept of disease.
- The sequence of events in the spectrum of disease can be interrupted by early diagnosis and treatment or by preventive measures which if introduced at a particular point will prevent or retard the further development of the disease. The concept of spectrum of disease provides for inclusion of all cases, both subclinical and clinical, in the study of disease.

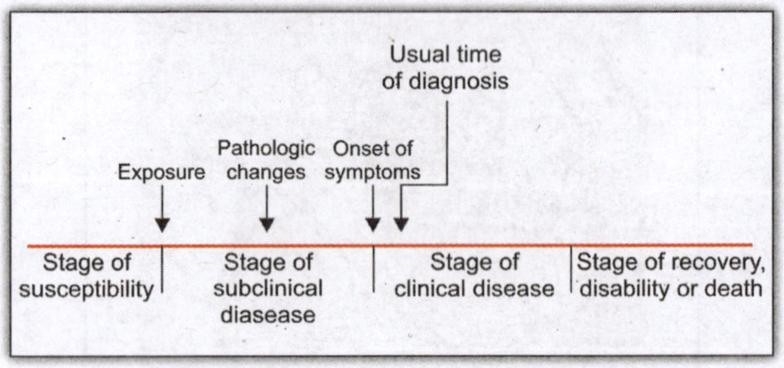

Fig: Natural history of disease timeline

40. Ans. (a) NAAT

Ref: Technical and Operational guidelines for TB control in India - 2016

Cartridge Based Nucleic Acid Amplification Test (CB NAAT): The CB NAAT is known as the GeneXpert in most countries other than India. This is the preferred first diagnostic test in children and people with TB and HIV co-infection.

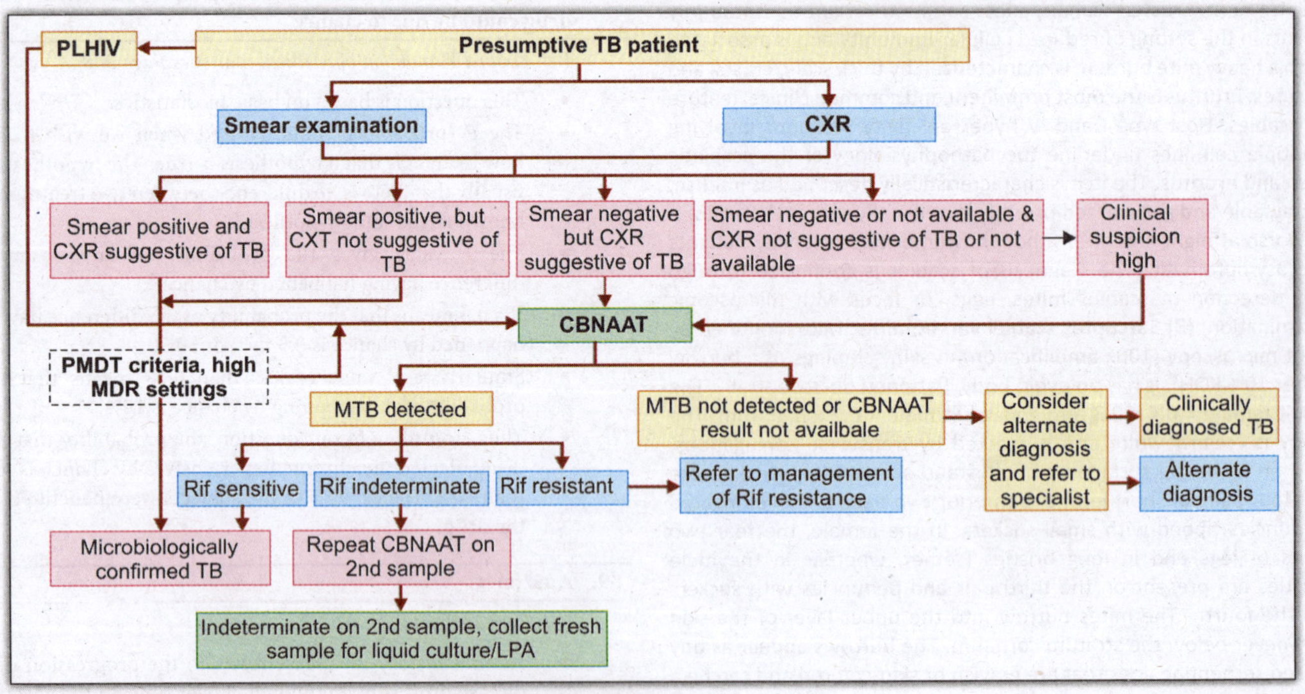

Fig: Diagnostic algorithm of pulmonary TB

41. Ans. (b) Endemic, sporadic, epidemic

Ref: Park 24th ed page 98

In disease 1: We see a continuous trend. Thus we can call this endemic.
In disease 2: No trend can be seen, it can be sporadic increase.
In disease 3: There is an abrupt increase in cases, within a week, we can label it epidemic.

Some Important Definitions

Term	Description	Example
Epidemic	The "unusual" occurrence in a community or region of disease, specific health-related behavior or other health-related events clearly in excess of "expected occurrence". The amount of disease occurring in the past, in the absence of an epidemic, defines the "expected" frequency.	Cholera, chickenpox. Modern "slow" epidemics-Coronary disease
Endemic	It refers to the constant presence of a disease or infectious agent within a given geographic area or population group, without importation from outside; may also refer to the "usual" or expected frequency of the disease within such area or population group.	Common cold
Hyperendemic	The disease is constantly present at a high incidence and/or prevalence rate and affects all age groups equally.	
Holoendemic	"Holoendemic" a high level of infection beginning early in life and affecting most of the child population, leading to a state of equilibrium such that the adult population shows evidence of the disease much less commonly than do the children.	Malaria
Sporadic	The cases occur irregularly, haphazardly from time to time, and generally infrequently. The cases are so few and separated widely in space and time that they show little or no connection with each other, nor a recognizable common source of infection. A sporadic disease may be the starting point of an epidemic when conditions are favorable for its spread.	Polio, tetanus, herpes-zoster and meningococcal meningitis.
Pandemic	An epidemic usually affecting a large proportion of the population, occurring over a wide geographic area such as a section of a nation, the entire nation, a continent or the world.	Influenza pandemics of 1918 and 1957, cholera El Tor in 1962 (still continuing) & acute hemorrhagic conjunctivitis in 1971 and 1981.

42. Ans. (b) Incidence remains the same and prevalence increases

Ref: Park 24th ed page 66

See table of Risk, Incidence and Prevalence in PSM AIIMS May 2016 (see page no. 599-600)

Indirect repeat PSM AIIMS NOV 2015 (Options were in single parameter that is prevalence or incidence decrease or increase) The new treatment is not going to affect the number of new cases. That is, treatment has no effect on the disease incidence. But if we increase survival by new treatment, we ultimately increase number of people living with disease in the community and thus we increase prevalence.

43. Ans. (d) High sensitivity low specificity

Ref: Park 23rd ed page 141, Lange Epidemiology 4th ed ch 6

NOTE

This question can be solved by application of ROC curve. Precision and accuracy are not the same as sensitivity and specificity.

Summary

Lesser the area under overlapping curves greater is the sensitivity and lesser is the specificity

Conventional analyses of diagnostic accuracy by using 2 × 2 table consider the sensitivity and the specificity of a diagnostic test as the primary indices of accuracy since these indices are considered to be independent of the prior probability of disease. However, using a single sensitivity and a single specificity as measures of accuracy is problematic since these measures depend on a diagnostic criterion. ROC analysis has become a popular method for evaluating the accuracy of medical diagnostic systems. The most desirable property of ROC analysis is that the accuracy indices derived from this technique are not distorted by fluctuations caused by the use of arbitrarily chosen decision criteria or cut-offs.

ROC Curve

The ROC curve is a fundamental tool for diagnostic test evaluation. In a receiver operating characteristic (ROC) curve the true positive rate (Sensitivity) is plotted in function of the false positive rate (100-Specificity). The area under a receiver operating characteristic (ROC) curve can be used to assess the performance of a diagnostic test. This curve derives its name from its first application—measuring the ability of radar operators to distinguish radar signals from noise. For the purposes of diagnostic testing, a graph is constructed with sensitivity (sometimes labeled as the true-positive rate) on the vertical axis, and 1 – specificity (sometimes labeled as the false-positive rate) on the horizontal axis. This idea point indicates the diagnostic test has a sensitivity of 100% and specificity of 100%. It is also called perfect classification. Diagnostic test with 50% sensitivity and 50% specificity can be visualized on the diagonal determined by coordinate (0, 0) and coordinates (1, 0). The interpretation of ROC curve is similar to a single point in the ROC space, the closer the point on the ROC curve to the ideal coordinate, the more accurate the test is. The closer the points on the ROC curve to the diagonal, the less accurate the test is.

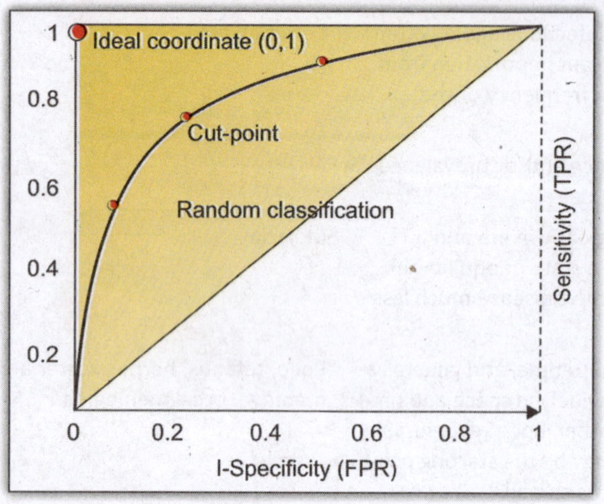

Fig: ROC Space: shadow area represents better diagnostic classification

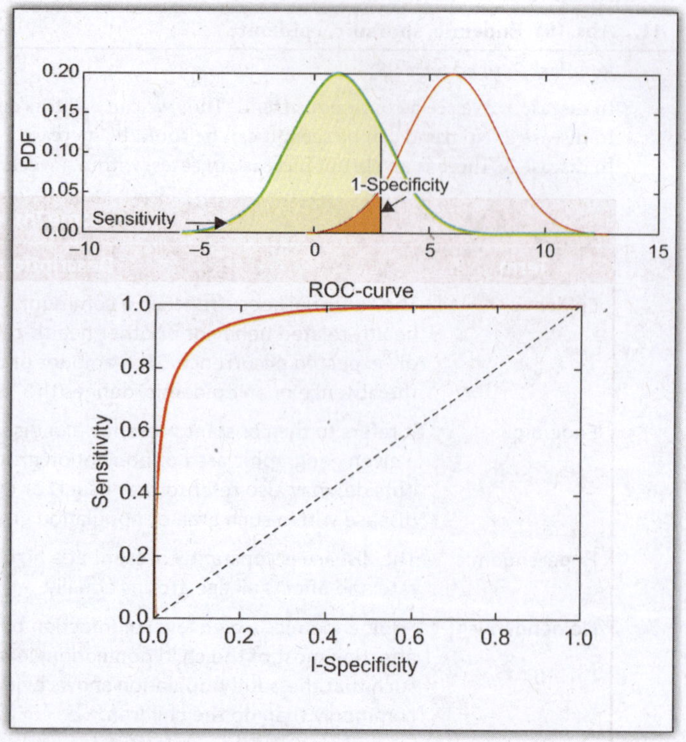

Fig: Top: Probability density functions for two distributions showing areas of sensitivity and 1-specificity. Bottom: Corresponding ROC-curve

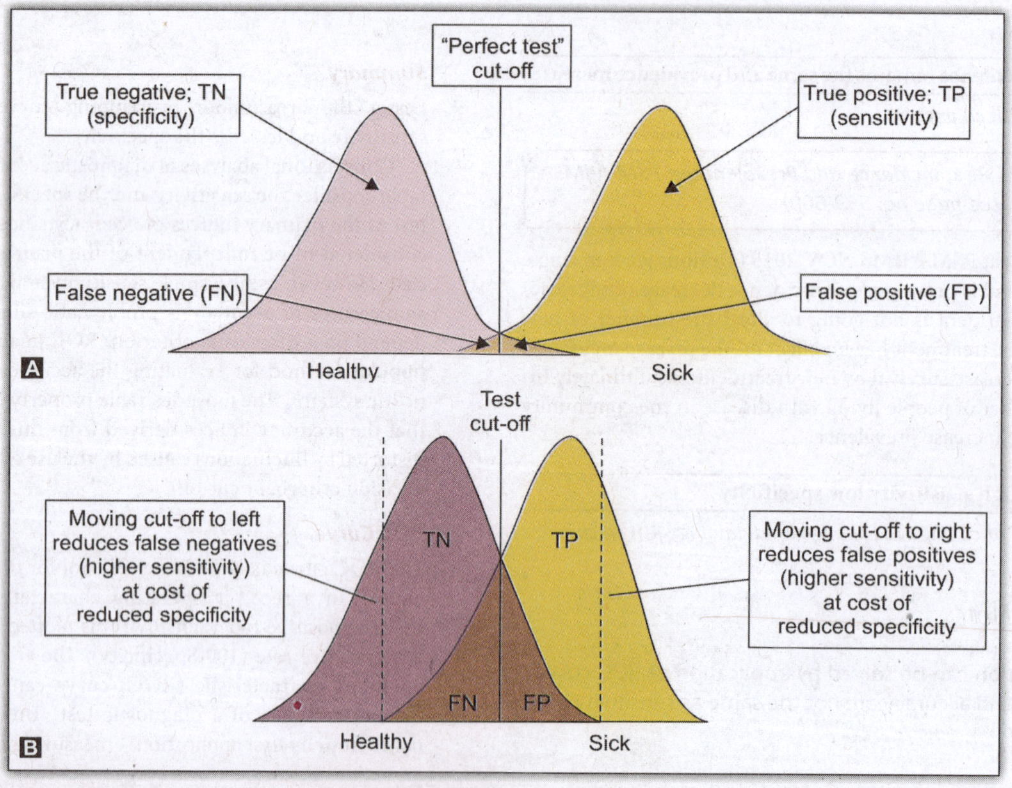

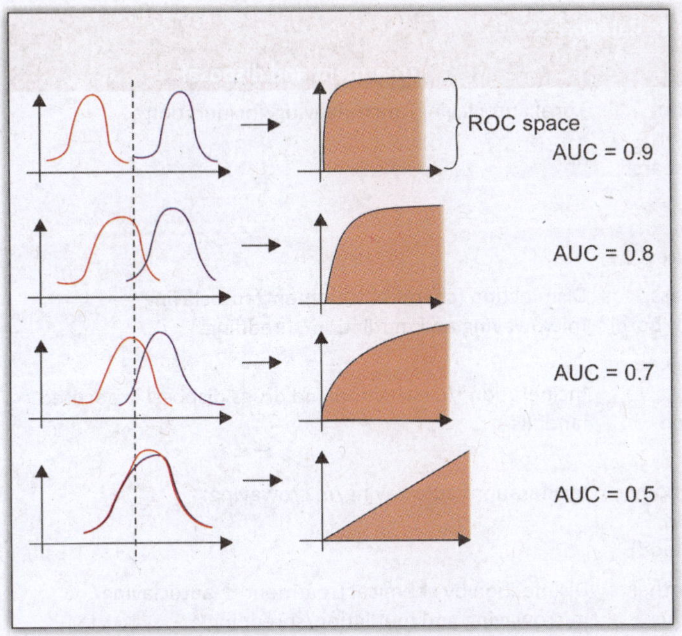

From the above discussion and particularly from the above graph it is clear that lesser the area under overlapping curves greater is the sensitivity and lesser is the specificity

Table: AUC (Area under curve) classification for diagnostic test

AUC Range	Classification
0.9 < AUC < 1.0	Excellent
0.8 < AUC < 0.9	Good
0.7 < AUC < 0.8	Worthless
0.6 < AUC < 0.7	Not good

44. Ans. (d) Soiled plastic waste

Ref: Park 24th ed page 830

The picture is of Red Colored Biomedical waste container.

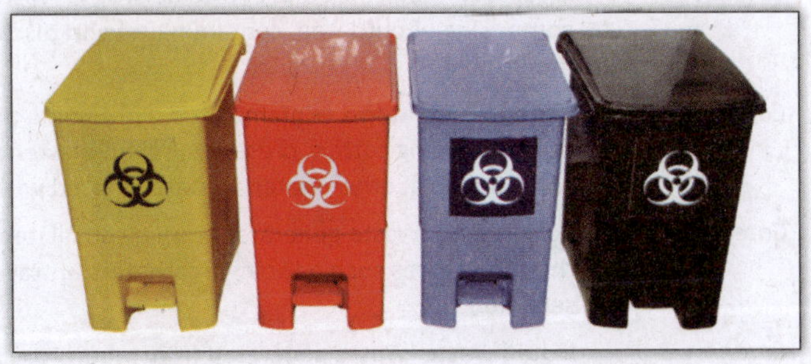

Fig: Types of Biomedical waste containers

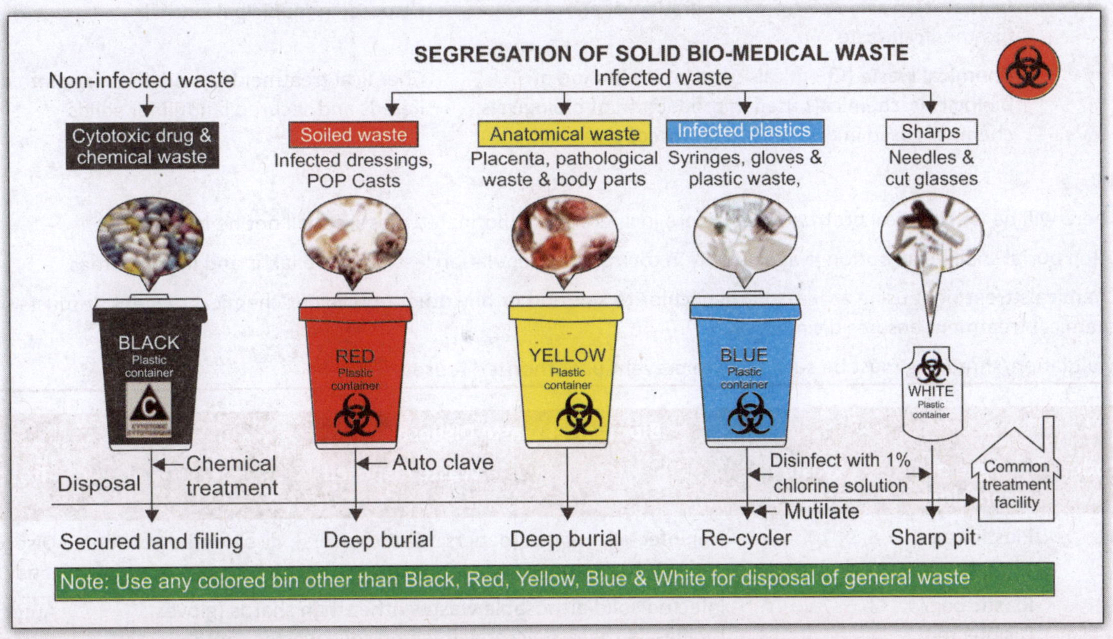

Biomedical Waste Categories		
Category	**Waste category**	**Treatment and disposal**
Category 1	**Human Anatomical Waste** (human tissues, organs, body parts)	Incineration@/deep burial*
Category 2	**Animal Waste** (Animal tissues, organs, body parts carcasses, bleeding parts, fluid, blood and experimental animals used in research, waste generated by veterinary hospitals, colleges, discharge from hospitals, animal houses)	Incineration@/deep burial*

Contd...

Biomedical Waste Categories		
Category	**Waste category**	**Treatment and disposal**
Category 3	**Microbiology and biotechnology waste** (Wastes from laboratory cultures, stocks or micro-organisms live or vaccines, human and animal cell culture used in research and infectious agents from research and industrial laboratories, wastes from production of biologicals, toxins, dishes and devices used for transfer of cultures)	Local autoclaving/micro-waving/incineration@
Category 4	**Waste sharps** (needles, syringes, scalpels, blade, glass, etc. that may cause puncture and cuts. This includes both used and unused sharps)	Disinfection (chemical treatment/autoclaving/ microwaving and mutilation/shredding##
Category 5	**Discarded medicines and cytotoxic drugs** (Waste comprising of outdated, contaminated and discarded medicines)	Incineration@/destruction and drugs disposal in secured landfills
Category 6	**Soiled waste** (items contaminated with blood, and body fluids including cotton, dressings, soiled plaster casts, lines, bedding, other material contaminated with blood)	Incineration@autoclaving/microwaving
Category 7	**Solid waste** (Waste generated from disposal items other than the sharps such a tubings, catheters, intravenous sets etc.)	Disinfection by chemical treatment@@ autoclaving/ microwaving and mutilation/shredding##
Category 8	**Liquid waste** (Waste generated from laboratory and washing, cleaning, housekeeping and disinfecting activities)	Disinfection by chemical treatment@@ and discharge into drains
Category 9	**Incineration ash:** Ash from incineration of any bio-medical waste	Disposal in municipal landfill
Category 10	**Chemical waste** (Chemicals used in production of biologicals, chemicals used in production of biologicals, chemicals used in disinfection, as insecticides, etc.)	Chemical treatment@@ and discharge into drains for liquids and secured landfill for solids

Footnote:

@	There will be no chemical pretreatment before incineration. Chlorinated plastics shall not be incinerated.
*	Deep burial shall be an option available only in towns with population less than five lakhs and in rural areas.
@@	Chemicals treatment using at least 1% hypochlorite solution or any other equivalent chemical reagent. It musts be ensured that chemical treatment ensures disinfection.
##	Multilation/shredding must be such so as to prevent unauthorized reuse.

Biomedical Waste Disposal

Color code	Type of container	Waste category	Waste disposed	Treatment options
Black bag	Plastic bag	5, 9, 10	Noninfectious waste (papers, plastic covers), discarded medicines and cytotoxic drugs	Disposal in secure land fills
Red bag	Plastic bag/ Disinfected container	3, 6, 7	Infected solid disposable wastes other than sharps (gloves, tunings, catheters, iv sets), infected solid wastes contaminated with blood and body fluids (dressing, plaster, linen), microbiology/Biotech waste (vaccines, cultures)	Autoclave, microwave, chemical treatment
Yellow bag	Plastic bag	1, 2, 3, 6	Human anatomical waste Animal waste, Microbiology/Biotech waste (vaccines, cultures), Infected solid wastes contaminated with blood and body fluids (dressing, plaster, linen)	Incineration
Blue bag	Plastic bag/ Puncture proof container	4, 7	Solid sharps (needles, syringes, scalpels, blades), infected solid disposable wastes other than sharps (gloves, tunings, catheters, iv sets)	Autoclave, microwave, chemical treatment, destruction and shredding

45. Ans. (c) Chi-square test

Ref: Park 23rd ed page 852

Incidence of depression will be in nominal form, i.e. depression present or absent, whatever may be the value of the scale used for each patient. The other variable is number of male and female babies. Thus the comparison is best made through Chi square test.

Summary Table of Statistical Tests

Level of measurement	Sample Characteristics					Correlation
	1 Sample	2 Sample		K sample (i.e., >2)		
		Independent	Dependent	Independent	Dependent	
Categorical or nominal	x^2 or binomial	x^2	Mcnamara's x^2	x^2	Cochran's Q	
Rank or ordinal	x^2	Mann Whitney U	Wilcoxon Matched Pairs Signed Ranks	Kruskal Wallis H	Friedman's ANOVA	Spearman's rho
Parametric (Interval and ration)	z test or t test	t test between groups	t test within groups	1 way ANOVA between groups	1 way ANOVA (within or repeated measure)	Pearson's
		Factorial (2 way) ANOVA				

46. Ans. (c) Mean anywhere between 300 to 400

Ref: Oxford Handbook of Medical Statistics page 182

In a normal distribution bell shaped curve without any skew (if the given histogram is converted to a curve) the mean will anyway lie at the midpoint, i.e. between 300 and 400

Mean CD4 count = Total values/Total population

Total values will be given by: Mid points of histogram X Height of Histogram column

CD4 Count	Mid-point (X)	Number of people (n)	X n
0 – 100	50	5	250
100 – 200	150	10	1500
200 – 300	250	25	6250
300 – 400	350	35	12250
400 – 500	450	20	9000
500 – 1600	1050	5	5250
Total		100	34500

Mean = $x_1.n_1+x_2.n_2+\ldots\ldots$

$n_1 + n_2 + \ldots\ldots$

= 34500/100 = 345

Hence, the answer is option (C) Mean anywhere between 300 to 400

AIIMS NOVEMBER 2016

47. Ans. (a) There is a positive correlation between two groups

Ref: With text

Let us first know the difference between Correlation and agreement.

NOTE

- The figure and case is taken directly from a Study done at St Stephen's Hospital Tis Hazari, Delhi "Evaluation of pulse-oximetry oxygen saturation taken through skin protective covering. James J, Tiwari L, Upadhyay P, Sreenivas V, Bhambhani V, Puliyel JM - BMC Pediatr (2006)
- This is the graph of Regression analysis not Bland and Altman plot, However since Bland and Altman plot is often preceded by a Regression analysis some people confuse it to be a part of Bland and Altman plot because it is often used as step one of agreement measurement

In clinical measurement comparison of a new measurement technique with an established one is often needed to see whether they agree sufficiently for the new to replace the old. Such investigations are often analysed inappropriately, notably by using correlation coefficients. The use of correlation is misleading. **A high correlation does not necessarily imply that there is good agreement between the two methods**. Correlation studies the relationship between one variable and another, not the differences, and it is not recommended as a method for assessing the comparability between methods.

Correlation	Agreement
• Correlation studies the relationship between two variables not the difference	• Agreement studies the difference between the two variables
• Calculated by Regression analysis plot	• Calculated by Bland and Altman plot

Contd...

Correlation	Agreement
• Perfect correlation if the points lie along any straight line.	• Perfect agreement only if the points in Fig 1 lie along the line of equality
• Change in scale of measurement does not affect the correlation, If we were to plot calipers measurement against half calipers measurement, for skin fold thickness the correlation would be 1.0	• Change in scale of measurement affects the agreement. If we were to plot calipers measurement against half calipers measurement the two measurements would not agree. Since one is twice the other
Test of significance (P value) may show that the two methods are correlated	The test of significance is irrelevant to the question of agreement.

(Ref: Bland JM, Altman DG. (1986). Statistical methods for assessing agreement between two methods of clinical measurement. Lancet, i, 307-310.)

Altman and Bland (BandA) proposed an alternative analysis, based on the quantification of the agreement between two quantitative measurements by studying the mean difference and constructing limits of agreement. The BandA plot method only defines the intervals of agreements, it does not say whether those limits are acceptable or not. Acceptable limits must be defined a prior, based on clinical necessity, biological considerations or other goals. The Bland-Altman plot or difference plot, is a graphical method to compare two measurements techniques. In this graphical method the differences (or alternatively the ratios) between the two techniques are plotted against the averages of the two techniques.

The resulting graph is a scatter plot XY, in which the Y axis shows the difference between the two paired measurements (A-B) and the X axis represents the average of these measures ((A+B)/2). In other words, the difference of the two paired measurements is plotted against the mean of the two measurements. BandA recommended that 95% of the data points should lie within ± 2s of the mean difference. This is the most common way to plot the BandA method, but it is also possible to plot the differences as percentages or ratios, and one can use the first method or the second one, instead of the mean of both methods.

Method comparisons of two measurements/methods presented as:

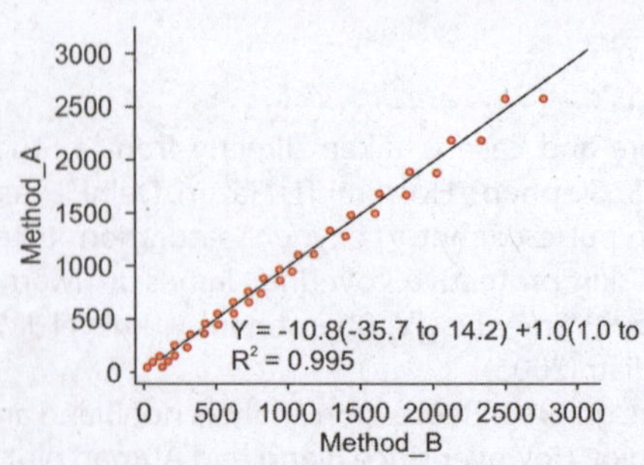

Fig: Regression analysis: We have perfect agreement only if the points in fig 1 lie along the line of equality, but we will have perfect correlation if the points lie along any straight line.

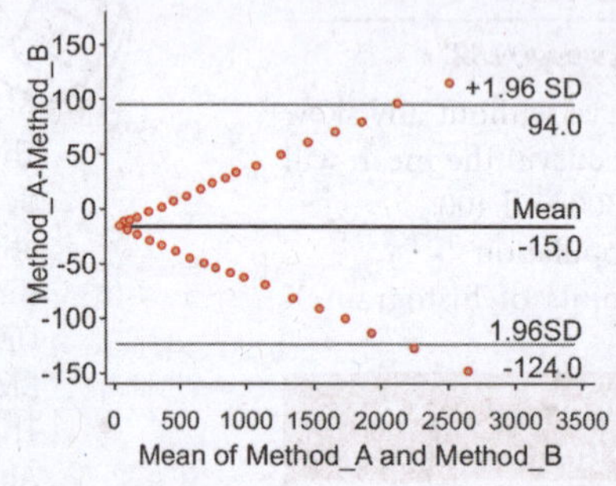

Fig: Bland and Altman plot where differences are presented as units

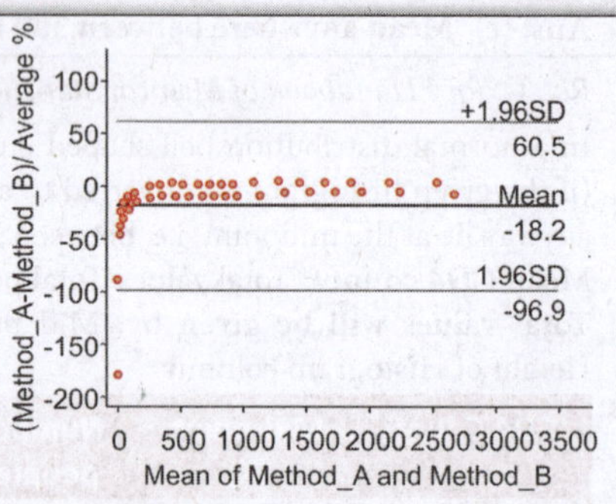

Fig: Bland and Altman plot where differences are presented as percentage

(Ref: Evaluation of pulse-oximetry oxygen saturation taken through skin protective covering. James J, Tiwari L, Upadhyay P, Sreenivas V, Bhambhani V, Puliyel JM - BMC Pediatr 2006)

Background

The hard edges of adult finger clip probes of the pulse oximetry oxygen saturation (POOS) monitor can cause skin damage if used for prolonged periods in a neonate. Covering the skin under the probe with Micropore surgical tape or a gauze piece might prevent such injury. The study was done to see if the protective covering would affect the accuracy of the readings.

Methods

POOS was studied in 50 full-term neonates in the first week of life. After obtaining consent from their parents the neonates had POOS readings taken directly (standard technique) and through the protective covering. Bland-Altman plots were used to compare the new method with the standard technique. A test of repeatability for each method was also performed.

Results

The Bland-Altman plots suggest that there is no significant loss of accuracy when readings are taken through the protective covering. The mean difference was 0.06 (SD of 1.39) and 0.04 (SD 1.3) with Micropore and gauze respectively compared to the standard method. The mean difference was 0.22 (SD 0.23) on testing repeatability with the standard method.

Conclusion

Interposing Micropore or gauze does not significantly affect the accuracy of the POOS reading. The difference between the standard method and the new method was less than the difference seen on testing repeatability of the standard method.

48. Ans. (a) Cross sectional study

Ref: Park 23rd ed page 62

NOTE

In the same question prevalence of anything can be asked like for example Prevalence of Hypertension on measuring BP. However if any intervention is done like Giving Typhoid prophylaxis or Antihypertensive then it will be a field trial

This study will involve investigation of all the residents of the 3 villages to look for the typhoid carriers, and there is no other intervention involved. It cannot be labeled as a field trial, as field trial is a type of Experimental/Intervention studies with healthy people as the unit of the study.

It is a Cross sectional study design as these are also called as prevalence studies

Classification of Epidemiological Studies	
Observational studies	**Experimental/interventional studies**
Descriptive studies Analytical studies • Ecological • Cross sectional (prevalence study) • Case control • Cohort	Randomized control trials Field trials Community trials

Descriptive study is limited to a description of the occurrence of a disease in a population. An analytical study goes further by analyzing relationship between health status and other variables. Experimental or intervention studies involve an active attempt to change a disease determinant or the progress of a disease, and are similar in design to experiments in other sciences.

Cross Sectional Studies

- Simplest form of observational study
- Based on single examination of a cross section of a population at one point of time, the result of which can be projected on the whole population provided the sampling is done correctly
- It is also known as **prevalence study**.
- Although a cross-sectional study provides information about disease prevalence, it provides very little information about the natural history of disease or about the rate of occurrence of new cases (incidence). In short, ***Incidence can be obtained from "longitudinal" studies, and prevalence from "cross-sectional" studies***.
- Most useful in chronic diseases such as hypertension.
- Tells us about distribution of disease in a population rather than etiology.

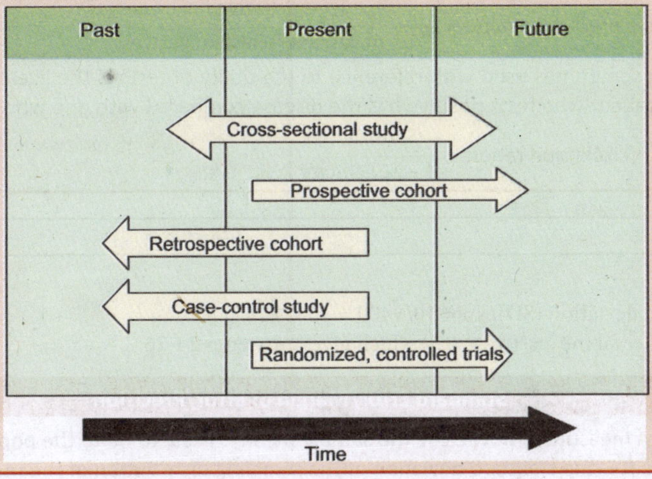

49. Ans. (d) 80/100

Ref: Park 23rd ed page 139

The working examples of the question with all possible calculations are shown in the following table. All possible calculations are potential questions.

Patients with Ovarian Cancer by Histopath				
		Disease positive	**Disease negative**	
Screening by CA 125	Test Outcome Positive	**True Positive** (TP) = 60	**False Positive** (FP) = 40	**Positive predictive value** = TP/(TP + FP) = 60/(60 + 40) **= 60%**
	Test Outcome Negative	**False Negative** (FN) = 20	**True Negative** (TN) = 80	**Negative predictive value** = TN/(FN + TN) = 80/(20 + 80) **≈ 80%**
		Sensitivity = TP/(TP + FN) = 60/(60 + 20) ≈ 75%	**Specificity** = TN/(FP + TN) = 80/(40 + 80) = 67%	

Sensitivity: The term sensitivity was introduced by Yerushalmy in 1940s as a statistical index of diagnostic accuracy. It has been defined as the **ability of a test to identify correctly all those who have the disease, that is "true-positive"**. A 90 per cent sensitivity means that 90 per cent of the diseased people screened by the test will give a "true-positive" result and the remaining 10 per cent a "false-negative" result.

$$\text{Sensitivity} = \frac{\text{True positives}}{\text{True positives + False negatives}}$$

Specificity: It is defined as the ability of a test to identify correctly those who do not have the disease that is, "true-negatives". A 90 per cent specificity means that 90 per cent of the non- diseased persons will give "true-negative" result, 10 per cent of non-diseased people screened by the test will be wrongly classified as "diseased" when they are not.

$$\text{Specificity} = \frac{\text{True negatives}}{\text{True negatives + False positives}}$$

Positive predictive value: The PPV of a test is a proportion that is useful to clinicians since it answers the question: 'How likely is it that this patient has the disease given that the test result is positive?' Predictive value" reflects the **diagnostic power of the test**. The predictive accuracy depends upon sensitivity, specificity and disease prevalence. The "predictive value of a positive test" indicates the probability that a patient with a positive test result has, in fact, the disease in question. *The more prevalent a disease is in a given population, the more accurate will be the predictive value of a positive screening test*. The predictive value of a positive result falls as disease prevalence declines.

$$\text{Positive predictive value} = \frac{\text{True positives}}{\text{True positives + False positives}}$$

Negative predictive value: The NPV of a test answers the question: 'How likely is it that this patient does not have the disease given that the test result is negative?'

$$\text{Negative predictive value} = \frac{\text{True negatives}}{\text{True negatives + False negatives}}$$

Likelihood ratio: A final term sometimes used with reference to the utility of tests is the likelihood ratio. This is defined as how much more likely is it that a patient who tests positive has the disease compared with one who tests negative.

$$\text{Likelihood ration} = \frac{\text{Sensitivity}}{1 - \text{Specificity}}$$

50. Ans. (b) 24–26

Ref: Park 23rd ed page 850

Standard error (SD) = Standard deviation (SD)/√n = 10/√400 = 10 ÷ 20 = 0.5

SE = 0.5 So 95% Confidence interval means + (2 × 0.5) which gives answer as 24-26

Standard Error/Margin of Error/Precision

Standard error of the mean: A measure of how close the sample mean is likely to be to the population mean. A measure of precision of the sample mean. It is the standard deviation of the sampling distribution of the mean. Standard error is equal to the standard deviation divided by square root of sample size.

The SEM provides a measure of the precision of our estimate. The variability of the distribution is measured by the standard deviation of the estimates; this is known as the standard error of the mean (often denoted by SEM). If we know the population standard deviation (σ), then the standard error of the mean is given by:

$$\text{SEM} = \sigma/\sqrt{n}$$

Contd...

Standard Error/Margin of Error/Precision

Standard error of the proportion: The standard error of a reported proportion or percentage p measures its accuracy, and is the estimated standard deviation of that percentage. It can be estimated from just p and the sample size, n, if n is small relative to the population size, using the following formula

$SEP = \sqrt{\frac{p(1-p)}{n}}$ Where P = Proportion

Confidence Interval and Limit

Confidence intervals are ranges of values within which we estimate the true mean to be. Confidence intervals are always associated with probability levels. A range of values within which we are fairly confident the true population value lies.
For example, a 95% CI means that we can be 95% confident that the population value lies within those limits. In a normal distribution, 68% of the values fall within 1 standard deviation of the mean. So, if X is a normal random variable, the 68% confidence interval for X is -1SD <= X <= 1SD. This is demonstrated in the following diagram.

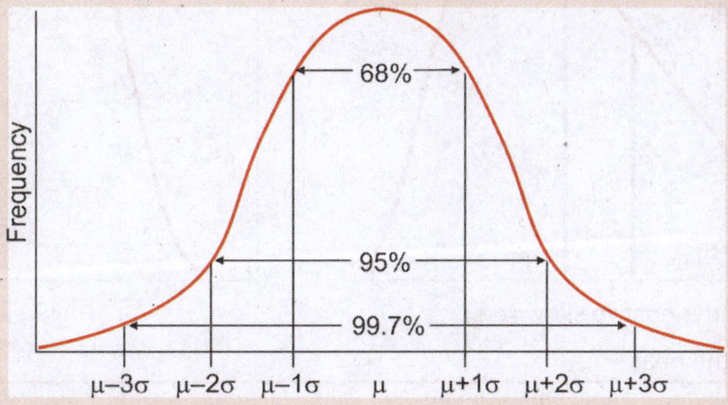

The confidence interval is the sample proportion plus or minus the margin of error (standard error of proportion)

$CI = \hat{p} \pm Z\sqrt{\frac{\hat{p}(1-\hat{p})}{n}}$ Where Z = z score i.e. 1.96 or 2 for 95% CI

Also Power = (1- β), CI = (1-α) where α and β are Type 1 and Type 2 errors respectively

Standard deviation and confidence intervals – what is the difference?
Standard deviation tells us about the variability (spread) in a sample. The CI tells us the range in which the true value (the mean if the sample were infinitely large) is likely to be
The four commonly used confidence intervals for a normal distribution are:

- 68% of values fall within 1 standard deviation of the mean (-1SD <= X <= 1SD)
- 90% of values fall within 1.65 standard deviations of the mean (-1.65 SD ⇐ × ⇐ 1.65SD)
- 95% of values fall within 1.96 standard deviations of the mean (-1.96 SD ⇐ × ⇐ 1.96 SD) Note: Many people take it as 2SD to make it simple but that is not accurate.
- 99% of values fall within 2.58 standard deviations of the mean (-2.58 SD ⇐ × ⇐ 2.58 SD)

Confidence limits: The upper and lower values of a confidence interval. Confidence limit is equal to the sample mean plus or minus the Z score multiplied by standard error. 95% confidence limit is conventionally used in medical research.

51. Ans. (d) 1 = Mode, 2 = Median, 3 = Mean

Ref: Park 23rd ed page 847

Measure of Central Tendency

An entire distribution can be characterized by one typical measure that represents all the observations - measure of central tendency, these measures includes Mean, Median and Mode

Mean	The arithmetic average of a distribution of values; calculated as the sum of the individual values divided by the number of observations.
Median	A measure of central tendency of a distribution; calculated as the mid-point of the distribution when individual values are ordered from the smallest to the largest. When distribution has odd number of elements, the median is the middle one. When distribution is
Mode	A measure of central tendency of a distribution; it is the value that occurs most frequently within the distribution. It is easy to see on the frequency polygon at the **highest point of the curve**. If there are two modes in a distribution then the distribution is **Bimodal**, if more than two modes are there in a distribution then it is **Multimodal**.

Contd...

Measure of Central Tendency

"Many textbooks", teach a rule of thumb stating that **the mean is right of the median under right skew, and left of the median under left skew**. But this rule fails with surprising frequency. It can fail in multimodal distributions, or in distributions where one tail is long but the other is heavy. Most commonly, though, the rule fails in discrete distributions where the areas to the left and right of the median are not equal. However for exam point of view you just have to remember the

Rule of thumb

- In normal distribution curve: **Mean = Median = Mode**
- When the histogram is **Negative skewed (left-skewed)** the mean is to the left thus Mean<Median<Mode
- When the histogram is **positive skewed (right-skewed)**, the mean is to the right: Mean>Median>Mode

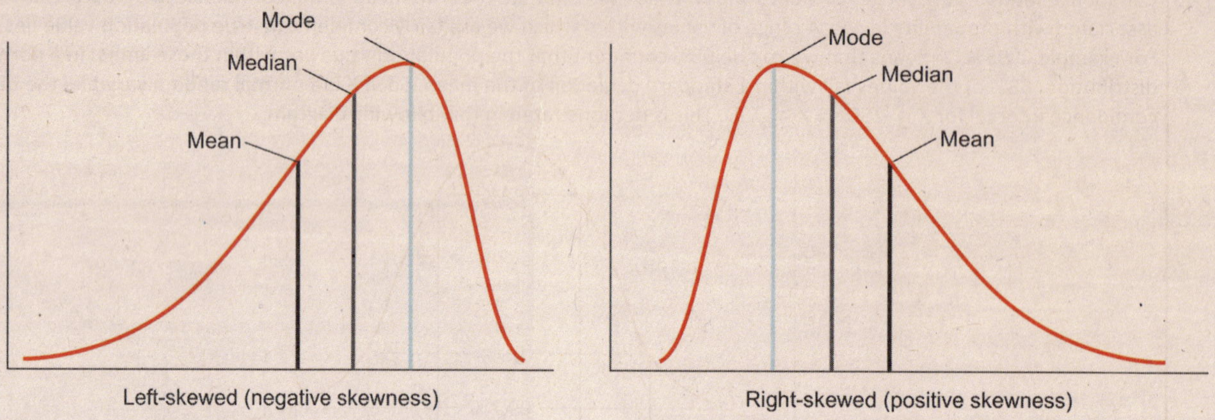

Note: See the tail not the peak

52. Ans. (d) Receptor operator curve

Ref: Receiver-Operating Characteristic Analysis for Evaluating Diagnostic Tests and Predictive Models Available at: http://circ.ahajournals.org/content/115/5/654

Conventionally, a standard way of describing the accuracy of a diagnostic test is the two-by-two table. This is performed when the test results are recorded as dichotomous outcomes (positive/negative results). Conventional analyses consider the sensitivity and the specificity of a diagnostic test as the primary indices of accuracy since these indices are considered to be independent of the prior probability of disease.

However, using a single sensitivity and a single specificity as measures of accuracy is problematic since these measures depend on a diagnostic criterion (i.e. cut-off) for positivity which is often chosen arbitrarily. Also, when evaluating a continuous-scale diagnostic test, we need to account for the changes of specificity and sensitivity when the test threshold varies.

For example, one observer may choose a lenient threshhold and the other may choose a stringent threshhold for positivity. (Cut off values for Diagnosis of diabetes, hypertension, etc.) ROC analysis outsmarts this arbitrariness.

ROC analysis is used in clinical epidemiology to quantify how accurately medical diagnostic tests (or systems) can discriminate between two patient states, typically referred to as "diseased" and "nondiseased". An ROC curve is a plot of sensitivity on the y axis against (1_specificity) on the x axis for varying values of the threshold t.

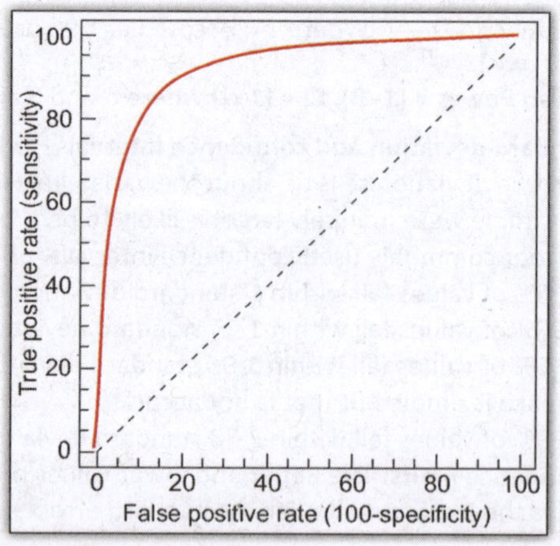

53. Ans. (c) There is no increase in risk because for the occurrence of the effect

Ref: Park 23rd ed page 73, 78, 89

Relative risk (RR) = Incidence among exposed/Incidence among non exposed = $\frac{A/(A+C)}{B/(B+D)}$

Odds ratio (cross product ratio): Measure of strength of association between risk factor and outcome = AD/BC

- OR=1 Exposure does not affect odds of outcome
- OR>1 Exposure associated with higher odds of outcome
- OR<1 Exposure associated with lower odds of outcome

54. Ans. (a) Confirmed case of extrapulmonary tuberculosis with cough of any duration

Ref: Revised National TB Control Programmes, Technical and Operational Guidelines for tuberculosis control in India, 2016. Central TB division, Directorate General of health Sciences, MoHFW, New Delhi, India. Available from: http://tbcindia.gov.in/showfile.php?lid=3216

Definitions of Presumptive TB

- **Presumptive Pulmonary TB** refers to a person with any of the symptoms and signs suggestive of TB including cough >2 weeks, fever > 2 weeks, significant weight loss, haemoptysis, any abnormality in chest radiograph. Note: In addition, contacts of microbiologically confirmed TB Patients, PLHIV, diabetics, malnourished, cancer patients, patients on immune-suppressants or steroid should be regularly screened forsign and symptomsof TB
- **Presumptive Extra Pulmonary:** TB refers to the presence of organ specific symptoms and signs like swelling of lymph node, pain and swelling in joints, neck stiffness, disorientation, etc and/or constitutional symptoms like significant weight loss, persistent fever for O2 weeks, night sweats.
- **Presumptive paediatric TB** refers to children with persistent fever and/or cough for more than 2 weeks, loss of weight'/no weight gain and/or history of contact with infectious TB cases**. 'History of unexplained weight loss or no weight gain in past 3 months; loss of weight is defined as loss of more than 5% body weight as compared to highest weight recorded in last 3 months. "In a symptomatic child, contact with a person with any form of active TB with in last 2 years may be significant
- **Presumptive DR TB** refers to those TB patients who have failed treatment with first line drugs, paediatric TB non responders, TB patients who are contacts of DR-TB (or Rif resistance), TB patients who are found positive on any follow-up sputum smear examination during treatment with first line drugs, previously treated TB cases, TB patients with HIV co-infection.

55. Ans. (C) Height in cm to cube of weight in Kg

Ref: Park 23rd ed page 399, IAP Textbook of Pediatrics 4th ed page 82

Indices of Obesity	
Body mass index	Weight (kg)/height² (m)
Ponderal index	Height (cm)/cube root of body wt (kg)
Broca's index	Height in cm – 100
Lorentz formula	$\text{Height (cm)} - 100 - \frac{\text{Height (cm)} - 150}{2\text{ (women) }4\text{ (men)}}$
Corpulence index	$\frac{\text{Actual weight}}{\text{Desired weight}}$

AIIMS MAY 2016

56. Ans. (a) 4–16

Ref: Park 22nd ed page 794

See Table of Confidence Interval and Limit" in PSM AIIMS Nov 2016 (see page no. 585)
See Table of Standard Error/Margin of Error/Precision in PSM AIIMS Nov 2016 (see page no. 584-585)

If prevalence of disease is 10%, simple proportion will be P = 10
Standard error of proportion will be

$$\text{SEP} = \sqrt{\frac{p(1-p)}{n}} = \sqrt{\frac{10 \times 90}{100}} = 3$$

Now for 95% Confidence interval we know that
Confidence interval = proportion (prevalence) ± 2 SE

$$\text{CI} = 10 \pm (2 \times 3) = 10 \pm 6 = 4 \text{ to } 16$$

57. Ans. (b) Negatively skewed

Ref: Fundamental Statistics for the Behavioral Sciences 7th edition David C. Howell, High Yield Statistics page 67

See Table of Measure of Central Tendency in PSM AIIMS Nov 2016 (see page no. 585-586)

The left-skewed shape of the distribution suggests a randomly selected newborn will have an Apgar score at the high end of the scale. There is a small chance of getting a baby with a score of 5 or lower. They are cut off by a ceiling at 10, and are somewhat negatively skewed

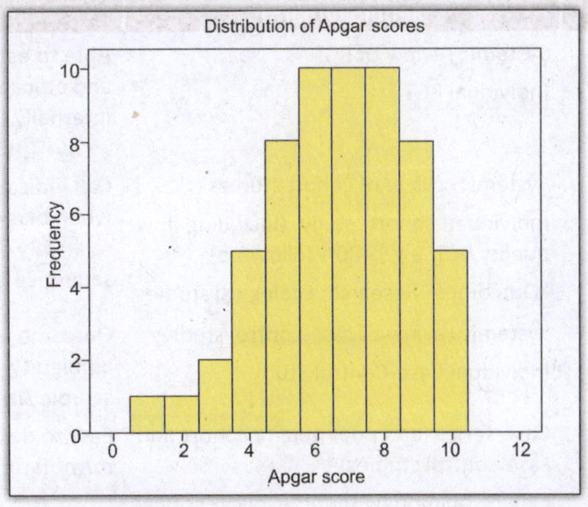

58. Ans. (c) 900

Ref: Park 22nd ed page 792

See Table of Confidence Interval and Limit" in PSM AIIMS Nov 2016 (see page no. 585)

NOTE

Words Margin of Error, Standard error and Precision are used interchangeable

If relative precision is 20%, absolute precision will be ME = 20% of 10 = 2

We know that Confidence interval = 1 – α = 1 – 5/100 = 95%

For 95 % CI we know that Z score is 1.96 (or 2 for simplification)

Sample size $N = p(1 - p) Z^2/ME^2$

$= 10 (100 - 10) \times (2 \times 2)/(2 \times 2) = 900$

Sample Size
Sample size N = p (1–p) Z^2/ME^2 Where Z = Z score, p = proportion, ME = Margin of error or Standard error, This formula is derived from **Standard error of the proportion** (Margin of error) which is calculated as $SEP = \sqrt{\frac{p(1-p)}{n}}$ Where P = Proportion

Factors Affecting Sample Size Requirement	
Factor	**Effect on Sample Size Required**
Decrease acceptable type I error	Increase
Decrease acceptable type II error	Increase
Decrease variability of outcome measures	Decrease
Decrease expected differences in outcome and between groups	Increase

59. Ans. (a) Case control study

Ref: Park 22nd ed page 76

Case control study is lower to RCT and Cohort Study in the pyramid of Level of Evidence however both RCT and Cohort study are time consuming while Case control study takes much less time as it id from Effect to cause.

Levels of Evidence

Level	Therapy/prevention, aetiology/harm	Advantages	Disadvantages	Grade of Recommendation
1a 1b	Systemic review of RCT Individual RCT	**Able to establish cause effect** and efficacy, Internally valid results	Assumes ideal conditions, Can be done only for potentially beneficial regimens, Expensive	A
2a 2b 2c	Systemic review of cohort studies Individual cohort study (including low quality RCT; e.g., <80% follow-up) "Outcomes" Research; Ecological studies	Can indicate cause to effect when bias are under control, relatively easier, Establishes sequence of events	**Cause to effect is only indicated not established,** requires larger sample size	B
3a 3b	Systemic review of case-control studies Individual Case-Control Study	Outcome is predefined so no ambiguity, **Quick results,** Small sample size sufficient	Sequence of events not established, High likelihood of survival and recall bias	
4	Case-series (and poor quality cohort and case-control studies)	Easy to do, Helps in **formulating Hypothesis**	Do not reflect cause effect relationship	C
5	Expert opinion without explicit critical appraisal, or based on physiology, bench research or "first principles"		Do not reflect cause effect relationship	D

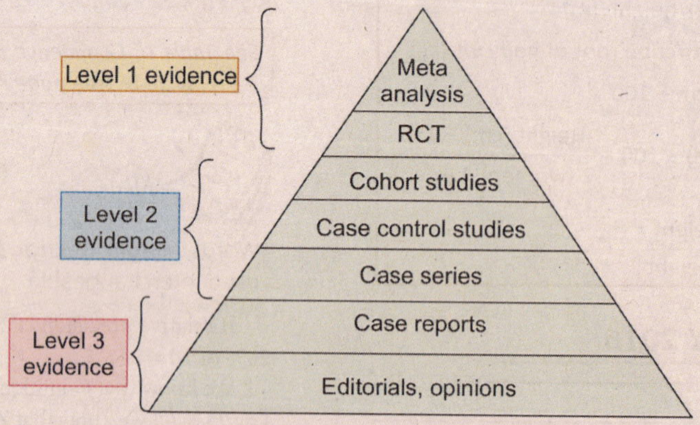

Evidence Pyramid

Hierarchy of study designs by the level of evidence for cause effect relationship

Contd...

Levels of Evidence				
Level	Therapy/prevention, aetiology/harm	Advantages	Disadvantages	Grade of Recommendation

Footnote:
- RCT is best (individual study) study to establish cause effect relationship
- The case-control study is often the best approach to study rare diseases
- The cohort study design is particularly useful for studying rare exposures or clinical interventions in a nonrandomized fashion
- RCT is considered the best study design to study causation.
- **As a rule of thumb:** Higher is the type of study in Evidence pyramid higher is the sample size. Hence sample size required for RCT is higher than Case control study

60. Ans. (b) Stratified random sampling

Ref: Park 23rd ed page 850

Stratified random sampling divides Heterogeneous population into homogenous subgroups which otherwise influence the outcome of the study.

Note that in clustered random sampling Heterogeneous population is subdivided into Heterogenous subgroups only, matching the population.

Sampling Methods

1. Probability or Random Sampling Methods
- Every element has a known equal and non zero probability of being sampled
- Involves random selection at some point.

	Simple Random Sampling	Systematic Random Sampling	Stratified Random Sampling	Cluster Sampling (Aka- Block Sampling)
Population	Homogenous	Homogenous	Heterogeneous	Heterogeneous
Use of random number table	Required	Not required	Required	Required
Method	Each item in the population has the same probability of being selected as part of the sample as any other item.	Every nth element from the list is selected as the sample	Divide population into homogenous subgroups. Random or systematic samples are then taken from each subgroup.	Divide population into groups called clusters (heterogenous subgroups matching the population). A random sample is then taken from within one or more selected clusters.
Advantages	Simple, Easy to analyze. Provides greatest number of possible samples	More precise than simple random sampling as more evenly spread over population	More precision because heterogeneous population is split into homogeneous strata	**Reduced field costs**, Applicable where no complete list of units is available
Disadvantages	if population heterogeneous estimates have large variance	If list has periodic arrangement, sample collected may not be an accurate representation of entire population	Complicated, Problems if strata not clearly defined	Complicated (**Two staged process**), of all probability sampling cluster sampling is **least representative of whole population**, High sampling error

2. Nonprobability or Nonrandom Sampling
- Used when it cannot be ensured that each item has an equal chance of being selected or when selection is based on expert knowledge of population
- Not everyone has the equal probability of being a sample
- Some elements of the population have *no* chance of selection
- Because it's non-random, **bias** is almost certainly introduced.

Convenience, Haphazard or Accidental sampling	**Judgmental, Purposive or biased sampling**	**Quota sampling**	**Snowball sampling**	**Volunteer sampling**
Members of the population are chosen based on their relative ease of access. To sample friends, co-workers, or shoppers at a single mall, are all examples of convenience sampling. Such samples are biased because researchers may unconsciously approach some kinds of respondents and avoid others	The researcher chooses the sample based on who they think would be appropriate for the study.	Quota sampling is a type of stratified sampling in which selection within the strata is non-random. A quota is established (say 65% women) and researchers are free to choose any respondent they wish as long as the quota is met.	The first respondent refers a friend. The friend also refers a friend, and so on. Such samples are biased because they give people with more social connections an unknown but higher chance of selection	It usually involves individuals who agree to participate in research, sometimes for payment.

61. Ans. (b) Type II error

Ref: High Yield Biostatistics page 46

This type of question may be asked in two forms. One in the form of Null hypothesis which states that Type II error is **Accenting null hypothesis when its false"**, Other in the form of Alternate or Research Hypothesis which states that Type II error is when **"We fail to observe a difference when in reality there is a difference"**. You need to remember both.

Hypothesis Testing	
We often gather sample data in order to assess how much evidence there is against a specific hypothesis about the population. We use a process known as hypothesis testing (or significance testing) to quantify our belief against a particular hypothesis.	
The **null hypothesis (H 0)** is a hypothesis which the researcher tries to disprove, reject or nullify. The 'null' often refers to the common view of something, while the alternative hypothesis is what the researcher really thinks is the cause of a phenomenon.	The **Alternative/research hypothesis** is our working hypothesis -- our prediction, or what we expect to happen. It is also called the alternative hypothesis - because it is an alternative to the null hypothesis
We usually test the **null hypothesis (*H0*)** which assumes *no effect* (e.g. the difference in means equals zero) in the *population*. For example, if we are interested in comparing smoking rates in men and women in the population, the null hypothesis would be: *H*0: smoking rates are the same in men and women in the population We then define the **alternative hypothesis (*H1*)** which holds if the null hypothesis is not true. The alternative hypothesis relates more directly to the theory we wish to investigate. So, in the example, we might have: *H*1: the smoking rates are different in men and women in the population.	

Types of Error	
Type 1 error	**Type II error**
Alpha error	*Beta error*
False negative	*False positive*
Rejecting null hypothesis when its true	*Accenting null hypothesis when its false*
• There is no real difference however we find a difference • An example of this would be if a test shows that a woman is pregnant (H0: she is not) when in reality she is not, or telling a patient he is sick (H0: he is not), when in fact he is not	• We fail to observe a difference when in reality there is a difference • An example of this would be if a test shows that a woman is not pregnant (H0: she is not), when in reality, she is

Tabulated Relations between Truth/Falseness of the Null Hypothesis and Outcomes	Null hypothesis (H_0) is true	Null hypothesis (H_0) is false
Reject null hypothesis	Type I error False positive	Correct outcome True Positive
Fail to reject null hypothesis	Correct outcome True Negative	Type II error False negative

62. Ans. (b) Blood group (A, B, AB, O)

Ref: Medical Statistics Made easy by M Harris and G Taylor page 98, Medical Statistics from A to Z 2nd ed by B.S. Everitt page 39

Types of Variables	
Continuous variable: (AKA Interval variable)	A variable which can take any value within a given range, for examples include weight, height, temperature and blood pressure. For such a variable, equal-sized differences on different parts of the scale are equivalent
Covariate	A covariate is a continuous variable that is not of primary interest but is measured because it may affect the outcome and may therefore need to be included in the analysis.
Discrete variable	A variable where the data can only be certain values, usually whole numbers, for example the number of children in families. Compare this with continuous variable
Categorical variable	A variable that gives the appropriate label of an observation after allocation to one of several possible categories, for example gender: male or female; marital status: married, single or divorced; blood group: A, B, AB or O. Categorical variables separate observations into groups. The categories are often given numerical labels, but for this type of data these have no numerical significance
Categorizing continuous variables	A procedure common in medical research in which continuous variables are converted into categorical variables by grouping values into two or more categories, for example age might become 'young' (<40) and 'old' (≥40)

63. Ans. (b) Drug inventory

Ref: Textbook of Hospital Administration By Sonu Dr Goel page 35, Park 23rd ed page 73, 78

Modern Techniques of Drug Inventory Control

Based of criteria of selection there are different analysis methods as follows:

ABC (Always Better Control) analysis	Based on annual consumption
VED (Vital, Essential, Desirable) Analysis	Criticality for production
Sparce, Difficult, Easy (SDE) analysis	Availability
High Medium Low (HML) analysis	Weight Cost permit
Fast Slow moving, Nonmoving (FSN) analysis	Consumption rate
Government source Ordinary Local Foreign (GOLF) Analysis	Based on source of supply
SOS (Seasonal Off Seasonal)	Availability

NOTE

A combination of ABC and VED analysis takes the best of both the methods to help in efficient Inventory control. This method categorized inventory into three groups

ABC Analysis		
A items	**B items**	**C items**
Tight control	Moderate control	Ordinary control measures
Rigid estimates of requirement	Purchase based on rigid requirements	Purchase based on usage estimates
Strict and close watch	Reasonably strict watch and control	Control exercised by storekeeper
Safety stock should be low	Safety stocks moderate	Safety stocks high
Management of items at top managerial levels	Management be done at middle levels	Management be done at lower levels
10% of items	***20% of items***	***70% of items***
70% of cost	***20% of cost***	***10% of cost***

VED Analysis		
Vital	**Essential**	**Desirable**
When out of stock, completely hinders the functioning of the hospital	When out of stock, moderate amount of disruption of hospital functioning	Do not cause any major effect on functioning of the hospital
E.g. Oxygen supply	E.g. IV Fluids	E.g. Vitamin E
The classification of items under VED is hospital/setup specific and shall be done by Hospital management, Officer Incharge of PHC/CHC		

64. Ans. (a) Give immunization to all eligible children in the village

Ref: Park 23nd ed page 449, http://www.mohfw.nic.in/showfile.php?lid=656

Administration of Vaccination is not done by ASHA neither is she trained for the same. ASHA helps in Immunization by keeping records, arrange, assist, maintaining cold chain etc.

ASHA (Accredited Social Health Activist)	
One of the key components of the National Rural Health Mission is to provide every village in the country with a trained female community health activist ASHA or Accredited Social Health Activist. Selected from the village itself and accountable to it, the ASHA will be trained to work as an interface between the community and the public health system. Their role is very important in initiating community based interventions for behavior change through IEC for prevention and control of various noncommunicable diseases, e.g. diabetes, cardiovascular diseases, stroke, cancers, mental health, deafness etc	
Selection of ASHA	ASHA must be the **resident of the village** a woman (married/widow/divorced) preferably in the age group of **25 to 45 years** with formal education up to **8th class in Tribal areas and 10 class in Nontribal areas**, having communication skills and leadership qualities. The general norm of selection will be **one ASHA for 1000 population**. In tribal, hilly and desert areas the norm could be relaxed to one ASHA per habitation. The target is to select and train at least 40 per cent of ASHAs In the first year. Rest of the ASHAs can be selected and trained during second and third year. At present about one lac ASHAs have been already selected and are being trained
Training of ASHA	• **Total training period of 23 days training in five episodes (modules) spread over a period of 12 months.** • Module 1 may be of 7 days, modules 2–5 are of 4 days. • However, it is clarified that ASHA training is a continuous one and that she will develop the necessary skills and expertise through continuous on the job training. • After a period of 6 months of her functioning in the village it is proposed that she be sensitized on HIV/AIDS issues including STI, RTI, prevention and referrals and also trained on new born care.

Contd...

ASHA (Accredited Social Health Activist)	
	• A cascade model of training is proposed. At most peripheral level, Block trainers (who are the members of identified block training teams) would have to spend at least the same number of days in acquiring the knowledge and skills as ASHAs. The block teams would be trained by a district trainer's team. (Or Master trainers) who are in turn trained by the state training team
Role and responsibility of ASHA	ASHA will be a health activist In the community who will create awareness on health. Her responsibilities will be as follows: • ASHA will take steps to **create awareness** and provide information to the community on determinants of health such as nutrition, basic sanitation and hygienic practices, healthy living and working conditions, information on existing health services, and the need for timely utilization of health and family welfare services • She will **counsel women** on *birth preparedness, importance of safe delivery, breast-feeding and complementary feeding, immunization, contraception* and prevention of common infections including reproductive tract infection/sexually transmitted infection and care of the young child. • ASHA will **mobilize the community** and facilitate them in accessing health and health related services available at the anganwadi/subcenter/primary health centers, such as *immunization, ante natal check-up, postnatal check-up", supplementary nutrition, sanitation* and other services being provided by the government. • She will work with the *village health and sanitation committee* of the gram panchayat to develop a *comprehensive village health plan*. • She will arrange **escort/accompany pregnant women and children** requiring treatment/admission to the nearest pre-identified health facility i.e. primary health center/community health center/First Referral Unit. • ASHA will **provide primary medical care for minor ailments** such as diarrhea, fevers, and first-aid for minor injuries. She will be a provider of directly observed treatment short-course **(DOTS)** under revised national tuberculosis control program. • She will also act as a **depot holder** for essential provisions being made available to every habitation like oral rehydration therapy, iron folic acid tablet, chloroquine, disposable delivery kits, oral pills and condoms etc. A drug kit will be provided to each ASHA. Contents of the kit will be based on the recommendations of the expert/technical advisory group set up by the government of India, and include both AYUSH and allopathic formulations. • Her role as a provider can be enhanced subsequently. States can explore the possibility of graded training to her for providing newborn care and management of a range of common ailments, particularly childhood illnesses. • She will *inform about the births and deaths* in her village and any unusual health problems/*disease outbreaks in the community* to the sub-center/primary health center. • She will **promote construction of household toilets** under total sanitation campaign

Role of ASHA in prevention and control of NCDs (Non communicable diseases)	• Educate women, men and adolescents regarding the determinants of NCD's and various associated risk factors like unhealthy diet, physical inactivity, intake of Tobacco and Alcohol and Stress, essentiality of Iodine etc.
	• Promoting a healthy life style during her regular interactions with the community. \\
	• Assist ANM/LHV in:
	  ▪ Organizing camps/village health days on NCD themes
	  ▪ Screening of people at high risk
	  ▪ Advising patients to consult appropriate levels of health care system for diagnosis and treatment
	• Arrange follow up visits.

Role and integration with Anganwadi	Anganwadi worker will guide ASHA in performing following activities: • Organizing Health Day once/twice a month. On health day, the women, adolescent girls and children from the village will be mobilized for orientation on health related issues such as importance of nutritious food, personal hygiene, care during pregnancy, importance of antenatal checkup and institutional delivery, home remedies for minor ailment and importance of immunization etc. AWWs will inform ANM to participate and guide organizing the Health Days at anganwadi center • **AWWs and ANMs will act as resource persons for the training of ASHA** • IEC activity through display of posters, folk dances etc. on these days can be undertaken to sensitize the beneficiaries on health related issues. • Anganwadi worker will be depot holder for drug kits and will be issuing it to ASHA. The replacement of the consumed drugs can also be gone through AWW • AWW will update the list of eligible couples and also the children less than one year of age in the village with the help of ASHA • ASHA will support the AWW in mobilizing pregnant and lactating women and infants for nutrition supplement. She would also take initiative for bringing the beneficiaries from the village on specific days of immunization, health check-ups/health days etc. to anganwadi centers.

Contd...

ASHA (Accredited Social Health Activist)	
Role and integration with ANM:	Auxiliary Nurse Midwife (ANM) will guide ASHA in performing following activities: • She will hold weekly/fortnightly meeting with ASHA and discuss the activities undertaken during the week/ fortnight. She will guide her in case ASHA had encountered any problem during the performance of her activity • AWWs and ANMs will act as resource persons for the training of ASHA • ANMs will inform ASHA regardin date and time of the outreach session and will also guide her for bringing the beneficiary to the outreach session • ANM will participate and guide in organizing the Health Days at anganwadi center • She will take help of ASHA in updating eligible couple register of the village concerned • She will utilize ASHA in motivating the pregnant women for coming to sub-center for initial check-ups. She will also help ANMs in bringing married couples to sub-centers for adopting family planning • ANM will guide ASHA in motivating pregnant women for taking full course of iron and folic acid tablets and tetanus toxoid injections etc. • ANMs will orient ASHA on the dose schedule and side effects of oral pills • ANMs will educate ASHA on danger signs of pregnancy and labor so that she can timely identify and help beneficiary in getting further treatment • **ANMs will inform ASHA on date, time and place for initial and periodic training schedule.** She will also ensure that during the training ASHA gets the compensation for performance and also TA/DA for attending the training.
New initiatives	The following are the major decisions of **Mission Steering Group**; taken in June 2011: • **Home delivery of contraceptives** (condoms, Oral contraceptive pills, emergency contraceptive pills) by ASHA; • **Conducting District Level Household Survey (DLHS)** – 4 in 26 States/UTs where the Annual Health Survey (AHS) is not being done • Modifications in the scheme for **promotion of menstrual hygiene** covering 152 districts and nearly 1.5 crores of adolescent girls in 20 states • Differential financial approach for comprehensive healthcare by which allocation of Untied Funds and Rogi Kalyan Samiti grants will be made based on the case load and services provided by the health facility • Involving ASHA in **Home-Based Newborn Care** • Revision in the criterion of allocation of funds to the states under NRHM based on the performance of the states against the monitorable targets and implementation of specific reform agenda in the health sector • Expansion of Village Health and Sanitation Committees to include nutrition in its mandate and renaming it as Village Health, Sanitation and Nutrition Committee (VHSNC) • Partial modification of the centrally sponsored scheme for development of AYUSH hospitals and dispensaries for mainstreaming of AYUSH under NRHM.
Payments	ASHA is paid ₹ 250 for conducting home visits for the care of newborn and Postpartum mother. The schedule of payment is as follows: • Six visits in case of Institutional delivery (day 3, 7, 14, 21, 28, 42) • Seven visits in case of Home delivery (day 1, 3, 7, 14, 21, 28, 42) The payments are made on 45th day (using the state mechanism of JSY payments). Excerpts from the Mission Steering Group Minutes (June, 2011): The proposal as recommended by the Empowered Program Committee proposed incentive of ₹250 for a set of six home visits to assess the new born as well as postpartum care of mother was approved by MSG. MSG also decided that the incentive amount would be paid one time after 45 days of delivery subject to the following: • Ensuring the birth weight is recorded in the Maternal and child protection (MCP) card • Ensuring the newborn is immunized with BCG, first dose of OPV and DPT, and entering into the MCP card • Ensuring birth registration • Both mother and child are safe till 42nd day of delivery • HBNC incentive is applicable per newborn, thus in cases of twins or triplets the incentive amount for ASHA would be two times of the regular HBNC incentive of ₹250 (i.e, ₹500) or three times of ₹250 (i.e. ₹750) respectively

65. Ans. (c) Weight for age

Ref: Park 22nd ed page 506, http://unicef.in/PressReleases/250/ India-adopts-new-child-growth-standards

The World Health Organization (WHO) released a new international growth standard statistical distribution in 2006, which describes the growth of children ages 0 to 59 months

Growth Monitoring and promotion of children from birth to five years is one of the important activities of Anganwadi Center (AWC) under Integrated Child Development Scheme (ICDS) program.

In order to introduce New WHO Child Growth Standards, a National Workshop on the Adoption of New WHO Child Growth Standards was organized jointly by the Ministry of Women and Child Development (MWCD) and Ministry Health and Family Welfare (MHFW), Government of India, with WHO and UNICEF collaboration in New Delhi on 8-9 February 2007. Govt announced that, In all Anganwadi centers, nutritional status of the child will be assessed against **weight for age** there will be separate charts for girls and boys.

Basis of Recommendations

- Limitations of the existing Child Growth Standards used in the country.
- Clear evidence of the accuracy of the New WHO Child Growth Standards and the availability of gender disaggregated data
- Guiding Principle that the new standards are the **"golden standards"** for the child – in the best circumstances and environment – the Right of the Child in India
- Implementing the new standards is feasible and an opportunity to revamp the ICDS
- System for improvement in quality and convergence with NRHM.
- This is a powerful entry point for accelerating reduction in under-nutrition and promoting early child development.

66. Ans. (c) Primary health centers

Ref: Park 22nd ed page 847, http://health.bih.nic.in/Docs/Guidelines/Guidelines-PHC-2012.pdf

Psychiatrist is not Posted at Primary Health Centers

Apart from one medical officer all other staff at PHC are technical and Paramedical. At present, a PHC is manned by a Medical Officer supported by 14 paramedical and other staff.

Primary Health Center (PHC)

A new approach to health care came into existence in 1978, following an international conference at **Alma-Ata** (USSR). This is known as **"primary health care"**. The Alma-Ata Conference defined primary health care as follows:- **"Primary health care is essential health care made universally accessible to individuals and acceptable to them, through their full participation and at a cost the community and country can afford"**

Elements of primary health care: Although specific services provided will vary in different countries and communities, the Alma-Ata Declaration has outlined 8 essential components of primary health care:

- Education concerning prevailing health problems and the methods of preventing and controlling them
- Promotion of food supply and proper nutrition;
- An adequate supply of safe water and basic sanitation
- Maternal and child health care, including family planning
- Immunization against major infectious diseases
- Prevention and control of locally endemic diseases
- Appropriate treatment of common diseases and injuries
- Provision of essential drugs

PHC is the first contact point between village community and the Medical Officer. The PHCs were envisaged to provide an integrated curative and preventive health care to the rural population with emphasis on preventive and promotive aspects of health care. The PHCs are established and maintained by the State Governments under the Minimum Needs Programme (MNP)/Basic Minimum Services Program (BMS).

Objectives of IPHS for PHCs	• To provide comprehensive primary health care to the community through the Primary Health Centers. • To achieve and maintain an acceptable standard of quality of care. • To make the services more responsive and sensitive to the needs of the community
Population covered	A typical Primary Health Center covers a population of 20,000 in hilly, tribal, or difficult areas and 30,000 populations in plain areas
Number of beds	6 indoore/observation beds per PHC
Referral to and from	It acts as a referral unit for 6 Sub-Centers and refer out cases to CHC (30 bedded hospital) and higher order public hospitals located at sub-district and district level
Types	From Service delivery angle, PHCs may be of two types, depending upon the delivery case load – Type A and Type B. • **Type A PHC:** PHC with delivery load of less than 20 deliveries in a month • **Type B PHC:** PHC with delivery load of 20 or more deliveries in a month
Essential (Minimum Assured Services)	• **OPD services:** A total of 6 hours of OPD services out of which 4 hours in the morning and 2 hours in the afternoon for six days in a week • 24 hours emergency services • Referral services. • In-patient services (6 beds) • Antenatal care, Intranatal care, Postnatal care and Newborn care • Care of the child including Vaccination and Vitamin A prophylaxis (IMNCI) • **Family welfare** (Contraception, Tubectomy, NSV) • Management of Reproductive Tract Infections/Sexually Transmitted Infections

Contd...

Primary Health Center (PHC)	
	• **Nutritional services**: Diagnosis of and nutrition advice to malnourished children, pregnant women, Diagnosis and management of anemia and vitamin A deficiency, Coordination with ICDS • **School health:** Screening of general health, assessment of Anemia/Nutritional status, visual acuity, hearing problems, dental check up, Immunization, Micronutrient (Vitamin A and IFA) management, De-worming and Mid-day meals in coordination with the school and HRD • **Adolescent Health Care:** To be provided preferably through adolescent friendly clinic for 2 hours once a week on a fixed day. • Promotion of Safe Drinking Water and Basic Sanitation • Prevention and control of locally endemic diseases like malaria, Kala-azar, Japanese Encephalitis etc. • Collection and reporting of vital events • National health programs
Desirable services	• MTP using Manual Vacuum Aspiration (MVA) technique • Medical Method of Abortion with linkage for timely referral to the facility approved for 2nd trimester of MTP • Health promotion at schools • Testing of water quality using H2S - Strip Test (Bacteriological) • Mainstreaming of AYUSH • Maternal death review

MANPOWER

Staff	Type A		Type B	
	Essential	Desirable	Essential	Desirable
Medical Officer–MBBS	1		1	1*
Medical Officer–AYUSH		1*		1*
Accountant cum Data Entry operator	1		1	
Pharmacist	1		1	
Pharmacist AYUSH		1		1
Nurse-midwife (Staff-Nurse)	3	+1	4	+1
Health worker (Female)	1*		1*	
Health Assistant (Male)	1		1	
Health Assistant (Female)/Lady Health Visitor	1		1	
Health Educator		1		1
Laboratory Technician	1		1	
Cold Chain and Vaccine Logistic Assistant		1		1
Multi-skilled Group D worker	2		2	
Sanitary worker cum watchman	1		1	+1
Total	**13**	**18**	**14**	**21**

67. Ans. (a) A, B

Ref: Park 22nd ed page 170

RNTCP

Treatment Categories

Category of Treatment	Type of Patient	Regimen
New Cases **Category I** **Supplied in Box**	New sputum smear positive New sputum smear negative New extra pulmonary New others	$2\ (HRZE)_3 + 4\ (HR)_3$
Previously Treated **Category II** **Supplied in Blue Box**	Sputum smear positive Relapse Sputum smear positive Failure Sputum smear positive treatment after default Others	$2\ (HRZES)_3 + 1\ (HRZE)_3 + 5\ (HRE)_3$

Contd...

Note that according to previous classification of DOTS regimens, Sputum negative was placed in Cat III and seriously ill sputum negative was placed in Cat I. However, according to the new classification, there are only 2 categories- New and Previously treated. Hence, the answer is Cat I

Chemoprophylaxis of Tuberculosis

The dose of **INH** for chemoprophylaxis is **10 mg/kg** (instead of earlier recommended dosage of 5 mg/kg) administered daily for 6 months. Isoniazid chemoprophylaxis is not recommended for all persons infected with tubercle bacilli. Because of the small but significant risk of **isoniazid hepatotoxicity**, chemoprophylaxis is reserved for only those at the highest risk of tuberculosis activation (**not suitable for Mass chemoprophylaxis**). TB preventive therapy should be provided to:

All asymptomatic contacts (under 6 years of age) of a smear positive case, after ruling out active disease and irrespective of their BCG or nutritional status.
Chemoprophylaxis is also recommended for all HIV infected children who either had a known exposure to an infectious TB case or are tuberculin skin test (TST) positive (~5 mm induration) but have no active TB disease.
All TST (Mantoux) positive children who are receiving immunosuppressive therapy (e.g. children with nephrotic syndrome, acute leukemia, etc).
A child born to mother, who was diagnosed to have TB · in pregnancy, should receive prophylaxis for 6 months, provided congenital TB has been ruled out. BCG vaccination can be given at birth even if INH chemoprophylaxis is planned.

Sputum AFB: New guidelines, effective from 1st April 2009

- Every patient with cough for 2 weeks or more should have sputum sample examined for AFB.
- Ideally, a sputum specimen should have a volume of 3-5 ml
- The number of specimen required for diagnosis of smear positive pulmonary TB is two, with one of them being a morning sputum specimen. Two sputum specimens are collected over one, or two consecutive days. Of the two sputum specimens, one is collected on the spot and the other is an early morning specimen collected at home by the patient
- One specimen positive out of the two is enough to declare a patient as smear positive TB.
- The spot sputum specimen, irrespective of whether it is collected prior or after the morning specimen, should be recorded as specimen "a" (first specimen) in the laboratory register and the laboratory form for sputum examination. The morning specimen is always recorded as specimen "b", i.e. second specimen, in the laboratory form for sputum examination and the laboratory register. The space for the "c" specimen should be left blank (earlier 3 specimens were to be collected)

Diagnostic algorithms for Pulmonary TB

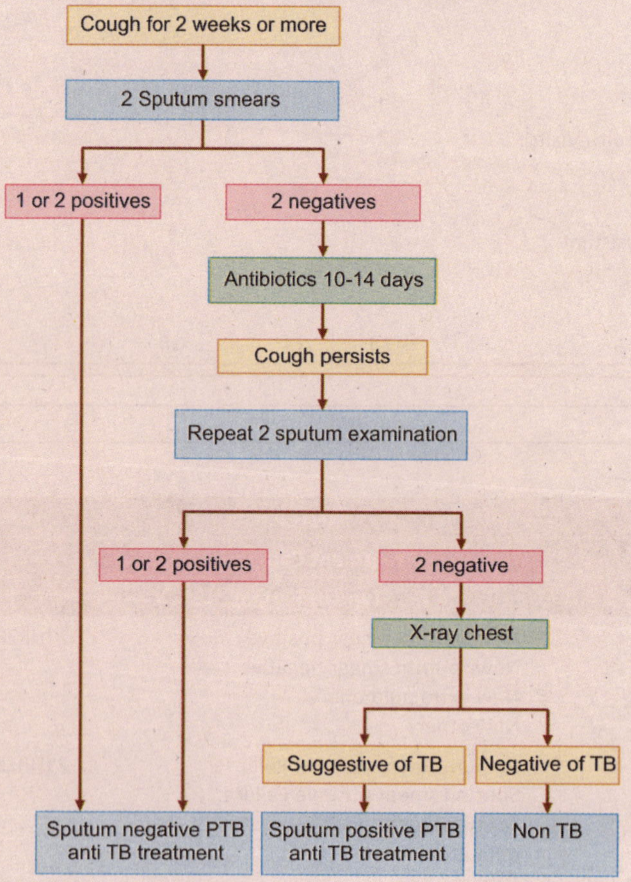

Contd...

Five Components of DOTS
Element 1: Political commitment with increased and sustained financing (including both political will at all levels, and establishing a centralized and prioritized system of TB monitoring, recording and training)
Element 2: Case detection through quality-assured bacteriology (sputum smear microscopy)
Element 3: Standardized treatment, with supervision and patient support (directly observed by a healthcare worker or community health worker for at least the first two months)
Element 4: A regular drug supply
Element 5: A standardized recording and reporting system that allows assessment of treatment results for accountability

Measurement of Epidemiological Indices of TB

INDEX	TEST
Prevalence of infection	It is the percentage of individuals who show a positive reaction to the standard **tuberculin test**. Represents a cumulative experience of a population to **recent and remote infection.** BCG vaccination gives false positive hence a problem in identifying true prevalence.
Incidence of infection (Annual Infection Rate/Tuberculin conversion Index)	It is the percentage of population under study who will be newly infected by Mycobacterium tuberculosis among the noninfected of the preceding survey during the course of one year. It reflects the annual risk of being infected (or reinfected) in a given community. Determines the attacking force of tuberculosis in a community. One of the best indicators for evaluating the tuberculosis problem and its trend. The higher the rate, the greater the problem
Prevalence of infection	Tuberculin test: not validated for diagnosis of the disease and has little value as case finding tool
Incidence of infection	Determines the attacking force of infection, given by tuberculin conversion index
Prevalence of disease	Percentage of people whose sputum is positive for AFB. **Best tool to determine the case load, case rate of community**
Incidence of disease	No. Of new sputum positive cases/1000
Prevalence of suspect cases	Chest X-ray

Therefore test of choice to diagnose TB in community is sputum for AFB, but for determining prevelance of infection is mantoux.

AFB Testing

Number of bacilli	Result reported
No AFB per 100 oil immersion fields	0
1-9 AFB per 100 oil immersion fields	Scanty (or number AFB seen)
10-99 AFB per 100 oil immersion fields	+ (1+)
1-10 AFB per oil immersion field	++ (2+)
>10 AFB per oil immersion field	+++ (3+)

NIKSHAY- To monitor Revised National Tuberculosis Program (RNTCP) effectively, a web enabled and case based monitoring application called NIKSHAY has been developed by National Informatics Center (NIC). This is used by health functionaries at various levels across the country in association with Central TB Division (CTD), Ministry of Health and Family Welfare. NIKSHAY covers various aspects of controlling TB using technological innovations.

This software was launched in **May 2012** and has following functional components:

- Master management
- User details
- TB Patient registration and details of diagnosis, DOT provider, HIV status, follow-up, contact tracing

Outcomes:

- Details of solid and liquid culture and DST, LPA, CBNAAT details.
- MDR-TB patient registration with details.
- Referral and transfer of patients.
- Private health facility registration and TB notification.
- Mobile application for TB notification.
- SMS alerts to patients on registration.
- SMS alerts to program officers.
- Automated periodic reports: (a) Case finding, (b) Sputum conversion, (c) Treatment outcome.

68. Ans. (a) Goiter are classified into three grades not visible, palpable, visible

Ref: Park 22nd ed page 578, http://pbhealth.gov.in/presentation_idd.pdf, http://nrhm.gov.in/images/pdf/programmes/ndcp/niddcp/revised_guidelines.pdf

IDD endemic area is defined as the prevalence of IDD is above 10 per cent in the population (ICMR) or above 5% in children aged 6-12 (MOHFW/WHO). Later being more commonly used because school survey is easy to perform.

Total goiter rate: Percentage of children aged 6-12 with palpable or visible goiter. This is an indicator of iodine deficiency, which causes brain damage and mental retardation. Currently, the prevalence of goiter is quantified using the total goiter rate (TGR), which is equivalent to the number of **goiters of grades 1 and 2** detected in a population divided by the total number of individuals examined. In addition to inspection and palpation, goiter can also be detected by using ultrasonography and is most often measured in **school-age children (6–12 years of age)** because of this population's accessibility and high physiologic vulnerability.

The first recommendations for defining endemic goiter were made during the 1973 consultation. It was agreed that an area would be arbitrarily defined as endemic with respect to goiter if **TGR > 10% of its population** was found to be goitrous on appropriate survey. In 1994, this recommendation was revised and it was recommended that a **TGR (sum of goiter grades 1 and 2) of 5% or more in primary school children (age range approximately 6–12 years)**

Classification of Goiter by Palpation

Grade	Characteristic
0	No palpable or visible goiter.
1	A goiter that is palpable but not visible when the neck is in the normal position (i.e. the thyroid gland is not visibly enlarged). Nodules in a thyroid that is otherwise not enlarged fall into this category.
2	A swelling in the neck that is clearly visible when the neck is in a normal position and is consistent with an enlarged thyroid gland when the neck is palpated.

NOTE

For TGR only grade 1 and 2 are considered

IDD Survey has have 4 compulsory members (Including RMO/MO) + 1 ASHA/Link Worker from identified cluster. The survey is done by **cluster sampling**. Team composition in each district is as follows:

- District Epidemiologist (for Goiter examination)
- Block Level RMO/MO (for Goiter examination)
- Block Level LHV/ANM
- Block Level BEE/SI
- ASHA/Link worker from identified cluster

Role of MO/RMOs

- Identification of around 90 children of 6-12 yrs age group from School and community in a cluster (total 30 clusters)
- Goiter Examination in each identified child.

NOTE

- Government of India launched the National Goiter Control Programme in 1962; which was renamed as National Iodine deficiency Disorders Control Programme (NIDDCP) in the year 1992.
- Ministry of Health and Family Welfare, Government of India, issued a notification banning the sale of noniodized salt for direct human consumption throughout the country under the Prevention of Food Adulteration (PFA) Act to be effective from 17th May 2006
- The IDD control goal in India was to reduce the prevalence of IDD (i.e. total goiter rate) below 10 per cent in the entire country by 2012

69. Ans. (c) 100 mg of elemental iron and 500 microgram of folic acid to pregnant women biweekly for a year

Ref: Park 22nd ed page 596, http://www.nrhmhp.gov.in/sites/default/files/files/Iron%20plus%20initiative%20for%206%20months%20-5%20years.pdf

Under National Iron+ Initiative, the following age groups are covered for lifelong supplementation of Iron from the age of 6 month onwards:

National Iron Plus Initiative

The National Iron+ Initiative guidelines have four objectives:

- To bring to the attention of program managers of health and health-related activities the serious consequences of anemia on health and the physical, mental and economic productivity of individuals and populations
- To develop protocols for iron folic acid (IFA) supplementation across the life cycle (preventive strategy)
- To define a protocol for minimum standard treatment for facility-based management of mild, moderate and severe anemia segregated by levels of care (curative strategy)
- To broadly identify platforms for the delivery of services and indicate the roles of the service providers.

Contd...

IFA Supplementation Programme and Service Delivery			
Age group	**Intervention/Dose**	**Regime**	**Service delivery**
6 months to 5 years (preschool)	1 ml of IFA syrup containing 20 mg of elemental iron and 100 mcg of folic acid	Biweekly throughout the period 6–60 months of age and de-worming for children 12 months and above	Inclusion in MCP card Through ASHA/ANM
5–10 years (Class I to V)	Tablets of 45 mg elemental iron and 400 mcg of folic acid	Weekly throughout the period 5–10 years of age and biannual de-worming	In school through teachers and for out of school children through Anganwadi center (AWC)
10–19 years (Adolescents)	100 mg elemental iron and 500 mcg of folic acid	Weekly throughout the period 10–19 years of age and Biannual de-worming	In school through teachers and for those out of school through AWC
Pregnant and lactating women	100 mg elemental iron and 500 mcg of folic acid	1 tablet daily for 100 days, starting after the first trimester, at 14–16 weeks of gestation. To be repeated for 100 days post-partum	ANC/ANM/ASHA Inclusion in MCP card
Women in reproductive age (WRA) group	100 mg elemental iron and 500 mcg of folic acid	Weekly throughout the reproductive period	Through FHW during house visit for contraceptive distribution

70. Ans. (b) Incidence will decrease if a new drug is effective in reducing mortality from the disease

Ref: Park 23rd ed page 61

Option (A)

Incidence in is a measure of the probability of occurrence of a given medical condition in a population within a specified period of time.

Option (B)

Incidence is not influenced by the duration of disease (Park). Do not get confused by the formula of Prevalence (P) = Incidence × Duration. If a new drug decreases death the prevalence is also decreasing, incidence remains constant.

Option (C)

Incidence is Absolute risk of developing a disease

Option (D)

Prevention decreases incidence of any disease or accident or misshapen. Its a age old saying, no medical science.

Risk, Prevalence and Incidence

INCIDENCE

Incidence rate is defined as "the number of new cases occurring in a defined population during a specified period of time". Incidence in is a measure of the probability of occurrence of a given medical condition in a population within a specified period of time. I.e. **Absolute risk** of developing a disease. It is given by the formula:

$$\text{Incidence} = \frac{\text{Number of new cases occuring in the population in a given period of time}}{\text{Total number of people in the same population during the same period of time}} \times 1{,}000 \text{ population}$$

The incidence rate refers:

- Only to new cases
- During a given period
- In a specified population or "population at risk", unless other denominators are chosen
- It can also refer to new spells or episodes of disease arising in a given period of time, per 1000 population.
- It is not influenced by duration of disease
- The use of incidence is generally restricted to acute conditions

PREVALENCE: Refers specifically to all current cases (old and new) existing at a given point of time or over a period of time in a given population. The number of people who have a disease or condition at a given point in time in a defined population **(point prevalence)**, or the total number of people known to have had the condition at any time during a specified period **(period prevalence)**.

PREVALENCE = INCIDENCE × DURATION

Contd...

Risk, Prevalence and Incidence

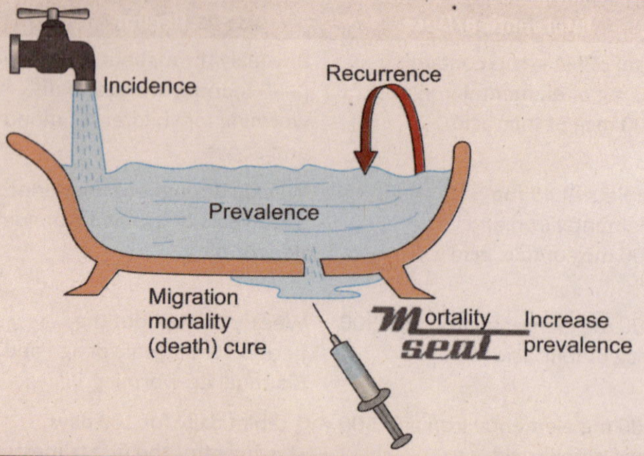

Characteristics of Risk, Prevalence, and Incidence Rate

Characteristic	Risk	Prevalence	Incidence Rate
What is measured	Probability of disease	Percentage of population with disease	Rapidity of disease occurrence
Units	None	None	Cases/person-time
Time of disease diagnosis	Newly diagnosed	Existing	Newly diagnosed
Synonyms	Cumulative incidence	—	Incidence density

AIIMS NOVEMBER 2015

71. Ans. (c) Sand fly, Visceral leishmaniasis

Ref: Park 23rd ed page 775, 304, www.nvbdcp.gov.in, Operational Guidelines on Kala-azar Elimination - 2015

Sand Fly

The leishmaniasis are caused by 20 species pathogenic for humans belonging to the genus Leishmania, a protozoa transmitted by the bite of a tiny 2 to 3 millimeter-long insect vector, the phlebotomine sandfly. Only the female sandfly transmits the protozoa, infecting itself with the Leishmania parasites contained in the blood it sucks from its human or mammalian host in order to obtain the protein necessary to develop its eggs. The insect vector of leishmaniasis, the phlebotomine sandfly, is found throughout the world's inter-tropical and temperate regions.

- Body: Brownish, Less than 5 mm length, Hairy body and wings
- Mandibles: well developed in females, absent in males
- Palps: Pendulous, 5 segments
- Long antennae
- Wings: Hairy, venation more or less parallel, held erect above the body
- Most active in night, shade and twilight
- Six genera: New world: Lutzomyia, Brumptomyia, Warileya and Old world: Phlebotomus, Sergentomyia, Chinius

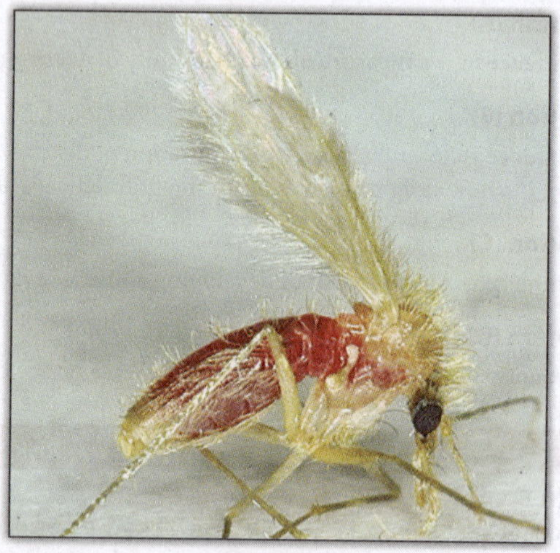

Fig: Sandfly

72. Ans. (b) Stem and leaf plot

Ref: Statistics: An Interactive Text for the Health and Life Sciences by Goteti Bala Krishnamurty, Patricia Kasovia-Schmitt, David J. Ostroff Page 117, Essentials of Inferential Statistics - By Malcolm O. Asadoorian, Demetrius Kantarelis Page 49

Option (A)

Box whiskers plot: A box-and-whiskers plot or box plot is a virtual representation of the distribution of data set. It displays a five—number summary for a variable (minimum, maximum, first and third quartiles, and median). It consists of a rectangle (the box) with one end at the **lower (or first) quartile Q_1** and the other end at the **upper (or third) quartile Q_3**. Usually, the lower quartile is calculated as the median of the lower half of the ordered data list and is referred to as the **lower hinge.** The upper quartile is calculated as the median of the upper half of the ordered data list and is referred to as the **upper hinge.** The line parallel to the ends cut the box at the median.

Q_1: The first quartile is the middle (the median) of the lower half of the data set. One-fourth (25%) of the data lies below the first quartile, and three-fourths (75%) lies above.	**Q_2:** The second quartileis another name for the median of the entire set. One-half (50%) of the data lies below the second quartile, and one-half (50%) lies above.	**Q_3:** The third quartile is the middle (the median) of the upper half of the data set. Three-fourths (75%) of the data lies below the third quartile and one-fourth (25%) lies above.

Construction of the Box and Whiskers plot requires that a box is drawn such that

- Ends of the box are at Q_1 and Q_3
- A vertical line is drawn within the box which indicated median which is measure of center
- Lines drawn from left end of box to minimum value and from right end of box to maximum value, these lines are called **Whiskers**
- Symmetry is reflected if the median is at the middle of the box.
- Skewness is reflected if the median is closer to one end of the box.
  - If Q_2 is closer to Q_3 = Positive or Right skew
  - If Q_2 is closer to Q_1 = Negative or Left Skew
- Length of the box = Interquartile range (IQR) = Q_3- Q_1

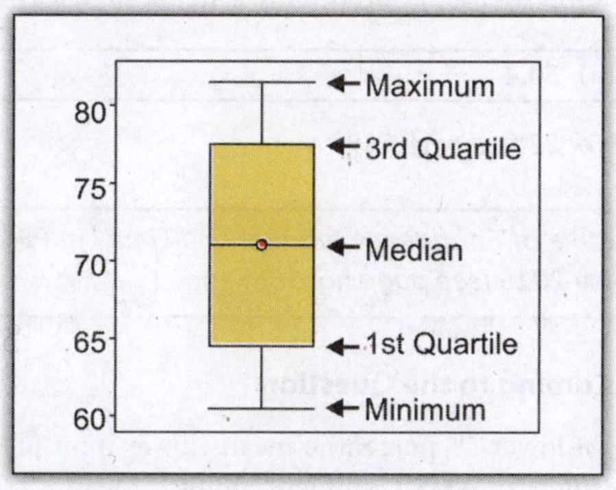

Option (B) Stem and Leaf Plot

A stem and leaf plot is one way of graphically displaying information about a frequency distribution. As with a frequency table, data are ordered from minimum to maximum observation, but in the stem and leaf plot we save some work by not writing down the complete numbers every time they occur. The stem (all but the last digit) is written only once followed by the leaf (Last digit). For example in 61, the stem is 6 and the leaf is 1. Hence in the stem and leaf plot of the question the 2nd row represents; 12, 18, 13, 19 and 15.

0	9
1	2, 8, 3, 9, 5
2	0, 3, 9, 2
3	9, 8, 2, 5, 7, 8, 8
4	9, 3, 2, 6
5	8, 9, 0, 3, 5
6	6, 7, 5
7	1

Option (C) Forest Plot

A forest plot, also known as a **blobbogram,** is a graphical display of estimated results from a number of scientific studies addressing the same question, along with the overall results. It was developed for use in medical research as a means of **graphically representing a meta-analysis** of the results of randomized controlled trials.

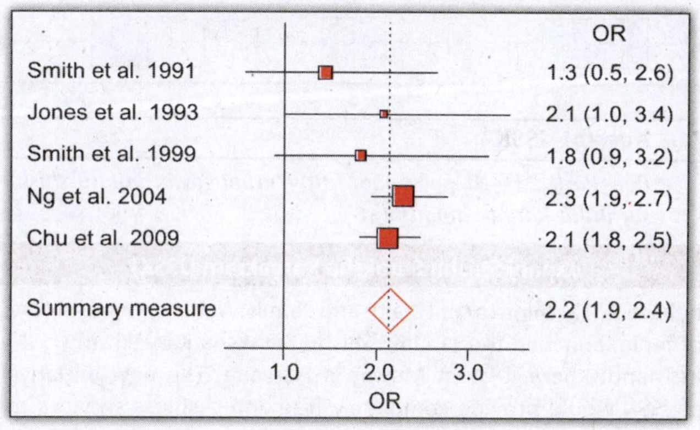

Option (D) Funnel Plot

A funnel plot is a graph designed to check for the existence of publication bias; funnel plots are commonly used in systematic reviews and meta-analyses. In the absence of publication bias, it assumes that the largest studies will be plotted near the average, and smaller studies will be spread evenly on both sides of the average, creating a roughly funnel-shaped distribution. Deviation from this shape can indicate **publication bias.** An example funnel plot showing no publication bias. Each dot represents a study (e.g. measuring the effect of a certain drug); the y-axis represents the size of the study (e.g. number of experimental subjects) and the x-axis shows the study's result (e.g. the drug's measured average effect).

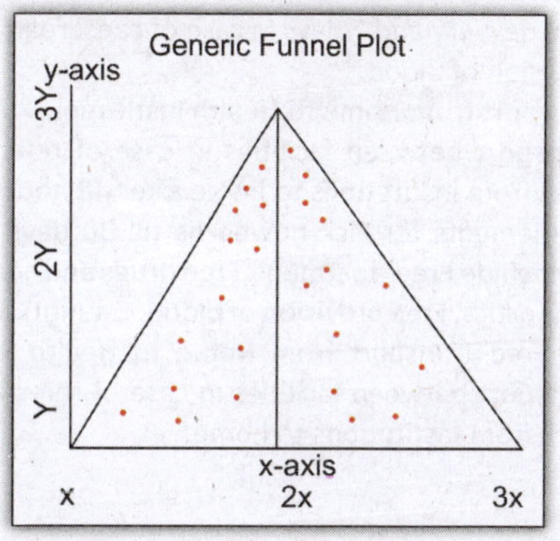

73. Ans. (b) 1-Normal Distribution, 2- Negative skewed, 3- Positive skewed

Ref: Statistics: An Interactive Text for the Health and Life Sciences by Goteti Bala Krishnamurty, Patricia Kasovia-Schmitt, David J. Ostroff Page 117, Essentials of Inferential Statistics - By Malcolm O. Asadoorian, Demetrius Kantarelis Page 49

See previous question for details of Box whiskers plot

Skewness is reflected if the median is closer to one end of the box.

- If Q_2 is closer to Q_3 = Positive or Right skew
- If Q_2 is closer to Q_1 = Negative or Left Skew

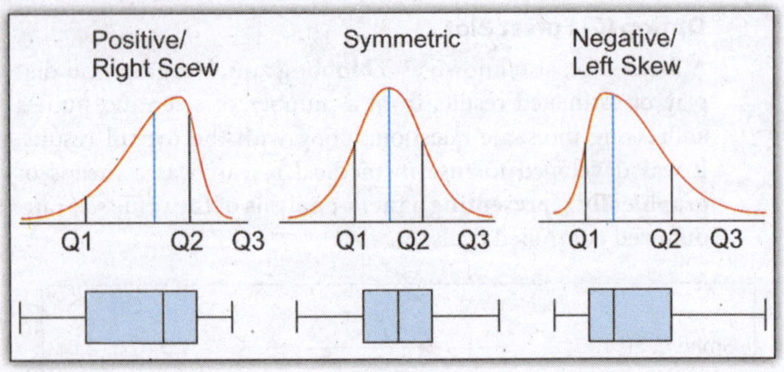

74. Ans. (b) JSSK

Ref: Park 23rd ed page 456, http://nrhm.gov.in/janani-shishu-suraksha-karyakram.html

Janani Shishu Suraksha Karyakram (JSSK)

In June 2011, Ministry of Health and Family Welfare, Government of India launched the Janani –Shishu Suraksha Karyakram (JSSK) at Mandi Khera, District Mewat in Haryana. The new initiative of JSSK would provide completely free and cashless services to **pregnant women** including normal deliveries and caesarean operations and sick new born **(up to 30 days after birth)** in Government health institutions in both rural and urban areas.

Janani-Shishu Suraksha Karyakram *supplements the cash assistance given to a pregnant woman under Janani Suraksha Yojana* and is aimed at mitigating the burden of out of pocket expenses incurred by pregnant women and sick newborns

The following are the Free Entitlements for pregnant women:

- Free and Cashless Delivery
- Free C-Section
- Exemption from User Charges
- Free Drugs and Consumables
- Free Diagnostics
- Free Diet during stay in the health institutions – 3 days in case of normal delivery and 7 days in case of caesarean section
- Free Provision of Blood
- Free Transport from Home to Health Institutions
- Free Transport between facilities in case of referral as also Drop Back from Institutions to home after 48 hours stay.
- Free Entitlements for Sick newborns till 30 days after birth similarly include Free treatment, Free drugs and consumables, Free diagnostics, Free provision of blood, Exemption from user charges, Free Transport from Home to Health Institutions, Free Transport between facilities in case of referral and Free drop Back from Institutions to home.

Contd...

Janani Shishu Suraksha Karyakram (JSSK)

The following are the Free Entitlements for Sick newborns till 30 days after birth. This has now been expanded to cover sick infants:

- Free treatment
- Free drugs and consumables
- Free diagnostics
- Free provision of blood
- Exemption from user charges
- Free Transport from Home to Health Institutions
- Free Transport between facilities in case of referral
- Free drop Back from Institutions to home

75. Ans. (d) Can get cashless benefit in all enlisted hospitals showing smart card and fingerprints

Ref: http://www.rsby.gov.in/about_rsby.aspx

Indirect repeat AIIMS Nov 2013, Nov 2012

See Table of Rashtriya Swasthya Bima Yojana (RSBY) in PSM (see volume II)

76. Ans. (a) Prevalence increase

Ref: Park 23rd ed page 61

See table of Risk, Prevalence and Incidence in PSM AIIMS May 2016 (see page no. 599-600)

If a drug is not curing the disease and just relieving its symptoms that means the duration of disease is increased. Prevalence being total number of old and new cases in a given population over a period of time is hence increased.

77. Ans. (a) 50.4

Ref: Park 22nd ed page 789

See table of Confidence Interval and Limit" in PSM AIIMS Nov 2016 (see page no. 585)

Now Coming to the Question

Value of lower 5th percentile means lower limit of 95% confidence interval, AKA Confidence limit = Mean – 1.96 SD = 70 – (1.96 × 10) = 70 – 19.6 = 50.4

78. Ans. (b) Sampling distribution

Ref: Basic Tools of Research: Sampling, Measurement, Distributions, and Descriptive Statistics chapter 9 page 120- 124, http://www.cios.org/readbook/rmcs/ch09.pdf

Types of Distribution		
Population distribution	Represents the distribution of all units (many or most of which will remain unobserved during our research). A population distribution is made up of all the classes or values of variables which we would observe if we were to conduct a census of all members of the population.	For instance, if we wish to determine whether voters "Approve" or "Disapprove" of a particular candidate for president, then all individuals who are eligible voters constitute the population for this variable. If we were to ask every eligible voter his or her voting intention, the resulting two-class distribution would be a population distribution
Sample distribution	Distribution of the observations that we actually make, after drawing a sample from the population. A sample is simply a subset of all the units of analysis which make up the population. They are only estimates of the population values.	For instance, a group of voters who "Approve" or "Disapprove" of a particular presidential candidate constitute a small subset of all those who are eligible voters (the population). Since the observed values in the three samples are not identical, the means, variances, and standard deviations are different among the samples, as well. These numbers are not identical to the population parameters. The difference between any population parameter value and the equivalent sample statistic indicates the error we make when we generalize from the information provided by a sample to the actual population values. This brings us to the third type of distribution
Sampling distribution	Which is a description of the accuracy with which we can make statistical generalization, using descriptive statistics computed from the observations we make within our sample. A sampling distribution is a statement of the frequency with which values of statistics are observed or are expected to be observed when a number of random samples is drawn from a given population. This is a kind of "second-order" distribution. Whereas the population distribution and the sample distribution are made up of data values, the sampling distribution is made up of values of statistics computed from a number of sample distributions. There are three reasons for constructing sampling distributions of means. In a nutshell, these sampling distributions give us insight into sampling error; they give insight into probability; and they allow us to test hypotheses.	Figure illustrates the population which consists of a set of scores (5, 6, 7, 8 and 9) which distribute around a parameter mean of 7.00. From this population we can draw a number of samples. Each sample consists of three scores which constitute a subset of the population. The sample scores distribute around some statistic mean for each sample. For sample A, for instance, the scores are 5, 6 and 7 (the sample distribution for A) and the associated statistic mean is 6.00. For sample B the scores are 5, 8 and 8, and the statistic mean is 7.00. Each sample has a statistic mean. It is extremely important that a clear distinction is kept between the concepts of sample distribution and of sampling distribution. A sample distribution refers to the set of scores or values that we obtain when we apply the operational definition to a subset of units chosen from the full population. Such a sample distribution can be characterized in terms of statistics such as the mean, variance, or any other statistic. A sampling distribution emerges when we sample repeatedly and record

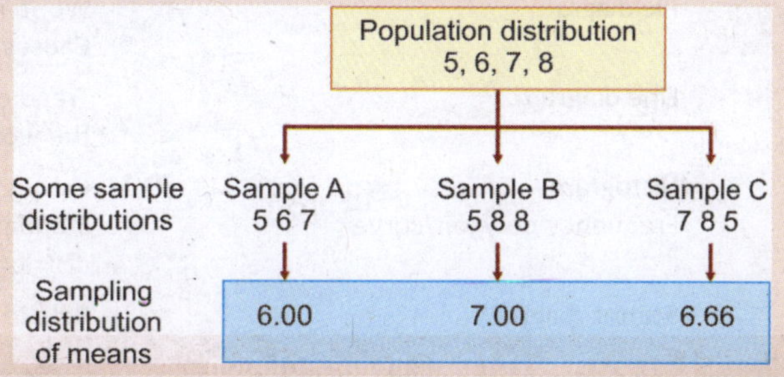

	Distribution Type		
	Population Distribution	Sample Distribution	Sampling Distribution
Distribution consists of:	Individual observations (X)	Individual observations (X)	Statistics e.g., $\bar{X}$
Central tendency	M (Parameter)	$\bar{X}$ (statistic)	$\bar{X}$ (statistic of statistics)
Dispersion	Population variance (parameter σ^2)	Sample variance (statistic) *variance*	Sample variance of means (statistic of statistics) *sampling variance*
	Population standard deviation (parameter)	Sample standard deviation (statistic)	Standard error of means (statistic of statistics)
	s	sd	std error

79. **Ans. (a) Venn diagram**

Ref: Medical Statistics from A to Z 2nd ed page 242

Venn Diagram

A graphical representation of the extent to which two or more quantities or concepts are mutually inclusive and mutually exclusive. An example is shown in figure

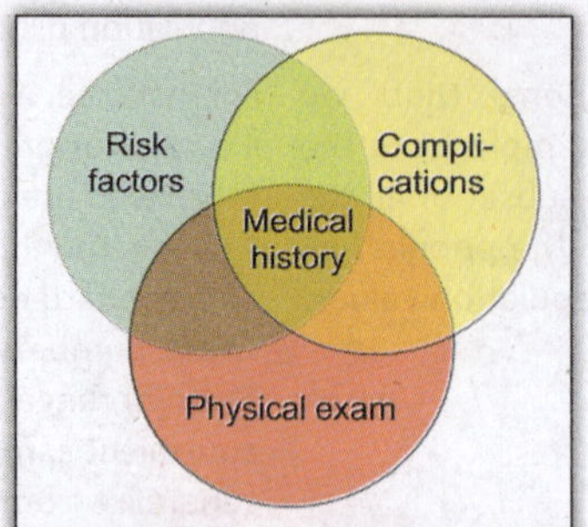

Venn diagram

Presentation of Data	
Qualitative Data	**Quantitative Data**
Bar Pictogram Pie Spot map Mode and Median	Histogram Frequency polygram Frequency curve Cumulative frequency curve (AKA- Ogive) Line chart Scatter diagram Stem and leaf plots Dot plot Whisker or box plot Mean

Data	Method	Example
Comparison of magnitude (Qualitative data)	Bar diagram	Females per 1000 males Mean age at marriage
	Pie diagram	World Population Causes of PPH
Trends over time (Quantitative data)	Line diagram	Trend of malaria cases reported throughout the world
Distribution of frequency (Quantitative data)	Histogram Frequency polygon/curve	Frequency distribution of BP Standard Normal curve (e.g.: for distribution of MCHC %)
Association	Scatter diagram	Relation between height and age
Types of Data Representation		
Pictograph A pictograph uses an icon to represent a quantity of data values in order to decrease the size of the graph. A key must be used to explain the icon.	**Advantages** Easy to read Visually appealing Handles large data sets easily using keyed icons	**Disadvantages** Hard to quantify partial icons Icons must be of consistent size Best for only 2-6 categories Very simplistic
Pie chart A pie chart displays categorical data as a percentage of the whole by using a circle. Each pie section should have a label and percentage. A total data number should be included.	**Advantages** Visually appealing Shows percent of total for each category	**Disadvantages** No exact numerical data Hard to compare 2 data sets "Other" category can be a problem Total unknown unless specified Best for 3 to 7 categories Use only with discrete data

Contd...

Histogram A histogram displays discrete or continuous data in ordered columns. Each column represents a group defined by a quantitative variable such as time, inches, temperature, etc.	**Advantages** Visually strong Can compare to normal curve Usually vertical axis is a frequency count of items falling into each category	**Disadvantages** Cannot read exact values because data is grouped into categories More difficult to compare two data sets Use only with continuous data
Bar graph A bar graph displays discrete data in separate columns. A double bar graph can be used to compare two data sets. Each column represents a group defined by a categorical variable	**Advantages** Visually strong Can easily compare two or three data sets	**Disadvantages** Graph categories can be reordered to emphasize certain effects Use only with discrete data
Line graph A line graph plots continuous data as points and then joins them with a line. To show the trend of event with passage of time	**Advantages** Can compare multiple continuous data sets easily Interim data can be inferred from graph line	**Disadvantages** Use only with continuous data
Frequency Polygon A frequency polygon can be made from a line graph by shading in the area beneath the graph. It can be made from a histogram by joining midpoints of each column.	**Advantages** Visually appealing	**Disadvantages** Anchors at both ends may imply zero as data points Use only with continuous data

80. Ans. (b) Iron and vitamin C

Ref: Ghai 8th ed page 153, Park 23th ed page 545 table 22

Nutritive Value of Milks (value per 100 g)

	BUFFALO	COW	GOAT	HUMAN
Fat (g)	6.5 (max)	4.1	4.5	3.4 (min)
Protein (g)	4.3 (max)	3.2	3.3	1.1 (min)
Lactose (g)	5.1	4.4	4.6	7.4 (Max)
Calcium (mg)	210 (max)	120	170	28 (min)
Iron (mg)	0.2 (70% absorption)	0.2 (30% absorption)	0.3	
Vitamin C (mg)	1	2	1	3
Minerals (g)	0.8	0.8	0.8	0.1
Water (g)	81	87	86.8	88 (max)
Energy (kcal)	117 (max)	67	72	65 (min)

OP Ghai gives data per cup which is for practical purposes for calculation of Nutritional status of child during clinical assessment. This table (value per 100 g) from PARK is for all theoretical purposes like Entrance exams until specifically asked in per cup

Footnote:

- Maximum milk output (**730 ml/day**) is seen between **5-6 months**
- Chief protein of milk is **Casein**
- Animal milk contains nearly 3 times as much proteins as human milk
- Human milk contains greater amount of tryptophan and sulfur containing amino acids (especially cysteine) than the animal milk proteins
- Milk is a good source of retinol and vitamin D
- Carbohydrate in all milk is Lactose or milk sugar
- Human milk is **more sweeter** (contains more sugar than animal milks)
- Milk is particularly **rich in calcium**. The calcium/phosphorus ratio is high in breast milk, so that the uptake of calcium is better than cow's milk
- Milk is a **poor source of iron**, *However the coefficient of uptake of the iron in breast milk may be as high as 70%, whereas it is only 30% for cow's milk and infant formulas*
- Milk is a ***good source of all vitamins except vitamin C***
- Proteins of animal origin are found in milk, meat, eggs, cheese, fish and fowl. These proteins contain all the essential amino acids in adequate amounts and are called as **reference proteins**

81. Ans. (c) 0.60

Ref: Park 23rd ed page 852

From the discussion in the table it is clear that the correlation coefficient does not depends on the sample and its size. I.e. If correlation coefficient of 4 data set is 0.6 independently, the new Correlation coefficient will be the same.

Correlation Coefficient

In statistics correlation coefficient is a measure of the linear correlation between two variables X and Y, giving a value between ***+1 and –1 inclusive, where 1 is total positive correlation, 0 is no correlation, and –1 is total negative correlation.*** There are several correlation coefficients. The most popular coefficient is **Pearson's correlation coefficient**. The correlation coefficient is the slope (b) of the regression line (imaginary) when both the X and Y variables have been converted to z-scores. It characterizes the degree of linear dependence between variables. It is defined as

$$\frac{\sum_i (x_i-\bar{x})(y_i-\bar{y})}{\sqrt{\sum_i (x_i-\bar{x})^2}\sqrt{\sum_i (y_i-\bar{y})^2}}$$

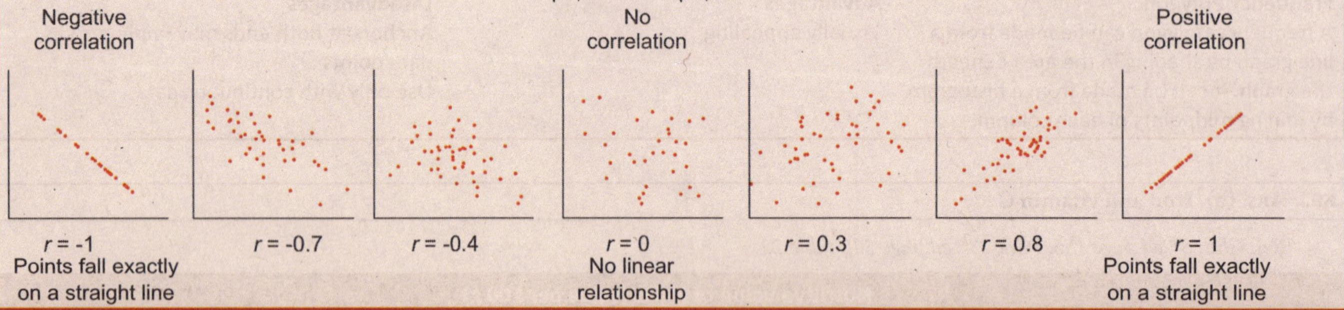

Correlation Coefficient of Different Data Set

The image shows scatter plots of **Anscombe's quartet**, a set of four different pairs of variables created by Francis Anscombe. The four y variables have the same mean (7.5), variance (4.12) and correlation (0.816). However, as can be seen on the plots, the distribution of the variables is very different. The first one (top left) seems to be distributed normally, and corresponds to what one would expect when considering two variables correlated and following the assumption of normality. The second one (top right) is not distributed normally; while an obvious relationship between the two variables can be observed, it is not linear. In this case the Pearson correlation coefficient does not indicate that there is an exact functional relationship: only the extent to which that relationship can be approximated by a linear relationship. In the third case (bottom left), the linear relationship is perfect, except for one outlier which exerts enough influence to lower the correlation coefficient from 1 to 0.816. Finally, the fourth example (bottom right) shows another example when one outlier is enough to produce a high correlation coefficient, even though the relationship between the two variables is not linear.

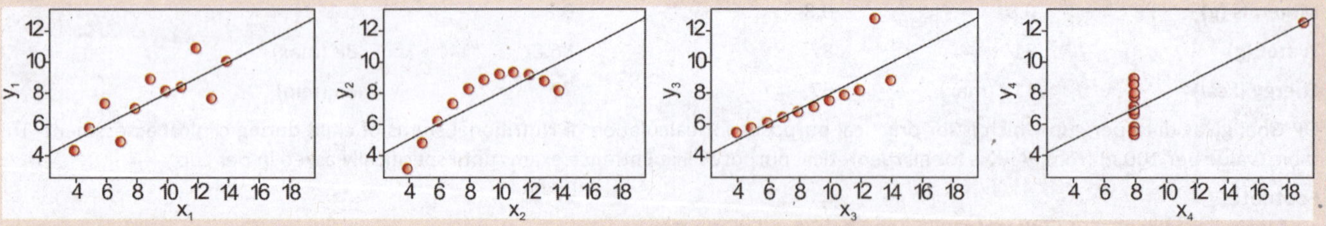

82. Ans. (d) RCT

Ref: Medical Biostatistics 3rd ed By Abhaya Indrayan page 44 table 2.2, Park 23rd ed page 75

See Table of Levels of Evidence in PSM AIIMS May 2016 (see page no. 588-589)

The randomized clinical trial is the most effective way to determine whether a cause-and-effect relationship exists between an intervention and a predefined outcome.

83. Ans. (b) Leprosy

Ref: Park 23rd ed page 322

Repeat AIIMS Nov 2018 PSM (see page no. 562)

84. Ans. (d) Increase external validity of the trial

Ref: Park 23rd ed page 82

Randomization increases internal validity not external validity.

Controlling Bias

Bias can be controlled by Randomization, Blinding, Matching and Standardization

The best method of ensuring comparability, in such cases, is by **randomization** or random allocation. Where random allocation is not possible (as in case control and cohort studies) what is known as "**matching**" is done for selected characteristics that might confound the interpretation of results. Another alternative is **standardization** which usually has a limited application to a few characteristics such as age, sex and parity.

Randomization is a statistical procedure by which the participants are allocated into groups- "study" and "control", to receive or not to receive an experimental, preventive or therapeutic procedure, maneuver or intervention.

- With randomization, the determination of assignment to treatment group is based on probability alone and is not influenced by the preference of the physician or patient.
- The purpose of randomization is to **achieve "equality"** of baseline characteristics of treatment groups, so that the comparison of treatments is considered fair.
- Randomization is an attempt to **eliminate Selection bias** and allow for **comparability**.
- Selection bias decreases Internal validity, hence by eliminating selection bias Randomization **increases Internal validity**
- Randomization is the heart of Randomized control trials.
- It will give the greatest confidence that "like" can be compared with "like"
- The advantages of proper randomization in RCTs include:
  - "It eliminates bias in treatment assignment, " specifically selection bias and allocation bias (confounding).
  - "It facilitates blinding (masking) of the identity of treatments from investigators, participants, and assessors."
  - "It permits the use of probability theory to express the likelihood that any difference in outcome between treatment groups merely indicates chance."

Blinding/Masking: An RCT may be blinded, (also called "masked") by "procedures that prevent study participants, caregivers, or outcome assessors from knowing which intervention was received." Unlike allocation concealment, blinding is sometimes inappropriate or impossible to perform in an RCT; for example, if an RCT involves a treatment in which active participation of the patient is necessary (e.g., physical therapy), participants cannot be blinded to the intervention. Traditionally, blinded RCTs have been classified as **"single-blind, " "double-blind, " or "triple-blind";**

MATCHING is a statistical technique which is used to evaluate the effect of a treatment by comparing the treated and the non-treated units in an observational study or quasi-experiment (i.e. when the treatment is not randomly assigned). The goal of matching is, for every treated unit, to find one (or more) non-treated unit (s) with similar observable characteristics against whom the effect of the treatment can be assessed. By matching treated units to similar non-treated units, matching enables a comparison of outcomes among treated and non-treated units to estimate the effect of the treatment reducing bias due to confounding.

Standardization: Rates are only comparable if the populations upon which they are based are comparable. And it is cumbersome to use a series of age specific death rates. The answer is "age adjustment" or "age standardization", which removes the confounding effect of different age structures and yields a single standardized or adjusted rate, by which the mortality experience can be compared directly.
Standardization is carried out by one of two methods - direct or indirect standardization. Both the methods begin by choosing a "standard population", not the age-structures of the populations.

- **Direct standardization:** First, a "standard population" is selected. The next step is to apply to the standard population, the age-specific rates of the population whose crude death rate is to be adjusted or standardized. As a result, for each age group, an "expected" number of deaths (or events) in the standard population is obtained; these are added together for all the age groups, to give the total expected deaths. The final operation is to divide the "expected" total number of deaths by the total of the standard population, which yields the standardized or age-adjusted rate
- **Indirect standardization:** The simplest and most useful form of indirect standardization is the Standardized Mortality Ratio (SMR). Standard mortality ratio is a ratio (usually expressed as a percentage) of the total number of deaths that occur in the study group to the number of deaths that would have been expected to occur if that study group had experienced the death rates of a standard population (or other reference population).

Standardized rates: These are obtained by direct or indirect method of standardization or adjustment, e.g., age and sex standardized rates.
Age-standardized rate: A rate is the number of new cases or deaths per 100 000 persons per year. An age-standardized rate is the rate that a population would have if it had a standard age structure. Standardization is necessary when comparing several populations that differ with respect to age because age has a powerful influence on the risk of cancer. A random variable (x) is said to have been standardized when it has. been adjusted so that its mean is zero and its standard deviation is 1. Standardization can be effected by subtracting the mean of x, from x and dividing the resulting difference by σ, the standard deviation of x.

Validity and Reliability

Validity (accuracy) refers to the credibility or believability of the research. Validity of an assessment is the degree to which it measures what it is supposed to measure.

- **Internal validity** is the extent to which the results of an investigation accurately reflect the true situation of the study population.
- **External validity** is the extent to which the results of a study are applicable to other populations

Reliability refers to the repeatability of findings. If the study were to be done a second time, would it yield the same results? If so, the data are reliable.

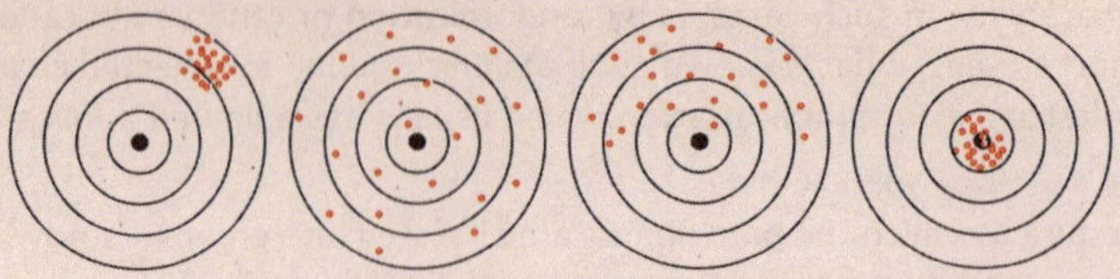

Reliable not valid | Valid not reliable | Neither reliable nor valid | Both reliable and valid

The figure above shows four possible situations.

- In the first one, you are hitting the target consistently, but you are missing the center of the target. That is, you are consistently and systematically measuring the wrong value for all respondents. This measure is reliable, but no valid (that is, it's consistent but wrong).
- The second shows hits that are randomly spread across the target. You seldom hit the center of the target but, on average, you are getting the right answer for the group (but not very well for individuals). In this case, you get a valid group estimate, but you are inconsistent. Here, you can clearly see that reliability is directly related to the variability of your measure.
- The third scenario shows a case where your hits are spread across the target and you are consistently missing the center. Your measure in this case is neither reliable nor valid.
- Finally, we see that you consistently hit the center of the target. Your measure is both reliable and valid

Note: If data are valid, they must be reliable. If people receive very different scores on a test every time they take it, the test is not likely to predict anything. However, if a test is reliable, that does not mean that it is valid. For example, we can measure strength of grip very reliably, but that does not make it a valid measure of intelligence or even of mechanical ability. Reliability is a necessary, but not sufficient, condition for validity.

85. Ans. (a) Sensitivity 90%, Specificity 95%

Ref: Park 23rd ed page 125

$$\text{Sensitivity} = \frac{\text{True positives}}{\text{True positives + False negatives}}$$

$= 27/27 + 3 = 27/30 = 90\%$

$$\text{Specificity} = \frac{\text{True negatives}}{\text{True negatives + False positives}}$$

$= 95/95 + 5 = 95\%$

Sensitivity and Specificity

		Patients with bowel cancer (as confirmed on endoscopy)		
		Disease Positive	**Disease Negative**	
Fecal Occult Blood Screen Test Outcome	Test Outcome Positive	**True Positive** (TP) = 20	**False Positive** (FP) = 180	**Positive predictive value** = TP/(TP + FP) = 20/(20 + 180) = **10%**
	Test Outcome Negative	**False Negative** (FN) = 10	**True Negative** (TN) = 1820	**Negative predictive value** = TN/(FN + TN) = 1820/(10 + 1820) ≈ **99.5%**
		Sensitivity = TP/(TP + FN) = 20/(20 + 10) ≈ **67%**	**Specificity** = TN/(FP + TN) = 1820/(180 + 1820) = **91%**	

Contd...

Sensitivity and Specificity		
	Patients with bowel cancer (as confirmed on endoscopy)	
	Disease Positive	Disease Negative

Worked example: Suppose the fecal occult blood (FOB) screen test is used in 2030 people to look for bowel cancer:

Sensitivity: The term sensitivity was introduced by Yerushalmy in 1940s as a statistical index of diagnostic accuracy. It has been defined as the **ability of a test to identify correctly all those who have the disease, that is "true-positive"**. A 90% sensitivity means that 90 per cent of the diseased people screened by the test will give a "true-positive" result and the remaining 10% a "false-negative" result.

$$\text{Sensitivity} = \frac{\text{True positives}}{\text{True positives + False negatives}}$$

Specificity: It is defined as the ability of a test to identify correctly those who do not have the disease that is, "true-negatives". A 90% specificity means that 90% of the non-diseased persons will give "true-negative" result, 10% of non-diseased people screened by the test will be wrongly classified as "diseased" when they are not.

$$\text{Specificity} = \frac{\text{True negatives}}{\text{True negatives + False positives}}$$

Positive predictive value: The PPV of a test is a proportion that is useful to clinicians since it answers the question: 'How likely is it that this patient has the disease given that the test result is positive?' Predictive value" reflects the **diagnostic power of the test**. The predictive accuracy depends upon sensitivity, specificity and disease prevalence. The "predictive value of a positive test" indicates the probability that a patient with a positive test result has, in fact, the disease in question. *The more prevalent a disease is in a given population, the more accurate will be the predictive value of a positive screening test.* The predictive value of a positive result falls as disease prevalence declines.

$$\text{Positive predictive value} = \frac{\text{True negatives}}{\text{True negatives + False positives}}$$

Negative predictive value: The NPV of a test answers the question: 'How likely is it that this patient does not have the disease given that the test result is negative?'

$$\text{Negative predictive value} = \frac{\text{True negatives}}{\text{True negatives + False positives}}$$

Likelihood ratio: A final term sometimes used with reference to the utility of tests is the likelihood ratio. This is defined as how much more likely is it that a patient who tests positive has the disease compared with one who tests negative.

$$\text{Likelihood ration} = \frac{\text{Sensitivity}}{1 - \text{Specificity}}$$

86. Ans. (a) Primaquine is contraindicated in pregnancy and infants

Ref: http://pib.nic.in/newsite/PrintRelease.aspx?relid=108346, http://nvbdcp.gov.in/Doc/National-Drug-Policy-2013.pdf

Recall Bias

There was no separate question like "Primaquine is contraindicated in". Primaquine was just the part of this question.

Option (A)

Pregnant women with uncomplicated *P. falciparum* should be treated as follows: 1st Trimester: Quinine, 2nd and 3rd Trimester: ACT

Note

Primaquine is contraindicated in pregnant woman, infants and individuals with G6PD deficiency

Option (B)

Presumptive treatment with chloroquine is no more recommended.

Option (C)

P. falciparum cases should be treated with ACT (Artesunate 3 days + Sulfadoxine- Pyrimethamine 1 day). This is to be accompanied by single dose primaquine preferably on day 2.

Option (D)

P. vivax cases should be treated with chloroquine for three days and Primaquine for 14 days. Primaquine is used to prevent relapse but is contraindicated in pregnant women, infants and individuals with G6PD deficiency.

AIIMS MAY 2015

87. Ans. (d) Student's T-test

Ref: Biostatistics BY Mahajan 7th ed page 134, Park 22nd ed page 795

Weight is a quantitative data. Comparing quantitative data of 2 groups will require Student T- Test or Z test depending on sample size.

Statistical Tests

Qualitative Data		Quantitative Data			
Fischer's test Small sample size >20% of cells have expected values <5	**Chi Square Test** Large sample size <20% of cells have expected values <5	**Z-test** (2 sample groups) Sample is large (n>100)	**Student 't' Test** (2 sample groups) Sample is small		**ANOVA** More than 2 sample groups
			Paired 't' test Same Sample (e.g. Before and After)	**Unpaired 't' test** 2 independent samples	

88. Ans. (c) Life expectancy at birth, knowledge and decent standard of living

Ref: Park 23rd ed page 17

Human Development Index

Human development index (HDI) is defined as a composite index combining indicators representing three dimensions:

- **Knowledge** (mean years of schooling and expected years of schooling. Before the year 2009, the indicators used were **adult literacy rate** Max 100, Min 0 and **gross enrolment ratio)** Max 100, Min 0, combined Primary Secondary and Tertiary education/gross enrolment)
  Education Index = 2/3 Adult literacy Index + 1/3 Gross enrolment Index
- **Decent standard of living (Income)**; (GNI per capita in purchasing power parity in US dollars, Max 40000, Min 0)
- **Longevity** (life expectancy at birth, Max 85, Min 25)
  HDI = 1/3 Education Index + 1/3 GDP Index + 1/3 Life expectancy Index

The HDI is a more comprehensive measure than per capita income. Income is only a means to Human development, not an end. Nor is it a sum total of human lives. Thus by focusing on areas beyond income and treating income as a proxy for a decent standard of living, the HDI provides a more comprehensive picture of human life than income does. **HDI measures development of a country as a whole while HPI measures the extent of deprivation and proportion of a society that is left out of progress.**

The HDI **values range between 0 and 1.** The HDI value for a country shows the distance that it has already travelled towards maximum possible value to 1, and also allows comparisons with other countries.

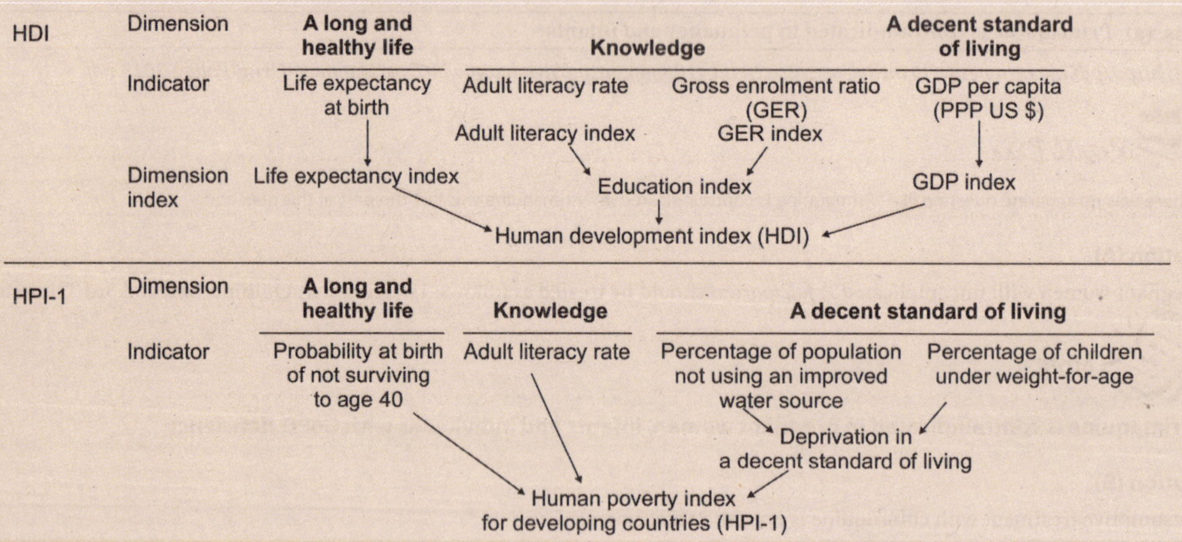

89. Ans. (a) 81-89

Ref: Park 22nd ed page 793

See Table of Confidence Interval and Limit" in PSM AIIMS Nov 2016

Option (A) and (B) at very close. The examiner want you to calculate precise and not approximately. Since we know CI of 95% CI is easy to calculate because we can add and subtract 2 (1.96 to be precise) SD from mean. But for 90% CI the usually we don't remember the Z score which is 1.645

Measure of Variability	
Variability is the property of having a spread of values, which may arise from random sources (viz. the operation of chance) or from systematic influences (viz. bias). There are three important measures of variability	
Range	Simplest measure of variability. It is the difference between lowest and highest scores in the distribution. It therefore responds to these scores only
Variance	Calculating variance (and SD) involves the use of deviation scores. Variance is represented by symbol σ^2 for population and s^2 for sample. The deviation score of an element is found by subtracting the distribution mean ($\bar{x}$) from the element (X). Variance of a distribution is the mean of the squares of all the deviation scores. Variance is therefore obtained by: Finding the deviation scores of all the elements ($x = X - \bar{x}$) Squaring each deviation scores (to eliminate minus) Obtaining mean of these $\sigma^2 = \frac{\Sigma x^2}{N}$ Variance is expressed in square units of measurement limiting its usefulness as a descriptive term
Standard deviation	A measure of the spread of scores away from the Mean. Standard deviation remedies this problem as it is the square root of variance, hence it is expressed in same same unit of measurement as the original data. Standard deviation is expressed as SD or σ. SD is useful in Normal distribution, because the proportion of elements in normal distribution is a constant for a given number of SD above and below the mean of the distribution
Z score of the element is expressed as the location of the element in a normal distribution in terms of how many standard deviation it lies above and below the mean of the distribution. A Z-score of 0 means the score is the same as the mean. A Z-score can also be positive or negative, indicating whether it is above or below the mean and by how many standard deviations. Z-score is represented by Z which is 1.645 for a 90% confidence interval, 1.96 for a 95% confidence interval, 2.58 for a 99% confidence interval	

Z score for 90% Confidence interval is 1.645

$$CI = Mean + 1.645\ SD = 85 + (1.645 \times 2.5)$$
$$= 85 + 4.11 = 80.89 \text{ to } 89.11$$

Confidence Interval: ±4.11

Range for the true population mean: 80.89 to 89.11

(Data confirmed from Online Confidence interval calculators: https://www.mccallum-layton.co.uk/tools/statistic-calculators/confidence-interval-for-mean-calculator/#confidence-interval-for-mean-calculator)

90. Ans. (d) Ministry of health and family welfare

Ref: Park 23rd ed page 660, http://www.fssai.gov.in/

Food Safety and Standards Authority of India (FSSAI) has been established under **Food Safety and Standards Act, 2006** which consolidates various acts and orders that have hitherto handled food related issues in various Ministries and Departments. FSSAI has been created for laying down science based standards for articles of food and to regulate their manufacture, storage, distribution, sale and import to ensure availability of safe and wholesome food for human consumption. **Ministry of Health and Family Welfare**, Government of India is the Administrative Ministry for the implementation of FSSAI. The Chairperson and Chief Executive Officer of Food Safety and Standards Authority of India (FSSAI) have already been appointed by Government of India. The Chairperson is in the rank of Secretary to Government of India.

91. Ans. (d) Selection bias

Ref: Park 23rd ed page 73

Bias
Bias is any systematic error in the determination of the association between the exposure and disease. A statistic is biased if it is calculated in such a way that it is systematically different from the population parameter of interest. The following lists some types of, or aspects of, bias which should not be considered mutually exclusive
• **Confounding bias:** In statistics, a confounding variable (also confounding factor, lurking variable, a confound, or confounder) is an extraneous variable in a statistical model that correlates (positively or negatively) with both the dependent variable and the independent variable. This bias is removed by matching in case control studies.

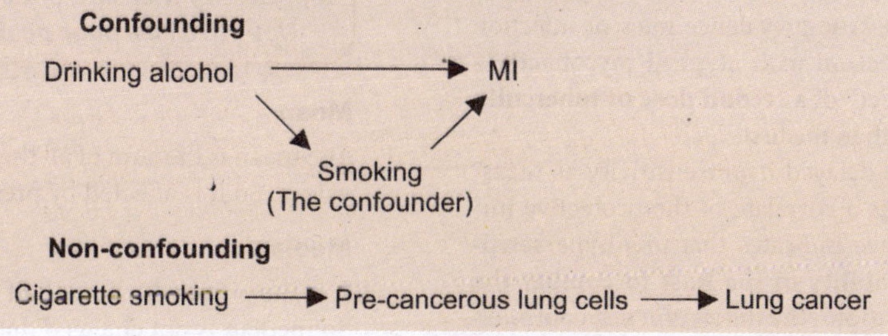

Contd...

Bias

- **Selection bias**: The error introduced when the study population does not represent the target population. Examples of selection bias are:
  - **Sampling bias** is systematic error due to a non-random sample of a population. It is mostly classified as a subtype of selection bias, sometimes specifically termed *sample selection bias*, but some classify it as a separate type of bias.
  - ***Healthcare access bias:*** when the patients admitted to an institution do not represent the cases originated in the community
  - **Berksonian bias**: first described by Berkson in 1946 for case-control studies. It is produced when the probability of hospitalization of cases and controls differ.
  - ***Neyman bias* (synonyms: *incidence-prevalence bias, selective survival bias*):** This type of bias can occur in cross-sectional and case-control studies when asymptomatic, mild, clinically resolved, or fatal cases are inadvertently excluded from the case group because the selected cases are examined sometime after the disease process has already begun (i.e. looking at prevalent versus incident cases).
  - **Healthy worker effect:**
  - **Volunteer bias** is another type of selection bias. It is due to the fact that those individuals who take part in epidemiologic studies tend to be systematically different from those who do not.
  - **Loss to follow-up bias** is a form of selection bias that may occur when there are significant losses to follow-up in ongoing cohort and experimental studies. If the final sample is systematically different from the original or target population with regard to exposure frequency or outcome susceptibility, then spurious associations can result
- **Information/Observation bias/Measurement Bias:** occurs when information is collected differently between two groups, leading to an error in the conclusion of the association. When information is incorrect, there is misclassification. Examples of Information Bias are:
  - **Memory/Recall bias:** When cases and control are asked questions about their past history, it may be more likely for the cases to recall the existence of certain event or factors than the control who are healthy persons. Recall bias is a type of measurement bias that is very common in case-control studies. It can be reduced using blinding
  - **Interviewer bias:** Interviewer knows the status of the subjects before the interview process. Interviewer may probe differently about exposures in the past if he or she knows the subjects as cases. Interviewer bias is a type of measurement bias that can arise in all types of epidemiologic studies. It can be reduced using blinding
  - **Lead time bias** is the bias that occurs when two tests for a disease are compared, and one test (the new, experimental one) diagnoses the disease earlier, but there is no effect on the outcome of the disease—it may appear that the test prolonged survival, when in fact it only resulted in earlier diagnosis when compared to traditional methods.
  - ***Hawthorne effect:*** described in the 1920s in the Hawthorne plant of the Western Electric Company (Chicago, IL). It is an increase in productivity—or other outcome under study—in participants who are aware of being observed
  - **Surveillance bias/Detection bias:** The group with the known exposure or outcome may be followed more closely or longer than the comparison group.
  - **Misclassification bias:** When subjects are erroneously classified with respect to either exposure or disease status.
    - Differential misclassification occurs when the level of misclassification differs between the two groups.
    - Random or Non-differential misclassification occurs when the level of misclassification does not differ between the two groups

92. Ans. (c) High percentage of immunized people

Ref: Park 23rd ed page 186

The validity of tuberculin test, like all medical tests, is subject to variability. It is limited by lack of specificity. Apart from **errors associated with the mode of administration,** reading of results and the test material used, there are other factors such as cross-reactions due to sensitization by other mycobacteria, which should be taken into account. In **countries with a high coverage of BCG,** which also produces tuberculin hypersensitivity, tuberculin test has lost its sensitivity as an indicator of the "true" prevalence of infection. The true prevalence rates of infection may be exaggerated by **infection with atypical mycobacteria** as well as the **"boosting effect" of a second dose of tuberculin** producing a larger reaction than the first.

It is often assumed that delayed hypersensitivity as measured by tuberculin testing is a correlate of the protective immune response. But evidence indicates that this **hypersensitivity is irrelevant to the ability of the host to combat the disease.** Despite these limitations, the tuberculin test continues to be the only tool for measuring the prevalence of tuberculous infection in a community. It has been aptly said that tuberculin test "must be approached with respect, administered with care, read with deliberation and interpreted with sentient discrimination".

93. Ans. (b) Increased mean, no change in median

Ref: Park 23rd ed page 847, Medical Statistics Made Easy, (2003), Page 10, 12

See Table of Measure of Central Tendency in PSM AIIMS Nov 2016 (see page no. 585-586)

Mean

The mean is the sum of all the values, divided by the number of values. So it is affected by presence of extreme values.

Median

It is the point which has half the values above, and half below. So median is not changed due to presence of extreme values.

94. Ans. (d) Injury prevention

Ref: http://www.med.uottawa.ca/sim/data/Injury_Prevention_Haddon_e.htm

William Haddon

Made a useful contribution to thinking about how injuries occur and how to prevent them. The "Haddon Matrix" is a table showing the host, agent and environmental factors involved, set against the time sequence of an incident. The cells of the matrix illustrate the range of risk or protective factors involved; Haddon emphasized the multidisciplinary nature of potential interventions.

To illustrate, for a motor vehicle collision:

	Host (Person Affected)	Agent or Vehicle	Physical Environment	Social Environment
Pre-event (→ primary prevention)	Driving skill; Time pressures (in a rush to get home?); Inebriated?	Car design and handling; Anti-lock brakes, etc.; Maintenance of car	Road design; Speed limits	Reliance on private, rather than public transportation raises traffic load; Compliance with seatbelt laws
During the event (→ secondary prevention)	Wearing seatbelt?	Air bags working? Size of car and crash resistance	Weather conditions; ice on road?	Quality of emergency assistance; Assistance from bystanders
Post-event (→ tertiary prevention)	Ability to call for help (phone available?); Knows first aid?	Tendency of car to catch on fire	Emergency vehicle access to collision site	Continued funding for emergency services

95. Ans. (c) 50

Ref: Medical Statistics Made Easy, (2003), Page 13

NOTE

There are three Q (Quartile - Q1, Q2, Q3) dividing the data into 4 equal parts 25% each. In the present question the examiner probably want to ask data above 3rd Quartile. The 4th quartile (if any) is the same as the 100th percentile (and is equal to the maximum value in the range).

Q1 = marks the 1st quartile = 25th percentile
Q2 = marks the 2nd quartile = 50th percentile (Mdn)
Q3 = marks the 3rd quartile = 75th percentile
Q4 = marks the 4th quartile = 100th percentile

Interquartile Range

The Interquartile Range is used to indicate the variability around the Median (which shows central tendency). It is the difference between the 1st and 3rd quartile (Q3-Q1), and covers the scores falling within the middle 2 quartiles (center 50%) of the distribution.

In Quartile system, the data is divided into 4 quarters, so the number of patients between 3rd and 4th quartile would be equal to one quarter of total no of patients. So number of patients will be: 200/4 = **50**

96. Ans. (a) District level health survey

Ref: Park 23rd ed page 849, https://data.gov.in/resources/child-immunization-children-age-12-23-months-dlhs-iv/download

There are currently 4–5 nationwide surveys capturing data on immunization, which include National Family Health Survey (NFHS), District Level Household Survey (DLHS), Coverage Evaluation Survey (CES) of UNICEF, and Multi-Indicator Cluster Survey (UNICEF). They vary in their methodology and questionnaire used for data collection. There is wide variation in the reports of the surveys. (Ref: Indian Pediatr 2009;46: 991–992)

District Level Household and Facility Survey (DLHS-4)

The District Level Household and Facility Survey (DLHS-4) is a nationwide survey which was conducted during 2012–13. The ever-married women's questionnaire contained information on women's characteristics, maternal care, immunization and childcare, contraception and fertility preferences, reproductive health including knowledge about HIV/AIDS. The village questionnaire contained information on availability of health, education and other facilities in the village, and whether the facilities are accessible throughout the year.

District Level Household and Facility Survey (DLHS-3)

The District Level Household and Facility Survey (DLHS-3) is a nationwide survey covering 601 districts from 34 states and union territories of India. This is the third round of the district level household survey which was conducted during December 2007 to December 2008. Data was collected from 7,20,320 households from 28 States and 6 Union Territories of India during 2007–08. From these households, 6,43,944 ever-married women aged 15–49 years and 1,66,620 unmarried women aged 15–24 years were interviewed.

97. Ans. (c) Exposure to laboratory detection of disease

Ref: Park 23rd ed page 99, 346

Terms Related to Natural History of Diseases

- **Incubation period:** Time interval between invasion of an infectious agent and appearance of first sign or symptom of the disease in question. During the incubation period, the infectious agent undergoes multiplication in the host. When a sufficient density of the disease agent is built up in the host, the health equilibrium is disturbed and the disease becomes overt. Also of interest to the epidemiologist is the median incubation period, defined as the time required for 50 per cent of the cases to occur following exposure.
- **Window period:** The period before antibodies are produced is the "window period" during which, although the person is particularly infectious because of the high concentration of virus in the blood, he will test negative on the standard antibody blood test. Though the body's immune system reacts to the invasion.
- **Serial interval:** Time between onset of primary case and secondary case.
- **Generation time:** Interval of time between receipt of infection by a host and maximum infectivity of the host.
- **Communicable period:** Time in which infectious agent is transferred directly or indirectly from one host to another.
- **"Lead time"** is the advantage gained by screening, i.e., the period between diagnosis by early detection and diagnosis by other means. A is usual outcome of the disease, and B is outcome to be expected when the disease is detected at the earliest possible moment. The benefit of the program are therefore B-A.
- **Isolation** is the oldest communicable disease control measure. It is defined as "separation, for the period of communicability of infected persons or animals from others in such places and under such conditions, as to prevent or limit the direct or indirect transmission of the infectious agent from those infected to those who are susceptible, or who may spread the agent to others"
- **Quarantine** has been defined as "the limitation of freedom of movement of such well persons or domestic animals exposed to communicable disease for a period of time not longer than the longest usual incubation period of the disease, in such manner as to prevent effective contact with those not so exposed"

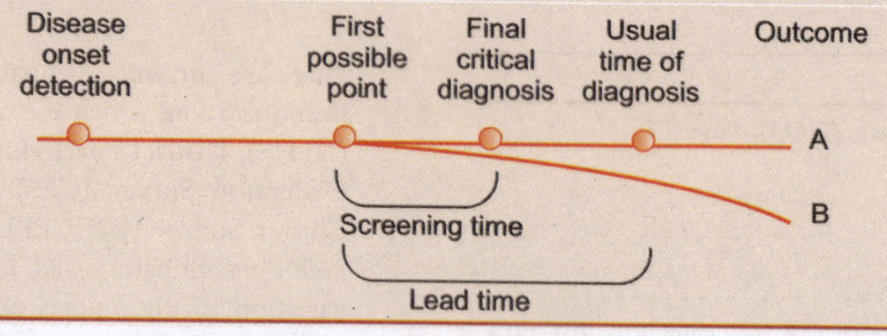

98. Ans. (c) Tuberculosis

Ref: Park 23rd/page 429, http://nikshay.gov.in/abourtbikshay.htm,ww.nhp.gov.in

See Table of RNTCP in PSM AIIMS May 2016 (see page no. 595)

99. Ans. (a) True positive

Ref: Park 23rd ed page 125, 139

See Table of Sensitivity and Specificity in PSM AIIMS Nov 2015 (see page no. 608-609)

100. Ans. (a) Testicular carcinoma

Ref: Park 23rd ed page 137, https://www.up todate.com/contents/screening-for-testicular-cancer

To date, no biomarkers for testicular cancer have been used as screening tests. Although serum levels of alpha fetoprotein (AFP) and/or the beta subunit of human chorionic gonadotropin (beta-hCG) are elevated in 80 to 85 percent of men with nonseminomatous testicular cancer, neither serum beta-hCG nor AFP alone or in combination have sufficient sensitivity or specificity to be used for screening or diagnosis.

A 2011 systematic review found no randomized trials comparing screening versus no screening for testicular cancer. The low incidence and high cure rate of testicular cancer make it unlikely that screening for testicular cancer would appreciably decrease the cancer mortality rate. In addition, most tumors currently diagnosed are Stage I so there is limited potential that screening would spare treatment-related morbidity associated with more advanced disease. The potential harms of screening for testicular cancer include false-positive results, anxiety, and adverse effects of diagnostic tests or procedures.

Screening Test	
Prescriptive screening	**Prospective screening**
• It is defined as the presumptive identification of unrecognized disease which does not arise from a patient's request. • In other words, people are screened primarily for their own benefit, e.g. neonatal screening, bacteriuria in pregnancy, breast cancer, cervical cancer, diabetes, PKU etc. • Prescriptive screening is also known as case detection.	• It is screening of the people for benefit of others • Eg-screening of immigrants from infectious diseases such as tuberculosis and syphilis to protect the home population and screening for streptococcal infection to prevent rheumatic fever. • Prospective screening is also called as control of disease.

Types of Screening

Three types of screening, have been described:

- **Mass screening:** Mass screening simply means the screening of a whole population or a sub-group, as for example, all adults. It is offered to all, irrespective of the particular risk individual may run of contracting the disease in question (e.g., tuberculosis). Mass screening for disease received enthusiastic support in the past. However, when a number of mass screening procedures were subjected to critical review, there appeared to be little justification for their use in many instances. Indiscriminate mass screening, therefore, is not a useful preventive measure unless it is backed up by suitable treatment that will reduce the duration of illness or alter its final outcome
- **High risk or selective screening:** Screening will be most productive if applied selectively to high-risk groups, the groups defined on the basis of epidemiological research. For example, since **cancer cervix** tends to occur relatively less often in the upper social groups, screening for cancer cervix in the lower social groups could increase the yield of new cases. Epidemiologists have extended the concept of screening for disease to screening for "risk factors", as these factors apparently antedate the development of actual disease. For example, elevated serum cholesterol is associated with a high risk of developing coronary heart disease.
- **Multiphasic screening:** It has been defined as the application of two or more screening tests in combination to a large number of people at one time than to carry out separate screening tests for single diseases.

Criteria of Disease Screening	
Criteria of disease	• The disease should be an important public health problem and prevalence should be high • The natural history should be understood • The disease must have a latent period during which it can be detected before symptoms appear. Examples include pre-cancerous lesions • The latent period between first signs and overt disease should be long enough that screening significantly advances the detection of disease. • There is a test which can detect disease prior to onset of symptoms and signs • There is evidence that early detection of disease will reduce mortality and morbidity • The expected benefit outweighs cost • There is an agreed policy on whom to call patients
Criteria of Diagnosis and Treatment	• Facilities need to be adequate • There is an available, effective, acceptable, and safe treatment; • Early treatment should be more effective than later
Criteria of screening test	• Should be sensitive (and ideally also specific), and have good predictive value *(see below)* • Simple and cheap; • Safe and acceptable • Reliable
Sensitivity of a screening test = True positive/True positive + false negative	

101. Ans. (a) Give post-exposure prophylaxis to the bitten person and watch dog for 10 days

Ref: Park 23rd ed page 279, http://www.who.int/rabies/human/postexp/en/

PARK says "*Post-exposure prophylaxis may be discontinued if the suspected animal is proved by appropriate laboratory examination to be free of rabies or, in the case of domestic dogs, cats or ferrets, the animal remains healthy throughout a 10 day observation period starting from the date of the bite.*" But waiting for 10 days and then starting the vaccine in case the dog doesn't look healthy is not advisable.

Post-Exposure Prophylaxis of Rabies		
Categories of Dog Bite		
Category 1	Touching or feeding animals, licks on the skin	No treatment required
Category 2	Nibbling of uncovered skin, minor scratches or abrasions without bleeding, licks on broken skin	Immediate vaccination, immediate washing and flushing of all bite wounds and scratches.
Category 3	Single or multiple transdermal bites or scratches, contamination of mucous membrane with saliva from licks; exposure to bat bites or scratches	Immediate vaccination and administration of rabies immune globulin, immediate washing and flushing of all bite wounds and scratches.

Note: Treatment may be discontinued if the animal involved (dog or cat) remains healthy throughout an observation period of 10 days; or if the animal is killed humanely and found to be negative for rabies by laboratory examination. But waiting for 10 days and then starting the vaccine in case the dog doesn't look healthy is not advisable.

Regimen of PEP of Rabies

Regimen	Days	Doses
Standard WHO Intramuscular regimen (5 dose regimen)	0, 3, 7, 14, 28	One dose each at day 0, 3, 7, 14, 28
Reduced Multisite Intramuscular regimen (4 dose regimen)	0, 7, 21	Two dose on each arm on day 0, one dose each at day 7 and 21 (2+1+1)
Alternative 4 dose Intramuscular regimen	0, 3, 7, 14	One dose each day
2 site intradermal regimen	0, 3, 7, 28	2 dose on different sites on each day (2+2+2+2)
Intradermal schedules: 8 site (20th ed park, no such schedule in 22nd ed)	0, 7, 28, 90	on 8 sites at day 0, on 4 sites at day 7, on one site at day 28 and 90 (8-0-4-0-1-1)
Postexposure prophylaxis in already immunized (Intramuscular)	0, 3	One dose each day (previously 0, 3, 7)
Alternative Post exposure prophylaxis in already immunized (Intradermal)	0	4 doses equally distributed on right and left deltoid or thigh on day 0

Footnote:
- Sometimes it is also written as 2-2-2-0-0-2 (as there are no doses on day 14 and 21)
- Antirabies serum is given in Class III bites (Single or multiple transdermal bites or scratches, licks on broken skin, Contamination of mucous membranes with saliva, exposure to bats).
- It is found to prolong the incubation period.
- Passive immunization in rabies may be given by:
  - Horse Anti-rabies serum: 40 IU/kg body wt (up to max 3000 units), infiltrated in the wound, and the rest given IM
  - Human Rabies Immunoglobulin: (Preferred) 20 IU/kg body wt infiltrated in the wound, and the rest given IM
- These are followed by Active Immunization against Rabies.

102. Ans. (a) Secular

Ref: Park 23rd ed page 65-66

Diseases Trends and Fluctuations		
Short-term fluctuations	Point source epidemic, Continuous common source epidemic, Propagated epidemics Se Next Appendix TYPES OF EPIDEMICS for details	
Periodic fluctuations	Seasonal trends	Occurrence of a particular disease in increased frequency in a particular season. E.g. diarrhea in early spring or summer, pneumonia in winters etc.
	Cyclic trends	Some disease occur in cycles over a short periods of time which may be days, weeks, months or years. *This is mainly due to changes in **herd immunity**.* Over the time the herd immunity gets lost and there is sudden increase in disease, after which it again builds up, only to fall over a period of time. E.g. is measles which occurred every 2-3 years or rubella which occurred after every 6-9 years. Influenza pandemics occur after 7-9 years. Noncommunicable diseases such as accidents occur more frequently on weekends.
Long-term fluctuations or secular trends		• *Implies change in frequency of disease over a long period of time* • E.g. increased incidence of diabetes in India due to life style modification over years. • Secular trend implies consistency in change. • *Line diagrams* are used to show trend of events with passage of time, hence can be used to demonstrate secular trends.

Ear, Nose & Throat

9

AIIMS NOVEMBER 2018

1. A 50-year-old male presents to ENT OPD with complaints of vertigo and nausea while getting up in morning from bed or taking turns on bed. What could be cause for this?
- a. BPPV
- b. Labyrinthitis
- c. Meniere's disease
- d. Vestibular neuronitis

2. A 16-year-old male complains of nasal obstruction. A mass is seen in the nasopharynx with minimal extension into sphenoid sinus. What is the stage of nasopharyngeal fibroma?
- a. Ia
- b. Ib
- c. IIa
- d. IIb

AIIMS MAY 2018

3. Best surgery to relieve intractable vertigo in Meniere's disease is?
- a. Labyrinthectomy
- b. Vestibular neurectomy
- c. Endolymphatic sac decompression
- d. Intratympanic gentamycin

4. A 12-year-old adolescent male presents with unilateral mass in nose with recurrent spontaneous bleeding. On examination, a pink mass covered with mucosa is found in the nasopharynx. Which of the following is not to be done?
- a. Biopsy is done for diagnosis
- b. CECT is done
- c. Endoscopy surgery can be done
- d. Angioembolization can be performed

5. A patient was administered cold water in right ear and nystagmus was seen in the opposite eye. Which of the following is correct assessment?
- a. Slow component to left
- b. Fast component to right
- c. Slow component to right
- d. Fast component to left

6. Identify the marked structure in the given picture:
- a. Malleus
- b. Incus
- c. Stapes
- d. Lateral SCC

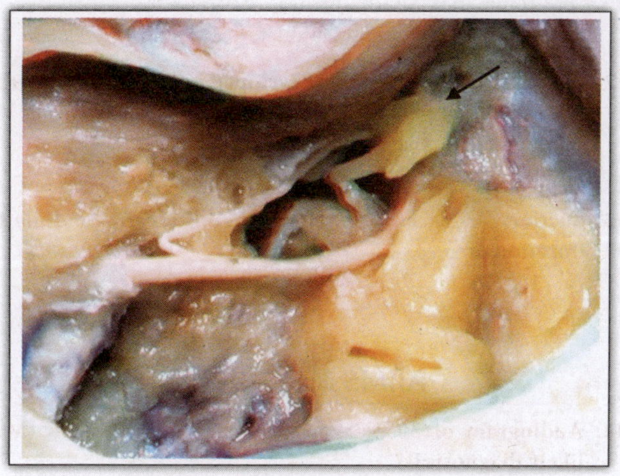

7. Gelle's test is done for?
- a. Otosclerosis
- b. Senile deafness
- c. Serous otitis media
- d. Traumatic deafness

AIIMS NOVEMBER 2017

8. Identify lateral semicircular canal in the given picture of mastoidectomy?
- a. 1
- b. 2
- c. 3
- d. 4

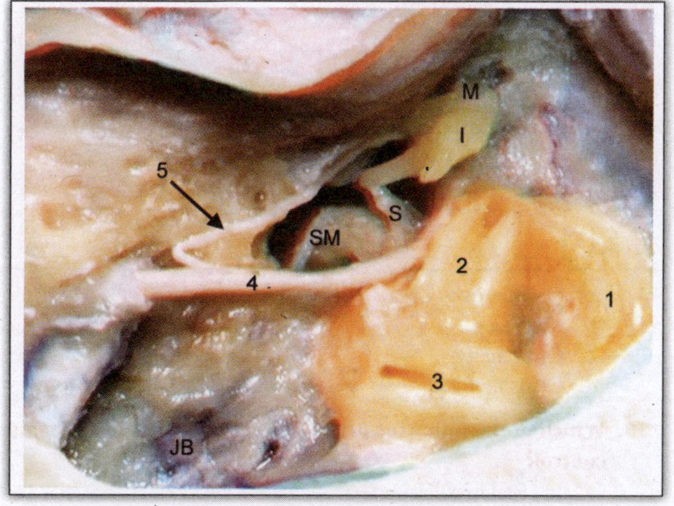

9. Which of the following is not a branch of external carotid artery in Kiesselbach's Plexus?
- a. Anterior and posterior ethmoid artery
- b. Greater palatine artery
- c. Septal Branch of superior labial artery
- d. Sphenopalatine artery

10. Which of the following sinus keeps growing till adulthood?
- a. Sphenoid
- b. Frontal sinus
- c. Ethmoid
- d. Maxillary

11. Target sign is seen in which of the following:
- a. Mastoid injury
- b. Spontaneous CSF Rhinorrhea
- c. Traumatic CSF Rhinorrhea
- d. Stone in submandibular duct

12. A worker in steel industry developed noise induced hearing loss. Which of the following structure is damaged?
- a. Crista ampullaris
- b. Cupula
- c. Inner hair cells
- d. Macula

13. Suction for tracheal secretions should ideally be done for duration of?
- a. 10–15 sec
- b. 30 sec
- c. 60 sec
- d. 3 minutes

AIIMS MAY 2017

14. Audiogram of 30-year-old female is shown below. Most likely diagnosis is?

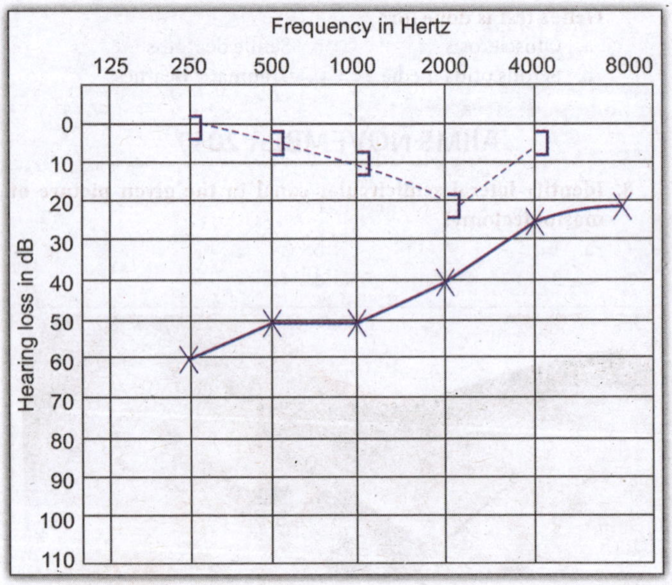

- a. Otosclerosis
- b. Ménière's
- c. Ototoxicity
- d. Otitis media

15. Which of the following arteries is never ligated in epistaxis control?
- a. Internal maxillary artery
- b. External carotid artery
- c. Internal carotid artery
- d. Anterior ethmoidal artery

16. A 5-year-old child presents with gradually progressive hoarseness in voice for the last 3 months and difficulty in breathing for the last 2 weeks. Most likely diagnosis is?
- a. Respiratory papillomatosis
- b. Acute epiglottitis
- c. Croup
- d. Vocal cord nodule

17. Identify the line shown in the picture?

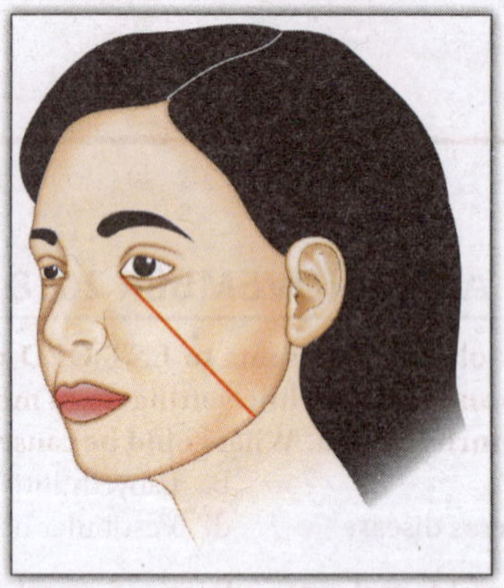

- a. Sebileau's lines
- b. Ohngren's line
- c. Donaldson line
- d. Frankfurt line

AIIMS NOVEMBER 2016

18. Membrane potential of endocochlear cells is?
- a. +45 mV
- b. –45 mV
- c. +80 mV
- d. –80 mV

19. Stapedial reflex centre is?
- a. Lateral lemniscus
- b. Medial geniculate ganglion
- c. Inferior colliculus
- d. Superior olivary nucleus

20. Spiral ganglion innervates which of the following cell in the following picture?

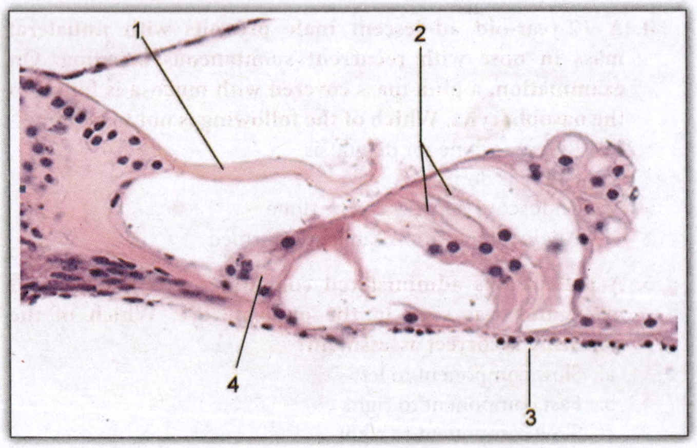

- a. 1
- b. 2
- c. 3
- d. 4

21. Patient got maxillofacial injury with compromised airway and desaturation. Patient is brought to casualty and one doctor is performing this procedure as shown in the picture. What is the procedure?
- a. Tracheostomy
- b. Cricothyroidotomy
- c. Percutaneous tracheostomy
- d. Laryngofissure

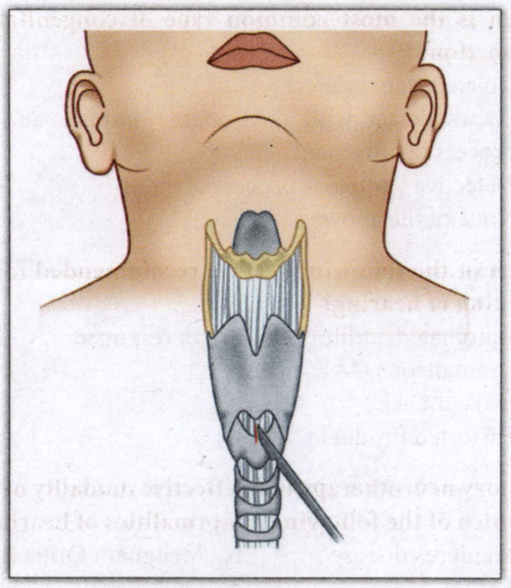

22. Identify the danger space in the following diagram?

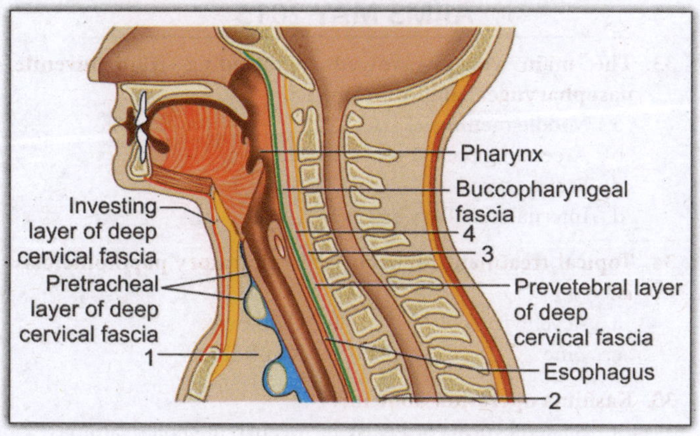

a. 1
b. 2
c. 3
d. 4

23. According to WHO, threshold of profound hearing loss in children is?

a. 71 dB
b. 81 dB
c. 91 dB
d. 101 dB

AIIMS MAY 2016

24. All of the following instruments are commonly used intonsillectomy EXCEPT:

a. Bipolar cautery
b. Conduction wand
c. Harmonic scalpel
d. Microdebrider

25. A 5-month-old male child present with 3 months history of change of voice. Fiberoptic laryngoscopy picture is shown below. The diagnosis is?

a. Multiple respiratory nodules
b. Respiratory papillomatosis
c. Carcinoma larynx
d. Hemangioma

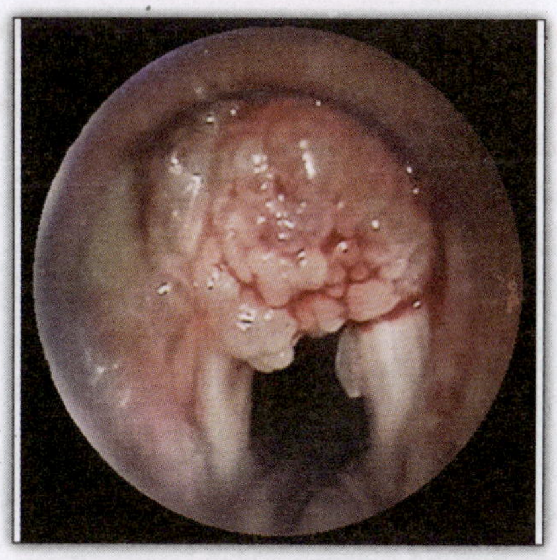

26. In the picture shown below, identify the area marked as 6?

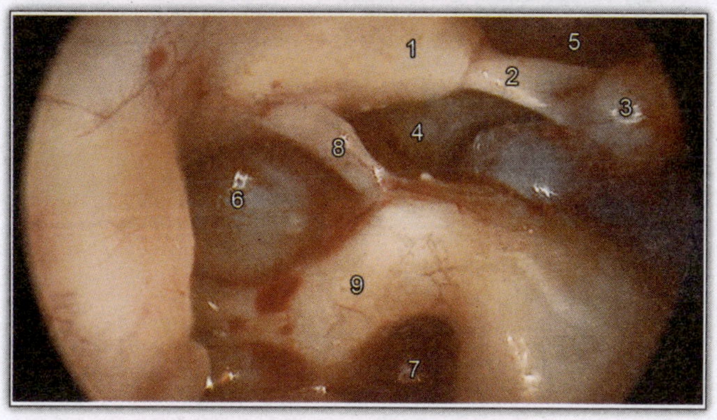

a. Facial recess
b. Fossa incudis
c. Sinus tympani
d. Pyriform fossa

27. A patient returned back with following audiometry report shown below. Interpret the audiogram and arrive at the most probable diagnosis?

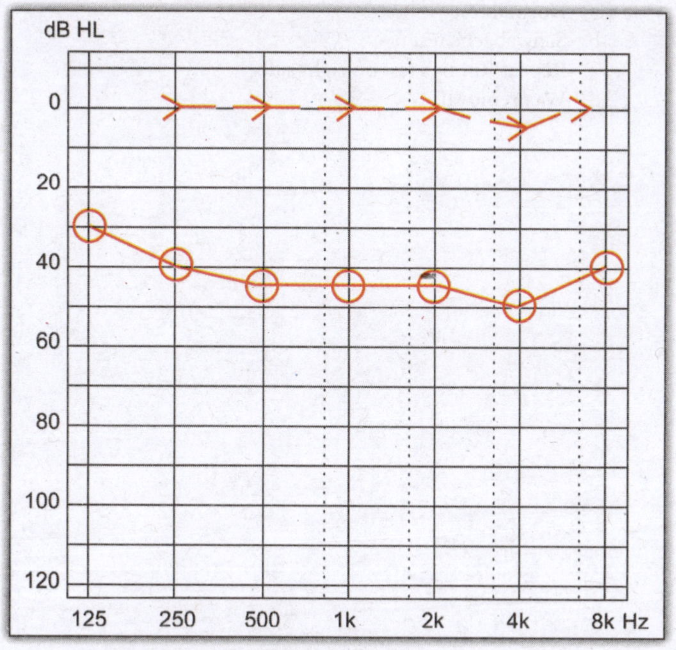

a. Conductive hearing loss right ear
b. Conductive hearing loss left ear
c. SN hearing loss right ear
d. SN hearing loss left ear

28. A 45-year-old male with history of nasal congestion, stiffness and anosmia for 6 months. On examination the patient had a nasal mass with mucin discharge. CT scan was done as shown below. What is the probable diagnosis?

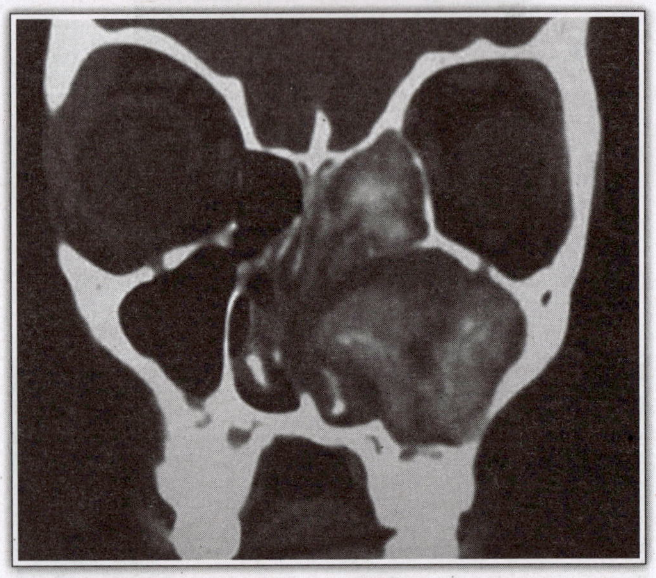

a. Antrochoanal polyp
b. Ethmoidal polyp
c. Maxillary carcinoma
d. Allergic fungal sinusitis

AIIMS NOVEMBER 2015

29. A patient presents to your clinic for evaluation of defective hearing. Rinnie's test shows air conduction greater than the bone conduction on both sides with Weber test lateralized to right ear. What is the next logical step?

a. Normal test
b. Schwabach's test
c. Repeat Rinnie's test on right side
d. Wax removal

30. Which is the most common type of congenital ossicular dysfunction?

a. Isolated stapes defect
b. Stapes defect with fixation of footplate and lenticular process involvement
c. Defective lenticular process of incus
d. None of the above

31. Which of the following tests is recommended for neonatal screening of hearing?

a. Automated auditory brainstem response
b. Spontaneous OAE
c. Evoked OAE
d. Distorted product OAE

32. Auditory neurotherapy is an effective modality of treatment for which of the following abnormalities of hearing?

a. Meniere's disease
b. Malignant Otitis Externa
c. CSOM
d. Otosclerosis

AIIMS MAY 2015

33. The main vessel involved in bleeding from juvenile nasopharyngeal angiofibroma is?

a. Middle meningeal artery
b. Ascending pharyngeal artery
c. Facial artery
d. Internal maxillary artery

34. Topical treatment for recurrent respiratory papillomatosis is?

a. Acyclovir
b. Cidofovir
c. Zinc
d. Ranitidine

35. Kashima operation done for?

a. Bilateral vocal cord palsy
b. Recurrent cholesteatoma
c. Atrophic rhinitis
d. CSOM

36. Eustachian tube function is best assessed by?

a. Politzer test
b. VEMP
c. Rhinomanometry
d. Tympnometry

ANSWERS WITH EXPLANATIONS

AIIMS NOVEMBER 2018

1. Ans. (a) BPPV

Ref: Dhingra 6th Ed Pg 45

The clinical picture is typical of BPPV

Peripheral Vestibular Disorders				
	Meniere's disease	BPPV	Labyrinthitis	Vestibular Neuronitis
Pathology	Distension of endolymphatic system due to increased volume of endolymph	Otoconial debris (crystals of calcium carbonate) is released from the degenerating macula of the utricle. When it settles on the cupula of posterior semicircular canal in a critical head position, it causes displacement of the cupula and vertigo	Inflammation of labyrinth	Inflammation of vestibular nerve
Vertigo	Present, sudden onset, lasts for a few minutes to 24 hours or so.	Present in a critical position by sudden movement, typically change in position. The vertigo is fatigable on assuming the same position repeatedly but can be induced again after a period of rest.	Present severe vertigo of sudden onset with no cochlear symptoms. Attacks may last from a few days to 2 or 3 weeks	Severe vertigo present
Hearing loss	**Fluctuating hearing loss.**	Absent	Unilateral	sensorineural hearing loss
Other symptoms	Tinnitus, sense of pressure in the involved ear, nausea, Vomiting, ataxia, nystagmus. vagal disturbances → abdominal cramps, diarrhea, cold sweats, pallor, Bradycardia. Tullio phenomenon	Nausea, vomiting. No neurologic deficit	Tinnitus Nausea vomiting	

2. Ans. (b) Ib

Ref: Atlas of Head and Neck Pathology by Bruce M. Wenig 3rd Ed Pg 448

Nasopharyngeal fibroma is also known as Juvenile nasal angiofibroma.

Radkowski staging is commonly used for classification of nasopharyngeal angiofibroma. As seen from table below, the sphenoid sinus is involved. The stage is thus Ib according to Radkowski classification.

Modified (Radkowski) Staging of Nasopharyngeal Angiofibroma)	
Stage	Extent of disease
IA	Limited to posterior nares and/or nasopharyngeal vault
IB	Tumor involving the posterior nares and/or nasopharyngeal vault withinvolvement of at least one paranasal sinus
IIA	Minimal lateral extension into pterygomaxillary fossa
IIB	Full occupation of pterygomaxillary fossa with or without superior erosion orbital bones
IIC	Extends into the infratemporal fossa or extension posterior to the pterygoid plates
IIIA	Erosion of base of skull (middle cranial fossa/base of pterygoids) - minimal intracranial extension
IIIB	Extensive intracranial extension with or without extension into cavernous sinus

AIIMS MAY 2018

3. Ans. (c) Endolymphatic sac decompression

Ref: Cumming's 6th ed page 2558

Recall Bias

We are not sure about the language of the question; Definitive surgery/Best surgery will change the answer

Summary

- Definitive surgery for treatment of intractable vertigo in Meniere's disease is Labyrinthectomy as it treats almost all patients
- Best surgery for treatment of Intractable vertigo in Meniere's disease withintact hearing is Endolymphatic sac decompression

Surgery is reserved for patients withintractable vertigo which fails to resolve on medical therapy.

Option (A) Labyrinthectomy

Surgical destruction of the bony and membranous relieves vertigo in virtually all patients but also causes irreversible hearing loss in all patients. Thus, it is only indicated in individuals withintractable symptoms despite medical therapy who already have poor or complete hearing loss on the affected side.

Option (B) Vestibular Neurectomy

Involves surgical lysis of the vestibular nerve. It relieves vertigo in 90 to 95 percent of patients and is associated with a low risk (10-20%) of sensorineural hearing loss. However, vestibular neurectomy requires general anesthesia with craniotomy and overnight monitoring in an intensive care unit and is associated with significantly more morbidity than labyrinthectomy. Since the widespread adoption of intratympanic gentamicin treatment for patients who fail noninvasive therapies, vestibular neurectomy has become a very infrequent treatment choice. It is reserved for those patients who have failed noninvasive therapies and who still have a level of hearing in the affected ear that they are unwilling to risk to intratympanic gentamicin.

Option (C) and (D)

A less invasive alternative to surgery is Intratympanic Gentamycin. Labyrinthectomy and Vestibular neurectomy most reliably relieves the vertigo in Meniere's disease but they fail to preserve the residual hearing function of the affected ear. Ideal procedure should restore the normal function or at least preserve the residual function of the affected ear. ***Two operative procedures proposed to achieve this goal are Cochleosacculotomy and Endolymphatic sac decompression.*** The nondestructive surgical procedures include endolymphatic sac procedures (decompression or shunting or both) and sacculotomy. They are associated with a low risk of sensorineural hearing loss and are commonly performed for Meniere disease in patients withintact hearing.

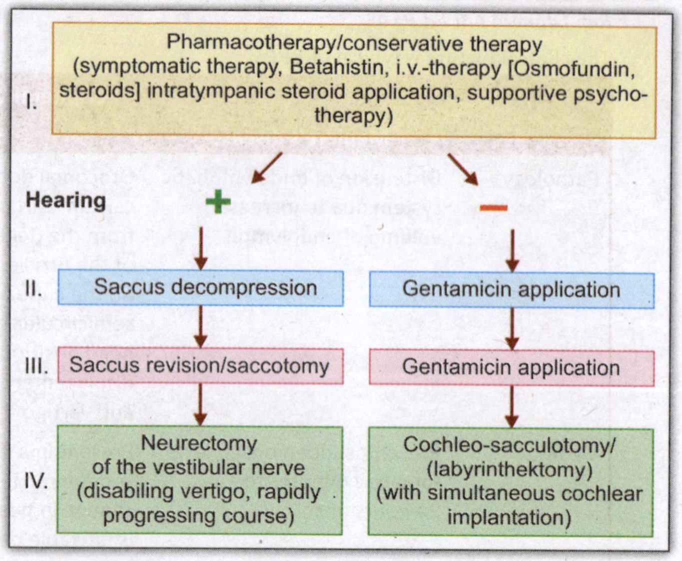

Fig: Bochum step-wise therapeutic scheme for patients with Meniere's disease

4. Ans. (a) Biopsy is done for diagnosis

Ref: Dhingra 6th ed page 246, KJ Lee's Essential Otolaryngology 11th ed page 873

Clue to Diagnosis

- **Adolescent male:** Nasopharyngeal Angiofibroma is predominantly seen in adolescent males in the second decade of life, it is thought to be testosterone dependent.
- **Unilateral nasal mass:** Nasopharyngeal angiofibroma presents with mass in the nasopharynx. Tumor is sessile, lobulated or smooth and obstructs one or both choanae. It is pink or purplish in colour. Consistency is firm but digital palpation should never be done until at the time of operation.
- **Recurrent nasal bleeding:** Profuse and recurrent epistaxis. This is the most common presentation of Nasopharyngeal angiofibroma

The most probable diagnosis is juvenile nasal angiofibroma. A biopsy in this case can cause torrential bleeding.

Juvenile Nasopharyngeal Angiofibroma AKA: Nasopharyngeal Fibroma	
Epidemiology	It is a rare tumor, though it is the commonest of all benign tumors of nasopharynx.
Etiology	The exact cause is unknown. As the tumor is predominantly seen in adolescent males in the second decade of life, it is thought to be testosterone dependent.
Site of origin	The site of origin of the tumor is still a matter of dispute. Earlier it was thought to arise from the roof of nasopharynx or the anterior wall of sphenoid bone but now it is believed to arise from the ***posterior part of nasal cavity close to the superior margin of sphenopalatine foramen.***

Contd...

Feeding vessel	**Internal maxillary artery > Ascending pharyngeal artery**
Pathology	Angiofibroma, as the name implies, is made up of ***vascular and fibrous tissues:*** the ratio of the two components may vary. *Mostly, the vessels are just endothelium-lined spaces with no muscle coat. This accounts for the severe bleeding as the vessels lose the ability to contract and also the bleeding cannot be controlled by application of adrenaline.*
Extensions	Nasopharyngeal fibroma is a ***benign tumor but locally invasive*** and destroys the adjoining structures. It may extend into: • **Nasal cavity** causing nasal obstruction, epistaxis and nasal discharge • **Paranasal sinuses:** Maxillary, sphenoid and ethmoid sinuses can all be invaded. • **Pterygomaxillary fossa, infratemporal fossa and cheek.** • **Orbits** giving rise to proptosis and ***"frog-face deformity"***. It enters through the inferior orbital fissure and also destroys apex of the orbit. It can also enter the orbit through superior orbital fissure. • **Cranial cavity.** Anterior cranial fossa (through ethmoid roof or cribriform plate). **Middle cranial fossa is the most common**. There are two routes of entry: a. By erosion of floor of middle cranial fossa, anterior to foramen lacerum. The tumor lies lateral to carotid artery and cavernous sinus. b. Through sphenoid sinus, into the sella. Tumor lies medial to carotid artery.
Clinical features	• **Age and sex.** Tumor is seen **almost exclusively in males** in the age group of 10–20 years. • **Profuse and recurrent epistaxis.** This is the **most common presentation** • **Progressive nasal obstruction and denasal speech** due to mass in the postnasal space. • **Conductive hearing loss and serous otitis media** due to obstruction of eustachian tube. • **Mass in the nasopharynx.** Tumor is sessile, lobulated or smooth and obstructs one or both choanae. It is pink or purplish in colour. Consistency is firm but ***digital palpation should never be done*** until at the time of operation. • **Others:** Broad nasal bridge, proptosis, swelling of cheek, infratemporal fossa or involvement of **2nd, 3rd, 4th, 6th cranial nerves** will depend on the extent of tumor
Investigations	• **Soft tissue lateral film of nasopharynx** shows soft tissue mass in the nasopharynx • **X-rays of paranasal sinuses** and base of skull may show DNS, opacification of sinuses, anterior bowing of posterior wall of maxillary sinus, destruction of medial antral wall, erosion of greater wing of sphenoid or pterygoid plates, widening of lower lateral margin of superior orbital fissure. • **CT scan of the head with contrast enhancement** is now the investigation of choice. It has replaced conventional radiographs. It shows the extent of tumor, bony destruction or displacements. Anterior bowing of the posterior wall of maxillary sinus (often called the ***Holman Miller or Antral sign***) is pathognomonic of angiofibroma. 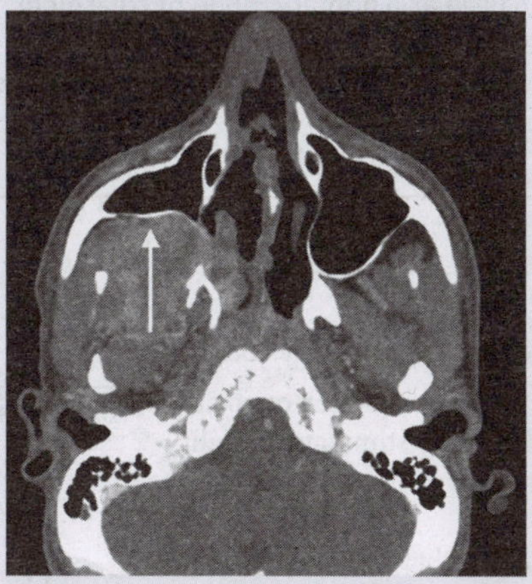 • **Magnetic resonance imaging (MRI)** is complementary to CT scans, when soft tissue extensions are present intracranially, in the infratemporal fossa or into the orbit. • **Carotid angiography** shows extension of tumor, its vascularity and feeding vessels. It is done when embolization is planned before operation. • **Biopsy of the tumor is attended with profuse bleeding and is therefore avoided**
Surgery	***Surgical excision is now the treatment of choice.*** Various approaches to angiofibroma, depending on origin and extensions, are listed below: • **Wilson's Approach (Transpalatine approach)** For tumors confined to nasopharynx • Transpalatine + Sublabial (**Sardana's approach**)

Contd...

<table>
<tr><td></td><td>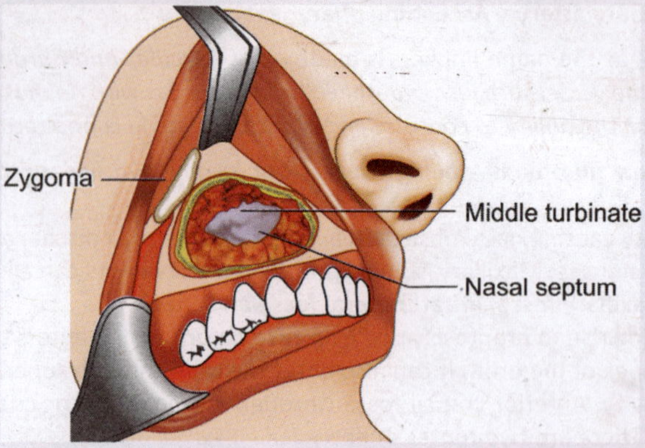

- **Extended lateral rhinotomy** (Via facial incision or Via degloving approach): for larger tumors involving nasal cavity, paranasal sinuses

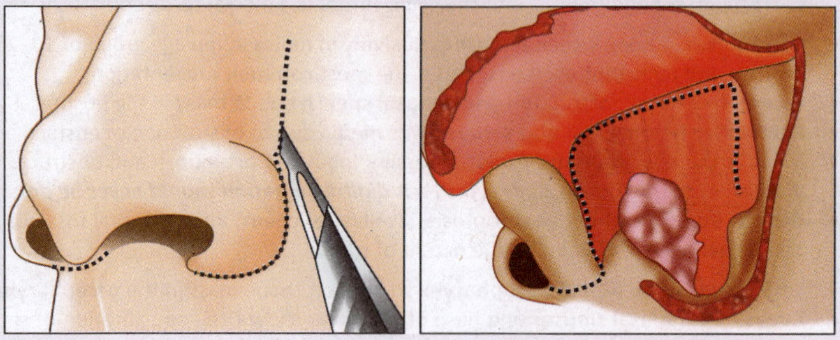

- Extended Denker's approach
- Intracranial-extracranial
- Infratemporal fossa
- Endoscopic</td></tr>
<tr><td>Other therapy</td><td>Radiotherapy has been used as a primary mode of treatment. A dose of 3000 to 3500 cGy in 15-18 fractions is delivered in 3–3.5 weeks.
Chemotherapy. Recurrent and residual lesions have been treated by chemotherapy, doxorubicin, vincristine and dacarbazine in combination</td></tr>
<tr><td>Recurrence</td><td>30–50% within 2–3 years postsurgery</td></tr>
</table>

5. Ans. (d) Fast component to left

Ref: Dhingra 6th ed page 43, 448, Ballinger 17th ed page 138

Applying simple Mnemonic COWS, i.e. cold water opposite side warm water same side implies that stimulating right cochlea with cold water will lead to a nystagmus to opposite side i.e. left side.

Nystagmus to left side also implies that fast component is towards left as nystagmus side is based on the direction of fast component. This nystagmus will be same in both the eyes whether you test left or right eye. Hence "Fast component to left" should be chosen as the answer.

Ballenger's 17th ed page 138; "*A warm caloric test transmits* ***heat to the lateral semicircular canal,*** *causing endolymph to rise and flow toward the cupula (ampullopetal flow). This is stimulatory to the lateral canal and nystagmus is generated with the fast phase beating toward the tested ear. The cool caloric stimulus effectively cools endolymph, making it more dense and causing it to fall away from the cupula (ampullofugal flow), which is inhibitory. This generates nystagmus away from the tested ear. The mnemonic devices, COWS (cold-opposite, warm-same), is a simple way to remember the association*"

6. Ans. (a) Malleus

Ref: Ballenger's Otorhinolaryngology: Head and Neck Surgery - Page 3, Dhingra 5th ed page 401, Gray's Anatomy 41st Ed Pg 638

NOTE

- Same dissection picture was given in AIIMS NOV 2016, but different structure (Lateral semicircular canal was asked.
- Endoscopic view of Middle ear was not given, But post mastoid air cell removal dissection pic was given in the question.

The diagram shows Malleus, which is the largest ossicle and is mallet shaped.

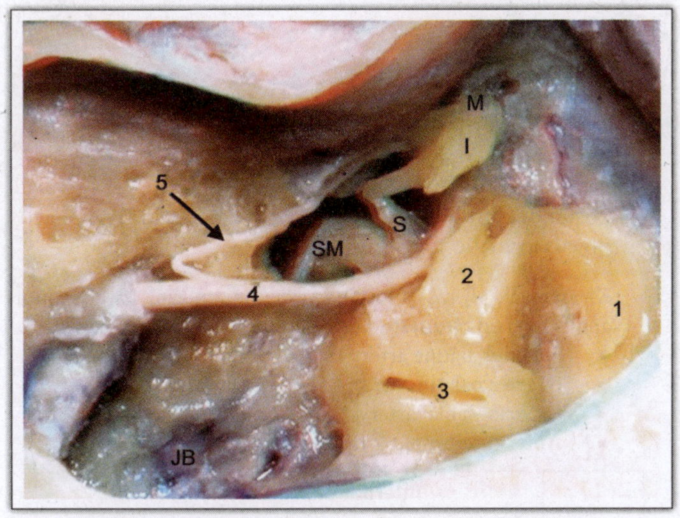

Fig: Mastoidectomy: Post mastoid air cell removal labelled

1 = Superior semicircular canal

2 = Lateral semicircular canal- Lateral semicircular canal can be identified acute angled from facial nerve, as the facial nerve passes in a dorsal direction between the lateral semicircular canal and the stapes

3 = Posterior semicircular canal

4 = VII cranial nerve

5 = Chorda tympani

M = malleus, I = incus, S = stapes

SM: stapedius muscle

JB: jugular bulb

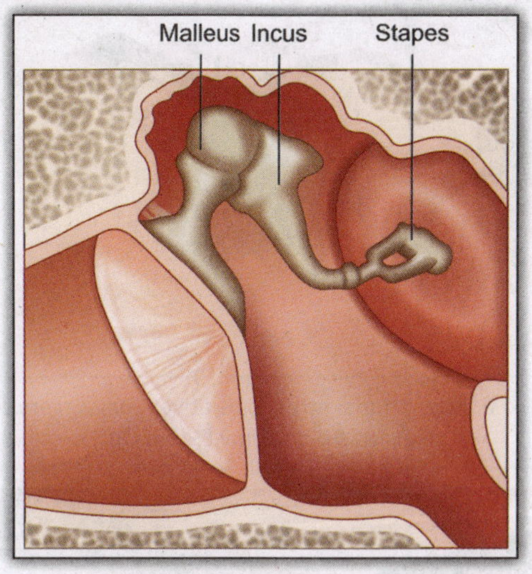

Fig: Middle ear ossicles illustration

EAR Ossicles			
	Malleus	Incus	Stapes
Derived from	1st arch	1st arch	Dual origin: Suprastructures: 2nd arch. Footplate: otic capsule (Hence most vulnerable to developmental anomaly)
Development period	4 – 26 weeks	15 – 25 weeks	15 – 25 weeks
Size & weight	Largest ear ossicle 8–9 mm long, 25 mg	In between malleus and stapes, Heaviest ossicle = 27 mg	Smallest bone of human body, 3 mm long, 3 mg
Shape	Mallet	Anvil	Stirrup
Parts	Has a head, neck, handle (manubrium) and anterior and lateral processes.	Body, long process, short process, lenticular process	Head, neck, two limbs (processes or crura) and a base (footplate)
Attachments/ Articulations	Tympanic membrane and Incus	Articular facet of incus joints with head of malleus while lenticular process articulates with head of the stapes	Head articulates with lenticular process of incus, footplate is attached to rim of the fenestra vestibuli.

7. Ans. (a) Otosclerosis

Ref: Dhingra 6th edition page 22

Gelle's Test	
Positive	Normal persons and in those with sensorineural hearing loss.
Negative	When ossicular chain is fixed or disconnected

- A vibrating tuning fork is applied over the mastoid process; if it is heard, the air in the external auditory canal is compressed, by means of a SIEGLE'S SPECULUM into the canal and a hand bulb, thereby fixing the stapes in the oval window; if the AMPLITUDE OF SOUND is not changed, the hearing loss is thought to be conductive; a test of the mobility of the ossicles.
- If patient hears it same, it may be due to fixed ossicles, e.g otosclerosis

AIIMS NOVEMBER 2017

8. Ans. (b) 2

Ref: Ballenger's Otorhinolaryngology: Head and Neck Surgery - Page 3, Dhingra 5th ed page 401

Lateral semicircular canal can be identified acute angled from facial nerve, as the facial nerve passes in a dorsal direction between the lateral semicircular canal and the stapes

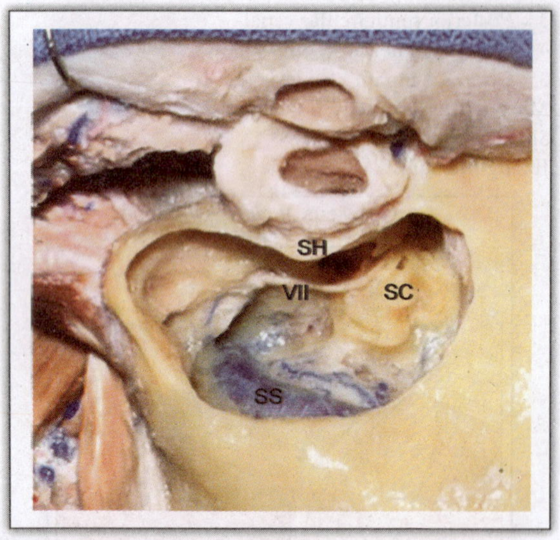

CC 4.0 International http://operativeneurosurgery.com

Fig: Mastoidectomy (Zoom Out)

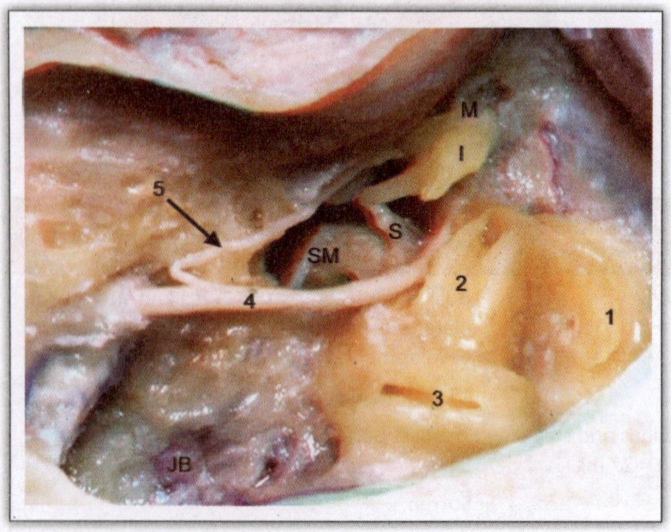

Fig: Mastoidectomy: Postmastoid air cell removal labelled

1 = Superior semicircular canal

2 = Lateral semicircular canal- Lateral semicircular canal can be identified acute angled from facial nerve, as the facial nerve passes in a dorsal direction between the lateral semicircular canal and the stapes

3 = Posterior semicircular canal

4 = VII cranial nerve

5 = Chorda tympani

M = malleus, I = incus, S = stapes

SM: stapedius muscle

JB: jugular bulb

9. Ans. (a) Anterior and posterior ethmoid artery

Ref: Ballenger's 17th ed page 459, Dhingra 6th ed page 176

NOTE

- Anterior and posterior ethmoid artery are branches of ophthalmic artery which are in turn branches of internal carotid artery.
- Posterior ethmoidal artery does not take part in Kiesselbach plexus formation.

Kiesselbach plexus is located over the anterior nasal septum and is formed by anastomosis between

- Sphenopalatine artery (Septal branch)
- Greater palatine artery (Septal branch)
- Superior labial artery (Septal branch)
- Anterior ethmoid arteries

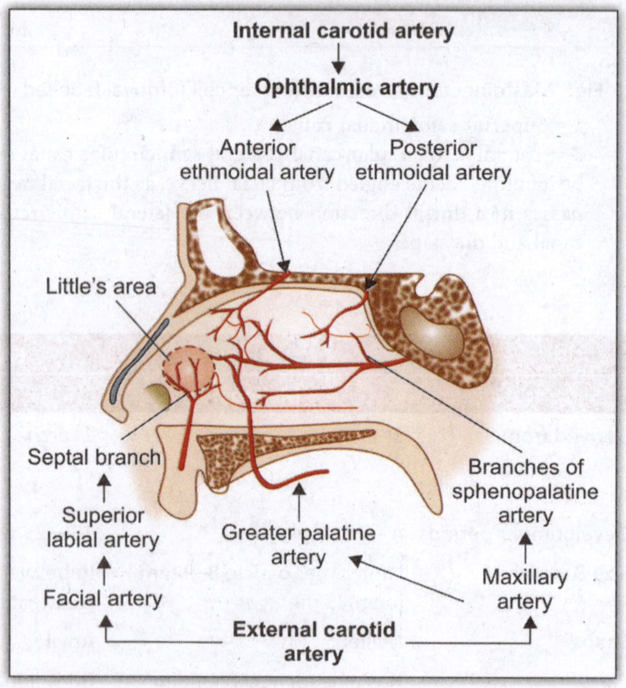

Fig: Blood supply of nasal septum

10. Ans. (b) Frontal sinus

Ref: Cummings Pediatric Otolaryngology 2015 ed page 64, Ballenger's 17th ed page 456, Scott Brown 7th ed page 1318 -22, Dhingra 6th ed page 189

There is difference of data of age in different text books. We have researched and made this table with most agreeable data which matches most reliable textbooks.

Cummings states "By the age of 16 years, the maxillary sinus reaches full size. The ethmoid sinuses are present at birth and have attained adult size by the early teens. The frontal sinus can be distinguished from the ethmoids around age 5 years and demonstrates a variable growth rate until reaching adult size in late puberty. The sphenoid sinus is the last to develop and is present radiologically at approximately age 6 years. Growth of the sphenoid sinus continues well past puberty into the early adult years. Shah and coworkers reviewed 91 scans in 66 patients (16 obtained serially over time) between birth and 12 years of age and demonstrated periods of significant growth in the paranasal sinuses in children. **The ethmoid sinuses were the first to fully develop, followed by the maxillary, sphenoid and frontal sinuses."**

Ballinger state "Frontal recess expands and grows cephalad after birth to form the frontal sinus which becomes radiologically apparent at years 7 to 12. The left and right frontal sinuses develop independently, thus accounting for their asymmetry" (frontal recess is a part of frontal sinus only) **Scott Brown States** "*The configuration of the sinuses and the frontal recess is subject to considerable variation. Diverticula and septation are not uncommon. The frontal recess, although frequently a narrow hourglass segment, may have a longer, more tortuous path encroached upon by adjacent anterior ethmoidal cells. These variations are a direct consequence of the sinus' embryological development* ***as it is the last to complete its growth, in early adulthood***".

Paranasal Sinuses

Paranasal sinus (PNS)	Status at birth	1st radiological evidence	Best radiological view	Adult size	Drains into	Comments
Maxillary	Present	4–5 months after birth (Can be seen at birth). Two growth spurts 1–4 years and 7–12 years	Waters' view/ Occipito-mental/ nose-chin Position	16 years	Middle meatus	Largest PNS, capacity of 15 mL in an adult, Antrum of Highmore
Ethmoid	Present	1st radio evidence at 1 year. Two growth spurts 0–3 years and 7–12 years	Caldwell view	Adult size by 12 years. (Early teens)	Anterior and middle Ethmoid= middle meatus, Posterior Ethmoid= Superior meatus	Adult vol 14 mL, Number varies from 3 to 18
Frontal	Absent	1st radio evidence at 5 years (distinguish itself from ethmoid). Growth spurt at 7–12 years	Caldwell view	Adult size by 20 years. Last sinus to pneumatize	Middle meatus	Adult volume 6-7 mL
Sphenoid	Absent	6 years (Last to start developing)	Water's view with open mouth	Adult size by 15 years	Sphenoethmoidal recess	Adult vol 7.5 mL, 2.2 cm x 2 cm x 2.2 cm

Footnotes:

- Most superior sinus: **Frontal**
- Most posterior sinus: **Sphenoid**
- Largest sinus: **Maxillary**
- M/c sinusitis in **children**: Ethmoidal sinusitis.
- M/c sinusitis in **adults**: Maxillary sinusitis
- Maxillary sinus is also known as **Antrum of Highmore**.
- Both the maxillary and ethmoidal sinuses are present at birth but only the ethmoidal sinuses are pneumatized.
- Order of development/first radiological appearance of sinuses: **Maxillary> Ethmoid> Frontal > Sphenoid** (Cummings Pediatric Otolaryngology 2015 ed page 64)
- Order of development/adult size of sinus/first to fully develop: **Ethmoid> Maxillary> Sphenoid >Frontal** (Cummings Pediatric Otolaryngology 2015 ed page 64)
- **Streptococcus pneumoniae** is the most common organism implicated to acute sinusitis in in both adults and children.
- In children with cystic fibrosis, most common organism implicated to sinusitis is **staphylococcus aureus**.
- Chronic sinusitis is most commonly associated with **S. aureus** and α hemolytic streptococci
- **Aspergillus mucormycosis** is the most common organism implicated to fungal sinusitis with maxillary sinus most frequently involved
- ***Wagner's granulomatosis*** is the most common granulomatous sinusitis with maxillary sinus most commonly involved.
- Acute sinusitis almost always involves single sinus, with ethmoid sinus being most common in children and maxillary in adults.
- Maxillary sinus is the most common location of chromic sinusitis in both children and adults closely followed by ethmoid sinus.
- (Note: To be more particular "Anterior ethmoid cells" are most common site of chronic sinusitis in children but comparing sinuses as a whole maxillary becomes more common than ethmoid)
- **Mucous retention cyst** (different from mucocele) is most commonly found at maxillary sinus.
- Most common site of **mucocele** is frontal sinus (60%), least common at sphenoid sinus.
- "The sinuses commonly affected by mucocele in the order of frequency, are the Frontal > Ethmoidal > Maxillary > Sphenoidal"
- **Squamous cell carcinoma** is the most common malignant tumor of sinuses with **maxillary sinus** most commonly involved (80%)
- Most common site of **adenocarcinoma** of sinus is **ethmoid sinus.**
- **Brain abscess** is the most common intracranial complication of sinusitis (as a whole)

Contd...

- **Meningitis** is the most common intracranial complication of acute sinusitis.
- **Orbital complication** is the most common extracranial an overall complication of sinusitis
- **Orbital cellulitis** most commonly involve, Ethmoidal sinus
- **Osteomas of paranasal sinuses:** Most commonly seen in **frontal sinus** followed by ethmoidal and maxillary
- **Complications of maxillary wash:**
  - Cheek swelling
  - Orbital injury and cellulitis
  - Puncture of posterior antral wall
  - Bleeding
  - Sudden death due to air embolism

11. Ans. (c) Traumatic CSF Rhinorrhea

Ref: Dhingra 6th ed page 164

Traumatic CSF rhinorrhea is blood mixed and shows double target sign when collected on a piece of filter paper. It shows central red spot due to blood and peripheral lighter halo due to CSF. While spontaneous CSF Rhinorrhea is not blood mixed.

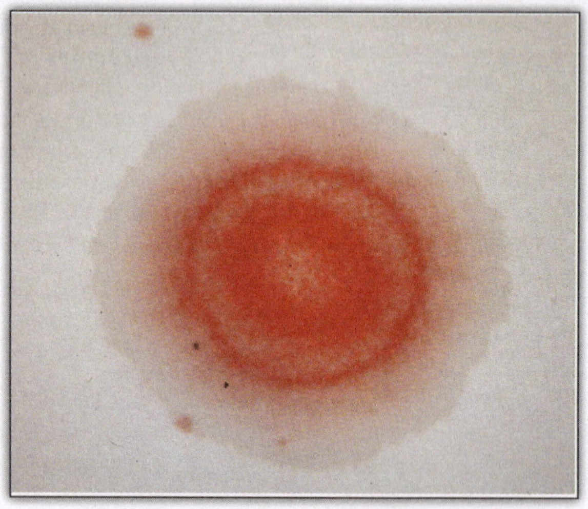

12. Ans. (c) Inner hair cell

Ref: Ballenger's 17th ed page 266-7, Dhingra 6th ed page 35

Hearing loss associated with exposure to noise has been well known in occupations like boiler makers, iron- and coppersmiths and artillery men. Hearing loss caused by excessive noise can be divided into two groups:

1. **Acoustic trauma:** Permanent damage to hearing can be caused by a single brief exposure to very intense sound. Such noise can arise from an explosion, gun fire (140–170 dB) or a powerful cracker (140 dB). Such brief and loud noises mechanically damage organ of Corti, tear Reissner's membrane, rupture hair cells and allowing mixing of perilymph and endolymph.
2. **Noise-induced hearing loss (NIHL):** is due to chronic exposure to less intense sounds than seen in acoustic trauma and is mainly a hazard of noisy occupations.

Ballenger says "Assessment of noise-induced histopathology reveals that many cell types in the cochlea can be compromised by sound overexposure (Figure). Hair cell stereocilia damage, evidence of swelling and vacuolization in the inner hair cell (IHC) area, hair cell loss, collapse of supporting cells, strial compromise, fibrocyte loss and neuronal loss all have been identified in noise-exposed ears"

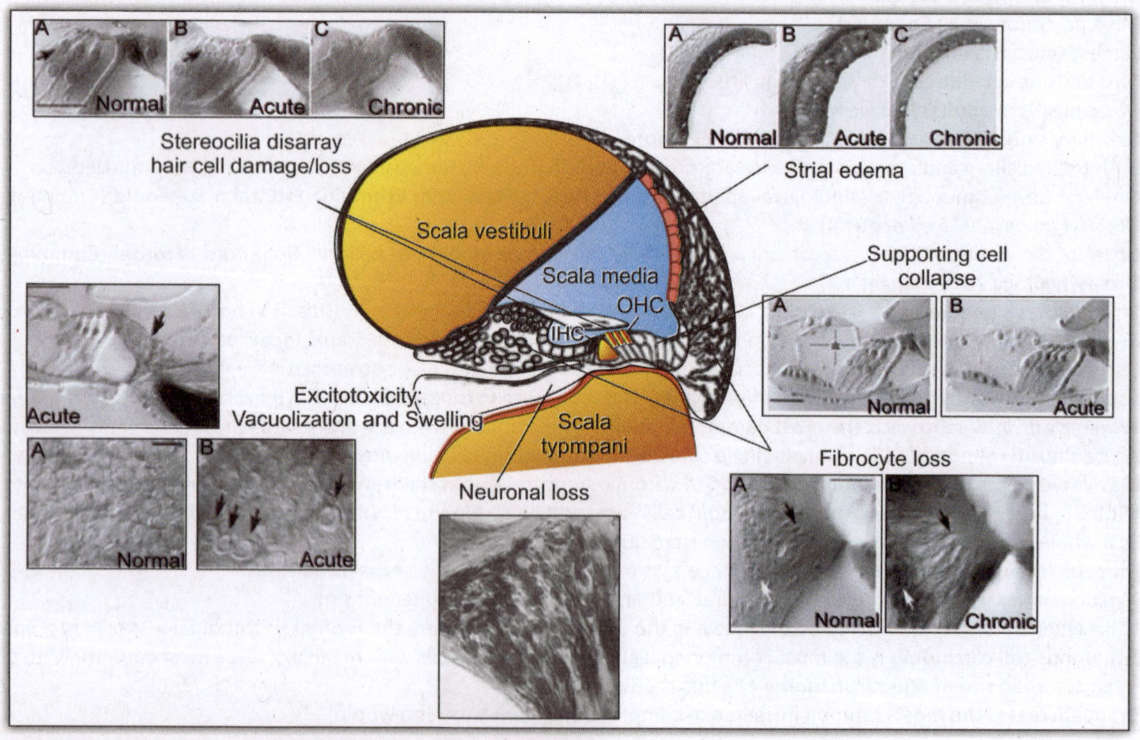

Noise induced hearing loss usually affects:

- Hair cell stereocilia damage
- Swelling and vacuolization in the inner hair cell (IHC) area
- Inner hair cell loss
- Damage to supporting cells
- Strial degeneration
- Loss of fibrocytes and
- Neuronal degeneration

Noise Trauma Depends on Several Factors

- Frequency of noise. A frequency of 2000–3000 Hz causes more damage than lower or higher frequencies.
- Intensity and duration of noise.
- Continuous vs interrupted noise. Continuous noise is more harmful.
- Susceptibility of the individual.
- Pre-existing ear disease.

NOTE

- The 85 dB maximum limit for 8 hours is recommended by the WHO and ACGIH (Association Advancing Occupational and Environmental Health) for most of the countries
- In India- A noise of 90 dB, 8 hour a day for 5 days per week is the maximum safe limit as recommended by Ministry of Labour, Govt. of India, Model Rules under Factories Act. No exposure in excess of 115 dB (A) is t be permitted. No impulse noise of intensity greater than 140 dB (A) is permitted.

13. Ans. (a) 10–15 sec

Ref: https://www.hopkinsmedicine.org/tracheostomy/living/suctioning.html

Steps for Suctioning Tracheal Secretions

- Wash your hands.
- Turn on the suction machine and connect the suction connection tubing to the machine.
- Use a clean suction catheter when suctioning the patient.
- Lay the patient flat on his/her back with a small towel/blanket rolled under the shoulders. Some patients may prefer a sitting position which can also be tried.
- Wet the catheter with sterile/distilled water for lubrication and to test the suction machine and circuit.
- Carefully insert the catheter into the tracheostomy tube.
- Allow the catheter to follow the natural curvature of the tracheostomy tube.
- The least traumatic technique is to pre-measure the length of the tracheostomy tube then introduce the catheter only to that length.
- Place your thumb over the suction vent (side of the catheter) intermittently while you remove the catheter.
- Do not leave the catheter in the tracheostomy tube for more than **5–10 seconds**
- Allow the patient to recover from the suctioning and to catch his/her breath. Wait for at least 10 seconds.
- Suction a small amount of distilled/sterile water with the suction catheter to clear any residual debris/secretions.
- Turn off suction machine and discard catheter.

AIIMS MAY 2017

14. Ans. (a) Otosclerosis

Ref: Scott Brown 7th edition page 3185, Dhingra 6th ed page 29

NOTE

It was a handmade graph in the examination

The audiogram is typical of otosclerosis.
Symbols used in audiogram:

MNEMONIC

- For 1st and 2nd symbols remember the mnemonic: Cross the Square from Left side
- For 3rd and 4th symbols - Note that the Open end of symbols > and] represents the ear side.
- Red for Right

Modality	Ear	
	Right	Left
AC unmasked	O	X
AC masked	△	□
BC unmasked	<	>
BC masked	[	]
No response	↙O	X↘

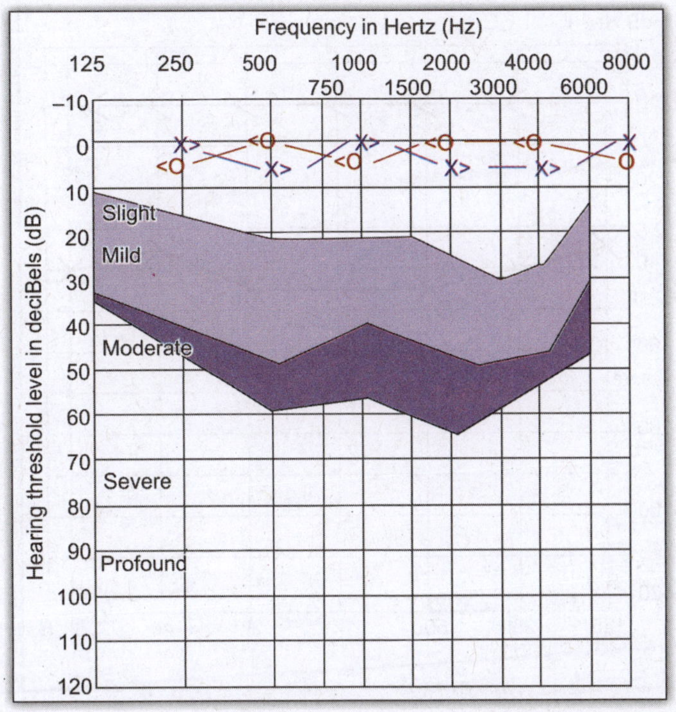

Fig: Normal Audiogram: The air bone (AB) conduction gap is less than 10–15 dB. The shaded area below the lines represents the imaginary mild moderate Hearing loss. Severe and profound hearing loss are lebelled more lower down in case the audiometric lines lies in that area. See the symbols used in audiogram above

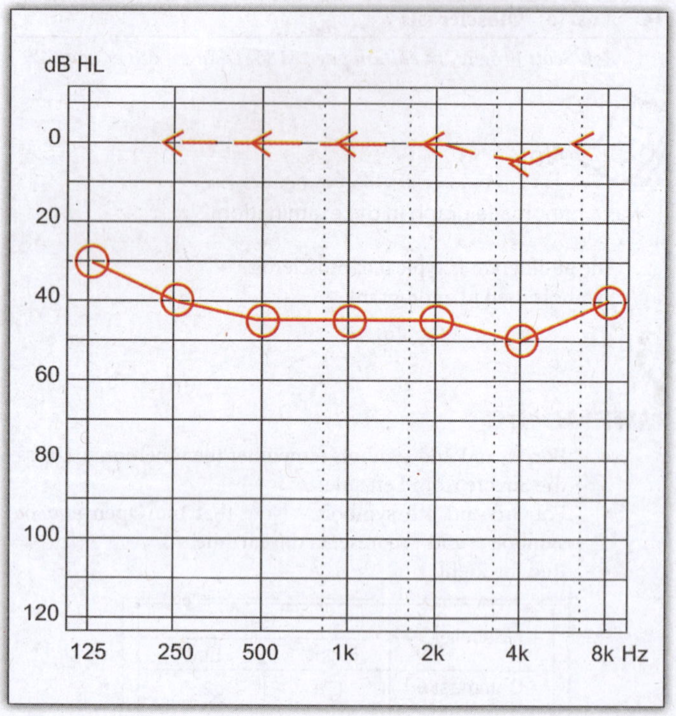

Fig: Conductive hearing loss of right ear: Difference between bone conduction and air conduction is more than 20 db which tells it is conductive loss. Red colour of lines on the graph and symbols tell it is right side

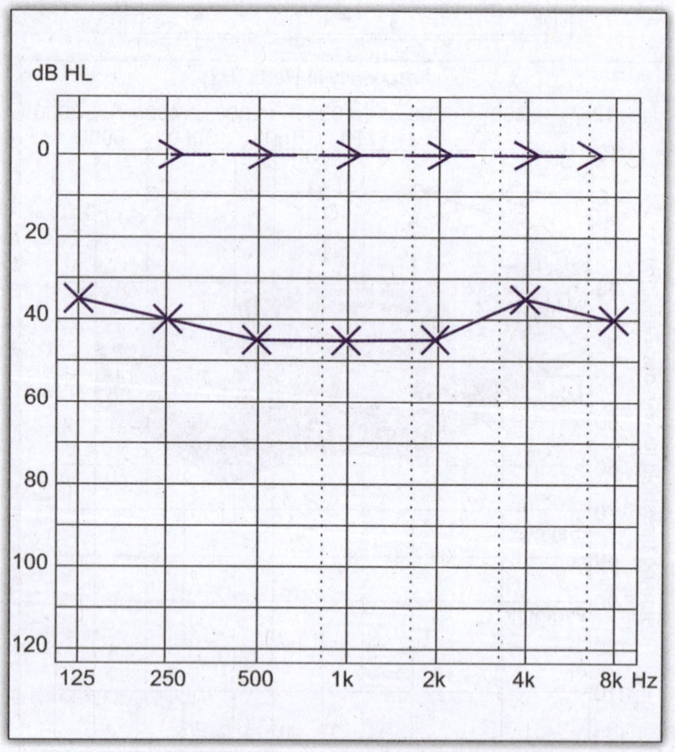

Fig: Conductive hearing loss of left ear

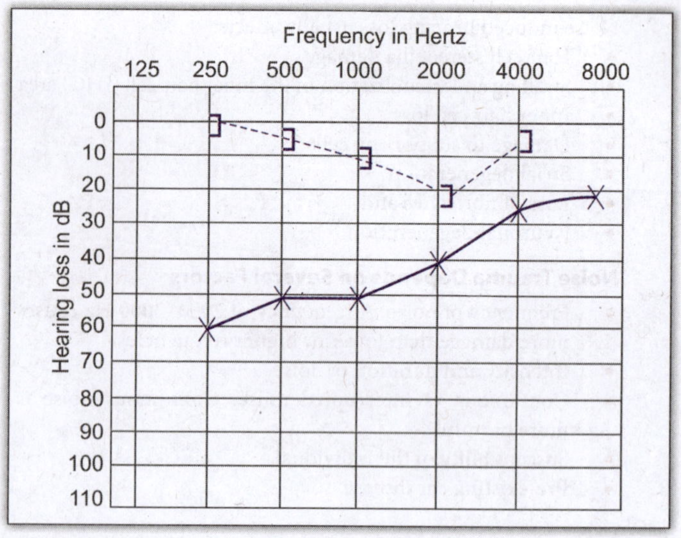

Fig: Conductive hearing loss due to Otosclerosis: There is typically an apparent lowering in the bone conduction hearing threshold by about 5 dB at 500 Hz. 10 dB at 1000 Hz, 15–20 dB at 2000 Hz and 5 dB at 4000 Hz. This peculiar configuration in the bone conduction hearing level, most marked (i.e., notched) at 2000 Hz is termed as **CARHART'S NOTCH**. If the notch in the bone conduction level is not duplicated by the air conduction curve, then it is a true Carhart's notch

Cumming's 5th ed: "This is not a true depression in bone conduction, but rather an artifact caused by a lack of the normal contribution of the mobile ossicular chain to bone conduction. This depression improves after the mobility of the ossicular chain is restored e.g. after stapedectomy"

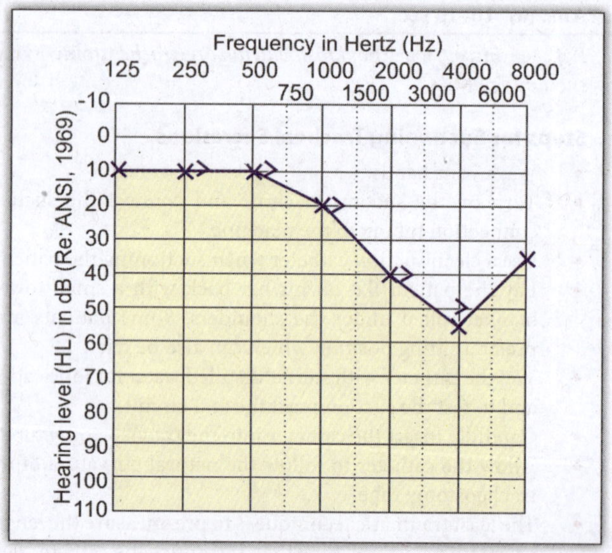

Fig: Sensory neural hearing loss: There is no air bone gap and both air conduction and bone conduction have come down. Hence it is sensory neural loss. Blue colour and symbols tell it is left side. Carhart's notch must be differentiated from **Boiler's notch** which is due to noise induced hearing loss. Boiler's notch is seen at 4 khz and is seen both in air conduction as well as bone conduction, in contrast to Carhart's notch which is seen at 2 khz and is only seen in bone conduction

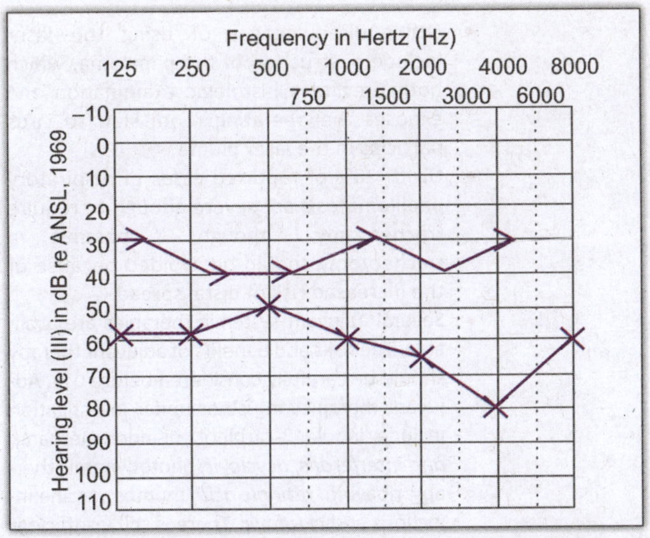

Fig: Mixed hearing loss: there is air bone gap more than 20 db and bone conduction has also come down. Colour and symbols indicate left side

15. Ans. (c) Internal carotid artery

Ref: Scott Brown 7th ed vol 2 page 1602

Internal carotid can never be ligated in any case as it will lead to hemiplegia or other even more severe intracranial complications of stroke within few minutes.

Scott says *"Endoscopy identifies the source of posterior epistaxis in over 80 percent of cases." Ligation should be performed as close as possible to the likely bleeding point; thus, the hierarchy of ligation is:*

- Sphenopalatine artery
- Internal maxillary artery
- External carotid artery
- Anterior/posterior ethmoidal artery.

Blood Supply of Nasal Septum

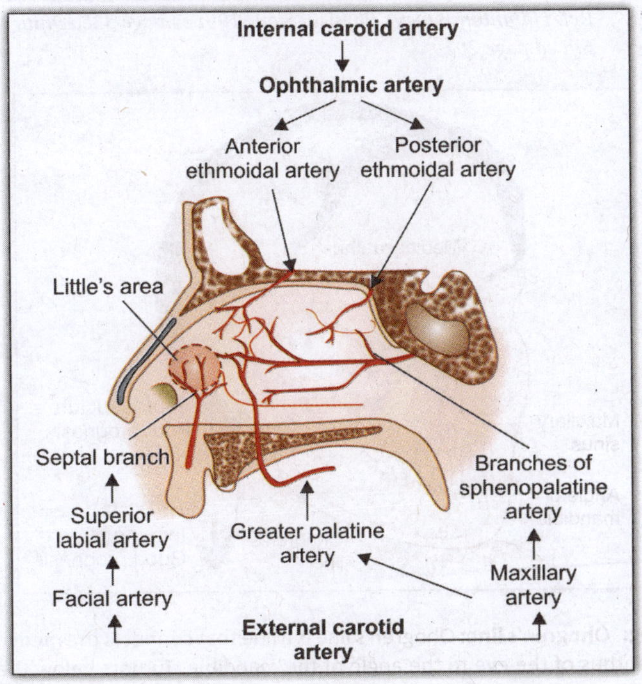

16. Ans. (a) Respiratory papillomatosis

Ref: Scott Brown 7th ed vol 1 page 1176, Dhingra 6th ed page 305, Current Otolaryngology 2nd ed Chapter 32

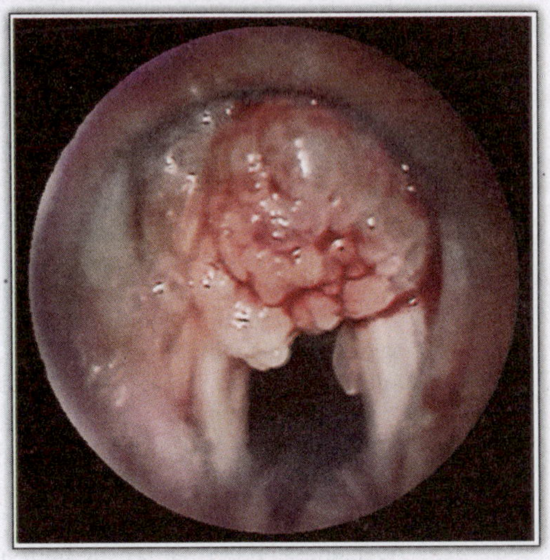

Fig: Respiratoy Papillomatosis

Respiratory Papillomatosis: Typical description and image is of **respiratory papilomatosis**. History of maternal genital infection or papillomas is frequently mentioned. Exuberant tissue resembling miniature clusters of grapes may be seen, especially on the anterior part of the true vocal folds, the false folds and the epiglottis

Recurrent Respiratory Papillomatosis (RRP)	
Definition	Rare condition characterized by recurrent growth of benign papillomas in the respiratory tract, most commonly in the larynx.
Essentials of diagnosis	1. Hoarse voice 2. Gradual onset of stridor 3. Recurrent disease requiring multiple surgical procedures. 4. Viral etiology
Etiology	Papillomatosis is caused by infection with human papillomavirus (HPV), the most commonly identified subtypes being **HPV-6 and HPV-11** (HPV-11 is more aggressive and more prone to malignant changes). The same HPV subtypes are responsible for genital warts and there is a recognized association between maternal genital warts and respiratory papillomatosis.
Epidemiology	• Mean age ages of 2 and 5 years, but papillomas can present in any age group. • There is no difference in incidence between males and females.
Risk factors	• The **first-born, vaginally delivered child** of a teenage mother is associated with an increased chance of developing respiratory papillomatosis. • Genital Condylomas of mother during pregnancy are considered the most important risk factor for acquiring JoRRP by vertical HPV transmission from mother to child.

Contd...

	• Cesarean delivery was *not* found to be protective against respiratory papillomatosis • In adults viral transmission may occur during oral sex, but this remains unproven. Reactivation of a latent HPV infection acquired in childhood is another possible cause.
Types	The disease is categorized as juvenile-onset (JoRRP) if it develops before the age of 18 and adult-onset (AoRRP) for cases that develop after the age of 18. • **Juvinile Onset:** because of diffuse involvement of the larynx, usually manifests in infancy or childhood as hoarseness and stridor. This form of papillomatosis is often aggressive and rapidly recurrent • **Adult-Onset** papillomas are occasionally solitary or at least more localized than juvenile-onset lesions and also less aggressive
Clinical features	The clinical course is highly variable, with frequent relapses and may be lifelong. • Hoarseness, abnormal cry, or both are the **most common** presenting symptoms of respiratory papillomatosis. • If the disease is untreated, then a gradual progression to dyspnea, stridor and eventually, complete airway obstruction can occur. • Stridor and airway obstruction are rarely the first symptoms.
Malignant transformation	The malignant transformation from benign nonkeratinizing squamous papillomas to squamous cell carcinoma can occur in children, but is rarely seen. Malignant transformation most commonly occurs in the distal bronchopulmonary tree and the prognosis is universally poor.
Evaluation	If the diagnosis of respiratory papillomatosis is suspected, then a histopathologic confirmation is required. At microlaryngoscopy, the papillomas are seen to be **firm, irregular, exophytic lesions that bleed easily** on manipulation. Examination should include tracheobronchoscopy to determine whether distal spread has occurred.
Treatment	• The **primary treatment modality** for respiratory papillomatosis is surgery. The aims of treatment are to maintain an adequate airway while avoiding tracheotomy, preserving the voice and controlling the papilloma. • The most widely accepted means of surgical ablation of respiratory papilloma is with the **CO_2 laser**. Because respiratory papillomatosis typically requires multiple procedures to maintain the airway, there is a significant risk of scarring and web formation due to repeated thermal damage caused by the laser. For this reason, it is advisable to leave small amounts of the papilloma in sites where scarring is likely to occur, such as the anterior commissure.

Contd...

	• Other disadvantages of using the laser include destruction of the papilloma, which both precludes histologic examination and exposes the operating room staff to virus particles in the laser plume. • Up to 20% of reported cases of respiratory papillomatosis are severe enough to require **tracheotomy**, although, if possible, a tracheotomy should be avoided because of the increased risk of distal spread. • Several adjuvant systemic therapies are available. The risks and benefits of adjuvant therapy should be carefully considered before use. Adjuvant therapies in use or under investigation include indole 3-carbinol, di-indolymethane, ***alfa interferons, acyclovir***, photodynamic therapy, ribavirin, ***retinoic acid***, mumps vaccine injections and ***cidofovir***. There is still insufficient evidence on the effectiveness of antiviral therapy. The ideal dose, frequency and duration of cidofovir therapy are yet to be known. • Maximum total dose of cidofovir should not exceed ***3 mg/kg***. • Due to high toxicity of cidofovir, analysis of laboratory parameters like morphology with blood smear, urea, creatinine, ALT, AST and bilirubin levels before the treatment, 1 day and 4 weeks after the injection. All papillomas should be examined histopathologically to exclude any dysplastic features or malignant transformation.

Option (B) and (C): Both are infective pathologies and child will present with toxic features like severe pain, fever, difficulty in breathing and sometimes stridor.

Option (D): Vocal nodule is rarely seen in children and never causes respiratory difficulty.

17. Ans. (b) Ohngren's line

Ref: Hamilton Bailey's Physical Signs 19th ed page 338, Dhingra 6th ed page 207

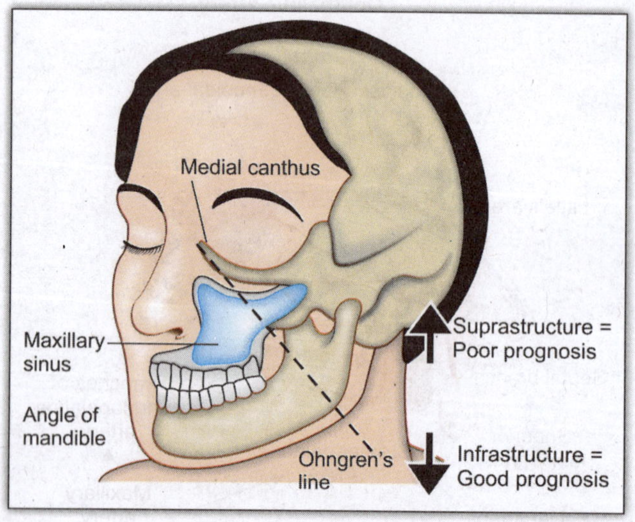

Fig: Ohngren's line: Ohngren's line is a line that connects the medial canthus of the eye to the angle of the mandible. Tumors below the line are considered infrastructure and carry a better prognosis, while tumors above this line are considered suprastructure and carries poor prognosis

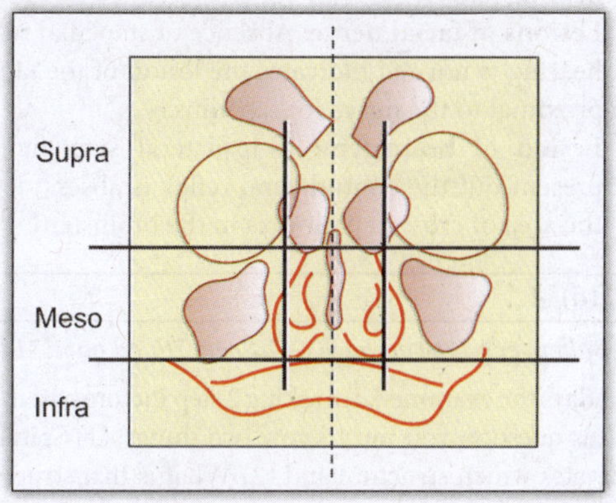

Fig: Sebileau's lines dividing the sinonasal area in regions and sites. Horizontal Sebileau's line in the Lederman's classification divides the structure into superior structure, mesostructure and inferior structure

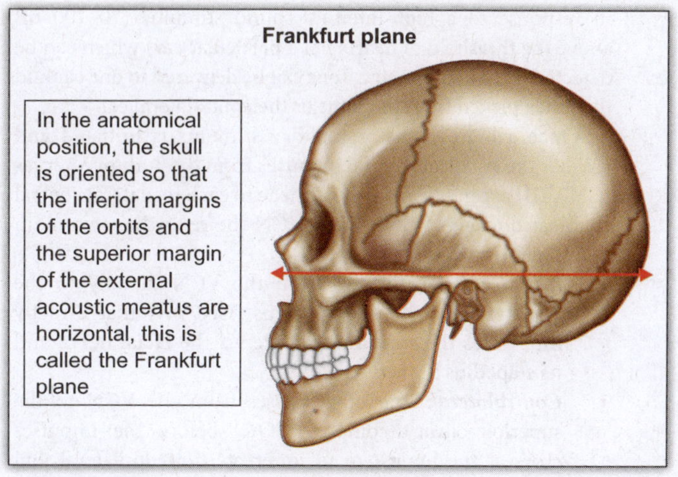

Fig: Frankfurt Line/Plane: A craniometric surface between the inferior borders of the bony orbits and the upper margin of the auditory meatus. It passes through the two orbitales and the two tragions and is commonly used as a reference surface in orthodontic diagnosis and treatment planning

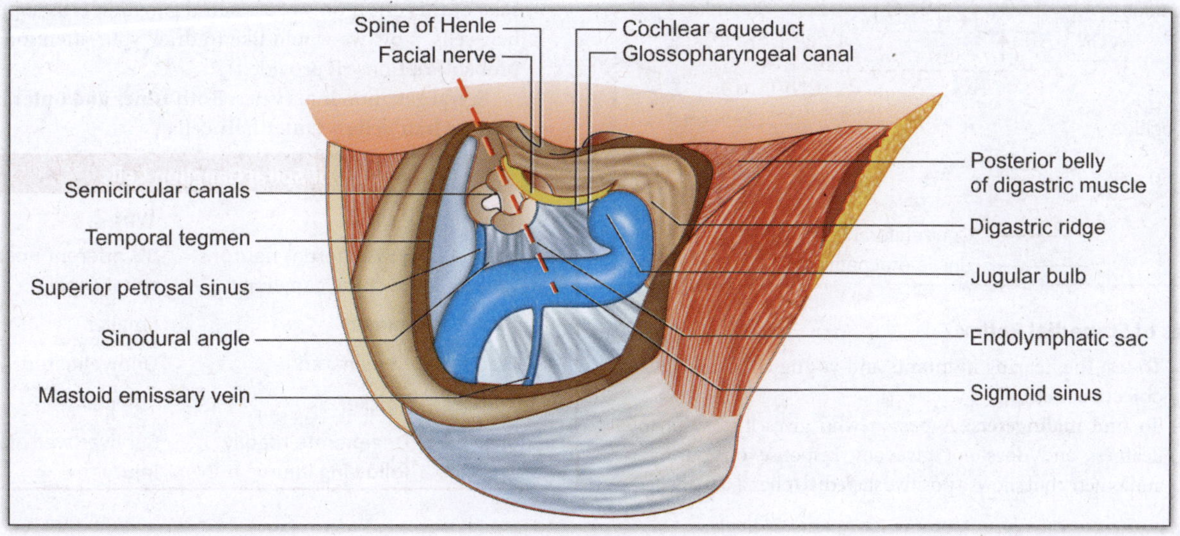

Fig: Donaldson's line: Line drawn along the horizontal semicircular canal, bisecting posterior SSC. It is landmark of endolymphatic surgery. (See dotted lines)

AIIMS NOVEMBER 2016

18. Ans. (c) + 80 mV

Ref: Cumming's 5th ed vol 1 page 2073, Guyton 12th ed page 637-638, Ganong 22nd ed chapter 9

"It is known that K^+ carries the major portion of the receptor current in vivo, as indicated by three observations:

- The high concentration of K^+ in endolymph;
- The reversal potential of the transducer current is the same as the endocochlear potential; and
- That the concentration of K^+ found in perilymph increases after stimulation.

As a result of the combined positive endocochlear potential (+80 mV) and the negative intracellular potential of hair cells (−40 to −60 mV), a large potential gradient (greater than 120 mV) is established across the apical hair cell membrane"

So important points extracted are:

- Positive endocochlear potential (+80 mV)
- Negative intracellular potential of hair cells (−40 to −60 mV)
- Potential gradient (greater than 120 mV)

19. Ans. (d) Superior olivary nucleus

Ref: Cumming's 5th ed vol 1 page 1848

Acoustic/Stapedial Reflex

The acoustic reflex, also known as the stapedius reflex refers to a bilateral involuntary muscle contraction of the stapedius muscle in response to a high-intensity sound stimulus (70–100 dB above the threshold of hearing of a particular ear) which can be detected by tympanometry. Tone can be delivered to one ear and the reflex picked from the same or the contralateral ear.

Once a high intensity auditory stimulus is initiated and reaches the cochleae, neural impulses from the auditory nerves (CN VIII) ascend from both cochleae to each ipsilateral ventral cochlear nucleus (VCN). From VCN the reflex has two main neural pathways:

- ***Ipsilateral:*** One passes from the VCN directly to the ipsilateral facial motor nucleus (CN VII) that directly innervates the stapedius muscle via the facial nerve and its stapedius branch
- ***Contralateral:*** The other passes from the VCN to the superior olivary complex (SOC) before the impulses cross at the brainstem to innervate both ipsilateral and contralateral facial motor nuclei to supply stapedius muscle

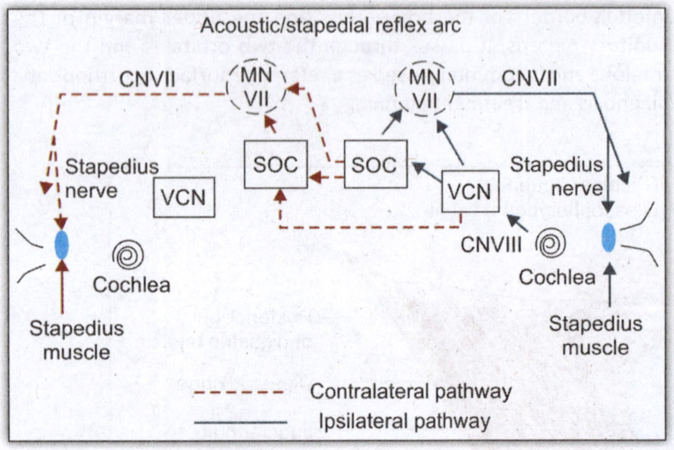

Uses of Stapedial Reflex

- To test the hearing in infants and young children. It is an objective method
- **To find malingerers:** A person who gives history of total deafness and does not give any response on pure tone audiometry but shows a positive stapedial reflex is a malingerer.
- **To detect cochlear pathology:** Presence of stapedial reflex at lower intensities, e.g. 40 to 60 dB than the usual 70 dB indicates recruitment and hence a cochlear type of hearing loss.
- **Lesions of facial nerve:** Absence of stapedial reflex when hearing is normal indicates the lesion of the facial nerve, proximal to the nerve to stapedius.
- **Lesion of brainstem:** If ipsilateral stapedial reflex is present but the contralateral reflex is absent, lesion is in the area of crossed pathways in the brainstem.

20. Ans. (d) 4

Ref: Ballenger's 17th ed page 6-7, Scott 7th ed page 3149,

Nowadays the examiners are asking 2 step Picture based questions. For this question you must know two things; (1) Spiral ganglion innervates which structure and (2) What is that structure in the picture (which is well explained in the figure)

Ninety-five percent of afferent fibres of spiral ganglion supply the inner hair cells and are called as Type 1 spiral gangflion cell, while only 5% supply the outer hair cells and are called as Type 2 spiral ganglion cells.

Hence Inner hair cells should be the ANSWER for the sake of this question as 95% spiral ganglion cells supply Inner hair cells. Now we would like to draw your attention to other probable options (if provided)

Spiral ganglion innervates: **Both Inner and outer hair cells > Inner hair cells > Outer hair cells**

Types of Spiral Ganglion Cells

	Type 1	**Type 2**
Number	95% afferent neurons of spiral ganglion	5% afferent nuerons of spiral ganglion
Size	Larger	Smaller
Myelination	Myelinated	Unmyelinated
Distal process	Thicker	Thinner
Response to injury	Degenerate readily following injury	Survives well after injury

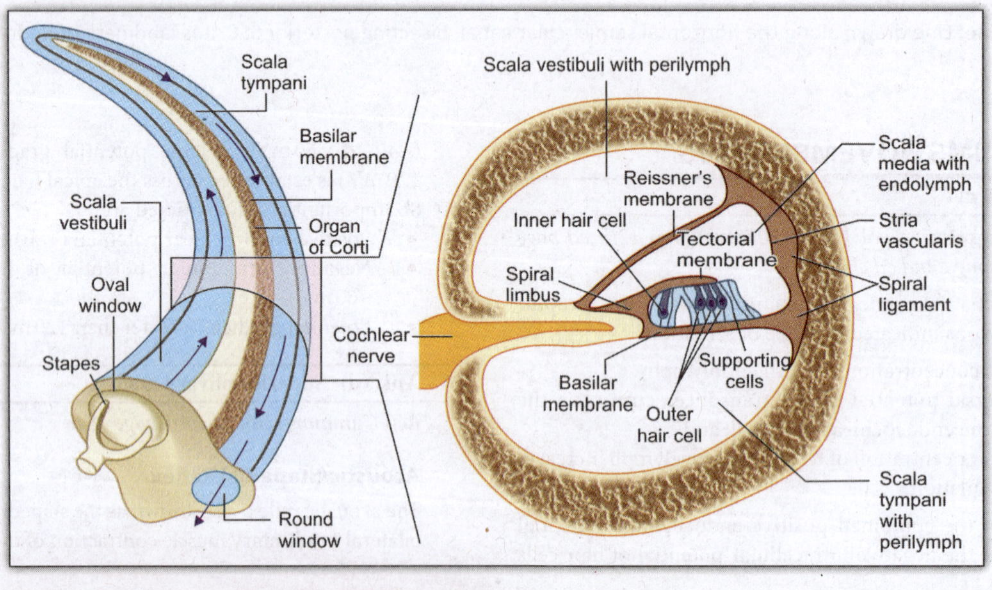

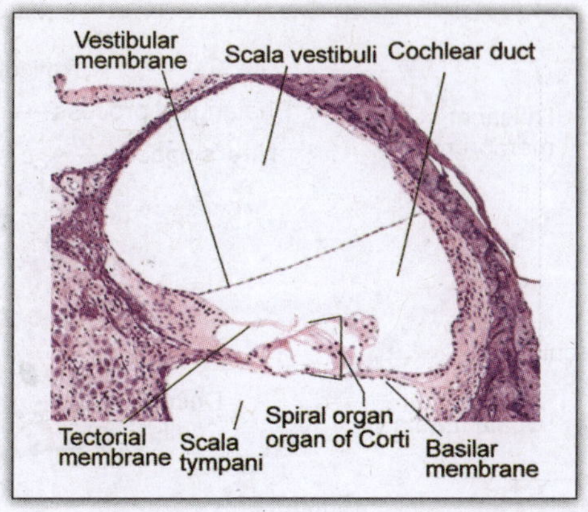

Fig: Cross section of cochlear duct: Representation above, Histological below (with labelling)

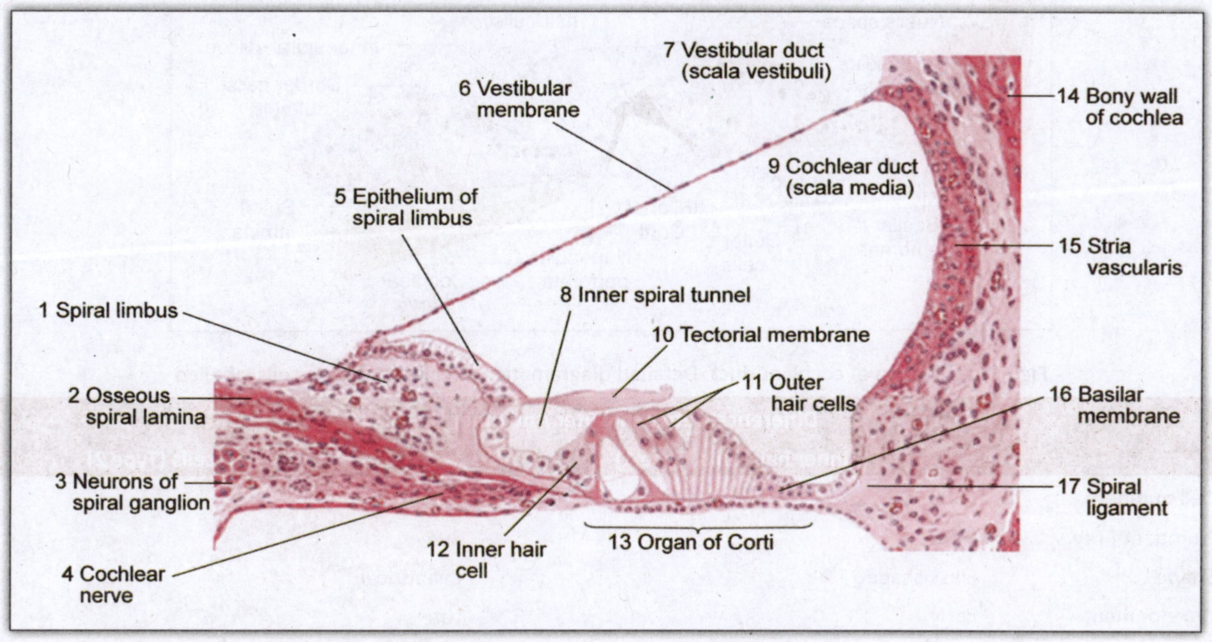

Fig: Cross section of scala media (with labelling)

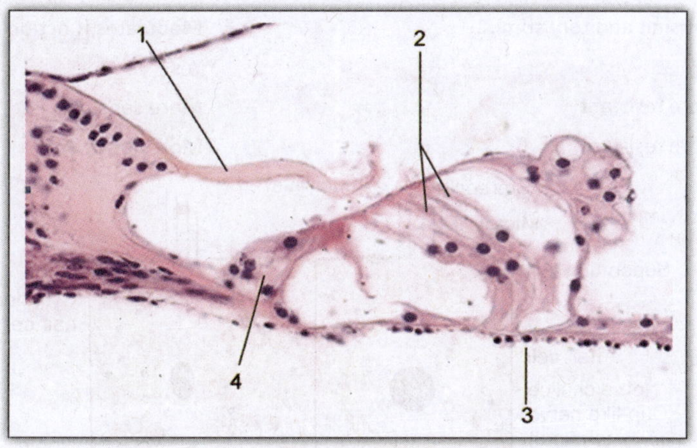

Fig: Cross section of Organ of Corti: (High power)

1. Tectorial membrane
2. Outer hair cell
3. Basillar membrane
4. Inner hair cell

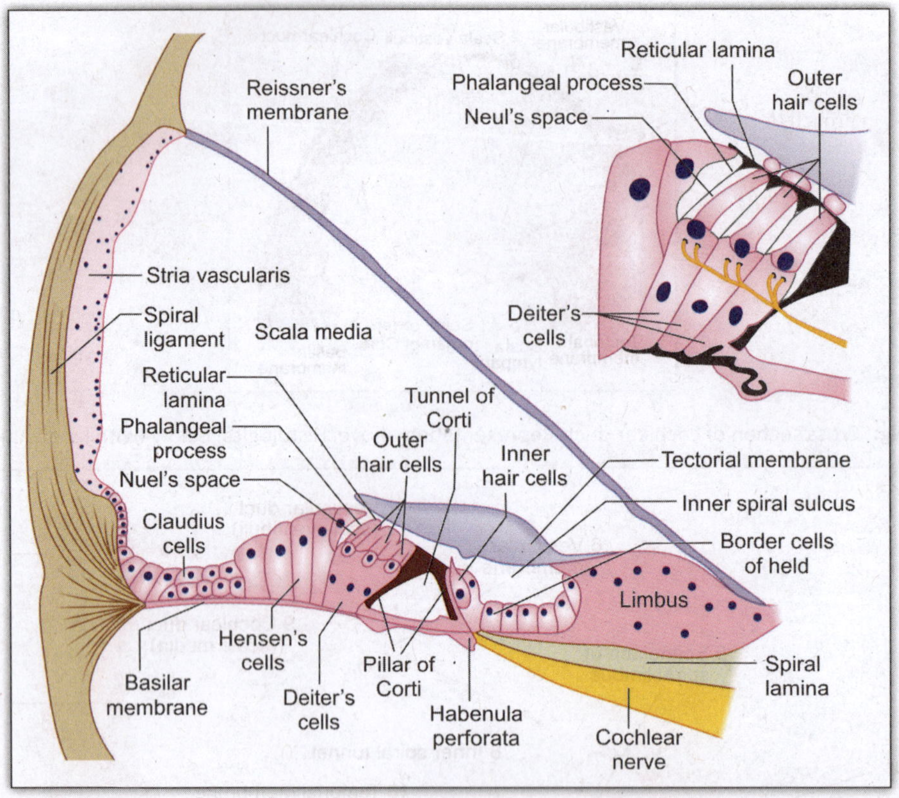

Fig: Cross section of cochlear duct: Detailed diagramatic with all supporting cells labelled

Difference Between Outer And Inner Hair Cells

	Inner hair cells (Type 1)	Outer hair cells (Type 2)
Cell numbers	3500	12000
Number of rows	Single	3–4
Shape	Flask shape	Cylindrical
Development	Early	Late
Nerve supply	Mainly afferent fibers (95% afferent fibers of spiral ganglion)	Mainly efferent fibers (Only 5% afferent fibers of spiral ganglion)
Function	Transmit auditory stimuli	Modulates function of inner hair cell
OAE generation	No	Yes
Ototoxicity	More resistant	More sensitive
High intensity sound	More resistant	More sensitive

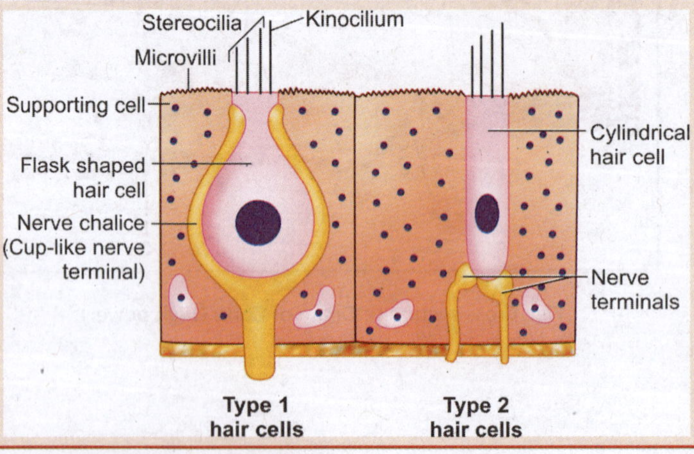

21. Ans. (b) Cricothyroidotomy

Ref: Head & Neck Surgery otolaryngology edited by Byron J. Bailey, Jonas T. Johnson, Shawn D. Newlands 4th ed Vol 1 Page 809

In this case, first approach for securing airway should be intubation, but sometimes in case of facial trauma and bone injuries, it becomes impossible to intubate. In such cases we opt for tracheostomy. But if the casuality or operation theatre or surgeon is not in position for urgent tracheostomy, we tend to do the procedure shown in figure called as cricothyroidotomy or mini tracheostomy.

Since more and more image based questions are being asked, we are giving details of all the procedures asked so that you can easily differentiate by viewing at it to differentiate use following important points:

Option (A)

Tracheostomy: Incision is given over trachea, can be both vertical or horizontal over skin, but when trachea in incised, usually vertical incision or criss cross incision is given. point to note that it is done at the level of 2nd or 3rd tracheal cartilage.

Option (B)

Cricothyroidotomy: Horizontal incision mostly. Plus it is given in between thyroid and cricoid cartilage.

Option (C)

Percutaneous tracheostomy: The site of incision is same as traditional tracheostomy but the size is very small. The incision is made just to introduce the guide wire. It is usually done in elective cases in adults only.

Option (D)

Laryngofissure: Incision given over thyroid cartilage, done for accessing the inner part of larynx.

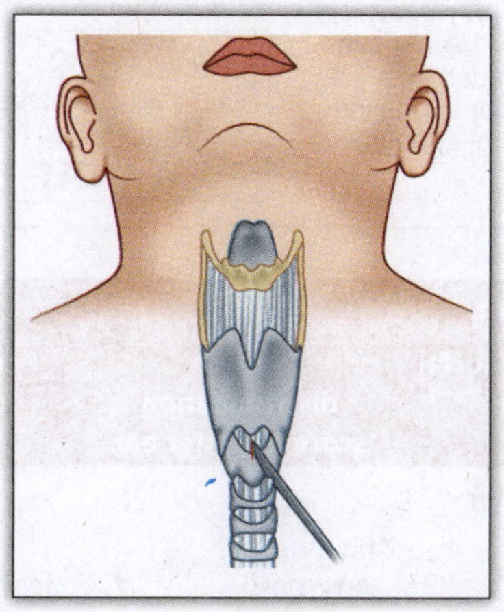

Fig: Cricothyroidotomy incision betwwen the thyroid cartilage and cricoid cartilave over the cricothyroid membrane. Surgical cricothyroidotomy provides a definitive airway (a cuffed tube in the trachea) if tracheal intubation is not possible. Technique for a surgical cricothyroidotomy is:

- Using a scalpel, make a transverse skin incision, then carefully incise through the cricoid membrane
- Enlarge the hole using artery forceps or the handle of the scalpel, rotate through 90 degrees
- Insert a size 6 cuffed tracheal or tracheostomy tube
- Inflate the cuff, check the position and ventilate

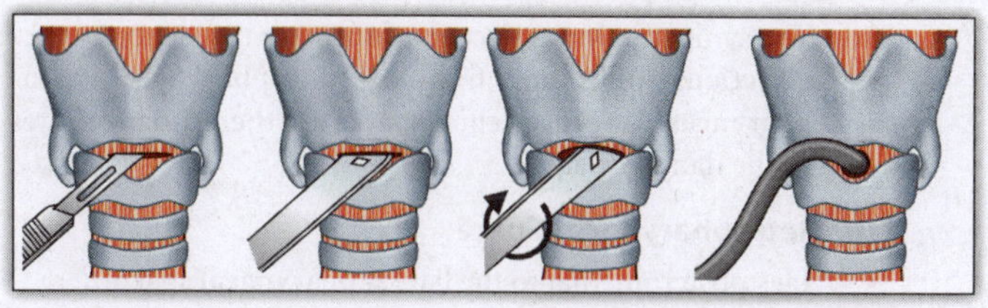

22. Ans. (c) 3

Ref: Cumming 6th ed page 166

NOTE

In 2015, the anatomy of the alar fascia was revisited. The authors revealed that the alar fascia originated as a well defined midline structure at the level of C1 and does not reach the base of the skull. It is suggested that the area between C1 and the base of the skull is a potential entry into the danger space

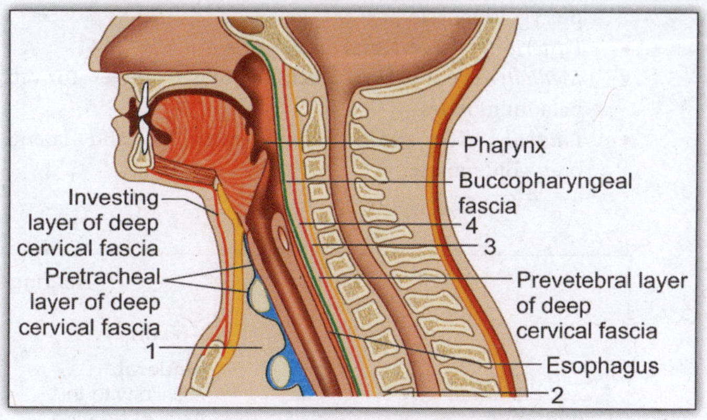

Fig: Sagittal section of neck

1. Pretracheal space
2. Prevertebral space
3. **Danger space/Alar space/Space 4** (Grodinsky and Holyoke). Between Alar fascia anteriorly and prevertebral fascia posteriorly and extends from the cranial base above to the level of the diaphragm. Name originates from the risk that an infection in this space can spread directly to the thorax. There exists a midline raphe in this space so some infections of this space appear unilateral.
4. **Retropharyngeal space** (Between Buccopharyngeal fascia anteriorly and Alar layer of Prevertebral fascia posteriorly)

Danger Space

Cumming's gives following limited, but very very important points

- So named because of the potential for rapid inferior spread of infection to the posterior mediastinum through its loose areolar tissue as it extends from the skull base to the diaphragm.
- Lies between the retropharyngeal and prevertebral spaces.
- The alar layer forms its anterior border and the prevertebral layer forms its posterior border.
- Laterally, the transverse processes of the vertebrae enclose the danger space.

- The sympathetic trunk courses through this space.
- Infectious infiltration from the retropharyngeal, parapharyngeal, or prevertebral spaces are the primary routes to the danger space.

The Retropharyngeal Space

- Lies posteromedial to the lateral pharyngeal space.
- Bounded anteriorly by the superior pharyngeal muscle and its investing fascia and posteriorly by the alar layer of prevertebral fascia.
- Begins at the skull base and extends inferiorly to the level of C7 or T1, where the alar and buccopharyngeal layers of fascia fuse.

Parapharyngeal Space

- Also called the *lateral pharyngeal* or *pharyngomaxillary space*
- An inverted pyramid shaped having base at the skull base and apex at the junction of the posterior belly of the digastric muscle and greater cornu of the hyoid bone.
- *Anteriorly:* Pterygomandibular raphe and medial pterygoid muscle
- *Posteriorly:* Prevertebral fascia
- *Medially:* The superior constrictor, tensor and levator veli palatini muscles
- *Laterally:* The parotid gland, mandible and lateral pterygoid muscle
- The styloid process divides the space into two compartments:
  - The anterior prestyloid compartment, contains fat, muscle (styloglossus and stylopharyngeus), lymph nodes, deep lobe of the parotid, internal maxillary artery, inferior alveolar, lingual and auriculotemporal nerves.
  - The posterior post-styloid compartment contains neurovascular structures: carotid artery, internal jugular vein, sympathetic chain and cranial nerves IX, X, XI and XII

The Prevertebral Space

- Enclosed by the prevertebral fascia, vertebral bodies and transverse processes.
- Extends from the clivus of the skull base to the coccyx.
- Contains dense areolar tissue.
- In addition to the paraspinous, prevertebral and scalene muscles, it contains the vertebral artery and vein, brachial plexus and phrenic nerve.
- Spread to the prevertebral space are:
  - From infection of the vertebral bodies
  - Penetrating injuries
  - Tuberculosis of the spine may breach the space and form a Pott's abscess.

23. Ans. (b) 81 dB

Ref: http://www.who.int/pbd/deafness/hearing_impairment_grades/en/, *http://www.rehabcouncil.nic.in/writereaddata/hi.pdf*

Hearing loss grades

26–40 dB — **Slight/mild**: A child with this level of hearing loss will have trouble hearing and understanding soft speech, speech from a distance or speech against a background of noise

41–60 dB — **Moderate**: A child with this level of hearing loss will have difficulty hearing regular speech, even at close distances.

61–80 dB — **Severe**: A child with this level of hearing loss may only hear very loud speech or loud sounds in the environment, such as a fire truck siren or a door slamming. Most conversational speech is not heard.

Over 81 dB — **Profound**: A child with this level of hearing loss may perceive loud sounds as vibrations.

Grades of Hearing Impairment

Grade of impairment	WHO 1980	WHO 2008	Ministry of social justice	Speech discrimination score of better ear	Percentage of disability
No impairment	25 dB or better (better ear)	25 dB or better (better ear)	25 dB or better (better ear)		
Mild impairment	26–40 dB (better ear)	26–40 dB (better ear)	26–40 dB (better ear)	80–100%	<40%
Moderate impairment	41–55 dB (better ear)	41–60 dB (better ear)	41–60 dB (better ear)	50–80%	40–50%
Moderately severe	56–70 dB (better ear)	**Removed from WHO 2008**	**No such category**		
Severe impairment	71–90 dB (better ear)	61–80 dB (better ear)	61–70 dB (better ear)	40–50%	51–70%
Profound impairment including deafness	91 dB or greater (better ear)	81 dB or greater (better ear)	71–90 dB (better ear)	<40%	71–100%

Contd...

Footnote

- Hearing impairment was initially classified in seven categories as per **Goodman's** (1965)
- As per Ministry of Social Justice and Empowerment, Procedure for calculating hearing disability is based on **pure tone thresholds** as well as **speech discrimination score** in order to arrive at the percentage of the disability
- The minimum degree of disability should be 40% in order to be eligible for any concessions/benefits (for children, it starts at 31 dB)
- **Disabling hearing loss:** Refers to hearing loss greater than 40 dB in the better hearing ear in adults and greater than 30 dB in the better hearing ear in children.
- The audiometric ISO values are averages of values at 500, 1000, 2000, 4000 Hz.

AIIMS MAY 2016

24. Ans. (c) Harmonic scalpel

Ref: Scott Brown 7th ed page 3576, Dhingra 6th ed page 430

All of the above are used of tonsillectomy. Least common is Laser tonsillectomy. Amongst the options provided Harmonic scalpel is least commonly used.

In May 2005 the Royal College of Surgeons of England published the data from the National Prospective Audit of Tonsillectomy (NPTA). Most common surgical techniques observed were cold steel dissection combined with bipolar diathermy for hemostasis (35%), followed by bipolar diathermy forceps (30%), followed by coblation (5%).

Cummings 5th edition 2796 says "More recently, however, dissection with electrocautery has become the most popular and common technique. Other current techniques are the Coblator, the Microdebrider, the ultrasonic Harmonic Scalpel, bipolar electrocautery and, less frequently, CO_2 or KTP laser tonsillectomy. A 2007 survey of pediatric otolaryngologists showed monopolar cautery to be by far the most common method of tonsillectomy, favored by 53% of the respondents. Coblation at 16% was the second most common method, cold dissection combined with electrocautery was third at 10%, followed by bipolar electrocautery at 6%"

Lesser common modalities have not been considered in the above 2 datas. Hence Harmonic scalpel and Microdebrider are both new lesser common modalities, both are Intracapsular approach, Harmonic scalpel is hot approach while Microdebrider is cold approach. Cost of Harmonic scalpel is far more than Microdebrider.

As per American Society of Pediatric Otolaryngology (ASPO) survey 2007:

Microdebrider is used in for obstructive indication in 27% and for infection as primary indication 11%. While Harmonic scalpel was used by 1/113 respondents that is less than 1% and 0/113 respondents used Laser tonsillectomy.

Types and Techniques of Tonsillectomy

- The techniques of Tonsillectomy can be broadly divided into 2 major categories: extracapsular (total tonsillectomy, subcapsular) and intracapsular (partial tonsillectomy). Intracapsular is also known as "subtotal,"
- The traditional technique of 'cold' dissection/Cold steel dissection was introduced about one hundred years ago. In this technique, the tonsils are dissected with metal instruments by blunt dissection. Any subsequent bleeding may be controlled by packing the tonsillar fossae with gauze dressings or ligating bleeding vessels.
- About 40 years ago, diathermy techniques were first introduced. In the last two decades, use of these 'hot' techniques has increased dramatically in routine practice and diathermy is now the most frequently used method
- Extracapsular tonsillectomy involves dissecting lateral to the tonsil in the plane between the tonsillar capsule and the pharyngeal musculature and the tonsil is generally removed as a single unit. Partial tonsillectomy, or tonsillotomy, involves removal of most of the tonsil, while preserving a rim of lymphoid tissue and tonsillar capsule in the most recent iteration of this older technique. Preservation of this margin of tissue, this "biologic dressing," may promote an easier recovery, with lower hemorrhage rates and better recovery of diet and activity reported in comparison with traditional monopolar tonsillectomy techniques

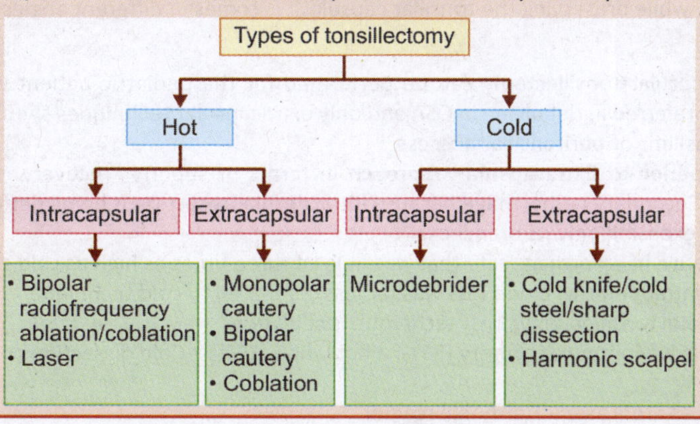

Contd...

Technique	Type	Advantages	Disadvantages
Cold knife/Cold steel/Sharp dissection (with ligature or cautery) Historically most commonly used method, Gold standard (6 fold increase in use from 2002–2007 (2.7– 15.9%) by ASPO survey (84% academic settings)	**Cold-Extracapsular:** In this technique, the tonsil and capsule are dissected from surrounding tissue using scissors, knife, or t dissector and the inferior pole is amputated with a tonsil snare.	Low post OP pain (Higher side with cautery), Low secondary hemorrhage risk (Higher side with cautery)	Higher intraop blood loss (lesser in cautery) Long operative time (shorter in cautery)
Monopolar electrocautery (53% use Cumming's)	**Hot-Extracapsular:** Lately Most common and most popular technique worldwide	Quick operative time, Minimal intraoperative bleeding	High risk of secondary hemorrhage Longer recovey Higher Post OP pain
Bipolar electrocautery (6% use Cumming's)	**Hot-Extracapsular**	Miniamal intraoperative bleeding, Limited post OP morbidity	Longer operative time, Higher secondary hemorrhage rate.
Harmonic scalpel (ASPO survey: 1/113 respondents, i.e. <1% use)	**Cold-Extracapsular:** uses ultrasonic energy to vibrate its blade at 55 kHz/second. The vibration transfers energy to the tissue, providing simultaneous cutting and coagulation	Less tissue damage, Less post operative pain compared to cautery, No additional instrument is needed for haemostasis	Long operative time, Variable intraoperative hemostasis
Bipolar radiofrequency ablation (AKA- Cold ablation or Coblation or coagulation wand or conduction wand, PlasmaBlade). 2nd most common method (16% use Cumming's)	**Hot-Intracapsular (MC)> Extracapsular:** Radiofrequency bipolar current is conducted accross the electrodes accross the tip of the conduction wand. Conductive saline solution is converted into an ionized plasma layer, resulting in molecular dissociation with minimal thermal energy transfer. Best technique in terms of results	The heat generated varies from 40–80°C, much lower than that of electro cautery 400–600 °C Relatively quick operative time, Minimal intraoperative bleeding, mixed post op morbidity results. Haemostasis can usually be performed with the coblation wand alone. Suction is built in the want itself	Mixed post op morbidity results, High secondary hemorrhage rates
Laser KTP 512 > CO_2 (ASPO survey 2007: Use 0/120 respondents)	**Hot-Intracapsular**	Can be done in coagulopathy patient	Anterior pillar must be sacrifised. Use is practically limited to patients with coagulopathies or hypertension
Microdebrider (Powered intracapsular tonsillectomy) introduced by Dr Peter Koltai in 2003 ASPO survey 2007: –27% use for obstructive indication –11% use for infection as primary indication	**Cold-Intracapsular:** MC intracapsulat technique. Microdebrider is a powered rotary shaving device with continuous suction. A partial tonsillectomy is completed with the removal of approximately 90% to 95% of the tonsil, while preserving the tonsillar capsule	Best post op results (0.7% versus 2.8% of coblation and 3.1% of electrocautery, It spares the adjacent mucosa (Mucosal sparing), Removes tissue real fast, Visualization is good since blade comes in different angles	Technically more difficult.

Footnote:

- Either extracapsular or intracapsular tonsillectomy can be performed for the pediatric patient with obstructive sleep apnea, but intracapsular tonsillectomy is preferred in debulking in OSA and only extracapsular techniques should be used for patients undergoing tonsillectomy as a result of tonsillitis or peritonsillar abscess.
- **Intracapsular approach is superior to Extracapsular approach** in terms of superior recovery outcomes. Intracapsular approach causes less intraoperative and Secondary hemorrhage because intracapsular resection is being performed distal to the arborization of primary tonsillar blood vessel, exposing only its branches.
- Hot technique had a postoperative haemorrhage rate that was at least three times as high as cold steel tonsillectomy without the use of a 'hot' technique, however intraoperative blood loss was far less compared to cold technique
- Extracapsular (also known as total tonsillectomy) best technique is coblation
- Most commonly used technique is Monopolar cautery (53%) > Coblation (16%) > Cold dissection combined with electrocautery (10%) > Bipolar electrocautery (6%)
- Least commonly used techniques are: Laser > Harmonic scalpel
- Frequency of use of Intracapsular also known as subtotal tonsillectomy: Microdebrider or powered instrument or shaver> bipolar radiofrequency ablation > Carbon dioxide laser

25. Ans. (b) Respiratory papilomatosis

Ref: Cummings 5th ed ch 62, Dhingra 6th ed page 305–306

See AIIMS May 2017 ENT for details of Respiratory Papillomatosis (see page no. 631)

26. Ans. (c) Sinus tympani

Ref: Dhingra 6th ed page 6, 126

Boundaries of Sinus Tympani

Above: Ponticulus
Below: Subiculum
Laterally: Facial nerve with facial canal
Importance: Cholesteatoma may lie hidden in this space which can be missed during surgery.

About Other Options

Pyriform fossa is in laryngopharynx adjacent to laryngeal inlet, not in ear.

Incudal fossa is a part of epitympanum which is seen during atticotomy after cortical mastoidectomy. This acts as marker for various surgeries like cortical mastoidectomy, atticotomy, facial recess approach to middle ear, cochlear implant etc.

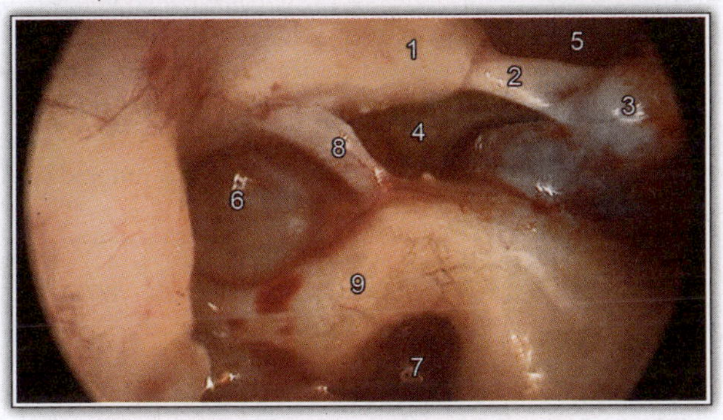

Fig: Endoscopic view of middle ear cavity

1. Pyramid
2. Stapedius tendon
3. Head of stapes
4. Posterior tympanic sinus
5. Facial recess (area above stapes)
6. Sinus tympani
7. Round window niche
8. Ponticulus
9. Subiculum

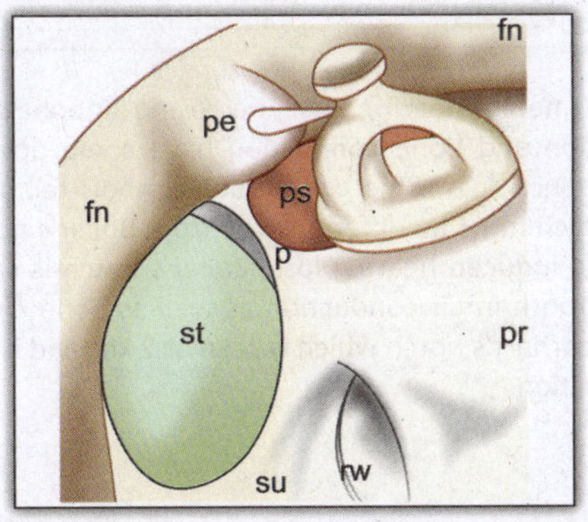

Fig: Diagramatic representation of the Endoscopic view of middle ear

Fn = Facial nerve
St = Sinus tympani
Rw = Round window
P = Ponticulus
Pe = Pyramid
Ps = Posterior tympanic sinus

27. Ans. (a) Conductive hearing loss right ear

Ref: Scott Brown 7th ed page 1156

Symbols used in Audiogram:

MNEMONIC

- For 1st and 2nd symbols remember the mnemonic: **Cross the Square from Left side**
- For 3rd and 4th symbols - Note that the Open end of symbols > and] represents the ear side.
- **Red for Right**

Modality	Ear	
	Right	Left
AC unmasked	O	X
AC masked	△	□
BC unmasked	<	>
BC masked	[	]
No response	O↙	X↘

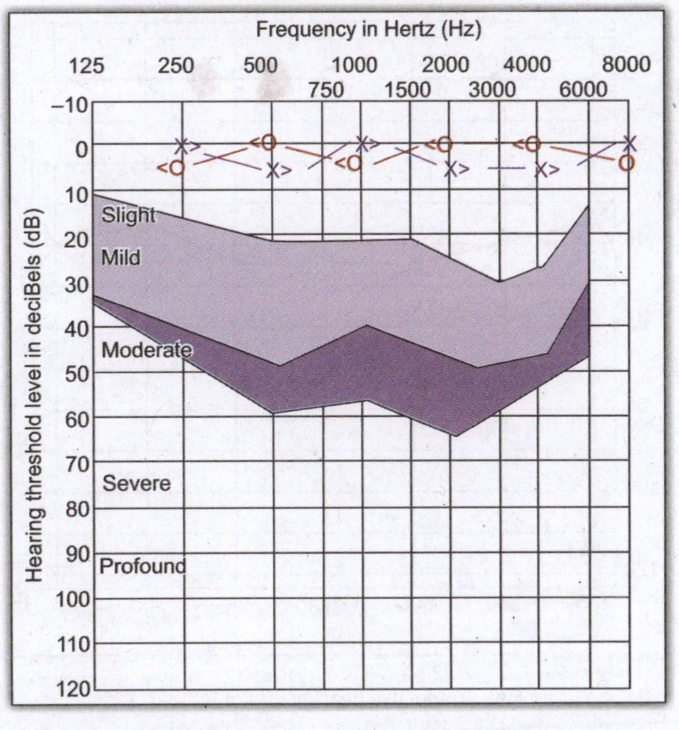

Fig: Normal audiogram: The Air Bone (AB) conduction gap is less than 10–15 dB. The shaded area below the lines represents the imaginary mild moderate Hearing loss. Severe and profound hearing loss are lebelled more lower down in case the audiometric lines lies in that area. See the symbols used in audiogram above

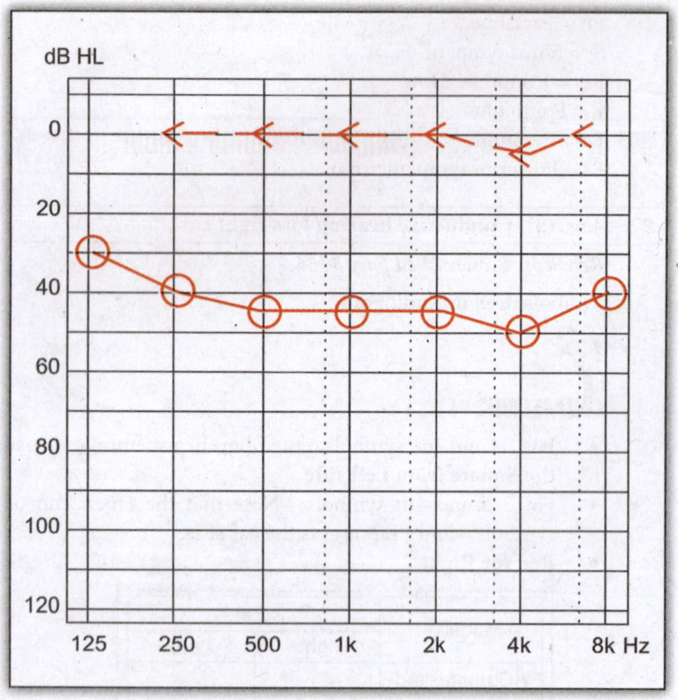

Fig: Conductive hearing loss of right ear: Difference between bone conduction and air conduction is more than 20 db which tells it is conductive loss. Red colour of lines on the graph and symbols tell it is right side

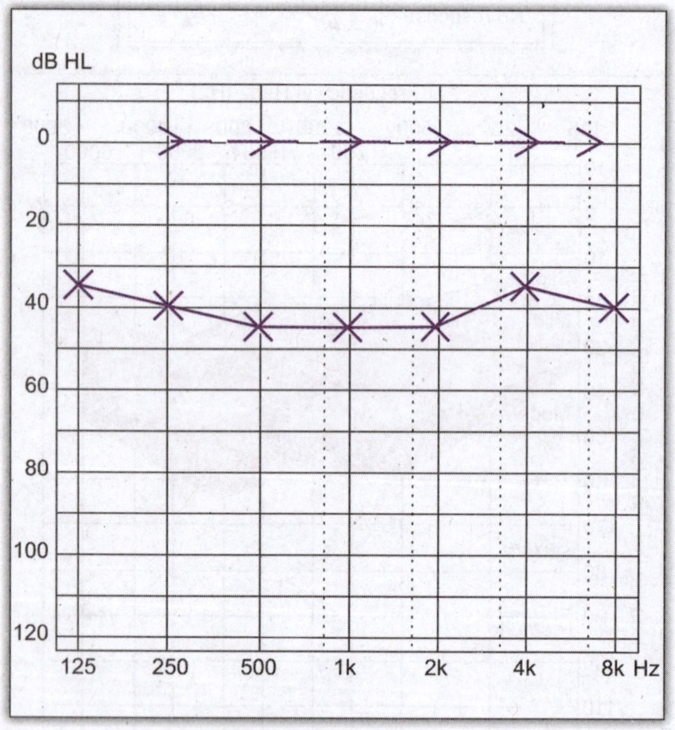

Fig: Conductive hearing loss of left ear

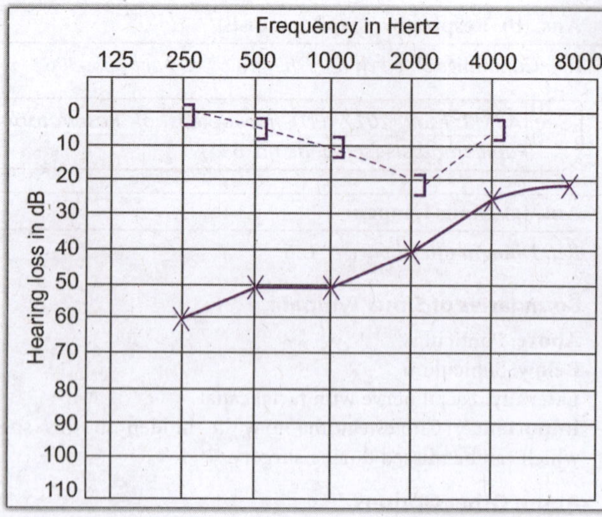

Fig: Conductive hearing loss due to Otosclerosis: There is typically an apparent lowering in the bone conduction hearing threshold by about 5 dB at 500 Hz. 10 dB at 1000 Hz, 15-20 dB at 2000 Hz and 5 dB at 4000 Hz. This peculiar configuration in the bone conduction hearing level, most marked (i.e., notched) at 2000 Hz is termed as CARHART'S NOTCH. If the notch in the bone conduction level is not duplicated by the air conduction curve, then it is a true Carhart's notch

Cumming's 5th ed: "This is not a true depression in bone conduction, but rather an artifact caused by a lack of the normal contribution of the mobile ossicular chainto bone conduction. This depression improves after the mobility of the ossicular chain is restored eg after stapedectomy"

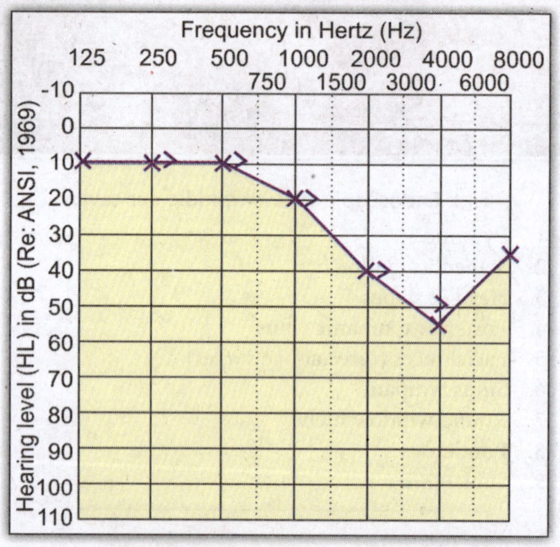

Fig: Sensory neural hearing loss: There is no air bone gap and both air conduction and bone conduction have come down. Hence it is sensory neural loss. Blue colour and symbols tell it is left side. Carhart's notch must be differentiated from Boiler's notch which is due to noise induced hearing loss. Boiler's notch is seen at 4 khz and is seen both in air conduction as well as bone conduction, in contrast to carhart's notch which is seen at 2 khz and is only seen in bone conduction

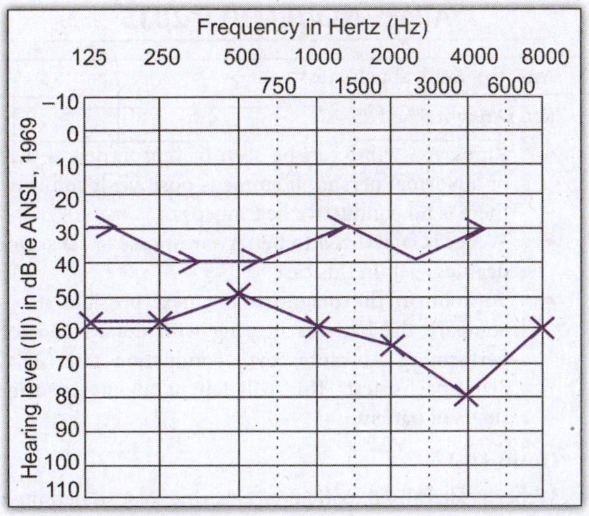

Fig: Mixed hearing loss: There is air bone gap more than 20 db and bone conduction has also come down. Colour and symbols indicate left side

28. Ans. (d) Allergic fungal sinusitis

Ref: Scott Brown 7th ed page 2734, Dhingra 6th ed page 173-175

A heterogenous opacity of the maxilla with some bony destruction but without any orbital or Lateral wall of maxilla involvement points towards Allergic Fungal sinusitis. One should keep in mind one thing: "WE DIAGNOSE AND TREAT PATIENT, NOT INVESTIGATIONS". So always read history, keep in mind the age and sex of patient, look for clues in examination and then strengthen your diagnosis with investigations.

Mucin discharge is characteristic of Allergic fungal sinusitis while Mucous discharge is most likely to be polyps.

NOTE

If bony destruction is absent carcinoma is ruled out and fungal lesion becomes less likely

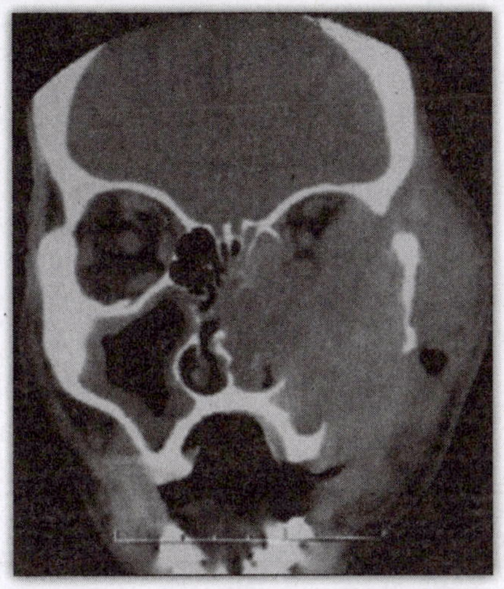

Fig: CT PNS Maxillary Carcinoma will show extensive destruction but the lesion will not be heterogenous, with possible destruction of outer wall. Invasion of orbital cavities and opposite side cavities should be noted. Age, if given is a great help in diagnosis but not confirmatory

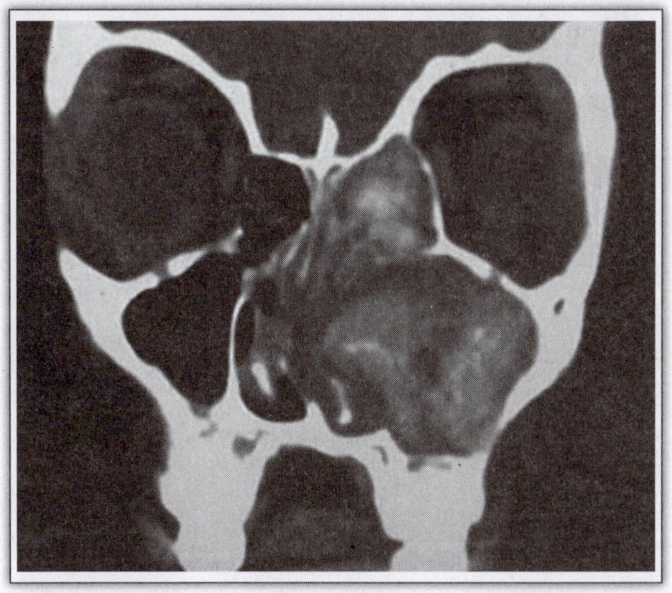

Fig: CT PNS - Fungal sinusitis: Heterogenous lesion, evidence of destruction present, but not as extensive as in carcinaoma. Outer wall of maxilla is usually preserved. Orbital cavities are usually not involved

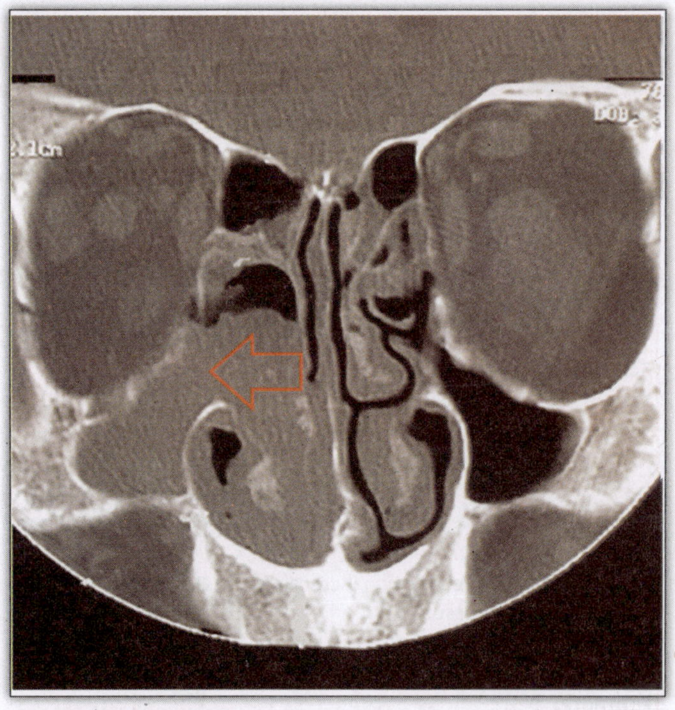

Fig: CT PNS - Antrochoanal polyp: homogenous mass, usually unilateral. Maxillary ostium may be widened (arrow), this is not bone destruction. No evidence of bone destruction. All cavity outlines well preserved

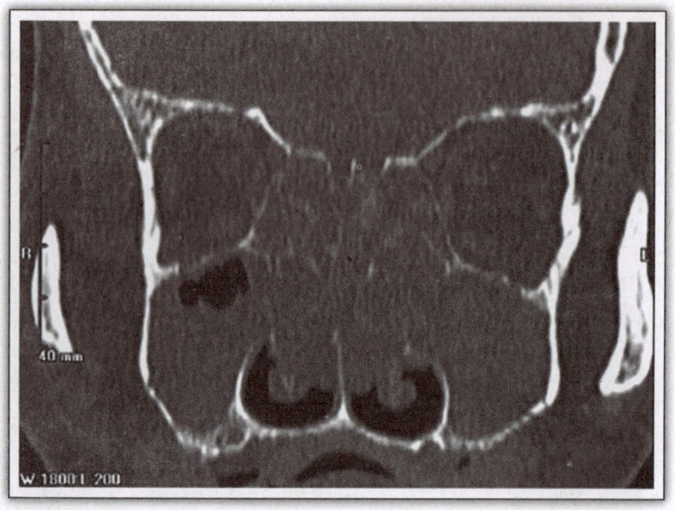

Fig: CT SCAN PNS - Ethmoidal polyps: usually bilateral, homogenous mass, no bone destruction all sinuses involved.

AIIMS NOVEMBER 2015

29. Ans. (b) Schwabach's test

Ref: Dhingra 5th ed 25-27

- Rinne AC > BC can be seen in sensoryneural deafness or a Normal person. If rinnie is positive, it confirms that there is no conductive hearing loss.
- Weber is lateralized to better ear in case of sensorineural deafness, left in this case.
- To confirm the diagnosis the next possible step is to compare the patients hearing with ourself (doctor) by performing Absolute Bone conduction test (ABC) or Schwabach's test. This will tell us about sensorineural status of patient.

Option (A)

Weber is lateralised, patient c/o hearing loss, so definitely not normal.

Option (C)

Doesn't make any sense, unless doctor has done it with improper way. And repeating the test wont help.

Option (D)

Wax removal can be thought off if patient had conductive deafness. Students should keep in mind that usually wax wont cause any deafness. And if at all it is occludine the canal completely, it will lead to conductive deafness.

Tuning Fork Tests

	Conductive deafness	Sensorineural	Comments
Rinne's test	BC > AC Negative (minimum air-bone gap of 15-20 dB.)	AC > BC Positive (Also in normal persons)	• False negative is seen in Unilateral total hearing loss • Negative Rinne for 256, 512 and 1024 Hz indicates a minimum AB gap of 15,30, 45 dB respectively.
Weber's test	Lateralised to the worse ear	Lateralised to the better ear	Not lateralized (Equal on both sides) in normal individuals
Absolute bone conduction (ABC)	ABC same as examiner	The patient hears the fork for a shorter duration	ABC is same as examiner in normal individual and conductive deafness
Schwabach's test	Lengthned	Shortened	Schwabach's test is the same as ABC but meatus is not occluded
Bing's test	Pt will appreciate no change (Bing negative)	Hears louder when ear canal is occluded and softer when the canal is open (Bing positive) (Also positive in normal persons)	• Test of bone conduction & examines the effect of *occlusion of ear* canal on hearing. • A vibrating tuning fork placed on the mastoid while the examiner alternately closes and opens the ear canal by pressing on the tragus inward
Gelle's test	No change on increasing pressure (Seen when ossicular chain is fixed or disconnected)	Decreased hearing on increasing pressure, Positive (Also in normal persons)	Test of bone conduction examines the effect of *increased air pressure* in ear canal on the hearing

Footnote:
- Most commonly used tuning fork is 512 Hz, because of longer tone decay and distinct sound

30. Ans. (b) Stapes defect with fixation of footplate and lenticular process involvement

Ref: Nelson 20th ed page 3071

Congenital Stapes ankylosis with other ossicular anomaly is the most commom class of Congenital ossicular malformation. Only Option (B) lies in class 2 as lenticular pocess is a part of Incus.

Teunissen's Classification of Ossicular Anomalies		
Class	**Anomaly**	**%**
I	Congenital stapes ankylosis without other deformity i.e. Isolated stapes ankylosis	30.6%
II	Congenital Stapes ankylosis with other ossicular anomaly	38.1%
III	Congenital anomaly of Ossicular chain with mobile footplate • IIIa Ossicular discontinuity • IIIb Epitympanic fixation	21.6%
IV	Congenital Aplasia or dysplasia of round or oval window Aplasia or dysplasia with crossing facial nerve Aplasia or dysplasia with persistent stapedial artery	9.7%

Footnote
- Most common congenital ossicular anomaly: **Incus + Sapes anomaly > Isolated stapes anomaly**
- Stapes represent approximately 40% of all congenital ossicular lesions. Stapes develops from dual origin and therefore has the greatest potential for malformation
- Congenital stapes footplate fixation is the most common isolated ossicular anomaly (approximately 40% of all congenital ossicular malformations)
- **Triple ossicular malfomations** are rare and are mostly associated withinner ear malformations
- Malleus anomalies are least amongst the ossicles. **Epitympanum fixation of head of malleus** is most common malleus anomaly
- Congenital stapes disorder is frequently related to **facial nerve anomalies**
- Surgical experience in patients with stapes ankylosis (Class I) and stapes ankylosis combined with ossicular anomaly (Class II) has been favorable, with a 73% rate of postoperative air-bone gap <20 dB
- In contrast, patients with mobile footplates, ossicular discontinuity, epitympanic fixation (Class III), or dysplasia of either the round or oval windows (Class IV) are poor surgical candidates
- A high-resolution CT scan of the temporal bones may define the ossicular anomaly as well as the anatomy of the facial nerve and inner ear structures

EAR Ossicles			
	Malleus	**Incus**	**Stapes**
Derived from	1st arch	1st arch	Dual origin: Suprastructures: 2nd arch. Footplate: otic capsule (Hence most vulnerable to developmental anomaly)
Development period	4 – 26 weeks	15 – 25 weeks	15 - 25 weeks
Size & weight	Largest ear ossicle 8–9 mm long, 25 mg	In between malleus and stapes, Heaviest ossicle = 27 mg	Smallest bone of human body, 3 mm long, 3 mg
Shape	Mallet	Anvil	Stirrup
Parts	Has a head, neck, handle (manubrium) and anterior and lateral processes	Body, long process, short process, lenticular process	Head, neck, two limbs (processes or crura) and a base (footplate)
Attachments/ Articulations	Tumpanic membrane and Incus	Articular facet of incus joints with head of malleus while lenticular process articulates with head of the stapes	Head articulates with lenticuar process of incus, footplate is attached to rim of the fenestra vestibuli

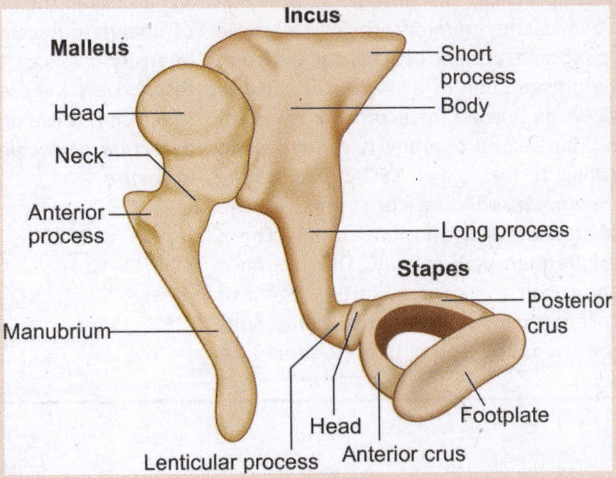

31. Ans. (c) Evoked OAE

Ref: Dhingra 6th ed page 119, Nelson 20th ed page 3075-79, Cummings 5th edition ch- 190-1

NOTE

If transient otoacoustic emissions (TOAEs) or transient evoked otoacoustic emissions (TEOAEs) is provided as option it is better answer

Evoked OAE are preferable over spontaneous as do not depend upon CNS.

Otoacoustic Emissions (OAE)

Definition	Otoacoustic emissions (OAE) are sounds produced by motile elements of cochlear outer hair cells. These sounds can be recorded easily. These sounds were first identified and reported by **Kemp in 1978.**
Uses	The main function of OAE tests is to assess the function of cochlear hair cells. These tests could be used: • To screen children and neonates for hearing disabilities • Estimate hearing sensitivity within a limited range of frequencies • To differentiate sensory and neural components in sensorineural hearing loss • To rule out malingering (functional hearing loss)

Types of OAE

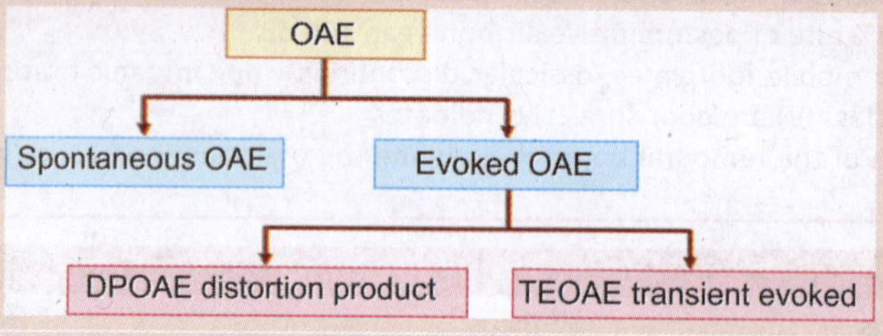

Spontaneous otoacoustic emissions (SOAEs)-Sounds emitted without an outside acoustic evoking stimulus (ie, spontaneously).

The clinical value of this signal is limited, as this is not present in all normal ears. The absence of spontaneous otoacoustic emission does not imply cochlear dysfunction. Measurement of these potentials is difficult and highly cumbersome. They do not have any diagnostic/ prognosic value as it is not a consistent feature in all normal ears

Evoked otoacoustic emissions (EOAEs) are used widely for newborn hearing screening. EOAEs are acoustic signals generated by the cochlea in response to auditory stimulation. They are a physiologically vulnerable indicator of cochlear status, specifically outer hair cells. EOAE generation is independent of neural activity, so EOAE testing measures cochlear status independent of CNS status

Types of EOAE

Transient otoacoustic emissions (TOAEs) or transient evoked otoacoustic emissions (TEOAEs) - Sounds emitted in response to an acoustic evoking stimuli of very short duration; usually clicks but can be tone-bursts. TEOAEs provide information over a broad frequency range (approximately 500 to 6000 Hz). Since it was first described by Kemp it is also known as ***Kemp echos***. The time delay between the stimulus and response allows the examiner to isolate these responses. The probe used to record transient otoacoustic emission has two openings, one for the presentation of a single stimulus like a click and the other opening which is used to record the transient evoked otoacoustic emission. The second opening is connected to a microphone to enable recording to take place. ***TEOAE are usually used to screen neonates for hearing disabilities.*** These impulses can be recorded only in response to short and transient stimuli. These impulses have a very limited frequency specificity. The presence of these emissions suggest the cochlear sensitivity in the region of 20–40 dB or better. Clicks are commonly used as stimuli, sometimes tone burst stimuli can also be used. The stimulus used should be 80–85 dB sound pressure level.

Distortion product otoacoustic emissions (DPOAEs) occur in response to 2 simultaneous tones of different frequencies and provide frequency-specific information across a broad range of frequencies. A common way to record them is to present the ear with two continous signals called the primary tones and analyse the spectrum of sounds detected at the external auditory canal. The intensity levels of the signals used are 55 dB and 65 dB respectively. These emissions have greater frequency specificity. These potentials are useful in detection of ***early detection of cochlear damage i.e. due to noise or drug exposure***

Screening of Pediatric Population for Hearing

Hearing test of newborn	Hearing tests for infants	Hearing tests for older children
• **OAE:** Used as a screening test of hearing in neonates and to test hearing in uncooperative or mentally challenged individuals after sedation. Sedation does not interfere with OAEs. Help to distinguish cochlear from retrocochlear hearing loss especially auditory neuropathy. OAEs are absent in cochlear lesions) They detect ototoxic effects earlier than pure-tone audiometry. • **aABR** (Automated Auditory Brain Stem Response)	• **Auditory Brain Stem Response (ABR):** Most common diagnostic hearing test for infants < 6 months of age. It is similar to the aABR, but it provides more information and must be given by a specialist. Also known as **Brainstem evoked response audiometry (BERA).** It is an objective test. It is a special kind of EEG. It is also called the "auditory brainstem response" test (ABR). Time taking process. Child *needs to be sedated* or calm. Used for confimation of diagnosis or localisation of sensorineural hearing loss, but definitely not used for screening.	• **Visual reinforcement audiometry (VRA):** This test is used in children between 6 months and 2½ years of age • **Conditioned play audiometry (CPA):** Children between 2½ and 4 years of age • **Conventional audiometry:** Children ages 4 years and older

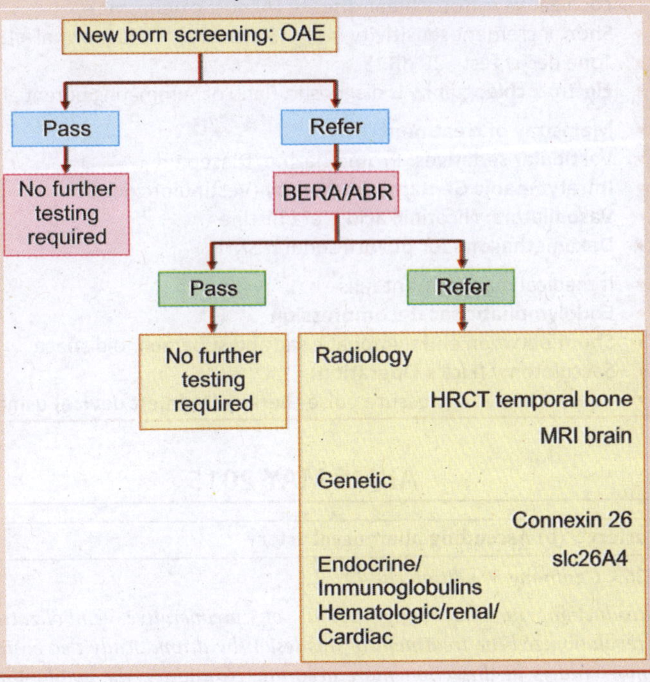

32. Ans. (a) Meniere's disease

Ref: Scott-Brown's 7th ed page 3570, Dhingra 6th ed page 100-104

From the options provided only Meniere's disease involves vestibular system. Auditory Neurotherapy or Neurofeedback or Neurobiofeedback acts primarily on the Vestibular system.

Recent Advances in Otolaryngology: Head & Neck Surgery, Volume 3 By Anil K Lalwani, Markus HF Pfister page 276: **Earlier studies showed a high effectiveness of a free-field auditory neurofeedback training to reduce the body sway in patients with different peripheral vestibular disorders**

Meniere's Disease, AKA Endolymphatic Hydrops

Definition	Disorder off inner ear where endolymphatic system is distended due to increased volume of endolymph
Triad	• *Unilateral fluctuating sensorineural deafness* • *Episodic Vertigo* • *Tinnitus (not pulsatile)*
Clinical features	Clinical triad as above Commonly affects **35–60 year** More common in **Male** Associated with **Syphilis**

Contd...

Meniere's Disease, AKA Endolymphatic Hydrops	
	Disease is usually **unilateral** There is also sense of **fullness** or pressure in the ear
Genetics	A Meniere's disease gene linked to **chromosome 12pl2.3.**
Tullio phenomenon (some cases of Meniere's disease shows Tullio)	• Subjective vertigo & Nystagmus (in loud/noise sound) • Recruitment (intolerance to loud/amplified sounds) • Diplacusis (distortion of sound) • Tinnitus- Roaring type • Aural fullness
Lermoyez syndrome	A variant of Meniere's disease with reversal of symptoms. SNHL improves suddenly during attacks of vertigo
Cochlear hydrops	Only cochlear symptoms are present. There is no vertigo.
Investigations	• **Pure tone audiometry:** Show sensorineural hearing loss with Early; loss of lower frequencies (rising type curve) and Late; higher frequencies involves, flat or falling curve • **Speach audiometry:** Discrimination score 55-85%. Indicates cochlear nature of disease, differentiate cochlear vs retrocochlear disease (Acoustic neuroma) • Short increment sensitivity index (SISI score) >70% (normal <15%) • Tone decay test >20 dB • **Electrocochleography** is diagnostic. Ratio of Summating potential to action potential (SP/AP ratio) >30%
Medical management	• **Mainstray of treatment** • **Vestibular sedatives:** Promethazine, Diazepam • **Intratympanic Gentamycin therapy** (Vestibulotoxic) • **Vasodilators:** Nicotinic acid, Beta histine • **Dexamethasone** for pt with sudden SNHL
Surgical management	• If medical management fails • **Endolymphatic sac decompression** • **Shunt** between endolymphatic sac and subarachnoid space • Sacculotomy **(Fick's Operation)** • Intermittent low pressure pulse therapy **(Meniett device)** using myringotomy and ventillation tube

AIIMS MAY 2015

33. Ans. (d) Internal maxillary artery > (b) Ascending pharyngeal artery

Ref: Dhingra 5th ed page 262-263, Cumming 5th edition ch- 49

Cumming says: *"The introduction in the early 1970s of preoperative embolization, which is commonly performed 48 hours before surgery, has revolutionized the treatment of this lesion by dramatically decreasing intraoperative bleeding and therefore making the assessment of tumor borders at dissection more accurate. Nowadays, the availability of* ***intra-arterial digital subtraction angiography, microcatheters and embolic agents such as polyvinyl-alcohol particles*** *makes superselective embolization of feeding vessels even easier. Furthermore, angiography provides a detailed map of the lesion's vascular supply, showing connections with the internal carotid artery, the vertebral artery and branches of the contralateral carotid system. Although the currently available methods of embolization provide excellent devascularization of feeding vessels from the* ***internal maxillary artery and its branches*** *as well as from the* ***ascending pharyngeal artery****, control of major vascularization from the internal carotid artery is demanding".*

Reading above lines from above mentioned source, authors conclude that first choice should be internal maxillary artery, followed by ascending pharyngeal artery.

	Commonly Treated Tumors	Uncommonly Treated Tumors
Tumors treated by embolisation	Meningioma Paraganglioma Juvenile angiofibroma Haemangiopericytoma	Schwannoma Carcinoid Alveolar sarcoma Thyroid carcinoma Granular cell myoblastoma Capillary haemangioma Esthesioneuroblastoma Neurinoma
Ref: Scott brown 7th edition p-734		

Juvenile Nasopharyngeal Angiofibroma AKA: Nasopharyngeal Fibroma	
Epidemiology	It is a rare tumor, though it is the most common of all benign tumors of nasopharynx
Etiology	The exact cause is unknown. As the tumor is predominantly seen in adolescent males in the second decade of life, it is thought to be testosterone dependent
Site of origin	The site of origin of the tumor is still a matter of dispute. Earlier it was thought to arise from the roof of nasopharynx or the anterior wall of sphenoid bone but now it is believed to arise from the ***posterior part of nasal cavity close to the superior margin of sphenopalatine foramen***
Feeding vessel	Internal maxillary artery > Ascending pharyngeal artery
Pathology	Angiofibroma, as the name implies, is made up of ***vascular and fibrous tissues:*** the ratio of the two components may vary. *Mostly, the vessels are just endothelium-lined spaces with no muscle coat. This accounts for the severe bleeding as the vessels lose the ability to contract and also the bleeding cannot be controlled by application of adrenaline*
Extensions	Nasopharyngeal fibroma is a *benign tumor but locally invasive* and destroys the adjoining structures. It may extend into: • **Nasal cavity** causing nasal obstruction, epistaxis and nasal discharge • **Paranasal sinuses:** Maxillary, sphenoid and ethmoid sinuses can all be invaded • **Pterygomaxillary fossa, infratemporal fossa and cheek.** • **Orbits** giving rise to proptosis and *"frog-face deformity"*. It enters through the inferior orbital fissure and also destroys apex of the orbit. It can also enter the orbit through superior orbital fissure • **Cranial cavity.** Anterior cranial fossa (through ethmoid roof or cribriform plate). Middle cranial fossa is the most common. There are two routes of entry: ▪ By erosion of floor of middle cranial fossa, anterior to foramen lacerum. The tumor lies lateral to carotid artery and cavernous sinus ▪ Through sphenoid sinus, into the sella. Tumor lies medial to carotid artery
Clinical features	• **Age and sex.** Tumor is seen almost exclusively in males in the age group of 10-20 years • **Profuse and recurrent epistaxis.** This is the most common presentation • **Progressive nasal obstruction and denasal speech** due to mass in the postnasal space • **Conductive hearing loss and serous otitis media** due to obstruction of eustachian tube • **Mass in the nasopharynx.** Tumor is sessile, lobulated or smooth and obstructs one or both choanae. It is pink or purplish in co lour. Consistency is firm but *digital palpation should never be done* until at the time of operation • Others: Broad nasal bridge, proptosis, swelling of cheek, infratemporal fossa or involvement of 2nd, 3rd, 4th, 6th cranial nerves will depend on the extent of tumor
Investigations	• **Soft tissue lateral film of nasopharynx** shows softtissue mass in the nasopharynx • **X-rays of paranasal sinuses** and base of skull may show DNS, opacification of sinuses, anterior bowing of posterior wall of maxillary sinus, destruction of medial antral wall, erosion of greater wing of sphenoid or pterygoid plates, widening of lower lateral margin of superior orbital fissure • **CT scan of the head with contrast enhancement** is now the investigation of choice. It has replaced conventional radiographs. It shows the extent of tumor, bony destruction or displacements. Anterior bowing of the posterior wall of maxillary sinus (often called the ***Holman Miller or Antral sign***) is pathognomic of angiofibroma • **Magnetic resonance imaging (MRI)** is complementary to CT scans, when soft tissue extensions arepresent intracranially, in the infratemporal fossa orinto the orbit 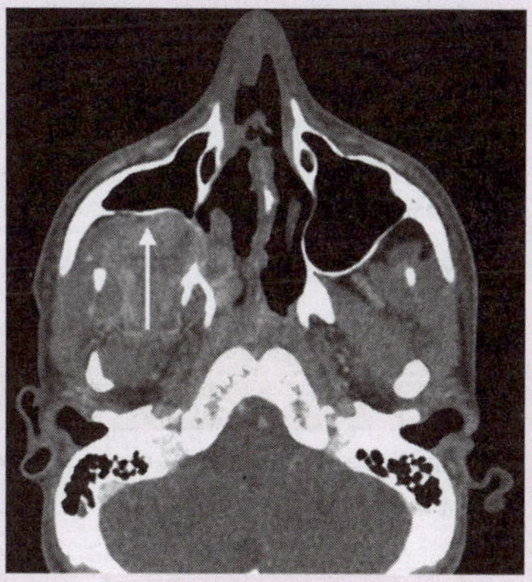 • **Carotid angiography** shows extension of tumor, its vascularity and feeding vessels. It is done whenembolisation is planned before operation • Biopsy of the tumoris attended with profuse bleeding and is therefore avoided

Contd...

Surgery	***Surgical excision is now the treatment of choice.*** Various approaches to angiofihroma, depending onorigin and extensions, are listed below. • **Wilson's Approach (Transpalatine approach)** For tumors confined to nasopharynx • Transpalatine + Sublabial (**Sardana's approach**) 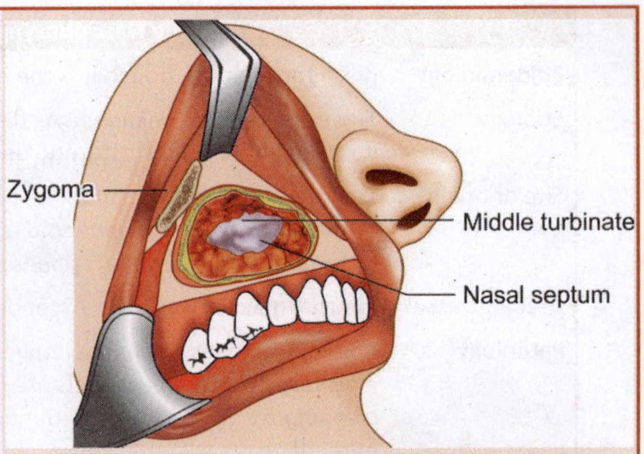
	• **Extended lateral rhinotomy** (Via facial incision or Via degloving approach): for larger tumors involving nasal cavity, paranasal sinuses • Extended Denker's approach • Intracranial-extracranial • Infratemporal fossa • Endoscopic 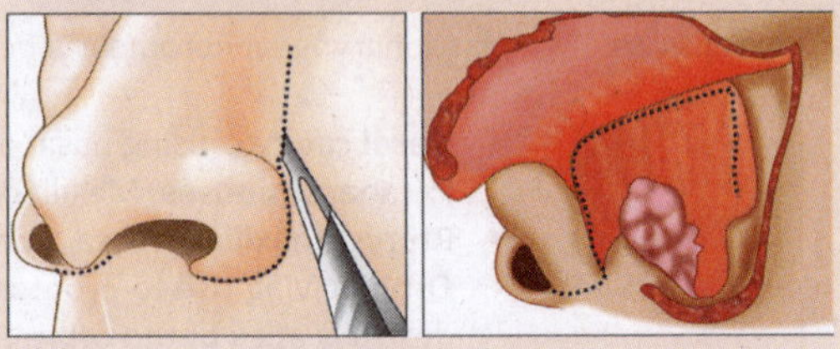
Other therapy	**Radiotherapy** has been used as a primary mode of treatment. A dose of 3000 to 3500 cGy in 15–18 fractions is delivered in 3–3.5 weeks **Chemotherapy.** Recurrent and residual lesions have been treated by chemotherapy, doxorubicin, vincristine and dacarbazine in combination
Recurrence	30–50% within 2–3 years postsurgery

34. Ans. (b) Cidofovir

Ref: Dhingra 6th ed page 305, Current Otolaryngology 2nd ed Chapter 32

See AIIMS May 2017 ENT for details of Respiratory Papillomatosis (see page no. 631)

Cummings 5th ed ch 240 says: "Intralesional administration of cidofovir, an acyclic nucleoside phosphate, has shown promise in treating severe cases of RRP (**recurrent respiratory papillomatosis**) in pediatric patients. Other adjuvant therapies (e.g., photodynamic therapy, acyclovir, ribavirin, isotretinoin, indole 3-carbinol) are infrequently used"

Current Otolaryngology 2nd ed Chapter 32 says "Both Acyclovir and Cidofovir can be used. However, There is still insufficient evidence on the effectiveness of antiviral therapy"

35. Ans. (a) Bilateral vocal cord palsy

Ref: Byron head and neck surgery 4th edition ch-61, Dhingra 6th ed page 300

Laryngeal Nerve Lesions	
Lesion	**Symptoms**
Superior Laryngeal Nerve (Ext LN + Internal LN)	• **External LN** supplies cricothyroid muscles which is adductor & tensor. Tensors, including vocalis give quality to voice. So in Superior LN lesion ***voice is weak & husky, loss of timber*** (poor quality voice not suitable in singing) • **Internal LN** is sensory to larynx above Vocal cord. So a lesion of Internal LN causes ***aspiration pneumonia and death***
Recurrent Laryngeal Nerve (U/L complete section)	Speech is not affected much. Vocal cord in half abducted position or sometimes called ***cadaveric position***
Recurrent Laryngeal Nerve (U/L partial section)	Vocal cord is in ***adducted*** (midline) position of affected side
Recurrent Laryngeal Nerve (B/L complete section)	Both Vocal cords are in midway between abduction & adduction breathing is impaired since rima glottidis is partially closed

Contd...

Recurrent Laryngeal Nerve (B/L partial section)	• Acute breathlessness - dyspnoea & stridor. Both Vocal cords are adducted *(B/L abductor palsy)*. Emergency cricothyroidotomy or tracheostomy is necessary • **Abductor paralysis**: Vocal cord midline, normal voice but respiratory difficulty. B/L Abductor paralysis is treated by Tracheostomy, Arytenoidectomy, or Transverse Cordectomy (**Kashima Operation**). Rx of choice is Vocal Cord lateralisation (***Type- II thyroplasty)*** • **Adductor paralysis:** Vocal cord lateral, change in voice but no respiratory difficulty, prone for aspiration. Rx of choice is Vocal Cord medialisation ***(Type- I thyroplasty)***. Injection of teflon in VC is also effective • **Adductor spasm:** Strained and croacky voice with spasmodic dysfunction

Causes of Vocal Cord Paralysis	
Surcical Causes of Vocal Cord Paralysis	
Surgery or procedure	**Mechanism of nerve injury or relevant anatomy**
Anterior cervical spine	Retraction; stretch injury of RLN (right more common)
Esophagectomy	RLN injury in tracheoesophageal groove
Carotid endarterectomy	Vagal injury during dissection
Mediastinoscopy	RLN injury, usually left
Coronary artery bypass grafting	• Retraction or direct injury to vagus or RLN during internal mammary artery harvest for grafting • Hypothermic nerve injury form ice cardioplegia
Pulmonary resection	Usually left upper lobe or RLN injury
Endotracheal intubation	Possible pressure neuropraxia from compression of anterior rami of RLN caused by a high-riding endotracheal cuff in the subglottis
Causes of Unilateral Vocal Fold Immobility	
Cause	**Percentage**
Malignancy (nonlaryngeal)	24.7
Iatrogenic (surgical trauma)	23.9
Idiopathic	19.6
Nonsurgical trauma	11.1
Intubation	7.5
Neurologic	7.9
Thoracic aortic aneurysm	4.3
Pulmonary or mediastinal tuberculosis	1.1
Causes of Bilateral Vocal Fold Paralysis (BVFP)	
Iatrogenic	82.8
Malignancy	8.6
Neurologic	3.8
Intubation	2.7
Idiopathic	2.2
Causes of Bilateral Vocal Fold Immobility (BVFI)	
Iatrogenic	25.7
Malignancy	17
Neurologic	12.8
Intubation	15.4
Idiopathic	12.8
External trauma	11.1
Rheumatoid arthritis or inflammatory disease	3.4
Radiation therapy	1.7

Transverse Cordotomy

"Perhaps the most widely used surgical procedure for the treatment of BVFP, endoscopic CO_2 laser transversecordotomy (TC) is an excellent surgical option. Originally described by **kashima** in 1991, this technique is technically less demanding than an endoscopic laser arytenoidectomy and appears to result in comparable airway enlargement. The goal is to detach as much of the thyroarytenoid (TA) muscle from the arytenoid cartilage as possible. The TA muscle retracts anteriorly and heals over several weeks, leaving a rounded tear-shaped opening anterior to the arytenoid"

36. Ans. (d) Tymponometry

Ref: Dhingra 5th ed page 30, 65-66, Cumming 5th edition ch-133

Eustachian Tube Tests

- Valsalva's maneuver
- Politerisation
- Toynbee's test
- Eustachian tube catheterization
- Tympanometry (impedance audiometry)
- Sachhrine or methylene blue test
- Sonotubometry

Test number 1 to 4 only tell anatomical patency, where as 5 to 7 tell functional status of Eustachian tube

Option (A)

Politzer test: Test for Eustachian tube function. But it is a **subjective test.** Done in those who can not perform valsalve especially children. Politzer bag is introduced in one nostril and other is closed. Patient id told to swallow and asked if he feels air entry in ear

Option (B)

Vemp: Test of vestibular function. See details of VEMP in ENT May 2012

Option (C)

Rhinomanometry: Measurement of nasal pressure and flow

Option (D)

Tympanometry: "Specifically, tympanometry provides an estimation of intratympanic pressure, eustachian tube function, tympanic membrane integrity and mobility and continuity of the ossicular chain. Acoustic admittance is optimal when the same air pressure is present on both sides of the tympanic membrane. The peak of the tympanogram reflects the resting pressure in the middle ear. Because the eustachian tube serves to ventilate the middle ear space, the tympanogram peak also provides information regarding eustachian tube function; a negative tympanogram pressure peak almost invariably indicates that the eustachian tube is not adequately ventilating the middle ear space because of eustachian tube obstruction caused by inflammation, infection, a mass lesion, or neuromuscular dysfunction"

Ophthalmology

10

AIIMS NOVEMBER 2018

1. Identify the marked layer in the given picture?

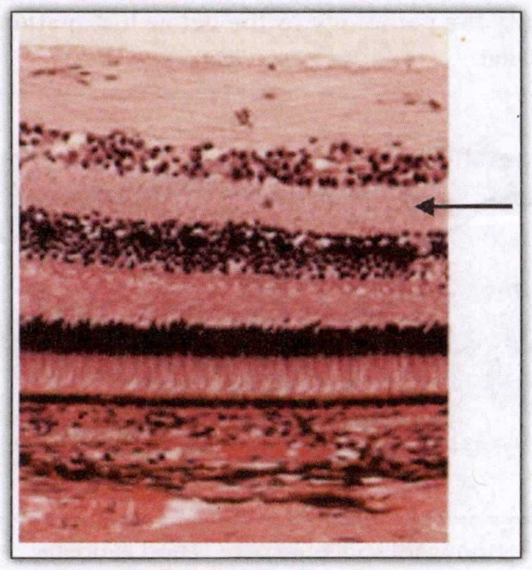

a. Outer plexiform layer
b. Inner plexiform layer
c. Outer limiting membrane
d. Inner limiting membrane

2. Most common ocular feature seen in sturge weber Syndrome is?

a. Retinitis pigmentosa b. Glaucoma
c. Uveitis d. Keratitis

3. A patient presents with following clinical picture. What is the most likely diagnosis?

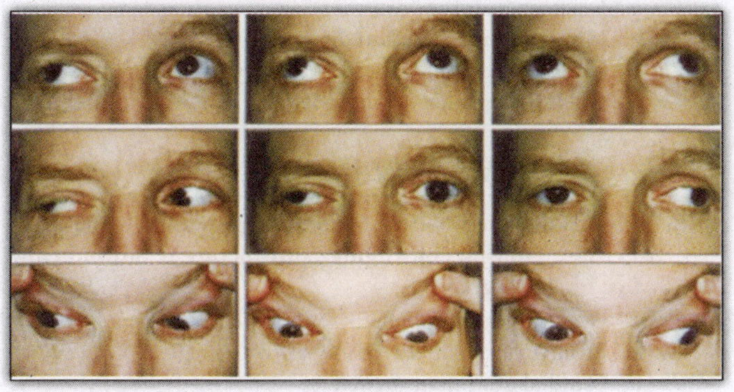

a. Internuclear ophthalmoplegia
b. Oculomotor nerve palsy
c. Lateral rectus paralysis
d. Trochlear nerve palsy

4. The angle in minutes subtended by the largest alphabet of Snellens chart on a person's eye who is reading it from a distance of 6 meters? ***(AIIMS Nov 2018, May 2016)***

a. 1 min b. 5 min
c. 10 min d. 50 min

5. A 2-year-child presents with complaints of bilateral proptosis and photophobia. On examination, his eyes were found to be as shown in given image. What is most likely diagnosis?

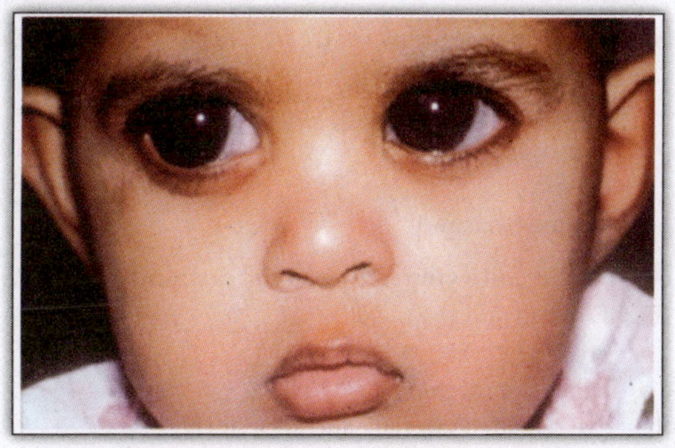

© Baiyeroju A, Bowman R, Gilbert C, Taylor D - Community eye health (2010)

Fig: Congenital glaucoma

a. Congenital glaucoma
b. Retinoblastoma
c. Megalocornea
d. Congenital endothelial dystrophy

6. A 33-year-old man presents with pain and watering of right eye for 36 hours. On examination, there is a 3 × 2 mm greyish white corneal ulcer with elevated margins, surrounded by feathery finger like infiltration into the adjacent corneal stroma. Minimal hypopyon is also observed. Most likely causative organism is? ***(AIIMS Nov 2018, May 2016)***

a. Aspergillus spp.
b. Pseudomonas spp.
c. Herpes simplex virus
d. Acanthamoeba spp

7. A patient of diabetic macular edema presents with glaucoma. Which of the following drug should be prescribed at last?

a. Prostaglandin analogue
b. Beta blockers
c. Pilocarpine
d. Alpha agonist

8. A patient was prescribed following spectacles. Identify condition for which they are prescribed:

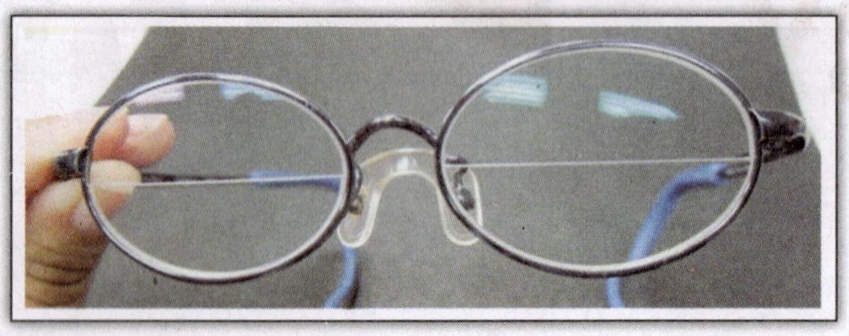

a. Bifocals for pediatric pseudophakia
b. Bifocals for presbyopia
c. Bifocals for adult aphakia
d. Progressive glasses for presbyopia

AIIMS MAY 2018

9. All are Ophthalmological manifestations of dengue virus EXCEPT:

a. Cataract
b. Maculopathy
c. Vitreous haemorrhage
d. Optic neuropathy

10. Most appropriate adjuvant treatment in fungal corneal ulcer is:

a. Atropine eye drop
b. Lignocaine eye drop
c. Pilocarpine
d. Dexamethasone

11. All of the following are seen in oculomotor nerve palsy EXCEPT:

a. Ptosis
b. Dilatation of pupil
c. Eye deviated laterally and superiorly
d. Absence of light reflex

12. Nucleus of upward gaze is:

a. Paramedian Pontine Reticular formation
b. Nucleus Raphe magnus
c. Cuneiform nucleus
d. Interstitial nucleus of Cajal

13. All of the following are uses of Stenopeic slit EXCEPT:

a. To find the cylindrical axis
b. Fincham test
c. For performing iridectomy
d. Corneal tattooing

14. A female patient with history of arthritis presented to ophthalmologist with a complain of sudden painless loss of vision. She had undergone cataract surgery for the same eye one year back. The fluorescein angiography picture of the eye is given. What is most likely diagnosis:

a. AMRD
b. Cystoid macular edema
c. Chloroquine toxicity
d. Macular dystrophy

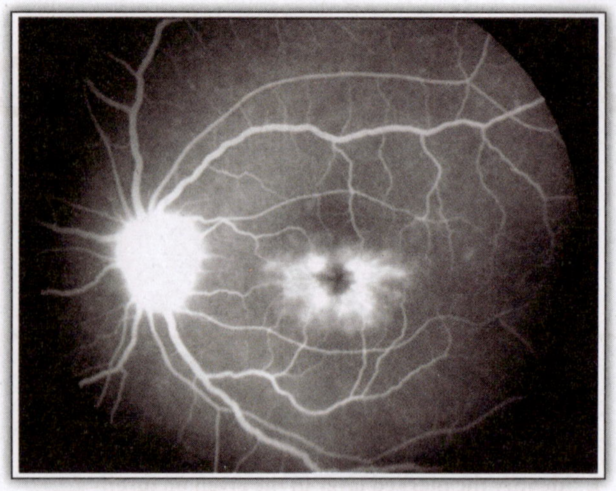

15. Identify the pathology in the below histopathology picture of retina:

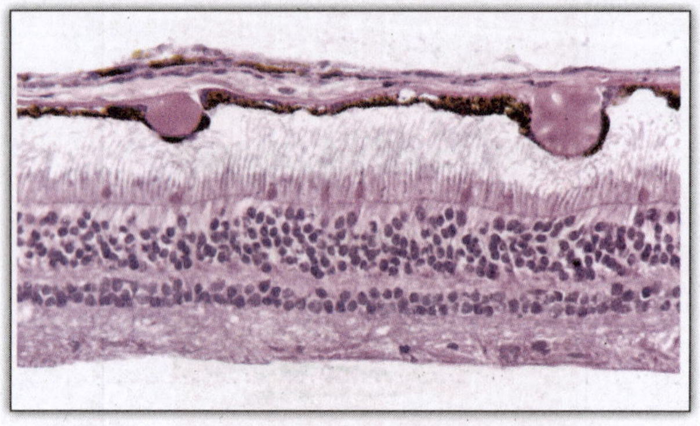

a. Cotton wool spots
b. Hard exudates
c. Drusen
d. Microaneurysm

16. A 55-year-old male with history of cataract surgery 1 year back now came with the chief complaints of glare when driving in the night. On examination visual acuity is Right- 6/12, Left- 6/9. What is the probable diagnosis:

a. Age related macular degeneration
b. Posterior subcapsular cataract
c. Cystoid macular edema
d. Corneal degeneration

17. NARP syndrome is:

a. Lysosomal storage disorder
b. Mitochondrial function disorder
c. Glycogen storage disorder
d. Golgi body transport disorder

AIIMS NOVEMBER 2017

18. A 65-year-old male with diabetes now presents with decrease in vision. Fluorescein Angiography picture is shown below. Most likely diagnosis is:

a. Nonproliferative diabetic retinopathy
b. Proliferative diabetic retinopathy
c. Familial dominant drusen
d. Birdshot retinopathy

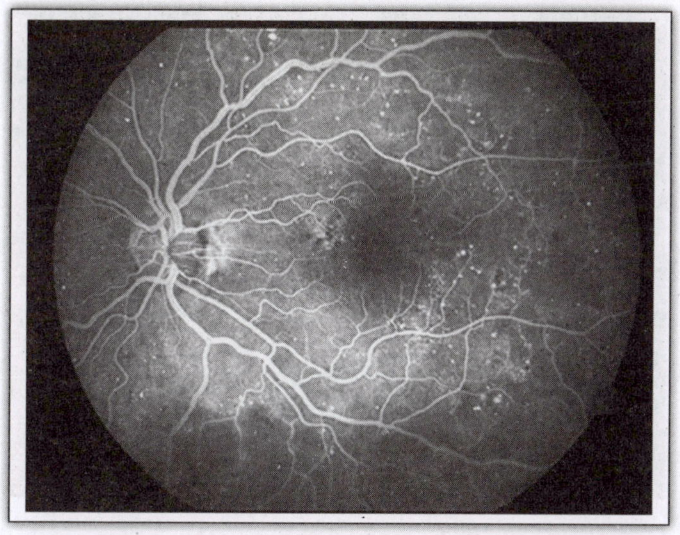

19. Identify the refractive error from the following diagram?

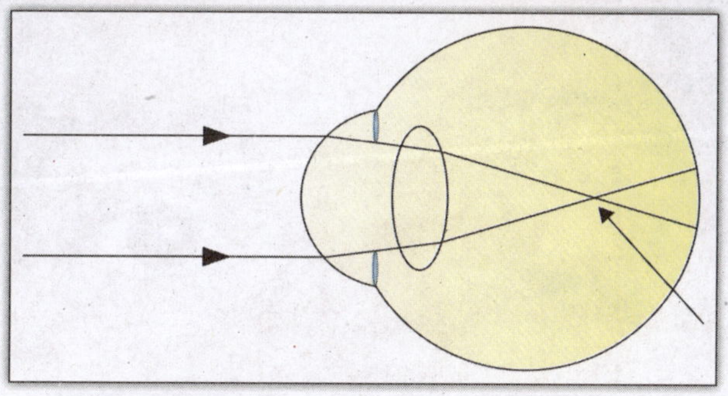

a. Hypermetropia
b. Myopia
c. Astigmatism
d. Presbyopia

20. A patient post cataract surgery developed endophthalmitis after 5 days. All can be done EXCEPT:

a. Topical antibiotics
b. Intravenous antibiotics
c. Intravitreal antibiotics
d. Pars Plana Vitrectomy

21. Most common tumour of lacrimal gland is?

a. Pleomorphic adenoma
b. Non Hodgkin's Lymphoma
c. Mucoepidermoid carcinoma
d. Adenoid cystic carcinoma

22. A glaucoma patient presenting with bulging of cornea. Most likely diagnosis is?

a. Keratoconus
b. Keratomalacia
c. Staphyloma
d. Granular dystrophy

23. Which nerve palsy leads to the following condition in the picture?

a. II
b. III
c. IV
d. VI

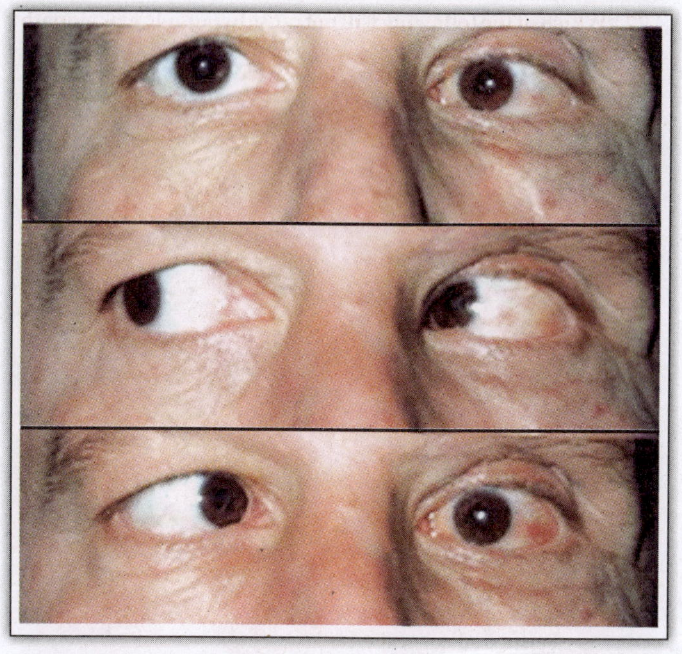

24. Identify the condition given in the following Picture?

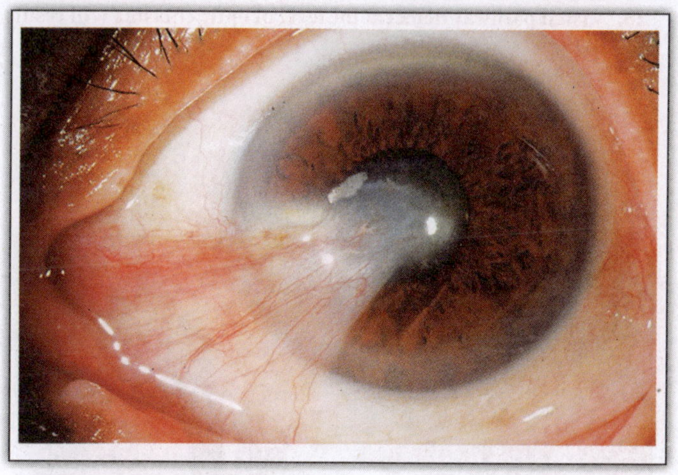

a. Pterygium
b. Pinguecula
c. Corneal ulcer
d. Xerophthalmia

25. A patient comes with ptosis and hypotropia of left eye. Ptosis gets resolved on administration of a IV drug. Patient is most likely suffering from?

a. Myasthenia gravis
b. Tolosa hunt syndrome
c. 3rd nerve palsy
d. Congenital ptosis

AIIMS MAY 2017

26. A 2 weeks old infant had conjunctivitis, which later developed into respiratory distress and pneumonia. Chest X-ray showed bilateral lung infiltrates. WBC count 14,300/dl. Which of the following is the most likely organism?

a. Chlamydia trachomatis
b. H. influenzae
c. N. gonorrhoeae
d. Streptococcus pneumoniae

27. Which of the following will not cause hypotonic maculopathy in the given image?

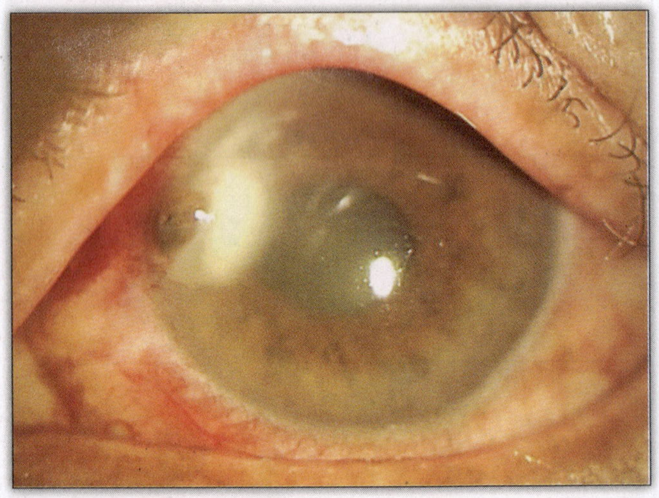

a. Suprachoroidal haemorrhage
b. Cyclodialysis of uvea
c. Perforated corneal ulcer
d. Overflowing bleb

28. Visual pathway defect at the level of optic chiasma will result in?

a. Binasal hemianopia
b. Bitemporal hemianopia
c. Central scotoma
d. Bilateral hemianopia

29. Identify the test shown below?

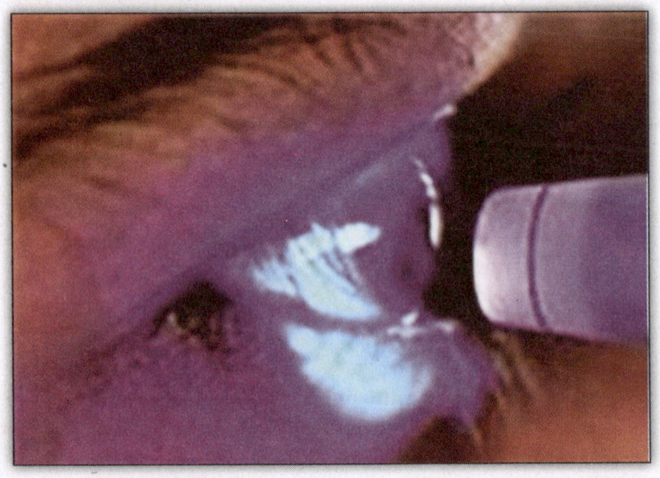

a. Tonometry
b. Laser interferometry
c. Pachymetry
d. Refractometer

30. A 60-year-old with cataract surgery. After 1 year he came with complaints of diminished vision and shows the following finding. Diagnosis?

a. Irvine-gass syndrome
b. After cataract
c. UGH syndrome
d. End-ophthalmitis

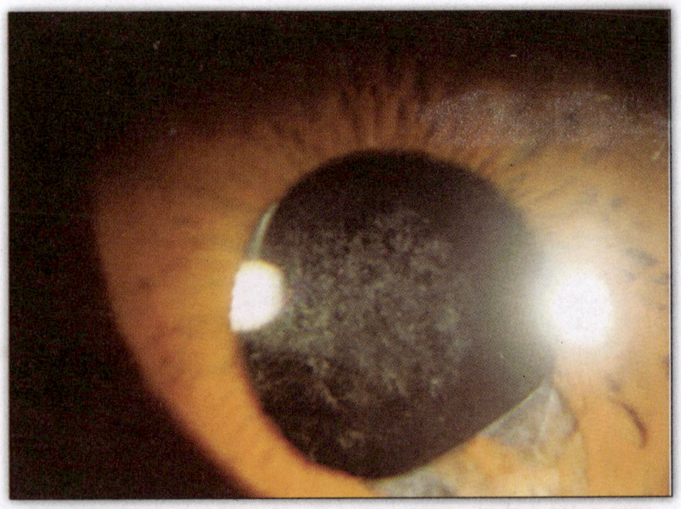

31. Identify the finding given in the picture?

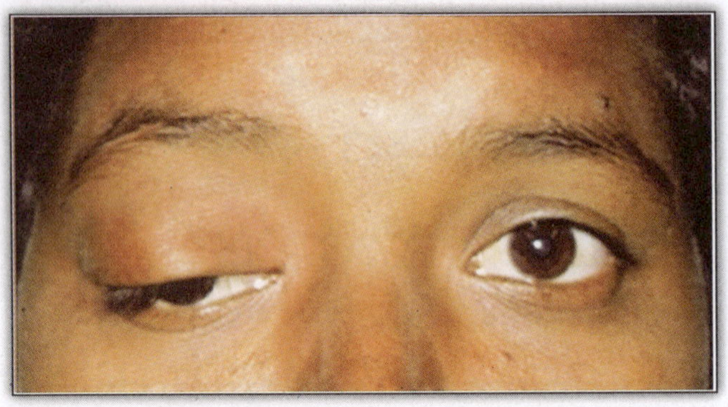

a. Ptosis of right eye
b. Entropion of right eye
c. Lagophthalmos right eye
d. Ectropion left eye

AIIMS NOVEMBER 2016

32. Identify the pathology from the given picture?

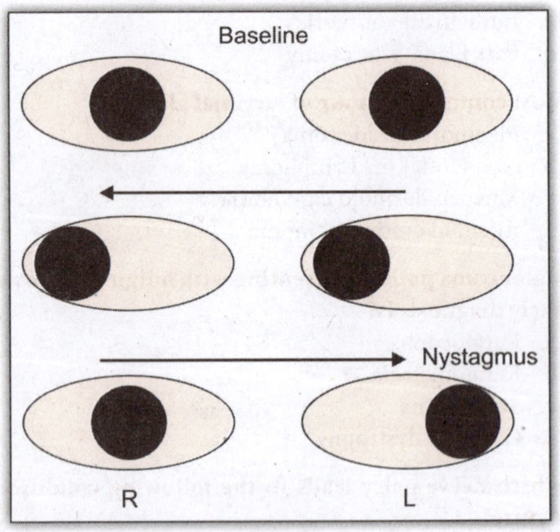

a. Internuclear ophthalmoplegia
b. Horizontal gaze palsy
c. 3rd nerve palsy
d. Superior oblique palsy

33. Maximum refractive power is of?

a. Anterior surface of cornea
b. Posterior surface of cornea
c. Anterior surface of lens
d. Posterior surface of lens

34. Which of the following is not a criteria of Blindness as per NPCB?

a. Diminution of field vision to 20 degrees or less in better eye
b. Vision 6/60 or less with best possible spectacle correction in better eye
c. Vision 4/60 or less with best possible spectacle correction in better eye
d. Inability of person to count fingers from distance of 6 meters or 20 feet

35. You are using a Rabbit for ophthalmological drug testing, what is the ideal weight of this Rabbit?

a. 2–4 kg
b. 4–6 kg
c. 6–10 kg
d. 10–12 kg

36. You are using an indirect ophthalmoscopy for retinal examination. What is the power of anterior lens used in indirect ophthalmoscope?

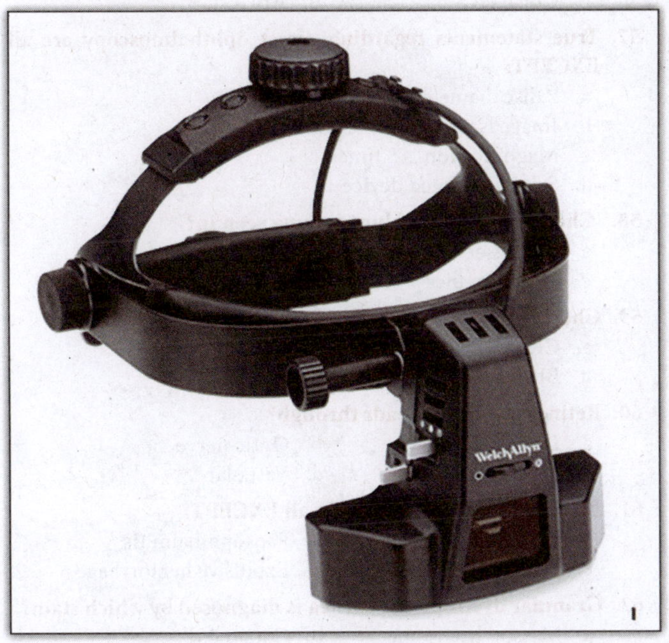

a. +20 D
b. +58 D
c. +78 D
d. +90 D

37. Laser assisted cataract removal done using laser of how much frequency?

a. 10^{-15}
b. 10^{-12}
c. 10^{-9}
d. 10^{-6}

38. A farmer had history of stick injury to his eye 10 days back. Presented to you with difficulty in vision, redness, photophobia and eye pain. Examination reveals corneal ulcer with fuzzy margins and collection as shown below. Next line of management is?

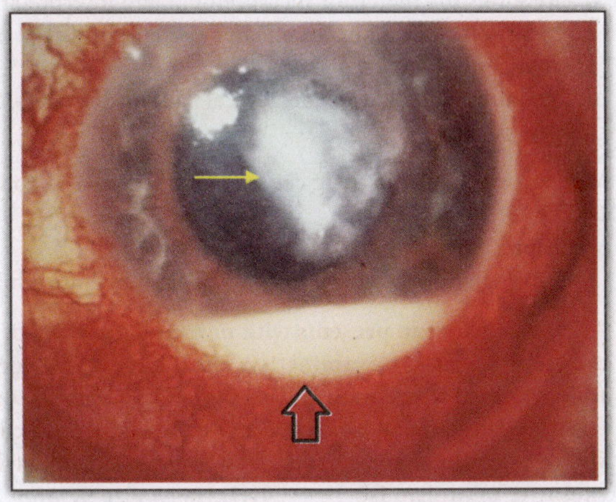

a. Topical natamycin and drainage of hypopyon
b. Topical natamycin and corneal scraping for culture
c. Topical Ceftazidime 1.5% + IV Antibiotic and corneal scraping culture
d. Topical antibiotic drops + topical steroid

39. A young male has sudden painless diminution of vision of left eye. On examination, the right eye power is 6/6. left eye 3/6. Fundus and ocular coherence tomography as shown. Which layer of retina is detached?

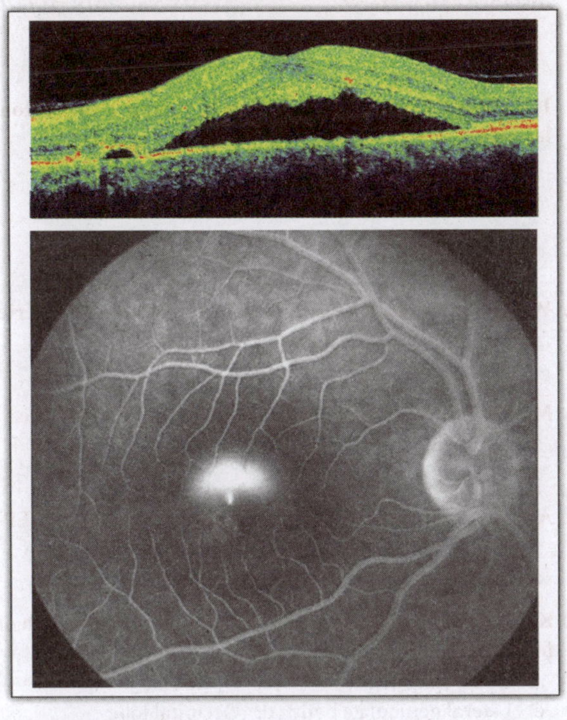

a. Retinal pigment epithelium
b. Neurosensory retina
c. Outer nuclear layer
d. Inner nuclear layer

AIIMS MAY 2016

40. Phenol red thread test is used for dry eye, true is?
a. Colour change on contact with tears to assess the volume of tears
b. Requires pH meter for measurement and interpretation
c. Measures ocular surface mucin deficiency if thread colour changes to blue
d. Requires instillation of topical anesthesia before the procedure

41. Which antiglaucoma drug causes black deposits in conjunctiva?
a. Alpha blocker b. Adrenaline
c. Prostaglandins d. Carbonic anhydrase inhibitors

42. A 33-year-old man presents with pain and watering of right eye for 36 hours. On examination, there is a 3 × 2 mm greyish white corneal ulcer with elevated margins, surrounded by feathery finger like infiltration into the adjacent corneal stroma. Minimal hypopyon is also observed. Most likely causative organism is? *(AIIMS Nov 2018, May 2016)*
a. Aspergillus spp. b. Pseudomonas spp.
c. Herpes simpex virus d. Acanthamoeba spp

43. Which of the following organisms produce corneal ulcer resembling fungal ulcers?
a. Nocardia asteroids b. Klebsiella species
c. Mycobateria d. Chlamydia

44. The angle in minutes subtended by the largest alphabet of Snellen's chart on a person's eye who is reading it from a distance of 6 meters? *(AIIMS Nov 2018, May 2016)*
a. 1 min b. 5 min
c. 10 min d. 50 min

45. Immediately after photodynamic therapy, the colour of lesion?
a. Remains unchanged b. Becomes yellow
c. Becomes grey d. Becomes white

AIIMS NOVEMBER 2015

46. Wavelength of ND-YAG laser used in refractive surgeries is?
a. 193 nm b. 451 nm
c. 532 nm d. 1064 nm

47. Most common fungal ocular infection in HIV AIDS is?
a. Aspergillosis b. Cryptococcosis
c. Coccidioidomycosis d. Candidiasis

48. All present in benign intracranial hypertension EXCEPT:
a. Papilledema b. Proptosis
c. 6th nerve palsy d. Normal size ventricles

49. Key hole defect in visual field is due to lesion of which of the following?
a. Optic chiasmsa b. Optic disc
c. Lateral geniculate body d. Occipital lobe

50. Which drug had similar action on dilator pupillae as that of pilocarpine's action on sphincter pupillae?
a. Timolol b. Epinephrine
c. Cocaine d. Hydroxyamphetamine

AIIMS MAY 2015

51. Which nerve is involved in loss of corneal sensation?
a. Supratrochlear nerve b. Infraorbital nerve
c. Nasociliary nerve d. Supraorbital nerve

52. Which of the following topical agents causes heterochromia iridis?
a. Latanoprost b. Prednosolone
c. Timolol d. Olapatadine

53. In right trochlear nerve (Right superior oblique) palsy, all are present EXCEPT:
a. Right hypertropia
b. Diplopia on upper gaze and adduction
c. Right extorsion d. Right head tilt

54. Vitreous humor has higher concentration of what compared to blood?
a. Glucose b. Sodium
c. Potassium d. Ascorbate

55. High Molecular weight proteins found in cataractous lens seen only in humans is?
a. HM 1 and 2 b. HM 2 and 3
c. HM 1 and 3 d. HM 3 and 4

56. Universal marker of limbal stem cells is?
a. Elastin b. Keratin
c. Collagen d. ABCG2

57. True statements regarding direct ophthalmoscopy are all EXCEPT:
a. 2 disc diameter field of vision
b. Image is virtual and erect
c. Magnification is 5 times
d. Self illuminated device

58. Cherry spot due to blunt trauma seen in?
a. Berlins oedema b. Tay sachs
c. Niemann pick d. CRVO

59. Cherry red spot and Hollen horst plaques are seen in?
a. CRAO b. CRVO
c. BRAO d. BRVO

60. Retinoblastoma spreads through?
a. Lymphatics b. Optic nerve
c. Direct invasion d. Vascular

61. Evisceration of eye is done in all EXCEPT:
a. Malignancy b. Pan-ophthalmitis
c. Trauma d. Expulsive hemorrhage

62. Granular dystrophy of cornea is diagnosed by which stain?
a. Masson trichrome b. Congo red
c. PAS d. Colloid iron

63. Multifocal ERG is used to assess the function of?
a. Rods b. Macular cones
c. Gangilion cells d. Bipolar cells

64. Whorl like Corneal Deposits are seen in all EXCEPT:
a. Amiodarone b. Chlorpromazine
c. Indomethacin d. Quinine/Chloroquine

65. Painful unilateral dimness of vision with after images, flashes of light is seem in?
a. Retrobulbar neuritis b. Ocular ischaemic syndrome
c. CRAO d. Papilledema

ANSWERS WITH EXPLANATIONS

AIIMS NOVEMBER 2018

1. Ans. (b) Inner plexiform layer

Ref: Khurana 6th ed page 265

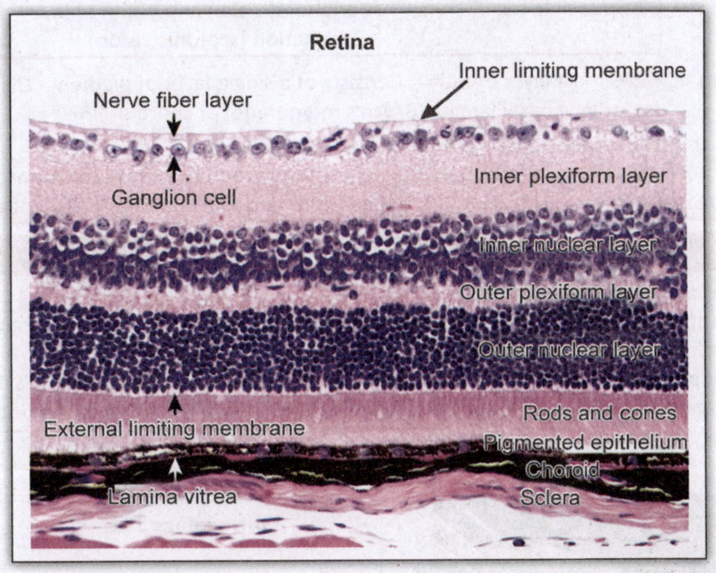

Fig: Layers of Retina (labelled). Retina consists of 3 types of cells and their synapses arranged in ten layers.

Layers of Retina		
1	Inner limiting membrane	Innermost layer of retina and is essentially a basement membrane. It separates the retina from vitreous and is formed by the union of terminal expansions of the Muller's fibres
2	Nerve fiber layer (Stratum Opticum)	Consists of axons of the ganglion cells, which pass through the lamina cribrosa to form the optic nerve.
3	Ganglion cell layer	Consists of cell bodies of ganglion cells (2nd order neurons of visual pathway). There are two types of ganglion cells. 1. **Midget ganglion cells** are present in the macular region and the dendrite of each such cell synapses with the axon of single bipolar cell. 2. **Polysynaptic ganglion cells** lie mainly in the peripheral retina and each cell may synapse with up to a hundred bipolar cells.
4	Inner Plexiform layer	Consists of connections between the axons of bipolar cells and dendrites of the ganglion cells and processes of amacrine cells.
5	Inner Nuclear Layer	Contains cell bodies of bipolar cells (majorly), cell bodies of horizontal amacrine and Muller's cellsand capillaries of central artery of retina. *The bipolar cells is the 1st order neurons of visuaL pathway.*
6	Outer Plexiform Layer	Consists of connections of rod spherules and cone pedicles with the dendrites of bipolar cells and horizontal cells.
7	Outer Nuclear Layer	Contains nuclei of rods and cones
8	External Limiting membrane	Fenestrated membrane, through which passes the processes of rods and cones.

Contd...

Layers of Retina

9	Inner/outer segment Junction (Photoreceptor layer- Rods and Cones)	Rods and cones (photoreceptors) arranged in a palisade manner.

Photoreceptors

	Rods	Cones
Number	120 millions	6.5 millions.
Photosensitive substance	Rhodopsin	Photopsin
Responsible for	Peripheral vision and vision of low illumination (scotopic vision)	Central vision (photopic vision) and colour vision.

10	Retinal Pigment Epithelium	Outermost layer of retina. Consists of a single layer of pigment cells. Firmly adherent to the underlying basal lamina (Bruch's membrane) of choroid

Mnemonic = In new generation improved interns opt only Externship to Rule PGME
In (Inner limiting) New (Nerve fiber layer) Generation (Ganglion layer) Improved (Inner plexiform) Interns (Inner Nuclear) Opt (Outer Plexiform) Only (Outer Nuclear) Externship (External limiting) to Rule (Rods and Cones) PGME (Pigment epithelium layer)

Faq Retinal Layers

- **Microaneurysms** are present mainly in inner nuclear layer.
- **Cotton wool spots** are present in nerve fibre layer. It is seen more commonly in hypertensive retinopathy
- Normal retinal vasculature is found in between outer plexiform and inner nuclear layer
- Soft exudates or Cotton wool spots are small yellowish type, irregular margins, due to axonal debris. It's due to axonal transport blockage.
- Hard exudates are slightly large, sharp margins, due to lipid deposits. Hard exudates are mostly in outer plexiform layer

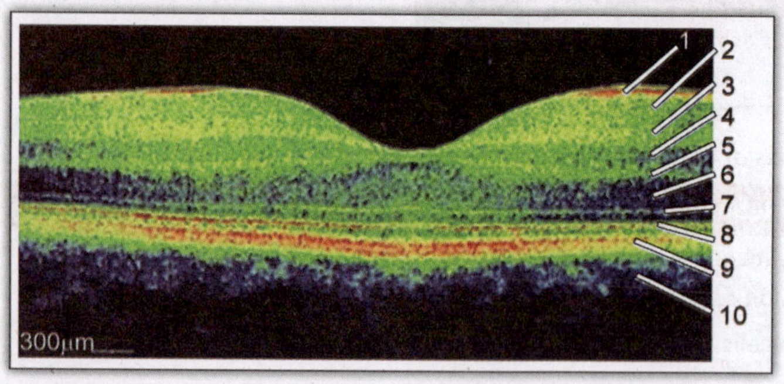

Fig: Normal optical coherence tomography of retinal layers **1.** Nerve fiber layer; **2.** Ganglion cell layer **3.** Inner plexiform layer; **4.** Inner nuclear layer; **5.** Outer plexiform layer; **6.** Outer nuclear layer; **7.** External limiting membrane; **8.** Inner/outer segment junction; **9.** Retinal pigment epithelium; **10.** Larger choroidal vessels

2. Ans. (b) Glaucoma

Ref: With Text

Glaucoma associated with phakomatosis is seen in Sturge-Weber syndrome (50% cases) and Von Recklinghausen's neurofibromatosis (25% cases). (Ref: Khurana 6th ed page 228)

Ocular Features of Sturge Weber Syndrome

Sturge Weber syndrome (encephalotrigeminal angiomatosis) is a congenital, sporadic phacomatosis. Ocular features may include ipsilateral glaucoma, episcleral haemangioma, iris heterochromia and diffuse choroidal haemangioma

Glaucoma ipsilateral to the facial hemangioma develops in about 30% and in 60% of these IOP elevation occurs before the age of 2 years and may result in buphthalmos. In the remainder, glaucoma may develop at any time from infancy to adulthood. The pathogenesis includes trabeculodysgenesis in infants and raised episcleral venous pressure associated with episcleral hemangioma in older patients. **(Ref: Kanski's 8th Edition page 394)**

3. Ans. (b) Oculomotor nerve Palsy

Ref: Kanski's Clinical Ophthalmology 8th Edition page 823

The given picture shows right 3rd (Oculomotor) nerve palsy. In the primary gaze right eye is down and out. In Right gaze abduction of right eye is complete but in left gaze adduction of right eye is limited. Elevation and depression are also restricted.

NOTE

The examiner may give a 3 gaze eye position or a more comprehensive 9 gaze eye position in the examination. For basic interpretation a 3 gaze eye position is generally enough to make a diagnosis. In case a 9 gaze eye positions (3 rows) are given in the picture, see the middle row first.

Signs of 3rd Nerve Palsy Include

- Abduction and depression in primary position: due to unopposed action of the lateral rectus and superior oblique muscles. The intact superior oblique muscle also causes intorsion of the eye at rest, which increases on attempted downgaze.
- Normal abduction as lateral rectus is intact.
- Limited adduction due to medial rectus weakness.
- Limited elevation due to weakness of the superior rectus and inferior oblique.
- Limited depression due to weakness of inferior rectus
- Varying degree of ptosis
- In complete 3rd nerve involvement, dilated pupil and defective accommodation due to parasympathetic palsy

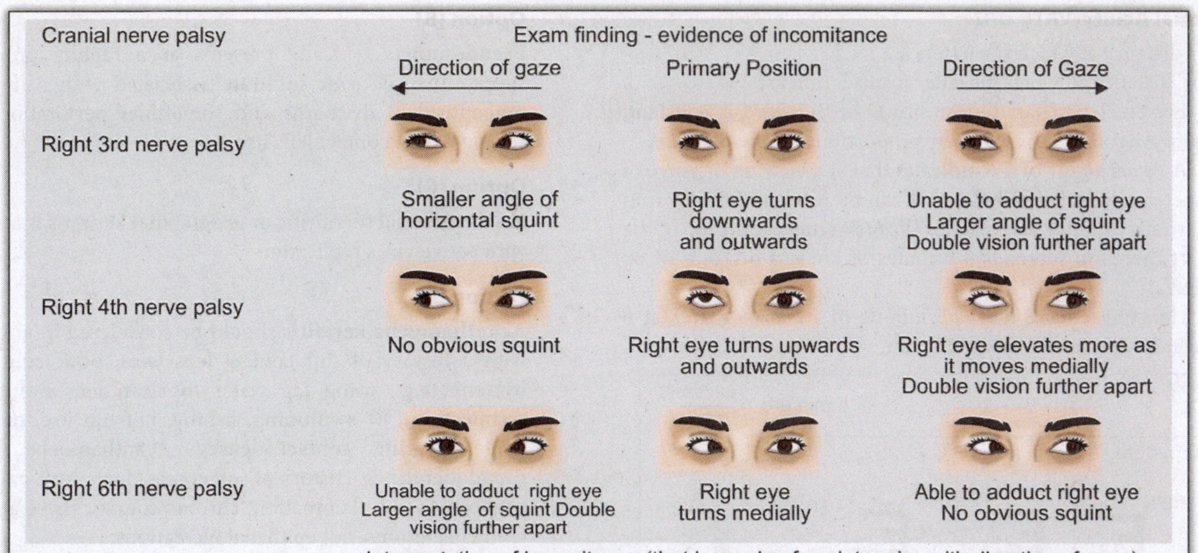

Interpretation of incomitance (that is, angle of squint varies with direction of gaze)

NOTE

Pupil sparing palsy/ pupil involving palsy: Surgical Causes like aneurysm and compressive lesions always involve pupil. Medical causes of third nerve palsy like DM and Hypertension cause pupil sparing third nerve palsy

MNEMONIC In primary gaze see the deviation of eye DUM; Downward and Outward = 3rd nerve, Upward and Outward = 4th nerve, Medially = 6th nerve

4. Ans. (c) 50 min

Ref: Parson's 22nd ed page 97

Snellen's test: The distant central visual acuity is usually tested by Snellen's test . *The fact that two distant points can be visible as separate only when they subtend an angle of 1 minute at the nodal point of the eye, forms the basis of Snellen's test.* It consists of a series of black capital letters on a white board, arranged in lines, each progressively diminishing in size. *The lines comprising the letters have such a breadth that they will subtend an angle of 1 min at the nodal point.* Each letter of the chart is so designed that it fits in a square, the sides of which are five times the breadth of the constituent lines. **Thus, at the given distance, each letter subtends an angle of 5 min at the nodal point of the eye**

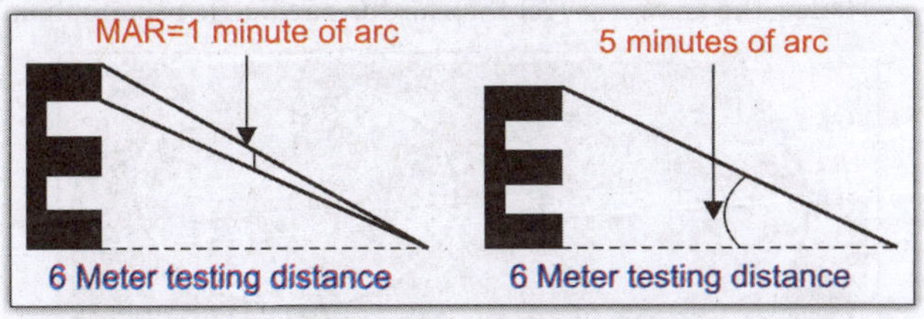

Fig: Each letter is in 5 rows: Each row subtends an angle of 1 min at nodal point of eye and each letter subtends an angle of 5 min at nodal point of eye at the given distance. MAR= Minimum angle of resolution.

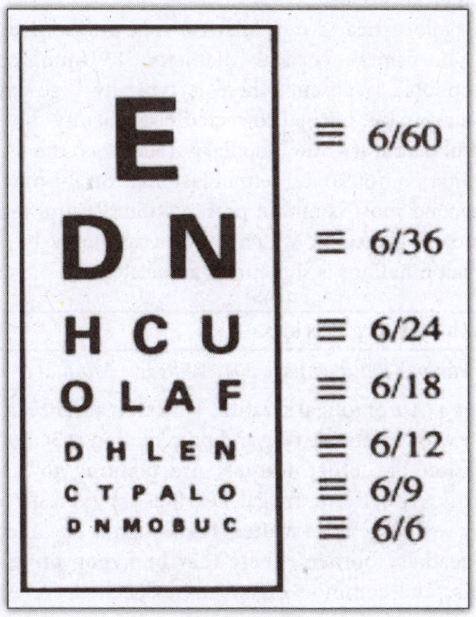

Fig: Snellen standard chart seen at 6 meters: If only top letter can be read the VAS is 6/60. If patient can read top 4 lines then VA is 6/18. A normal person should be able to read top 7 lines i.e. VA = 6/6

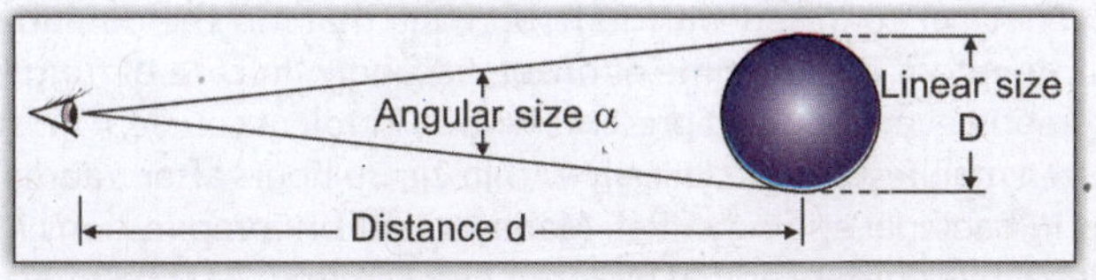

Visual Acuity(VA) = d/D

d = distance at which the letters are read

D = Distance at which the letter forms 5 min arc

For Snellen's chart Linear size D of the word is constant, hence Angular size is inversely proportional to the distance.

A visual acuity of 6/6 indicates that at a viewing distance of 6 meters, the smallest letter that can be resolved forms 5 min of arc at a distance of 6 meters. The 6/60 letters at the top of the chart therefore subtends 5 minutes of arc at a distance of 60 metres.

Hence if letter E makes 5 minute of arc at 60 meter, at 6 meter it will make an arc of 50 min.

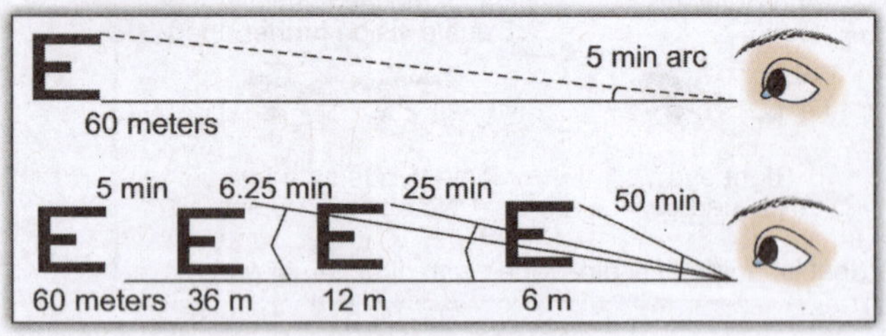

5. Ans. (a) Congenital glaucoma

Ref: Kanski's Clinical Ophthalmology 8th Edition Pg .385,235499

(For Image please refer Qs. No. 5 Page No. 653)

Congenital glaucoma usually presents as corneal haze, large (Buphthalmos) or asymmetrical eyes, watering, photophobia or blepharospasm which is noticed either by the parents or a health professional.

Megalocornea is rare bilateral non-progressive condition with horizontal corneal diameter 13 mm or greater. Photophobia is absent .There is typically high myopia and astigmatism but normal corrected visual acuity.

Leukocoria (white pupillary reflex) is the commonest presentation (60%) of retinoblastoma. Strabismus (20%) is the second most common presentation. Painful red eye with secondary glaucoma which may occasionally be associated with buphthalmos is sometimes associated.

6. Ans. (b) Aspergillus spp.

Ref: Parson's 22nd ed page 201, Wills Eye Manual 6th ed page 73

This is a case of fungal keratitis. However, absence of history of injury with vegetative twig and presentation at 36 hours creates confusion but other features are pointing towards fungal keratitis. Mycotic or fungal keratitis are typically seen after injury with vegetative matter. The slough is dry in appearance with feathery borders. There may be hypopyon and satellite lesions. The common organisms associated are Aspergillus, Fusarium or Candida albicans.

NOTE

Do not get confused with 36 hours. One that it is the duration of symptom not the time of onset. Secondly "In case of fungal keratitis, even though it presents with an indolent course, it most often manifests itself clinically within 24–36 hours after trauma, as in bacterial etiology" (Ref: Management of Complications in Refractive Surgery edited by Jorge Alió, Dimitri T. Azar page 37)

Option (B)

Pseudomonas typically presents as a rapidly progressive, suppurative, necrotic infiltrate associated with a hypopyon, mucopurulent discharge and sometimes perforation in the setting of soft contact lens use

Option (C)

HSV epithelial (dendritic or geographic) keratitis is associated with active virus replication

Option (D)

Acanthamoeba keratitis should be considered in any patient with a history of soft contact lens wear, poor contact lens hygiene (e.g., using tap water to clean lenses, infrequent disinfection), or swimming, fishing, hot-tub use, or trauma while wearing contact lenses. Acanthamoeba keratitis pseudodendrites: History of soft contact lens wear, pain out of proportion to inflammation, chronic course. These are raised epithelial lesions, not epithelial ulcerations.

7. Ans. (a) Prostaglandin analogue

Ref: Yanoff Ophthalmology 5th edition pg.1121

The use of beta-blockers should be avoided in patients with diabetes because symptoms of hypoglycemia may be masked. Other contraindications of beta blockers include asthma, severe chronic obstructive pulmonary disease, bradycardia, second or third degree heart block and congestive heart failure.

Macular edema can develop during treatment with any PGF2α analogue, especially in aphakic patients; a watch should be kept to detect it early (KDT 7th ed page 155)

Beta-blockers are also preferred in conditions such as ocular inflammation and cystoid macular oedema, or where there is a history of herpes simplex keratitis. (Kanski 8th ed page 332)

8. Ans. (a) Bifocals for pediatric pseudophakia

Ref: Pediatric eye disease: color atlas and synopsis by Richard. W. Hertle Pg 223

- The catch in this question is that the spectacle has a nasal rest.
- Nasal rest is often provided in paediatric spectacles so as to protect the nasal bridge.
- The shape and proportions of the skull of a young child are rounder than that of an adult; the nares together with the nasal bridge are not fully formed and so, unable to support eyeglasses as in an adult. This either transfers the role of support to the glabella or requires the use of thick silicone nose pads in the form of a strap or saddle.
- The small pupillary distance and undeveloped **nasal bridge** require specially designed frames.

Hence, the answer is (A) Bifocals for paediatric pseudophakia.

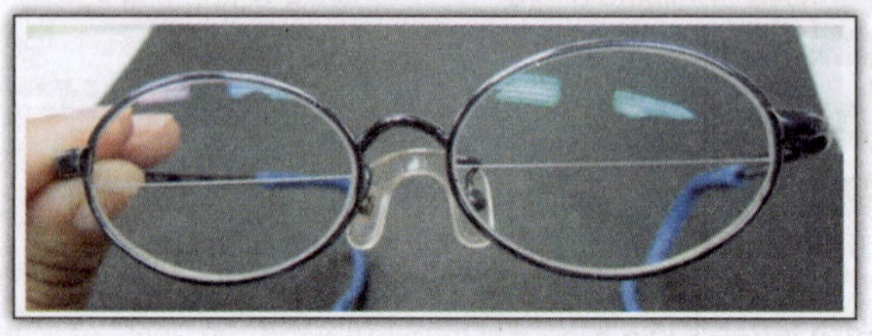

Fig: Bifocal lens with pediatric nose rest

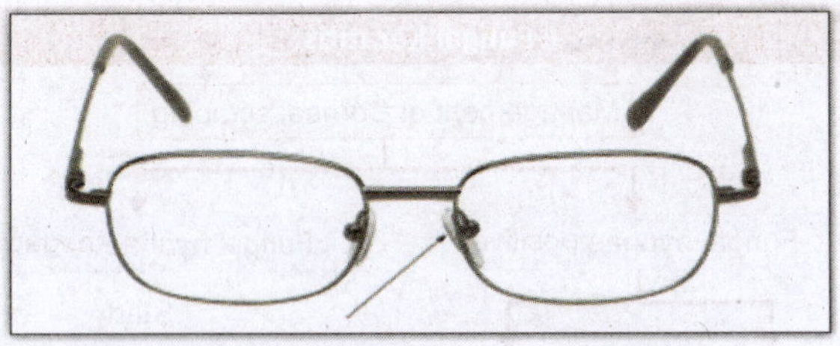

Fig: Nose rest of adult spectacles (arrow)

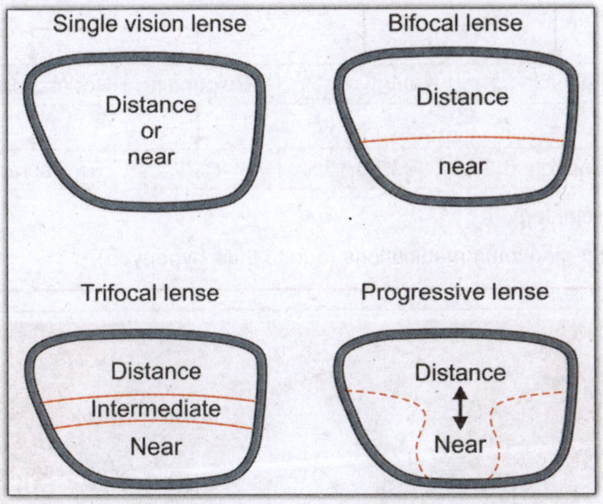

Fig: Types of lens

AIIMS MAY 2018

9. Ans. (a) Cataract

Ref: Intraocular Inflammation by Manfred Zierhut Pg 1154

Ophthalmic Complications of Dengue

- Small, intraretinal, whitish lesions, with localized retinal and retinal pigment epithelium (RPE) disturbances
- Small dot hemorrhages
- Macular edema
- Vascular occlusion
- Vascular sheathing around the macula and the papillomacular bundle
- Optic neuritis and disc hemorrhage
- Subconjunctival haemorrhage
- Uveitis

10. Ans. (a) Atropine eye drop

Ref: Parson's 22nd Ed Pg 155

Atropine eye drop can be used as adjunctive treatment In fungal corneal ulcer

Fungal Keratitis	
Types	• **Yeasts** (e.g. genus Candida), ovoid unicellular organisms that reproduce by budding, are responsible for most cases of fungal keratitis in temperate climates. • **Filamentous fungi** (e.g. genera Fusarium and Aspergillus), multicellular organisms that produce tubular projections known as hyphae. They are the most common pathogens in tropical climates. Aspergillus is the commonest in India.

Contd...

Fungal Keratitis	
Predisposing factors	• Common predisposing factors are chronic ocular surface disease, long-term use of topical steroids (often in conjunction with prior corneal transplantation), contact lens wear, systemic immunosuppression and diabetes. • Filamentary keratitis may be associated with trauma, often relatively minor, involving plant matter or gardening/agricultural tools.
Clinical features	The diagnosis is often delayed unless there is a high index of suspicion and often infection will initially have been presumed to be bacterial. • Presentation is with a gradual onset of pain, grittiness, photophobia, blurred vision and watery or mucopurulent discharge. **Symptoms are in general less than in bacterial ulcer of same size.** • Signs: ▪ **Candida keratitis:** ♦ Yellow-white densely suppurative infiltrate ♦ A collar-stud/button morphology may be seen in case of Yeast ▪ **Filamentous keratitis:** ♦ A grey or yellow-white stromal infiltrate with indistinct **fluffy margins.** ♦ Progressive infiltration, often with satellite lesions. ♦ Feathery branch-like extensions or a ring-shaped infiltrate may develop. ♦ Rapid progression with necrosis and thinning can occur. ♦ Penetration of an intact Descemet membrane may occur and lead to endophthalmitis without evident perforation. ▪ An epithelial defect is not invariable and is sometimes small when present. ▪ Other features include anterior uveitis, hypopyon, endothelial plaque, raised IOP, scleritis and sterile or infective endophthalmitis.
Diagnosis	Samples for laboratory examination should be acquired before commencing antifungal therapy • **Staining** Gram and Giemsa staining are both about 50% sensitive Periodic acid-Schiff (PAS) and Grocott–Gömöri methenamine-silver (GMS) stains may also be used, but are more commonly performed on histological sections. • **Culture:** Corneal scrapes should be placed on Sabouraud dextrose agar, although most fungi will also grow on blood agar or in enrichment media. If applicable, contact lenses and cases should be sent for culture. • **Corneal biopsy** is indicated in the absence of clinical improvement after 3–4 days and if no growth develops from scrapings after a week. A 2–3 mm block should be taken, using a technique similar to the scleral block excision during trabeculectomy. The excised block is sent for culture and histopathological analysis. • **Confocal microscopy** is rarely available, but may permit identification of organisms in vivo.

Contd...

Fungal Keratitis	
Management	• **General measures** ▪ Hospital admission should be considered for patients who are not likely to comply or are unable to self-administer treatment. hospital admission is usually required. ▪ It should also be considered for aggressive disease particularly if involving an only eye. ▪ Discontinuation of contact lens wear is mandatory. ▪ A clear plastic eye shield should be worn between eye drop instillation if significant thinning (or perforation) is present. Removal of the epithelium over the lesion may enhance penetration of antifungal agents. It may also be helpful to regularly remove mucus and necrotic tissue with a spatula. • **Topical treatment** should initially be given hourly for 48 hours and then reduced as signs permit. Because most antifungals are only fungistatic, treatment should be continued for at least 12 weeks. **Natamycin 5%** drops (especially for filamentous fungi) or amphotericin B 0.15% drops (especially for Candida), initially q1–2h around the clock, then taper over 4 to 6 weeks • A broad-spectrum antibiotic should also be considered to address or prevent bacterial co-infection. • **Cycloplegia:** (cyclopentolate 1%, homatropine 2% or atropine 1%) are used to prevent the formation of posterior synechiae and to reduce pain • **Subconjunctival fluconazole** may be used in severe cases • **Systemic antifungals** may be given in severe cases, when lesions are near the limbus, or for suspected endophthalmitis. Options include voriconazole 400 mg b.d. for one day then 200 mg b.d., itraconazole 200 mg daily, reduced to 100 mg daily, or fluconazole 200 mg b.d. • **Tetracycline** (e.g. doxycycline 100 mg b.d.) may be given for its anticollagenase effect when there is significant thinning. • IOP should be monitored using a Tono-Pen. • Superficial keratectomy can be effective to de-bulk the lesion. • Therapeutic keratoplasty (penetrating or deep anterior lamellar) is considered when medical therapy is ineffective or following perforation.
Penetrating Keratoplasty	• **Inspite Of Intensive Antifungal Therapy If:** ▪ ncreasing Hypopyon ▪ Central To Peripheral Corneal Involvement ▪ Impending /Frank Perforation ▪ Scleral Involvement • Therapeutic PK With/Without Scleral Graft With Amphotericin B Wash • Use: Debulk Fungal Load ▪ Reestablish Integrity Of Globe ▪ Absolute Diagnosis Of Fungal Etiology • Optical PK for corneal opacity in healed corneal ulcer

Contd...

Fungal Keratitis

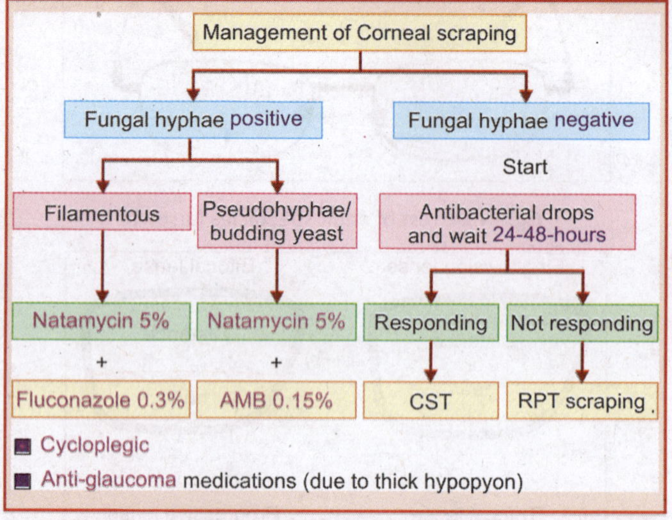

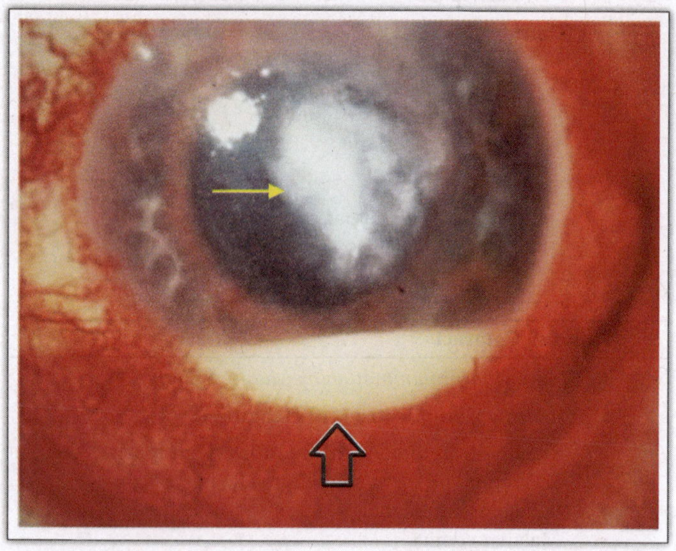

Fig: Fungal ulcers are indolent and have a gray infiltrate with **irregular edges (Yellow arrow)**, often a **hypopyon (Black arrow)** marked inflammation of the globe, superficial ulceration and **satellite lesions** (usually infiltrates at sites distant from the main area of ulceration)

11. Ans. (c) Eye deviated laterally and superiorly

Ref: Yanoff's 4th Ed Pg 924, Kanski's 8th Edition page 823

Oculomotor (3rd) nerve palsy would lead to eye position Down and Out position because Superior Oblique and Lateral rectus are spared.

Signs of 3rd Nerve Palsy Include

- Abduction and depression in primary position: due to unopposed action of the lateral rectus and superior oblique muscles. The intact superior oblique muscle also causes intorsion of the eye at rest, which increases on attempted downgaze.
- Normal abduction as lateral rectus is intact.
- Limited adduction due to medial rectus weakness.
- Limited elevation due to weakness of the superior rectus and inferior oblique.

- Limited depression due to weakness of inferior rectus
- Varying degree of ptosis
- In complete 3rd nerve involvement,dilated pupil and defective accommodation due to parasympathetic palsy

Extraocular muscles supplied by: **Mnemonic SO4-LR6-O3** (The letters represent the extraocular muscles and numbers represent their respective cranial nerve. SO4- Superior Oblique, Lateral rectus = LR6- lateral rectus by 6th cranial nerve, O3 -Others by third cranial nerve

Syndromes Associated with Third Nerve Palsy

- Benedicts syndrome- Ipsilateral third nerve palsy and tremor and ataxia
- Weber's Syndrome – Ipsilateral third nerve palsy and a contralateral hemiplegia

Pupil Sparing Palsy/Pupil Involving Palsy

Surgical Causes like aneurysm and compressive lesions always involve pupil. Medical causes of third nerve palsy like DM and Hypertension cause pupil sparing third nerve palsy

12. Ans. (d) Interstitial nucleus of Cajal

Ref: Yanoff's 4th Ed Pg 916

Structures in the Control of the vertical Gaze Include

- Rostral Interstitial nucleus of the Medial Longitudinal Fasciculus
- Interstitial nucleus of Cajal
- Posterior Commissure

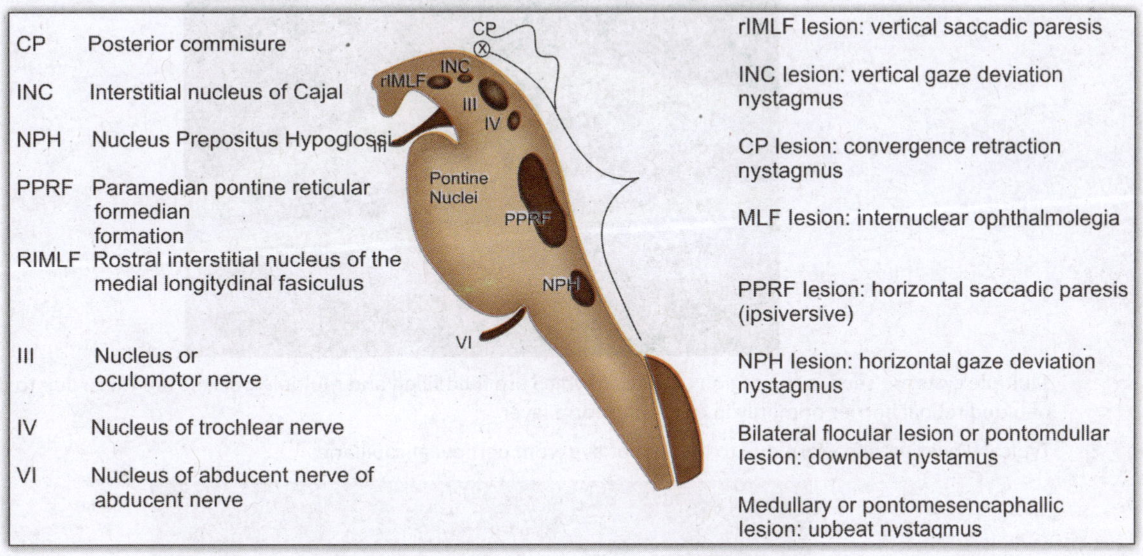

Fig: Supranuclear centers for control of eye movements

13. Ans. (d) Corneal Tattooing

Ref: Yanoff's 4th Ed Pg 51, Textbook of Ophthalmology By HV Nema 6th Ed Pg 241

Stenopaic Slit is Used in

- **Axis of the cylinder:** Stenopic slit is used to measure astigmatism and is a part of trial frame
- **Fincham test**: It differentiates angle closure glaucoma with cataract. The coloured halos in glaucoma must be differentiated from those found in acute purulent conjunctivitis and early cataractous changes. In conjunctivits, the halos can be eliminated by irrigating the discharge. The halos of glaucoma and immature cataract may be differentiated by Fincham's test in which a stenopaeic slit is passed across the pupil. During this test glaucomatous halo remains intact, while a halo due to cataract is broken up into segments. Emsley-Fincham stenopaeic-slit test demonstrating breaking up of halos due to immature cataract into different segments.
- **Optical iridectomy:** It helps the ophthalmologist to know the axis at which optical iridectomy to be done where there would be maximum gain of vision in cases of non homogenous corneal opacity

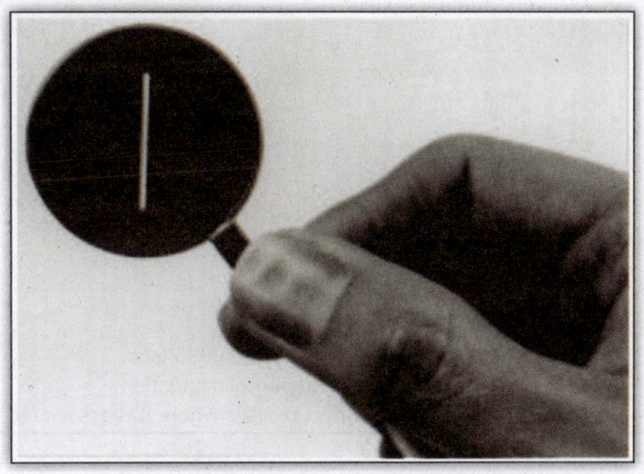

14. Ans. (b) Cystoid macular edema

Ref: Kanski 8th Ed Pg 295, Khurana 6th ed page 214

Hints to Diagnosis

- Painless loss of vision
- H/O Arthritis

- H/O Cataract surgery
- Fluorescein angiography picture shows early hyperfluorescent spots due to leakage that progress to a characteristic petaloid pattern (***Flower petal pattern***) of dye accumulation within microcystic spaces in the outer plexiform layer.

Cystoid Macular Edema	
Etiology	Post operative inflammation, Diabetes, Epinephrine, Uveitis, Retinitis pigmentosa, Vein occlusion
Pathogenesis	Accumulation of fluid in the outer plexiform and inner nuclear layers of the retina with the formation of cyst-like changes
Clinical features	Frequent complication of cataract surgery. in most cases it is clinically insignificant, does not produce any visual problem and undergoes spontaneous regression. In few cases, a significant CME typically produces visual diminution one to three months after cataract extraction
Fundoscopy	Honeycomb appearance
OCT Picture of cystoid macular edema	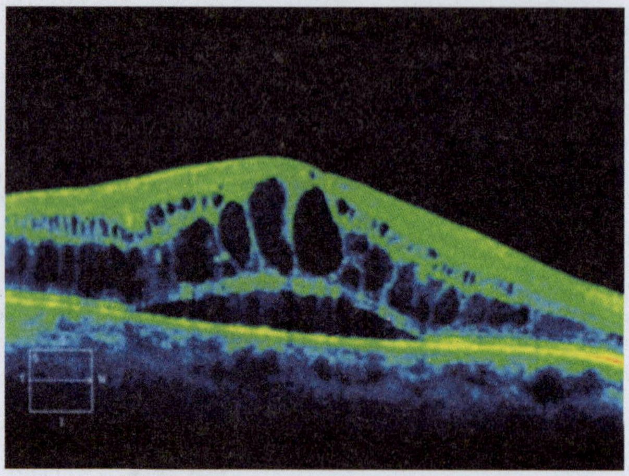 Multiple cysts are seen in the region of macula which are fluid filled and multiple pockets are there due to disruption of blood retinal barrier primarily in outer plexiform layer
Fluorescein angiography	Typical flower petal pattern due to leakage of dye from perifoveal capillaries. 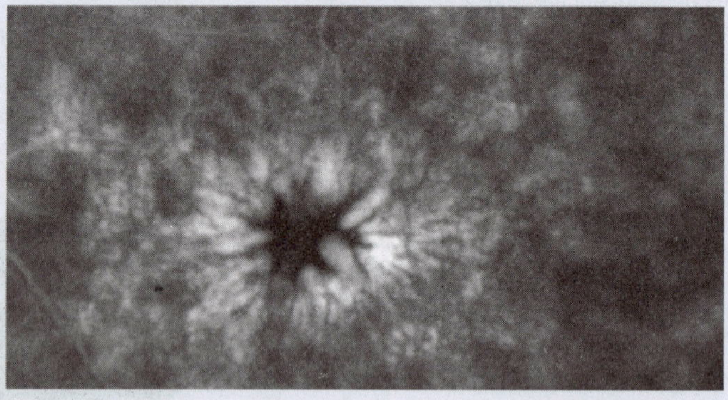
Treatment	• Wait and watch • Topical NSAIDS • Anti VEGF • Intravitreal steroids • Carbonic anhydrase inhibitors • Macular grid photocoagulation • Vitrectomy (in cases where it is associated with vitreomacular traction

15. Ans. (c) Drusen

Ref: Kanski 8th Ed Pg 602, Khurana 6th ed page 267 The image seen in the following picture is of drusen.

The image seen in the following picture is of drusen

Drusens are characteristic of Dry ARMD

Drusens are intrapapillary refractile bodies, which lie deep to the surface of the disc tissue in childhood and emerge out by the early teens. Thus, in children they present as pseudo papilloedema and by teens they can be recognised ophthal moscopically as waxy pea-like irregular retractile bodies.

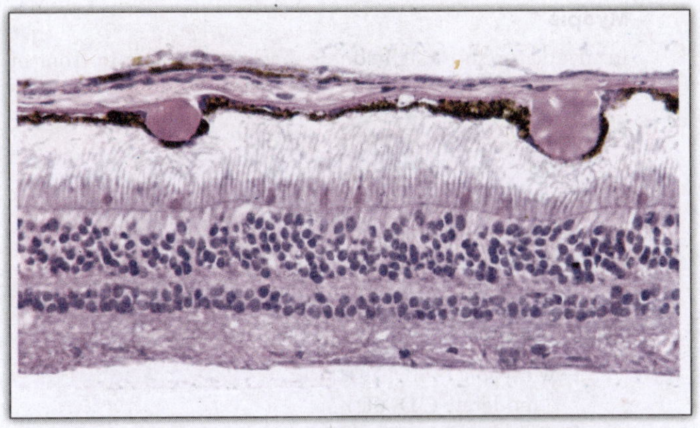

Fig: Histological section shows drusen forming between the RPE and Bruch's membrane in an early AMD case.

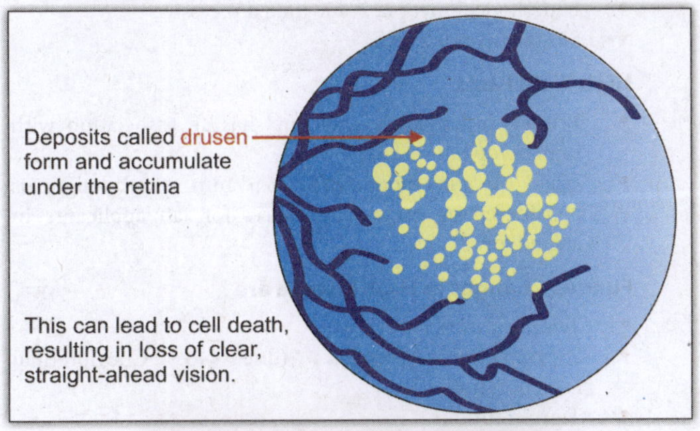

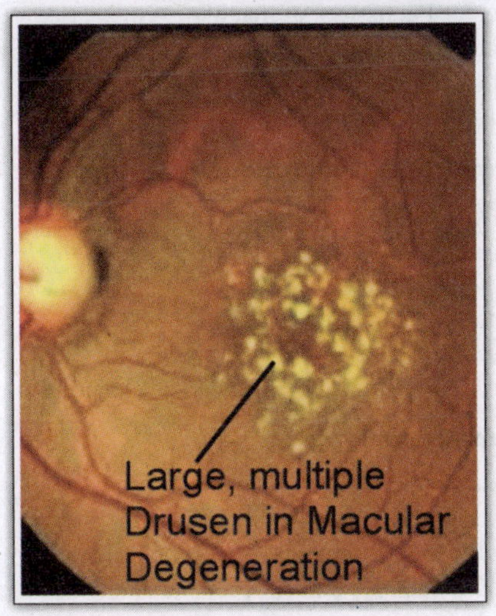

FAQs Regarding Retinal Layers

- Microaneurysms: Inner nuclear layer
- Cotton wool spots: Nerve fibre layer
- Normal retinal vasculature: In between outer plexiform and inner nuclear layer.
- Hard exudates: Outer plexiform layer
- Central serous retinopathy: Splitting at RPE level
- Dot & Blot hemorrhage: Inner nuclear layer > outer plexiform layer
- Wet ARMD: Abnormal vessels start forming in Bruch's membrane of choroid

16. Ans. (b) Posterior Subcapsular cataract

Ref: Kanski 8th Ed Pg 270

Clinical Features of Posterior Subcapsular Cataract

Posterior subcapsular cataracts (PSC) are opacities located in posterior cortical layer, directly under the posterior capsule. This type of cataract tends to occur in younger patients than cortical or nuclear sclerotic cataracts. As these types of opacities are more near to the visual axis so the visual disturbances are more pronounced

Clinical Features

- Glare
- Difficulty with near greater than distance vision (typically, but many patients may notice the opposite)
- Often rapidly diminishing vision

17. Ans. (b) Mitochondrial function disorder

Ref: Kanski 7th ed chapter 15, Clinical Pediatric Neurology Ronald B. David Pg 304

NARP Syndrome	
Full form	Neuropathy, Ataxia, & Retinitis Pigmentosa
Inheritance	Maternally inherited
Defect	Mitochondrial mutations
Clinical features	Multisystem disorder characterised by developmental delay, retinitis pigmentosa, ataxia, sensory polyneuropathy, muscle weakness, epilepsy and dementia
Investigations	MRI → Moderate diffuse cerebral and cerebellar atrophy and symmetric lesions of the basal ganglia
Leigh syndrome	>95% of mtDNA molecules are mutant More severe clinical, neuroradiologic and neuropathologic picture

AIIMS NOVEMBER 2017

18. Ans. (a) Non Proliferative Diabetic Retinopathy

Ref: Parson 22nd ed page 307, Khurana 6th ed page 517, 518

Fluorescein Angiography is done to identify the retinal vessels pattern- Leakage or Pooling

Contraindication: Renal Insufficiency or allergy to fluorescein

Procedure: we put sodium fluorescein dye 5 mL, 10 %, in antecubital vein

Take fundus photo with yellow green filter at various time intervals

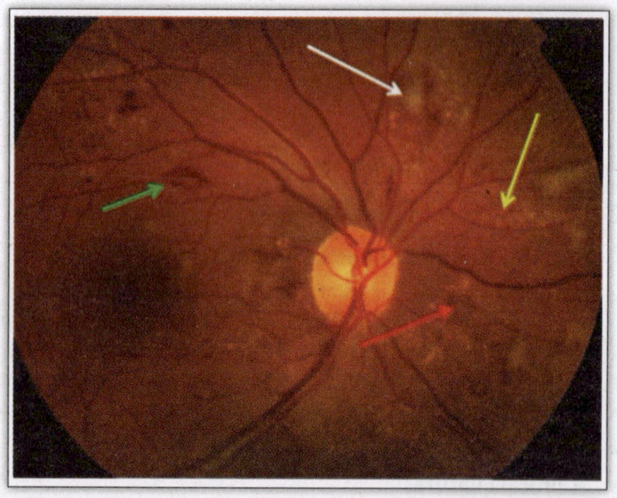

Fig: Non proliferative diabetic retinopathy (Moderate): Fundus with exudate (yellow arrow), microaneurysms (red arrow), cotton wool spot (white arrow), nerve fibre layer haemorrhage (green arrow)

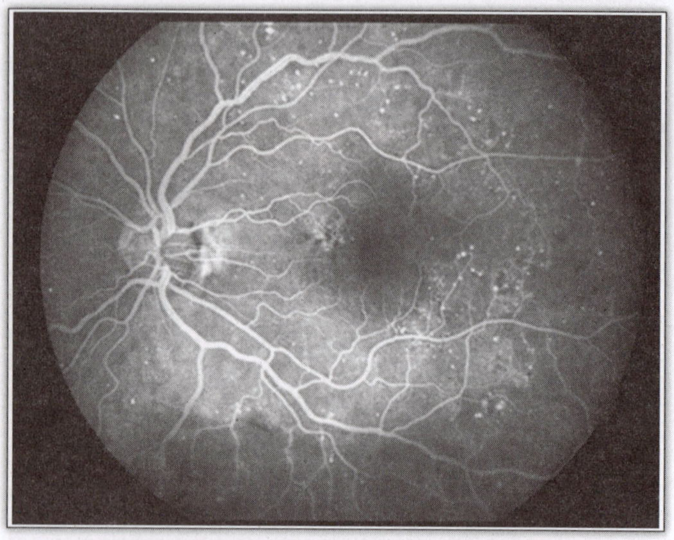

Fig: Non proliferative diabetic retinopathy (Moderate): Fluorescein Angiogram showing micro aneurysms

19. Ans. (b) Myopia

Ref: Parson 22nd ed page 68, Khurana 6th ed page 32

In myopia or short sightedness the rays converge in front of retina as shown in the given picture hence the answer is Myopia.

Myopia

In myopia or short sightedness the rays converge in front of retina

Types

- Axial
- Curvatural
- Positional
- Index
- Accomodation

Epidemiology

- Low myopia (< 3D, 29%)
- 7 % moderate (3D–6D)
- Pathological Myopia > 6D

Genetics

- Pathological myopia 2% X-linked recessive
- Simple myopia is AD

High Yield Facts

- Primary open angle glaucoma has an association with high myopia.
- High Myopia more than 26.5 mm Axial length is considered as exclusion criteria for jab applicants in armed forces

Fundus Changes in High Myopia are

- Temporal crescent
- Supratraction crescent (due to Chorioretinal Degeneration)
- Tigroid fundus
- Foster Fuchs spot at macula
- Lattice degeneration and snail track degeneration
- Posterior staphyloma
- Ring scotoma may be seen

Hypermetropia (Farsightedness)

- The rays converge behind the retina
- Size of eyeball is small
- Smaller cornea
- Shallow ant chamber
- Pseudopapillitis shot silk appearance
- Predisposition to primary angle closure glaucoma

Hypermetropia Types

- Axial
- Curvatural
- Index hypermetropia
- Positional Hypermetropia
- Aphakia

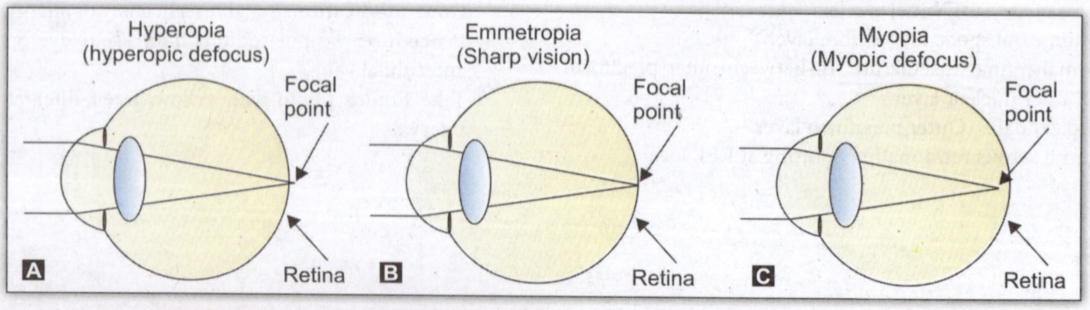

20. Ans. (b) Intravenous antibiotics

Ref: Parson 22nd ed page 235, Khurana 6th ed page 170-172

Intravenous antibiotics have no role in management of endophthalmitis. All clinical trials have shown the results are not superior of adding intravenous antibiotics in the management of Endophthalmitis.

Endophthalmitis	
Definition	**Infection of uveal tissue with involvement of vitreous**
Most common cause	Postoperative endophthalmitis
Postoperative endophthalmitis	• Delayed/Post Yag: MC cause- P. acnes > Fungal • MC in total- Coagulase Negative Staphylococci • MC-Post traumatic- Bacillus Cereus • MC cause in AIDS Patients: Candida
Clinical features	• Hypopyon and anterior segment inflammation • USG posterior segment suggestive of mild to moderate amplitude spikes • Exudates and associated corneal edema can be noted • Lids and conjunctiva may be swollen • Amaurotic cat's eye reflex (yellowish white reflex) can be seen through pupil
Treatment	• Intravitreal antibiotics • Pars plana vitrectomy • Topical fortified antibiotics • Cycloplegics • Anti glaucoma medications
Prevention	• Hand scrub • Sterilization of instruments

21. Ans. (b) Non Hodgkin's Lymphoma

Ref: Roy and Fraunfelder's Current Ocular Therapy by Frederick Hampton Roy, Frederick W. Fraunfelder, Frederick T. Fraunfelder 6th ed page 294, Orbital Imaging By F. Allan Midyett, Suresh Kumar Mukherji Page 192

Recall Bias

Some recallers think that most common epithelial tumor of lacrimal gland was asked. In that case Pleomorphic adenoma will be the correct answer.

Lacrimal gland tumors account for approximately 10% of all orbital tumors. Lacrimal gland tumors can arise from cells of epithelial origin (20%), such as acinar or ductal elements, or from non epithelial cells (80%), such as inflammatory, neural, vascular, or fatty elements. Epithelial tumors are evenly divided into benign (55%) and malignant lesions (45%). Pleomorphic adenoma is most common benign tumor while Adenoid cystic carcinoma is most common malignant tumor. Most common epithelial neoplasm of Lacrimal gland overall is also Pleomorphic adenoma

Adenoid cystic carcinoma is the most common malignant tumor of the lacrimal gland accounting for approximately 50% of malignant lacrimal gland tumors and 25% of all lacrimal gland tumors

Non-Hodgkin's lymphomas (NHLs) are among the most common primary tumors occurring in the ocular adnexa. Primary lacrimal gland lymphoma (LGL) is relatively rare. The mucosa-associated lymphoid tumor (MALT) subtype of extranodal marginal zone lymphoma is the most frequent histological subtype.

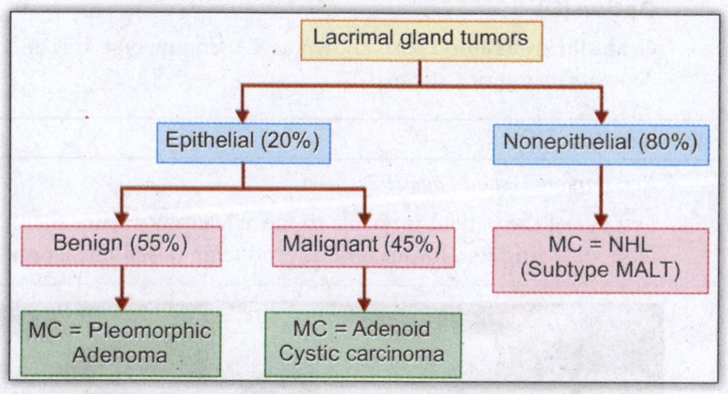

22. Ans. (c) Staphyloma

Ref: Parson 22nd ed page 229, Vaughan and Asbury's General Ophthalmology 17th Ed ch 7, Khurana 6th ed page 153

Option (A)

Keratoconus is a progressive disorder in which the cornea assumes a conical shape secondary to stromal thinning and protrusion Associations of Keratoconus:

- **Systemic disorders:** Down, Turner, Ehlers Danlos and Marfan syndromes, atopy, osteogenesis imperfecta, mitral valve prolapse and mental retardation.
- **Ocular associations** include vernal keratoconjunctivitis, blue sclera, aniridia, ectopia lentis, Leber congenital amaurosis, retinitis pigmentosa and persistent eye rubbing.

Option (B)

Keratomalacia refers to corneal necrosis due to vitamin A deficiency.

Option (C)

Staphyloma results from localised bulging of weak and thin outer tunic of the eyeball (cornea, sclera or both) with an incarceration of Uveal tissue. *Most commonly the disease causing weakening of the globe is accompanied by raised intraocular pressure and both contribute to the development of Staphyloma.*

Staphyloma		
Type	**Description**	**Etiology**
Anterior staphyloma	Bulging of cornea	Sloughing corneal ulcer forming "Pseudocornea", Seconday glaucoma
Intercalary staphyloma	Bulge in limbal area lined by root of iris. From limbus to 2 mm behind the limbus	Healing of a perforating injury or a peripheral corneal ulcer, secondary angle closure glaucoma, Marginal corneal ulcer, Anterior scleritis
Ciliary staphyloma	Bulge of weak sclera lined by ciliary body about 2–3 mm away from the limbus	Perforating injury, scleritis and absolute glaucoma
Equatorial staphyloma	Bulge of sclera lined by the choroid in the equatorial region	Pathological myopia
Posterior staphyloma	Bulge of weak sclera lined by the choroid behind the equator, most commonly near the optic nerve head	Pathological myopia, posterior scleritis and perforating injuries. (MC Staphyloma in Myopia)

Option (D)

Granular dystrophy: Also known as 'Groenouw type I, is an autosomal dominant dystrophy characterised by milky-granular hyaline deposits in anterior stroma.

23. Ans. (d) VI

Ref: Parson 21st ed page 397

Left eye of the patient is unable to move laterally, Hence there is lateral rectus palsy. Lateral rectus is supplied by 6th nerve. It can be a false localizing sign for the lesions producing raised intracranial tension.

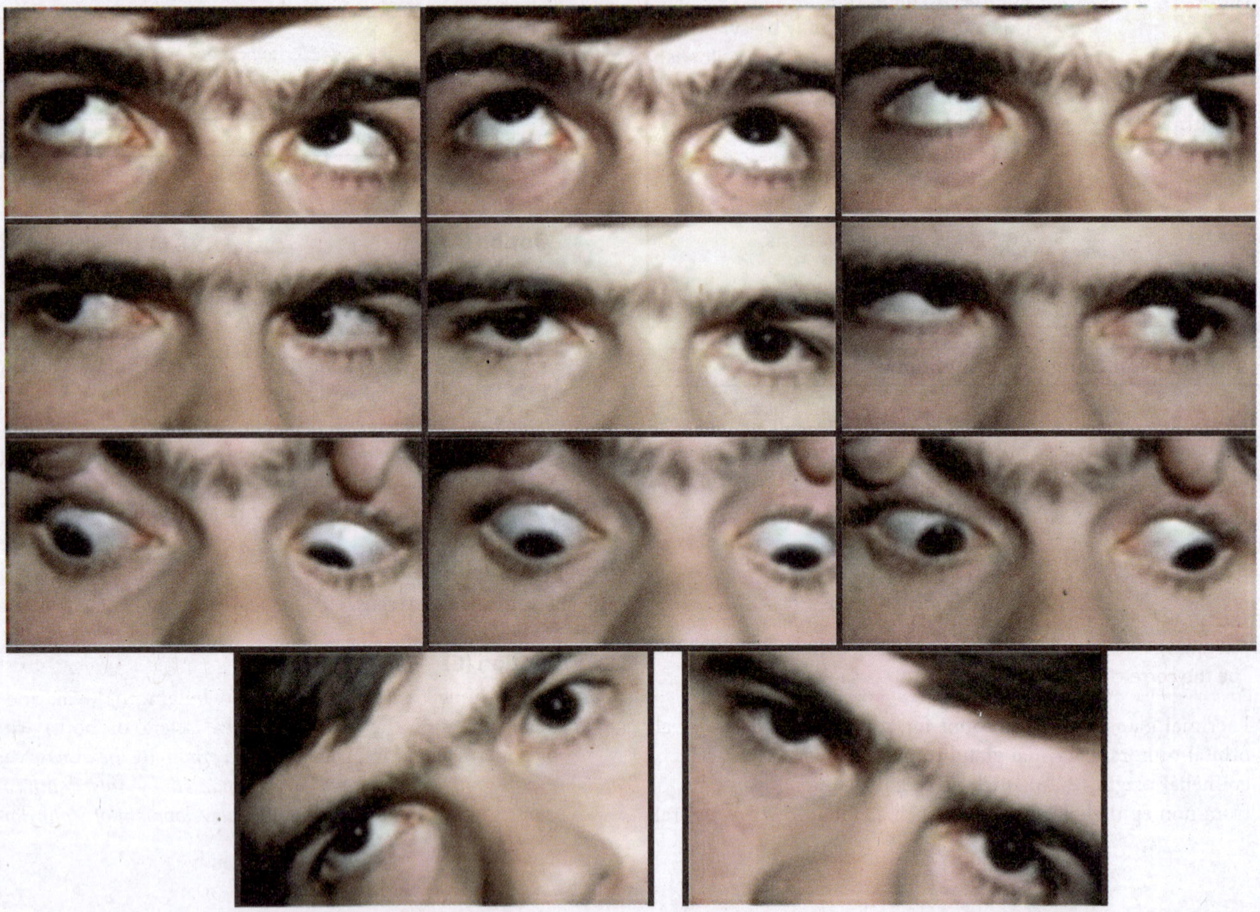

Fig: Right superior oblique muscle (6th-Trochlear nerve) palsy: There is a right hypertropia in primary position that increases in left gaze and with head tilt to the right. Mnemonic- WOOG = worse on opposite gaze, that is not there on left head tilt. So patient would like to have left head tilt. So remember mnemonic BOOT- Better on opposite tilt

3rd, 4th and 6th Cranial Nerve Palsy

	3rd (Oculomotor) nerve palsy	Superior oblique muscle (6th-Trochlear nerve) palsy	6th cranial nerve (abducent) palsy
Causes	Posterior circulation aneurysm Brainstem lesions Microvascular ischemia Cavernous sinus disease	Posterior circulation aneurysm Brainstem lesions Microvascular ischemia Cavernous sinus disease	Posterior circulation aneurysm, Brainstem lesions, Microvascular ischemia, Cavernous sinus disease, Elevated intracranial pressure, Superior orbital fissure syndrome
Clinical features	• Diplopia: Horizontal and vertical • Abduction and depression in primary position: due to unopposed action of the lateral rectus and superior oblique muscles. The intact superior oblique muscle also causes intorsion of the eye at rest,which increases on attempted downgaze	• Diplopia- oblique/tortional diplopia worse on downward gaze • Combination of Elevation, extorsion, esotropia (Since superior oblique does depression, intorsion, abduction)	• Diplopia (uncrossed, horizontal diplopia) on lateral gaze to the ipsilateral side worse at distance • Head turn towards the paralyzed side • Esotropia (one or both eyes turns inward) i.e. convergent squint in long standing LR Palsy
	• Normal abduction as lateral rectus is intact. • Limited adduction due to medial rectus weakness. • Limited elevation due to weakness of the superior rectus and inferior oblique. • Limited depression due to weakness of inferior rectus • Varying degree of ptosis • In complete 3rd nerve involvement, dilated pupil and defective accommodation due to parasympathetic palsy	• Ipsilateral hypertropia • The hypertropia is greater when they look to the opposite side • Hypertropia is greater when they tilt their head toward the same side • Spontaneous tilt of head to the contralateral side to compensate for diplopia • Diagnosis is based on either Head tilt or Parks Bielschowsky three step test	• Headache vomiting pain if a/w lesions causing raised Intracranial tension

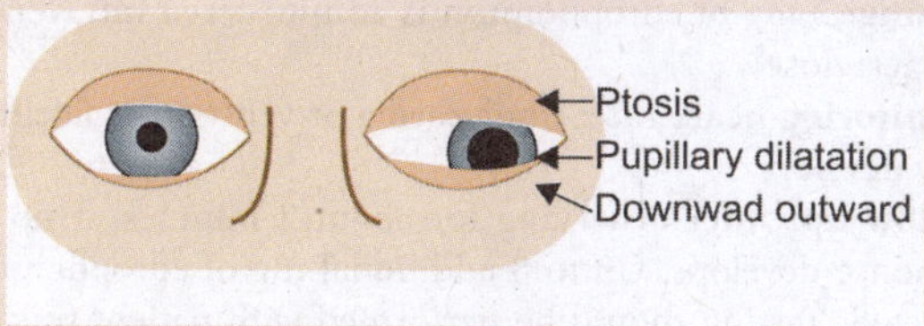

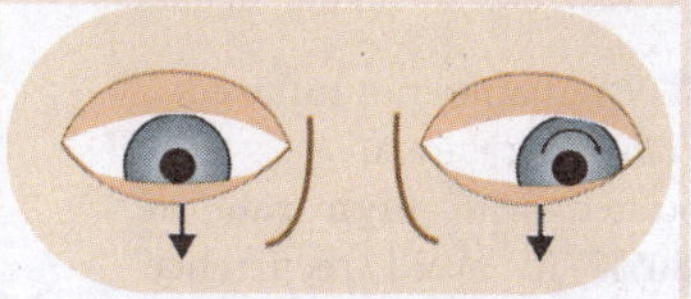
Extosion on downward gaze

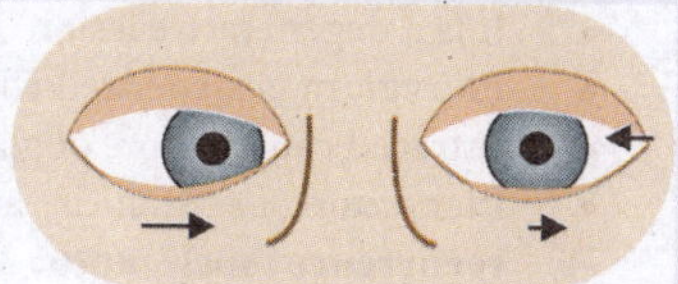
Lateral gaze palsy

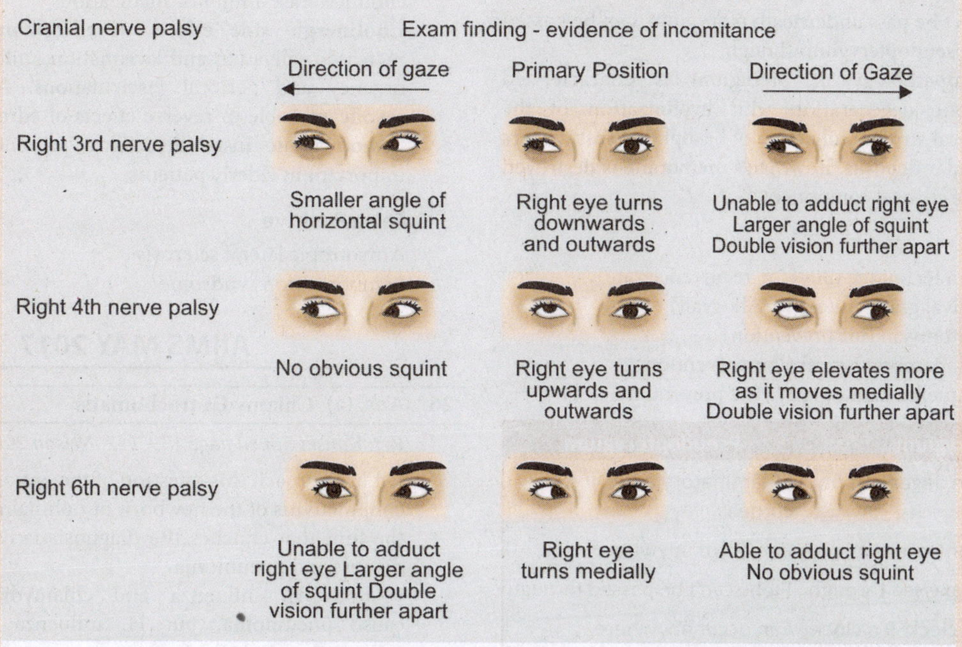

Interpretation of incomitance (that is, angle of squint varies with direction of gaze)

Mnemonic: In primary gaze see the deviation of eye DUM; Downward and Outward = 3rd nerve, Upward and Outward = 4th nerve, Medially = 6th nerve

24. Ans. (a) Pterygium

Ref: Khurana 6th ed page 87

This triangular encroachment of the conjunctiva over the cornea is known as Pterygium

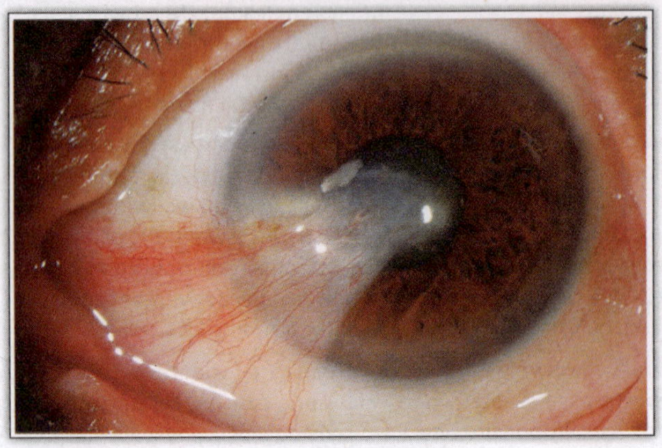

© JM Varas (Creative Commons)

Fig: Pterygium

Pterygium

- Pterygium is a growth onto the cornea, usually nasally, of fibrovascular tissue that is continuous with the conjunctiva. It occurs in the palpebral fissure area, more often nasally than temporally, although either or both ("double" pterygium) occur.
- It is a degenerative lesion
- Pterygium is associated with UV radiation not infrared.
- Infrared causes more of glass blowers cataract.
- Pterygium excision is associated with **high rate of recurrence such upto 30-80%.** To avoid recurrence autograft of conjunctiva, mitomycin c, 5- fluorouracil can be used.
- Probe can't be pass underneath pterygium, can be passed through pseudopterygium though.
- The histopathology of pterygium is characterized by elastotic degeneration with hyalinization of the conjunctival stroma, collection of basophilic elastic fibers and granular deposits. Bowman's membrane is destroyed within the corneal component

Treatment:

- Bare sclera technique (30–80% recurrence rate)
- Conjunctival graft (Autograft/Allograft)
- Use of mitomycin (for prevention)
- Amniotic membrane graft (For prevention)
- Partial Lamellar keratoplasty (For prevention)

Pterygium	Pseudopterygium
Stromal tissue degeneration	Inflammatory adhesion to cornea
More common nasally	Can occur anywhere
Probe can be passed through	Probe can't be passed through
Mostly at 3 o clock -9 o clock position	Can occur anywhere
History of old age or UV exposure	History of chemical, thermal injury

25. Ans. (a) Myasthenia Gravis

Ref: Parson 20th ed page 455, Newsom-Davis, J. (1993). Myasthenia gravis and the Lambert-Eaton myasthenic syndrome. Prescribers' Journal 33(5): 205-11

This is a case of myasthenia gravis and IV Edrophonium is given here. Most myasthenic muscles respond in 30 to 45 seconds after injection; Improvement in strength that may persist for up to 5 minutes. Edrophonium (Tensilon) Testing is readily performed at the bedside. It is not as sensitive, or specific, as the serological and electrophysiological studies

NOTE

There was a doubt that there was unilateral ptosis given in the question asked in the exam. Remember Asymmetric ptosis is there in 70 percent of Myasthenia gravis patients according to Critical Care Study Guide: Text and Review by Gerard J. Criner, Gilbert E. D'Alonzo

Edrophonium (Tensilon) Testing

Action: The drug inhibits acetylcholinesterase and Prolongs presence of neurotransmitter, acetylcholine, in the Neuromuscular junction. Its advantage is that it is rapid onset and short acting drug

Method

Dosing: 2 mg of edrophonium is administered intravenously as a test dose

Monitoring heart rate: Bradycardia or ventricular fibrillation may develop

Follow-up: After observing for about 2 minutes, if no clear response develops. Up to 8 additional mg of edrophonium is injected. Testing should be performed with patient free of all cholinesterase-inhibitor medications

Cholinergic side effects of edrophonium: May include increased salivation and lacrimation, mild sweating, flushing, urgency and perioral fasciculations. Atropine should be readily available to reverse effects of edrophonium in case of hemodynamic instability. Extra precautions are especially important in elderly patients

False Positive

Amyotropic lateral sclerosis

Lambort eaton syndrome

AIIMS MAY 2017

26. Ans. (a) Chlamydia trachomatis

Ref: Kanski 7th ed page 139-142, Nelson 20th ed page 1495, 3037

Let us approach this question of the options, all four can cause conjunctivitis of the newborn or ophthalmia neonatorum. But the hint that clinches the diagnosis is history of respiratory distress and pneumonia.

Both H. influenza and chlamydia trachomatis can cause pneumonia, but H. influenza causes ophthalmia neonatorum only in immunocompromised cases. The child in question has a WBC count of 14300/dL which means he is immunocompetent. Thus our answer of choice here is option (A) chlamydia trachomatis.

Ophthalmia Neonatorum

It is conjunctivitis happening in first one month of life.

Causes of Ophthalmia Neonatorum and its Treatment		
Time of on-set of disease	**Etiology**	**Treatment**
2-4 hours	Chemical	Erythromycin ointment
<48 hours	N. gonorrhoeae	Ceftriaxone
48-72 hours	Staph aureus, Streptococcus, Haemophilus influenzae	Bacitracin, Gentamycin, Tobramycin

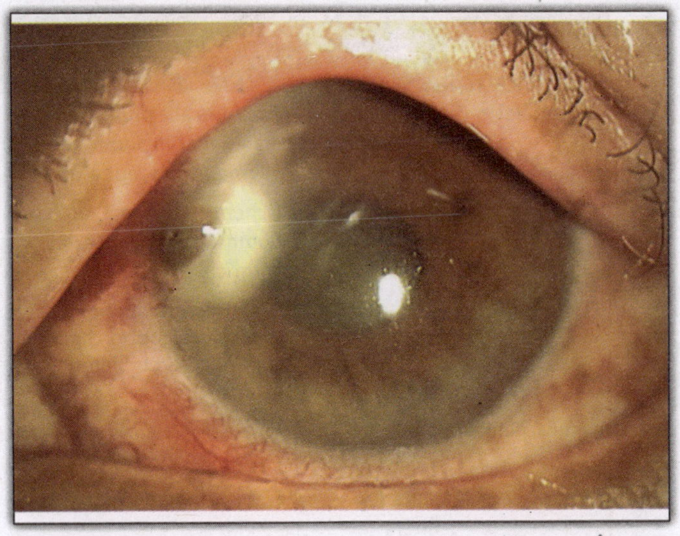

Fig: Corneal ulcer with perforation on superionasal area

27. Ans. (a) Suprachoroidal haemorrhage

Ref: Kanski's clinical ophthalmology 8th edn page 637

The image shows corneal ulcer with perforation, however, this question can be solved without the image provided.

Hypotony Maculopathy

Hypotony maculopathy is low intraocular pressure associated with chorioretinal folds near macula, optic nerve head edema and vessel tortuosity. Most common cause is filtering surgery.

Causes of Hypotonic Maculopathy			
Postoperative hypotony	**Traumatic hypotony**	**Bilateral hypotony**	**Miscellaneous forms of hypotony**
• Mitomycin C toxicity of the ciliary body • Overfiltration • Bleb leak • Wound leak • Iridocyclitis • Cyclodialysis • Ciliochoroidal detachment • Retinal detachment	• Scleral perforation/corneal perforation • Retinal detachment • Cyclodialysis • Iridocyclitis • Ciliochoroidal detachment	• Osmotic dehydration • Diabetic coma • Uremia • Myotonic dystrophy	Ciliary body hypoperfusion from vascular occlusive disease

Clinical Presentation of Hypotonic Maculopathy

Patients afflicted with hypotony maculopathy typically present with loss of central vision and distortions as well as a relative hyperopia due to reduction of the anterior-posterior diameter of the eye. On clinical examination, optic nerve swelling associated with folding of the retina and choroid in the posterior pole may be noted. The macular folds often radiate outward from the fovea.

Fluorescein angiography can also demonstrate chorioretinal folds and differentiate choroidal folds from retinal folds. Characteristic findings include an irregular increase in background choroidal fluorescence, producing a series of hyperfluorescent streaks corresponding to the crests of the choroidal folds. The troughs of the folds appear hypofluorescent. There is also some leakage from the optic nerve capillaries but usually not from the retinal capillaries.

28. Ans. (b) Bitemporal hemianopia

Ref: Kanski's clinical ophthalmology 8th ed page 820

Visual Field Defects		
Site	**Causes**	**Defect**
Optic nerve	Neuritis, neuropathy	Complete blindness, light reflex absent (B/L and consensual), near and accommodation reflex present
Proximal part of optic nerve		Ipsilateral blindness, contralateral hemianopia ipsilateral direct light reflex & contralateral indirect absent, near and accommodation reflex present

Contd...

Visual Field Defects

Site	Causes	Defect
Central lesions of the chiasma	Tumours like pituitary, craniopharyngioma, mets, 3rd ventricle glioma, hydrocephalus and arachnoiditis	Bitemporal hemianopia Bitemporal hemianopic loss of light reflex
Lateral chiasmal lesions	Ischemic lesions of carotid or postr. Communicating arteries, distention of 3rd ventricle	Binasal hemianopia Binasal hemianopic paralysis of papillary reflex
Optic tract	Syphilitic meningitis or gumma, TB & tumours of optic thalamus, aneurysm of superior cerebellar or posterior cerebral arteries	Incongrous homonymous hemianopia Contralateral hemianopic papillary reaction (Wernicke's reaction)
Lateral geniculate body		Homonymous hemianopia Sparing of papillary reflex
Optic radiation – Superior fibers	Parietal lobe defects	Inferior quadrantic hemianopia or **pie on the floor** defect
Optic radiation – Inferior fibers	Temporal lobe defects	Superior quadrantinopia or **pie on the roof/sky** defect, light reflexes are normal, no optic atrophy
Anterior optic cortex/lobe (sparing the posterior tip)	Posterior cerebral artery lesions	**Key hole defect;** bilateral congruous homonymous hemianopia with macular sparing, normal light reflex and no optic atrophy
Posterior tip of occipital cortex (lobe)	Head injury	Congruous homonymous hemianopia with macular defects. Normal light reflex and no optic atrophy

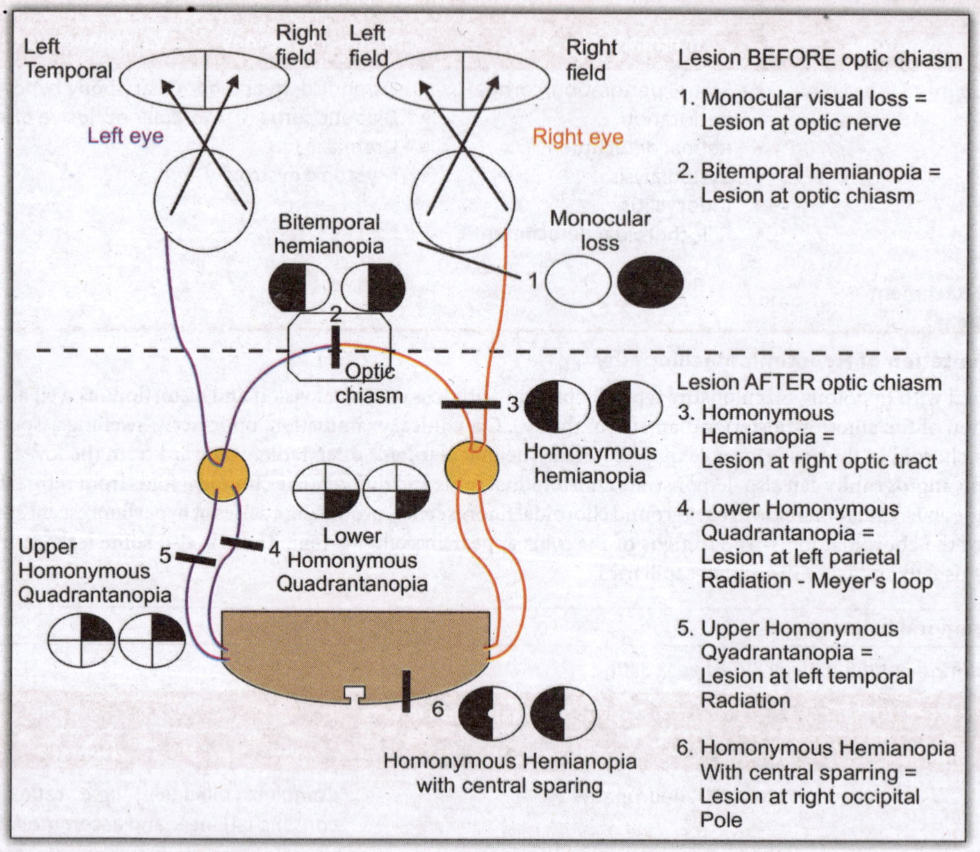

29. Ans. (a) Tonometry

Ref: Kanski's clinical ophthalmology 8th edn page 307–308. A.K. Khurana comprehensive ophthalmology 6th edn, page 510–511

Option (A)

The test seen in the picture is of Goldmann Applanation tonometry. Intraocular pressure is measured by an instrument called as Tonometer.

Option (B) Laser interferometry

Used to detect the maximum visual potential of the eye.

Option (C) Pachymetry

Used to measure corneal thickness.

Option (D)

Refractometry is the analytical method of measuring substances' refractive index.

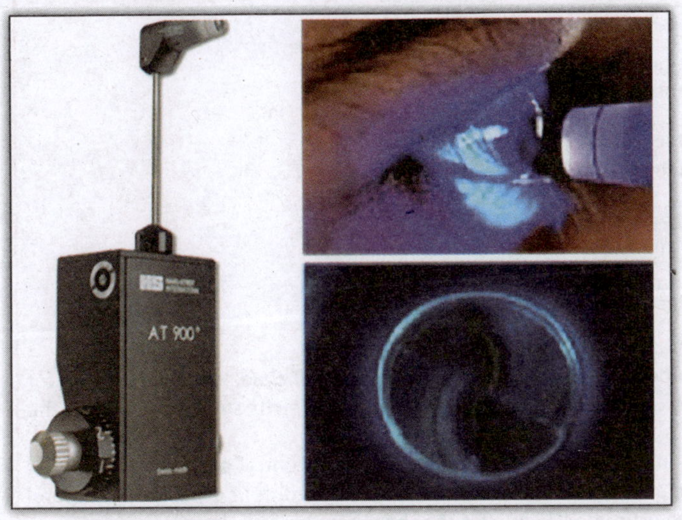

Fig: Goldmann tonometer and its application

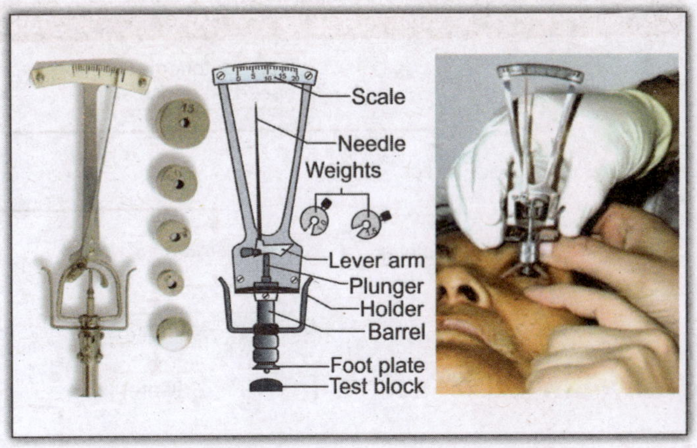

Fig: Schiotz tonometer and its application

Goldmann Applanation Tonometer Technique

- Most commonly used tonometer
- Consists of a double prism mounted on a slit lamp
- The prism applanates the cornea for surface area of diameter 3.06 mm
- The eye is anesthetised and tear film is stained with fluorescein
- Patient is made to sit in front of the slit lamp
- Cornea and biprisms are illuminated by cobalt light from slit lamp
- The biprism is advanced until such a time it touches the cornea
- The applanation force is provided until inner ends of two semicircles meet
- This is the end point
- IOP is measured by multiplying dial readings by 10

Schiotz Tonometer and its Application

Technique of Using a Schizont Tonometer

- **The cornea is anesthetised**
- Patient is asked to fix his eye on a target
- The foot plate is kept on the cornea
- It is customary to start with weight of 5.5 gms
- The reading is noted on a scale
- A conversion table is needed to convert the readings

Advantages of schizont tonometry is that it is cheap, easy to use and handy

Disadvantages are that it gives false readings when there is scleral rigidity as in high myopes or after scleral surgery

Tonometer
The intraocular pressure (IOP) is measured with the help of an instrument called tonometer
A tonometer uses certain physical principles to measure pressure within the globe. Basically, the force necessary to deform a globe is directly related to the pressure within that globe. Three styles of tonometer currently are in use. Indentation, or high-displacement, tonometers utilize a plunger to indent the cornea by a variable amount. This indentation displaces a significant volume of intraocular fluid at the time of corneal deformation and results in a near doubling of the IOP. Conversion tables, in turn, estimate the original IOP from the indentation tonometric value obtained. Applanation, or low-displacement, tonometers raise IOP negligibly, because they subject the eye to sufficient force only to flatten the cornea. The amount of force required to achieve a constant degree of corneal flattening is converted into IOP values. Noncontact tonometers flatten the cornea using a puff of air and the time required to flatten the cornea is correlated to estimated IOP. Each form of tonometer has a place in the examination of eyes

Contd...

Tonometer

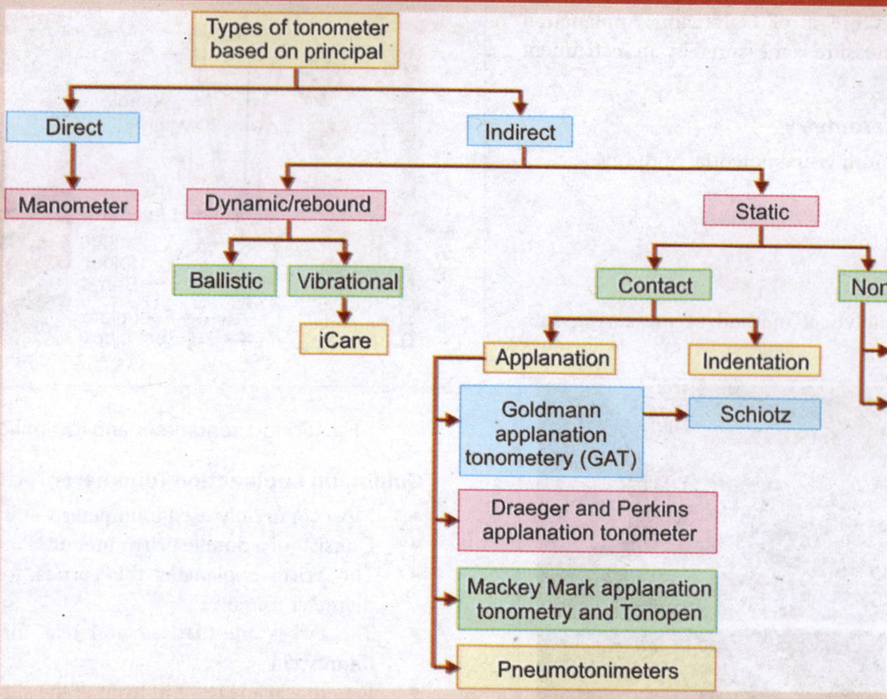

Footnote:

- **Goldmann applanation tonometry (GAT)** is a ***Gold standard*** Tonometer and is based on ***Imbert–Fick principle***, which states that for an ideal, dry, thin-walled sphere, the pressure (P) inside the sphere equals the force (F) necessary to flatten its surface divided by the area (A) of flattening (i.e. $P = F/A$)
- **Pneumotonometers** are also based on the principle of applanation but, instead of using a prism, the central part of the cornea is flattened by a jet of air. Contact is not made with the subject's eye and topical anaesthesia is not required, so it is particularly useful for screening in the community. Pneumotonometer may be used to estimate IOP in eyes that have scarred and irregular corneas
- **Perkins** applanation tonometer uses a Goldmann prism adapted to a small light source
- **Schiotz tonometer** uses the principle of indentation tonometry, in which the extent of corneal indentation by a plunger of known weight is measured; it is now seldom used in clinical practice
- **Rebound/dynamic tonometry** (e.g. **iCare**) involves a 1.8 mm plastic ball attached to a wire; deceleration of the probe upon contact with the cornea is proportional to IOP. Because only a very small force is applied to the cornea a topical anaesthetic is not required. The instrument can be used for **self-monitoring** and screening in the community.
- **Drager and Perkins** are type of Goldman that can be used **without slit lamp**.
- In LASIK **Dynamic Contour Tonometer** is the application of choice.
- **Tonopen is a hand held tonometer** used for measuring IOP in diseased cornea and in children. Reichert tonopen based on Mackay Marg principle. It can measure extremes of IOP as well as in scarred or irregular corneas.
- **Mackay Marg/tonopen used for irregular corneas**

30. Ans. (b) After cataract

Ref: Kanski's clinical ophthalmology 8th edn page 294; A.K. Khurana comprehensive ophthalmology 6th edn, page 215

This is after cataract. This picture shows a cluster of Elschnig pearls that have formed behind the lens after cataract surgery. Remember if the question asks immediate vision loss post cataract surgery differentials are:

- Endophthalmitis
- Toxic anterior chamber syndrome (TASS)
- **Macular edema**

If there is a gradual vision loss post cataract surgery then the answer has to be

- After cataract or
- Posterior capsular opacification

Let us rule out options.

Option (A) Irvin Gass Syndrome

It is development of cystoids macular edema after cataract surgery. It is most common cause of visual loss/blurring in the postoperative period.

Option (C) UGH Syndrome

Uveitis glaucoma hyphaema syndrome: Complication seen with ACIOL > PCIOL lenses due to iris chaffing and pigment dispersion associated with hyphaema and inflammation in anterior chamber leading to high IOP. It can cause vision loss and mimic the presentation of endophthalmitis, but there is no vitritis.

Option (D) Endophthalmitis

It is inflammation of vitreous accompanied by uveal involvement. Can be seen in postoperative period at any time. It causes photophobia, pain and lacrimation and on fundus examination there is inflammation.

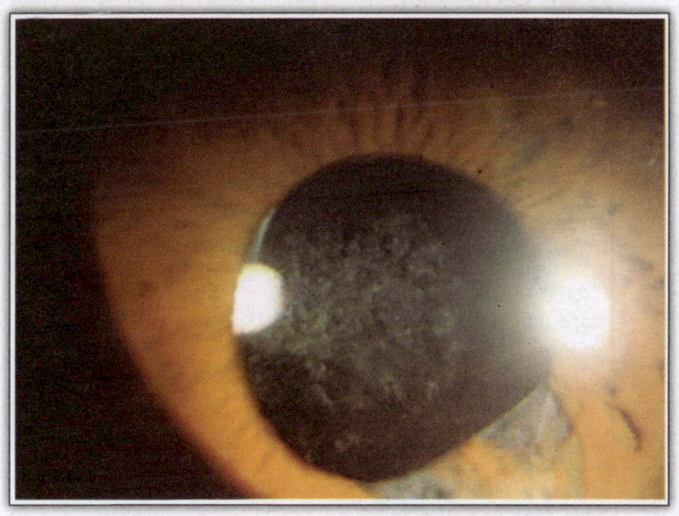

Fig: After cataract: This picture shows a cluster of Elschnig pearls that have formed behind the lens after cataract surgery. These grape-like clusters form from residual lens epithelial cells that migrate along the remaining capsular bag. They can be seen with a microscope and are usually visually insignificant

After Cataract

After Cataract can be of two types:

1. Anterior capsular opacification
2. **Posterior capsular opacification:** Posterior capsular opacification can be of two types: Soemeering Ring and Elsching pearls

Prevention

- Polishing of posterior capsule intra-operatively
- Using of square edge design IOL

Treatment: NdYAG Laser

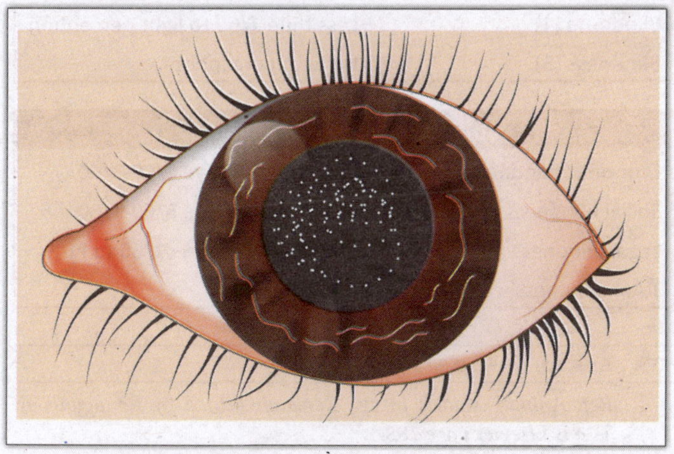

Fig: Elschnig Pearls results from proliferation of lens epithelium on the posterior capsule several months post cataract extraction.

31. Ans. (a) Ptosis of right eye

Ref: Kanski's clinical ophthalmology 8th edn page 40–42; A.K. Khurana comprehensive ophthalmology 6th edn, page 379

The picture shown is ptosis.

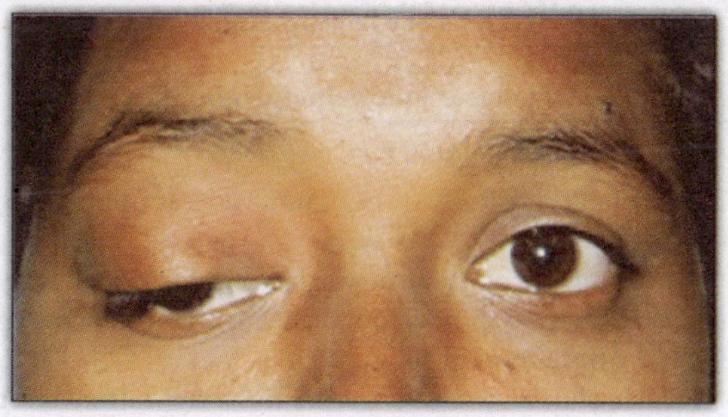

Fig: Ptosis of right eye

Ptosis

- Ptosis is Drooping of eyelid.
- Ectropion is eversion and entropion is inversion of eyelid
- Lagophthalmos is inability to close the eyelid seen in facial nerve palsy or tumors

Differential Diagnosis

Lugophthalmos, Ectropion, Entropion

Remember

Lagophthalmos is tested when the patient looks down, Ptosis is seen as drooping in primary position

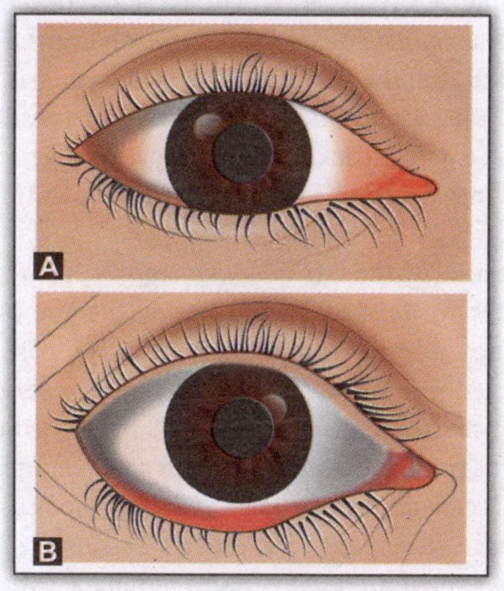

Figs A and B: **A.** Entropion—eyelid turned in; **B.** Ectropion—eyelid turned out

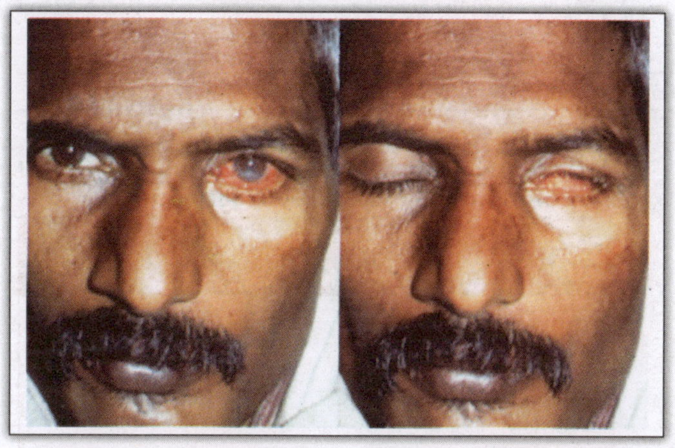

Fig: Classically you can observe that in left side image when the patient tries to close the eye, he is not able to close it fully. That is called Lagophthalmos

32. Ans. (a) Internuclear ophthalmoplegia

Ref: Yanoff 4th Ed page 919

The figure is classically of right intranuclear ophthalmoplegia (INO)

Internuclear ophthalmoplegia is characterized by paresis of eye adduction in horizontal gaze but not in convergence. It can be unilateral or bilateral.

During horizontal gaze, the **medial longitudinal fasciculus** (MLF) on each side of the brain stem enables abduction of one eye to be coordinated with adduction of the other. The MLF connects the following structures:

- 6th cranial nerve nucleus (which controls the lateral rectus, responsible for abduction)
- Adjacent horizontal gaze center (paramedian pontine reticular formation)
- Contralateral 3rd cranial nerve nucleus (which controls the medial rectus, responsible for adduction)

The MLF also connects the vestibular nuclei with the 3rd and 4th cranial nerve.

Internuclear ophthalmoplegia results from a lesion in the MLF. In young people, the disorder is commonly caused by multiple sclerosis and may be bilateral. In the elderly, internuclear ophthalmoplegia is typically caused by stroke and is unilateral. Rarely, the cause is Arnold-Chiari malformation, neurosyphilis, Lyme disease, tumor, head trauma, nutritional disorders (e.g. Wernicke encephalopathy, pernicious anemia), or drug intoxication (e.g. with tricyclic antidepressants or opioids).

If a lesion in the MLF blocks signals from the horizontal gaze center to the 3rd cranial nerve, the eye on the affected side cannot adduct (or adducts weakly) past the midline. The affected eye adducts normally in convergence because convergence does not require signals from the horizontal gaze center. This finding distinguishes internuclear ophthalmoplegia from 3rd cranial nerve palsy, which impairs adduction in convergence (this palsy also differs because it causes limited vertical eye movement, ptosis and pupillary abnormalities).

During horizontal gaze to the side opposite the affected eye, images are horizontally displaced, causing diplopia; nystagmus often occurs in the abducting eye. Sometimes vertical bilateral nystagmus occurs during attempted upward gaze.

33. Ans. (a) Anterior surface of cornea

Ref: Yanoff's 4th Ed page 38, 250, Guyton 13th ed page 639

About two third of the 59 diopters of the refractive power of eye is provided by the anterior surface of the cornea.

Refractive Index of Eye

	Refractive index	Refractive power
Eye		59 D
Cornea	1.37	40 D
Anterior surface of cornea	1.37	48 D
Posterior surface of cornea	1.37	–5D
Lens	1.39 (1.38 in the peripheral cortex to 1.41 in the central nucleus of the lens)	15 D
Anterior capsular surface of lens	1.364–1.381	5D
Posterior capsular surface of lens	1.338–1.357	8D
Aqueous humour	1.33	
Vitreous humour	1.34	

Contd...

34. Ans. (c) Vision 4/60 or less with best possible spectacle correction in better eye

Ref: Khurana 4th ed page 444

Blindness is defined under following headings: NPCB Criteria

- Inability of a person to count fingers from a distance of 6 meters or 20 feet
- **Technical definition:** Vision 6/60 or less with the best possible spectacle correction.

Diminution of field vision to 20 or less in better eye

WHO Classification of Blindness

Category (Grade)	Level
Normal vision (0)	6/6 to 6/18
Low vision (1)	Less than 6/18 to 6/60
Low vision (2)	Less than 6/60 to 3/60
Blindness (3)	Less than 3/60 to 1/60
Blindness (4)	Less than 1/60 to light perception
Blindness (5)	No light perception

Other Classification of Blindness

Economic blindness	Vision in better eye 6/60-3/60
Social blindness	Vision in better eye 3/60-1/60
Legal blindness	Vision in better eye <1/60 to PL
Total blindness	No PL

35. Ans. (a) 2–4 kg

Ref: Animal Models in eye Research Edited by Panagiotis A. Tsonis Elsevier page 188

Pharmacological Testing in Rabbit Eye

Rabbit	Age	Weight
NZA/Flemish giant	Very young	2 kg
NZA	Young	2.5–3.5 kg
NZA	Adult	3–4 kg

36. Ans. (a) + 20 D

Ref: Yanoff's 4th Ed page 69

> **NOTE**
>
> If the 20D is not in option mark the one that is lowest power.

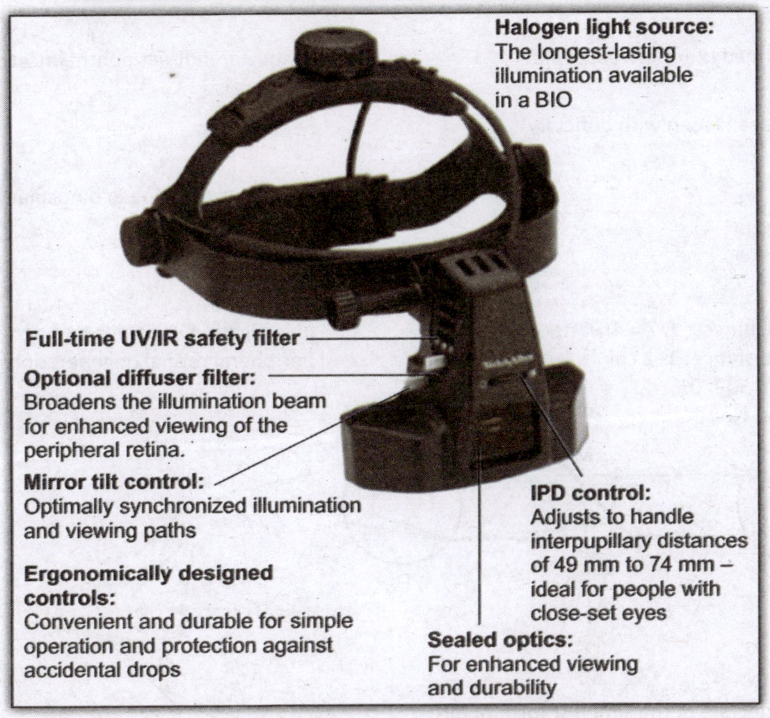

Fig: Indirect Ophthalmoscope labelled

Ophthalmoscopy		
	Direct ophthalmoscopy	Indirect ophthalmoscopy
Magnification	About 15 times	3 times if 20 D lens is used and 4 times if 14 D condensing lens is used 5 times when a +13D condensing lens is used
Condensing lens	Not required	Required
Illumination	Not so bright, so not useful in hazy media	Bright, so useful in hazy media
Examination distance	As close to the patient's eye as possible	At an Arm's length
Diameter of the field of observation view	Smaller (about 10° in diameter) About 2 disc dioptres (DD) 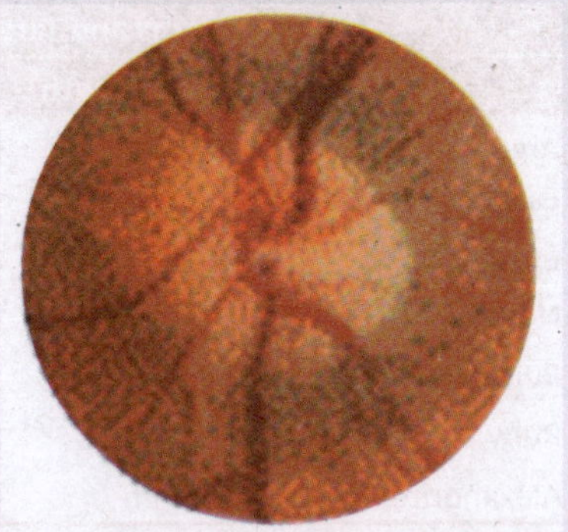	Wider (about 37° in diameter) About 8 disc dioptres (DD) 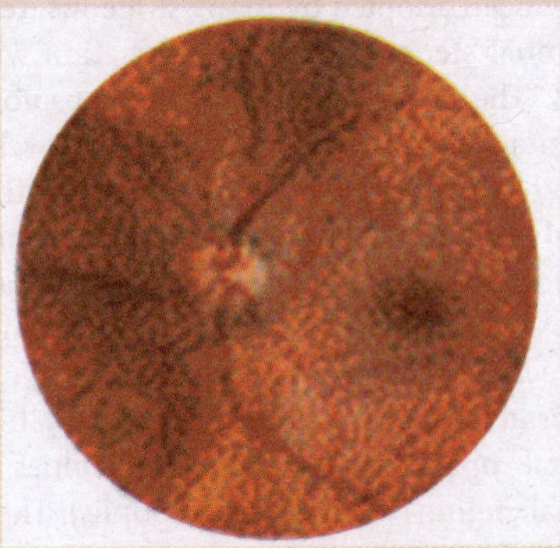

Contd...

Ophthalmoscopy		
	Direct ophthalmoscopy	**Indirect ophthalmoscopy**
Brightness	There is relatively low brightness	There is relatively greater brightness
Structures seen	Central retina only	Peripheral retina seen *(by using a scleral depressor in addition to the indirect ophthalmoscopy itself)*
Image of the fundus that is seen	Virtual & erect image	Real & inverted image
Stereopsis	Image formed is not stereoscopic	Binocular indirect ophthalmoscopy provides better stereopsis
Retina anterior to the equator	Not well seen (seen with difficulty)	Seen better
Scleral indentation	Difficult	Can be easily done in binocular indirect ophthalmoscopy
Visualization in hazy media	Poor	Better
Other comments	Image brightness: 1/2 = 4 watts Working distance: 1–2 cm Area seen: 50–70% Stereopsis: None	Investigation of choice to diagnose retinal detachment, ROP, peripheral retinal degenerations—Done in dilated pupil
Optics	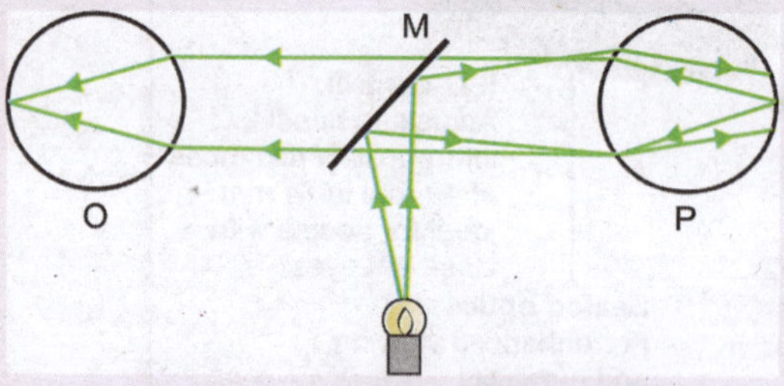 Optical principle of the simplest form of direct ophthalmoscope (O, observer's eye; P, patient's eye; M, semi-silvered mirror)	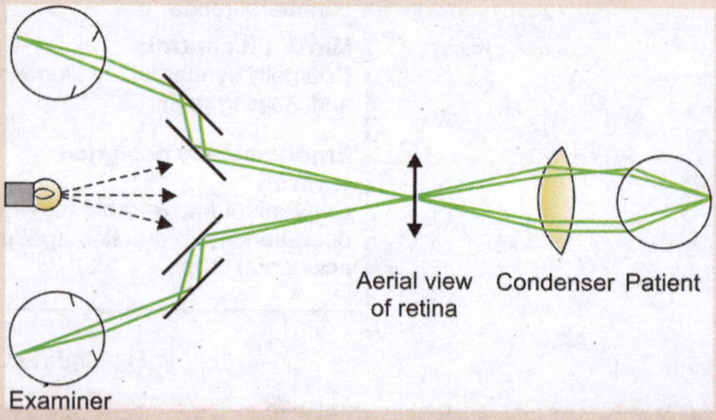 The light source mounted above and between the examiner's eyes illuminates the condenser, which images the source at the periphery of the patient's pupil. The illumination does not overlap the observation beam. The condenser lens is handheld; it forms an inverted aerial image of the retina

37. Ans. (a) 10-15

Ref: Kanski 8th ed page 285, Yanoff's 4th ed page 304

Femtosecond lasers (**femtosecond** is the SI unit of time equal to **10^{-15}**), used in refractive surgery for several years, have recently been adopted by many surgeons, replacing several of the manual steps of phacoemulsification with an automated process. The corneal incisions, the capsulorhexis and initial fragmentation of the crystalline lens, as well as astigmatism-relieving incisions, can all be performed with the laser.

- **Advantages** include greater precision and integrity of incisions, reduced phacoemulsification energy and possibly improved refractive outcomes due to more precise capsulorhexis placement.
- **Disadvantages** include substantially higher cost, longer total operating time and difficulties with technically challenging cases (e.g. small pupils). There is a substantial learning curve.
- Uses are:
  - Laser assisted cataract surgery
  - Refractive surgery
  - Keratoplasty
  - Intracorneal ring segments

Wavelengths and Targets of Lasers

Laser	Wavelength	Target Chromophore
Argon	488, 514 nm	Melanin, hemoglobin
Excimer	193 nm	LASIK, photoablative
Frequency-doubled Nd:YAG/KTP	532 nm	Vascular (LP); melanin/tattoo pigment (QS)
Pulsed dye	585–600 nm	Vascular
Ruby	694 nm	Melanin/tattoo pigment
Alexandrite	755 nm	Melanin/tattoo pigment

Contd...

Wavelengths and Targets of Lasers		
Laser	**Wavelength**	**Target Chromophore**
Diode	800 nm	Melanin, hemoglobin
Nd:YAG	1064 nm	Hemoglobin (LP), melanin/ tattoo pigment (QS)
Erbium: YAG	2940 nm	Water
Carbon dioxide	10600 nm 9.2 micron	Water

Lasers in Ophthalmology		
Mechanism	**Laser**	**Uses**
Photocoagulation [continuous mode or very rapidly pulsed (thermal) mode]	Argon laser (Workhorse of this group) krypton red laser Diode laser Frequency doubled Nd YAG, thermal mode Nd:YAG laser	• Retinal photocoagulation-diabetic retinopathy • Grid pattern photocoagulation: Clinically significant macula edema • Trabeculoplasty—Glaucoma • Laser iridotomy—Angle closure glaucoma • Sealing of retinal holes • Retinopathy of prematurity • Treatment of both benign (e.g. choroidal hemangioma) and malignant (e.g. choroidal melanoma and retinoblastoma) intraocular tumors
Photodisruption	Q-switched Nd YAG laser	• Posterior Capsulotomy—after cataract anterior capsular contraction • Laser iridotomy—Angle closure glaucoma • Anterior laser vitreolysis
Photo evaporation	Co_2 laser Holmium laser	• Lid tumors and lesions • Blood less incision over skin and sclera
Photoablation/ Photodecomposition	EXCIMER laser	• Phototherapeutic keratotomy (PTK)—corneal opacities • LASIK (laser-assisted in situ keratomileusis)—refractive errors, Laser epithelial keratectomy [LASEK]

38. Ans. (b) Topical natamycin and corneal scraping for culture

Ref: Kanski 8th ed page 180, Yanoff's 4th ed Pg 219

This is a typical case of fungal keratitis

See table of Fungal Keratitis" in AIIMS MAY 2018 Ophthalmology) (see page no. 664)

NOTE

Natamycin is the only commercially available topical antifungal agent; all others must be compounded from intravenous solutions with sterile techniques. (*Ref: Will's Eye manual 6th ed Page 74*)

39. Ans. (a) Retinal Pigment Epithelium

Ref: Yanoff's 4th Ed page 607, Kanski 8th ed page 581

- Retinal pigment epithelium would be better answer here than neurosensory retina.
- Neurosensory retina is basically what the 9 layer of retina combination is said.
- Outer plexiform split is seen in cystoid macular edema

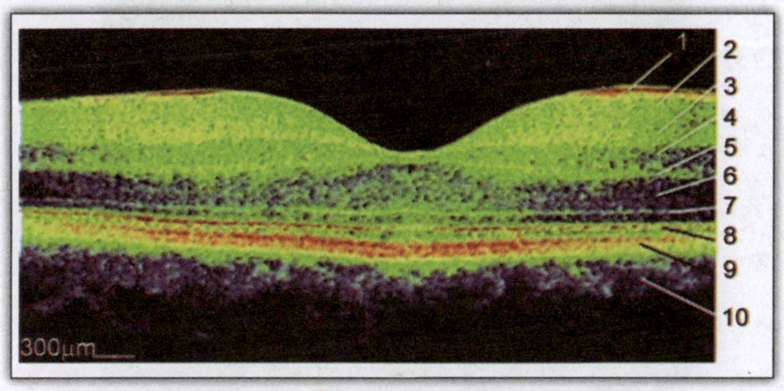

Fig: Normal Optical Coherence Tomography- Figure Legends: 1. Nerve fiber layer, 2. Ganglion cell layer, 3. Inner Plexiform layer, 4. Inner Nuclear Layer, 5. Outer Plexiform Layer, 6. Outer Nuclear Layer, 7. External Limiting membrane, 8. Inner/outer segment Junction , 9. Retinal Pigment Epithelium, 10. Larger Choroidal vessels

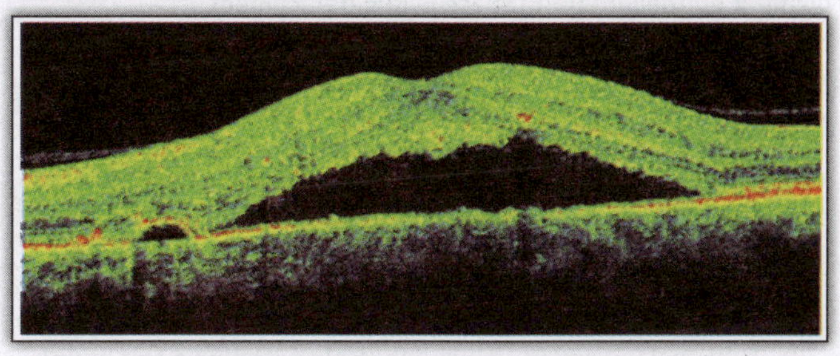

Fig: Detached Retinal pigment epithelium: Optical coherence tomography (OCT) is a safe, non-invasive, fast, reliable test that provides high resolution, cross-sectional images of the retina and vitreoretinal interface. It is an increasingly important tool for the diagnosis and monitoring of a wide range of vitreoretinal conditions. Current commercial OCT machines use a near infrared broadband light source (not a laser) to illuminate the retina. Familiarity with the appearance of a normal macular OCT scan is important to confidently identify pathological changes

Features to Note (From Anterior to Posterior) Include

- The anterior signal originates from the inner limiting membrane (ILM) and retinal nerve fibre layer (RNFL).

This has a smooth, relatively flat outline peripherally and a characteristic central dip at the fovea (referred to as the foveal pit).

- Posterior to the ILM/RNFL, subtle changes in reflectance are seen as alternating bands of hyper- (lighter) and hypo- (darker) reflectance representing the ganglion cell bodies, the inner plexiform, inner nuclear, outer plexiform and outer nuclear layers.
- Posterior to the outer nuclear layer, a series of three adjacent and increasingly hyper-reflective lines may be visible, representing the external limiting membrane (ELM), photoreceptor inner segment/outer segment junction (IS/OS junction) and RPE.
- A focal elevation of the ELM and IS/OS junction lines beneath the foveal pit is normally present. The ELM and IS/OS junction lines are often absent in SD-OCT scans of suboptimal image quality and in older TD-OCT scans.
- The signal posterior to the RPE arises from the choroid as patchy areas of high reflectivity.

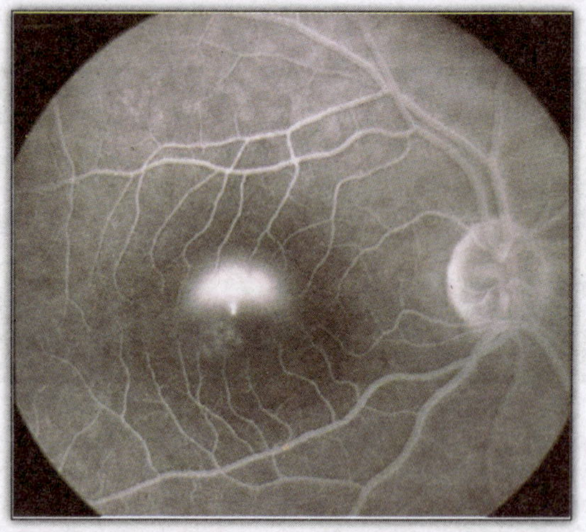

Fig: Hyperfluorescence caused by pooling of dye in the sub-retinal pigment epithelium (RPE) space in RPE detachment

Central Serous Retinopathy (CSR)

A type of choroidoretinopathy, caused due to excessive leakage from choriocapillaries. RPE is closest to choroidal capillaries, which get leaky in central cerous retinopathy (CSR).

History

Young anxious male coming to OPD with a chief complaint of central scotoma/blurred vision acute onset and says this happens quite often to him but resolves itself in a few months. Ink Blot Appearance (more common) and Honeycomb Appearance are seen in CSR on FA.

Associations

Also note CSR has been associated with:

- Central scotoma
- Type A personalities, males, it is more common
- Ask about the use of steroids from patient
- Hyperopic shift

Management

- Wait and observe
- Laser the leaky areas seen in FA
- PDT experimentally used

AIIMS MAY 2016

40. Ans. (a) Colour change on contact with tears to assess the volume of tears

Ref: Kanski 8th ed page 127, Yanoff 4th Ed page 277

Phenol red thread test is the test to detect dry eye severity. Phenol red thread test uses a thread impregnated with a pH-sensitive dye. The end of the thread is placed over the lower lid and the length wetted (the dye changes from yellow to red in tears) is measured after 15 seconds. A value of 6 mm is abnormal. It is comparable to the Schirmer test but takes less time to perform. Its main advantage that

- Less time consuming (15 sec)
- Anesthesia of cornea is not done
- On the contact of tear strip with the tear it turns red
- Can assess volume of tear film
- Can be done in children
- Reflex tearing is minimal
- Differentiates between aqueous deficient and non aqueous deficient eye

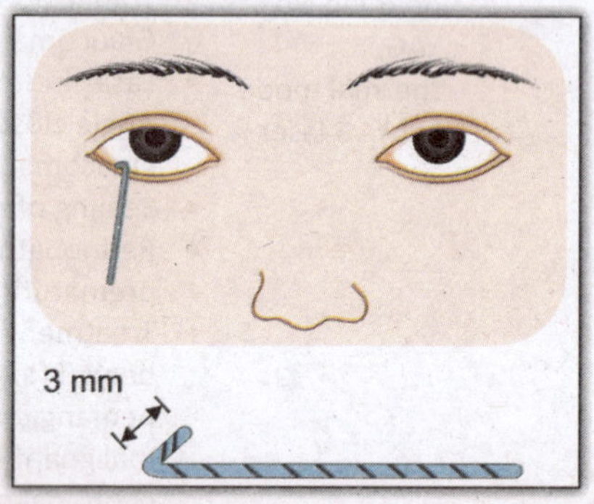

Diagnostic Tests for Dry Eye Disease

Test	Normal value
Tear film break-up time (TBUT)	>10 sec
Schirmer test with anesthesia	>5 mm in 5 min
Phenol red thread test	>5 mm in 15 sec
Tear Meniscus height	0.1- 0.6 mm
Tear film Osmolarity	<316 mOsm/L
Tear film matrix metalloproteinase-9 concentration	<40 ng/mL

41. Ans. (b) Adrenaline

Ref: Glaucoma Identification and co-management: Alicja R. Rudnicka. page 155, Goodman's and Gilman's The 12th Ed page 1788

- Black deposits on conjunctiva are seen after the use of adrenaline
- Adrenochrome deposits on forniceal conjunctiva occur due to alpha agonists on conjunctiva.
- Heterochromia iridis is seen after use of PG analogues
- Chronic use of epinephrine (adrenaline) to treat glaucoma has been associated with black adenochrome deposits on the conjunctiva and contact lenses used by the patients.
- Latanoprost – causes Iris pigmentation and not conjunctival pigmentation

42. **Ans. (a) Aspergillus spp.**

Ref: Parson's 22nd ed page 201, Wills Eye Manual 6th ed page 73

(Repeat AIIMS NOV 2018 Ophthalmology)
(see page no. 662)

43. **Ans. (a) Nocardia asteroids**

Ref: Yanoff 4th ed page 264

Nocardia infections also tend to follow trauma, especially if there is soil contamination. The ulcer is typically superficial, with irregular gray-white infiltrates and an undermined necrotic edge. The base might assume a cracked windshield appearance. Nocardia keratitis often resembles fungal infection, with a filamentous-appearing border and satellite lesions. Infection appears to be indolent and the anterior chamber reaction is often minimal. However, more severe anterior chamber reaction and hypopyon can rarely be seen.

44. **Ans. (d) 50 min**

Ref: Parson's 22nd ed page 97

Repeat AIIMS NOV 2018 (See for detailed explanation)
(see page no. 661)

The 6/60 letters at the top of the chart therefore subtends 5 minutes of arc at a distance of 60 metres. Hence if letter E (largest letter) makes 5 minute of arc at 60 meter, at 6 meter it will make an arc of 50 min.

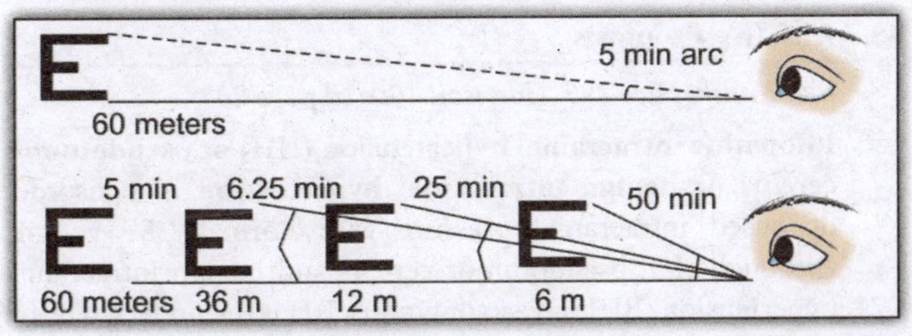

45. **Ans. (a) Remain unchanged**

Ref: Retina: 5th Edition Stephen J. Ryan Pg 1601, Yanoff's 4th Ed Pg 589, Rooks textbook of Dermatology 9th ed page 22.2

As sub-threshold laser is used to laser in PDT therapy, there should not be any change in the lesion color immediately. Photodynamic therapy can be used in both ophthalmology and dermatology. It is not associated with immediate change of colour of lesion either in ophthalmology or in dermatology. However, at 1 day after PDT, a circular hypopigmented retina with well demarcated borders is observe at the site of photodynamic therapy.

Photodynamic therapy (PDT) is a new laser technique for treatment of choroidal neovascularization and various tumors in the eye. In this technique, a special laser-activated dye is used to cause damage selectively to abnormal blood vessels, while minimizing damage to the nearby retinal tissue. A photosensitizing dye such as verteporfin is first injected intravenously into the patient. The dye preferentially accumulates in neovascular and neoplastic tissue, possibly because the dye binds with low-density lipoproteins (LDL). Cells with high mitotic activity, such as neovascular and neoplastic tissue, have high expression of LDL receptors and the LDL-bound dye may thereby be taken in the cells via receptor-mediated endocytosis. The dye in and of itself causes no significant damage to the neovascular tissue, but upon activation with wavelength-matched laser energy, PDT-mediated tissue destruction occurs by several mechanisms. Direct destruction to cell membranes occurs via lipid peroxidation and protein damage through oxygen and free radical intermediates. Vascular endothelial damage causes platelet aggregation and vessel thrombosis. Direct damage to nuclear components, as well as apoptotic mechanisms, have also been reported. In tumors, PDT may produce increased levels of cytokines, enhancing killing activity of cytotoxic T-lymphocytes.

Verteporfin was approved recently by the Food and Drug Administration for treatment of choroidal neovascularization secondary to age-related macular degeneration and myopic degeneration. In these conditions, verteporfin at a dosage of 6 mg/m^2 of patient body surface area is infused intravenously over 10 minutes. After allowing 5 minutes for the dye to accumulate in the neovascular tissue, laser light at a wavelength of 689 nm is then applied for 83 seconds at an intensity of 600 mW/cm^2; to give a total light dose of 50J/cm^2.

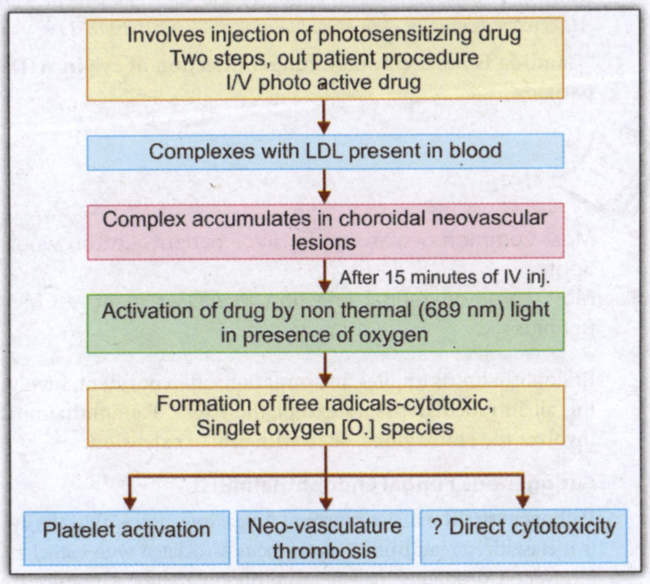

PDT Used in Dermatology

Photodynamic therapy (PDT) is a new form of photo-therapy used for skin cancers and precancers such as superficial basal cell carcinoma less than 2 mm thick intraepidermal carcinoma erythro-plasia of Queyrat and actinic keratoses. Selective tumour destruction is achieved by incorporating the photosensitizer in the target (malignant) tissue and then activating it with either a laser or non-laser light source. A promising combination is the naturally occurring porphyrin precursor, amino- laevulinic acid (ALA) and irradiation with a red light. The water-soluble ALA (20% in Unguentum M) is applied topically, under occlusion, to the tumour. After 4 h or so, when the ALA has been selectively absorbed by the tumour, the area is exposed to the light for 15 – 60 min. The activated ALA converts molecular oxygen to cytotoxic singlet oxygen and free radicals, which in turn cause ischaemic necrosis of the tumour by damaging cell membranes, especially those in the walls of blood vessels. PDT is carried out in an outpatient setting and its potential advantages over standard treatments include:

- Non-invasiveness
- Ability to treat many lesions at once

- Rarely causes ulceration and leads to a good cosmetic result
- Good patient acceptability
- Useful for treating tumours on sites that present surgical difficulty, e.g. the taut skin of the finger.

AIIMS NOVEMBER 2015

46. Ans. (d) 1064 nm

Ref: Kanski 7th ed ch 10, Vaughan and Asbury's General Ophthalmology 17th ed ch 24

See table of Lasers Used in Ophthalmology in AIIMS Nov 2016 (see page no. 681)

47. Ans. (d) Candidiasis

Ref: Ryan's Retina 5th ed page 733, Kanski 7th ed page 499, Santos C, Parker J, Dawson C. Bilateral fungal corneal ulcer in a patient with AIDS related complex. Am J Ophthalmol. 1986 Jul;102:118-119

"Candida is most common fungal infection of eye in AIDS patients"

NOTE

- Most Common ocular sign in HIV + patient- Cotton wool Spots
- Most common retinal infection in AIDS Patient – CMV Retinitis

Endophthalmitis implies inflammation, often purulent, involving all intraocular tissues except the sclera. Panophthalmitis involves the entire globe, often with orbital extension.

Endogenous Fungal Endophthalmitis

Pathogenesis: The major source of fungal infection within the eye is metastatic spread from a septic focus associated with catheters, intravenous drug abuse, parenteral nutrition and chronic lung disease such as cystic fibrosis. Neutropenia following immunosuppression and AIDS are also major risk factors. Approximately 75% of isolates are Candida spp.; other pathogens include Cryptococcus spp., Sporothrix schenckii and Blastomyces spp.

Presentation is dependent on the location and intensity of the inflammatory focus. Peripheral lesions may cause few or no visual disturbance while central lesions or those resulting in severe vitritis will manifest earlier. The progression is, however, much slower than in bacterial endophthalmitis and bilateral involvement is common.

Signs

- Anterior uveitis is uncommon in the early stages but may become prominent later.
- One or several creamy white chorioretinal lesions with overlying vitritis
- Floating 'cotton ball' colonies in the vitreous
- Chronic endophthalmitis characterized by severe vitreous infiltration and abscess formation

Course is relatively chronic and may result in retinal necrosis and retinal detachment associated with severe proliferative vitreoretinopathy.

Investigations involving vitreous biopsy and smears and cultures may be required to confirm the diagnosis and test the sensitivity of the organisms to antifungal agents.

Medical treatment is indicated for systemic disease and ocular disease without vitreous involvement.

- Oral fluconazole 100–200 mg/day (400–800 mg for disseminated disease) for 3–6 weeks. It can be used in conjunction with flucytosine (100 mg/kg/day) and has good ocular penetration.
- Oral, intravenous or intravitreal voriconazole to treat cases resistant to fluconazole. Good intraocular levels are achieved.
- Intravenous amphotericin has relatively poor ocular penetration.

Pars plana vitrectomy combined with intravitreal injection of amphotericin 5–10 μg in 0.1 mL is indicated in the presence of vitreous involvement.

48. Ans. (b) Proptosis

Ref: Kanski page 795, Harrison 19th ed page 203

Idiopathic intracranial hypertension (IIH) or pseudotumor cerebri or benign intracranial hypertension is a disorder of raised intracranial pressure with normal CSF volume Although IIH, pseudotumor cerebri and benign intracranial hypertension (BIH) are synonymous, IIH is the preferred term.

Clinical Features

- Raised ICP without any identifiable cause, i.e. No apparent cause on imaging, hydrocephalous, obstruction of CSF outflow. Venntricles are normal size
- **Obese young adult women** are most commonly affected
- **Papilledema**, with headache in 90% cases, which may lead to progressive optic atrophy and blindness.
- Patient presents with Headache and Diplopia (mostly due to 6th cranial nerve palsy)

Causes of Idiopathic Intracranial Hypertension

Systemic diseases	Endocrine risk factors	Drugs
• Familial Mediterranean fever • Hypertension • Anemia • Multiple sclerosis • Polyangiitis overlap syndrome • Psittacosis	• Female sex • Reproductive age group • Menstrual irregularity • Obesity • Recent weight gain • Adrenal insufficiency	• **Amiodarone**, • Antibiotics (e.g. nalidixic acid, penicillin and tetracycline) carbidopa, levodopa • Chlordecone, **corticosteroids** (topical and systemic) cyclosporine, danazol • Growth hormone

Contd...

Causes of Idiopathic Intracranial Hypertension		
Systemic diseases	**Endocrine risk factors**	**Drugs**
• Chronic renal disease • Reye syndrome • Sarcoidosis • Systemic lupus erythematosus • Thrombocytopenic purpura • Chronic respiratory insufficiency	• Cushing disease • Hypothyroidism • Excessive thyroxine replacement in children (i.e. low thyrotropin levels)	• Indomethacin, ketoprofen • Lead • Leuprolide acetate, levonorgestrel implants • Lithium • Oral contraceptives, oxytocin perhexiline • Phenytoin • Vitamin A (>100,000 u/day)/retinoic acid

Treatment

- **Acetazolamide** appears to be the most effective agent for lowering ICP
- In the event of intolerance to acetazolamide, furosemide may be used as a replacement diuretic
- **Headache prophylaxis**: Headaches can often be controlled with amitriptyline, propranolol, or other commonly prescribed migraine prophylaxis agents. Topiramate is also an excellent choice, in that one of its side effects is weight loss
- **Corticosteroids are effective in lowering ICP in patients whose IIH has an inflammatory etiology**. In addition, they may be used as a supplement to acetazolamide to hasten recovery in patients who present with severe papilledema. Because of their significant adverse effects, corticosteroids should not be considered as a long-term solution for IIH patients.
- If conservative management fails and visual field loss is progressive, a shunt is performed to prevent blindness.

49. Ans. (c) Lateral geniculate body > (D) Occipital lobe

Ref: Dejong 7th Ed page 175, Walsh and Hoyts' Neuroophthalmology 6th Ed page 112

Both lateral geniculate body and occipital lobe lesion causes homonymous hemianopia. Occipital lobe lesion pesents with homonymous hemianopia with macular sparing, which is sometimes referred to as keyhole defect. However lateral geniculate body lesion causing sectoranopia ae true keyhole defects. Bilateral occipital lobe lesions may occur from a single or from consecutive events and may cause bilateral homonymous scotomas, usually with some macular sparing ("ring" scotomas) that respects the vertical midline. In some cases there may be "tunnel" or "keyhole" fields with bilateral complete homonymous hemianopias except for macular sparing

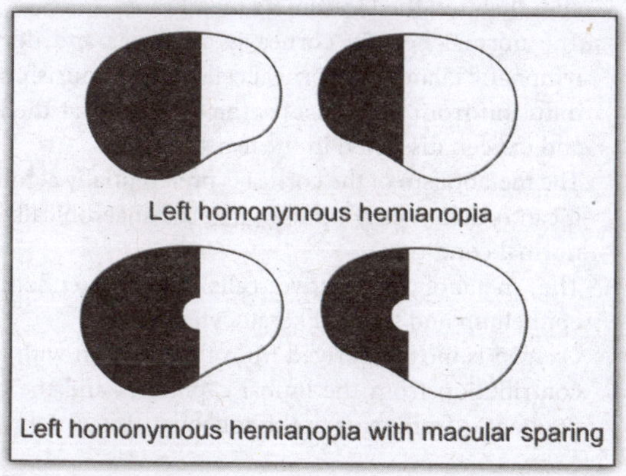

Field Defects in Lateral Geniculate Body

A lesion of the left LGN may be associated with two different vascular lesions.

Dejong States

LGB lesions are rare and usually due to vascular disease. They cause acontralateral homonymous hemianopia that is somewhat incongruous, occasionally with a wedge shaped or hour glass pattern along the horizontal meridian pointing to fixation (**sectoranopia or keyhole defect**) and splits the macula. The unusual patternis due to the organization of the LGB and to its dual blood supply. Etiiologies of the LGB lesion include ischemia, AVM, neoplasm, demyelinating disease and trauma.

Defect of LGB	Artery Involved	Figure
Horizontal sectoranopia (Right for example)	Posterior choroidal artery occlusion (left for example)	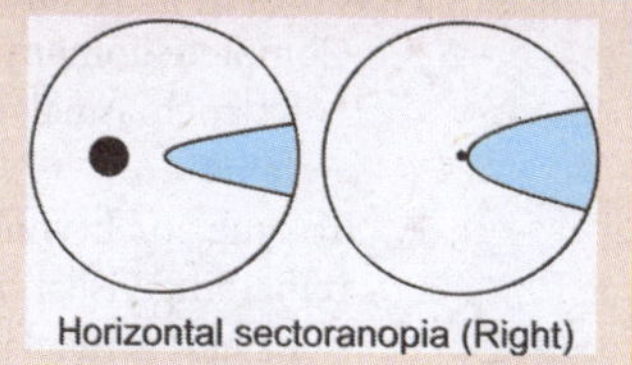
Quadruple sectoranopia AKA; Sector sparing Homonymous hemianopia (Right for example)	Anterior choroidal artery occlusion (left for example)	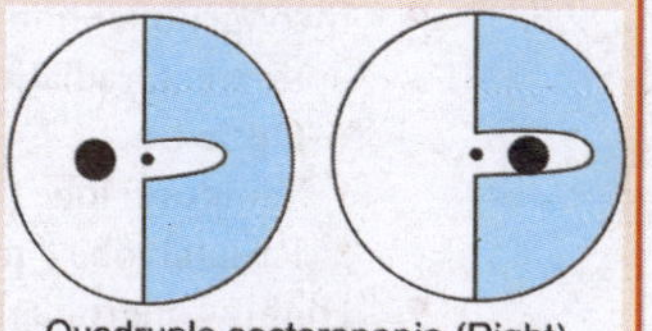

Differential Diagnosis of Visual Kidd Deficits

- **General Depression**
  - Cataract (diffuse depression from cataracts may improve with dilation)
  - Corneal disease (shows no improvement with dilation)
  - Other media opacities
  - Some optic neuropathies
- **Enlarged Blind Spot**
  - Optic nerve disease
    - Papilledema and big blind spot syndrome
    - Drusen of the optic nerve head
    - Congenital optic nerve lesion (coloboma. staphyloma)
    - Optic neuritis
  - Retinal disease
    - Multiple evanescent white dot syndrome (MEWDS)
    - Acute zonal occult outer retinopathy (AZOOR)
  - High myopia

- **Arcuate, altitudinal, Nasal Step. Nasal Depression**
  - Optic nerve disease
    - Glaucoma
    - Papilledema
    - Drusen of the optic nerve head
    - Other optic neuropathies (AION. optic neuritis, etc.)
  - Branch artery occlusion
- **Crosses the Vertical and Horizontal Meridians**
  - **Retinal disease**
    - Ring scotomas, peripheral depression, "scalloped" field loss
  - Optic neuropathy
    - Generalized depression, sparing of central vision C
  - Fatigue, poor testing ability
  - Malingering
    - I Peripheral depression, square visual fields, spiraling or crossed isopters, inconsistent patterns of loss
- **Central or Centrocecal Defects**
  - Maculopathy (visual acuity often more affected than visual field)
  - Optic neuropathies of all types
- **Bitemporal Defects**
  - Superior bitemporal defects (pituitary adenoma)
  - Inferior bitemporal defects (craniopharyngioma, hypothalamic tumor)
- **Homonymous Hemianopsia**
  - Complete homonymous hemianopsia
    - Retrochiasmal defect with no further localizing value
  - Tongue- or keyhole-shaped homonymous defect, or remaining visual field
    - Lateral geniculate lesion
  - Incongruous homonymous hemianopsia (anterior optic tract, radiations)
    - Optic tract
    - Temporal lobe ("pie in (the sky" delect)
    - Parietal lobe ("pie on the floor" defect)
  - Highly congruous homonymous hemianopsia
    - Occipital lobe lesion

      a. "Cookie cutter" punched-out lesion
      b. Macular sparing
      c. Temporal crescent
      d. Tatokinetic dissociation

50. Ans. (b) Epinephrine

Ref: Kanski 7th ed page 385-386

Option (A)

Timolol is a beta blocker

Option (B)

Epinephrine acts on dilator muscles causing the pupil to dilate analogous to pilocarpine action on sphinctor pupillae

Option (C)

Cocaine prevents the reuptake of epinephrine, but don't have analogous to pilocarpine action.

Option (D)

Hydroxyamphetamine paralyzes the muscle causing dilation so its action cannot be said analogous to pilocarpine

AIIMS MAY 2015

51. Ans. (c) Nasociliary nerve

Ref: Gray's 40th ed page 667-668, Anatomy and Physiology of Eye 2nd ed Dr AK Khurana Pg 24

Cornea is supplied by nasociliary nerve and has the highest amount of sensory endings. It is affected in herpetic or any other viral disease causing decreased or abnormal corneal sensations. The nasociliary branch of the ophthalmic branch (V_1) of the 5th cranial nerve (trigeminal nerve) supplies the sensory innervations to cornea.

NOTE

- If the nasolacrimal nerve is written in option, please note there is no this kind of nerve, it woud be a spelling mistake
- Infraorbital nerve damage can cause sensation loss over cheek, supraorbital nerve supplies the brow and frontal region of head
- If loss of corneal reflex is question, mark oculomotor nerve as answer

Anatomy of Cornea

The transparent cornea comprises 1/6 of the anterior eyeball. Its curvature is greater than the rest of the globe and the junction of the cornea with the sclera, anatomically called the limbus.

Anatomical Dimensions of the Normal Cornea

	Corneal diameter (mm)		Radius of curvature in mm
	Horizontal	Vertical	
Anterior surface	11.7	10.6	7.8
Posterior surface	11.7	11.7	6.5
Corneal thickness	Central 0.5-0.6	Peripheral 1.2	

- The cornea consists of three layers: (i) the epithelium; (ii) the substantia propria or stroma and (iii) the endothelium.
- Between the epithelium and stroma lies the Bowman's layer or membrane and between the stroma and endothelium, the Descemet's membrane.
- The normal healthy cornea is avascular and devoid of lymphatic channels. Corneal cells derive nourishment by diffusion from the aqueous, the capillaries at the limbus and oxygen dissolved in the tear film
- The metabolism of the cornea is preferentially aerobic and it can function only up to 6–7 hours anaerobically under normal conditions.
- The metabolically active cells are the endothelium, epithelium and stromal keratocytes.
- Oxygen is mostly derived from the tear film with a small contribution from the limbal capillaries and the oxygen gradient is from tears to the aqueous.

- Glucose supply for corneal metabolism is mainly (90%) derived from the aqueous and supplemented by the limbal capillaries.
- The cornea is supplied by nerves which originate from the small ophthalmic division of the trigeminal nerve, mainly by the long ciliary branches of the nasociliary nerves which run in the perichoroidal space and pierce the sclera a short distance posterior to the limbus. Here they form an annulus from which branches travel radially to enter the corneal stroma.
- The cornea is the most important refractive surface of the eye. Its refractive index is 1.38 (1.376) and the anterior surface is the main refractive surface.
- The tear film is important in maintaining a healthy normal environment for the corneal epithelial cells. The tear film consists of an inner mucin laver which lines the hydrophobic epithelium and makes it 'wettable', an aqueous layer and a superficial lipid laver which decreases evaporation.
- The cornea is normally avascular, but may be invaded by new blood vessels from the limbus in case of infection and inflammation.
- The transparency of the cornea is due to its relatively dehydrated state, absence of blood vessels and pigment, uniform refractive index of all the layers and uniform spacing of the collagen fibrils in the stroma. The collagen fibrils are separated by a distance which is less than the wavelength of light so that any irregularly refracted rays of light are eliminated by destructive interference.

High Yielding Facts

- Factors contributing to the maintainence of transparency of cornea – Lack of vasculature, dehydrated state of cornea maintained by endothelial pump, regular arrangement of corneal fibres having diameter less than the wavelength of light and keratocytes inhibition of scattering.
- *Dua Layer*- New Sub-stromal layer discovered by Indian Ophthalmologist: Dr Harminder S Dua.

52. Ans. (a) Latanoprost

Ref: Clinical Ocular Pharmacology by Jimmy D. Bartlett 5th Ed Pg 143

One iris may have a different colour from the other (heterochromia iridium), or parts of the same iris, usually a sector, may differ in colour from the remainder (heterochromia iridis) The blue iris is due to the absence of pigment in the iris stroma, the pigment in the retinal epithelium being seen through the translucent stroma.

Causes of Heterochromia Iridis

- Congenital
- Fuchs' heterochromic iridocyclitis
- Siderosis
- Latanoprost, a PG analogue can cause heterochromia iridis in patients.

NOTE

- The Friends with Benefits star, Mila Kunis has complete Heterochromia iridis, one eye brown and the other greenish hazel.
- Pakistani-American, David Coleman Headley (born Daood Sayed Gilani), convicted terrorist in the 2008 Mumbai attacks, also had heterocrhomia.

Side Effects of PG Analogues	
Ocular	**Systemic**
• Hyperchromia Iridis • Growth of Eyelashes • Periocular Pigmentation • Cystoid Macular Edema • Anterior Uveitis • Transient Hyperemia • Burning/Stinging (More With Bimatoprost) • Reactivation of herpetic keratitis	• Flu like syndrome • Dysponea and Asthma • Myalgias • Headache • **Contraindications** • Hypersensitivity to the drug or preservative • Patients with active ocular inflammation

To be used with caution: Cystoid macular edema in aphakics and pseudophakics, concurrent NSAID use.

53. Ans. (d) Right head tilt

Ref: Kanski 7th ed page 833-834

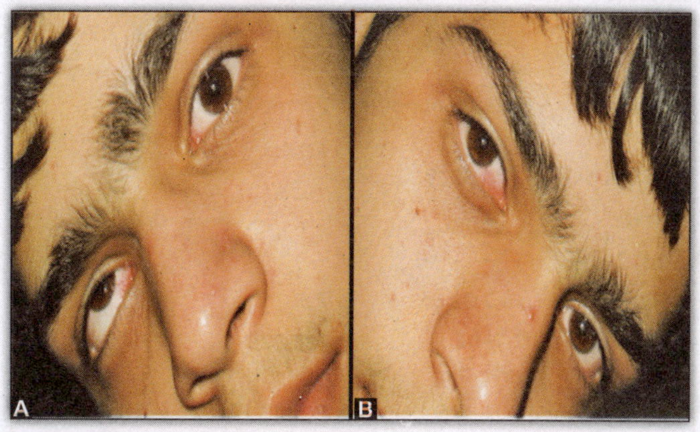

Source: Dr Vineet Sehgal

Right Superior Oblique Palsy

On right head tilt there is elevation and slight esotropia (Fig A) Mnemonic- WOOG = worse on opposite gaze, that is not there on left head tilt (Fig B). So patient would like to have left head tilt. So remember mnemonic BOOT- Better on opposite tilt

Right Trochlear Nerve Palsy- Superior Oblique Palsy

- Superior Oblique action is Intorsion, Depression in adduction, better Intorter on Abduction.

- Patients complain of diplopia – vertical, diagonal or torsional
- If the principal complaint is torsion - B\L palsy should be suspected
- Compensatory head posture
- Facial Asymmetry
- Chin down in bilateral palsies
- Combination of Elevation, Extorsion, Esotropia (Since SO does Depression, Intorsion, Abduction)
- Diagnosis is based on either Head tilt or Park three step test

54. Ans. (d) Ascorbate

Ref: Yanoff 4th ed page 1339

Chemical Composition of Human Aqeuous Humor, Vitreous, Blood			
Ingredient	**Aqeuous humor**	**Vitreous humor**	**Plasma**
Sodium	162.9	144	142
Potassium	2.2-3.9	5.5	4
Calcium	1.8	1.6	1.8
Magnesium	1.1	1.3	1.5
Chloride	131.6	177	103
Bicarbonate	20.15	15	28
Phosphate	0.62	0.4	4
Lactate	2.5	7.8	0.3 – 1.3
Glucose (mmol/kg)	2.7-3.7	3.4	3.9- 7.9
Ascorbate	1.06 mmol/l	2 mmol/L	23-85 micromol/l
Glutathione	0.0019	–	
Citrate	–	–	0.135
Acetate	–	–	
PH	7.38	7.5	7.35
Osmolality (mOsm/kg)	304	288-323	295
Refractive index	1.336	1.3341	–
Water	99.1%	99%	
Solid	1.1%		
Protein	5–16 mg% (much less than plasma)		6–7 g %
Amino acid	5 mg/kg water		

All concentrations are expressed in mmol/l or mEq/l of solution.
1 millimoles= 1000 miicromoles
Collagen type 2 is most common type of collagen in the vitreous.
Hyaluronic acid is also in maximum concentration in the aqueous humor

55. Ans. (d) HM 3 and 4

Ref: Biochemistry of the eye by David R. Whikehart Pg 28; Mishra G, Das GB, Behera HN. *Possible role of lens collagen in cataractogenesis.* Indian J Ophthalmol. *1997; 45: 227-231*

Type 4 collagen is mostly synthesized by lens epithelial cells so should be answer of choice. An age-related increase in the total collagen in lens capsule from individuals indicates an enhanced synthesis and/or decreased degradation, followed by its incorporation into fibres, a fact supported by higher level of salt-soluble, acid-soluble and insoluble collagens. This view is further corroborated by the observation that the lens capsule increases in thickness with age and this accretion process appears to be due completely to uniform assembly of three types of collagen (I, III and IV), a process possibly intrinsic to aging and that these collagens may not be present in the human capsule in the early decades. So the best option is (D) (HM 3 and 4)

Note

- Post lens capsule is thinner than anterior.
- Posterior polar cataract occurs in younger people than senile cataract. Chances of posterior capsule rupture are more in cataract surgery than in normal cataract.
- Various proteins in the lens are—Insoluble albuminoids (12.5 %), Alpha Crytallins (31.7 %), Beta Crystallins (53.4%), Gamma Crystallins (1.5 %).

56. Ans. (d) ABCG2

Ref: Stem Cells: From Bench to Bedside By Ariff Bongso, Eng Hin Lee, P- 435; Marzieh Ebrahimi, Ehsan Taghi-Abadi and Hossein Baharvand Limbal Stem Cells in Review J Ophthalmic Vis Res. 2009; 4: 40–58

ABCG2 transporter has been identified as a molecular determinant for bone marrow stem cells and it has been proposed as a universal marker for stem cells from a variety of sources

Limbal Stem Cell Markers

- **ABCG2:** ATP binding cassette protein 2 is also considered universal marker for stem cells
- P63
- DNP63a
- Bmi-2
- iNTEGRIN a9

Palisadt's of Vogue in the basal layer of limbal epithelium are storage sites of stem cells.

Conditions Causing Limbal Stem Cell Deficiency

- Chemical or thermal injury
- Multiple surgeries or cryotherapies of the limbus
- Steven Jhonson syndrome
- Contact lens induced keratopathy
- Severe microbial infection
- Aniridia
- Keratitis associated with Multiple endocrine deficiencies

- Neurotropic keratopathy
- Pterygium or pseudopterygium
- Idiopathic keratopathy

57. Ans. (c) Magnification is 5 times

Ref: Khurana 5th ed page 600

See table of OPHTHALMOSCOPY in AIIMS NOV 2016 Ophthalmology (see page no. 680)

58. Ans. (a) Berlins oedema

Ref: Kanski 7th ed page 682-683, Khurana 6th Ed page- 432

Blunt trauma is a very hot topic in AIIMS and you all should know about it.

Blunt Tauma of the Eye	
Corneal	**Corneal abrasion** • Involves a breach of the epithelium (stained by fluorescein). • If over the pupillary area, vision may be grossly impaired. **Acute corneal oedema** • Secondary to focal or diffuse dysfunction of the corneal endothelium. • Commonly associated with folds in **Descemet membrane** and stromal thickening • Usually clears spontaneously **Tears in Descemet membrane** • Usually vertical and most commonly arise as the result of birth trauma
Anterior chamber	**Hyphaema** • Hyphaema (haemorrhage into the anterior chamber) is a common complication. The **source of the bleeding is the iris or ciliary body** • Characteristically, the red blood cells sediment inferiorly with a resultant 'fluid level', except when the hyphaema is total. • Treatment is aimed at prevention of secondary haemorrhage and control of any elevation of intraocular pressure that may result in corneal blood staining
Anterior uvea	**Pupil** • The iris may momentarily be compressed against the anterior surface of the lens by severe anteroposterior force, with resultant imprinting of pigment from the pupillary margin. • Transient miosis accompanies the compression, evidenced by the pattern of pigment corresponding to the size of the miosed pupil resulting in formation of **Vossius ring**. • Damage to the iris sphincter may result in traumatic mydriasis, which can be temporary or permanent; the pupil reacts sluggishly or not at all to both light and accommodation. • Radial tears in the pupillary margin are common
Anterior uvea	**Iridodialysis** • Dehiscence of the iris from the ciliary body at its root. • The pupil is typically D-shaped and the dialysis is seen as a dark biconvex area near the limbus. • May be asymptomatic if covered by the upper lid; if exposed in the palpebral aperture, uniocular diplopia and glare sometimes ensue and may necessitate surgical repair of the dehiscence. • Traumatic aniridia (360° iridodialysis) is rare; in a pseudophakic eye, the detached iris may be ejected through a cataract surgical incision. **Trauma to ciliary body** ***Angle recession*** refers to the tear between longitudinal and circular muscle fibres of the ciliary body. It is characterized by deepening of the anterior chamber and widening of the ciliary body band on gonioscopy. Later on it is complicated by glaucoma.
Intraocular pressure	• Elevation can occur for a variety of reasons including hyphaema (above) and inflammation. • In contrast, the ciliary body may react to severe blunt trauma by temporary cessation of aqueous secretion (**'ciliary shock'**) resulting in hypotony; it is important for an occult open injury to be excluded as the cause of the hypotony. • Tears extending into the face of the ciliary body (**angle recession**) are associated with a risk of later glaucoma.
Lenticular	**Cataract** • Common sequel to blunt trauma. • Postulated mechanisms include traumatic damage to the lens fibres themselves and minute ruptures in the lens capsule with influx of aqueous humour, hydration of lens fibres and consequent opacification.

Contd...

Blunt Tauma of the Eye	
	• A ring-shaped anterior subcapsular opacity may underlie a Vossius ring. Commonly opacification occurs in the **posterior subcapsular cortex** along the posterior sutures, resulting in a **flower-shaped ('rosette')** opacity which may subsequently disappear, remain stationary or progress to maturity. **Subluxation** • Secondary to tearing of the suspensory ligament. • A subluxated lens tends to deviate towards the meridian of intact zonule; the anterior chamber may deepen over the area of zonular dehiscence, if the lens rotates posteriorly. • The edge of a subluxated lens may be visible under mydriasis and trembling of the iris **(iridodonesis)** or lens **(phakodonesis)** may be seen on ocular movement. Subluxation of magnitude sufficient to render the pupil partly aphakic may result in uniocular diplopia; lenticular astigmatism due to tilting may occur.
	Dislocation • Due to 360° rupture of the zonular fibres is rare and may be into the vitreous, or less commonly, into the anterior chamber an underlying predisposing condition should be suspected.
Globe rupture	• Rupture of the globe may result from severe blunt trauma. • The rupture is **usually anterior, in the vicinity of the Schlemm canal,** with prolapse of structures such as the lens, iris, ciliary body and vitreous • **An anterior rupture may be masked by extensive subconjunctival haemorrhage.** • An occult posterior rupture can be associated with little visible damage to the anterior segment • Gentle **B-scan ultrasonography** may demonstrate a posterior rupture, but CT or MR may be necessary • MR is not performed if there is a risk of ferrous intraocular foreign body
Vitreous	**Vitreous haemorrhage** • Often in association with posterior vitreous detachment. • **Pigment cells ('tobacco dust')** may be seen floating in the anterior vitreous and though not necessarily associated with a retinal break, should always prompt a careful retinal assessment
Retina	**Berlin's edema or Commotio Retina:** • Caused by concussion of the sensory retina resulting in cloudy swelling which gives the involved area a grey appearance. • Commotio most frequently affects the **temporal fundus** • If the macula is involved, a **'cherry-red spot' may be seen at the fovea.** • Severe involvement may be associated with intraretinal haemorrhage, sometimes affecting the macula. • The prognosis in mild cases is good with spontaneous resolution within 6 weeks. • Sequelae to more severe commotio may include progressive pigmentary degeneration and macular hole formation. **Retinal breaks and detachment** • Trauma is responsible for about 10% of all cases of retinal detachment (RD) and is the **most common cause in children,** particularly boys. • A great variety of breaks may develop in traumatized eyes either at the time of impact or subsequently: ▪ **Dialysis** is a **break occurring at the ora serrata** and is caused by traction of the relatively inelastic vitreous gel along the posterior aspect of the vitreous base with tearing of the retina. This may be associated with avulsion of the vitreous base, giving rise to a **'bucket-handle' appearance** which comprises a strip of ciliary epithelium, ora serrata and the immediate post-oral retina into which basal vitreous gel remains inserted. Traumatic dialyses occur most frequently in the **superonasal and inferotemporal quadrants**. Although they occur at the time of injury they do not inevitably result in RD. In cases that detach, subretinal fluid frequently may not develop until several months later and progression is typically slow. ▪ **Equatorial breaks** are less frequent and are due to direct retinal disruption at the point of scleral impact. ▪ **Macular holes** may occur either at the time of injury or following resolution of commotio retinae
Choroid	**Choroidal rupture** • Involves the **choroid, Bruch membrane and retinal pigment epithelium (RPE)** • It may be direct or indirect. • **Direct ruptures** are located **anteriorly** at the site of impact and run parallel with the ora serrata. • **Indirect ruptures** occur opposite the site of impact. • A fresh rupture may be partially obscured by subretinal haemorrhage,which may break through the internal limiting membrane with resultant subhyaloid or vitreous haemorrhage. • Weeks to months later, on absorption of the blood, a white crescentic vertical streak of exposed underlying sclera concentric with the optic disc becomes visible. -The visual prognosis is poor if the fovea is involved. • An uncommon late complication is **choroidal neovascularization** which may result in haemorrhage, scarring and further visual deterioration

Contd...

Blunt Tauma of the Eye	
Optic nerve	**Traumatic optic neuropathy (TON)** • Presents following ocular, orbital or head trauma as sudden visual loss which cannot be explained by other ocular pathology. It occurs in up to 5% of cases of facial fracture. • Vision is often very poor from the outset, with only perception of light (PL) in around 50%. • Typically the only objective finding is an afferent pupillary defect; the optic nerve head and fundus are initially normal, with pallor developing over subsequent days and weeks. It is important to exclude potentially reversible causes of traumatic visual loss such as compressive orbital haemorrhage. **Optic nerve avulsion** is rare and typically occurs when an object intrudes between the globe and the orbital wall, displacing the eye. Fundus examination shows a striking cavity where the optic nerve head has retracted from its dural sheath, There is no treatment

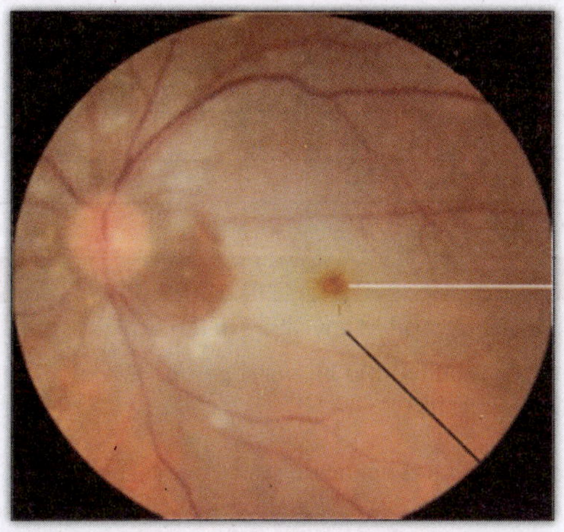

Fig: Berlin's edema or commotio retina: It follows post blunt trauma and manifests as pale retina due to retinal edema (Black arrow), with a Cherry Red Spot in the central foveal region (White arrow)

59. Ans. (a) CRAO

Ref: Kanski 7th ed page 559, Khurana 6th ed page 269

It is a clinical sign seen in the context of thickening and loss of transparency of posterior pole of the retina. The CRS is visualised as a bright to dull red spot at the centre of macula, surrounded and accentuated by a greyish white or yellowish halo.

Please do not get confused in this question. Hollenhorst plaque can be seen in CRVO and BRVO also but it does not cause Cherry red spot in CRVO.

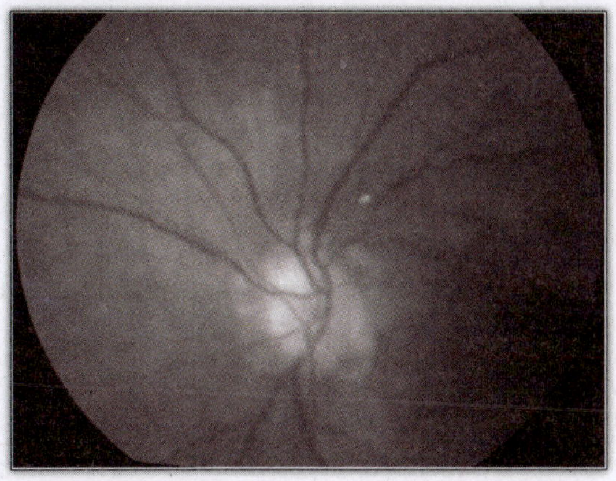

Fig: Hollenhorst plaque in the superonasal vessel

- Its colour is due to the pigment epithelium and choroid. Hollenhorst plaque is basically a cholesterol emboli in the vessel that can cause vascular occlusion
- Occlusion of the central retinal artery is associated with "cherry-red spot". The fundoscopy reveals a diffuse retinal arteriole constriction often with visible emboli or blood flow segmentation.
- The fovea retains its blood supply via the choroidal circulation while the surrounding retina appears milky white due to infarction, intracellular oedema, cellular necrosis and cellular debris accumulation.

The CRS is associated with

- Inherited metabolic conditions
- Central Retinal Artery Occlusion (CRAO)
- Orbital contusion
- Orbital ischemia due to vasospasm.
- Methanol Poisoning
- Quinine poisoning

In metabolic disorders, it is seen more consistently in certain conditions like Tay Sachs disease, Sandhoff's disease and Sialidosis (evident in most cases by the time psychomotor retardation and mental deterioration set in). It may be seen in many cases of Infantile Niemann Pick disease type IA and GM_1 Gangliosidosis and occasionally in Metachromatic leukodystrophy. Other conditions associated with CRS include: Farber's disease, Goldberg's disease, Gaucher's disease (infantile form), Hurler's syndrome, Mucopolysaccharidosis VII, Hallervorden Spatz syndrome, Batten-Mayou-Vogt-Spielmeyer syndrome, Spranger's disease, Cryoglobulinemia and Leber's congenital amaurosis.

NOTE

- Krabbe disease rarely present with cherry red spot
- Type 1 GM 1 Gangliosidoses have cherry red spot but not Type 2 GM1 Gangliosidoses

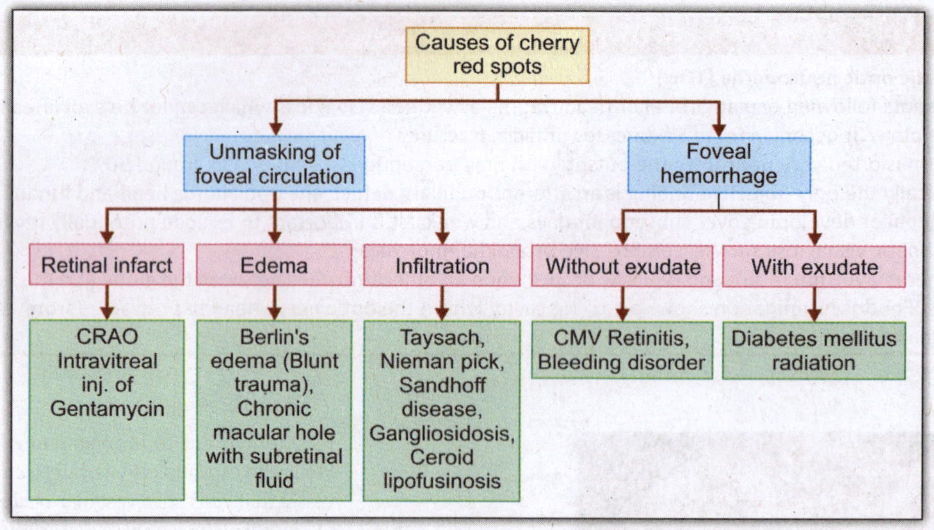

60. Ans. (b) Optic nerve

Ref: Kanski's 7th ed page 510-517, Khurana 5th ed page 300-306, Parson's 21th ed page 368-370

Retinoblastoma	
Retinoblastoma is a tumor of retinal cells, the RB cells can disperse in vitreous and get deposited anywhere in the ocular tissue.	
Epidemiology	• It is the most common primary intraocular malignancy of childhood in all racial groups (3% of all childhood cancers) Even so, it is rare, occurring in about 1 : 17 000 live births • Affects infants and children. • Retinoblastoma affects boys and girls with equal frequency and has noknown racial predilection.
Genetics	• **Autosomal Dominant** • **Germinal (heritable, 40%)** and somatic (nonheritable, 60%) forms. • Inherited as an autosomal dominant trait. • A gene responsible for the childhood eye tumor retinoblastoma was identified in 1986 on **chromosome 13q14.** • Among individuals who inherit a mutant copy of the retinoblastoma gene, 90% sustain a second hit to the remaining normal copy of the gene and develop a tumor. Approximately 10% of individuals who inherit a mutant copy of the gene do not sustain a second mutation and do not develop a tumor.

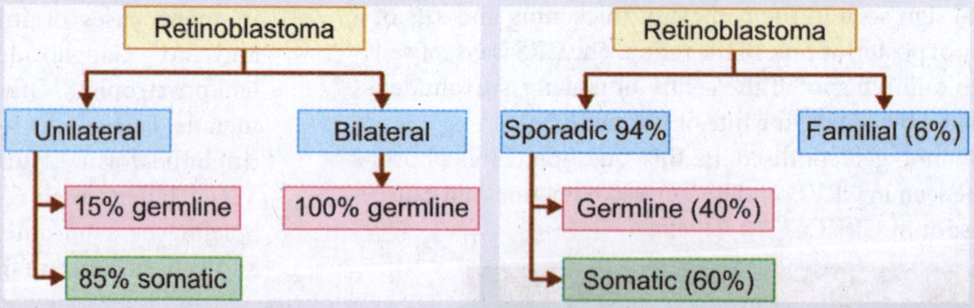

Clinical features	• Most common presentation is a white glow in the pupil (**leukokoria or Cat's reflex- 60%**) followed by strabismus (20%) is the most common manifestation of RB • Unilateral (60–70%) or **bilateral (30–40%)** ocular involvement; most unilateral cases are unifocal and most bilateral cases are multifocal in both eyes.
Pathology	It is characterized by **Flexner winterstiener rosette, homer – wright rosette**
Spread	The metastasis of the tumor can be through optic nerve as it is the communication cable between Retina and rest of body. **Patterns of tumour spread** • Growth pattern may be endophytic (into the vitreous), with seeding of tumour cells throughout the eye or exophytic (into the subretinal space), causing retinal detachment • Optic nerve invasion, with spread of tumour along the subarachnoid space to the brain

Contd...

	• Diffuse infiltration of the retina, without exophytic or endophytic growth. • Metastatic spread is to regional nodes, lung, brain and bone. Direct spread is not a case. Lymphatics can occur when it is in adnexal tissue like lids etc. Hematogenous can be there but it is more common in choroidal tumors like ocular melanoma
Management	• Chemotherapy is indicated in **Group B-D** RB tumors. (Internantional Classification of Intraocular Retinoblastoma *Murphee et al*) • Please note if there is Assymetrical Bilateral Involvement of the eyes and one eye is Group E, treatment is always aimed at treating the worse eye: So do an enucleation then followed by treating the other eye.

Tumors of Eye FAQ		
Most common	**Children**	**Adult**
Intraocular malignancy	Retinoblastoma	Metastasis > Melanoma of choroid
Primary orbital malignancy	Rhabdomyosarcoma	
Soft tissue malignancy	Rhabdomyosarcoma	
Tumor of orbital/periorbital area	Capillary Hemangioma	
Benign orbital tumor		Cavernous Hemangioma
Cause of orbital metastasis	Neuroblastoma	Breast carcinoma
Choroidal malignancy	Metastatic	Metastatic
Site of metastasis	Choroid > iris and ciliary body	Choroid > iris and ciliary body
Epithelial tumor of lacrimal gland	Pleomorphic adenoma	Pleomorphic adenoma
Peripheral neural tumor of orbit	Plexiform neuroma	Plexiform neuroma
Eyelid tumor	Basal cell carcinoma	Basal cell carcinoma

61. Ans. (a) Malignancy

Ref: Kanski 8th ed page 113, Khurana 6th Ed page 173

Option (A)

Evisceration provides disrupted and incomplete material for histology and should not be undertaken in the presence of suspected intraocular malignancy.

Option (B)

Panophthalmitis is infection of all coats of eye is a contraindication of enucleation but evisceration can be done

Option (C)

Severe trauma to eye with displaced globe is an indication where we can do evisceration, so that some globe remains intact and the shape of the eye can be maintained. Patient gets a mental satisfaction that some part of globe is there and we can put silicon implant inside.

Option (D)

Choroidal hemorrhage: The modality of choice is to close the globe. Evisceration is theoretically curable but otherwise not done

Ophthalmologic Surgeries			
	Evisceration	**Enucleation**	**Exenteration**
Definition	Removal of contents of eyeball/ globe except sclera. Since extraocular muscles are part of orbit, its intact.	Surgical removal of the entire globe (including sclera). Since extraocular muscles are part of orbit its intact. But it requires cutting the six extraocular muscles as well as the optic nerve	Removal of the entire orbit including the globe, soft tissue and orbital contents like lacrimal system, Extraocular muscles, Optic nerve etc. The eyelid can be spared, depending on the extent of the tumor.
Indication	As for enucleation, except for intraocular tumors or risk of sympathetic ophthalmitis **Blind painful or unsightly eyes -** Evisceration is procedue of choice	• **Blind painful eye;** can be managed by enucleation but Evisceration is procedure of choice • Intraocular tumor (when other modalities fail or inappropriate) • Severe trauma with risk of sympathetic ophthalmitis	• Cutaneous tumors with orbital invasion • Lacrimal gland malignancies • Extensive conjunctival malignancies • Other orbital malignancies • Orbital Mucormycosis

Contd...

Ophthalmologic Surgeries			
	Evisceration	**Enucleation**	**Exenteration**
		• Phthisis bulbi • Microphthalmia • Endophthalmitis/ panophthalmitis • Cosmetic deformity	
Contraindication	• Evisceration provides disrupted and incomplete material for histology and should not be undertaken in the presence of suspected intraocular malignancy. • Treatment of severe ocular trauma with a ruptured globe, where sympathetic ophthalmia is a concern	Infective endophthalmitis with secondary orbital cellulitis	
Anaesthesia	Done with a regional nerve block without general anesthesia	Done with a regional nerve block without general anesthesia. General anesthesia can be used, if required.	Done under general anaesthesia
Comments	Prosthesis mobility is good because Extraocular muscles are intact	Prosthesis mobility is comparable to Evisceation. Less post-operative pain and swelling with enucleation as compared with evisceration.	Prosthesis mobility is poor because extraocular muscles are removed
	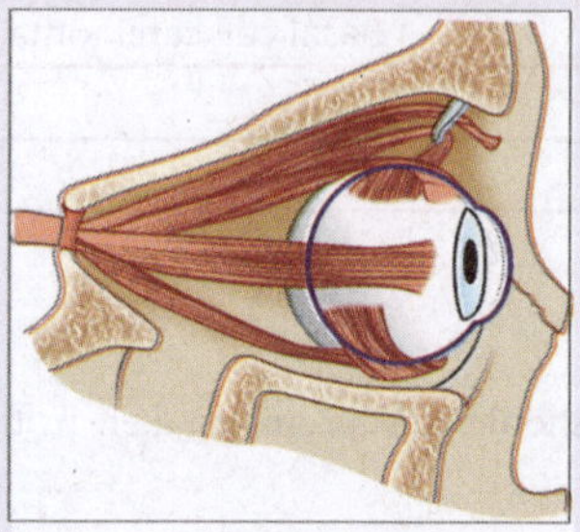 Evisceration	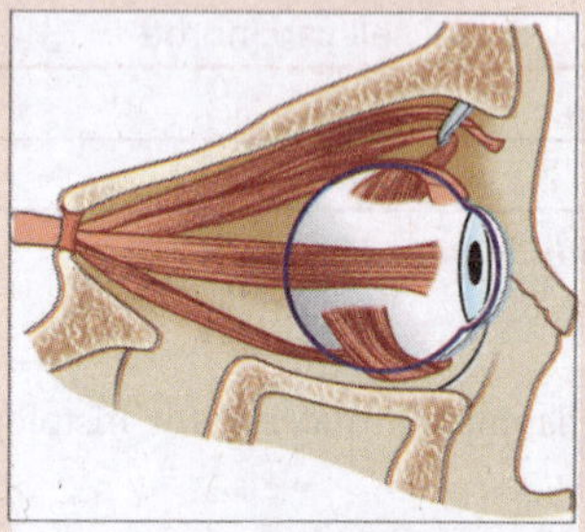 Enucleation	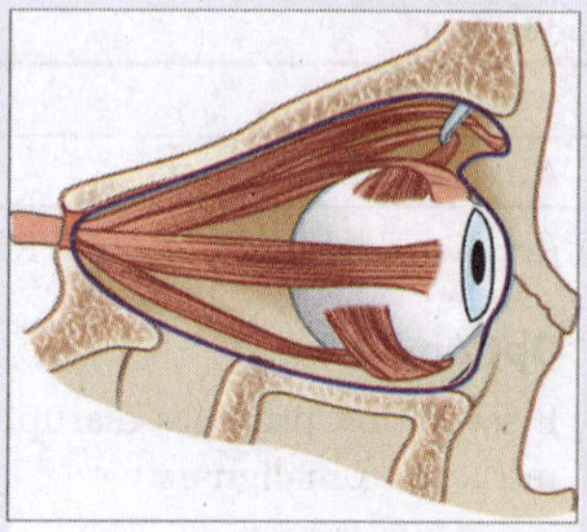 Exenteration

62. Ans. (a) Masson trichrome

Ref: Kanski 8th ed page 216, Khurana 6th ed page 128

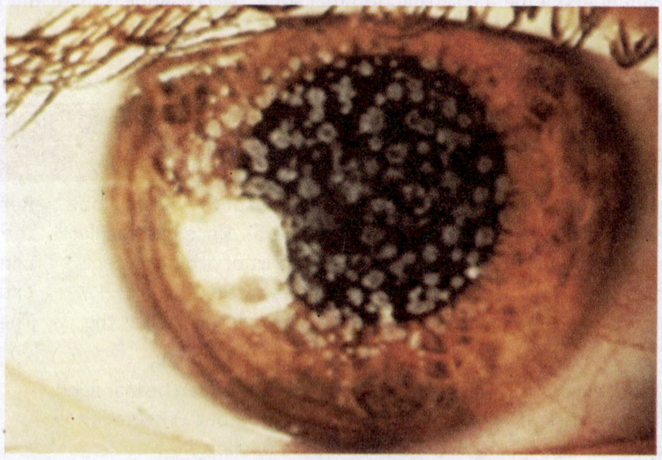

Fig: Granular Dystrophy: B/L Small, discrete, sharply demarcated, grayish-white opacities, DROP, CRUMB, RING shaped may resemble 'snowflakes', can take form of 'christmas tree' & often described as 'popcorn' type

- Initially stroma is clear between lesion with periphery remain free.
- Vision not affected early & impairment, is rare before 5th decade
- Light Microscope: Eosinophilic, hyalinedeposits in stroma & beneath epithelium; stains bright red with MASSON'S TRICHROME.

Corneal Dystrophies					
	Inheritance	Age of onset	Pattern	Comments	Treatment
Epithelium					
Epithelial basement membrane dystrophy (AKA; Cogan's microcystic dystrophy)	AD	Variable	Map, Dot , Fingerprints	**Most common** of all corneal dystrophies seen in working age adults. Most cases are asymptomatic. 10% develop recurrent corneal erosions and severe disabling pain.	Bandage Soft contact lens, Hypertonics, Cuettage, Phototherapeutic keratotomy, Anterior stromal puncture
Meesmann's (Juvenile epithelial dystrophy)	AD	1st decade	Epithelial microcytes	In most cases, condition is asymptomatic and does not require treatment.	Bandage Soft contact lens, Keratoplasty
Bowman's					
Reis Buckler	AD	1st decade	Ring shaped dystrophy	Progressive recurrent corneal erosions that usually result in diffuse anterior scarring.	Bandage Soft contact lens, Keratoplasty
Stromal					
Macular	AS	1st decade	Dense grey opacity in the central cornea	Due to accumulation of **mucopolysaccharides** owing to a local enzyme deficiency. Marked defective vision in early life, which usually requires penetrating keratoplasty.	Bandage Soft contact lens, Keratoplasty
Granular	AD	1st or 2nd decade	Milky granular Hyaline, Drop/ ring shaped deposits with clear stroma in between	Slowly progressive and usually asymptomatic	Bandage Soft contact lens, Keratoplasty
Lattice (AKA; **Biber-Haab-Dimmer** dystrophy)	AD	1st decade	Branching spider-like **amyloid** deposits, sparing the periphery	It appears at the age of 2 years, but the occurrence of recurrent erosions and progressive clouding of central cornea is apparent by the age of 20 years. Soon, visual acuity is impaired. Usually penetrating keratoplasty is required by the age of 30 40 years.	Bandage Soft contact lens, Keratoplasty
POSTERIOR (Endothelium & Descemet membrane)					
Posterior Polymorphous Corneal Dystrophy (PPMD)	AD	1st decade	Variable lesion; vesicles, curvilinear lines or geographical opacities at Descemet membrane	Very slowly progressive and thus usually asymptomatic	Bandage Soft contact lens, Hypertonics, Keratoplasty
Fuchs' epithelial endothelial dystrophy (late hereditary endothelial dystrophy).	AD	4-5th decade (F> M)	Guttata / corneal edema	**Slowly progessive, Bilateral** • **Stage of cornea guttata:** beaten-metal' appearance. Asymptomatic stage	Bandage Soft contact lens, Hypertonics, Keratoplasty, DSAEK- Descement's automated endothelial keratoplasty

Contd...

Corneal Dystrophies

	Inheritance	Age of onset	Pattern	Comments	Treatment
				• **Oedematous stage or stage of endothelial decompensation:** stromal oedema, blurring vision • **Stage of bullous keratopathy:** Epithelial oedema with formation of bullae, which when rupture cause pain, decreased visual acuity. • **Stage of scarring:** Epithelial bullae are replaced by scar tissue and cornea becomes opaque and vascularized.	
Cornea Guttata of vogt	AD	Old age (F> M)	Drop like excrescences involving the entire posterior surface of Descemet's membrane.	Cornea guttata may occur independently or as a part of early stage of Fuch's dystrophy.	It rarely affects the vision and hence treatment is usually not required.

Footnote:

Most important Corneal Dystrophies to remember are Stromal Dystrophies, which can be remembered by

MNEMONIC

- **M**arilyn—**M**acular Dystrophy
- **M**onroe—**M**ucopolysaccharide
- **A**lways—**A**lcian Blue stain
- **G**ets—**G**ranular Dystrophy
- **H**er—**H**yaline
- **M**an in—**M**asson Trichrome stain
- **L**os—**L**attice Dystrophy
- **A**ngeles—**A**myloid
- **C**alifornia—**C**ongo Red

Stains used and Patterns for Histopathological Diagnosis of the Stromal Corneal Dystrophies

Technique	Granular	Lattice	Macular
PAS (Periodic acid Schift)		+	+
Aician blue			+
Trichrome Masson	+	+	
Congo red (under polarization)		+	

Note: Lattice Dystrophy- Shows green birefringence with polarizing microscope

Footnote:

- Macular dystrophy is least found but most severe
- It is the only dystrophy with AR inheritance pattern.
- Cogan map print dot is most common corneal dystrophy
- Granular dystrophy is most common stromal dystrophy

63. Ans. (b) Macular cones

Ref: The Retina and Its Disorders by Joseph C. Besharse page 706

Multifocal electroretinography (MFERG) is an investigation that can simultaneously measure multiple electroretinographic responses at different retinal locations.

- It is basically used to identify macular toxicity and dystrophies, such as drug toxicities and foveal dystrophies. In Mf ERG there is a HILL region corresponding to the sensitivities which is decreased in macular diseases.
- Done after light adaptation for 15 minutes and fully dilated pupil.

Clinical Applications

ARMD, DR, MH, CSR, ERM, RVO, Drug induced toxicity, monitoring of therapy, Congenital Retinal Dystrophies, Acquired retinopathies (white dot syndromes)

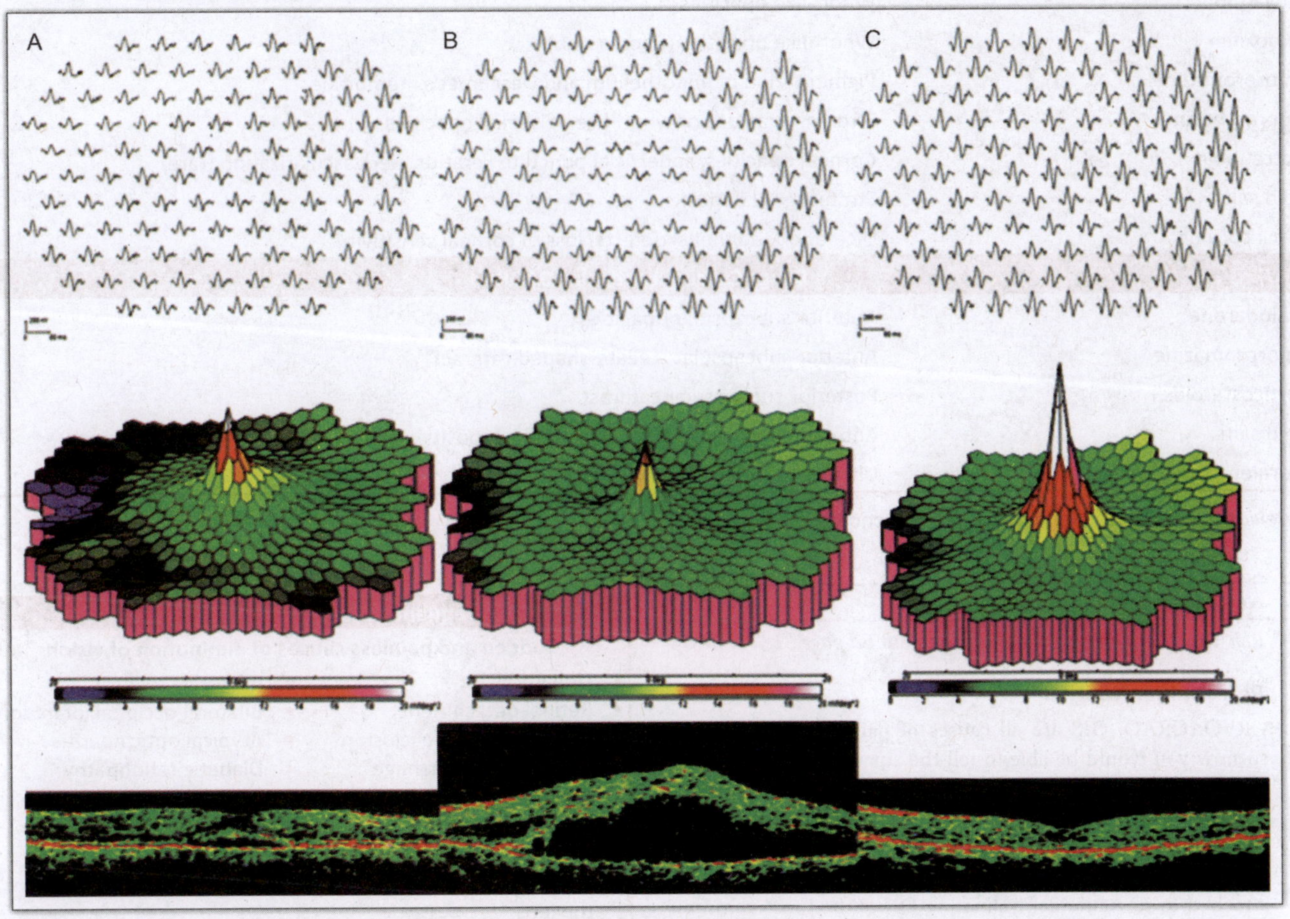

Fig: The decrease in the height of the hill corresponds to the macular pathology correspondingly seen in the OCT image showing macular edema

> **NOTE**
> - *Electro-Oculogram:* Arden ratio > 1.85 is normal, clinically its used to diagnose Best Disease
> - Supernormal ERG occurs in- Early siderosis bulbi, Albinism, Subtotal circulatory disturbances of retina

64. Ans. (b) Chlorpromazine

Ref: Clinical Ocular Pharmacology by Jimmy D. Bartlett 2nd Ed Pg 704, 803

Cornea Verticillata, also called vortex keratopathy, are type of fine, golden brown or gray opacities that are always bilateral at the level of the basal epithelium

Drugs That Can Alfeci the Cornea and Crystalline Lens

Drug	Adverse effect
Drugs Causing Corneal OADRs	
Corticosteroids	Decreased epithelial wound healing increased risk for infection (decreased tear lysozyme)
Chloroquine and hydroxychloroquine	Whorl-like epithelial opacities (also termed vortex keratopathy or corned verticillata)
Amiodarone	Whorl-like opacities
Atovaquone	Whorl-like opacities
Tamoxifen	Whorl-like opacities (uncommon)
Chlorpromazine	Pigmentation of endothelium and Descemet's membrane.
Indomethacin	Stromal opacities or whorl-like epithelial opacities
Isotretinoin	Corneal opacities, superficial punctate keratitis, neovascularization (rare)
Gold salts	Stromal gold deposits
Crack cocaine	Ulceration, epithelial defects, loss of corneal sensitivity
Drugs Causing Lenticular OADRs	
Amiodarone	Anterior subcapsular opacities
Chlorpromazine	Anterior subcapsular steliate-shaped cataract
Corticosteroids	Posterior subcapsular cataract
Gold salts	Anterior capsular or subcapsular gold deposits
Psoralen (8-methoxypsoralen)	Ultraviolet-induced cataract

Abbreviation: OADR- Ocular adverse drug reactions.

65. Ans. (a) Retrobulbar neuritis

Ref: Yanoff 4th ed page 946, Khurana 6th Ed page 318

Retrobulbar Neuritis

CRVO, CRAO, OIS are all causes of painless loss of vision so now you would be able to tell the answer. Now coming to Retrobulbar neuritis, there is a saying that neither the patient nor the patient is able to see. Optic nerve is almost normal most of the times, sometimes rarely hyperfluorescence on FA. There is pain in movement as some fibres of superior rectus is attached to it. Acute demyelinating ON is the most common cause of unilateral painful visual loss in a young adult. The diagnosis of ON is made clinically and consists of a classic triad of visual loss, periocular pain and dyschromatopsia.

Frequent Causes of Decreased Vision

Causes of gradual, painless and progressive diminution of vision	
• **Age less than 40 years** • Refractive error • Keratoconus • Corneal dystrophy • Developmental cataract • Juvenile glaucoma • Retinitis pigmentosa • Compressive optic neuropathy • Hereditary macular degeneration	• **Age more than 40 years** • Presbyopia • Age-related cataract • Chronic simple glaucoma (primary open-angle glaucoma*) • Dry type of age-related macular degeneration • Diabetic retinopathy • Corneal dystrophies • Retinitis pigmentosa • Drug-induced maculopathy or optic neuropathy

Contd...

Frequent Causes of Decreased Vision

Sudden and painless causes of diminution of vision	
• Unilateral • Retinal detachment • Retinal vascular occlusion • Vitreous haemorrhage • Retinal haemorrhage • Exudative age-related macular degeneration • Subluxation or dislocation of the lens	• Bilateral • Bilateral occipital infarction • Atypical optic neuritis • Diabetic retinopathy • Grade IV hypertensive retinopathy with macular star • Toxic optic neuropathy • Posterior uveitis
Diminution of vision associated with pain and/or an acute red eye	
Uveitis Endophthalmitis Corneal ulcer Retrobulbar neuritis Acute angle-closure glaucoma	

Since dearranged light reflex and dark adaptation time is due to optic nerve dysfunction it can be seen as sluggish response and increased adaptation time.

Some High Yielding Points about Optic Neuritis

- Optic neuritis treatment trial ONTT, a landmark trial, told i.v methyl prednisolone can be given in acute optic neuritis, oral prednisolone not to be given.
- CHAMPS trial- Avonex- Interferon Beta- 1a, is indicated in Optic neuritis.
- Dyschromatopsia can be the initial complaint in optic neuritis, initial defect is blue yellow.
- Papillitis is usually unilateral, Papilledema is usually bilateral.

Medicine

11

AIIMS NOVEMBER 2018

1. Which of the following enzymes is specific for alcoholic hepatitis?

a. ALP　　b. ALT
c. GGT　　d. LDH

2. Dotted lines in the Transpulmonary pressure vs volume graph as shown below indicates which diseases? ***(AIIMS Nov 2018, 2015)***

a. Asthma　　b. COPD
c. Bronchiectasis　　d. Interstitial fibrosis

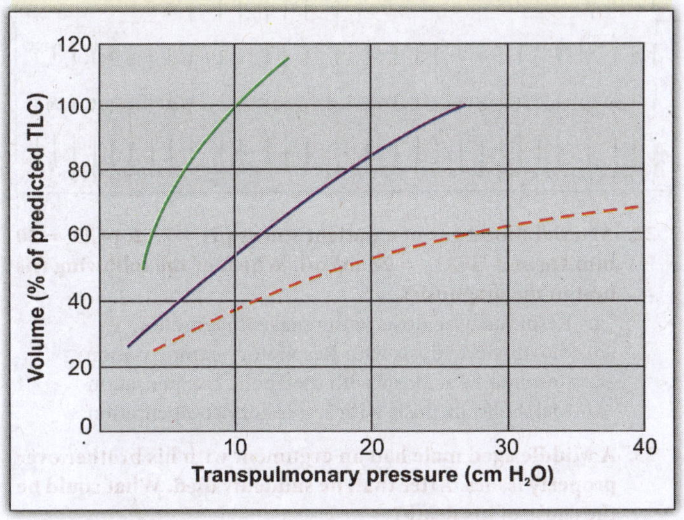

3. A female was started on anti epileptic drug after she had complaint of seizures during sleep. She has no history of seizures for last 6 months and her CT/MRI are also normal. She wants to stop taking medications. What would be done ?

a. Life long treatment
b. Stop drug and follow up with EEG every 6 months
c. Stop treatment
d. Continue for 2 years

4. A 40-year-old female with syphilis comes to OPD. She has problem walking in straight line with eyes closed and she stamp off on walking. Identify tract involved?

a. Spinocerebellar tract
b. Dorsal column tract
c. Lateral Spinothalamic tract
d. Vestibulospinal tract

5. What is the difference between RIFLE & KDIGO criteria in differentiating a tubular injury?

a. Uosm
b. Urinary Na
c. Urinary NGAL
d. FeNa (UNa × Scr / SNa × Ucr)

6. Patient had recurrent optic neuritis of both eyes with extensive transverse myelitis. Visual acuity in right eye is 6/60 and visual acuity in left eye 6/18. Patient showed 50% response to steroids. Diagnosis is?

a. Neuromyelitis optica (NMO)
b. Subacute combined degeneration of spinal cord (SACD)
c. Posterior cerebral artery stroke
d. Neurosyphilis

7. Which of the following is not useful in measuring cardiac output?

a. Transthoracic echocardiogram
b. Central venous catheter
c. Thermodilution pulmonary catheter
d. Continuous cardiac output pulmonary catheter

8. ECG with "mean" axis of 90°. In which lead there would be the maximum voltage of R wave? ***(AIIMS Nov 2018, May 2018)***

a. aVF　　b. III
c. aVL　　d. aVR

9. Patient presents with recent onset breathlessness and ECG is taken. ECG is shown below. What is the diagnosis?

a. Atrial Fibrillation
b. PSVT
c. AMI
d. MAT

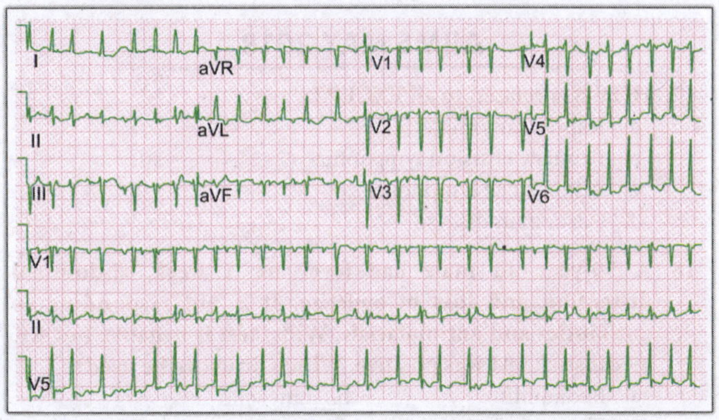

10. Relative bradycardia is uncommon in?

a. Malaria b. Factitious fever
c. Typhoid d. Brucellosis

11. How do you differentiate tamponade from tension pneumothorax?

a. Low volume pulse b. Breath sounds present
c. Distended veins d. No response to IV fluids

12. A patient came with a Chest trauma and Tachypnea (RR >40) and after checkup he had hypertension (BP- 90/60) and hyperresonant note on involved side. He is able to speak sentences in words. Next management will be?

a. Secure Airway
b. Needle insertion in 2nd intercostal space
c. IV Fluids
d. Chest X ray

13. A patient presents with tamponade. You ask intern to document his blood pressure. What intern should advise patient to do while documenting blood pressure ?

a. Breath normally
b. Rapid and shallow breaths
c. Slow and deep breaths
d. To hold breaths

14. A patient who is a known case of CKD has complaints of vomiting. His ABG reports are as follows: pH - 7.40, pCO2 - 40, HCO3 – 24. Na -140, chloride–100. Which of the following is the correct interpretation?

a. No acid base disorder
b. Normal anion gap metabolic acidosis
c. High anion gap metabolic acidosis
d. High anion gap acidosis with metabolic alkalosis

15. Which of the following is not done before ABG:

a. Allen's test
b. Heparin to rinse the syringe
c. Flexion of wrist
d. Poking at 45° angle

16. A female Patient presents with left sided weakness since 1 hour and left sided facial weakness with BP - 160/90. CT scan does not show any intracranial hemorrhage. What is the best next step?

a. Start thrombolysis
b. Give loading dose of aspirin and clopidogrel
c. Lower BP
d. Wait and watch as CT is normal

AIIMS MAY 2018

17. HHV 8 is related to all EXCEPT:

a. Kaposi sarcoma
b. Primary effusion lymphoma
c. Adult T cell lymphoma
d. Castleman disease

18. A 50-year-old male had fever for 1 week, abdominal distention and loss of appetite. It is not responding to antibiotics and antimalarials. Widal test is negative but RK 39 dipstick test was positive. Which drug can be used?

a. Bedaquiline b. Linezolid
c. Fluconazole d. Amphotericin B

19. A 50-year-old man who is a known hypertensive and diabetic, fell unconscious in the morning. He was taken to emergency department and examined. BP 180/100 mm Hg, pulse 120/min and bilateral plantar extensor. What is the next step in the line of management?

a. Take CT b. Start mannitol
c. Measure blood sugar d. Start thrombolysis

20. Middle aged woman with Menorrhagia, cold intolerance presents in emergency with altered sensorium, non pitting edema. On examination her Rectal temperature 32 degree C, bradycardia and hypotension. Most likely diagnosis is?

a. Septic shock b. Cardiogenic shock
c. Myxedema coma d. Hypothermia

21. Patient presents with recent onset breathlessness and ECG is taken. ECG is shown below. What is the diagnosis?

(AIIMS Nov 2018, May 2018)

a. Atrial Fibrillation b. PSVT
c. AMI d. MAT

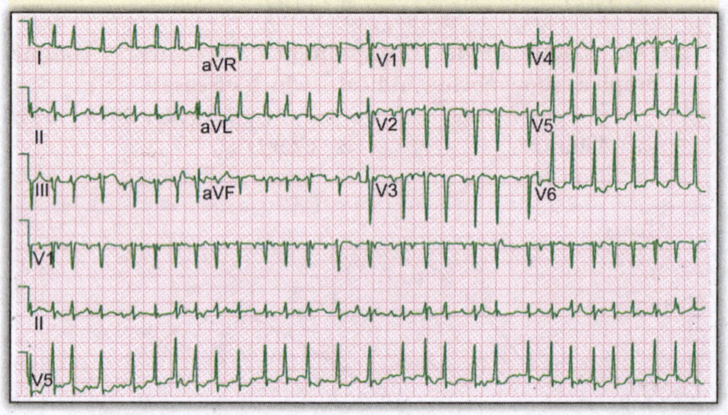

22. Arterial Blood gas of a patient shows pH = 7.12, pCO_2 = 50 mm Hg and HCO_3- = 28 mEq/l. Which of the following fits best in the diagnosis?

a. Respiratory acidosis with renal compensation
b. Metabolic acidosis with Respiratory compensation
c. Respiratory acidosis with metabolic compensation
d. Metabolic alkalosis with respiratory compensation

23. A Middle aged male had an argument with his brother over property issues. After that, he suddenly died. What could be the cause of his death?

a. Dilated cardiomyopathy
b. Takotsubo cardiomyopathy
c. Right atrial arrhythmia
d. Chronic ischemic cardiomyopathy

24. Which of the following is common cause of Ventilator acquired pneumonia?

a. Klebsiella
b. Acinetobacter
c. Mycobacterium tuberculosis
d. Proteus

25. Which of the following drug is commonly used for community acquired pneumonia caused by S. aureus?

a. Vancomycin
b. Cefoperazone
c. Cefazolin
d. Azithromycin

26. A patient from North eastern region comes with history of fever and body ache. Antigen test is positive for falciparum malaria. What will be the treatment?

a. Chloroquine
b. Mefloquine
c. Artemether plus lumefantrine
d. Sulfadoxine plus pyrimethamine

27. Most common form of arthritis is?

a. Rheumatoid arthritis b. Psoriatic arthritis
c. Seronegative arthritis d. Osteoarthritis

28. Triad of skin lesions asymmetric mononeuritis complex and eosinophilia are seen in?

a. Cryoglobulinemic vasculitis
b. Polyarteritis nodosa
c. Churg Strauss syndrome
d. Giant cell arteritis

29. Which of the following is not a component of Syndrome Z?

a. Obstructive Sleep Apnea
b. Blood pressure more than 130/85 mm Hg
c. Fasting Triglyceride more than 150 mg/dL
d. LDL more than 100 mg/dL

30. A patient presented with headache and fever for 7 days. While doing a lumbar puncture, it was noticed that the opening CSF pressure increased on jugular vein compression and became normal on relieving the pressure on jugular vein. What is the interpretation of this?

a. Subdural blockage b. Subarachnoid blockage
c. Arachnoid villi blockage d. Patent subarachnoid space

31. An old lady came with diarrhea had she was given rapid fluids and sodium correction. During the course of recovery she become paraplegic, comatose and mute. Which of the following is cause of the CNS symptoms?

a. It is a normal sequelae of hypernatremia
b. Rapid correction of hyponatremia
c. Slow correction of hyponatremia
d. Brainstem infarct

AIIMS NOVEMBER 2017

32. While taking history from a patient's attendant, which of the following is of no significance?

a. Educational status
b. Blood relation
c. His observation capacity
d. Duration of stay in hospital with patient

33. All of the following are reduced in iron deficiency anaemia EXCEPT:

a. Serum ferritin b. Serum iron
c. Transferrin saturation d. TIBC

34. A man came from high altitude, presents with Hypertension and develops itching and fatigue. On physical examination splenomegaly was present. WBC 21000, platelets 350000, Eosinophil 5%. What test to order next?

a. Philadelphia chromosome
b. Bone marrow Biopsy
c. Erythropoietin levels
d. JAK mutation

35. A patient comes to Emergency Department with fever and headache. On examination he has neck stiffness. CSF analysis shows following findings; Opening pressure – Increased, Proteins- Mild increased, Glucose – Normal, Lymphocytes - Increased. Most likely diagnosis ?

a. TB meningitis
b. N. Gonorrhea meningitis
c. Cryptococcus meningitis
d. Coxsackie meningitis

36. What is the most likely diagnosis of the following ECG?

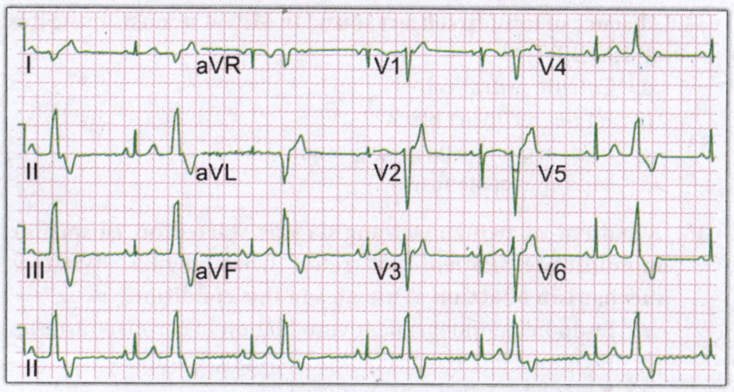

a. Ventricular bigeminy b. Electrical alternans
c. P pulmonale d. Improper calibration

37. A 53-year-old patient was admitted complains of dyspnea. On examination he has Puffy face with engorged veins over the chest. SVC obstruction is suspected. Chest X-ray shows widening of mediastinal. What is the next step?

a. Total blood count with peripheral smear
b. CT Thorax
c. Start cyclophosphamide
d. Urgent referral to RT

38. Normal anion gap metabolic acidosis seen in all EXCEPT:
(AIIMS Nov 2017, DNB December 2011, December 2010, June 2009, 2006, 2004)

a. Proximal RTA
b. Pancreatitis
c. Hyperchloremic diarrhea
d. Salicylate poisoning

39. A patient has Right upper limb BP of 180/95 mm Hg and Left upper limb Bp of 130/90 mm Hg. He also has early diastolic murmur in right 2 Intercostal space. Which of the following would be least likely associated with these findings?

a. Supravalvular aortic stenosis
b. Coarctation of aorta
c. Takayasu arteritis
d. Aortic dissection

40. Which of the following is the test for Immediate memory?

a. Serial (100–7) subtraction test upto 5 steps
b. Serial (20–1) subtraction test upto 5 steps
c. Digit span forward upto 7 digits with 2 skips allowed
d. Digit span backwards upto 5 digits with 2 skips allowed

41. All of the following are associated with SAAG >1 gm% in Ascitic fluid analysis EXCEPT:

a. Liver cirrhosis b. Liver metastasis
c. Liver failure d. Tubercular peritonitis

42. **All of the following are seen in tumor lysis Syndrome EXCEPT:**
a. Hyperuricemia b. Hypercalcemia
c. Hyperkalemia d. Hyperphosphatemia

43. **A patient comes with sudden onset palpitations. ECG showed a narrow complex tachycardia without P waves and with a rate of 160 BPM. His Blood pressure is 96/68 mm Hg. What is the next management ?**
a. Carotid body massage b. Adenosine
c. Beta blocker d. Defibrillator

44. **Absence of loud first heart sound in Mitral stenosis indicates all EXCEPT:**
a. Calcific mitral valve
b. 1st degree heart block
c. Presence of aortic regurgitation
d. Mild mitral stenosis

45. **A patient of prinzmetal angina was started on isosorbide mononitrate. Patient got relief from angina. What is mechanism of action of nitrates in this condition?**
a. Endothelial independent vasodilation of coronary arteries
b. Increased left ventricular end diastolic volume
c. Reduced cardiac contractility
d. Decreased diastolic perfusion pressure

46. **A person presents in emergency department with complaint of headache and says it is the worst headache of his life. Which investigation would you perform next?**
a. NCCT b. Lumbar puncture
c. MRI d. Angiography

47. **Which of the following is not used in emergency management of hyperkalemia?**
a. Nebulised salbutamol
b. IV Insulin and dextrose
c. IV calcium gluconate
d. Inj. Magnesium sulphate

48. **A patient presents with anaphylactic shock. What will be the treatment of choice?**
a. Adrenaline 1 mg 1:10000 by intravenous route
b. Adrenaline 0.5 mg 1:1000 by intramuscular route
c. Atropine 3 mg by intravenous route
d. Adenosine 6 mg followed by 12 mg IV

49. **A friend of yours had 5 episodes of loose stools 2 hours after having lunch at hotel you were staying on a road trip. On examination he is afebrile but has mild dehydration and tachycardia. As a physician what would you do?**
a. Start only ORS
b. Give ciprofloxacin only
c. Give him ciprofloxacin and tinidazole
d. Give ciprofloxacin, tinidazole and ORS

AIIMS MAY 2017

50. **A 40-year-old male with history of fall and one episode of vomiting near an alcoholic shop. He was brought to casualty, he was awake with open eyes and had unrelieved retrograde amnesia. Which of the following is the most likely cause?**
a. Concussion b. Drunkenness
c. Diffuse axonal injury d. Cerebral venous thrombosis

51. **A 56-year-old came to casualty with history of massive hemoptysis. His routine investigation chest X-ray was normal. Which of the following is not done to prevent hemoptysis?**
a. Bronchial artery embolization
b. Pulmonary artery embolization
c. Bronchoscopic ligation
d. Resection of affected lung lobe

52. **A 20-year-old female came with complaints of headache, vomiting and decrease in movement of right leg. In the past she had episodes of violent and aggressive behaviour and abdominal pain. Which of the following is the most probable diagnosis?**
a. Conversion disorder b. AIDP with migraine
c. Right side paralysis d. Acute intermittent porphyria

53. **A female comes with elevated TSH with subnormal level of free T4?**
a. Primary hyperthyroidism
b. Secondary hypothyroidism
c. Primary hypothyroidism
d. Subclinical hypothyroidism

54. **A lady delivered a normal vaginal delivery and was discharged. On third day she came back with fever, tachycardia and seizures. Fundus showed papilledema with no focal deficits. Diagnosis?**
a. Meningitis b. Acute migraine
c. Cortical vein thrombosis d. Subarachnoid haemorrhage

55. **A middle aged man presented with frontal bossing and large tongue and he had spade shaped hands. Which of the following tests will you do for diagnosis?**
a. Thyroid hormone assay b. Serum prolactin
c. Insulin like growth factor d. Serum testosterone

56. **A 12-year-old patient comes with history of bilateral ascending muscle weakness, along with areflexia. There is no history of trauma. Which of the following should be evaluated first?**
a. Serum potassium b. Serum calcium
c. Serum magnesium d. Serum sodium

57. **A young girl with the diagnosis of acute promyelocytic leukaemia (APML) was treated medically. She developed fever and tachypnea and chest X-ray shows pulmonary infiltrates. Which is the drug she should be given next?**
a. Doxorubicin b. Methotrexate
c. Dexamethasone d. Cytarabine

58. **What is the acute management for the condition shown in the following ECG?**

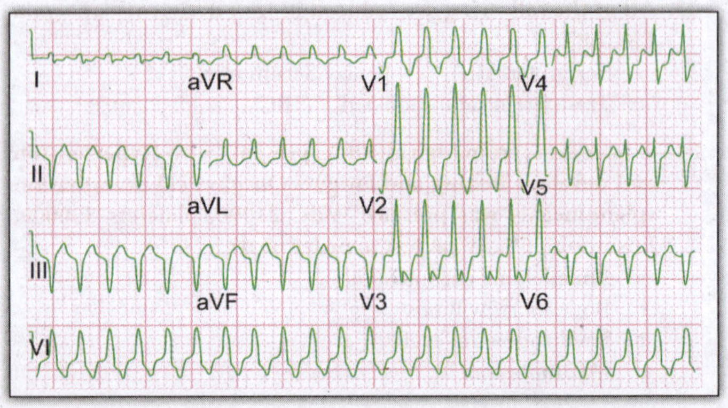

a. $MgSO_4$
b. DC cardioversion
c. Lignocaine
d. Diltiazem

59. Definition of PUO includes all of the following EXCEPT:
a. Fever persisting for more than 3 weeks
b. Two fever spikes more than 38.3°C
c. Undiagnosed after one week of investigation
d. No history of immunocompromised state

60. Window period for thrombolytic therapy in case of stroke is?
a. 1.5 hour
b. 2.5 hours
c. 3.5 hours
d. 4.5 hours

61. A 40-year-old female currently on a drug for psychiatric illness and hypertension presents with NYHA class III heart failure with dyspnea, pedal edema and K levels of 5.5 mEq/L and creatinine 2.5 mg%. Which of the following drug is best avoided?
a. Spironolactone
b. Amitriptyline
c. Enalapril/Lisinopril
d. Digoxin

62. Which of the following is not a feature of Myasthenia Gravis?
a. Ptosis
b. Normal pupillary reflex
c. Muscle fatigue
d. Absent deep tendon reflexes

63. A 70-year-old smoker with brain metastasis with BP - 150/100 mm Hg, was admitted and started on antihypertensive drug thiazide. There are no neurological signs of pedal edema. Serum electrolytes were normal at admission, after starting of treatment developed hyponatremia comes confused and drowsy, his Sr. Na-123, urine-Na increased, Sr.osmol-285, Urine-osmol-350. Most likely cause of hyponatremia is?
a. SIADH
b. Cerebral salt wasting
c. Diuretic induced hyponatremia
d. Pseudohypoaldosteronism

64. What complication of stroke does not require any treatment?
a. Spasticity
b. Neglect
c. Dysphagia
d. Fever

65. All of the following is seen in CURB 65 score EXCEPT:
a. Respiratory rate of >30/min
b. Confusion and blood urea greater than 7 mmol/L
c. SBP less than or equal to 100 mm Hg, DBP less than or equal to 60 mm Hg
d. Age > 65

AIIMS NOVEMBER 2016

66. A 82-year-old lady with diabetes and hypertension presented with severe constipation. Her relatives brought her for check up. She also gives recent history of depression, Agitated at times and does irrelevant talking. Heart rate was 58/min. BP was found 150/100 around on supine position and 122/90 upon standing. She is having constipation for past 3 days and her intestine was loaded with hard stools. She was on beta blockers, imipramine, haloperidol and isaphgul. Which is most appropriate for her?
a. Change beta blockers to ACE inhibitors and calcium channel blockers as she has resting bradycardia and add bisacodyl for constipation
b. Change imipramine and haloperidol to Fluoxetine plus Resperidone as they are causing postural hypotension. And add bisacodyl for constipation
c. Stop all medication and manual removal of impacted stool and bisacodyl
d. Only add Bisacodyl for constipation and continue rest of the medication

67. Which of the following set of first and second line treatment of Seizure is incorrect?

	Seizure	1st line	Alternative
a.	Absence seizure	Lamotrigine, Ethosuximide	Carbamazepine, valproate
b.	Myoclonic	Valproate, Lamotrigine	Clonazepam
c.	Generalized tonic clonic seizure (GTCS)	Valproate Carbamazepine	Lamotrigine Topiramate
d.	Partial seizure	Lamotrigine Gabapentin	Carbamazepine

68. Centripetal distribution of rash is seen in all EXCEPT:
a. Measles
b. Epidemic typhus
c. Typhoid
d. Secondary Syphilis

69. If a patient has worm infestation with no systemic Complaints. What should be the cut off absolute eosinophil count to call it as hyper eosinophilia syndrome?
a. 500
b. 1000
c. 1500
d. 2000

70. A 40-year-old presents with complaints for vomiting since three days. On examination signs of dehydration was present. His blood gas analysis shows the following findings pH-7.22, HCO_3^- = 9 mEq, pCO_2 = 21 mm Hg. Most likely diagnosis is?
a. Metabolic acidosis
b. Respiratory alkalosis
c. Mixed Metabolic acidosis and respiratory alkalosis
d. Mixed Metabolic acidosis with metabolic alkalosis

71. A 75 kg weight patient with a diagnosis of acid base imbalance with pH = 6.5, pCO_2 = 30 mm Hg, pO_2- 90 mm hg and HCO_3– = 6 m Eq. Calculate the base deficit?
a. 200 m Eq/L
b. 300 m Eq/L
c. 400 m Eq/L
d. 500 m Eq/L

72. A 42-year-old person came with complaints of weakness on the right side and loss of sensation on left side. On examination both upper limb and lower limb of right side had decreased tone and signs of Horner's syndrome on right side. He had dysarthria and difficulty in swallowing. In addition there was hemisensory loss of touch, pain and temperature on the left side of the body. What is most likely diagnosis?
a. Right posterior inferior cerebellar artery occlusion
b. Right anterior inferior cerebellar artery occlusion
c. Right superior cerebral artery occlusion
d. Basilar artery occlusion

73. DLCO decreased in all EXCEPT:
a. Pulmonary vascular disease
b. Emphysema
c. Interstitial lung disease
d. Polycythemia

74. A patient of lung carcinoma has serum calcium of 16 mg/dL. He is weak and lethargic. Most immediate step of management is?

a. IV phosphate
b. Bisphosphonate
c. Subcutaneous calcitonin
d. IV fluids with furosemide

75. In a patient on metformin, All are risk factor of Lactic acidosis EXCEPT:

a. Renal dysfunction
b. Liver diseases
c. Smoking
d. Advance age

76. Cerebellar lesion produces all EXCEPT:

a. Ataxic gait
b. Past pointing
c. Resting tremor
d. Nystagmus

77. Which of the following is not associated with MEN 1 syndrome?

a. Posterior pituitary tumor
b. Foregut carcinoid
c. Parathyroid hyperplasia
d. Pancreatic neuroendocrine tumor

78. The following ECG picture is showing?

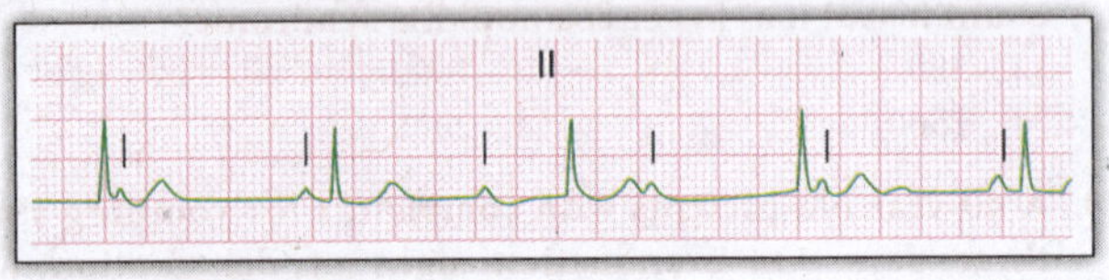

a. Sinus arrest
b. Trifascicular block
c. 2: 1 block
d. Complete heart block

79. A 68-year-old man with history of type 2 Diabetes mellitus on insulin, Hypertension and on Anticoagulant for atrial fibrillation comes with altered sensorium. Which of the following investigation is not required in emergency?

a. NCCT head
b. Lumbar puncture
c. Random blood sugar
d. 12 lead ECG

80. Sjögren syndrome feature are all EXCEPT:

a. High phosphate in saliva
b. High salivary sodium
c. Increased salivary IgA
d. Saliva secretion less than 0.5 mL

81. Most suitable test for Intestinal malabsorption is?

(AIIMS Nov 2016, May 2010)

a. D-xylose
b. Stool fat estimation
c. NBT- PABA
d. Schilling test

82. Continuous murmur can be heard in all EXCEPT:

a. Pulmonary AV fistula
b. Coronary AV fistula
c. Patent ductus arteriosus
d. VSD with AR

83. In a patient of Jaundice and with liver enzyme panel, AST 86.5 U and ALT- 81 U. USG suggestive of Liver cirrhosis. Viral markers were done as in the table below. Which of the following is your next step in management?

Test	Result
HBsAg	Negative
Anti HBsAg	Negative
Anti HBeAg	Negative
Anti HbCAg IgG	Positive
Anti HbCAg IgM	Negative
Anti HCV	Positive
Anti HEV	Negative

a. Anti-HBS
b. HCV RNA- RT PCR
c. HBV DNA estimation
d. Liver biopsy

84. Which of the following is/are features of airway obstruction?

a. Impaired speech
b. High pitch sound
c. Impaired alveolar ventilation
d. All are true

85. In patient with iron deficiency anemia following statement is correct about iron supplementation?

a. Test dose is required for giving IV iron
b. Once target hemoglobin of >12 mg/dl is achieved oral iron is discontinued
c. Most common side effect of oral iron therapy is gastric intolerance and it should be managed by giving IV iron
d. Parenteral iron supplementation is required in a patient with hemoglobin of less than 7 mg/dl

86. A chronic binge alcoholic and smoker comes with history of fatigue, cough and purulent sputum with postural variation. Chest X-ray was done, as seen in picture. What will be the next step in management?

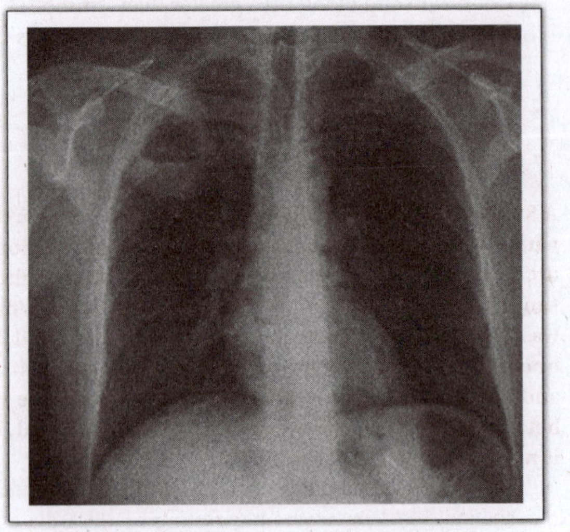

a. Gemcitabin and paclitaxel
b. IV Clindamycin
c. Lobectomy
d. ATT

AIIMS MAY 2016

87. A 16-year-old patient with history of trauma to the right side of chest came to the emergency with hypotension (BP 90/60 mm Hg) and severe dyspnea. On examination breath sounds were absent on right hemithorax with tracheal deviation towards left side, percussion note was hyper resonant. The next line of management for this patient is?

a. Immediate needle thoracotomy
b. Intercostal chest tube insertion
c. Emergent trachestomy
d. Start vasopressors for low BP

88. A 52-year-old female known Asthamatic, came to emergency department with increased breathlessness, cough and wheezing for 2 days. On examination PR 144/min, BP 96/64 mm Hg, RR -30/min with SPO_2 – 76%. Arterial Blood gas analysis showed PO_2 50 mm Hg, PCO_2 70 mm Hg and pH – 7.2. The next step is?

a. Intubation with low tidal volume mechanical ventilation
b. Continuous positive pressure ventilation
c. IV diuretics with digoxin
d. High flow oxygen through non rebreathing face mask

89. On emergency duty, a second year medicine resident asks you to perform an ABG, all are true regarding ABG EXCEPT:

a. Radial artery is the preferred site
b. Preloaded syringe with 0.3 mL heparin prior to drawing blood
c. Normal levels of HCO_3, $PaCO_2$, pH does not exclude acid base imbalance
d. Different side is chosen if modified allens test is positive on the side

90. pH of 7.30 and $PaCO_2$ of 35 mm Hg is suggestive of?

a. Metabolic alkalosis
b. Respiratory alkalosis
c. Respiratory acidosis
d. Metabolic acidosis

91. Tourniquet test is useful in monitoring of patients with?

a. Swine flu
b. Dengue fever
c. Zika viral disease
d. Chikungunya

92. The most important parameter to monitor during dengue haemorrhagic fever is?

a. Platelet count
b. Hemoglobin
c. Total leukocyte count
d. Hematocrit

93. In a patient with post tuberculous bronchiectasis which of the following is correct clinical finding?

a. Bibasilar crackles
b. Mixed fine and coarse crackles
c. Tubular breathing
d. Both early and late inspiratory crackles

94. A young patient presents with history suggestive of tuberculosis. On examination he has pleural effusion. You will send the sample for all of the following parameter for pleural fluid analysis EXCEPT:

a. Gene Xpert
b. LDH
c. Albumin
d. ADA

95. A 40-year-old patient with head injury. Best strategy of the following to decreasing the ICT is?

a. Administer nimodipine
b. Oxygen supplementation by mechanical ventilation
c. Prevent increase in pCO_2 levels
d. Administer sedative

96. A doctor performed deep tendon reflex as shown in picture below. With regards to this picture which of the following statement is correct?

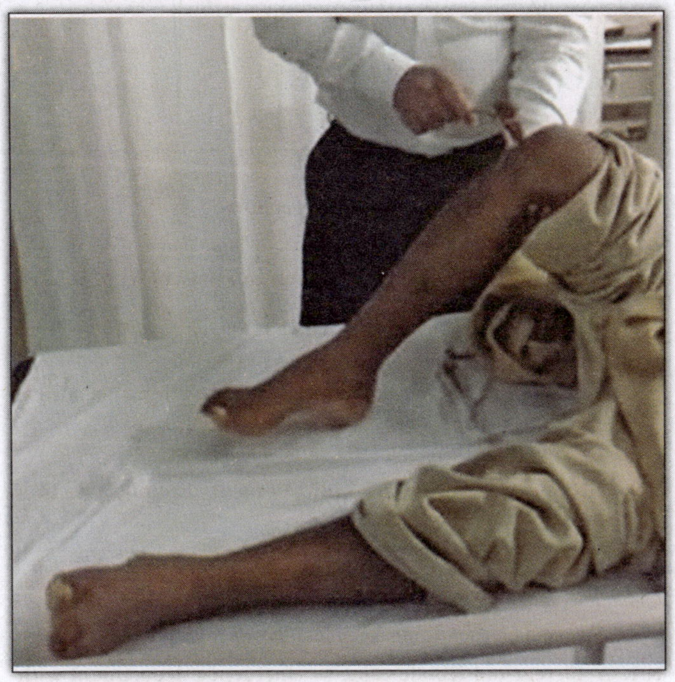

a. Deep tendon reflex is always brisk in case of motor neuron disease
b. The examiner is doing the test wrongly
c. Deep tendon reflex is always absent in case of peripheral neuropathy
d. Root value of this reflex is L1, L2, L3

97. A 52-year-old diabetic male patient complaints of palpitations. On examination his Systolic BP was 70 mm Hg. His ECG was recorded in emergency as below. The immediate next step of management is?

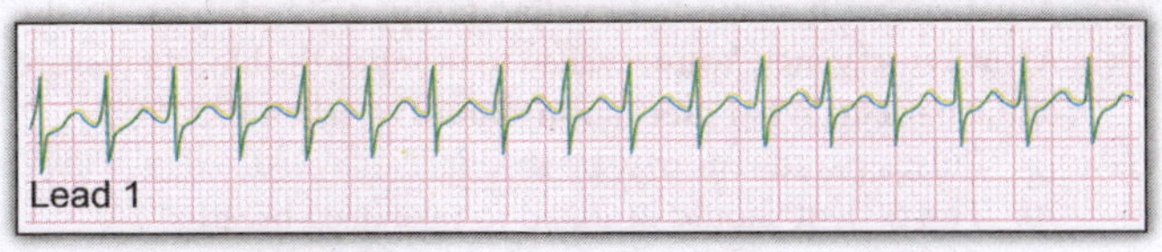

a. Primary PCI
b. Cardioversion
c. IV amiodarone
d. Adenosine

MEDICINE • Questions

98. A 76-year-old male came to AIIMS emergency department with complaints of retrosternal pain for 6 hours. The following is the ECG of the patient. The appropriate next line of management of this patient is?

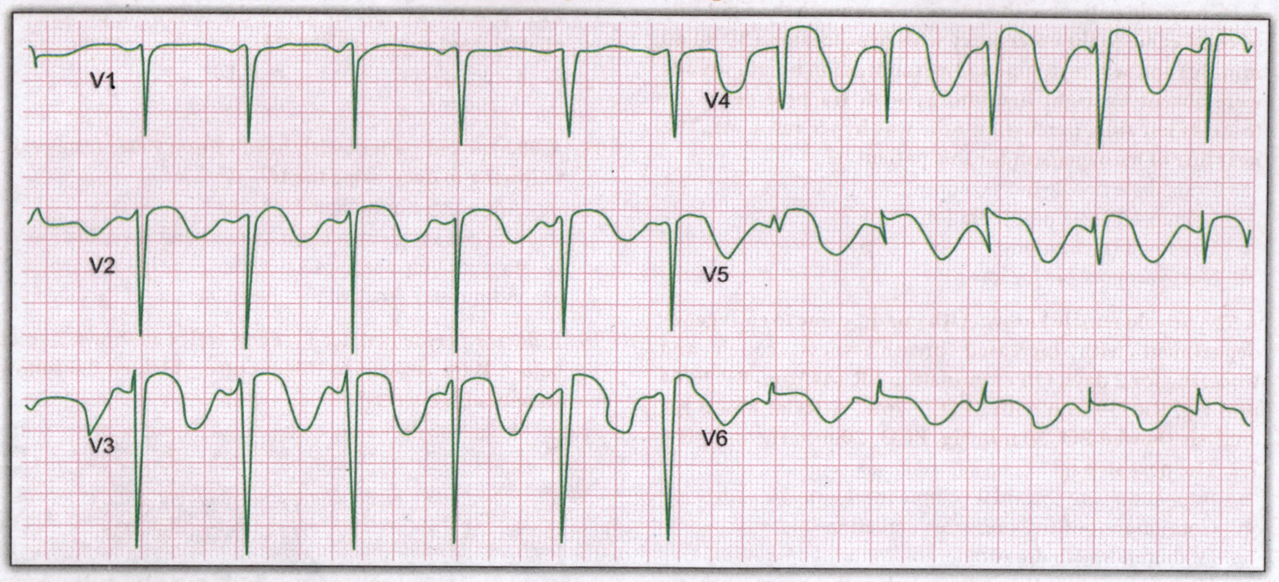

a. Abciximab
b. Thrombolysis
c. Primary percutaneous intervention
d. Low molecular weight heparin

99. The following are clinical findings in a patient with isolated aortic stenosis EXCEPT:
a. The left ventricular impulse is displaced laterally
b. Pulsus bisferiens is the hallmark finding
c. Systemic arterial pressure is usually within the normal limits in early stages
d. A thrill is palpabale over carotid arteries

100. All of the following are indications of thrombolysis in a stroke patient EXCEPT:
a. Age >18 years
b. Blood pressure >185/100 mm Hg despite treatment
c. CT Brain showing edema <1/3rd of MCA territory
d. Acute ischemic stroke of less than 3 hours onset

101. A 40-year-old female came to emergency department with complaints of acute onset of breathlessness after a prolonged air travel for 16 hours. On clinical examination pulse rate 115/min, BP 90/60 mm Hg, SO_2 80% and sinus tachycardia on ECG. Bedside echo suggestive of right ventricular dilatation with interventricular septum deviated to left. What is the primary treatment modality?
a. Intravenous plasminogen activator
b. Intravenous unfractionated heparin
c. Thrombectomy
d. IVC filter

102. A patient with suspected cardiac tamponade presents to the AIIMS emergency. You are asked to monitor the blood pressure of the patient. What precaution should be taken EXCEPT:
a. Pulsus paradoxus may be absent
b. The patient should be asked to take deep breaths
c. Cuff pressure slowly deflated until the 1st koratkoff sound is heard only during expiration
d. The blood pressure cuff is inflated 20 mm Hg above systemic pressure

103. A patient with disseminated malignancy receiving palliative care presents with nausea, vomiting and altered sensorium. You made a provisional diagnosis of hypercalcemia which was confirmed by investigations. The next line of management is?
a. IV fluids
b. IV steroid
c. Thiazide diuretics
d. IV bisphosphanates

104. All of the following are true regarding lumbar puncture EXCEPT:
a. The needle is inserted at a slightly cephalad angle
b. In lateral recumbent position, the bevel of the needle should face up
c. The legs should be straightened during measurement of opening pressure
d. The needle is inserted at L1-L2 intervertebral space

105. A person employed in Glass factory to polish glasses complaints of numbness of hands, generalized weakness of limbs, constipation and frequent episode of pain abdomen. X-ray showed linear radiopaque lines on metaphysis of knee and wrist joints. Which of the following tests ordered will diagnose?
a. Serum Mercury level
b. ALA in urine
c. RBC cholinesterase levels
d. Vitamin D levels

106. L-asparaginase is useful in the treatment of?
a. ALL
b. AML
c. CML
d. CLL

107. All are true about the procedure performed by the instrument shown in the image below EXCEPT:

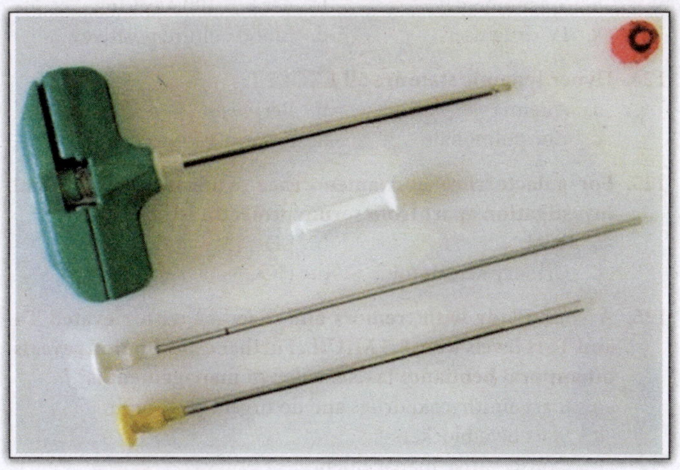

a. The procedure may be done in both lateral or prone positions
b. Useful for the diagnosis of infiltrative and granulomatous disorders
c. Platelet count <40,000/mm^3 is a contraindication
d. Breath holding is not necessary during this procedure

AIIMS NOVEMBER 2015

108. Identify the following instrument?

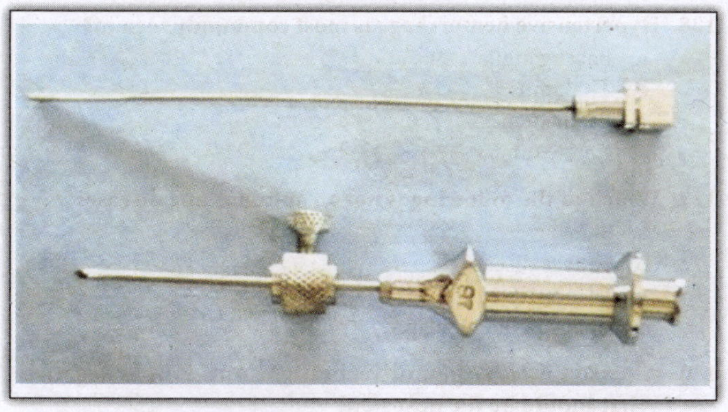

a. Bone marrow biopsy needle
b. Seldinger's needle
c. Pleural biopsy needle
d. Trucut needle

109. Older male adult presenting with chronic sinusitis not subsiding with antihistaminics, along with nasopharyngeal ulcers, cavitary lung lesion, glomerulonephritis, pneumonitis and purpura. Diagnosis and next step will be?
a. Systemic fungal infections, biopsy
b. Miliary tuberculosis, mantoux
c. Wegener's granulomatosis, ANCA and evaluate for vasculitis
d. Multiple metastasis

110. As per WHO, In which condition investigations for latent TB is not required?
a. Patient is chronic alcoholic
b. Patient has silicosis
c. Patient on routine hemodialysis
d. Patient on anti TNG therap

111. Glucocorticoids are not used in which of the following condition?
a. CML
b. Hodgkin's Lymphoma
c. Kaposi sarcoma
d. Multiple myeloma

112. Glucocorticoids deficiency causes all EXCEPT:
a. Hyperkalemia
b. Fever
c. Weight loss
d. Postural hypotension

113. Most specific sign in metabolic encephalopathy is?
a. Asterixis
b. Abulia
c. Akinetic mutism
d. Apraxia

114. A 46-year-old lady comes with history of chest pain and diaphoresis for past one day. ECG was done and following picture was obtained. BP was 150/90 mm Hg. Which of the following should not be used as treatment?

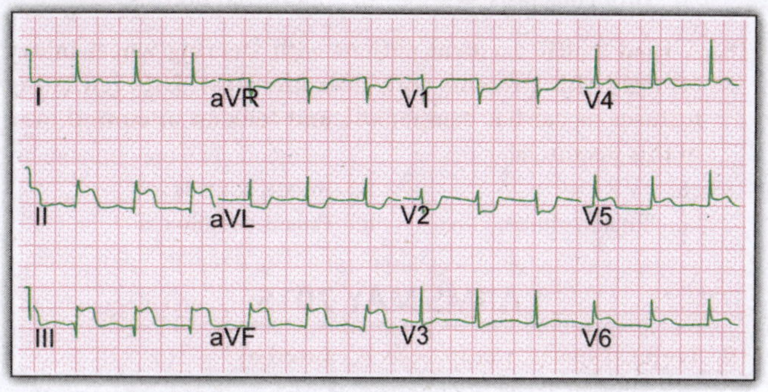

a. Aspirin
b. Thrombolytics
c. Morphine
d. Statins

115. Identify the condition in the given ECG?

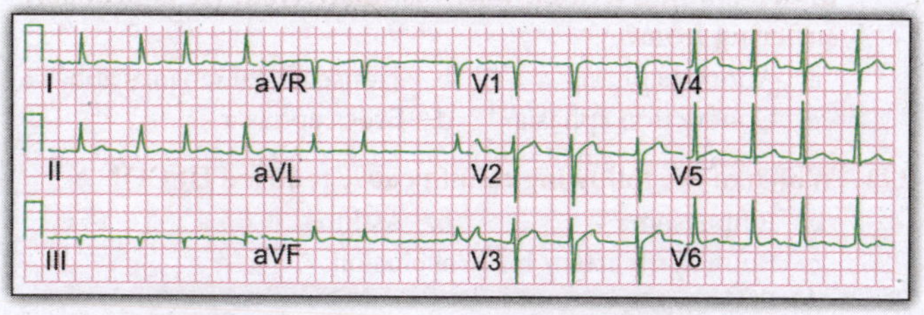

a. PSVT
b. Sinus rhythm
c. Atrial fibrillation
d. Ventricular tachycardia

116. A patient presented to the emergency with following ECG. Which drug is used for treatment are all EXCEPT:

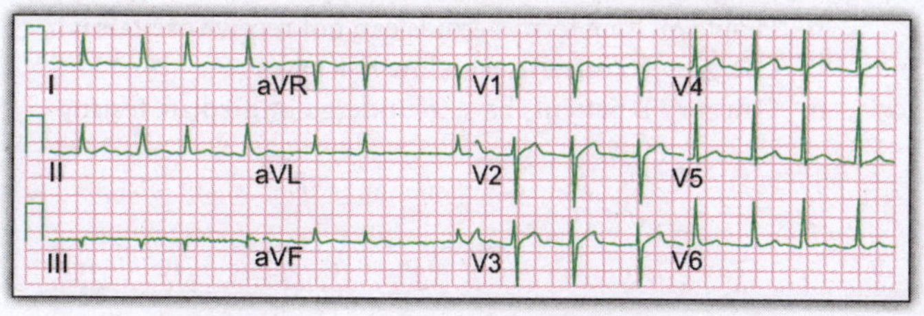

a. Metoprolol
b. Adenosine
c. Amiodarone
d. Diltiazem

117. Dotted lines in the transpulmonary pressure vs volume graph as shown below indicates which diseases?: *(AIIMS Nov 2018, 2015)*

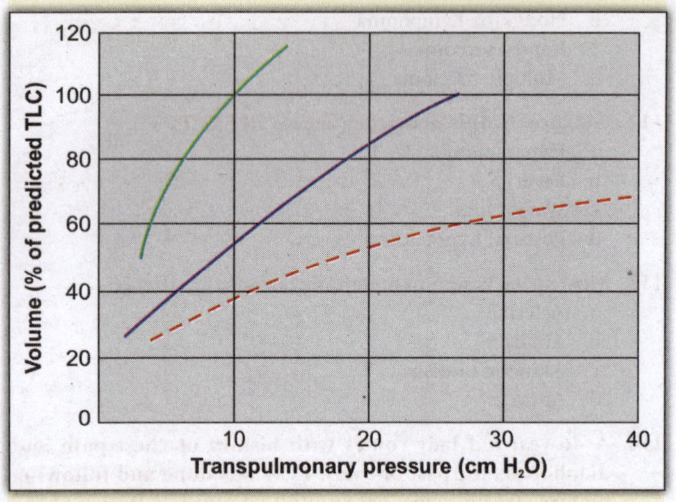

a. Asthma b. COPD
c. Bronchiectasis d. Interstitial fibrosis

118. A road traffic accident patient with steering wheel injury on right side presents with breathlessness. Differentiating features of cardiac tamponade and tension pneumothorax in this person is?

a. JVP b. Breath sounds
c. Pulse volume d. Pulsus paradoxus

AIIMS MAY 2015

119. Tropical spastic paraparesis is caused by?

a. Human T-cell lymphotropic virus
b. Hep B virus c. HIV
d. Ebstein barr virus

120. A man comes with aphasia. He is unable to name things and repetition is poor. However comprehension, fluency and understanding written words is unaffected. He is probably suffering from?

a. Anomic aphasia b. Transcortical sensory aphasia
c. Conduction aphasia d. Broca aphasia

121. Which of the following cannot cause reduced DLCO?

a. Emphysema b. Asthma
c. Pulmonary artery HTN/occlusion
d. Pneumonia

122. Which of the following statements is true regarding H1N1?

a. Pregnant woman with sore throat can be started immediately on oseltamivir without diagnostic testing under category B
b. People on long term steroids can not receive oseltamivir
c. Category B concerns with low risk cases
d. Category B patients have to undergo immediate testing

123. Which of the following is not a part of duke criteria for infective endocarditis?

a. Splenomegaly b. Fever > 100.4 celsius
c. IV drug user d. Blood culture positive

124. Hyperdynamic state are all EXCEPT:

a. Anemia b. Beri beri
c. Cor pulmonale d. Arterio-venous fistula

125. For galactorrhea and amenorrhea syndromes, additional investigation apart from serum prolactin is?

a. TSH b. LH
c. Urinary ketosteroids d. HCG

126. A young lady with tremors and diarrhea with elevated T4 and TSH levels were 8.5 MIU/L. Further examination reveals bitemporal hemianopia. Next step of management is?

a. Start antithyroid drugs and do urgent MRI brain
b. Start beta blockers
c. Conservative management
d. Start antithyroid drugs and wait for symptoms to resolve

127. A middle aged man comes with RTA and bleeding from the scalp. He is unconscious. A card in his pocked reveals that he is a known diabetic on Glimipiride + Metformin 2 tablets twice daily. What should be the next step?

a. Send blood for tests, start iv glucose and send to CT
b. Start normal saline and send to CT
c. Dextrose solution, CT scan
d. Airway, CT scan, Blood sugar if <70 start dextrose

128. Hypertensive hemorrhage is most commonly seen in?

a. Basal ganglia
b. Thalamus
c. Brain stem
d. Cerebrum

129. Which of the following is not an autoimmune disease?

a. SLE
b. Graves disease
c. Ulcerative colitis
d. Rheumatoid arthritis

130. A person is HBsAg positive, but IgM Anti-HBc is negative. What should be the next step?

a. Repeat test after 6 months
b. Check HBeAg, if positive start interferon
c. Check HBV DNA load
d. Reassure patient that he does not have any disease

131. A girl comes with Sydenham's chorea and acute rheumatic fever is suspected. Other major criteria of rheumatic fever are absent. No evidence of sore throat. Best investigation to prove rheumatic etiology is? *(AIIMS May 2015, Nov 2014)*

a. Antistreptolysin-S b. Antistreptolysin-O
c. PCR for M protein d. Throat culture

AIIMS NOVEMBER 2018

1. Ans. (b) ALT

Ref: Harrison 19th Ed Pg 2053

Summary

- ALT is more sensitive for viral hepatitis
- AST is more sensitive for Alcoholic hepatitis
- Elevated alkaline phosphatase is seen in cholestasis

Laboratory Tests in Alcoholic Hepatitis

Patients with alcoholic hepatitis typically have:

1. **Moderate elevations of the AST and ALT** (typically less than 300 int. unit/L, rarely higher than 400 IU/L, except in patients with alcoholic foamy degeneration (a histologic variant of alcoholic hepatitis)
2. Disproportionate increase of AST i.e. **AST: ALT ratio** ≥2 (rarely seen in other liver diseases). Lower elevation of the serum ALT relative to the AST is due to hepatic deficiency of pyridoxal 5'-phosphate in alcoholics, which is a cofactor for the enzymatic activity of ALT. Hence, the altered ratio reflects a failure to appropriately increase the ALT, rather than a disproportionate elevation in AST. The primary features that differentiate alcoholic hepatitis from other causes of acute hepatitis include a history of heavy alcohol use and an AST: ALT ratio of ≥2. An AST: ALT ratio of ≥2 is rarely seen in other forms of liver disease
3. An elevated serum bilirubin
4. An elevated gamma-glutamyl transferase (GGT)
5. A leukocytosis with a predominance of neutrophils
6. An elevated international normalized ratio (INR) due to impaired production of coagulation factors by the inflamed liver

2. Ans. (d) Interstitial fibrosis

Ref: Ganong 25th ed page 629

The figure is of pressure-volume curves of lungs and chest wall (slope = compliance; note low compliance at extreme volumes)

- **Compliance** is developed due to the tendency for tissue to resume its original position after an applied force has been removed. Compliance of the lung and chest wall is measured as the slope of the curve, or, as a change in lung volume per unit change in airway pressure ($\Delta V/\Delta P$).
- After an expiration during quiet breathing (e.g. at the FRC), the lungs have a tendency to collapse and the chest wall has a tendency to expand. The interaction between the recoil of the lungs and recoil of the chest can be measured through a spirometer that has a valve just beyond the mouthpiece.
- The mouthpiece contains a pressure-measuring device. After the person inhales a given amount, the valve is shut, closing off the airway.
- The respiratory muscles are then relaxed while the pressure in the airway is recorded. The procedure is repeated after inhaling or actively exhaling various volumes. The curve of airway pressure obtained in this way, plotted against volume, is the pressure-volume curve of the total respiratory system
- The pressure is zero at a lung volume that corresponds to the volume of gas in the lungs at FRC (relaxation volume).
- As can be noted from Figure, this relaxation pressure is the sum of slightly negative pressure component from the chest wall and a slightly positive pressure from the lungs
- It is normally measured in the pressure range where the relaxation pressure curve is steepest and normal values are ~0.2 L/cm H_2O in a healthy adult man.
- However, compliance depends on lung volume and thus can vary. In an extreme example, an individual with only one lung has approximately half the ΔV for a given ΔP.
- **Compliance** is also slightly greater when measured during deflation than when measured during inflation. Consequently, it is more informative to examine the whole pressure-volume curve.

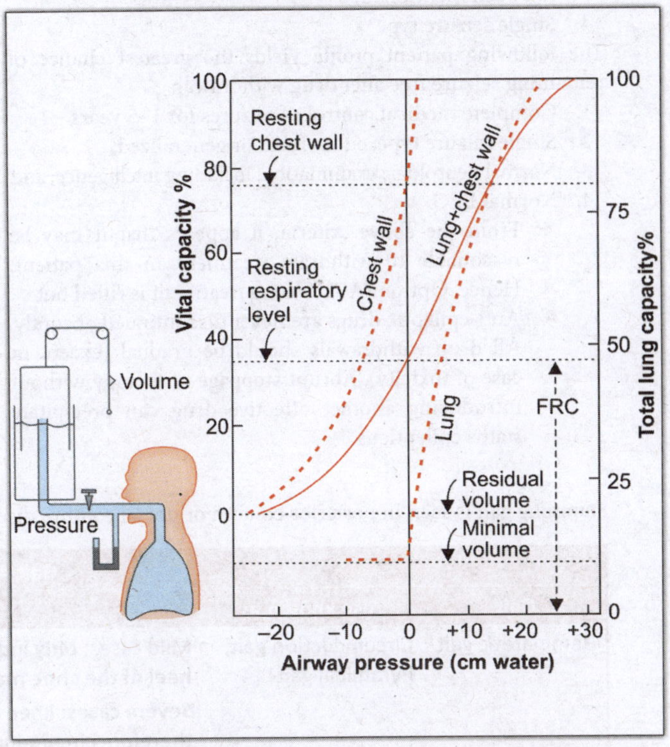

- *The curve is shifted downward and to the right (compliance is decreased) by pulmonary edema and interstitial pulmonary fibrosis.*
- **Pulmonary fibrosis** is a progressive restrictive airway disease in which there is stiffening and scarring of the lung. *The curve is shifted upward and to the left (compliance is increased) in emphysema.*

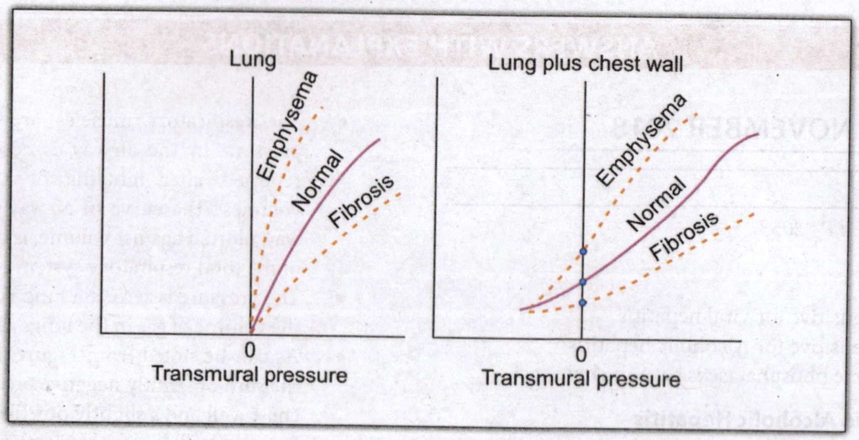

3. Ans. (b) Continue for 2 years

Ref: Harrison's 19th Ed page 2556

Following are the favourable features of epilepsy in the above patient:

1. Complete medical control
2. Normal CT/MRI
3. Patient has normal intelligence (mental retardation has not been mentioned)
4. Single seizure type

The following patient profile yields the greatest chance of remaining seizure free after drug withdrawal:

1. Complete medical control of seizures for 1–5 years
2. Single seizure type, either focal or generalized;
3. Normal neurologic examination, including intelligence; and
4. Normal EEG.

- From the above criteria, it appears that it may be reasonable to withdraw treatment in this patient. Hence, Option (A) Life long treatment is ruled out
- Anti-epileptic drugs are never discontinued abruptly. All drug withdrawals should be gradual (except in case of toxicity). Abrupt stoppage of therapy without introducing another effective drug can precipitate status epilepticus.
- Hence, Option (B) Stop drug and follow up with EEG every 6 months and Option (C) Stop treatment are ruled out.
- Now, the appropriate seizure free interval is unknown and undoubtedly varies for different forms of epilepsy. However **it seems reasona ble to attem pt withdrawal of therapy after 2 years in a patient** who meets all of the above criteria, is motivated to discontinue the med ication and clearly understands the potential risks and benefits.
- In most cases it is preferable to reduce the dose of the drug gradually over 2–3 months.
- Most recurrences occur in the first 3 months after discontinuing therapy and patients should be advised to avoid potentially dangerous situations such as driving or swimming during this period.
- Overall, about 70% of children and 60% of adults who have their seizures completely controlled with antiepileptic drugs can eventually discontinue therapy.

4. Ans. (b) Dorsal column tract

Ref: Harrison's 19th Ed Pg 1136, Kumar and Clark's 8th ed page 1087

Stamping gait is seen in posterior column or dorsal column diseases. History of syphilis points towards Tabes dorsalis

Gait Abnormalities			
Gait	**Also known as**	**Description**	**Found in**
Hemiparetic gait	Circumduction gait, Pyramidal gait	Mild cases: **only indication of paresis may be that the ball/ heel of the shoe may be worn more on the affected side** **Severe cases:** knee extended, ankle plantar flexed. Patient therefore circumducts the affected leg to ambulate	Hemiplegia (upper motor neuron disease)
Ataxic gait	Broad based gait	Patient spreads legs apart to widen the base to compensate for the imbalance while standing or walking	Cerebellar sign, alcoholism
Lurching gait	Jack knife gait, Gluteus Maximus Lurch	The trunk lurches back on the stance phase side hyperextending	Gluteus maximus weakness
	Trendelenburg's gait, Gluteus medius lurch	The trunk shifts over the side of the weak muscle in stance phase to minimise the fall of the swing phase side of the pelvis.	Hip dislocation Coxa vara Short limb Unilateral superior gluteal nerve injury

Contd...

Gait Abnormalities			
Gait	Also known as	Description	Found in
Waddling gait	Myopathic gait	The patient uses circumduction to compensate for gluteal weakness	Muscular dystrophy Bilateral superior gluteal nerve injury
Shuffling gait	Festinating gait	Short steps, appears to shuffle his or her legs rather than put them forward. Steps and pace may vary with a tendency for the patient to accelerate	Parkinson's disease (extrapyramidal)
Stepping gait	High-stepping, slapping	High steps as if climbing stairs while walking on a level surface, trying to avoid injury to the feet (from dragging them) by stepping high	Peripheral neuropathies (bilateral foot drop)
Stamping gait		This resembles high stepping gait but due to sensory loss in the feet rather than motor disturbance. Broad base, lifts the leg suddenly, raising them too high and then bringing them down forcibly with a stamp and often heel first. Due to loss of position sense	Tabes dorsalis (Dorsal column, AKA Posterior column)
Spastic gait	Scissoring gait	Legs are held in adduction at the hip and the thighs rub against each other as the patient walks	Cerebral diplegia (cerebral palsy)
Charlie Chaplin gait	Out toe gait	'Spread-eagle' or frog leg position	Tibial torsion
Antalgic gait		Patient favours the affected painful extremity and walks, putting weight on the normal leg	Limb pain

5. Ans. (c) Urinary NGAL (Most suitable)

Ref: Brenner and Rector's The Kidney, 8th ed. Ch 29

Recall bias: Either the question or options was not recalled properly. ***The KDIGO criteria differ from the RIFLE classification in that the KDIGO criteria only utilize changes in serum creatinine and urine output, not changes in GFR for staging,*** with the exception of children under the age of 18 years, for whom an acute decrease in eGFR to <35 mL/min/1.73 m^2 is included in the criteria for stage 3 AKI. However GFR is not provided in the option. Secondly the question mentions about differentiating Tubular injury and both RIFLE and KDIGO can not differentiate between types of AKI. Taking this into consideration we assume that the examiner want to ask the ***Marker of Tubular injury, which is Urinary NGAL***

Acute kidney injury (AKI), previously called acute renal failure (ARF), is a common clinical problem. Although measurement of the serum creatinine concentration is widely used for the detection of AKI, it does not permit early diagnosis of acute tubular necrosis (ATN), since tubular injury precedes a significant rise in serum creatinine. Investigational biomarkers have been evaluated in patients with possible ATN in an attempt to detect tubular injury at an earlier stage.

Urinary neutrophil gelatinase-associated lipocalin (NGAL) an iron-transporting protein rapidly accumulating in the kidney tubules and urine after nephrotoxic and ischemic insults, has been put forward as an early, sensitive, non-invasive biomarker for acute kidney injury (AKI). NGAL shows promise as a biomarker to help diagnose early Acute tubular necrosis. ***Furthermore, NGAL can differentiate prerenal disease from Acute tubular necrosis.***

Novel Biomarkers of Acute Renal Failure		
Marker	Substrate—Test	Comments
SSAT	Rat kidney—RT-PCR and Northern blot	SSAT was able to distinguish ARF with tubular injury from ARF without ATN
CYR61	Kidney and urine—Western blot	CYR61 is upregulated in kidneys with IRI—able to distinguish prerenal from intrarenal ARF
IL-18	Urine—ELISA	IL-18 elevated in human kidney ATN (native and transplanted kidneys)
NHE3	Urine—semiquantitative immunoblotting	NHE3 differentiated prerenal from intrarenal ischemic ATN from other intrarenal causes of ARF
Urine Proteome pattern	Urine—mass spectroscopy	Humans following cardiopulmonary bypass surgery—markers at 2 and 6 hours postoperative highly sensitive and highly predictive of AKI
KIM-1	Urine, kidney—multiple methods	Specific for *ischemic* ARF/ATN when compared with other forms of kidney disease
Gro-α, KC	Urine, blood—ELISA	Gro-α correlates well with renal recovery from AKI/DGF in transplant, early increase in urine and blood well before rise in serum creatinine in ARF models

Novel Biomarkers of Acute Renal Failure		
Marker	**Substrate—Test**	**Comments**
NGAL	Blood, urine—western blot and ELISA	NGAL sensitive, specific and predictive marker of ARF in blood and urine of patients after cardiopulmonary bypass
Actin, IL-6 and IL-8	Urine—dot immunoblot and ELISA	All three markers predicted prolonged ARF following renal transplantation in humans
CYR61, cysteine-rich protein 61; DGF, delayed graft function; Gro-α, human growth-related oncogene-α; IL-6, interleukin-6; IL-8, interleukin-8; IL-18, interleukin-18; KC, keratinocyte-derived chemokine; KIM-1, kidney injury molecule 1; NGAL, neutrophil gelatinase-associated lipocalin; NHE3, Na^+/H^+ exchanger isoform 3; SSAT, spermidine/spermine *N*1-acetyltransferase		

Criteria for Acute Kidney Injury			
	Rifle	**Akin**	**Kdigo**
Diagnostic criteria*			
		↑serum creatinine of ≥0.3 mg/dL or ≥50% within 48 hours OR Urine output of <0.5 mL/kg/hour for >6 hours	↑serum creatinine of ≥0.3 mg/dL within 48 hours or ≥50% within 7 days OR Urine output of <0.5 mL/kg/hour for >6 hours
Staging criteria			
Risk (RIFLE) or stage 1 (AKIN/KDIGO)	↑serum creatinine of 50 to 99% OR Urine output of <0.5 mL/kg/hour for 6 to 12 hours	↑serum creatinine of ≥0.3 mg/dL or 50 to 100% OR Urine output of <0.5 mL/kg/hour for 6 to 12 hours	↑serum creatinine of ≥0.3 mg/dL or 50 to 99% OR Urine output of <0.5 mL/kg/hour for 6 to 12 hours
Injury (RIFLE) or stage 2 (AKIN/KDIGO)	↑serum creatinine of 100 to 199% OR Urine output of <0.5 mL/kg/hour for 12 to 24 hours	↑ serum creatinine of >100 to 200% OR Urine output of <0.5 mL/kg/hour for 12 to 24 hours	↑serum creatinine of 100 to 199% OR Urine output of <0.5 mL/kg/hour for 12 to 24 hours
Failure (RIFLE) or stage 3 (AKIN/KDIGO)	↑serum creatinine of ≥200% OR ↑ serum creatinine by >0.5 mg/dL to >4.0 mg/dL OR Urine output of <0.3 mL/kg/hour for >24 hours or anuria for >12 hours OR Initiation of renal replacement therapy	Increase in serum creatinine of >200% OR Increase in serum creatinine by >0.5 mg/dL to ≥4.0 mg/dL OR Urine output of <0.3 mL/kg/hour for >24 hours or anuria for >12 hours OR Initiation of renal replacement therapy	Increase in serum creatinine of ≥200% OR ↑serum creatinine of ≥0.3 mg/dL to ≥4.0 mg/dL¶ OR Urine output of <0.3 mL/kg/hour for ≥24 hours or anuria for ≥12 hours OR Initiation of renal replacement therapy
Loss (RIFLE)	Need for renal replacement therapy for >4 weeks		
End stage (RIFLE)	Need for renal replacement therapy for >3 months		

RIFLE: Risk, injury, failure, loss, ESRD; AKIN: Acute Kidney Injury Network; KDIGO: Kidney Disease: Improving Global Outcomes; ESRD: end-stage renal disease.

* AKIN and KDIGO provided both diagnostic and staging criteria. RIFLE provided a graded definition of AKI that is implicit in the staging criteria.

In patients <18 years, stage 3 AKI is also defined by KDIGO as a decrease in estimated glomerular filtration rate (eGFR) to <35 mL/min/1.73 m^2.

6. Ans. (a) Neuromyelitis optica (NMO)

Ref: Harrison's 19th Ed Pg 2673

Recurrent bilateral optic neuritis with Transverse myelitis point towards a diagnosis of Neuromyelitis Optica (NMO) also known as Devic's disease.

Neuromyelitis Optica/Devic's Disease	
Incidence	Women>Men (>3:1) Typically begins in begins i n childhood o r early adulthood More common in Asian and african population

Neuromyelitis Optica/Devic's Disease	
Diagnosis	**Required**: 1. Optic neuritis 2. Acute transverse myelitis **Supportive (2 of 3 criteria required)** 1. Longitudinally extensive cord lesion extending over 3 or more vertebral segments 2. Brain MRI normal or not meeting criteria for multiple sclerosis 3. Aquaporin-4 seropositivity
Clinical Signs and Symptoms	**Optic Neuritis**: Attacks can be **bilateral** (rare in Multiple Sclerosis → MS) or unilateral; **Myelitis:** can be severe and **transverse** (rare in MS) and is typically longitudinally extensive involving three or more contiguous vertebral segments. Also in contrast to MS progressive symptoms do not occur in NMO. Endocrinopathy, intractable hiccoughs or vomiting (lower brainstem), encephalopathy, seizures.
Radiological Features	**Brain:** In approximately half of cases, there are lesions involving the hypothalamus the lower brainstem, lower medulla; or the cerebral hemispheres. Large MRI lesions in the cerebral hemispheres can be asymptomatic, sometimes have a "cloud-like" appearance and are often not destructive (unlike MS) and can resolve completely. **Spinal cord:** MRI lesions typically consist of focal enhancing areas of swelling and tissue destruction, extending over **three or more spinal cord segments**, and on axial sequences, these are centered on the gray matter of the cord.
Pathology	The pathology of NMO is a distinctive astrocytopathy with inflammation a loss of astrocytes and an absence of staining of the water channel protein aquaporin-4 by immunohistochemistry, plus thickened blood vessel walls, demyelination and deposition of antibody and complement. CSF findings include pleocytosis greater than that observed in MS, with neutrophils and eosinophils present in some cases; OCBs are uncommon, occurring in fewer than 30% of NMO patients
Anti-aquaporin 4 antibody	• Aquaporin-4 is localized to the foot processes of astrocytes in close • Apposition to endothelial surfaces, as well as at paranodal regions near nodes of Ranvier. • A highly specific autoantibody directed against aquaporin-4 is present in the sera of approximately 2/3rd of patients. • Seropositivity indicates very high risk for future relapses; >50% chances of relapse within 1 year if untreated.
Treatment	• **Acute:** **High-dose glucocorticoids** (solumedrol 1–2 g/d for 5–10 days followed by a prednisone taper). **Plasma exchange** (typically 7 qod exchanges of 1.5 plasma volumes) has also been used empirically for acute episodes that fail to respond to glucocorticoids. • **Prophylaxis** Given the unfavorable natural history of untreated NMO, prophylaxis against relapses is recommended for most patients using the following regimens: Mycophenylate mofetil (250 mg bid gradually increasing to 1000 mg bid); OR B cell depletion with anti-CD20 monoclonal antibody (rituximab); OR Combination of glucocorticoids (500 mg IV methylprednisolone daily for 5 days; then oral prednisone 1 mg/kg per day for 2 months followed by slow taper) plus azathioprine (2 mg/kg per day started on week 3). Use of IFN-ß is ineffective and paradoxically may increase the risk of NMO relapses.
Confusion with Multiple Sclerosis	• When MS affects individuals of African or Asian ancestry there is a propensity for demyelinating lesions to involve predominantly the optic nerve and spinal cord, an MS subtype termed opticospinal MS. • Some individuals with opticospinal MS are seropositive for aquaporin-4 antibodies, suggesting that such cases represent an NMO spectrum disorder

7. Ans. (b) Central venous catheter

Ref: Miller's 8th Ed Pg 1387

Measurement of cardiac output provides a global assessment of the circulation and in combination with other hemodynamic measurements (heart rate, arterial blood pressure, CVP, pulmonary artery pressure and wedge pressure), it allows calculation of additional important circulatory variables, such as systemic and pulmonary vascular resistance and ventricular stroke work.

Cardiac Output Monitoring	
Invasive methods	
Thermodilution technique: PA Catheter/Swan Ganz catheter with thermistor	• The indicator-dilution method of measuring blood flow is based on the premise that, when an indicator substance is added to circulating blood, the rate of blood flow is inversely proportional to the change in concentration of the indicator over time. • If the indicator is a temperature, the method is known as thermodilution. • A dextrose or saline solution that is colder than blood is injected through the proximal port of the catheter in the right atrium. • The cold fluid mixes with blood in the right heart chambers and the cooled blood is ejected into the pulmonary artery and flows past the thermistor on the distal end of the catheter. • The thermistor records the change in blood temperature with time; the area under this curve is inversely proportional to the flow rate in the pulmonary artery, which is equivalent to the cardiac output. For example, if the cardiac output is low, cooling will take more time, there will be longer delay from time of injection till blood reaches the thermistor. • In adults, an injectate volume of 10 mL should be used, whereas in children, an injectate volume of 0.15 mL/kg is recommended
Continuous Thermodilution Cardiac Output Monitoring	• Warm instead of cold thermal indicator is used. • Small quantities of heat are released from a 10-cm thermal filament incorporated into the right ventricular portion of a PAC, about 15 to 25 cm from the catheter tip and the resulting thermal signal is measured by the thermistor at the tip of the catheter in the pulmonary artery. • The cardiac output is derived from cross correlation of the measured pulmonary artery temperature with the known sequence of heating filament activation • Updated every 30 seconds and value of cardiac output is averaged over 3- 6 minutes
Transpulmonary Thermodilution Cardiac Output	• Icecold saline is injected into a central venous line while the change in temperature is measured in a large peripheral artery (femoral, axillary, or brachial artery) via a special arterial catheter equipped with a thermistor. • Because the measurement lasts over several cardiac cycles, respiratory effects on stroke volume are averaged and eliminated, in contrast to standard thermodilution • Other indices measured are **Extravascular lung water** (indicator of pulmonary edema, helps guide fluid administration in acute lung injury), **global end-diastolic volume, intrathoracic blood volume and cardiac function index**, calculated using cardiac output and the intrathoracic blood volume (gives left ventricular ejection fraction).
Lithium Dilution Cardiac Output Monitoring	• Following an IV bolus injection of a small dose of lithium chloride, an ion-selective electrode attached to a peripheral arterial catheter measures the lithium dilution curve, to derive cardiac output. • This is an accurate technique compared with standard thermodilution or electromagnetic flowmetry. • The lithium indicator can be injected through a peripheral intravenous catheter with similar measurement accuracy, thus eliminating the need for a central venous line. • Can also be used in children. • Contraindications: patients taking lithium, or those who have just received nondepolarizing neuromuscular blockers (because these blockers also alter the lithium sensor electrode measurement).
Non invasive methods	
Esophageal and transthoracic Doppler	Cardiac output can be intermittently measured by the **Doppler technique during transthoracic or transesophageal echocardiography.** **Esophageal Doppler:** The transducer is incorporated into the tip of a probe resembling a standard esophageal stethoscope and allows continuous monitoring of cardiac output. **Principle:** Doppler shift of the interrogated blood flow in the descending thoracic aorta is measured. **Position:** Into the esophagus to a depth of approximately 35 cm from the incisor teeth (T5-T6 vertebral interspace or 3rd sternocostal junction→ esophagus & descending aorta lie in close proximity and run parallel to each other at this location) and is adjusted to optimize the audible Doppler flow sound from the descending aorta. **Measurement:** The ultrasound transducer is mounted at a fixed angle that is anatomically defined and known by the cardiac output computer. This angle is then used to correct the resulting Doppler shift frequency to provide an accurate velocity measurement.
Bioimpedance Cardiac Output Monitoring	• Based on changes in electrical impedance of the thoracic cavity occurring with ejection of blood during cardiac systole. **$SV = \rho L^2 / Z_0^2$ X VET X max dZ/dt** where SV = stroke volume ρ = specific resistivity of blood

Contd...

Cardiac Output Monitoring	
	L = thoracic length Z_o = basal thoracic impedance VET = ventricular ejection time max dZ/dt = maximum rate of impedance change during systolic upstroke • For performing the measurements, disposable electrodes are applied to the skin surface along the sides of the neck and lateral aspect of the lower thorax and a continuous small electrical current is applied across the chest. • Patient height, weight and gender are used to calculate the volume of the thoracic cavity. • Bioimpedance cardiac output is computed for each cardiac cycle and continuously displayed as an average value over several heart beats • Unreliable in critically ill patients, including those with sepsis, pulmonary edema, aortic regurgitation and cardiac pacing
Partial CO_2 Rebreathing Cardiac Output Monitoring	• **Principle:** Uses the change in CO_2 production and end-tidal CO_2 concentration in response to a brief, sudden change in minute ventilation. • **Method:** With a specially designed breathing system and monitoring computer, this measurement is easily performed in any tracheally intubated patient. Every 3 minutes, a computer-controlled pneumatic valve intermittently increases dead space for a 50-second period, thereby causing partial rebreathing of exhaled gases. Changes in end-tidal CO_2 in response to the rebreathing maneuver are used to calculate cardiac output by a differential version of the Fick equation for carbon dioxide. This method measures pulmonary capillary blood flow as an indicator of total cardiac output. • **Fick's equation:** $Q=\dot{V}co_2/(C\underline{v}co_2—Caco_2)$ where $Q^{\cdot}$ = cardiac output $V^{\cdot} CO_2$ = rate of carbon dioxide elimination $CVCO_2$ = carbon dioxide content of mixed venous blood $Caco_2$ = carbon dioxide content of arterial blood • Requires tracheal intubation, Contraindicated in raised intracranial Pressure, Ventilation may have an unpredictable influence.
Pulse Contour Cardiac Output Monitoring (not completely noninvasive)	• Continuous measurement of cardiac output is derived from the analysis of the arterial pulse pressure waveform. It determines stroke volume from computerized analysis of the area under the arterial pressure waveform recorded from an arterial catheter or even a noninvasive finger blood pressure waveform. • Pulse contour methods offer the potential for noninvasive, continuous, beat-to-beat cardiac output monitoring. • Also, the change in stroke volume from beat to beat (termed stroke volume variation→ SVV) can be used to evaluate volume status in ventilated • Patients (however, the patient must be mechanically ventilated with tidal volume of 8 mL/kg and should not have arrhythmia for evaluation of SVV). In conditions like tachycardia,dysrhythmia and low volume states, the waveform is not very discernable and analysis of cardiac output may not be reliable. 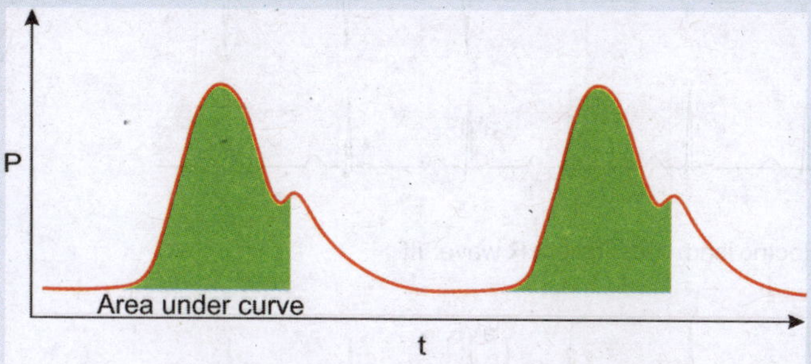 **Arterial waveform and cardiac output**

8. Ans. (a) aVF

Ref: Rapid Review of ECG Interpretation -by Tariq Azeem, Michael Vassallo, Nilesh J Samani Page 15

- In calculating the mean QRS axis, you are looking for the general direction or toward which lead axis is the QRS complex predominantly oriented.
- Now, +90° mean axis means the heart is more or less vertical. This means, in the above scenario, the electrical axis of the heart will produce the strongest positive deflection in a lead that represents the vertical axis, i.e, aVF. In other words, R wave will appear to to have maximum voltage in aVF.
- Also note that since the mean axis is perpendicular to the to the lead with the smallest QRS complex, if in the above question you are asked about the smallest QRS, it will be present in Lead I.

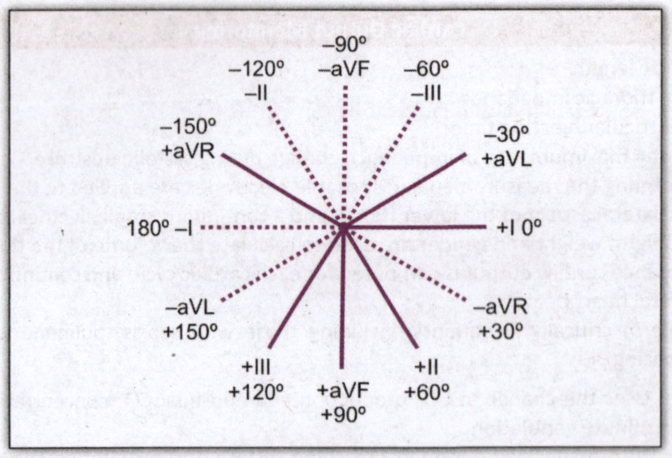

–90°
–aVF
–120°
–II
–60°
–III
–150°
+aVR
–30°
+aVL
180° –I
+I 0°
–aVL
+150°
–aVR
+30°
+III
+120°
+aVF
+90°
+II
+60°

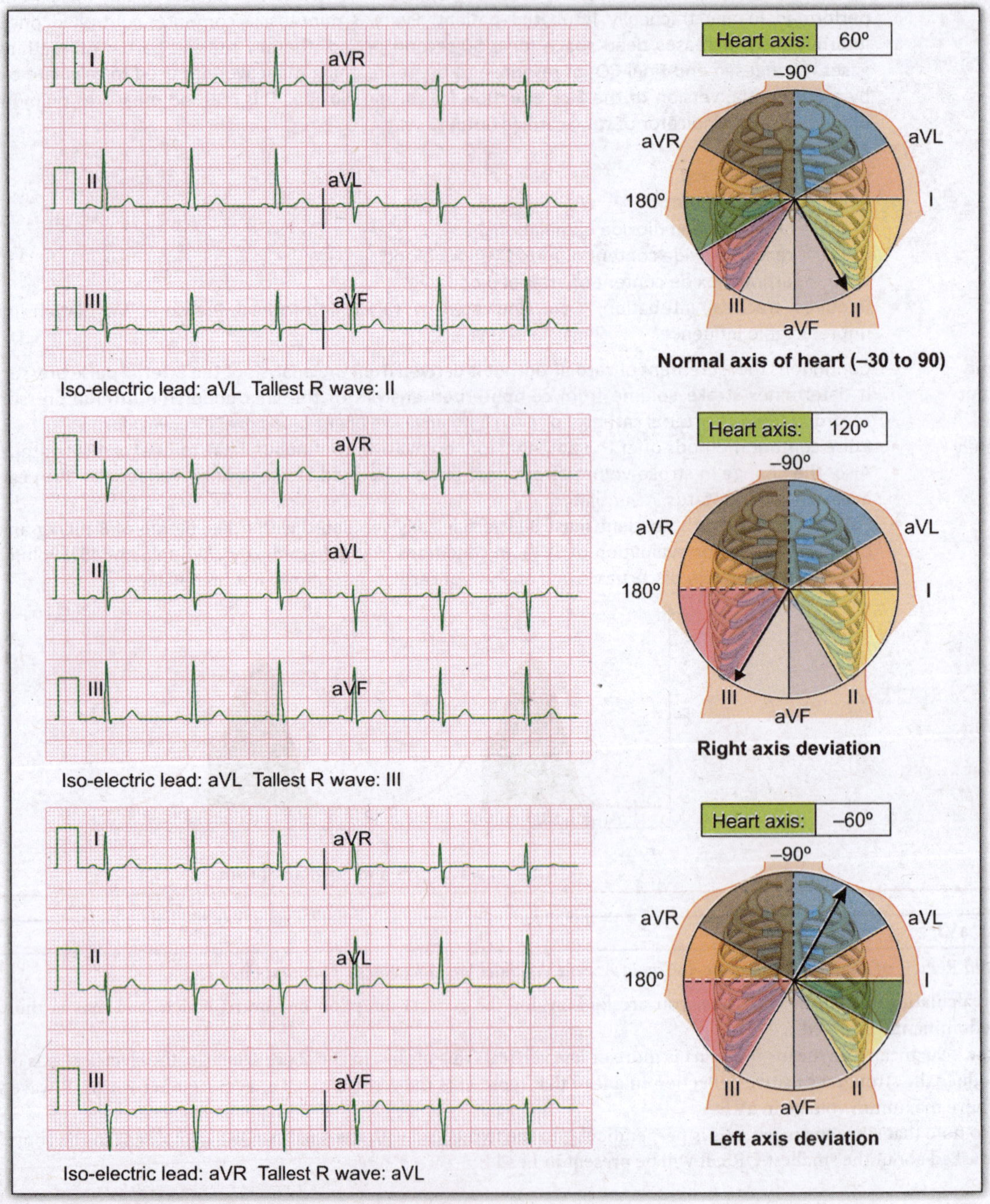

I
aVR
II
aVL
III
aVF
Heart axis: 60°
–90°
aVR
aVL
180°
I
III
II
aVF
Normal axis of heart (–30 to 90)
Iso-electric lead: aVL Tallest R wave: II
I
aVR
II
aVL
III
aVF
Heart axis: 120°
–90°
aVR
aVL
180°
I
III
II
aVF
Right axis deviation
Iso-electric lead: aVL Tallest R wave: III
I
aVR
II
aVL
III
aVF
Heart axis: –60°
–90°
aVR
aVL
180°
I
III
II
aVF
Left axis deviation
Iso-electric lead: aVR Tallest R wave: aVL

9. Ans. (d) MAT

Ref: Introduction to ECG Interpretation by Frank G. Yanowitz Pg 23

Looking at the ECG we know that the rate indicates tachycardia.

A rough algorithmic guide for diagnosis of tachycardia is as below:

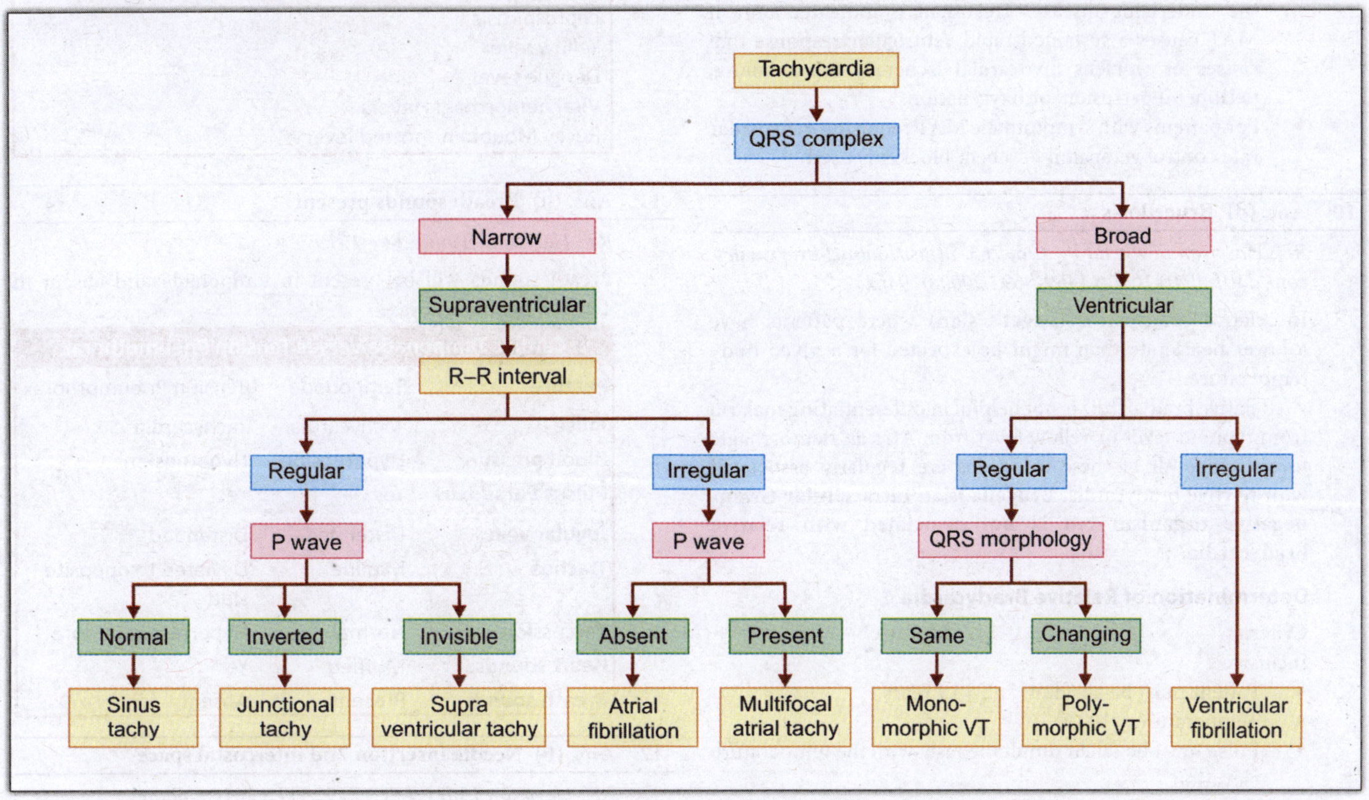

From the ECG asked, we can say that this is a narrow complex tachycardia with irregular RR interval and P wave is present. Moreover, P wave has different morphologies.

Thus, diagnosis is Multifocal atrial tachycardia.

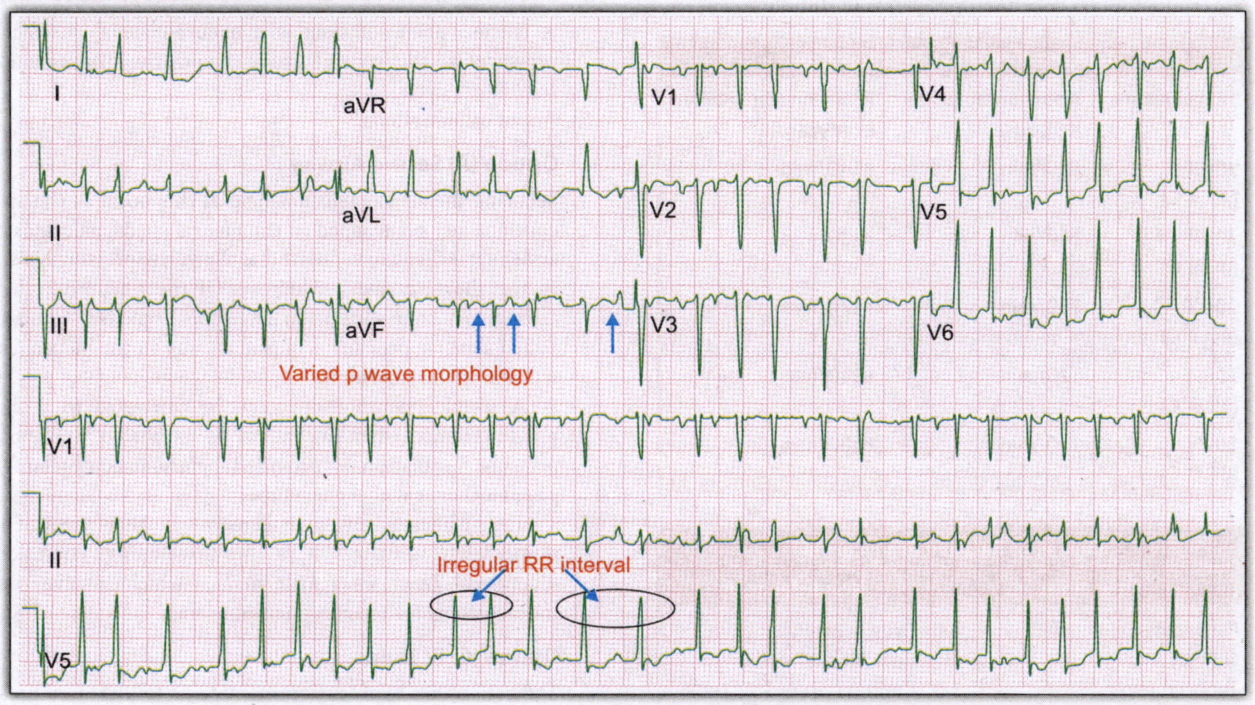

- MAT is an irregular SVT with a heart rate of > 100 bpm distinguished by at least 3 P-wave morphologies.
- It is often associated with COPD and congestive heart failure.
- Therapy in patients with MAT should be aimed at treating the underlying disease. Treatment is indicated only if MAT causes a sustained rapid ventricular response that causes or worsens myocardial ischemia, heart failure, peripheral perfusion, or oxygenation.
- For patients with symptomatic MAT requiring ventricular rate control verapamil or a beta-blocker is used

10. Ans. (d) Brucellosis

Ref: Harrison's 19th Ed Pg 126, 763, https://onlinelibrary.wiley.com/doi/full/10.1046/j.1469-0691.2000.0194f.x

In relative bradycardia **(Faget's sign)** where patients have a lower heart rate than might be expected for a given body temperature.

Relative bradycardia is not helpful in differentiating malaria from typhoid fever or yellow fever from African hemorrhagic fevers, since all of these infections are regularly associated with relative bradycardia. **Brucella is an intracellular Gram-negative organism but is not associated with relative bradycardia.**

Determination of Relative Bradycardia

Criteria:

Inclusive

- Patient must be an adult, i.e., ≥ 13 years
- Temperature ≥ 102°F
- Pulse must be taken simultaneously with the temperature elevation

Exclusive

- Patient has no arrhythmia, second-/third-degree heart block or pacemaker-induced rhythm
- Patient no on B-blocker, verapamil, or diltiazem

Temperature-pulse Relationships

Temperature	Appropriate pulse response	Pulse rate in relative bradycardia
106°F (41.1°C)	150/min	<140/min
105°F (40.6°C)	140/min	<130/min
104°F (40.7°C)	130/min	<120/min
103°F (39.4°C)	120/min	<110/min
102°F (38.9°C)	110/min	<100/min

Causes of Relative Bradycardia

Infectious	Non-infectious
Psittacosis	Drug fever
Q fever	Beta blocker use
Typhoid fever	Central nervous system lesions
Typhus	

Causes of Relative Bradycardia

Infectious	Non-infectious
Babesiosis	Malignant Lymphoma
Malaria	Factitious fever
Leptospirosis	
Yellow fever	
Dengue fever	
Viral hemorrhagic fevers	
Rocky Mountain spotted fever	

11. Ans. (b) Breath sounds present

Ref: Harrison's 19th Ed Pg 1719

Breath sounds will be present in tamponade and absent in Tension pneumothorax

Cardiac Tamponade Versus Tension Pneumothorax

Feature	Tamponade	Tension Pneumothorax
Pulse	Tachycardia	Tachycardia
Blood pressure	Hypotension	Hypotension
Pulsus Paradoxus	Yes	Yes
Jugular vein	Distended	Distended
Trachea	Midline	Deviated to opposite side
Percussion	Normal	Hyperresonant note
Heart sounds	Muffled	Yes
Breath sounds	Present	Absent

12. Ans. (b) Needle insertion 2nd intercostal space

Ref: Harrison 19th Ed Pg 1719, ATLS 2018 Updates

(See Table of "Chest Trauma" in AIIMS Nov 2016 Surgery) (see page no. 669)

A tension pneumothorax is a pneumothorax in which the pressure in the pleural space is positive throughout the respiratory cycle.

About other options:

Option (A) Secure Airway

Securing the airway will not help at this point as the air will continuously get trapped in the pleural space making it more and more difficult to ventilate due to positive pressure resistance in the thoracic cavity. Moreover, if the pneumothorax has an internal communication (e.g:bronchopleural fistula), the added positive pressure will find its way in the pleural cavity, worsening the condition.

A simple pneumothorax can be converted to a tension pneumothorax when a patient is intubated and positive pressure ventilation is provided before decompressing the pneumothorax with a chest tube.

The principle of management is that treatment is immediately initiated if a life-threatening condition is identified—***Treat what kills first***, —which involves needle thoracostomy for tension pneumothorax.

Option (C) IV Fluids

The patient has hypotension mainly due to increased pressure in the thoracic cavity, which is impeding the preload as well as afterload. Administration of IV fluids will not be very useful. On the other hand, immediate relief of the precipitating cause by needle insertion in 2nd ICS will serve as most effective, definitive and immediate treatment in this scenario.

Option (D) Chest X-ray

The clinical picture is highly suggestive of tension pneumothorax, which is an emergency life-threatening condition. Shifting the patient to the X-ray room is time consuming and tension pneumothorax as well as haemodynamics will worsen by that time.

13. Ans. (a) Breathe normally

Ref: Harrison's 19th Ed Pg 1574

- Paradoxical Pulse is an important clue to the presence of cardiac tamponade consisting of a greater than normal (10 mmHg) inspiratory decline in systolic arterial pressure.
- When severe, it may be detected by palpating weakness or disappearance of the arterial pulse during inspiration, but usually sphygmomanometric measurement of systolic pressure **during slow respiration is required.**

Measurement of Pulsus Paradoxus

- For patients without an indwelling arterial catheter, pulsus paradoxus must be measured by the clinician using a manually-operated sphygmomanometer; an automated blood pressure machine can not accurately measure pulsus paradoxus. Alternatively, in patients with continuous invasive arterial blood pressure monitoring, pulsus paradoxus can be measured directly from the invasive blood pressure recordings.
- To measure pulsus paradoxus, a manually-operated sphygmomanometer is employed for blood pressure measurement in the standard fashion except that the cuff is deflated more slowly than usual. During deflation, the first Korotkoff sounds are audible with heart beats occurring only during expiration. With further cuff deflation, Korotkoff sounds become audible on all heart beats throughout the respiratory cycle. The difference between the systolic pressure at which the first Korotkoff sounds are heard during expiration and the pressure at which they are heard throughout the respiratory cycle quantifies pulsus paradoxus. Pulsus paradoxus can also be quantified by an invasive arterial measurement and may also be observed by respirophasic variation of the pulse oximetry waveform. Pulsus paradoxus primarily reflects the inspiratory decline in left ventricular stroke volume. Thus, when measured via an intra-arterial cannula, pulsus paradoxus appears as a decline in both systolic and pulse pressures; the change in diastolic pressure is minimal.
- Since the depth of respiration influences the severity of pulsus, the patient should not be instructed to change his/her breathing pattern during this evaluation (i.e. to breathe deeply in the middle of the examination); any spontaneous change in respiration between observations must be taken into account. The magnitude of respiratory effort-related changes may be exaggerated in obese patients and those with pulmonary disease.

14. Ans. (c) High anion gap acidosis with metabolic alkalosis

Ref: Paul Marino's ICU book 4th Ed Ch 31.11

- This is a tricky question. pH is apparently normal, however we need to trace each value and check if it adequately fits, since all components are interrelated in an ABG. Only then we can comment if the patient is normal or the body is attempting to correct the primary disorder.
- **Clinical parameters and clues:** The patient is a case of chronic kidney disease and hence is most likely to have metabolic acidosis. However, the vomiting may have caused loss of H^+ ions and hence metabolic alkalosis.

Quick Key

Note that the question mentions values of major electrolytes, hence it is worthwhile to calculate Anion gap in the beginning itself so that we have some hint towards diagnosis, as pH is normal. It will save us some time.

Na – (Cl + HCO_3) = Anion gap (AG)

140 - (100 + 24) = 16

This points towards High anion gap metabolic acidosis, we can make further calculations in this direction. Moreover, the pH is normal in the presence of metabolic acidosis, which points towards the presence of compensatory alkalosis which has corrected the pH.

Now to Completely Analyse the ABG Step by Step

Interpretation of ABG	
Step 1	Look at the pH. Is the patient acidemic (H < 7.35) or Alkalemic (pH > 7.45)
Step 2	Is it a primary metabolic or respiratory disturbance?
	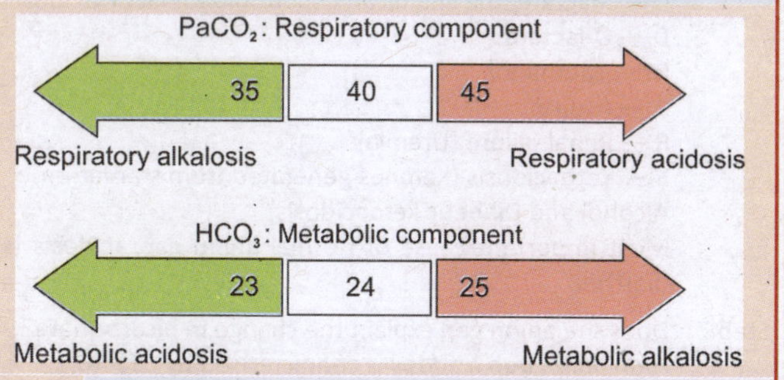
	Acidemia: With HCO_3 <22 mmol/L= Metabolic. With pCO_2 >45 mm Hg = Respiratory **Alkalemia:** With HCO_3 >26 mmol/L = Metabolic With PCO_2 <35 mm Hg = Respiratory **Note:** For ease of calculation normal pH= 7.4, pCO_2 is 40 and HCO_3 is 24 Go to step 3 and 4 if Respiratory and step 5 to 7 if metabolic
Step 3	If there is a primary respiratory disturbance, is it acute? Expected Δ pH = 0.08 × Δ pCO_2/10 (For respiratory acidosis (pCO_2–40) = ΔPCO_2) (For respiratory alkalemic (40–PCO_2) = ΔPCO_2) If not acute go to step 4, if yes –also consider steps 5–7

Contd...

Interpretation of ABG	
Step 4	For a respiratory disorder is renal (Metabolic) compensation appropriate? Respiratory acidosis: < 24 hrs: $\Delta (HCO_3) = 1/10 \times \Delta PCO_2$ > 24 hrs: $\Delta (HCO_3) = 4/10 \times \Delta PCO_2$ Respiratory alkalosis: 1–2 hrs: $\Delta (HCO_3) = 2/10 \times \Delta pCO_2$ > 2 days: $\Delta (HCO_3) = 5/10 \times \Delta pCO_2$ Where Δ = Change in
Step 5	If the disturbance is metabolic is the respiratory compensation appropriate? For metabolic acidosis: Expected $pCO_2 = [1.5 \times (HCO_3)] + 8 \pm 2$ For metabolic alkalosis: Expected $pCO_2 = [0.7 \times (HCO_3)] + 21 \pm 1.5$ If Actual pCO_2 > Expected pCO_2 = Hidden respiratory acidosis If Actual PCO_2 < Expected pCO_2 = Hidden respiratory alkalosis
Step 6	If there is metabolic acidosis, is there an anion gap? Anion gap (AG) is imperial in etiological diagnosis of metabolic acidosis. Na – (Cl + HCO_3) = Anion gap (Usually < 12). If gap is more than 12, patient has an High anion gap acidosis **Mnemonic** proposed by The Lancet as per the latest trend is: G — Glycols (ethylene glycol & propylene glycol) O — Oxoproline, a metabolite of paracetamol L — L-lactate, the chemical responsible for lactic acidosis D — D-lactate M — Methanol A — Aspirin R — Renal failure (Uremia) K — Ketoacidosis (Ketones generated from starvation, Alcohol and Diabetic ketoacidosis) Most important cause of normal anion gap acidosis is diarrhea.
Step 7	Does the anion gap explain the change in bicarbonate? *High anion gap acidosis* is characterised by 2 factors: 1. Low HCO_3, 2. Increased anion gap Rise in anion gap = Fall in HCO_3. i.e, Anion gap excess= HCO_3 deficit (AG-12) = (24- HCO_3) Thus, (AG-12)/(24- HCO_3)= 1 This ratio is also known as the Gap-Gap ratio. In high AG metabolic acidosis, Gap-Gap ratio should be 1. *Mixed disorders*: • Mixed metabolic acidosis: i.e, there are 2 primary causes of metabolic acidosis. If the 2nd cause of acidosis is a normal AG (e.g, hyperchloremic acidosis), the picture will be as follows: AG excess < HCO_3 deficit Thus gap-gap ratio <1 shows mixed metabolic acidosis- where 1 cause has a high AG, while the 2nd cause has normal AG.

Contd...

Interpretation of ABG
• Mixed metabolic alkalosis with metabolic acidosis New HCO_3 is being added in the presence of high AG. Hence, HCO_3 deficit (24- HCO_3) is now decreased. Thus, AG excess> HCO_3 deficit. Thus, high AG metabolic acidosis with Gap-gap ratio >1 means superimposed metabolic alkalosis.
Note: Anion gap (AG) is imperial in etiological diagnosis of metabolic acidosis. Na – (Cl + HCO_3) = Anion gap (Usually < 12). If gap is more than 12, patient has an High anion gap acidosis **Mnemonic** = GOLDMARK G — Glycols (ethylene glycol & propylene glycol) O — Oxoproline, a metabolite of paracetamol L — L-lactate, the chemical responsible for lactic acidosis D — D-lactate M — Methanol A — Aspirin R — Renal failure (Uremia) K — Ketoacidosis (Ketones generated from starvation, Alcohol and Diabetic ketoacidosis) Most important cause of normal anion gap acidosis is diarrhea.

Step - 1: pH is in the normal range

Step - 2: pCO_2 – 40 - normal

HCO_3 – 24 - normal

Thus, so far neither the disturbance nor the primary component can be pointed out.

Step - 3: $\Delta pH = 0.08 \times \Delta pCO_2 / 10$

$\Delta pH = 0$, $\Delta pCO_2 = 0$. There is no acute respiratory component

Step - 4: Also meets the same fate since $\Delta pH = 0$, $\Delta pCO_2 = 0$

There is no chronic respiratory component

Step - 5: For metabolic acidosis:Compensation = Expected $pCO_2 = [1.5 \times (HCO_3)] + 8 \pm 2$

Thus, $[1.5 \times (24)] + 8 = 44$, while pCO_2 is 40.

Thus actual pCO_2 < Expected pCO_2.

We must expect hidden respiratory alkalosis, so indeed there is metabolic acidosis which has been compensated by respiratory component.

We have now come to a diagnosis of Metabolic acidosis with hidden respiratory alkalosis.

Step - 6: Calculation of anion gap

Na – (Cl + HCO_3) = Anion gap (AG)

Thus, anion gap = 140 - (100 + 24) = 16

This is a case of high anion gap metabolic acidosis with hidden respiratory component.

Step - 7: Anion gap excess = (AG-12) = 16–12 = 4

HCO3 deficit = 24–24 = 0

Thus,

AG excess> HCO_3 deficit

Hence, there is metabolic alkalosis as well.

Thus, the final diagnosis is High anion Gap metabolic acidosis with superimposed metabolic alkalosis with hidden respiratory alkalosis.

15. Ans. (c) Flexion of wrist

Ref: Miller's Anaesthesia 8th Ed page 1350, Objective Anaesthesia Review: A Comprehensive Textbook for the Examinees By Atul P Kulkarni, JV Divatia, Vijay P Patil, RP Gehdoo 3rd ed page 323, www.uptodate.com

Radial artery of non dominant hand is the ideal site of arterial puncture due to following reasons

1. Small, superficial, easily accessible
2. Easily compressible in case of bleeding
3. No nearby nerve
4. Good collaterals with ulnar artery

Steps for collection of an arterial blood gas sample:

a. As for all procedures, the equipment necessary should be brought to the bedside prior to the procedure. This **includes:**
   1. Non sterile gloves
   2. Antiseptic skin solution (e.g. chlorhexidine and povidone-iodine are solutions)
   3. ABG kit
   4. 2 × 2 inch sterile gauze
   5. Adhesive bandage
   6. Plastic hazard bag with ice (if not provided in the kit)
   7. Sharp object contain
b. **Preparation of syringe:** Heparinize the syringe. See AIIMS 2016 Medicine for further details.
c. **Perform Allen's test**: See AIIMS 2016 Medicine for further details.
d. **Positioning and Procedure:**

The patient should be lying down or sitting with the arm well-supported and the clinician should also be seated if possible. Sterile precautions should ideally be taken.

The area is first thoroughly cleaned and draped.

The wrist is placed in extension by putting a rolled towel underneath.

The needle is introduced at an angle of about 45 degrees after palpating the radial artery with the other hand. Blood is then collected by puncturing the underlying radial artery.

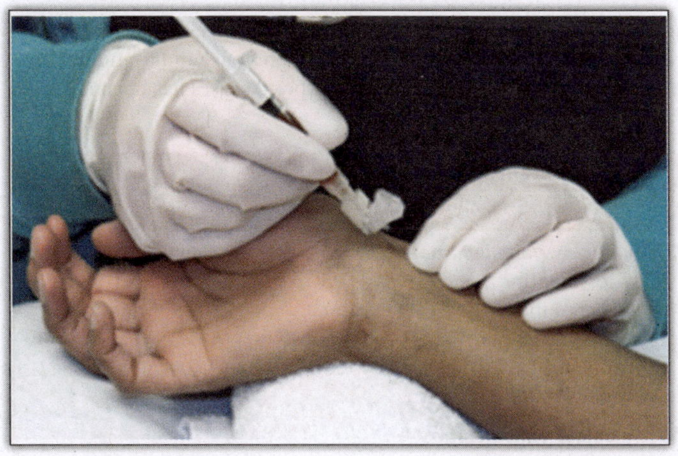

e. **Pressure:** AFter withdrawal of the sample, Apply pressure to the site for at least 5 minutes (normal clotting time) or more if patient has prolonged clotting time
f. Keep ABG sample in an ice bag sample unless it is going to be analyzed within 10–15 minutes

16. Ans. (a) Start Thrombolysis (Most suitable)

Ref: Harrison 19th ed page 2562, 2018 AHA/ASA Stroke Early Management Guidelines

> **NOTE**
>
> Ideally MRI should be performed before starting thrombolysis but if option is not provided and intracranial hemorrhage is ruled out in CT scan then thrombolysis can be considered.

The patient here comes with clinical suspicion of stroke. Thrombolysis is done for ischemic stroke while measures to lower down BP is done for hemorrhagic stroke. Since CT scan shows no evidence of intracranial hemorrhage Thrombolysis is the next best step.

Intravenous thrombolysis is usually practiced within the window period of 4.5 hours (Hacke W, 2008; ECASS III). (Ref: Neurological Practice: An Indian Perspective edited by Noshir H. Wadia, Satish V Khadilkar 2nd ed Page 175)

Clinical studies showing the effectiveness of intravenous (IV) rt-PA (recombinant tissue plasminogen activator) in arterial ischemic stroke (AIS) have selected patients based on brain CT. In this case the purpose of imaging was to exclude an intracranial hemorrhagic lesion.

MRI is the best investigation to show early signs of ischemia and visualize intracranial hemorrhage. This should be performed as the first line examination. If MRI is available as a first line investigation it should be accessible in the emergency settings and short protocols should be preferred. If urgent access to MRI is not available, a cerebral CT should be performed".

Indication of Thrombolysis in Stroke

- Clinical diagnosis of Stroke
- Onset of symptoms to time of drug administration ≤3 h
- CT scan showing no hemorrhage or edema of >1/3 of the MCA territory
- Age ≥18 years
- Consent by patient or surrogate

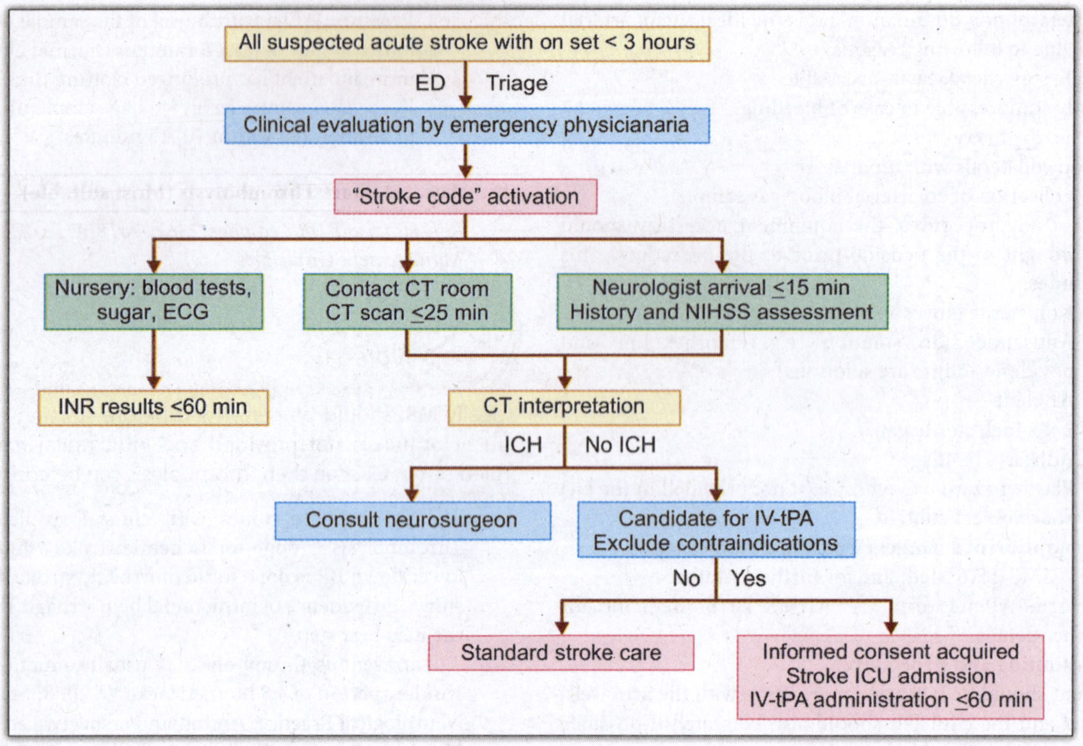

Fig: Flowchart of stroke code

AIIMS MAY 2018

17. Ans. (c) Adult T cell lymphoma

Ref: Harrison 19th ed page 923

HHV-8, which infects B lymphocytes, macrophages and both endothelial and epithelial cells, appears to be causally related not only to KS but also to a subgroup of AIDS-related B cell body cavity–based lymphomas (primary effusion lymphomas) and to multicentric Castleman's disease, a lymphoproliferative disorder of B cells. The association of HHV-8 with several other diseases has been reported but not confirmed. (Harrison)

Sites of Predilection for Human Herpes Virus (HHV)

HHV	Site	Disease
HHV-1 /Herpes simplex virus (HSV-1)	Trigeminal ganglia, Temporal lobe in Encephalitis	**Mostly above waist lesions** • Gingiostamatitis • Keratoconjunctivitis • Eczema herpaticum • Encephalitis (MC in Temporal lobe) • Herpetic whitlow
HHV-2/HSV-2	Sacral ganglia	**Mostly below waist lesions** • Genital herpes • Aseptic meningitis • Neonatal infections
HHV-3/Varicella Zoster Virus	Sensory ganglia	Chicken pox, Zoster
HHV-4 /Epstein Barr Virus	Lymphoid tissue	**Infectious Mononucleosis**, Burkitt's lymphoma
HHV-5/Cytomegalovirus	Salivary glands, Kidney	**Petechiae, Hepatosplenomegaly and jaundice (MC),** CMV mononucleosis, Hemorrhagic retinitis in Immunocompromised pts, **intrauterine infection (MC cause), complicates organ transplant (MC pathogen)**, pneumonia in transplant pts
HHV-6/Human B cell Lymphotropic virus	Lymphoid tissue	Roseola infantum/6th disease/Exanthema subitum, Focal Encephalitis

Contd...

Sites of Predilection for Human Herpes Virus (HHV)		
HHV	**Site**	**Disease**
HHV-7/R K virus	Lymphoid tissue	
HHV- 8	Lymphoid tissue	Primary effusion lymphoma Multicentric Castleman's disease Kaposi sarcoma in AIDS

18. Ans. (d) Amphotericin B

Ref: Harrison's 19th Ed Pg 1390

The catch in the question is RK39 test positive. Diagnosis is visceral Leishmaniasis or Kala Azar.

Visceral Leishmaniasis	
Causative organism	Leishmania donovani
Vector	Sandfly
Affected areas	India and neighboring Nepal, Bangladesh, Sudan and Brazil
Life cycle	

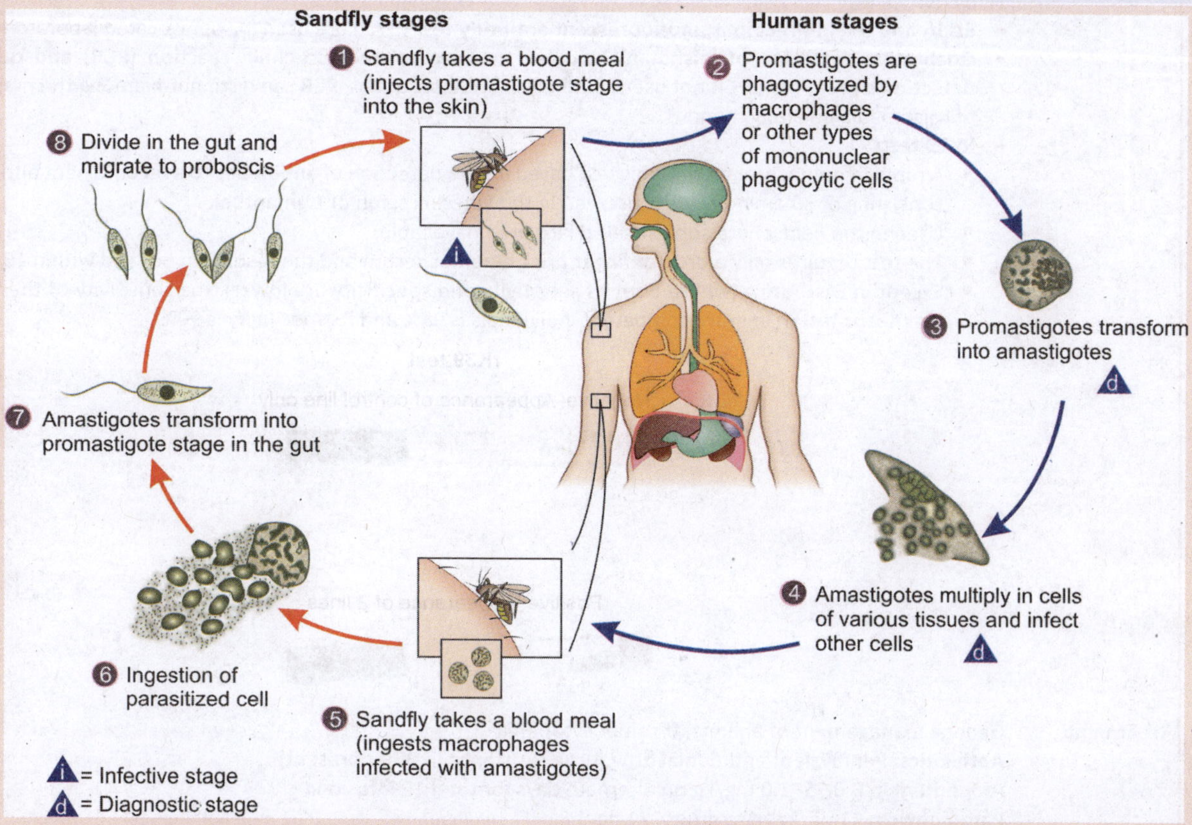

Leishmaniasis is transmitted by the bite of infected female phlebotomine sandflies. The sandflies inject the infective stage (i.e., promastigotes) from their proboscis during blood meals (1). Promastigotes that reach the puncture wound are phagocytized by macrophages (2) and other types of mononuclear phagocytic cells. Promastigotes transform in these cells into the tissue stage of the parasite (i.e., amastigotes) (3), which multiply by simple division and proceed to infect other mononuclear phagocytic cells (4). Parasite, host and other factors affect whether the infection becomes symptomatic and whether cutaneous or visceral leishmaniasis results. Sandflies become infected by ingesting infected cells during blood meals (5), (6). In sandflies, amastigotes transform into promastigotes, develop in the gut (7) (in the hindgut for leishmanial organisms in the Viannia subgenus; in the midgut for organisms in the Leishmania subgenus) and migrate to the proboscis (8).

Contd...

Visceral Leishmaniasis	
Clinical features	• Abrupt onset of moderate- to high-grade fever with rigor, chills. Fever may continue for several weeks with decreasing intensity and the patient may become afebrile for a short period before experiencing another bout of fever. • The spleen may be palpable by the 2nd week of illness and, may become hugely enlarged. • Hepatomegaly (usually moderate) • Lymphadenopathy is common in most endemic regions of the world except the Indian subcontinent, where it is rare. • Weight loss, weakness, hyperpigmentation of skin • Hypoalbuminemia, pedal edema and ascites. • Anemia, may become severe enough to cause congestive heart failure. • Epistaxis, retinal hemorrhages and gastrointestinal bleeding are associated with thrombocytopenia. • Secondary infections such as measles, pneumonia, tuberculosis, bacillary or amebic dysentery, gastroenteritis, Herpes zoster, chickenpox, boils in the skin and scabies • Untreated, the disease is fatal in most patients, including • 100% of those with HIV co-infection.
Laboratory diagnosis	**Gold standard:** Demonstration of amastigotes in smears of tissue aspirates. Sensitivity of splenic smears> bone marrow > Lymph node aspirates Culture of tissue aspirates increases sensitivity. Serology: • **ELISA and the indirect immunofluorescent antibody test (IFAT)** are used in sophisticated laboratories. • **Qualitative detection of leishmanial nucleic acid by polymerase chain reaction (PCR) and quantitative detection by real-time PCR** not used routinely in endemic are as. PCR can distinguish among the major species of Leishmania infecting humans. • **RK39 test:** ▪ A rapid immunochromatographic test based on the detection of antibodies to a recombinant antigen (rK39) consisting of 39 amino acids conserved in the kinesin region of L. infantum. ▪ Used in the field where sophisticated labs are unavailable ▪ The test requires only a drop of finger prick blood or serum and the result can be read within 15 minutes. ▪ Except in East Africa (where both its sensitivity and specificity are lower), the sensitivity of the rK39 rapid diagnostic test in immunocompetent individuals is 98% and its specificity is 90%. 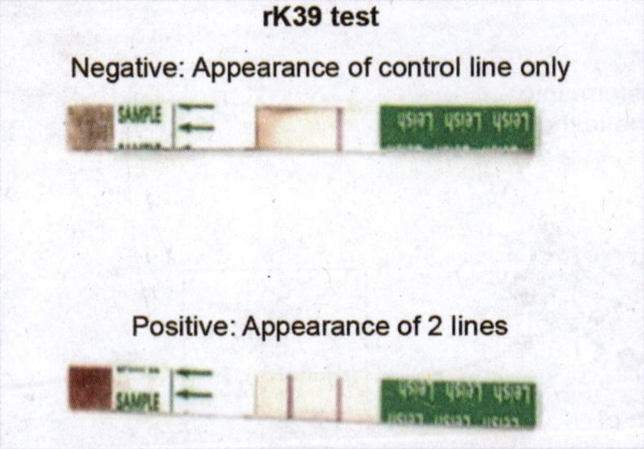
Treatment	General management of anemia, thrombocytopenia **Antibiotics:** Pentavalent antimonial drug (drug resistance in Bihar present) **Amphotericin B** 0.75–1.0 mg/kg on alternate days for total 15 infusions **Paromomycin** 11mg/kg base drug X 21 days **Miltefosine** (first oral drug approved): 2–11 years: 2.5 mg/kg X 28 days <25 kg 50 mg OD X 28 days >25 kg 50 mg BD X 28 days

19. Ans. (c) Measure blood sugar

Ref: Textbook of Clinical Neuropsychiatry and Behavioral Neuroscience By David P. Moore 3rd Ed Pg 216

- The presentation of the patient does not pinpoint to a definite diagnosis. However, THE NEXT STEP has been asked:

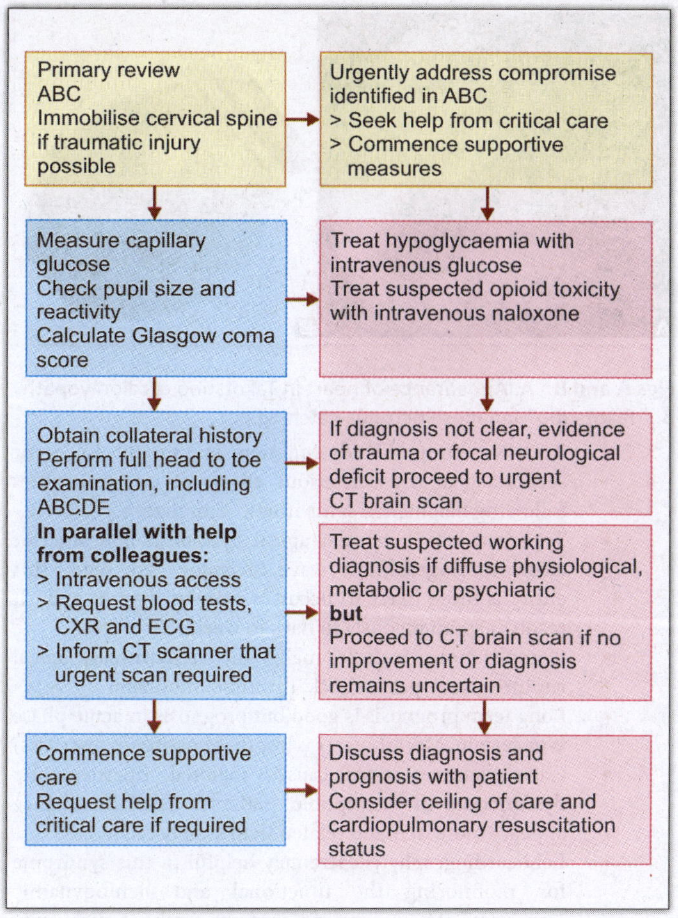

20. Ans. (c) Myxedema coma

Ref: Harrison's 19th Ed Pg 2290, 2293

- This is a classical case of Myxedema coma.
- Classical feature includes
  - Decreased mental status
  - Hypothermia
  - Bradycardia
  - Hyponatremia
  - Hypoglycemia
  - Hypotension
  - Precipitating illness

The hallmarks of myxedema coma are decreased mental status and hypothermia, but hypotension, bradycardia, hyponatremia, hypoglycemia and hypoventilation are often present as well. Puffiness of the hands and face, a thickened nose, swollen lips and an enlarged tongue may occur secondary to nonpitting edema with abnormal deposits of albumin and mucin in the skin and other tissues (myxedema). The possibility of a precipitating infection or other acute illness should always be considered;

- Clinical features of hypothyroidism: puffy face with edematous eyelids and nonpitting edema, yellowish skin, alopecia, Bradycardia, reduced stroke volume, diastolic hypertension, Oligomenorrhea or menorrhagia, constipation, weight gain, pericardial effusion, conductive hearing loss, carpal tunnel nerve entrapment.
- Advanced cases of hypothyroidism are accompanied by an edematous appearance known as myxedema.
- This condition is mistaken for edema, but is caused by the intradermal accumulation of proteins.
- Myxedema coma is a loss of brain function as a result of severe, long standing hypothyroidism. This condition is mostly seen in elderly patients and tends to occur more often in women. The condition carries very high mortality.
- Clinical manifestations include reduced level of consciousness, sometimes associated with seizures, as well as the other features of hypothyroidism.
- Hypothermia can reach 23°C (74°F). There may be a history of treated hypothyroidism with poor compliance, or the patient may be previously undiagnosed.
- Myxedema coma almost always occurs in the elderly and is usually precipitated by factors that impair respiration, such as drugs (especially sedatives, anesthetics, antidepressants), pneumonia, congestive heart failure, myocardial infarction, gastrointestinal bleeding, or cerebrovascular accidents.
- Sepsis should also be suspected. Exposure to cold may also be a risk factor.
- Hypoventilation, leading to hypoxia and hypercapnia, plays a major role in pathogenesis; hypoglycemia and dilutional hyponatremia also contribute to the development of myxedema coma

Treatment

- **Levothyroxine administered as a single IV bolus of 500 mcg**, as a loading dose followed by 50–100 mcg/d.
- If suitable **IV preparation is not available**, the same initial dose of levothyroxine can be given by **nasogastric tube** (though absorption may be impaired in myxedema).
- An alternative is to give **liothyronine (T3) intravenously or via nasogastric tube**, in doses ranging from **10 to 25 mcg every 8–12 h**. This treatment has been **advocated because T4 to T3 conversion is impaired** in myxedema coma. However, excess liothyronine has the potential to **provoke arrhythmias.**
- Another option is to combine **levothyroxine (200 mcg) and liothyronine (25 mcg)** as a single, **initial IV bolus** followed by daily treatment with levothyroxine (50–100 mcg/d) and liothyronine (10 mcg every 8 h).
- **Supportive therapy** should be provided to correct any associated metabolic disturbances. **External warming** is indicated only **if the temperature is <30°C**, as it can result in cardiovascular collapse.
- **Space blankets** to prevent further heat loss.
- **Parenteral hydrocortisone (50 mg every 6 h)** should be administered, because there is impaired adrenal reserve in profound hypothyroidism.
- Any precipitating factors should be treated, including the early use of broad-spectrum antibiotics, pending the exclusion of infection.
- **Ventilatory support** with regular blood gas analysis is usually needed during the first 48 hours. Hypertonic saline or IV glucose may be needed if there is severe hyponatremia or hypoglycemia; hypotonic IV fluids should be avoided because they may exacerbate water

retention secondary to reduced renal perfusion and inappropriate vasopressin secretion. The metabolism of most medications is impaired and sedatives should be avoided if possible or used in reduced doses.

21. Ans. (d) MAT

Ref: Introduction to ECG Interpretation by Frank G. Yanowitz Pg 23

Repeat AIIMS NOV 2018 General Medicine (See for explanation) (see page no. 717)

22. Ans. (c) Respiratory acidosis with metabolic compensation

Ref: Harrison's 19th Ed Pg 316

See table of "interpretation of ABG" in AIIMS NOV 2018 General Medicine (see page no. 720)

Let us go step by step.

pH → 7.12 → suggests acidosis

pCO_2 → 50 → suggests acidosis, in the direction of pH

HCO_3^- → 28 → suggests alkalosis, in the opposite direction of pH

The trend which goes in the direction of pH is usually the primary culprit. **This is respiratory acidosis with metabolic compensation.**

Let us Complete the Diagnosis

In acute acidosis, HCO_3 increases by 1 meq/L for every 10 mm Hg increase in $PaCO_2$.

In chronic acidosis, the HCO_3 increases by 3.5 meq/L for each 10 mm Hg increase in $PaCO_2$

In our case,

pCO_2 difference is 50–40 = 10 (normal pCO_2 → 35–45, for calculation, 40)

HCO_3 difference is 28–24 = 4 (normal HCO_3 →22-26, for calculation, 24)

So, for every 10 mm Hg increase in pCO_2, there is 4 mEq increase in HCO_3. (Note: The compensation is never complete.)

This is chronic respiratory acidosis with metabolic compensation.

Causes of respiratory acidosis mainly consist of hypoventilation.

23. Ans. (b) Takotsubo cardiomyopathy

Ref: Braunwald's 9th Ed Ch 15, Harrison's 19th Ed Pg 1565

- The above event was preceded by a stressful situation followed by sudden death. No other history is given. So, we shall assume that the patient had no genetic syndrome and no chronic cardiac disease.
- **Takotsubo cardiomyopathy/Apical ballooning syndrome/stress induced cardiomyopathy:**
- Emotional stress can precipitate severe reversible LV dysfunction that is accompanied by chest pain, pulmonary edema and cardiogenic shock in patients without coronary disease (Takotsubo syndrome).
- The name "Takotsubo" is derived from a Japanese pot that is used to catch octopus.

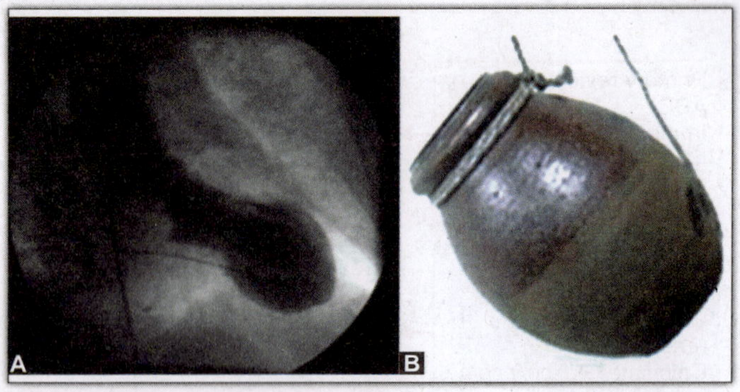

Figs A and B: A. Appearance of heart in Takotsubo cardiomyopathy B. "Takotsubo" Japanese octopus-catching pot

- In this setting, LV dysfunction is thought to occur secondary to the deleterious effects of catecholamines following heightened sympathetic stimulation.
- Transient left ventricular apical dyskinesis and anterior electrocardiographic T wave inversions are seen. This entity is more likely to occur in women than in men. It resolves spontaneously in days to weeks.
- Complications include malignant arrhythmias, apical rupture, cardiogenic shock, thromboembolism.
- Long term prognosis is good but prognosis in acute phase is uncertain. Mortality rate is low (but possible in few cases)
- Catecholamine surge causes regional microvascular dysfunction in susceptible patients. The disturbance appears more demand related than supply related.
- Echocardiography is extremely helpful in this syndrome for monitoring the functional and hemodynamic responses to treatment.Contrast echocardiography shows relatively normal perfusion in apical ballooning, indicating that wall motion abnormalities in apical ballooning are more demand related (such as increased catecholamine level) than supply related .
- Nuclear cardiac imaging shows apical perfusion defects in the setting of angiographic normal coronaries.

24. Ans. (b) Klebsiella

Ref: Harrison 19th Ed Page 809-812

NOTE

In absence of Pseudomonas aeruginosa and Staph aureus in options the third best answer will be Klebsiella

Ventilator-associated pneumonia (VAP) is **pneumonia** that develops 48 hours or longer after mechanical **ventilation** is given by means of an endotracheal tube or tracheostomy.

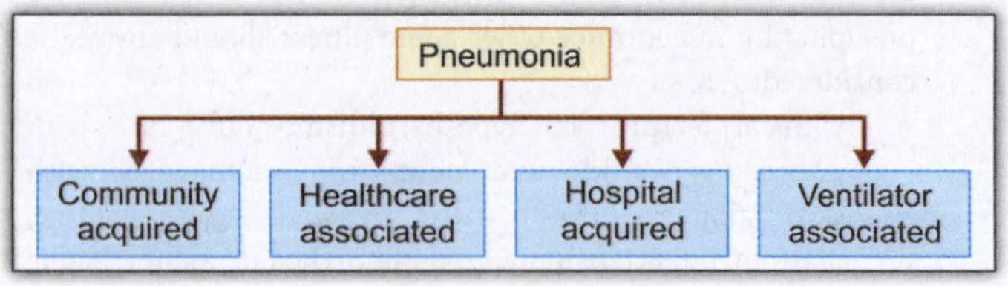

The most common cause of Ventilator associated pneumonia is Pseudomonas aeruginosa followed by Staph aureus. *(Ref: Paul Marino ICU book 4th Ed Ch 29)*

VAP pathogens are S. aureus (24.1 percent), P. aeruginosa (16.6 percent), Klebsiella species (10.1 percent), Enterobacter species (8.6 percent), Acinetobacter baumannii (6.6 percent) and E. coli (5.9 percent). However the incidence of Staph aureus have decreased now.

NOTE

35% OF VAP develops superinfection and most frequently by Pseudomonas aeruginosa, Staphylococcus aureus and Klebsiella spp.

25. Ans. (a) Vancomycin

Ref: Harrison's 19th Ed Table 153-2

- S. aureus pneumonia is well known to complicate influenza infection.
- However **Methicillin Resistant S.aureus (MRSA) has been reported as the primary etiologic agent of community acquired pneumonia (CAP).** Two important developments have led to this problem: the spread of MRSA from the hospital setting to the community and the emergence of genetically distinct strains of MRSA in the community.
- The former circumstance is more likely to result in HCAP (Healthcare associated Community Acquired Pneumonia),whereas the novel community-acquired MRSA (CA-MRSA) strains may infect healthy individuals with no association with health care.
- While this entity is still relatively uncommon, complications such as necrotizing pneumonia can occur.

Microbiology of Community Acquired Pneumonia

Outpatients	Non-ICU	ICU
Streptococcus pneumonia	*S. pneumonia*	*S. pneumonia*
Mycoplasma pneumonia	*M. pneumonia*	*Staphylococcus aureus*
Haemophilus influenzae	*Chlamydia pneumonia*	*Legionella* spp.
C. pneumonia	*H. influenzae*	Gram-negative bacilli
Influenza A and B viruses, adenoviruses, respiratory syncytial viruses, parainfluenza viruses	*Legionella spp.*	*H. influenzae*
	Influenza A and B viruses, adenoviruses, respiratory syncytial viruses, parainfluenza viruses	

Empirical Treatment of Community Acquired Pneumonia

Outpatient

- Previously healthy and no antibiotics in past 3 months
  - A macrolide (clarithromycin [500 mg PO bid] or azithromycin [500 mg PO once, then 250 mg qd]) Or
  - Doxycycline (100 m g PO bid)
- **Comorbidities or antibiotics in past 3 months:** Select an alternative from a different class
  - A respiratory fluoroquinolone (moxifloxacin [400 mg PO qd, gemifloxacin [320 mg PO qd], levofloxacin [750 mg PO qd]) or
  - **A ß-lactam (preferred:** High-dose amoxicillin [1 g tid] or amoxicillin/clavulanate [2 g bid; alternatives: ceftriaxone [1–2 g IV qd], cefpodoxime [200 mg PO bid, cefuroxime [500 mg PO bid]) plus a macrolide
- In regions with a high rate of "high-level" pneumococcal macrolide resistance consider alternatives listed above for patients with comorbidities

Inpatients, Non-ICU

A respiratory fluoroquinolone (e.g. moxifloxacin [400 m g PO or IV qd] or levofloxacin [750 mg PO or IV qd])
A ß-lactam (e.g. ceftriaxone [1–2 g IV qd, ampicillin [1–2 g IV q 4–6 h], cefotaxime [1–2 g IV q8hl ertapenem [1 g IV qd]) plus a macrolide (e.g. oral clarithromycin or azithromycin [as listed above] or IV azithromycin [1 g once, then 500 mg qd])

Inpatients, ICU

- A ß-lactam (e.g. ceftriaxone 2 g IV qd, ampicillin-sulbactam [2 g IV q8h] or cefotaxime [1–2 g IV q8h]) plus either azithromycin or a fluoroquinolone (as listed above for inpatients, non-ICU)

Special Concerns

If Pseudomonas is a consideration

- An antipseudomonal ß-lactam (e.g piperacillin/tazobactam [4.5 g IV q6h, cefepime [1–2 g IV q 12h, imipenem [500 mg IV q6h, meropenem [1 g IV q8h]) plus either ciprofloxacin (400 mg IV q 12 h) or levofloxacin (750 mg IV qd)
- The above ß-lactams plus an aminoglycoside (amikacin [15 mg/kg qd] or tobramycin [1.7 mg/kg qd]) plus azithromycin
- The above ß-lactams plus an aminoglycoside plus an antipneumococcal fluoroquinolone

If CA-MRSA is a consideration

- Add linezolid (600 mg IV q 12 h) or vancomycin (15 mg/kg q 12 h initially, with adjusted doses)

26. Ans. (c) Artemether plus lumefantrine

Ref: Guidelines for Diagnosis and Treatment of Malaria in India 3rd Edition (NATIONAL VECTOR BORNE DISEASE CONTROL PROGRAMME DELHI)

- Artemisinin combination therapy (ACT) should be given to all the confirmed P. falciparum cases found positive by microscopy or RDT.ACT consists of an artemisinin derivative combined with a long-acting antimalarial (amodiaquine, lumefantrine, mefloquine, piperaquine or sulfadoxine-pyrimethamine).
- In the **northeastern states** (Arunachal Pradesh, Assam, Manipur, Meghalaya, Mizoram, Nagaland and Tripura), due to the recent reports of late treatment failures to the current combination of artesunate + sulfadoxine-pyrimethamine in P. falciparum malaria, the presently recommended ACT in national drug policy is fixed dose combination (FDC) of Artemether-lumefantrine (AL).

Co-formulated Tablet AL	Total dose of AL (Twice Daily for 3 day)	No. of Tablets in the Packing	Administration (Twice daily for 3 days) Tablets
5–14 kg (>5 months to <3 years)	20 mg/120 mg	6	1
12–24 kg (≥3 to <9 years)	60 mg/240 mg	12	2
25–34 kg (≥9 to <14 years)	60 mg/360 mg	18	3
≤34 kg (≤14 years)	80 mg/480 mg	24	1
Not recommended during the first trimester of pregnancy and for children weighing <5 kg.			

27. Ans. (d) Osteoarthritis

Ref: Davidson 22nd Ed Pg 1060

Davidson 22nd Ed Pg 1060 says:

"Osteoarthritis (OA) is by far the most common form of arthritis."

- It is characterised by focal loss of articular cartilage with new bone proliferation and remodelling of the joint contour. Inflammation is not a prominent feature.
- OA preferentially targets certain small and large joints; the knee and hip are the principal large joints involved
- It is strongly associated with ageing and is a major cause of pain and disability in older people. Up to 45% of all people develop knee OA and 25% hip OA at some point during life.

28. Ans. (c) Churg Strauss syndrome

Ref: Davidson 22nd Ed 1117-1119

Churg-Strauss syndrome (CSS) is a small-vessel vasculitis associated with eosinophilia. Some patients have a prodromal period for many years, characterised by allergic rhinitis, nasal polyposis and late-onset asthma that is often difficult to control. ***The typical acute presentation is with a triad of skin lesions (purpura or nodules), asymmetric mononeuritis multiplex and eosinophilia.*** Pulmonary infiltrates and pleural or pericardial effusions due to serositis may be present. Up to 50% of patients have abdominal symptoms provoked by mesenteric vasculitis.

Diagnosis

- Patients with active disease have raised levels of ESR and CRP and an eosinophilia.
- Although antibodies to MPO or PR3 can be detected in up to 60% of cases, CSS is considered to be a distinct disorder from the other ANCA-associated vasculitides.
- Biopsy shows a small-vessel vasculitis with eosinophilic infiltration of the vessel wall.

Management

- High-dose steroids and cyclophosphamide, followed by maintenance therapy with low-dose steroids and azathioprine, methotrexate or MMF.

29. Ans. (d) LDL more than 100 mg/dL

Ref: Obstructive Sleep Apnea in Adults-advances in cardiology vol 46 By Jaffrey R. Borer Page 113

The association of Obstructive Sleep Apnea and metabolic syndrome has been termed 'syndrome Z'. It refers to the association of the 5 following components:

1. Obesity (especially central adiposity, waist circumference >102 cm in men and >88 cm in women)
2. Raised blood pressure (≥ 130/85 mm Hg)
3. Elevated glucose (fasting glucose >6.1 mmol/l)
4. Elevated triglyceride levels (triglycerides ≥ 1.7 mmol/l or ≥150 mg/dL)
5. Low HDL cholesterol levels (HDL cholesterol <50 mg/dL)

30. Ans. (d) Patent Subarachnoid space

Ref: Inderbir Singh Neuroanatomy 10th Ed Pg 239

Pressure on jugular veins increases pressure in the subarachnoid space. This indicates that the space is in continuation. This is also known as the Queckenstedt test.

Queckenstedt's Test	
Indications	To check for patency of subarachnoid space, as in spinal stenosis; clinical subarachnoid block, tumor or thrombosis with normal opening pressure of CSF.

Contd...

Queckenstedt's Test	
Contra-indications	Raised intracranial pressure
Procedure	The patient lies in lateral decubitus position. A lumbar puncture is done and the opening pressure is measured. Both jugular veins are compressed and then released and subsequent changes in CSF pressure are observed
Mechanism	Jugular compression causes an increase in the intracranial blood volume. CSF is displaced caudally and increases the volume of the dural sac. The latter becomes more distended with a consequent increase in both the CSF pressure and the venous pressure
Result in normal individuals	Normally, upon compression of jugular veins, CSF pressure rapidly rises and with the release of pressure on jugular veins, CSF pressure rapidly falls → Indicates patent subarachnoid space
Block in Subarachnoid space	In the presence of a spinal block, there is no rise of CSF pressure with jugular vein compression (or a pressure rise is low or delayed).
Note: Tobey-Ayer-Queckenstedt sign is used in the diagnosis of unilateral and bilateral **lateral sinus thrombophlebitis**. In cases where the lateral sinus is obstructed on one side, compression of the **jugular vein** on the intact side causes a rise in **CSF** pressure, whereas compression of the obstructed side does not raise the CSF pressure.	

31. Ans. (b) Rapid correction of hyponatremia

Ref: The ICU book by Paul Marino 4th Ed page 668 , Irwin and Rippe's Intensive Care Medicine by 6th Ed Pg 1972

Rapid correction of Serum sodium can cause Central Pontine myelinosis. Hence, utmost care and monitoring is required during correction of hyponatremia.

Treatment of Hyponatremia

- **Mild cases:** Treatment of underlying cause and fluid restriction
- The management of hyponatremia is determined by the ECV and the presence or absence of neurological symptoms.
- Symptomatic hyponatremia (mostly plasma [Na] < 120 mEq/L) requires a more rapid increase in the plasma [Na] than asymptomatic cases and this is accomplished with hypertonic saline (3% NaCL).

Rate of Correction

Rapid correction of the plasma [Na] (i.e., >10–12 mEq/L in 24 hrs) can produce an **osmotic demyelinating syndrome** (sometimes called central pontine myelinolysis) characterized by **dysarthria, quadriparesis, "locked-in syndrome" over a period of days and loss of consciousness**. The following measures are recommended for avoiding osmotic demyelination:

Comparison of the United States and European Guidelines

Subject	United states guideline	European guideline
Acute or symptomatic hyponatremia	**Severe symptoms:** Bolus 3% NaCl (100 mL over 10 min × 3 as needed)	**Severe symptoms:** Bolus 3% NaCl (150 mL over 20 min 2–3 times as needed)
	Moderate symptoms: Continuous infusion 3% NaCl (0.5–2 mL/kg per h)	Moderate symptoms: Bolus 3% NaCl (150 mL 3% over 20 min once)
Chronic hyponatremia SIAD	Fluid restriction (First line) Demeclocycline, urea, or vaptan (second line)	Fluid restriction (First line) Urea or loop diuretics + oral Nacl (second line) Do not recommend or recommend against vaptan Recommend against lithium or demeclocycline
Hypovolemic hyponatremia	Isotonic saline	Isotonic saline or balanced crystalloid solution
Hypovolemic hyponatremia	Fluid restriction Vaptans	Fluid restriction Recommend against vaptan
Correction rates	Minimum: 4–8 mmol/L per d, 4–5 mmol/L per d, 8 mmol/L per d (high risk of ODS)	No minimum
	Limits: 10–12 mmol/L per d, 8 mmol/L per d (high risk of ODS)	Limit: 10 mmol/L per d
Management of overcorrection	Baseline $S_{Na} \geq 120$ mmol/L: probably unnecessary	Start once limit is exceeded

Contd...

Comparison of the United States and European Guidelines		
Subject	United states guideline	European guideline
	Baseline S_{Na} < 120 mmol/L: start relowering with electrolyte-free water or desmopressin after correction exceeds 6–8 mmol/L per d	Consult an expert to discuss infusion containing electrolyte-free water (10 mL/kg) with or 2 μg desmopressin iv
Do not recommend when S_{Na} < 130 mmol/L "recommend against" when S_{Na} < 125 mmol/L In liver cirrhosis, restrict to patients where potential benefit outweigh risk of worsened liver function		

AIIMS NOVEMBER 2017

32. Ans. (c) His observation capacity

Ref: Textbook of Psychiatry By Sujata Sethi 1st ed page 9, Essentials of Mental Health Nursing By BT Basavanthappa page 114

Observation skills of informant is a Subjective criteria and there is not way to measure the same.

Informant's Ability to report depends on following factor:

- **Age:** Children are poor informant
- **Sex:** Informant of same sex as patient are more reliable
- **Educational status:** Educated informant better visualize the details of illness, treatment and prognosis
- **Biological relationship:** Blood relatives are likely to give accurate information
- **Presence in previous episode:** Person present at the time of previous episode is likely to give more accurate detail
- **Length of stay with the patient:** A person (friend, relative or Colleague) staying with the patient is likely to give more accurate information. A relative might not be staying with the patient due to outstation job and hence might not be a good informant.
- **History of drug abuse or mental illness of the informant:** Such informant is not a reliable informant

33. Ans. (d) TIBC

Ref: Harrison 19th ed page 628, Robbins 9th ed page 455

Total Iron binding capacity is Increased not reduced in Iron deficiency anemia. Serum Iron, Serum Ferritin and Transferrin saturation all are reduced in iron deficiency anemia

Types of Microcytic Anemia				
	Iron deficiency (Sideropenic anemia)	Thalassemia	Sideroblastic anemia	Anemia of chronic disease
Peripheral smear	Microcytic hypochromic	Microcytic hypochromic	Microcytic hypochromic	Normocytic normochromic (Microcytic hypochromic can be seen)
Serum iron	Low	Normal	Normal	Low
TIBC	High	Normal	Normal	Low
Tansferrin Saturation %	↓ (< 20%)	N/↑	N/↑	↓
Serum Ferritin (μg/l)	↓ (Best/most specific and sensitive marker of Fe deficiency anemia)	↑	↑ (reflects degree of iron overload)	N/↑
Hemoglobin pattern on electrophoresis	Normal	Abnormal with β thalassemia; can be normal with α thalassemia	Normal	Normal
RDW	High	Normal	High	
MCV	Normal (pre latent and latent) or low (stage 3)	Low	Low	
Bone marrow	Normoblastic		Prussian blue stain of RBC in marrow shows ringed sideroblasts	

Footnote:

- Transferrin saturation, which is normally 25–50%, is obtained by the following formula: **serum iron x 100 ÷ TIBC**
- The serum iron level represents the amount of circulating iron bound to transferrin
- TIBC is an indirect measure of the circulating transferrin. (Hence plasma transferrin is increased in Iron deficiency anemia)
- **RDW= Red cell distribution width** is a quantitative measure of the variation in red cell size and the higher the values, the more heterogeneous the RBC population size (i.e., anisocytosis). The upper limit of normal values for RDW is 14.6%.
- ***RDW is particularly useful in characterizing microcytic anemia***, allowing to distinguish between uncomplicated iron deficiency anemia (high RDW, normal to low MCV) and uncomplicated heterozygous thalassemia (normal RDW, low MCV)

34. Ans. (c) Erythropoietin levels

Ref: Harrison 19th ed page 399, 672

Hint to Diagnosis

- High altitude
- Hypertension
- Itching/Pruritus
- Splenomegaly

Polycythemia is defined as an increase in the hemoglobin above normal. Features of the clinical history that are useful in the differential diagnosis include smoking history; current living at high altitude; or a history of congenital heart disease, sleep apnea, or chronic lung disease.

Manifestations range from digital ischemia to Budd- Chiari syndrome with hepatic vein thrombosis. Abdominal vessel thromboses are particularly common Neurologic symptoms such as vertigo, tinnitus, headache and visual disturbances may occur. **Hypertension** is often present. Patients with polycythemia vera may have **aquagenic pruritus** and symptoms related to **hepatosplenomegaly**. Patients may have easy bruising, epistaxis, or bleeding from the gastrointestinal tract. Peptic ulcer disease is common Polycythemia can be spurious (related to a decrease in plasma volume; Gaisbock's syndrome), primary, or secondary in origin. The secondary causes are all associated with increases in EPC levels

Option (A)

Philadelphia chromosome is seen in CML. Originally, this was recognized by the presence of a shortened chromosome 22 (22q-), designated as the Philadelphia chromosome, that arises from the reciprocal t(9;22). Splenomegaly and Fatigue are only matching symptoms of CML in this question.

Option (D)

JAK 2 mutation is confirmed only after checking Erythropoietin level for confirming the diagnosis of Polycythemia vera

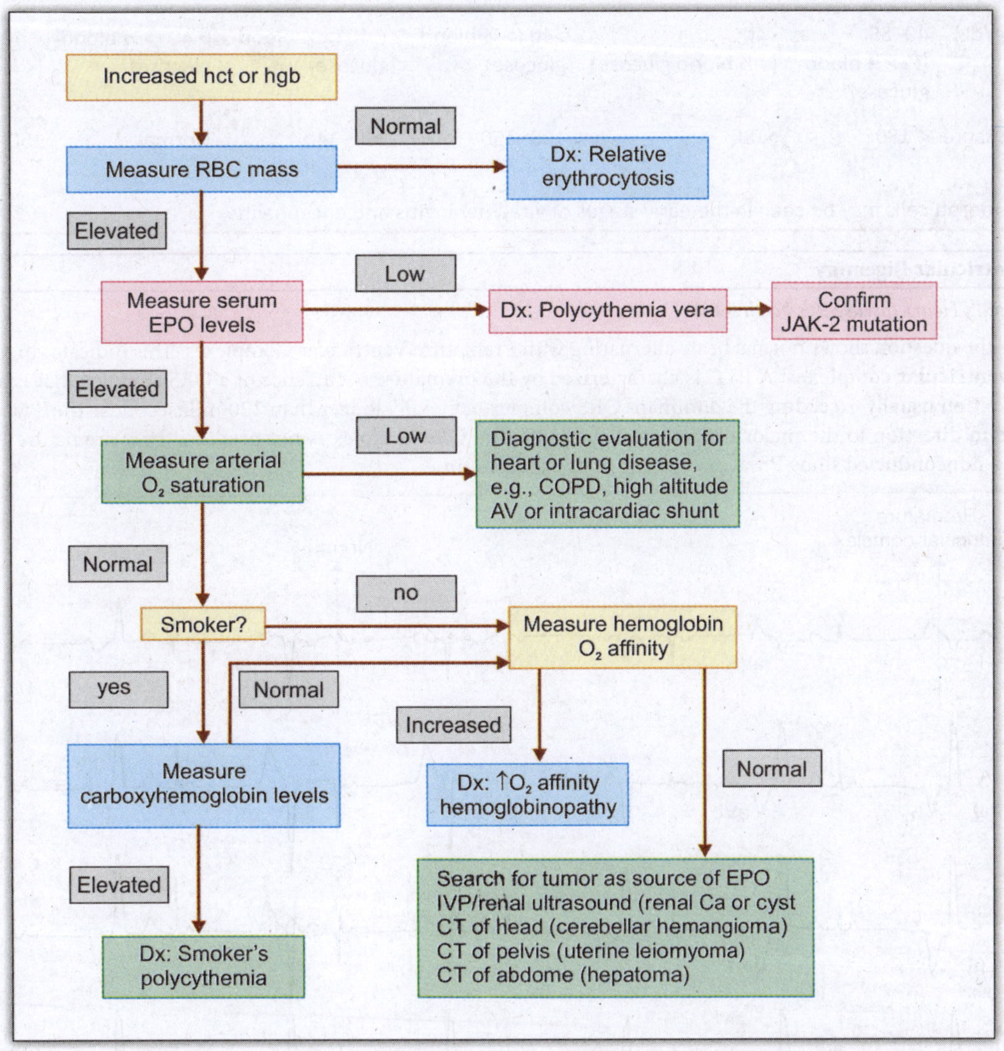

35. Ans. (d) Coxsackie meningitis

Ref: Harrison 19th ed page 766

A cerebrospinal fluid (CSF) profile with lymphocytic pleocytosis and a normal glucose concentration is consistent with viral meningitis and can often be treated as outpatients if appropriate contact and monitoring can be ensured

Typical CSF Changes in Meningitis

	Normal	Pyogenic/Bacterial	Viral	Fungal	Parasitic	Tuberculosis
Appearance	Crystal-clear	Turbid/purulent	Clear/turbid	Turbid/viscous	Turbid/viscous	Turbid/viscous
Gram's stain	Negative	Positive in> 60% cases	Negative	Rarely positive	Negative	Occasionally positive
Culture	Negative	Positive in> 80%	Negative	Rarely positive	Negative	Occasionally positive
WBC count (/µL)	<5	10–10000	25–500	40–600	150–2000	25–100
Differential WBC	60–70% Lymphocytes	> 80% Polymorphs	Predominantly Lymphocytes	Lymphocytes or PMNs depending on organism	↑ Eosinophils	Predominantly Lymphocytes
Protein (mg/dL)	15–45	>100	20–80	150–300	50–200	100–200
Glucose (mg/dL)	40–85 (⅔ > ½ blood glucose)	<40 (< ½ blood glucose)	>40 (> ½ blood glucose)	> 40 (> ½ blood glucose)	> 40 (> ½ blood glucose)	< 40 (< ½ blood glucose)
Opening pressure (mmH_2O)	< 180	>180	100–350	160–340	Normal	150–280

*Some polymorph cells may be seen in the early stages of viral meningitis and encephalitis

36. Ans. (a) Ventricular Bigeminy

Ref: Braunwald's Heart disease 9th ed ch 39

The figure in the question shows normal beats alternating with Premature Ventricular Complexes. This indicates bigeminy.

Premature ventricular complexes: A PVC is characterized by the premature occurrence of a QRS complex that is abnormal in shape and has a duration usually exceeding the dominant QRS complex, generally longer than 120 milliseconds. The T wave is usually large and opposite in direction to the major deflection of the QRS. The QRS complex is not preceded by a premature P wave but can be preceded by a nonconducted sinus P wave occurring at its expected time.

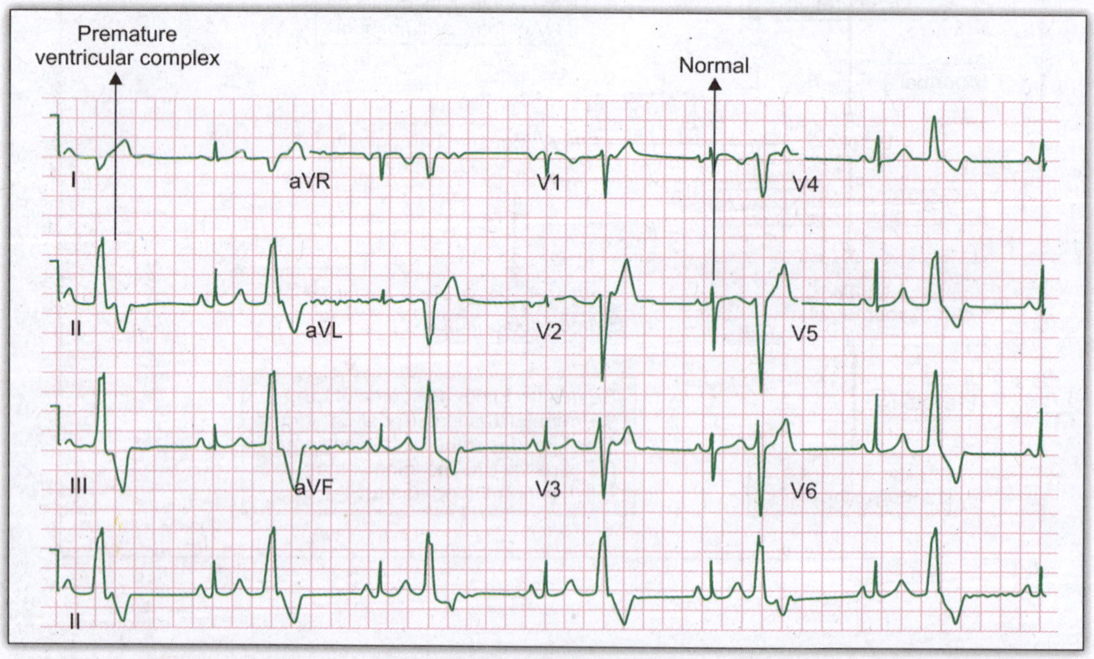

The term bigeminy refers to pairs of complexes and indicates a normal and premature complex; trigeminy indicates a premature complex that follows two normal beats; a premature complex that follows three normal beats is called quadrigeminy and so on.

TYPES OF PVCs
Infrequent PVCs: Less than five PVCs/min
Frequent PVCs: Five or more PVCs/min
Isolated PVCs (Beats): PVC. occurring singly.
Group Beats, Bursts, Salvos: PVC, occuring in groups of two or more.
Paired PVCs (Couplet): Two PVCs in a row.
Ventricular Tachycardia: Three or more PVCs in a row.
Ventricular Bigeminy: PVC. alter-nating with the QRS complexes of the underlying rhythm.
Ventricular Trigeminy/Ventricular Quadrigeminy: PVCs following may two or three QRS complexes of the underlying rhythm, respectively.
R-on-T Phenomenon: A PVC occurring during the downslope of the preceding T wave (vulnerable period of ventricular repolarization.)

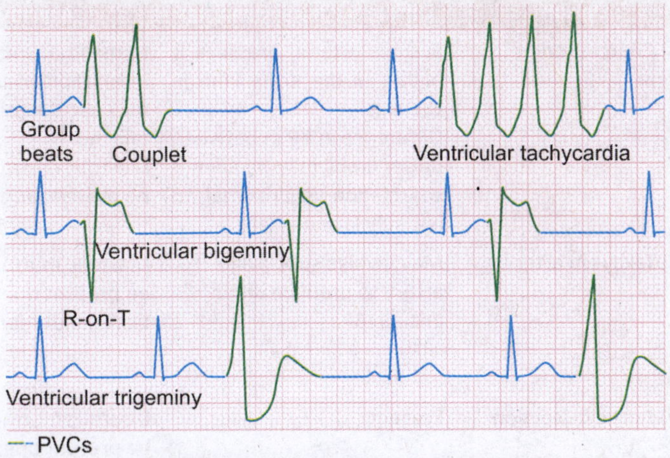

37. Ans. (b) CT Thorax

Ref: Harrison 19th ed page 1788

Superior vena cava syndrome (SVCS) is the clinical manifestation of superior vena cava (SVC) obstruction, with severe reduction in venous return from the head, neck and upper extremities. Malignant tumors, such as lung cancer, lymphoma and metastatic tumors are responsible for the majority of SVCS cases. In young adults, malignant lymphoma is a leading cause of SVCS. Patients with SVCS usually present with neck and facial swelling (especially around the eyes), dyspnea and cough. Other symptoms include hoarseness, tongue swelling, headaches, nasal congestion, epistaxis, hemoptysis, dysphagia, pain, dizziness, syncope and lethargy. Bending forward or lying down may aggravate the symptoms. The characteristic physical findings are dilated neck veins; an increased number of collateral veins covering the anterior chest wall; cyanosis; and edema of the face, arm and chest.

The diagnosis of SVCS is a clinical one. ***The most significant chest radiographic finding is widening of the superior mediastinum, most commonly on the right side.*** However, a normal chest radiograph is still compatible with the diagnosis if other characteristic findings are present. ***Computed tomography (CT) provides the most reliable view of the mediastinal anatomy.*** The diagnosis of SVCS requires diminished or absent opacification of central venous structures with prominent collateral venous circulation. Magnetic resonance imaging (MRI) has no advantages over CT.

38. Ans. (d) Salicylate poisoning

Ref: Harrison 19th ed page 318

Anion gap (AG) is imperial in etiological diagnosis of metabolic acidosis.

Na – (Cl + HCO_3) = Anion gap (Usually < 12).

If gap is more than 12, patient has an High anion gap acidosis

MNEMONIC = GOLDMARK

G — Glycols (ethylene glycol and propylene glycol) **O** — Oxoproline, a metabolite of paracetamol **L** — L-lactate, the chemical responsible for lactic acidosis **D** — D-lactate **M** — Methanol **A** — Aspirin **R** — Renal failure (Uremia) **K** — Ketoacidosis (Ketones generated from starvation, Alcohol and Diabetic ketoacidosis)

Most important cause of normal anion gap acidosis is diarrhea.

39. Ans. (b) Coarctation of aorta

Ref: Harrison 19th ed page 1525

Important findings in this patient are:

- Difference in BP between right and left upper limb (>10 mm Hg)
- Early diastolic murmur in right 2nd ICS

Let us discuss optionwise through this comparative table

Option	Difference in BP Readings	Murmur	Remarks
(A)Supravalvular aortic stenosis	Systolic blood pressure is higher in the right arm than in the left arm, by around 30 mm Hg.	Midsystolic ejection murmur best over right 1st ICS.	• Localized or diffuse narrowing of the ascending aorta originating just above the level of the coronary arteries at the superior margin of the sinuses of Valsalva • Usually congenital • Most commonly associated cardiac defect in Williams-Beuren syndrome • Aortic regurgitation may be present

Contd...

Option	Difference in BP Readings	Murmur	Remarks
(B) Coarctation of aorta	Systolic arterial pressure is higher in the arms than in the legs. Difference in BP in between upper limbs may be seen if coarctation is proximal to left subclavian artery	Midsystolic murmur. Interscapular area may elicit continuous murmur. Diastolic murmur may be present due AR	• Most commonly distal to the origin of the left subclavian artery near the insertion of the ligamentum arteriosum frequent in patients with gonadal dysgenesis (e.g., Turner syndrome). Also in fetal hydantoin syndrome • AR can be easily a manifestation of Coarctation as Bicuspid AV is seen in most cases.
(C) Takayasu arteritis	May involve subclavian artery to produce difference in BP	Diastolic murmur May be present due to aortic regurgitation	Inflammatory stenotic disease involves medium and large sized arteries with a predilection for aortic arch and its branches and also pulmonary arteries. Subclavian artery involvement may cause claudication of involved arm.
(D) Aortic dissection	Present	Diastolic murmur May be present due to aortic regurgitation	

Footnote:
- **Causes of BP difference in both upper limbs:** Atherosclerotic or inflammatory subclavian artery disease, supravalvular aortic stenosis, aortic coarctation,aortic dissection.
- **Williams-Beuren syndrome(chromosome 7):** "elfin" facies, low nasal bridge, cheerful demeanor, mental retardation with retained language skills and love of music, supravalvular aortic stenosis and transient hypercalcemia

We conclude that since site of coarctation is rarely proximal to left subclavian (thus difference in BP between upper and lower limbs is more common), coarctation of aorta is the answer.

40. Ans. (c) Digit span forward upto 7 digits with 2 skips allowed

Ref: Harrison 19th ed page 168, Clinician's Guide To Neuropsychological Assessment by Rodney D. Vanderploeg 2nd Ed Pg 507

Memory Tests

- **Immediate and working memory** is assessed by tests of attention including the digit span. Attention is the ability to focus and direct cognitive processes and to resist distraction; concentration is the ability to focus and sustain attention over a period of time. The most elementary assessment of attention is accomplished through the digit span test.
  - **Digit span test:** The examiner recites number digits at the rate of one number per second and asks the patient to repeat back the number sequence in exactly the same order. The string of digits increases in length. A normal span is seven digits plus or minus two digits for adults, regardless of age or educational level. Spelling simple words backward or stating the months of the year in reverse are other simple tests of attention and concentration.
  - More complex tests are Trailmaking Test (Trails A), symbol-copying tasks (e.g., Digit Symbol) and letter-cancellation tasks.
- **Recent memory** involves the learning of new material.
  - Testing orientation to time and place and asking the patient about events of the day are useful to assess recent memory.
  - Asking patient to remember 3–4 words, having them repeat them to ensure normal attention/immediate memory and then ask them to recall the words after 5 to 10 minutes of distraction. Normal older adults should be able to remember 3–4 words without cues and up to eight words with cues.
  - The **"three-words three-shapes" memory test** is another test of recent memory. In this test, patients are asked to copy 3 words (e.g. justice, parliament, Press) along with three abstract shapes.
- **Remote memories** can be tested by asking for the names of Indian Prime Ministers in reverse order as far back as the patient can remember, or by asking about important historical events and dates. The patient can also be asked about details of personal life such as his or her birth date, the names and ages of children and grandchildren and work history, assuming independent verification is available

Option (A) and (B)

Harrison 19th ed page 2537 states- Calculation ability is assessed by having the patient carry out a computation that is appropriate to the patient's age and education (e.g. serial subtraction of 7 from 100 or 3 from 20; or word problems involving simple arithmetic)

41. Ans. (d) Tubercular peritonitis

Ref: Harrison 19th ed page 287

- The serum-ascites albumin gradient (SAAG) is useful for distinguishing ascites caused by portal hypertension from nonportal hypertensive ascites.
- The SAAG reflects the pressure within the hepatic sinusoids and correlates with the hepatic venous pressure gradient.
- The SAAG is calculated by subtracting the ascitic albumin from the serum albumin and does not change with diuresis.
- A SAAG $\geq$ 1.1 g/dL reflects the presence of portal hypertension and indicates that the ascites is from an increased pressure in the hepatic sinusoids.
- Possible causes include cirrhosis, cardiac ascites, sinusoidal obstruction syndrome (venoocclusive disease),

massive liver metastasis, or hepatic vein thrombosis (Budd-Chiari syndrome).

- **A SAAG <1.1 g/dL indicates that the ascites is not related to portal hypertension as in tuberculous peritonitis, peritoneal carcinomatosis, or pancreatic ascites**

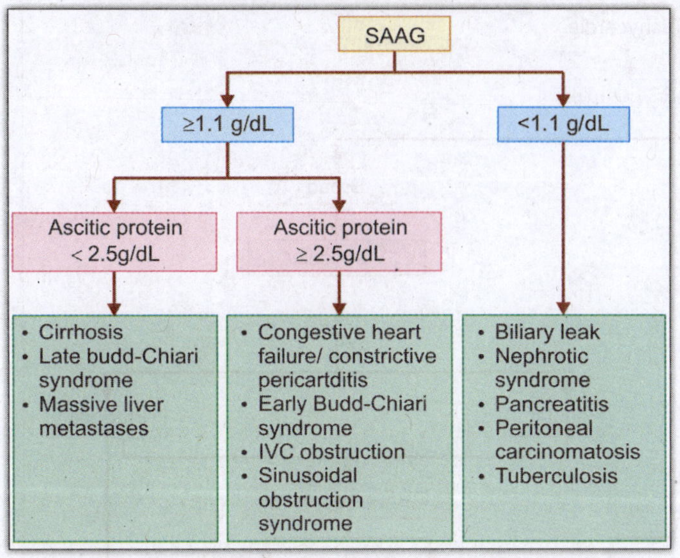

42. Ans. (b) Hypercalcemia

Ref: Harrison's 19th ed page 1795, The ICU book by Paul Marino 4th Ed Ch 36

Tumor Lysis Syndrome

- Tumor lysis syndrome (TLS) is characterized by hyperuricemia, hyperkalemia, hyperphosphatemia and hypocalcemia and is caused by the destruction of a large number of rapidly proliferating neoplastic cells. Acidosis may also develop. Acute renal failure occurs frequently.
- TLS is most often associated with the treatment of Burkitt's lymphoma, acute lymphoblastic leukemia and other rapidly proliferating lymphomas, but it also may be seen with chronic leukemias and, rarely, with solid tumors and also with chronic lymphocytic leukemia after treatment with nucleosides like fludarabine.
- TLS has been observed with administration of glucocorticoids, hormonal agents such as letrozole and tamoxifen and monoclonal antibodies such as rituximab and gemtuzumab.
- TLS usually occurs during or shortly (1–5 days) after chemotherapy. Rarely, spontaneous necrosis of malignancies causes TLS.
- Hyperuricemia may be present at the time of chemotherapy. Effective treatment kills malignant cells and leads to increased serum uric acid levels from the turnover of nucleic acids. Owing to the acidic local environment, uric acid can precipitate in the tubules, medulla and collecting ducts of the kidney, leading to renal failure.
- Lactic acidosis and dehydration may contribute to the precipitation of uric acid in the renal tubules. The finding of uric acid crystals in the urine is strong evidence for uric acid nephropathy. The ratio of urinary uric acid to urinary creatinine is >1 in patients with acute hyperuricemic nephropathy and <1 in patients with renal failure due to other causes.
- **Hyperphosphatemia**, which can be caused by the release of intracellular phosphate pools by tumor lysis, produces a reciprocal **depression in serum calcium**, which causes severe neuromuscular irritability and tetany. Deposition of calcium phosphate in the kidney and hyperphosphatemia may cause renal failure.
- Potassium is the principal intracellular cation and massive destruction of malignant cells may lead to hyperkalemia. Hyperkalemia in patients with renal failure may rapidly become life-threatening by causing ventricular arrhythmias and sudden death.
- The likelihood that TLS will occur in patients with Burkitt's lymphoma is related to the tumor burden and renal function.
- Hyperuricemia and high serum levels of lactate dehydrogenase (LDH >1500 U/L), both of which correlate with total tumor burden, also correlate with the risk of TLS.
- In patients at risk for TLS, pretreatment evaluations should include a complete blood count, serum chemistry evaluation and urine analysis. High leukocyte and platelet counts may artificially elevate potassium levels ("pseudohyperkalemia") due to lysis of these cells after the blood is drawn.
- In these cases, plasma potassium instead of serum potassium should be followed. In pseudohyperkalemia, no electrocardiographic abnormalities are present.
- In patients with abnormal baseline renal function, the kidneys and retroperitoneal area should be evaluated by sonography and/or CT to rule out obstructive uropathy. Urine output should be watched closely.

Prevention and treatment of Tumor lysis syndrome

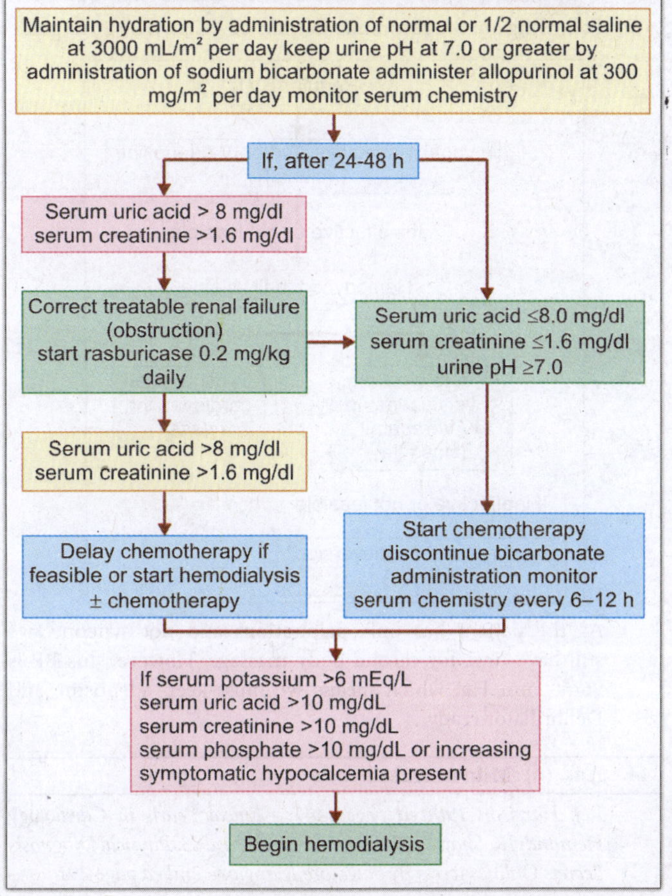

43. Ans. (a) Carotid body massage

Ref: Harrison 19th ed page 1479, 2015 ACC/AHA/HRS Guideline for the Management of Adult Patients With Supraventricular Tachycardia: Executive Summary

The above ECG picture is suggestive of Supraventricular tachycardia.

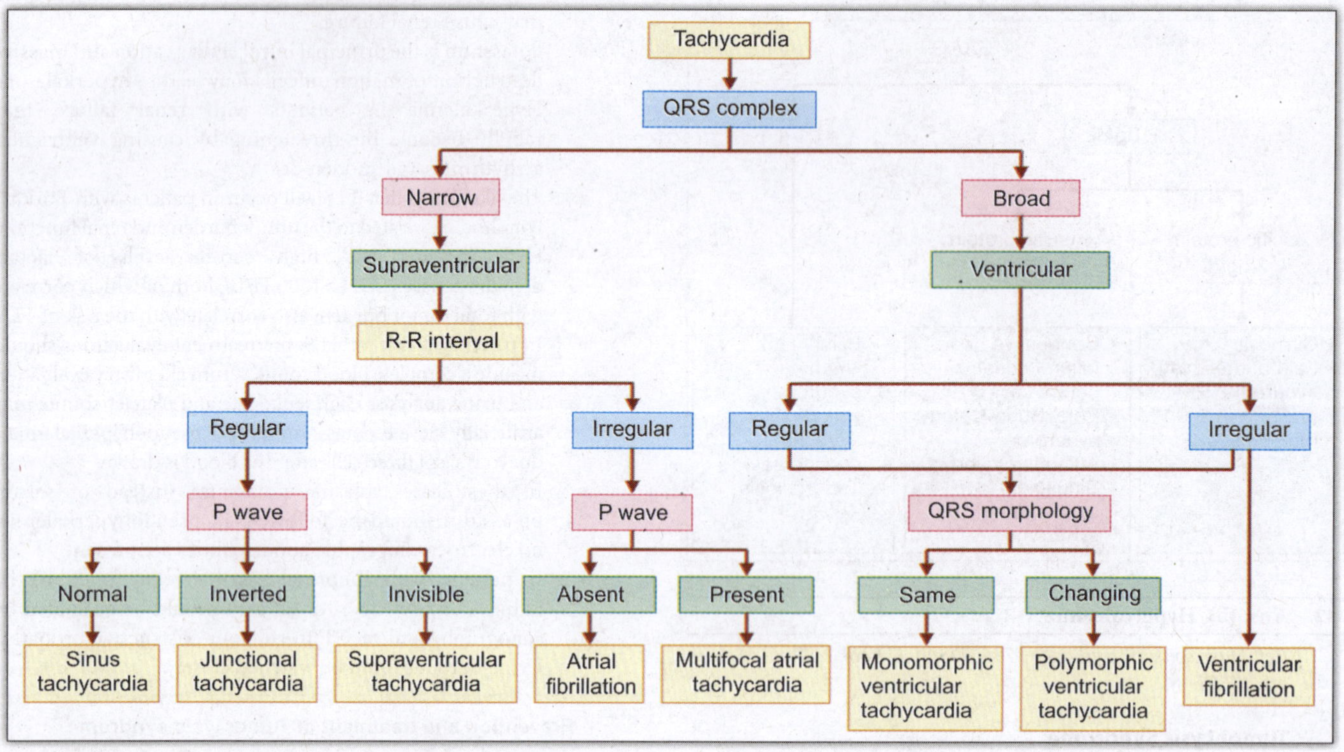

Following are the recommendations of ACC/AHA 2015 guidelines for acute treatment of SVT of unknown mechanism:

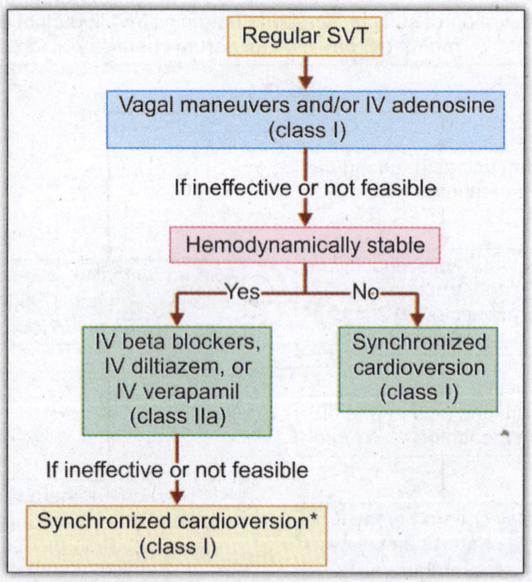

As the patient has only palpitations and not syncope, we still have time for carotid body massage. However, his BP is 96/68 mm Hg, which means we must keep adenosine and Defibrillator ready.

44. Ans. (d) Mild mitral stenosis

Ref: Harrison 19th ed page 1447, Clinical Pearls in Cardiology Hemanth IK, Shafeeq Mattummal 1st ed Page 83, Physical Diagnosis Secrets Online Access By Salvatore Mangione 2nd ed page 291

A loud first heart sound occurs when the leaflets are wide open at the end of ventricular diastole and shut forcefully at the beginning of ventricular systole. Loud S1 is associated with Early Mitral stenosis not Mild Mitral stenosis. All early might not be mild and all Mild might not be early.

Other than calcific mitral stenosis, a soft S1 is usually heard in either early closure of the mitral valve (aortic regurgitation) or late closure (prolonged P-R interval). Alternatively, a soft or absent S1 can result from inadequate left ventricular contraction because of congestive heart failure, myocardial infarction or Left bundle branch block.

Most clinically significant abnormalities of S1 are related to its intensity or loudness rather than its split. When compared to the second heart sound, the first heart sound is longer in duration but it is lower in pitch. The important factors that influence the intensity of the first heart sound are the following:

- **Duration of the PR interval:** Short PR interval (WPW syndrome) causes loud S1, whereas long PR interval (e.g. first degree heart block) produces soft S1.
- **Atrioventricular Pressure gradient:** A large atrioventricular pressure gradient (Mitral stenosis) produces loud S1.
- **Rate of rise of ventricular pressure during systole:** A rapid rate of rise of ventricular pressure due to increased force of ventricular contraction (Eg. Hyperdynamic circulatory state- Eg Aortic Regurgitation) produces Loud S1. A slow rate of rise of left ventricular pressure (Left ventricular dysfunction) produces soft S1

- **Mobility and thickening of the valve cusp:** A mobile and thickened valve cusp produces loud S1 (Early mitral stenosis with uncalcified valve cusp). S1 becomes softer in the later stages of MS when the leaflets are rigid and calcified
- **Factors that decreases the conduction of sound:** Thick chest wall, pleural effusion, Emphysema.

45. Ans. (a) Endothelial independent vasodilation of coronary arteries

Ref: KDT 7th ed page 541, Goodman Gillman's 12th ed page 749

Variant/Prinzmetal/Vasospastic Angina (Uncommon form)

- They are due to recurrent localized (occasionally diffuse) coronary vasospasm which may be superimposed on arteriosclerotic coronary artery disease. Attacks occur at rest or during sleep and are unpredictable.
- The relaxant effect on larger coronary vessels is the principal action of nitrates benefiting variant angina (Prinzmetal) by counteracting coronary spasm.
- Other mechanisms of nitrate action are:
- Preload reduction
- Afterload reduction
- Redistribution of coronary flow

46. Ans. (a) NCCT

Ref: Harrison 19th ed page 107, 1777, Bailey 26th Ed Pg 321

"Worst headache of the life" is a typical textbook description of a SAH. Acute, severe headache with stiff neck but without fever suggests subarachnoid hemorrhage

In a case of headache a careful neurologic examination is an essential first step in the evaluation. In most cases, patients with an abnormal examination or a history of recent onset headache should be evaluated by a computed tomography (CT) or magnetic resonance imaging (MRI) study. In some circumstances, a lumbar puncture (LP) is also required, unless a benign etiology can be otherwise established.

SAH Clinical Features

- The location of the headache is often occipital or cervical.
- There may be associated nausea, vomiting and photophobia.
- Patients may experience transient loss of consciousness and collapse.
- There may be a history of less severe headache some days prior to the ictus the warning or sentinel headache.
- Physical examination may be normal or may include Meningism with neck stiffness and photophobia.
- The development of a third nerve palsy in the context of a sudden severe headache may be due to SAH from a ruptured posterior communicating artery aneurysm, because of the proximity of this nerve and artery.
- Patients may have an altered level of consciousness. A Cushing's response (hypertension and bradycardia) may be seen in patients with altered consciousness secondary to raised ICP
- Focal neurological deficits in the limbs at presentation suggest a focal intracerebral haematoma or vascular dissection. Patients in the more severe grades are more likely to exhibit the systemic complication of SAH: cardiac tachyarrhythmias and neurogenic pulmonary oedema.

Diagnosis of Subarachnoid Haemorrhage

Investigation	When	Remarks
CT scan (non contrast - NCCT)	Within 48 hours	• First investigation of choice. • Positive in aneurysmal SAH in 95% of cases within 48 hours. • Sensitivity falls off rapidly with increased time from ictus as blood is cleared from the subarachnoid space. • The extent and location of subarachnoid blood on NCCT help locate the underlying aneurysm, identify the cause of any neurologic deficit and predit delayed vasospasm. • A positive CT scan precludes a lumbar puncture.
Lumbar puncture	Suspicious history but negative CT scan	Rarely if the hemorrhage is small or below the foramen magnum the head CT scan can be normal. Therefore LP may be required to definitively diagnose SAH. Lumbar puncture prior to an imaging procedure is indicated only, if a CT scan is not available First breakdown product in blood is oxyhaemoglobin, which appears from around 2–12 hours; Bilirubin appears later and a **bilirubin peak** is diagnostic of SAH. False negatives: if the lumbar puncture is performed within 12 hours of the ictus. False positives: in the presence of a traumatic tap or increased serum bilirubin. A traumatic tap (fresh procedure-related blood in the sample) does not exclude an SAH – it means that the lumbar puncture may not give a useful result.
CT angiogram/formal cerebral angiogram	Highly suspicious history negative lumbar puncture	Localises aneurysm

47. Ans. (d) Inj. Magnesium sulphate

Ref: Harrison's 19th Ed Pg 308, The ICU book by Paul Marino 3rd Ed Pg 620

Similar question was asked in AIIMS Nov 2014 (Medicine) where hyperkalemia was not directly given but ECG interpretation was given and "drug not used was asked".

MgSO4 is used in digitalis induced Hyperkalemia only. Beta-2-adrenergic agonists can be effective in the acute treatment of hyperkalemia, lowering the serum potassium concentration by 0.5 to 1.5 mEq/L. beta-2-adrenergic receptors, can be given as 10 to 20 mg in 4 mL of saline by nebulization over 10 minutes (which is 4 to 8 times the dose used for bronchodilation)

Acute management of Hyperkalemia

Condition	Treatment	Commnet
ECG changes or serum K>7 mEq/L	Calcium gluconate (10%): 10 mL IV over 3 minutes; can repeat in 5 minutes	Response lasts only 20 to 30 minutes. *Do not* give bicarbonate after
ECG changes and circulaory compromise	Calcium chloride (10%): 10 mL IV over 3 minutes	Calcium chloride contains 3 times more calcium than calcium gluconate.
AV block refractory to calcium treatment	• 10 U regular insulin in 500 mL of 20% dextrose: infuse over 1 hours • Transvenous pacemaker	Insulin—dextrose treatment K by 1 mEq/L for 1 to 2 hours
Digitalis cardiotoxicity	• Magnesium sulfate: 2 g as IV bouls • Digitalis specific antibodies if necessary	*Don not* use calcium for the hyperkalemia of digitalis toxicity
After acute phase or when no ECG changes	Kayexalate: Oral does of 30 g in 50 mL of 20% sorbitol, or rectal dose of 50 g in 200 mL 20% sorbitol as a retention	Oral dosing is preferred. Enemas poorly toler ated by patients and nurses.

Hyperkalemia Management Rapid Overview

Clinical features

Signs and symptoms are uncommon and tend to occur only when the serum potassium exceeds 7.0 meq/L; symptoms can include muscle weakness and ventricular arrhythmias

There are two major mechanisms of hyperkalemia:

- Increased potassium release from cells (eg, severe hyperglycemia, rhabdomyolysis, succinylcholine)
- Reduced potassium excretion in urine, most often due to hypoaldosteronism or renal failure

Contd...

Pseudohyperkalemia, which is most often due to hemolysis of the blood specimen, is the most common cause of a reported elevation in serum potassium and must be excluded. It does not reflect true hyperkalemia and does not produce ECG changes

Electrocardiogram manifestations

Large interpatient variability exists in the relationship between the serum potassium and ECG changes; at a given serum potassium, ECG changes are more common with acute elevations and less common with chronic elevations (e.g. chronic kidney disease)

Careful cardiac monitoring and serial ECGs are essential

ECG findings commonly progress as follows:

Peaked T waves

Prolonged PR and QRS intervals and small P waves

Loss of P wave, further prolongation of QRS interval (**"sine wave" pattern**) and conduction delay that can manifest as bundle branch or AV nodal block

Ventricular fibrillation or asystole can result

Management

Confirm the patient is truly hyperkalemic (i.e., exclude pseudohyperkalemia)

Obtain electrocardiogram and, if signs of hyperkalemia are seen, place patient on cardiac monitor

The specific therapies that follow are listed according to their rapidity of action; the choice among them varies according to the severity of ECG changes and muscle weakness

Stabilize cardiac membranes with calcium:

Give for hyperkalemia with significant ECG findings (eg, widening of the QRS complex or loss of P waves, peaked T waves) or severe arrhythmias thought to be caused by hyperkalemia

Give adults **calcium chloride** 500 to 1000 mg (5 to 10 mL of 10 percent solution) by IV infusion slowly over 2 to 3 minutes, preferably via a central line; or give **calcium gluconate** 1000 mg (10 mL of 10 percent solution) also infused slowly; may be given peripherally in large vein; time to onset is immediate

Calcium treatment may be repeated after 5 minutes if ECG changes persist; patient must be on cardiac monitor when receiving calcium; calcium can exacerbate digoxin toxicity

Give children **calcium gluconate** (10 percent solution) 0.5 mL/kg

Since the effect of calcium is transient, patients with hyperkalemia also require treatments to shift potassium into cells and to remove potassium

Shift potassium into cells:

Give insulin and glucose to hyperkalemic patients with ECG changes OR serum potassium ≥6.5 to 7 meq/L

Contd...

Insulin and glucose: Give IV bolus of regular insulin 10 units with 50 mL of a 50 percent glucose solution; give children regular insulin 0.2 units per gram of glucose, give glucose 1 g/kg; time to onset is 10 to 20 minutes; after insulin and glucose bolus therapy, start dextrose infusion; monitor fingerstick glucose closely
Beta-2 agonist: May give albuterol 10 to 20 mg in 4 mL saline nebulized over 10 minutes (may use metered dose inhaler); pediatric dose 0.1 to 0.3 mg/kg; time to onset is 20 to 30 minutes; IV albuterol or epinephrine are alternatives
Sodium bicarbonate: Provides minimal effect on shifting potassium intracellularly, even in acidemic patients; may give 150 meq in one liter of 5 percent dextrose in water at 250 mL/hour; do not give in same IV as calcium
Since the effect of shifting potassium into the cells is transient, treatments to remove potassium are also required
Remove potassium
Cation exchange resin (sodium polystyrene sulfonate): Give 15 to 30 grams of sodium polystyrene sulfonate (without sorbitol) orally; pediatric dose is 1 g/kg; although less preferable, sodium polystyrene sulfonate may be given as a retention enema (dose is 50 g) without sorbitol; time to onset is approximately 1 to 2 hours; may repeat dose after 4 to 6 hours based upon repeat serum potassium; sorbitol can cause intestinal necrosis and should be avoided; do not give sodium polystyrene sulfonate or sorbitol to post-operative or renal transplant patients
Loop or thiazide diuretic: Provides only limited short-term effect; may give furosemide 20 to 40 mg IV; pediatric dose is 1 to 2 mg/kg IV; higher dose may be required with renal insufficiency; fluid losses must be replaced unless the patient is volume expanded
Hemodialysis: Can be used if the conservative measures listed above fail, if hyperkalemia is severe, if the patient has renal failure, or if the patient has marked tissue breakdown and is releasing large amounts of potassium from injured cells

48. Ans. (b) Adrenaline 0.5 mg 1: 1000 by intramuscular route

Ref: With text

This is a controversial question with different textbooks giving different statements.

Katzung 12th ed page 145 states

"The syndrome of bronchospasm, mucous membrane congestion, angioedema and severe hypotension usually responds rapidly to the parenteral administration of epinephrine, **0.3–0.5 mg (0.3–0.5 mL of a 1:1000 epinephrine solution).** Intramuscular injection may be the preferred route of administration, since skin blood flow (and hence systemic drug absorption from subcutaneous injection) is unpredictable in hypotensive patients. In some patients with impaired cardiovascular function, intravenous injection of epinephrine may be required."

KDT 7th Ed Pg 87 states

"Inject adrenaline ***0.5 mg (0.5 ml of 1 in 1000 solution for adult, 0.3 ml for child 6-12 years and 0.15 ml for child upto 6 years) i.m.***; repeat every 5–10 min in case patient does not improve or improvement is transient. This is the only life saving measure. Adrenaline should not be injected i.v. (can itself be fatal) unless shock is immediately life threatening. If adrenaline is to be injected i.v., it should be diluted to 1:10,000 or 1:100,000 and infused slowly with constant monitoring."

KDT 7th Ed Pg 138 states

"Adrenaline 0.5 mg injected promptly i.m. is the drug of choice in anaphylactic shock"

Harrison 19th ed page 2117

An IV infusion should be initiated to provide a route for administration of 2.5 mL epinephrine, diluted 1:10000, 5-10 min interval, volume expanders such as normal saline and vasopressor agents such as dopamine if intractable hypotension occurs.

Finally, ***World Allergy Organisation 2015 guidelines*** state that

"There were no overdoses with IM injection, versus an overdose rate of 13 % after IV bolus administration. These data support the safety of the IM route and suggest need for extreme caution when IV bolus doses are administered" Also, the options do not mention infusion of IV dose. Hence our answer is option (B) Adrenaline 0.5 mg 1:1000 by intramuscular route.

Uses of Adrenaline

USE	DOSE	ROUTE
Laryngeal edema	1: 100 (10 mg/mL) 0.25 mg in 2 mL saline	Nebulizer
Anaphylaxis	1:1000 (1 mg/mL), 0.3–0.5 mg with repeated doses as required at 5- to 20-min intervals for a severe reaction	IM
Asystole or PEA (Pulseless Electrical Activity)	1: 10,000 (0.1 mg/mL) 10mL (1 mg) every 3–5 min	IV
Anaphylactic shock	1:1000- 0.3- 0.5 mg (1mg/mL)	IM (Preferred)
	1:1,00,000 infusion @5–15 mcg/min	IV infusion
Local anesthetics	1:200000 (more commonly) or 1:100000	Infiltration
Control of bleeding	1 in 10000	
Cardiac arrest	1 mg every 3–5 min	IV

Note:

- In case of anaphylaxis IM route is preferred, Because in anaphylaxis IV route might not be possible due to collapsed veins and IM route is safer (no everdose rate). Subcutaneuos absorption May not be possible
- 1:1000 regular 1 mg Adrenaline that comes in 1 ampule

49. Ans. (a) Start only ORS

Ref: CMDT 2017 page 1305

The mainstay of treatment of diarrhea is Rehydration Therapy. If person is able to take orally well the rehydration should be done orally and when he is not able to it is has to be done parentally.

About antibiotics: They should be used only in case of bacterial diarrhea as unnecessary use leads to antibiotic abuse. Also there is an entity called as "antibiotic induced diarrhea" which can set in when antibiotics are used when not needed.

In the index case there is no fever or blood in stools so possibility of bacterial infection is least likely.

AIIMS MAY 2017

50. Ans. (a) Concussion

Ref: With Text

With history of fall, concussion and diffuse axonal injury are more probable outcomes.

The retrograde amnesia involves an inability to recall experiences that occurred before the onset of the amnesic state. Relatively recent events are more vulnerable to retrograde amnesia than are more remote and more extensively consolidated events.

Option (A)

A brief period of both retrograde and anterograde amnesia is characteristic of concussion and it recedes rapidly in alert patients. Memory loss spans the moments before impact but may encompass the previous days or weeks (rarely months). With severe injuries, the extent of retrograde amnesia roughly correlates with the severity of injury (Ref: Harrison 19th ed page 4S7e-1)

Option (B)

Just standing near an alcohol shop does not makes you an alcoholic. Harrison States "Fortunately, very few alcoholics (perhaps as few as 1 in 500 for the full syndrome) develop Wernicke's (ophthalmoparesis, ataxia and encephalopathy) and Korsakoff's (retrograde and anterograde amnesia) syndromes" (Ref: Harrison 19th ed page 2724)

Option (C)

Diffuse axonal injury is associated with severe head trauma and may be seen on CT as multiple areas of punctate hemorrhage in deep white matter and corpus callosum. DAI is associated with poor prognosis. (Ref: Blueprints Neurology 3rd ed page 120)

Option (D)

Cerebral venous thrombosis is most frequently observed in the superior sagittal and transverse sinuses and is associated with headache and increased intracranial pressure. (Harrison 19th ed page 2194)

51. Ans. (c) Bronchoscopic ligation

Ref: Harrison 19th ed page 246, Schwartz 9th ed ch 19

Summary

Bronchoscopic interventions are done in massive hemoptysis but does not includes ligation. Ligation is not possible by bronchoscopy.

For the most part, the treatment of hemoptysis will vary based on its etiology. However, large-volume, life-threatening hemoptysis generally requires immediate intervention regardless of the cause. The ***first step is to establish a patent airway*** usually by endotracheal intubation and subsequent mechanical ventilation. The volume of the hemoptysis is also important not only in determining the cause, but in gauging the urgency for further diagnostic and therapeutic maneuvers. ***Massive hemoptysis is defined as hemoptysis of greater than 200–600 cc in 24 hours.*** Massive hemoptysis should be considered a medical emergency.

Option (A)

It is generally employed when there is persistent brisk hemoptysis despite correction of coagulopathy and after bronchoscopy. The bronchial arteries should be the first vessels studied in most patients with massive hemoptysis because they are the most common source of bleeding. Severe hemoptysis from bronchial arteries can be treated with angiographic embolization of the culprit bronchial artery. This intervention should only be entertained in the most severe and life-threatening cases of hemoptysis because there is a risk of unintentional spinal-artery embolization and consequent paraplegia with this procedure.

Option (B)

The pulmonary arteries are generally studied only if bronchial arteriography does not identify a bleeding source or if there is a high suspicion for arteriovenous malformation (AVMs) or pulmonary embolism. Overall, the pulmonary arteries are the bleeding source in fewer than 10% of patients with massive hemoptysis.

Option (C)

As large-volume hemoptysis usually arises from an airway lesion, it is ideal to identify the site of bleeding by either chest imaging or bronchoscopy (more commonly rigid rather than flexible). Endobronchial lesions can be treated with a variety of bronchoscopically directed interventions, including cauterization and laser therapy. ***There are a variety of bronchoscopic techniques that may control pulmonary hemorrhage, but none have been indisputably proven to be of benefit. They include balloon tamponade, iced saline lavage, topical medications, laser therapy and electrocautery***

Option (D)

In extreme conditions, surgical resection of the affected region of lung is considered

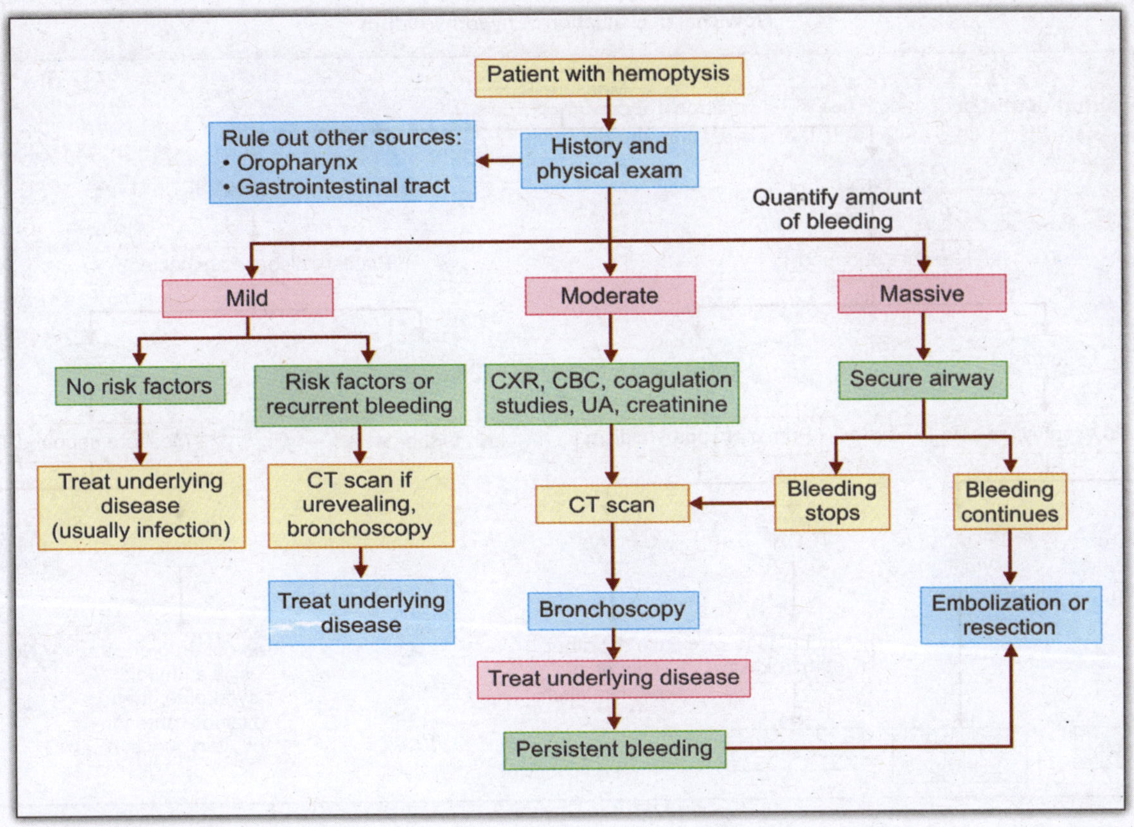

NOTE

Blood products in massive hemoptysis: Patients with massive hemoptysis should be suspected for coagulation abnormalities. Those who are receiving an anticoagulant or have an elevated prothrombin time, partial thromboplastin time, or international normalized ratio should receive fresh frozen plasma. Those who are thrombocytopenic should receive a platelet transfusion. Patients who are uremic or taking an antiplatelet agent (e.g. aspirin, clopidogrel) or transfused platelets. Finally, the administration of recombinant factor VIIa should be considered.

52. Ans. (d) Acute intermittent porphyria

Ref: Harrison's 19th Ed Pg 2527, CMBT 2017 page 1676

Indirect Repeat Medicine AIIMS May 2013 (See for details of porphyria)

53. Ans. (c) Primary hypothyroidism

Ref: Harrison 19th ed page 2292

Flow chart: Evaluation of hypothyroidism

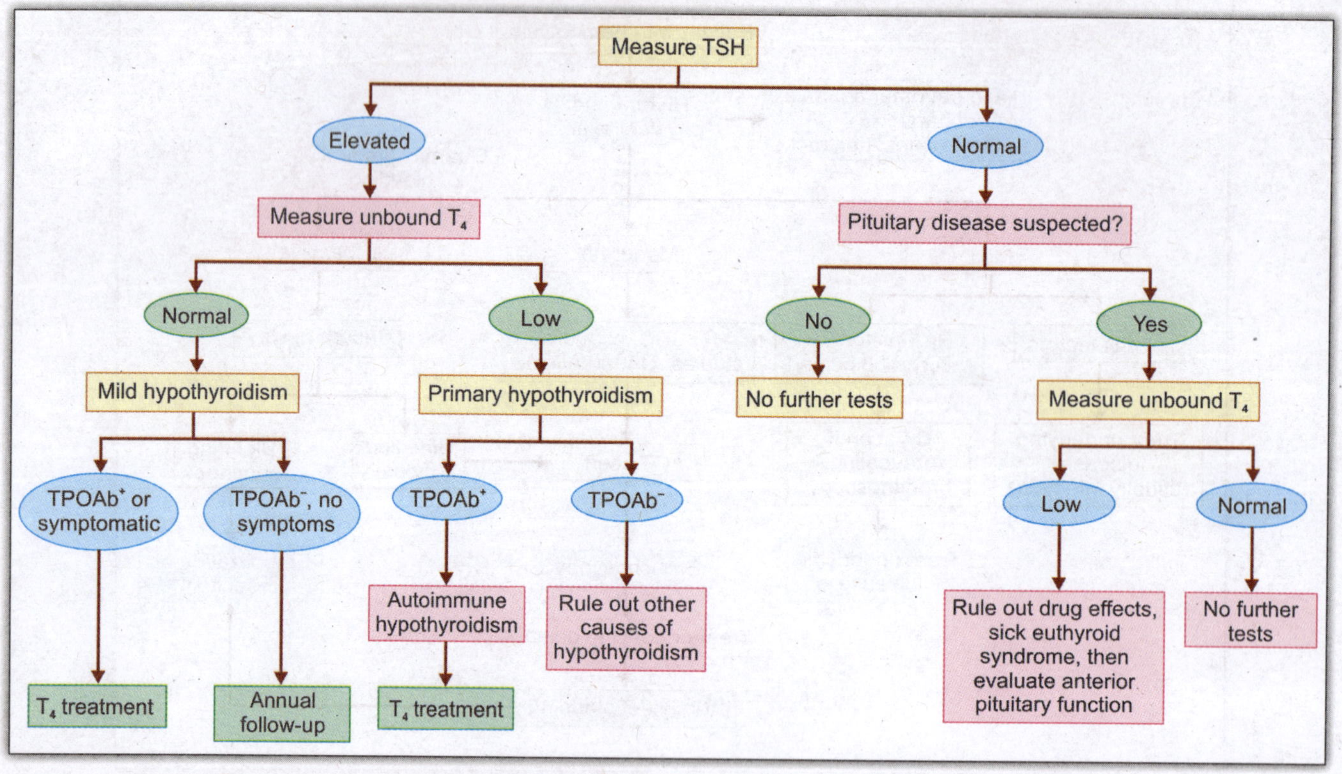

Thyroid Function Tests Assessment

Assessment	Serum TSH	Serum free T4	Serum T3
Euthyroid	Normal	Normal	Normal
Euthyroid hyperthyroxinemia	Normal	Normal or high	Normal or high
Euthyroid hypothyroxinema	Normal	Normal or low	Normal or low
Euthyroid: T3 therapy	Normal	Low	Normal or high
Euthyroid: thyroid extract therapy	Normal	Low-normal or low	Normal or high
Primary hypothyroidism	High	Low	Normal or low
Subclinical hypothyroidism	High	Normal	Normal
Hyperthyroidism	Low	High or normal	High
Subclinical hyperthyroidism	Low	Normal	Normal
TSH-mediated hyperthyroidism	Normal or high	High	High
Central hypothyroidism	Normal or low*	Low or low-normal	Low or normal

T3: triiodothyronine; T4: thyroxine; TSH: thyroid-stimulating hormone.
* In central hypothyroidism, serum TSH may be low, normal, or slightly high.

54. Ans. (c) Cortical vein thrombosis

The following differential diagnoses must come to our mind for a postpartum patient with headache and seizure.

- Eclampsia
- Cortical venous thrombosis
- Pituitary hemorrhage/Sheehan's syndrome

However, eclampsia is not given in the options. There is no other specific history pointing towards eclampsia either.

Option (A)

Meningitis would be associated with fever, neck rigidity/photophobia and presence of early papilledema usually goes against acute bacterial/viral meningitis.

Option (B) Acute migraine

The history of fever and seizures does not go with the diagnosis of migraine.

Option (C) Cortical vein thrombosis

Points in favour are predisposing factor in the form of prothrombotic state, history of headache, papilledema, seizures.

- Cerebral venous thrombosis is more common in women than men, with a female to male ratio of 3:1. The imbalance may be due to the increased risk of CVT associated with pregnancy and puerperium and with oral contraceptives
- The major risk factors for CVT in adults are prothrombotic conditions, oral contraceptives, pregnancy and the puerperium, malignancy, infection and head injury.
- Symptoms and signs of CVT can be grouped in three major syndromes:

- Isolated intracranial hypertension syndrome (headache with or without vomiting, papilledema and visual problems)
- Focal syndrome (focal deficits, seizures, or both)
- Encephalopathy (multifocal signs, mental status changes, stupor, or coma)

- Headache (of gradual, acute, or thunderclap onset) is the most frequent symptom occurring in almost 90% of patients. It is associated with fever, nausea, vomiting, seizures, raised ICT.
- It may be with or without vomiting, papilledema and visual problems. In other cases, headache may be accompanied by focal neurologic deficits, focal or generalized seizures and encephalopathy with altered mental status or coma. It may occur without focal neurological deficits.
- Parenchymal brain lesions, including brain swelling, edema, venous infarction, or hemorrhagic venous infarction, may occur secondary to venous occlusion.
- Brain MRI in combination with magnetic resonance (MR) venography is the most sensitive examination technique for demonstrating the thrombus and the occluded dural sinus or vein. Head CT scan is normal in up to 30% of CVT cases and most of the findings with CVT are nonspecific.

55. Ans. (c) Insulin like growth factor

Ref: Harrison 19th ed page 2270, CMT 2017, Page. 1114-1116

Acromegaly

- The diagnosis of acromegaly should be suspected in individuals who present with the typical clinical features of growth hormone (GH) excess, which include the enlargement during adulthood of the jaw (macrognathia), hands and feet, which result in increasing shoe and glove size and the need to enlarge finger rings.
- The facial features become coarse, with enlargement of the nose and frontal bones as well as the jaw and the upper incisors may become spread apart. Despite the prominence of these findings at the time of diagnosis, the rate of change is so slow that few patients seek care because their appearance had changed.
- Other features include cardiovascular disease, sleep apnea, type 2 diabetes, arthropathies, carpal tunnel syndrome and problems directly related to the pituitary tumor size (headache, visual loss).
- Once a patient is suspected to have acromegaly, the first step is biochemical testing to confirm the clinical diagnosis, followed by radiologic testing to determine the cause of the excess growth hormone (GH) secretion. The cause is a somatotroph adenoma of the pituitary in over 95% of cases.

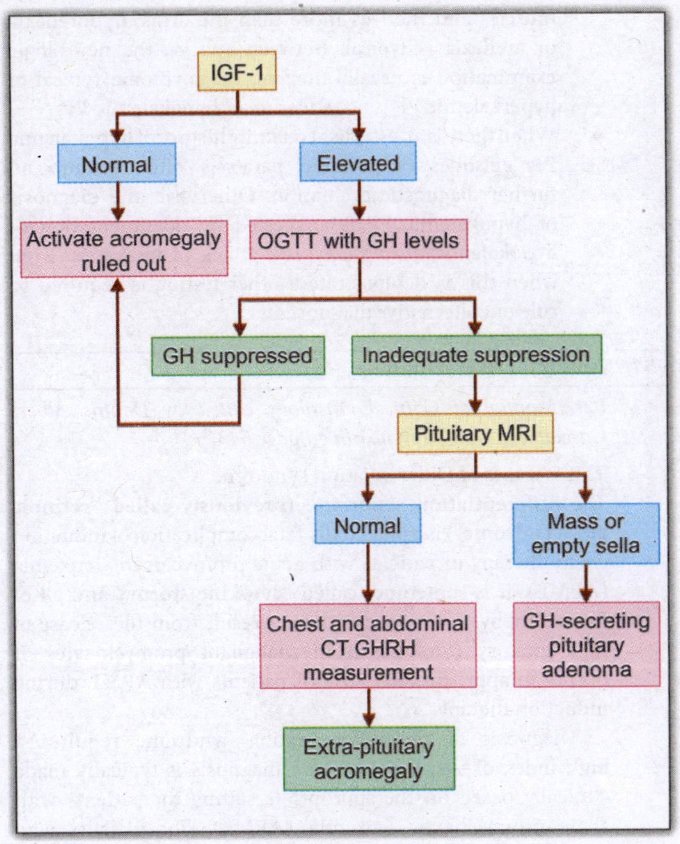

56. Ans. (a) Serum potassium

Ref: Harrison 19th edition 462-e 16

This is a case of Hypokalemic periodic paralysis (Bilateral muscle weakness, no history of trauma, young age)

- Hypokalemic periodic paralysis is a rare inherited neuromuscular disorder, related to a defect in muscle ion channels and manifest by episodes of painless muscle weakness that may be triggered by rest after vigorous exercise, stress, or a high-carbohydrate meal.
- Hypokalemic PP, attacks begin in late childhood or teenage years. These attacks vary in frequency and duration. Intervals of weeks to months are common, but some patients experience several attacks per week. Attacks typically last several hours, but the duration can range from minutes to days. Attacks may be triggered by rest after vigorous exercise, stress, or a high-carbohydrate meal, often after a delay of several hours. These events are often associated with an increased release of epinephrine or insulin, both of which cause movement of potassium into cells and low potassium blood levels.
- Neurologic examination during an attack demonstrates weakness, usually affecting proximal more than distal

muscles and the legs more than the arms; hyporeflexia or areflexia is typical. Between attacks, the neurologic examination is usually normal; the myotonia typical of hyperkalemic PP is not a feature of hypokalemic PP.

- When there is an established family history of hypokalemic PP, episodes of periodic paralysis often require no further diagnostic evaluation. Otherwise, the diagnosis of hypokalemic PP is suggested by documentation of hypokalemia during a typical attack of weakness. Even when this is demonstrated, other testing is required to rule out alternative diagnoses.

57. Ans. (c) Dexamethasone

Ref: Manual of Clinical Oncology edited by Dennis Albert Casciato, Mary C. Territo 6th ed page 543

This is a case of Differentiation syndrome.

The **differentiation syndrome (previously called "retinoic acid syndrome")** is a potentially fatal complication of induction chemotherapy in patients with acute promyelocytic leukemia (APML). It is sometimes called **"cytokine storm,"** and all of the pathophysiologic consequences result from the release of inflammatory cytokines from malignant promyelocytes. It occurs in approximately 25% of patients with APML during induction therapy.

Diagnosis of the differentiation syndrome requires a high index of suspicion, but the diagnosis is typically made clinically based on the appropriate setting for patients with acute promyelocytic leukemia (APML). For patients who develop fever and/or dyspnea following differentiation induction for APL, oxygen saturation should be assessed and a chest radiograph obtained. Funduscopic examination may demonstrate papilledema from brain swelling; this is a medical emergency.

Clinical features: The differentiation syndrome is a clinical diagnosis based upon a constellation of findings. Any three or more of the following signs in the absence of other causes are sufficient to make the diagnosis and ***institute glucocorticoids***:

- Fever
- Weight gain (from capillary leak and soft tissue edema)
- Respiratory distress
- Radiographic opacities
- Pleural or pericardial effusion
- Hypotension
- Renal failure (usually from hypotension, although disseminated intravascular coagulation may also be present)

The majority of patients will have a combination of dyspnea, fever and radiographic opacities.

Pulmonary hemorrhage is a rare complication of the differentiation syndrome. ***As glucocorticoid therapy and transfusions are the main treatments, an invasive procedure is not usually warranted to make this diagnosis.***

A rapid improvement in respiratory status with initiation of glucocorticoids supports the diagnosis of differentiation syndrome. A lung biopsy is rarely needed, unless the patient fails to improve and noninvasive studies are unrevealing.

58. Ans. (b) DC cardioversion

Ref: Harrison 19th ed page no 1494

A wide complex tachycardia (WCT) represents a unique clinical challenge for two reasons:

- Diagnosing the arrhythmia is difficult—Although most WCTs are due to VT, the differential diagnosis includes a variety of SVTs. Diagnostic algorithms to differentiate these two etiologies are complex and imperfect
- Urgent therapy is often required—Patients may be unstable at the onset of the arrhythmia or deteriorate rapidly at any time, particularly if the WCT is VT

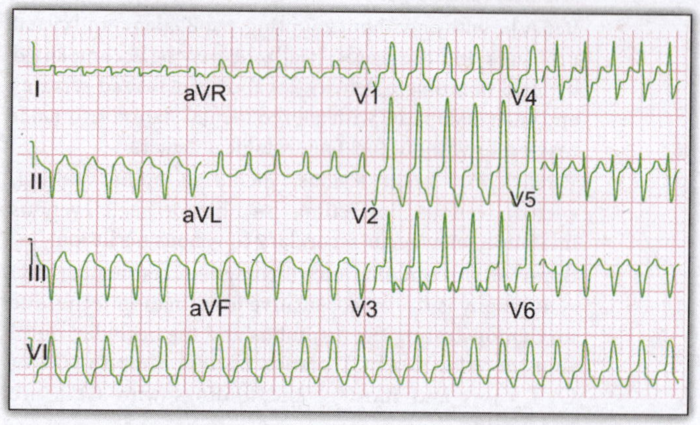

This is a ECG of wide QRS complex tachycardia. QRS complex duration ≥120 ms, rate ≥100 bpm

Acute Management of Sustained Ventricular Tachycardia

- VT that does not cause hemodynamic decompensation can be treated medically to achieve acute termination by the intravenous administration of amiodarone, lidocaine, or procainamide, followed by an infusion of the successful drug.
- Lidocaine is often ineffective; amiodarone, sotalol and procainamide appear to be superior.
- Initial management follows advanced cardiac life support (ACLS) guidelines.
- If hypotension, impaired consciousness, or pulmonary edema is present, QRS synchronous electrical cardioversion should be performed, ideally after sedation if the patient is conscious.
- For **stable tachycardia**, a trial of adenosine is reasonable, as this may clarify a supraventricular tachycardia with aberrancy.
- Patients with WCT who are **hemodynamically unstable and pulseless**, should be managed according to standard advance cardiac life support (ACLS) resuscitation algorithms, with immediate high-energy countershock and cardiopulmonary resuscitation (CPR). Patients should initially be treated with a synchronized (if possible) 120 to 200 Joule shock from a biphasic defibrillator or a 360 Joule shock from a monophasic defibrillator; if synchronization is not possible, then an unsynchronized countershock should be delivered, typically at higher energy doses.
- For patients with WCT who are **hemodynamically unstable, but still responsive** with a discernible blood pressure and pulse, we recommend urgent cardioversion (with procedural sedation when feasible).

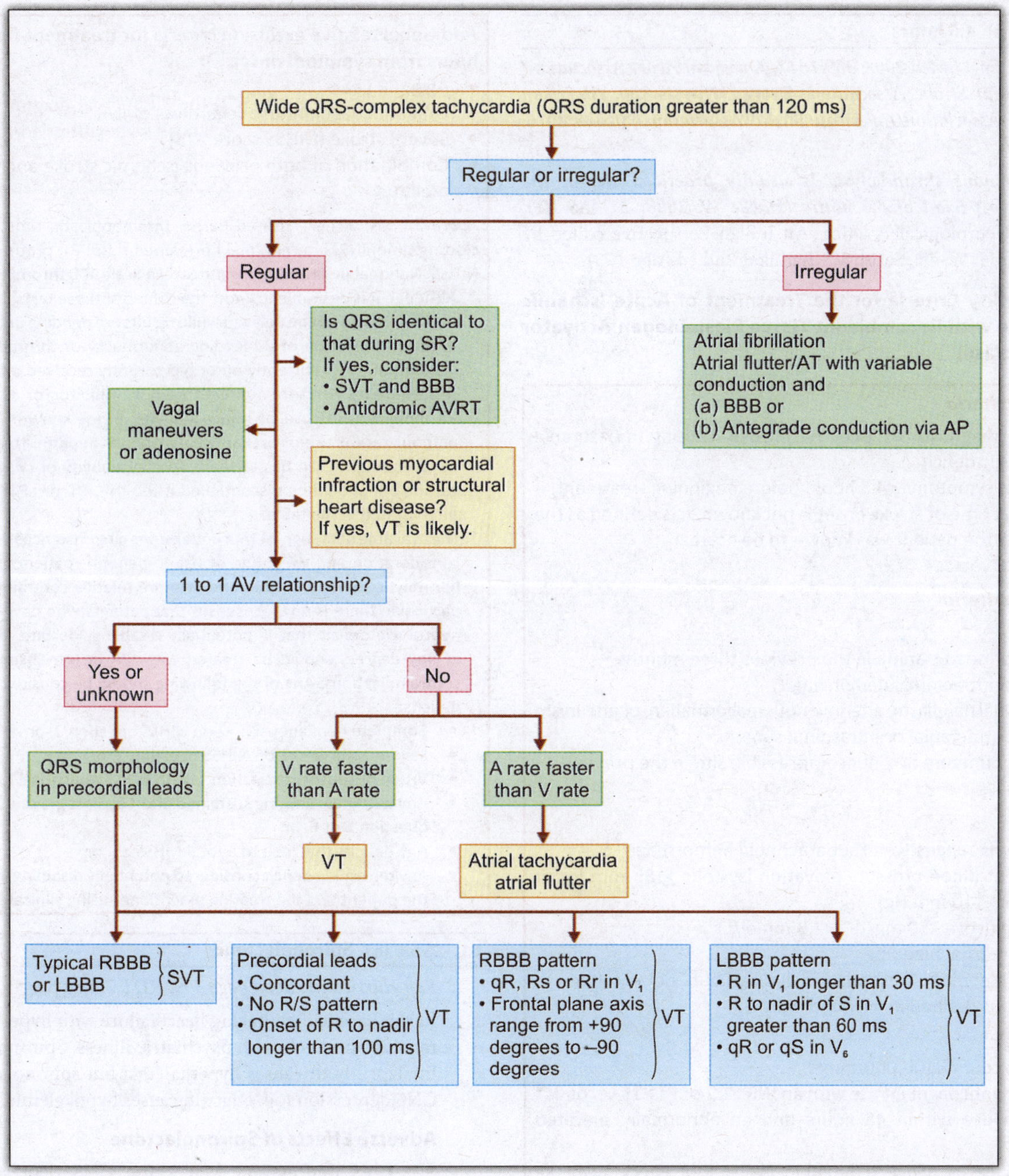

59. Ans. (b) Two fever spikes more than 38.3°C

Ref: Harrison 19th ed page no 135

Accordingly, FUO is now defined as:

- Fever >38.3°C (101°F) on at least two occasions
- Illness duration of ≥3 weeks
- No known immunocompromised state
- Diagnosis that remains uncertain after a thorough history-taking, physical examination and the following obligatory investigations:
  - Determination of erythrocyte sedimentation rate (ESR) and C-reactive protein (CRP) level
  - Platelet count
  - Leukocyte count and differential
  - Measurement of levels of hemoglobin, electrolytes, creatinine, total protein, alkaline phosphatase, alanine aminotransferase, aspartate aminotransferase, lactate dehydrogenase, creatine kinase, ferritin, antinuclear antibodies and rheumatoid factor
  - Protein electrophoresis
  - Urinalysis
  - Blood cultures and urine culture
  - Chest X-ray
  - Abdominal ultrasonography
  - Tuberculin skin test (TST)

60. Ans. (d) 4.5 hours

Ref: N Engl J Med 2008; 359:1317, American Heart Association/ American Stroke Association. Stroke 2013; 44:870, American Heart Association/American Stroke Association. Stroke 2016; 47:581

Intravenous thrombolysis is usually practiced within the window period of 4.5 hours (Hacke W, 2008; ECASS III). (Ref: Neurological Practice: An Indian Perspective edited by Noshir H. Wadia, Satish V Khadilkar 2nd ed Page 175)

Eligibility Criteria for the Treatment of Acute Ischemic Stroke with Recombinant Tissue Plasminogen Activator (Alteplase)

Inclusion criteria

- Clinical diagnosis of ischemic stroke causing measurable neurologic deficit
- Onset of symptoms <4.5 hours before beginning treatment; if the exact time of stroke onset is not known, it is defined as the last time the patient was known to be normal
- Age ≥ 18 years

Exclusion criteria

Historical

- Stroke or head trauma in the previous three months
- Previous intracranial hemorrhage
- Intracranial neoplasm, arterimienous malformation, or aneurysm
- Recent intracranial or intraspinal surgery
- Arterial puncture at 2 noncompressible site in the previous seven days

Clinical

- Symptoms suggestive of subarachnoid hemorrhage
- Persistent blood pressure elevation (systolic ≥185 mm Hg or diastolic ≥110 mm Hg)
- Serum glucose <50 mg/dL (<2.8 mmol/L)
- Active internal bleeding
- Acute bleeding diathesis, including but not limited to conditions defined in 'Hematologic'

Hematologic

- Platelet count <100,000/mm^3*
- Current anticoagulant use with an INR >1.7 or PT >15 seconds*
- Heparin use within 48 hours and an abnormally elevated aPTT*
- Current use of a direct thrombin inhibitor or direct factor Xa inhibitor with evidence of anticoagulant effect by laboratory, tests such as aPTT INR, ECT, TT. or appropriate factor Xa activity assays

Head CT scan

- Evidence of hemorrhage
- Extensive regions of obvious hypodensity consistent with irreversible injury

Relative exclusion criteria¶

- Only minor and isolated neurologic signs
- Rapidly improving stroke symptoms
- Major surgery or serious trauma in the previous 14 days
- Gastrointestinal or urinary, tract bleeding in the previous 21 days
- Myocardial infarction in the previous three months

Contd...

Additional relative exclusion criteria for treatment from 3 to 4.5 hours from symptom onset

- Age >80 years
- Oral anticoagulant use regardless of INR
- Severe stroke (NIHSS score >25)
- Combination of both previous ischemic stroke and diabetes mellitus

Abbreviations: aPTT, activated partial thromboplastin time; ECT, ecarin clotting time; INR, international normalized ratio; PT, prothrombin time; NIHSS, National Institutes of Health Stroke Scale; TT, thrombin time.

* Although it is desirable to know the results of these tests, thrombolytic therapy should not be delayed while results are pending unless (1) there is clinical suspicion of a bleeding abnormality or thrombocytopenia, (2) the patient is currently on or has recently received anticoagulants (e.g. heparin, warfarin, a direct thrombin inhibitor, or a direct factor Xa inhibitor), (3) use of anticoagulants is not known. For patients without recent use of oral anticoagulants or heparin, treatment with intravenous tPA can be started before availability of coagulation test results but should be discontinued if the INR, PT, or aPTT exceed the limits stated in the table.

¶ The available data suggest that under some circumstances—with careful consideration and weighting of risk-to-benefit—patients may receive fibrinolytic therapy despite one or more relative contraindications. In particular, there is now consensus that patients who have a persistent neurologic deficit that is potentially disabling, despite improvement of any degree, should be treated with tPA in the absence of other contraindications. Any of the following should be considered disabling deficits:

- Complete hemianopsia: ≥2 on NIHSS question 3, or
- Severe aphasia: ≥2 on NIHSS question 9, or
- Visual or sensory extinction: ≥1 on NIHSS question 11, or
- Any weakness limiting sustained effort against gravity: ≥2 on NIHSS question 5 or 6, or
- Any deficits that lead to a total NIHSS >5, or
- Any remaining deficit considered potentially disabling in the view of the patient and the treating practitioner using clinical judgement.

61. Ans. (a) Spironolactone

Ref: Harrison 19th ed page 309, KDT 7th ed page 523

In this case patient having heart failure with hyperkalemia and renal dysfunction with psychiatric illness. Spironolactone and Enalapril both causes hyperkalemia but spironolactone cause CNS depression too. Digoxin causes hypokalemia.

Adverse Effects of Spironolactone

- **CNS depression:** May cause CNS depression, which may impair physical or mental abilities; patients must be cautioned about performing tasks which require mental alertness (e.g. operating machinery or driving).
- **Fluid/electrolyte imbalance:** Fluid and electrolyte imbalance (e.g. hypomagnesemia, hyponatremia, hypochloremic alkalosis, hyperkalemia, acidosis, elevated BUN) may occur; close medical supervision and dose evaluation are required. Patients with heart failure, renal disease, or cirrhosis may be particularly susceptible. Watch for and correct electrolyte disturbances; adjust dose to avoid dehydration.
- **Gynecomastia:** Related to dose and duration of therapy; typically is reversible following discontinuation of therapy but may persist (rare).

- **Hyperkalemia:** Hyperkalemia may occur; risk of hyperkalemia is increased with renal impairment, excessive potassium intake and patients taking certain drugs (e.g. ACE inhibitors, angiotensin-II blockers, NSAIDs). Monitor closely for hyperkalemia; increases in serum potassium are dose related and rates of hyperkalemia also increase with declining renal function. The concurrent use of larger doses of ACE inhibitors (e.g. ≥ lisinopril 10 mg daily in adults) also increases the risk of hyperkalemia (ACCF/AHA [Yancy 2013]). Dose reduction or interruption of therapy may be necessary with development of hyperkalemia. Use is contraindicated in patients with hyperkalemia; use caution in conditions known to cause hyperkalemia.

Disease-related Concerns

- **Adrenal vein catheterization:** Discontinue use prior to adrenal vein catheterization.
- **Heart failure:** When evaluating a heart failure patient for spironolactone treatment, eGFR should be >30 mL/minute/1.73 m^2 or creatinine should be ≤2.5 mg/dL (men) or ≤2 mg/dL (women) with no recent worsening and potassium <5 mEq/L with no history of severe hyperkalemia (ACCF/AHA [Yancy 2013]). Serum potassium levels require close monitoring and management if elevated. The manufacturer recommends to discontinue or interrupt therapy if serum potassium >5 mEq/L or serum creatinine >4 mg/dL. The ACCF/AHA recommends considering discontinuation upon the development of serum potassium >5.5 mEq/L or worsening renal function with careful evaluation of the entire medical regimen. Avoid routine triple therapy with the combined use of an ACE inhibitor, ARB and spironolactone. Instruct patients with heart failure to discontinue use during an episode of diarrhea or dehydration or when loop diuretic therapy is interrupted (ACCF/AHA [Yancy 2013]).
- **Hepatic impairment:** Use with caution in patients with hepatic impairment; minor alterations of fluid and electrolyte balance may precipitate hepatic coma.
- **Renal impairment:** Risk of hyperkalemia is increased with declining renal function and with the concurrent use of larger doses of ACE inhibitors (e.g. ≥ lisinopril 10 mg daily in adults) (ACCF/AHA [Yancy 2013]). Use with caution in patients with mild renal impairment; contraindicated with anuria, acute renal insufficiency, or significant impairment of renal excretory function.

Hyperkalemia: May occur with ACE inhibitors; risk factors include renal dysfunction, diabetes mellitus, concomitant use of potassium-sparing diuretics, potassium supplements and/or potassium-containing salts. Use cautiously, if at all, with these agents and monitor potassium closely.

62. Ans. (d) Absent deep tendon reflex

Ref: Harrison 19th ed page no 2702

The diagnosis is suspected on the basis of weakness and fatigability in the typical distribution described below, without loss of reflexes or impairment of sensation or other neurologic function.

Diagnosis of Myasthenia Gravis
History
Diplopia, ptosis, weakness
Weakness in characteristic distribution
Fluctuation and fatigue: Worse with repeated activity, improved by rest
Effects of previous treatments
Physical examination
Ptosis, diplopia
Motor power survey: Quantitative testing of muscle strength
Forward arm abduction time (5 minutes)
Vital capacity
Absence of other neurologic signs
Laboratory testing
Anti-AChR radioimmunoassay: 85% positive in generalized MG; 50% in ocular MG; definite diagnosis if positive; negative result does not exclude MG. 40% of AChR antibody–negative patients with generalized MG have anti-MuSK antibodies.
Repetitive nerve stimulation: Decrement of >15% at 3 Hz: highly probable
Single-fiber electromyography: Blocking and jitter, with normal fiber density; confirmatory, but not specific
Edrophonium chloride (Tensilon) 2 mg + 8 mg IV; highly probable diagnosis if unequivocally positive
For ocular or cranial MG: Exclude intracranial lesions by CT or MRI

63. Ans. (a) SIADH

Ref: Harrison 19th ed page 299

In this case scenerio patient having hyponatremia with increased urinary sodium and normal serum osmolality with lung malignancy.

SIADH should be suspected in any patient with hyponatremia, hypoosmolality and a urine osmolality above 100 mosmol/kg. In SIADH, the urine sodium concentration is usually above 40 meq/L, the serum potassium concentration is normal, there is no acid-base disturbance and the serum uric acid concentration is frequently low.

Flow chart: Diagnostic approach to hyponatremia

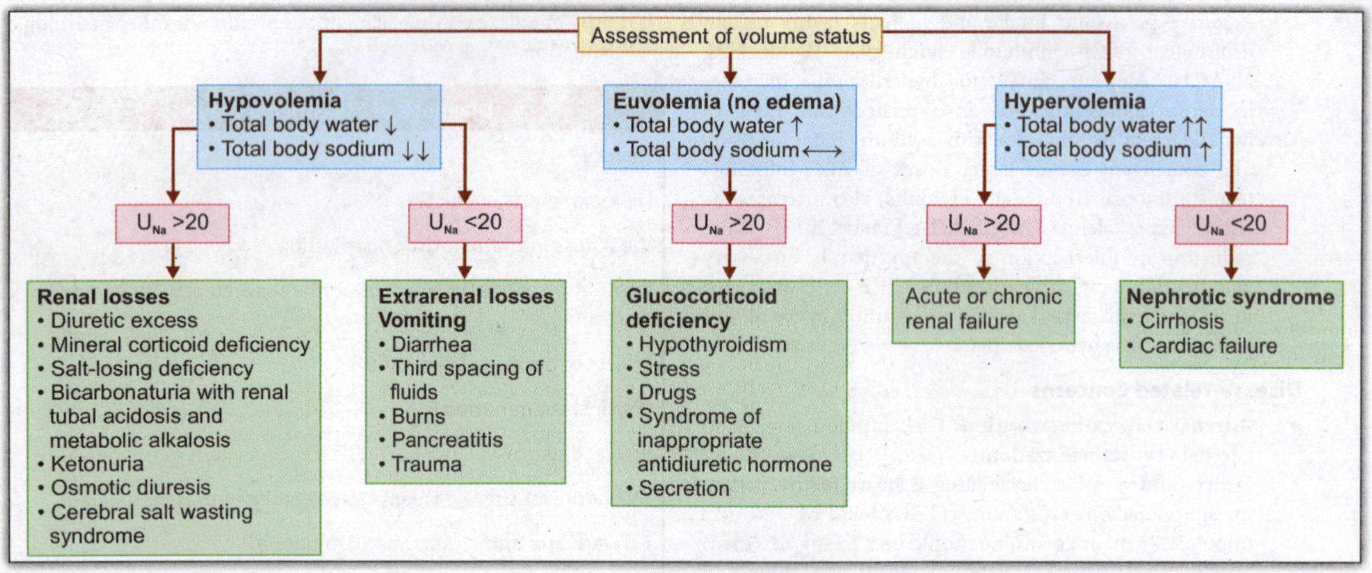

Source: S Kumar, T Berl: Diseases of water metabolism, in Atlas of Diseases of the Kidney, RW Schrier [ed]. Philadelphia, Current Medicine, Inc, 1999; with permission

64. Ans. (a) Spasticity

Ref: Bradley's neurology By Robert B. Daroff, Joseph Jankovic, John C Mazziotta, Scott L Pomeroy 7th Ed page 797

Spasticity is seen in 20% of hemiplegic patients. Spasticity per se does not produce weakness and other aspects of motor control. During rehabilitation the most visually striking signs of UMN syndrome tends to be treated and sometimes overtreated. These includes hyperreflexia, plantar flexion, dystonic postures, rigidity and contractures that may accompany weakness.

65. Ans. (c) SBP less than or equal to 100 mm Hg, DBP less than or equal to 60 mm Hg

Ref: Harrison 19th ed page 806-807

CURB-65 Pneumonia Severity Score
Confusion (based upon a specific mental test or new disorientation to person, place, or time)
Urea (blood urea nitrogen in the United States) >7 mmol/L (20 mg/dL)
Respiratory rate ≥30 breaths/minute
Blood pressure (systolic <90 mm Hg or diastolic <60 mm Hg)
Age ≥65 year, 1 point is assigned for each criterion that is met. Generally hospital favors admission for patients with a score of 1 or 2, although patients with a score of 1 due to being ≥65 years of age who do not have major comorbidities do not necessarily require admission. For patients with a score of 3 to 5, hospitalization is indicated and the patient should be assessed for possible intensive care unit admission, especially if the score is 4 or 5.

AIIMS NOVEMBER 2016

66. Ans. (b) Change imipramine and haloperidol...

Ref: Harrison 19th ed page 2710, 2722

The issue in this case is diabetes, hypertension, depression, bradycardia, orthostatic hypotension and constipation. Now have a look on her drug chart and side effects .

Beta blockers	Relative contraindication includes COPD, AV conduction disturbances, severe bradycardia, raynauds phenomenon side effects includes fatigue, reduces exercise intolerance, intermittent claudication, left ventricular failure sudden discontinuation may lead to ischemia
Imipramine	Anticholinergic dry mouth, constipation, urinary retention, blurred vision sweating, tremors, postural hypotension, cardiac conduction delay, sedation, weight gain
Haloperidol	No anticholinergic side effects, extrapyramidal side effects
Isaphgul	It is a soluble fibre-side effects Gastrointestinal: Abdominal cramps, constipation, diarrhea, esophageal obstruction, intestinal obstruction Hypersensitivity: Anaphylaxis (upon inhalation in susceptible individuals) Ophthalmic: Allergic conjunctivitis (rhinoconjunctivitis) Respiratory: Bronchospasm

As patient is having anticholinergic side effects of imipramine. So switching over to SSRI fluoxentine is good option. For constipation adding stool softener is good choice

67. Ans. (a) Absence seizure

Ref: Harrison 19th ed page 2552 table 445-8, KDT 7th ed page 421

Recall Bias

Different versions of the options of this questions has emerged. But one thing was sure that Absent seizure was mismatched. It is advised to remember the Original table from Harrison.

Note

Table from Harrison talks about only first line drug and alternatives, while table from KDT talks about first line, second line and then alternatives. Also the two tables are bit different and its hard to remember both. We suggest to read Harrison over KDT as its more updated and universal.

Selection of Antiepileptic Drugs

Generalized onset Tonic-Clonic	Focal	Typical absence	Atypical absence, myoclonic, atonic
First-Line			
Valproic acid Lamotrigine Topiramate	Lamotrigine, Carbamazepine Oxcarbazepine, Phenytoin Levetiracetam	Valproic acid Ethosuximide	Valproic acid Lamotrigine Topiramate
Alternatives			
Zonisamide, Phenytoin Carbamazepine, Oxcarbazepine Phenobarbital, Primidone Felbamate	Topiramate, Zonisamide Valproic acid, Tiagabine Gabapentin, Lacosamide Phenobarbital, Primidone Felbamate	Lamotrigine Clonazepam	Clonazepam Felbamate

68. Ans. (b) Epidemic typhus > (A) Measles

Ref: Harrison 19th edition page 1297,128,129

Centrifugal rash (starts from face of trunk centrally and moves to extremities peripherally) are Dengue fever, Variola (Small pox), Rubeola (measles), Rubella, Infectious mononucleosis, Endemic typhus

Centripetal rash (Starts from Extremities peripherally and moves to trunk and face centrally) is seen in varicella (chickenpox), Atypical measles, Rocky mountain spotted fever

Note

- The synchronous nature of the rash and its centrifugal distribution distinguish smallpox from chickenpox, which has a centripetal distribution
- Rocky Mountain spotted fever have centripetal rash compared to centrifugal rash of endemic typhus. The spotted fever group resembles typhus clinically; however, unlike the rash in other rickettsial diseases, the rash of the spotted fever group usually appears first on the extremities, moves centripetally and involves the palms and soles. (Jawetz)

Option (A)

Measles Enanthem: Approximately 48 hours prior to onset of the exanthem, patients may develop an enanthem characterized by Koplik's spots; these are 1 to 3 mm whitish, grayish, or bluish elevations with an erythematous base, typically seen on the buccal mucosa opposite the molar teeth, though they can spread to cover the buccal and labial mucosa

Measles Exanthem: The exanthem of measles arises approximately two to four days after onset of fever; it consists of an erythematous, maculopapular, blanching rash, which classically begins on the face and spreads ***cephalocaudally and centrifugally*** to involve the neck, upper trunk, lower trunk and extremities. The palms and soles are rarely involved. The cranial to caudal progression of the rash is characteristic of measles but is not pathognomonic

CMDT states: Typical Measles presents with maculopapular, brick-red; begins on head and neck; spreads downward and outward (centrifugal), in 5–6 days rash brownish, desquamating. While atypical measles presents with Centripetal rash.

Nelson 19th ed ch 243 states; Children who had received the original formalin-inactivated measles vaccine at times developed a more severe form of disease called atypical measles. Patients had onset of high fever and headache followed by the appearance of a maculopapular rash on the extremities that become petechial and purpuric and progressed in a centripetal direction.

Option (B)

Epidemic typhus is a potentially lethal, louse-borne, exanthematous disease caused by Rickettsia prowazekii. The rash of epidemic typhus classically begins several days after the onset of symptoms, appearing as a red macular or maculopapular eruption on the trunk that later spreads centrifugally to the extremities sparing the palms and soles,. (CMDT and Uptodate)

Option (C)

Typhoid: Typhoid fever usually presents with abdominal pain, fever and chills approximately 5 to 21 days after ingestion of the causative microorganism. Classic manifestations include relative bradycardia, pulse temperature dissociation and "rose spots" (faint salmon-colored macules on the trunk and abdomen).

Option (D)

Rash is the most characteristic finding of secondary syphilis. The rash is classically a diffuse, symmetric macular or papular eruption involving the entire trunk and extremities, including the palms and soles. Although involvement of the palms and soles is an important clue to the diagnosis of secondary syphilis, localized lesions can also occur. Cutaneous lesion of secondary syphilis are symmetrically distributed polymorphic, non pruritic and are abundant on the central part of the body, as compared to the extremities (called "centripetal distribution").

69. Ans. (c) 1500

Ref: Harrison 19th ed page 442

The hypereosinophilic syndromes (HES) are a group of disorders marked by the sustained overproduction of eosinophils, in which eosinophilic infiltration and mediator release cause damage to multiple organs. Although these disorders had long been considered idiopathic (e.g. as in the "idiopathic hypereosinophilic syndrome," IHES), etiologies for some forms of HES have been described.

Hypereosinophilia: Hypereosinophilia (HE) in the peripheral blood is defined as an absolute eosinophil count (AEC) $>1.5 \times 10^9$/L (or >1500 cells/microL) on two examinations separated in time by at least one month **and/or** pathologic confirmation of tissue HE.

For these purposes, **tissue** HE is defined by:

- On bone marrow section, a percentage of eosinophils that exceeds 20 percent of all nucleated cells **and/or**
- Tissue infiltration that is extensive in the opinion of a pathologist (hematoxylin-eosin, May-Grunwald-Giemsa and Wright-Giemsa are the recommended stains for visualizing eosinophils in tissue section) **and/or**
- Marked deposition of eosinophil granule proteins in tissue (in the absence or presence of major tissue infiltration by eosinophils). This is demonstrated by immunofluorescence and usually performed in expert centers. There is also a novel monoclonal antibody that recognizes eosinophil peroxidase, which can detect both tissue eosinophils and eosinophil degranulation.

Hypereosinophilic syndrome: A hypereosinophilic syndrome (HES) is defined by the association of HE (as defined above), with eosinophil-mediated organ damage and/or dysfunction, provided other potential causes for the damage have been excluded.

- The term "HES" can therefore be used to qualify any condition characterized by eosinophilic infiltrates and associated complications, **including situations where the cause of HE is identified** (e.g. restrictive cardiac disease occurring in the setting of parasitic infections [Löffler's endocarditis]).
- In contrast, the term "HES" should **not** be used when the clinical manifestations and underlying organ damage found in a hypereosinophilic patient can be explained by a mechanism **other than** HE. As an example, a patient with cardiovascular risk factors presenting with persistent HE and thoracic pain that is shown to be secondary to coronary artery occlusion, should not be diagnosed as HES, unless another clinical manifestation can be attributed to eosinophilic tissue infiltration. Eosinophilia is the presence of >500 eosinophils per Lit of blood and is common in many settings besides parasite infection.

70. Ans. (a) Metabolic acidosis

Ref: Harrison 19th ed page 316, Practical Guidelines of fluid therapy by Sanjay Pandey 2nd ed page 196, 200; Anaesthesia Review Course 3rd Ed Pg 329

pH is low so patient is having acidosis. Low HCO_3^- is suggestive of metabolic acidosis. pCO_2 is also suggestive of compensation.

Expected compensation (fall in pCO_2) will be

$pCO_2 = (HCO_3 \times 1.5) + 8 = 13.5 + 8 = 21.5$

So expected pCO_2 matches actual CO_2 suggestive of simple acid base disorder.

Interpretation of ABG	
Step 1	Look at the pH Is the patient acidemic (H <7.35) or Alkalemic (pH > 7.45)
Step 2	Is it a primary metabolic or respiratory disturbance?

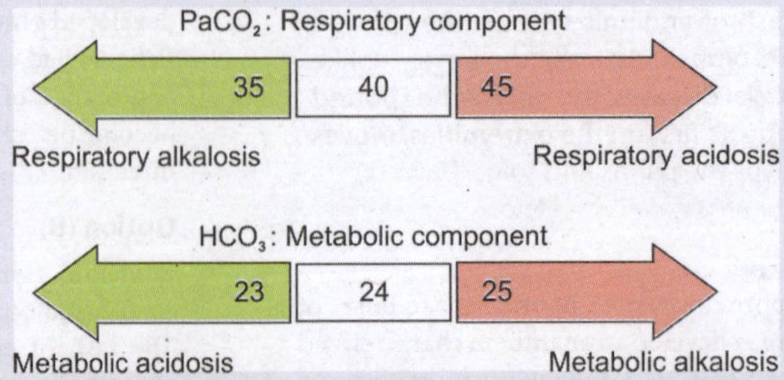

Contd...

Interpretation of ABG

Acidemia:
With HCO_3 <22 mmol/L= Metabolic
With pCO_2 > 45 mm Hg = Respiratory
Alkalemia:
With HCO_3 >26 mmol/L = Metabolic
With PCO_2 <35 mm Hg = Respiratory
Note: For ease of calculation normal pH = 7.4, pCO_2 is 40 and HCO_3 is 24
Go to step 3 and 4 if respiratory and step 5 to 7 if metabolic.

Step 3

If there is a primary respiratory disturbance, is it acute?
Expected Δ pH = $0.08 \times \Delta pCO_2/10$
(For respiratory acidosis (pCO_2–40) = ΔPCO_2)
(For respiratory alkalemic (40–PCO_2) = ΔPCO_2)
If not acute go to step 4, if yes –also consider steps 5–7.

Step 4

For a respiratory disorder is renal (Metabolic) compensation appropriate?
Respiratory acidosis:
<24 hrs: $\Delta (HCO_3) = 1/10 \times \Delta PCO_2$
> 24 hrs: $\Delta (HCO_3) = 4/10 \times \Delta PCO_2$
Respiratory alkalosis:
1–2 hrs: $\Delta (HCO_3) = 2/10 \times \Delta pCO_2$
>2 days: $\Delta (HCO_3) = 5/10 \times \Delta pCO_2$
Where Δ = Change in

Step 5

If the disturbance is metabolic is the respiratory compensation appropriate?
For metabolic acidosis: Expected $pCO_2 = [1.5 \times (HCO_3)] + 8$
For metabolic alkalosis: Expected $pCO_2 = [0.7 \times (HCO_3)] + 21$
If Actual pCO_2 > Expected pCO_2 = Hidden respiratory acidosis
If Actual PCO_2 < Expected pCO_2 =Hidden respiratory alkalosis

Step 6

If there is metabolic acidosis, is there an anion gap?
Anion gap (AG) is imperial in etiological diagnosis of metabolic acidosis.
Na – (Cl + HCO_3) = Anion gap (Usually <12).
If gap is more than 12, patient has an High anion gap acidosis

MNEMONIC **Proposed by the Lancet as per the latest trend is: GOLDMARK**

G — Glycols (ethylene glycol & propylene glycol)
O — Oxoproline, a metabolite of paracetamol
L — L-lactate, the chemical responsible for lactic acidosis
D — D-lactate
M — Methanol
A — Aspirin
R — Renal failure (Uremia)
K — Ketoacidosis (Ketones generated from starvation, Alcohol and Diabetic ketoacidosis)
Most important cause of normal anion gap acidosis is diarrhea.

Step 7

Does the anion gap explain the change in bicarbonate?
High anion gap acidosis is characterised by 2 factors:
Low HCO_3 2. Increased anion gap
Rise in anion gap = Fall in HCO_3.
i.e, Anion gap excess= HCO_3 deficit
(AG-12) = (24- HCO_3)
Thus, (AG-12)/(24- HCO_3)= 1.
This ratio is also known as the Gap-Gap ratio.
In high AG metabolic acidosis, Gap-Gap ratio should be 1.
Mixed disorders:

a. **Mixed metabolic acidosis**: i.e, there are 2 primary causes of metabolic acidosis. If the 2nd cause of acidosis is a normal AG (e.g, hyperchloremic acidosis), the picture will be as follows:
AG excess < HCO_3 deficit

Contd...

Interpretation of ABG
Thus gap-gap ratio <1 shows mixed metabolic acidosis- where 1 cause has a high AG, while the 2nd cause has normal AG. b. **Mixed metabolic alkalosis with metabolic acidosis** New HCO_3 is being added in the presence of high AG. Hence, HCO_3 deficit (24- HCO_3) is now decreased. Thus, AG excess> HCO_3 deficit. Thus, high AG metabolic acidosis with Gap-gap ratio >1 means superimposed metabolic alkalosis.

Prediction of Compensatory Responses on Simple Acid-base Disturbances

Disorder	Expected compensation	Range of values		
		pH	HCO_3	PCO_2
Metabolic acidosis	$PCO_2 = (1.5 \times HCO_3^-) + 8$	Low	Low (P)	Low (S)
Metabolic alkalosis	Rise in $PCO_2 = 0.75 \times$ Rise in $[HCO_3^-]$	High	High (P)	High (S)
Respiratory alkalosis		High	Low (S)	Low (P)
Acute	Fall in $[HCO_3^-] = 0.2 \times$ Fall in PCO_2			
Chronic	Fall in $[HCO_3^-] = 0.4$ Fall in PCO_2			
Respiratory acidosis		Low	High (S)	High (P)
Acute	Rise in $[HCO_3^-] = 0.1 \times$ Rise in PCO_2			
Chronic	Rise in $[HCO_3^-] = 0.4 \times$ Rise in PCO_2			

P = Primary change, S = secondary change
If actual change = Expected change, the disorder is simple
If actual change > Expected change, the disorder is mixed
Same direction rule: Compensatory changes are in same direction as primary change. i.e. Decreased HCO_3 leads to decreased PCO_2 and increased HCO_3 leads to increased PCO_2. If changes are in opposite direction think of mixed disorder.

Mixed acid base disorders

Disorder	Findings	Common causes
Metabolic acidosis + Respiratory acidosis	Low pH, $\downarrow HCO_3$, $\uparrow pCO_2$	Cardiac arrest (Hypoventillation + Lactic acidosis) Shock with Respiratory failure DKA with respiratory disease
Metabolic acidosis + Respiratory alkalosis	Normal pH, $\downarrow HCO_3$, $\downarrow pCO_2$	Salicylate intoxication Gram negative sepsis Liver failure
Metabolic alkalosis + Respiratory acidosis	Normal pH, $\uparrow HCO_3$, $\uparrow pCO_2$	COPD with diuretics Metabolic alkalosis with severe hypokalemia and respiratory weakness leads to hypoventilation
Metabolic alkalosis + Respiratory alkalosis	$\uparrow$pH, $\uparrow HCO_3$, $\downarrow pCO_2$	Liver failure with vomiting Patient on ventilator with continuous nasogastric aspiration
Metabolic acidosis + Metabolic alkalosis	Near normal pH and HCO_3	Diabetic ketoacidosis with vomiting Vomiting with severe volume depletion causing lactic acidosis
Respiratory acidosis + Respiratory alkalosis		Do not co exist

71. Ans. (d) 500 Eq/L

Ref: Harrison 19 ed page 315

See table of Interpretation of ABG in previous questions. (see page no. 752)

As pH is low this patient is having acidemia. Low HCO_3 is suggestive of metabolic acidosis. Low PCO_2 is suggestive of compensation.

Expected compensation (fall in PCO_2) will be = $HCO_3 \times 1.5 + 8 = 6 \times 1.5 + 8 = 17$

So expected PCO_2 will be 40 – 17 = 23. However actual PCO_2 is 30, that is higher than expected, suggestive of respiratory acidosis.

Hence this patient is having patient **metabolic acidosis and respiratory acidosis.**

When blood pH drops below 7.15 such a severe acidemia can be life threatening. When HCO_3 level falls below 10 mEq/L. It needs urgent treatment.

Amount of HCO_3 required (Base deficit) = 0.4 × Wt in kg × (Desired HCO_3 - Actual HCO_3)

In this case total amount of bicarbonate needed will be 0.4 × 75 × (24–6) = 540 meq. 500 is the close answer.

72. Ans. (a) Right posterior inferior cerebellar artery occlusion

Ref: Harrison 19th ed page 2576

- Lateral medullary syndrome (occlusion of any of five vessels may be responsible—vertebral, posterior inferior cerebellar, superior, middle, or inferior lateral medullary arteries)

On side of Lesion

- Pain, numbness, impaired sensation over one-half the face: *Descending tract and nucleus fifth nerve*
- Ataxia of limbs, falling to side of lesion: *Uncertain—restiform body, cerebellar hemisphere, cerebellar fibers, spinocerebellar tract*
- Nystagmus, diplopia, oscillopsia, vertigo, nausea, vomiting: *Vestibular nucleus*
- Horner's syndrome (miosis, ptosis, decreased sweating): *Descending sympathetic tract*
- Dysphagia, hoarseness, paralysis of palate, paralysis of vocal cord, diminished gag reflex: *Issuing fibers ninth and tenth nerves*
- Loss of taste: *Nucleus and tractus solitarius*
- Numbness of ipsilateral arm, trunk, or leg: *Cuneate and gracile nuclei*
- Weakness of lower face: *Genuflected upper motor neuron fibers to ipsilateral facial nucleus*

On opposite Side Lesion

- Impaired pain and thermal sense over half the body, sometimes face: *Spinothalamic tract.*

73. Ans. (d) Polycythemia

Ref: Harrison 19th ed page 306-e

Diffusing capacity (DLCO) This test uses a small (and safe) amount of carbon monoxide (CO) to measure gas exchange across the alveolar membrane during a 10-sec breath hold. CO in exhaled breath is analyzed to determine the quantity of CO crossing the alveolar membrane and combining with hemoglobin in red blood cells. This "single-breath diffusing capacity" (DLCO) value increases with the surface area available for diffusion and the amount of hemoglobin within the capillaries and it varies inversely with alveolar membrane thickness. Thus, DLCO decreases in diseases that thicken or destroy alveolar membranes (e.g., pulmonary fibrosis, emphysema), curtail the pulmonary vasculature (e.g. pulmonary hypertension), or reduce alveolar capillary hemoglobin (e.g. anemia). Single-breath diffusing capacity may be elevated in acute congestive heart failure, asthma, polycythemia and pulmonary hemorrhage.

Polycythemia is a cause of increased diffusion state of body.

Obstructive versus Restrictive Lung Disease

	Restriction due to increased lung elastic recoil (Pulmonary fibrosis)	Restriction due to chest wall abnormalities (Moderate obesity)	Restriction due to respiratory muscle weakness (Myasthenia gravis)	Obstruction due to airway narrowing (Acute asthma)	Obstruction due to decreased elastic recoil (Severe emphysema)
TLC	60%	95%	75%	100%	130%
FRC	60%	65%	100%	104%	220%
RV	60%	100%	120%	120%	310%
FVC	60%	92%	60%	90%	60%
FEV1	75%	92%	60%	35% pre b.d 75% post b.d	35% pre b.d 38% post b.d
Raw	1.0	1.0	1.0	2.5	1.5
DLCO	60%	95%	80%	120%	40%
	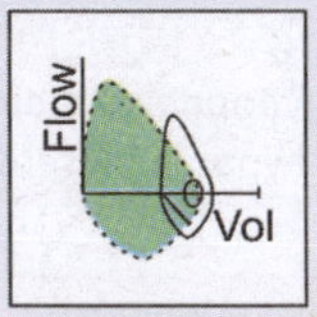	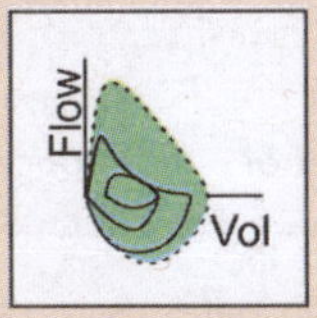	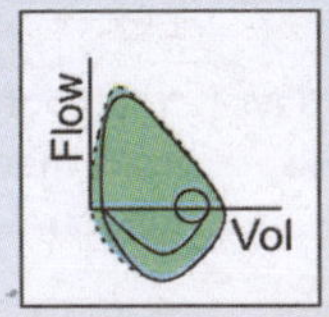	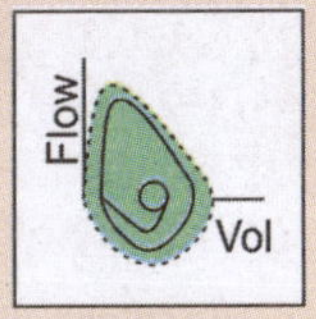	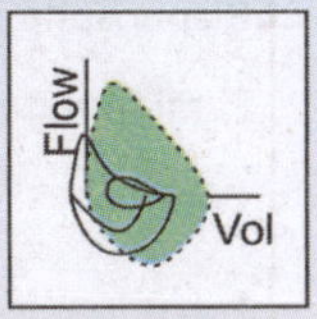

Key: Pulmonary function values are expressed as percent of normal predicted values, except for raw, which is expressed as cm H_2O/L/s (normal <2 cm H_2O/L/s). The figures at the bottom of each column show typical configuration of flow-volume loops in each condition, including the flow-volume relationship during tidal breathing. b.d., bronchodilator; DLCO, diffusion capacity of lung for carbon monoxide; FEV1, forced expiratory volume in one second; FRC, functional residual capacity; FVC, forced vital capacity; Raw, airways resistance; RV, residual volume; TLC, total lung capacity.

Algorithm for Pulmonary Function Test Interpretation

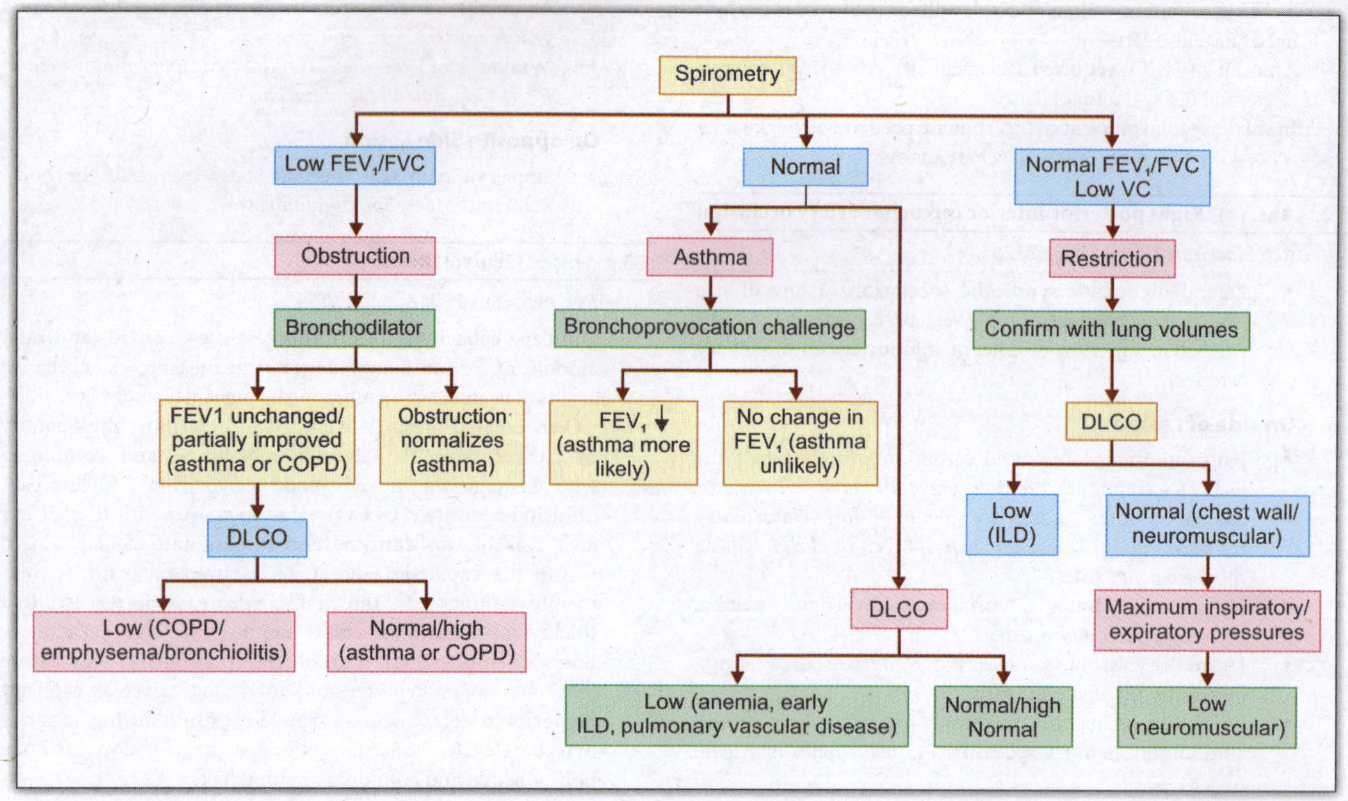

COPD: Chronic obstructive pulmonary disease; DLCO: Diffusing capacity for carbon monoxide; FEV_1: Forced expiratory volume in one second; FVC: Forced vital capacity; VC: Vital capacity; ILD: Interstitial lung disease

74. Ans. (d) IV Fluids with furosemide

Ref: Harrison's 19th page 2490

The patient is having hypercalcemia due to paraneoplastic syndrome of lung cancer.

Therapies for Severe Hypercalcemia

Treatment	Onset of action	Duration of action	Advantages	Disadvantages
Most useful therapies				
Hydration with saline	Hours	During infusion	Rehydration invariably needed	Volume overload
Forced diuresis; saline plus loop diuretic	Hours	During treatment	Rapid action	Volume overload, cardiac decompensation, intensive monitoring, electrolyte disturbance, inconvenience
Bisphosphonates				
Pamidronate	1–2 days	10–14 days to weeks	High potency; intermediate onset of action	Fever in 20%, hypophosphatemia, hypocalcemia, hypomagnesemia, rarely jaw necrosis
Zolendronate	1–2 days	>3 weeks	Same as for pamidronate (may last longer)	Same as pamidronate above
Calcitonin	Hours	1–2 days	Rapid onset of action; useful as adjunct in severe hypercalcemia	Rapid tachyphylaxis

Contd...

Special use therapies				
Phosphate Oral	24 hours	During use	Chronic management (with hypophosphatemia); low toxicity if P <4 mg/dL	Limited use except as adjuvant or chronic therapy
Glucocorticoids	Days	Days, weeks	Oral therapy, antitumor agent	Active only in certain malignancies, vitamin D excess and sarcoidosis; glucocorticoid side effects
Dialysis	Hours	During use and 24–48 hours afterward	Useful in renal failure; onset of effect in hours; can immediately reverse life-threatening hypercalcemia	Complex procedure, reserved for extreme or special circumstances

75. Ans. (c) Smoking

Ref: Harrison 19th ed page 2413

Clinically significant lactic acid accumulation almost always occurs in the presence of comorbid conditions, such as:

- Renal insufficiency (serum creatinine concentration above 1.4 mg/dL [124 μmol/L] in women and 1.5 mg/dL [132 μmol/L] in men), or low creatinine clearance.
- Concurrent liver disease or alcohol abuse
- Heart failure
- History of lactic acidosis
- Decreased tissue perfusion or hemodynamic instability
- Hypoxic states or serious acute illness
- Do not initiate metformin treatment in patients 80 years of age and older unless measurement of creatinine clearance (CrCl) demonstrates that renal function is not reduced because these patients are more susceptible to developing lactic acidosis

76. Ans. (c) Resting tremor

Ref: Harrison 19th ed page 2538, Guyton 13th page 730

Intention Tremor is a feature of cerebellar lesion, not the resting tremor.

Resting tremor is seen in Parkinson's disease

Clinical Abnormalities of the Cerebellum

Sign/Symptom	Definition	Lesion
Dysmetria	Inability to judge distance or scale	Vestibulocerebellum & spinocerebellum, spinocerebellar tracts
Ataxia	Unsteady and clumsy motion of the limbs or torso	Vestibulocerebellum & spinocerebellum, spinocerebellar tracts
Asynergia	Failure of components of complex multiple joint movements in coordinated fashion	Cerebrocerebellum
Past Pointing	Pointing beyond the finger in the finger-nose test	# Cerebrocerebellum
Intention tremor	Inability to coordinate fine motor activities, tremor is slow (at 2-4 cycles per second) and is present only during movement	Cerebrocerebellum Ipsilateral to symptomatic limb
Dysarthria	Motor speech disorder due to lack of coordination of muscles of speech	# Cerebrocerebellum
Dysdiadochokinesis	Inability to perform rapid alternating movements e.g. inability to rapidly flip the hands	Spino cerebellum
Nystagmus	Involuntary left-right eye movements	Vestibulocerebellum (flocculonodular lobes)

Usually must involve one or more of the deep cerebellar nuclei-the dentate, interposed, or fastigial nuclei

77. Ans. (b) Foregut carcinoid

Ref: Harrison 19th ed page 1928, 2340

Clinical diagnosis means two of the three endocrine organs (parathyroid, pancreas/duodenum or pituitary) or has a family history of MEN 1 and one of the endocrine organ tumors.

Men Syndrome			
Feature	**MEN 1**	**MEN 2A**	**MEN 2B**
Eponym	Wermer syndrome	Sipple syndrome	Williams Pollock syndrome, Gorlin Vickers syndrome, Wagenmann Froboese syndrome
Gene	MEN 1 gene encodes for **Menin**, found on the long arm of chromosome **11q13**, mutation in 70-90%	RET, Receptor tyrosine kinase 10q11.2	RET, Receptor tyrosine kinase 10q11.2
Entero-Pancreatic tumors	Total 40–80% Gastrinoma (25%) Insulinoma (20%) VIPoma Glucagonoma PPoma	—	—
Pituitary adenoma	30–60%	—	—
Parathyroid hyperplasia	80–90%	10–25%	—
Medullary thyroid carcinoma	—	90%	>90%
Pheochromocytoma	—	>50%	> 50%
Associated abnormalities Mucosal neuromas Marfanoid habitus Medullated corneal nerve fibers Megacolon	—	—	40–50%
Gene(s)	**MEN 1**	**RET**	**RET**
Approx. prevalence	1 in 35,000 (1 in 20,000 to 1 in 40,000)	1 in 40,000	1 in 40,000

Footnote:
- Primary hyperparathyroidism is the most common manifestation of MEN1
- Hyperparathyroidism is the earliest manifestation of the syndrome in most MEN1 patients.
- Enteropancreatic tumors are the second most common manifestation of MEN1
- Gastrinomas are the most common enteropancreatic tumors observed in MEN1 patients
- Insulinomas are the second most common enteropancreatic tumors in patients who suffer from MEN1. Unlike gastrinomas, most insulinomas originate in the pancreas bed, becoming the most common pancreatic tumor in MEN1

78. Ans. (d) Complete heart block

Ref: Harrison 19th ed 278e-10, Leo Schamroth page 375

Recall Bias

Most of the students recalled it as 2:1 Block. However we have strong first hand information that it was a complete heart block. Still we advise you to read about all options carefully for future ECG

NOTE

In the examination, single ECG lead was given just like the picture in this question

Patients with third degree (complete) AV block will have evidence of atrial (P waves) and ventricular (QRS complexes) activity that are independent of each other on the surface ECG. The p wave bear no relationship to the QRS complexes.

AV block is characterized by a delay or interruption in conduction of the atrial impulse through the specialized AV conducting system. There are three degree

First-degree AV block: Delayed conduction from the atrium to the ventricle (defined as a prolonged PR interval of >200 milliseconds) without interruption in atrial to ventricular conduction. In first degree heart block all P waves are followed by QRS complexes.

Second -degree AV block: In second degree AV block, some atrial impulses fail to reach the ventricles. Wenckebach described progressive delay between atrial and ventricular contraction and the eventual failure of a P wave to reach the ventricles. Mobitz subsequently divided second degree AV block into two subtypes, as determined by the findings on the electrocardiogram (ECG).

1. **Mobitz type I second degree AV block**, in which progressive PR interval prolongation precedes a non-conducted P wave. The first P wave after block conducts to the ventricle with a shorter PR interval compared with the last P wave before block.

Electrocardiogram (ECG) showing mobitz type I (Wenckebach) Atrioventricular (AV) block

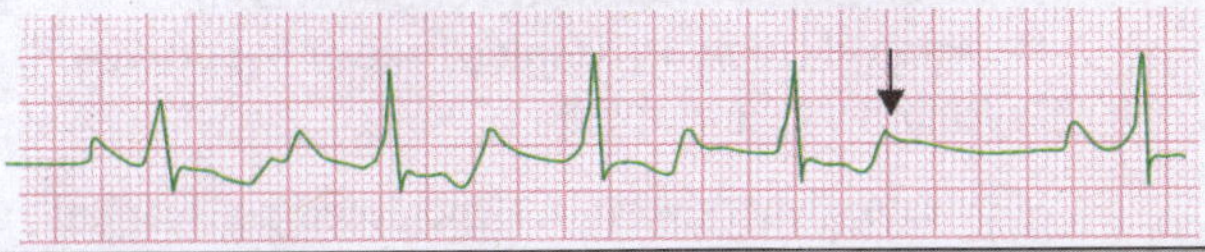

Single lead electrocardiagram (ECG) showing Mobitz type I (Wenckebach) second degree AV block with 5:4 conduction. The characteristics of this arrhythmia include: a progressively increasing PR interval until a P wave is not conducted (arrow); a progressive decrease in the increment in the PR interval; a progressive decrease in the RR interval; and the RR interval that includes the dropped beat (0.96 sec) is less than twice the RR interval between conducted beats (0.53 to 0.57 sec).

2. **Mobitz type II second degree AV block**, in which the PR interval remains unchanged prior to a P wave that fails to conduct to the ventricle.

Mobitz type II second degree atrioventricular (AV) block

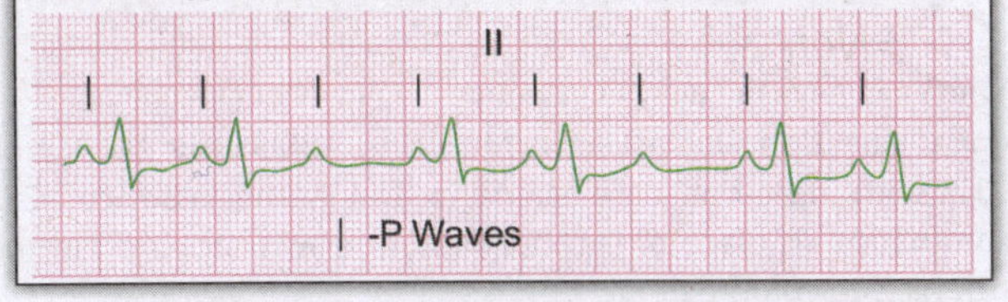

The third and sixth P waves are not conducted through the AV node (there is no associated QRS complex). The PR interval is constant prior to and after the non-conducted beats.

High-grade AV block, in which two or more consecutive P waves are non-conducted. In contrast to third degree or complete heart block, however, some P waves continue to be conducted to the ventricle

Single-lead electrocardiogram (ECG) showing sinus rhythm with third degree (complete) AV block

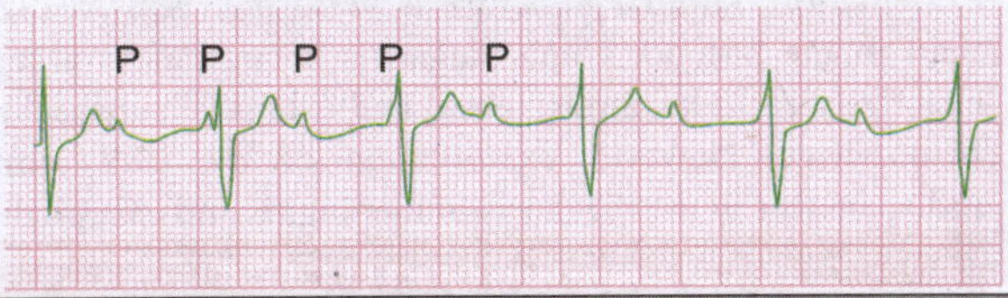

Sinus rhythm with third degree (complete) heat block. There is indapendent atrial (as shown by the P waves) and ventricular activity, with respective rate of 83 and 43 beats per minute. The wide QRS complexes may represent a junctional escape rhythm with underlying bundle branch block or an idioventricular pacemaker.

Type of Arrhythmia	P Waves	QRS Complexes	Other Findings	Ventricular Response to Carotid Sinus Massage	Treatment
First-degree AV block	60-100 Regular Contour Normal (Upright and uniform)	60-100 Regular Normal contour (0.06–0.10 sec)	PR Interval: Prolonged (> 0.20 sec)	Gradual slowing caused by sinus	None
Type I second-degree AV block **(Mobitz I heart block Wenckebach)**	60–100 Regular (Intermittent blocked P waves) Blocked P follows dropped QRS, more P waves than QRS Normal contour	30-100 Irregular Normal contour	PR Interval: Progressively longer until one P wave is blocked and a QRS is dropped	Slowing caused by sinus slowing and an increase in AV block	None, unless symptomatic; atropine
Type II second-degree AV block **(Mobitz II heart block)**	60–100 Regular, more P waves than QRS Normal contour	30–100 Conduction ratio (P waves to QRS complexes) is commonly 2:1, 3:1, 4:1, or variable Irregular Abnormal, >0.12 sec	PR interval normal or prolonged but constant prior to & after blocked P wave	Gradual slowing caused by sinus slowing	Pacemaker
Complete AV block	60–100 Regular (but atria and ventrical acts independently), Normal contour, may be superimposed in QRS or T wave	40–60 if escape focus is junctional, <40 if escape focus is ventricular. Fairly regular, Contour Abnormal, 0.06 to 0.1 sec if junctional, > 0.12 sec if ventricular	PR Interval: Varies greatly	None	Pacemaker

79. Ans. (b) Lumbar puncture

Ref: Harrison's 19th Ed table 328-1, page 1775, Advanced Medical Life Support: An Assessment-based Approach page 61

NOTE

Similar question was asked in Medicine AIIMS Nov 2013, Nov 2012 with different case scenario but same essence. CSF examination in place of Lumbar Puncture was provided in the options (see volume II)

This patient is having diabetes, hypertension, atrial fibrillation with altered sensorium The two strong possibilities are drug induced hypoglycemia and atrial fibrillation leading to a stroke. So random blood sugar, ECG and a NCCT head is warranted in emergency. Lumbar puncture is not an emergency investigation in this case.

Harrison 19th ed page 1775: The studies that are most useful in the diagnosis of coma are chemical toxicologic analysis of blood and urine, cranial CT or MRI, EE.g. and CSF examination. Lumbar puncture is performed less frequently than in the past for coma diagnosis because neuroimaging effectively excludes intracerebral and extensive subarachnoid hemorrhage. However, examination of the CSF remains indispensable in the diagnosis of meningitis and encephalitis.

Causes of Decreased Level of Consciousness

MNEMONIC AEIOU-TIPS

A	Alcohol (Intoxication or withdrawal), Anaphylaxis, Acute Myocardial infarction
E	**Encephalopathy** (Hepatic, Uremic, Hypertensive, Hypoxic) **Endocrinopathy** (Hypothyroidism, Hyperthyroidism), **Electrolyte imbalance** (Hyponatremia, Hypernatremia, Hypercalcemia)
I	Insulin
O	Opiates, Oxygen (Hypoxia)
U	Uremia
T	**Trauma** **Temperature:** (Hypothermia, Hyperthermia) **Toxins:** (Anticholinergic, Hallucinogens, Cocaine)
I	Infection (Sepsis, Meningitis, CNS infection), Intracranial (Tumour/Haemorrhage or hypertension)
P	Psychiatric, Post ictal state
S	Substrate: Hyperglycemia, Hypoglycemia, Thiamine Seizure, Stroke, Shock

Contd...

Vital signs as a clue to diagnosis of altered mentation

Fever/Hyperthermia	Infection, heatstroke, neuroleptic malignant syndrome, thyroid storm
Hypothermia	Exposure, sepsis, myxedema, coma
Tachycardia	Sepsis, hypovolemia, sympathomimetic, toxidrome, anticholinergic toxidrome
Bradycardia	Inreased intracranial pressure, beta-blocker overdose, calcium-channel blocker over dose, hypoxia
Hypertension	Sympathomimetic toxidrome, intracranial hemorrhage
Hypotension	Sepsis, hypovolemia, opiate toxidrome, sedative hypnotic toxidrome
Tachypnea	Acidosis (diabetic ketoacidosis, lactic acidosis), aspirin overdose, hypoxia
Hypoxia	Pneumoniam, pulmonary embolus, congestive heatrt failure

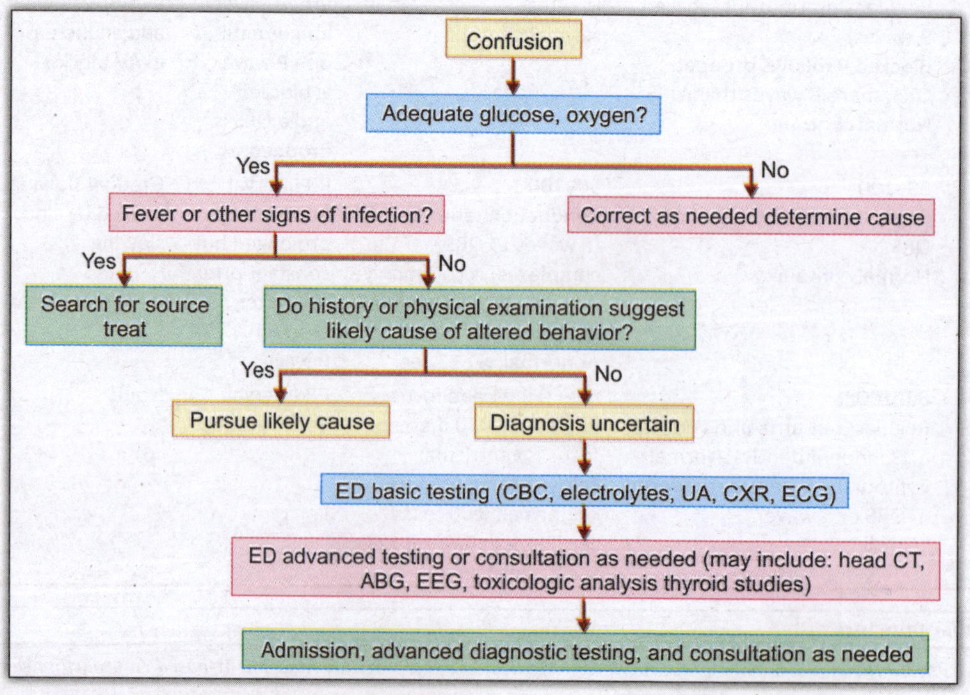

80. Ans. (a) High phosphate in saliva

Ref: Harrison 19th ed page 2166

Sjögren's syndrome is a chronic, slowly progressive autoimmune disease characterized by lymphocytic infiltration of the exocrine glands resulting in xerostomia and dry eyes. Saliva from patients with Sjögren syndrome has elevated levels of sodium, chloride, lactoferrin and IgA, but these findings are not specific.

Diagnosis and Differential Diagnosis

Primary Sjögren's syndrome is diagnosed if

- The patient presents with eye and/or mouth dryness
- Eye tests disclose keratoconjunctivitis sicca
- Mouth evaluation reveals the classic manifestations of the syndrome and/or
- The patient's serum reacts with Ro/SS-A and/or La/SS-B autoantigens.

Labial biopsy is needed when the diagnosis is uncertain or to rule out other conditions that may cause dry mouth or eyes or parotid gland enlargement.

Sialometry: This is a test which measures salivary flow rate. Collection devices are placed over various salivary glands while saliva flow is stimulated with citric acid. It evaluates stimulated and unstimulated saliva flow rates for a set period of time. **A flow rate of 0.5 L or less in one minute for stimulated saliva or a flow rate of 0.5 L or less in 5 min for unstimulated saliva is indicative of xerostomia.** However, this test cannot differentiate between various causes of xerostomia.

81. Ans. (a) D-xylose

Ref: Harrison 19th ed page 1938

Option (A)

Urinary D-Xylose test: The urinary D-xylose test for carbohydrate absorption provides an assessment of proximal small-intestinal mucosal function. D-xylose, a pentose, is absorbed almost exclusively in the proximal small intestine. The D-xylose test is usually performed by giving 25 g D-xylose and collecting urine for 5 hours. An abnormal test (<4.5 g excretion) primarily reflects the presence of duodenal/jejunal mucosal disease. The D-xylose test can also be abnormal in patients with blind loop syndrome (as a consequence primarily of abnormal intestinal mucosa) and, as a false-positive study, in patients with large collections of fluid in a third space (i.e., ascites, pleural fluid). The ease of obtaining a mucosal biopsy of the small intestine by endoscopy and the false-negative rate of the D-xylose test have led to its diminished use. When small-intestinal mucosal disease is suspected, a small-intestinal mucosal biopsy should be performed.

Option (B)

Stool fat estimation: Most malabsorption syndromes are associated with steatorrhea, an increase in stool fat excretion to >6% of dietary fat intake. Some malabsorption disorders are not associated with steatorrhea. Establishing the diagnosis of steatorrhea and identifying its specific cause are often quite difficult. The "gold standard" remains a timed quantitative stool-fat determination. From a practical standpoint, stool collections are invariably difficult and often incomplete, as nobody wants to handle stool. A qualitative test-Sudan III staining-has long been available to document an increase in stool fat. *This test is rapid and inexpensive but, as a qualitative test, does not establish the degree of fat malabsorption and is best used as a preliminary screening study.*

Option (C)

NBT-PABA test is the most widely used test of pancreatic exocrine insufficiency

Option (D)

Schilling test is performed to determine the cause of cobalamin malabsorption.

82. Ans. (d) VSD with AR

Ref: Braunwald heart disease 9th ed Table 12-5, Algappan 4th ed page 104

Braunwald enumerates following causes of Continuous Murmur

- PDA
- Coronary AV fistula
- Ruptured sinus of Valsalva aneurysm
- Aortic septal defect
- Cervical venous hum
- Anomalous left coronary artery
- Proximal coronary artery stenosis
- Mammary souffle of pregnancy
- Pulmonary artery branch stenosis
- Bronchial collateral circulation
- Small (restrictive) ASD with MS
- Intercostal AV fistula

In the above list both option (A) Pulmonary AV fistula and option (D) VSD with AR are not enlisted. However the classification in Algappan is comprehensive and clarifies the confusion.

Classification of Continuous Murmurs

High pressure to low pressure shunts

- Systemic to pulmonary communication
- Patent ductus arteriosus
- Aortopulmonary window
- Tricuspid atresia
- Pulmonary atresia
- Anomalous origin of left coronary artery from pulmonary artery

Systemic to right heart connection

- Coronary arteriovenous fistula
- Rupture of sinus of Valsalva.
- Left atrium to right atrium connection
- Lutembacher syndrome (atrial septal defect + acquired MS).

Arteriovenous fistula

- Systemic
- Pulmonary

Venovenous shunts

Portosystemic shunts.

Contd...

Normal flow through constricted arteries	
• Coarctation of aorta • Peripheral pulmonary artery stenosis carotid stenosis • Coeliac artery stenosis • Mesenteric artery stenosis • Renal artery stenosis	
Increased flow through normal vessels	
Venous (Diastolic accentuation) • Cervical venous hum • Umbilical vein (Cruveilhier-Baumgarten murmur).	Arterial (Systolic accentuation) • Mammary souffle • Uterine souffle • Hepatoma • Nephroma Thyrotoxicosis.

Regarding Option (D) VSD with AR (Ref: Pediatric Cardiology for Practitioners
By Myung K. Park 6th ed page 170)
Aortic regurgitation complicating VDS is an important clinical entity in congenital heart disease. AR is a late manifestation of VSD. A **"To and fro murmur" (To-Systolic, Fro Diastolic)** is seen in VSD with AR. It is differentiated from continuous murmur by a distinct reduction in the intensity of murmur towards the end systole and a different murmur appear in diastole. While, a continuous murmur is a single murmur that peaks around sound heart sound, overlaps the second heart sound and spills well into diastole.

83. Ans. (b) HCV RNA- RT PCR

Ref: Harrison 19th ed page 2014

Anti HbCAg IgG and Anti HCV are positive signifying Hepatitis C infection.
Initial diagnostic evaluation for chronic HCV typically begins with an antibody test. **A reactive or indeterminate/equivocal antibody test should be followed by HCV RNA testing.** For patients who have a greater likelihood of false negative antibody testing (e.g. immunocompromised patients or those suspected of having acute hepatitis C), HCV RNA testing should be sent at the same time as antibody testing when there is a high level of suspicion for infection.
HCV RNA detection and quantification are essential tools in the diagnosis and management of individuals with chronic HCV infection. HCV RNA assays are used to confirm the presence or absence of infection and to quantify the amount of HCV RNA present and may be used to guide decisions regarding duration of treatment with certain regimens.

84. Ans. (d) All are true

Ref: Harrison 19th ed page 1661, Essentials of Ear, Nose & Throat By Mohan Bansal page 359

Central airway obstruction: Central airway obstruction (CAO) refers to the obstruction of airflow in the trachea and mainstem bronchi.
Upper airway obstruction: Upper airway obstruction (UAO) refers to the obstruction of flow in the portion of the airway that extends from the mouth through the length of the trachea and therefore also includes the nasopharynx and larynx. Some conditions that involve this region of the airway may also involve the proximal trachea (e.g. laryngeal, esophageal, or nasopharyngeal cancer), such that CAO and UAO can coexist.
Lower airway obstruction: Airflow obstruction due to chronic obstructive lung diseases including asthma, bronchiectasis and chronic obstructive pulmonary disease (COPD) involves the smaller bronchi in the lower airway distal to the mainstem bronchi and is not typically associated with CAO or UAO.

- The clinical manifestations typically depend upon the degree of luminal obstruction, as well as the location and length of time that obstruction has been present.
- Patients with minor obstruction are often asymptomatic since airflow limitation is mild. Symptoms and signs develop when airflow impairment reaches a critical threshold.
- The clinical manifestations of impaired airway may include dyspnea and stridor, voice change (hoarseness), cough, Wheeze, local pain, restlessness, indrawing of intercostals, suptaclavicular, suprasternal space and drooling.
- Many patients with acute airway compromise have acute onset tachypnea, tachycardia, inspiratory stridor, or wheeze (e.g. patients with acute foreign body aspiration)
- Patients may also present with additional signs and symptoms of the underlying disorder. As examples:
  - Patients with cancer, may also present with constitutional symptoms (e.g. weight loss), hoarseness or hemoptysis (laryngeal or lung cancer), dysphagia (esophageal cancer) and chest pain
  - A smoker or a patient with COPD may have dyspnea, sputum retention, or recurrent infections that may suggest underlying tracheobronchomalacia.
  - Patients with endotracheal or tracheostomy tubes who develop acute shortness of breath or stridor during weaning, following removal of an airway, or capping of a tracheostomy tube should prompt a thorough airway inspection for subglottic or tracheal stenosis)
  - **Laryngeal stridor:** It is a high pitched, crowing sound better heard during inspiration, e.g. obstruction of the larynx by foreign body, laryngeal oedema

85. Ans. (a) Test dose is required for giving IV iron

Ref: Harrison 19th edition 629

Option (A)

In administering intravenous iron dextran, anaphylaxis is a concern. Anaphylaxis is much rarer with the newer preparations. Generalized symptoms appearing several days after the infusion of a large dose of iron caninclude arthralgias, skin rash and low grade fever. These may be dose-related, but they do not preclude the further use of parenteral iron in the patient. To date, patients with sensitivity to iron dextran have been safely treated with other parenteral iron preparations. If a large dose of iron dextran is to be given (>100 mg), the iron preparation should be diluted in 5% dextrose in water or 0.9% NaCI solution. The iron solution can then be infused over a 60–90 minutes period (for larger doses). *Although a test dose (25 mg) of parenteral iron dextran is recommended, in reality a slow infusion of a larger dose of parenteral iron solution will afford the same kind of early warning as a separately injected test dose.*

Option (B)

The goal of therapy in individuals with iron deficiency anemia is not only to repair the anemia, but a l so to provide stores of at least 0.5-1 9 of iron. Sustained treatment for a period of 6-12 months after correction of the anemia will be necessary to achieve this.

Option (C)

- Oral supplements are the only form of iron available to many patients, especially those in resource-poor settings.
- For many patients, oral iron may be more cost effective due to the lack of need for monitored infusion.
- Use of oral iron avoids the need for IV access and monitored infusion.
- Use of oral iron eliminates the potential for infusion reactions and/or anaphylaxis.
- Oral supplements are generally used for infants, children and adolescents.

Strategies to improve tolerability: Interventions to reduce the side effects of oral iron and improve tolerability include the following:

- Reducing the dose (e.g. to once daily) or increasing the interval (e.g. to every other day).
- Making dietary modifications (e.g. taking iron with food or milk), although this may reduce absorption.
- Switching to a formulation with a lower amount of elemental iron.
- Switching from a tablet to a liquid, for which it is easier to titrate the dose

Option (D)

Parenteral iron is not given for rapid rise of Hb as the rise in Hb is the same with oral, IM and IV iron. Indications for parenteral iron: (a) Noncompliant patient (b) Nontolerance to oral iron (c) Malabsorption syndrome (celiac disease, Whipple's disease, bacterial overgrowth) (d) Ongoing blood loss like surgery, Variceal bleeding, Trauma

86. Ans. (b) IV Clindamycin

Ref: Harrison 19th ed page 815

Chest X-ray suggestive of thick walled cavity with an air fluid level and the history is also suggestive of infective etiology, so diagnosis is lung abscess.

For primary lung abscesses, the recommended regimens are

- Clindamycin (600 mg IV three times daily; then, with the disappearance of fever and clinical improvement, 300 mg PO four times daily) or
- IV-administered β-lactam/β-lactamase combination, followed—once the patient's condition is stable—by orally administered amoxicillin-clavulanate.

This therapy should be continued until imaging demonstrates that the lung abscess has cleared or regressed to a small scar. Treatment duration may range from 3 weeks to as long as 14 weeks.

AIIMS MAY 2016

87. Ans. (a) Immediate needle thoracotomy

Ref: Harrison 19th ed page 1719

Traumatic Pneumothorax

- Traumatic pneumothorax can result from both penetrating and nonpenetrating chest trauma.
- Traumatic pneumothorax should be treated with tube thoracostomy unless they are very small. If a hemopneumothorax is present, one chest tube should be placed in the superior part of the hemithorax to evacuate the air and another should be placed in the inferior part of the hemithorax to remove the blood.
- Iatrogenic pneumothorax is a type of traumatic pneumothorax that is becoming more common.
- The leading causes are transthoracic needle aspiration, thoracentesis and the insertion of central intravenous catheters.
- Most can be managed with supplemental oxygen or aspiration, but if these measures are unsuccessful, a tube thoracostomy should be performed.

88. Ans. (a) Intubation with low tidal volume mechanical ventilation

Ref: Harrison 19th ed page 1679

This patient is suffering from acute exacerbation of bronchial asthma with type 2 respiratory failure ABG suggestive of respiratory acidosis with haemodynamic compromise (tachycardia hypotension and hypoxia) so ideal step is to intubate the patient and start mechanical ventilation.

Acute Severe Asthma

- A high concentration of oxygen should be given by face mask to achieve oxygen saturation of >90%.
- The mainstay of treatment are high doses of SABA given either by nebulizer or via a metered-dose inhaler with a spacer. In severely ill patients with impending respiratory failure, IV β2-agonists may be given. A nebulized anticholinergic may be added if there is not a satisfactory response to β2-agonists alone, as there are additive effects. In patients who are refractory to inhaled therapies, a slow infusion of aminophylline may be effective, but it is important to monitor blood levels, especially if patients have already been treated with oral theophylline.
- Magnesium sulfate given intravenously or by nebulizer is effective when added to inhaled β2-agonists and is relatively well tolerated but is not routinely recommended.
- **Prophylactic intubation may be indicated for impending respiratory failure, when the pCO_2 is normal or rises.**
- **For patients with respiratory failure, it is necessary to intubate and institute ventilation. These patients may benefit from an anesthetic such as halothane if they have not responded to conventional bronchodilators.** Sedatives should never be given because they may depress ventilation.
- Antibiotics should not be used routinely unless there are signs of pneumonia.

The following measures are designed to limit dynamic hyperinflation:

- Ventilate with low tidal volumes (6 mL/kg) using the lung protective ventilation protocol in.
- Maximize the time for expiration by:

- Preventing rapid respiratory rates (with sedation, if possible, or neuromuscular paralysis, if necessary) and
- Maintaining inspiratory:expiratory ratio of 1:2 or higher

89. Ans. (d) Different side is chosen if modified allen test is positive on the side

Ref: Miller's Anaesthesia 8th Ed page 1350, Objective Anaesthesia Review: A Comprehensive Textbook for the Examinees By Atul P Kulkarni, JV Divatia, Vijay P Patil, RP Gehdoo 3rd ed page 323, www.uptodate.com

Summary

Different side is chosen if modified allen test is negative (not positive) on the side

Option (A)

Radial artery of non dominant hand is the ideal site of arterial puncture due to following reasons

- Small, superficial, easily accessible
- Easily compressible in case of bleeding
- No nearby nerve
- Good collaterals with ulnar artery

Option (B)

Heparin is available in 10 units/mL, 100 units/mL, 1000 units/mL, 5000 units/mL and 10,000 units/mL.

Ref: Roberts and Hedges' Clinical Procedures in Emergency Medicine By James R. Roberts, Jerris R. Hedges 6th ed page 370:

Precoated blood gas plastic syringes (with dry lithium heparin) are commonly used and allow a longer shelf life and ready. Such devices are designed to minimize sampling error as a result of heparin. If necessary, prepare a regular syringe with 1-2 mL of a heparinized saline solution (1000 1U/ml) drawn into the syringe to coat the barrel and needle. Fully eject the heparin through the needle immediately before skin puncture to minimize heparin related errors. Although the syringe may appear devoid of heparin, enough heparin remains in the needle and syringe to provide anticoagulation.

Ref: AACN Procedure Manual for High Acuity, Progressive and Critical Care By AACN 7th ed page 531

If prepackaged ABG kits are not available, draw 0.5 mL of 1:1000 dilution heparin in a 3 mL syringe pull back the plunger to coat the syringe with heparin and push out the excess heparin and air from the syringe.

Ref: Objective Anaesthesia Review: A Comprehensive Textbook for the Examinees By Atul P Kulkarni, JV Divatia, Vijay P Patil, RP Gehdoo 3rd ed page 323

Very little heparin is actually needed in the sample to prevent clotting; 0.05 to 0.10 mL of a dilute solution (1000 units/mL) will anticoagulate 1 mL of blood without affecting pH, PCO_2, PO_2

Hence 3 mL syringe = 3 mL blood to be drawn, requires just 0.15- 0.3 mL of 1:1000 diluted heparin

Option (C)

The starting point in any evaluation should be the hydrogen ion concentration or pH. However, a normal value does not exclude an acid–base disorder

Option (D)

Ref: Ruppel's Manual of Pulmonary Function Testing By Carl Mottram 10th ed page 158, The Allen Test: A Historical Literature Review and Recommendation Respiratory Care Education Annual Volume 21, Fall 2012, 57-66

NOTE

Positive Allens test denotes inadequate collateral circulation whereas Positive Modified Allen's seat denotes adequate collateral circulation.

The Original Allen Test was first described by Edgar Van Nuys Allen in Mayo's Clinics in 1920 to assist the diagnosis of. It is performed with the patient sitting, with his/her hands supinated on the knees. Standing at the patient's side with your fingers around his/her wrist, **compress the radial artery.** Check for the return of color with flush in the thumb nail. Compression of the radial arteries allows the examiner to assess the adequacy of ulnar blood flow. The test is repeated by occluding Ulnar artery to test Radial artery. This test was modified by Ryan, the procedure of which is as follows:

- Instruct the patient to clench his/her fist, or if the patient is unable, you may close the hand tightly.
- Using your fingers, apply occlusive pressure to **both the ulnar and radial arteries simultaneously**. This maneuver obstructs blood flow to the hand. Allow a few minutes for the blood to drain from the hand while the patient opens and closes his/her hands several times.
- While applying occlusive pressure to both the arteries, have the patient relax his/her hand. Blanching of the palm and fingers should occur. If it does not, you have not completely occluded the arteries with your fingers.
- Release the pressure on the ulnar artery while keeping the radial artery occluded. Normal skin color should return to the ulnar side of the palm in 1-2 seconds, followed by quick restoration of normal color to the entire palm. The usual values are:
  - <7 sec is normal
  - 8-14 sec is borderline
  - >15 sec in the hand and >10 sec in the foot is taken as abnormal and radial artery puncture is contraindicated.
- This normal flushing of the hand is considered to be a positive modified Allen's test which denotes that the ulnar artery is patent and has good blood flow. A negative modified Allen's test is one in which the hand does not flush within the specified time period.

Positive: Ulnar flow sufficient to hand—Radial artery can be cannulated.

Negative: Ulnar flow not sufficient- Radial artery cannot be cannulated.

Arterial blood Gases (ABGs) are frequently used for the following:

- Identification and monitoring of acid-base disturbances
- Measurement of the partial pressures of oxygen (PaO_2) and carbon dioxide ($PaCO_2$)
- Assessment of the response to therapeutic interventions (e.g. insulin in patients with diabetic ketoacidosis)

- Detection and quantification of the levels of abnormal hemoglobins (e.g. carboxyhemoglobin and methemoglobin)
- Procurement of a blood sample in an acute emergency setting when venous sampling is not feasible (most tests can be performed from an arterial sample)

Absolute contraindications for ABG sampling Include the following:
- Local infection or distorted anatomy at the puncture site (e.g. previous surgical interventions, congenital or acquired malformations, burns, aneurysm, stent, arteriovenous fistula, vascular graft)
- Severe peripheral vascular disease of the artery selected for sampling
- Active Raynaud's syndrome (particularly sampling at the radial site)
- Negative modified Allen test

If a contraindication is present, in many cases an alternative site or consideration for using venous blood should be sought for sampling.

The initial step in percutaneous needle puncture is locating a palpable artery. ***Common sites include the radial, femoral, brachial, dorsalis pedis, or axillary artery.*** There is no evidence that any site is superior to the others. However, the radial artery is used most often because it is accessible and more comfortable for the patient than the alternative sites. The radial artery is also typically used for outpatients, while all sites can be used for inpatients who require an ABG.

As for all procedures, the equipment necessary should be brought to the bedside prior to the procedure. This includes:
- Non sterile gloves
- Antiseptic skin solution (e.g. chlorhexidine and povidone-iodine are solutions)
- ABG kit OR a pre-heparinized 3 mL ABG syringe with a 22 to 25-gauge needle and syringe cap (containing diluted heparin {1000 U/cc} in a quantity 0.05–0.1 U/mL of blood (0.15-0.3 Units in 3 mL syringe)
- 2 × 2 inch sterile gauze
- Adhesive bandage
- Plastic hazard bag with ice (if not provided in the kit)
- Sharp object contain

90. Ans. (d) Metabolic acidosis

Ref: Harrison 19th ed page 316, Practical Guidelines of fluid therapy by Sanjay Pandey 2nd ed page 196, 200

See table of Interpretation of ABG in Medicine AIIMS Nov 2016 (see page no. 752)

pH is low so patient is having acidosis

As pCO_2 is low it can not be respiratory acidosis, Hence it is metabolic acidosis

91. Ans. (b) Dengue fever

Ref: Harrison 19th ed page 1310, Park 22nd ed page 229, http://www.cdc.gov/dengue/training/cme/ccm/page73112.html

The tourniquet test is part of the new WHO case definition for dengue. The test is a marker of capillary fragility and it can be used as a triage tool to differentiate patients with acute gastroenteritis, for example, from those with dengue. Even if a tourniquet test was previously done, it should be repeated if
1. It was previously negative
2. There is no bleeding manifestation

Procedure

- Take the patient's blood pressure and record it, for example, 100/70
- Inflate the cuff to a point midway between SBP and DBP and maintain for 5 minutes. (100 + 70) ÷ 2 = 85 mm Hg
- Reduce and wait 2 minutes.
- Count petechiae below antecubital fossa. (A positive test is 10 or more petechiae per 1 square inch)

The tourniquet test has variable sensitivity and specificity. Using a cut off of ≥20 petechiae/square inch increases specificity, but loses sensitivity. The tourniquet test is
- More likely to be positive near time of defervescence
- Less likely to be positive in patients with shock

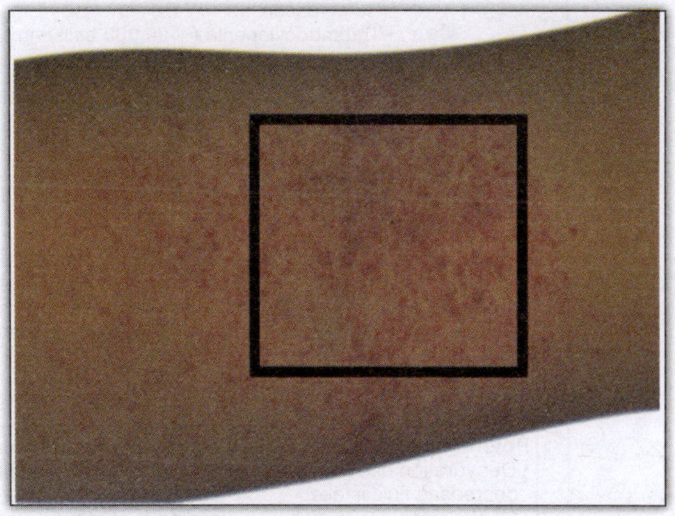

92. Ans. (d) Hematocrit

Ref: Harrison 19th ed page 1310, Park 23rd ed page 259

Dengue hemorrhagic fever occurs where multiple types of dengue virus are simultaneously or sequentially transmitted. Second dengue infections are relatively mild in the majority of instances, ranging from an inapparent infection through an undifferentiated upper respiratory tract or dengue-like disease, but may also progress to dengue hemorrhagic fever.

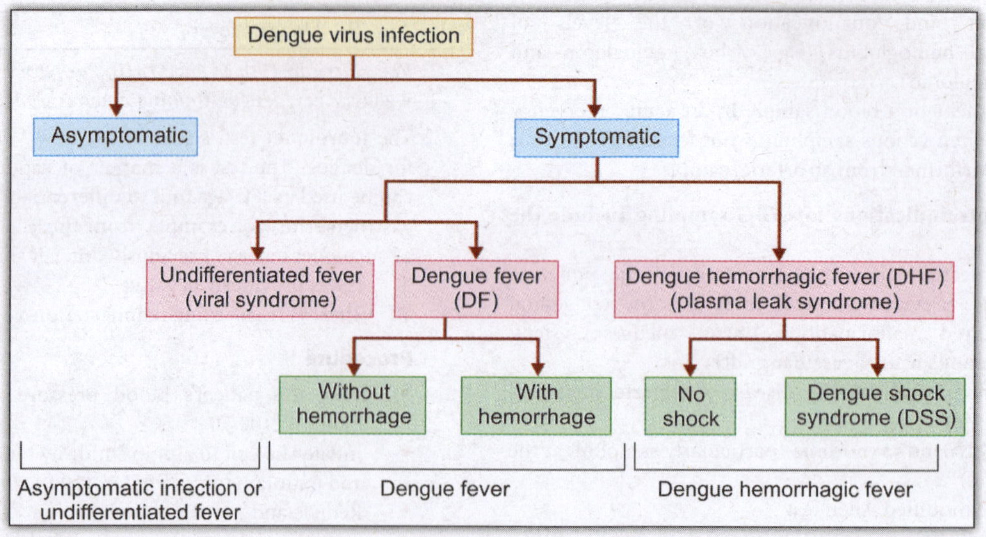

There are three phases of DHF: the Febrile Phase; the Critical (Plasma Leak) Phase; and the Convalescent (Reabsorption) Phase.

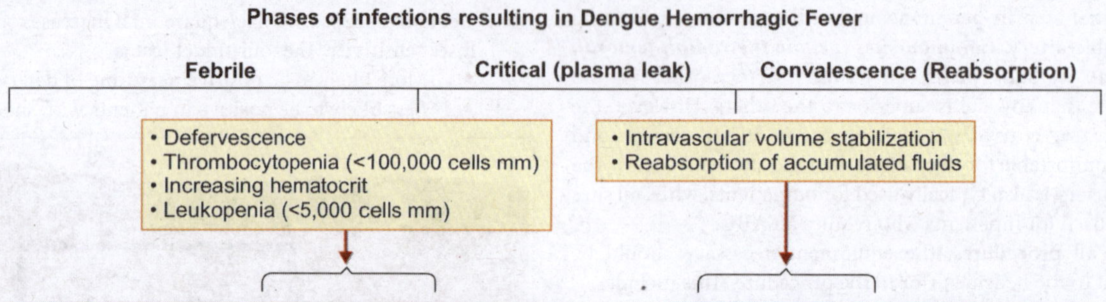

Fever last 2-7 days	Plasma leak lasts 24-28 hours	Reabsorption lasts 2-4 days
Hallmark features: • High fever and symptoms consistent with either Dengue fever	**Hallmark features:** • Normal or subnormal temperatures. • Varying degrees or plasma leak into pleural and peritoneal spaces. • Varying degrees of hemorrhage. • Risk of developing shock and death.	**Hallmark features:** • Resolution of plasma leakage and hemorrhage • Stabilization of vital sings. • Reabsorption of accumulated fluids; including leaked plasma and administered intravascular fluids • Improved appetite and sense of well-being
Potential complications: • Dehydration due to decreased fluid intake • Convulsions due to high fever • Rarely, severe hemorrhage	**Potential complications:** • Unrecognized severe plasma leakage or hemorrhage leading to shock • Intracranial bleed • Metabolic abnormalities (e.g., hypoglycemia, hyponafremia, hypocalcemia, metabolic acidosis) • Coagulopathy (e.g., abnormal INR or PTT) • Fulminant hepatic failure • Prolonged shock leading to death	**Potential complications:** • Intravascular fluid overload due to continual aggressive volume resuscitation during convalescence phase.

The World Health Organization criteria for dengue hemorrhagic fever are fever, minor or major hemorrhagic manifestations, thrombocytopenia (≤100,000/mm³, Platelets rarely fall below 100,000/mm³) and objective evidence of increased capillary permeability (hematocrit increased by ≥20%), serosal effusion (by chest radiography or ultrasonography), or hypoalbuminemia. Dengue shock syndrome criteria include those for dengue hemorrhagic fever as well as hypotension or narrow pulse pressure (≤20 mm Hg).

Nelson states: **The most common hematologic abnormalities during dengue hemorrhagic fever and dengue shock syndrome is hemoconcentration with an increase of >20% in hematocrit.**

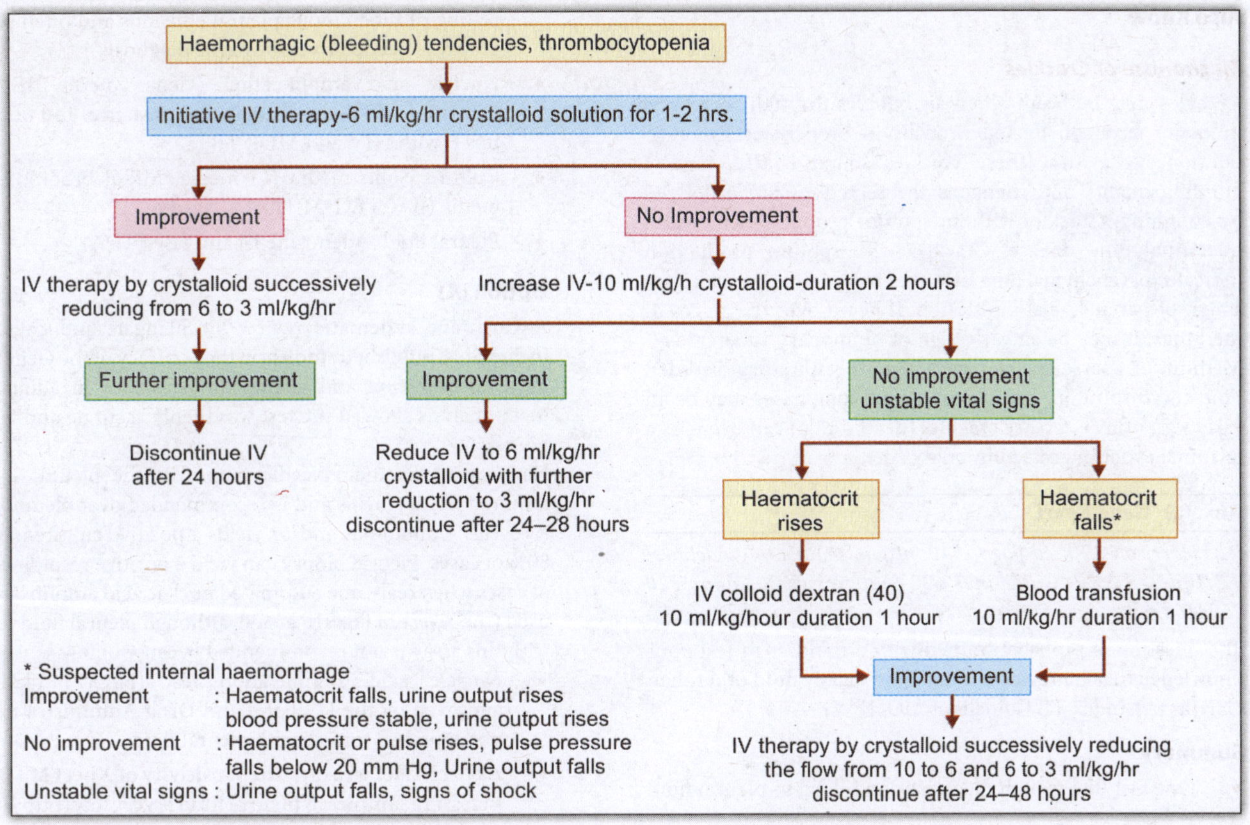

93. Ans. (d) Both early and late inspiratory crackles

Ref: Macleod's clinical examination 13th ed page 154, Manual of Practical Medicine Alagappan 4th ed page 206

Note

The clinical findings of Bronchiectasis of any cause will be more or less similar.

Crackles are interrupted non-musical sounds and result from collapse of peripheral airways on expiration. On inspiration, air rapidly enters these distal airways and the alveoli and small bronchi open abruptly, producing the crackling noise. Early inspiratory crackles suggest small airways disease and can occur in bronchiolitis. In pulmonary oedema crackles occur in mid-inspiration. Fine late inspiratory crackles, which sound similar to rubbing hair between your fingers, are characteristic of pulmonary fibrosis. Bronchiectasis can cause crackles throughout inspiration and expiration.

Option (A)

The crackles which originate at the bases of both the lungs, are known as bibasilar or bibasal crackles, or bilateral basilar crackles. Apart from heart failure, a few basilar crackles can be heard in normal lungs after prolonged shallow breathing and clears off after few deep breaths.

Option (B)

Pulmonary edema causes fine crackles at the base of lung while Bronchiectasis causes coarse crackles

Crackles Types

1. Fine—They are less loud, short in duration and arise from the alveoli. e.g. Early stage of Pneumonia/Consolidation, Fibrosing alveolitis
2. Coarse—They are low pitched, loud and arise from the bronchus and bronchioles. e.g. Resolving pneumonia, bronchiectasis and lung abscess.

Option (C)

Tubular breathing is seen in consolidation

Option (D)

See the table below

Causes of Crackles	
Phase of inspiration	**Cause**
Early inspiratory	Small airways disease, as in bronchiolitis
Middle inspiratory	Pulmonary oedema
Late Inspiratory	Pulmonary fibrosis (fine) Pulmonary oedema (medium) Bronchial secretions in COPD, pneumonia, lung abscess, tubercular lung cavities (coarse)
Biphasic	Bronchiectasis (coarse)

Also Know

Mechanism of Crackles

Crackles may be heard when air bubbles through secretions in major bronchi, dilated bronchi in bronchiectasis or in pulmonary cavities. These crackles sound coarse, have a gurgling quality and change if the secretions are dislodged by coughing. Crackles without sputum production indicates interstitial lung disease. Crackles with sputum production indicates parenchymal lung disease. Fine localised crackles are a sign of parenchymal infiltration. If heard over the apices of the lungs, it may be an early sign of pulmonary tuberculosis. Medium or coarse crackles are a sign of respiratory disorder. Fine end inspiratory crackles over both lung bases may be an early sign of LVF. Coarse crackles (death rattle) can occur as a terminal event in gross pulmonary edema.

94. Ans. (a) Gene Xpert

Ref: Harrison 19th ed page 1110, http://icmr.nic.in/guidelines/TB/Index-TB%20Guidelines%20-%20green%20colour%202594164.pdf

The question is probably framed with a mindset to test your knowledge that Gene Xpert is not done for any fluid other than CSF (as per Index TB Guidelines MOHFW)

Summary

- One test that is both diagnostic and done in pleural fluid is ADA
- Single most effective diagnostic test of TB is Nucleic acid amplification (Gene Xpert), which also gives information about Resistance. But Pleural fluid is not the right sample for it.
- LDH is routinely done as a part of Light's criteria to differentiate transudative vs Exudative fluid, but not diagnstic to TB
- Total protein not Albumin is a part of Light's criteria. However Pleural fluid analysis cantains many parameterswhich are not part of 3 point Light's criteria. Differentiate transudative vs Exudative fluid, but not diagnstic to TB

Tuberculous pleural effusion is an exudative, lymphocyte-predominant pleural effusion that occurs as a result of a delayed hypersensitivity reaction to mycobacteria or mycobacterial antigens in the pleural space. The fluid is straw colored and at times hemorrhagic; it is an exudate with a protein concentration >50% of that in serum (usually ~4–6 g/dL), a normal to low glucose concentration, a pH of ~7.3 (occasionally <7.2) and detectable white blood cells (usually 500–6000/μL).

Out of the Options provided only Option (A) Gene Xpert and Option (D) ADA are diagnostic tests for Tuberculosis. But the question is not about the Diagnostic test. They have simply asked what we will ask in Pleural fluid. Read Following lines from Davidson.

Ref: Davidson 22nd ed page 693

Diagnostic Tests of Tuberculosis are

- Tuberculin skin test: Low sensitivity and speciticity. Useful only in primary and deep seated infection
- Stain (Z N stain, Auramine fluorescence): Acid-fast bacilli (AFB) stains and AFB cultures are of low yield in the setting of tuberculous pleural effusions and often pleural biopsy is needed to confirm the diagnosis.
- Nucleic acid amplification (Gene Xpert, RIF test): Diagnosis of TB plus Rifampicin resistance. Test of choice in TB with HIV and MDR TB
- Culture: Solid media (LJ media, Middlebrook), Liquid media (BACTEC, MJIT)
- Pleural fluid: Adenosine Deaminase (ADA)

Option (A)

A Cochrane systematic review by Steingart and colleagues included 18 published studies on the accuracy of the GeneXpert for PTB detection and rifampicin resistance in adults. The meta-analysis showed the test was highly accurate and fast (in hours)

Harrison states that: Needle biopsy of the pleura is often required for diagnosis and is recommended over pleural fluid; it reveals granulomas and/or yields a positive culture in up to 80% of cases. Pleural biopsy can yield a positive result in ~75% of cases when real-time automated nucleic acid amplification is used (the Xpert MTB/RIF assay), although pleural fluid testing with this assay is not recommended because of low sensitivity.

- Nucleic acid amplification test (NAAT) platforms approved by the US Food and Drug Administration are not approved for use with pleural fluid.
- As per WHO website: **The sensitivity of Xpert MTB/RIF in testing samples of pleural fluid is very low** (http://apps.who.int/iris/bitstream/10665/112469/1/9789241506700_eng.pdf)
- One that Gene Xpert is a costly test and secondly Pleural fluid is not the right sample for it.

Option (B)

There is no confusion in LDH as its a part of Light's criteria

Light's Criteria: Determination of transudate versus exudate source of pleural effusion. Fluid is exudate if one of the following Light's criteria is present:

- Effusion protein/serum protein ratio greater than 0.5
- Effusion lactate dehydrogenase (LDH)/serum LDH ratio greater than 0.6
- Effusion LDH level greater than two-thirds the upper limit of the laboratory's reference range of serum LDH

Option (C)

Total serum protein not Albumin is included in Light's criteria. However Lights criteria is not the only criteria to be considered. Albumin is also independentely taken into consideration. Also practically pleual fluid panel includes Albumin. Read following table

Ref: Textbook of Pulmonary Medicine By D Behera 2nd ed page 1564

Differentiation between transudative and exudative effusions		
Character	Exudates	Transudates
Pleural fluid LDH level*	>200 or >2/3rd of serum	<200 or <2/3rd of serum

Contd...

Differentiation between transudative and exudative effusions		
Fluid: Serum LDh*	>0.6	<0.6
Fluid Serum Protein*	>05	<0.5
Pleural fluid cholesterol	>5.5 mg/dl	<5.5 mg/dl
Serum pleural albumin gradiant	>1.2 mg/dl	<1.2 mg/dl
Fluid: Serum billirubin	=/> 0.6	<0.6
* Commonly used criteria		

Test sensitivity and specificity for exudate		
	Sensitivity, %	Specificity, %
Light's criteria	98	83
Protein/serum protein ratio >0.5	85	84
LDH/serum LDH ratio >0.6	90	82
LDH >2/3 upper limits of serum normal	82	89
Pleural-fluid cholesterol level >60 mg/dL	54	92
Pleural-fluid cholesterol level >43 mg/dL	75	80
Pleural-fluid/serum cholesterol ratio >0.3	89	81
Serum/pleural-fluid albumin level ≤1.2 g/dL	87	92

Option (D)

The diagnosis of TB is established by demonstrating high levels of TB markers in the pleural fluid (adenosine deaminase >40 IU/L or interferon >140 pg/mL).

95. Ans. (c) Prevent increase in pCO_2 levels

Ref: Harrison 19th ed page 1780

NOTE

First step or next step i not asked in the question. The examiner is particular about Best strategy

Interventions to lower ICP are ideally based on the underlying mechanism responsible for the elevated ICP. For example, in hydrocephalus from SAH, the principal cause of elevated ICP is impairment of CSF drainage. In this setting, ventricular drainage of CSF is likely to be sufficient and most appropriate. In head trauma and stroke, cytotoxic edema may be most responsible and the use of osmotic agents such as mannitol or hypertonic saline becomes an appropriate early step.

Emergent treatment of elevated ICP is most quickly achieved by intubation and hyperventilation, which causes vasoconstriction and reduces cerebral blood volume. In order to avoid provoking or worsening cerebral ischemia, hyperventilation is best used for short periods of time until a more definitive treatment can be instituted

Hyperventilation: Use of mechanical ventilation to lower $PaCO_2$ to 26 to 30 mm Hg has been shown to rapidly reduce ICP through vasoconstriction and a decrease in the volume of intracranial blood; a 1 mmHg change in $PaCO_2$ is associated with a 3 percent change in CBF. Hyperventilation also results in respiratory alkalosis, which may buffer post-injury acidosis. The effect of hyperventilation on ICP is short-lived (1 to 24 hours). Following therapeutic hyperventilation, the patient's respiratory rate should be tapered back to normal over several hours to avoid a rebound effect. Therapeutic hyperventilation should be considered as an urgent intervention when elevated ICP complicates cerebral edema, intracranial hemorrhage and tumor. Hyperventilation should not be used on a chronic basis, regardless of the cause of increased ICP.

Stepwise Approach to Treatment of Elevated Intracranial Pressure

Insert ICP monitor—ventriculostomy versus parenchymal device

General goals: maintain ICP <20 mm Hg and CPP 60 mm Hg

For >20–25 mm Hg for >5 minutes

- Drain CSF via ventriculostomy (if in place)
- Elevate head of the bed; midline head position
- **Osmotherapy**—mannitol 25–100 g q4h as needed (maintain serum osmolality <320 mosmol) or hypertonic saline (30 mL, 23.4% NaCl bolus)
- **Glucocorticoids**—dexamethasone 4 mg q6h for vasogenic edema from tumor, abscess (avoid glucocorticoids in head trauma, ischemic and hemorrhagic stroke)
- **Sedation** (e.g., morphine, propofol, or midazolam); add neuromuscular paralysis if necessary (patient will require endotracheal intubation and mechanical ventilation at this point, if not before)
- **Hyperventilation**—to $PaCO_2$ 30–35 mm Hg
- **Pressor therapy**—Phenylephrine, dopamine, or norepinephrine to maintain adequate MAP to ensure CPP 60 mm Hg (maintain euvolemia to minimize deleterious systemic effects of pressors)
- **Consider second-tier therapies for refractory elevated ICP**
  - High-dose barbiturate therapy ("pentobarb coma")
  - Aggressive hyperventilation to $PaCO_2$ <30 mm Hg
  - Hypothermia
  - Hemicraniectomy

96. Ans. (b) The examiner is doing the test wrongly

Ref: Macleods Clinical examination 13th ed page 262

Option (A) False

Deep tendon reflex are Hyperactive (not Brisk) in Motor neuron disease.

Reflex Pattern with Different Neurological Disorders				
Site or type of lesion	Muscle stretch reflex	Superficial reflex	Pathological reflex	Associated movements
Neuromuscular junction	N or ↓	Normal	Absent	Normal
Muscle	Usually N, May be ↓	Normal	Absent	Normal
Peripheral nerve	↓ Or Absent	N, ↓ or Absent in the distribution of nerve	Absent	Normal
Corticospinal tract (Upper motor neuron)	Hyperactive (↑)	↓ Or Absent	Present	Pathologic associated movement present
Extrapyramidal	Usually normal	N or Slightly ↑	Absent	Normal associated movement absent
Cerebellum	Pendular	Normal	Absent	Normal
Psychogenic	N or ↑ especially in range of response	N or ↑	Absent	Normal or Bizzare

Option (B) True

The examiner is doing the test wrongly. The quadriceps should have been exposed completely.

Option (C) False

Deep tendon refle are decreased or absent in case of peripheral neuropathy

Option (D) False

The patellar reflex is mediated by the femoral nerve (L2-L4) not L1, L2, L3.

Knee Jerk

The patellar reflex is contraction of the quadriceps femoris muscle, with resulting extension of the knee, in response to percussion of the patellar tendon. A firm tap on the tendon draws the patella down, stretching the quadriceps and provoking reflex contraction. If the reflex is brisk, the contraction is strong and the amplitude of the movement is large. If the examiner places one hand over the muscle and with the other hand taps the patellar tendon just below the patella, He/ she can palpate the contraction as well as observe the rapidity and range of response. Palpation helps in judging the latency between the time of the stimulus and the resulting response.

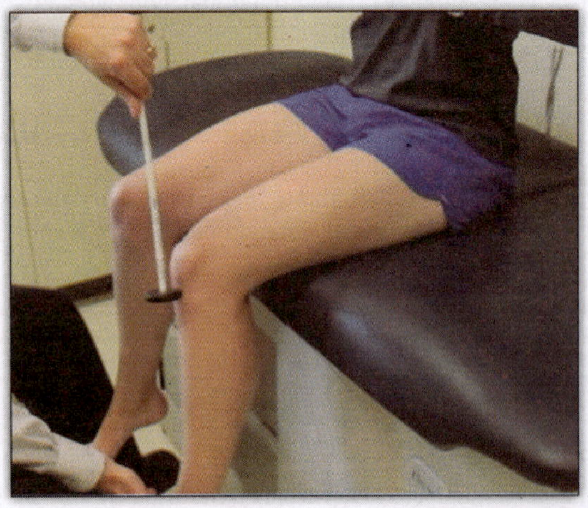

Fig: The patient may sit in a chair with the knees slightly extended and the heels resting on the floor or sit on an examination table with the legs dangling. If the patient is lying in bed, the examiner should partially flex the knee by placing one hand beneath it and then tap the tendon. The responses on the two sides can be compared by lifting both knees simultaneously, supporting them on one forearm as the patient's heels rest lightly on the bed, before tapping the tendons. If the patient is wearing loose pajamas, the examiner can suspend both legs by holding the pajamas, as she uses the other hand to strike the tendon.

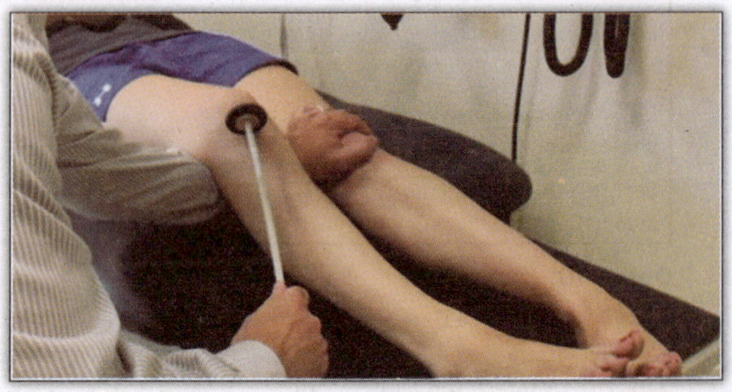

Fig: Another technique is having the patient sit with one leg crossed over the other and tapping the patellar tendon of the uppermost leg, but this method does not facilitate side-to-side comparison.

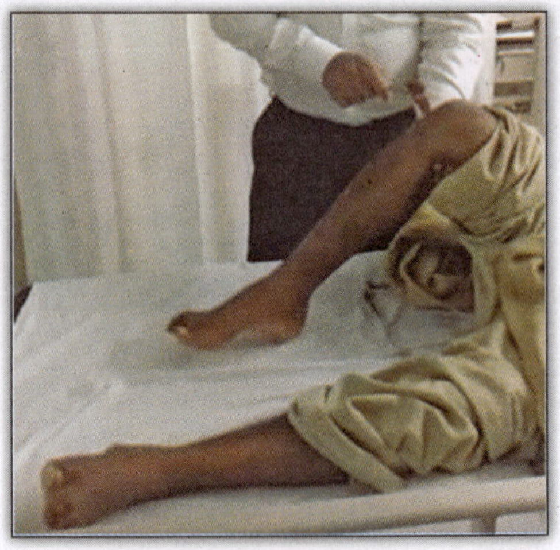

Fig: Incorrect method of doing Knee jerk. As quadriceps (Thigh) should have been exposed completely.

97. Ans. (b) Cardioversion

Ref: Harrison 19th ed page 1483, A Primer of ECG By K P Mishra, Braunwald's Heart Disease: A Textbook Of Cardiovascular Medicine 8th Ed. Table 35-1

This is a case of SVT with shock

Hint to diagnosis

- BP of 70 mm Hg points towards shock
- In ECG notice the metronomic regularity with a rate of 170 beats/min (Tachycardia). No P waves are visible because they are "buried" in the QRS or t wave due to simultaneous atrial and ventricular stimulation

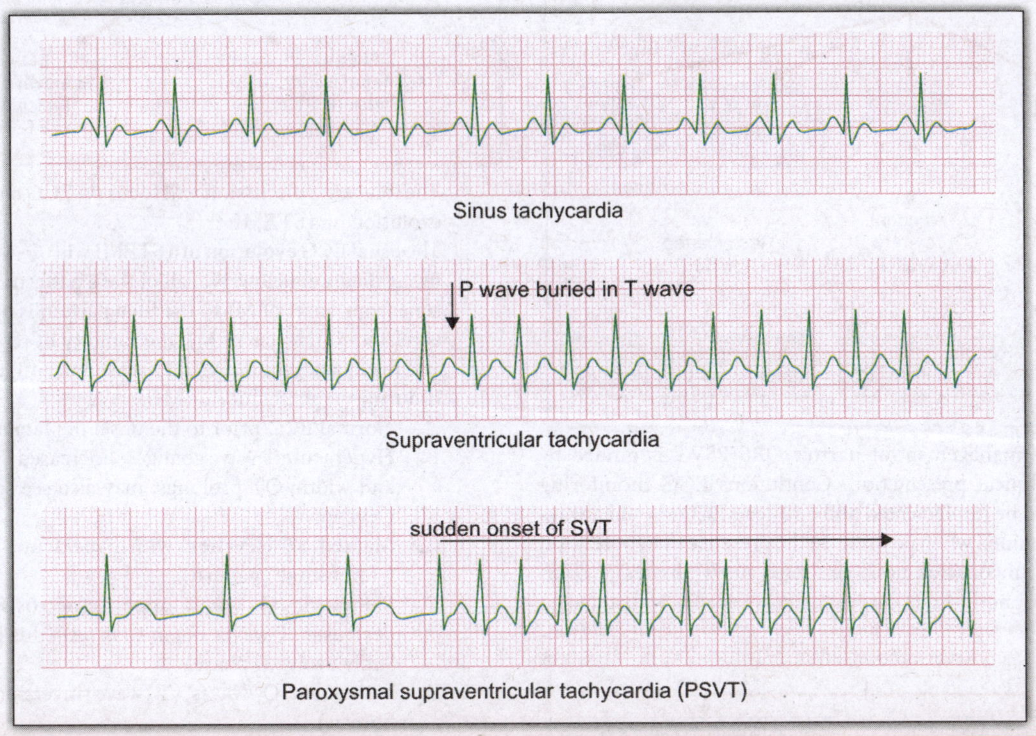

Type of arrhythmia	P waves Trate (beats/min) Rhythm Contour	QRS complexes Trate (beats/min) Rhythm Contour	Other findings	Ventricular response to carotid sinus massage	Treatment
AV nodal reentry (SVT/ PSVT)	150-250 Very regular except at onset and termination Retrograde; difficult to see; lost in T wave or QRS complex	150-250 Very regular except at onset and termination Contour Normal (0.06–0.10 sec)	Sudden onset of SVT that stop suddenly is PSVT, PR Interval: Usually not possible to measure. AV Nodal Reentrant Tachycardia (AVNRT) is MC PSVT	Abrupt slowing caused by termination of tachycardia, or no effect	Vagal stimulation adenosine, verapamil, digitalis, propranolol, DC shock, pacing

Classification of Tachycardia

- Rapid heart rhythms can be divided clinically into ***narrow complex*** **and *wide complex***.
- **Narrow complex tachycardias**, which are always supraventricular in origin, include sinus, paroxysmal supraventricular tachycardias (PSVTs), atrial fibrillation and atrial flutter.
- **Wide complex tachycardias** include ventricular tachycardia and any of the supraventricular tachycardias with aberrant ventricular conduction or conduction down a bypass tract.
- **Narrow complex tachycardias**, in turn, can also be divided based on regularity.
- Sinus tachycardia, atrial tachycardia or atrial flutter with pure 1:1 or 2:1 conduction, atrioventricular nodal reentrant tachycardia (AVNRT) and atrioventricular reentrant tachycardia (AVRT) are regular, but atrial fibrillation and atrial flutter or atrial tachycardia with variable degrees of atrioventricular (AV) block are irregular.

Cardiac Rhythm Disturbances

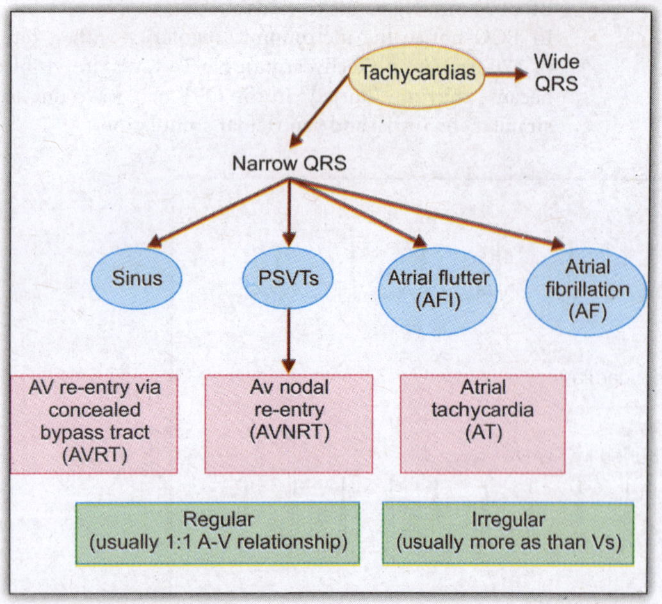

- Acute management of narrow QRS PSVT is guided by the clinical presentation. Continuous ECG monitoring should be implemented and a 12-lead ECG should always be obtained when possible. In the presence of hypotension with unconsciousness or respiratory distress, QRS-synchronous direct current cardioversion is warranted.

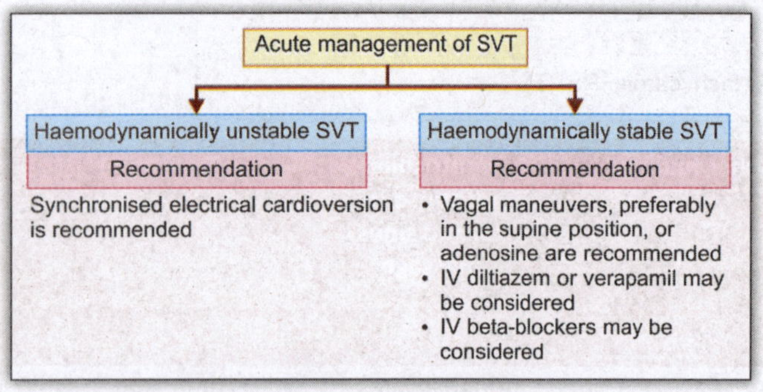

98. Ans. (c) Primary percutaneous intervention

Ref: Harrison 19th ed page 1604

This is a ECG of ST segment elevated myocardial infarction

Myocardial Ischemia/Infarction/Acute Coronary Syndrome:

On the left side no myocardial necrosis occurs but there is either **subendocardial** ischemia manifested by reversible ST segment **depression** or **transmural** ischemia manifested by reversible ST segment **elevation**. On the right are two types of myocardial infarction, one manifested by ST segment elevation (**STEMI**) and one manifested by no ST segment elevation (**NonSTEMI**). Either of these can evolve into Q-wave or non-Q-wave MIs.

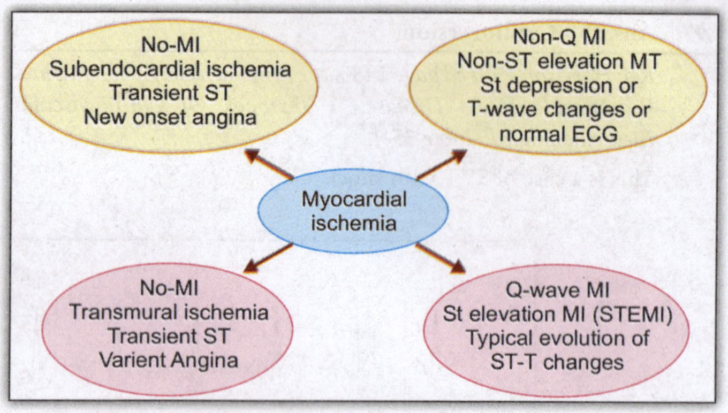

The following discussion will focus on ECG changes during the evolution of a STEMI:

The usual ECG evolution of a STEMI with Q-waves is illustrated in the diagram below. Not all of the 6 patterns may be seen; the time from onset of MI to the final pattern is quite variable and is related to the size of MI, the rapidity of reperfusion (if any) and the location of the MI. (This example might be seen in lead II during an acute inferior MI)

A. Normal ECG prior to the onset of plaque rupture
B. Hyperacute T wave changes - increased T wave amplitude and width; QT prolongs; may also see some ST segment elevation
C. Marked ST elevation with hyperacute T wave changes ("tombstone" pattern)
D. Pathologic Q waves appear (necrosis), ST elevation decreases, T waves begin to invert (this is also called the "fully evolved" phase)
E. Pathologic Q waves, T wave inversion (necrosis and fibrosis)
F. Pathologic Q waves, upright T waves (fibrosis)

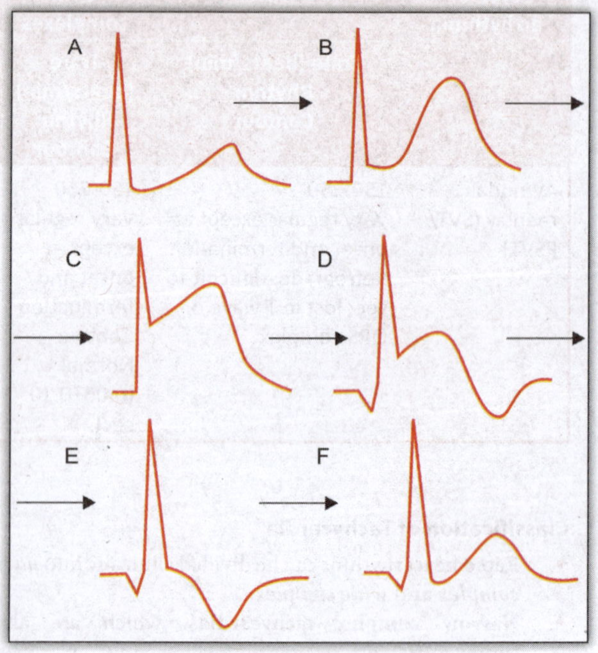

MI on the Basis of Thickness of Wall Involved

Subendocardial ischemia	Transmural or epicardial ischemia
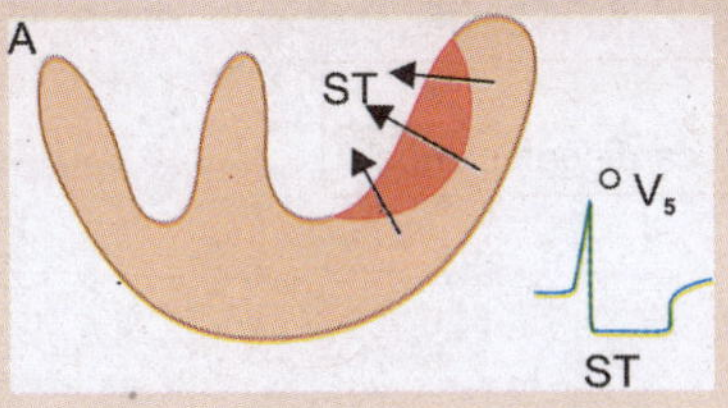	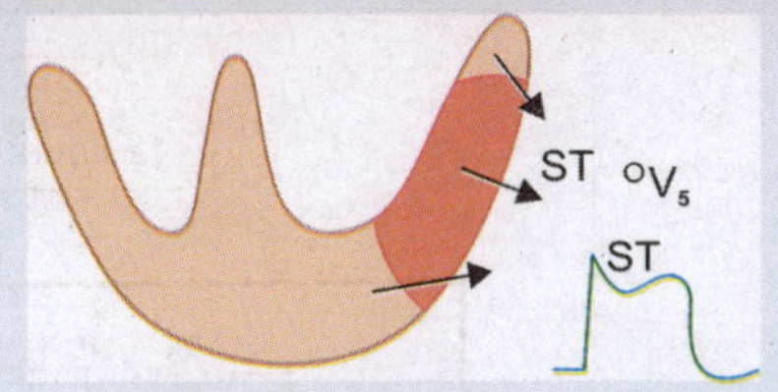
With **predominant subendocardial ischemia**, the resultant ST vector will be directed toward the inner layer of the affected ventricle and the ventricular cavity. Overlying leads therefore will record ST depression.	With ischemia involving **transmural or epicardial injury,** the ST vector will be directed outward. Overlying leads will record ST elevation.

- PCI, usually angioplasty and/or stenting without preceding fibrinolysis, referred to as *primary PCI*, is effective in restoring perfusion in STEMI when carried out on an emergency basis in the first few hours of MI.
- It has the advantage of being applicable to patients who have contraindications to fibrinolytic therapy but otherwise are considered appropriate candidates for reperfusion.
- It appears to be more effective than fibrinolysis in opening occluded coronary arteries and, *when performed by experienced operators in dedicated medical centers*, is associated with better short-term and longterm clinical outcomes.
- Compared with fibrinolysis, primary PCI is generally preferred when the diagnosis is in doubt, cardiogenic shock is present, bleeding risk is increased, or symptoms have been present for at least 2–3 hours when the clot is more mature and less easily lysed by fibrinolytic drugs

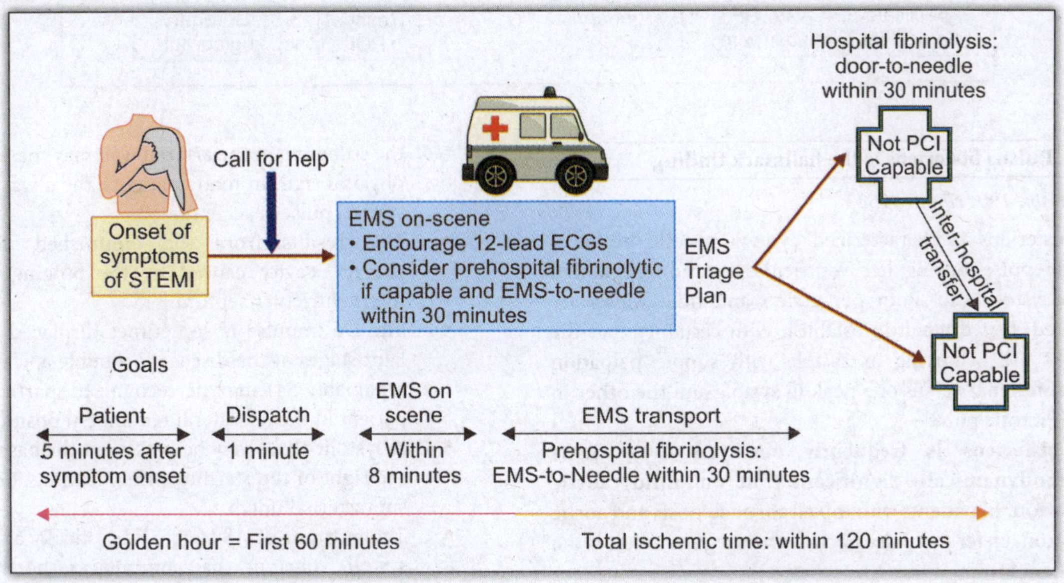

Primary percutaneous coronary intervention (PCI) is the preferred reperfusion strategy for most patients with acute ST elevation myocardial infarction (STEMI). When timely primary PCI is not available, early fibrinolysis should be carried out.

Following recommendations for the use of fibrinolytic therapy in patients with acute STEMI:

- For patients within 12 hours of the onset of STEMI who have no absolute contraindications to fibrinolytic therapy and for whom reperfusion with primary PCI cannot be performed within the recommended time, Fibrinolytic therapy as opposed to no reperfusion therapy.
- For symptomatic patients who present after 12 (**but before 24**) hours of symptom onset and when PCI is not readily available, fibrinolytic therapy as opposed to no reperfusion therapy.
- Prehospital as opposed to in-hospital administration of fibrinolytic therapy for patients with acute STEMI in whom a decision has been made to not use primary PCI as the reperfusion strategy.

This recommendation applies only to patients in health-care settings where prehospital administration of fibrinolytic therapy is feasible.

- Irrespective of whether fibrinolytic therapy is given prehospital or in the hospital (emergency department), it should be started within 30 minutes after the diagnosis of STEMI is made.

- Recommend a fibrin-specific agent instead of streptokinase
- Tenecteplase instead of alteplase or reteplase).
- Early transfer to a PCI center after fibrinolysis should be recommended to decide whether rescue or elective PCI are necessary.

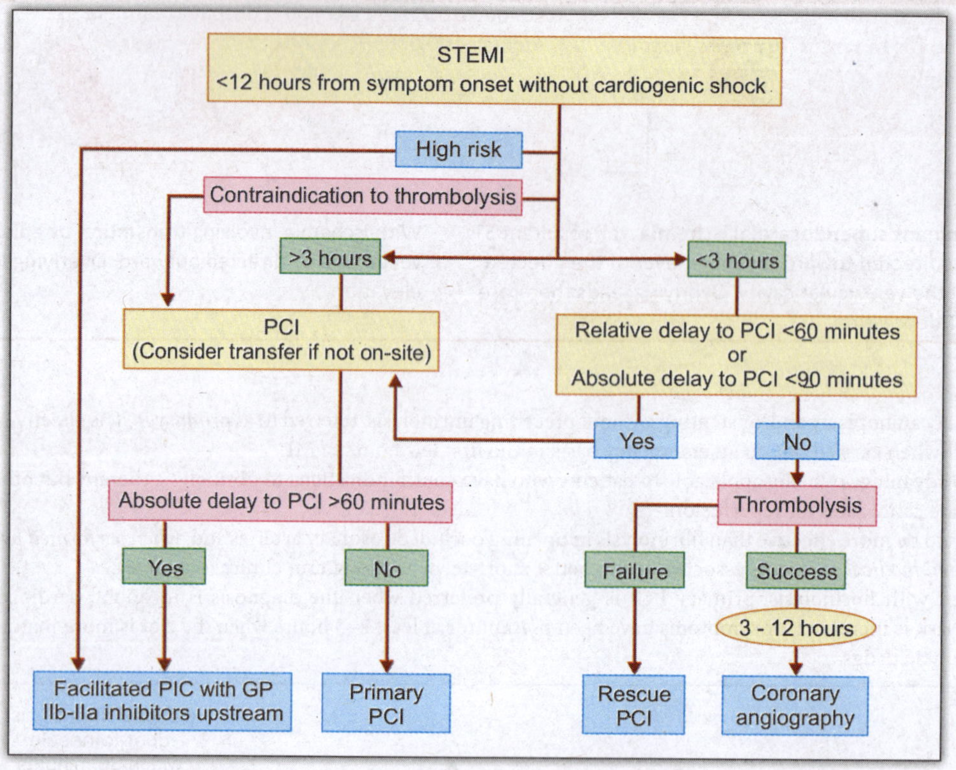

99. Ans. (b) Pulsus bisferiens is the hallmark finding

Ref: Harrison 19th ed page 1531

Pulsus bisferiens is characterized by two systolic peaks of the aortic pulse during left ventricular ejection separated by a midsystolic dip. Both percussion and tidal waves are accentuated. It is difficult to establish with certainty that the two peaks are occurring in systole with simple palpation (pulsus bisferiens) versus one peak in systole and the other in diastole (dicrotic pulse).

Pulsus bisferiens is frequently observed in patients with hemodynamically significant (but not mild) aortic regurgitation. In patients with mixed aortic stenosis and aortic regurgitation, bisferiens pulse occurs when regurgitation is the predominant lesion.

Physical Findings of Aortic Stenosis

- The rhythm is generally regular until late in the course; at other times, AF should suggest the possibility of associated mitral valve disease. The systemic arterial pressure is usually within normal limits. In the late stages, however, when stroke volume declines, the systolic pressure may fall and the pulse pressure narrow. The carotid arterial pulse rises slowly to a delayed peak (*pulsus parvus et tardus*).
- A thrill or anacrotic "shudder" may be palpable over the carotid arteries, more commonly the left. In the elderly, the stiffening of the arterial wall may mask this important physical sign. In many patients, the *a* wave in the jugular venous pulse is accentuated.
- This results from the diminished distensibility of the RV cavity caused by the bulging, hypertrophied interventricular septum.
- The LV impulse is sometimes displaced laterally in the later stages of the disease. A double apical impulse (with a palpable S4) may be recognized, particularly with the patient in the left lateral recumbent position.
- A systolic thrill may be present at the base of the heart to the right of the sternum when leaning forward or in the suprasternal notch.
- The murmur of AS is characteristically an ejection (mid) systolic murmur that commences shortly after the S1, increases in intensity to reach a peak toward the middle of ejection and ends just before aortic valve closure. It is characteristically low-pitched, rough and rasping in character and loudest at the base of the heart, most commonly in the second right intercostal space.
- It is transmitted upward along the carotid arteries. Occasionally it is transmitted downward and to the apex, where it may be confused with the systolic murmur of mitral regurgitation (MR) (Gallavardin effect).

100. Ans. (b) Blood pressure >185/100 mm Hg despite treatment

Ref: Harrison 19th ed page 2562

Administration of Intravenous Recombinant Tissue Plasminogen Activator (RTPA) for Acute Ischemic Stroke

Indication	Contraindication
Clinical diagnosis of stroke	Sustained BP >185/110 mm Hg despite treatment
Onset of symptoms to time of drug administration <3 hours	Platelets <100,000; HCT <25%; glucose <50 or >400 mg/dL
CT scan showing no hemorrhage or edema of >1/3 of the MCA territory	Use of heparin within 48 h and prolonged PTT, or elevated INR
Age >18 years	Rapidly improving symptoms
Consent by patient or surrogate	Prior stroke or head injury within 3 months; prior intracranial hemorrhage
	Major surgery in preceding 14 days
	Minor stroke symptoms
	Gastrointestinal bleeding in preceding 21 days
	Recent myocardial infarction
	Coma or stupor
Administration of rtPA	
Intravenous access with two peripheral IV lines (avoid arterial or central line placement)	
Review eligibility for rtPA	
Administer 0.9 mg/kg IV (maximum 90 mg) IV as 10% of total dose by bolus, followed by remainder of total dose over 1 hours	
Frequent cuff blood pressure monitoring	
No other antithrombotic treatment for 24 hours	
For decline in neurologic status or uncontrolled blood pressure, stop infusion, give cryoprecipitate and reimage brain emergently	
Avoid urethral catheterization for >2 hours	

101. Ans. (a) Intravenous plasminogen activator

Ref: Harrison 19th edition page 1634

This is a cae of massive pulmonarty thromboembolism.

For patients with massive PE and hypotension, replete volume with 500 mL of normal saline. Additional fluid should be infused with extreme caution because excessive fluid administration exacerbates. RV wall stress, causes more profound RV ischemia and worsens LV compliance and filling by causing further interventricular septal shift toward the LV. Dopamine and dobutamine are first-line inotropic agents for treatment of PE-related shock. Maintain a low threshold for initiating these pressors.

PE Management

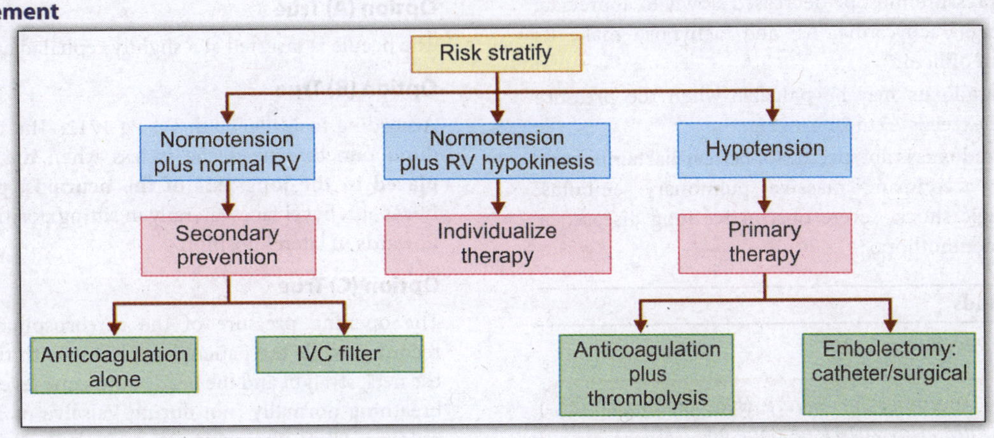

Fibrinolysis

Successful fibrinolytic therapy rapidly reverses right heart failure and may result in a lower rate of death and recurrent PE by

- Dissolving much of the anatomically obstructing pulmonary arterial Thrombus
- Preventing the continued release of serotonin and other neurohumoral factors that exacerbate pulmonary hypertension and
- Lysing much of the source of the thrombus in the pelvic or deep leg veins, thereby decreasing the likelihood of recurrent PE.

The preferred fibrinolytic regimen is 100 mg of recombinant tissue plasminogen activator (tPA) administered as a continuous peripheral intravenous infusion over 2 hours. The sooner thrombolysis is administered, the more effective it is. However, this approach can be used for at least 14 days after the PE has occurred. Contraindications to fibrinolysis include intracranial disease, recent surgery and trauma. The overall major bleeding rate is about 10%, including a 1–3% risk of intracranial hemorrhage. Careful screening of patients for contraindications to fibrinolytic therapy.

Inferior Vena Caval (IVC) Filters

The two principal indications for insertion of an IVC filter are

- Active bleeding that precludes anticoagulation and
- Recurrent venous thrombosis despite intensive anticoagulation.

Prevention of recurrent PE in patients with right heart failure who are not candidates for fibrinolysis and prophylaxis of extremely high-risk patients are "softer" indications for filter placement

Pulmonary Embolectomy

The risk of major hemorrhage with systemically administered fibrinolysis has prompted a renaissance of interest in surgical embolectomy, an operation that had almost become extinct.

102. Ans. (b) The patient should be asked to take deep breaths

Ref: Macleod clinical examination 13th ed page 111, Alagappan Manual of practical medicine 4th ed page 195

This question is a trap. In normal individual the sytolic B.P. drops by 2-4 mm Hg with normal inspiration and up to 10 mm Hg during deep inspiration so you should not tell the patient to take deep breaths. This is a common practical question asked during MD exams. Rest of the options are Hoax

- A more than 10 mm Hg fall in systolic pressure with inspiration (pulsus paradoxus) is considered pathologic and a sign of pericardial or pulmonary disease and can also occur in obesity and pregnancy without clinical disease.
- Pulsus paradoxus is measured by noting the difference between the systolic pressure at which the Korotkoff sounds are first heard (during expiration) and the systolic pressure at which the Korotkoff sounds are heard with each beat, independent of respiratory phase. Between these two pressures, the sounds are heard only intermittently (during expiration).
- The cuff pressure must be decreased slowly to appreciate the finding. Tachycardia, AF and tachypnea make its assessment difficult.
- Pulsus paradoxus may be palpable when the pressure difference exceeds 15 to 20 mm Hg.
- Pulsus paradoxus is not specific for pericardial tamponade and can accompany massive pulmonary embolus, hemorrhagic shock, severe obstructive lung disease, or tension pneumothorax.

103. Ans. (a) IV fluids

Ref: Harrison 19th ed page 2481

See table of "Therapies for Severe Hypercalcemia" in Medicine AIIMS Nov 2016 (see page no. 754)

Humoral Hypercalcemia of Malignancy

- The management of HHM begins with removal of excess calcium in the diet, medications, or IV solutions. Saline rehydration (typically 200–500 mL/h) is used to dilute serum calcium and promote calciuresis; exercise caution in patients with cardiac, hepatic, or renal insufficiency.
- Forced diuresis with furosemide (20–80 mg IV in escalating doses) or other loop diuretics can enhance calcium excretion but provides relatively little value except in life-threatening hypercalcemia.
- When used, loop diuretics should be administered only after complete rehydration and with careful monitoring of fluid balance.
- Oral phosphorus (e.g., 250 mg Neutra-Phos 3–4 times daily) should be given until serum phosphorus is >1 mmol/L (>3 mg/dL). Bisphosphonates such as pamidronate (60–90 mg IV), zoledronate (4–8 mg IV) and etidronate (7.5 mg/kg per day PO for 3–7 consecutive days) can reduce serum calcium within 1–2 days and suppress calcium release for several weeks.
- Bisphosphonate infusions can be repeated, or oral bisphosphonates can be used for chronic treatment. Dialysis should be considered in severe hypercalcemia when saline hydration and bisphosphonate treatments are not possible or are too slow in onset.
- Previously used agents such as calcitonin and mithramycin have little utility now that bisphosphonates are available. Calcitonin (2–8 U/kg SC every 6–12 hours) should be considered when rapid correction of severe hypercalcemia is needed. Hypercalcemia associated with lymphomas, multiple myeloma, or leukemia may respond to glucocorticoid treatment (e.g., prednisone 40–100 mg PO in four divided doses).

104. Ans. (d) The needle is inserted at L1-L2 intervertebral space

Ref: Harrison 19th edition page 443e-2

Option (A) True

The needle is inserted at a slightly cephalad angle 15°.

Option (B) True

According to Miller's 8th Ed Pg 1712: The incidence of post dural puncture headache is less when the **needle bevel is placed in the long axis of the neuraxis, parallel to dural fibres**- i.e, bevel faces laterally in sitting position, while it faces upwards in lateral position.

Option (C) True

The opening pressure of the cerebrospinal fluid (CSF) is recorded while the patient is reclining with the legs extended, the neck straight and the head at the same level as the spine and breathing normally (not during Valsalva maneuver or breath holding) **(Ref: Blueprints Neurology By Frank W. Drislane 4th ed Page 8)**

Option (D)

False: The needle is inserted at L3-L4 intervertebral space (Not L1-L2)

Lumbar Puncture

Indications:

- For the diagnosis of various types of Meningitis.
- C S F pressure study
- Spinal anesthesia
- Myelography
- Intrathecal administration of the drugs
- Sub-Arachnoid haemorrhage
- CNS Malignancy
- Demyelinating diseases
- Guillain-Barré syndrome
- Unexplained Coma

Precaution: Patients with an altered level of consciousness, a focal neurologic deficit, new-onset seizure, papilledema, or an immunocompromised state are at increased risk for potentially fatal cerebellar or tentorial herniation following LP. Neuroimaging should be obtained in these patients prior to LP to exclude a focal mass lesion or diffuse swelling

Contraindications:

Absolute contraindications: Patient refusal, patient's inability to maintain stillness during the needle puncture and raised intracranial pressure, which may theoretically predispose to brainstem herniation.

Relative contraindications: Intrinsic and idiopathic coagulopathy, skin or soft tissue infection at the proposed site of needle insertion, severe hypovolemia; and lack of anesthesiologist experience.

Legal contraindication: The often-cited relative contraindication of preexisting neurologic disease (e.g., lower extremity peripheral neuropathy) is not usually based on medical criteria but rather on legal considerations

Complications:

- CSF leakage
- Infections
- Injury to spinal cord, paralysis
- Patients with coagulation defects including thrombocytopenia are at increased risk of post-LP spinal subdural or epidural hematomas,either of which can produce permanent nerve injury and/or paralysis.

Patient positioning:

- **The lateral decubitus** position is the most commonly used because it allows easier administration, less dependent on assistant and allow more accurate measurement of the opening pressure.
- **The sitting position** when low lumbar and sacral levels of sensory anesthesia are adequate for the surgical procedure (perineal and urologic operations), or when obesity or scoliosis makes identification of midline anatomy difficult in the lateral position
- **The prone position** should be chosen when the patient is to be maintained in that position during the surgical procedure (rectal, perineal, or lumbar procedures)

The procedure should be performed on a firm surface; if the procedure is to be performed at the bedside, the patient should be positioned at the edge of the bed and not in the middle. The patient is asked to lie on his or her side, facing away from the examiner and to "roll up into a ball." The neck is gently anteflexed and the thighs pulled up toward the abdomen; the shoulders and pelvis should be vertically aligned without forward or backward tilt.

Site of puncture: The spinal cord terminates at approximately the L1 in adults and L3 in infacts Although the spinal cord ends at the lower border of L1 in adults, the subarachnoid space continues to S2. LP is therefore performed at or below the ***L3–L4 interspace.*** A useful anatomic guide is a line drawn between the posterior superior iliac crests, which corresponds closely to the level of the L3–L4 interspace. The interspace is chosen following gentle palpation to identify the spinous processes at each lumbar level. A line joining both iliac crests **(Tuffier's line)** passes across the spine of L4 and is a reliable landmark for locating the **L3/4 interspace**, which is usually easily defined and is the one most often used. or sometimes the L4-5 space.

Note: The incidence of post dural puncture headache is less when the **needle bevel is placed in the long axis of the neuraxis, parallel to dural fibres**- i.e, bevel faces laterally in sitting position, while it faces upwards in lateral position.

Procedure: Sterilize the skin over the lumbar spine and raise a skin weal with lidocaine 1% over the appropriate interspace. Inject 2–3 ml more lidocaine into the subcutaneous tissue. Insert the needle or introducer in the midline in slightly cephalad angle (15 degrees) Feedback from the needle tip will monitor the progress of the needle through the supraspinous and interspinous ligaments, the ligamentum flavum and sometimes the dura mater. If bone is contacted, withdraw the needle to the subcutaneous tissue and redirect slightly cephalad in the first instance. Puncture of the dura is usually obvious and when the stylet is removed CSF should flow freely.

The first snap or giveway or loss of resistance is seen after puncture of ligamentum flavum. This first loss of resistance is used for identifying epidural space. When trying to put an epidural catheter, we do not go any further in. The second loss of resistance is due to puncture of the dura and is used for identifying the subarachnoid space. Once we feel the second giveway, we withdraw the stylet and look for CSF.

During lumbar puncture the needle passes through the following structures in that sequence

- Skin
- Subcutaneous tissue
- Supraspinatous ligament
- Interspinous ligament
- Ligamentum flavum (First snap/ loss of resistance)
- Dura matter
- Arachnoid matter
- Subarachnoid space (Target)

Contd...

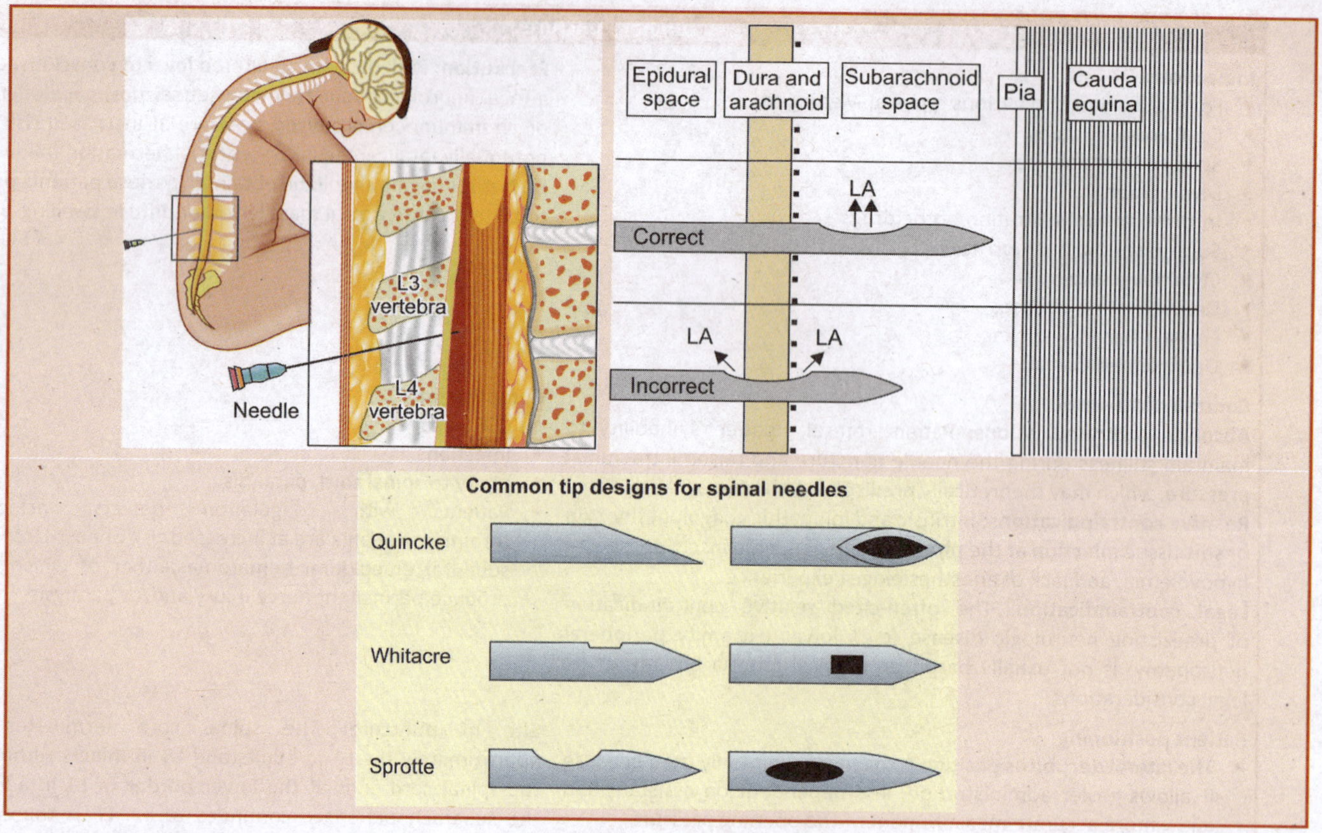

105. Ans. (b) ALA in urine

Ref: Harrison 19th edition 472-e, Rapid Review Biochemistry By John W. Pelley, Edward F. Goljan 3rd ed Page 109

Glass blowers and painters are most likely to suffer from heavy metal poisoning, mist likely Lead poisoning.

Lead Poisoning Lead inhibits two steps in the heme synthetic pathway: ALA dehydratase and ferrochelatase. Consequently, the substrates of these two enzymes, ALA and protoporphyrin accumulate in lead poisoning. Urinary measurement of ALA is a sensitive measure of lead poisoning. Whole blood (Not serum) Lead levels are diagnostic test of Lead poisoning, However Urinary ALA levels can be used as screening

An increased level of urinary delta-ALA may indicate:

- Lead poisoning

Porphyria (Several Types)

Lead Poisoning				
Main sources	**Metabolism**	**Toxicity**	**Diagnosis**	**Treatment**
Automobile batteries, lead crystal, ceramics, lead paint, glass making, plumbing, soldering; environmental exposure to paint chips, firing ranges (from bullet dust), food or water from improperly glazed ceramics, lead pipes; contaminated herbal remedies, candies; exposure to the combustion of leaded fuels.	Absorbed through ingestion or inhalation; organic lead (e.g., **tetraethyl lead**). 95–99% sequestered in RBCs—thus measure lead in whole blood (not serum). Distributed widely in soft tissue, with half- life- 30 days; 15% of dose sequestered in bone with half-life of >20 years. Excreted mostly in urine, ***Interferes with mitochondrial oxidative phosphorylation, ATPases, calcium-dependent messengers***; enhances oxidation & cell apoptosis.	Anemia; mental retardation; and deficits in language, motor function, balance, hearing, behavior, peripheral neuropathy (mainly motor), hypertension, ECG conduction delays, interstitial nephritis and CRF, diminished sperm counts, spontaneous abortions.	Abdominal pain, irritability, lethargy, anorexia, anemia, Fanconi's syndrome, pyuria, azotemia in children with blood lead level (BPb) >80 μg/dL; may also see epiphyseal plate **"lead lines"** on long bone X-rays. Noticeable neurodevelopmental delays at BPb of 40–80 μg/dL; may also see symptoms associated with higher BPb levels. Physical exam may reveal a **"lead line"** at the gingiva-tooth border, pallor, wrist drop and cognitive dysfunction (e.g., declines on the mini-mental status exam); lab tests may reveal a **normocytic, normochromic anemia**, basophilic stippling, an **elevated blood protoporphyrin level** (free erythrocyte or zinc) and motor delays on nerve conduction.	Correction of exposure sources. In the highly exposed individual chelation is recommended with oral **DMSA (succimer);** if acutely toxic, hospitalization and IV or IM chelation with ethylenediamine tetraacetic acid calcium disodium **(CaEDTA)** may be required, with the addition of dimercaprol to prevent worsening of encephalopathy. Correction of dietary deficiencies in iron, calcium, magnesium and zinc will lower lead absorption and may also improve toxicity. Vitamin C is a weak but natural chelating agent. Calcium (1200 mg at bedtime)

106. Ans. (a) ALL

Ref: KDT 7th ed page 868

- L-asparaginase was introduced on the basis of a qualitative difference observed between normal cells and those from childhood lymphoblastic leukemia-the leukaemia cells are deficient in L-asparagine synthase and depend on the supply of L-asparagine from the medium.
- The enzyme L-asparaginase (from E. coli) degrades L-asparagine to L-aspartic acid, depriving leukaemic cells of an essential metabolite-may cause cell death. However, the clinical response to L-asparaginase has been disappointing.
- Though remission is induced in acute leukaemia, it is short lasting. Thus, it is now used when other drugs have failed to induce rernission. It is ineffective in solid tumours.
- Many of the typical adverse effects of anticancer drugs are not seen with L-asparaginase (no leucopenia, alopecia or mucosal damage); but it produces liver damage, pancreatitis and CNS symptoms (due to defective protein synthesis). Being a foreign protein, it produces allergic reactions in a significant percentage of patients

107. Ans. (c) Platelet count <40,000/mm³ is a contraindication

Ref: Manual of Practical medicine By R Alagappan 4th ed page 810

Bone marrow biopsy needle was asked for identification in AIIMS NOV 2015 and now they have asked about the procedure.

Option (A)

True. Bone marrow aspiration from Iliac crest can be done in lateral and Prone position.

Option (B)

True: A variety of infiltrative (myelophthisic) processes including granulomatous and metastatic deposits may be (Ref: API Textbook of Medicine 9th Ed page 925)

Option (C)

The contraindications of splenic aspiration are INR more than 2.5 and platelet count 40,000/mm³. Bone marrow aspiration is usually without any risk. However if platelet count is <20,000/mm³ sternal puncture is avoided. (Ref: IAP Textbook of Pediatrics By A Parthasarathy Page 265, Paniker 7th ed page 56)

The only absolute contraindications to performing a bone marrow biopsy are the presence of severe hemophilia, severe disseminated intravascular coagulopathy, or other related severe bleeding disorders. Thrombocytopenia, regardless of severity, is not a contraindication. However, depending on the circumstances, platelet transfusion to insure a platelet count >20,000/microL may be warranted prior to the procedure (Harrison, Uptodate)

Option (D)

True: Breath holding is not required in Bone marrow aspiration.

Bone Marrow Biopsy Needle

There are 3 types of needles that can be used. They have a stylet and the length of the needle to be inserted into the marrow cavity can be adjusted with the use of a guard.

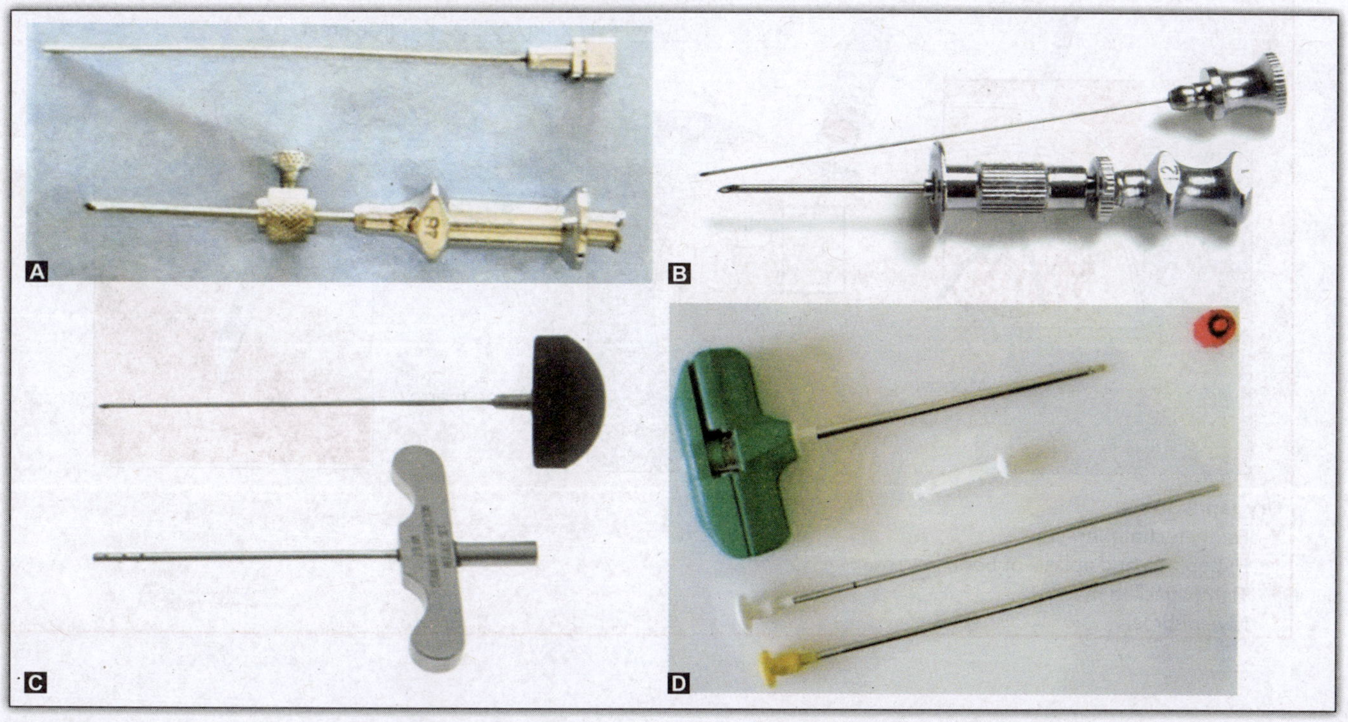

Figs A to D: A. Salah's needle; with side screw; **B.** Klima needle; with central screw, Mostly used for Sternal puncture; **C.** Islam Bone marrow aspiration/ trephine needle: Dome shaped handle and T bar for stability and control; **D.** Modern Jamshidi bone aspiration/ trephine needle

Trephine Biopsy

- Simpler than aspiration
- Can be done in outpatient or bedside
- Valuable in case of previous dry tap

Bone Marrow Biopsy

- Indications:
- Aplastic anemia and Myelosclerosis
- Megaloblastic anemia
- Leukemia
- Storage diseases
- Tumours –primary/ Secondaries
- Multiple myeloma
- Parasitic diseases e.g. Malaria, Leishmania
- Iron content study
- Bone marrow transplantation

Contraindications:

- Deep penetration of bone leading to Injury to Aorta
- Haemorrhage
- Infection
- Shock

Complications:

Bone marrow aspiration is usually without any risk. However if platelet count is < 20,000/mm^3 sternal puncture is avoided.

Site: The procedure can be done at any one of the following sites.

- Sternal body or manubrium
- Posterior iliac crest
- Tibia (medial aspect just below the tibial tubercle)
- Spinous process of vertebra
- Site of bone infiltration or tumour.

Note: The posterior iliac crest and tibia are the preferred sites in children.

Procedure: Under strict aseptic precautions.

- Local anaesthesia is infiltrated from the skin upto the periosteum
- **Position:** For iliac crest both lateral and Prone (face down) position can be done
- First the guard of the needle is adjusted so that only a further 5 mm can be advanced into the marrow. The bone marrow needle is then pushed into the skin, subcutaneous tissues up to the periosteum.
- The needle is advanced into the periosteum at right angles and a clockwise counter clock wise motion until a sensation of decreased resistance is felt when the marrow cavity is entered. The stylet is removed, a 10 or 20 mL syringe is attached to the needle and with sharp suction up to 0.5 mL of marrow is aspirated into the syringe to avoid mixing with peripheral blood. While aspirating, patient experiences an intense suction pain indicating the needle is in the marrow
- A drop of aspirate is placed on the slides to get a pure bone marrow smear.

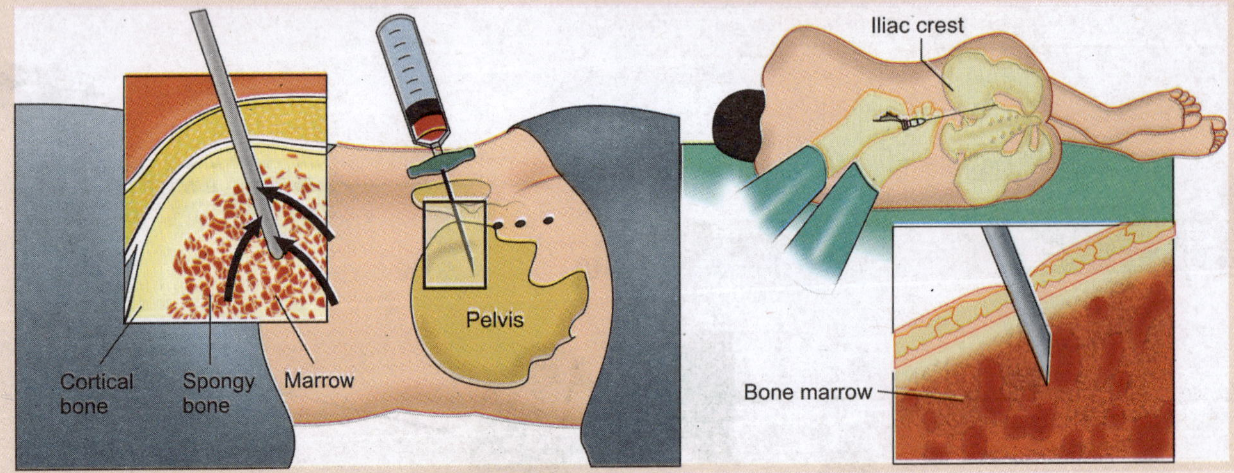

Dry Tap

- Faulty technique
- Hypoplasia and aplasia of bone marrow
- Tightly packed marrow
- Myelofibrosis

AIIMS NOVEMBER 2015

108. Ans. (a) Bone marrow biopsy needle

Ref: Manual of Practical medicine By R Alagappan 4th ed page 810

See details of bone marrow biopsy needle in Previous Question AIIMS May 2016 General Medicine (see page no. 777)

109. Ans. (c) Wegener's granulomatosis, ANCA and evaluate for vasculitis

Ref: Harrison 19th ed page 2182, Robbins 9th ed page 511

This patient presenting with chronoic sinusitis, nasopharygeal ulcers, glomerulonephritis, pneumonitis and purpura pointing towards a vasculties. Clinical presentation is classical of Wegner's.

Granulomatosis with polyangiitis (Wegener's) is a distinct clinicopathologic entity characterized by granulomatous vasculitis of the upper and lower respiratory tracts together with glomerulonephritis. In addition, variable degrees of disseminated vasculitis involving both small arteries and veins may occur.

Pathology and Pathogenesis

- The histopathologic hallmarks of granulomatosis with polyangiitis (Wegener's) are necrotizing vasculitis of small arteries and veins together with granuloma formation, which may be either intravascular or extravascular.
- Lung involvement typically appears as multiple, bilateral, nodular cavitary infiltrates, which on biopsy almost invariably reveal the typical necrotizing granulomatous vasculitis.
- Upper airway lesions, particularly those in the sinuses and nasopharynx, typically reveal inflammation, necrosis and granuloma formation, with or without vasculitis. In its earliest form, renal involvement is characterized by a focal and segmental glomerulitis that may evolve into a rapidly progressive crescentic glomerulonephritis.
- Granuloma formation is only rarely seen on renal biopsy. In contrast to other forms of glomerulonephritis, evidence of immune complex deposition is not found in the renal lesion of granulomatosis with polyangiitis (Wegener's).
- In addition to the classic triad of disease of the upper and lower respiratory tracts and kidney, virtually any organ can be involved with vasculitis, granuloma, or both.
- The immunopathogenesis of this disease is unclear, although the involvement of upper airways and lungs with granulomatous vasculitis suggests an aberrant cell-mediated immune response to an exogenous or even endogenous antigen that enters through or resides in the upper airway.
- Chronic nasal carriage of *Staphylococcus aureus* has been reported to be associated with a higher relapse rate of granulomatosis with polyangiitis (Wegener's); however, there is no evidence for a role of this organism in the pathogenesis of the disease.

Kidney: Glomerulonephritis

Ear/nose/throat: Sinusitis, Nasal disease, Otitis media, Hearing loss, Subglottic stenosis, Ear pain, Oral lesions

Lung, Pulmonary infiltrates, Pulmonary nodules, Hemoptysis, Pleuritis

Eyes: Conjunctivitis, Dacryocystitis, Scleritis, Proptosis, Eye pain, Visual loss, Retinal lesions, Corneal lesions, Iritis

Clinical and Laboratory Manifestations/Diagnosis

- The diagnosis of granulomatosis with polyangiitis (Wegener's) is made by the demonstration of necrotizing granulomatous vasculitis on tissue biopsy in a patient with compatible clinical features.
- Pulmonary tissue offers the highest diagnostic yield, almost invariably revealing granulomatous vasculitis.
- Biopsy of upper airway tissue usually reveals granulomatous inflammation with necrosis but may not show vasculitis. Renal biopsy can confirm the presence of pauci-immune glomerulonephritis.
- The specificity of a positive antiproteinase-3 ANCA for granulomatosis with polyangiitis (Wegener's) is very high, especially if active glomerulonephritis is present. However, the presence of ANCA should be adjunctive and, with rare exceptions, should not substitute for a tissue diagnosis.
- False-positive ANCA titers have been reported in certain infectious and neoplastic diseases.

110. Ans. (a) Patient is chronic alcoholic

Ref: Guidelines on the management of latent tuberculosis infection by WHO 2015, http://apps.who.int/iris/bitstream/10665/136471/1/9789241548908_eng. df?ua=1&ua=

Systematic Testing and Treatment of Ltbi (Latent Tb Infection)

Should be performed in	Should be considered	Not recommended
• People living with HIV • Adult and child contacts of pulmonary TB cases • Patients initiating anti-tumour necrosis factor (TNF) treatment • Patients receiving dialysis • Patients preparing for organ or haematologic transplantation • Patients with silicosis.	• Prisoners • Health workers • Immigrants from high TB burden countries • Homeless persons and illicit drug users.	• Diabetes • People with harmful alcohol use • Tobacco smokers • Underweight people provided they are not already included in the above recommendations

- Either interferon-gamma release assays (IGRA) or Mantoux tuberculin skin test (TST) should be used to test for LTBI.
- Treatment options recommended for LTBI include: 6-month isoniazid, or 9-month isoniazid, or 3-month regimen of weekly rifapentine plus isoniazid, or 3–4 months isoniazid plus rifampicin, or 3–4 months rifampicin alone. (Strong recommendation, moderate to high quality of evidence).

111. Ans. (c) Kaposi sarcoma

Ref: Harrison 19th ed page 1268

NOTE

The examiner is probable trying to ask about the cancer where Glucocorticoids are not used as a curative agent. Because glucocorticoids are used in palliative treatment of Metastatic lung cancer, Metastatic bladder cancer, Mesothelioma and Kaposi's sarcoma, along with chemotherapy to prevent skin rashes and to Blunt hypersensitivity (Ref: Glucocorticoid Signaling: From Molecules to Man edited by Jen-Chywan Wang, PhD, Charles Harris, MD, PhD page 327 table 1.1)

Kaposi's sarcoma is a multicentric neoplasm consisting of multiple vascular nodules appearing in the skin, mucous membranes and viscera. The course ranges from indolent, with only minor skin or lymph node involvement, to fulminant, with extensive cutaneous and visceral involvement.

Management of AIDS-Associated Kaposi's Sarcoma

- Observation and optimization of antiretroviral therapy
- Single or limited number of lesion
- Radiation
- Intralesional vinblastine
- Cryotherapy

Extensive Disease

- Initial therapy
- Interferon α (if CD4+ T cells >150/L)
- Liposomal daunorubicin

Subsequent Therapy

- Liposomal doxorubicin
- Paclitaxel
- Combination chemotherapy with low-dose doxorubicin, bleomycin and vinblastine (ABV)
- Targeted radiation

112. Ans. (a) Hyperkalemia

Ref: Harrison 19th ed page 2325

Sign and Symptoms of Glucocorticoid Deficiency	Signs and Symptoms of Mineralocorticoid Deficiency	Sign and Symptoms of Adrenal Androgen Deficiency
• Fatigue, lack of energy • Weight loss, Anorexia • Myalgia, Joint pain • Fever • Normochromic anemia, lymphocytosis, eoisnophilia • Slightly increased TSH • Hypoglycemia • Low blood presure, postural hypotension • Hyponatremia (due to loss of feedback inhibition of AVP release	• Abdominal pain, nausea, vomiting • Dizziness, postural hypotension • Salt craving • Low blood pressure, postural hypotension • Increased serum creatinine • Hyponatremia • Hyperkalemia	• Lack of energy • Dry and itchy skin (in women) • Loss of libido • Loss of axillary and pubic hair (in women)

113. Ans. (a) Asterixis

Ref: Harrison 19th ed page 1782, Nelson 17th ed table 361.1

- Encephalopathy is characterized by day–night reversal, asterixis, tremor, dysarthria, delirium, drowsiness and ultimately coma also occurs late except when precipitated by an acute hepatocellular insult or an episode of gastrointestinal bleeding
- Asterixis is a disorder of motor control characterized by irregular myoclonic lapses of posture affecting various parts of the body independently. These lapses are caused by involuntary 50- to 200-msec silent periods appearing in muscles (even antagonistic groups of muscles) which are tonically active. That is, the silent periods and postural lapses occur in muscles that have been contracting for a time whether or not there has been slow shortening or lengthening but probably do not occur during or immediately after a sudden movement at a joint. What constitutes a sudden as opposed to a slow movement remains to be defined.
- **When bilateral asterixis is present, one cannot rule out the possibility of a focal lesion, but it is almost always due to a metabolic encephalopathy (with a wide variety of possible causes).** Unilateral asterixis is due to a localized lesion, perhaps otherwise not clinically evident, in the contralateral cerebral hemisphere.
- This episodic dysfunction within neural circuits which are normally concerned with maintenance of sustained

or tonic muscle contraction may be released by focal lesions only in specific CNS areas (such as ventrolateral thalamus) or by a more generalized neurochemical imbalance (metabolic encephalopathies of various kinds). The system, a lesion or metabolic dysfunction which produces asterixis, is presumably an anatomically and/or pharmacologically distinct one.

Stages of Hepatic Encephalopathy				
	Stage I	Stage II	Stage III	Stage IV
Symptoms	Periods of lethargy, euphoria; reversal of day-night sleeping; may be alert	Drowsiness, inappropriate behavior, agitation, wide mood swings, disorientation	Stupor but arousable, confused, incoherent speech	Coma IVa responds to noxious stimuli IVb no response
Signs	Trouble drawing figures, performing mental tasks	Asterixis fetor hepaticus, incontinence	Asterixis, hyperreflexia, extensor reflexes, rigidity	Areflexia, no Asterixis, flaccidity
EEG	Normal	Generalized slowing, ϴ waves	Markedly abnormal, triphasic waves	Markedly abnormal bilateral slowing, δ waves, electric-cortical silence

114. Ans. (b) Thrombolytics

Ref: Harrison 19th ed page 1605

The ECG represents Posterior and inferior wall MI

Similar question was asked in Medicine AIIMS MAY 2016 (See for details of STEMI MANAGEMENT)

Primary percutaneous coronary intervention (PCI) is the preferred reperfusion strategy for most patients with acute ST elevation myocardial infarction (STEMI). When timely primary PCI is not available, early fibrinolysis should be carried out.

For localization of Myocardial infarction remember this simple chart. Clearly in our case the ST elevation is seen in Lead II, III and aVF; Hence Inferior wall MI

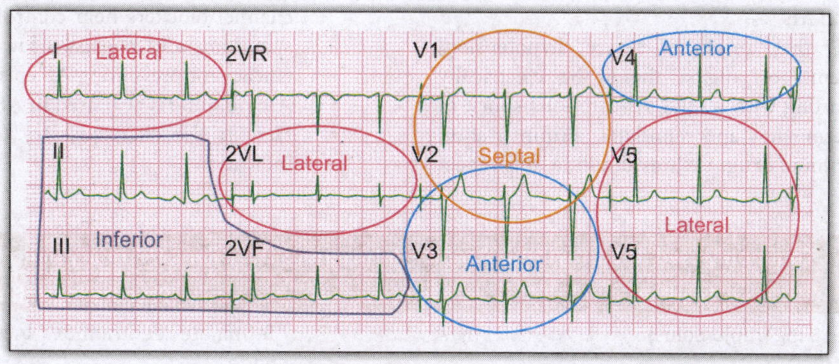

115. Ans. (c) Atrial fibrillation

Ref: Harrison 19th ed page 2090

In this ECG you can eaily make out there is fine or absent p wave with a varying RR interval. Pulse is irregularly irregular suggestive of atrial fibrillation.

Atrial fibrillation (AF) is characterized by disorganized, rapid and irregular atrial activation with loss of atrial contraction and with an irregular ventricular rate that is determined by AV nodal conduction.

AF is associated with the following changes on ECG

- Lack of discrete P waves
- Fibrillatory or f waves are present at a rate that is generally between 350 and 600 beats/minute; the f waves vary continuously in amplitude, morphology and intervals.
- Ventricular response follows no repetitive pattern; the variability in the intervals between QRS complexes is often termed "irregularly irregular."
- The ventricular rate (especially in the absence of AV nodal blocking agents or intrinsic conduction disease) usually ranges between 90 to 170 beats/min.

The QRS complexes are narrow unless AV conduction through the His Purkinje system is abnormal due to functional (rate-related) aberration, pre-existing bundle branch or fascicular block, or ventricular preexcitation with conduction down the accessory pathway.

Atrial Fibrillation

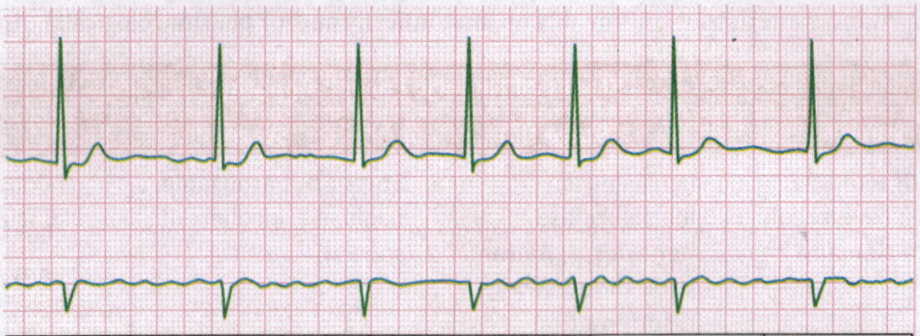

Heart rate	Rhythm	P wave	PR interval (in seconds)	QRS (in seconds)
A: 350–650 bpm V: Slow to rapid	Irregular	Fibrillatory (fine to course)	N/A	<.12

116. Ans. (b) Adenosine

Ref: Harrison's 19th edition page 1487 -1488

The ECG represents Atrial fibrilation. See previous question for details of ECG og AF. Adenosine is used in SVT/PSVT not Atrial fibrillation.

- Treatment for AF is primarily guided by patients' symptoms, the hemodynamic effect of AF, the duration of AF if there are persistent risk factors for stroke and underlying heart disease. Oral anticoagulation in high-risk patients with AF.
- New-onset AF that produces severe hypotension, pulmonary edema, or angina should be electrically cardioverted starting with a QRS synchronous shock of 200 J, If AF terminates and reinitiates, administration of an antiarrhythmic drug, such as ibutilide and repeat cardioversion may be considered. Acute rate control can be achieved with beta blockers and/or the calcium channel blockers verapamil and diltiazem administered either intravenously or orally Digoxin may be added, particularly in heart failure.
- Patients who remain in AF chronically, the goal of rate control is to alleviate and prevent symptoms and prevent deterioration of ventricular function from excessive rates. β-Adrenergic blockers, calcium channel blockers and digoxin are used. β-Adrenergic blockers and calcium channel blockers help control ventricular rate, improve symptoms and possess a low-risk profile, but have low efficacy for preventing AF episodes.
- Amiodarone is also used in AF.
- Here is the chart just try to remember the primary indication

Commonly used Antiarrhythmic Agents—Intravenous Dose Range/Primary Indication

Drug	Loading	Maintenance	Primary indication	Class
Adenosine	6–18 mg (rapid bolus)	N/A	Terminate reentrant SVT involving AV node	—
Amiodarone	15 mg/min for 10 min, 1 mg/min for 6 h	0.5–1 mg/min	AF, AFL, SVT, VT/VF	III
Digoxin	0.25 mg q2h until 1 mg total	0.125–0.25 mg/d	AF/AFL rate control	—
Diltiazem	0.25 mg/kg over 3–5 min (max 20 mg)	5–15 mg/h	SVT, AF/AFL rate control	IV
Esmolol	500 μg/kg over 1 min	50 μg/kg per min	AF/AFL rate control	II
Ibutilide	1 mg over 10 minutes if over 60 kg	N/A	Terminate AF/AFL	III
Lidocaine	1–3 mg/kg at 20–50 mg/min	1–4 mg/min	VT	IB
Metoprolol	5 mg over 3–5 min x 3 doses	1.25–5 mg q6h	SVT, AF rate control; exercise-induced VT; long QT	II
Procainamide	15 mg/kg over 60 minutes	1–4 mg/min	Convert/prevent AF/VT	IA
Quinidine	6–10 mg/kg at 0.3–0.5 mg/kg/min	N/A	Convert/prevent AF/VT	IA
Verapamil	5–10 mg over 3–5 minutes	2.5–10 mg/h	SVT, AF rate control	IV

117. Ans. (d) Interstitial fibrosis

Ref: Ganong 25th ed page 629

Repeat AIIMS Nov 2018 Medicine (see page no. 709)

118. Ans. (b) Breath sounds

Ref: Harrison 19th ed page 1573, 1719

Breath sounds is absent in pneumothorax but it is present in cardiac tamponade. JVP is elevated in pneumothorax and cardiac tamponade as well. Pulsus paradoxus is classical seen in cardiac tamponade but also in pneumothorax cardiac tamponade and pneumothorax both can have low volume pulse.

Cardiac Tamponade

- The accumulation of fluid in the pericardial space in a quantity sufficient to cause serious obstruction to the inflow of blood to the ventricles results in cardiac tamponade.
- The three most common causes of tamponade are neoplastic disease, idiopathic pericarditis and renal failure.
- Tamponade may also result from bleeding into the pericardial space after cardiac operations, trauma and treatment of patients with acute pericarditis with anticoagulants.
- The three principal features of tamponade (Beck's triad) are hypotension, soft or absent heart sounds and jugular venous distention with a prominent x descent but an absent y descent.

Pneumothorax

- Characteristic physical findings of a large pneumothorax include decreased chest excursion, diminished breath sounds, absent fremitus and hyperresonance to percussion on the affected side.
- Subcutaneous emphysema may be present. Labored breathing and hemodynamic compromise (e.g. tachycardia, hypotension) may suggest a possible tension pneumothorax, which necessitates emergency decompression.
- Tracheal deviation from the midline is a rare and typically late finding in pneumothorax.
- Systemic blood pressure is not constant but varies slightly from heart beat to heart beat and between inspiration and expiration.
- Normally, the systolic blood pressure decreases by less than 10 mmHg during inspiration, but a decline of this magnitude is not detectable on examination of the peripheral pulse.
- Moderate to severe cardiac tamponade and occasionally constrictive pericarditis, induce hemodynamic changes that enhance the inspiratory fall in systolic blood pressure.
- This exaggerated drop in systemic blood pressure during inspiration is termed pulsus paradoxus. Pulsus paradoxus resulting from cardiac pathology, pulsus paradoxus can be seen in non-cardiac conditions, including
  - Asthma and chronic obstructive pulmonary disease
  - Obstructive sleep apnea
  - Tension pneumothorax
  - Pulmonary embolism
  - Right ventricular myocardial infarction
  - Bilateral pleural effusion
  - Restrictive cardiomyopathy
  - Marked obesity
  - Hypovolemic shock
  - Pectus excavatum
  - Extrinsic cardiac compression

AIIMS MAY 2015

119. Ans. (a) Human T-cell lymphotropic virus

Ref: Harrison 19th ed page 163, 697, 707

Human T-cell Lymphotropic Virus

Human T-lymphotropic virus (HTLV-I) is a retrovirus

Two well-recognized disease associations are caused by the virus:

- Adult T cell leukemia-lymphoma (ATL) and
- HTLV-I-associated myelopathy (HAM), also known as tropical spastic paraparesis (TSP) occurs after a shorter latency (1-3 years) and is most common in individuals who acquire the virus during adulthood from transfusion or sex.

Four Distinct Clinical forms of ATL are Recognized

- Acute
- Lymphomatous
- Chronic
- Smoldering

- HTLV-I associated myelopathy/tropical spastic paraparesis is characterized by an insidious onset of slowly progressive weakness and spasticity of one or both legs, together with hyperreflexia, ankle clonus, extensor plantar responses and lumbar pain.
- Other disease manifestations include neuropathy, infiltrative skin disorders, uveitis and rheumatologic and pulmonary disorders.
- The diagnosis of HTLV-I infection is generally based upon serologic testing with ELISA followed by a confirmatory Western blot test.
- No therapy is of proven benefit in HAM/TSP but corticosteroids may slow progression and reduce disability.

120. Ans. (c) Conduction aphasia

Ref: Harrison 19th ed 178 Dejong 7th Ed page 102

Speech output is fluent but contains many phonemic paraphasias, comprehension of spoken language is intact and repetition is severely impaired. Naming elicits phonemic paraphasias and spelling is impaired. Reading aloud is impaired, but reading comprehension is preserved. The lesion sites spare the functionality of Broca's and Wernicke's areas but may induce a disconnection between the two.

Clinical Features of Aphasias and Related Conditions					
Type of aphasia	**Etiology**	**Comprehension**	**Repetition of spoken language**	**Naming**	**Fluency**
Wernicke's (AKA- fluent or jargon aphasia) (Mnemonic: Wer-nicke is wordy but non sence)	Infarction of Wernicke's area due to inferior division of the middle cerebral artery	Impaired (without meaningful content)	Impaired (Mild to severe)	Impaired	Preserved or increased (paraphasic)
Broca's (Mnemonic: Broca is broken)	Infarction of Broca's area due to superior division of the middle cerebral artery	Preserved (except grammar)	Impaired (Mod to severe)	Impaired	Decreased, Non-fluent, effortful, slow
Global	Combined dysfunction of Broca's & Wernicke's areas from involvement of entire middle cerebral artery	Impaired	Impaired	Impaired	Decrease, non fluent
Conduction	Functional disconnection between Broca's & Wernicke's areas. Lesion is present in arcuate fasciculus, connection between Broca's & Wernecke's areas.	Preserve	Impaired	Impaired	Preserved, fluent
Nonfluent (motor) transcortical	Disconnects intact language network from prefrontal areas, involves anterior watershed zone between ACA & MCA or the supplementary motor cortex in the territory of ACA	Preserved	Preserved	Impaired	Impaired, nonfluent
Fluent (sensory) transcortical	Disconnects intact core of language network from other temporoparietal association areas. Involve temporoparietal cortex posterior to Wernicke's area (MC)	Impaired	Preserved	Impaired	Preserved, fluent
Isolation/Mixed transcortical (combination of the two transcortical aphasias)	Broca's & Wernicke's spared, but damage to surrounding frontal, parietal & temporal cortex due to anoxia, CO poisoning, or complete watershed zone infarct	Impaired	Echolalia	Impaired	No purposeful speech, non fluent
Anomic (single MC language disturbance in head trauma, metabolic encephalopathy, & Alzheimer)	Lesion sites can be anywhere within Lt hemisphere language network, including the middle and inferior temporal gyri	Preserved	Preserved	Impaired	Preserved except for word-finding pauses
Pure word deafness A.K.A Auditory verbal agnosia (AVA)	B/L or Lt-MCA strokes affecting the superior temporal gyrus interrupting the flow of information from the auditory association cortex to Wernicke's area.	Impaired only for spoken language	Impaired	Preserved	Preserved

Contd...

Clinical Features of Aphasias and Related Conditions					
Type of aphasia	**Etiology**	**Comprehension**	**Repetition of spoken language**	**Naming**	**Fluency**
Pure alexia usually have Rt hemianopia. Can understand & speak, name objects in Lt visual hemifield	Combination of damage to Lt occipital cortex & posterior sector of corpus callosum due to vascular lesion in PCA	Impaired only for reading	Preserved	Preserved	Preserved

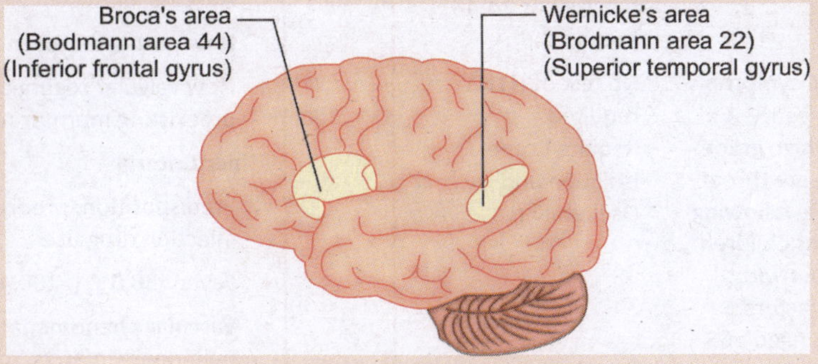

ACA = Anterior cerebral artery
MCA = Middle cerebral artery
PCA = Posterior cerebral artery

121. Ans. (b) Asthma

Ref: Harrison 19th ed page 1662

See table of Obstructive Vs Restrictive Lung Disease in Medicine AIIMS Nov 2016

A test of the diffusing capacity of the lungs for carbon monoxide (DLCO, also known as transfer factor for carbon monoxide or TLCO), is one of the most clinically valuable tests of lung function. The DLCO measures the ability of the lungs to transfer gas from inhaled air to the red blood cells in pulmonary capillaries.

Diffusing Capacity

- This test uses a small (and safe) amount of carbon monoxide to measure gas exchange across the alveolar membrane during a 10-second breath hold.
- Carbon monoxide in exhaled breath is analyzed to determine the quantity of CO absorbed by crossing the alveolar membrane and combining with hemoglobin in red blood cells.
- This "single-breath diffusing capacity" [diffusion capacity of the lung for carbon monoxide (DL_{CO})] value increases with the surface area available for diffusion and the amount of hemoglobin within the capillaries and varies inversely with alveolar membrane thickness.
- Thus, DL_{CO} decreases in diseases that thicken or destroy alveolar membranes (e.g., pulmonary fibrosis, emphysema), curtail the pulmonary vasculature (e.g., pulmonary hypertension), or reduce alveolar capillary hemoglobin (e.g., anemia).
- Single-breath diffusing capacity may be elevated in acute congestive heart failure, asthma, polycythemia and pulmonary hemorrhage

Increased DLCO: Disorders to consider when the DLCO is near or above the upper limit of the normal range include the following:

- Obesity
- Asthma
- High altitude
- Polycythemia
- Pulmonary hemorrhage
- Left-to-right intracardiac shunting
- Mild left heart failure (due to increased pulmonary capillary blood volume)
- Exercise just prior to the test session (due to increased cardiac output)
- Supine position; Mueller maneuver (inhalation against closed glottis decreases intrathoracic pressure and increases blood return to the lung

Clinical significance of DLCO

- Evaluation of emphysema
- Evaluation for presence of interstitial lung disease
- Monitoring of known interstitial lung disease
- Differential diagnosis of lung volume restriction
- Detection of pulmonary vascular disease
- Pulmonary disability/impairment

122. Ans. (a) Pregnant woman with sore throat can be started immediately on oseltamivir without diagnostic testing under category B

Ref: http://nrhmchd.gov.in/Disease_updates/H1N1_risk_guide 2015.pdf, Harrison 19th edition page 1210

Ministry of Health and Family Welfare Guidelines on categorization of Seasonal Influenza A H1N1 (Revised on 11.02.2015)	
Category	**Management**
Category A: Patients with mild fever plus cough/sore throat with or without bodyache, headache, diarrhoea and vomiting	No H1N1 testing required, No Oseltamivir required. Treat symptomatic, reassess at 24-48 hours
Category B: Signs and symptoms mentioned under Category-A plus: • If the patient has high grade fever and severe sore throat • One or more of the following high risk conditions Children with mild illness but with predisposing risk factors. Pregnant women, Aged >65 years or older, Patients with lung diseases, heart disease, liver disease kidney disease, blood disorders, diabetes, neurological disorders, cancer and HIV/AIDS, Patients on long term cortisone therapy.	No test of H1N1 required Require home isolation and Oseltamivir
Category C: Signs and symptoms of Category-A and B, Plus 1 or more of the following: Breathlessness, chest pain, drowsiness, fall in blood pressure, sputum mixed with blood, bluish discolouration of nails	Require testing, immediate hospitalization and treatment.

123. Ans. (a) Splenomegaly

Ref: Harrison 19th ed page 816

Modified Duke Criteria for Diagnosis of Infective Endocarditis

The Duke Criteria for the Clinical Diagnosis of Infective Endocarditis
Major Criteria
• Positive blood culture
Typical microorganism for infective endocarditis from two separate blood cultures
Viridans streptococci, *Streptococcus gallolyticus*, HACEK group, *Staphylococcus aureus*, or
Community-acquired enterococci in the absence of a primary focus, or
Persistently positive blood culture, defined as recovery of a microorganism consistent with infective endocarditis from:
Blood cultures drawn >12 hours apart; or
All of 3 or a majority of >4 separate blood cultures, with first and last drawn at least 1 hours apart
Single positive blood culture for *Coxiella burnetii* or phase I IgG antibody titer of >1:800
• Evidence of endocardial involvement
Positive echocardiogram[b]
Oscillating intracardiac mass on valve or supporting structures or in the path of regurgitant jets or in implanted material, in the absence of an alternative anatomic explanation, or
Abscess, or
New partial dehiscence of prosthetic valve, *or*
New valvular regurgitation (increase or change in preexisting murmur not sufficient)
Minor Criteria
• Predisposition: predisposing heart condition or injection drug use
• Fever >38.0°C (>100.4°F)
• Vascular phenomena: major arterial emboli, septic pulmonary infarcts, mycotic aneurysm, intracranial hemorrhage, conjunctival hemorrhages, Janeway lesions
• Immunologic phenomena: glomerulonephritis, Osler's nodes, Roth's spots, rheumatoid factor
• Microbiologic evidence: positive blood culture but not meeting major criterion as noted previously[c] or serologic evidence of active infection with organism consistent with infective endocarditis

124. Ans. (c) Cor pulmonale

Ref: Manual of practical medicine Alagappan 4th ed page 83

High Output States	
Systemic	Anaemia, pyrexia, beriberi, thyrotoxicosis, pheochromocytoma, arteriovenous fistula
Cardiac	Aortic regurgitation Patent ductus arteriosus High output cardiac failure
Volume	Hypovolemia, hypotension
Drugs	Atropine, Nifedipine, Beta Agonists—Salbutamol, Thyroxine, Catecholamines, Nicotine, Caffeine

125. Ans. (a) TSH

Ref: Harrison 19th ed page 2267

Galactorrhea

- *Galactorrhea*, the inappropriate discharge of milk-containing fluid from the breast, is considered abnormal if it persists longer than 6 months after childbirth or discontinuation of breast-feeding.
- Postpartum galactorrhea associated with amenorrhea is a self-limiting disorder usually associated with moderately elevated PRL levels.
- Galactorrhea may occur spontaneously, or it may be elicited by nipple pressure. In both men and women, galactorrhea

may vary in color and consistency (transparent, milky, or bloody) and arise either unilaterally or bilaterally.

- Mammography or ultrasound is indicated for bloody discharges (particularly from a single nipple), which may be caused by breast cancer.
- Galactorrhea is commonly associated with hyperprolactinemia.
- Acromegaly is associated with galactorrhea in about one-third of patients.
- Treatment of galactorrhea usually involves managing the underlying disorder (e.g., replacing T4 for hypothyroidism, discontinuing a medication, treating prolactinoma).

Laboratory Investigation

- Basal, fasting morning PRL levels (normally <20 μg/L) should be measured to assess hypersecretion. Both falsepositive and false-negative results may be encountered. In patients with markedly elevated PRL levels (>1000 μg/L), reported results may be falsely lowered because of assay artifacts; sample dilution is required to measure these high values accurately.
- Falsely elevated values may be caused by aggregated forms of circulating PRL, which are usually biologically inactive (macroprolactinemia).
- **Hypothyroidism should be excluded by measuring TSH and T4 levels**

126. Ans. (a) Start antithyroid drugs and do urgent MRI brain

Ref: Harrison 19th ed page 2298

TSH-producing macroadenomas are rare but are often large and locally invasive when they occur. Patients usually present with thyroid goiter and hyperthyroidism, reflecting overproduction of TSH. Diagnosis is based on demonstrating elevated serum free T4 levels, inappropriately normal or high TSH secretion and MRI evidence of a pituitary adenoma.

Treatment: TSH-Secreting Adenomas

- The initial therapeutic approach is to remove or debulk the tumor mass surgically, usually using a transsphenoidal approach.
- Total resection is not often achieved as most of these adenomas are large and locally invasive. Normal circulating thyroid hormone levels are achieved in about two-thirds of patients after surgery.
- Thyroid ablation or antithyroid drugs (methimazole and propylthiouracil) can be used to reduce thyroid hormone levels.
- Somatostatin analogue treatment effectively normalizes TSH and α subunit hypersecretion, shrinks the tumor mass in 50% of patients and improves visual fields in 75% of patients; euthyroidism is restored in most patients.
- Because somatostatin analogues markedly suppress TSH, biochemical hypothyroidism often requires concomitant thyroid hormone replacement, which may also further control tumor growth.
- *TSH-secreting pituitary adenoma* is a rare cause of thyrotoxicosis. It can be identified by the presence of an inappropriately normal or increased TSH level in a patient with hyperthyroidism, diffuse goiter and elevated T4 and T_3 levels.
- Elevated levels of the α-subunit of TSH, released by the TSH-secreting adenoma, support this diagnosis, which can be confirmed by demonstrating the pituitary tumor on MRI or CT scan.
- A combination of transsphenoidal surgery, sella irradiation and octreotide may be required to normalize TSH, because many of these tumors are large and locally invasive at the time of diagnosis. Radioiodine or antithyroid drugs can be used to control thyrotoxicosis

127. Ans. (d) Airway, CT scan, Blood sugar if <70 start dextrose

Ref: Harrison 19th ed page 457e

ABCs and C-Spine

- The unconscious patient's airway, breathing and circulation should be quickly assessed and concurrently treated (see the Airway, Ventilation and Sedation protocol).
- Ensuring patency of the airway is an overriding initial priority to allow oxygenation and ventilation. The patient's cervical spine should be immobilized if there is a possibility of injury.
- A rapid initial survey should follow, looking for injury or other notable physical findings of the head and neck, chest, abdomen and extremities.
- Intravenous (IV) access should be established quickly. Bedside blood glucose testing should be performed in all unconscious patients.
- If the blood glucose is <70 mg/dL, 50 mL of 50% dextrose should be administered intravenously. Thiamine (100 mg) should be given intravenously with the dextrose in patients at risk for nutritional deficiency (e.g., chronic ethanol users, bariatric surgery patients, with malabsorption states).
- If there is clinical suspicion of opioid toxicity (e.g., history of illicit drug use, apnea or bradypnea, small pupils), naloxone 0.4–2 mg IV should be administered and repeated as needed, up to 4 mg. Other antidotes, such as physostigmine, may be administered for anticholinergic toxicity in selected patient.
- Patients who are comatose from the moment of injury require immediate neurologic attention and resuscitation.
- After intubation, with care taken to immobilize the cervical spine, the depth of coma, pupillary size and reactivity, limb movements and Babinski responses are assessed.
- As soon as vital functions permit and cervical spine X-rays and a CT scan have been obtained, the patient should be transported to a critical care unit.
- Hypoxia should be reversed and normal saline used as the resuscitation fluid in preference to albumin.

128. Ans. (a) Basal ganglia

Ref: Harrison 19th ed page 2582

Causes of Intracranial Hemorrhage

Hypertensive ICH usually results from spontaneous rupture of a small penetrating artery deep in the brain.

- The most common sites are the basal ganglia (especially the putamen), thalamus, cerebellum and pons.

- The small arteries in these areas seem most prone to hypertension-induced vascular injury.
- When hemorrhages occur in other brain areas or in nonhypertensive patients, greater consideration should be given to other causes such as hemorrhagic disorders, neoplasms, vascular malformations and cerebral amyloid angiopathy.
- The hemorrhage may be small, or a large clot may form and compress adjacent tissue, causing herniation and death. Blood may also dissect into the ventricular space, which substantially increases morbidity and may cause hydrocephalus.

Causes of Intracranial Hemorrhages

Cause	Location
Head trauma	Intraparenchymal: frontal lobes, anterior temporal lobes; subarachnoid
Hypertensive hemorrhage	Putamen, globus pallidus, thalamus, cerebellar hemisphere, pons
Transformation of prior ischemic infarction	Basal ganglion, subcortical regions, lobar
Metastatic brain tumor	Lobar
Coagulopathy	Any
Drug	Lobar, subarachnoid
Arteriovenous malformation	Lobar, intraventricular, subarachnoid
Aneurysm	Subarachnoid, intraparenchymal, rarely subdural
Amyloid angiopathy	Lobar
Cavernous angioma	Intraparenchymal
Dural arteriovenous fistula	Lobar, subarachnoid
Capillary telangiectasias	Usually brainstem

Contd...

129. Ans. (c) Ulcerative colitis

Ref: Harrison 19th ed page 2124

Out of all these ulcerative colitis the most appropriate answer. In absence of any better answer, Ulcerative colitis becomes the answer of choice.

Harrison states that; IBD is currently considered an inappropriate immune response to the endogenous commensal microbiota within the intestines, with or without some component of autoimmunity. Mechanisms of tissue injury in autoimmune diseases can be divided into antibody-mediated and cell-mediated processes. Representative examples are listed:

Mechanisms of Tissue Damage in Autoimmune Diseases

Effector	Mechanism	Target	Disease
Autoantibody	Blocking or inactivation	α Chain of the nicotinic acetylcholine receptor Phospholipid–β alpha$_2$-glycoprotein 1 complex Insulin receptor Intrinsic factor	Myasthenia gravis Antiphospholipid syndrome Insulin-resistant diabetes mellitus Pernicious anemia
	Stimulation	TSH receptor (LATS) Proteinase-3 (ANCA) Epidermal cadherin$_1$ Desmoglein 3	Graves' disease Granulomatosis with polyangiitis (Wegener's) Pemphigus vulgaris
	Complement activation Immune-complex formation Opsonization	α_3 Chain of collagen IV Double-stranded DNA Ig Platelet GpIIb:IIIa	Goodpasture's syndrome Systemic lupus erythematosus Rheumatoid arthritis Autoimmune thrombocytopenic purpura
		Rh antigens, I antigen	Autoimmune hemolytic anemia
	Antibody-dependent cellular cytotoxicity	Thyroid peroxidase, thyroglobulin	Hashimoto's thyroiditis
T cells	Cytokine production	?	Rheumatoid arthritis, multiple sclerosis, type 1 diabetes mellitus
	Cellular cytotoxicity	?	Type 1 diabetes mellitus

130. Ans. (c) Check HBV DNA load

Ref: Harrison 19th ed page 2032, http://apps.who.int/iris/bitstream/10665/154590/1/9789241549059_eng.pdf

Lab findings are consistent with chronic hepatitis. Singe IgM AntiHBc is negative this is a chromic infection. Next step will be check the viral load before starting the therapy

On 12 March 2015 WHO today issued its first-ever guidance for the treatment of chronic hepatitis B

Algorithm of WHO Recommendations of the Management of Persons with chronic Hepatitis B Infections

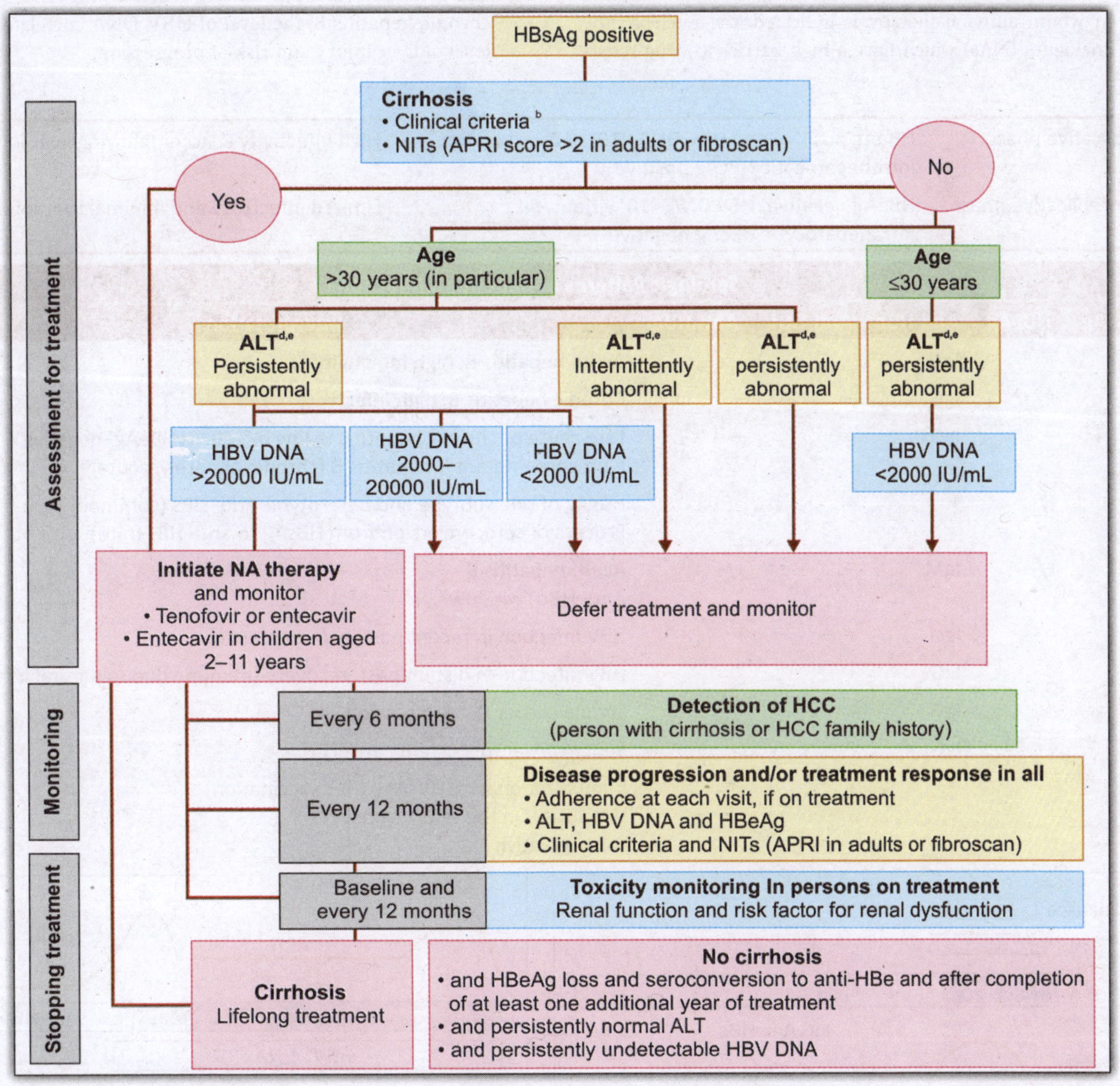

NITs = Noninvasive tests, ALT = alanine aminotransferase, APRI = Aspartase aminotransferase-to-platelet ratio index

APRI (aspartate aminotransferase [AST]-to-platelet ratio index) is recommended

as the preferred non-invasive test (NIT) to assess for the presence of cirrhosis

(APRI score >2 in adults) in resource-limited settings. Transient elastography

(e.g. FibroScan) or FibroTest may be the preferred NITs in settings where they

are available and cost is not a major constraint.

- All adults, adolescents and children with Chronic Hepatitis B and clinical evidence of compensated or decompensated cirrhosis (or cirrhosis based on APRI score >2 in adults) should be treated, regardless of ALT levels, HBeAg status or HBV DNA levels.
- Treatment is recommended for adults with Chronic Hepatitis B who do not have clinical evidence of cirrhosis (or based on APRI score ≤2 in adults), but are aged more than 30 years (in particular) and have persistently abnormal ALT levels and evidence of highlevel HBV replication (HBV DNA >20,000 IU/mL), regardless of HBeAg status.
- ALT levels fluctuate in persons with chronic hepatitis B and require longitudinal monitoring to determine the trend. Upper limits for normal ALT have been defined

as below 30 U/L for men and 19 U/L for women, though local laboratory normal ranges should be applied.

- Where HBV DNA testing is not available, treatment may be considered based on persistently abnormal ALT levels, but other common causes of persistently raised ALT levels such as impaired glucose tolerance, dyslipidaemia and fatty liver should be excluded.
- In all adults, adolescents and children aged 12 years or older in whom antiviral therapy is indicated, the nucleos(t)ide analogues (NAs) which have a high barrier to drug resistance (tenofovir or entecavir) are recommended. Entecavir is recommended in children aged 2–11 years. (Strong recommendation, moderate quality of evidence). NAs with a low barrier to resistance (lamivudine, adefovir or telbivudine) can lead to drug resistance and are not recommended.

Harrison states: Chronic HBV infection can occur in the presence or absence of serum hepatitis B e antigen (HBeAg) and generally, for both HBeAg-reactive and HBeAg negative chronic hepatitis B, the level of HBV DNA correlates with the level of liver injury and risk of progression.

Replicative phase	HBeAg positive and HBV DNA $>10^5-10^6$ virions/mL, intrahepatocytic HBcAg positive	High infectivity & accompanying liver injury
Nonreplicative phase	HBeAg negative, HBV DNA $<10^3$ virions/mL, intrahepatocytic HBcAg negative	Limited infectivity and minimal liver injury

Serologic Patterns of Hepatitis B Infection

HBsAg	HBeAg	Anti-HBc	Anti-HBs	Anti-HBe	Interpretation
+	+	IgM	–	–	Acute hepatitis B, high infectivity
+	+	IgG	–	–	Chronic hepatitis B, high infectivity
+	–	IgG	–	+	Late acute or chronic hepatitis B, low infectivityHBeAg–negative ("precore–mutant") hepatitis B (chronic or, rarely, acute)
+	+/–	+	+	+/–	HBsAg of one subtype and heterotypic anti–HBs (common) Process of seroconversion from HBsAg to anti–HBs (rare)
–	+/–	IgM	–	+/–	Acute hepatitis B Anti–HBc "window"
–	–	IgG	+	+	HBV infection in recent past, convalescence
–	–	IgG	+	–	HBV infection in distant past, recovery (Immune due to natural infection)
+	--	IgG	-	-	Simple carrier (Healthy carrier)
+	+	IgG	-	-	Super carrier (persistent carrier)
–	–	–	+	–	Immunization with HBsAg (after vaccination) Hepatitis B in the remote past (?) False–positive

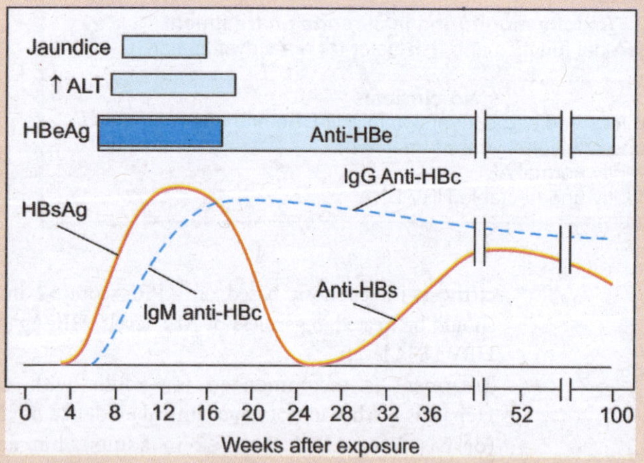

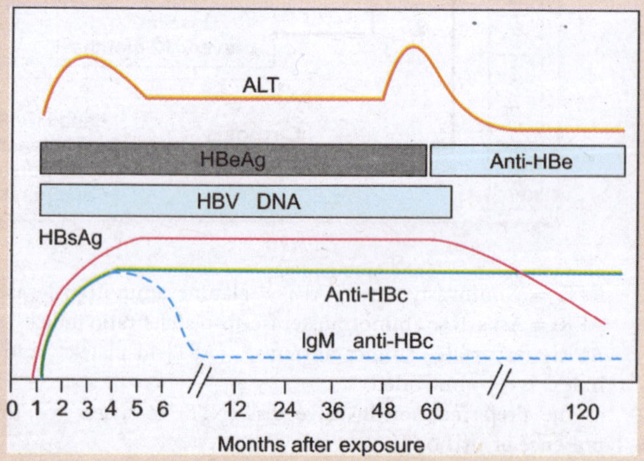

Footnote

- First virologic marker detectable in serum within 1–12 weeks, usually between 8–12 weeks, is HBsAg
- Anti-HBc is first antibody marker to appear in HBV infection and is readily demonstrable in serum, beginning within the first 1–2 weeks after the appearance of HBsAg and preceding detectable levels of anti-HBs by weeks to months.
- After HBsAg disappears, antibody to HBsAg (anti-HBs) becomes detectable in serum and remains detectable indefinitely thereafter.

Contd...

- The titer of HBsAg bears little relation to the severity of clinical disease. Indeed, an inverse correlation exists between the serum concentration of HBsAg and the degree of liver cell damage.
- Principal clinical usefulness of HBeAg is as an indicator of relative infectivity
- Markers of replication: HBeAg, HBV DNA (viral load): 2,000 IU/mL in his blood (= 10,000 copies/ml) HBeAg is a qualitative marker and HBV DNA a quantitative marker of this replicative phase, during which all three forms of HBV circulate, including intact virions.
- Pre-S1 and pre-S2 proteins are also expressed during periods of peak replication, but assays for these gene products are not routinely available
- Because HBcAg is intracellular and, when in the serum, sequestered within an HBsAg coat, naked core particles do not circulate in serum and, therefore, HBcAg is not detectable routinely in the serum of patients with HBV infection.
- Window period: Time gap between disappearance of HBsAg and the appearance of anti-HBs. During this "gap" or "window" period, anti-HBc may represent the only serologic evidence of current or recent HBV infection
- Most instances of isolated anti-HBc represent hepatitis B infection in the remote past. Rarely, however, isolated anti-HBc represents low-level hepatitis B viremia, with HBsAg below the detection threshold; occasionally, isolated anti-HBc represents a cross-reacting or false-positive immunologic specificity
- Anti-HBc of the IgM class (IgM anti-HBc) predominates during the first six months after acute infection, whereas IgG anti-HBc is the predominant class of anti-HBc beyond six months.
- After immunization with hepatitis B vaccine, which consists of HBsAg alone, anti-HBs is the only serologic marker to appear
- Based on serological markers, hepatitis B carriers have classified into two types: super carriers and simple carriers. Super carriers have high titres of HBsAg and HBV DNA in their blood along with HBeAg.
- The simple carrier patient continues to shed HBsAg and the super carrier continues to shed HBsAg and HBeAg beyond the 24th week/6 months from the start of infection.

131. Ans. (b) Antistreptolysin -O

Ref: Harrison 19th ed page 2152

With the exception of chorea and low-grade carditis, both of which may become manifest many months later, evidence of a preceding group A streptococcal infection is essential in making the diagnosis of ARF.

Because most cases do not have a positive throat swab culture or rapid antigen test, serologic evidence is usually needed. The most common serologic tests are the antistreptolysin O (ASO) and anti-DNase B (ADB) titers.

Where possible, age-specific reference ranges should be determined in a local population of healthy people without a recent group A streptococcal infection.

World Health Organization Criteria 2002–2003 for the Diagnosis of Rheumatic Fever and Rheumatic Heart Disease (Based on the 1992 Revised Jones Criteria)

Diagnostic categories	Criteria
Primary episode of rheumatic fever[a]	Two major or one major and two minor manifestations plus evidence of preceding group A streptococcal infection
Recurrent attack of rheumatic fever in a patient without established rheumatic heart disease	Two major or one major and two minor manifestations plus evidence of preceding group A streptococcal infection
Recurrent attack of rheumatic fever in a patient with established rheumatic heart disease[b]	Two minor manifestations plus evidence of preceding group A streptococcal infection[c]
Rheumatic chorea Insidious onset rheumatic carditis[b]	Other major manifestations or evidence of group A streptococcal infection not required
Chronic valve lesions of rheumatic heart disease (patients presenting for the first time with pure mitral stenosis or mixed mitral valve disease and/or aortic valve disease)[d]	Do not require any other criteria to be diagnosed as having rheumatic heart disease
Major manifestations	Carditis Polyarthritis Chorea Erythema marginatum Subcutaneous nodules
Minor manifestations	**Clinical:** Fever, polyarthralgia **Laboratory:** Elevated ESR or leukocyte counte **Electrocardiogram:** Prolonged P-R interval

World Health Organization Criteria 2002–2003 for the Diagnosis of Rheumatic Fever and Rheumatic Heart Disease (Based on the 1992 Revised Jones Criteria)	
Diagnostic categories	**Criteria**
Supporting evidence of a preceding streptococcal infection within the last 45 days	Elevated or rising anti-streptolysin O or other streptococcal antibody, *or* A positive throat culture, *or* Rapid antigen test for group A streptococcus, *or* Recent scarlet fever[e]

Footnote

a- Patients may present with polyarthritis (or with only polyarthralgia or monoarthritis) and with several (three or more) other minor manifestations, together with evidence of recent group A streptococcal infection. Some of these cases may later turn out to be rheumatic fever. It is prudent to consider them as cases of "probable rheumatic fever" (once other diagnoses are excluded) and advise regular secondary prophylaxis. Such patients require close follow-up and regular examination of the heart. This cautious approach is particularly suitable for patients in vulnerable age groups in high incidence settings.

b- Infective endocarditis should be excluded.

c- Some patients with recurrent attacks may not fulfill these criteria.

d- Congenital heart disease should be excluded.

e- 1992 Revised Jones criteria do not include elevated leukocyte count as a laboratory minor manifestation (but do include elevated C-reactive protein) and do not include recent scarlet fever as supporting evidence of a recent streptococcal infection.

Pediatrics

12

AIIMS NOVEMBER 2018

1. A 5-year-old male child presents to OPD having coarse facies with hepatosplenomegaly, hearing impairment, frontal head enlargement and thickening of cardiac valves. What is the most likely diagnosis?

a. Hurler's syndrome
b. Fragile X syndrome
c. Hunter's syndrome
d. Tay-Sachs disease

2. Maximum steroid produced by fetal adrenal?

a. DHEA-S
b. Cortisol
c. Corticosterone
d. Progesterone

3. A video of sick neonate is shown in the video. What is the most likely diagnosis? (Scan the given QR code from your mobile to watch the video. Install a QR code scanner if not done already).

a. Focal clonic seizure
b. Multifocal clonic seizure
c. Multifocal tonic clonic seizure
d. Focal tonic seizure

4. Video of a child having respiratory distress is shown in the video. The Silverman score is? (Scan the given QR code from your mobile to watch the video. Install a QR code scanner if not done already).

a. 7
b. 8
c. 9
d. 10

5. Which of the following is true statement regarding Turner's syndrome?

a. Turner syndrome with webbed neck is 3 times more likely to develop CVS defects than non-webbed neck
b. Coarctation of aorta is more likely in non-webbed neck patients
c. Male turner (Noonan syndrome) is much more likely to have CVS defects
d. Turner syndrome with webbed fingers and toes is likely to be associated with visceral anomalies

AIIMS MAY 2018

6. A child underwent Kasai portoenterostomy. What else is seen in this child?

a. Midgut malrotation
b. Renal agenesis
c. Aberrant hepatic artery
d. Omphalocele

7. A 2-year-old child with history of skull trauma with parietal bone linear fracture now comes with increased swelling. What is most likely diagnosis?

a. Hygroma
b. Contusion
c. Chronic abscess
d. Growing fracture

8. A young girl comes with presenting complaint of frequent dropping of objects. There is no memory lapses and no Generalized tonic clonic seizure. Her maternal cousin was diagnosed for seizure. What is her most likely diagnosis?

a. Juvenile myoclonic seizure
b. Absence seizure
c. Febrile seizure
d. Choreoathetoid epilepsy

9. **What does 'A' depict in the following image of serum immunoglobulin levels in a paediatric patient?**

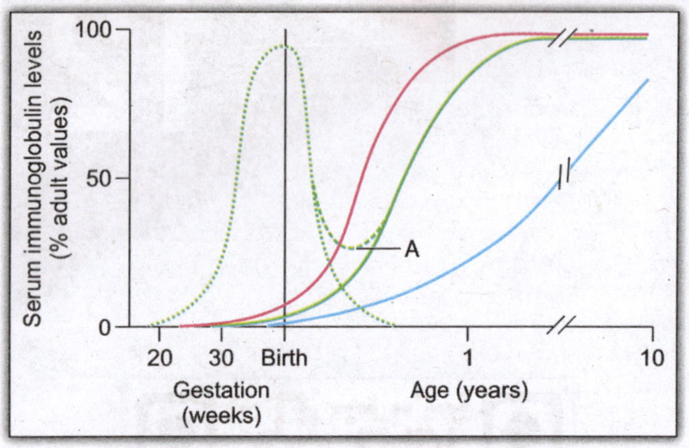

a. IgM
b. IgG
c. Maternal and neonatal IgM
d. Maternal and neonatal IgG

10. **Which of the following is the correct order of suction during Neonatal resuscitation?**
a. Mouth, Nose, Trachea
b. Nose, Mouth, Trachea
c. Nose, Trachea, Mouth
d. Mouth, Trachea, Nose

11. **A child swallowed a battery and he was brought to the ER by his parents and X-ray was done which showed it to be present in stomach. What is the next step in management?**
a. Surgical removal
b. Do endoscopic retrieval immediately
c. Give the child antiemetic immediately
d. Reassure and repeat X-ray 5 days later

12. **A 3-year-old child's development milestone is said to be delayed if he fails to?** ***(AIIMS May 2018, Nov 2017)***
a. Hold spoon
b. Catch a ball
c. Hopping on one foot
d. Draw a square

13. **A 13-month-old child comes to you completely unimmunized. According to National Immunization programme which vaccine would you give?**
a. BCG DPT Hep B OPV IPV
b. DPT Hep B Measles OPV
c. DPT BCG Penta OPV
d. Measles BCG DPT OPV Penta

14. **A 3-day-old neonate presented with recurrent bilious vomiting and abdominal distension. Which of the following will be the next step in management of the given patient?**
a. USG abdomen
b. Exploratory laparotomy
c. CECT abdomen with oral contrast
d. Gastrografin swallow with follow through

15. **You have been called to declare brain death of a 12-year-old child in PICU. All of the following are signs of brain death EXCEPT:**
a. Normal BP without pharmacological support
b. Positive spinal reflexes on stimulation
c. Dilated pupils
d. Decorticate and decerebrate posturing

16. **A 3-year-old child presented with umbilical discharge as shown in the image, with no palpable mass in the abdomen. What is the best step?**

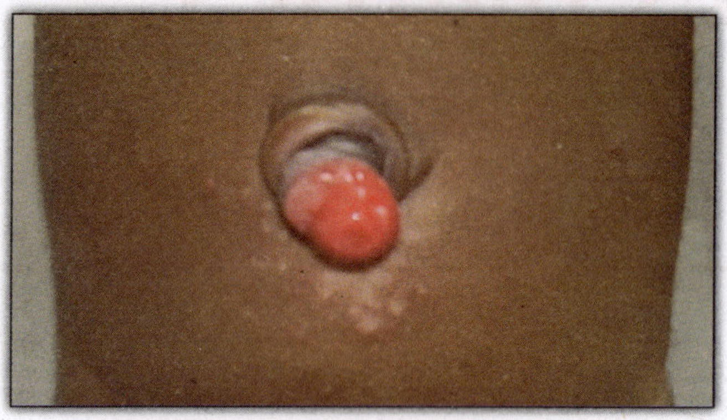

a. USG abdomen
b. Diagnostic laparotomy and proceed
c. MRI abdomen
d. CT

17. **All of the following are false with respect to CMV in children EXCEPT:**
a. Ganciclovir resistance is due to mutation in UL97 gene - DNA polymerase
b. CMV can be cultured in vitro in mammalian cells of animal origin like MDCK line
c. Commonest manifestation of CMV associated disease in HIV seropositive patients is watery diarrhea
d. Ganciclovir resistant CMV strains show cross resistance to Foscarnet

18. **After the delivery of an infant of a diabetic mother, blood glucose of the infant was 60 mg/dL. Which other investigation is to be done?**
a. Serum potassium
b. Serum calcium
c. CBC
d. Serum chloride

19. **Which of the following is a causative protein for viral diarrhea in children?**
a. NSP 1
b. NSP 4
c. VP 4
d. VP 7

AIIMS NOVEMBER 2017

20. **A neonate present with congenital hydrocephalus, chorioretinitis and periventricular calcifications on CT Brain. He was diagnosed to have Congenital CMV infection. Best sample to be sent for PCR to detect CMV infection is?**
a. CSF
b. Urine
c. Blood
d. Liver Biopsy

21. **A child presents with Kinky hairs, Intellectual disabilities and seizures. What is most likely diagnosis?**
a. Down's syndrome
b. Menkes disease
c. Pompe's disease
d. Niemann Pick disease

22. **The acronym of APGAR stands for?**
a. Appearance, Pallor, Grimace, Activity, Respiration
b. Appearance, Pulse, Grimace, Activity, Respiration
c. Activity, Pulse, Grimace, Anxiety, Respiration
d. Activity, Pallor, Grimace, Appearance, Respiration

23. **A child presents with hypotonia, seizure and craniofacial abnormalities. It was confirmed to be Zellweger syndrome. Which of the following accumulates in brain?**
   a. Glucose b. Lactic acid
   c. Triglycerides d. Very long chain fatty acid

24. **A 3-year-old child's development milestone is said to be delayed if he fails to?** *(AIIMS May 2018, Nov 2017)*
   a. Hold spoon b. Catch a ball
   c. Hopping on one foot d. Draw a square

25. **A 4-day-old baby presents with bilirubin 18 mg but feeding well. What will be the next line of management?**
   a. Stop breast feed and phototherapy
   b. Continue breastfeed and phototherapy
   c. Exchange transfusion
   d. Only observe, as it is Physiological Jaundice

26. **Hutchinson's triad in congenital syphilis includes?**
   a. Hutchinson teeth, interstitial keratitis, eighth nerve deafness
   b. Hutchinson teeth, eighth nerve deafness, strawberry tongue
   c. Interstitial keratitis, eighth nerve deafness, mulberry teeth
   d. Keratoconjunctivitis sicca, eighth nerve deafness, mulberry teeth

27. **A 18-month-old child comes to immunization clinic for the first time i.e. he has never got any vaccine. Which of the following vaccine you would give to him?**
   a. Pentavalent vaccine only
   b. Pentavalent vaccine + BCG + OPV
   c. DPT + OPV only
   d. DPT + OPV + MMR

28. **Dried blood spot (DBS) assay is done for?**
   a. HIV b. Inborn error of metabolism
   c. Hepatitis d. Cataract

AIIMS MAY 2017

29. **A 18-month-old child comes to subcenter with history of breathlessness, fever and cough. On examination weight was 15 kg, respiratory rate was 46/min, and there was no chest indrawing. Which is the most appropriate management?**
   a. IV antibiotics at PHC and observe
   b. Give first dose of IV antibiotics & refer to higher center
   c. Oral cotrimoxazole for 5 days and send home
   d. Home remedies

30. **Which of the following is true regarding congenital CMV infection?**
   a. Diagnosed only by persistent presence of IgM antibody after 6 months
   b. It is the most common cause of non-syndromic sensorineural hearing loss
   c. All babies born are symptomatic
   d. Mothers of developing countries who transmit the virus are usually symptomatic

31. **Which of the following is not seen in fetal alcohol syndrome?**
   a. Microcephaly
   b. Macrocephaly
   c. Holoprosencephaly
   d. Thinning of corpus callosum

32. **A 5-year-old child comes to hospital with history of loose stools but no history of fever or blood in stools. Mother says he is irritable and drinks water if given. On examination eyes sunken and skin pinch test – the skin retracted within two seconds but not immediately. What will be the appropriate management?**
   a. Administer the first dose of IV antibiotic and immediately refer to higher center
   b. Give oral antibiotics and ORS and ask the mother to continue the same and visit again next day
   c. Consider severe dehydration start IV fluids, IV antibiotics and refer to higher center
   d. ORS with zinc for 14 days

AIIMS NOVEMBER 2016

33. **A newborn is to be kept in warmer, what is ideal labour room temperature for neonate?**
   a. 25–28°C b. 28–30°C
   c. 32–35°C d. 35–37°C

34. **A child with history of difficulty in walking picture of lower limb is given below. What is the most likely diagnosis?**
   a. Muscular dystrophy b. Congenital myotonia
   c. Peripheral neuropathy d. Myasthenia

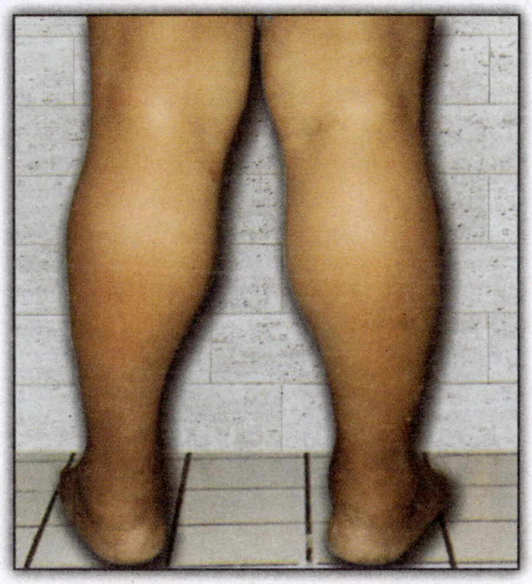

35. **Neonate with jaundice on day 1, how will you manage?**
   a. Only observe, as it is physiological jaundice
   b. Start Phototherapy
   c. Exchange transfusion
   d. LFT and Coombs test

36. **A 2-month-old child with birth weight of 3200 g was brought to subcenter with history of fever for past 2 days and diarrhea. On examination the weight of the child is 2800 g, otherwise he is active, accepting oral feeds. Skin when pinched is not going back with more than 10 pustules. Oral mucosa is dry what to do by sub center?**
   a. Administer the 1st dose of IV antibiotic and then immediately refer to higher center
   b. Start IV antibiotics and IV fluid and then immediately refer to higher center
   c. Send child home with few packets of ORS and call after 2 days
   d. Refer to higher center with mother giving frequent ORS sips to child

37. **What medication taken in excess during pregnancy can cause the condition given in the picture?**

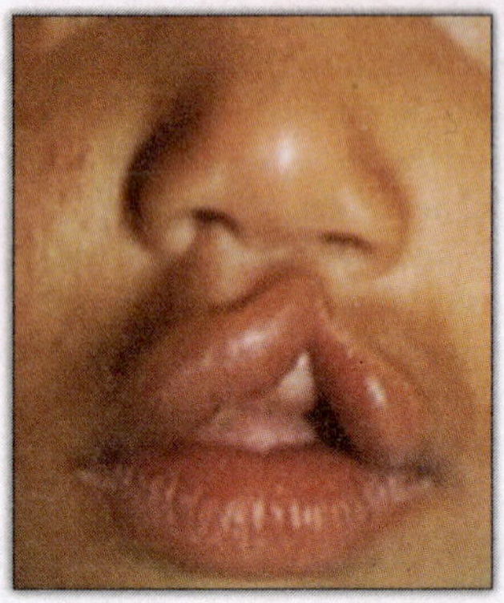

a. Folic acid b. Isotretinoin
c. Niacin d. Thiamine

38. **A neonate presented with cicatrizing skin lesion all over the body with hypoplasia off all limbs. Ophthalmological examination reveals chorioretinitis. MRI of brain showed diffuse cerebral atrophy. Which of the following test is most likely to be positive in this case?**

a. Anti VZV antibodies b. Anti-toxoplasma antibodies
c. Anti-rubella antibodies d. Anti HCMV antibodies

39. **A newborn born to a mother infected with CMV in first trimester did not have any symptoms or signs of infection. IgM Anti HCMV antibody was positive. Which of the following is not a long term complication in this child?**

a. Hearing loss b. Seizures
c. Mental retardation d. Liver failure

40. **Palivizumab is a humanized monoclonal antibody used against which virus?**

a. RSV b. HCV
c. Influenza d. Parainfluenza

AIIMS MAY 2016

41. **A 5-year-old presents comes to casualty with sepsis and shock. His heart rate is 145/min, respiratory rate – 30/min, blood pressure – 60/40 mm Hg. The most appropriate step is administration of?**

a. 10 mL/kg of 6% HES b. 20 mL/kg of 0.9% NS
c. 20 mL/kg of 0.45% NS d. 5 mL/kg of 5% albumin

42. **A 6-year-old child presents with bed wetting at night. There is no history of any day time symptoms. The urine microscopy is normal, the specific gravity of urine is 1.020 and other investigations are normal. What should be advised?**

a. Reassurance and revisit after 6 months
b. CT pelvis c. USG kidney and bladder
d. Refer to child psychiatrist

43. **Family members of a 3-month-old baby are insisting on introduction of cereals into diet. The mother came to you for advice regarding the same. Which of the following is most likely to happen on the introduction of cereals in this child?**

a. Increased the risk of gastroesophageal reflux
b. Increase the risk of GI infections
c. Promote development of oral motor skills
d. Increases the risk of food allergy

44. **A 4-year-old admitted in ward with pneumonia. He develops sudden onset of breathlessness. X-ray was done as shown below. What is the next step in management?**

a. Intercostal drainage tube insertion
b. Emergency needle thoracotomy
c. Decrease mechanical ventilation
d. Increase mechanical ventilation

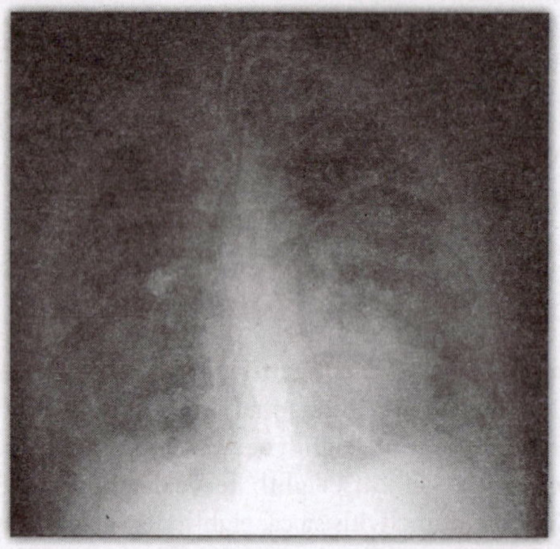

45. **A 14-year-old admitted in ward with pneumonia. He develops sudden onset of breathlessness. A chest X-ray was done and right pleural effusion is seen as shown below. Which of the following additional finding is not seen?**

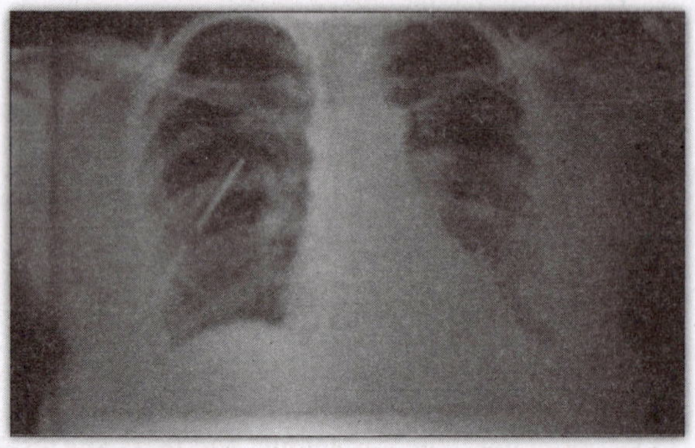

a. Pleural effusion b. Pneumothorax
c. In situ chest drain d. Mediastinal shift

46. **A 5-year-old male child presented with pain and restriction in the neck and right shoulder region with following image. The most likely diagnosis is?**

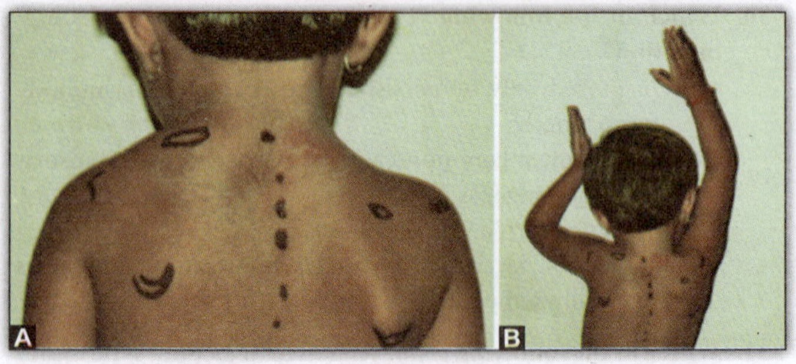

a. Ankylosing spondylitis
b. Long thoracic nerve palsy
c. Fasioscapulohumeral dysplasia
d. Klippel Feil syndrome

47. **A 4-month-old infant with tetralogy of Fallot presents with fever and a loose stool, which of the following is compatible is tetrology spells?**
   a. Oxygen saturation <75% in room air
   b. Inability to hear a murmur
   c. Hepatomegaly
   d. S3 gallop rhythm

AIIMS NOVEMBER 2015

48. **Identify the congenital defect seen in the following picture?**

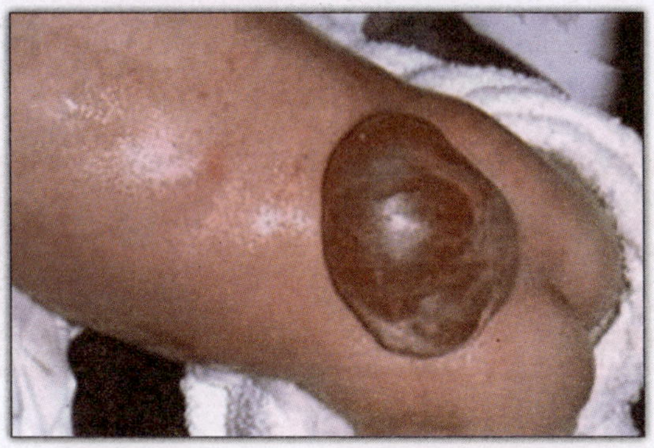

   a. Meningocele b. Meningomyelocele
   c. Teratoma d. Cystic hygroma

49. **A 3.5 kg male infant born at term after an uncomplicated pregnancy and delivery develops respiratory siatress shortly after birth and requires mechanical ventilation. The chest radiograph reveals a normal cardiothymic silhouette but a diffuse ground glass appearance to the lung fields. Surfactant replacement fails to improve gas exchange. Over the first week life, the hypoxemia worsens. Results of routine culture and echocardiographic findings are negative. A term female sibling died at 1 month of age with "respiratory distress" Which of the following is the most likely diagnosis? *(AIIMS Nov 2015, May 2011)***
   a. Neonatal pulmonary alveolar proteinosis
   b. Meconium aspiration syndrome
   c. Total anomalous pulmonary venous return
   d. Disseminated herpes simplex infection

50. **A 2-year-old child was brought to the emergency department at 3 AM. The child presented with fever and cough. On examination, respiratory rate was 36/min, temperature was 39°C and saturation on the pulse oximetry was 96%. The child had barking cough and stridor only on crying. Otherwise, the child was hydrated, able to drink and consolable. The next step in the management would be? *(AIIMS Nov 2015, May 2013)***
   a. Single dose Dexamethasone
   b. Nebulize racemic epinephrine
   c. Complete blood count and culture
   d. Nasal washing for respiratory sentitium virus

51. **A 1-year-old baby complaint of watery stool 8-10 times per day for 9 days. Other than zinc supplementation, what else should be given?**
   a. ORS alone
   b. ORS with probiotic
   c. ORS with antibiotic
   d. IV infusion with Ringer lactate

52. **In a 24-months-old baby presented with severe acute malnutrition. Which of the following cannot be used as diagnostic criteria for severe acute malnutrition?**
   a. Weight for height b. Mid upper arm circumference
   c. Height for age d. Pitting edema

53. **First sign of puberty in female is?**
   a. Growth spurt b. Breast bud
   c. Menarche d. Pubic and axillary hairs

54. **Under nutrition is defined as?**
   a. Weight for age <2SD b. Weight for height <2SD
   c. Weight for age <3SD d. Weight for height <3SD

55. **A 9-year-old girl with progressive difficulties in combing hair and climbing steps upwards, growers sign positive, maculopapular pigmentation over back of hands. Next step for diagnosis will be? *(AIIMS Nov 2015, May 2011)***
   a. Nerve conduction studies b. Rheumatoid factor
   c. Electromyography d. Creatine Kinase levels

AIIMS MAY 2015

56. **Regarding Japanese encephalitis vaccine, what is not true?**
   a. Booster doses are given after 1 year and repeated every 3 years
   b. In endemic areas vaccination is given to cover children between one to nine years age group
   c. Not given for infants less than 6 months
   d. Two primary doses given to children in the one to three year age group

57. **A male child with coarse facies, macroglossia, thick lips with hepatosplenomegaly presents with copious mucus discharge from nose. Probable underlying diagnosis is?**
   a. Hurler disease
   b. Beckwith Wiedemann syndrome
   c. Proteus syndrome
   d. Hypothyroidism

58. **An infant at 7 months with history of vomiting and failure to thrive. Patient improved with IV glucose. After one month returns with same complaints. On evaluation found to have high blood ammonia but no ketones. Also he has high urinary glutamine, alanine and uracil. Which is the likely enzyme defect/deficiency?**
   a. CPS1 b. Ornithine transcarbamylase
   c. Arginase deficiency d. Argininosuccinate lyase

59. **A 10-year-old child with edema and decreased urine output. On evaluation, serum albumin is 2.5 g/dL, S. Creatinine is 0.5 mg/dL, urine protein is 3+ with no RBC/WBC or casts. Pathological change expected is? *(AIIMS May 2015, 2014)***
   a. Minimal change disease b. Interstitial nephritis
   c. IgA nephropathy d. FSGS

60. **Fluid of choice in infant diarrhea?**
   a. ORS b. Salt water
   c. Sugar water d. Dextrose

61. **A 1-month-old newborn presents with conjugated hyperbilirubinemia, intrahepatic cholestasis and high alkaline phosphatase. Eosinophilic, PAS positive cytoplasmic granules are seen in liver biopsy specimen. Diagnosis is?**
   a. Alpha 1 antitrypsin deficiency
   b. Congenital hepatic fibrosis
   c. Extrahepatic biliary atresia
   d. Ductal plate defect

ANSWERS WITH EXPLANATIONS

AIIMS NOVEMBER 2018

1. Ans. (a) Hurler's syndrome

Ref: Nelson 20th ed page 5738-5739

Similar question with different set of clinical features of Hurler's syndrome is asked in AIIMS Pediatrics May 2015

Hurler is characterized by:

- Inguinal hernia
- Hepatosplenomegaly
- Coarse facial features
- Corneal clouding
- Large tongue
- Prominent forehead
- Joint stiffness
- Short stature
- Skeletal dysplasia
- Cardiomyopathy, valvular heart disease
- Recurrent URTI (copious mucus discharge, obstructive airway disease).

Recognition Pattern of Mucopolysaccharidoses

Manifestations	Mucopolysaccharidosis Type						
	Type I-H hurler disease	Type I-S scheie disease	Type II hunter	Type III sanfilipppo disease	Type IV morquio disease	Type VI ma-roteaux-Lamy disease	Type VII sly disease
Mental deficiency	+	-	±	+	-	-	±
Coarse facial features	+	(+)	+	+	-	+	±
Corneal clouding	+	+	-	-	(+)	+	±
Visceromegaly	+	(+)	+	(+)	-	+	+
Short stature	+	(+)	+	-	+	+	+
Joint contractures	+	+	+	-	-	+	+
Dysostosis multiplex	+	(+)	+	(+)	+	+	+
Leucocyte inclusions	+	(+)	+	+	-	+	+
Mucopolysaccharidura	+	+	+	+	+	+	+

Note: All mucopolysaccharidosis are Autosomal recessive except Hunter's disease, which is X linked recessive

2. Ans. (a) DHEA-S

Ref: Nelson 20th Ed Pg 2700

- ***Major steroid products of the mid gestation fetal adrenal gland are DHEA and DHEA sulfate (DHEAS)***
- Steroid synthesis in the fetal adrenal varies during gestation.
- Shortly after the fetal adrenal gland forms (8–10 weeks), it efficiently secretes cortisol, which is able to negatively feedback on the fetal pituitary and hypothalamus to suppress ACTH secretion.
- This is a critical time for differentiation of the external genitalia in both sexes; to prevent virilization, the female fetus must not be exposed to high levels of androgens of adrenal origin, and placental aromatase activity must remain low during this time to minimize conversion of testosterone to estradiol in male fetuses, which would interfere with masculinization.
- After 12 weeks 3-beta-hydroxysteroid dehydrogenase activity in the fetal adrenal gland decreases and steroid sulfo kinase activity increases.
- Thus, the ***major steroid products of the mid gestation fetal adrenal gland are DHEA and DHEA sulfate (DHEAS)*** and, by 16α-hydroxylation in the liver, 16α-hydroxy DHEAS. Aromatase activity increases in the placenta at the same time, and steroid sulfatase activity is high as well.
- Thus, the placenta uses DHEA and DHEAS as substrates for estrone and estradiol and 16α-OH DHEAS as a substrate for estriol.

3. Ans. (b) Multifocal clonic seizure

Ref: IAP Textbook of Pediatrics page 456, Clinical Pediatric Neurology: A Signs and Symptoms Approach By Gerald M. Fenichel 6th ed page 2

The video shows clonic movement of multiple body parts and does not shows and Extension of limbs hence its Multifocal Clonic seizure.

Different Seizure Patterns:

- **Subtle seizures** does not show any tonic or clonic movement of the limbs. EEG does not show any epileptiform waveforms. Subtle seizures may manifest as eyelid blinking, fluttering or buccal-lingual movement. Subtle seizures lasting for brief duration need not be treated. There may be pedaling or automatic movements because of subcortical neuronal discharges.

- **Focal Clonic seizures:** Repeated irregular clonic limb movements (1-3 movements/sec) of one limb or both limbs on one side.
- **Multifocal clonic seizure:** Migratory jerky movements are noted in first limb then another. The migration appear random and does not follow expected pattern of epileptic spread (Jacksonian march)
- **Myoclonic seizures:** Repeated flexion and extension movements of arms, legs or all limbs.
- **Tonic seizures** are characterized by extension of extremities and axial muscles. It is usually associated with apnea and upward movement of eyes

4. Ans. (b) 8

Ref: Ghai 7th ed page 143

Silverman scoring calculation in the given case is

1. Audible grunt without stethoscope= 2
2. Nasal flare = 2
3. See saw upper chest movement = 2
4. Xiphoid retractions just visible = 1
5. Lower chest retractions just visible = 1

Hence the total score is 8

Assessment of Severity of Respiratory Distress

Silverman Anderson Score Interpretation

Score	0	1	2
Upper Chest Retractions	Synchronized	Lag on inspiration	See-saw movement
Lower Chest Retractions	None	Just visible	Marked
Xiphoid Retractions	None	Just visible	Marked
Nasal Flaring	None	Minimal	Marked
Expiratory Grunting	None	Stethoscope only	Naked eye and ear

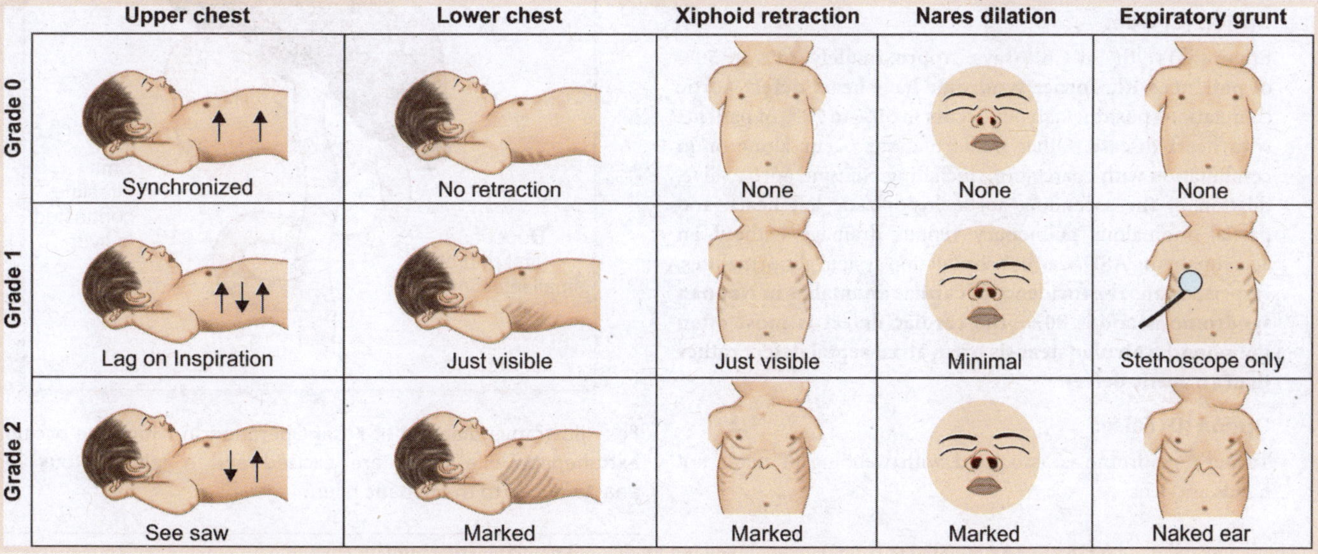

Normal babies have a cumulative score close to "0". Severely depressed babies score close to "10"

Score 0-3 = Mild respiratory distress – O2 by hood

Score 4-6 = Moderate respiratory distress - CPAP

Score > 6 = Impending respiratory failure

Downe's Score and Its Interpretation

RDS Score	0	1	2
Cyanosis	None	Cyanotic in air	Cyanotic in 40% O_2
Retractions	None	Mild	Severe
Grunting	None	Audible with stethoscope	Audible without stethoscope
Air entry-make baby cry and listen to breath sounds while baby cries	Clear	Delayed or decreased	Barely audible
Respiratory rate	60	60 to 80	80 or apneic episodes

- An RD score of 4 or more for at least 2 hours during the first 8 hours of life denotes clinical RD and requires assessment of the infant by a physician.
- An RD score of 6 or more is an indication for ventilatory assistance.

5. **Ans. (c) Male turner (Noonan syndrome) is much more likely to have CVS defects**

Ref: Nelson 20th Ed Pg 2745

The incidence of cardiac anomalies in Noonan syndrome is about 80%, and thus these patients have more likelihood of having CVS defects as compared to Turner's syndrome (20–50%).

Let us go option wise:

Option (A) False:

The presence of neck webbing and increased thoracic anterior-to-posterior diameters are useful predictors for cardiovascular abnormalities. Coarctation is 8 times more common in Turner's syndrome patients with webbed neck than those without webbed neck. **(Ref: Critical Heart Disease in Infants and Children by David G. 2nd ed page 627). Note:** Earlier 1984 study demonstrated 3 fold risk of developing CVS defect in Webbed neck turner syndrome.

Option (B) False:

Among patients with Turner syndrome, those with webbed necks have a much greater chance of having coarctation of the aorta than do those without webbed necks.

Option (C) True:

Braunwald's 9th Ed Ch 8 says: **Approximately 20% to 50% of patients with Turner syndrome have heart defect.** Aortic coarctation (postductal type) occurs in 50% to 70% of patients with heart disease. Other malformations occur alone or in combination with coarctation, including bicuspid aortic valve, dilation of the ascending aorta, hypoplastic left heart, and partial anomalous pulmonary venous drainage without an accompanying ASD, Cardiac conduction system abnormalities, Hypertension. **The incidence of cardiac anomalies in Noonan syndrome is about 80%. The cardiac defect is most often pulmonary valvular stenosis or an atrial septal defect rather than an aortic defect.**

Option (D) False:

Turner's syndrome is associated with webbing of neck, not hands and feet.

AIIMS MAY 2018

6. **Ans. (a) Midgut malrotation**

Ref: Nelson 20th Ed Pg 1933, Bailey 26th ed page 121

- Kasai portoenterostomy is done for the treatment of biliary atresia.
- Biliary Atresia should be considered in any infant who remains jaundiced after 2 weeks of age.
- The extrahepatic bile ducts are occluded causing obstructive jaundice and progressive liver fibrosis in early infancy.
- Most patients with biliary atresia (85–90%) are normal at birth and have a postnatal progressive obliteration of bile ducts; the embryonic or fetal-onset form manifests at birth and is associated with ***other congenital anomalies (situs inversus, polysplenia, intestinal malrotation, complex congenital heart disease)*** within the polysplenia spectrum (biliary atresia splenic malformation)

Kasai Portoenterostomy:

- Biliary atresia is treated by a Kasai portoenterostomy in which the occluded extrahepatic bile ducts are excised and a jejunal Roux loop is anastomosed to the hepatic hilum.
- Effective bile drainage is more likely if the operation is performed before 8 weeks of age and may obviate the subsequent need for liver transplantation.

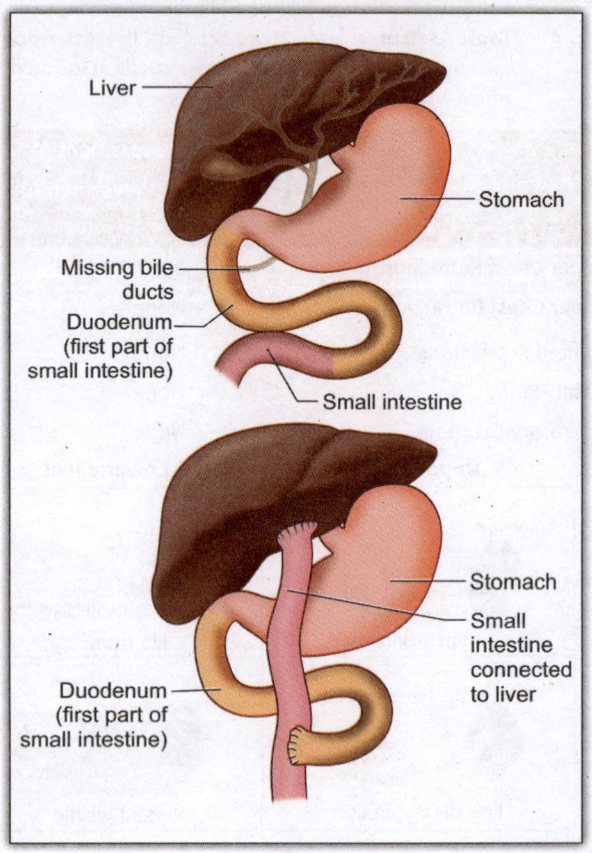

Fig: Illustrative diagram of Kasai Operation in which the occluded extrahepatic bile ducts are excised and a jejunal Roux loop anastomosed to the hepatic hilum

7. **Ans. (d) Growing fracture**

Ref: Oski's essential Pediatric 2nd Ed Pg 234

Described above is most likely a case of Growing fracture wherein, there occurs herniation of underlying tissue through torn dura at fracture site in the skull.

Hints to Diagnosis:

Age of the child: <3 years

Bone involved: Parietal bone

More About Growing Fracture:

- Diastatic skull fractures are traumatic separations of cranial bones at one or more suture sites. Most frequently, they affect the lambdoid suture and occur in the first 4 years of life.
- Such fractures should be followed closely in children **younger than 3 years** because they can become sites of so-called **growing fractures.**

- Growing skull fractures are caused by **herniation of tissue through torn dura and an accompanying fracture (linear or diastatic) into the overlying scalp**.
- Such fractures occur most often in the **parietal region**.
- The herniating tissue is either solid brain parenchyma or cystic in nature, usually a porencephalic cyst (communicating with a lateral ventricle) or (less often) a leptomeningeal cyst.

Clinical Approach to Diagnosis of Scalp Swellings in Childhood

Transillumination	Scalp swelling	
	Diffuse	Focal
Increased	Caput succedaneum	Porencephalic
Decreased	Subgaleal hematoma	Cephalhematoma

Major Varieties of Skull Fracture in Childhood

Fracture	Comments
Linear	More common especially in children <2 yrs, mostly temporoparietal. May overlie intracranial pathological conditions (e.g.: epidural hemorrhage) and hence require further imaging (if above sagittal suture or temporal bone). If present in infants and young children, possibility of neglect and infliction of injury must be ruled out.
Depressed	Either continuity of the bony calvaria is disrupted or the skull may simply be indented, resulting in a ping-pong or pond fracture unaccompanied by a break in the cranial vault
Compound/Open skull	Fractures have a direct communication between a scalp laceration and the fracture site. These fractures are called penetrating if a tear in the dura is also present. These fractures are of urgent concern because of the danger of complicating infection.
Basal	Two main varieties of basal fractures are frontobasal and petrous. Because of the anatomic complexity of the base of the skull, only approximately, of basal skull fractures can be recognized on standard skull radiography. Although the addition of multiplanar tomography and thin-section CT substantially increases the frequency with which such fractures can be demonstrated radiographically, usually the firm diagnosis of basal skull fracture depends on the recognition of coexisting signs. This diagnosis can often be inferred, if not confirmed, by coexisting sips that include hemorrhage in the nose, nasopharynx, or middle ear; overlying the mastoid bone (Battle sign); or around the eyes raccoon eyes.).
Diastatic	Diastatic skull fractures are traumatic separations of cranial bones at one or more suture sites. Most frequently, they affect the lambdoid suture and occur in the first 4 years of life. They may lead to a growing fracture

8. Ans. (a) Juvenile myoclonic seizure

Ref: Nelson 20th Ed Pg 2836

- Juvenile myoclonic epilepsy **(Janz syndrome)** is the most common generalized epilepsy in young adults.
- Linked to mutation in many genes including CACNB4, CLCN2, EJM2,3,4,5,6,7,9; GABRA1; GABRD; Myoclonin1/EFHC1.
- Typically, it starts in early adolescence. Clinical manifestations are myoclonic jerks in the morning, often causing the patient to **drop things;** generalized tonic-clonic or clonic-tonic-clonic seizures upon awakening; and juvenile absences.
- Sleep deprivation, alcohol (in older patients) and photic stimulation or rarely, certain cognitive activities can act as precipitants.

9. Ans. (d) Maternal neonatal IgG

Ref: Nelson's 20th Ed Pg 911

The "A" marked in the figure represents Maternal and neonatal IgG. Maternally transferred IgG has mostly been catabolized by 6 months. A physiological trough is seen between 3 and 6 months as the neonate starts synthesis of IgG slowly.

- Maternal IgG is actively transported across the placenta to the fetal circulation from the fourth month of gestational life, although maximum transfer takes place during the final 2 months.
- At birth, the infant has a serum IgG at least equal to that of the mother; at first, catabolism of maternal IgG is only partly compensated by IgG synthesized by the newborn child.
- The period between 3 and 6 months of age represents a phase of "physiological hypogammaglobulinemia".
- The normal infant is not unduly susceptible to infection because functioning antibody is present despite the low IgG level, and T-cell function is intact.
- However, the trough in IgG is more severe and the risk of sepsis much greater if the gift of IgG acquired from the mother is severely reduced, as in extremely premature infants born around 28 weeks' gestation or earlier.

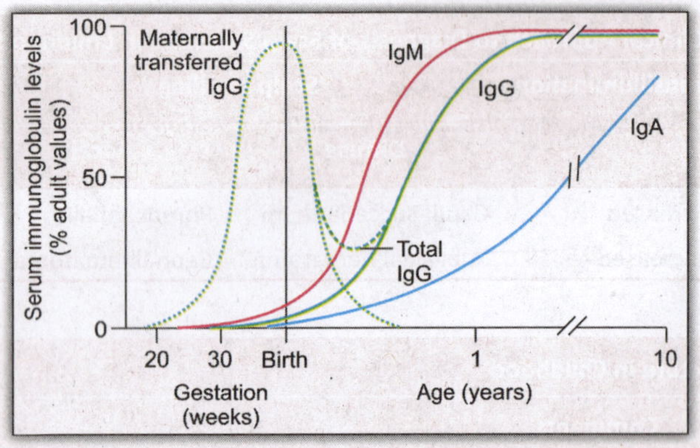

Fig: Serum Immunoglobulin levels in relation to age. Maternally transferred IgG has mostly been catabolized by 6 months. As the neonate synthesizes IgG the level rises slowly but a physiological trough of IgG is seen between 3 and 6 months

10. Ans. (a) Mouth, Nose, Trachea

Ref: Merenstein & Gardner's Handbook of Neonatal Intensive Care By Sandra Lee Gardner 7th Ed Pg 58,61; Ghai 8th Ed Pg 127

- The oropharynx in the neonate carries a bulk of secretions.
- Nasal suctioning often causes a reflex cough/sneeze/cry.
- If **suctioning** is necessary to clear the airway, it must be done after oral suctioning to minimize the possibility of aspiration of oropharyngeal content. This may be followed by tracheal suctioning in some cases.
- National resuscitation algorithm 2015 update

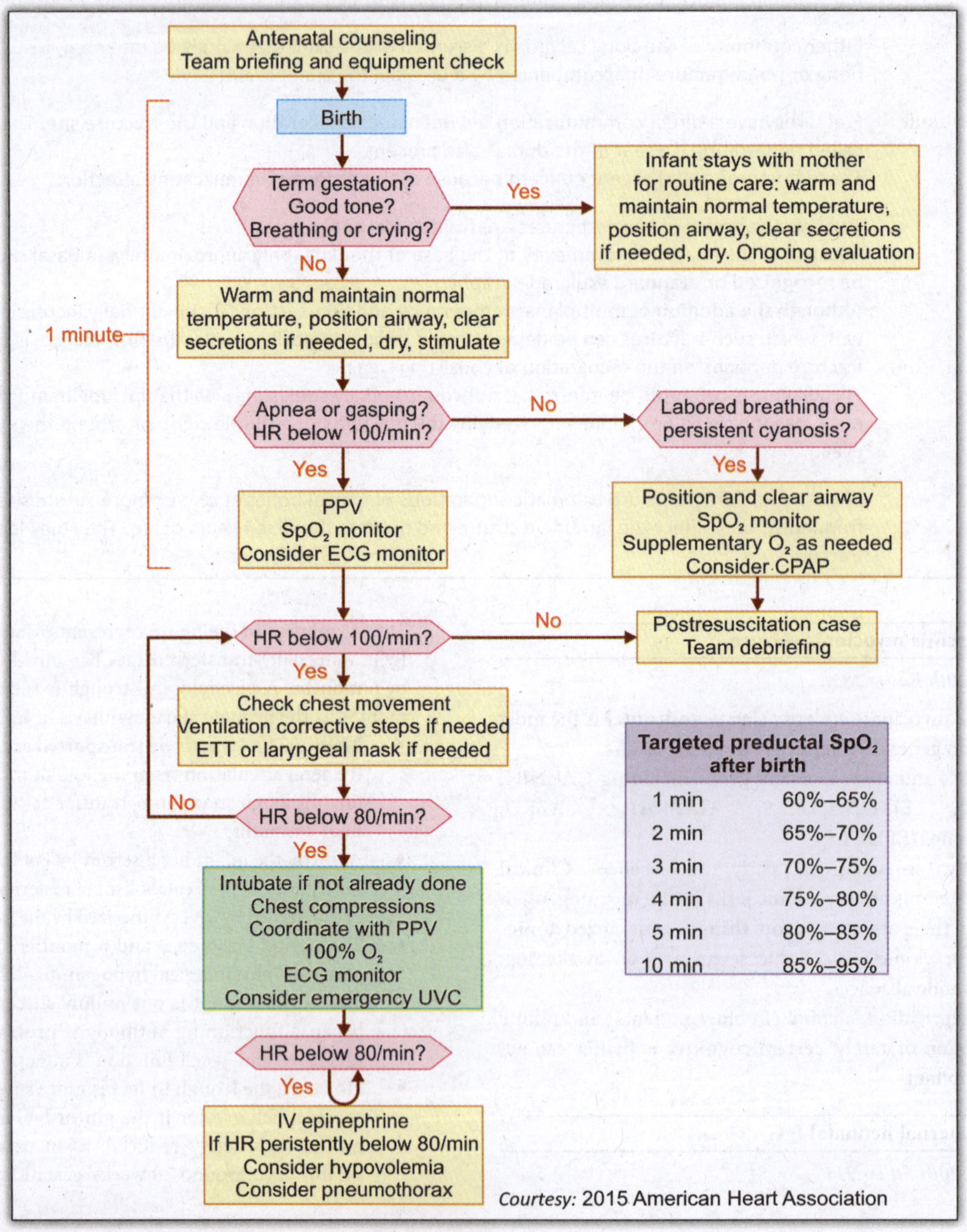

Targeted preductal SpO_2 after birth	
1 min	60%–65%
2 min	65%–70%
3 min	70%–75%
4 min	75%–80%
5 min	80%–85%
10 min	85%–95%

Courtesy: 2015 American Heart Association

11. Ans. (d) Reassure and repeat X-ray 5 days later

Ref: Pediatric Emergency Medicine Secrets by Steven M. Selbst 3rd Ed Pg 52; NBIH Triage and Treatment Algorithm for Battery Ingestions 2013 task force guidelines, T. Litovitz, N. Whitaker, L. Clark, N.C.White, M. Marsolek Emerging battery-ingestion hazard: clinical implications Pediatrics, 125 (6) (2010), pp. 1168-1177

Now, in the above question, the age of the child is not mentioned. However, since the most common age group is 1-4 yrs old, we shall assume that the age of the child belongs to this age group.

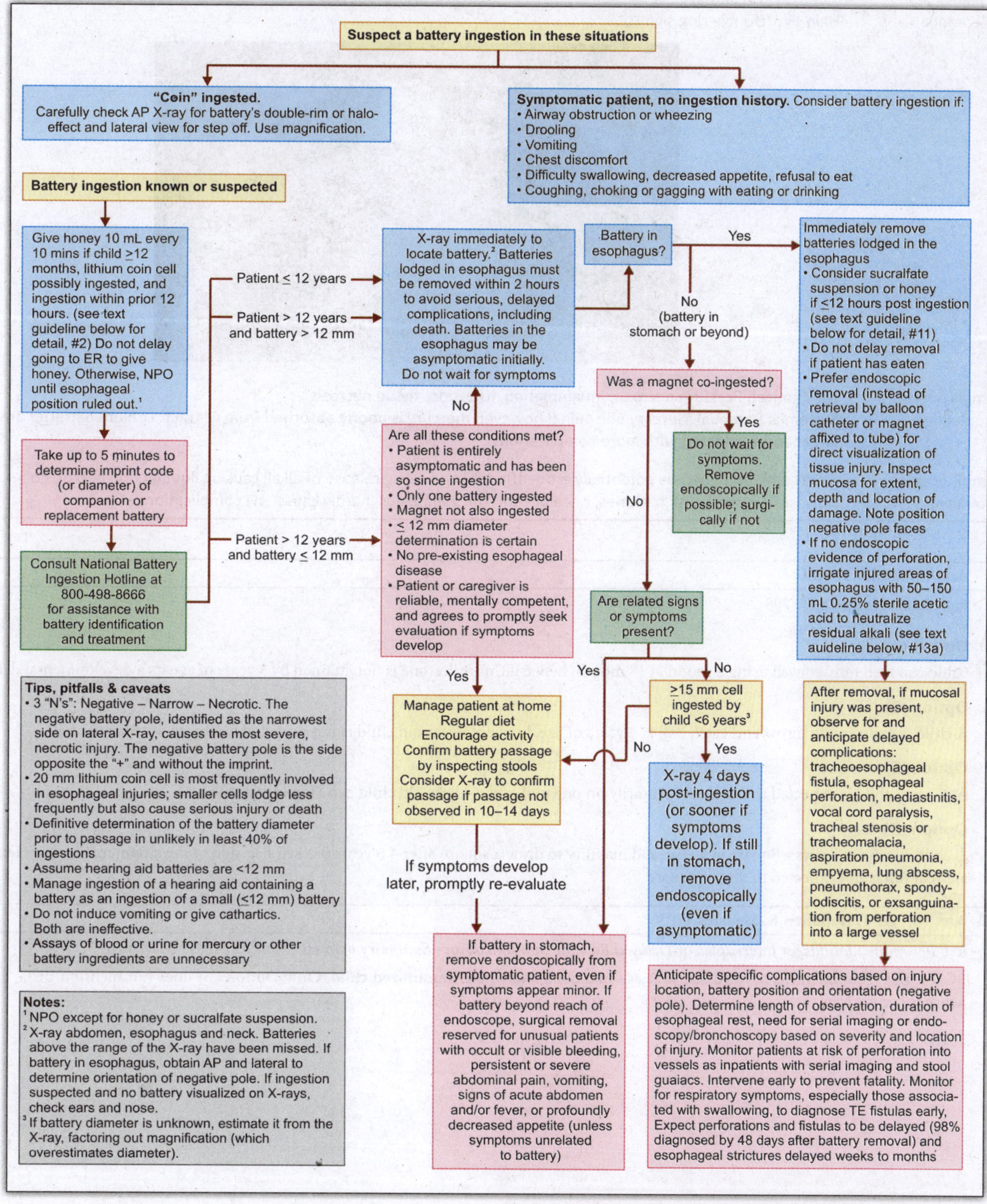

Battery Ingestion In Children	
Age group	**Most common in 1-4 yr old**
Types of battery	Shape: Disk (more common), cylindrical Content: Lithium/Mercuric oxide/ Zn/manganese dioxide/Silver oxide/Cupric oxide etc.
Radiological appearance	"Step off" on lateral view Halo sign/Double ring sign 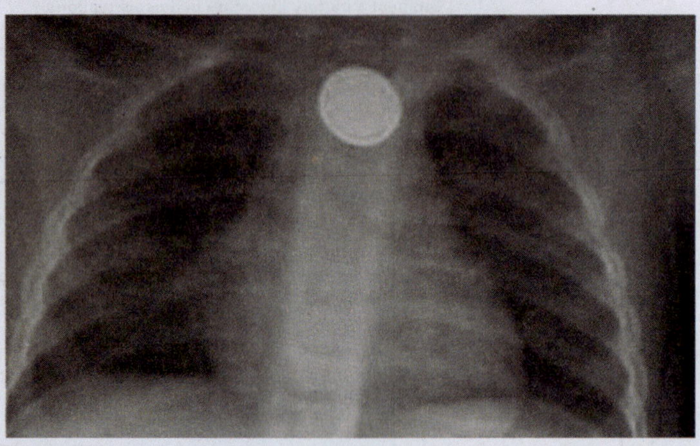
Complications (Esophagus)	**Mechanical:** Pressure necrosis, inflammation, irritation, tissue necrosis **Systemic:** Potential Mercury poisoning, however, mercury is poorly absorbed from GI tract. Lithium batteries are larger and associated with more complications
Complications (Stomach)	Acidic environment may potentially erode the seal and cause release of alkali causing liquefaction necrosis of mucosa. However, disk batteries, once beyond the esophagus, hardly cause any complications.

12. Ans. (a) Holds spoon

Ref: Nelson 20th ed page 798

Option (A)

Child can feed himself well using a spoon at 18 month, hence if this milestone is not attained by 3 years of age its a developmental delay

Option (B)

A child is expected to throw and catch ball at 4 years of age, hence a 3 year old child is not expected to Throw or catch the ball.

Option (C)

At 3 years child is expected to stand momentarily on one foot and a 4 year old child can Hop on one foot.

Option (D)

A child normally draws a Square at 4 year and inability to draw a square after 4.5 years is a red flag sign of developmental delay. Hence a 3 year old is not expected to draw a square.

13. Ans. (b) DPT, Hepatitis B, Measles, OPV

Ref: Recommendations for Interrupted or Delayed Routine Immunization - Summary of WHO Position Papers March 2017

BCG is not recommended beyond one year age in a completely non-immunized child. Only Option (B) does not mention BCG, and hence is the answer.

Antigen		Age of 1st Dose	Dose in Primary Series (min interval between doses)**	Interrupted Primary Series***	Does for those who start vaccination late		Booster
					If ≤ 12 months of age	If > 12 months of age	
Recommendations for all immunization programs							
BCG		As soon as possible after birth	1 dose	NA	1 dose	Not recommended	Not recommended
Hepatitis B		As soon as possible after birth (<24 hours)	Birth dose <24 hours plus 2-3 doses with DTP (4 weeks)	Resume without repeating previous dose	3 doses	3 doses	Not recommended
Polio	bOPV + IPV	6 weeks (see footnote for birth dose)	4 doses (IPV dose to be given with bOPV dose from 14 weeks of age) (4 weeks)	Resume without repeating previous dose	4 doses (IPV to be given with 1st dose of bOPV)	4 doses (IPV to be given with 1st dose of bOPV)	Not recommended
	IPV/bOPV Sequential	8 weeks (IPV 1st)	1-2 doses IPV and 2 doses bOPV (4 weeks)	Resume without repeating previous dose	1-2 doses IPV and 2 doses bOPV	1-2 doses IPV and 2 dose bOPV	Not recommended
	IPV	8 weeks	3 doses (4 weeks)	Resume without repeating previous dose	3 doses	3 doses	If the primary series begins <2 months of age, booster to be given at least 6 months after the last dose
DTP-containing vaccine		6 weeks (min)	3 doses (4 weeks)	Resume without repeating previous dose	3 doses	3 doses with interval of at least 4 weeks between 1st & 2nd dose, and 6-12 months between 2nd & 3rd dose (If >7 yrs use only aP containing vaccine; if >4 years Td containing vaccine is preferred and should only be used for >7 yrs)	3 boosters: 12-23 months (DTP-containing vaccine); 4-7 years (Td containing); and 9-15 years (Td containing) if >7 yrs use only aP containing vaccine If tetanus vaccination started during adolescence or adulthood only 5 doses required for lifelong protection

Table: Recommendations* for Interrupted or Delayed Routine Immunization - Summary of WHO Position Papers

Contd...

Recommendations* for Interrupted or Delayed Routine Immunization - Summary of WHO Position Papers

Antigen		Age of 1st Dose	Dose in Primary Series (min interval between doses)**	Interrupted Primary Series***	Does for those who start vaccination late: If ≤ 12 months of age	Does for those who start vaccination late: If > 12 months of age	Booster
Haemophilus Influenzae type b	Option 1	6 weeks (min)	3 doses (4 weeks)	Resume without repeating previous dose	3 doses	1 dose >5 yrs not recommended if healthy	None
	Option 2		2-3 doses (8 weeks if 2 doses; 4 weeks if 3 doses)		2-3 doses		At least 6 months (min) after last dose
Pneumococcal (Conjugate)		6 weeks (min)	3 doses with DTP (4 weeks) or 2 doses (8 weeks)	Resume without repeating previous dose	2-3 doses	1-2 yrs: 2 doses 2-5 yrs at high-risk: 2 doses	Booster at 9-15 months if following 2 dose schedule Another booster If HIV+ or preterm neonate
Rotavirus	Rotarix	6 weeks (min)	2 doses with DTP (4 weeks)	Resume without repeating previous dose	2 doses	>24 months limited benefits	Not recommended
	Rota Teq	6 weeks (min)	3 doses with DTP (4 weeks)	Resume without repeating previous dose	3 doses	>24 months limited benefits	Not recommended
Measles		9 or 12 months (6 months min, see footnote)	2 doses (4 weeks)	Resume without repeating previous dose	2 doses	2 doses	Not recommended
Rubella		9 or 12 months	1 dose with measles containing vaccine	NA	1 dose	1 dose	Not recommended
HPV		As soon as possible from 9 years of age (females)	2 doses (5 months)	If 1st dose given before 15 years of age resume without repeating previous dose)	NA	Girls: 9-14 years 2 doses (see footnote)	Not recommended

*For some antigens the WHO position paper does not provide a recommendation on interrupted or delayed schedules at this present time. When the position paper is next revised this will be included. In the meantime, some of the recommendations are based on expert opinion.

Recommendations* for Interrupted or Delayed Routine Immunization - Summary of WHO Position Papers							
Antigen		Age of 1st Dose	Dose in Primary Series (min interval between doses)**	Interrupted Primary Series***	Does for those who start vaccination late		Booster Dose
					If ≤ 12 months of age	If > 12 months of age	
Recommendations for certain regions							
Japanese Encephalitis	**Inactivated Vero cell-derived vaccine**	6 months	2 (4 weeks) generally	Resume without repeating previous dose	2 doses (generally)	2 doses (generally)	Note recommended
	Live attenuated	8 months	1	NA	1 dose	1 dose	
	Live recombinant vaccine	9 months	1	NA	1 dose	1 dose	
Yellow Fever		9-12 months	1 doses with measles containing vaccine	NA	1 dose	1 dose	Note recommended
Tick-Borne Encephalitis	**FSME-Immun & Encepur**	≥1 year	3 doses (1st to 2nd 1-3 mos; 2nd to 3rd 12 mos)	Resume without repeating previous dose	3 doses	3 doses	At least 1 booster
	TBE_Moscow & EnceVir	≥3 years	3 doses (1st to 2nd 1-7 mos; 2nd to 3rd 12 mos)	Resume without repeating previous dose	3 doses	3 doses	Every 3 years
Recommendations for some high-risk populations							
Typhoid	**VI PS**	2 years (min)	1 dose	NA	Not recommended	1 dose	Every 3 years
	Ty 21a	Capsules 5 years (min) (see footnote)	3-4 doses (1 day) (see footnote)	If interruption between doses is <21 days resume without repeating previous dose; If >21 days restart primary series	Not recommended	>5 years: 3-4 doses	Every 3-7 years
Cholera	**Dukoral (WC-rBS)**	2 years (min)	2-5 yrs: 3 doses ≥ 6 yrs: 2 doses (≥ 7 days)	If interval since last dose ≥ 6 weeks restart primary series	Not recommended	2-5 years: 3 doses > 6 yrs: 2 doses	2-5 yrs: every 6 months. If booster is delayed > 6 months the primary series must be repeated > 6 yrs: every 2 years. If booster is delayed > 2 yrs the primary series must be repeated
	Shanchol and mORCVAX	1 year (min)	2 doses (2 weeks)	Resume without repeating previous dose	Not recommended	2 doses	After 2 years

Contd...

Recommendations* for Interrupted or Delayed Routine Immunization - Summary of WHO Position Papers							
Antigen		Age of 1st Dose	Dose in Primary Series (min interval between doses)**	Interrupted Primary Series***	Does for those who start vaccination late		Booster Dose
					If ≤ 12 months of age	If > 12 months of age	
Meningococcal	MenA conjugate (5µg)	9-18 months	1	NA	2 doses if < 9 months with 8 weeks interval	1 dose of 5 µg up to 24 months	Note recommended
	MenC conjugate	2-11 months	2 (8 weeks min)	Resume without repeating previous dose	2 doses	1 dose	2-11 months of age after 1 years
		>12 months	1	NA			
	Quadrivalent conjugate	9-23 months	2 (12 weeks min)	Resume without repeating previous dose	2 doses	1 dose	
		≥2 years	1	NA			
Hepatitis A		1 year (min)	At least 1 dose		Not recommended	At least 1 dose	Not recommended
Rabies		As required	3 doses (1st to 2nd 7 days; 2nd to 3rd 14-21 days)	Resume without repeating previous dose; Interval between last two doses should be 14 days minimum	3 doses	3 doses	Only if occupation puts a frequent or continual risk of exposure
Dengue (CYD-TDV)		9 years (min)	3 doses (6 months)	Resume without repeating dose	Not recommended	3 doses ≥ 9 years	Not recommended
Recommendations for immunization programs with certain characteristics							
Mumps		12-18 months	2 doses with measles containing vaccine (4 weeks)	Resume without repeating previous dose	Not recommended	2 doses	Not recommended
Seasonal Influenza (Inactivated tri- and qudrivalent)		6 months (min)	< 9 yrs: 2 doses (4 weeks) ≥ 9 yrs: 1 dose	Resume without repeating previous dose	2 doses	< 9 yrs: 2 doses ≥ 9 yrs: 1 dose	Revaccinate annually 1 dose only
Varicella		12-18 months	1-2 (4 weeks - 3 months, depending on manufacturer)	Resume without repeating previous dose	Not recommended	1-2 doses	

Pentavalent vaccine provides protection to a child from 5 life-threatening diseases – Diphtheria, Pertussis, Tetanus, Hepatitis B and Hib. DPT (Diphtheria + Pertussis + Tetanus) and Hep B are already part of routine immunization in India; Hib vaccine is a new addition. Together, the combination is called Pentavalent.

14. Ans. (d) Gastrografin swallow with follow through

Ref: Nelson 20th ed 1801-1803

This is a case of intestinal obstruction mostly due to Jejunal Atresia. A child of Jejunal Atresia presents with Bilious vomiting and abdominal distension on 1st day of life. The diagnosis is suggested by the presence of a "Triple bubble sign" on plain abdominal radiographs

Why not Duodenal Atresia? *The hallmark of duodenal obstruction is bilious vomiting without abdominal distention, which is usually noted on the 1st day of life. The diagnosis is suggested by the presence of a "Double-bubble sign" on plain abdominal radiographs* (Nelson)

Duodenal vs Jejunal Atresia

	Duodenal atresia	Jejunal atresia
Bilious vomiting	Present	Present
Abdominal distension	Absent	Present
Radiograph	Double bubble sign	Triple bubble sign
Age of presentation	1 day of life	First day of life

Nelson states that: **"Bile-stained emesis suggests intestinal obstruction beyond the duodenum, but may also be idiopathic. Abdominal X-rays (kidney-ureter-bladder [KUB] and cross-table lateral views) should be performed in neonates with persistent emesis and in all infants with bile-stained emesis to detect air-fluid levels, distended bowel loops, characteristic patterns of obstruction (double bubble: duodenal atresia), and pneumoperitoneum (intestinal perforation). A contrast swallow roentgenogram with small bowel follow through is indicated in the presence of bilious emesis"**

The clinical presentation of intestinal obstruction varies with the cause, level of obstruction, and time between the obstructing event and the patient's evaluation. The classic symptoms of obstruction include nausea and vomiting, abdominal distention, and obstipation. Obstruction high in the intestinal tract involving the duodenum or proximal jejunum results in large-volume, frequent, bilious emesis

15. Ans. (d) Decorticate and decerebrate posturing

Ref: Nelson 20th ed 514

Brain dead criteria are different for different age group. Criteria for brain death in infants younger than 1 wk of age have not been delineated but should be at least as stringent as for those 1 wk–2 mo of age. It is often very difficult to diagnose brain death in premature infants; the wait period should be at least 72 hr. The standard wait period for adults is 6 hours.

- **Children 1 wk–2 mo of age:** fulfillment of the set criteria 2 separate examinations at least 48 hr apart, or 1 clinical examination followed by an isoelectric EEG at least 48 hr later
- **Children 2 mo–1 yr:** Fulfillment of the set clinical criteria in 2 separate examinations, at least 24 hours apart, or 1 clinical examination followed by an isoelectric EEG or negative results of a cerebral blood flow study at least 24 hours later
- **Children >1 yr:** Fulfillment of the set clinical criteria in 2 separate examinations at 12 hours apart

Brain Dead criteria in Children

Prerequisites	• A recognized cause of coma, sufficient to explain the irreversible cessation of all brain function • Potentially reversible causes of coma must be excluded: ▪ Sedatives and neuromuscular blocking drugs ▪ Hypothermia ▪ Metabolic and endocrine disturbances: ◆ Severe electrolyte disturbances ◆ Severe hypo- or hyperglycemia ▪ Uncontrolled hypotension ▪ Surgically remediable intracranial conditions ▪ Any other sign that suggests a potentially reversible cause of coma
Clinical evaluation	• **Absence of higher brain function:** *Lack of consciousness, voluntary movement or responsiveness except for spinal reflexes; no decorticate or decerebrate posturing, no convulsions* • **Absence of brainstem function** ▪ Absence of sympathetic and parasympathetic regulation of the pupils- Pupils in mid position or dilated, showing neither direct nor indirect reaction to light ▪ Disruption of the pathways controlling eye movement in the brainstem- Absence of spontaneous eye movement, absence of reaction to injection of iced water into the ear (vestibulo-ocular reflex), absence of doll's eye phenomenon (oculocephalic reflexes) ▪ Disruption of the afferent trigeminal and efferent facial nerve pathways- Absence of blink response to (careful) corneal stimulation ▪ Disruption of afferent and efferent pathways of cranial nerves IX and X in the medulla oblongata- Absence of gag response ▪ Absence of vagal efferent activity- No significant increase of heart rate on administration of intravenous atropine or on pressure applied to the eyeballs (oculocardiac reflex) ▪ Disruption of the respiratory control centers of the medulla oblongata- No respiratory movement (as assessed by observation ± capnography)
Confirmatory test	• Confirmation of absence of higher brain function- Electrocerebral silence on EEG during at least 30 minutes • Confirmation of complete infarction of the brain and brainstem by confirmation of absence of blood flow by Four-vessel contrast angiography or radionuclide imaging

16. Ans. (a) USG abdomen

Ref: Nelson 20th ed 891, SRB Manual of Surgery 4th ed page 786, Fundamentals of Pediatric Surgery by Peter Mattei Pg 541

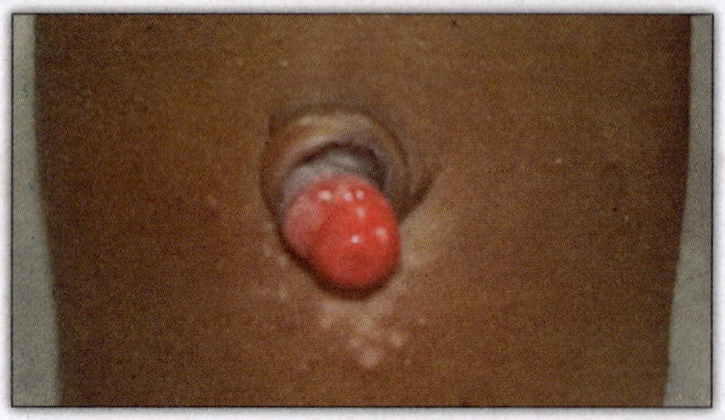

The given picture shows a reddish umbilical mass. ***Differential diagnosis of Reddish umbilical mass is Umbilical polyp, Umbilical granuloma and patent Vitellointestinal duct.*** This may have underlying remnant of vitellointestinal duct in 30–60% of cases and need evaluation by ultrasonography or laparoscopy. (Ref: Pediatric Surgery: A Quick Guide to Decision-making By Subhasis Roy Choudhury Page 135)

Umbilical granuloma must be differentiated from umbilical polyp, a rare anomaly resulting from persistence of all or part of the omphalomesenteric duct or the urachus. The tissue of the polyp is firm and resistant, is bright red, and has a mucoid secretion. If the polyp is communicating with the ileum or bladder, small amounts of fecal material or urine may be discharged intermittently. Histologically, the polyp consists of intestinal or urinary tract mucosa. Treatment is surgical excision of the entire omphalomesenteric or urachal remnant. (Nelson)

- Umbilical anomalies may be associated with Meckel's diverticulum. Although the treatment is mostly surgical, an imaging of the abdomen is warranted to rule out any connections with the bowel or any other structure.
- Umbilical polyps do not regress with silver nitrate cauterization (unlike umbilical granuloma) and should be surgically excised.

17. Ans. (a) Ganciclovir resistance is due to mutation in UL97 gene - DNA polymerase

Ref: Nelson 20th Ed Pg 1541, Harrison 19th Ed Pg 215e-7

Option (A) Ganciclovir resistance is due to mutation in UL97 gene - DNA polymerase - TRUE

- Ganciclovir is a nucleoside analog with structural similarity to acyclovir.
- Like acyclovir, ganciclovir must be phosphorylated for antiviral activity, which is targeted against the viral polymerase.
- The gene responsible for ganciclovir phosphorylation is not TK but rather the virally encoded UL97 phosphotransferase gene.
- Cidofovir is used against CMV isolates that are resistant to ganciclovir because of UL97 phosphotransferase mutations.

Option (B) CMV can be cultured in vitro in mammalian cells of animal origin like MDCK line - FALSE

- Human fibroblasts are used for virus isolation attempts. Humans are the only known host for CMV
- Madin-Darby Canine Kidney (**MDCK**) cells are a heteroploid cell culture. CMV can only be cultivated in diploid cell cultures.

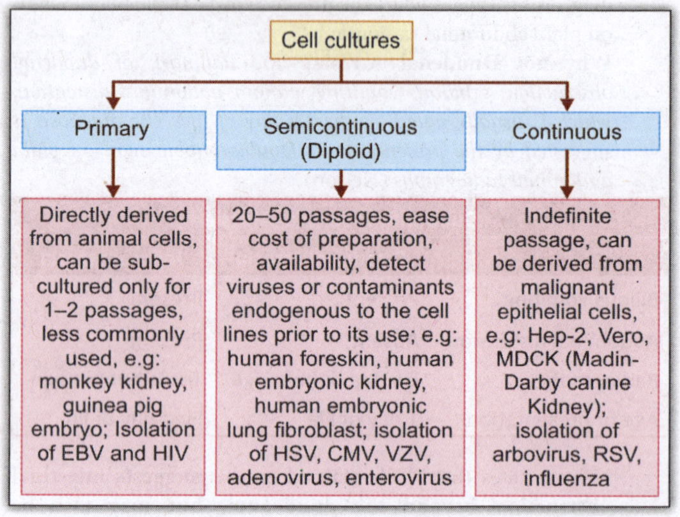

Option (C) Commonest manifestation of CMV associated disease in HIV seropositive patients is watery diarrhea-FALSE

Retinitis is the most common manifestation of CMV disease in HIV infected children.

Other manifestations are GI disorders (esophagitis, colitis, hepatitis), pulmonary manifestations (interstitial pneumonia), neurological disease(subacute focal encephalopathy, myelitis, polyradiculopathy)

Option (D) Ganciclovir resistant CMV strains show cross resistance to Foscarnet - FALSE

- Resistance has been noted in CMV isolates obtained after therapy with ganciclovir, especially those from patients with AIDS or from patients receiving prolonged ganciclovir therapy after organ transplantation.
- Such resistance may develop through a mutation in either the viral UL97 gene or the viral DNA polymerase. **Ganciclovir-resistant isolates are usually sensitive to Foscarnet** or may be sensitive to cidofovir, depending on the mechanism of resistance

18. Ans. (b) Serum calcium

Ref: Nelson's 20th Ed Pg 897

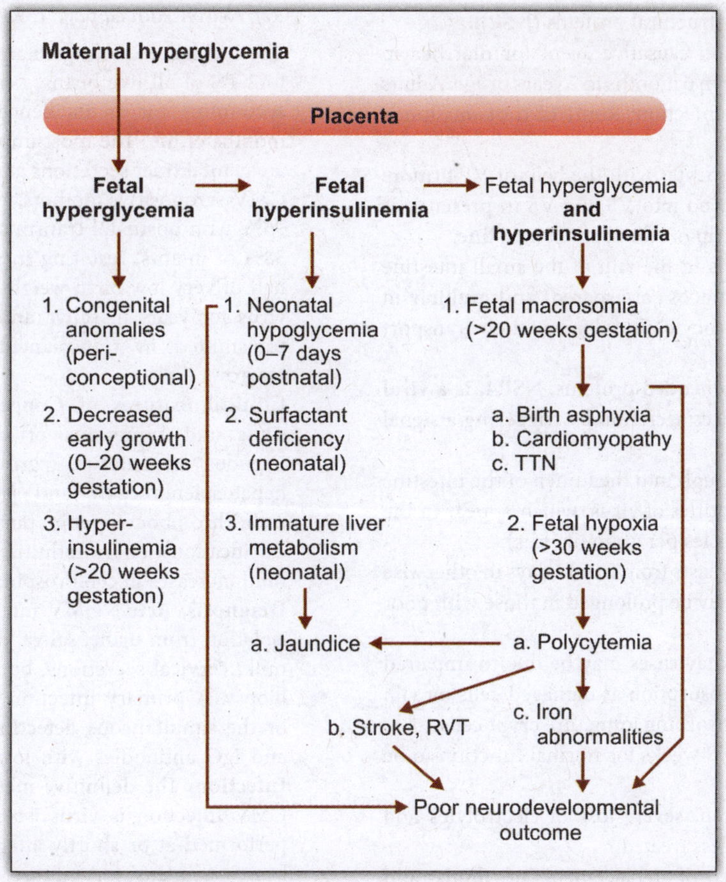

Anomalies in Infants of Diabetic Mothers	
Congenital cardiac anomalies	Transposition of Great Vessels, Double Outlet Right Ventricle, Ventricular Septal Defect, Tricuspid Atresia, Truncus Arteriosus, Patent Ductus Arteriosus
Other congenital anomalies	Neural tube defects, neural tube defects, hydronephrosis, renal agenesis and dysplasia, duodenal or anorectal atresia, situs inversus, double ureter, and holoprosencephaly, small left colon syndrome
Hypoglycemia	The infants tend to be jumpy, tremulous, and hyperexcitable during the 1st 3 days of life, although hypotonia, lethargy, and poor sucking may also occur. Early appearance of these signs is more likely to be related to hypoglycemia and later appearance related to hypocalcemia; these abnormalities may also occur together.
Hypomagnesemia	Diabetes, by causing maternal magnesium depletion, may decrease transfer of magnesium to the fetus. The consequent hypomagnesemia in infants causes secondary hypoparathyroidism and hypocalcemia.
Hypocalcemia	Due to PTH abnormalities
Tachypnea	During the 1st 2 days of life and may be a manifestation of hypoglycemia, hypothermia, polycythemia, cardiac failure, transient tachypnea, or cerebral edema from birth trauma or asphyxia. Higher incidence of respiratory distress syndrome due to an antagonistic effect of insulin on stimulation of surfactant synthesis by cortisol.
Cardiac complications	Cardiomegaly is common, heart failure may occur. Asymmetric septal hypertrophy may occur and become manifested similar to idiopathic hypertrophic subaortic stenosis. Inotropic agents worsen the obstruction and are contraindicated
Other complications	Increased incidence of hyperbilirubinemia, polycythemia, and renal vein thrombosis, stroke Renal vein thrombosis should be suspected in infants with a flank mass, hematuria, and thrombocytopenia.

19. Ans. (b) NSP 4

Ref: Jawetz 26th Ed Pg 546-548

- Viruses have 2 types of proteins - structural proteins (viral proteins VP) and nonstructural proteins (NSP).
- Rotavirus is a common causative agent for diarrhea in children, especially from 6 months to 2 years of age. Adults may have subclinical infection. Route of transmission is feco-oral.
- Rotavirus enters enterocytes with the help of VP4 (more rapid when V4 is cleaved into V5 and V8 in presence of trypsin) targeting the tip of villi in small intestine.
- Rotaviruses infect cells in the villi of the small intestine (gastric and colonic mucosa are spared) and multiply in the cytoplasm of enterocytes and damage their transport mechanisms.
- One of the rotavirus-encoded proteins, **NSP4, is a viral enterotoxin** and induces secretion by triggering a signal transduction pathway.
- Damaged cells may slough into the lumen of the intestine and release large quantities of virus, which appear in the stool (up to 1012 particles per gram of feces).
- Viral excretion usually lasts from 2 to 12 days in otherwise healthy patients but may be prolonged in those with poor nutrition.
- Diarrhea caused by rotaviruses may be due to impaired sodium and glucose absorption as damaged cells on villi are replaced by non absorbing immature crypt cells.
- It may take from 3 to 8 weeks for normal function to be restored
- In infants and children, severe loss of electrolytes and fluids may be fatal unless treated.
- Management consists of replacement of fluids and restoration of electrolyte balance either intravenously or orally as feasible.
- Live attenuated oral pentavalent (human-bovine) and monovalent vaccines are available and effective.

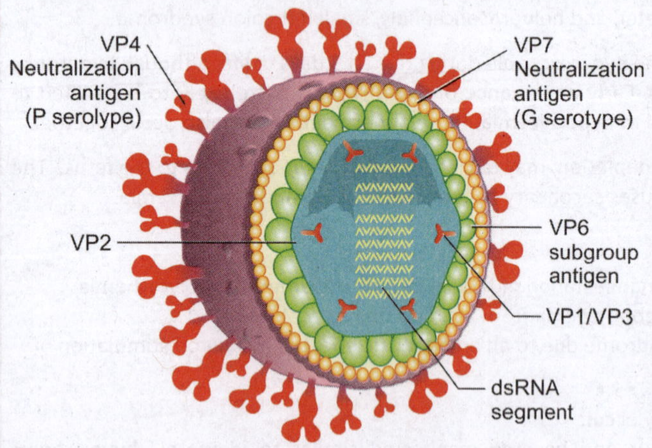

Structure of Rotavirus

20. Ans. (b) Urine

Ref: Nelson 20th ed page 1593

The incidence of congenital CMV infection ranges from 0.2 to 2.4% of all live births. Perinatal transmission is common, accounting for an incidence of 10–60% through the 1st 6 months of life. The most important perinatal sources of virus are genital tract secretions at delivery and breast milk. Among CMV-seropositive mothers, virus is detectable in breast milk in 96%, with postnatal transmission occurring in approximately 38% of infants, resulting in symptomatic infection in nearly half of very low birth weight infants. Infected infants excrete virus for years in saliva and urine. CMV infection may be transmitted in transplanted organs (kidney, heart, bone marrow).

Clinical features of Congenital CMV: The characteristic signs and symptoms of clinically manifested infections include intrauterine growth restriction, prematurity, hepatosplenomegaly and jaundice, blueberry muffin like rash, thrombocytopenia, purpura, microcephaly, intracranial calcifications, chorioretinitis, sensorineural hearing loss, and mild increases in cerebrospinal fluid protein.

Diagnosis: Active CMV infection is best confirmed by virus isolation from urine, saliva, bronchoalveolar washings, breast milk, cervical secretions, buffy coat, and tissues obtained by biopsy. A primary infection is confirmed by seroconversion or the simultaneous detection of immunoglobulin M (IgM) and IgG antibodies with low functional avidity. **Congenital Infection:** The definitive method for diagnosis of congenital CMV infection is virus isolation or PCR, which should be performed at or shortly after birth. Urine and saliva are the best specimens for culture. Infants with congenital CMV infection may excrete CMV in the urine for several years. An IgG antibody test is of little diagnostic value because a positive result also reflects maternal antibodies, although a negative result excludes the diagnosis of congenital CMV infection.

21. Ans. (b) Menkes disease

Ref: Nelson 18th ed Ch 599.5, 661

Menkes Kinky-hair Syndrome (Trichopoliodystrophy)

- Menkes disease (kinky hair disease) is a progressive neurodegenerative condition inherited as a sex-linked recessive trait. Males with this X-linked recessive trait are born to an unaffected mother after a normal pregnancy.
- Symptoms begin in the 1st few months of life and include **hypothermia, hypotonia, poor feeding, seizures, and failure** to thrive.
- The facies are distinctive, with chubby, rosy cheeks and kinky, colorless, friable hair.
- Hair is normal to sparse at birth but is replaced by short, fine, brittle, light-colored hair. Microscopic examination of the hair shows several abnormalities, including trichorrhexis nodosa (fractures along the hair shaft) and pili torti (twisted hair).

- The skin is hypopigmented and thin cheeks typically appear plump, and the nasal bridge is depressed.
- Progressive psychomotor retardation is noted in early infancy. Severe mental retardation and optic atrophy are constant features of the disease.
- Menkes gene **ATP7A** gene codes for a copper transporting **P-type ATPase.** Mutations in the, encoding a copper transporting ATPase protein, cause Menkes kinky hair syndrome.
- The, and mutations in the protein are associated with low serum copper and ceruloplasmin levels as well as a defect in copper absorption and transport across the intestines.
- Death occurs by 3 years of age in untreated patients.
- Parenteral administration of copper is helpful if begun in the 1st 2 month of life.
- Copper-histidine therapy may be effective in preventing neurologic deterioration in some patients with Menkes disease, particularly when treatment is begun in the neonatal period or, preferably, with the fetus. Copper-histidine is given subcutaneously in a dose of 50–150 μg elemental copper/kg/24 hr for the duration of the child's life. The serum copper and ceruloplasmin levels return to the normal range within 2–3 weeks of commencing therapy.

22. Ans. (b) Appearance, Pulse, Grimace, Activity, Respiration

Ref: Nelson 20th ed page 798, http://www.acog.org/Resources-And-Publications/Committee-Opinions/Committee-on-Obstetric-Practice/The-Apgar-Score

This Question was asked twice in this paper

Apgar Score

A useful clinical tool to identify those neonates who require resuscitation as well as to assess the effectiveness of any resuscitative measures is the Apgar scoring system (Apgar, 1953). As shown in each of the five easily identifiable characteristics—**heart rate, respiratory effort, muscle tone, reflex irritability, and color**—is assessed and assigned a value of 0 to 2. The total score, based on the sum of the five components, is determined 1 and 5 minutes after delivery.

	Score of 0	Score of 1	Score of 2	Component of acronym
Skin color/Complexion	Blue or pale all over	Blue at extremities body pink (acrocyanosis)	No cyanosis body and extremities pink	Appearance
Pulse rate	Absent	<100	≥100	Pulse
Reflex irritability	No response to stimulation	Grimace/feeble cry when stimulated	Cry or pull away when stimulated	Grimace
Muscle tone	None	Some flexion	Flexed arms and legs that resist extension	Activity
Breathing (respiratory effort)	Absent	Weak, irregular, gasping	Strong, lusty cry	Respiration

Factors Affecting the Apgar Score

False-Positive (No Fetal Acidosis or Hypoxia; Low Apgar)	False-Negative (Acidosis; Normal Apgar)
Immaturity	Maternal acidosis
Analgesics, narcotics, sedatives	High fetal catecholamine levels
Magnesium sulfate	Some full-term infants
Acute cerebral trauma	
Precipitous delivery	
Congenital myopathy	
Congenital neuropathy	
Spinal cord trauma	
Central nervous system anomaly	
Lung anomaly (diaphragmatic hernia)	
Airway obstruction (choanal atresia)	
Congenital pneumonia and sepsis	
Previous episodes of fetal asphyxia (recovered)	
Hemorrhage-hypovolemia	

Footnote:
- APGAR scoring is done at 1 min and 5 min. Thereafter **EXPANDED APGAR** is done at every 5 min interval till 20 min if required. Sometimes additional APGAR scoring is also done at 7 min if required.
- Respiratory effort not Respiratory rate is a part of APGAR scoring system[Q]
- Neonatal Encephalopathy and Neurologic Outcome, Second Edition, published in 2014 by the College in collaboration with the American Association of Pediatrics, defines a 5-minute APGAR score of 7–10 as reassuring, a score of 4–6 as moderately abnormal, and a score of 0–3 as low in the term infant and late-preterm infant

Contd...

- A low score may be due to a number of factors, including drugs given to the mother during labor and immaturity
- The APGAR score was not designed to predict neurologic outcome. Indeed, the score is normal in most patients in whom cerebral palsy subsequently develops, and the incidence of cerebral palsy is low in infants with APGAR scores of 0–3 at 5 minutes (but higher than in infants with APGAR scores of 7–10)
- The **APGAR score and umbilical artery blood pH both predict neonatal death.** An APGAR score of 0–3 at 5 minutes is uncommon but is a better predictor of neonatal death (in both term and preterm infants) than an umbilical artery pH of 7.0 or less; the presence of both variables increases the relative risk of neonatal mortality in term and preterm infants

23. Ans. (d) Very Long chain fatty acid

Ref: Nelson 20th ed page 685, Harper 30th ed page 241, 614

There are four disorders of Peroxisome Import
- Zellweger syndrome
- Neonatal adrenoleukodystrophy
- Infantile Refsum disease
- Rhizomelic chondrodysplasia punctata (RCDP)

Peroxisomal Disorder can be diagnosed by measurement of plasma VLCFA (Very long chain fatty acid), which is the most commonly used assay. Whereas plasma VLCFA levels are elevated in many patients with peroxisomal disorders, this is not always the case. The most important exceptions are RCDP (Rhizomelic chondrodysplasia punctata), in which VLCFA levels are normal, but plasma phytanic acid levels are increased and red blood cell plasmalogen levels are reduced

Newborn infants with Zellweger syndrome show striking and consistent, recognizable abnormalities. Of central diagnostic importance are the typical facial appearance (high forehead, unslanting palpebral fissures, hypoplastic supraorbital ridges, and epicanthal folds severe weakness and hypotonia, neonatal seizures, and eye abnormalities (cataracts, glaucoma, corneal clouding, Brushfield spots, pigmentary retinopathy, and nerve dysplasia). Because of the hypotonia and "mongoloid" appearance, Down syndrome may be suspected. Infants with Zellweger syndrome rarely live more than a few months

24. Ans. (a) Holds spoon

Ref: Nelson 20th ed page 798

Option (A)

Child can feed himself well using a spoon at 18 month, hence if this milestone is not attained by 3 years of age its a developmental delay

Option (B)

A child is expected to throws and catches ball at 4 years of age, hence a 3 year old child is not expected to throw or catch the ball.

Option (C)

At 3 years child is expected to stand momentarily on one foot and a 4 year old child can Hop on one foot.

Option (D)

A child normally draws a square at 4 year and inability to draw a square after 4.5 years is a red flag sign of developmental delay. Hence a 3 year old is not expected to draw a square.

25. Ans. (b) Continue breastfeed and phototherapy

Ref: Nelson 20th ed page 65-70, 640, Ghai 8th ed page 173, IAP Textbook of Pediatrics 4th ed page 78, Manual of Neonatal care Cloherty 7th ed page 332

At 4th day (96 hours) 18 mg/dL bilirubin is high risk hence Phototherapy has to be initiated. But it is below critical level of 25 mg/dL hence Exchange transfusion is not indicated. Since Phototherapy causes dehydration stopping Breastfeeding is not recommended by IAP

Three determinants in this question are:
- Is the Jaundice Pathological or Physiological
- When to initiate therapy
- What therapy should be initiated

Physiological Jaundice: About 60 to 70 percent of healthy newborn babies are likely to develop physiological jaundice which may cause undue anxiety to the parents. Physiological jaundice appears between 24 and 72 hours of age, its maximum intensity is seen on the 4th to 5th days of life, and the peak serum bilirubin level does not exceed 15 mg/dL

The management of neonatal hyperbilirubinemia is focused on prevention of hyperbilirubinemia, defined as total serum or plasma bilirubin (TB) >95th percentile on the hour-specific Bhutani nomogram. The decision of when to initiate therapy and the choice of intervention are based on the probability of developing severe hyperbilirubinemia using hour-specific TB values, gestational age (GA), and the presence or absence of risk factors.

Option (C)

Exchange transfusion: If despite phototherapy and other supportive measures, the bilirubin level is approaching 20 mg/dL, exchange blood transfusion is mandatory to prevent brain damage.

Indications for Exchange Blood Transfusion

Early indications in infants with Rh-HDN	Jaundice due to any cause
• Cord hemoglobin of 10 g/dL or less • Cord bilirubin of 5 mg/dL or more • Unconjugated serum bilirubin of more than 10 mg/dL within 24 hours or rate of rise of more than 0.5 mg/dL per hour	• Exchange at lower bilirubin levels in the presence of perinatal distress factors (Asphyxia, respiratory distress, sepsis, hypothermia, etc.) • Unconjugated serum bilirubin of 20 mg/dL or more in a term baby • In preterm babies, serum bilirubin of more than 1.0 mg/ 100 g weight of the infant (i.e., 10 mg/dL for 1000 g and 15 mg/dL for 1500 g and so on)

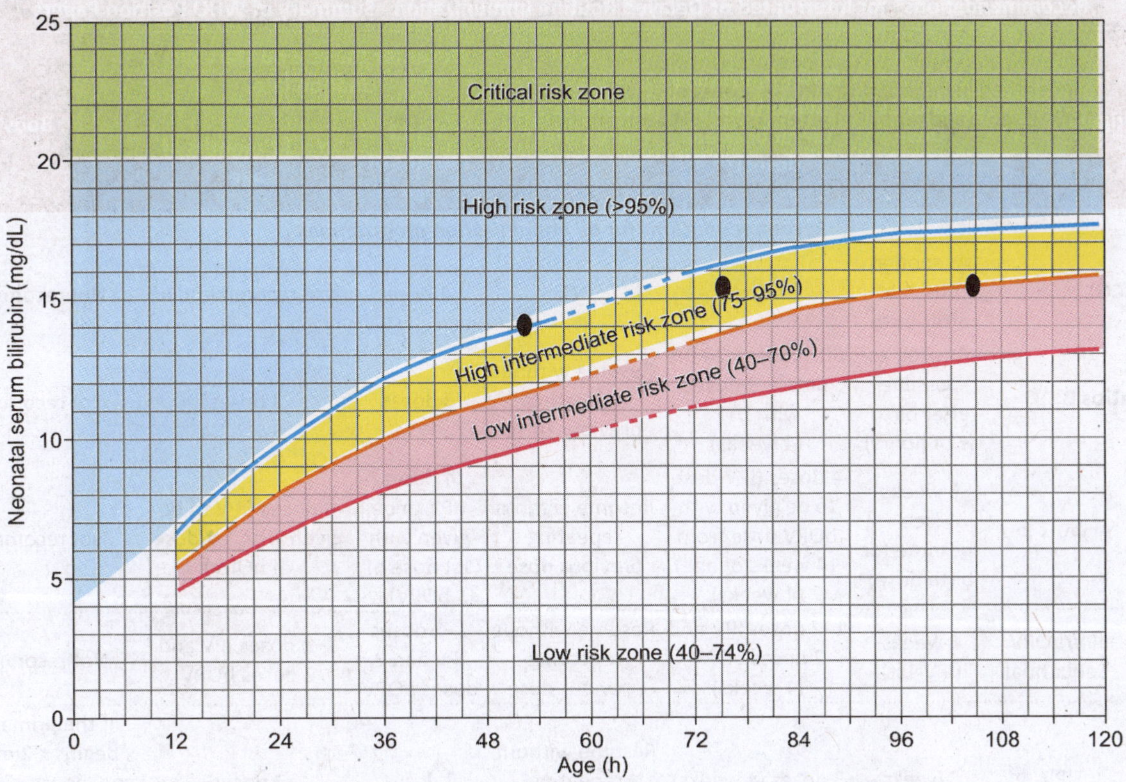

Hour-specific Bilirubin risk chart for term and near-term infants

Adapted and revised (April 2003) based on IHC data (12-54 h) and from Bhutani VK et al. Pediatr 199; 103:6–14 and J Perinat 2001;21:S76-S28 (72-120 h)

26. Ans. (a) Hutchinson teeth, interstitial keratitis, eighth nerve deafness

Ref: Ghai 8th ed page 273, Shafer's Textbook of Oral Pathology 6th ed Page 324, Harrison 19th ed page 1137

NOTE

Mulberry molars was not described in the original article of Hutchinson, hence it was not the part of original Hutchinson triad. But later many textbooks started quoting Mulberry Molars as part of triad. Hence for the Purpose of this question Mulberry molar is not the part of triad. (Ref: J. Hutchinson: Report on the effects of infantile syphilis in marring the development of the teeth. Transactions of the Pathological Society of London, 1858, 9: 449-456.)

Hutchinson's triad is named after Sir Jonathan Hutchinson. It is a common pattern of presentation for congenital syphilis, and consists of three phenomena: interstitial keratitis, Hypoplasia of Incisors (Hutchinson incisors) and Molars (Mulberry molars), and eighth nerve deafness (SNHL)

Hutchinson teeth, which are the peg or barrel-shaped upper central incisors that erupt during the 6th year of life. Mulberry molars, the abnormal 1st lower (6 years) molars characterized by a small biting surface and an excessive number of cusps.

27. Ans. (d) DPT + OPV + MMR

Ref: Ghai 8th ed page 207, Park 24th ed page 132, WHO Recommendations for interrupted or delayed Routine Immunization (March 2017)

Pentavalent vaccine provides protection to a child from 5 life-threatening diseases—Diphtheria, Pertussis, Tetanus, Hepatitis B and Hib. DPT (Diptheria + Pertussis + Tetanus) and Hep B are already part of routine immunization in India; Hib vaccine is a new addition. Together, the combination is called Pentavalent. Basically, BCG is the only vaccine which is not recommended if the child is more than 1 year of age. Also note that Haemophilus influenzae B is not recommended if the child is healthy and > 5 years old.

Recommendations* for Interrupted or Delayed Routine Immunization - Summary of WHO Position Papers

Antigen		Age of 1st Dose	Doses in Primary Series (min interval between doses)**	Interrupted primary series***	Doses for those who start vaccination late: If ≤ 12 months of age	Doses for those who start vaccination late: If > 12 months of age	Booster
Recommendations for all immunization programmes							
BCG[1]		As soon as possible after birth	1 dose	NA	1 dose	Not recommended	Not recommended
Hepatitis B[2]		As soon as possible after birth (<24 hours)	Birth dose <24 hrs plus 2–3 doses with DTP (4 weeks)	Resume without repeating previous dose	3 doses	3 doses	Not recommended
Polio[3]	bOPV + IPV	6 weeks (see footnote for birth dose)	4 doses (IPV dose to be given with bOPV dose from 14 weeks of age) (4 weeks)	Resume without repeating previous dose	4 doses (IPV to be given with 1st dose of bOPV)	4 doses (IPV to be given with 1st dose of bOPV)	Not recommended
Polio[3]	IPV/bOPV Sequential	8 weeks (IPV 1st)	1–2 doses IPV and 2 doses bOPV (4 weeks)	Resume without repeating previous dose	1–2 doses IPV and 2 doses bOPV	1–2 doses IPV and 2 doses bOPV	Not recommended
Polio[3]	IPV	8 weeks	3 doses (4 weeks)	Resume without repeating previous dose	3 doses	3 doses	If the primary series begins < 2 months of age, booster to be given at least 6 months after the last dose
DTP-containing vaccine[4]		6 weeks (min)	3 doses (4 weeks)	Resume without repeating previous dose	3 doses	3 doses with interval of at least 4 weeks between 1st & 2nd dose, and 6–12 months between 2nd and 3rd dose (if >7 years use only aP containing vaccine; if > 4 years Td containing vaccine is preferred and should only be used for >7 yrs)	3 boosters: 12–23 months (DTP- containing vaccine); 4–7 years (Td containing); and 9–15 yrs (Td containing) (if > 7 yrs use only aP containing vaccine) If tetanus vaccination started during adolescence or adulthood only 5 doses required for lifelong protection
Haemophilus influenzae type b[5]	Option 1	6 weeks (min)	3 doses (4 weeks)	Resume without repeating previous dose	3 doses	1 dose >5 yrs not recommended if healthy	None
Haemophilus influenzae type b[5]	Option 2	6 weeks (min)	2–3 doses (8 weeks if 2 doses; 4 weeks if 3 doses)	Resume without repeating previous dose	2–3 doses	1 dose >5 yrs not recommended if healthy	At least 6 months (min) after last dose
Pneumococcal (Conjugate)[6]		6 weeks (min)	3 doses with DTP (4 weeks) or 2 doses (8 weeks)	Resume without repeating previous dose	2–3 doses	1–2 yrs: 2 doses 2–5 yrs at high-risk: 2 doses	Booster at 9–15 months if following 2 dose schedule Another booster if HIV+ or preterm neonate
Rotavirus[7]	Rotarix	6 weeks (min)	2 doses with DTP (4 weeks)	Resume without repeating previous dose	2 doses	>24 months limited benefits	Not recommended

Contd...

Recommendations* for Interrupted or Delayed Routine Immunization - Summary of WHO Position Papers						
Antigen	Age of 1st Dose	Doses in Primary Series (min interval between doses)**	Interrupted primary series***	Doses for those who start vaccination late		Booster
				If ≤ 12 months of age	If > 12 months of age	
Rota Teq	6 weeks (min)	3 doses with DTP (4 weeks)	Resume without repeating previous dose	3 doses	>24 months limited benefits	Not recommended
Measles[8]	9 or 12 months (6 months min, see footnote)	2 doses (4 weeks)	Resume without repeating previous dose	2 doses	2 doses	Not recommended
Rubella[9]	9 or 12 months	1 dose with measles containing vaccine	NA	1 dose	1 dose	Not recommended
HPV[10]	As soon as possible from 9 years of age (females)	2 doses (5 months)	If 1st dose given before 15 years of age resume without repeating previous dose	NA	Girls: 9–14 years 2 doses (see footnote)	Not recommended

* For some antigens the WHO position paper does not provide a recommendation on interrupted or delayed schedules at this present time. When the position paper is next revised this will be included. In the meantime, some of the recommendations are based on expert opinion.

** See Table 2: Summary of WHO Position Papers - Recommended Routine Immunizations for Children for full details (www.who.int/immunization/documents/position papers/).

*** Same interval as primary series unless otherwise specified.

28. Ans. (b) Inborn error of metabolism

Ref: Nelson 20th ed page 1022, 1053

One emerging technique in the field of bioanalysis and drug discovery is the dried blood spot (DBS) analysis, which is also successfully used for neonatal screening of inborn errors of metabolism using targeted metabolomics—one of the most widely adopted clinical metabolomics applications to date.

AIIMS MAY 2017

29. Ans. (c) Oral cotrimoxazole for 5 days and send home

Ref: Ghai 8th ed page 759, IMNCI protocol, http://apps.who.int/iris/bitstream/10665/137319/1/9789241507813_eng.pdf

NOTE

That WHO has revised the classification of Childhood Pneumonia.

Indirect repeat AIIMS NOV 14, MAY 2014, NOV 2013 (Straight forward question was asked, whether or not child has Pneumonia?)

See table of CHILDHOOD PNEUMONIA in Pediatrics AIIMS NOV 2014

In 18-month-old child respiratory rate of 46/min is fast breathing. As per new guidelines of childhood pneumonia, fast breathing is categorized along with pneumonia for the sake of treatment plan.

- Children with fast breathing were classified as having "pneumonia" and were given an oral antibiotic (at that time **oral cotrimoxazole**) to take at home for **five days.**
- Children who had chest indrawing with or without fast breathing were classified as having **"severe pneumonia"** and were referred to the closest higher-level health facility for treatment with injectable penicillin.
- Children who had any general danger signs were classified as having **"severe pneumonia or very severe disease".** These children received a first dose of oral antibiotic and were then urgently referred to a higher-level health facility for further evaluation and treatment with parenteral antibiotics.

30. Ans. (b) It is the most common cause of non-syndromic sensorineural hearing loss

Ref: Nelson 20th ed Page 1592

Option (A) False

The diagnosis of congenital CMV infections requires the recovery of replicating virus and/or viral nucleic acids within the 1st 3 weeks of life. Sources of virus and viral nucleic acids include urine, saliva, and blood. Methods of detection include routine virus culture combined with immunofluorescence and polymerase chain reaction. IgM even at birth to 6 months will be suggestive of congenital CMV. Beyond 6 months it is said to be not of congenital origin.

Option (B) True

Hearing loss is the most common long-term sequela associated with congenital CMV infection. The most common congenital cause of nonhereditary and non syndromic deafness is cytomegalovirus (CMV).

NOTE

Nonsyndromic and Nonhereditary words are interchangeably used by many text to describe hearing loss but there is a minor difference. Syndromic hearing loss is always due to genetic alteration and with additional clinical features. Nonsyndromic lacks additional clinical features but can still have genetic alteration, i.e. it can be hereditary or nonhereditary.

Option (C) False

Congenital infection with CMV can present with symptomatic infections in approximately **10% of infected newborns, whereas 90% of infected infants will have no clinical manifestations** of infection in the newborn period. Severe multiorgan disease is infrequent and occurs less than 5% of infants with congenital CMV infections. The clinical findings of infants with symptomatic congenital CMV infections can include hepatosplenomegaly, petechial rashes, jaundice, and in some cases microcephaly. These findings were utilized for natural history studies to classify infants as having symptomatic or asymptomatic infections; however, several authors have included intrauterine growth restriction as a finding of symptomatic congenital CMV infection. Laboratory findings include direct hyperbilirubinemia, elevation of hepatic transaminases, thrombocytopenia, anemia, and abnormal findings on cranial ultrasonography. If cerebrospinal fluid is obtained, there can be evidence of encephalitis with elevation of mononuclear cell number and in some cases, elevation of cerebrospinal fluid protein. A small number of symptomatically infected infants (<10%) will be found to have chorioretinitis.

Option (D) False

Mother transmitting the disease usually are asymptomatic usually whether it is developed or developing nation.

31. Ans. (b) Macrocephaly

Ref: Nelson 20th ed Page 895

See Table of TERATOGENS in Pediatrics AIIMS Nov 2016 (see page no. 824-825)

Microcephaly not macrocephaly is seen in Fetal Alcohol syndrome

Option (B)

Holoprosencephaly (HPE) is a cephalic disorder in which the prosencephalon (the forebrain of the embryo) fails to develop into two hemispheres. It is not mentioned in association with fetal alcohol syndrome in Nelson. But other books clearly mentions it in severe cases of fetal alcohol syndrome

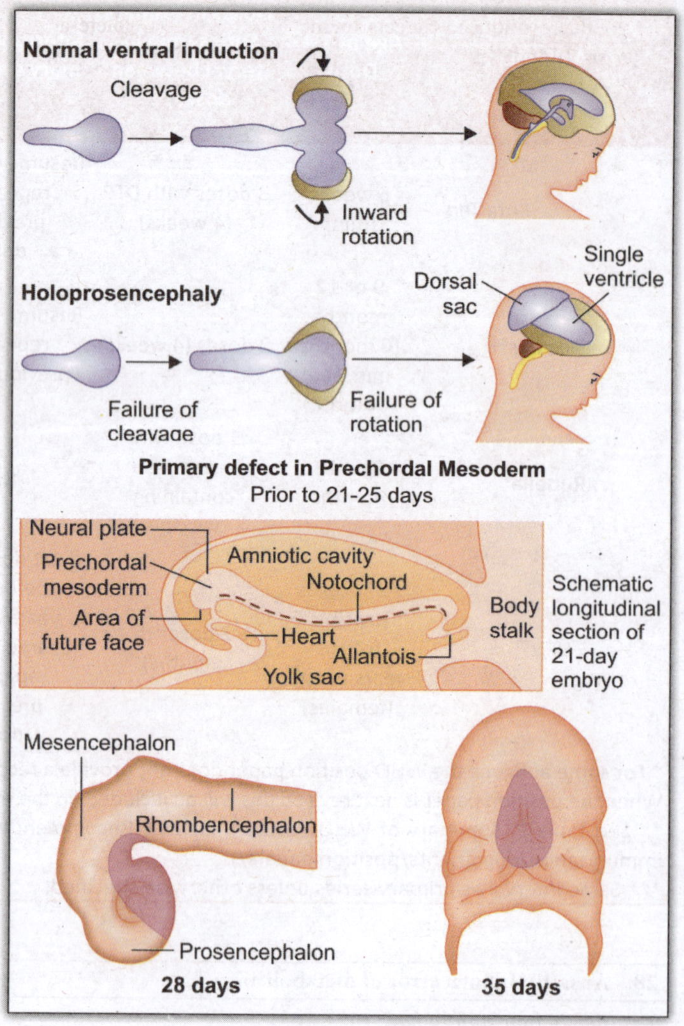

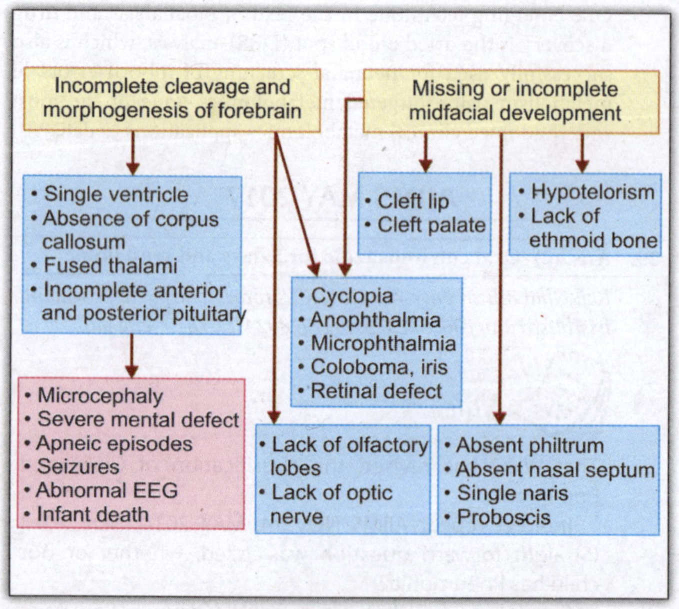

Fig: Developmental pathogenesis of sequence

Option (D)

Reduced brain volume and thinning is corpus callosum is not clinical feature but CT/MRI finding of Fetal alcohol syndrome. Ethanol-induced defects to the CC include complete agenesis (nondevelopment), hypoplasia (underdevelopment), and spatial displacement. Complete agenesis of the CC is the most severe manifestation of this defect and occurs with greater frequency among fetal alcohol-exposed individuals than other developmentally disabled groups.

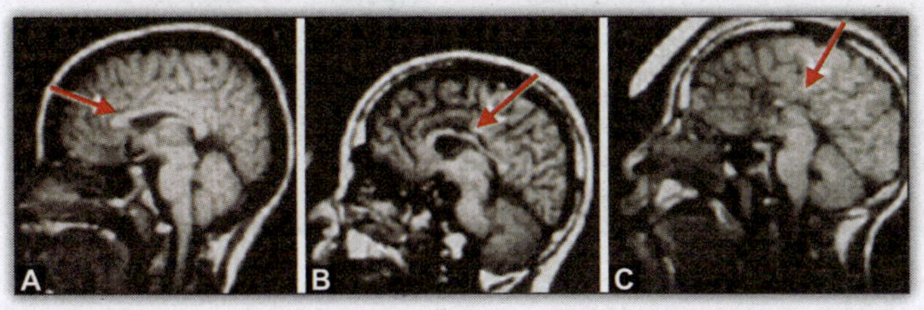

Fig: The brain of a normal individual (A) and two with FAS (B, C) shows permanent loss of the tissue indicated by the arrows (portions of the corpus callosum)

32. Ans. (d) ORS with zinc for 14 days.

Ref: Nelson 20th Ed page 1869-74, Ghai 8th ed page 293-294

Similar question was asked in Pediatrics AIIMS Nov 2015.

The *mainstay of treatment of diarrhea is* ***Rehydration Therapy***. If child is able to take orally well the rehydration should be done orally and when he is not able to, has to be done parentally.

Zinc supplementation is the only adjunct therapy that has proven benefit in reducing the severity and duration of non-cholera diarrheal illnesses. Various strains of probiotics have been studied for the treatment of acute onset diarrhea but reports in various literature suggest a moderate clinical improvement of diarrhea with strains of Lactobacillus GG and Saccharomyces boulardii with no adverse effects attributed to probiotic treatments. The efficacy is strain- and dose dependent. *Further research is needed to establish specific treatment guidelines for the use of probiotics in the pediatric population.*

About antibiotics: They should be used only in case of bacterial diarrhea as unnecessary use leads to antibiotic abuse. Also there is an entity called as "antibiotic induced diarrhea" which can set in when antibiotics are used when not needed.

In the index case there is no fever or blood in stools so possibility of bacterial infection is least likely.

AIIMS NOVEMBER 2016

33. Ans. (a) 25–28°C

Ref: http://apps.who.int/iris/bitstream/10665/63986/1/WHO_RHT_MSM_97.2.pdf

Thermal Protection of a Newborn: A Practical Guide

- The guidelines are field tested in 8 Countries: Brazil, China, India, Indonesia, Kazakhstan, Nepal, Mozambique and Zimbabwe
- A newborn regulates body temperature much less efficiently than adult
- The **temperature inside mother's womb is 38°C (100.4°F).** At birth, the newborn finds himself in a much colder environment and starts loosing heat immediately.
- Baby loses heat in 4 different ways. Evaporation, conduction, convection and radiation. Heat loss is mainly due to evaporation of the amniotic fluid from the baby's body surface. Most cooling occurs in first minute after birth.
- If a naked baby is exposed to an environmental temperature of 23°C (73.4°F) at birth, suffers the same heat loss as a naked adult at 0°C (32°F)
- There is no single environmental temperature ideal for all size, gestational age and condition of newborn babies.
- In general, most newborn at birth, if left wet and naked cannot cope up with environmental temperature of less than 32°C (89.6°F), But if the baby is immediately dried, put skin to skin with mother and covered, the deliver, room temperature can be kept as low as **25–28°C** (77–82.4°F)
- The room temperature of birth/delivery room should be kept warm (At least 25°C/77°F)
- It is more difficult to determine the upper limit of optimum temperature, except for the wet baby at birth the optimum maximum environmental temperature is 35°C (95°F)
- Optimum room temperature of delivery room is very warm by adult standards, therefore adults should not determine the delivery room temperature as per their own comfort
- In cases of **mild hypothermia** (body temperature 36.0–36.4°C/96.8–97.5°F), the baby can be rewarmed by skin-to-skin contact, in a warm room **(at least 25°C/77°F).**
- In cases of **moderate hypothermia** (body temperature 32–35.9°C/89.6–96.6°F) the clothed baby may be rewarmed: under a radiant heater; in an incubator at **35–36°C** (95–96.8°F); by using a heated water-filled mattress; in a warm room: the temperature of the room should be **32–34°C**/89.6–93.2°F (more if the baby is small or sick)
- The term **Warm chain** is given to the set of 10 interconnected steps and interventions to minimize heat loss and hypothermia in a newborn at birth and first day of life.

The Warm Chain

- Warm delivery room
- Immediate drying
- Skin-to-skin contact
- Breast-feeding
- Bathing and weighing postponed
- Appropriate clothing/bedding
- Mother and baby together
- Warm transportation
- Warm resuscitation
- Training and awareness raising

34. Ans. (a) Muscular dystrophy

Ref: Nelson 20th Ed page 2960-2963

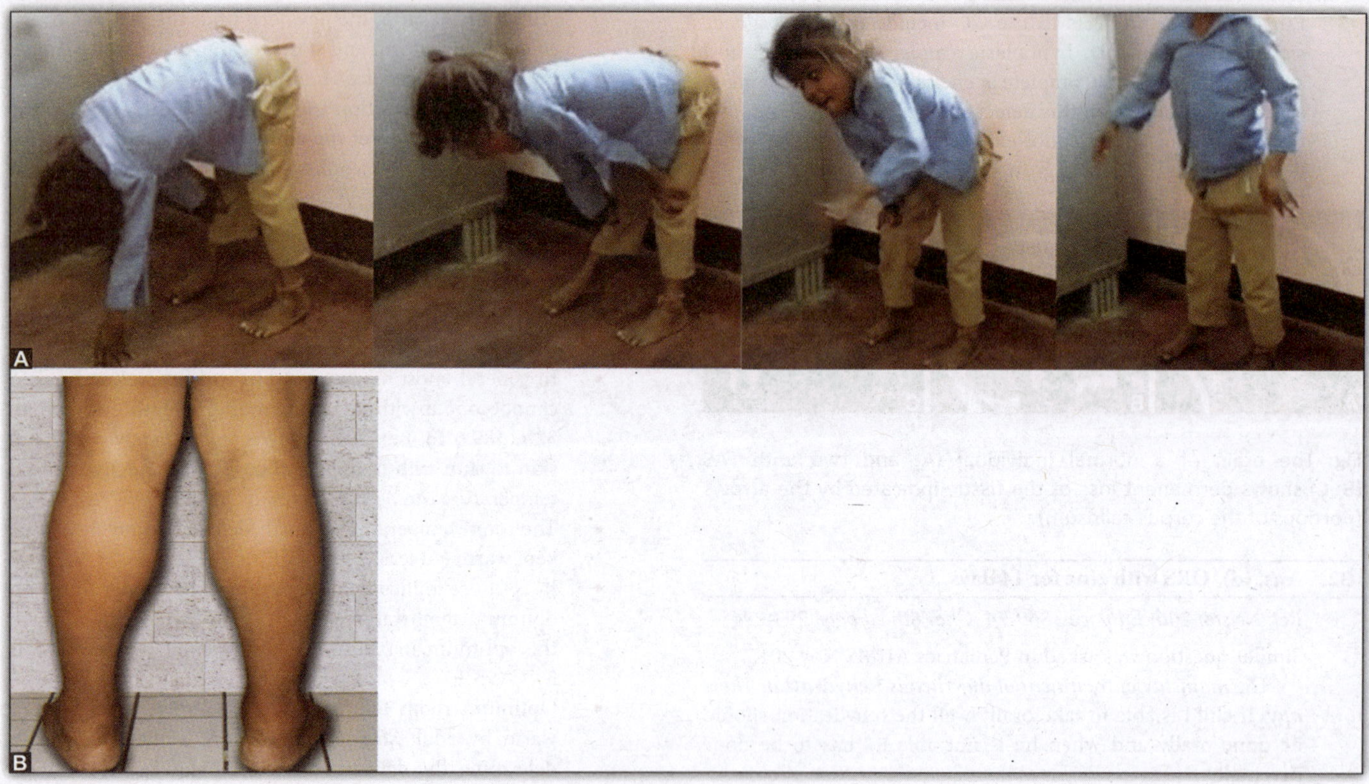

Credit: Senanayake HM, Dedigama AD, De Alwis RP, Thirumavalavan K

Fig: (A) Gower's sign: Gower's sign is pathognomonic in patients with Duchenne muscular dystrophy. These patients, when rising, 'climb up' their thighs using their hands in order to overcome the weakness of the pelvic girdle and paravertebral muscles. Gowers' sign is a screening test for muscle weakness, typically seen in Duchenne muscular dystrophy but also seen in numerous other conditions; **(B) Pseudohypertrophy of calf**

Muscular Dystrophy

A muscular dystrophy is distinguished from all other neuromuscular diseases by four obligatory criteria:

1. It is a primary myopathy
2. It has a genetic basis
3. The course is progressive
4. Degeneration and death of muscle fibers occur at some stage in the disease.

This definition excludes neurogenic diseases such as spinal muscular atrophy, nonhereditary myopathies such as dermatomyositis, non-progressive and non-necrotizing congenital myopathies such as congenital muscle fiber–type disproportion (CMFTD), and nonprogressive inherited metabolic myopathies.

Duchene muscular dystrophy (DMD) is the most common hereditary neuromuscular disease affecting all races and ethnic groups. Duchene recognized most of the characteristic clinical features in 1861: hypertrophy of the calves, progressive weakness, intellectual impairment, and proliferation of connective tissue in muscle

Incidence	1 : 3,600 live born infant boys.
Inheritance	X-linked recessive trait. The abnormal gene is on the **X chromosome** at the Xp21 locus and is one of the largest genes identified.
Deficiency	**Dystrophin deficiency:** Dystrophin is expressed in brain and retina, as well as in striated and cardiac muscle, though the level is lower in brain than in muscle. This distribution may explain some of the CNS manifestations.
Clinical features	• **Gower's sign positive:** A maneuver performed by a patient with weak knee and thigh flexors on changing from the sitting to the standing position. Consists of first flexing the trunk at the hips, then placing the hands on the knees, and then extending the trunk by using the hands to walk up the legs. Evident by age 3 years and is fully expressed by age 5–6 years

Contd...

Muscular Dystrophy	
	• **Intellectual impairment** occurs in all patients, although only 20–30% have an IQ <70. • **Cardiomyopathy,** including persistent tachycardia and myocardial failure, is seen in 50–80% of patients with this disease. The severity of cardiac involvement does not necessarily correlate with the degree of skeletal muscle weakness. • Enlargement of the calves **(pseudohypertrophy)** and wasting of thigh muscles are classic features. After the calves, the next most common site of muscular **hypertrophy is the tongue**, followed by muscles of the forearm. Fasciculations of the tongue do not occur. • Progressive muscle weekness. Proximal muscles and neck flexors are involved more. Leg involvement more severe than arm. • Contractures of heels and iliotibial tract by 6 years of age. • Progressive scoliosis and chest deformity. • Death occurs usually at about 18–20 years of age
Becker muscular dystrophy	Becker muscular dystrophy is the same DMD, with a genetic defect at the same locus, but clinically it follows a milder course. In Becker muscular dystrophy, boys remain ambulatory until late adolescence or early adult life. Calf pseudohypertrophy, cardiomyopathy, and elevated serum levels of creatine kinase (CK) are similar to those of patients with Duchenne dystrophy. Learning disabilities are less frequent. The onset of weakness is later in Becker than in Duchenne dystrophy. Death often occurs in the mid to late 20s; fewer than half of patients are still alive by age 40 years; these survivors are severely disabled.

35. Ans. (d) LFT and Coombs test

Ref: Nelson 20th ed page 65-70, 640, Ghai 8th ed page 173, IAP Testbook of Pediatrics 4th ed page 78, Manual of Neonatal care Cloherty 7th ed page 332,

Three determinants in this question are:

1. Is the Jaundice Pathological or Physiological
2. When to initiate therapy
3. What therapy should be initiated

Summary

Practically speaking no intervention is initiated before knowing the Bilirubin levels. Secondly Bhutani Chart is the standard chart used worldwide now a days. Other charts like Maisels chart are no more used.

Option (A)

While evaluating a case of hyperbilirubinemia in jaundice the most important question which needs to be answered it whether it is physiological or pathological.

Causes of Neonatal Jaundice

Within 24 hours	2nd–3rd day	3rd day to 1 week
Erythroblastosis Fetalis Concealed Hemorrhage Sepsis **Congenital Infections:** Syphilis Cytomegalovirus Rubella Toxoplasmosis	Usually **Physiological** **May Represent A More Severe Form:** Familial Non-Hemolytic Icterus (Crigler-Najjar Syndrome) Early-Onset Breast-Feeding jaundice	Bacterial Sepsis Urinary Tract Infection Syphilis Toxoplasmosis Cytomegalovirus Enterovirus

Physiological Jaundice

About 60 to 70 percent of healthy newborn babies are likely to develop physiological jaundice which may cause undue anxiety to the parents. Physiological jaundice appears between 24 and 72 hours of age, its maximum intensity is seen on the 4th to 5th days of life, and the peak serum bilirubin level does not exceed 15 mg/dL.

Physiological Jaundice	Pathological Jaundice

The serum UCB level of most newborn infants rises to >2 mg/dL in the first week of life. This level usually rises in full-term infants to a peak of 6 to 8 mg/dL by 3 to 5 days of age and then falls. A rise to 12 mg/dL is in the physiologic range. In premature infants, the peak may be 10 to 12 mg/dL on the fifth day of life, possibly rising >15 mg/dL without any specific abnormality of bilirubin metabolism. Levels <2 mg/dL may not be seen until 1 month of age in both full term and premature infants. This "normal jaundice" is attributed to:
• **Increased bilirubin production** due to:
  ▪ Increased RBC volume per kilogram and decreased RBC survival (90 days versus 120 days) in infants compared with adults.
  ▪ Increased ineffective erythropoiesis and increased turnover of nonhemoglobin heme proteins.
• **Increased enterohepatic circulation** caused by high levels of intestinal-glucuronidase, preponderance of bilirubin monoglucuronide rather than diglucuronide, decreased intestinal bacteria. And decreased gut motility with poor evacuation of bilirubin-laden meconium.
• **Defective uptake of bilirubin from plasma** caused by decreased ligandin and binding of ligandin by other anions.
• **Defective conjugation** due to decreased UGT activity.
• **Decreased hepatic excretion** of bilirubin.
	Nonphysiologic jaundice may not be easy to distinguish from physiologic jaundice. The following situations suggest nonphysiologic hyperbilirubinemia and require evaluation
	• **Onset of jaundice before 24 hours of age.**
	• Any elevation of serum bilirubin that requires phototherapy.
	• A rise in serum bilirubin levels of >0.2 mg/dL/hr.
	• Signs of underlying illness in any infant (vomiting, lethargy, poor feeding, excessive weight loss, apnea, tachypnea, or temperature instability).
	• Jaundice persisting after 8 days in a term infant or after 14 days in a premature infant.
	In addition to this detailed evaluation as discussed below will help us to distinguish physiological from non-physiological jaundice.

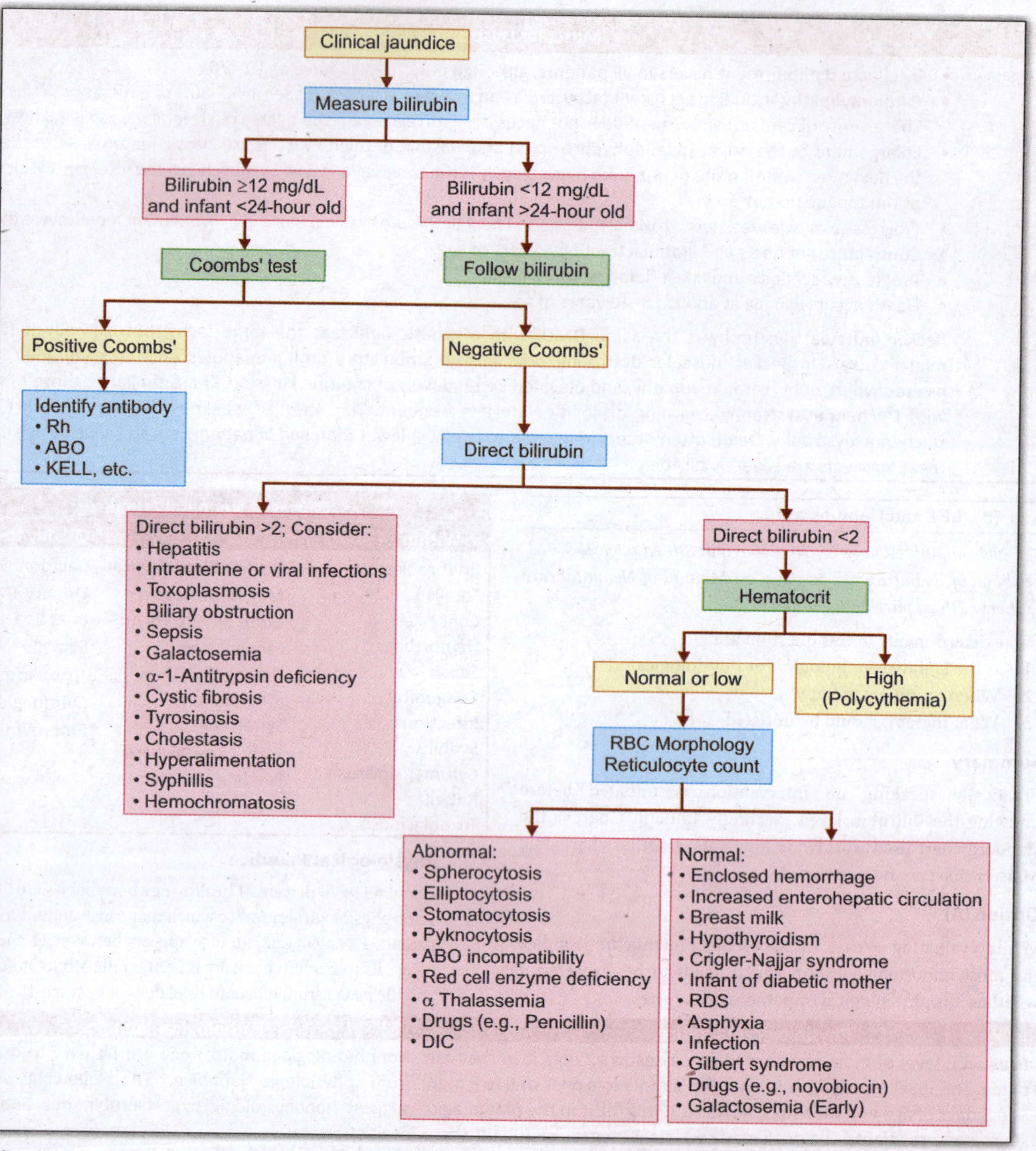

Option (B)

Intensive phototherapy results in a decline of Total Bilirubin of at least 2 to 3 mg/dL (34 to 51 micromol/L) within 4 to 6 hours. A decrease in TB can be measured as soon as two hours after initiation of treatment. In infants ≥35 weeks gestational age (GA), 24 hours of intensive phototherapy can result in a 30 to 40 percent decrease in the initial TB. With conventional phototherapy, a decline of 6 to 20 percent can be expected in the first 18 to 24 hours.

Phototherapy exposes the infant's skin to light of a specific wavelength, which reduces TB by the following three mechanisms:

- **Non reversible structural isomerization to lumirubin:** Lumirubin, a more soluble substance than bilirubin, is excreted without conjugation into bile and urine. This is probably the principal mechanism by which phototherapy reduces the TB concentration.
- **Photoisomerization to a less toxic bilirubin isomer**
- **Photo-oxidation to polar molecules**

Discontinuation

Discontinue phototherapy when the Total Bilirubin has reached 12 to 14 mg/dL (205 to 239 micromol/L)

The management of neonatal hyperbilirubinemia is focused on prevention of hyperbilirubinemia, defined as total serum or plasma bilirubin (TB) >95th percentile on the hour-specific **Bhutani nomogram**. The decision of when to initiate therapy and the choice of intervention are based on the probability of developing severe hyperbilirubinemia using hour-specific TB values, gestational age (GA), and the presence or absence of risk factors.

The American Academy of Pediatrics has released recommendations to standardize phototherapy in newborns with hyperbilirubinemia.

Group	Age	Phototherapy Cut off Bilirubin	Exchange Transfusion Cut off Bilirubin
Group 1: Gestation ≥38 weeks and medically well	12 hours	9 mg/dL	17.70 mg/dL
	24 hours	11.60 mg/dL	19.00 mg/dL
Group 2: Gestation ≥ 38 weeks and clinical risk factors	12 hours	7.60 mg/dL	15.10 mg/dL
	24 hours	9.80 mg/dL	16.60 mg/dL
Group 2: Gestation 35 to 37.9 weeks and medically well	12 hours	7.60 mg/dL	15.10 mg/dL
	24 hours	9.80 mg/dL	16.60 mg/dL
Group 3: Gestation 35 to 37.9 weeks and clinical risk factors	12 hours	5.80 mg/dL	13.40 mg/dL
	24 hours	7.80 mg/dL	15.00 mg/dL

Online calculators are available to check cut off levels of bilirubin as per age and risk group for starting intervention

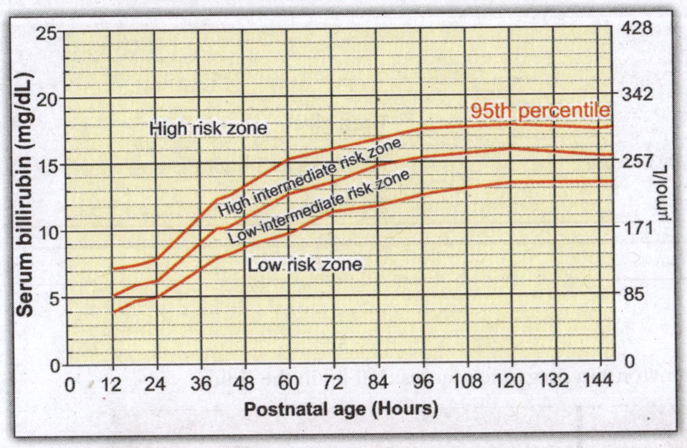

Option (C)

If despite phototherapy and other supportive measures, the bilirubin level is approaching 20 mg/dL, exchange blood transfusion is mandatory to prevent brain damage.

Indications for Exchange Blood Transfusion	
Early indications in infants with Rh-Hdn	**Jaundice due to any cause**
• Cord hemoglobin of 10 g/dL or less • Cord bilirubin of 5 mg/dL or more	• Exchange at lower bilirubin levels in the presence of perinatal distress factors (Asphyxia, respiratory distress, sepsis, hypothermia, etc.)
• Unconjugated serum bilirubin of more than 10 mg/dL within 24 hours or rate of rise of more than 0.5 mg/dL per hour	• Unconjugated serum bilirubin of 20 mg/dL or more in a term baby • In preterm babies, serum bilirubin of more than 1.0 mg/100 g weight of the infant (i.e., 10 mg/dL for 1000 g and 15 mg/dL for 1500 g and so on)

Option (D)

Just on the basis of the day of origin of jaundice, one cannot be sure its Physiological or pathological. Evaluation is required. Hence LFT and Coombs test is the answer.

36. Ans. (b) Start IV antibiotics and IV fluid and then immediately refer to higher center

Ref: IAP Testbook of Pediatrics 4th ed page 200, 1522, Park 23rd ed page 457-460

Presence of 10 or more skin pustules or a large boil indicates a possible serious bacterial infection.

IMNCI-Integrated Management of Neonatal and Childhood Illnesses		
IMNCI bacterial infection classification		
Bacterial infection	**Signs**	**Treatment**
Possible serious bacterial infection	Convulsions or fast breathing (>60 breaths/min) or severe chest indrawing or nasal flaring or grunting or bulging fontanelle or 10 or more skin pustules or a big boil or if axillary temperature 37.5°C or above (or feels hot to touch) or temperature less than 35.5°C (or feels cold to touch) or lethargy or unconsciousness or less than normal movement	Referred urgently to the hospital after being given the first dose of intramuscular ampicillin plus gentamicin, treatment to prevent hypoglycemia, and advice to the mother on keeping the young infant warm while arranging referral, and on the way to the hospital
Local bacterial infection	Umbilicus red or draining pus or pus discharge from the ear or <10 skin pustules	This infant may be treated at home with oral antibiotics but should be seen in follow-up after two days.
No serious or local bacterial infection	Nil	Nil
IMNCI child dehydration classification		
Dehydration	**Signs**	**Treatment**
Severe dehydrarion	If two or more of following is present, lethargic or unconscious Sunken eyes, not able to drink or feed properly, skin pinch goes back slowly (>2 sec)	Fluids according to **Plan C** Refer urgently to hospital Give ORS on the way, continue breast feeding Keep child warm
Some dehydration	If two or more of following is present, restless or irritable sunken eyes Eagerly drinks and thirsty Skin pinch goes back slowly (>2 sec)	Fluids according to **Plan B** Continue breast feeding and feeding Follow up in 2 days if needed
No dehydration	No visible signs	Fluids according to **Plan A** follow up in 5 days

Treatment Plans of Dehydration						
PLAN A: Home based treatment						
AGE	Amount of ORS to give after each loose stool or other culturally appropriate ORT fluids				Amount of ORS to provide for use at home	
<2 years	50-100 mL				500 mL/day	
2-10 years	100-200 mL				1000 mL/day	
>10 years	As much as wanted				2000 mL/day	
Plan B: Give 75 mL/kg ORS in first 4 hours						
Approx amount of ORS to be given in first 4 hours						
Age	<4 months	4–11 months	12–23 months	2–4 years	5–14 years	>15 years
Approx. weight in kg	<5 kg	5–8 kg	8–11 kg	11–16 kg	16–30 kg	>30 kg
ORS in mL	200–400	400–600	600–800	800–1200	1200–2200	>2200
Local measure in glass	1–2	2–3	3–4	4–6	6–11	12–20

Plan C
1. Start fluids immediately
2. Best fluid ringer lactate
3. Give 100 mL/kg of chosen solution divided as follows:

Age	First give	Then give
<12 months	30 mL/kg in 1st hour	70 mL/kg in 5 hours
12 months to 5 years	30 minutes	2½ hours

37. Ans. (b) Isotretinoin

Ref: Nelson 19th ed ch 85, 307, KDT 7th ed page 89, 414

The picture shown is unilateral incomplete cleft lip.

Smoking, isotretinoin (Retinoic acid) and anticonvulsants (Phenytoin) in pregnancy causes cleft lip in the child.

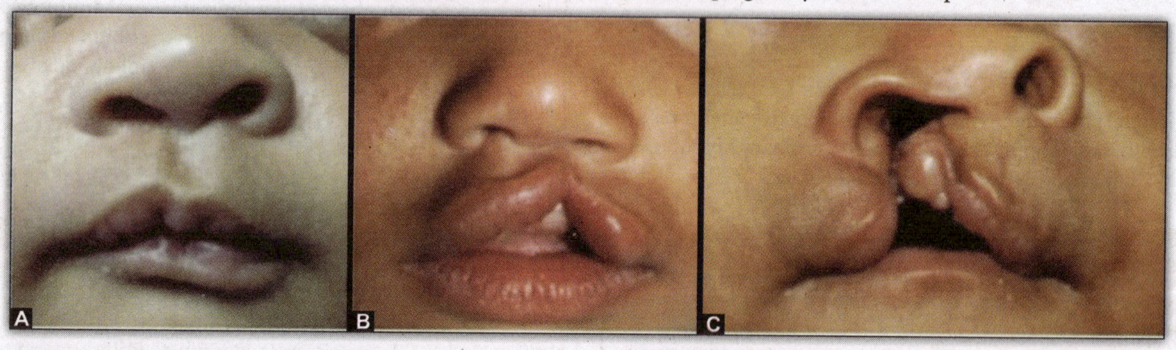

Credit: Shkoukani MA, Chen M, Vong A

Fig: Unilateral cleft lip. (A) Microform type, (B) incomplete type, (C) complete type CLP is traditionally classified by phenotype, which can have variable expression ranging from microform to complete clefting, and may involve the alveolar ridge and palate. Phenotypes have been correlated with specific genetic linkage patterns, suggesting a possible correlation. CLP and CP are embryologically distinct processes from disruption at different stages of development and possess unique epidemiologic and genetic features

Teratogens		
Teratogen	**Critical period**	**Embryopathy/fetopathy**
Thalidomide	34-51 days after LMP	External ear deformity (earliest), Phocomelia (MC-four groups: 4-limb phocomelia, Upper limb phocomelia, predominantly upper-limb phocomelia, predominantly lower limb defects), facial hemangioma, esophageal atresia, TOF, renal agenesis

Contd...

Teratogens		
Teratogen	**Critical period**	**Embryopathy/fetopathy**
Retinoic acid (Aka-accutane, isotretinoin)	3-5 weeks	**Accutane Embryopathy (AKA- Retinoic acid embryopathy;** cranio-facial abnormalities (cleft lip/palate), Microtia/Anotia (deafness), Missing jaw or one that is too small, Disorders of jaw formation (split jaw), Disorders of formation of aortic arch, Thymic aplasia/hypoplasia, Deformities in the CNS (MC- hydrocephalus)
Diethylstilboestrol		Vaginal adenosis, erosions of the cervix and vagina carcinoma
Alcohol		**Fetal alcohol syndrome:** ASD, VSD, LBW, microcephaly, maxillary hypoplasia, flat nasal bridge, micrognathia, microphthalmia, hypoplastic upper lip, broad lower lip.
Cocaine		Addiction in the child, retarded growth, to malformations of the circulatory system
Phenytoin		**Fetal hydantoin syndrome:** VSD, ASD, coarctation of aorta, PDA, Hypoplastic phalanges, Syndactyly, cleft palate, cleft/hare lip, microcephaly – caused by arene-oxide metabolite
Valproate		Neural tube defects, coarctation of aorta, hypoplastic left side of heart, aortic stenosis, pulmonary atresia, VSD
Lithium	3-8 weeks	Ebstein anomaly (mc), cleft palate in experimental animals
Streptomycin	4-8 weeks	Damage of the 8th cerebral nerve-deafness
Warfarin	1st trimester	Hypoplastic nasal bridge, chondrodysplasia
	2nd trimester	CNS malformation
	3rd trimester	Risk of bleeding
Rubella	1st trimester	Congenital Rubella Syndrome (CRS) **CVS**: PDA, Pulmonary artery stenosis, VSD, Myocarditis. **CNS**: Chronic meningitis, Parenchymal necrosis, Vasculitis with calcification. **Eye:** Microphthalmia, Cataract, Iridocyclitis, Ciliary body necrosis, Glaucoma, Retinopathy. **Ear:** Cochlear hemorrhage, Endothelial necrosis. **Lung:** Chronic mononuclear interstitial pneumonitis. **Liver:** Hepatic giant cell transformation, Fibrosis, Lobular disarray, Bile stasis. **Kidneys:** Interstitial nephritis. **Adrenals:** Cortical cytomegaly. **Bone**: Malformed osteoid, Poor mineralization of osteoid, Thinning cartilage. **Spleen, lymph nodes:** Extramedullary hematopoiesis. **Thymus:** Histiocytic reaction, Absence of germinal centers. **Skin:** Erythropoiesis in dermis
Cytomegalovirus	Spontaneous miscarriage in 1st trimester, anomalies from 2nd trimester. Risk is greatest with maternal primary CMV infection (30%) and much less likely with recurrent infection (<1%)	90% subclinical. 5% mild forms. Another 5% **Cytomegalic inclusion disease** (hepatosplenomegaly, jaundice, mental retardation, microcephaly, cerebral atrophy, hydrocephaly, cerebellar hypoplasia, intracranial/ Periventricular calcifications, seizures, IUGR, prematurity, blueberry muffin like rash, thrombocytopenia, purpura, chorioretinitis, atrophy of the eyes, sensorineural hearing loss (Asymptomatic congenital CMV infection is the leading cause of sensorineural hearing loss)
Herpes Simplex Viral	As a rule, HSV occurs in late pregnancy	Mental deficiency, microcephaly, myocardiopathy, spasticity, retinal dysplasia
Varicella (Chicken Pox)	In 2% fetus, till 20th week	**Congenital Varicella Syndrome**: 6–12 weeks of gestation appear to have maximal interruption with limb development; fetuses infected at 16–20 weeks may have eye and brain involvement. **Skin**: Cicatricial skin lesions, hypopigmentation. **Eye:** Microphthalmia, cataracts, chorioretinitis, optic atrophy. **Brain:** Encephalitis, microcephaly, hydrocephaly, calcifications, aplasia of brain. **Damage to Cervical or Lumbosacral Cord:** Hypoplasia of an extremity, motor and sensory deficits, absent deep tendon reflexes, anisocoria, horner syndrome, Anal/urinary sphincter dysfunction
Toxoplasmosis (Toxoplasma Gondi)		Cerebral calcification, microcephaly, microphthalmia, chorioretinitis, microphthalmia, hydrocephalus
Congenital Syphilis		Mental deficiency, hydrocephalus, deafness, blindness, bone malformations, Hutchinson's teeth (pathognomonic)

38. Ans. (a) Anti VZV antibodies

Ref: Nelson 19th ed ch 250 Table 250-1

Cicatrizing skin lesion, Chorioretinitis, limb hypoplasia and cerebral atrophy points towards the diagnosis of Varicella (Chicken Pox). See table of teratogen in previous question for details

Rapid laboratory diagnosis of VZV is often important in high-risk patients and is sometimes important for infection control. VZV can be identified quickly by direct fluorescence assay of cells from cutaneous lesions, and by PCR amplification testing. Although multinucleated giant cells can be detected with nonspecific stains (Tzanck smear), they have poor sensitivity and do not differentiate VZV from herpes simplex virus infections. Infectious virus may be recovered using tissue culture methods; shell vial assays have decreased the time needed for culture from 7–10 days to 3–4 days. **VZV IgG antibodies can be detected by several methods and a 4-fold rise in IgG antibodies is also confirmatory of acute infection.** VZV IgG antibody tests can also be valuable to determine the immune status of individuals whose clinical history of varicella is unknown or equivocal. Testing for VZV IgM antibodies is not useful for clinical diagnosis because commercially available methods are unreliable and the kinetics of the IgM response are not well defined. Reliable VZV-specific IgM assays are available in certain reference laboratories, and a capture-IgM assay is available at the national VZV laboratory at centers for disease control.

39. Ans. (d) Liver failure

Ref: Nelson 19th ed ch 252

Hepatosplenomegaly is seen in Symptomatic Congenital CMV infection, but not as sequelae of Congenital CMV infection (Symptomatic or Asymptomatic)

NOTE

90% of congenital CMV infections are subclinical and in the question the newborn is asymptomatic, hence we are talking about the long-term sequelae of the asymptomatic group of the congenital CMV infection.

Most consistent sequelae of asymptomatic congenital CMV infection is sensorineural hearing loss. (Ref: Neurology of the Newborn By Joseph J. Volpe 5th ed page 859)

Most common and most severe sequelae of CMV infection are the CNS manifestations like Mental retardation, Seizures and sensorineural deafness (Ref: Fanaroff and Martin's Neonatal-Perinatal Medicine: Diseases of the Fetus and Infant 9th ed vol 1 By Richard J. Martin, Avroy A. Fanaroff, Michele C. Walsh page 847)

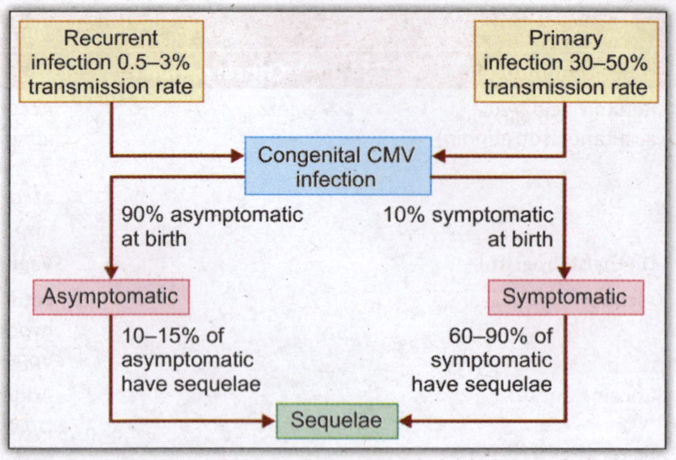

40. Ans: (a) RSV

Ref: Nelson 18th ed ch 170

Palivizumab (monoclonal antibody)is used for prophylaxis for infants and children <2 years of age with chronic lung disease (CLD) who have required medical therapy for CLD within 6 months of start of prophylaxis.

The major monoclonal antibody used in infectious diseases is palivizumab, which can prevent severe disease from respiratory syncytial virus (RSV) among children ≤24 months of age with chronic lung disease (CLD, also called bronchopulmonary dysplasia) or with a history of premature birth (<35 weeks).

Administration of palivizumab (15 mg/kg IM once a month), a monoclonal antibody against RSV, is recommended for protecting high-risk children against serious complications from RSV disease. Immunoprophylaxis reduces the frequency and total days of hospitalization for RSV infections in high-risk infants. Palivizumab is administered monthly from the beginning (October–December) to the end (March–May) of the RSV season.

Adverse events with palivizumab are uncommon. Serious adverse reactions to palivizumab primarily are rare cases of anaphylaxis and hypersensitivity reactions.

AIIMS MAY 2016

41. Ans. (b) 20 mL/kg of 0.9% NS

Ref: Nelson 20th ed chapter page 516-528, Ghai 8th ed page 718

In above question it is clearly mentioned that child is having shock and sepsis. Hence the diagnosis is already made as "**Septic shock**". Remember that in septic shock the first intervention is always "**fluids fluids and only fluids**" (remember in cardiogenic shock and anaphylactic shock is different hence diagnosis of type of shock becomes important). It has to be colloids and iso-osmolar which is Normal saline (0.9 % NS) and the dose is always 20 mL/kg.

Reason for 20 mL/kg-body is having 80 mL/kg of blood totally and the bolus is 25% of it as shock manifest only when deficit of 25% happens in vessels. Algorithm of shock is shown in figure below.

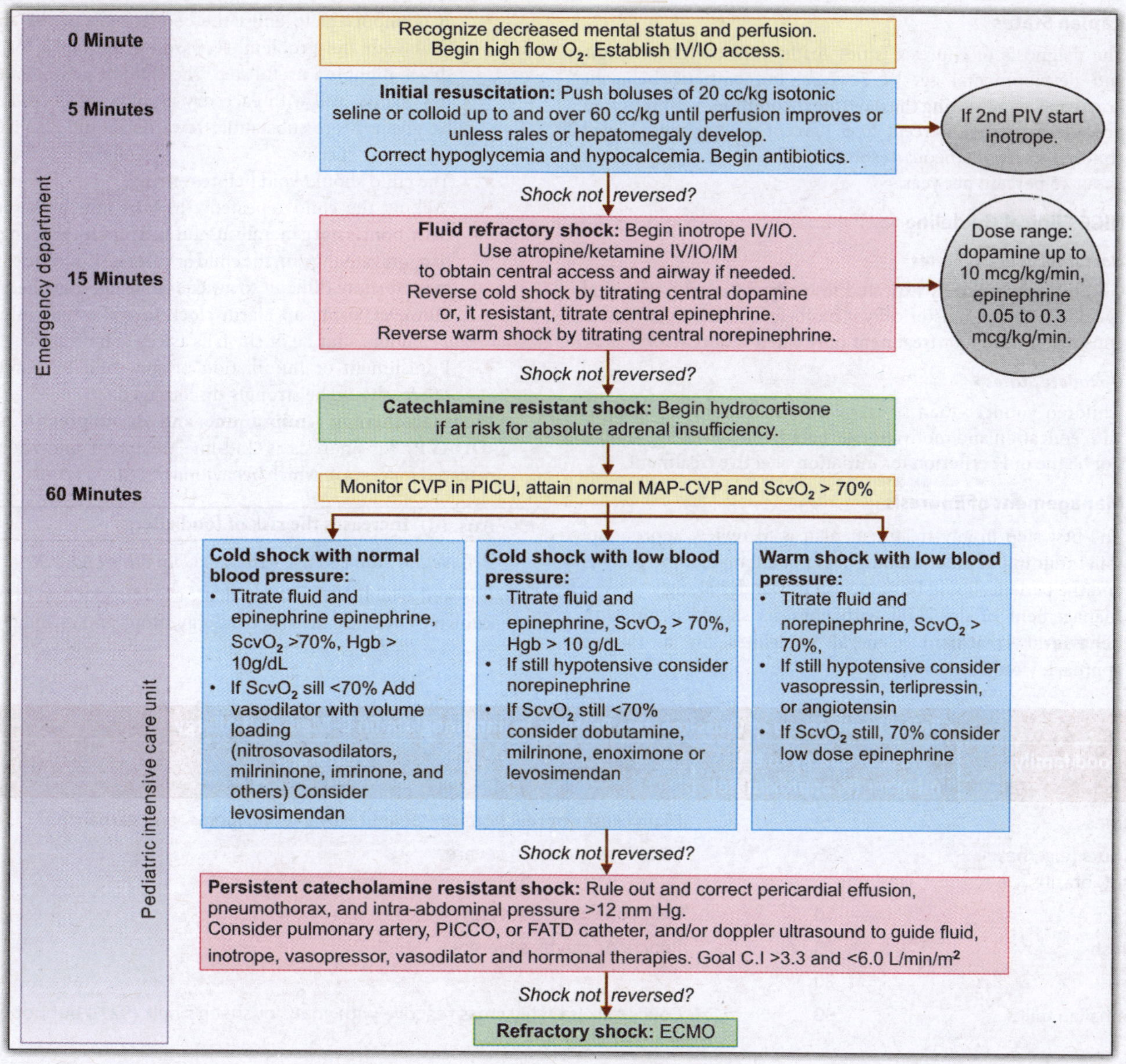

42. Ans. (a) Reassurance and revisit after 6 months

Ref: Kaplan 10th ed ch 47, Nelson 18th ed ch 22.3

Enuresis is defined as the voluntary or involuntary repeated discharge of urine into clothes or bed after a developmental age when bladder control should be established. Bed-wetting may be divided into the persistent (primary) type, in which the child has never been dry at night, and the regressive (secondary) type, in which a child who has been continent for 6 months or longer then begins to wet the bed. Primary enuresis represents approximately 90% of all cases. Further classification involves nocturnal enuresis (voiding urine at night), and diurnal enuresis (voiding urine while awake). **Primary nocturnal enuresis is the most common.**

The debate in this question is whether or not the condition is to be designated as Enuresis and if Enuresis then what should be done?

The clinical picture is consistent with the DSM IV TR criteria of enuresis. The age greater than 5 years is consistent with criteria 3. Normal urine microscopy and other tests is consistent with criteria 4. Only nocturnal or daytime bed wetting does not exclude enuresis.

DSM IV TR Criteria of Enuresis

- Repeated voiding of urine into bed or clothes (whether involuntary or intentional).
- The behavior is clinically significant as manifested by either a frequency of twice a week for at least 3 consecutive months or the presence of clinically significant distress or impairment in social, academic (occupational), or other important areas of functioning.
- Chronological age is at least 5 years (or equivalent developmental level).
- The behavior is not due exclusively to the direct physiological effect of a substance (e.g., a diuretic) or a general medical condition (e.g., diabetes, spina bifida, a seizure disorder).

Specify type:
Nocturnal only
Diurnal only
Nocturnal and diurnal

Now question arises weather or not this case requires an intervention?

Kaplan States

The diagnosis of enuresis is not made until the chronologic and developmental age of 5 years, but enuretic behavior nocturnally and during the daytime is common, with reported prevalence from 2 percent to 5 percent among school-aged children. A spontaneous resolution of nocturnal enuresis is about 15 percent per year.

NICE Clinical Guideline

Nocturnal Enuresis States

Children are generally expected to be dry by a developmental age of 5 years, and historically it has been common practice to consider children for treatment only when they reach 7 years.

Up todate States

Children younger than seven years usually can be managed with education and motivational therapy. However, age should not be the only criterion for initiation of active treatment.

Management of Enuresis

The first step in any treatment plan is to review appropriate toilet training. If toilet training was not attempted, the parents and the patient should be guided in this undertaking.

Management of the child with enuresis should begin with **behavioral treatment**. General guidelines for a 1st-line approach would be as follows:

- It is important to enlist the cooperation of the child to deal with the problem. Rewarding the child for being dry at night is a useful step. The child or parent can chart dry nights, and with each dry night, a small reward can be given. More substantial rewards should be given for increasing success.
- The child should void before retiring.
- Waking the child repeatedly to take him or her to the bathroom is not generally useful and may further engender or aggravate anger in the child or parents. Enuretic children may be more difficult to awaken than age-matched peers. However, using an alarm clock to wake the child once 2–3 hours after he or she falls asleep is indicated.
- Punishment or humiliation of the child by parents or others should be strongly discouraged.

Pharmacotherapy (imipramine and desmopressin acetate -DDAVP) for enuresis is 2nd-line treatment and should be reserved for cases in which behavioral treatment is unsuccessful.

43. Ans. (d) Increases the risk of food allergy

Ref: Nelson 20th ed Page 516-528, Ghai 8th ed page 90

It is well established concept that early introduction of food is known to increase the risk of allergy, atopy and asthma.

Clinical Implications of Cross-reactive Proteins in Immunoglobulin E–Mediated Allergy

Food family	Risk of allergy to ≥ 1 member (% approximate)	Feature(s)
Legumes	5	Main causes of reactions are peanut, soya, lentil, lupine, and garbanzo
Tree nuts (e.g., hazel, walnut, brazil)	35	Reactions are often severe
Fish	50	Reactions can be severe
Shellfish	75	Reactions can be severe
Grains	20	
Mammalian milks	90	Cow's milk is highly cross reactive with goat's or sheep's milk (92%) but not with mare's milk (4%)
Rosaceae (rock) fruits	55	Risk of reactions to more than three related foods is very low (<10%)
Latex-food	35	For individuals allergic to latex, banana, kiwi, and avocado are the main causes of reactions

Prevention of food allergy

- Exclusive breast feeding for 4-6 months
- Introduce solid (complementary) foods after 4-6 months of exclusive breast feeding
- Introduce low-risk complementary foods 1 at a time
- Introduce potentially highly allergenic foods (fish, eggs, peanut products, milk, wheat) soon after the lower-risk foods (no need to avoid or delay)
- Do not avoid allergenic foods during pregnancy or nursing
- Soy-based formulas do not prevent allergic disease

44. Ans. (c) Decrease mechanical ventilation

Ref: Nelson 18th ed ch 69, Ghai 8th ed page 393, Mechanical Ventilation in ARDS: 2014 Review http://pulmccm.org/main/2012/review-articles/mechanical-ventilation-in-ards-2012-update/

Findings in this Chest X-ray are:

- Bilateral diffuse fluffy infiltrates
- Right subclavian central line seen
- Tracheostomy tube seen
- ECG leads can be seen

People with acute respiratory distress syndrome (ARDS) are by definition severely hypoxemic, and nearly all require invasive mechanical ventilation. Yet mechanical ventilation itself can further injure damaged lungs (so-called ventilator-induced lung injury); minimizing any additional damage while maintaining adequate gas exchange ("compatible with life") is the central goal of mechanical ventilation in ARDS and acute lung injury.

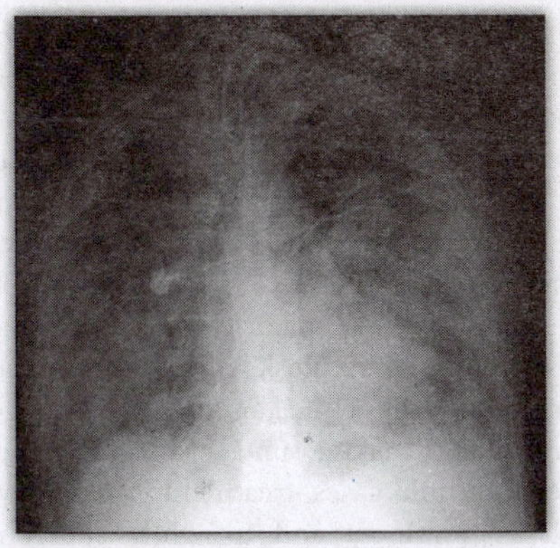

Fig: Acute Respiratory distress syndrome

Benefits of Low Tidal Volume Ventilation in ARDS

Low tidal volume ventilation (LTVV) reduces the damaging, excessive stretch of lung tissue and alveoli (so-called volutrauma), and is the standard of care for people with ARDS requiring mechanical ventilation. Although ARMA, the largest clinical trial supporting this paradigm, was criticized both for its design and for ethical concerns, its results (published in 2000 by ARDS Net), followed by two flawed but concordant meta-analyses including ten randomized trials total, have convinced most intensivist physicians that using low tidal volumes improves survival for people with ARDS. Taken together, the trials suggest that a strategy of low tidal volume ventilation (6-8 mL/kg ideal body weight) reduces absolute mortality by about 7-9%, as compared to using ≥ 10 mL/kg tidal volumes (~42% mortality in control groups vs. ~34% in the LTVV groups). This translates to a "number needed to treat" of between 11-15 people with ARDS to prevent one death by using LTVV.

How to use Low Tidal Volume Ventilation in ARDS

The protocol from the ARMA trial can serve as a guide to performing low tidal volume ventilation for mechanically ventilated patients with ARDS:

- Start in any ventilator mode with initial tidal volumes of 8 mL/kg predicted body weight in kg, calculated by: **[2.3 × (height in inches – 60) + 45.5 for women or + 50 for men]**.
- Set the respiratory rate up to 35 breaths/min to deliver the expected minute ventilation requirement (generally, 7-9 L/min)
- Set positive end-expiratory pressure (PEEP) to at least 5 cm H_2O (but much higher is probably better), and FiO_2 to maintain an arterial oxygen saturation (SaO_2) of 88-95% (paO_2 55-80 mm Hg). Titrate FiO_2 to below 70% when feasible (though ARDSNet does not specify this).
- Over a period of less than 4 hours, reduce tidal volumes to 7 mL/kg, and then to 6 mL/kg.

45. Ans. (b) Pneumothorax

Ref: Nelson 18th ed ch 410

Recall Bias

We were not able to get the exact picture asked in the exam. Some people thing it was bilateral. However it will not change the answer. Pneumothorax (if any initially) will not be seen due to in situ chest tube drain. Pleural effusion with pneumothorax is called Hydropneumothorax, and present with Air fluid levels which is not seen here.

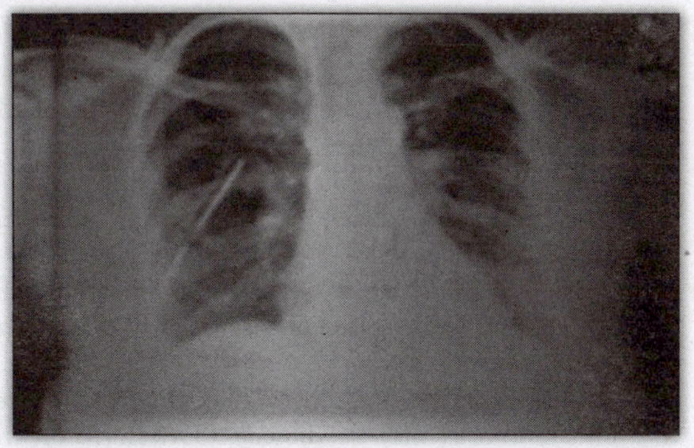

Fig: Right Pleural effusion: Chest X-ray PA view showing intercostal tube placed for pleural effusion. The chest tube is in correct place draining the effusion fluid with expanded right lung. Mediastinal shift (tracheal shift) is not very clearly visible in this picture is however likely to be present

Radiological Features of Pleural Effusion:

- CXR (PA film) – effusions up to 300 mL may not be visible.
- Blunting of the costophrenic angles.
- Blunting of cardiophrenic angle
- Eventually a **meniscus** shaped upper surface will be seen, on frontal films seen laterally and gently sloping medially (if a hydropneumothorax is present, no such meniscus will be visible). They may be large extending up to the apex and causing mediastinal shift away from the effusion.
- Look for differential increased density projected beneath the diaphragm. Elevated apex of the diaphragm laterally, in keeping with a subpulmonic effusion.
- Fluid within the horizontal or oblique fissures
- With large volume effusions, mediastinal shift occurs away from the effusion (note: if coexistent collapse dominates then mediastinal shift may occur towards the effusion)
- Always look for any additional findings like:
  - Subcutaneous emphysema
  - Signs of trauma (fracture)
  - Signs of chest tube blockage (lack of expansion, kinking)
  - Hydropneumothorax (Air fluid levels)

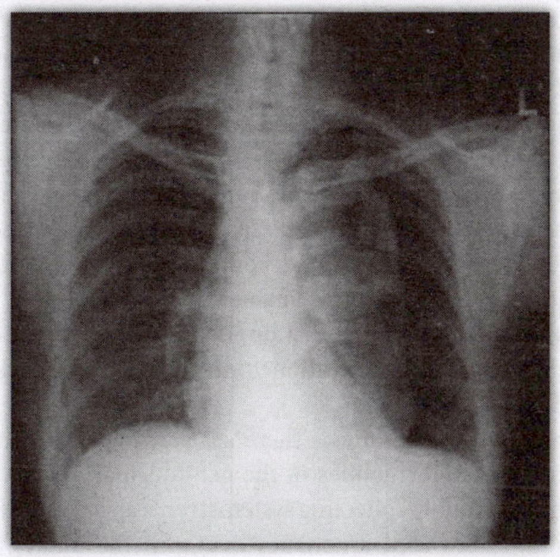

Fig: Left pneumothorax: Pneumothorax refers to the presence of gas (air) in the pleural space and on chest X-ray

Radiological Features of Pneumothorax

- Simple pneumothorax: visceral pleural edge visible (thin sharp white line) with dark area lacking vascular markings laterally. Loss of volume on the affected side (e.g. raised hemidiaphragm). A small pneumothorax may not be visualized on a standard inspiratory film. An expiratory film may be of benefit.
- Tension pneumothorax –this is a clinical and not a radiological entity. Radiological signs are similar to Simple pneumothorax
- Associated mediastinal shift to the opposite side is seen.
- Pneumothorax may be difficult to visualize on frontal films, particularly on supine films. Look for increased lucency over the costophrenic recess (the **deep sulcus sign**).

46. Ans. (d) Klippel-Feil syndrome

Ref: Nelson 18th ed ch 679

NOTE

That the figure B of arm raising was not provided in the exam

The clinical picture is consistent with **Sprengel's deformity** which is seen in **Klippel-Feil syndrome**.

Sprengel Deformity

Sprengel deformity, or congenital elevation of the scapula, is a disorder of development that involves a high scapula and limited scapulothoracic motion. The severity of the deformity depends on the location of the scapula and associated anomalies.

Embryology: Klippel-Feil syndrome involves the congenital fusion (failure of segmentation) of one or more cervical motion segments, and most patients have associated congenital anomalies of the cervical spine. These anomalies may occur at the craniocervical junction (occiput-C2), the subaxial spine (below C2), or both. The scapula originates in early embryogenesis at a level posterior to the 4th cervical vertebra, but descends during development to below the 7th cervical vertebra. Failure of this descent, either unilateral or bilateral, is the Sprengel deformity.

Clinical features: *The clinical triad of short neck, low hairline, and restriction of neck motion is seen in only about half of the patients.* The scapula in mild cases is simply rotated, with a palpable or visible bump corresponding to the superomedial corner of the scapula in the region of the trapezius muscle. Function is generally good. In moderate cases, the scapula is higher on the neck and connected to the spine with an abnormal omovertebral ligament or even bone. Shoulder motion, particularly abduction, is limited. In severe cases, the scapula is small and positioned on the posterior neck, and the neck may be webbed.

Associated Anomalies: There is a strong association with congenital abnormalities of the genitourinary tract (30–40%), including double collecting systems, renal aplasia, and horseshoe kidney. Associated anomalies occur in the auditory system, neural axis, cardiovascular system, and the musculoskeletal system. Sprengel deformity (congenital elevation of the scapula) is a common associated finding, and >50% of patients will develop scoliosis. Since congenital anomalies may exist in more than one region of the spine, radiographs of the thoracic and lumbosacral spine are routinely obtained. These cervical findings may also be seen in patients with Goldenhar syndrome, Mohr syndrome, VACTERL syndrome, and fetal alcohol syndrome. The majority of patients have associated anomalies of the musculoskeletal system, especially in the spine (including Klippel-Feil anomaly with congenital cervical vertebral fusions), making spinal evaluation important.

Treatment: In mild cases, treatment is generally unnecessary, although a prominent and unsightly superomedial corner of the scapula can be excised. In more severe cases, surgical repositioning of the scapula with rebalancing of parascapular muscles can significantly improve both function and appearance.

Syndromes associated with Sprengel's deformity include teratological conditions such as **inencephaly** (a triad of occipital defect, spina bifida of cervical vertebrae, and fixed retroflexion of the head) and the **Klippel-Feil syndrome**

The Cavendish Grade of Sprengel's Deformity

Grade	Indications
1	Very mild, shoulder level and deformity invisible when dressed
2	Mild, shoulders almost level, lump visible in web of the neck when dressed
3	Moderate, shoulder elevated 2 to 5 cm. Deformity easily visible.
4	Severe, superior angle of scapula near occiput, with or without neck webbing

The functional aspect of **Sprengel deformity** has been attributed to:

- A forward curvature of the superior angle of the scapula over the apex of the thorax
- Abutment of the medial scapular border against the spinous processes of adjacent vertebrae
- The omovertebral bone

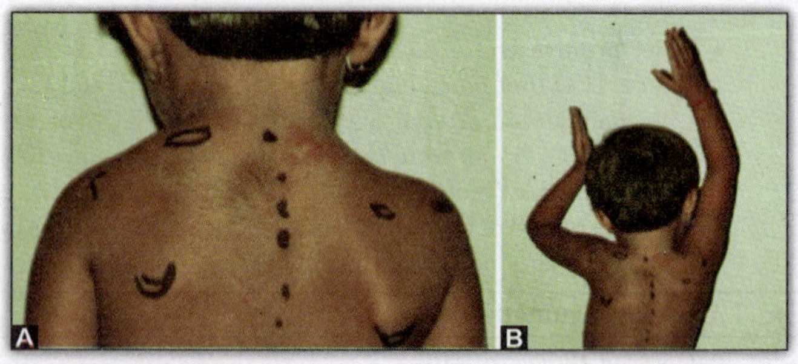

(*Source:* Kadavkolan AS, Bhatia DN, Dasgupta B, Bhosale PB - Int J Shoulder Surg 2011)

Fig: Sprengel deformity: (A) Cosmetic aspect of Sprengel's deformity is shown. The landmarks show marked elevation of the left scapula as compared with the right; **(B)** Functional aspect of Sprengel's deformity is shown. Marked restriction of abduction on the left side is seen as compared to the right

47. Ans. (b) Inability to hear a murmur

Ref: Nelson 20th ed page 2212-2213

Option (A)

Nelson says: The level of arterial oxygen saturation depends on the magnitude of the right-to-left shunt; in "pink tets," systemic saturation may be normal, whereas in a moderately cyanotic patient at rest, it is usually 75–85%. Growth and development may be delayed in patients with severe untreated tetralogy of Fallot, particularly when oxygen saturation is chronically <70%.

Option (B)

Paroxysmal hypercyanotic attacks (hypoxic, "blue," or "tet" spells) are a particular problem during the 1st-2nd year of life in children with Tetralogy of Fallot. The infant becomes hyperpneic and restless, cyanosis increases, gasping respiration ensue, and syncope may follow. The spells occur most frequently in the morning on initially awakening or after episodes of vigorous crying. **Temporary disappearance or a decrease in intensity of the systolic murmur** is usual as flow across the right ventricular outflow tract diminishes. The spells may last from a few minutes to a few hours. Short episodes are followed by generalized weakness and sleep.

Severe spells may progress to unconsciousness and, occasionally, to convulsions or hemiparesis. The onset is usually spontaneous and unpredictable. Spells are associated with reduction of an already compromised pulmonary blood flow, which, when prolonged, results in severe systemic hypoxia and metabolic acidosis. Infants who are only mildly cyanotic at rest are often more prone to the development of hypoxic spells because they have not acquired the homeostatic mechanisms to tolerate rapid lowering of arterial oxygen saturation, such as polycythemia.

Characteristic feature of cyanotic spell is
• Paroxysm of hyperpnoea (rapid and deep breathing) • Sudden marked increase in cyanosis • Irritability and prolonged crying • Decreased intensity of heart murmur

Option (C) and (D)

Hepatomegaly, peripheral edema and S3 gallop are signs of right sided heart failure which is rarely seen in TOF. Pulmonary edema and poor perfusion are signs of left sided heart failure.

Tetralogy of Fallot	
Tetralogy of Fallot is one of the conotruncal families of heart lesions in which the primary defect is an anterior deviation of the infundibular septum (the muscular septum that separates the aortic and pulmonary outflows).	
Components	• Obstruction to right ventricular outflow (pulmonary stenosis) • Ventricular septal defect (VSD) • Dextroposition of the aorta with override of the ventricular septum • Right ventricular hypertrophy
Pathophysiology	Obstruction of right ventricular outflow (pulmonary atresia with VSD) is classified as an extreme form of tetralogy of Fallot. The degree of pulmonary outflow obstruction varies, with the severity of the obstruction determining the degree of the patient's cyanosis. The VSD is usually nonrestrictive and large, is located just below the aortic valve, and is related to the posterior and right aortic cusps. Rarely, the VSD may be in the inlet portion of the ventricular septum (atrioventricular septal defect). The degree of right ventricular outflow obstruction determines the timing of the onset of symptoms, the severity of cyanosis, and the degree of right ventricular hypertrophy. When obstruction to right ventricular outflow is mild to moderate and a balanced shunt is present across the VSD, the patient may not be visibly cyanotic (acyanotic or "pink" tetralogy of Fallot). When obstruction is severe, cyanosis will be present from birth and worsen when the ductus begins to close.
Clinical features	• **Often, cyanosis is not present at birth,** but with increasing hypertrophy of the right ventricular infundibulum and patient growth, cyanosis occurs later in the 1st year of life. • **Dyspnea occurs on exertion**. Infants and toddlers play actively for a short time and then sit or lie down. Older children may be able to walk a block or so before stopping to rest. • Characteristically, children assume a **squatting position** for the relief of dyspnea caused by physical effort; the child is usually able to resume physical activity within a few minutes. These findings occur most often in patients with significant cyanosis at rest. • Paroxysmal hypercyanotic attacks (hypoxic, "blue," or "tet" spells) are a particular problem during the 1st 2 year of life. The infant becomes hyperpneic and restless, cyanosis increases, gasping respirations ensue, and syncope may follow. The spells occur most frequently in the morning on initially awakening or after episodes of vigorous crying.
	• Because **metabolic acidosis** develops when arterial PO_2 is <40 mm Hg, rapid correction (within several minutes) with intravenous administration of **sodium bicarbonate** is necessary if the spell is unusually severe and the child shows a lack of response to the foregoing therapy. Recovery from the spell is usually rapid once the pH has returned to normal. Repeated blood pH measurements may be necessary because rapid recurrence of acidosis may ensue. • For spells that are resistant to this therapy, drugs that increase systemic vascular resistance, such as **intravenous phenylephrine**, can improve right ventricular outflow, decrease the right-to-left shunt, and improve the symptoms. β-Adrenergic blockade by the intravenous administration of **propranolol** (0.1 mg/kg given slowly to a maximum of 0.2 mg/kg) is also useful. • The level of arterial oxygen saturation depends on the magnitude of the right-to-left shunt; in "pink tets," systemic saturation may be normal, whereas in a moderately cyanotic patient at rest, it is usually **75–85%.**

Contd...

Tetralogy of Fallot	
	• Growth and development may be delayed in patients with severe untreated tetralogy of Fallot, particularly when **oxygen saturation is chronically <70%**. Puberty may also be delayed in patients who do not undergo surgery. • The **pulse is usually normal**, as is venous and arterial pressure. The left anterior hemithorax may bulge anteriorly because of right ventricular hypertrophy. The heart is generally normal in size, and a substernal right ventricular impulse can be detected. In about half the cases, a systolic thrill is felt along the left sternal border in the 3rd and 4th parasternal spaces. The systolic murmur is usually loud and harsh; it may be transmitted widely, especially to the lungs, but is most intense at the left sternal border. The murmur is generally ejection in quality at the upper sternal border, but it may sound more holosystolic toward the lower sternal border. It may be preceded by a click. The murmur is caused by turbulence through the right ventricular outflow tract. It tends to become louder, longer, and harsher as the severity of pulmonary stenosis increases from mild to moderate; however, it can actually become less prominent with severe obstruction, especially during a hypercyanotic spell. Either the 2nd heart sound is single, or the pulmonic component is soft. Infrequently, a continuous murmur may be audible, especially if prominent collaterals are present.
Diagnosis	• Roentgenographically, the typical configuration as seen in the anteroposterior view consists of a narrow base, concavity of the left heart border in the area usually occupied by the pulmonary artery, and normal heart size. The hypertrophied right ventricle causes the rounded apical shadow to be uptilted so that it is situated higher above the diaphragm than normal. The cardiac silhouette has been likened to that of a **boot or wooden shoe ("coeur en sabot")** • The electrocardiogram demonstrates right axis deviation and evidence of right ventricular hypertrophy. A dominant R wave appears in the right precordial chest leads (Rs, R, qR, qRs) or an **RSR' pattern**. In some cases, the only sign of right ventricular hypertrophy may initially be a positive T wave in leads V3R and V1. The **P wave is tall and peaked or sometimes bifid** • **Two-dimensional echocardiography establishes the diagnosis** and provides information about the extent of aortic override of the septum, the location and degree of the right ventricular outflow tract obstruction, the size of the proximal branch pulmonary arteries, and the side of the aortic arch.
Complications	Complications are rare in TOF • **Cerebral thrombosis** (mostly <2 years age) • **Brain abscess** (less common than Cerebral vascular events because most patients are repaired early and brain abscess is seen in patients >2 years age) • **Bacterial endocarditis** • **Heart failure** is not a usual feature in patients with the tetralogy of Fallot. It may occur in a young infant with "pink" or acyanotic tetralogy of Fallot. As the degree of pulmonary obstruction worsens with age, the symptoms of heart failure resolve and eventually the patient experiences cyanosis, often by 6–12 months of age
Associated anomalies	• **PDA** may be present • A **right aortic arch** occurs in ≈20% of patients with the tetralogy of Fallot • **Multiple VSDs** are occasionally present and must be diagnosed before corrective surgery. • Tetralogy of Fallot may also occur with an **atrioventricular septal defect**, often associated with **Down syndrome.**
Treatment	Depending on the frequency and severity of hypercyanotic attacks, one or more of the following procedures should be instituted in sequence: • Placement of the infant on the abdomen in the **knee-chest position** while making certain that the infant's clothing is not constrictive • **Administration of oxygen** (although increasing inspired oxygen will not reverse cyanosis caused by intracardiac shunting) • Injection of **morphine subcutaneously** in a dose not in excess of 0.2 mg/kg Treatment of the tetralogy of Fallot depends on the severity of the right ventricular outflow tract obstruction. Infants with severe tetralogy require medical treatment and surgical intervention in the neonatal period. The modified **Blalock-Taussig shunt** is currently the most common aortopulmonary shunt procedure and consists of a Gore-Tex conduit anastomosed side to side from the subclavian artery to the homolateral branch of the pulmonary artery. **Corrective surgical therapy** consists of relief of the right ventricular outflow tract obstruction by removing obstructive muscle bundles and by patch closure of the VSD.

AIIMS NOVEMBER 2015

48. Ans. (a) Meningocele

Ref: IAP textbook of pediatrics 4th ed page 452, Ghai 8th ed page 575, Nelson 20th ed Page 2805

Based on just picture and no clinical findings it is very difficult to differentiate between meningocele and myelomeningocele. But the absence of nervous tissue points towards meningocele. At times it is difficult to appreciate the nervous tissue.

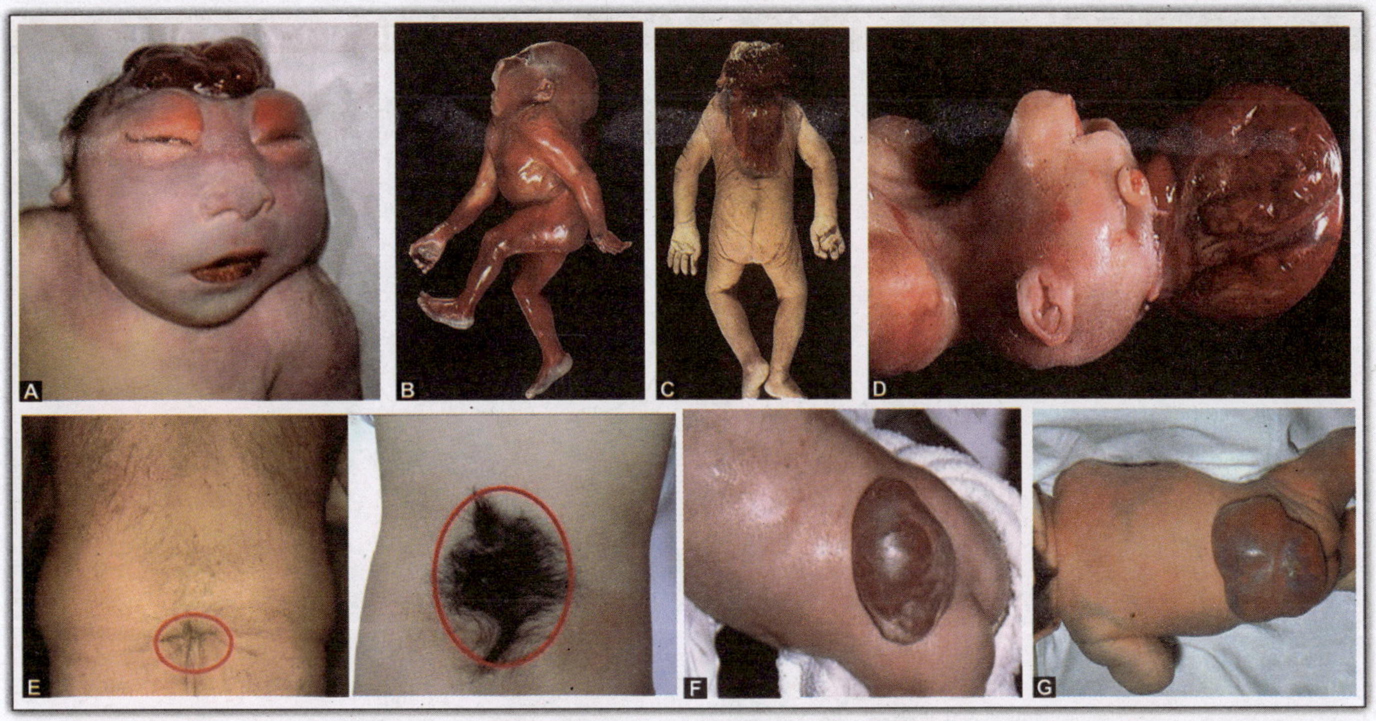

Figs A to G: **(A) Anencephaly:** Defect of cranial vault, frontoparietal region: partially degenerated brain tissue visible within the cranial bone defect. Severe swelling of palpebral, large appearing nose; **(B) Iniencephaly:** Imperfect formation of the base of the skull, with rachischisis and exaggerated lordosis of the spine. This is iniencephaly. The key features are: (1) imperfect formation of the base of the skull, (2) rachischisis, and (3) exaggerated lordosis of the vertebral column; **(C) Complete/total rachischisis** is demonstrated here in a case of iniencephaly. Craniospinal rachischisis is the failure of closure of most or all the neuraxis resulting in an absence/exposure of major portions of the brain and spinal cord; **(D) Exencephaly:** The cranial vault is not completely present, but a brain is present, because it was not completely exposed to amniotic fluid. Such an event is very rare. It may be part of craniofacial clefts with limb-body wall complex; **(E) Spina bifida occulta** is the simplest form of the spina bifida in which only the bony defect is present but no protrusion of meninges (protective layers covering the spinal cord) and the spinal cord. On right a dimple is shown on the lower back in the midline. A red circle is made around the dimple. It is also a common sign of spina bifida occulta. Due to a bony defect on the posterior side of vertebra, a space develops and skin is depressed at that point making a dimple on the skin. On left a tuft of hair on the lower back is one of the typical signs of spina bifida occulta. A red circle is made around the hair tuft on this picture; **(F) Meningocele:** Protrusion of the membranes that cover the spine and part of the spinal cord through a bone defect in the vertebral column containing CSF and lacks nervous tissue; **(G) Myelomeningocele:** A fluctuant midline mass that may transilluminate occurs along the vertebral column, usually in the lumbar region of a newborn baby with myelomeningocele. The skin is intact, and the placode-containing remnants of nervous tissue can be observed over the lesion, which is filled with cerebrospinal fluid

Neural Tube Defects

Neural Tube Defects (Dysraphism): This group of congenital anomalies of the CNS results from failure of the neural tube to close spontaneously. NTD are the most common malformations accounting for 0.5-1.3 cases/1000 live births with multifactorial etiology. Neural tube defects (NTDs) are a group of severe congenital abnormalities resulting from the failure of neurulation of multifactorial etiology around the 28th day of conception.

Cranial NTDs	Spinal NTDs	Craniospinal NTDs
Exencephaly Anencephaly Cranial meningocele Cranial myelomeningocele Encephalocele (myeloencephalocele) Spinal meningocele	Spina bifida occulta Lumbar dermal sinus Spina bifida aperta (spina bifida cystica) +/– posterior meningocele or myelomeningocele rachischisis Anterior meningocele/myelomeningocele Lateral meningocele/myelomeningocele Iniencephaly	Craniospinal rachischisis

Contd...

OPEN NTDs	CLOSED NTDs (Skin Covered)
Anencephaly Myelomeningocele (spina bifida) Myeloschisis Hemimyelomeningocele Hemimyelocele Craniorachischisis	Lipomyeloschisis Lipomyelomeningocele Meningocele Myelocystocele

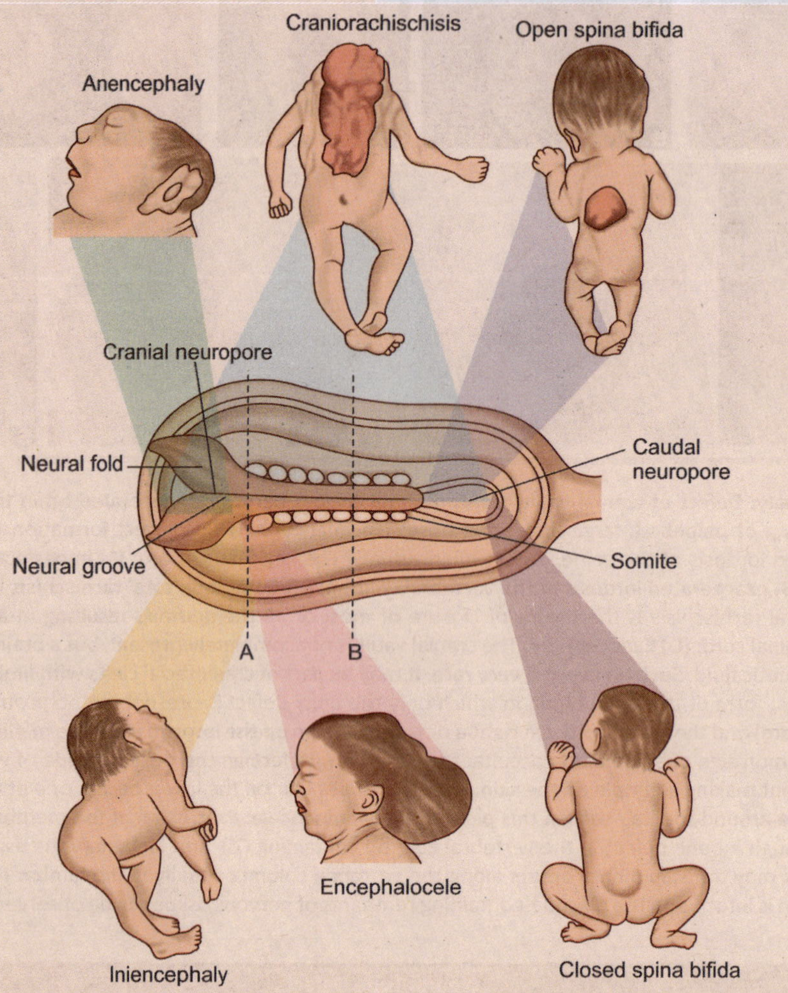

Types of Spina Bifida			
	Spina bifida occulta	Meningocele	Myelomeningocele
Incidence	5% of population	Most common type of spina bifida per 5000 live births	Most common type of spina bifida 1 per 800 live births
Location	Lumbosacral area is the most common location	Present along the length of spinal cord and skull. Lumbosacral area is the most common location	Present along the length of spinal cord, but not seen in skull. Lumbosacral area is the most common location
Clinical features	A mild form of spina bifida. Mostly asymptomatic & detected on X-ray. But may have a patch of hair, a lipoma or pigmentation of the low back	Cystic swelling in the skull or along the back bone. Contents of meningocele do not contain the spinal cord. Neurological deficits are rare.	Cystic swelling in the lower back. Sac consists of both meninges and spinal cord contents. Most common and most severe form of spina bifida. If not treated leads to irreversible neurological deficit.

Contd...

Types of Spina Bifida

Spina bifida occulta | **Meningocele** | **Myelomeningocele**

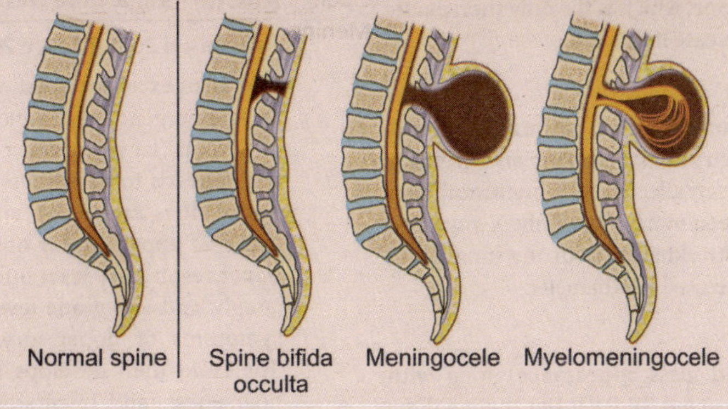

Footnote:
- Before surgical correction of the defect, the patient must be thoroughly examined with the use of plain roentgenograms, ultrasonography, and MRI to determine the extent of neural tissue involvement, if any, and associated anomalies, including diastematomyelia, tethered spinal cord, and lipoma.
- **Urologic evaluation,** usually including cystometrogram (CMG), will identify those children with neurogenic bladder who are at risk for renal deterioration.
- Those patients with leaking cerebrospinal fluid (CSF) or a thin skin covering should undergo immediate surgical treatment to prevent meningitis.
- A CT scan of the head is recommended for children with a meningocele because of the association with hydrocephalus in some cases.
- An **anterior meningocele** projects into the pelvis through a defect in the sacrum. Symptoms of constipation and bladder dysfunction develop due to the increasing size of the lesion.
- Female patients may have associated anomalies of the genital tract, including a rectovaginal fistula and vaginal septa. Plain roentgenograms demonstrate a defect in the sacrum, and CT scanning or MRI outlines the extent of the meningocele.

49. Ans. (a) Neonatal pulmonary alveolar proteinosis

Ref: Nelson 20th Ed page 2119

This is a very commonly asked question in AIIMS and one of the favorites. Though I really do not understand the logic behind this uncommon condition seen in a NICU still, things to be discussed in this question are:

Option (A)

Pulmonary Airway Proteinosis is a rare type of diffuse lung disease with intra-alveolar accumulation of pulmonary surfactant. It is of two types:

1. **Primary:** Disordered signaling of granulocyte-macrophage colony-stimulating factor (GM-CSF) leading to impaired alveolar macrophage maturation is the major underlying cause of primary PAP. Mostly autoantibodies to GM-CSF is seen which block binding of GM-CSF to its receptor, thereby ***inhibiting alveolar macrophage maturation and function and surfactant clearance***. Some children mutation in genes encoding both α and β subunits of the GM-CSF receptor forms the genetic basis for some cases. It is also reported in children with **lysinuric protein intolerance**, a rare AR disorder and also in **Niemann-Pick disease**.
2. **Secondary:** It may occur along with **infection**, particularly in **immunocompromised** individuals. However, it is **not clear** whether this phenotype results from a secondary infection or the underlying immunodeficiency. Environmental exposures to dust, silica, and chemicals and chemotherapeutic agents have also been associated.

The other way of classification is (a) fatal form which present shortly after birth called congenital PAP and (b) gradually progressive form which is seen in older infants and children. In congenital alveolar proteinosis as in above question there is an inherited disruption of pulmonary surfactant metabolism. Surfactant protein A and B makes a monolayer of dipalmitoylphosphatidylcholine which acts as a surface tension lowering agent. In congenital alveolar proteinosis protein B will be absent which will not let monolayer form and cause accumulation of surfactant leading to failure of expansion of alveoli and cardiorespiratory arrest.

Clinical presentation of infants and children will be dyspnea, fatigue, cough, weight loss, chest pain or hemoptysis. Later stages it will be cyanosis and clubbing. Boys are 3 times more commonly affected than girls. In newborns the presentation is severe enough and will cause respiratory distress shortly following birth with X-ray showing ground glass appearance. When surfactant administered it accumulates in lungs and causes more distress finally leading to hypoxia and death. Family history will be positive.

Diagnosis (gold standard) is established by histopathologic examination of lung biopsy specimens immunohistochemical staining reveals **abundant quantities of alveolar and intracellular surfactant proteins**. This is likely to change as molecular tests become available. Latex agglutination tests for the presence of anti–GM-CSF antibodies in BAL fluid or blood are highly sensitive and specific for the autoimmune forms of alveolar proteinosis.

Treatment

If untreated it have a stormy course leading to death. Palliative measure is to have a **bronchoalveolar lavage** repeatedly until **lung transplantation** can be done, which is the only therapeutic option but the recurrence of disease limits it too.

Option (B)

Meconium Aspiration Syndrome presents **within few hours of life** with tachypnea, chest retractions, cyanosis and grunting observed in infants who are severely affected. Also **pneumothorax and pneumomediastinum** is seen more commonly. **X-ray chest** shows patchy infiltrates with streaking of both the lung fields, flattening of diaphragm and increased AP diameter.

Option (C)

CHD which can have ground glass appearance along with small heart after birth is **obstructed TAPVR** but there will be **cyanosis** associated, with **murmur** along left sternal border and also gallop rhythm sometimes. (Do not confuse with Figure of 8 or snowman's heart X-ray as it will be seen in older children with unobstructed TAPVR.)

Option (D)

HSV infection in newborn period will be generally localized but even if it is disseminated it usually begin within the first week of neonatal life. The liver, adrenals, and other visceral organs are usually involved. Approximately two-thirds of infants also have encephalitis. Clinical findings include seizures, shock, respiratory distress, disseminated intravascular coagulation (DIC), and respiratory failure. A typical vesicular rash may be absent in as many as 20% of infants. Forty percent of the infants who survive have long-term morbidity.

50. Ans. (a) Single dose Dexamethasone

Ref: Nelson 20th Ed page 2033-34

This is an excellent question as it tests your knowledge and the ward/emergency experience too. Read following discussion.

Croup (laryngotracheobronchitis) is a medical emergency and it needs to be address immediately once it comes to your notice. It is caused by viral infection and is most common cause of upper airway obstruction in children. It starts with upper respiratory tract infection rhinorrhea, pharyngitis, mild cough, and low-grade fever for 1-3 days before the signs and symptoms of upper airway obstruction become apparent. The child then develops the characteristic "barking" cough, hoarseness, and inspiratory stridor. Symptoms are worse at night and often recur with decreasing intensity for several days and resolve completely within a week. Family history of URTI will be positive.

Examination reveals audible stridor, inflamed pharynx, tachypnea and respiratory distress with varying degree. Being a disease of upper airway alveolar gas exchange will be normal. Hypoxia and low oxygen saturation are seen only when there is complete airway obstruction. Croup is a clinical diagnosis and do not require any X-ray for diagnosis. However, if at all done radiographs of the neck can show the typical subglottic narrowing, or steeple sign, of croup on the posteroanterior view. This **steeple sign** could be absent in children with croup or it could be seen in normal children too.

Feature	Number of Points Assigned for this Feature					
	0	1	2	3	4	5
Chest wall retraction	None	Mild	Moderate	Severe	-	-
Stridor	None	With agitation	At rest	-	-	-
Cyanosis	None	-	-	-	With agitation	At rest
Level of consciousness	Normal	-	-	-	-	Disoriented
Air entry	Normal	Decreased	Markedly decreased	-	-	-

- A total score of ≤2 indicates ***mild*** croup. The characteristic barking cough and hoarseness may be present, but there is no stridor at rest.
- A total score of 3–5 is classified as ***moderate*** croup. It presents with easily heard stridor, but with few other signs.
- A total score of 6–11 is ***severe*** croup. It also presents with obvious stridor, but also features marked chest wall indrawing.
- A total score of ≥ 12 indicates impending respiratory failure. The barking cough and stridor may no longer be prominent at this stage.

85% of children presenting to the emergency department have mild disease; severe croup is rare (<1%).

In given scenario-child does not have retraction (at respiratory rate of 36/min it is very less likely) oxygen saturation is 96% which means no cyanosis (as cyanosis due to hypoxia is clinically visible only when oxygen saturation is <85%). Stridor is heard only on crying (with agitation). Child is looking well hydrated, able to drink and is consolable (not disoriented). Nothing is mentioned about air entry but given other parameters of respiratory rate, oxygen saturation, stridor on crying it is very obvious air entry is normal. Hence the scoring comes to be = 1. So it is a mild croup.

- The mainstay of therapy is airway management and treatment of hypoxia. ***Treatment of respiratory distress should take the priority before any testing.***
- Nebulized racemic epinephrine is an accepted treatment for ***moderate or severe croup***. The mechanism of action is believed to be constriction of the precapillary arterioles through the β-adrenergic receptors, causing fluid resorption from the interstitial space and a decrease in the laryngeal mucosal edema. The indications for the administration of nebulized epinephrine include moderate to severe stridor at rest, the possible need for intubation, respiratory distress, and hypoxia.
- The effectiveness of oral corticosteroids in viral croup is well established. Corticosteroids decrease the edema in the laryngeal mucosa through their anti-inflammatory action. Oral steroids are ***beneficial, even in mild croup***, as measured by reduced hospitalization, shorter duration of hospitalization, and reduced need for subsequent

interventions such as epinephrine administration. Most studies that demonstrated the efficacy of oral dexamethasone used a single dose of 0.6 mg/kg, a dose as low as 0.15 mg/kg may be just as effective. A single dose of oral prednisolone is less effective.

- Children with croup should be hospitalized for any of the following: progressive stridor, severe stridor at rest, respiratory distress, hypoxia, cyanosis, depressed mental status, poor oral intake, or the need for reliable observation.
- Antibiotics are not indicated in croup. Nonprescription cough and cold medications should not be used in children younger than 4 years of age.

Hence from above explanation it is clear that in the given case option c and d are the options for further testing are conveniently ruled out and since adrenaline nebulization is used only in moderate or severe croup it is also ruled out. Steroids are effective in mild moderate or severe croup it is the answer.

51. Ans. (a) ORS alone

Ref: Nelson 20th Ed page 1869-74, Ghai 8th ed page 293-294

This question could be taken as an incomplete question since there is no mention of hydration status, fever, characteristics of stools and other associated features which are necessary to make a diagnosis, which will enable you to initiate the treatment needed. However, it is one of the questions where the examiner wants to know something very particular. We can draw the following inferences from the given scenario.

- It is an **acute diarrhea**—since less than 14 days.
- Since it is 1-year-old child, it will be considered as **viral** diarrhea, as it is the **most common** etiology in children especially infants and toddlers. Since none other details are given it will be justified to considered everything as normal.

Now coming to the treatment part of diarrhea—the ***mainstay of treatment of diarrhea is rehydration therapy***. If child is able to take orally well the rehydration should be done orally and when he is not able to it is has to be done parentally. In given scenario it is to be considered that child is otherwise well and hence option d is ruled out because as the answer wanted is very specific by the examiner for option d to be the answer child should have feature of severe dehydration which are not mentioned in the scenario.

Coming back to the treatment of diarrhea, zinc supplementation is the only adjunct therapy that has proven benefit in reducing the severity and duration of non-cholera diarrheal illnesses. Various strains of probiotics have been studied for the treatment of acute onset diarrhea but reports in various literatures suggest a moderate clinical improvement of diarrhea with strains of Lactobacillus GG and Saccharomyces boulardii with no adverse effects attributed to probiotic treatments. The efficacy is strain- and dose dependent. ***Further research is needed to establish specific treatment guidelines for the use of probiotics in the pediatric population.***

About antibiotics—they should be used only in case of bacterial diarrhea as unnecessary use leads to antibiotic abuse. Also there is an entity called as "antibiotic induced diarrhea" which can set in when antibiotics are used when not needed.

52. Ans. (c) Height for age

Ref: Ghai 8th ed page 97, Consensus Statement of the Indian Academy of Pediatrics on Integrated Management of Severe Acute Malnutrition. Indian Pediatrics. Volume 50__APRIL 16, 2013;399-404

Indicators of Malnutrition

Indicator	Parameter	Interpretation
Stunting	Low height for age	Chronic malnutrition
Wasting	Low weight for height	Acute malnutrition
Underweight	Low weight for age	Both acute and chronic malnutrition

In children between the ages of 6 and 59 months, severe acute malnutrition (SAM) is defined as:

- ***Weight/height or Weight/length*** <3 Z score, using the WHO Growth Charts; OR
- Presence of ***visible severe wasting***; OR
- Presence of ***bipedal edema*** of nutritional origin; OR
- Mid- upper arm circumference (***MUAC***) <115 mm.

WHO Definitions: These indicators are used to measure nutritional imbalance resulting in undernutrition (assessed from underweight, wasting and stunting) and overweight. The percentage of children who have low weight for age (underweight) can reflect 'wasting' (i.e. low weight for height), indicating acute weight loss, 'stunting', or both.

Thus, 'underweight' is a composite indicator and may therefore be difficult to interpret.

- **Underweight:** Weight for age <–2 standard deviations (SD) of the WHO Child Growth
- **Standards median**
- **Stunting:** Height for age < –2 SD of the WHO Child Growth Standards median
- **Wasting:** Weight for height < –2 SD of the WHO Child Growth Standards median
- **Overweight:** Weight for height > +2 SD of the WHO Child Growth Standards median

Contd...

Z-score	Growth Indicators			
	Length/height-for-age	Weight-for-age	Weight-for-length/height	BMI-for-age
Above 3	*See note 1*		*Obese*	*Obese*
Above 2		*See note 2*	*Overweight*	*Overweight*
Above 1			*Possible risk of overweight*	*Possible risk of overweight*
0 (median)				
Below-1				
Below-2	*Stunted*	*Underweight*	*Wasted*	*Wasted*
Below-3	*Severely stunted*	*Severely underweight*	*Severely wasted*	*Severely wasted*

Wasting = Acute malnutrition
Stunting = Chronic malnutrition

53. Ans. (b) Breast bud

Ref: Nelson 20th Ed page 926-31

In girls, the breast bud (Thelarche) is usually the first sign of puberty (10–11 years), followed by the appearance of pubic hair 6–12 months later. The interval to menarche is usually 2–2.5 years but may be as long as 6 years. Peak height velocity occurs early (at breast stage II–III, typically between 11 and 12 years of age) in girls and always precedes menarche.

Stages of Puberty					
Adrenarche→	Gonadarche→	Thelarche→	Pubarche→	Menarche	Spermarche
Both males and females	Both males and females	Only females	Both males and females	Only females	Only males
7 years	8 years	11 years	12 years	12.5 years	11–15 years

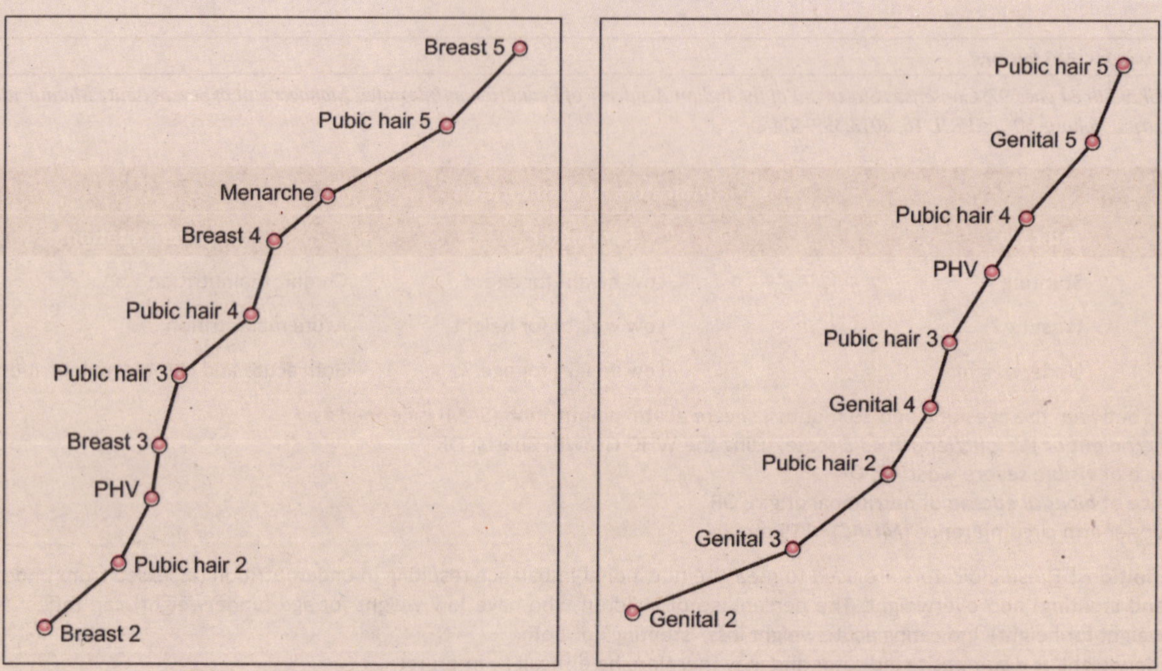

Pubertal events in female **Pubertal events in males**

(PHV, Peak height velocity)

Note:
- For Girls; peak height growth = Breast stage III and Axillary hair stage III
- For Boys; peak height growth = Genitalia (testes and penis) stage IV and Axillary hair stage IV.

Sexual Maturity Rating (SMR) for Girls		
Staging	Breast	Pubic hair staging
1	Prepubertal, papilla Elevation	No pigmented hair
2	Budding; larger areole; palpable and visible elevated contour	Pigmented hair, mainly labial
3	Enlargement of the breast and areola	Coarser, spread of pigmented hair over mons
4	Secondary mound of areola and papilla	Adult type but smaller area
5	Mature	Adult distribution

54. Ans. (b) Weight for height <2SD

Ref: Ghai 8th ed page 96, IAP textbook of pediatrics 4th ed page 138, http://www.who.int/nutrition/nlis_interpretation_guide.pdf

See Table of Indicators of Malnutrition Pediatrics Aiims Nov 2015 (see page no. 837)

NOTE

The question is about Undernutrition or malnutrition not underweight. Malnutrition is best assessed by Wasting i.e. Weight for age.

55. Ans. (d) Creatine Kinase levels

Ref: Nelson 20th Ed page 2960-2963

See Details of Muscular Dystrophy in AIIMS NOV 2016 Pediatrics (see page no. 820-821)

It is a case of proximal muscle weakness which is progressive. To answer this question we should come to the differential diagnosis of the given case and then only we can plan further investigations. So with progressive proximal muscle weakness and positive Gower's sign first DD clicked in my head was DMD but it is a girl child. DMD is more common in boys as it is X linked though it can occur in girls too. Now another added point is maculopapular pigmentation over back if hands so can it be some rheumatic cause? Answer is less likely. Since the main complaint is of proximal muscle weakness the only rheumatic condition causing it is dermatomyositis in which insidious onset of fever and rash with joint pain will be present. Hence my DDs in sequence of probabilities are:

- DMD
- Becker's
- Other muscular dystrophies
- Dermatomyositis

Another possibility of the given question could be neuropathy but they generally involve the distal muscles except SMA type 3.

Now for any muscular dystrophy the first investigation which is done is CPK as DMD and becker's are common and will show elevated level of CPK in range of 15000-35000 IU/L (normal is <160 IU/L) after seeing this and ruling out muscular dystrophies will go for nerve conduction study for any neuropathies, if suspected. Electromyography helps distinguish between demyelinating or hypomyelinating and axonal forms of neuropathies. Rheumatoid factor is done in case of proximal muscle weakness when dermatomyositis is thought of (which is very less likely in this child). Hence in the index case answer is (D) CK level estimation.

AIIMS MAY 2015

56. Ans. (b) In endemic areas vaccination is given to cover children between one to nine years age group

Ref: Nelson 18th ed ch 173, Park 23rd ed page 286

Japanese encephalitis vaccination: Vaccination of population at risk has been recommended. Currently, the three types of JE vaccines in large-scale use are:

- **The mouse brain-derived,** purified and inactivated vaccine, which is based on either the Nakayama or Beijing strains of the JE virus and produced in several Asian countries; The mouse—brain derived, inactivated vaccine has been used successfully to reduce the incidence of JE in a number of countries, and is likely to be used nationally and internationally for some more years.
- The cell culture-derived, inactivated JE vaccine based on the Beijing P—3 strain, and
- The cell culture-derived, live attenuated vaccine based on the SA 14-14-2 strain of the JE virus.

When **immunizing children 1—3 years of age** the mouse brain-derived vaccine provides adequate protection throughout childhood following 2 primary doses 4 weeks apart, and **boosters after 1 year and subsequently at 3-yearly intervals until the age of 10—15 years.** The vaccine is given subcutaneously in doses of 0.5 mL for children under 3 years and 1 mL for children more than 3 years of age. Protective immunity develops in about one month time after the second dose. The vaccine is best used in the inter epidemic period. It should be offered to the most vulnerable and high-risk groups. Equally good childhood protection is obtained by a single dose of the cell-culture based, live attenuated vaccine (SA-14-14-2) followed by a single booster given at an interval of about 1 year. **This vaccine is available in India and is an integral part of Universal Immunization Programme in 83 endemic districts in Uttar Pradesh, Assam, West Bengal and Karnataka targeting children in age group 1–15 years.** The importance of achieving long-term protection is underlined by the observation that in some areas an increasing proportion of the JE cases occur in individuals older than 10 years of age.

Given the most infrequent occurrence of JE in infancy and the likely interference with passively acquired maternal antibodies during the first months of life, **vaccination is not recommended for children before the age of 6 months.**

Vaccine name, strain, type, route, dosage, storage	Schedule of routine immunization	Schedule for catch-up Immunization from 4 months to 6 years	Schedule for catch up Immunization from 7 to 18 years	Contraindications and precautions	Adverse effects
Japanese encephalitis **inactivated mouse brain–derived vaccine (JE-MB** Nakayama NIH or Beijing-1 strains, Wild type. Stored at 2-80C, Diluent **Phosphate buffer solution (PBS)**	Routine immunization is not recommended. Only in endemic area as catch up	IAP recommendations: Only in endemic area as catch-up up to 15 years age. Live attenuated, cell culture derived SA-14-14-2 JE vaccine should be preferred 0.5 mL, SC, single dose. **JE-MB**; 3 primary doses at days 0, 7 and 28; alternatively 2 primary doses preferably 4 weeks apart. 0.5 mL for **1–3 years of age**; 1 mL for >3 years of age. **Booster doses** at 1 year then every 3 years	Contraindications • Previous anaphylaxis • Severe acute illness	Localized erythema, tenderness, and swelling. Mild systemic side effects (fever, chill, headache, rash, myalgia). Allergic hypersensitivity reactions. Neurologic symptoms; encephalitis, seizures, gait disturbances, and parkinsonism	• Least thermosensitive but reconstituted vaccine is heat and light sensitive • Recommended in visitors to high risk states if duration of stay is >4 weeks
Japanese Encephalitis inactivated Vero cell culture-derived vaccine (JE-VC) Inactivated SA14-14-2 strain (LAV-SA14-14-2 also available) Stored at 2-8°C	Routine immunization is not recommended. Only in endemic area as catch up	IAP recommendations: Only in endemic area as catch-up up to 15 years age. Live attenuated, cell culture derived SA-14-14-2 JE vaccine should be preferred 0.5 mL, SC, single dose. JE-VC; 2 doses at 0 and 28 days for ≥17 years, 0.5 mL IM	Contraindications • Previous Anaphylaxis • Severe acute illness	Local and systemic adverse events similar JE-MB. No serious hypersensitivity reactions or neurologic adverse events were identified among JE-VC	LAV- SA14-14-2 was used in pilot projects by Govt of India in hyperendemic districts of UP, West Bengal, Assam, Karnataka

57. Ans. (a) Hurler disease

Ref: Nelson 20th ed page 5738-5739

Similar question with different set of clinical features of Hurler's syndrome is asked in AIIMS Pediatrics Nov 2018 (see page no. 798)

Option (A) Hurler Disease

Hurler is characterized by

- Inguinal hernia
- Hepatosplenomegaly
- Coarse facial features
- Corneal clouding
- Large tongue
- Prominent forehead
- Joint stiffness
- Short stature
- Skeletal dysplasia
- Cardiomyopathy, valvular heart disease
- Recurrent URTI (copious mucus discharge, obstructive airway disease.)

Option (B) Beckwith-wiedemann Syndrome

Organomegaly (liver, kidney, adrenal and pancreas), macroglossia, omphalocele/umbilical hernia, hemihypertrophy, ear pits. Hypoglycemia.

Option (C) Proteus Syndrome

Café-au-lait spots, macrodactyly, leg length discrepancy, verrucous cutaneous lesions, angiomas of various types, thickening of bones, syndromic hemimegalencephaly and excessive growth of muscles without weakness. Histology demonstrates muscular dysgenesis.

Option (D)

Hypothyroidism will have macroglossia; can have coarse facial features but hepatosplenomegaly and copious nasal discharge.

Recognition Pattern of Mucopolysaccharidoses							
	Mucopolysaccharidosis type						
Manifestations	Type I-H Hurler disease	Type I-S Scheie disease	Type II Hunter	Type III Sanfilippo disease	Type IV Morquio disease	Type VI Maroteaux-Lamy disease	Type VII Sly disease
Mental deficiency	+	−	±	+	−	−	±
Coarse facial features	+	(+)	+	+	−	+	±
Corneal clouding	+	+	−	−	(+)	+	±
Visceromegaly	+	(+)	+	(+)	−	+	+
Short stature	+	(+)	+	−	+	+	+
Joint contractures	+	+	+	−	−	+	+
Dysostosis multiplex	+	(+)	+	(+)	+	+	+
Leucocyte inclusions	+	(+)	+	+	−	+	+
Mucopolysaccharidura	+	+	+	+	+	+	+
Note: All mucopolysaccharidosis are autosomal recessive except Hunter's disease, which is X linked recessive							

58. Ans. (b) Ornithine transcarbamylase

Ref: Nelson 20th ed page 669-675, Harper 28th ed page 242-246

In urea cycle enzyme defect most commonly, the affected infant becomes symptomatic during the 1st few days of life with signs and symptoms of hyperammonemia (refusal to eat, vomiting, lethargy, convulsion, and coma). Do not get confused with the age because first few days of life mentioned here is the age of onset and in the question 7 month age infant gives positive previous history and recurrence.

From the discussion below it is concluded that the given clinical picture is consistent with both Ornithine transcarbamoylase and CPS 1 deficiency. The two conditions are differentiated based on Orotic aciduria which is not provided in the question. Ornithine transcarbamylase deficiency is the most common urea cycle disorders in humans, hence the answer of choice.

Routine laboratory studies show no specific findings when hyperammonemia is due to defects of the urea cycle enzymes. Blood urea nitrogen is usually low. Serum pH is usually normal or mildly elevated. In infants with organic acidemias, hyperammonemia is commonly associated with severe acidosis. Clinical approach of hyperammonemia is discussed in following flow chart and table.

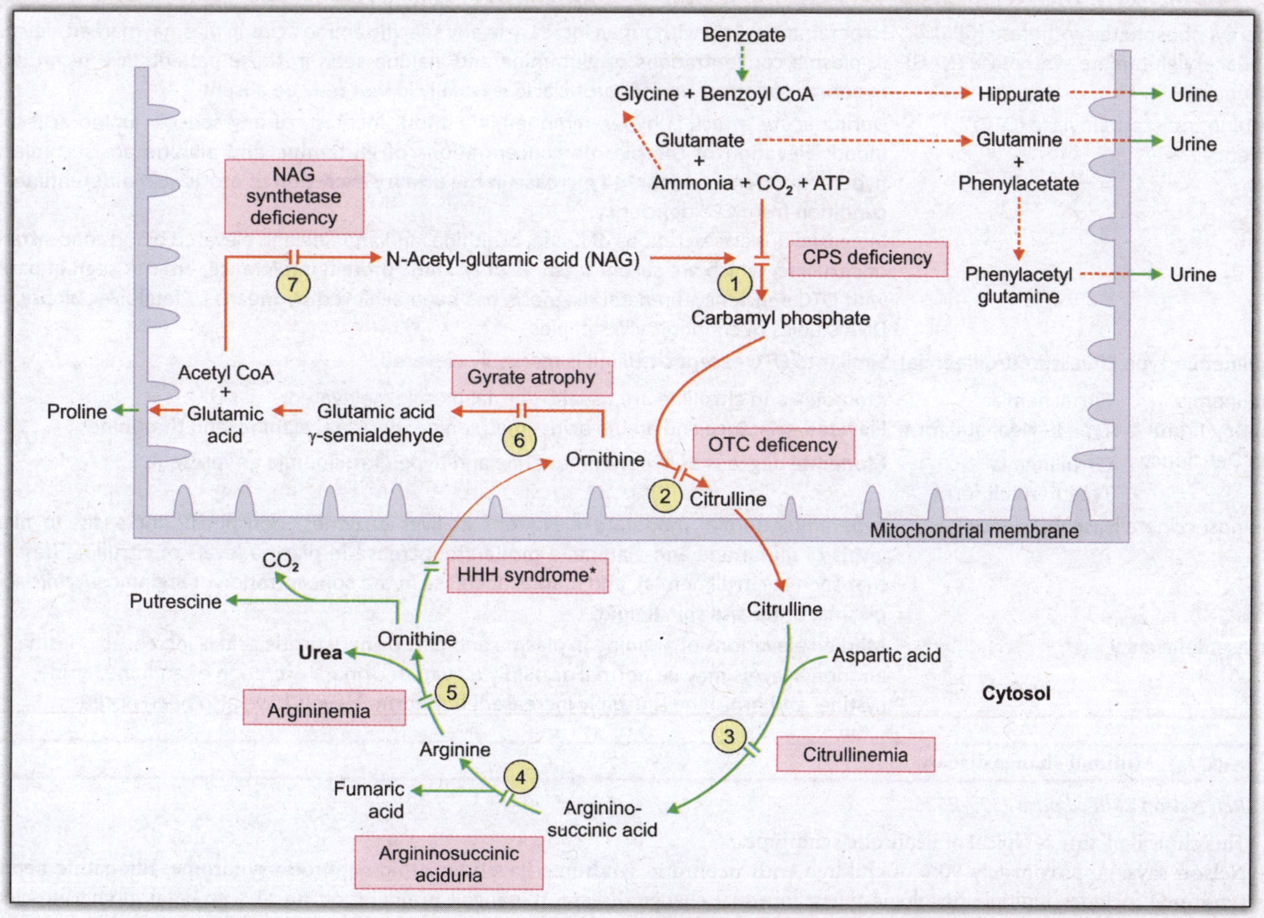

Clinical approach to a newborn infant with symptomatic hyperammonemia

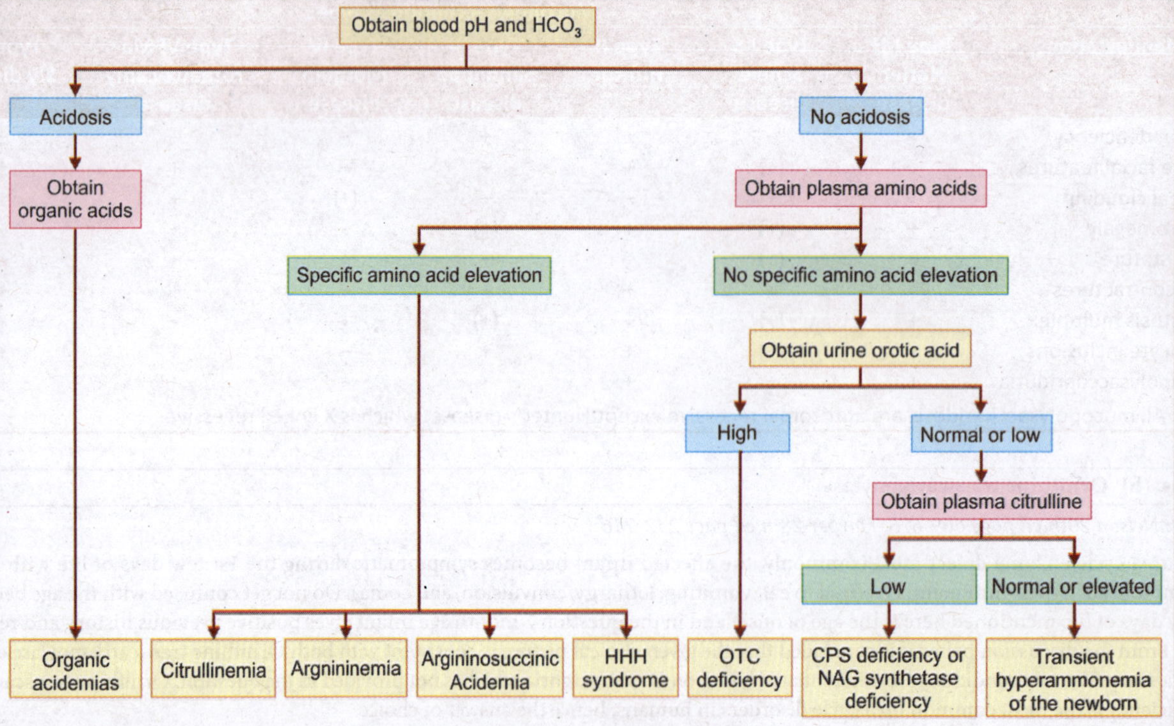

Abbreviations: CPS, carbamyl phosphate synthetase; HHH syndrome, hyperammonemia-hyperornithinemia-homocitrullinuria, NAG, *N*-acetylglutamate; OTC, ornithine transcarbamylase

Urea Cycle Defect	Lab Findings
Carbamyl phosphate synthetase (CPS) and N-acetylglutamate synthetase (NAG) deficiencies	Hyperammonemia without an increase in any specific amino acids in plasma; marked elevations in plasma concentrations of glutamine and alanine seen in these patients are secondary to hyperammonemia. Urinary orotic acid is usually low or may be absent
Ornithine transcarbamylase (OTC) deficiency	During acute attack is hyperammonemia without increase of any specific amino acid in the blood. Elevation of the plasma concentrations of **glutamine and alanine** are secondary to hyperammonemia. A **marked increase in the urinary excretion of orotic acid** differentiates this condition from CPS deficiency. Increased urinary excretions of lysine, ornithine, and arginine and elevated blood concentrations of citrulline, which are salient features of lysinuric protein intolerance, are not seen in patients with OTC deficiency. Prenatal diagnosis has been achieved by means of fetal liver biopsy or by DNA studies of chorionic villi samples
Citrullinemia Type I (Classic Citrullinemia)	Similar to OTC except citrulline is markedly elevated.
Citrullinemia Resulting From Citrin Deficiency — Citrullinemia Type II- Neonatal form	Ammonia and citrulline are usually normal or mildly elevated. Elevated galactose and amino acids- methionine, tyrosine, alanine, and threonine
Citrullinemia Resulting From Citrin Deficiency — Citrullinemia Type II- Adult form	Moderate degrees of hyperammonemia and hypercitrullinemia are present.
Argininosuccinate lyase deficiency	hyperammonemia, moderate elevations in liver enzymes, nonspecific increases in plasma levels of glutamine and alanine, a moderate increase in plasma levels of citrulline (less than that seen in citrullinemia), and marked increase in the concentration of argininosuccinic acid in plasma, urine and spinal fluid.
Arginase deficiency	Marked elevations of arginine in plasma and CSF. Urinary orotic acid is increased. Plasma ammonia levels may be normal or mildly elevated. Urinary excretion of arginine, lysine, cystine, and ornithine is usually increased, but normal levels have also been noted

59. Ans. (a) Minimal change disease

Ref: Nelson 20th ed page 2523-2526

This clinical picture is typical of nephrotic syndrome.

Nelson says: Approximately 90% of children with nephrotic syndrome have idiopathic nephrotic syndrome. Idiopathic nephrotic syndrome includes multiple histologic types: minimal change disease, mesangial proliferation, focal segmental glomerulosclerosis, membranous nephropathy and membranoproliferative glomerulonephritis.

In minimal change nephrotic syndrome (MCNS) (**approximately 85% of total cases of nephrotic syndrome in children**), the glomeruli appear normal or show a minimal increase in mesangial cells and matrix.

60. Ans. (a) ORS

Ref: Nelson's 20th ed page 1869-74

Dehydration is the principle concern of diarrhea and ORS is the fluid of choice for dehydration.

NOTE

Sugar containing water will cause osmotic diarrhea and salt water of whose concentration not properly predefined if given will cause electrolyte imbalance.

IMCI Child Dehydration Classification

Dehydration	Signs	Treatment
Severe dehydration	If two or more of following is present, lethargic or unconscious Sunken eyes, not able to drink or feed properly, skin pinch goes back slowly (>2 sec)	Fluids according to **Plan C** Refer urgently to hospital Give ORS on the way, continue breast feeding Keep child warm
Some Dehydration	If two or more of following is present, restless or irritable sunken eyes Eagerly drinks and thirsty Skin pinch goes back slowly (>2 sec)	Fluids according to **Plan B** Continue breast feeding and feeding Follow-up in 2 days if needed
No dehydration	No visible signs	Fluids according to **Plan A** Follow up in 5 days

Treatment Plans of Dehydration

Plan A: Home-based treatment

Age	Amount of ORS to give after each loose stool or other culturally appropriate ORT fluids	Amount of ORS to provide for use at home
<2 years	50–100 mL	500 mL/day
2–10 years	100–200 mL	1000 mL/day
>10 years	As much as wanted	2000 mL/day

Plan B: Give 75 mL/kg ORS in first 4 hours

Approx amount of ORS to be given in first 4 hours

Age	<4 months	4–11 months	12–23 months	2–4 years	5–14 years	>15 years
Approx. Weight in kg	<5 kg	5–8 kg	8–11 kg	11–16 kg	16–30 kg	>30 kg
ORS in mL	200–400	400–600	600–800	800–1200	1200–2200	>2200
Local measure in glass	1–2	2–3	3–4	4–6	6–11	12–20

Plan C

- **Start fluids immediately**
- **Best fluid ringer lactate**
- **Give 100 mL/kg of chosen solution divided as follows:**

Age	First give	Then give
<12 months	30 mL/kg in 1st hour	70 mL/kg in 5 hours
12 months to 5 years	30 minutes	2½ hour

61. Ans. (a) Alpha 1 antitrypsin deficiency

Ref: Nelson 20th ed page 1928-36, Robbins 9th ed page 847-851

See Table of Causes of Neonatal Jaundice in Pediatrics AIIMS NOV 2016 (see page no. 821)

The basic approach to neonatal cholestasis is important I felt as lot of MCQs has been directed to this topic.

Option (A)

Alpha at Deficiency

The characteristic liver biopsy finding has been described in the question is of alpha 1 antitrypsin deficiency.

Option (B)

Congenital Hepatic Fibrosis

It is usually associated with ARPKD and is characterized by peri-portal and peri-lobular fibrosis. Hepatocellular function is usually well preserved. Serum aminotransferase activities and bilirubin levels are usually normal in the absence of cholangitis and choledocholithiasis; serum alkaline phosphatase activity may be slightly elevated. The serum albumin level and prothrombin time are normal. Liver biopsy is rarely required for diagnosis, particularly in patients with obvious real disease. Given child have high alkaline phosphatase hence ruled out.

Option (C)

Extrahepatic biliary atresia—as question clearly mentions intrahepatic cholestasis it is straightforwardly ruled out.

Option (D)

Ductal plate defect: Ductal plate malformation refers to the persistence of excess embryonic bile duct structures in the portal tracts. Congenital hepatic fibrosis and Caroli disease likely result from an abnormality in remodeling of the embryonic ductal plate of the liver. Liver biopsy shows bile duct proliferation and ectasia, as well as progressive hepatic fibrosis.

α1 Antitrypsin Deficiency	
• α_1-Antitrypsin deficiency is an **autosomal recessive** disorder marked by very low levels of α_1-antitrypsin. The major function of this protein is the **inhibition of proteases, particularly neutrophil elastase, cathepsin G, and proteinase 3,** which are normally released from neutrophils at sites of inflammation. • α_1-Antitrypsin is a small **394–amino acid plasma glycoprotein synthesized predominantly by hepatocytes and also expressed in lungs.** • The normal α_1-antitrypsin PiM protein is secreted by the liver into the circulation at a rate of ≈**34 mg/kg/day**	
Genetics	• Conventional nomenclature identifies **normal variants as PiMM**; the **most common genotype is PiMM, occurring in 90% of individuals** (in the traditional sense, this would be the wild-type genotype). These individuals have normal blood levels of AAT. • The most common abnormal variants are called S and Z. Individuals homozygous for the Z mutation **(PiZZ) have low levels of AAT (about 15% of normal)** and these patients are susceptible to liver and/or lung disease, yet only a proportion (about 25%) of PiZZ patients develop disease manifestations. • The **most common clinically significant mutation is PiZ;** homozygotes for the PiZZ protein have only **10% of normal ATT.** • Rare variants termed ***Pi-null*** have no detectable serum α_1-antitrypsin Null variants have undetectable levels of AAT and are susceptible to premature lung disease. • Some *deficiency variants*, including the **PiS variant**, result in a moderate reduction in serum concentrations of α_1-antitrypsin without clinical manifestations.
Morphology	α_1-Antitrypsin deficiency is characterized by the presence of round-to-**oval cytoplasmic globular inclusions in hepatocytes,** which in routine HandE stains are acidophilic and indistinctly demarcated from the surrounding cytoplasm. They are strongly **periodic acid–Schiff (PAS)-positive and diastase-resistant**
Clinical features	• α_1-Antitrypsin deficiency leads to the development of **pulmonary emphysema**, because the activity of destructive proteases is not inhibited. With low levels of serum α1-antitrypsin, elastic tissue destruction is unchecked and emphysema results. It also causes **liver disease**, as a consequence of the accumulation of this protein in hepatocytes. In addition, **cutaneous panniculitis, arterial aneurysm, bronchiectasis, pancreatitis, and Wegener's granulomatosis** can occur in α_1-Antitrypsin deficiency. α_1-antitrypsin (α-AT) is an important cause of the *early onset of severe panacinar pulmonary emphysema in adults in the 3rd and 4th decades of life and an important cause of liver disease in children; it rarely causes lung disease in children.* **Smoking** greatly increases the risk of emphysema developing in mutant Pi types. In a minority of patients AAT deficiency appears initially as **neonatal cholestasis** • Finally, risk of **hepatocellular carcinoma** is significantly increased in patients with cirrhosis due to AAT deficiency
Laboratory findings	Serum immunoassay measures low levels of α_1-antitrypsin; normal serum levels are **180–280 mg/dL.**
Treatment	Treatment of α_1AT is nonspecific and supportive. Liver transplantation is curative. Recombinant AT administered IV has been used in patients with chronic lung disease due to 1AT deficiency but is of no benefit in patients with α_1AT liver disease.

Obstetrics & Gynecology

13

AIIMS NOVEMBER 2018

1. A pregnant woman suffering from RHD with prosthetic valve. When would you switch to heparin?

a. 32 weeks b. 36 weeks
c. 40 weeks d. At onset of labor

2. Before ovulation development of granules in a cell is dependent on?

a. Estrogen b. Progesterone
c. FSH d. LH

3. Which of the following heart sound may be normal finding during pregnancy?

a. S_3 b. S_4
c. Wide fixed splitting of S_2 d. Pericardial knock

4. Investigation of choice for vesicovaginal fistula is?

a. IVP b. Cystoscopy
c. 3 swab test d. X-ray

5. What should be the time of termination of pregnancy of a female withinsulin dependent diabetes?

a. 34 weeks b. 37 weeks
c. 38 weeks d. 40 weeks

6. Sentinel lymph node biopsy is most useful in which of the following female genital cancers?

a. Endometrium b. Cervix
c. Vagina d. Vulva

7. Levonorgestrel dose for emergency contraception as per WHO recommendation is?

a. 1.5 mg within 72 hours b. 3 mg within 72 hours
c. 1.5 μg within 72 hours d. 3 μg within 72 hours

8. All of the following are reversible long acting contraceptives EXCEPT:

a. Copper T b. Laparoscopic tubal ligation
c. LNG- IUS d. Implanon

9. Young female with history of spontaneous abortion and secondary amenorrhea since then. FSH 6 mIU/mL. What is the most probable cause of amenorrhea?

a. Ovarian failure b. Pituitary failure
c. Fresh pregnancy d. Uterine synechiae

10. In case of transformation of molar pregnancy to choriocarcinoma all of the following are associated EXCEPT: ***(AIIMS Nov 2018, AIPG 2010)***

a. High hCG levels b. Theca lutein cysts
c. Enlarged uterus d. Suburethral nodule

11. A 40-year-old female was diagnosed with CIN-III on PAP smear. What will be the management?

a. Conization
b. Colposcopy + LEEP
c. Hysterectomy
d. Trachelectomy

12. A 55-year-old postmenopausal lady comes with simple endometrial hyperplasia with atypia. What is the best management of this case?

a. Hysterectomy b. Mirena
c. Progestin d. Estrogen

13. Which of the following has to monitored in the fetus of a mother taking lithium?

a. Cardiac b. Urogenital
c. NTD d. Facial

14. Which of the following is not in quadruple test for antenatal detection of Down syndrome?

a. AFP b. β-hCG
c. Estradiol d. Inhibin B

15. Placenta grade 3, 35 + 3 weeks pregnancy and absent end diastolic flow in Doppler; next management is?

a. Dexamethasone and terminate after 48 hours
b. Terminate after 37 weeks
c. Talk with pediatrician and termination
d. Monitor and do nothing

16. Active management of third stage of labor includes all EXCEPT:

a. Ergometrine after anterior shoulder delivery
b. Uterine massage
c. Cord traction
d. Oxytocin infusion

AIIMS MAY 2018

17. A 76-year-old female comes with nonhealing ulcer of left labia measuring approximately 2 × 3 cm. There is no palpable inguinal lymphadenopathy. Histopathology shows squamous cell carcinoma. What is the most ideal management of this case?

a. Simple vulvectomy
b. Radical vulvectomy with unilateral lymph node dissection
c. Radical vulvectomy with bilateral lymph node dissection
d. Chemoradiation followed by tailored surgery

18. A term woman presents with nonprogress of labor for 15 hours and posted for C-Section. Which is the correct position of patient to be put up on operation table by nurse?

a. Prone Trendelenburg with legs in Stirrup
b. Supine with wedge under right hip
c. Semi Fowler
d. Supine position

19. While performing the Burch operation there was significant bleeding and pooling of blood in the space of Retzius. The source of bleeding cannot be visualized. What is the next step in management?

a. Call vascular surgeon
b. Give a generalized suture in the bleeding area
c. Lift endopelvic fascia by putting fingers in vagina
d. Placing surgical drain

20. Following are the features of the color of normal amniotic fluid during delivery.

a. Milky to yellowish green with mucus flakes
b. Amber colored
c. Clear colorless to pale yellow
d. Golden color

21. Identify the anomaly based on the picture below?

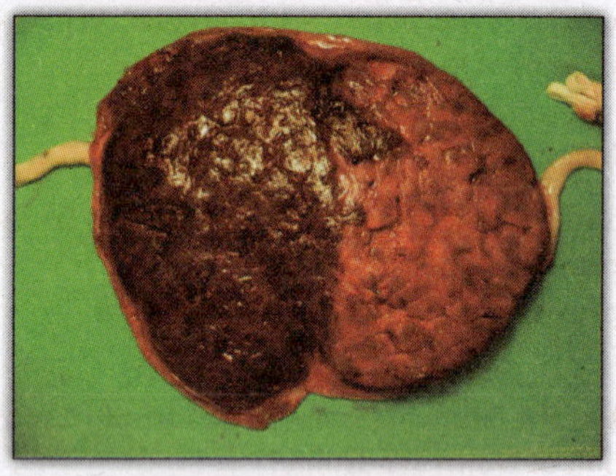

a. Twin-twin transfusion syndrome
b. Monochorionic diamniotic pregnancy
c. Monochorionic monoamniotic pregnancy
d. Dichorionic diamniotic pregnancy

22. A 25-year-old female having a 2-year-old child was started on Mala N for contraception. After the end of first strip, there was no withdrawal bleeding. What should be done?

a. Start next cycle of tablets from 5th day
b. Start next cycle from next day
c. Take two pills after 12 hours
d. Ask her to use another method of contraception
e. Urgent visit to hospital and check for pregnancy

23. Identify the test done in the picture given below?

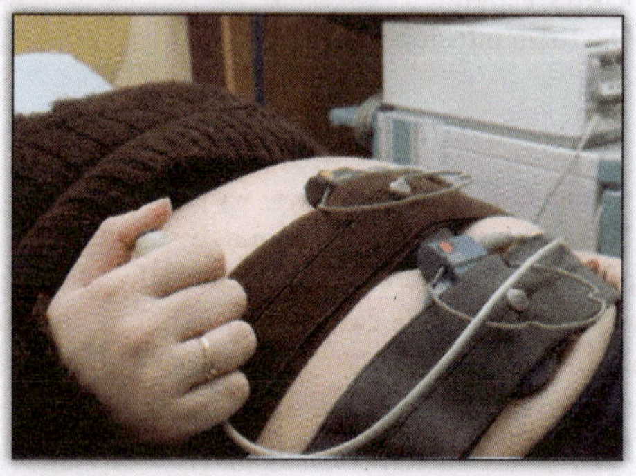

a. Non stress test
b. Amniocentesis
c. Amniotic fluid index
d. MCA Doppler

24. Identify the instrument shown below?

(AIIMS MAY 2018, Nov 2017)

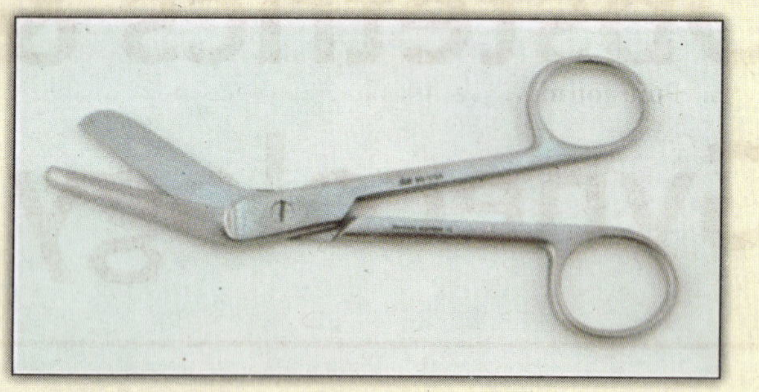

a. Mayo scissor
b. Episiotomy scissor
c. Suture remover
d. Curved scissors

25. All of the following are used testing lung maturity EXCEPT:

a. Blue cells in Nile blue test
b. Lecithin/Sphingomyelin ratio >2
c. Positive shake test
d. Elevated Phosphatidylglycerol

26. A woman is treated withinduced ovulation. Her ovary shows 8 follicles and estradiol level 800 pg/mL. What is to be done next?

a. Give cabergoline
b. Cancel cycle
c. Withhold HCG
d. Retrieve follicles

27. Women with history of double valve replacement 2 years back and history of Warfarin embryopathy in previous 2 pregnancies. Now she is 6 weeks pregnant. Course management in this pregnancy will be?

a. Warfarin should be replaced by heparin in 1 trimester
b. Start low molecular weight heparin
c. Heparin throughout the pregnancy
d. Use direct thrombin inhibitors

28. Craniopagus twins are attached by?

a. Head
b. Thorax
c. Head and legs
d. Head and Pelvis

29. A patient with G3 P2 L0 with previous history recurrent abortions in 2nd trimester, comes for preconception counseling. What will be the best next step?

a. Karyotyping
b. Hysteroscopy
c. Ultrasonography
d. Transvaginal sonography

30. A G3P2L0 woman with history of recurrent premature abortions at 30 and 32 weeks now comes with 9 weeks pregnancy. She has a history of conization one year back currently on follow up with no recurrence on PAP smear. What is the next step in management?

a. USG to see cervical length
b. Cervical Donald cerclage
c. Complete bed rest
d. Abdominal cerclage

31. Which of the following is absolute contraindication of CuT?

a. Previous history of Ectopic pregnancy
b. Anemia
c. Menorrhagia
d. Unmotivated person

32. **A 13-year-old girl comes with amenorrhea. On hysteroscopy uterus was present but Ovaries are absent. Lab reports shows raised FSH and reduced or nil estradiol. Karyotyping showed 46 XY. Most likely diagnosis is?**
   a. Pure gonadal dysgenesis b. Androgen insensitivity
   c. MRKH Syndrome d. Kallmann syndrome

33. **In postmenopausal women, indication for endometrial curettage is Endometrial thickness greater than?**
   a. 3 mm b. 5 mm
   c. 7 mm d. 8 mm

34. **The presence of fibronectin in cervical discharge at 34 weeks indicates?**
   a. Preterm labor b. Precipitate labor
   c. IUGR d. IUD

35. **A pregnant female delivered a baby with normal expulsion of intact placenta. After half an hour she started bleeding per vaginally. On examination, she was hypotensive and a boggy mass was palpated per abdomen. USG showed retained placental tissue. What is the likely diagnosis?** ***(AIIMS May 2018, 2016)***
   a. Placenta succenturiata b. Adenomyosis
   c. Placenta accreta d. Membranous placenta

36. **A 25-year-old with submucosal fibroid was undergoing myomectomy. The surgeon was using 1.5% glycine as irrigating fluid for the cavity. During the surgery the nurse informs the surgeon that there is 500 mL fluid deficit. What is the next step to be done?**
   a. Stop the surgery
   b. Change the fluid to normal saline
   c. Continue the surgery with careful monitoring of fluid status
   d. Give furosemide to the patient and continue the surgery

37. **Which of the following is the best parameter to assess in case of male infertility?** ***(AIIMS May 2018, 2017)***
   a. The number of sperm b. The morphology of sperms
   c. Motility of sperms d. Quantity of semen

AIIMS NOVEMBER 2017

38. **In confirmed case of Down's syndrome, what will be finding in 2nd trimester in triple test?**
   a. Low MSAFP, Low UE3 low, Low beta hCG
   b. Low MSAFP, Low UE3 and High beta hCG
   c. High MSAFP, High UE3 and Low beta hCG
   d. High MSAFP, Low UE3 and High beta hCG high

39. **A pregnant lady who is Nurse by profession needs how much extra calories in first trimester of pregnancy?**
   a. 300 kcal b. 500 kcal
   c. 600 kcal d. No extra calories

40. **A Multigravida with cervical dilation 6 cm and contraction every 10 min last for 20 sec. Which stage of labor she is in?**
   a. 1st stage b. 2nd stage
   c. 3rd stage d. 4th stage

41. **First reading on partogram should be placed at?**
   a. Left side of the action line
   b. Right side of the action line
   c. Left side of the alert line
   d. Right side of the alert line

42. **According to Naegele's rule, calculate EDD of a patient with LMP 9 January 2017.**
   a. 16/09/2017 b. 16/10/2017
   c. 16/11/2017 d. 9/10/2017

43. **An 18-year-old female presents with an ovarian mass, her serum biomarker are found to be normal except LDH, which is found to be elevated. The most likely diagnosis is?**
   a. Dysgerminoma
   b. Endodermal sinus tumor
   c. Malignant teratoma
   d. Mucinous cystadenocarcinoma

44. **For effective protection after unprotected intercourse one single tab of levonorgestrel 0.75 mg has already been taken, when is next dose to be taken?**
   a. 1 tab after 24 hours b. 1 tab after 12 hours
   c. 2 tab after 12 hours d. 2 tab after 24 hours

45. **Nonavalent HPV vaccine protects against which subtypes of HPV viruses?**
   a. 6, 11, 16, 18, 31, 33, 45, 48 and 52
   b. 6, 11, 16, 18, 31, 33, 45, 52 and 58
   c. 6, 11, 16, 18, 33, 45, 48, 52 and 58
   d. 6, 11, 16, 18, 33, 38, 45, 52 and 58

46. **A 60-year-old postmenopausal woman presents with history of bleeding PV. Biopsy showed Endometrial hyperplasia with atypia. Next line of management is?**
   a. Mirena b. Type 1 hysterectomy
   c. Oral progestins d. Dilatation and Curettage

47. **Drug of choice for gonococcal as well as nongonococcal mucopurulent cervicitis and urethritis is?**
   a. Cefixime 400 mg single oral dose
   b. Ceftriaxone 250 mg IM single dose
   c. Azithromycin 2 g oral single dose
   d. Ciprofloxacin 500 mg single oral dose

48. **A 26-year-old pregnant lady is diagnosed to have Hypertension during her pregnancy. How would you say that Hypertension is systemic hypertension and not pregnancy induced hypertension?**
   a. Hypertensive retinopathy
   b. Hypertension at 10 weeks of pregnancy
   c. Episode of seizure
   d. Proteinuria

49. **A 35-year-old female comes with history of postcoital bleed. What to do next?**
   a. PAP smear
   b. Hysteroscopy and then take biopsy
   c. Four quadrant biopsy
   d. Conisation
   e. Cryotherapy

50. **A couple with 2 children who are not able to conceive for over a year now present to OPD. Male partner is diagnosed to be having hypogonadotropic hypogonadism. Which of the following is not true?**
   a. Low LH and Low FSH b. Low testosterone
   c. Oligospermia d. High prolactin levels

51. **A 27-year-old female comes with history of infertility and she is being treated with Bromocriptine. What is disease she could be suffering from?**
   a. Hypogonadotropic hypogonadism
   b. Hyperprolactinemia
   c. Polycystic ovarian disease
   d. Pelvic Inflammatory disease

52. **An 18-year-old female with primary amenorrhea, infantile uterus and genotype 45XO/46XX comes to you. How you will treat her?**
   a. Bilateral gonadectomy
   b. Hormone replacement therapy
   c. Remove the clitoris
   d. Vulvoplasty

53. **Identify the name of meneuver shown in the picture?** ***(AIIMS May 2018, Nov 2017)***

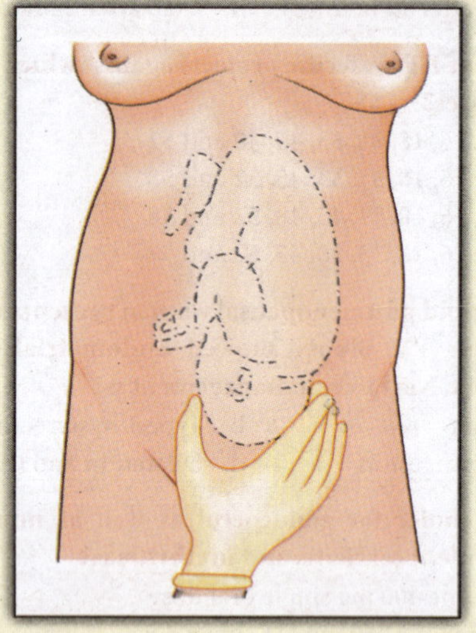

   a. Pelvic grip b. Pawlick's grip
   c. Fundal grip d. Lateral grip

54. **Identify the instrument shown below?** ***(AIIMS May 2018, Nov 2017)***

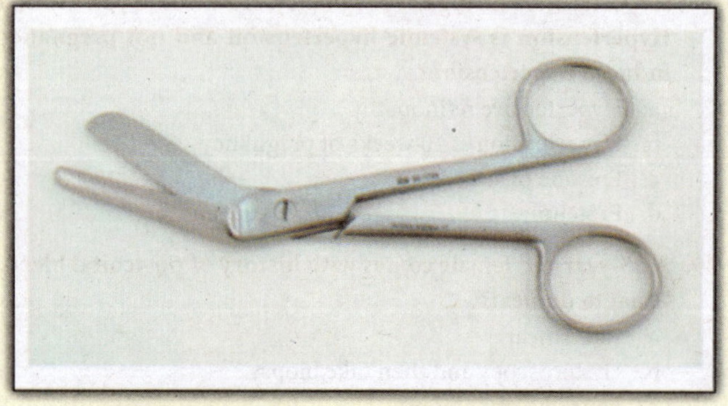

   a. Mayo scissor b. Episiotomy scissor
   c. Suture remover d. Curved scissors

AIIMS MAY 2017

55. **A woman withinfertility and bilateral cornual block on HSG. Best management?** ***(AIIMS May 2017, Nov 2011)***
   a. Tuboplasty b. IVF
   c. Hydrotubation d. Hysteroscopy and laparoscopy

56. **A 59-year-old female with history of ovarian carcinoma in the mother achieved menopause with smooth transition. She is on hormone replacement therapy. She developed abdominal pain and the right adnexal mass was palpable, non tender. On routine examination she has a 3 × 3 cm smooth cyst in her ovary. Which is the next step?**
   a. Do CA-125 levels, if normal advise regular check up
   b. Confirm USG findings by ordering CT scan
   c. Do an exploratory laparoscopy to visualize the nature of cyst
   d. Reassure and advise regular follow-up once in 6 months

57. **Which of the following fits into the criteria of severe variable deceleration, variations less than?**
   a. 70 beats per minute lasting for 60 seconds
   b. 80 beats per minute lasting for 60 seconds
   c. 90 beats per minute lasting for 60 seconds
   d. 100 beats per minute lasting for 60 seconds

58. **A 28-year-old female nearing her date has been admitted following regular contractions. The resident doctor did an examination and told the intern that the head is at +1 station. What is the exact position of head?**
   a. High up in the false pelvis
   b. Just above ischial spine
   c. Just below ischial spine
   d. At the perineum

59. **Which of the following is the best parameter to assess in case of male infertility?** ***(AIIMS May 2018, 2017)***
   a. The number of sperm b. The morphology of sperms
   c. Motility of sperms d. Quantity of semen

60. **A patient close to her due date and she experienced uterine contractions and was admitted in the hospital for observation. The resident was instructed to plot the partogram regularly. From what cm of cervical dilatation is partogram plotted in regular intervals?**
   a. 4 cm b. 5 cm
   c. 6 cm d. 8 cm

61. **A patient came to OPD with a twin pregnancy. She already had 2 first trimester abortion and she has a 3-year-old female child who was born at the end of ninth month of gestation. Which of the following is her accurate representation? G = gravid, P = para**
   a. G4P1 1+2+1 b. G5P1 2+0+1
   c. G4P1 0+1+2 d. G5P0 1+0+2

62. **Ureteric injury is most commonly associated with which of the following?**
   a. Anterior colporrhaphy b. Vaginal hysterectomy
   c. Wertheim hysterectomy d. Abdominal hysterectomy

63. **A 23-year-old female came with complaints of 4 months amenorrhea. The FSH and LH were elevated above the normal value, thyroid function test were normal. Which is the next step in management?**
   a. Give progesterone and stop after 10 days for withdrawal bleeding
   b. Check USG for polycystic ovaries
   c. Estimate serum estradiol values
   d. Do a urine pregnancy test

64. A pregnant lady was admitted for pregnancy induced hypertension for monitoring and bed rest. In supine position which of the following is a complication of the below representation?

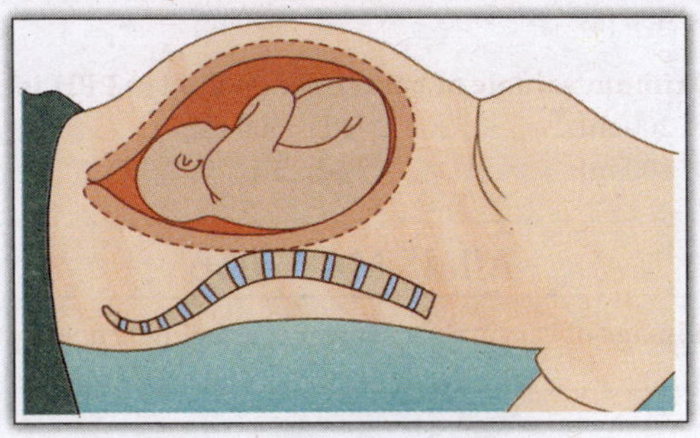

a. Abdominal aorta syndrome
b. Supine vena cava syndrome
c. Superior vena cava syndrome
d. Ascending aorta syndrome

65. Which of the following is a WHO guideline in second stage of labor?

a. Perform labor in lithotomy position
b. Give warm compress to the perineum
c. Manual support to perineum with deflexion of head
d. Do a routine episiotomy

66. Rh negative mother, ICT negative was given Anti D during 28 weeks of pregnancy. Which of the following is the ideal one?

a. Give another dose of Anti D 72 hours postpartum depending on the baby's blood group
b. Give another dose of Anti D 72 hours postpartum irrespective of baby blood group
c. No need additional dose since she is ICT negative
d. All of the above

67. A 32-year-old female came for routine PAP smear testing. The report came as carcinoma in situ. What is the next step?

a. Colposcopy and biopsy
b. Conization
c. Hysterectomy
d. HPV DNA testing

68. Drug of choice for strawberry vagina is?

a. Metronidazole b. Tetracycline
c. Doxycycline d. Fluconazole

69. Endometriotic lesion is due to which hormone effect?

a. High estrogen b. High progesterone
c. High cholesterol d. High levels of prolactin

AIIMS NOVEMBER 2016

70. An 18-year-old female presents with primary amenorrhea, with normal breast development and absent pubic hairs. On PV examination the vagina is normally developed but there is clitoromegaly. On USG gonads are visible in the inguinal canal. What is most likely diagnosis?

a. Gonadal dysgenesis
b. Partial androgen insensitivity
c. Complete androgen insensitivity
d. Mayer Rokitansky Kuster Hauser syndrome

71. A 30-year-old lady, G3P2 with 10 weeks intrauterine gestation comes to OPD with an IUCD and the tail of the IUCD is noted to be protruding from the cervical OS. The most appropriate course of action is?

(AIIMS Nov. 2016, May 2016)

a. Keep the IUCD in place and continue prophylactic antibiotics in place
b. Keep the IUCD in place without any treatment
c. Terminate the pregnancy because of high risk of infection
d. Remove the IUCD immediately and continue pregnancy

72. Which of the following is the drug of choice for precocious puberty in girls?

a. GnRH analog
b. Danazol
c. Medroxyprogesterone acetate
d. OCP e. Cyproterone acetate

73. All of the following are true regarding partogram EXCEPT:

a. Right side of alert line indicates immediate referral to FRU
b. Alert and action line are separated by a difference of 4 hours
c. Each small square in partogram is equal 1 hour
d. Partograph recording should be started once the cervical dilatation reaches 4 cm

74. Graphic evaluation of a labor is depicted below. What does the curve marked as C represent?

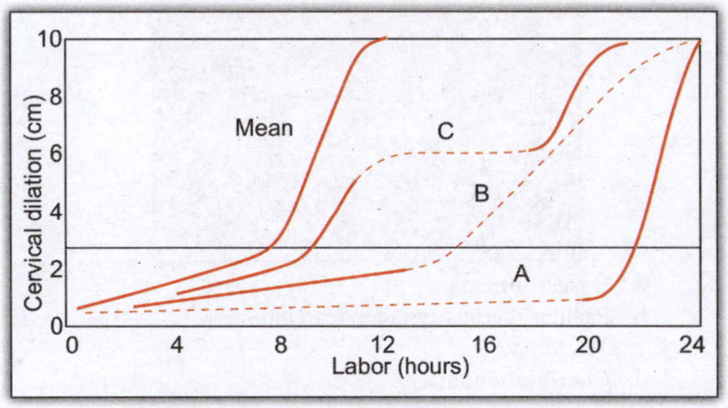

a. Normal labor in primigravida
b. Prolonged active phase of labor
c. Secondary arrest after progression of labor
d. Prolonged latent phase of labor

75. A 38 weeks primigravida presented with pain abdomen and mild uterine contractions. On examination the cervix is 2 cm dilated and 50% effaced. Heart rate of the patient is 86/min and Blood pressure is 126/76 mm Hg. What should next step?

a. Sedation
b. Observation
c. Induce labor by ARM
d. Give oxytocin to augment labor

76. For lung maturation in preterm delivery Inj betamethasone is given. Which of the following statement is correct?

a. Single dose of inj Betamethasone 24 mg
b. Inj Betamethasone 6 mg, 4 doses 12 hours apart
c. Inj Betamethasone 12 mg, 2 doses 12 hours apart
d. Inj Betamethasone 12 mg, 2 doses 24 hours apart

77. Which of the following statement is not correct regarding cervical cancer screening program guidelines as per WHO?

a. In female more than 65 years of age visual inspection of cervix is done as transformational zone is clearly visible
b. HPV test is done every 5 yearly in women aged between 30 to 49 years
c. PAP smear should be repeated yearly in women of reproductive age group
d. PAP smear can be repeated less frequently if it comes out negative for 3 consecutive years

78. First trimester screening test for Down's syndrome is?

a. AFP, PAPP-A b. Beta hCG, PAPP-A
c. Inhibin, PAPP-A d. Estradiol, PAPP-A

79. A 35-year-old female presents with adnexal mass. CA 125 and LDH raised and CA 19-9 normal. Tumor was resected with the gross and HPE image given below. What is the diagnosis?

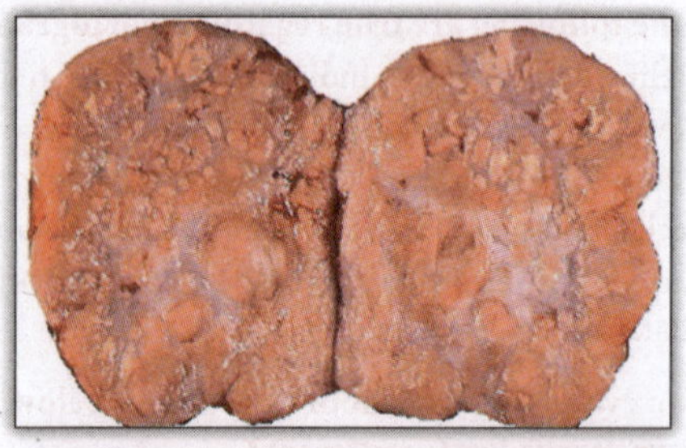

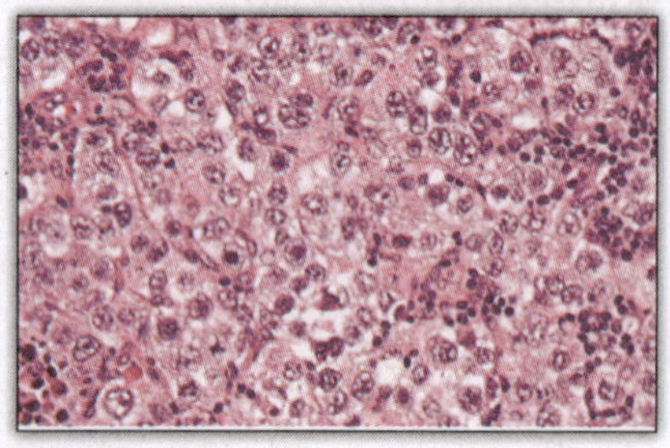

a. Dysgerminoma
b. Papillary serous cystadenocarcinoma
c. Teratoma
d. Choriocarcinoma

80. A 24-year-old female presents with right adnexal mass. Patient underwent laparotomy. The excised specimen picture is given below. Most likely diagnosis is?

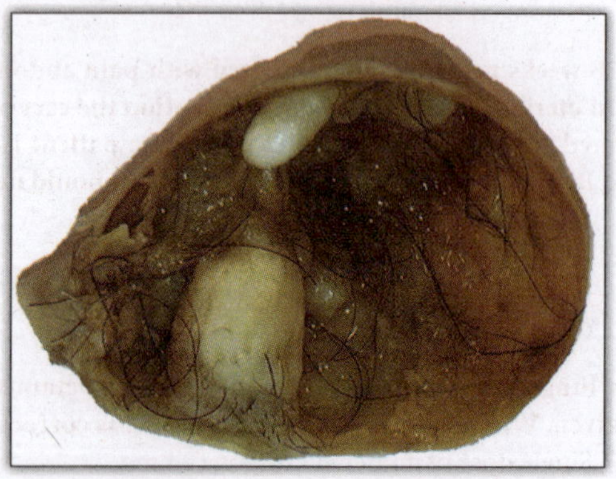

a. Mature teratoma b. Dysgerminoma
c. Granulosa cell tumor d. Mucinous cystadenoma

81. WHO recommendation of dose of Misoprostol for prevention of PPH is?

a. 200 μg b. 400 μg
c. 600 μg d. 800 μg

82. Maximum volume of bakri balloon used in PPH is?

a. 200 mL b. 500 mL
c. 800 mL d. 1 L

AIIMS MAY 2016

83. An image of cervical Pap smear is as below. The diagnosis is?

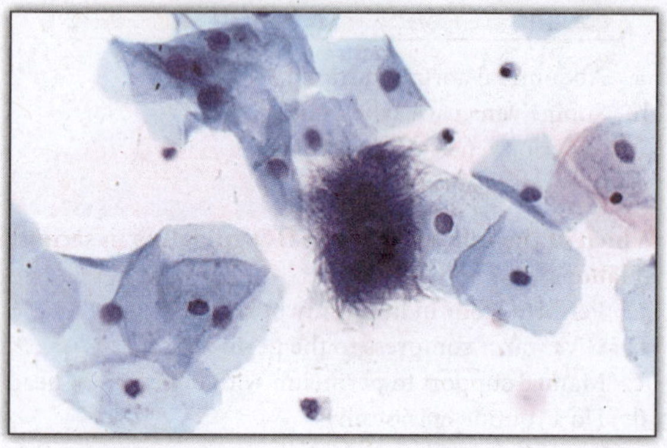

a. Actinomyces b. Candida
c. Trichomonas d. Herpes simplex type 2

84. At full term pregnancy all of the following parameters are raised EXCEPT:

a. Blood volume
b. Minute ventilation
c. Glomerular filtration rate
d. Cardiac output

85. A 25-year-old female visits OPD for infertility treatment. During evaluation, hysteroscopy was done and was diagnosed to have Asherman syndrome. Which of the following symptom the patient is most likely to have?

(AIIMS May 2016, Nov. 2015)

a. Dysmenorrhea b. Menorrhagia
c. Hypomenorrhea d. Oligomenorrhea

86. A 26-year-old female presents in OPD for dull aching lower abdomen pain. She had previous two normal vaginal deliveries. Her LMP was 3 weeks ago. On P/V examination a cystic mass was felt in the left fornix region, which on USG was found to be a left clear ovarian cyst of 5 cm. Which of the following is recommended for this patient?

a. Review after 2–3 months for ovarian cyst
b. CA 125
c. CT scan pelvis
d. Diagnostic laparoscopy

87. A 39-year-old female para 2, complains of severe progressive secondary dysmenorrhea. Pelvic examination revealed a tender diffuse enlarged uterus with no adnexal tenderness. Endometrium biopsy came normal. The diagnosis is:

a. Adenomyosis
b. Endometriosis
c. Endometritis
d. Leiomyoma

88. **The instrument shown in the picture is commonly used for?**

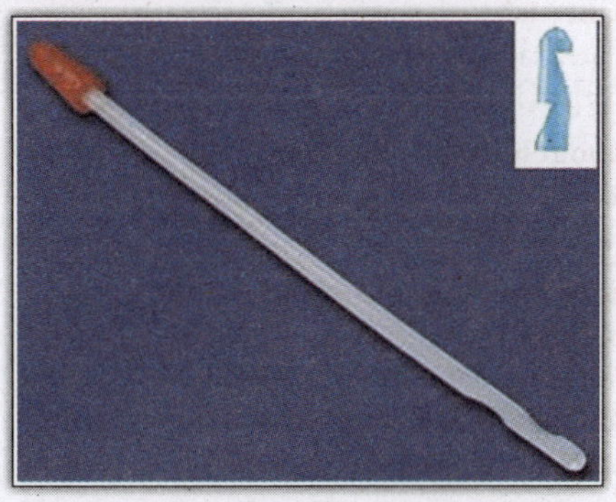

a. Endometrial curettage b. Fractional curettage
c. Endometrial biopsy
d. Instillation of dye in hysterosalpingoscopy

89. **A pregnant female delivered a baby with normal expulsion of intact placenta. After half an hour she started bleeding per vaginally. On examination, she was hypotensive and a boggy mass was palpated per abdomen. USG showed retained placental tissue. What is the likely diagnosis?**
(AIIMS May 2018, 2016)

a. Placenta succenturiata b. Adenomyosis
c. Placenta accreta d. Membranous placenta

90. **A mother brings her 19-year-old daughter to OPD with complaints of menarche not attained. On examination breast and pubic hair development is normal but with a blind vagina and uterus not felt. The most likely diagnosis is?**

a. XXY syndrome b. Mullerian agenesis
c. Gonadal dysgenesis d. Turner syndrome

91. **A 30-year-old lady, G3P2 with 10 weeks intrauterine gestation comes to OPD with an IUCD and the tail of the IUCD is noted to be protruding from the cervical OS. The most appropriate course of action is?**
(AIIMS Nov. 2016, May 2016)

a. Keep the IUCD in place and continue prophylactic antibiotics in place
b. Keep the IUCD in place without any treatment
c. Terminate the pregnancy because of high risk of infection
d. Remove the IUCD immediately and continue pregnancy

92. **A primigravida with 40 + 5 weeks was admitted in the labor room for induction. On per vaginal examination it was found cervix with 1 cm dilatation, 30% effaced and station at Vx -1, cervix is soft posterior. Bishop score is?**

a. 3 b. 5
c. 8 d. 0

93. **A primipara is in labor and episiotomy is about to be cut. Compared to median the advantage of mediolateral episiotomy is?**

a. Ease to repair b. Fewer breakdowns
c. Less extension of lesion d. Less blood loss

94. **A 28-year-old with G2A1 presents in OPD with 8 weeks gestation. She is a diabetic and says her blood sugar is under control. Which of the following is the most common birth defect associated with diabetes?**

a. Anencephaly b. Sacral agenesis
c. VSD d. Meningomyelocele

95. **A 30-year-old primigravida came to OPD with complaints of bleeding per vaginm associated with pain. On examination abdomen is soft and non-tender. Palpation-uterus is enlarged 12 weeks size, soft non-tender and no cervical excitation. The USG is as shown below. The most probable diagnosis is?**

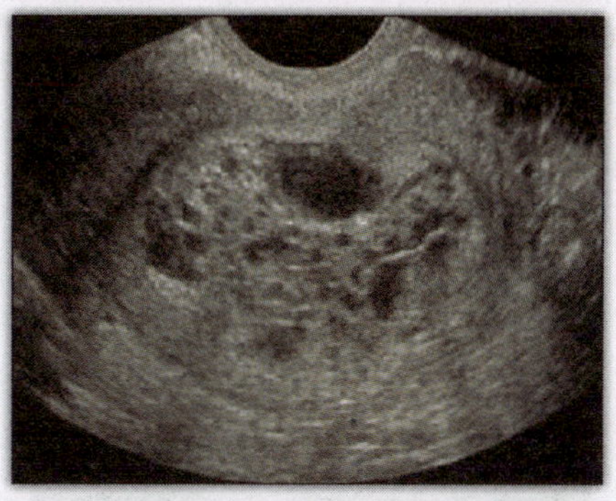

a. Hydatidiform mole b. Missed abortion
c. Blighted ovum d. Ectopic pregnancy

96. **An infertile couple comes to OPD with a normal HSG report and semen analysis showing azoospermia. Which of the following is used as diagnostic test to differentiate testicular failure from obstruction of vas deferens?**
(AIIMS May 2016, UPSC CMS 2004)

a. Estimation of FSH levels
b. Testicular FNAC c. Karyotyping
d. Testosterone levels in blood

AIIMS NOVEMBER 2015

97. **Following Fetal cardiotocograph indicates?**

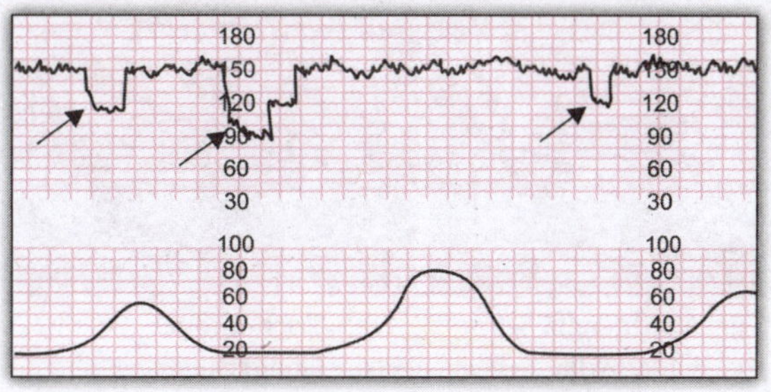

a. Cord compression b. Head compression
c. Uteroplacental insufficiency
d. Fetal distress

98. **Smallest anteroposterior diameter of pelvic inlet is?**

a. Anatomical conjugate b. Diagonal conjugate
c. Obstetrics conjugate d. Transverse diameter

99. **Beaded appearance of fallopian tubes and clubbing of fimbrial ends in an infertile woman in HSG is due to?**

a. Genital tuberculosis b. Endometrial polyp
c. Salpingitis isthmica nodosa
d. Asherman syndrome

100. **A 25-year-old female visits OPD for intertility treatment. During evaluation, hysteroscopy was done and was diagnosed to have Asherman syndrome. Which of the following symptom the patient is most likely to have?**
(AIIMS May 2016, Nov. 2015)

a. Dysmenorrhea b. Menorrhagia
c. Hypomenorrhea d. Oligomenorrhea

101. Modified biophysical profile includes?
- a. NST + Fetal tone
- b. NST + Amniotic fluid index
- c. NST + Fetal movement count
- d. NST + Fetal breathing movements

102. Identify the pathology shown in the following picture on laparoscopic examination?

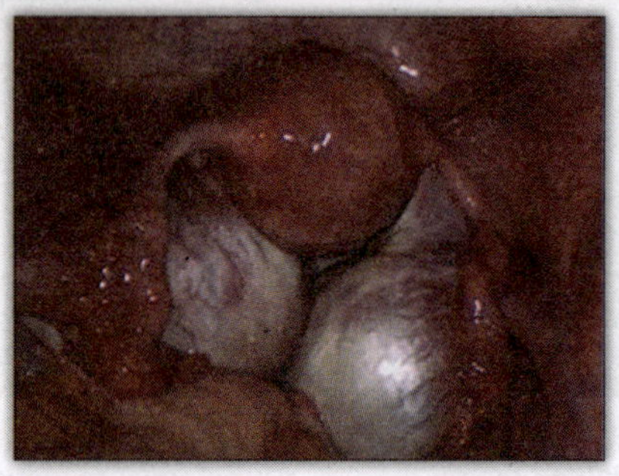

- a. Krukenberg tumor
- b. Endometrioma
- c. Dermoid cyst
- d. Serous cystadenoma

103. Appropriate treatment for fertility in a patient with Swyer syndrome is?
- a. IVF with donor oocyte
- b. IVF with surrogacy
- c. Androgen supplementation
- d. Gonadectomy

104. A 25-year-old female complaints of itching in genital area and vaginal discharge. Cervical smear shows the following picture. Identify the organism?

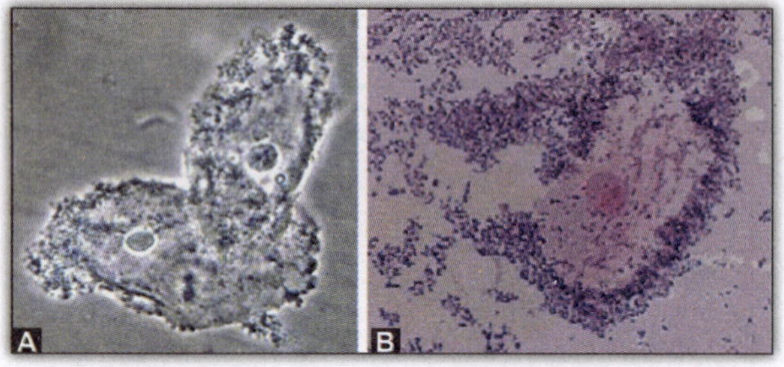

- a. Gardnerella
- b. Trichomonas
- c. Chlamydia
- d. Gonorrhea

105. Prophylaxis of folic acid taken by women on anticonvulsants?
- a. Any woman who can potentially be pregnant
- b. 3 months before planning pregnancy
- c. At confirmation of pregnancy
- d. After delivery

106. Dose of misoprostol for emergent management of PPH is?
- a. 400 mcg
- b. 600 mcg
- c. 800 mcg
- d. 1000 mcg

107. Time of prophylaxis for Rh disease/anti D in pregnancy is?
- a. 12 weeks
- b. 24 weeks
- c. 28 weeks
- d. 36 weeks

108. In a G3P2 Pregnant woman at 18 weeks gestation, previous children born with thalassemia, what should be the screening method of choice?
- a. Cordocentesis
- b. Chorionic villous sampling
- c. Amniocentesis
- d. NIPT (noninvasive prenatal testing)

109. Source of estrogen and progesterone in first two months of pregnancy is?
- a. Maternal steroid
- b. Placenta
- c. Corpus luteum
- d. Theca externa

110. True about hormone level in menopause is?
- a. Serum LH >20 IU/L
- b. Serum FSH >40 IU/L
- c. Estradiol <20 IU/L
- d. Progesterone <40 IU/L

111. Levonorgestrel is not used for?
- a. Endometriosis
- b. Premenstrual tension
- c. Emergency contraception
- d. Atypical endometrial hyperplasia

112. Identify the pathology shown in hysterosalpingography picture below?

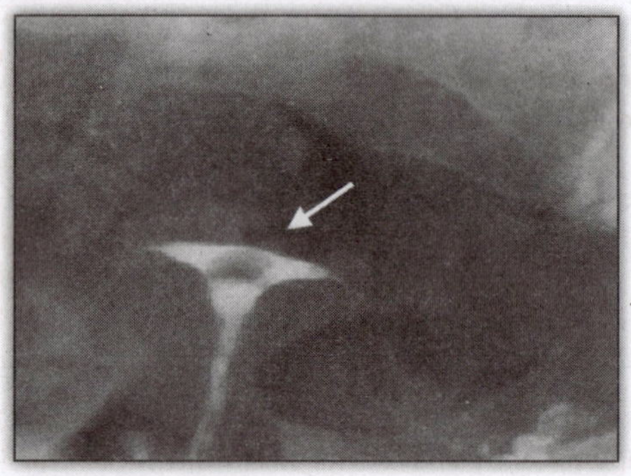

- a. Asherman syndrome
- b. Endometrial polyps
- c. Endometrial hyperplasia
- d. Intramural leiomyoma

113. Which of the following cannot be used as emergency contraceptive?
- a. IUCD
- b. Ulipristal acetate
- c. Levonorgestrel
- d. Desogestrel

114. Which of the following is drug of choice for pregnancy induced hypertension? ***(AIIMS Nov 2015, May 2015)***
- a. Atenolol
- b. α- methyldopa
- c. Enalapril
- d. Sodium nitroprusside

AIIMS MAY 2015

115. Which of the following is drug of choice for pregnancy induced hypertension? (AIIMS Nov. 2015, May 2015)
- a. Atenolol
- b. α- methyl dopa
- c. Enalapril
- d. Sodium Nitroprusside

116. Antihypertensive not used in pregnancy is? ***(AIIMS May 2015, 2014)***
- a. Enalapril
- b. Nifedipine
- c. Labetalol
- d. Hydralazine

117. A lady with abdominal mass was investigated. On surgery, she was found to have bilateral ovarian masses with smooth surface. On microscopy they revealed mucin secreting cells with signet ring shapes. Diagnosis?
- a. Dysgerminoma
- b. Krukenberg tumor
- c. Primary adenocarcinoma of the ovaries
- d. Dermoid cyst

118. According to the 2010 WHO criteria what are the characteristics of normal semen analysis?

a. Volume >1.5 mL, count >15 million/mL, Normal morphology >4% progressive motility >32%
b. Volume >2.0 mL, count >20 million/mL, Normal morphology >4% progressive motility >32%
c. Volume >1.5 mL, count >20 million/mL, Normal morphology >4% progressive motility >32%
d. Volume >2.0 mL, count >15 million/mL, Normal morphology >4% progressive motility >32%

119. Anticipated preterm delivery. Dose of dexamethasone given to mother is?

a. 12 mg 12 hourly 2 doses b. 12 mg 24 hourly 4 doses
c. 6 mg 24 hourly 2 doses d. 6 mg 12 hourly 4 doses

120. In a lady with history of birth of a previous child with neural tube defect, amount of folic acid to be given in microgram as secondary prophylaxis before next conception is?

a. 4 micrograms/day b. 40 micrograms/day
c. 400 micrograms/day d. 4000 micrograms/day

121. A lady underwent vaginal hysterectomy for Carcinoma cervix. Following the surgery after her urethral catheter was removed, she complained of urinary incontinence. On examination she had normal voiding as well as continuous incontinence. Methylene blue dye was instilled in her bladder through her urethra and she was given oral phenazopyridine dye. After some time her pad was checked and it showed yellow staining at the top portion, but not the middle or bottom. She is likely to have?

a. Ureterovaginal fistula b. Vesicovaginal fistula
c. Urethrovaginal fistula d. Vesicouterine fistula

122. What is the level of proteinuria to diagnose severe preeclampsia?

a. 20 mg b. 200 mg
c. 300 mg d. 3000 mg

123. Which of these is not a support of the uterus?

a. Urogenital diaphragm b. Pelvic diaphragm
c. Perineal body d. Rectovaginal septum

124. A 32-year-old P2 L2 lady comes 4 days/5 days after unprotected sexual intercourse. What will be your advice for contraception in this lady?

a. Levonorgestrel 0.75 mg
b. Copper IUD
c. 2 tablets of high dose OCP, repeated after 24 hours
d. Laparoscopic tubectomy

125. Carbetocin dose for PPH is?

a. 100 microgram IM b. 50 microgram IV
c. 150 microgram IV d. 200 mg

126. What are the cut off values in 2 hours OGTT for fasting and at 1 hour and 2 hours after meals respectively?

a. 92, 182, 155 b. 92, 180, 153
c. 95, 180, 155 d. 92, 180, 155

127. A G6+P0+L0 lady with history of recurrent missed abortions at 14-16 weeks comes to you with a missed abortion at 12 weeks. Which of the following tests is not warranted?

a. Lupus anticoagulant
b. Anticardiolipin AB
c. VRDL of father and mother
d. Fetal karyotype

128. A 10-year-old girl presents with a mass in lower abdomen involving umbilical and the hypogastrium. On examination it is cystic and mobile and the examiner is unable to insinuate fingers between the mass and the pelvic bone. What is the likely diagnosis?

a. Duplication of small intestine
b. Mesenteric cyst
c. Omental cyst
d. Ovarian cyst

129. A young lady with 6 weeks amenorrhea had nausea and vomiting with severe abdominal pain. Her BP was 100/80 mm Hg. Examination revealed a 5 × 5 cm adnexal mass. What is the plan of management?

a. Plan for immediate laparoscopic surgery
b. Send beta hCG
c. Methotrexate
d. Give IV fluids, keep NPO and observe for 4-5 days

130. A 16-year-old girl presented to the gynecology OPD with primary amenorrhea. On examination she was found to have Tanner's stage V breasts and no pubic and axillary hair and normal stature. She was prescribed OCP 2 years back for 6 months, but failed to produce menstrual bleeding. What is the likely diagnosis?

a. Androgen insensitivity
b. Turner's syndrome
c. Cryptomenorrhea
d. Mayer rokitansky kuster hauser syndrome

131. In Galactorrhea Amenorrhea syndrome, apart from serum prolactin, which other investigation should be advised?

a. TSH b. LH
c. hCG d. Urinary Ketosteroids

132. A 16-year-old girl came for evaluation of primary amenorrhea. She was having hirsutism, irregular bleeding and infertility, diagnosed as PCOS. Which of the following drugs should not be given? ***(AIIMS May 2015, Nov. 2013)***

a. Spironolactone b. Tamoxifen
c. OCPs d. Clomiphene citrate

ANSWERS WITH EXPLANATIONS

AIIMS NOVEMBER 2018

1. Ans. (b) 36 weeks

Ref: With text

Women with mechanical valve prosthesis must be anticoagulated and when not pregnant, warfarin is recommended. Although most effective to prevent mechanical valve thrombosis, warfarin is teratogenic and can cause miscarriage, stillbirths and fetal malformation. **The European Society of Cardiology favors warfarin anticoagulation until 36 weeks, at which time heparin is given until delivery.** Heparin is discontinued just before delivery. Anticoagulant therapy with warfarin or heparin may be restarted 6 hours following vaginal delivery (Ref: William's 24th ed page 2067)

The patient taking warfarin should discontinue it as soon as pregnancy is diagnosed and replace by heparin 5000 units twice daily subcutaneously up to **12th week**. This is then replaced by warfarin tablet 3 mg. daily to be taken at the same time each day and continued up to **36 weeks.** Thereafter it is replaced by heparin up to **7 days postpartum**. Warfarin is then to be continued. (Ref: Dutta 7th ed page 277)

American College of Chest Physicians Guidelines for Anticoagulation of Pregnant Women with Mechanical Prosthetic Valves

For pregnant women with mechanical heart valves, any one of the following anticoagulant regimens is recommended:

- Adjusted-dose *LMWH* twice daily throughout pregnancy. The doses should be adjusted to achieve the manufacturer's peak anti-Xa level 4 hours after subcutaneous injection.
- Adjusted-dose *UFH* administered every 12 hours throughout pregnancy. The doses should be adjusted to keep the midinterval aPTT at least twice control or attain an anti-Xa heparin level of 0.35 to 0.70 U/mL.
- LMWH or UFH as above until 13 weeks' gestation with warfarin substitution until close to delivery when LMWH or UFH is resumed.

In women judged to be at very high risk of thromboembolism and in whom concerns exist about the efficacy and safety of LMWH or UFH as dosed above—some examples include older generation prosthesis in the mitral position or history of thromboembolism. Warfarin is suggested throughout pregnancy with replacement by UFH or LMWH close to delivery (36wks). In addition, low-dose aspirin—75 to 100 mg daily—should be orally administered.

2. Ans. (a) Estrogen

Ref: William's 24th Ed Pg 82

During preovulation phase estrogen levels are highest.

Uterine Cycle or Menstrual Cycle

The Uterine Cycle or *menstrual cycle* is a repeating series of changes in the structure of the endometrium. The uterine cycle averages 28 days in length, but it can range from 21 to 35 days in healthy women of reproductive age. We can divide the Endometrial cycle into three phases

	From 1st to 4th day. Menstrual bleeding indicates end of one cycle and beginning of next cycle. On day 28 endometrium begins of degenerate due to withdrawal of hormonal support and menstruation starts. Two third of endometrial tissue is lost
Proliferative phase	From 5th to 14th day of menstrual cycle. Proliferative phase (estrogenic phase) *begins* with *regeneration* of the *endometrium* and lasts until ovulation. Endometrium stops growing but becomes more vascular and glandular due to the rising level of estrogens.
Luteal or Secretory phase	Secretory phase (progestogenic phase) begins with ovulation and ends with menstruation. From 15th to 28th day. Progesterone peaks on 21st day. Corpus luteum (CL) produces estrogen and progesterone, which prepare the endometrium for implantation

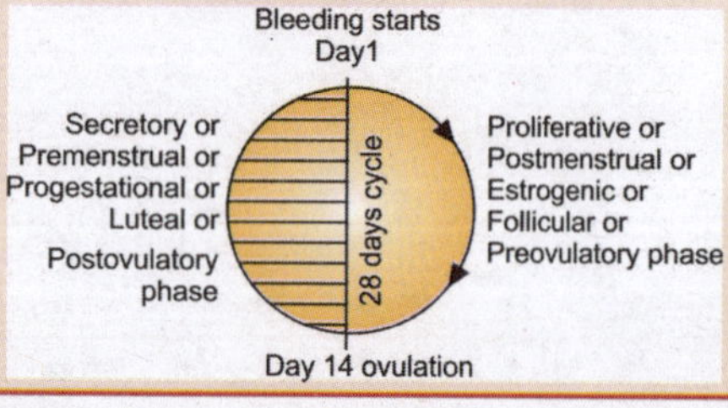

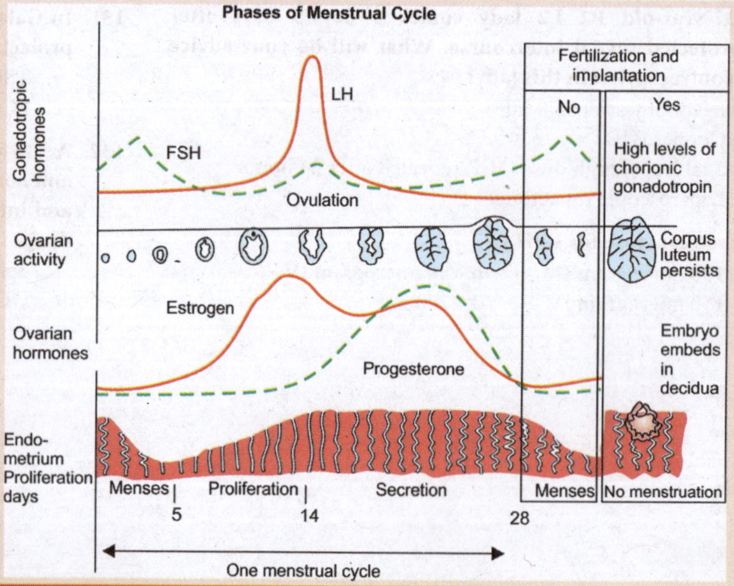

Contd...

Uterine Cycle or Menstrual Cycle
Footnote: 1. The endometrial surface is re-epithelialized within 4 to 7 days after the beginning of menstruation 2. Even during menses, increasing estrogen levels produced by the ovary begin the healing process and the endometrium begins to regenerate and prepare for the next cycle 3. Progesterone peaks on 21st day of menstrual cycle

3. Ans. (a) S_3

Ref: William's 24th ed page 136, Dutta's 8th Ed page 60

Many of the normal cardiac sounds are modified during pregnancy. Cutforth and MacDonald documented that:

- An exaggerated splitting of the first heart sound and increased loudness of both components
- No definite changes in the aortic and pulmonary elements of the second sound
- A loud, easily heard third sound.

In 90 percent of pregnant women, they also heard a systolic murmur that was intensified during inspiration in some or expiration in others and that disappeared shortly after delivery. A soft diastolic murmur was noted transiently in 20 percent and continuous murmurs arising from the breast vasculature in 10 percent.

4. Ans. (b) Cystoscopy

Ref: Shaw's 15th ed page 184- 186, ACOG vol 2 part 2 page 611, Novak's 14th ed page 886

See Table of "URINARY FISTULAS" in AIIMS MAY 2015 (OBG) (see page no. 909)

Vesicovaginal fistula: There is a communication between the bladder and the upper third of the anterior vaginal wall The site of fistula, size and relationship to bladder trigone are identified with cystoscopy. Hence, cystoscopy not only definitively identifies vesicovaginal fistula, but also gives its anatomical parameters

5. Ans. (c) 38 weeks

Ref: Dutta 8th Ed Pg 327, ACOG Practice Bulletin 190 Gestational Diabetes (February 2018)

- Dutta 8th Ed Pg 327 says:

"Elective delivery (induction or Caesarean section) is considered in patients requiring insulin or with complications (macrosomia) at around 38 weeks."

NOTE

That the time of termination for gestational diabetes mellitus is 39 weeks.

Gestational Diabetes ACOG 2018 Guidelines – Termination of Pregnancy

Status	Termination
Controlled on diet	≥39 weeks Expectant management up to 40 weeks 6 days is appropriate with antepartum testing
Well controlled on medication	Deliver at 39 weeks 0 days to 39 weeks 6 days
Poorly controlled	Expert guidance supports earlier delivery but data lacking regarding precise timing • Delivery between 37 weeks 0 days and 38 weeks 6 days may be justified • Delivery between 34 weeks 0 days and 36 weeks 6 days reserved for (1) failure of in-hospital glycemic control or (2) abnormal fetal testing
Estimated fetal weight ≥4500	Counsel regarding risks and benefits of a scheduled cesarean section

6. Ans. (d) Vulva

Ref: Novak 14th ed page 1562-1563

Sentinel lymph node detection has become an integral part of the management strategy for breast cancer and melanoma. **Studies have suggested that the sentinel lymph nodes can be identified in most cases of Vulva carcinoma.**

7. Ans. (a) 1.5 mg within 72 hours

Ref: Shaw 15th ed page 237, https://www.who.int/news-room/fact-sheets/detail/emergency-contraception

WHO recommends emergency Contraceptive Pills (ECPs) with LNG taken as a single dose of 1.5 mg, or alternatively, LNG taken in 2 doses of 0.75 mg each, 12 hours apart.

Postcoital/Emergency Contraceptives
Also called Postcoital or Morning after pills. It prevents pregnancy by interfering with postovulatory events and are therefore known as interceptions. Oral pills are recommended within 72 hours of unprotected intercourse.

Contd...

Indications:
- Unprotected intercourse
- Condom rupture
- Sexual assault
- Missed pills
- Misplaced IUCD

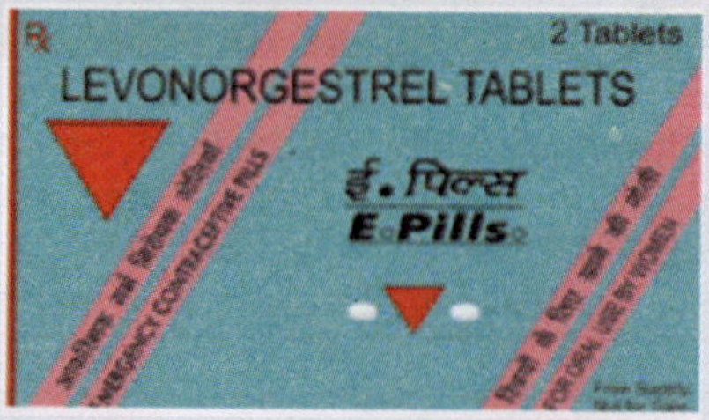

Drug	Dose	Pregnancy rate (%)
1. * **Levonorgestrel (Plan B)**	0.75 mg stat and after 12 hours Or 1.5 mg (2 Tab. stat dose)	0-1
2. * **Ethinyl estradiol 50 µg + Levonorgestrel 0.25 mg** (Yuzpe regimen/ method or OCPs method)	2 tab stat (100 µg of ethinyl estradiol plus 0.50 mg of LNG) and 2 after 12 hours	0–2
3. **Ethinyl estradiol** (Estrogen high dose), Now replaced by LNG	2.5 mg BD × 5 days	0–0.6
4. **Mifepristone (RU-486)** (Effective up to 49 days of LMP)	100 mg single dose	0-0.6
5. **Copper IUDs Insertion** (Gold standard but now not recommended)	Within 5 days	0-0.1
6. * **Ulipristal acetate** (synthetic progesterone hormone receptor modular, attaches to progesterone receptor and prevents/delays ovulation and suppresses endometrium, prevents implantation)	A 30 mg tablet should be taken within 5 days	0-1

Footnote:
1. **Plan B** contains 0.75 mg LNG taken 1 tab stat and 1 tab after 12 hours Or 1.5 mg (2 Tab. stat dose)
2. **Preven** tablet contains 0.05 mg ethinyl estradiol + 0.25 mg levonorgestrel, two tablets 12 hours apart within 72 hours of unprotected intercourse

* **WHO recommends** only 3 types of emergency contraception. Ulipristal acetate (UPA), Levonorgestrel (LNG) and ethinyl estradiol plus LNG (Yuzpe method)

8. Ans. (b) Laparoscopic tubal ligation

Ref: Dutta's 7th Ed Pg 475

- Amongst the given options, the best choice would be laparoscopic tubal ligation. Rest all are surely reversible.
- Although recanalization procedures are available, they are difficult and they may not be able to return fertility.
- **Also know:**
- **Long acting reversible contraceptives:** (1) intrauterine devices (IUDs) and (2) the etonogestrel single-rod contraceptive implant.
- Implanon is a progestin only delivery system containing 3 Ketodesogestrel (etonogestrel). It is a long-term (up to 3 years) reversible contraception.

9. Ans. (d) Uterine synechiae

Ref: Shaw 15th ed page 293, Step-Up to USMLE Step 1: A High-Yield, Systems-Based Review for the USMLE Step 1 by Samir Mehta page 225

With history of spontaneous abortion it can be presumed that Curettage would have been done. History of instrumentation and normal FSH levels points towards Uterine synechiae (Asherman syndrome).

Secondary amenorrhea is defined as the absence of menses for 6 months or the length of three cycles after establishment of regular cycles.

Option (A)

Ovarian failure: Women with hypooestrogenic amenorrhea have either ovarian failure or hypothalamic-pituitary dysfunction. **Serum concentrations of FSH and LH of more than 40-50 mIU/mL are diagnostic of ovarian failure.** Serial assessments may be necessary because of the pulsatile nature of pituitary gonadotropin secretion.

In women with FSH and LH values less than 5 mIU/mL, measurements of thyroid function tests (T3, T4 and TSH) and serum cortisol concentrations are important to exclude panhypopituitarism involving other tropic hormones additionally.

Option (C)

Pregnancy is the first thing to be ruled out in case of secondary amenorrhea. In the question Pregnancy test was given but can be presumed that its negative as FSH levels are given

Option (D)

Uterine synechiae (Asherman syndrome) usually result from destruction of large areas of endometrium by curettage (MTP). A hysterosalpingogram may show characteristic multiple filling defects, but hysteroscopy is more accurate for diagnosis. With subsequent pregnancy, the amount of remaining endometrium may be insufficient to support the pregnancy and abortion may ensue. ***Women with normal laboratory results and a history of uterine instrumentation should be evaluated for intrauterine adhesions (Asherman syndrome).***

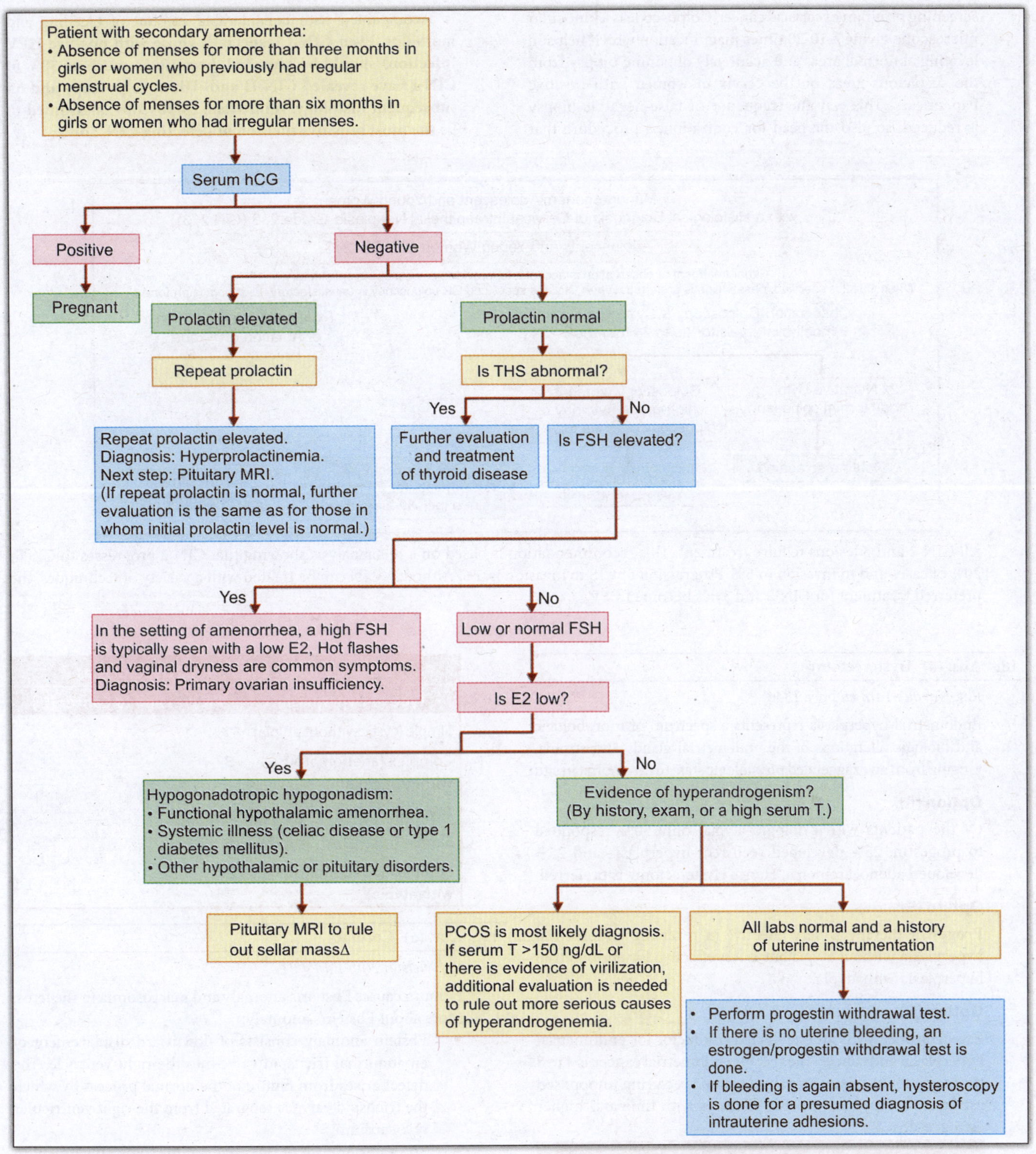

10. Ans. (d) Suburethral nodule

Ref: Novak 14th ed page 1591

Locally invasive GTT develops in about 15% of patients after evacuation of a complete mole and infrequently after other gestations. These patients usually present with the following symptoms:

- Irregular vaginal bleeding
- Theca lutein cysts
- Uterine subinvolution or asymmetric enlargement
- Persistently elevated serum hCG levels

11. Ans. (b) Colposcopy + LEEP

Ref: Novak 14th ed page 581, Shaw 15th ed page 413

Colposcopy, first introduced by Hinselmann in 1927, enjoys a universal place and its value is recognized in the integrated screening program of cervical cancer. Colposcope is a binocular microscope giving a 10-20 times magnification which helps in locating abnormal areas and accurately obtaining biopsy from the suspicious areas on the cervix in women with positive Pap smears. This way the frequency of false-negative biopsy is reduced, so also the need for conization, a procedure that is accompanied with considerable amount of bleeding and morbidity. **Even CIN-I (especially those with positive HPV infection) should be screened, because as much as 50% of CIN-I have revealed CIN-II and -III on colposcopy and on subsequent histology. Immediate colposcopy is assumed to be the most sensitive method of detecting CIN 2 or 3**

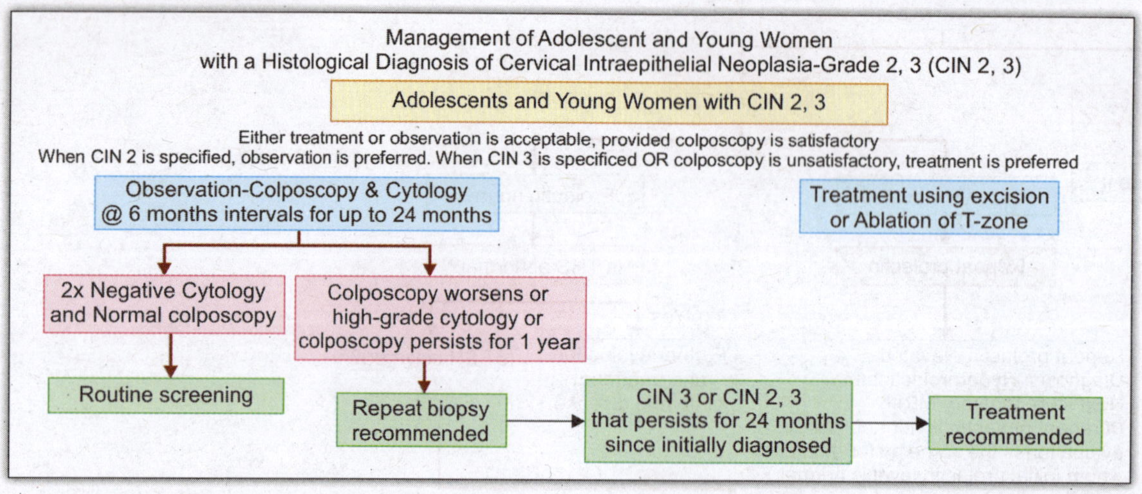

All CIN 2 and 3 lesions require treatment. This recommendation is based on a metaanalysis showing that CIN 2 progresses to CIS in 20% of cases and to invasion in 5%. Progression of CIS to invasion is 5%. Although CIN can be treated with a variety of techniques, the preferred treatment for CIN 2 and 3 has become LEEP

12. Ans. (a) Hysterectomy

Ref: Novak's 14th ed page 1346

Endometrial hyperplasia represents a spectrum of morphologic and biologic alterations of the endometrial glands and stroma, ranging from an exaggerated physiologic state to carcinoma in situ

Option (A)

Of the patients with cytologic atypia, only 50% responded to progestin, 25% developed recurrent hyperplasia and 25% developed adenocarcinoma, Hence Hysterectomy is preferred

Option (C)

Progestin therapy is very effective in reversing endometrial hyperplasia without atypia but is less effective for endometrial hyperplasia with atypia.

Option (D)

Estrogen therapy is an established risk factor for endometrial hyperplasia and cancer. The risk for endometrial cancer is 4 to 8 times greater in postmenopausal women receiving unopposed estrogen therapy and the risk increases with time and higher estrogen doses.

Endometrial Hyperplasia	
Causes	1. PCOS 2. Granulose/Theca cell tumor 3. ↑ ACTH 4. Estrogen treatment

Contd...

Classification of Endometrial Hyperplasias	
Type of Hyperplasia	**Progression to Cancer (%)**
Simple (cystic without atypia)	1
Complex (adenomatous without atypia)	3
Atypical	
Simple (cystic with atypia)	8
Complex (adenomatous with atypia)	29

13. Ans. (a) Cardiac

Ref: Nelson 20th Ed Pg 812

Lithium causes Ebstein's anomaly and macrosomia in the fetus. More about Ebstein's anomaly:

- Ebstein anomaly consists of downward displacement of an abnormal tricuspid valve into the right ventricle. The defect arises from failure of the normal process by which the tricuspid valve is separated from the right ventricular myocardium.
- The anterior cusp of the valve retains some attachment to the valve ring, but the other leaflets are adherent to the wall of the right ventricle.
- The right ventricle is thus divided into 2 parts by the abnormal tricuspid valve: the first, a thin-walled "atrialized" portion, is continuous with the cavity of the right atrium; the second, often smaller portion consists of normal ventricular myocardium.

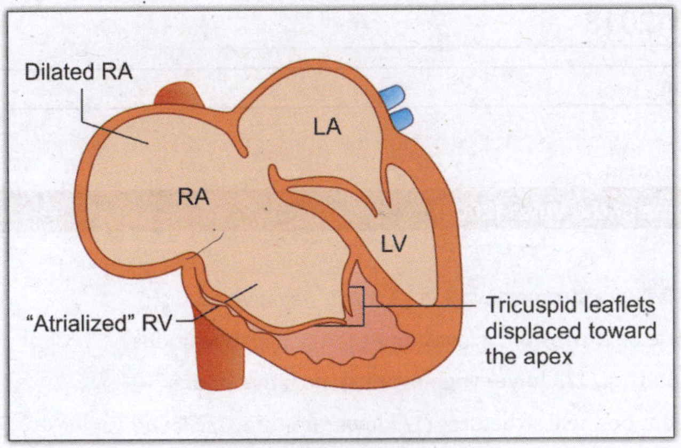

Fig: Ebstein's anomaly

14. Ans. (d) Inhibin B

Ref: William's 24th ed page 599 table 14-5

Inhibin A not Inhibin B is part of Quadruple test for Down's syndrome.

Neither Inhibin A not Inhibin B are part of Triple test for Down's syndrome

Triple test: AKA- Kettering test or the Bart's test

- ↓MSAFP, ↓ UE3 (unconjugated estriol), ↑ Total hCG
- Also called triple screen
- It is a combined biochemical test which includes MS-AFP, hCG and UE3
- Maternal age in relation to confirmed gestation age is also taken into account
- The test is for screening, not for diagnosis.
- Usually done between 15-18 weeks (16 weeks optimum).

Genetic diseases	β-hCG	MS-AFP	UE3
Down's syndrome	↑	↓	↓
Turner's syndrome	↑	↑	↓
Edward syndrome	↓	↓	↓

Quadruple test: Triple test + **DIA** (Dimeric Inhibin A ↑). Also called tetra screen, Quad test, or Quad screen.

	β-hCG	MS-AFP	UE3	DIA
Down's syndrome	↑	↓	↓	↑
Edward's syndrome	↓	↓	↓	↓

15. Ans. (c) Talk with pediatrician and termination

Ref: RCOG guidelines Clinical Practice Guideline Fetal Growth Restriction - Recognition, Diagnosis & Management 2017

Absent end-diastolic flow on Doppler is an ominous sign and indicates placental insufficiency, which demands urgent management. Flow in the umbilical artery(ies) should be in the forward direction in normal circumstances. If placental resistance increases, the diastolic flow may reduce, later becoming absent and finally reverses.

"In cases of absent end diastolic flow, delivery should be considered no later than 34 weeks gestation. Earlier delivery may be indicated in cases of poor interval growth, or a deterioration of sonographic variables"

Thus, the next step would be to consult the pediatrician for neonatal well-being and resuscitation and termination of pregnancy.

Doppler Patterns of Umbilical Artery

Normal flow

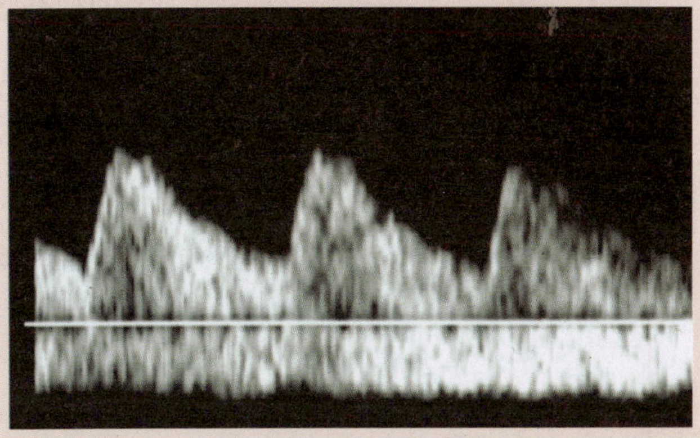

Absent End-diastolic flow

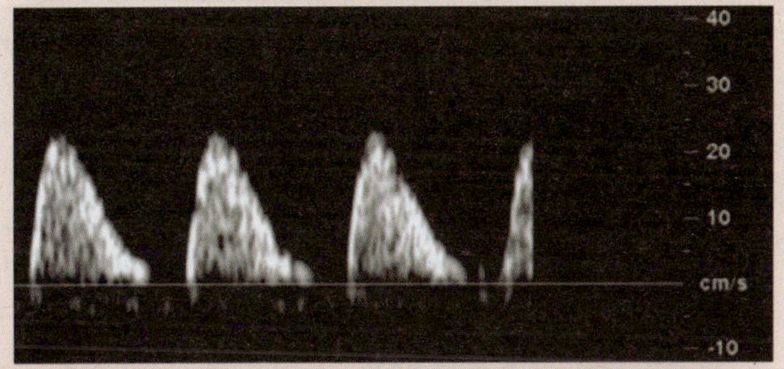

Reversed End-Diastolic flow

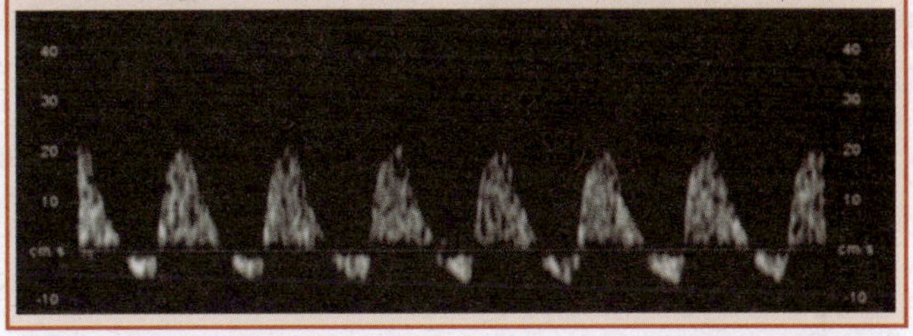

16. Ans. (a) Ergometrine infusion after anterior shoulder delivery.

Ref: Danforth's Obstetrics and Gynecology 10th ed ch 2; William's 24th Ed Pg 444-446, Dutta's obstetrics 8th ed pg no 386, WHO recommendations

See details of Active Management of Third stage of Labor (AMTSL) in OBG AIIMS May 2013 (see volume II)

Active Management of Third stage of Labor (AMTSL) as a prophylactic intervention is composed of a package of three components or steps:

- Administration of a uterotonic (preferably oxytocin) immediately **after** birth of the baby
- Controlled cord traction (CCT) to deliver the placenta; and
- Massage of the uterine fundus after the placenta is delivered.

17. Ans. (c) Radical vulvectomy with bilateral lymph node dissection

Ref: Dutta's 7th Ed Pg 277

The above description suggests Stage IB disease according to FIGO system.

Figo Staging of Carcinoma of the Vulva (2009)	
Stage I	**Tumor confined to the vulva**
IA	Tumor confined to the vulva or perineum, ≤2 cm in size with stromal invasion ≤1 mm*, negative nodes
IB	Tumor confined to the vulva or perineum, >2 cm in size or with stromal invasion >1 mm*, negative nodes
Stage II	**Tumor of any size with adjacent spread (1/3 lower urethra, 1/3 lower vagina, anus), negative nodes**
Stage III	Tumor of any size with or without extension to adjacent perineal structures (1/3 lower urethra, 1/3 lower vagina, anus) with positive inguinofemoral lymph nodes
IIIA	Tumor of any size with positive inguinofemoral lymph nodes • With 1 lymph node metastasis (≥5 mm) or • 1–2 lymph node metastasis(es) (<5 mm)
IIIB	• 2 or more lymph nodes metastases (≥5 mm) • 3 or more lymph nodes metastases (<5 mm)
IIIC	Positive node(s) with extracapsular spread
Stage IV	**Tumor invades other regional (2/3 upper urethra, 2/3 upper vagina), or distant structures**
IVA	Tumor invades any of the following: • 2/3 upper urethra, 2/3 upper vagina, bladder mucosa, rectal mucosa, or fixed to pelvic bone or • Fixed or ulcerated inguinofemoral lymph nodes
IVB	Any distant metastasis including pelvic lymph nodes

*The depth of invasion is defined as the measurement of the tumor from the epithelial-stromal junction of the adjacent most superficial dermal papilla to the deepest point of invasion

Surgical Treatment of Vulvar Cancer

Stage	Treatment
Microinvasive (Stage IA)	Wide local excision (tumor free margin at least 1 cm) with/without ipsilateral groin lymphadenectomy
Early invasive stage (Stage I B/II)	• Radical vulvectomy with bilateral inguinal lymphadenectomy → ideal surgery but causes major morbidity. • Radical local excision (Margins-1-3 cm) is an alternative in this case • For positive deep nodes: External radiation to pelvis and groin >Pelvic lymphadenectomy • Negative Sentinel lymph node biopsy can help avoid extensive lymphadenectomy.
Advanced vulvar cancer (stage III to IV) or if the general condition is poor and/or in presence of medical diseases	**The following principles may be adopted:** **Two stage operation is preferred.** Total vulvectomy followed by at a later date, bilateral inguinofemoral lymphadenectomy. Total vulvectomy followed by full pelvic and groin irradiation (megavoltage therapy). Stage III cases with resectable tumors may under undergo radial surgery and postoperative pelvic and growth irradiation. Neoadjuvant chemotherapy—followed by surgery, radiotherapy or both. Technically inoperable or recurrent lesion • Chemotherapy (cisplatin, bleomycin, 5-1,11) can be used as radiation sensitizer. • Chemoradiation therapy may be combined as primary therapy or following surgical excision of the tumor. • Radiotherapy can be used as a primary therapy for advanced disease.

Note:
Lesions with an invasion of more than 1 mm have a higher chance of lymph node involvement.

18. Ans. (b) Supine with wedge under right hip

Ref: Miller's 8th Ed page 2344

The gravid uterus compresses the Inferior Vena Cava in supine position. This decreases venous return to the heart. The mother is going to be taken up for a C-section and will require Spinal anesthesia for conduction of the surgery.

After administration of spinal anesthesia, due to vasodilatation, the venous return will further fall. Moreover, there has been non progress of labor so the patient is likely to be dehydrated and exhausted.

Under such circumstances, there will be a profound fall in BP and decreased venous return due to gravid uterus will further complicate the above situation.

By placing a wedge under the right hip, the gravid uterus will not compress the IVC and hypotension will not be compounded.

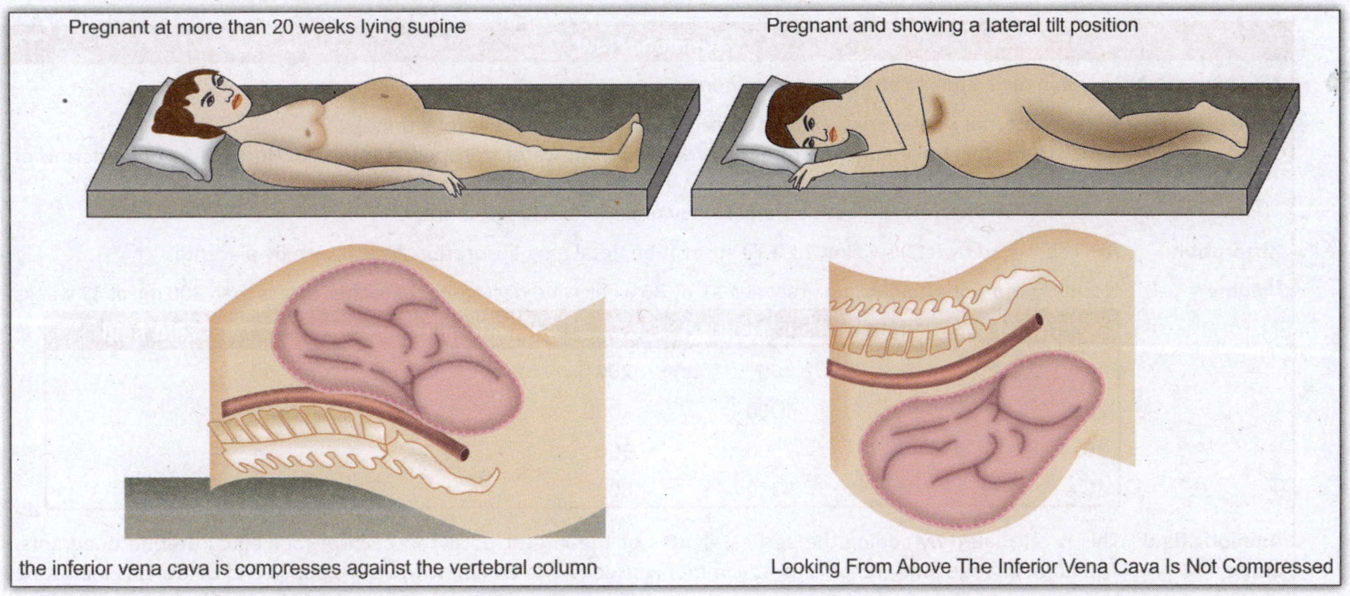

19. Ans. (c) Lift endopelvic fascia by putting fingers in vagina

Ref: William's 23rd Ed Pg 1940, Atlas of Pelvic Anatomy and Gynecologic Surgery Michael S. Baggish, 4th Ed Pg 405, Te Linde's Operative Gynecology 11th Ed

Burch colposuspension (also referred to as retropubic urethropexy) is an effective procedure for the treatment and prevention of stress urinary incontinence (SUI).

It is a surgical **procedure** in which the neck of the bladder is suspended from nearby ligaments with sutures

In the Burch procedure, the endopelvic fascia adjacent to the mid and proximal urethra at the bladder neck is attached to the pectineal (Cooper's) ligaments on the posterior surface of the superior pubic ramus.

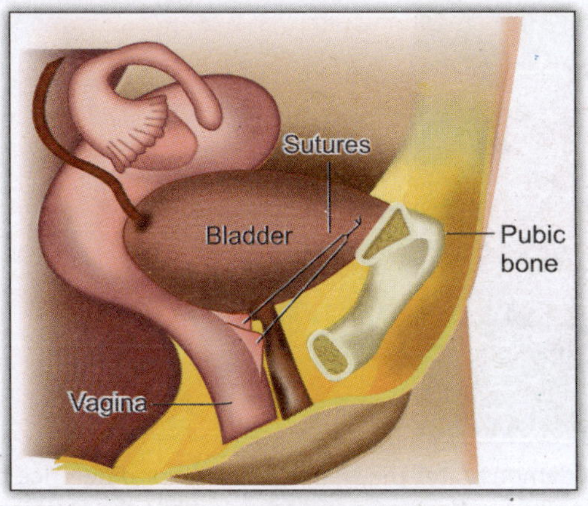

Fig: Burch procedure

After the retropubic space is reached, the index and middle fingers of the surgeon's nondominant hand are place in the vagina. The space of Retzius or retropubic space is a potential space containing much areolar tissue between the back of the pubic bone and the anterior portion of the bladder.

Surrounding the bladder is a visceral bladder capsule that contains the rich network of perivesical venous sinuses (Santorini plexus) that are very fragile and bleed easily when surgery is performed in this space. Centrally over the urethra is the deep dorsal vein of the clitoris that feeds into these venous channels.

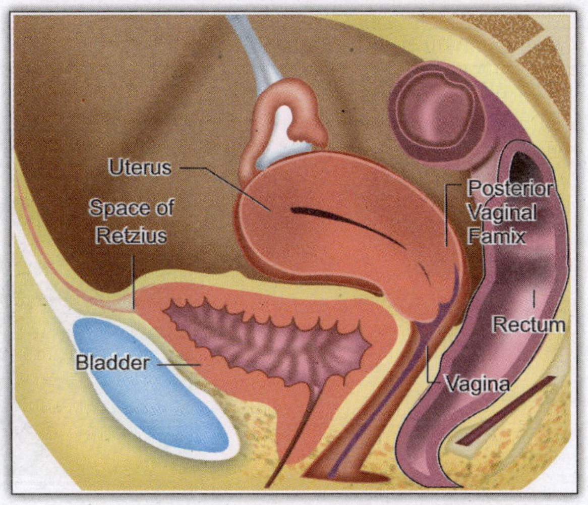

Fig: Space of retzius

Dissection in this area may bring laceration of vessels within the Santorini plexus of paravaginal veins and a risk for significant bleeding.

This is controlled easily with upward pressure from the vaginal fingers. Identified vessels can be sealed with electrosurgical coagulation, ligation, or placement of vascular clips

Nonabsorbable sutures of (3–4) polyglycolic acid are placed on the lateral fornices (paravaginal tissue) lateral to the bladder base and the bladder neck fixed to the ipsilateral iliopectineal ligament on either side.

20. Ans. (c) Clear colorless to pale yellow

Ref: Dutta 8th Ed Pg 43

In early pregnancy, amniotic fluid is colorless, but near term it becomes pale straw colored due to the presence of exfoliated lanugo and epidermal cells from fetal skin. It may look turbid due to the presence of vernix caseosa.

Amniotic Fluid		
Nile blue sulphate test in AF is done to see fetal lung maturity.		
Source	Mixed maternal & fetal origin (main source of amniotic fluid AFP is fetal urine) • ***1st trimester:*** Large component of AF is derived from water transport across skin. Horny layer of epidermis of is absent before 20th week. • ***2nd & 3rd trimester***: Fetal urine (fetal kidney origin), fetal lungs, amnion	
Absorption	AF is absorbed by fetal swallowing + GI absorption, fetal lung absorption & clearance by placenta.	
Volume	Normally, amniotic fluid volume reaches 1 L by 36 weeks and decreases thereafter to less than 200 mL at 42 weeks	
Amniotic fluid index	This is calculated by adding the vertical depths of the largest pocket in each of four equal uterine quadrants. The normal range for AFI that is most commonly used is **5 to 24 cm**, with values above and below this indicating hydramnios and oligohydramnios, respectively. (Williams) Polyhydramnios: AFI >24 cm Oligohydramnios: AFI <5 cm	
Color of Amniotic fluid	Normal	In early pregnancy= colorless Near term= pale straw colored
	Meconium stained	Meconium stained
	Golden	Due to ↑↑ bilirubin (Rh-incompatibility)
	Green/pea-souped	Due to bile pigments
	Greenish yellow (*saffron*)	In postmaturity
	Dark colored/Tobacco	IUD

Weeks' gestation	Fetus (g)	Amniotic fluid (mL)	Percent fluid
16	100	200	50
28	1000	1000	45
36	2500	900	24
40	3300	800	17

21. Ans. (a) Twin-twin transfusion syndrome

Ref: Dutta's 7th Ed Pg 240

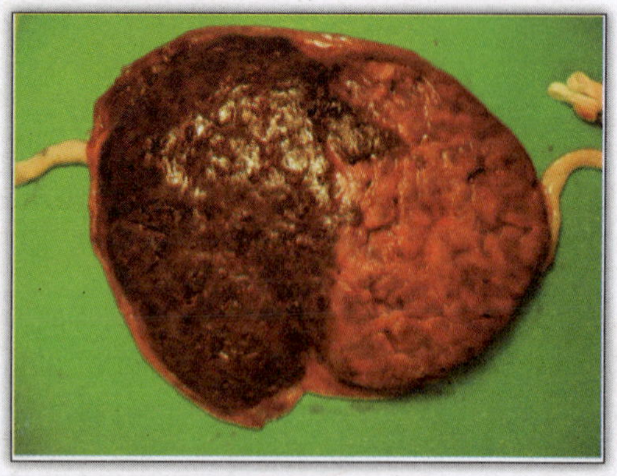

Fig: Single placenta with two umbilical cord. The maternal side of the placenta demonstrates the characteristic color difference between both placental shares suggestive of Twin to twin transfusion syndrome. The donor side is more pale and shaggy, while the recipient side is dark red, congested appearance

- The above picture is of twin-to-twin transfusion syndrome.
- **Hints to diagnosis:**
  - Single placenta with two umbilical cords
  - Vascular anastomoses can be seen between the vessels of two umbilical cords.
- Twin to twin transfusion syndrome is a clinicopathological state, exclusively met within monozygotic twins, where one twin appears to bleed into the other through some kind of placental vascular anastomosis.
- Clinical manifestations of twin transfusion syndrome occur when there is hemodynamic imbalance due to unidirectional deep arteriovenous anastomoses.
- As a result the receptor twin becomes larger with hydramnios, polycythemic, hypertensive and hypervolemic, at the expense of the donor twin which becomes smaller with oligohydramnios, anemic, hypotensive and hypovolemic.
- The donor twin may appear "stuck" due to severe oligohydramnios.
- Difference of hemoglobin concentration between the two, usually exceeds 5 g% and estimated fetal weight discrepancy is 25% or more.

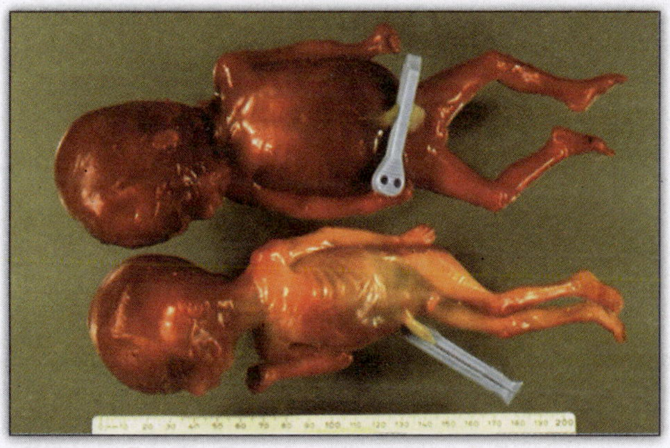

Fig: Twin-twin transfusion syndrome can develop via blood flow between the fetuses. In this condition, there is diminished blood flow to one twin (the "donor") and increased blood flow to the other twin (the "recipient"). The pale appearing donor is smaller and may die for lack of sufficient blood flow. More commonly, the larger plethoric recipient may die from congestive heart failure

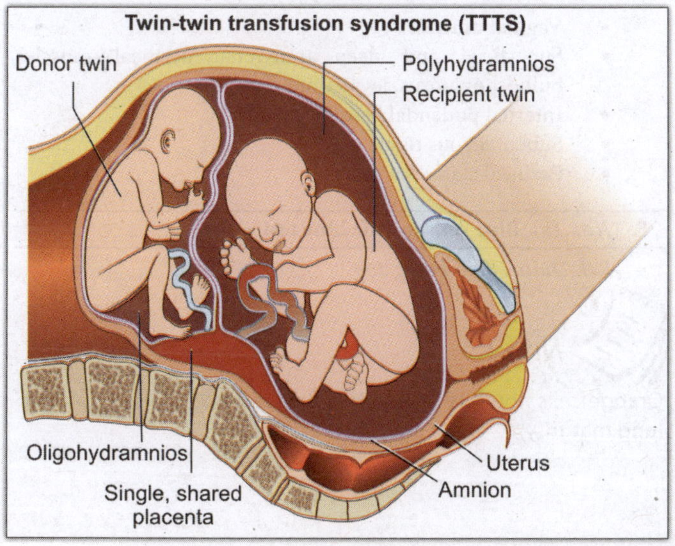

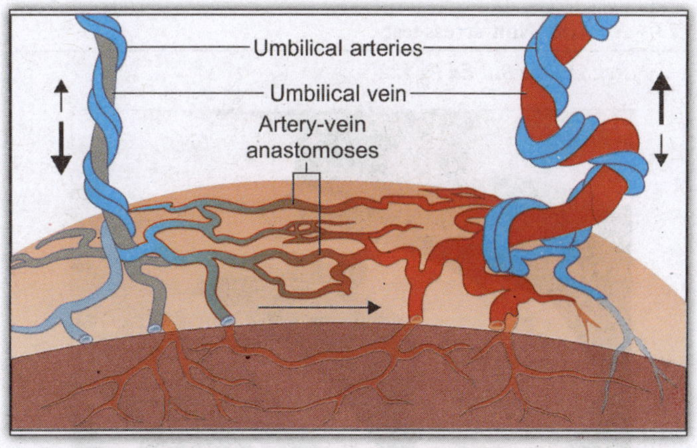

22. Ans. (E) Urgent visit to hospital and check for pregnancy >(B) Start next cycle from next day

Ref: William's 23rd Ed Ch 5 Pg 246

Recall Bias

Some students believe that option (E) Urgent visit to hospital and check for pregnancy was provided in the options. In that case it will be the best answer. In absence of Option (E) the next best answer will be Option (B) Start next cycle from next day

- Mala-N is a combined oral contraceptive that contains Levonorgestrel (0.15 mg) + Ethinyl estradiol (30 mcg). It is distributed by the government channel free of cost.
- A strip of Mala-N contains 21 tablets of contraceptive plus 7 iron tablets as placebo.
- "If withdrawal bleeding does not follow during the week of placebo pills, a woman should continue the pills but seek medical attention to exclude pregnancy."
- Hence, if exclusion of pregnancy is amongst the options, that should be the answer. However, the second best answer would be to continue the pills from the next day.

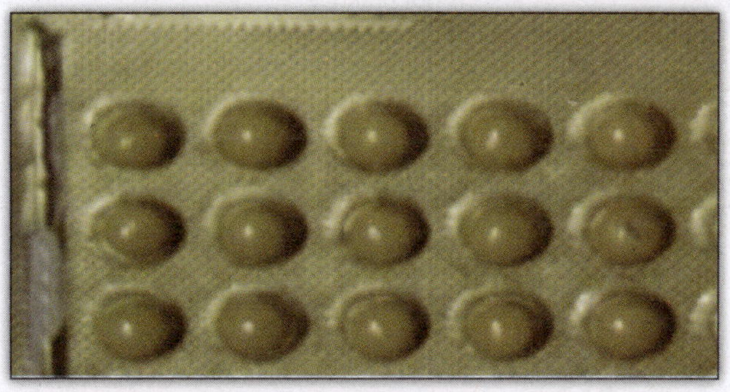

Fig: MALA-N: Hormonal pills for 3 weeks are followed by Red ones (placebo or iron) for 1 week.

Missed Combined Oral Contraceptive Pills	
Missed one dose	Double dose for next day
Several doses missed	Next dose doubled and effective barrier technique for next week. Continue the remainder of pills for the month. Alternatively, a new pack can be started with a barrier method as additional contraception for a week

23. Ans. (a) Non-stress test

Ref: Dutta's 8th Ed Pg 122

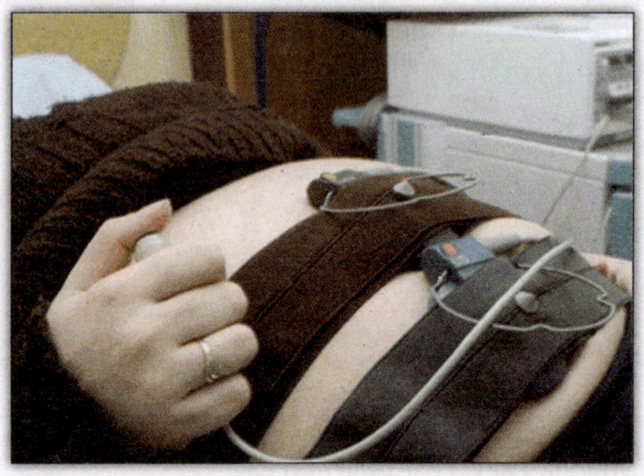

- The above figure shows the equipment and procedure for Non-stress test.
- The non-stress test describes fetal heart rate acceleration in response to fetal movement as a sign of fetal health.
- This test involves the use of Doppler-detected fetal heart rate acceleration coincident with fetal movements perceived by the mother.
- The mother lies down and has a belt placed around her abdomen with a transducer positioned over the fetal heartbeat, called an external fetal heart rate monitor. It continuously records the fetal heart rate (FHR) in graphical form.
- In most external FHR monitoring systems, the FHR is measured by focusing an ultrasound beam on the fetal heart from a small Doppler ultrasound device
- The mother is given a button in her hand, which she is supposed to click every time she feels fetal movement.

Non-Stress Test (NST)

- Most widely used primary screening testing method for assessment of antenatal fetal well-being.
- It is based on FHR acceleration in response to fetal movement (Perceived by mother) as a sign of fetal health.
- In this test continuous electronic monitoring of the FHR along with recording of fetal movements is done.
- These days only NST in used. If NST is non-reassuring then decide to deliver the baby immediately.
- Fetal scalp blood sampling to assess fetal hypoxia is an obsolete practice now a day.

Indications	• ↓ Fetal movement or loss of fetal movement • IUGR • Pregnancy induced hypertension • Diabetes mellitus • Severe heart disease • Severe chronic pulmonary disease • Postmaturity
Interpretation	• ***Normal NST:*** >2 accelerations that peak at >15 bpm above baseline, all occurring within 20 minutes of beginning of test. If no spontaneous FM during initial 20 minutes, continue the test for another 20 minutes & now FM is provoked by external manipulation. • ***Abormal NST:*** If no acceleration with spontaneous or repeated external stimuli during a 40 minutes period, test is not reactive. • If test is reactive repated every week. • If non reative- Repeate after 24 hours. If still not reactive CST done.

24. Ans. (b) Episiotomy scissor

Ref: William's 24th ed page 550

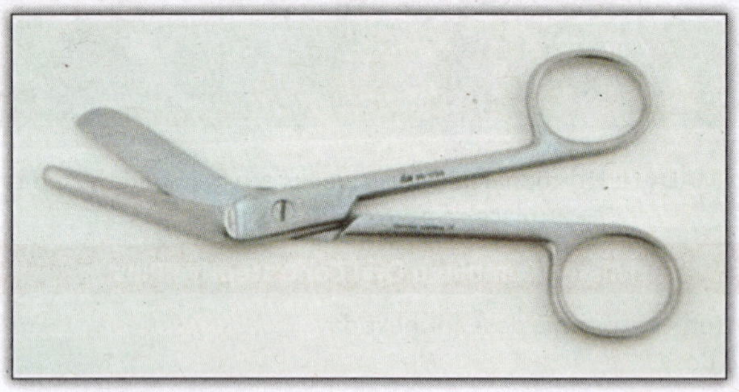

Episiotomy Scissor

Angulation in the scissor: To prevent extension of pelvic tears in to the anal margins (OASIS/CPT) obstetric anal sphincter injuries/complete perineal tear.

Structures Cut in Episiotomy

- Vaginal mucosa
- Superficial and deep transverse perineal muscles, bulbospongiosus, levator ani muscles.
- Internal pudendal blood vessels
- Subcutaneous tissue
- Perineal skin

25. Ans. (a) Blue cells in Nile blue test

Ref: Dutta's 8thh Ed Pg 369

NOTE

Orange cells not Blue cells in Nile Blue test is suggestive of fetal lung maturity

Fetal Lung Maturity	
• Confirmation of lung maturation reduces the incidence of respiratory distress syndrome (RDS) in the newborn. • The risk of RDS is high for infants that are delivered preterm (<37 weeks). • RDS is caused by the deficiency of pulmonary surfactant, which is synthesized by the type-II alveolar cells • Surfactant is packaged in lamellar bodies → discharged in the lung alveoli → carried in the pulmonary fluid → carried into the amniotic fluid.	
Shake test or Bubble test (Clement's)	• Bedside test, rapidly performed with a fair degree of accuracy. • Test is based on the ability of pulmonary surfactant to form a foam or bubble, on shaking which remains stable for at least 15 minutes. • Increasing dilutions of amniotic fluid are mixed with 96% ethanol, shaken for 15 seconds and inspected after 15 minutes for the presence of a complete ring of bubbles at the meniscus. If it is present, the test is ***positive*** and indicates maturity of the fetal lungs.
Lecithin/Sphingomyelin (L/S) ratio	Amniotic fluid L/S ratio *at 31–32 weeks is 1; at 35 weeks L/S ratio is 2.* ***L/S ratio >2 indicates pulmonary maturity.***
Foam Stability Index (FSI)	• It is based on surfactant detection by **shake test**. • FSI is calculated by utilizing serial dilutions of amniotic fluid to quantitate the amount of surfactant present. • FSI >47 virtually excludes the risk of RDS.
Fluorescence polarization	Presence of 55 mg of surfactant per g of albumin indicates fetal lung maturity.
Amniotic fluid turbidity	During 1st & 2nd trimesters, amniotic fluid is yellow and clear. At term it is turbid due to vernix.
Nile blue sulphate test in amniotic fluid	Estimation of phosphatidylglycerol (PG) I or phosphatidylcholine (>500) in amniotic fluid especially in mother with DM is the most reliable test to assess fetal lung maturity. ***Orange colored cells >50% suggests pulmonary maturity***- exfoliated fat containing cells from sebaceous glands of the fetus obtained from the centrifuged amniotic fluid are stained with 0.1% Nile blue sulfate.

26. Ans. (d) Retrieve follicles

Ref: Novak's 13th ed pg 419

- Ovarian dysfunction is the most common indication for the use of medications to induce ovulation to increase chances of conception naturally or by IVF.
- Commonly, multiple follicles are stimulated during induction of ovulation. These predispose to multiple pregnancies as well as Ovarian Hyperstimulation syndrome (OHSS).
- The cycle is monitored using USG and Serum Estradiol levels. The course of the cycle is guided by the aforementioned parameters, decisions like cancellation of cycle, continuation of cycle, retrieval of follicles are taken based on the same.
- Following is a rough guide to the course of events in an ovulation induction cycle:

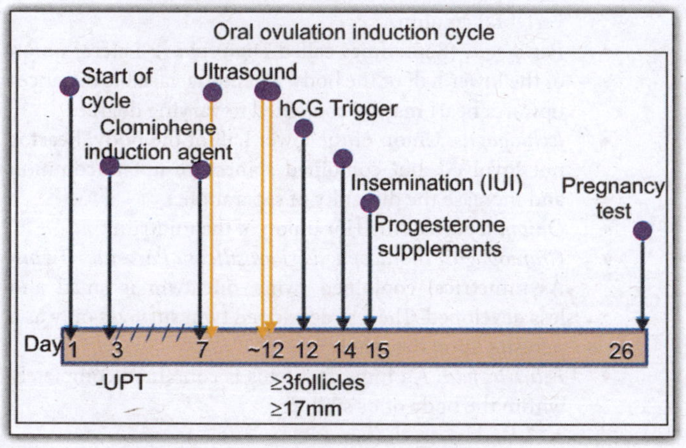

Fig: Ovulation induction

NOTE

Gonadotropins are given for 8–10 days before hCG injection trigger.

Follicle retrieval/intercourse/Intrauterine Insemination is done 36 hours posthCG injection.

- Transvaginal ultrasound and serum estradiol measurements are performed every 1 to 3 days to evaluate follicular size, number and quality. Follicles can be predicted to grow 1 to 2 mm per day and follicular development is believed to be adequate when maximal follicular diameter exceeds 18 to 19 mm.
- When hMG is used, the serum estradiol level roughly corresponds to 150 to 250 pg/mL per mature follicle (Speroff's 8th Ed Pg 1318 says 200-400 pg/mL).
- However, serum estradiol levels may not be as closely correlated with the number of mature follicles when recombinant FSH is used.
- In general, the serum estradiol level can be expected to double every 24 hours if the same dosage of gonadotropins is maintained. Therefore, the main reasons for following the estradiol levels are as follows:
  - To detect missed spontaneous ovulation or premature luteinization, which may be reflected by a drop in serum estradiol levels
  - To identify patients at risk for OHSS.
- Estradiol levels approaching 800 to 1000 pg/mL indicate increased risk for OHSS. A decrease in gonadotropin dosage should be considered and monitoring is mandated in 24 hours.

- Withholding gonadotropin in this situation is referred to as "coasting" and is usually followed by a more than 25% decrease in serum estradiol while the follicle numbers and diameters increase. If follicle numbers increase and are excessive, the cycle should be cancelled
- Estradiol levels in the range of 1,500 to 2,000 pg/mL indicate that treatment should absolutely be stopped because of the high risk for OHSS. All medications should be discontinued and hCG should not be administered.
- The patient should be asked to abstain from intercourse until menses occurs because she may spontaneously ovulate. Under these conditions, ovulation and intercourse may lead to increased risk for multiple gestations.

Let's discuss the options:

- **Give cabergoline:** Cabergoline is a dopamine agonist given in hyperprolactinemia. This option is false
- **Cancel cycle:** The serum Estradiol levels are 800 pg/mL which are borderline for the risk of OHSS. However, the levels are not so high (1,500 to 2,000 pg/mL) so as to completely cancel the cycle. This option is false
- **Withhold hCG:** As seen in the figure above, the number of follicles is >3. Thus, hCG injection is in fact indicated at this stage. This option is false
- **Retrieve follicles:** Estradiol levels are also 800 pg/mL. At this stage, further gonadotropins should be stopped to avoid the risk of OHSS. Also, Number of follicles is >3, hCG trigger is indicated. Monitoring and retrieval of follicles is thus indicated. This option is correct amongst the given options.

27. Ans. (a) Warfarin should be replaced by heparin in 1 trimester

Ref: With Text

Women with a mechanical valve prosthesis must be anticoagulated and when not pregnant, warfarin is recommended. Although most effective to prevent mechanical valve thrombosis, warfarin is teratogenic and can cause miscarriage, stillbirths and fetal malformation. **The European Society of Cardiology favors warfarin anticoagulation until 36 weeks, at which time heparin is given until delivery**. Heparin is discontinued just before delivery. Anticoagulant therapy with warfarin or heparin may be restarted 6 hours following vaginal delivery (Ref: William's 24th ed page 2067)

The patient taking warfarin should discontinue it as soon as pregnancy is diagnosed and replace by heparin 5000 units twice daily subcutaneously up to **12th week**. This is then replaced by warfarin tablet 3 mg. daily to be taken at the same time each day and continued up to **36 weeks.** Thereafter it is replaced by heparin up to **7 days postpartum**. Warfarin is then to be continued. (Ref: Dutta 7th ed page 277)

Dewhurst 9th Ed Pg 91 says:

Warfarin is associated with warfarin embryopathy (chondrodysplasia punctata) if given during the period of organogenesis (6–12 weeks' gestation) and with fetal intracerebral hemorrhage in the second and third trimesters. The risk is higher with Warfarin doses of >5 mg.

There are three basic options for anticoagulation management.

1. Continue warfarin throughout pregnancy, stopping only for delivery. This is the safest option for the mother (lowest risk of thrombosis)
2. Replace warfarin with high-dose LMWH from 6 to 12 weeks' gestation to avoid warfarin embryopathy but continue until prior to delivery when LMWH is used again.
3. Use high-dose LMWH throughout pregnancy.

American College of Chest Physicians Guidelines for Anticoagulation of Pregnant Women with Mechanical Prosthetic Valves

For pregnant women with mechanical heart valves, any one of the following anticoagulant regimens is recommended:

- Adjusted-dose *LMWH* twice daily throughout pregnancy. The doses should be adjusted to achieve the manufacturer's peak anti-Xa level 4 hours after subcutaneous injection.
- Adjusted-dose *UFH* administered every 12 hours throughout pregnancy. The doses should be adjusted to keep the mid interval aPTT at least twice control or attain an anti-Xa heparin level of 0.35 to 0.70 U/mL.
- LMWH or UFH as above until 13 weeks' gestation with warfarin substitution until close to delivery when LMWH or UFH is resumed.

In women judged to be at very high risk of thromboembolism and in whom concerns exist about the efficacy and safety of LMWH or UFH as dosed above—some examples include older generation prosthesis in the mitral position or history of thromboembolism. Warfarin is suggested throughout pregnancy with replacement by UFH or LMWH close to delivery (36 weeks). In addition, low-dose aspirin—75 to 100 mg daily—should be orally administered.

28. Ans. (a) Head

Ref: Plastic Surgery Secrets Plus E-Book by Jeffrey Weinzweig 2nd Ed Pg 269; Coran Pediatric surgery 7th Ed Pg 1728

- *Craniopagus:* Cranial union only. Simple cases may involve only scalp and calvarium, whereas more complete cases involve scalp, calvarium, dura, venous sinuses and brain
- *Pygopagus:* Posterior union of the buttocks
- *Thoracopagus:* Anterior union of the upper portion of the trunk. This form of conjoining is the most common type of conjoined twinning
- *Cephalopagus:* Anterior union of the upper half of the body with two faces on opposite sides of a conjoined head (extremely rare); the heart may be involved
- *Rachipagus:* Dorsal union of the trunk with fused vertebral columns
- *Parapagus* (Sometimes called *Diprosopus*): Lateral union of the lower half of the body, extending variable distances upward; heart may be conjoined to varying degrees
- *Ischiopagus:* Union of the lower half of the body; heart is not involved, but conjoined spines are not uncommon and increase the difficulty of separation
- *Omphalopagus:* Anterior union of the midtrunk
- *Craniopagus/Thoracopagus Parasiticus Parasitic Twins:* Asymmetrical conjoined twins; one twin is small and less developed. The less developed twin survives only as a parasite upon the other.
- *Fetus-in-fetu:* An imperfect fetus is contained completely within the body of its sibling.

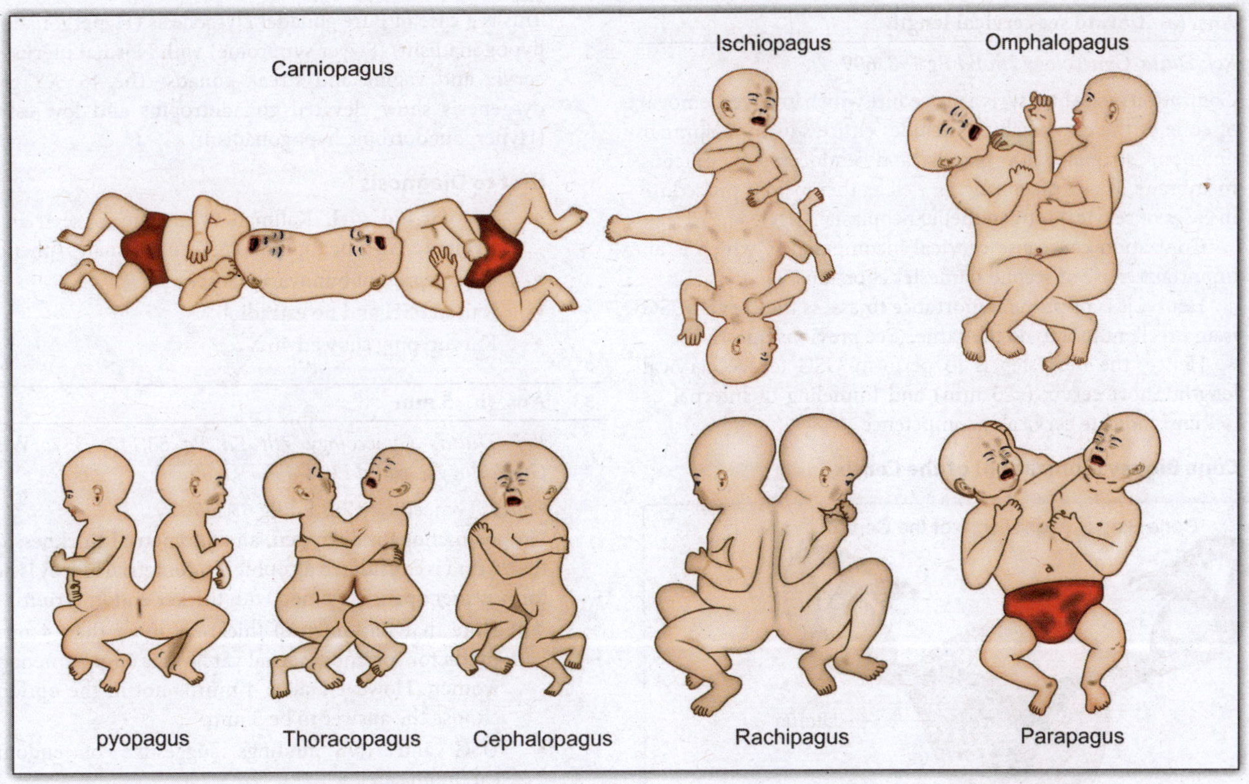

29. Ans. (d) Transvaginal sonography

Ref: Novak 14th ed page 415, Dutta's 8th Ed Pg 196

RCOG guidelines 2011 (The Investigation and Treatment of Couples with Recurrent First trimester and Second-trimester Miscarriage) say that:

"All women with recurrent first-trimester miscarriage and all women with one or more second-trimester miscarriages should have a pelvic ultrasound to assess uterine anatomy"

Although transvaginal ultrasonographic examination can be more helpful than transabdominal ultrasonography in ascertaining details of pelvic anatomy, the use of the vaginal probe may not be possible in a young girl or one who has not used tampons or had intercourse. Direct communication between the clinician and the radiologist can be helpful in identifying candidates for transvaginal ultrasonographic examination (Ref: Novak 14th ed page 415)

To decide between transvaginal and transabdominal ultrasound.

- The most common cause of second trimester abortions is anatomic abnormalities- mainly cervical incompetence and uterine anomalies.
- Uterine anomalies, Cervical length and other factors for diagnosing cervical incompetence are better seen in transvaginal ultrasound.

Hence, (D) Transvaginal sonography is the answer.

About other options:

Option (A) Karyotyping

After the first trimester, both the abortion rate and the incidence of chromosomal anomalies decrease. Hence, Karyotyping at this stage is not likely to be very useful at this stage, since we are dealing with recurrent second trimester abortions.

Option (B) Hysteroscopy

Hysteroscopy can be done subsequently to diagnose uterine anomalies; however, it is not the next step.

Recurrent Abortions

Loss of 3 or more consecutive pregnancies, affects 1% of couples trying to conceive.

1st trimester abortion	2nd trimester abortion
• Genetic factors/Chromosomal (Most common 1st trimester causes) • Poorly controlled diabetic • Presence of thyroid autoantibodies/Hypothyroidism • Luteal phase defect (LPD) with less production of progesterone • Hypersecretion of luteinizing hormone as seen in PCOD cases • Infection in the genital tract • Inherited thrombophilia/ Lupus anticoagulant • Presence of autoantibodies • Unexplained	**Anatomic abnormalities (10-15%):** Congenital/Acquired • ***Congenital abnormalities: Defective Mullerian fusion***- such as double uterus, septate or bicornuate uterus. • **Acquired anomalies** are: ▪ Intrauterine adhesions ▪ Uterine fibroids ▪ Endometriosis ▪ Cervical incompetence **Other causes:** ***Chronic maternal illness***- uncontrolled diabetes with arteriosclerotic changes, hemoglobinopathies, Chronic renal disease. Inflammatory bowel disease, systemic lupus erythematosus. ***Infection***- Syphilis, toxoplasmosis and listeriosis may be responsible in some cases. *Unexplained.*

30. Ans. (a) USG to see cervical length

Ref: Dutta' Gynecology 7th Ed Pg 198, 609

Conization (cone biopsy) is a procedure which involves removal of cone of the cervix which includes entire squamocolumnar junction, stroma with glands and endocervical mucous membrane. It is a diagnostic as well as therapeutic procedure in cases of cervical intraepithelial neoplasia (CIN).

Conization can cause cervical incompetence, which is an important cause of second trimester abortions.

Hence, it is of prime importance to assess the cervix. USG is an excellent tool to do the same. (See previous question)

Hence, the next step is to perform USG to see cervical length. Short cervix (<25 mm) and funneling of internal os (>1 cm) indicate cervical incompetence.

Cone Biopsy (Conization) of the Cervix

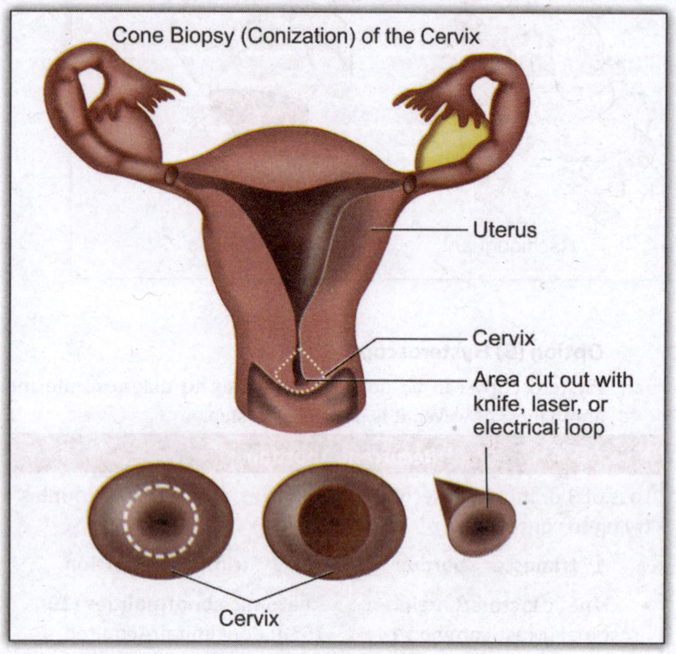

Fig: Conization of cervix

31. Ans. (a) Previous history of ectopic pregnancy

Ref: William's Gynecology 23rd Ed page 263

Contraindications of IUCD	
Absolute contraindications	**Relative contraindications**
• Pregnancy • Current PID- Pelvic inflammatory disease • Previous Ectopic • Malignancy of female genital tract	• Anemia • Menorrhagia • Unmotivated person • Past PID • Fibroid or congenital malformations of Uterus

32. Ans. (a) Pure gonadal dysgenesis

Ref: Williams 24th ed page 149, Shaw's 15th ed page 111, Speroff 8th ed page 374-376

See Table of "CAUSES OF PRIMARY Amenorrhea" in AIIMS NOV 2016 (see page no. 882)

This is a case of Pure gonadal Dysgenesis (Hypergonadotropic hypogonadism) (Swyer syndrome) with Normal uterus, tubes, cervix and vagina and streak gonads. The 46, XY gonadal dysgenesis show elevated gonadotropins and low estrogens (Hypergonadotropic hypogonadism)

Hint to Diagnosis

- **13-year-old girl:** Kallman syndrome is seen in Male >Female. All other options are seen in females (phenotype)
- Uterus present but ovaries absent
- Raised FSH and no estradiol
- Karyotyping showed 46 XY

33. Ans. (b) 5 mm

Ref: Dutta's Gynecology 7th Ed Pg 63,117, 357; William's Gynecology 23rd Ed Fig 8-4

Dutta's Gynecology 7th Ed Pg 63,117 says

"In postmenopausal women, an endometrial thickness of less than 5 mm is considered atrophic. Endometrial biopsy is needed for postmenopausal women with thicker endometrium."

- Note that Endometrial thickness more than 4 mm is a predictor for endometrial carcinoma in postmenopausal women. However, since 4 mm is not in the options, we choose the answer to be 5 mm.
- USG and TVS findings suggestive of endometrial carcinoma are:
- Endometrial thickness >4 mm.
- Hyperechoic endometrium with irregular outline.
- Increased vascularity with low vascular resistance.
- Intrauterine fluid.

34. Ans. (a) Preterm labor

Ref: Dutta' Obstetrics 8th Ed Pg 366

- The presence of fibronectin in cervical discharge between 24–34 weeks indicates Preterm labor.
- Fibronectin is a glycoprotein that binds the fetal membranes to the decidua. Normally it is found in the cervicovaginal discharge before 22 weeks and again after 37 weeks of pregnancy.
- Presence of fibronectin in the cervicovaginal discharge between 24 weeks and 34 weeks is a predictor of preterm labor. When the test is negative it reassures that delivery will not occur within next 7 days.

Predictors of Preterm Labor		
Clinical predictors	**Biophysical predictors**	**Biochemical predictors**
• History of prior preterm birth; • Multiple pregnancy; • Presence of genital tract infection; • Symptoms of preterm labor	• Uterine contractions >4/hr; • Bishop score >4; • Cervical length (TVS) 5.25 mm	• Fetal fibronectin (fFN) in cervicovaginal discharge • Others IL-6, IL-8, TNF-alpha.

35. **Ans. (a) Placenta succenturiata**

Ref: William's Obstetrics 23rd Ed Ch 27

This is a case of placenta succenturiata. The accessory lobe of placenta has been retained succenturiate lobe of placenta

Succenturiate Lobe of Placenta

- Two lobes of placenta attached to each other with marginal insertion of the umbilical cord. If both the lobes of such placenta are nearly similar in size it is known as *bilobate placenta, bipartite placenta* or *placenta duplex*. However , when the size of the lobes is not similar and one lobe is smaller as shown in the figure it is known as succenturiate lobe
- The accessory lobe may sometimes be retained in the uterus after delivery and may cause serious hemorrhage.
- One or more small accessory lobes—succenturiate lobes—may develop in the membranes at a distance from the main placenta. These lobes have vessels that course through the membranes.
- If these vessels overlie the cervix to create a vasa previa, they can cause dangerous fetal hemorrhage if torn. An accessory lobe may also be retained in the uterus after delivery and cause postpartum uterine atony and hemorrhage.
- In some cases, an accompanying vasa previa may cause dangerous fetal hemorrhage at delivery.
- A twofold higher incidence of succenturiate lobes in twin placentas.

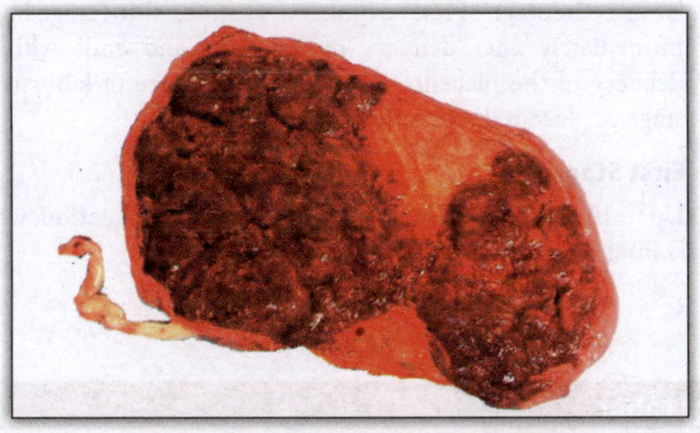

Fig: Succenturiate Lobe of placenta

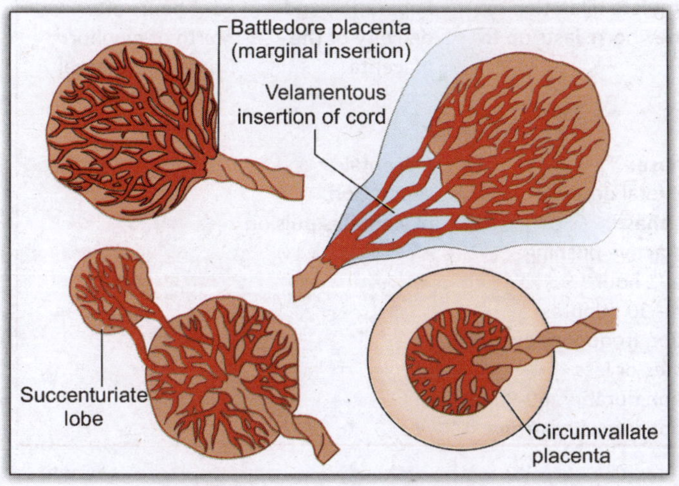

Fig: Anomalies of placenta

36. **Ans. (c) Continue the surgery with careful monitoring of fluid status**

Ref: Novak's 14th Ed page 795

- For operative hysteroscopy, low-viscosity, nonconductive fluids such as 1.5% glycine and 3% sorbitol are used most often. These fluids are used for irrigation in hysteroscopic procedures as distention of the endometrial cavity is necessary to create a viewing space.
- These solutions can be used with electricity because there are no electrolytes to disperse the current and impede the electrosurgical effect. Both 1.5% glycine and 3% sorbitol are inexpensive and are readily available in 3-L bags suitable for continuous-flow hysteroscopy.
- Because each fluid is hypotonic, extravasation into the systemic circulation can be associated with fluid and electrolyte disturbances. Therefore, uterine "absorption" must be monitored continuously by collecting outflow from the sheath and subtracting it from the total infused volume.
- Absorbed volumes greater than 1 L mandate the measurement of electrolyte levels.
- If there is more than 2 L of extravasated fluid, the procedure should be stopped. Excessive circulating sorbitol may cause hyperglycemia and large volumes of glycine may elevate levels of ammonia in the blood

37. **Ans. (b) The morphology of sperms**

Ref: Speroff 8th ed pg no 1270-1271, Novak's Gynecology 15th ed page 1142

Repeat AIIMS MAY 2017 OBG (See for explanation) (see page no. 878)

AIIMS NOVEMBER 2017

38. **Ans. (b) Low MSAFP, Low UE3 and High beta hCG**

Ref: Williams 24th ed page 290

Triple test can detect 60–70% cases of Down's syndrome

Triple test

- Also called triple screen, the Kettering test or the Bart's test.
- It is a combined biochemical test which includes MS-AFP, hCG and UE3 (unconjugated estriol).
- Maternal age in relation to confirmed gestation age is also taken into account
- The test is for screening, not for diagnosis.
- Usually done between 15–18 weeks (16 weeks optimum).

Genetic diseases	β-hCG	MS-AFP	UE3
Down's syndrome	↑	↓	↓
Turner's syndrome	↑	↑	↓
Edward syndrome	↓	↓	↓

Tests for Down's syndrome	
1st trimester	↑ hCG, ↓ MSAFP, ↓ PAPP
2nd trimester	• **Triple test** (↓ MSAFP, ↓ UE3, ↑ Total hCG) • **Quadruple test** (↓ MSAFP, ↓ UE3, ↑ Total hCG, ↑ Inhibin A) • **USG (sonographic marker/Soft sign)** ▪ *↑ nuchal fold thickness (Nuchal translucency)* ▪ *↓ Femur length and humerus* ▪ *Nasal bone absence or hypoplasia* ▪ *Shortened frontal lobe or brachycephaly* ▪ *Short ear length* ▪ *Echogenic bowel and intracardiac focus* ▪ *Mild renal pelvis dilation* ▪ *Widened iliac angle* ▪ *Widened gap between first and second toes- "sandal gap"* ▪ *Clinodactyly, hypoplastic mid-phalanx of fifth digit* ▪ *Single transverse palmar crease*

39. Ans. (d) No extra calories

Ref: With Text

At first look this question appears to be a repeat question from Preventive and social medicine. Supplementary Nutrition is given to the children (6 months – 6 years) and pregnant and lactating mothers under the Integrated Child Development Services (ICDS) Scheme. However since first trimester was specifically mentioned in the question we had a second look. PSM books including PARK and ICDS does not differentiate on the basis of Trimester however Obstetric books do mention trimester wise. Going through the below text from Williams it is clear that the answer is (D) No extra calories

William's obstetrics 24th ed page 51; Analysis by the World Health Organization (2004) estimates that the additional total pregnancy energy demands associated with normal pregnancy are approximately 77,000 kcal or 85 kcal/day, 285 kcal/day and 475 kcal/day during the first, second and third trimester, respectively.

William obstetrics 24th ed page 178; Pregnancy requires an additional 80,000 kcal, mostly during the last 20 weeks. To meet this demand, a caloric increase of 100 to 300 kcal per day is recommended during pregnancy (American Academy of Pediatrics and the American College of Obstetricians and Gynecologists, 2012). This intake increase, however, should not be divided equally during the course of pregnancy. The Institute of Medicine (2006) recommends adding **0, 340 and 452 kcal/day** to the estimated nonpregnant energy requirements in the first, second and third trimesters, respectively.

40. Ans. (a) 1st Stage

Ref: Danforth's Obstetrics and Gynecology 10th ed ch 2; William's 24th Ed Pg 444-446, Dutta's obstetrics 8th ed pg no 386

The first stage begins when spaced uterine contractions of sufficient frequency, intensity and duration are attained to bring about cervical thinning, or effacement. This labor stage ends when the cervix is fully dilated—about 10 cm—to allow passage of the term-sized fetus. The first stage of labor, therefore, is the stage of cervical effacement and dilatation.

The second stage begins when cervical dilatation is complete and ends with delivery. Thus, the second stage of labor is the stage of fetal expulsion. Last, the third stage begins immediately after delivery of the fetus and ends with the delivery of the placenta. Thus, the third stage of labor is the stage of placental separation and expulsion.

First Stage

Up to 10 cm dilation is called as full/complete dilatation, which is First Stage of Labor irrespective of parity

Stages and Phases of Labor

	First stage	Second stage	Third stage	Fourth stage
Description	0 to 10 cm dilatation (full dilatation)	From complete dilatation to birth of newborn, lasts up to 1 hour	Separation and delivery of the placenta	1-4 hours after birth of newborn; time of maternal physiological adjustment
Phases	**Latent phase:** 0-3 cm dilatation Effacement 0-40% Nullipara – 9 hours Multipara – 5 to 6 hours Contraction frequency every 5-6 minutes Contraction duration 40-45 sec Contraction intensity mild	**Pelvic phase:** Period of fetal descent **Perineal phase:** Period of active pushing. Nullipara -1 hour Multipara- 30 minutes Contraction frequency every 2-3 minutes or less Contraction duration 60-90 sec Contraction intensity strong	Placental separation, placental expulsion	

Contd...

Stages and Phases of Labor				
	First stage	Second stage	Third stage	Fourth stage
	Active phase: 4–7 cm dilatation Effacement 40–80% Nullipara – 6 hours Multipara – 4 hours Contraction frequency every 2–5 minutes Contraction duration 45–60 sec Contraction intensity moderate **Transition phase:** 8–10 cm dilatation Effacement 80–100% Nullipara – 1 hours Multipara – 30 minutes Contraction frequency every 1–2 minutes Contraction duration 60–90 sec Contraction intensity strong			

41. Ans. (c) Left side of the alert line

Ref: Sheila Balakrishnan 2nd edition pg 121; William's 24th ed page 452, Dutta 6th ed p- 528

See Table of PARTOGRAPH in AIIMS NOV 2016 (see page no. 886)

Prolonged labor is diagnosed, once the alert line is crossed, i.e. shift to right. There is considered an indication for intervention. If the patient is in peripheral hospital, once the alert line is crossed from left to right, it is an indication for referral to higher center.

42. Ans. (b) 16/10/2017

Ref: Dutta's 8th ed page 108, 734, William's 24th ed page 172

Naegele's formula: Provided the periods are regular, it is very useful and commonly practiced means to calculate the expected date. Its prediction range is about 50% with 7 days on either side of EDD. If the interval of cycles is longer, the extra days are to be added and if the interval is shorter, the lesser days are to be subtracted to get the EDD.

Calculation of the expected date of delivery (EDD): This is done according to Naegele's formula by adding 9 calendar months and 7 days to the first day of the last normal (28 day cycle) period. Alternatively, one can count back 3 calendar months from the first day of the last period and then add 7 days to get the expected date of delivery; the former method is commonly employed.

Example: The patient had her first day of last menstrual period on 9th January. By adding 9 calendar months it comes to 9th October and then add 7 days, i.e. 16th October, which becomes the expected date of delivery.

NOTE

For IVF pregnancy date of LMP is 14 days prior to date of embryo transfers (266 days).

Naegele's rule is based on 28 days regular cycle. If the interval of cycles is longer, the extra days are to be added and if the interval is shorter, the lesser days are to be subtracted to get the EDD. Examples: (1) If she is having 40days cycle regularly, to get corrected EDD, add 12 days (40–28) with the EDD calculated from LMP. (2) If she is having 21 days cycle regularly, to get corrected EDD, subtract 7 days (28–21) with the EDD calculated from LMP.

43. Ans. (a) Dysgerminoma

Ref: Shaw's Gynecology 16th ed page 821, Novak's Gynecology 15th ed page 1223

Option (A) Dysgerminoma

Dysgerminoma (MC malignant germ cell tumor, MC malignant tumor diagnosed during pregnancy)	• 30–40% of germ cell tumors • Unilateral in 85–90% of cases	• Female counterpart of the seminoma • Most radiosensitive (but surgery is the preferred treatment) • Tumor with lymphocytic infiltration, LDH +ve, ALP +ve

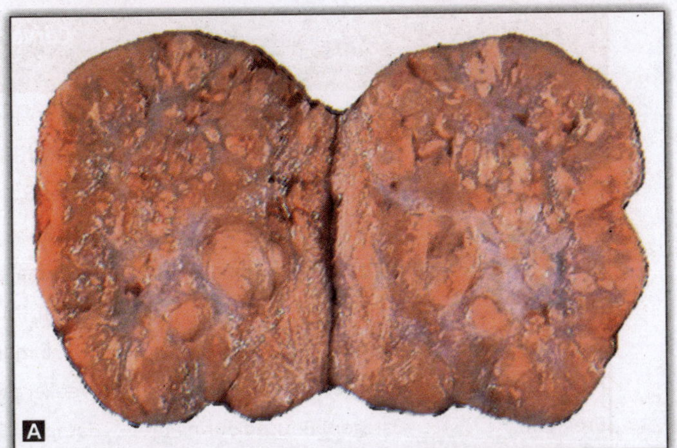

A

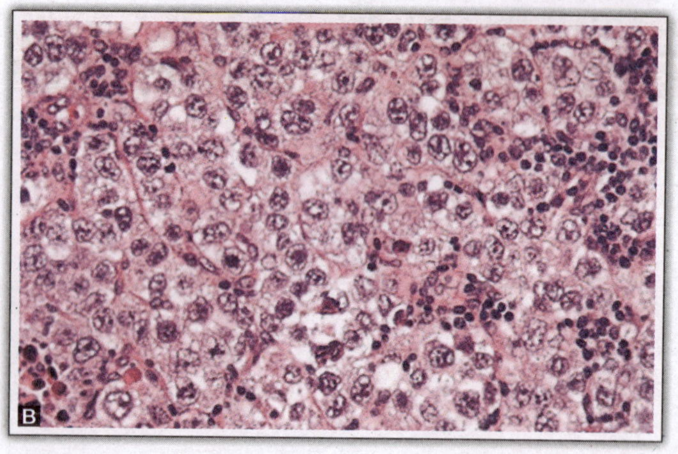

Figs A and B: **A. Dysgerminoma gross:** The size of dysgerminomas varies widely, but they are usually 5 to 15 cm in diameter. Ovarian dysgerminoma that has been sectioned into two halves. Firm and encapsulated. The cut surface of the tumor is solid with some cystic areas and necrosis, fleshy, lobulated and a yellow-white to gray-pink appearance; **B. Dysgerminoma Microscopy:** Histopathology of the biopsy specimen: Sheet or cords of Round, polygonal large uniform tumor cells with vesicular nuclei and clear or finely granular cytoplasm that is eosinophilic, separated by scanty fibrous septa, which are often extensively infiltrated with lymphocytes, plasma cells and granulomas with epithelioid cells and multinucleated giant cells. Mitotic figures are seen in varying numbers, although they are usually numerous

Option (B)

Endodermal sinus tumor is AFP positive

Option (C)

Malignant Teratoma is AFP positive

Option (D)

Mucinous cystadenocarcinoma s epithelial tumor and is negative for all biomarkers including LDH and ALP

44. Ans. (b) 1 tab after 12 hours

Ref: Shaw 16th ed page 609, William's 24th ed page 1484, Dutta 7th ed page 551

Postcoital/emergency contraceptives

Drug	Dose	Pregnancy rate (%)
• **Levonorgestrel** (Progesterone only pills)	0.75 mg stat and after 12 hours Or 1.5 mg (2 Tab.stat dose)	0-1
• **Ethinyl estradiol 50 μg + Norgestrel 0.25 mg** (Yuzpe method or OCPs method)	2 tab stat and 2 after 12 hours	0–2
• **Ethinyl estradiol** (Estrogen high dose), Now replaced by LNG	2.5 mg BD × 5 days	0–0.6
• **Mifepristone (RU-486)** (Effective up to 49 days of LMP)	100 mg single dose	0-0.6
• **Copper IUDs Insertion** (Gold standard but now not recommended)	Within 5 days	0-0.1
• **Ulipristal acetate** (synthetic progesterone hormone receptor modular, attaches to progesterone receptor and prevents/delays ovulation and suppresses endometrium, prevents implantation)	A 30 mg tablet should be taken within 5 days	0-1

45. Ans. (b) 6, 11, 16, 18, 31, 33, 45, 52 and 58

Ref: Shaw's Gynecology 16th ed page 623, Novak's Gynecology 15th ed page 1203

Cervarix vs Gardasil

	Cervarix	Gardasil	Gardasil- 9
Valency	Bivalent vaccine	Quadrivalent vaccine	Nonavalent vaccine
Strains	HPV viruses Types 16 and 18	HPV viruses 6, 11, 16, 18	HPV viruses 6, 11, 16, 18, 31, 33, 45, 52 and 58
Protection	Types 16 and 18, 45 and 31	Types 6, 11, 16, 18	Types 6, 11, 16, 18, 31, 33, 45, 52 and 58
Age group	9 to 26 years	9 to 26 years	9 to 26 years
Gender use	Both male and females	Both male and Female	Both Males and females
Dose and Route	0.5 mL IM	0.5 mL IM	0.5 mL IM
Vaccine schedule	0, 2, 6 months	0, 2, 6 months	0, 2, 6 months
Immune response	Stronger and longer	Weaker and shorter	Weaker and shorter
Pregnancy	Category B- used during pregnancy only if clearly needed	Category B- used during pregnancy only if clearly needed	Category B- used during pregnancy only if clearly needed.

Contd...

Cervarix vs Gardasil			
	Cervarix	Gardasil	Gardasil- 9
FDA Approval	2009	2006	2014
Comments	More effective for Ca cervix AS04 adjuvant		

46. Ans. (b) Type 1 Hysterectomy

Ref: Shaw's 16th ed page 826, Novak's 15th ed page 1121, Novak's 14th ed page 466, 1347

If not specifically mentioned at 60 years of age the patient does not require fertility. Hence Type 1 Hysterectomy is the best answer.

All postmenopausal women with unexpected uterine bleeding patients should be evaluated for endometrial carcinoma. Approximately 5 to 10 percent of women with postmenopausal vaginal bleeding have endometrial cancer. For this reason, ***atypical endometrial hyperplasia should be treated by hysterectomy and not merely by ablative technique***.

Progestin therapy is very effective in reversing endometrial hyperplasia without atypia but is less effective for endometrial hyperplasia with atypia.

- For women with endometrial hyperplasia without atypia, ovulation induction, **cyclical progestin therapy** (e.g., medroxyprogesterone acetate, 10-20 mg/day for 14 days per month), or **continuous progestin therapy** (e.g., megestrol acetate, 20-40 mg/day) appear to be effective.
- In a younger woman who wishes to retain her fertility treatment of choice for endometrial hyperplasia is Medroxy Progesterone Acetate 30-40 mg/day for 6-12 months or MIRENA IUCD". Surprisingly, Mirena is not effective against endometrial hyperplasia caused by tamoxifen. Continuous progestin therapy with megestrol acetate (40-160 mg/day) is probably the most reliable treatment for reversing complex or atypical hyperplasia. Therapy should be continued for 2 to 3 months and endometrial biopsy should be performed 3 to 4 weeks after completion of therapy to assess response. Periodic endometrial biopsy or transvaginal ultrasonography is advisable in patients being monitored after progestin therapy for atypical hyperplasia because of the presence of undiagnosed cancer in 25% of cases, the 29% progression rate to cancer and the high recurrence rate after treatment with progestins.
- Oral, parenteral, or intrauterine delivery of progestins may be used in selected women with atypical endometrial hyperplasia who wish to maintain their fertility
- For women with atypical complex hyperplasia who no longer desire fertility, hysterectomy is recommended.

Normally a 1-year period of amenorrhea after the age of 40 is considered as menopause. However, vaginal bleeding occurring any time after 6 months of amenorrhea in a menopausal age should be considered as postmenopausal bleeding and investigated. In the majority of women, estrogen withdrawal at menopause causes endometrial atrophy and the endometrium is only **1-3 mm** in thickness. The postmenopausal endometrium measuring **more than 4 mm** is considered abnormal

Classification of Endometrial Hyperplasias	
Type of Hyperplasia	**Progression to Cancer (%)**
Simple (cystic without atypia)	1
Complex (adenomatous without atypia)	3
Atypical	
Simple (cystic with atypia)	8
Complex (adenomatous with atypia)	29

47. Ans. (c) Azithromycin 2 g oral single dose

Ref: Park 23rd ed page 332, Novak 14th ed page 150, 151

This question is on Syndromic management of STI.

Option (A) and (B)

- Ceftriaxone is not included by NACO in its syndromic management KIT, however CDC recommends it to be used as first line management.
- Ceftriaxone 250 mg IM in a single dose PLUS Azithromycin 1g orally in a single dose
- If ceftriaxone is not available: Cefixime 400 mg orally in a single dose PLUS Azithromycin 1 g orally in a single dose
- CDC states **"A 400-mg oral dose of cefixime should only be considered as an alternative cephalosporin regimen because it does not provide as high, nor as sustained, bactericidal blood levels as a 250-mg dose of ceftriaxone"**

Option (C)

Monotherapy with azithromycin 2 g orally as a single dose has been demonstrated to be 99.2% effective against uncomplicated urogenital gonorrhea. However, monotherapy is no longer recommended because of concerns over the ease with which N. gonorrheae can develop resistance to macrolides and because several studies have documented azithromycin treatment failures. However in absence of any other more suitable option, Azithromycin 2 g Oral is the best answer.

Syndromic Management of STI

A woman is liable to several infections in the lower genital tract most common of which are gonorrhea, chlamydia, trichomonal infection, monilial infection and bacterial vaginosis. The tests and cultures take time, are costly and invite more visits to the clinic, therefore, 'syndrome management' approach is implemented. This consists of giving multiple drug therapy in one sitting and comprises 1 g azithromycin, 2 g metronidazole and 150 mg fluaride. Only those who fail to respond or those who are resistant are subjected to detailed investigations. Advantages of this approach are

- Single visit.
- Cost-effective.
- Quicker treatment.

Syndromic Management of STI			
STI/RTI Syndromic diagnosis	Name of the Kit	Color code of Kit	Contents of the Kits (Name of the Drugs)
Urethral Discharge (UD) Cervicitis (CD) Ano-rectal Discharge (ARD) Painful Scrotal Swelling (PSS) Presumptive Treatment (PT)	Kit-1	Gray	1 tablet of Azithromycin (1 g)/2 tablets of Azithromycin (500 mg) and 1 tablet of cefixme (400 mg)
Vaginitis/Vaginal discharge (VD) (TV + BV + Candida)	Kit-2	Green	• Tab. Secnidazole 2 g orally, single dose OR Tab. Metronidazole/Tinidazole 500 mg orally, twice daily for 5 days. • Tab. Metoclopropramide 30 minutes before Tab. Secnidazole, to prevent gastric intolerance. • Treat for candidiasis with Tab Fluconazole 150 mg orally single dose OR local Clotrimazole 500 mg vaginal pessaries once.
Genital Ulcer Disease Non Herpetic (GUD-NH)	Kit-3	White	Injection Benzathine penicillin (2.4 MU) + 1 tablet Azithromycin (1 g) + distilled water (10 mL) +
Genital Ulcer Disease Non Herpetic (GUD-NH)- for patients allergic to penicillin	Kit-4	Blue	28 tablets/capsules of Doxycycline (100 mg) and 1 tablet of Azithromycin (1 g)/2 tablets of Azithromycin (500 mg)
Genital Ulcer Disease - Herpetic (GUD-H)	Kit-5	Red	21 tablets of Acyclovir (400 mg)
Lower Abdominal Pain (LAP/PID)	Kit-6	Yellow	1 tablet of cefixime (400 mg) 28 tablets of Metronidazole (400 mg) 28 tablets of Doxycycline (100 mg)
Inguinal bubo (IB)	Kit-7	Black	42 tablets of Doxycyline (100 mg) and 1 tablet of Azithromycin (1 g)

48. Ans. (b) Hypertension at 10 weeks of pregnancy

Ref: William's 24th ed page 729, 738, Dutta's 7th ed page 219

Hypertensive disorders in pregnancy (NHBPEP 2000 classification)	
Hypertension	BP ≥140/90 mm Hg measured 2 times with at least a 6-hour interval
Proteinuria	Urinary excretion of ≥0.3 g protein/24 hours specimen or 0.1 gm/L
Gestational hypertension	BP ≥140/90 mm Hg for the first time in pregnancy after 20 weeks, without proteinuria
Pre-eclampsia	Gestational hypertension with proteinuria
Eclampsia	Women with pre-eclampsia complicated with convulsions and/or coma
Chronic hypertension	Known hypertension before pregnancy or hypertension diagnosed first time before 20 weeks of pregnancy
Superimposed pre-eclampsia or eclampsia	Occurrence of new onset of proteinuria in women with chronic hypertension

The term, **'Pregnancy-induced hypertension (PIH)'** is defined as the hypertension that develops as a direct result of the gravid state.

It includes—**(i) gestational hypertension, (ii) preeclampsia and (iii) eclampsia** and gestational hypertension is hypertension detected after 20 weeks of pregnancy.

- Hypertensive retinopathy- it is a complication of hypertension that can be seen in preeclampsia
- Hypertension at 10 weeks of pregnancy-it is detected after 20 weeks hence hypertension at 10 weeks was already present before pregnancy.
- Episode of seizure-it is called as eclampsia which is pregnancy induced
- Proteinuria-gestational hypertension with proteinuria is preeclampsia.

49. Ans. (b) Hysteroscopy and the toke biopsy

Ref: With text

Option (A)

PAP Smear: The false negative rate of pap smear in the presence of invasive cancer is 50% and a negative pap test should never be relied on in a symptomatic patient

Option (B)

Hysteroscopy and then take biopsy

Causes of postcoital bleeding:

- **Uterine** - pregnancy, endometrial polyps, endometrial hyperplasia, endometrial carcinoma, leiomyomata
- **Cervical**-polyps, cervicitis, cervical erosion, cervical dysplasia or neoplasia
- **Vaginal**- trauma, infection, atrophy
- **Perineal**- vulvar lesions , hemorrhoids. (Netter's obstetrics and gynecology 3rd ed, pg no 120)

Also, Postcoital bleeding is frequently associated with endocervical polyps.(Women's health, American College of Physicians-Menstrual disorders 2006) In a 35-year-old women, polyps is a fair common occurrence(incidence 20-40%). We cannot be sure that the cause is cervical malignancy only. Doing a hysteroscopy will detect any cause of the bleeding whether vaginal, cervical or uterine. But, Vaginal bleeding is the most common symptom in cancer cervix, most often which is postcoital bleeding but may occur as irregular or postmenopausal bleeding.**(Ref: Novak's 15th ed pg 1365).** So taking a biopsy is an imperative step. The biopsy could be done after VIA or VILI.

Option (C)

Four quadrant biopsy-It is a type of cervical biopsy. The types of cervical biopsy are punch biopsy, wedge biopsy, ring biopsy (not done) and four quadrant biopsy from 3,6,9 and 12 o'clock positions. (Practical manual of gynecology 2nd edition by Amitava Pal and Rupali Modak). Cervical biopsy is done as a diagnostic modality for cervical cancer.

Option (D)

Cervical conization is an invasive procedure and is required to assess correctly the depth and the linear extent of involvement when microinvasion is suspected. Early invasion is characterized by a protrusion of malignant cells from the stromal epithelial junction. This focus consists of cells that appear better differentiated than the adjacent noninvasive cells and have abundant pink-staining cytoplasm, hyperchromatic nuclei and small- to medium-sized nucleoli **(Novak 14th ed page 1406)**

Option (E)

Cryotherapy destroys the surface epithelium of the cervix by crystallizing the intracellular water using nitrous oxide or carbon dioxide. Hence cryotherapy is indicated only for biopsy proven cases of abnormal epithelium. Cryotherapy is ideal only for small superficial lesions.

50. Ans. (d) High prolactin levels

Ref: Shaw 16th ed page page 431

Hypogonadotropic hypogonadism	Hypergonadotropic hypogonadism	Normogonadotropic hypogonadism
• Low LH, Low FSH • Low testosterone • Low testicular volume (Oligospermia), • Low Prolactin levels	• High LH, High FSH • Low testosterone • Low testicular volume (Oligospermia) • High prolactin levels	Normal LH and FSH, Normal testosterone, Normal testicular volume and Normal prolactin levels

51. Ans. (b) Hyperprolactinemia

Ref: Novaks 15th ed page 1107

Bromocriptine is an ergot alkaloid, a strong dopamine agonist, decreases prolactin levels within hours. Dose: 1.25 to 2.5 mg BD, Hence it is given in Hyperprolactinemia.

52. Ans. (a) Bilateral gonadectomy

Ref: Leon speroff endocrinology 8th ed page 461, Novak's gynecology, 15th ed page 1040

See Table of CAUSES OF PRIMARY AMENORRHEA in AIIMS NOV 2016 (see page no. 882)

This is a case of Mixed Gonadal Dysgenesis (Turner's syndrome). Hypergonadotropic hypogonadism- elevated gonadotropins, and low estrogens is seen. With Karyotyping already done 45XO/46XX, there is no risk of gonadoblastoma hence Hormone replacement is the best management.

Option (A)

Even in the presence of typical turner stigmata, a karyotype is indicated to eliminate the presence of Y chromosome. Presence of Y chromosome is associated with 12% risk of gonadoblastoma. If Y chromosome is identified, laparoscopic prophylactic gonadectomy is recommended to eliminate the risk of malignancy. **(Novak's gynecology 15th ed page 1008, 1009)** Now since there is no Y chromosome in this case as provided in the question that Karyotyping is done, Gonadectomy is of no use.

Option (B)

Hypergonadotropic hypogonadism.- elevated gonadotropins, and low estrogens is seen in Turners syndrome. With Karyotyping already done 45XO/46XX, there is no risk of gonadoblastoma hence Hormone replacement is the best management.

Option (C) and (D)

Removing Clitoris and Valvuloplasty will solve no purpose and is totally unnecessary.

53. Ans. (b) Pawlik's grip

Ref: William's 24th ed page 437

Abdominal Palpation in Pregnancy Leopold's Maneuver			
	Purpose	**Procedure**	**Findings**
First maneuver: **(Fundal grip)**	To determine the fetal part lying in the fundus. To determine the presentation	Using both hands feel the fetal parts lying in the fundus	Heal is round, firm, hand and moves independently from the body. Breech is less well defined and moves only in conjunction with the body
Second Maneuver **(Umbilical grip)**	To determine location of fetal back and to determine position	One hand is used to steady the uterus on one side, other hand moves slowly on the opposite side from top to lower segment with circular motion to feel the back of the fetus	Fetal back is smooth, hard and resistant surface. Knees and elbows of fetus is felt as angular nodulation
Third Maneuver **(Pawlik's grip)**	To determine engagement of presenting part	Using thumb and finger grasp the upper part of abdomen above pubic symphysis. Press in slightly and make gentle movements from side to side	Presenting part is not engaged if it is not movable.
Fourth Maneuver **(Pelvic grip)**	To determine the degree of flexion of the fetal head. To determine attitude or Habitus	Facing for part of the woman, palpate fetal head pressing downward about 2 inches above the inguinal ligament.	Good attitude if brow corroesponds to the side (2nd maneuvre) that contained the elbows and knees. Poor attitude- If examining fingers will meet an obstruction on the same side as fetal back (hyperextended head)

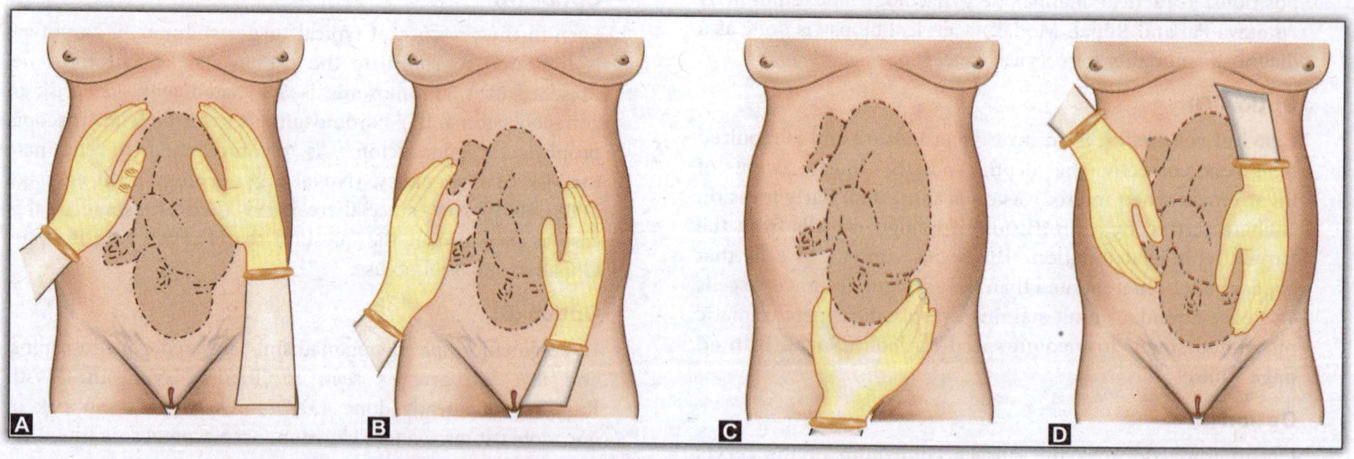

Figs A to D: Abdominal palpation: Leopold's maneuver; A. First maneuver (Fundal palpation); **B.** Second maneuver (Lateral palpation); **C.** Third maneuver (Pawlik's grip/second pelvic grip); **D.** Fourth maneuver (Pelvic palpation/first pelvic grip)

54. Ans. (b) Episiotomy scissor

Ref: William's 24th ed page 550

Repeat AIIMS MAY 2018 OBG (See for explanation) (see page no. 864)

AIIMS MAY 2017

55. Ans. (d) Hysteroscopy and Laparoscopy

Ref: Speroff 8th ed page 1108

HSG: Moderate sensitivity—65%

High specificity—83% in a typical infertile population

False negatives are much more common than false positives.

False-negative Causes

- Injection of contrast may cause "cornual spasm" misinterpreted as proximal tubal occlusion.
- Unilateral tubal patency and contralateral proximal occlusion may be due to catheter placement allowing contrast to take the path of least resistance.

False-positive Causes

- When contrast entering a widely dilated hydrosalpinx is diluted to yield a blush that is misinterpreted as evidence of tubal patency.
- Peritubular adhesions surrounding an otherwise normal and patent tube can sequester contrast as it escapes from the tube, resulting in a focal lobulation that can be misinterpreted as distal obstruction.

The clinical implications are that when HSG reveals obstruction there is still a relatively high probability (approximately 60%) that the tube is open, but when HSG demonstrates patency there is little chance the tube is actually occluded (approximately 5%).

- Laparoscopy is considered the gold standard for diagnosis of tubal and peritoneal diseases.
- Abnormal findings on HSG can be validated by direct visualization on laparoscopy.
- Chromopertubation involves the transcervical installation of a dye, such as methylene blue or indigo carmine. Tubal patency is assessed by direct laparoscopic visualization of the dye extruding through the fimbrial openings of the tubes.
- Along with laparoscopy hysteroscopy should also be done in the same sitting because in a case of infertility this will complete the examination.

56. Ans. (a) Do a CA 125 levels, if normal advise regular check up

Ref: RCOG Green-top Guideline No. 34, www.rcog.org.uk/globalassets/documents/guidelines/green-top-guidelines/gtg_34.pdf

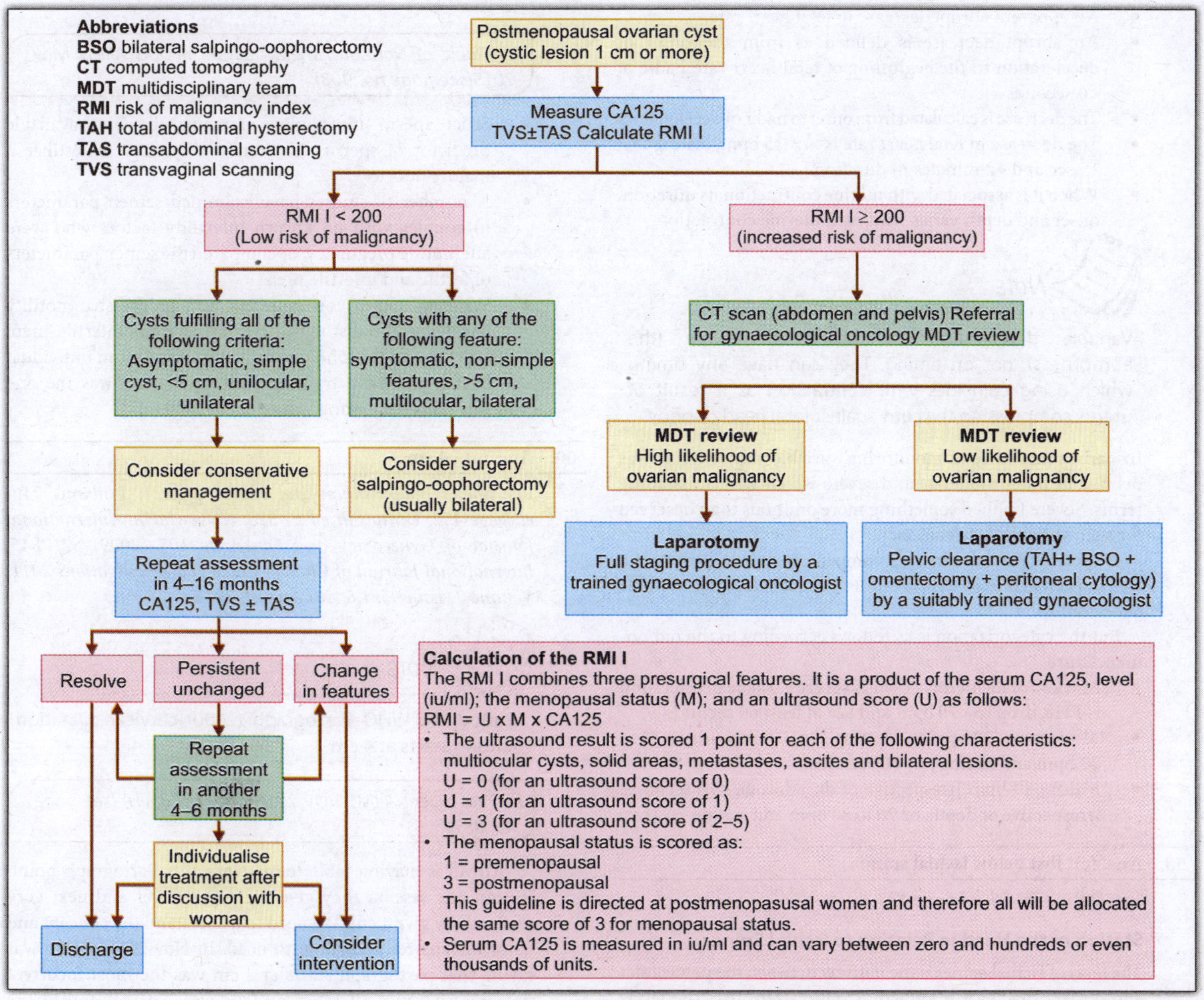

NOTE

There was a question in AIIMS MAY 2016 asking about the management of ovarian cyst in a young woman. Answer given has a flowchart showing the management of adnexal mass in a postmenopausal women as surgery. (Flowchart reference: Novak's gynae 15th ed pg 412).

Kindly do not get confused with that question because here the adnexal mass is a simple cyst and RCOG guidelines deal specifically with it. So the answer will not be surgery but CA 125 measurement.

57. Ans. (a) 70 beats per minute lasting for 60 seconds

Ref: William's 24th Ed page 98, 995 Fetal monitoring interpretation by Micki L.Cabbanis, Michael. G. Ross 2nd ed pg no 80

See Table of Fetal Monitor Pattern in OBG AIIMS NOV 2015 (see page no. 899)

Variable Deceleration is Defined as (as Per NICHD)

- An apparent abrupt decrease in fetal heart rate.
- An abrupt decrease is defined as from the onset of deceleration to the beginning of fetal heart rate nadir of <0 seconds.
- The decrease is calculated from onset to nadir of deceleration.
- The decrease in fetal heart rate is >/= 15 bpm, lasting >/= 15 sec and <2 minutes in duration.
- When it is associated with uterine contraction its duration, onset and depth varies with each uterine contraction.

NOTE

Variable deceleration are based on shape (the abruptness), not on timing. They can have any timing which using coincides with contraction as a result of uterus compressing the cord against fetal head or body.

In early years of fetal monitoring variable deceleration was defined as mild, moderate and severe which were misleading terms. Severe implied something more ominous than deserved for such variable deceleration.

A variable pattern can be a compensatory mechanism of a well oxygenated fetus. NICHD does not subcategorize variable deceleration.

But the categorization is as follows according to the old nomenclature.

- **Marked** or formerly known as **severe** variable deceleration is FHR drop to <70 bpm and last at least 60 seconds.
- **Moderate:** >70 bpm and lasting 30 to 60 seconds or 70 to 80 bpm and lasting >/= 60 seconds.
- **Mild:** >80 bpm irrespective of duration or <30 seconds, irrespective of depth, or 70 to 80 bpm and lasting <60 sec.

58. Ans. (c) Just below ischial spine

Ref: Dutta's obs 7th ed pg no 133

Station of the Head in Relation to Ischial Spines

The level of ischial spines is the halfway between the pelvic inlet and outlet. This level is known as station zero (0). The levels above and below the spines are divided into fifths to represent centimeters. The station is said to be 'O' if the presenting part is at the level of the spines. The station is stated in minus figures, if it is above the spines (–1 cm, –2 cm, –3 cm –4 cm and –5 cm) and in plus figures if it is below the spines (+1 cm, +2 cm, +3 cm, +4 cm and +5 cm).

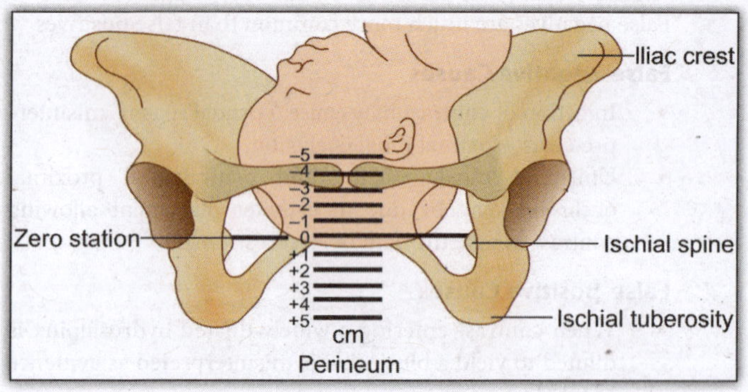

59. Ans. (b) The morphology of sperms

Ref: Speroff 8th ed pg no 1270-1271, Novak's Gynecology 15th ed page 1142

See Table of Normal Semen Analysis in OBG AIIMS May 2015(see page no. 908)

- Strict sperm morphology remains the best available predictor of sperm function (the capacity to fertilize a mature oocyte.
- A number of studies have examined semen parameters in couples with no known infertility factors who were attempting pregnancy, or compared the semen parameters of fertile and infertile men.
- Whereas sperm concentration and progressive motility had value for distinguishing fertile from infertile men, strict sperm morphology (as determined by an individual having extensive training and experience) was the one most discriminating value.

60. Ans. (a) 4 cm

Ref: Sheila Balakrishnan 2nd edition pg 121; William's 24th ed page 452, Dutta 6th ed p- 528, www.who.int, International Journal of Gynecology and Obstetrics 107 (2009) S21–S45, International Journal of Clinical Cases and Investigations 2011. Volume 3 (Issue 1), 1:6, 6th August, 2011

NOTE

In Modified WHO Partograph (2000) cervical dilatation plotting starts at 4 cm.

Indirect repeat AIIMS NOV 2016 (See for details) (see page no. 887)

AIIMS is playing table tennis with this Partograph point. Within one session they give 3 cm as answer and next very session they give 4 cm. We need to understand the concept and tailor the answer according to need. In Nov 2016 option was saying that partograph starts at 4 cm was the most incorrect statement because all other options were correct and in the original partograph plotting started at 3 cm cervical dilatation so 4 cm was chosen as the wrong statement. But here 3 cm is not in option and 4 cm is one option so we need it select 4 cm as answer.

61. Ans. (c) G4 P1 0+1+2

Ref: Dutta's 7th ed pg 94-95, 131

- **Gravida:** Gravida denotes a pregnant state both present and past, irrespective of the period of gestation. A woman *who delivers twins in first pregnancy is still a gravida one and para one.*
- **Parity:** Parity denotes a state of previous pregnancy beyond the period of viability.

NOTE

The 28th week is taken arbitrarily as the lower limit of fetal viability. (Dutta's Obs 7th ed pg 131)

- Infants now considered to be at the threshold of viability are those born at 22, 23, 24, or 25 weeks (American College of Obstetricians and Gynecologists, 2012a,b). (Williams obstetrics 24th ed pg no 1712).
- For all purposes we will consider 28 weeks as the period of viability being a developing country.

Past obstetric history is summarized by two methods.

Two digits (the first one relates with viable births and the second one relates with abortion) connected with a plus sign affixing the letter 'P'.

Thus P2+1 denote the patient had two viable births and one abortion.

It is also expressed by four digits connected by dashes.

PA–B–C–D, where

A denotes number of term (37 to 42 weeks) pregnancies

B – Number of preterm (28 to <37 weeks) pregnancies

C – Number of miscarriages (<28 weeks)

D – The number of children alive at present.

The given patient is pregnant for the fourth time hence is G4 and P1-0-2-1.

But, this option is not given and considering that the given options are what were actually present, there is a general use format called as G (gravida) P (para) L (live issues) A (abortions) format used in history taking and is widely practiced.

Our patient is G4, P1 (one girl delivered at term) 0 (no preterm deliveries)+1(one living issue)+2 (2 abortions).

62. Ans. (c) Wertheim hysterectomy

Ref: Shaw 15th ed pg no 184, 414

- 75% of ureteric injuries occur with gynecological procedures.
- 3/4th of which occur in abdominal procedures.
- 1–2% highest incidence is seen with extensive surgeries for invasive carcinoma.
- Incidence is higher for abdominal (1–2%) than with vaginal (0.1%) hysterectomy.
- The incidence of ureterovaginal fistula after laparoscopic hysterectomy appears to be 1% to 4%. (Novak's gynaec 15th ed pg no 870).

Hence risk of ureteric injury.

Laparoscopic Hysterectomy (1–4%) >Abdominal (1–2 %) >Vaginal Hysterectomy (0.1%)

Also, the risk is high when the surgery is undertaken for pelvic endometriosis, pelvic inflammatory disease, cervical and broad ligament, Wertheim hysterectomy when the ureter anatomy is distorted.

63. Ans. (c) Estimate serum estradiol values

Ref: Novak's 15th ed pg 1036

World Health Organization (WHO) Classes of Amenorrhea		
Group I	**Group II**	**Group III**
No evidence of endogenous estrogen production, normal or low FSH levels, normal prolactin levels and no lesion in the hypothalamic-pituitary region.	Evidence of estrogen production and normal levels of prolactin and FSH.	Elevated serum FSH indicating gonadal insufficiency or failure.

The given patient belongs to gonadal failure group.

Option (A)

Give progesterone and stop after 10 days for withdrawal bleeding and

Option (B)

Check USG for polycystic ovaries. It is not PCOS because in it LH/FSH ratio is increased. Also progesterone challenge test would be positive in anovulation cases, i.e. PCOS.

Option (C)

Women with hypoestrogenic amenorrhea have either ovarian failure or hypothalamic-pituitary dysfunction. Serum concentrations of FSH and LH of more than 40-50 mIU/mL are diagnostic of ovarian failure. Serial assessments may be necessary because of the pulsatile nature of pituitary gonadotropin secretion. Most women under the age of 40 years belonging to this category have premature ovarian failure. Overt primary ovarian insufficiency (POI) is defined as the presence of amenorrhea for 4 months or more accompanied by two serum FSH levels in the menopausal range for a woman who is less than 40 years of age. Serum estradiol values will be low in gonadal failure cases like premature ovarian failure. (Novak's 15th ed pg 1157)

Option (D)

Urine pregnancy test is of no use because FSH and LH would be normal in that case. Although our diagnosis is made before doing serum estradiol as FSH is high which would not be in PCOS still doing serum estradiol seems to be the most appropriate answer of the given options which would be normal in PCOS and low in premature ovarian failure.

64. Ans. (b) Supine vena cava syndrome

Ref: Williams 24th ed page 1369, Dutta 6th Ed page 52

Compression of vena cava by gravid uterus in supine position leads to opening of collaterals, however in some people when they fail to open, it leads to compromised venous return and hence hypotension. It is treated by turning patient to lateral position. It is not abdominal aorta, or superior vena cava or ascending aorta because we can see the uterus compressing the vessel which is inferior vena cava.

65. Ans. (c) Manual support to perineum with deflexion of head

Ref: WHO guidelines

http://apps.who.int/iris/bitstream/10665/63167/1/WHO_FRH_MSM_96.24.pdf

Option (A) Perform Labor in Lithotomy Position

The lithotomy position with the legs in stirrups was experienced as less comfortable and more painful and restricted in movement. Women who had given birth in that position would prefer the option of an upright position in the future. (WHO guidelines http://apps.who.int/iris/bitstream/10665/63167/1/WHO_FRH_MSM_96.24.pdf)

"During second-stage labor, pushing positions may vary. But for delivery, dorsal lithotomy position is the most widely used and often the most satisfactory. For better exposure, leg holders or stirrups are used." (Williams obs 24th ed pg 1080).

As understood it is not a guideline by WHO but is widely practized.

Option (B) Give Warm Compress to the Perineum

Another technique aiming at reducing the risk of trauma to the perineum, is massaging the perineum during the last part of the second stage of labor, thus attempting to stretch the tissues. The technique has never been properly evaluated, but there may be doubts about the benefit of the sustained rubbing of tissues that are already highly vascularized and edematous. Hence is not a guideline.

Option (C) Manual Support to Perineum with Deflexion of Head

Many textbooks describe the practice of guarding the perineum during delivery of the fetal head: the fingers of one hand (usually the right) support the perineum, while the second hand applies pressure to the fetal head to control the speed of crowning, thus trying to prevent or reduce damage to the perineal tissues. It is possible that by this maneuver a perineal tear may be prevented, but it is also conceivable that the pressure on the fetal head impedes the extension movement of the head and diverts it from the pubic arch to the perineum, thus increasing the chance of perineal damage. Because there have been no formal evaluations of this strategy or of the opposite: not touching the perineum or the head during this phase of delivery, it is impossible to decide which strategy is preferable. (WHO guidelines (http://apps.who.int/iris/bitstream/10665/63167/1/WHO_FRH_MSM_96.24.pdf)

"When the head distends the vulva and perineum enough to open the vaginal introitus to a diameter of 5 cm or more, a gloved hand may be used to support the perineum. The other hand is used to guide and control the fetal head to avoid expulsive delivery". (Willams obs 24th ed pg 1082)

"If expulsive efforts are inadequate or expeditious delivery is needed, the modified Ritgen maneuver may be employed. With this, gloved fingers beneath a draped towel exert forward pressure on the fetal chin through the perineum just in front of the coccyx. Concurrently, the other hand presses superiorly against the occiput. Originally described in 1855, the Ritgen maneuver allows controlled fetal head delivery. It also favors neck extension so that the head passes through the introitus and over the perineum with its smallest diameters."(Williams obs 24th ed pg 547).

Hence although not a guideline it is mentioned in all the standard texts to perform the perineum guard during the head delivery.

Option (D) Do a Routine Episiotomy

There is no reliable evidence that liberal or routine use of episiotomy has a beneficial effect, but there is clear evidence that it may cause harm. A restricted use of this intervention is recommended.

If we see the WHO guidelines none of the options is true but considering the standard texts most appropriate answer is (C) Manual support to perineum with deflexion of head >(A) Perform labor in lithotomy position.

66. Ans. (a) Give another dose of Anti D 72 hours postpartum depending on the baby's blood group

Ref: RCOG guidelines; William's 24th ed page 312, 643

Recommendation for RAADP (Routine Antenatal Anti D Prophylaxis)

- Anti-D immune globulin is given prophylactically to all Rh D-negative, unsensitized women at approximately 28 weeks and a second dose is given after delivery if the infant is Rh D-positive. (ACOG 2010)
- Following delivery, anti-D immune globulin should be given within 72 hours.
- Importantly, if immune globulin is inadvertently not administered following delivery, it should be given as soon as the omission is recognized, because there may be some protection up to 28 days postpartum.
- Anti-D immune globulin is also administered after pregnancy related events that could result in fetomaternal hemorrhage

67. Ans. (a) Colposcopy and biopsy

Ref: ASCCP guidelines, Novak's 15th ed page 574, 589

- The HSIL category includes CIN 2 and CIN 3 (moderate dysplasia, severe dysplasia and carcinoma in situ).
- Any woman with a cytologic specimen suggesting the presence of HSIL should undergo colposcopy and directed biopsy.
- This is because two-thirds of patients with this cytologic finding will have CIN2 or greater.
- After colposcopically directed biopsy and determination of the distribution of the lesion, excisional or ablative therapy that addresses the entire transformation zone should be performed.

68. Ans. (a) Metronidazole

Ref: Novak's gynae 15th ed page 560, KDT 7th ed page 83

Drug of choice for Trichomonas Vaginalis is Metronidazole or tinidazole, 2 g orally (single dose) or Metronidazole, 500 mg PO bid for 7 days.

Vaginitis and Bacterial Vaginosis				
	Normal vagina	Bacterial vaginosis	*Trichomonas vaginalis* vaginitis	*Candida albicans* vulvovaginitis
Microorganism	Lactobacilli	Gardenella vaginalis, hemophillus vaginosis, ureplasma ureolyticum, mycoplasma hominis, mobilincus	Trichomonas vaginalis	Candida albicans
Primary symptoms	None	Discharge with fishy odor, may have itching	Discharge, bad odor, may have itching, **Strawberry vagina**	Discharge; itching and burning of vulvar skin
Vaginal discharge	Slight, white, flocculent	Slightly increased, thin, homogeneous, white, gray, adherent with fishy odor	Profuse, yellow, green, frothy, adherent; cervical petechiae often present, with fishy odor (±)	Increased, white, curdy like **cottage cheese**
Inflammation of vulvar or vaginal epithelium	None	None (Hence vaginosis not vaginitis)	Erythema of vaginal and vulvar epithelium; colpitis macularis	Erythema of vaginal epithelium, introitus; vulvar dermatitis, fissures common
PH	<4.5	>4.5	>4.5	≤4.5
Amine ("fishy") odor with 10% KOH **(Whiff test)**	None	Present	May be present	None
Microscopy	Epithelial cells with lactobacilli	**Clue cells**; few leukocytes; no lactobacilli or only a few outnumbered by profuse mixed microbiota, nearly always including *G. vaginalis* plus anaerobic species on g's stain (Nugent's score ≥7)	By **hanging drop technique**, Leukocytes; motile trichomonads seen in 80–90% of symptomatic patients, less often in the absence of symptoms	KOH preparation showing budding yeasts and pseudohyphae in up to 80% of *C. albicans* culture positive persons with typical symptoms
Treatment	None	DOC- **Metronidazole** 500 mg PO bid for 7 days Metronidazole gel, 0.75%, one applicator (5 g) intravaginally once daily for 5 days, Clindamycin 2% cream, one full applicator vaginally each night for 7 days	• Metronidazole or tinidazole, 2 g orally (single dose) Metronidazole, 500 mg PO bid for 7 days • If recurrence metronidazole 2 g po for 5 days. • If refractory culture sensitivity for metronidazole and tinidazole	Azole cream, tablet, or suppository—e.g., miconazole (100-mg vaginal suppository) or clotrimazole (100-mg vaginal tablet) once daily for 7 days Fluconazole, 150 mg orally (single dose)
Usual management of sexual partner	None	None	Examination for STD; treatment with metronidazole, 2 g PO (single dose)	None; topical treatment if candidal dermatitis of penis is detected

69. Ans. (a) High estrogen

Ref: Robbin Basic Pathology 10th edition. Page. 721, Shaw's gynaec 15th ed pg 466

Whatever the initial genesis of endometriosis, its further development depends on the presence of hormones, mainly estrogen. Various facts proving it are:

- Pregnancy causes atrophy of endometriosis chiefly through high progesterone level.
- Regression follows oophorectomy and irradiation.
- Rarely seen before puberty and it regresses after menopause.
- Hormones with antioestrogenic activity also suppress endometriosis and are used therapeutically.

AIIMS NOVEMBER 2016

70. Ans. (b) Partial androgen insensitivity

Ref: Williams 24th ed page 149, Shaw's 15th ed page 111, Speroff 8th ed page 374-376

Similar question with different case scenario was asked in AIIMS MAY 2015 and AIIMS NOV 2011, see for differentiation. The girl is having gonads visible in inguinal canal which are undescended testis and since she is not responsive to androgens she is having no axillary or pubic hair but clitoromegaly points towards partial androgen insensitivity.

NOTE

Mutations in the androgen receptor (AR) cause resistance to androgen (testosterone, DHT) action or the *androgen insensitivity syndrome* (AIS).

Causes of Primary Amenorrhea					
Feature	**Mullerian agenesis/ MRKH syndrome**	**Androgen insensitivity syndrome (Testicular feminisation syndrome)**	**Mixed gonadal dysgenesis (Turner syndrome)**	**Pure gonadal dysgenesis (Hypergonadotropic hypogonadism) (Swyer syndrome)**	**Kallmann syndrome (Hypogonadotropic hypogonadism)**
Genotype	46; XX	46, XY	45, XO/Mosaic (45X/46XX ; 45XO/46XY)	46 XX or 46 XY karyotypes **(Swyer syndrome)**	Normal
Cause	Polygenic and multifactorial inheritance. HOX genes are essential for development of the müllerian tract in the embryonic period	Mutations in the androgen receptor (AR) cause resistance to androgen (testosterone, DHT) action or the *Androgen insensitivity syndrome* (AIS).	Aneuploidy	Streak gonads with no AMH or androgen production (mutation in SRY gene), gonads undergo premature degeneration	Failure of both olfactory axonal and GnRH neuronal migration from the olfactory placode in the nose.
Phenotype	Female	Female	Female	Female	Male > Female
Presentation	Amenorrhea or Cryptomenorrhea Mullerian agenesis or hypoplasia can be A. Vaginal B. Cervical C. Fundal D. Tubal E. Combined Uterine malformations causing spontaneous abortion, preterm labor, abnormal presentations and complications of labor (i.e., retained placenta)	Most patients present with- inguinal hernias (containing testes) in childhood or with primary amenorrhea in adulthood.	Primary amenorrhea, poor growth, short stature, webbed neck, low set ears, posterior hairline, short 4th metacarpal, cubitus valgus. Cardiac lesions (coarctation of aorta -MC) Could be more like normal in mosaic cases	For 46 XX: Ovarian development and subsequent internal and external genitalia development proceed normally. There could be minimal pubertal development and sometimes menstruation also. **For 46,XY** karyotype: Primary amenorrhea with delayed sexual maturation but normal growth and intellectual development.	Females present with primary amenorrhea, infantile sexual development, associated with anosmia or hyposmia with color blindness in men and cleft lip and palate, cerebellar ataxia, nerve deafness and abnormalities of thirst and vasopressin release in women.
Secondary sexual characteristics and physical characteristics.	**Present. Well developed** breasts and pubic hair (Tanner stage 4)	**Present but asynchronous.** Normal or ↑ breast development (due to aromatization of testosterone). Scanty pubic and axillary hair (tanner stage 1 or 2) Female psychosexual orientation	Infantile. Absent secondary sexual development	Normal müllerian structures. Normal uterus, tubes, cervix and vagina.	Normal according to genotype
Reproductive organs	Any transverse blockage of the müllerian system. Such outflow obstructions include imperforate hymen, transverse vaginal septum and hypoplasia or absence of the uterus, cervix, vagina and various uterine malformations; bicornuate, unicornuate, didelphys. Normal ovaries.	Short, blind vagina but no uterus (because MIS production is normal) Testes rather than ovaries are present in the abdomen or in inguinal hernias because of the presence of normally functioning genes on the Y chromosome.	Normal or hypoplastic uterus with tubes. **Streak ovaries** present.	Normal müllerian structures and **streak gonads** Female external genitalia, uterus, fallopian tubes. Minimal breast enlargement reflects peripheral aromatization of androgens	External phenotype and internal genitalia are according to the genotype. Adrenarche occurs despite the absence of gonadarche.

Contd...

Causes of Primary Amenorrhea					
Feature	Mullerian agenesis/ MRKH syndrome	Androgen insensitivity syndrome (Testicular feminisation syndrome)	Mixed gonadal dysgenesis (Turner syndrome)	Pure gonadal dysgenesis (Hypergonadotropic hypogonadism) (Swyer syndrome)	Kallmann syndrome (Hypogonadotropic hypogonadism)
Biochemical abnormalities	Gonadotropins are normal.	Gonadotropins and testosterone; ↓, ↑ or N depending on degree of androgen resistance and contribution of estradiol to feedback inhibition of hypothalamic pituitary gonadal axis. AMH/MIS levels: ↑or N	Hypergonadotropic hypogonadism. - elevated gonadotropins, and low estrogens	The 46,XY gonadal dysgenesis patients show elevated gonadotropins, and low estrogens (Hypergonadotropic hypogonadism)	Hypogonadotropic (Low GNRH) hypogonadism
Variant/ Associations	Associated with abnormal galactose metabolism. Absent, pelvic, or horseshoe kidney (15%), Double urinary collecting system (40%), skeletal abnormalities (5-12%)	PARTIAL AIS **(Reifenstein's Syndrome):**	**Noonan syndrome:** 46 XX/ XY, Autosomal dominant, Normal males and females with phenotype features of turner's syndrome. Normal gonads with normal fertility		
Management and treatment	**Hymenectomy** for imperforate hymen (cruciate incision), surgical correction depending on the abnormality and vaginoplasty before marriage.	**Gonadectomy** sometimes is performed, as there is a low risk of malignancy and estrogen replacement is prescribed. Alternatively, the gonads can be left in situ until breast development is complete. The use of graded dilators in adolescence is usually sufficient to dilate the vagina and permit sexual intercourse.	Sequential sex steroid treatment regimen, **Gonadectomy** if XY mosaic component present, soon after puberty	**Gonadectomy:** As early in life as possible because of the known risk of tumor development. Pulsatile administration of exogenous GnRH and clearly this is the most physiologic approach to ovulation induction.	Treatment of patients with a drug (naltrexone) which blocks opioid receptors restores normal function (ovulation and pregnancy). Also, induction of ovulation with exogenous gonadotropins is successful.
Fertility	Depending on the uterine malformation. **Oocyte donation, IVF** followed by surrogacy is a feasible option	Infertile	**Rare spontaneous pregnancy** with a high risk (30%) of congenital abnormalities. **IVF with donor oocyte** if normal uterus and **IVF with surrogacy** if hypoplastic uterus.	For women not seeking pregnancy, therapy with exogenous estrogen and progestin is indicated. **IVF with donor oocytes** since normal uterus.	

Androgen Insensitivity Syndrome				
Clinical features	Complete AIS	Partial AIS/Female	Partial AIS/Male (Reifenstein syndrome)	Minimal AIS
Gender	Female	Female	Male	Male
Genital appearance	Completely female external genitalia, short vagina	Clitoromegaly, narrow vagina, variable fusion of labia minora	Hypospadias, variable scrotum bifidum	Unambiguous male
Location of gonads	Mostly abdominal or inguinal	Mostly inguinal	Mostly scrotal	Scrotal
Pubertal development	Feminization	Breast development and slight virilization	Persistent gynecomastia and slight virilization	Gynecomastia and virilization
Secondary sexual hair	Sparse to absent	Sparse	Slightly diminished	Slightly diminished

Contd...

Spermatogenesis	Absent	Absent	Absent to severely impaired	Mostly severely impaired
AR gene mutations	Located throughout AR gene	Mostly DNA-binding and hormone binding domain	Mostly DNA-binding and hormone binding domain	Located throughout AR gene, in case of spino-bulbar muscular atrophy: within CAG repeat region of N-terminal region
Timing of gonadectomy	Postpubertal gonadectomy favored	Prepubertal gonadectomy favored	No gonadectomy, but surveillance recommended	No gonadectomy, but surveillance recommended

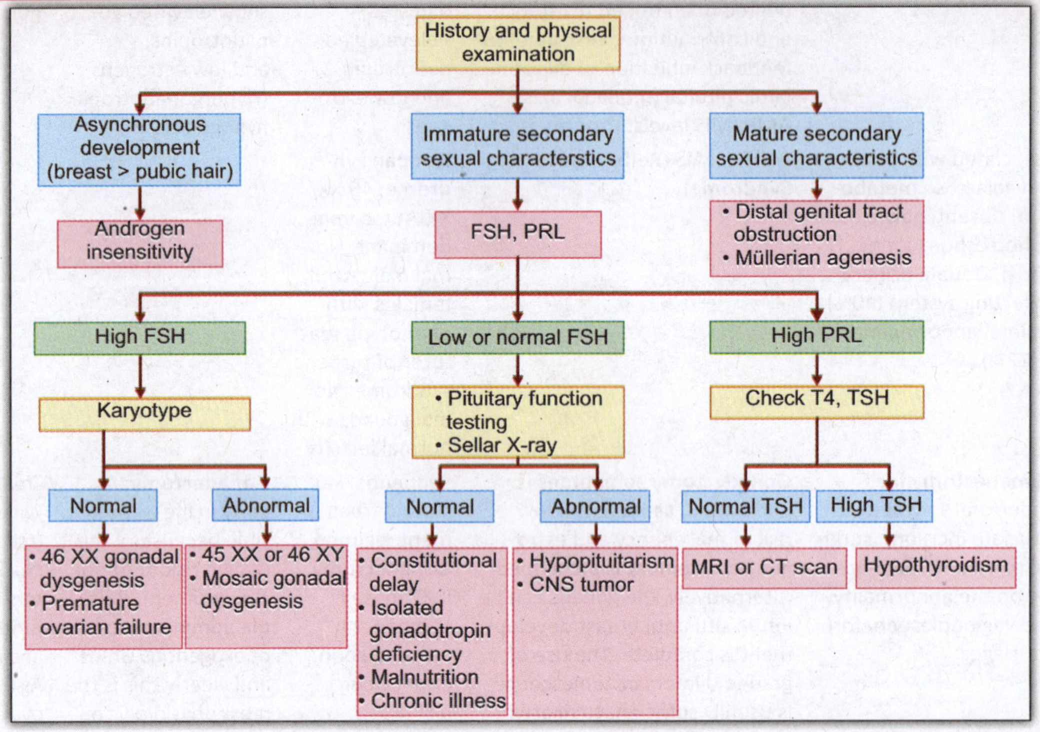

71. Ans. (c) Terminate the pregnancy because of high risk of infection

Ref: Novak's 14th ed page 375

A woman with an IUD in place who has amenorrhea should have a pregnancy test and pelvic examination.

- **If an intrauterine pregnancy is diagnosed and the IUD strings are visible, the IUD should be removed as soon as possible to prevent later septic abortion, premature rupture of the membranes and premature birth.**
- When the strings of the IUD are not visible, an ultrasound examination should be performed to localize the IUD. **If the IUD is present, therapeutic abortion, Ultrasound guided intrauterine removal of the IUD or continuation of the pregnancy with the device left in place if the patient wishes.** When pregnancy continues with an IUD in place, the patient must be warned of the symptoms of intrauterine infection.
- There is a very high risk of infection in developing countries like ours hence IUCD should be removed and pregnancy terminated.

William's: Until about 14 weeks, the tail may be visible through the cervix and if seen, it should be removed. This action reduces subsequent complications such as late abortion, sepsis and preterm birth (Alvior, 1973). Tatum and co-workers (1976) reported an abortion rate of 54 percent with the device left in place compared with a rate of 25 percent if it was promptly removed.

William's: Second-trimester abortion with an IUD in place is more likely to be infected (Vessey and associates, 1974). Sepsis may be fulminant and fatal. Pregnant women with a device in utero who demonstrate any evidence of pelvic infection are treated withintensive antimicrobial therapy and prompt uterine evacuation. Because of these risks, a woman should be given the option of early pregnancy termination if the device cannot be removed.

RCOG says **"Women with an intrauterine pregnancy with an IUD in situ should be advised to have the IUD removed before 12 completed weeks' gestation, whether or not they intend to continue the pregnancy".**

The NHS Clinical Knowledge Summary adds:

"The reason for recommending that a copper intrauterine device (IUD) not be removed if the gestational age is more than 12 weeks is that:

- It is believed that after this time, the gestational sac occupies the whole of the uterine cavity and removal would endanger the pregnancy.
- Threads are more likely to be visible in the first trimester than later; in the second trimester, threads are unlikely

to be visible unless the device is at the lower pole of the uterus or in the endocervical canal."

Each of the patients can prefer either termination of pregnancy or continue her pregnancy and thus, when a pregnant woman decides to continue her pregnancy, the IUD is removed if strings are visible (Ref: Pak J Med Sci. 2016;32(5):1087–1091) American college of Obsteticians and Gynecologists committee opinion No 672, Sept 2016

Management of IUD in Pregnancy

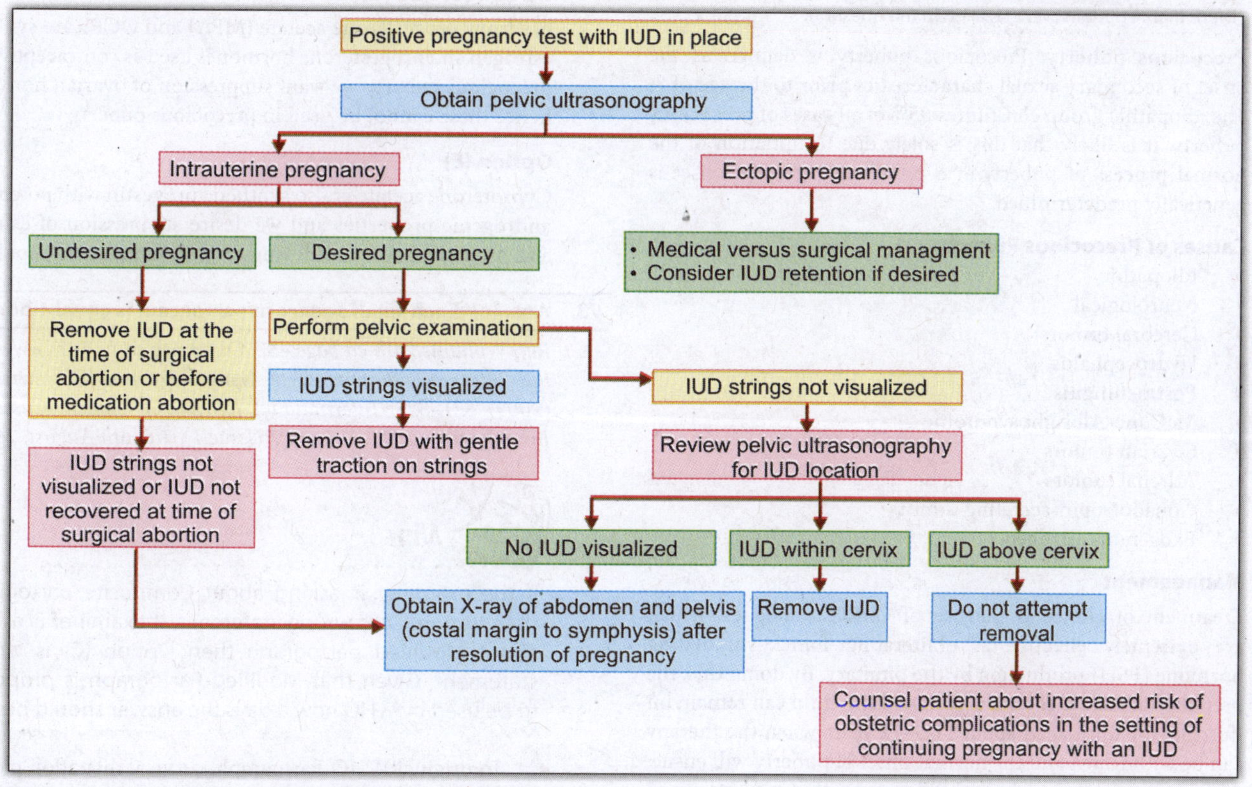

Management of Nonvisualized IUD

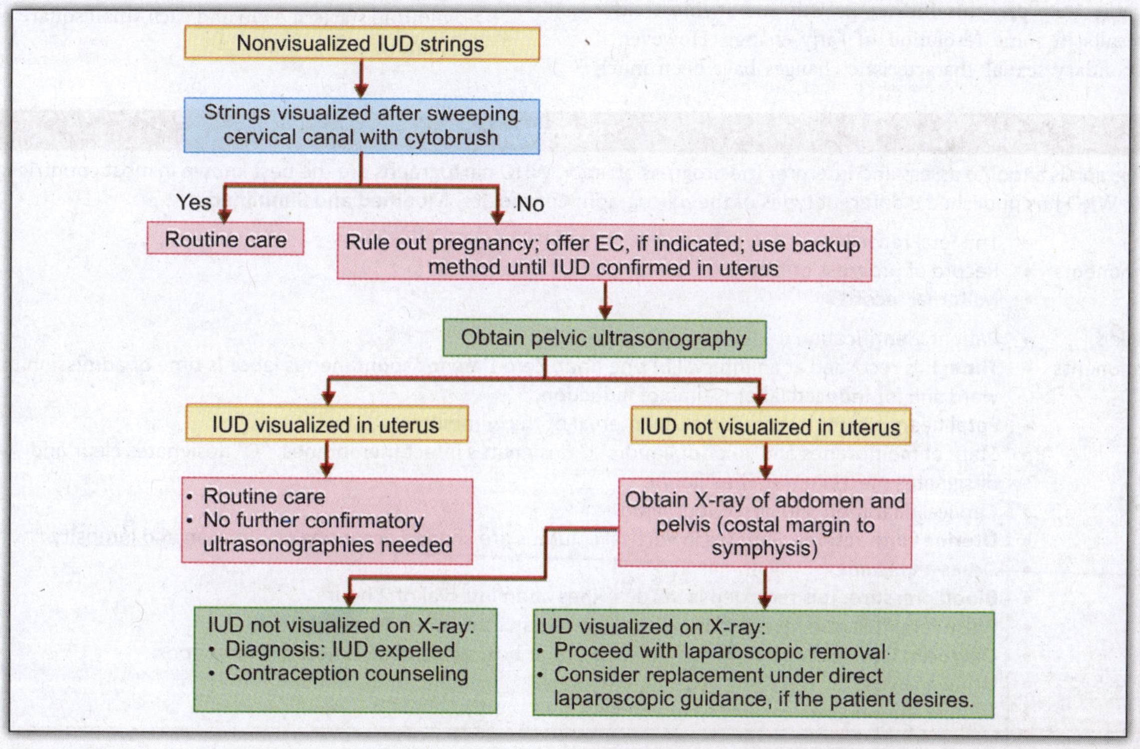

72. Ans. (a) GnRH analog

Ref: Shaw 15th ed page 56, Dewhurst's Textbook of Obstetrics and Gynecology 7 ed page 366

Recall Bias

More than 4 options were recalled in this question.

Precocious puberty: Precocious puberty is defined as the onset of secondary sexual characteristics prior to the age of 8. The idiopathic group constitutes 95% of all cases of precocious puberty. It is likely that this is solely due to initiation of the normal process of puberty at a premature age. The onset is genetically predetermined.

Causes of Precocious Puberty

- Idiopathic
- Neurological
- Cerebral tumors
- Hydrocephalus
- Postmeningitis
- McCune-Albright syndrome
- Ovarian tumors
- Adrenal tumors
- Gonadotropin-secreting tumors
- Exogenous estrogen

Management

Treatment of choice is the use of GnRH analogues, which are extremely effective at obliterating follicle-stimulating hormone (FSH) production by the pituitary. By doing this, the prepubertal state is re-established and the child can remain on this therapy until aged about 11.5–12 years when the therapy can be withdrawn and the normal onset of puberty will ensue. Any breast or pubic hair development that has occurred prior to the diagnosis will usually be reversible as the hypo-estrogenic state prevents further growth and in most cases this results in some resolution of early change. However, if the secondary sexual characteristic changes have been much greater and development is beyond Tanner stage 3, little effect can be expected by this therapy on the physical changes.

Option (B)

Danazol- is used in AUB, endometriosis, adenomyosis, mastalgia, autoimmune disorders

Option (C) and (D)

Medroxy progesterone acetate (MPA) and OCP's are synthetic estrogen and progesterone hormones used as contraceptives. In precocious puberty we want suppression of ovarian hormones hence these cannot be used in precocious puberty.

Option (E)

Cyproterone acetate is also synthetic progestin with potent anti androgenic properties and we desire suppression of estrogen and progesterone for achieving reversal in precocious puberty.

73. Ans. (c) Each small square in partogram is equal 1 hour

Ref: William's 24th ed page 452, Dutta 6th ed p- 528, www.who.int, International Journal of Gynecology and Obstetrics 107 (2009) S21–S45, International Journal of Clinical Cases and Investigations 2011. Volume 3 (Issue 1), 1:6, 6th August, 2011

NOTE

If the examiner is asking about Composite partograph then option (D) is wrong statement, If examiner is asking about Modified partograph then Option (C) is wrong statement. Given that Modified Partograph is proposed to be used by WHO now a days the answer should be (C)

- In original WHO Partograph, cervical dilatation plotting starts at 3 hours and each small square measures 1 hour.
- In Modified WHO Partograph (2000) cervical dilatation plotting starts at 4 cm and each small square measures 30 minutes

Partograph	
Partograph is a tool to assess and interpret the progress of labor. WHO partographs are the best known in most countries. Since the 1990, WHO has published 3 different types of the partograph; **Composite, Modified and Simplified.**	
Major Components	• The fetal record • Record of progress of labor • Maternal record
Detailed Components	• Patient identification • **Time:** It is recorded at an interval of one hour. Zero time for spontaneous labor is time of admission in the labor ward and for induced labor is time of induction. • **Fetal heart rate:** It is recorded at an interval of thirty minutes. • State of membranes and color of liquor: "I" designates intact membranes, "C" designates clear and "M" designates meconium stained liquor. • Cervical dilatation and descent of head • **Uterine contractions:** Squares in vertical columns are shaded according to duration and intensity. • Drugs and Fluids • **Blood pressure:** It is recorded in vertical lines at an interval of 2 hours. • **Pulse rate:** It is also recorded in vertical lines at an interval of 30 minutes. • **Oxytocin:** Concentration is noted down in upper box; while dose is noted in lower box. • Urine analysis • Temperature record

Contd...

Partograph	
Principles of WHO **Composite partograph** (1990)	• Latent phase = 8 hours • Active stage of labor starts at 3 cm cervical dilatation • During active stage, cervix should dilate at the rate of **1 cm per hour** (slope of alert line) • Action line is 4 hours to the right of and parallel to the alert line. • 1 square = 1 hour

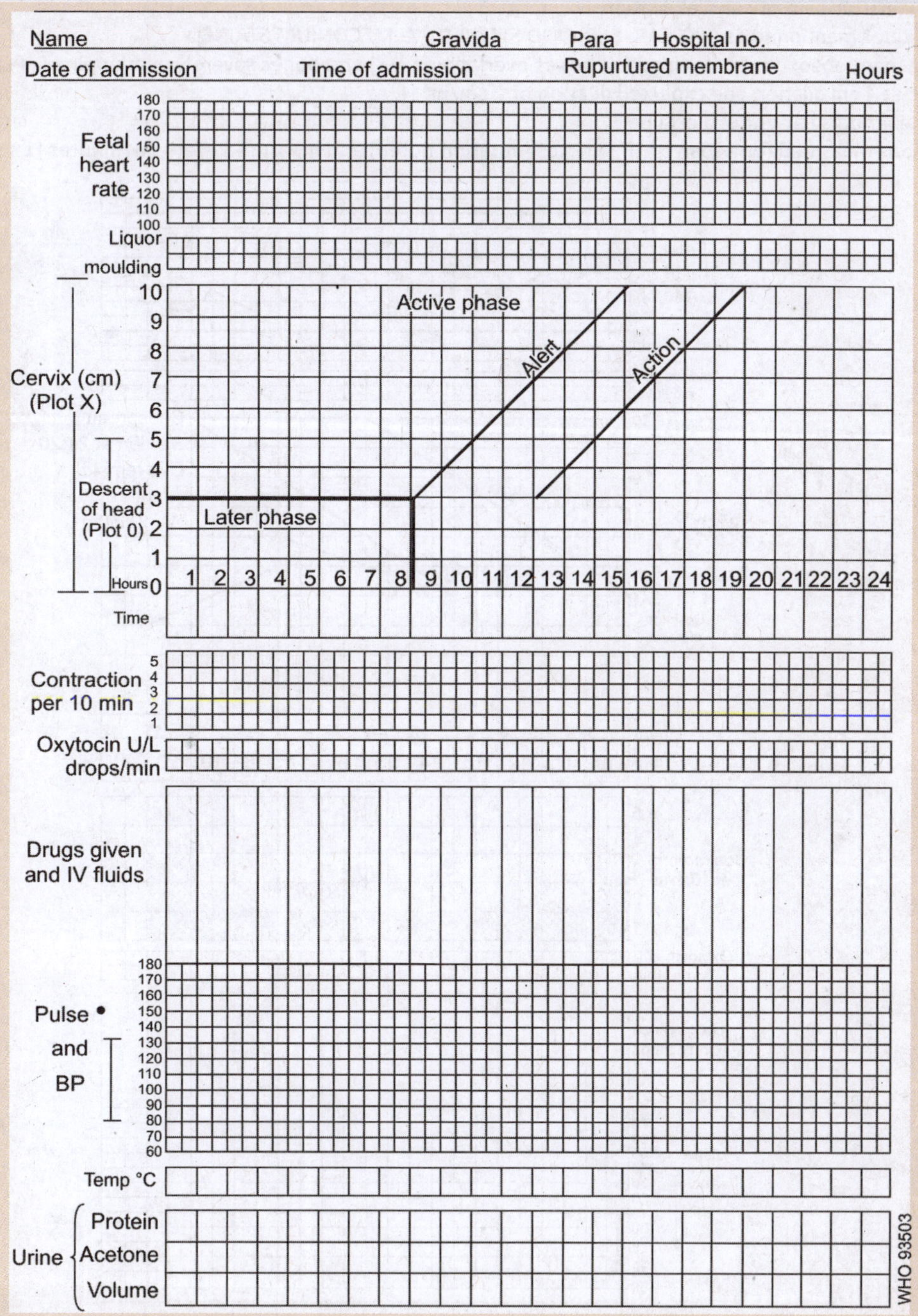

- Once labor is diagnosed, its progress is charted on a partogram by abdominal and vaginal examinations.
- Labor is considered normal as long as the progress of cervical dilatation is to the left of alert line.
- Prolonged labor is diagnosed, once the alert line is crossed i.e shift to right. There is considered an indication for intervention
- If the patient is in peripheral hospital, once the alert line is crossed, it is an indication for referral to higher center.
- Thus partogram can be used to identify an abnormal labor pattern and to indicate the correct time for intervention by means of alert and action lines

WHO Modified Partograph: WHO modified the partograph for use in hospitals in 2000. The latent phase was excluded in this partograph. The active phase commences at 4 cm dilatation. The other features are the same as the composite WHO partograph.

Contd...

Partograph

The reason for excluding the latent phase were that interventions are more likely if the latent phase is included and because staff reported difficulties in transferring from latent to active phase. The choice of 4 cm was made to reduce the risk of interventions in multiparous women with patulous cervices who were not yet in labor"

Changes in modified partogram by WHO:

- No latent phase
- Charting starts at 4 cm of cervical dilation
- Color of liquor mentioned as C- CLEAR, B- BLOOD STAINED, M- MECONIUM STAINED
- Moulding mentioned: bones touching (+), bones overlapping (++) and bones severely overlapping (+++)
- Alert line: at 4 cm dilation and expected dilation of 1 cm/hr
- Action line 4 hours to right of alert line
- Contractions measured for a span of 10 minutes (duration noted) and measured every 30 minutes (1 square = half hour)

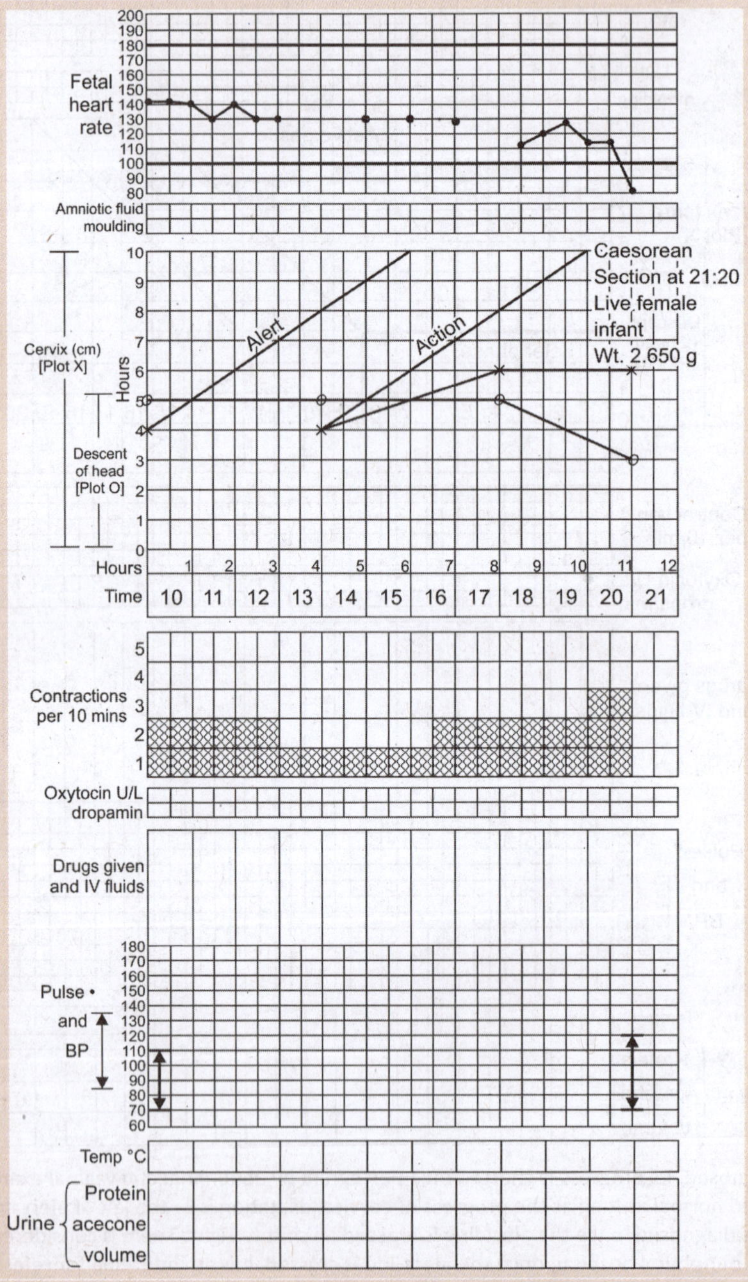

WHO Simplified Partograph: WHO further modified the paragraph for the third time, this time for use by skilled attendants in health centers. This simplified partograph is color coded. The area to the left of the alert line in the cervicograph is colored green, representing normal progress. The area to the right of the action line is colored red, indicating dangerously slow progress in labor. The area in between the alert and action line is colored amber, indicating the need for greater vigilance.

74. Ans. (c) Secondary arrest after progression of labor

Ref: Williams obstetrics 24th ed page 452, Dutta 7th ed page 402, 529

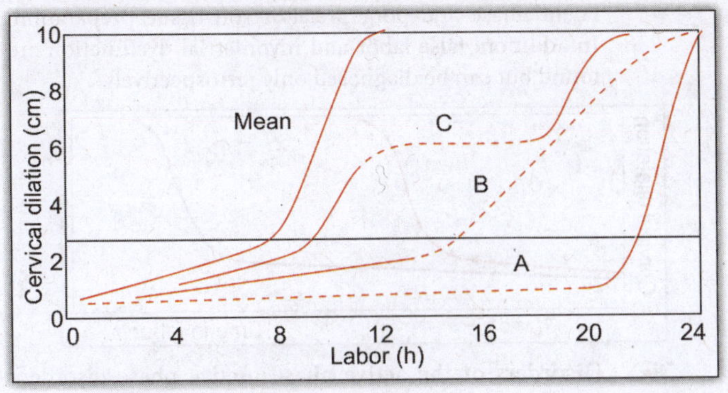

Legends

Mean curve represents the Friedmans curve of normal labor in primigravida

- Curve A in question represents prolonged latent phase.
- Curve B represents prolonged active phase.
- Curve C represents secondary arrest of labor.

Partograph

Partograph is a composite graphical record of key data (maternal and fetal) during labor, entered against time on a single sheet of paper. Freidman (1954) first devised it. Partograph is a composite graphical record of cervical dilatation and descent of head against duration of labor in hours.

Friedman Curve

In 1954 Emanuel Friedman conducted his now classic studies defining the spectrum of normal labor by evaluating the course of labor of 500 primigravidas. Sigmoid curve composite of the average dilatation curve for labor in nulliparous women. The curve is based on analysis of data derived from a large, nearly consecutive series of women. The norms established by his data, depicted as the **"Friedman curve"** as shown in the Figure 1.

The Zhang's curve (Figure 2) is different from the Friedman curve (Figure 1). Zhang's curves also demonstrate an increase in the rate of cervical dilation as labor progresses, but the increase is more gradual than that described by Friedman.

The Zhang research and ACOG have taken the position that the Friedman curve was no longer valid and is now outdated. ACOG and the Zhang research reached the decision that women were being incorrectly diagnosed with failure to dilate in labor, when they might be experiencing normal progressive labor. The ACOG changes lead to lower Cesarean rates.

As a result, ACOG published the Obstetric Care Consensus, "Safe Prevention of the Primary Cesarean Section Delivery," in March 2014, which recommended new guidelines for handling labor. The ACOG publication defined "arrest of labor" in the first stage and replaced the Friedman Curve with its 60 years of supporting evidence.

Graph	Friedman curve Figure 1	Zhang curve Figure 2	WHO curve Figure 3
Transition of latent to active phase at cervical dilatation of	3 to 4 cm cervical dilation	6 cm	4 cm in Original WHO. 3 cm in Modified WHO
Rate of cervical dilatation in active stage	1.2 cm/hour for nulliparous, 1.5 cm/hour for multiparous	Over 50% of patients did not dilate >1 cm/hour until 5-6 cm dilation (similar for Nulliparous and Multiparous)	1 cm/hour
Deceleration phase	Entering a deceleration phase at approx 9 cm	Not observed	Not observed
Prolonged 2nd stage	3 hours for nulliparas and 1 hour for multiparas		

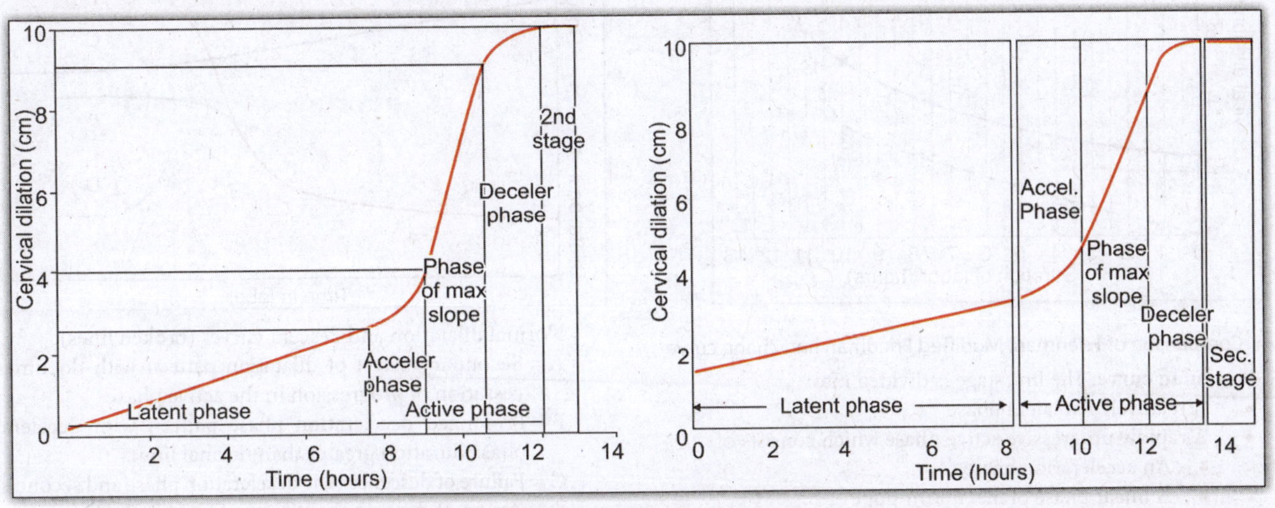

Fig. 1: Friedman curve (left) and modified Friedman curve (right)

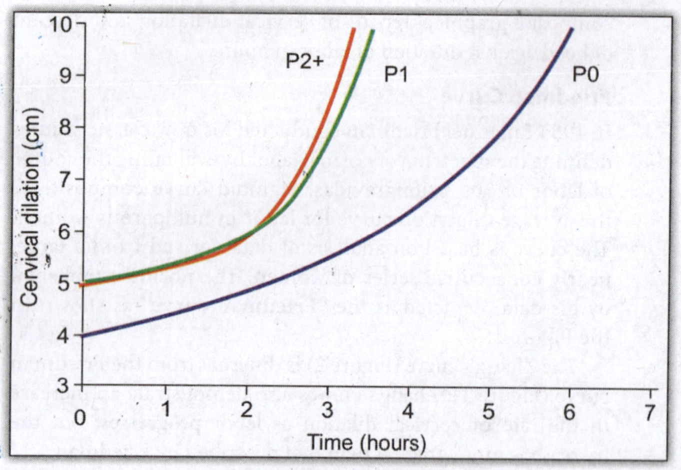

Fig. 2: Zhang curve

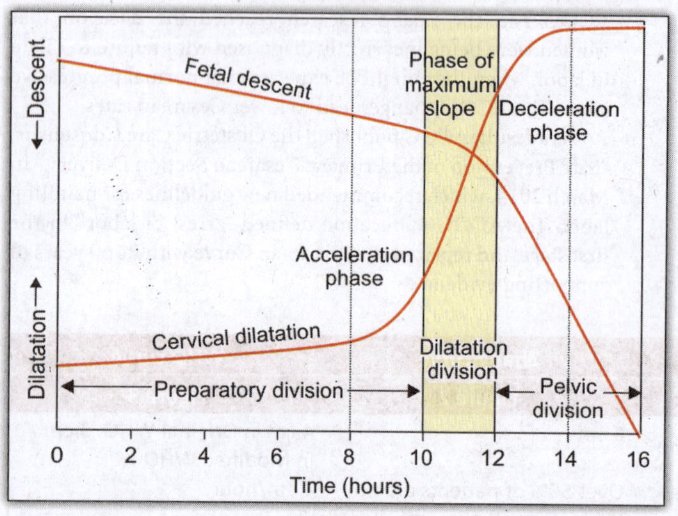

Fig. 3: Friedman curve with both dilatation curve and descent curve

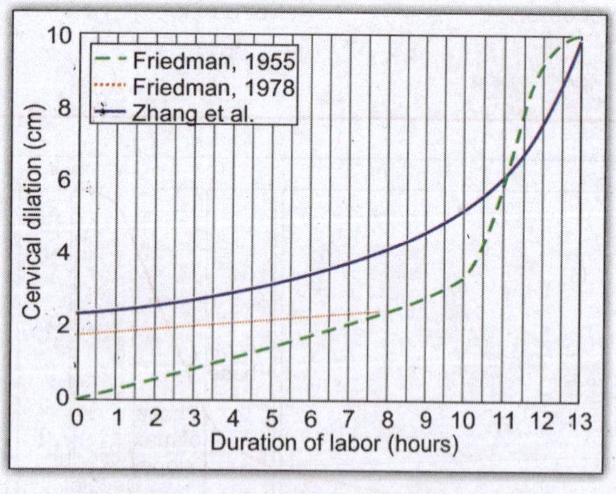

Fig. 4: Comparison of Friedman, Modified Friedman and Zhang curve

Friedman curve: The first stage is divided into:

- A relatively flat latent phase
- A rapidly progressive active phase which consists of
  - An acceleration phase
  - A linear phase of maximum slope
  - A deceleration phase.

- **Prolonged latent phase of labor:** Etiologic factors that appear to be responsible for the development of prolonged latent phase disorders in multiparas most often include excessive sedation administered during the course of the latent phase and poor prelabor soft-tissue preparation. In addition, false labor and myometrial dysfunction are found but can be diagnosed only retrospectively.

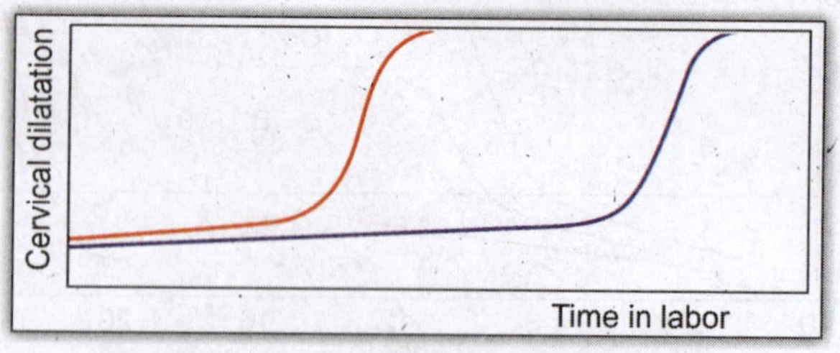

- **Disorders of the active phase:** Active phase disorders may be divided into:
  - **Protracted active phase:** When the rate of cervical dilatation is <1.2 cm/hour in a primipara and <1.5 cm/hour in a multipara. A protracted active phase may be due to—(i) Inadequate uterine contractions (ii) Cephalopelvic disproportion (iii) Malposition (OP) or malpresentation (brow) or (iv) Epidral anesthesia.
  - **Arrest disorder:** Arrest of dilatation is defined when no cervical dilatation occurs after 2 hours in the active phase of labor. It is commonly due to inefficient uterine contractions. No descent for a period of >1 hour is called arrest of descent. It is commonly due to CPD. **Secondary arrest** is defined when the active phase of labor (cervical dilatation) commences normally but stops or slows significantly for 2 hours or more prior to full dilatation of the cervix. It is commonly due to malposition or CPD.
- **Disorders of the second stage:** *(i) Protraction of descent:* when the descent of the presenting part is at <1 cm/hour in a nullipara or <2 cm/hour in a multipara. *(ii) Arrest of descent:* when no progress in descent is observed. It may be due to combination of several underlying abnormalities like CPD, malposition, malpresentation, inadequate uterine contradictions or asynclitism.

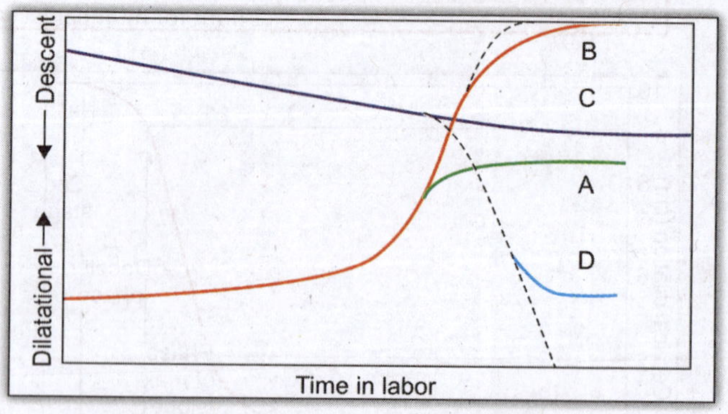

Normal dilatation and descent curves (broken lines).
A = Secondary arrest of dilatation pattern with documented cessation of progression in the active phase
B = Prolonged deceleration phase pattern with deceleration phase duration greater than normal limits
C = Failure of descent in the deceleration phase and second stage
D = Arrest of descent characterized by halted advancement of fetal station in the second stage.

75. Ans. (b) Observation

Ref: William's 24th ed ch 22

A partograph was designed by the World Health Organization (WHO) for use in developing countries.

Labor is divided into a latent phase, which should last no longer than 8 hours and an active phase. The active phase starts at 3 cm dilatation (4 cm in Modified WHO partograph) and progress should be no slower than 1 cm/hr. A 4-hour wait is recommended before intervention when the active phase is slow. Labor is graphed and analysis includes use of alert and action lines.

The patient is in latent phase of labor with no indication to accelerate labor. Although the management of labor is a subjective and protocol varies from hospital to hospital ; we will follow the management according to Partograph and hence the answer will be observation.

Also know regarding amniotomy: The American College of Obstetricians and Gynecologists (2013a) recommends the use of amniotomy to enhance progress in active labor, but cautions that this may increase the risks of infection and maternal fever.

76. Ans. (d) Inj Betamethasone 12 mg, 2 doses, 24 hours apart

Ref: William's 24th ed page 850, 1562, 1768, Nelson 20th ed page 852, Dutta 7th ed page 316, Royal College of Obstetricians and Gynaecologists Greentop Guidelines no.7 (https://www.rcog.org.uk/globalassets/documents/guidelines/gtg_7.pdf)

Antenatal Corticosteroids - Summary/FAQS

- A **single** course of antenatal corticosteroids (American College of Obstetricians and Gynecologists (2013 c) is recommended to women between 24 + 0 and 34 + 6 weeks of gestation who are at risk of preterm birth. No rescue dose is recommended.
- Antenatal corticosteroids should be given to all women for whom an elective caesarean section is planned prior to 38 + 6 weeks of gestation and also to women with multiple pregnancy at risk of imminent iatrogenic or spontaneous preterm delivery between 24 + 0 and 34 + 6 weeks of gestation.
- **Betamethasone 12 mg given intramuscularly in two doses 24 hours apart** or **dexamethasone 6 mg given intramuscularly in four doses 12 hours apart** are the steroids of choice to enhance lung maturation.
- A large non randomized retrospective study has suggested that infants exposed to antenatal betamethasone have less neonatal cystic periventricular leukomalacia than infants exposed to antenatal dexamethasone. Hence **betamethasone is the steroid of choice.**

77. Ans. (c) PAP smear should be repeated yearly in women of reproductive age group

Ref: http://www.asccp.org/asccp-guidelines, http://apps.who.int/iris/bitstream/10665/94830/1/9789241548694_eng.pdf

Guidelines for Prevention and Early Detection of Cervical Cancer

Population	Recommended screening method	Management of screen results	Comments
<21 years	No screening		HPV testing is not used for screening or management in this age group
21-29 years	Cytology alone every 3 years		HPV-Positive ASC-USb or cytology of LSIL or more severe: Refer to ASCCP Guidelines Cytology Negative or HPV-Negative ASC-USb: Rescreen with cytology in 3 years
30-65 years	HPV and Cytology "Cotesting" every 5 years (Preferred) or Cytology alone every 3 years (Acceptable) H	• HPV-Positive ASC-US or cytology of LSIL or more severe: treat according to ASCCP guidelines. • HPV Positive, Cytology Negative: Option 1-year 12-month follow-up with cotesting Option 2-year Test for HPV16 or HPV16/18 genotypes if HPV16 or HPV16/18 positive: refer to colposcopy If HPV16 or HPV16/18 negative: 12-month follow-up with cotesting • Cotest Negative or HPV-Negative ASC-US: Rescreen with cotesting in 5 years • HPV-Positive ASC-USb or cytology of LSIL or more severe: Refer to ASCCP Guidelines • Cytology Negative or HPV-Negative ASC-USb: Rescreen with cytology in 3 years	Screening by HPV testing alone is not recommended for most clinical settings.
>65 years	No Screening following adequate negative prior screening		Women with a history of CIN2 or a more severe diagnosis should continue routine screening for at least 20 years.
After hysterectomy	No screening		Applies to women without a cervix and without a history of CIN2 or a more severe diagnosis in the past 20 years or cervical cancer ever.
HPV Vaccinated	Follow age-specific recommendations (same as unvaccinated women)		

NOTE

No screening method is recommended annually.

Option (A)

VIA identifies disease in the ectocervix only when the transformation zone remains at least partially on the visually exposed part of the cervix. Since the transformation zone recedes to the endocervical canal in postmenopausal women, VIA is likely to be less accurate among these older women.

WHO Guidelines states that "VIA is appropriate to use in women whose transformation zone is visible (typically in those younger than 50). This is because once menopause occurs, the transformation zone, where most precancerous lesions occur, frequently recedes into the endocervical."

78. Ans. (b) Beta hCG and PAPP-A

Ref: William's 24th ed page 289

Down's syndrome	1st trimester	2nd trimester
Screening test	• Nuchal translucency + beta hCG + PAPP i.e combined test	• Triple test (hCG + AFP +UE_3) • Quadruple test (triple test + inhibin A)
Diagnostic test	CVS	Amniocentesis

79. Ans. (a) Dysgerminoma

Ref: Novaks Gynecology 14th ed page 1507

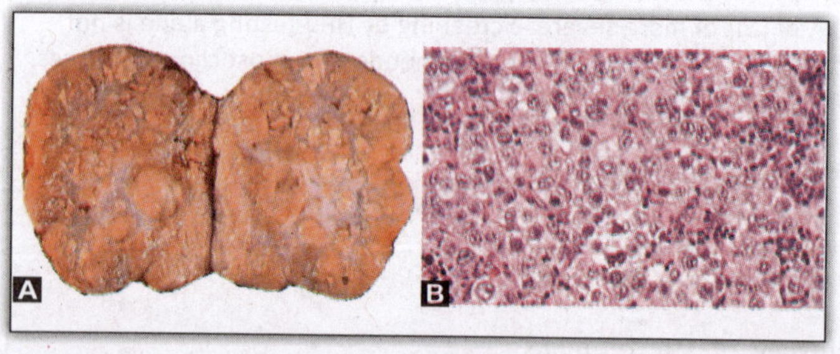

Figs A and B: A. Dysgerminoma Gross: The size of dysgerminomas varies widely, but they are usually 5 to 15 cm in diameter. Ovarian dysgerminoma that has been sectioned into two halves. Firm and encapsulated. The cut surface of the tumor is solid with some cystic areas and necrosis, fleshy, lobulated and a yellow-white to gray-pink appearance; **B. Dysgerminoma Microscopy:** Histopathology of the biopsy specimen: Sheet or cords of Round, polygonal large uniform tumor cells with vesicular nuclei and clear or finely granular cytoplasm that is eosinophilic, separated by scanty fibrous septa, which are often extensively infiltrated with lymphocytes, plasma cells and granulomas with epithelioid cells and multinucleated giant cells. Mitotic figures are seen in varying numbers, although they are usually numerous

80. Ans. (a) Mature teratoma

Ref: Novak's Gynecology 14th ed page 1512

The specimen shows the maturation of embryonal elements like hair and teeth hence it is mature teratoma (dermoid).

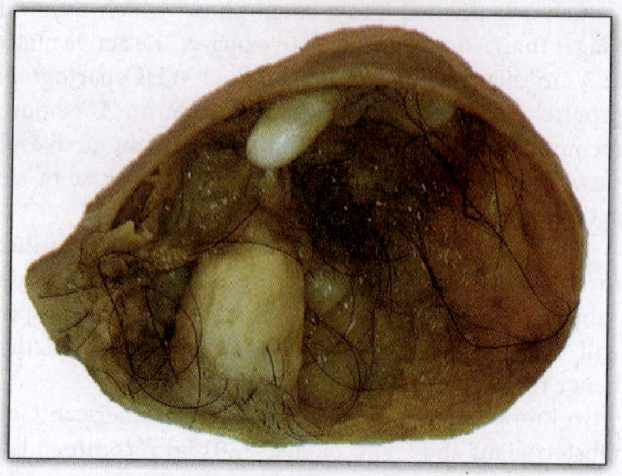

Fig: Mature/Benign Teratoma Gross: Characteristically they are unilocular cysts containing hair and cheesy sebaceous material. On section, they reveal a thin wall lined by an opaque, gray-white, wrinkled epidermis. From this epidermis, hair shafts frequently protrude. Within the wall, it is common to find tooth structures and areas of calcification. A variety of mature, well-differentiated tissue elements may be found from all three embryologic germ layers (ectoderm, mesoderm, endoderm). These tumors are often called "dermoid cysts" because they are mostly cystic and mostly contain ectodermal elements. The most common tissue element of these teratomas is skin, so large amounts of hair and sebum are produced, leading to a challenging cleanup problem in surgical pathology following dissection of these tumors. If these tumors are mostly solid, then they are often "immature" teratomas with less differentiated tissue and may behave more aggressively.

NOTE

Immature Malignant teratoma Gross: The tumors are bulky and have a smooth external surface. On section they have a solid (or predominantly solid) structure. There are areas of necrosis and hemorrhage. Hair, sebaceous material, cartilage, bone and calcification may be present

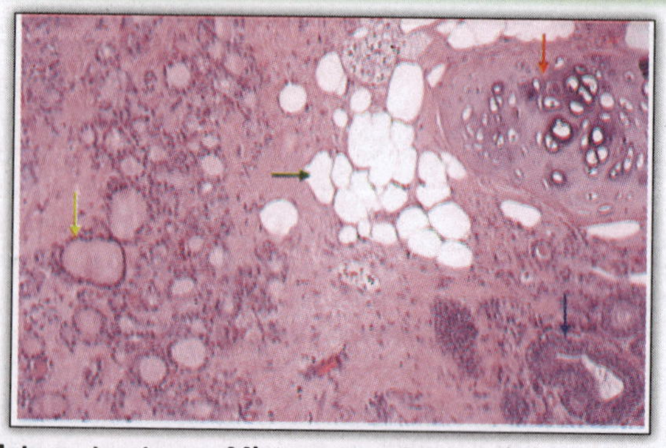

Fig: Mature teratoma Microscopy: Cyst wall is composed of stratified squamous epithelium and within there is cartilage (Red arrow) as well as adipose tissue (Green arrow) and even intestinal glands (Blue arrow) at the right, while at the left are a lot of thyroid follicles (Yellow arrow). The presence of abundant thyroid tissue within a mature teratoma can be termed struma ovarii.

81. Ans. (c) 600 µg

Ref: Williams 24th ed page 1130

Indirect repeat from AIIMS Nov 2015 (Dose of Misoprostol for Emergent Management of PPH was asked) (see page no. 903)

Misoprostol-Prostaglandin E1 Analogue

Although oxytocin is preferred for prevention and management of PPH, in resource-poor settings that lack oxytocin, misoprostol is used for hemorrhage prophylaxis and is given as a single oral 600 µg dose. Side effects include shivering in 30 percent and fever in 5 percent. Unlike some other prostaglandins, nausea or diarrhea is infrequent.

82. Ans. (b) 500 mL

Ref: William's 24th ed page 786

Although up to 800 mL can be been instilled, but we will go with 500 mL as according to most of the standard text.

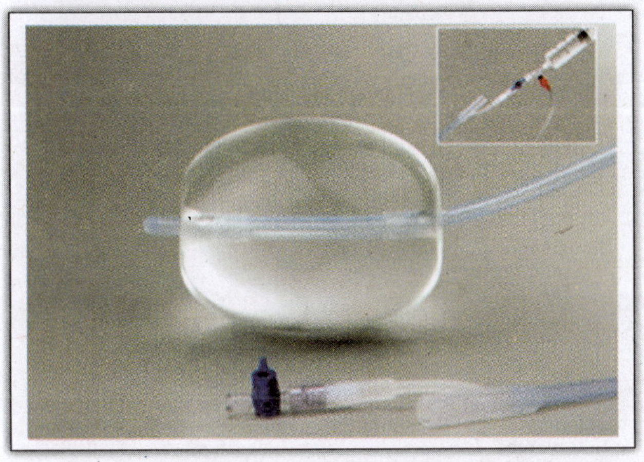

Fig: Bakri Postpartum Balloon

A Bakri Postpartum Balloon works on the principle of tamponade *(for uterine atony)* to stop bleeding. Success rate approximately 85 percent.

Procedure: Insertion requires two or three team members. The first performs abdominal sonography during the procedure. The second places the deflated balloon into the uterus and stabilizes it. The third member instills fluid to inflate the balloon, rapidly infusing at *least 150 mL* followed by further instillation over a few minutes for a total of *300 to 500 mL* to arrest hemorrhage.

Advantage: There is continuous drainage hence the risk of infection is reduced.

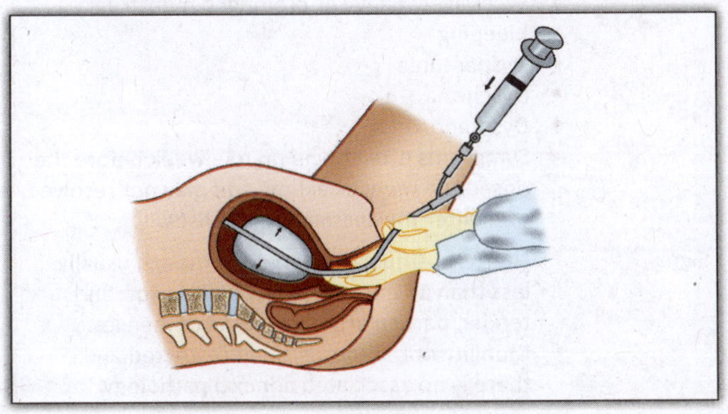

AIIMS MAY 2016

83. Ans. (a) Actinomyces

Ref: With text

Actinomyces can be detected by cervical cytology. Should actinomyces-like particles be found, removal of the IUD and treatment with oral penicillin is recommended. **(Novak 14th ed page 263)**

Actinomyces is an anaerobic g-positive filamentous, non-sporing bacterial infection often associated with IUCD. The incidence is 7% with IUCD worn for more than 2 years against 1% in non-users. The woman develops fever, abdominal pain, abnormal bleeding and discharge. Sulfur granules can be recognized. The infection is treated with 250,000 units/kg daily of penicillin IV in four doses for 2-6 weeks. Thereafter, oral 100 mg/kg daily in divided doses is administered for 3-12 months **(Datta gynecology 15th ed page 446)**

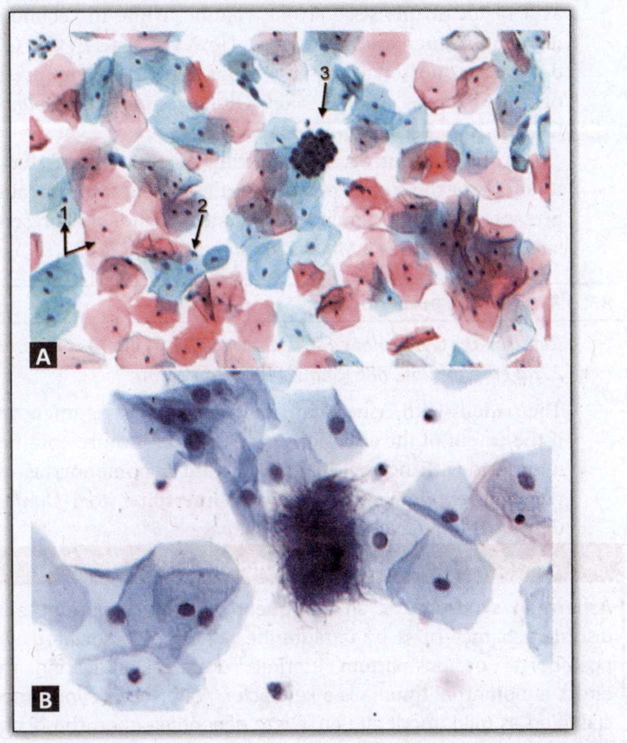

Figs A and B: A. Normal Cervical PAP Smear; Negative for intraepithelial lesion or malignancy. 1 – superficial squamous epithelial cells; 2 – intermediate squamous epithelial cells; 3 – endocervical (glandular) epithelial cells. The presence of infective agents and conditions such as Trichomonas, Herpes simplex virus, Candida and bacterial vaginosis may be detected in cervical samples; **B. Actinomyces** forms aggregates of long filamentous organisms **(Cotton ball cluster)** and perinuclear halo and is usually associated withintra-uterine contraceptive devices

84. Ans. (d) Cardiac output

Ref: William obstetrics 24th ed page 59

All four options/parameters are increased in pregnancy overall, but cardiac output is relatively decreased to some extent at the term. This decreased level is still higher than the prepregnant levels however in absence of no better option it Cardiac output should be the answer.

Option (A)

Blood volume is markedly raised. Starts to increase at 6th week ↑+ 30–40% i.e 1500 mL. (Nonpregnant = 4000 mL and Pregnant = 5500 mL). reaches maximum at 30–32 weeks and remains static till term.

Option (B)

Minute ventilation (Respiratory rate × Tidal volume).

Respiratory rate is unaffected in pregnancy while tidal volume increases by 40%. Hence minute ventilation is increased. At term, this translates into a 30% to 50% increase in minute ventilation.

Option (C)

GFR Glomerular filtration rate and renal plasma flow increase by 50%

Option (D)

Cardiac output: In first half of pregnancy cardiac output rises as a result of increased stroke volume, while in second half it is due to increased heart rate. However at term the CO is decreased due to decreased venous return due to pressure of gravid uterus on IVC. *(Ref: Obstetrics and Gynecology by Charles R. B. Beckmann with ACOG 6th ed page 43)*

Cardiac output decreases during the third trimester due to effects of the supine position in the patient at term causing pressure on IVC by gravid uterus and which is not present in lateral position. *(Ref: Miller's Anesthesia page 2204)*

85. Ans. (c) Hypomenorrhea

Ref: Novak's Gynecology 14th ed page 1505, Williams Gynecology 22nd ed page 754, 886, Shaw's 16th Ed Pg 250

The patient with Asherman syndrome may have amenorrhea if the extent of the adhesions is severe, but it more commonly manifests with normal menses or mild hypomenorrhea with recurrent spontaneous abortion or infertility. *(Ref: Danforth's Obstetrics and Gynecology 10th Ed page 815)*

Asherman's Syndrome

Asherman syndrome is an infrequently found acquired uterine disorder characterized by intrauterine adhesions associated with postabortal or postpartum uterine curettage, indicating that direct endometrial trauma is a key factor. Asherman's syndrome is classified as mild, moderate or severe depending upon the degree and extent of adhesion. Asherman syndrome is a risk factor of cervical pregnancy.

Causes	Excessive curettage, uterine infection or endometrial tuberculosis, transcervical resection of endometrium for dysfunctional uterine bleeding (DUB) and uterine packing in postpartum hemorrhage.
Clinical features	The woman presents with hypomenorrhea (most common), secondary amenorrhea, oligomenorrhea, dysmenorrhea, habitual abortion and infertility depending upon the extent of uterine cavity obliteration Asherman's syndrome may recur and require repeat hysteroscopic excision.
Diagnosis	The diagnosis is confirmed with hysterosalpingography (multiple filling defects) or hysteroscopy (more accurate)

Contd...

Asherman's Syndrome

Management	Hysteroscopy enables adhesiolysis. Reformation of adhesions is prevented by insertion of **IUCD** for 3 months and giving estrogen cyclically (21 days) for 3 months to develop endometrium or by inserting the Foley catheter into the uterine cavity for 7 days and giving estrogen. Lately many omit the insertion of IUCD. Resectoscope, scissor, laser or cautery is used to break up adhesions.

86. Ans. (a) Review after 2-3 months for ovarian cyst

Ref: Novak's gynecology 14th ed page 681

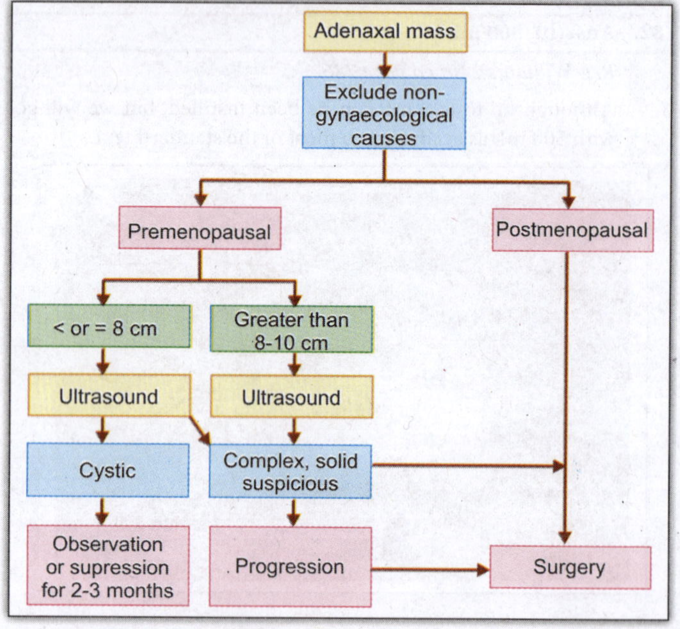

87. Ans. (a) Adenomyosis

Ref: Novak's Gynecology 14th ed page 521

Adenomyosis

- **Adenomyosis is defined as presence of endometrial tissue within the myometrium, at least 1 high-power field from the basis of the endometrium.**
- Adenomyosis, endometriosis and uterine leiomyomas frequently coexist; average age of symptomatic women is usually older than 40 years.

Symptoms	• Asymptomatic. • Excessively heavy or prolonged menstrual bleeding • Dyspareunia • Dyschezia • Dysmenorrhea • Symptoms often begin up to a week before the onset of a menstrual flow and may not resolve until after the cessation of menses.
Signs	• Uterus is diffusely enlarged, although usually less than 14 cm in size and is often soft and tender, particularly at the time of menses. • Mobility of the uterus is not restricted and there is no associated adnexal pathology.

Contd...

Adenomyosis	
Diagnosis	**Adenomyosis is a clinical diagnosis and can be confirmed only by pathology review.** Imaging studies, although helpful, are not definitive. Because of their cost are not recommended. The pathologic confirmation of suspected adenomyosis can be made only at the time of hysterectomy.
Management	The management of adenomyosis depends on the patient's age and desire for future fertility. Relief of secondary dysmenorrhea caused by adenomyosis can be ensured after hysterectomy but less invasive approaches can be tried initially. Nonsteroidal anti inflammatory agents, oral contraceptives and menstrual suppression using progestins have all been found to be useful. Treatment follows the same protocol as treatment for endometriosis.

88. Ans. (c) Endometrial biopsy

Ref: Manual of Obstetrics by Daftary 4th ed Page 478, Textbook of gynecology by sudha salhan page 516

Harvey Karman in the United States refined the technique of Vacuum or suction aspiration in the early 1970s with the development of the Karman cannula, a soft, flexible cannula that avoided the need for initial cervical dilatation and so reduced the risks of puncturing the uterus. The given instrument is Karman cannula that comes in various sizes mainly used for termination of pregnancy. The diameters of 4-6 are used for endometrial biopsy.

Material: Polypropylene

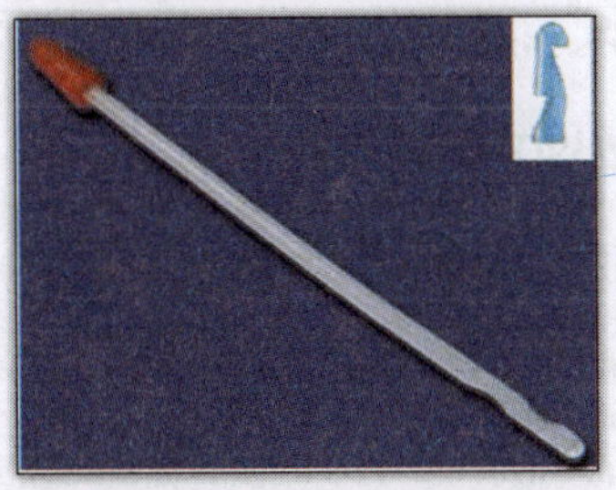

Fig: Karman cannula for endometrial biopsy

Sets of Manual Vacuum Aspiration

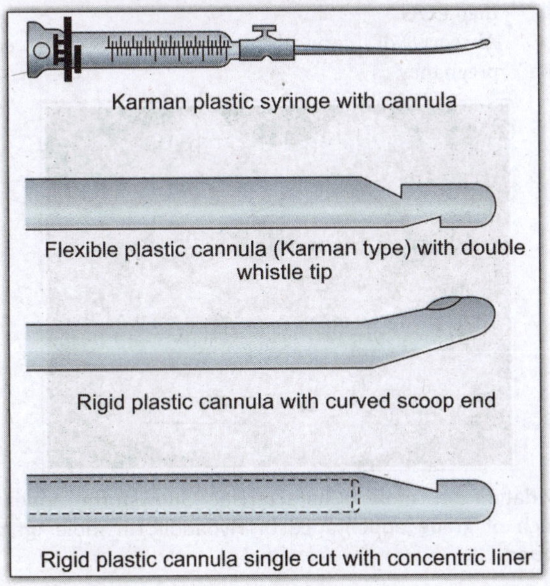

89. Ans. (a) Placenta succenturiate

Ref: Williams 24th ed page 251

Repeat AIIMS MAY 2018 OBG (See for explanation)

90. Ans. (b) Mullerian agenesis

Ref: Novak's gynecology 15th ed page 1005

Normal secondary sexual characters with blind vagina and absent uterus indicate towards diagnosis of Mullerian agenesis.

See OBG AIIMS NOV 2016 for discussion on Primary Amenorrhea

Similar Question on Mullerian Agenesis is asked in AIIMS MAY 2013 with slightly different language and options.

91. Ans. (c) Terminate the pregnancy because of high risk of infection

Ref: Novak's 14th ed page 375

Repeat AIIMS OBG NOV 2016 (See for explanation)

92. Ans. (b) 5

Ref: William's 24th edition page 1084

Bishop scoring system is used to assess the inducibility

Bishop Scoring Cervical Factor					
Bishop Score (B)	Effacement (Read-Effacement = (I)	Station (S)	Consistency (Hardness = H)	Dilatation (Opening = O)	Position (P)
0	0–30%	–3	Firm	Closed	Posterior
1	40–50%	–2	Medium	1–2	Mid position
2	60–70%	–1	Soft	3–4	Anterior
3	>80%	+1/+2		>/= 5	

93. Ans. (c) Less extension of lesion

Ref: William 24th ed page 551

Type of Episiotomy		
Characteristic	Midline	Mediolateral
Surgical repair	Easy	Difficult
Postoperative pain	Minimal	Common
Extensions	Common	Uncommon
Faulty healing	Rare	Common
Anatomical results	Excellent	Occasionally faulty
Blood loss	Less	More
Dyspareunia	Rare	Occasional

94. Ans. (c) VSD

Ref: Williams 24th ed page 965, 2327, Fernando arias 3rd ed page 445

Summary

- **Cardiovascular defects** are the most common birth defects associated with diabetic mothers amounting to more than half birth defects
- **Caudal regression (Sacral agenesis)** is the most specific birth defect associated with diabetic mothers.

Diabetes is the most common medical complication of pregnancy. Gestational diabetes mellitus is a type of diabetes mellitus. Gestational diabetes is defined as carbohydrate intolerance of variable severity with onset or first recognition during pregnancy. This definition applies whether or not insulin is used for treatment. Undoubtedly, some women with gestational diabetes have previously unrecognized overt diabetes.

Maternal and Fetal Effects of GDM

There has been an important shift in focus concerning adverse fetal consequences of gestational diabetes. Importantly, unlike in women with overt diabetes, **fetal anomalies are not increased**. Similarly, whereas pregnancies in women with overt diabetes are at greater risk for fetal death, this danger is not apparent for those who have only postprandial hyperglycemia (namely, class A_1 gestational diabetes)

- Fetal effects
  - Fetal demise (Increased perinatal mortality)
  - Macrosomia
  - Increased risk of low blood glucose (hypoglycemia), jaundice, high red blood cell mass (polycythemia) and low blood calcium (hypocalcemia) and magnesium (hypomagnesemia)
- Maternal effects
  - Increased frequency of hypertension
  - Increased frequency of cesarean delivery
  - Risk for cardiovascular complications associated with abnormal serum lipids, hypertension and abdominal obesity—the *metabolic syndrome*

Maternal and Fetal Effects of Overt Diabetes

- Fetal effects
  - First trimester abortion
  - Preterm delivery
  - Congenital malformations
  - Hydramnios
  - Macrosomia
  - Fetal demise
- Neonatal effects
  - Respiratory distress
  - Hypoglycemia
  - Hypocalcemia
  - Hyperbilirubinemia
  - Cardiac hypertrophy
  - Low risk of developing Type 1 diabetes
- Maternal effects
  - 10 fold increase in maternal death
  - Ketoacidosis, hypertension, preeclampsia and pyelonephritis
- With the possible exception of diabetic retinopathy, however, the long-term course of diabetes is not affected by pregnancy.

Congenital Malformations in Infants of Women with Overt Diabetes

Anomaly	Incidence
Cardiovascular	52%
Musculoskeletal	12%
Urogenital	9%
CNS	4%
Gastrointestinal	2%
Chromosomal	3%
Others	10%
Multiorgan	8%

NOTE

- Chromosomal aberrations are not seen in diabetes mellitus complicating pregnancy but congenital malformations are seen.
- Both chromosomal aberrations and congenital malformations are not seen in gestational diabetes.

95. Ans. (a) Hydatidiform mole

Ref: Williams 24th ed page 399

Hints in History

- Complaint of bleeding per vaginum with pain—H. mole usually presents with bleeding per vaginam with pain and passage of vesicles.
- Abdomen is soft and non tender and because fetal parts are not palpable.
- Uterine size is 12 weeks—although the period of amenorrhea is not given but in h.mole uterine size is usually greater than POG and in missed abortion it is less than POG.
- Absence of cervical excitation—rules out ectopic pregnancy.

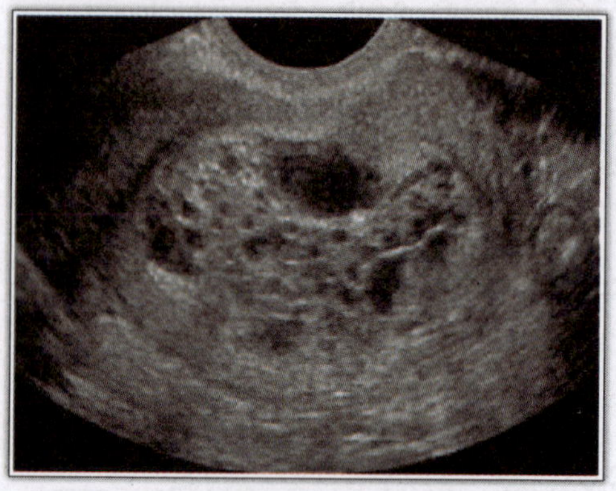

Fig: Hydatidiform mole: Characteristic Snowstorm appearance or bunch of grape appearance of Hydatidiform mole on pelvic ultrasound

Complete and Partial Hydatidiform Moles		
Feature	**Partial hydatidiform mole**	**Complete hydatidiform mole**
Karyotype	69XXY, Triploid, paternal and maternal origin	46XX, Diploid, mostly paternal origin
Immunohistochemistry		
hCG	Weak	>2.5 multiples of the median
Placental alkaline phosphatase	Strong	Weak
HPL	Variable	Weak
Pathology		
Fetus or amnion, fetal vessels	Present	Absent
Hydropic villi	Variable, often focal	Pronounced, generalized
Trophoblastic proliferation	Focal	Variable, often marked
Villous scalloping	Marked	Absent
Clinical		
Mole clinical diagnosis	Rare	Common
Uterus large for dates	Rare	30%-50%
Malignant sequelae	<5%	6%-36%
Persistent disease	20%	<5%
USG		
Theca lutein cysts	Uncommon	Common
	Focal swelling of the villous tissue and focal trophoblastic hyperplasia in the presence of embryonic or fetal tissue Increase in transverse diameter of gestational sac	Generalized swelling of the villous tissue and diffuse trophoblastic hyperplasia in the absence of embryonic or fetal tissue. Multiple hypoechoic areas corresponding to hydropic villi, at times described as a **"snowstorm pattern"**
$P^{57}kip^2$ ($P^{57}kip^2$ is a paternally imprinted gene which is maternally expressed. It is used in an immunostaining method to differentiate between complete and partial mole)	Positive	Negative

96. Ans. (b) Testicular FNAC

Ref: Novak's Gynecology 14th ed page 1722

NOTE

All four options help to differentiate between obstructive and nonobstructive azoospermia but testicular biopsy or FNAC is diagnostic.

Fine needle aspiration cytology (FNAC) of the testis is being increasingly used as a minimally invasive method of evaluating testicular function to differentiate a post-testicular, obstructive etiology of male infertility from an intrinsic testicular cause. When post-testicular azoospermia or severe oligospermia is demonstrated, surgical correction may be indicated.

Test	Primary testicular failure	Secondary testicular failure	Obstruction of vas deferens
FSH/LH levels	High	Low	Normal
Karyotyping	In syndromic cases like Klinefelters	In syndromic cases	Normal
Testosterone level	Low	Low	Normal
Testicular Biopsy/FNAC	Confirmatory diagnosis	Confirmatory diagnosis	Normal spermatogenesis

Male causes of infertility

Pretesticular (hormonal) (AKA-Hypogonadotropic hypogonadism, central or secondary hypogonadism)

2% of male causes of infertility
Disturbed hypothatorno pituitary axis,
INV- 1. Low ESN
2. Low 114
3. Low testosterone
4. Prolactin
5. Thyroid function tests
6. Karyotyping
7. Testicular biopsy
8. Seminal fluid analysis

Primary hypogonadotropic hypogonadism (HH)
Decreases sensitivity to GnRH
E.g Kallmann syndrome (Congenital.anosmia in addition to hypogonadism), idiopathic primary HH
Rx:1.Stop testosterone inj. already being admn.
2. hCG to stimulate Leydig cells to form testosterone
3. HMG for sertoli cell stimulation
4. Recombinant FSH
5. Pulsatile GnRH
6. intra cytoplasmic sperm In) (ICSI)

Secondary hypogonadotropic hypogonadism
GnRH decreased
E.g: Pituitary apoplexy. Head trauma. tumours
Inv: As per cause e.g: CT scan
Rx : 1. Removal of cause
2. Pulsatile GnRH therapy
3. FSH replacement

Testicular causes (Nonobstructive atoospeoms) (AKA hyperganadotropic hypogonadism) primary hypogonadism)

30-40% of male causes of infertility
A. Congenital: Anorchia, testicular dysgenesis, cryptorchidism, or genetic abnormalities—de Castillo syndrome (Sertoli cell only syndrome)
B. Acquired: Trauma. testicular torsion, orchitis, exogenous factors (e.g., medications, systemic diseases. varicocele 40% of male causes). or surgeries that damage the vascular structure of the testes
C. Idiopathic:
INV:Semen analysis followed by
1. High FSH. High LH, Low Testosterone
2. Karyotyping (Klinefelters' syndrome m.c)
3. If testis is not palpable, its presence is confirmed by admn of hCG & the resultant increase in testosterone levels
4. Antibody studies : for antisperm antibodies Rx. fertility restoration is generally not possible Sex hormones can be replaced as symptomatic measure e.g: a.Retrograde ejaculation:
1.Transrectal USG
2. Microscopic investigation of postcoital or po masturabatory urine Treatment :
1. Alpha Sympathomimetics
2. Urine centrifugation for retrieval of sperms
b. varicocoele : Inv: 1.USG
Rx. ligation of varice,
Other tests for sperm Analysis:
A. DNA assays:
i) Sperm chromatin structure assay: checking acid vulnerability of sperm DNADamaged DNA is more vulnerable to acids)
ii) Comet; Sperm DNA on gel electropneresis : Fragmented DNA is lighter and travels more.
iii) Terminal d-UTP Nick end labelling (TUNEL) identifies DNA strand breaks by incorporation of labelled d-UTP
B. Sperm penetration assay (Hamster egg penetration assay)

Post testicular (Obstructive azoospermis)

The obstruction can arise from the epididymis, vas deferens, or ejaculator duct and can be acquired or congenital.
a. Congenital: Cong.Bilateral absence of Vas deferens, Cystic fibrosis,Mullenan Prostatic cyst
b. Acquired: Gonorrhoea, Chlamydia. TB,Schistosormasis
c. Latrogenic: Vasectomy, Hydrocoele repair, Herniorrhaphy
Inv 1.Norrnal FSH
2.Normal LH
3.Normal Testosterone
4.Normal site of testis
Treatment :
1. Microsurgical anastomosis of vas deferens
2. Testicular exploration
3. Surgical sperm retrieval
4. Percutareous testicular or epidodynnal sperm aspiration
5. MESA. TESA
6. Sperm retreival is followed by in Vitro Fertilisation (IVF) or Intra Uterine Insemination (IUI)
7. ICSI
Note: Use of ICSI increases risk of imprinting disorders (Angelman syndrome) & Male offsprings are prone to developing microdeletions on Y chromosome

AIIMS NOVEMBER 2015

97. Ans. (a) Cord compression

Ref: William's 24th Ed page 98, 995, Evidence based color atlas of obstetrics and gynecology: Diagnosis and management page 110

The given graph is showing variable deceleration caused by cord compression. Hence, cord compression is the answer.

Fetal Monitor Pattern	Description	Management
Normal 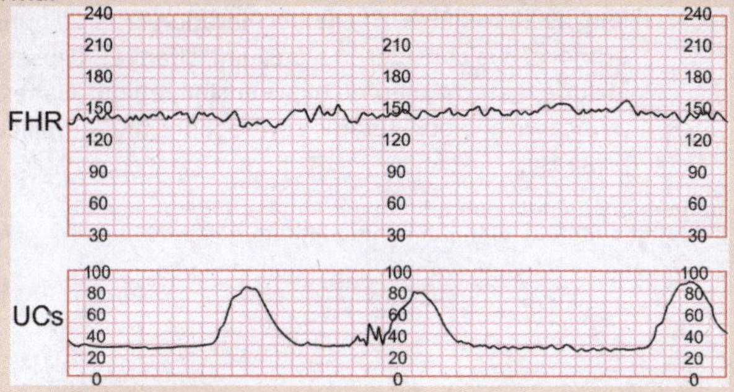	Upper graph; Normal fetal heart rate with moderate variability. Lower graph represents normal uterine contractions	
Early deceleration 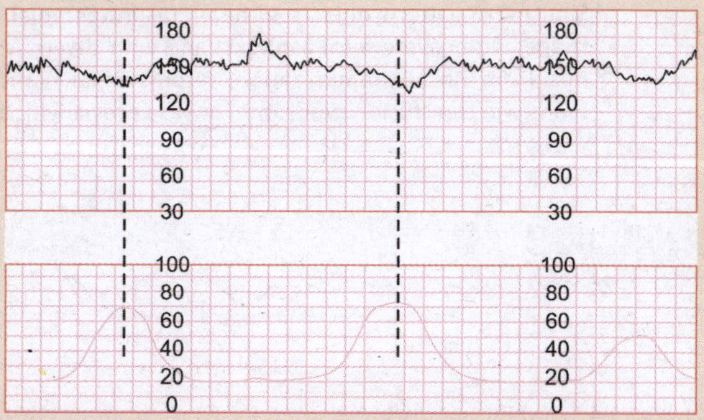	A decrease of FHR of more than 15 BPM for more than 15 sec but less than 2 minutes and can be episodic or periodic. Decrease in FHR starts at the start of contraction and nadir of deceleration coincides with the peak of contraction and recover fully by the end of contraction. Since these start very early after the contraction, it is termed as early deceleration. Caused by **Head compression**	Early decelerations during labor are usually due to head compression.it should be observed and p/v examination performed to see further associated factors like cord and hypoxia should be ruled out. In antenatal period early decelerations are always pathological. If present during labor watch for other ominous features.
Late deceleration 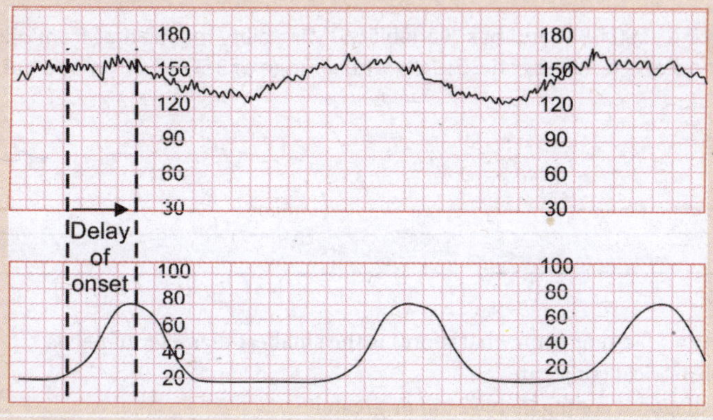	Onset of deceleration occurs after the onset of contraction and its nadir occurs after the peak of contraction. There must be presence of consecutive three contractions after normal heart rate for the diagnosis of same to be made. These are due to **uteroplacental insufficiency** and its persistence signifies bad fetal prognosis.	• Maternal position to left lateral • Stop oxytocin • 100% oxygen by mask • I.V. fluids to counter maternal hypotension • Uterine relaxant like terbutaline 0.25 mg subcutaneously • In persistent late declaration deliver the baby as soon as possible.
Variable deceleration 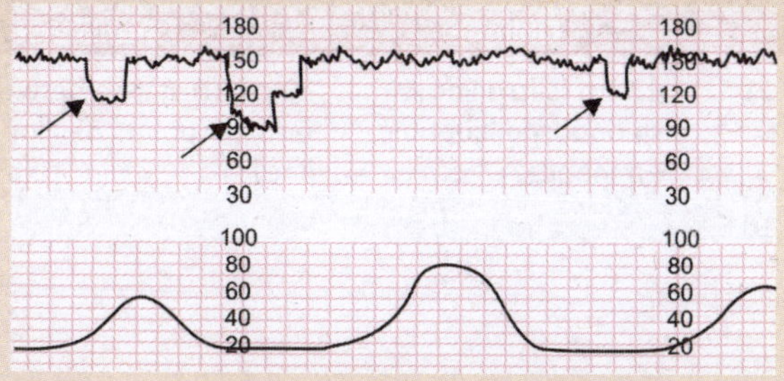	These can occur anytime during the contraction. These are variable in intensity duration and frequency. These are preceded by a short acceleration and a rapid deceleration and a short acceleration before returning to baseline. If associated with loss of variability than fetal acidosis is likely. Most common cause is **cord compression**.	• Change the maternal position. • Discontinue oxytocin. • p/v to rule out cord prolapsed. • Amnioinfusion if oligohydramnios. • 100% oxygen by a tight facial mask.

Contd...

Fetal Monitor Pattern	Description	Management
Prolonged decelerations 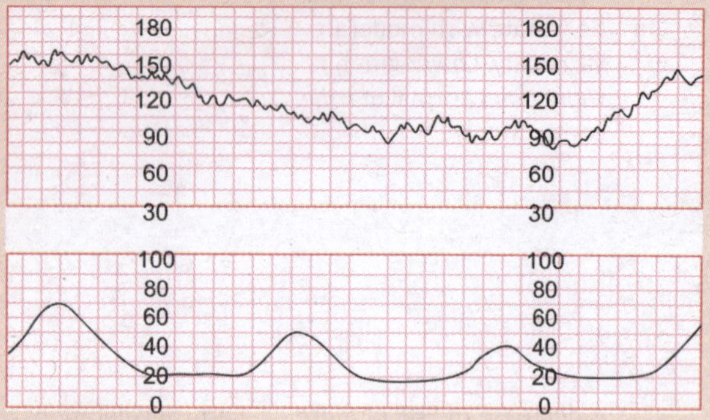	Prolonged decelerations last at least 2 minutes but not as long as 10 minutes. (If the deceleration lasts 10 minutes or more, it is considered a baseline change). Causes can include maternal supine hypotension, epidural anesthesia, paracervical block, tetanic contractions and umbilical cord prolapse.	
Sinusoidal pattern 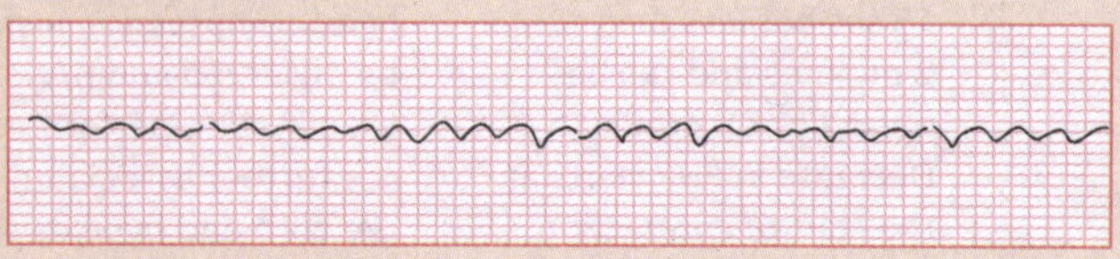	Sinusoidal pattern depicts either fetal **intracranial hemorrhage**, with severe **fetal asphyxia** and with severe fetal anemia from Rh alloimmunization, fetomaternal hemorrhage, twin-twin transfusion syndrome, or vasa previa with bleeding	

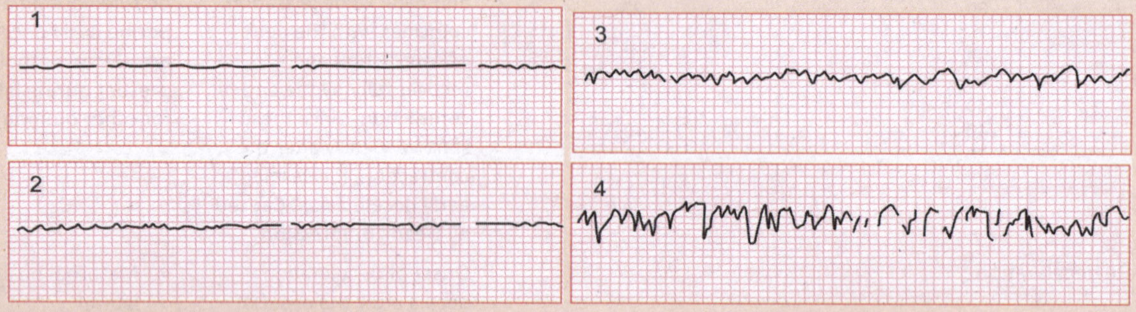

Variability: The normal fetal heart rate baseline is from 110 to 160 BPM and has "variability." Variability means that from one moment to the next, the fetal heart speeds up slightly and then slows down slightly, usually with a range of 3-5 BPM from the baseline.

1. Undetectable, absent variability
2. Minimal variability (Up to 5 beats/min)
3. Moderate variability (6–25 beats/min)
4. Marked variability (>25 beats/min)

98. Ans. (c) Obstetrics conjugate

Ref: Williams's 24th edition page 32, Dutta 7th ed page 89, 90

- Interspinous diameter (transverse diameter of midpelvis = 10 cm or somewhat more) is the smallest diameter of pelvis
- Shortest anteroposterior diameter of inlet of pelvis is obstetrical conjugate
- Pelvic inlet is an adequate size for a normal fetus if the diagonal conjugate is 12 cm or greater

Measurements of Pelvis	Anteroposterior		Oblique	Transverse
Inlet	**True/vera/anatomical conjugate:** = Diagonal conjugate -1.2 cm. Midpoint of sacral promontory to inner margin of upper border of pubic symphysis.	11	12 cm (sacroiliac joint to opposite iliopubic eminence	13 cm (Distance between two farthest points on iliopectineal line)
	Obstetric conjugate: = diagonal conjugate – 1.5. Midpoint of sacral promontory to bony projection on inner surface of symphysis pubis. ***(Smallest AP diameter)***	10.5		
	Diagonal conjugate: Midpoint of sacral promontory to lower border of pubic symphysis. Measured by PV examination.	12		

Contd...

Measurements of Pelvis				
	Anteroposterior		Oblique	Transverse
Mid pelvis	Plane of greatest dimension	12	12 cm	12 cm
	Plane of least dimension	10	10 cm	**Interspinous diameter:** 10 cm. *(Smallest diameter of pelvis)*
Outlet		13	12 cm	11 cm

 # All measurements in cm
Sacrocotyloid diameter (9.5.cm): Midpoint of sacral promontory to opposite illiopubic eminence. Space occupied by BPD while negotiating the brim in a flat pelvis.

99. Ans. (a) Genital Tuberculosis

Ref: Shaw's 16th Ed page 111

A hysterosalpingogram (HSG) is a fluoroscopic study performed by instilling radiopaque dye into the uterine cavity through a catheter to determine the contour of the endometrial cavity and patency of the fallopian tubes. Sensitivity and specificity of an HSG are approximately 65% and 85%, respectively. Abnormal findings include congenital malformations of the uterus, submucous leiomyomas, intrauterine synechiae (**Asherman's syndrome**), intrauterine polyps, salpingitis isthmica nodosa and proximal or distal tubal occlusion.

Option (C)

Salpingitis isthmica nodosa is a disease defined by an anatomic thickening of the proximal portion of the fallopian tubes at the junction with the uterus and is histologically characterized by multiple luminal diverticula. The etiology of this disease is not known; however, this pattern of tubal pathology increases the incidence of ectopic pregnancy by 52% in age- and race-matched controls. *(Ref: Danforth's Obstetrics and Gynecology 10th Ed page 73)*

Genital tuberculosis (TB) is an important cause of female infertility in the world, especially in developing countries. Majority of infertility cases are due to involvement of the fallopian tubes (92%–100%), endometrial cavity (50%) and ovaries (10%–30%).

Focus of genital tuberculosis is fallopian tubes, which almost always affects bilaterally but not symmetrically. This spreads to endometrium in half of the cases. If endometrium is involved, tubes

HSG Findings of Genital TB

- Hydrosalpinx with tubal blockage
- Blocked or lead pipe tubes
- Scarring leading to irregular uterine margins, pseudo unicornuate uterus of T shaped uterus
- Synechia as filling defect
- Venous and lymphatic intravasation of dyes

100. Ans. (c) Hypomenorrhea

Ref: Novak's Gynecology 14th ed page 1505, Williams Gynecology 22nd ed page 754, 886, Shaw's 16th Ed Pg 250

Repeat OBG AIIMS NOV 2016 (See for explanation)

101. Ans. (b) NST + Amniotic fluid volume

Ref: William's 24th ed page 707

Because the biophysical profile is labor intensive and requires a person trained in sonography; an abbreviated biophysical profile is used as a first-line screening test in singleton pregnancies.

- It includes a vibroacoustic nonstress test performed twice weekly and combined with amniotic fluid index determination for which <5 cm is considered abnormal.
- This abbreviated biophysical profile requires approximately 10 minutes to perform.
- The American College of Obstetricians and Gynecologists and the American Academy of Pediatrics (2012) have concluded that the modified biophysical profile test is as predictive of fetal well-being as other approaches to biophysical fetal surveillance.

USG Parameters done in Biophysical Profile	
Head circumference (HC)/ abdominal circumference (AC) ratio (HC/AC)	Normal: >1 before 32 weeks 1 from 32–34 weeks <1 after 34 weeks. Asymmetric IUGR: HC remains larger, elevated HC/AC Symmetric IUGR: HC/AC remains normal **AC is single most sensitive parameter to detect IUGR** Serial measurements of AC and fetal weight are more sensitive for IUGR
Femur length (FL)	Not affected in asymmetric IUGR FL/AC = 22 at all gestational ages from 21 weeks to term FL/AC >23.5 suggests IUGR
Amniotic fluid volume	Vertical pocket <2 cm suggests IUGR AFI (amniotic fluid index obtained by adding the largest pockets of all 4 quadreants): Normal = 5 to 25 <5 indicates oligohydramnios Reduced amniotic fluid: asymetrical IUGR
Doppler velocimetry	Elevated uterine artery systolic/diastolic (S/D) >2.6 and presence of diastolic notch shows IUGR See OBG 2013 Session 2 for details

102. Ans. (b) Endometrioma

Ref: Novak's 13th Ed page 388, Shaw's 15th Ed Page 471, Atlas of endometriosis 3rd ed page 47

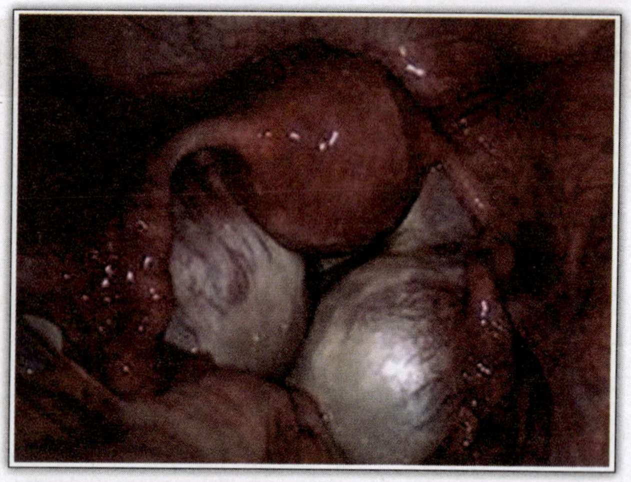

Fig: Endometrioma/chocolate cyst of ovary is a word used to describe endometriotic cyst of ovary. This is a laparoscopic picture showing bilateral endometrioma in the typical picture showing what is known as kissing ovaries.

Larger ovarian endometriotic cysts (endometrioma) are usually located on the anterior surface of the ovary and are associated with retraction, pigmentation and adhesions to the posterior peritoneum. These ovarian endometriotic cysts often contain a thick, viscous dark brown fluid (**Chocolate fluid**) composed of **hemosiderin** derived from previous intraovarian hemorrhage. Because this fluid may also be found in other conditions, such as in hemorrhagic corpus luteum cysts or neoplastic cysts, biopsy and preferably removal of the ovarian cyst for histologic confirmation are necessary for the diagnosis

103. Ans. (a) IVF with donor oocyte

Ref: Clinical gynecologic endocrinology and infertility by speroff 8th ed page 461-465

Recall Bias

We got many versions of this question from the recallers. We have settled this with the most common and most appropriate set of options.

See OBG AIIMS NOV 2016 for discussion on primary amenorrhea.

104. Ans. (a) Gardnerella

Ref: Shaw 15th ed page 131, Harrison 19th ed page 873

See Table of Vaginitis and Bacterial Vaginosis in AIIMS MAY 2017 OBG

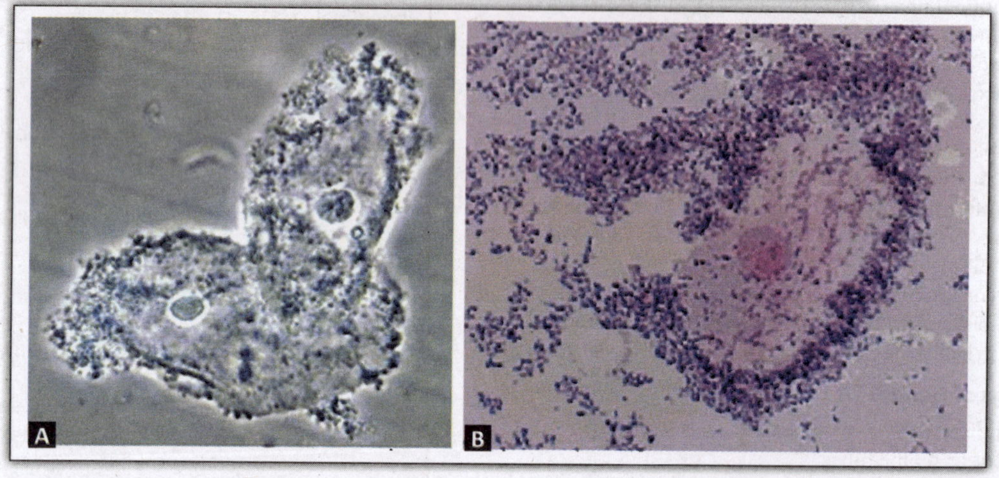

Figs A and B: A. Bacterial vaginosis: Normal saline wet mount showing two **clue cells** (original magnification × 400); **B. Bacterial vaginosis:** -g stain vaginal smear demonstrating how coccobacilli on the surfaces of vaginal epithelial cells create the characteristic granular appearance and indistinct borders of clue cells. Free floating clumps of **Gardnerella** are seen

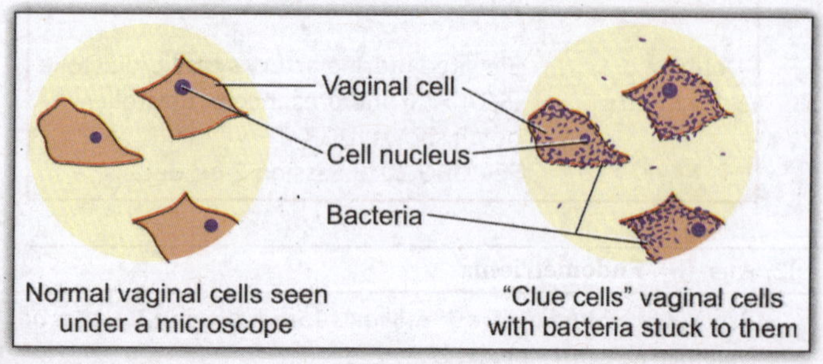

Amsel's criteria for bacterial vaginosis: (3 out of 4 should be present)

1. A fishy vaginal odor, which is particularly noticeable following coitus and vaginal discharge are present.
2. The pH of these secretions is higher than 4.5 (usually 4.7 to 5.7).
3. Whiff test/amine test positive (addition of 10% KOH to vaginal secretions produces fishy odor)
4. Presence of clue cells (>20% of epithelial cells)

105. Ans. (a) Any woman who can potentially be pregnant

Ref: Williams 24th ed page 1104, Nelson 20th ed page 2805

Summary

- Guidelines of Folic acid Prophylaxis are different for women planning pregnancy and women not planning pregnancy.
- Guidelines of High risk (Previous NTD, Family Histoy of NTD and on Anticonuilsants) differ on dose. Starting point and end point of the regimen is essentially similar in different risk categories.
- In women not planning any pregnancy recommendations is to take Folic acid throughout the reproductive age group.
- If women is planning pregnancy recommendations are divided into two school of thoughts; (a) Starting from >1 month preconception to end of first trimester (Conventionally) and (b) Starting from 3 month preconception to the end of first trimester.

Prophylactic Therapy

- A low risk women who is planning pregnancy should take 0.4 mg folic acid daily at least 1 month preconceptionally to 3 months pregnancy (first trimester).
- A woman with a prior child with a neural-tube defect can reduce the 2-5% recurrence risk by more than 70 percent with daily **4 mg folic acid supplements the month before conception** and during the first trimester. 4 mg should be given in all situations where the demand is high. Such conditions are: multiple pregnancies, patient having anticonvulsant therapy, hemoglobinopathies or associated chronic infection or disease.
- The Centers for Disease Control and Prevention has recommended that women of reproductive age (15-45 year) who are capable of becoming pregnant take supplemental folic acid (0.4 mg daily) to help prevent neural tube defects in their infants.
- Daily requirement of folic acid in a non-pregnant woman is 50–100 µg/day and during pregnancy is increased to 400 µg/day.
- Hernandez-Diaz and colleagues (2000) showed that fetuses who were exposed during embryogenesis to anticonvulsant medications that act as folic acid antagonists had a two- to threefold increased risk for oral clefts, cardiac defects and urinary tract abnormalities.
- Although periconceptional folate supplementation lowers the malformation rate (not eliminate), women with epilepsy should be given the fewest number of drugs possible during pregnancy as well as folic acid supplementation.

Folic Acid Prophylaxis

Prophylaxis	Dose	Starts	Ends
Normal Low risk prophylaxis	0.4 mg (400 µg) per day	≥1 month preconception	3 months (1st trimester)
Previous history of NTD and Family history of NTD	4 mg (4000 µg) per day	≥1 month preconception	3 months (1st trimester)

Contd...

Folic Acid Prophylaxis

Prophylaxis	Dose	Starts	Ends
On Anticonvulsants	4 mg (4000 µg) per day	≥1 month preconception	Throughout pregnancy

Footnote:
- 1 milligram (mg) = 1000 microgram (µg)
- Starting date and end date are applicable only when women are planning to get pregnant otherwise WHO and CDC recommends same dose daily for all women of reproductive age group (15-45 years)
- Society of Obstetricians and Gynaecologists of Canada 2015 guidelines recommends starting Folic acid 3 months preconception in all Risk categories of Prophylaxis, Dose being same.

106. Ans. (c) 800 mcg

Ref: Williams 24th ed page 1130

Similar question is asked in AIIMS Nov 2016 (Dose of Misoprostol for prevention of PPH is asked) (see page no. 893)

Recall Bias

Some students believe that prophylaxis of PPH was asked, in which case the answer would be 600 mcg

Misoprostol-Prostaglandin E1 Analogue

- Although oxytocin is preferred, in resource-poor settings that lack oxytocin, misoprostol is used for hemorrhage prophylaxis and is given as a single oral 600-µg dose.
- Side effects include shivering in 30 percent and fever in 5 percent. Unlike some other prostaglandins, nausea or diarrhea is infrequent.

107. Ans. (c) 28 weeks

Ref: William's 24th ed page 312, 643

Recommendation for RAADP (Routine Antenatal Anti D Prophylaxis)

- Anti-D immune globulin is given prophylactically to all Rh D-negative, unsensitized women at approximately 28 weeks and a second dose is given after delivery If the infant is Rh D-positive. (ACOG 2010)
- Following delivery, anti-D immune globulin should be given within 72 hours.
- Importantly, if immune globulin is inadvertently not administered following delivery, it should be given as soon as the omission is recognized, because there may be some protection up to 28 days postpartum.
- Anti-D immune globulin is also administered after pregnancy related events that could result in fetomaternal hemorrhage.

108. Ans. (a) Cordocentesis

Ref: William's obstetrics 24th page 615-620

There are three types of test, that can determine whether the unborn child has thalassemia

For thalassemia globin chain separation with gel electrophoresis is usual laboratory method of detection. Early and specific diagnosis by molecular methods has completely replaced cordocentesis. It is indicated if:

- Pregnant patient reports late in gestation
- CVS is inconclusive
- Previous studies of risk couple not available.

Since our patient has presented at 18 weeks for rapid testing we opt cordocentesis because termination of pregnancy is not legal beyond 20 weeks.

Prenatal Diagnosis			
	Cvs	Amniocentesis	Cordocentesis/Pubs
Time	Transcervical: 10–13 weeks Transabdominal 10 weeks to term.	15–20 weeks (early before 15 weeks)	18–20 weeks. (High failure rate if performed earlier)
Materials for study	Trophoblast cells	Fetal fibroblasts. Fluid for biochemical study.	Fetal blood cells
Karyotype Result	Direct preparation: 24–48 hours Culture: 10–14 days	Culture: Approx. 2 weeks	Culture: 24–48 hours
Accuracy	Accurate; may need amniocentesis for confirmation	Highly accurate	Highly accurate
Fetal loss	0.5–1%	0.5%- 1%)	1.4% 20-30% cord vessel bleeding 40% fetal maternal bleeding when placenta posterior, 5-10% fetal bradycardia.
Termination of pregnancy when Indicated	1st trimester: Safe	2nd trimester: Risky	2nd trimester: Risky
Maternal effects following termination of pregnancy	Very little	More traumatic; physically and psychologically	More traumatic; physically and psychologically

109. Ans. (c) Corpus luteum

Ref: William's 24th ed page 169, Ganong's 24th Ed Page 414

Uterine Cycle or Menstrual Cycle	
The Uterine Cycle or *menstrual cycle* is a repeating series of changes in the structure of the endometrium. The uterine cycle averages 28 days in length, but it can range from 21 to 35 days in healthy women of reproductive age. We can divide the Endometrial cycle into three phases	
Menses	From 1st to 4th day. Menstrual bleeding indicates end of one cycle and beginning of next cycle. On day 28 endometriun begins of degenerate due to withdrawal of hormonal support and menstruation starts. Two-third of endometrial tissue is lost
Proliferative phase	From 5th to 14th day of menstrual cycle. Proliferative phase (estrogenic phase) *begins* with *regeneration* of the *endometrium* and lasts until ovulation. Endometrium stops growing but becomes more vascular and glandular due to the rising level of estrogens.
Luteal or Secretory phase	Secretory phase (progestogenic phase) begins with ovulation and ends with menstruation. From 15th to 28th day. Progesterone peaks on 21st day. Corpus luteum (CL) produces estrogen and progesterone, which prepare the endometrium for implantation

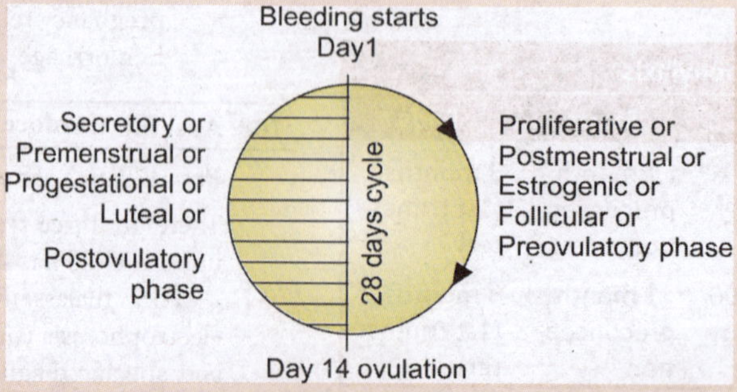

Contd...

Uterine Cycle or Menstrual Cycle

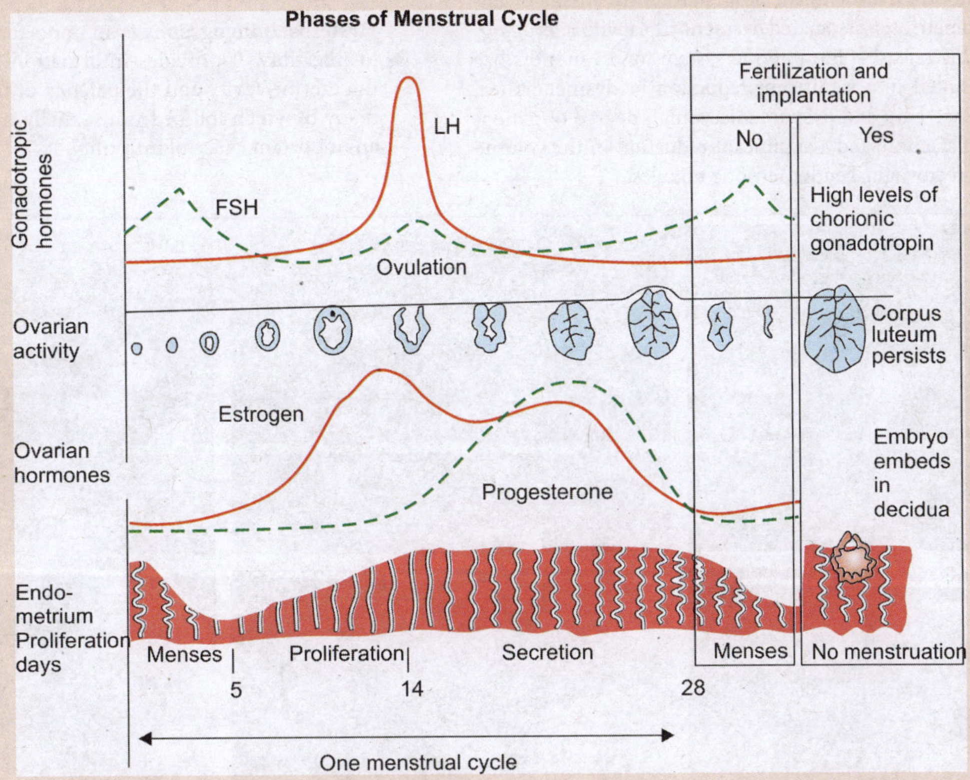

Footnote:
- The endometrial surface is reepithelialized within 4 to 7 days after the beginning of menstruation
- Even during menses, increasing estrogen levels produced by the ovary begin the healing process and the endometrium begins to regenerate and prepare for the next cycle
- Progesterone peaks on 21st day of menstrual cycle

110. Ans. (b) Serum FSH >40 IU/L

Ref: Novak's Gynecology 14th ed page 1952, Shaw's 15th ed page 62

Menopause

Menopause is defined retrospectively as the time of the final menstrual period followed by 12 months of amenorrhea. Postmenopause describes the period following the final menses.

- Mean age 51 years
- At the level of the ovary, there is a depletion of ovarian follicles, most likely secondary to apoptosis or programd cell death.
- The ovarian–hypothalamic–pituitary axis remains intact during the menopausal transition; thus, FSH levels rise in response to ovarian failure and the absence of negative feedback from the ovary.
- The menopausal transition is characterized by elevated FSH levels associated with variable cycle lengths and missed menses, whereas the postmenopausal period is marked by amenorrhea. The menopausal transition begins with variability in menstrual cycle length accompanied by rising FSH levels and ends with the final menstrual period.
- "Estrogens, progesterone and total androgen production is decreased after menopause, however FSH increases due to negative feedback of estrogen over FSH production by pituitary"

111. Ans. (b) Premenstrual tension

Ref: Novak's Gynecology 14th ed page 358, 680, 1658, William's 24th Ed page 701, Goodman Gilman 12th Ed page 1184

Mainly the progestin is used in premenstrual tension not levonorgestrel.

Uses of Levonorgestrel

- **Emergency contraception:** *Levonorgestrel 1.5 mg* (*Plan B*) is the most effective hormonal means of emergency contraception. Efficacy is greatest within 24 hours of intercourse but is still high at 5 days.
- **Atypical endometrial hyperplasia:** For women with abnormal uterine bleeding and histopathological diagnosis of atypical endometrial hyperplasia oral parenteral or intrauterine delivery of progestins may be used if they wish to retain their uterus.
  - *Levonorgestrel*-containing intrauterine devices also have been shown to reduce menstrual blood loss significantly and to result in improvements in

health-related quality of life that may be comparable to hysterectomy.

- **Endometriosis:** Local progesterone treatment of endometriosis–associated dysmenorrhea with a *levonorgestrel* releasing intrauterine system for 12 months has resulted in a significant reduction in dysmenorrhea, pelvic pain and dyspareunia; a high degree of patient satisfaction; and a significant reduction in the volume of rectovaginal endometriotic nodules.

112. Ans. (b) Endometrial polyps

Ref: Shaw's 16th Ed page 103

Hysterosalpingography is an important tool in the evaluation of infertility. It provides information regarding the shape of the uterine cavity and the patency of the tubes. Tubal factors, many of which follow from sexually transmitted diseases, are an important cause of infertility.

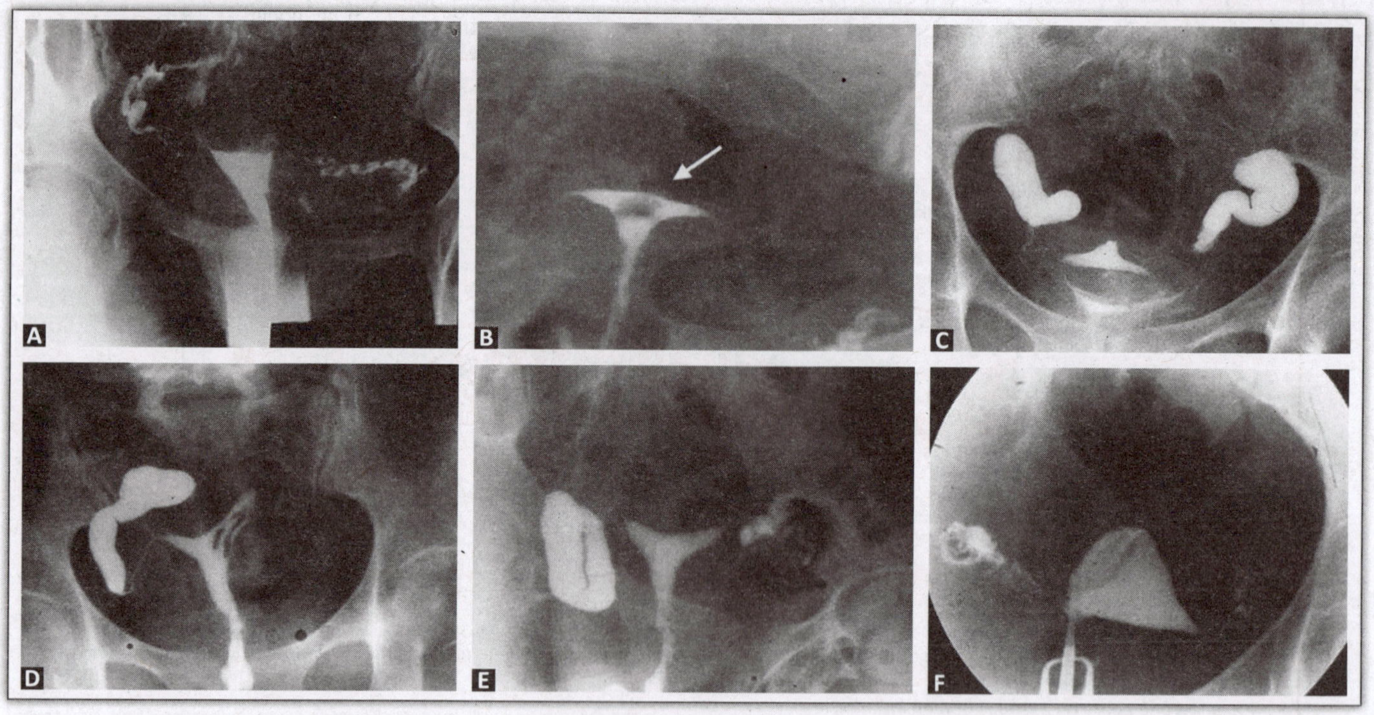

Figs A to F: A. Normal hysterosalpingogram: Shows normal filling and spillage of contrast media; **B. Endometrial polyps** are seen as filling defects of various size at the level of uterine cavity. This HSG shows a rounded fundal polyp; **C.** Displays bilateral hydrosalpinx and clubbing of the tubes with no evidence of any spillage into the peritoneal cavity. The uterine cavity in this HSG is normal; **D.** In the figure there is unilateral hydrosalpinx and evidence of adhesions within the uterine cavity consistent with **Asherman syndrome**. There is no filling of the other tube; **E.** One tube fills and has unilateral hydrosalpinx; the other shows loculation and minimal fluid accumulation. The uterine cavity here is normal; **F. Salpingitis isthmica nodosa:** characteristic "salt-and pepper" pattern of tubal filling and evidence of a diverticulum of the tube on one side

113. Ans. (d) Desogestrel

Ref: William's 24th ed page 1484; Dutta 7th ed page 551

Recall Bias

Ulipristal acetate was not asked as a separate question but as an option of this question

Emergency contraception with the copper T 380A IUD is highly effective up to 5 days after intercourse.

See Table of Postcoital/Emergency Contraceptives In OBG AIIMS Nov. 2017 (see page no. 872)

114. Ans. (b) α-methyl dopa

Ref: William's 23rd ed chapter 45

KDT 7th ed page 566: α-methyldopa is infrequently used now, except to treat hypertension during pregnancy wherein it has a long track record of safety, both for the mother as well as the foetus.

William's Says: The most commonly used drugs in pregnancy to treat hypertension are α-methyldopa

Because of its long-standing record of safety, -methyldopa is frequently used to control chronic hypertension during pregnancy. The drug has been extensively studied during pregnancy (Cockburn and associates, 1982; Montana and colleagues, 1992, 1993). In their review, Ferrer and colleagues (2000) concluded that its use in the first trimester has not been associated with any pattern of fetal anomalies. The results of treatment with labetalol are consistent with the view that the drug offers no advantages over -methyldopa (Sibai and colleagues, 1990a).

115. Ans. (b) α-methyldopa

Ref: William's 23rd ed chapter 45

Repeat AIIMS NOV 2015 OBG (See previous question for explanation) (see page no. 906)

116. Ans. (a) Enalapril

Ref: Williams 24th ed page 1005, KDT 6th ed page 909

ACE inhibitors are contraindicated used in pregnancy. Enalapril is an ACE inhibitor. This is a VITAL question you cannot miss.

Drugs Crossing Placenta			
ACE inhibitors	Kanamycin	Radioactive Iodine	Coumarins
Aminopterin	Leflunomide	Ribavirin	Cyclophosphamide
Androgens	Lithium	Streptomycin	Danazol
A-II antagonists	Methimazole	Tamoxifen	Diethylstilbestrol (DES)
Busulfan	Methotrexate	Tetracycline	Ethanol
Carbamazepine	Misoprostol	Thalidomide	Efavirenz
Chlorobiphenyls	Penicillamine	Tretinoin	Etretinate
Cocaine	Phenytoin	Tobacco	Isotretinoin
Corticosteroids	Valproic acid	Trimethadione	Warfarin

United States FDA Pharmaceutical Pregnancy Categories

Category	Description	Examples
Pregnancy Category A	Adequate and well-controlled human studies have failed to demonstrate a risk to the fetus in the first trimester of pregnancy (and there is no evidence of risk in later trimesters)	Inj. Mag. sulfate, Thyroxine
Pregnancy Category B	Animal reproduction studies have failed to demonstrate a risk to the fetus and there are no adequate and well-controlled studies in pregnant women OR Animal studies have shown an adverse effect, but adequate and well-controlled studies in pregnant women have failed to demonstrate a risk to the fetus in any trimester.	Penicillin V Amoxicillin Cefaclor Erythromycin Paracetamol Lignocaine, Brimonidine
Pregnancy Category C	Animal reproduction studies have shown an adverse effect on the fetus and there are no adequate and well-controlled studies in humans, but potential benefits may warrant use of the drug in pregnant women despite potential risks.	Morphine, Codeine Adropine, Corticosteroids Arenaline, Pilocarpine Thiopentone Bupivacaine Latanoprost, Dorzolamide
Pregnancy Category D	There is positive evidence of human fetal risk based on adverse reaction data from investigational or marketing experience or studies in humans, but potential benefits may warrant use of the drug in pregnant women despite potential risks.	Aspirin, Phenytoin, Carbamazepine, Valproate, Lorazepam
Pregnancy Category X	Studies in animals or humans have demonstrated fetal abnormalities and/or there is positive evidence of human fetal risk based on adverse reaction data from investigational or marketing experience and the risks involved in use of the drug in pregnant women clearly outweigh potential benefits.	Domperidone, Morphine Fluoroquinolones, Tetracycline, Doxycycline, Chloramphenicol, Streptomycin, Kanamycin, Tobramycin Tinidazole, Quinine, Sulfadoxine, Primaquine, Mebendazole, DEC Amphotericin –B, Itraconazole, Ketoconazole, Griseofulvin, Ganciclovir, Foscarnet, Amantadine, α-INF, ACE inhibitors, Angiotensin antagonist, Sulfonylurea, Acarbose, Metformin, Warfarin, Thalidomide, Alcohol, Radioactive iodine, Estrogen Isotretinoin, Cytotoxic drugs, Ergometrine

117. Ans. (b) Krukenberg tumor

Ref: Shaw's Textbook of Gynecology 15th ed page 425, Robbins 9th ed page 1032, Rosai and Akerman's Surgical Pathology 10th ed page 1607-08

History of Abdominal mass is consistent with GI Malignancy. Bilateral Ovarian mass in presence of GI Malignancy with histological features of **Signet ring appearance** is characteristic of Krukenberg's tumor.

The eponym Krukenberg tumor is used to designate an ovarian neoplasm, usually bilateral and nearly always metastatic origin. Most examples of Krukenberg tumors occur after the age of 40 years, but younger patients can also be affected. In the latter instance, a mistaken diagnosis of granulosa cell tumor or lipid cell tumor is often made.

The usual primary source of krukenberg tumors are stomach, large bowel, appendix and breast. Of these **diffuse gastric carcinoma (linitis plastica) used to be the most common,** but at present there is preponderance of cases originated from breast, at least in united states. The ovarian deposits can be accompanied by retroperitoneal lymph node metastasis and peritoneal implants

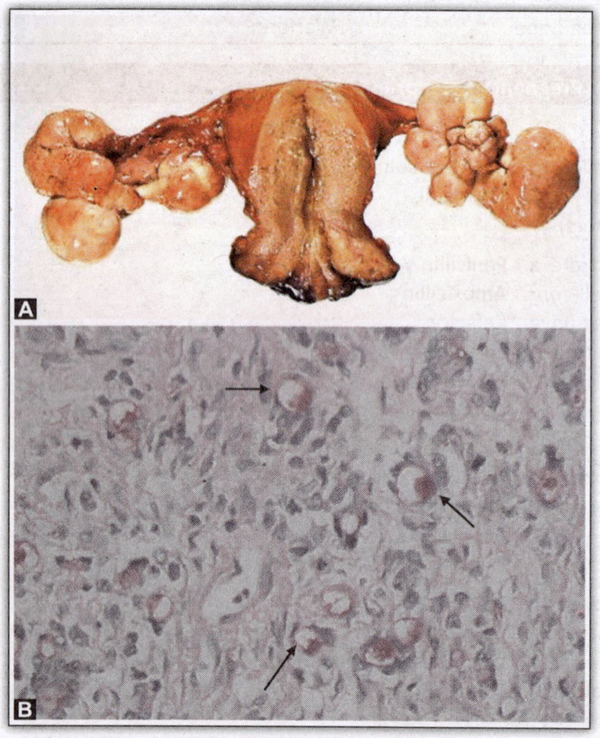

Figs A and B: A. Krukenberg tumor gross: Asymmetrical enlargement, lobular multinodular contour and either solid (mostly) or cystic consistency (30%); **B. Krukenberg tumor Microscopy:** Diffuse infiltration by signet ring cells containing abundant neutral and acidic (sialo mucin) vacuoles pushing the nucleus to one side. Tumor emboli are found in over 50% of the cases

118. Ans. (a) Volume >1.5 mL, count >15 million/mL, Normal morphology >4% progressive motility >32%

Ref: Speroff 8th ed pg no 1270-1271, Novak's Gynecology 15th ed page 1142

Normal Semen Analysis: World Health Organization

	1992 guidelines	2010 guidelines
Volume	2 mL	≥1.5 mL
Sperm concentration	20 million/mL	≥15 million/mL
Sperm motility	50% progressive or >25% rapidly progressive	≥32% progressive
Morphology (strict criteria/best parameter)	>15% normal forms	≥4% normal forms
White blood cells	<1 million/mL	<1 million/mL
Immunobead or mixed antiglobulin	<10% coated with antibodies	<50% reaction test

119. Ans. (d) 6 mg 12 hourly 4 doses

Ref: Nelson's 20th ed page 852, Dutta 7th ed page 316, Protocols for high risk pregnancies An evidence based approach 5th ed page 464; Williams 24th ed page 1562, 1768 and Royal College of Obstetricians and Gynaecologists Greentop Guidelines no. 7 (https://www.rcog.org.uk/globalassets/documents/guidelines/gtg_7.pdf)

Antenatal Corticosteroids - Summary/FAQS

- A **single** course of antenatal corticosteroids (American College of Obstetricians and Gynaecologists (2013 c) is recommended to women between 24 + 0 and 34 + 6 weeks of gestation who are at risk of preterm birth. No rescue dose is recommended.
- Antenatal corticosteroids should be given to all women for whom an elective caesarean section is planned prior to 38 + 6 weeks of gestation and also to women with multiple pregnancy at risk of imminent iatrogenic or spontaneous preterm delivery between 24 + 0 and 34 + 6 weeks of gestation.
- **Betamethasone 12 mg given intramuscularly in two doses 24 hours apart** or **dexamethasone 6 mg given intramuscularly in four doses 12 hours apart** are the steroids of choice to enhance lung maturation.
- A large nonrandomized retrospective study has suggested that infants exposed to antenatal betamethasone have less neonatal cystic periventricular leukomalacia than infants exposed to antenatal dexamethasone. Hence **betamethasone is the steroid of choice.**

120. Ans. (d) 4000 micrograms/day

Ref: Williams obstetrics 24th ed page 1104, Nelson 20th ed page 2805

See details of Folic Acid Prophylaxis in OBG AIIMS NOV 2015 (see page no. 903)

121. Ans. (a) Ureterovaginal fistula

Ref: Shaw's 15th ed page 184- 186, ACOG vol 2 part 2 page 611, Novak's 14th ed page 886

The given patient has undergone surgery for carcinoma cervix and uppermost portion of pad has yellow staining by urine (i.e. with phenazopyridine secreted in urine), it is ureterovaginal fistula.

Urinary Fistulas				
	Vesicovaginal fistula (VVF)	Ureterovaginal fistula	Urethrovaginal fistula	Vesicouterine fistula
Causes	*Obstructed labor* (MC cause in developing countries, manifests 3-5 days after delivery), *Pelvic surgery* (MC cause in developed countries), Bladder injury common during C-section if not emptied prior to it. May also be caused due to advanced genital cancers or radiation injuries	Hysterectomy (Max risk with Wertheim's hysterectomy)	Penetrating injury during fall or criminal abortion	Rare incidence. Caesarean section and repeat caesarean sections or uterine Rupture
Clinical features	Occurs 3-5 days after obstructed labor (due to ischemic necrosis), Continuous dribbling of urine from vagina, No normal urge for micturition	Continuous dribbling of urine from vagina, Normal urge for micturition	No continuous leakage, but when patient urinates, urine leaks from vagina and urethra	Cyclical hematuria, bladder continence is maintained
Methylene blue test, 3 swab test	Middle cotton plug is wet with dye and urine (blue in color)	Uppermost cotton plug is wet with urine but not with dye. Other 2 cotton swabs are dry	Lowermost cotton plug is wet with dye, other 2 are dye	Not useful
Investigation	Cystoscopy	Dye withindigo carmine demonstrates urinary extravasation and identifies the location of injury and Cystoscopy		Cystoscopy
Management of choice	Latzko repair/Layer technique/Chassar Moir technique Time of surgery: If it is due to obstructed labor-repair done after 3 months If due to surgery and recognized within 24 hours-immediate repair. If recognized later after 3-6 months If extensive loss of bladder tissue or repeated failure to heal-urinary diversion procedures should be considered.	**Boari Flap technique** (ureteroneocystostomy) As early as possible	Vaginal repair + Urethral reconstruction	Abdominal repair

Latzko procedure technique: Make a circumferential incision in the vagina 2 cm from the fistulous tract. Mobilize the vagina and close it over the fistulous tract with delayed absorbable sutures in double layer without disturbing the bladder mucosa.

122. Ans. (c) 300 mg

Ref: Hypertension in pregnancy (Report of the ACOG Task force on hypertension in pregnancy) obstetrics and gynecology, vol. 122, No. 5, November 2013, Danforth 10th ed page 264, William's 24th Ed page 181, Dutta 7th Ed page 224

In 2013, the American College of Obstetricians and Gynecologists removed proteinuria (if other severe preeclampsia features are present) as an essential criterion for diagnosis of preeclampsia. They also removed massive proteinuria (5 g/24 hours) and fetal growth restriction as possible features of severe disease because massive proteinuria has a poor correlation with outcome and fetal growth restriction is managed similarly whether or not preeclampsia is diagnosed.

Hence in absence of diagnostic requirement of 5 g as massive proteinuria for Severe preeclampsia, general definition of Proteinuria (>0.3 g = 300 mg) will suffice, provided that other criteria of severe Preeclampsia are present.

Classification of Hypertension in Pregnancy	
Definition of hypertension	
Mild:	Systolic blood pressure $\geq$140 mm Hg Diastolic blood pressure $\geq$90 mm Hg
Severe:	Systolic blood pressure $\geq$180 mm Hg Diastolic blood pressure $\geq$110 mm Hg
Chronic hypertension	
Hypertension with onset before pregnancy or before 20th week gestation Use of antihypertensive medications before pregnancy Persistence of hypertension beyond 12 weeks postpartum	

Contd...

Classification of Hypertension in Pregnancy
Preeclampsia
Hypertension that occurs after 20 weeks of gestation in a woman with previously normal blood pressure. Systolic blood pressure ≥140 mm Hg or diastolic blood pressure ≥90 mm Hg on two occasions at least 6 hours apart **Proteinuria,** defined as urinary excretion of **≥0.3 g protein** in a 24-hour urine specimen. This finding usually correlates with a finding of 1+ or greater on dipstick. Note edema is no longer a diagnostic criterion. Note a systolic rise of 30 mm Hg or a diastolic rise of 15 mm Hg is no longer a diagnostic criterion.
Eclampsia
New-onset grand mal seizures in a woman with preeclampsia that cannot be attributed to other causes. Superimposed preeclampsia—Eclampsia. Preeclampsia or eclampsia that occurs in a woman with a pre-existing chronic hypertension.
Gestational hypertension
• Hypertension detected for the first time after mid pregnancy. • Distinguished from preeclampsia by the absence of proteinuria. • Working diagnosis only during pregnancy.
Transient hypertension of pregnancy
• Gestational hypertension that resolves by 12 weeks postpartum. • If proteinuria develops in a patient with gestational hypertension, the diagnosis is preeclampsia. • If gestational hypertension does not resolve by 12 weeks postpartum, the diagnosis is chronic hypertension.

Classification of Preeclampsia	
Mild preeclampsia	**Severe preeclampsia**
Blood pressure ≥140/90 mm Hg but <160/110 mm Hg on two occasions at least 6 hours apart while the patient is on bed rest	Blood pressure ≥160 mm Hg systolic or ≥110 mm Hg diastolic on two occasions at least 6 hours apart while the patient is on bed rest
Proteinuria ≥300 mg/24 hours but <5 g/24 hours	Proteinuria of 5 g or higher in 24-hour urine specimen or 3+ or greater on two random urine samples collected at least 4 hours apart
Asymptomatic	Oliguria <500 mL in 24 hours Cerebral or visual disturbances Pulmonary edema or cyanosis Epigastric or right upper quadrant pain Impaired liver function Thrombocytopenia Fetal growth restriction

NOTE

AICOG in 2013 (a) Oliguria was also removed as a characteristic of severe disease. (b) Massive proteinuria >5 mg was removed from severe preeclampsia.

123. Ans. (d) Rectovaginal septum

Ref: Gray's anatomy 40th ed ch 77, 1333, BDC Vol 24th Edn Page 320, Shaw's 15th Ed Pg 331

The rectovaginal fascia (often called rectovaginal septum or sometimes fascia of Otto) is a thin structure separating the vagina and the rectum.

Supports of Uterus	
Primary supports of uterus	
Muscular or active supports:	• Pelvic diaphragm (formed by Levator ani muscle) • Perineal body • Urogenital diaphragm

Fibromuscular or mechanical support	• Uterine axis
	• Round ligament of uterus
	• **Major Ligaments; Triradiate ligament**
	  ▪ Pubocervical ligament
	  ▪ Uterosacral ligament
	  ▪ Cardinal ligaments (or Mackenrodt's ligament/lateral cervical ligament/transverse cervical ligament)

Secondary supports of uterus

- Broad ligament
- Utero vaginal fold of peritoneum
- Rectovaginal fold of peritoneum

Major ligaments; Triradiate ligament

Name	From	To	Comment
Uterosacral ligament (lies within recto-uterine folds)	Posterior cervix; pass back from the cervix and uterine body on both sides of the rectum	Anterior face of sacrum	**Chief support** Can be palpated laterally on vaginal and rectal examination. Keep uterus anteverted hence prevent retroversion
Cardinal ligaments (or Mackenrodt's ligament/ lateral cervical ligament/ transverse cervical ligament)	Side of the cervix and lateral fornix of the vagina	Ischial spines	**Chief support** Contains uterine artery and uterine vein. Close proximity to the ureters which can get damaged during ligation of the ligament during hysterectomy
Pubocervical ligament	Side of the cervix; passes forward from the anterior aspect of the cervix and upper vagina to diverge around the urethra	Posterior aspect of pubic symphysis	However it is a major ligament but not a chief support of uterus

Note:

- **Ligaments attached to cervix:** Cervix being the most fixed part of uterus, gives attachment to ligaments. There are three ligaments which forms a three spoked **Triradiate ligament**
- Peritoneum forms the ***weakest support of the uterus***
- The transverse cervical ligaments on either side and uterosacral ligaments at the back, form the **chief supports of the uterus.**
- The suspensory ligament of the ovary, also Infundibulopelvic ligament is a fold of peritoneum that extends out from the ovary to the wall of the pelvis. Some sources consider it a part of the broad ligament of uterus

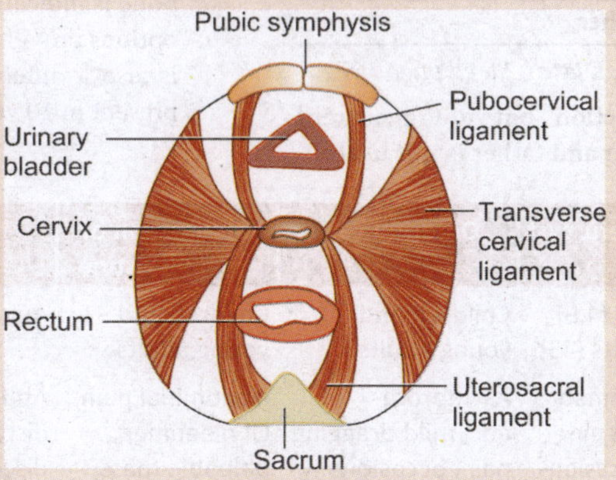

124. Ans. (b) Copper IUD

Ref: Williams 24th ed page 714, Dutta 7th Ed 551

See Details of Emergency Contraception in AIIMS Nov 2015 (see page no. 855 and 905)

Patient is a 32 years old lady with her family complete so long term contraception is a priority for her. And also, she has come after 4 days of intercourse. High dose oral contraceptive pill (OCP) and levonorgestrel 0.75 mg is effective up to 72 hours of intercourse, so in this case its effectiveness is doubtful.

Cu T disrupts implantation and can be put up to 5 days after the intercourse.

Laparoscopic tubectomy is the best long term management plan but it will not prevent this pregnancy.

125. Ans. (a) 100 microgram IM

Ref: Cochrane Database of Systematic Reviews 2012, Issue 4. Art. No.: CD005457. DOI: 10.1002/14651858.CD005457.pub4

Although textbooks are not yet mentioning the carbetocin dose for PPH, COCHRANE systematic review gives us the answer. Carbetocin is an oxytocin agonist.

For carbetocin and syntometrine: Four trials compared intramuscular carbetocin (100 mcg) and intramuscular syntometrine for women undergoing vaginal deliveries.

Comparison between carbetocin and syntometrine showed a lower mean blood loss in women who received carbetocin compared to syntometrine.

For carbetocin and oxytocin: Use of carbetocin resulted in a statistically significant reduction in the need for therapeutic uterotonics compared to oxytocin for those who underwent cesarean section, but not for vaginal delivery. Compared to oxytocin, carbetocin was associated with a reduced need for uterine massage following both caesarean delivery and vaginal delivery.

126. Ans. (b) 92, 180, 153

Ref: William's 24th ed page 1137, 2377

The recommended two-step approach begins with either universal or risk-based selective screening using a 50-g, 1-hour oral glucose challenge test.

Participants in the Fifth International Workshop Conferences on Gestational Diabetes endorsed universal screening. Screening should be performed between **24 and 28 weeks** gestation in those women not known to have glucose intolerance earlier in pregnancy. This *50-g screening test* is followed by a *diagnostic 100-g, 3-hour oral glucose tolerance test (OGTT)* if screening results meet or exceed a predetermined plasma glucose concentration.

Threshold Values for Diagnosis of Gestational Diabetes Mellitus

Plasma glucose at	Threshold cut off value (mg/dL)
Fasting	92
1 hour OGTT	180
2 hour OGTT	153

127. Ans. (c) VDRL of father and mother

Ref: William's 24th ed page 358-359, Dutta's 7th ed page 167

Syphilis causes congenital infection but not recurrent abortions. Hence VDRL of mother and father is not useful.

- Approximately half of miscarriages are *anembryonic*, that is, with no identifiable embryonic elements.
- The other 50 percent are *embryonic* miscarriages, which commonly display a developmental abnormality of the zygote, embryo, fetus, or at times, the placenta.

Option (A) and (B) Lupus Anticoagulant

Antiphospholipid syndrome—Includes Lupus anticoagulant (LA) Anticardiolipin antibodies (ACAS). Women with recurrent spontaneous pregnancy loss have a higher frequency of antiphospholipid antibodies compared with normal controls 5 to 15 versus 2 to 5 percent respectively. The *antiphospholipid antibody syndrome (APS)* is defined by these antibodies found together with various forms of reproductive losses along with substantively increased risks for venous thromboembolism.

Option (D) Karyotype

- Approximately half of miscarriages are *anaembryonic*. The other 50 percent are *embryonic* miscarriages, which commonly display a developmental abnormality of the zygote, embryo, fetus, or at times, the placenta.
- Of embryonic miscarriage, half of these—25 percent of all abortuses—have chromosomal anomalies and thus are *aneuploid abortions*. A small percentage of second trimester abortions are also aneuploid abortions.
- Hence the abortus is sent for karyotyping.

128. Ans. (d) Ovarian cyst

Ref: Shaw's 16th ed page 83, 448, Bailey 26th ed page 98

Inability to insinuate fingers between the mass and the pelvic bone is indicative of the mass being arising from Pelvis. In the options provided only Ovarian cyst is a pelvic mass. Pregnancy is also a differential of Pelvic mass by highly unlikely to be present in 10 years age.

Feature	Ovarian cyst	Mesenteric cyst	Omental cyst	Duplication of small intestine	Ascitis	Myoma	Pregnancy
Age group	Females, young	Children (4.9) and adults (45)	Children and young adults	Children and young adults	Any age	Females, usually >35-40	Reproductive
Clinical features	Menstrual disturbances,	Asymptomatic, mild dragging pain, occasionally intestinal obstruction	Asymptomatic, mild dragging pain, occasionally intestinal obstruction	Abdominal pain, GI bleeding, palpable mass, vomiting, bowel obstruction	Abdominal distention and discomfort (features of cause will be present)	Abnormal uterine bleeding, dysmenorrhea	Amenorrhea
Examination	Mobile, cystic, Arising from pelvis, dull note over cyst and resonant in flanks. Mass arising from pelvis, fingers not insinuated between mass and pelvic bone	Asymptomatic, thin walled freely mobile, soft mass located in mesentery near terminal ileum, not arising from pelvis	Asymptomatic, thin walled freely mobile, soft mass located in mesentery near terminal ileum, not arising from pelvis	Soft, compressible, mass at site of terminal ileum	Dull note over flanks, tympanitic on abdomen. Shifting dullness +nt	Midline pelvic mass depending on size and location	FHS and fetal movement present, Arising from pelvis. fingers not insinuated between mass and pelvic bone
Investigation	USG	USG, abdominal CT	USG, CT	USG	USG and according to pathology associated	USG	USG

129. Ans. (a) Plan for immediate laparoscopic surgery

Ref: Novak 15th ed page 627-633, Shaw 15th ed page 267, Williams 24th ed page 780, Dutta 7th Ed Pg 180-182

Shaw **says that in case of ruptured ectopic the patient should be immediately operated once the diagnosis is made and blood transfusion is given when it is earliest available. In expert hands laparoscopy is the surgery of choice.**

Ectopic Pregnancy	
Epidemiology	Most common in age group 20-30 years, Nulliparous.
Clinical features	Abdominal pain (100%) + Amenorrhea (75%) + Vaginal bleeding (70%) Vomiting, fainting attack, Pallor, Features of shock, Tense tumid and tender abdomen, Adnexal mass palpable (50% of cases)
Clinical features of tubal rupture	• Severe lower abdominal and pelvic pain that is frequently described as sharp, stabbing, or tearing. • Tenderness during abdominal palpation and also a tender adnexal mass could be present. Bimanual pelvic examination, especially cervical motion, causes exquisite pain. • Blood pressure will fall and pulse will rise only if bleeding continues and hypovolemia becomes significant.
USG	• Psuedogestational sac may be seen- centrally located, probably represents bleeding into the endometrial cavity by the decidual cast. Clots within may mimic a fetal pole. Identification of the double decidual sac sign (DDSS) is the best method of ultrasonographically differentiating true sacs from pseudo sacs. • Presence of an adnexal gestational sac with a fetal pole and cardiac activity is the most specific but least sensitive sign. • Presence of complex or solid adnexal mass. • Fluid in pouch of douglas • ***Blob sign***- Adnexal mass clearly separated from ovary • Rarely cardiac movement seen in unruptured pregnancy • ***Bagel's sign***- typical intact tubal ring is present
Doppler USG	Peritrophoblastic flow -high velocity low resistance flow.
Lab diagnosis	hCG quantification---*Doubling time for hCG* -—a 66% rise in the hCG level over 48 hours (85% confidence level) represents the lower limit of normal values for viable intrauterine pregnancies

130. Ans. (a) Androgen insensitivity

Ref: Williams 24th ed page 149, Shaw's 15th ed page 111, Novak's 14th Ed Pg 1037, 1451,1504

Recall Bias

Some people believe that absent uterus and gonads on USG was given in the question and there was no H/O OCP consumption. In that case the diagnosis will be same and even more definitive.

Different case scenario of AIS was asked in Nov 2011

See OBG AIIMS Nov 2016 for Discussion of Primary Amenorrhea (see page no. 883)

131. Ans. (a) TSH

Ref: Novaks 14th ed page 1017, Harrison's 19th Ed page 2267; Blueprints Obstetrics and Gynecology 5th ed page 228; Speroff clinical gynecologic endocrinology and infertility 6th ed page 183

Galactorrhea Amenorrhea Syndrome- Summary/FAQs

- Prolactin-secreting adenomas are the most common pituitary tumors.
- A high prolactin level is encountered in about 2/3 of women with no obvious cause of amenorrhea. And 1/3rd women with high prolactin levels have normal menses.
- Only 1/3 of women with high prolactin levels will have galactorrhea, probably because the low estrogen environment associated with the amenorrhea prevents a normal response to prolactin.
- As the prolactin concentration increases, a woman can progress sequentially from normal ovulation total anovulation and amenorrhea.
- The amenorrhea associated with elevated prolactin levels is due to prolactin inhibition of the pulsatile secretion of GnRH and low levels of FSH and LH are usually associated.
- Primary hypothyroidism also is associated with hyperprolactinemia because increased levels of thyrotropin–releasing hormone (TRH) stimulate secretion of prolactin.
- If both levels are elevated, hypothyroidism should be treated and prolactin levels can be checked after thyroid studies have normalised.
- Treatment: Transsphenoidal technique approaches via a sublabial incision (under the upper lip), with dissection under the nasal mucosa, removal of the nasal septum to expose the sphenoidal sinus and resection of the floor of the sphenoid sinus to expose the sella turcica.

NOTE

Amenorrhea and/or galactorrhea may precede the eventual full clinical expression of a tumor that secretes ACTH or growth hormone. If clinical criteria suggest Cushing's disease, ACTH levels and the 24-hour urinary levels of free cortisol should be measured and the rapid suppression test should be utilized. If acromegaly is suspected, growth hormone and the circulating level of IGF-I should be measured. Elevated gonadotropins in the presence of a pituitary microadenoma in a woman with amenorrhea are not a consequence of secretion by the tumor; another explanation must be pursued.

132. Ans. (b) Tamoxifen

Ref: Jeffcott 6th Ed page 205, Shaw's 15th ed, p 371, Novaks 15th Ed Pg 1076

Option (A)

Spironolactone decreases androgen production and competes with androgens at the androgen receptor level. Side effects include limited diuresis and dysfunctional uterine bleeding.

Option (C)

OCP's are used in PCOS patients to oppose the unopposed action of estrogen in the anovulatory cycles. Also, Oral contraceptives may be effective by decreasing ovarian androgen production as well as increasing circulating levels of sex hormone–binding globulin, leading to decreased free androgen circulation.

Option (D)

Clomiphene citrate is the primary ovulation inducing agent in patients with chronic anovulation and PCOS patients.

Rotterdam Criteria for Polycystic Ovarian Syndrome (PCOD) (2003)

- Oligo or anovulation
- Clinical or biochemical signs of hyperandrogenism
- Polycystic ovaries, with exclusion of other etiologies

At least 2 criteria should be present:

- **HAIR-AN syndrome** consists of hyperandrogenism (HA), insulin resistance (IR) and acanthosis nigricans (AN). It is a subset of polycystic ovary syndrome
- **SAHA syndrome** is characterized by seborrhea, acne, hirsutism and alopecia, frequently associated with polycystic ovary syndrome, cystic mastitis, obesity and infertility.

General Surgery

14

AIIMS NOVEMBER 2018

1. What is the method of breast examination depicted in the video?

a. Vertical strip method
b. Concentric method
c. Clockwise method
d. Quadrant method

2. Which is the most conspicuous sign of breast cancer?

a. Nipple retraction
b. Peau d'orange
c. Puckering
d. Both nipple retraction and puckering

3. Thyroid storm during surgery is due to? *(AIIMS Nov 2018, 2015)*

a. Recurrent laryngeal nerve injury
b. Inappropriate preoperative preparation
c. Rough handling during surgery
d. Removal of parathyroid

4. Identify the flap shown in the given image?

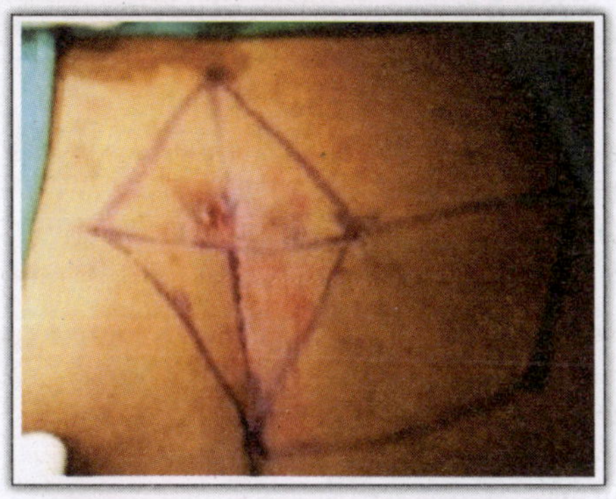

a. Rhomboid flap
b. Rotational flap
c. Bilobed flap
d. Free flap

5. What technique has been depicted in the given image?

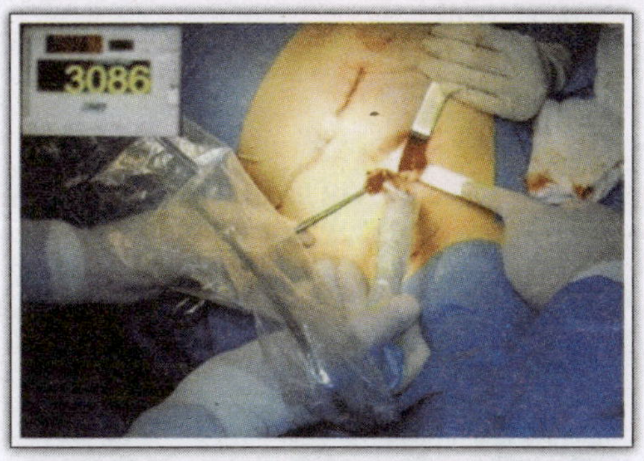

© Follacchio GA et al J. Exp. Clin. Cancer Res. (2015)

a. Brachytherapy
b. Ultrasonography
c. Sentinel lymph node biopsy
d. Lateral pectoral nerve block

6. While doing emergency laparotomy for an intestinal obstruction. Which structure will be first visualised by the surgeon to identify whether it is small or large intestine obstruction?

a. Ileum
b. Sigmoid colon
c. Cecum
d. Rectum

7. Color of the entry port of 16F Foley's catheter is?

a. Orange
b. Blue
c. Yellow
d. Black

8. Which is the best position for insertion of the tube shown in the picture? *(AIIMS Nov 2018, May 2018)*

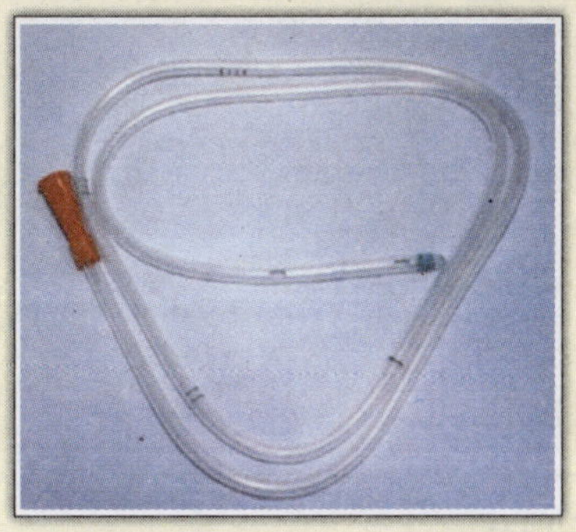

a. Sitting with neck flexed
b. Supine with neck flexed
c. Supine with neck extension
d. Prone with neck extended

9. The device shown in the Image is used in the management of which condition?

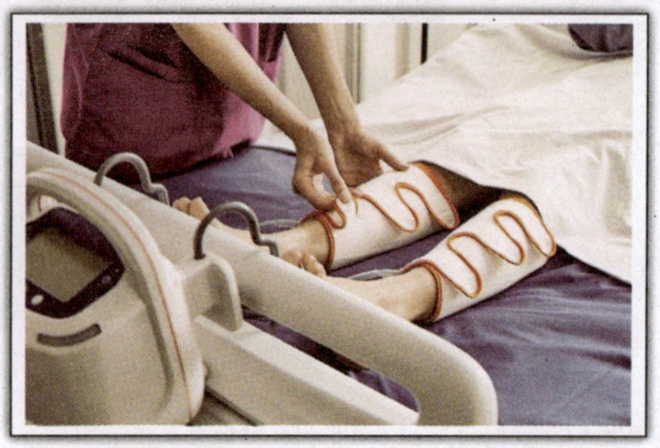

a. Varicose veins
b. Hypothermia
c. Cellulitis
d. DVT

10. The given instrument is used for harvesting the graft from healthy area in split skin thickness graft:

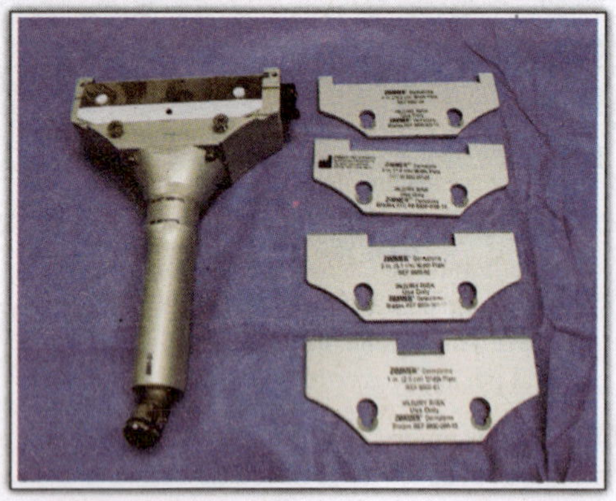

a. Silver's knife
b. Catlin amputating knife
c. Humby knife
d. Dermatome

11. Identify the given instrument.

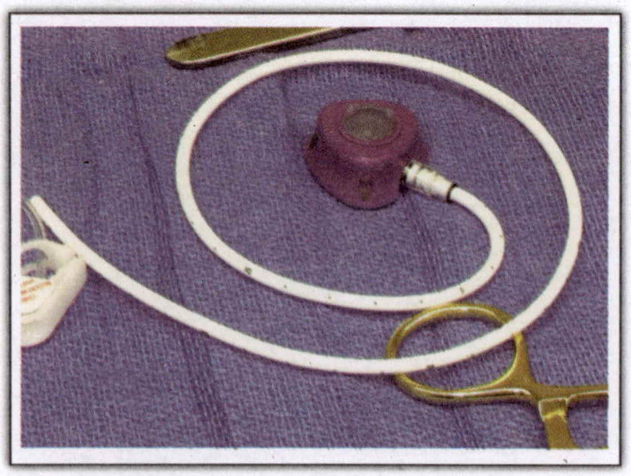

a. Gamma camera
b. Chemoport
c. IVC filter
d. Pacemaker

12. Calculate GCS for Intubated patient who is opening eyes on verbal command and moving his all four limbs spontaneously?

a. 7
b. 9
c. 10
d. 12

13. In a patient suffered massive hemorrhage in a Road Traffic accident and presents to emergency department with shock. Which of the following should not be done?

a. IV crystalloid 2 liters with in 2 minutes
b. Early tranexamic Acid recommended
c. Check coagulation with thromboelastography if available`
d. Fluid challenge

AIIMS MAY 2018

14. During a laparoscopic inguinal hernia repair, the triangle of doom refers to a triangular area bounded by?

a. Vas deferens medially, Medial Umbilical ligament laterally and Testicular vessels inferiorly
b. Medial Umbilical ligament medially, Lateral Umbilical ligament lateral and peritoneal fold inferiorly
c. Medial umbilical ligament medially, Testicular vessels laterally and peritoneal fold inferiorly
d. Vas deferens medially, Medial Umbilical ligament laterally and peritoneal fold inferiorly

15. Renal calculi most resistant to shock wave lithotripsy are?

a. Struvite
b. Cystine
c. Calcium oxalate monohydrate
d. Uric acid

16. Identify the pathology in the given picture?

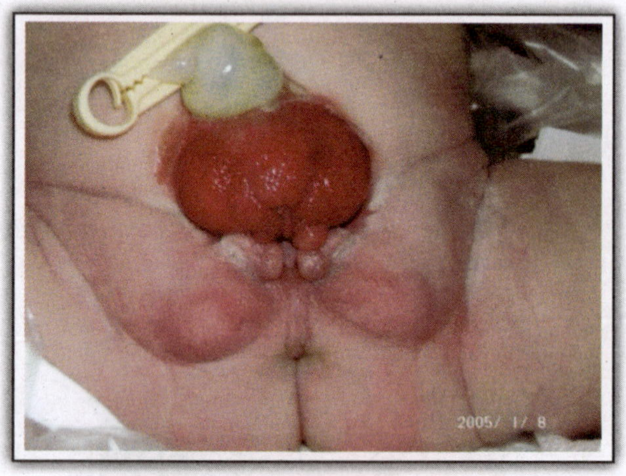

© Ebert AK

a. Gastroschisis
b. Bladder exstrophy
c. Omphalocele
d. Superior vesical fissure

17. Where is the second step of damage control resuscitation carried out?

a. In Emergency
b. In ICU
c. In OT
d. Prehospital resuscitation

18. Which is the best position for insertion of the tube shown in the picture? *(AIIMS Nov 2018, May 2018)*

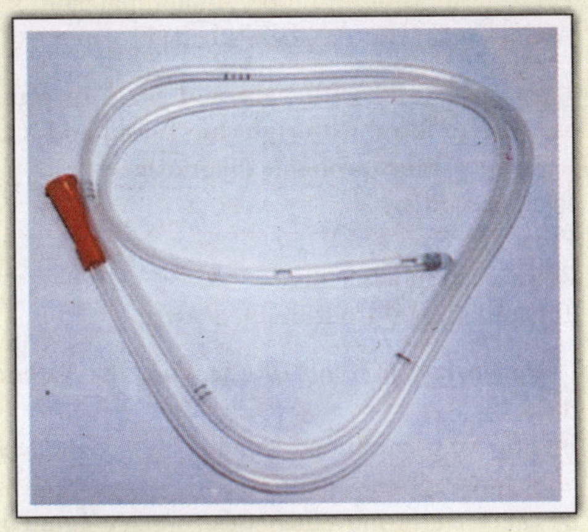

a. Sitting with neck flexed
b. Supine with neck flexed
c. Supine with neck extension
d. Prone with neck extended

19. In a breast cancer patient perilesional methylene blue dye is injected as shown in the picture for the purpose of?

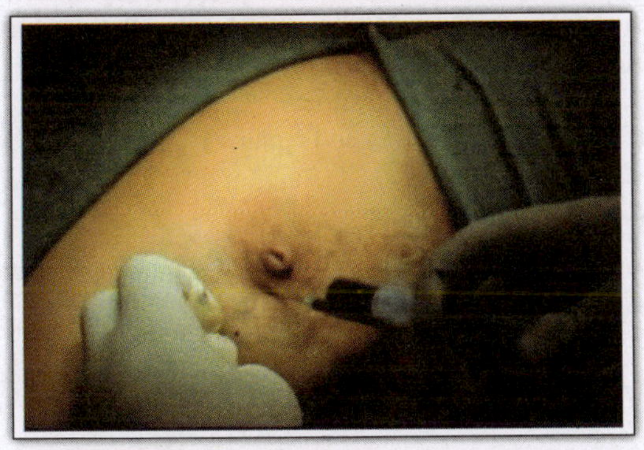

a. Sentinel lymph node biopsy
b. Tumor painting
c. Breast tattooing
d. Peri tumor marking with dye

20. A young male suffered RTA and presents with contusion of chest. On examination there is distended neck vein, BP-80/60 mmhg, Pulse -120 bpm, RR-20/ min and Right chest is resonant on percussion. What is most likely diagnosis?

a. Tension pneumothorax b. Hydrothorax
c. Cardiac tamponade d. Pleural effusion

21. Which of the following type of cancer is least likely to spread by lymphatic route?

a. Basal cell carcinoma
b. Malignant melanoma
c. Squamous cell carcinoma
d. Merkel cell carcinoma

22. An ulcer on the lateral border of tongue measuring approximately 2.5 × 3.5 cm and have indurations at the margins but no palpable lymph nodes in the neck. On histopathology it is diagnosed to have carcinoma of tongue. What will be the TNM staging?

a. T1 N0 M0 b. T2 N0 M0
c. T3 N0 M0 d. T4 N0 M0

23. In third degree hemorrhage, blood loss is approximately?

a. <15%
b. 15–30%
c. 30–40%
d. >40%

24. GCS score in an intubated patient with eye response to pain and abnormal flexion?

a. E2 Vt M4
b. E2 Vt M3
c. E2 V1 M4
d. E2 V1 M3

AIIMS NOVEMBER 2017

25. A 53-year-old man is admitted with a history of CVA 2 days ago. Patient is drowsy with minimal response and weakness of left side. CT picture is shown as in the figure. What will be your next line of management?

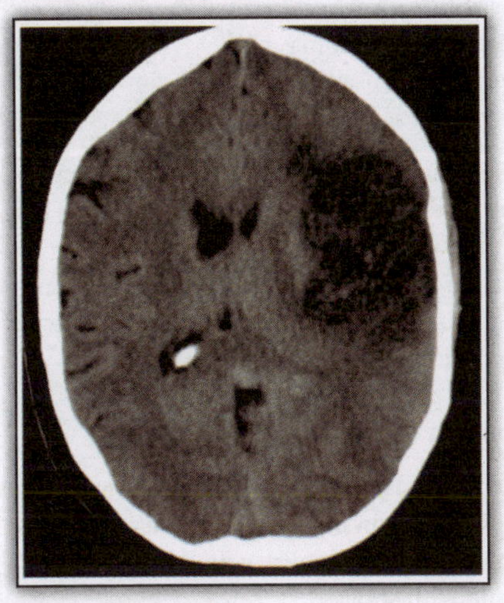

a. Aspirin and clopidogrel
b. Mannitol
c. Decompressive surgery
d. Mechanical thrombectomy

26. Which of the following is the best guide to measure fluid resuscitation in shock? *(AIIMS Nov. 2017, 2015)*

a. CVP
b. Urine output
c. Oxygen saturation
d. Systemic BP

27. Modified Shock Index formula is?

a. Heart rate/Systolic BP
b. Heart rate/Diastolic BP
c. Heart rate/Mean arterial pressure
d. Heart rate/Pulse rate

28. A person presents in emergency with history of traumatic head injury. On examination he was found to have moving all limbs spontaneously and obeys commands, uttering inappropriate words and opens eye on painful stimuli. His GCS would be?

a. 3
b. 10
c. 11
d. 13

29. **Elderly male presents with a ulcerative lesion on the dorsum of nose since 2 years as shown in the given picture, which bleeds on touch. What is most likely diagnosis?**

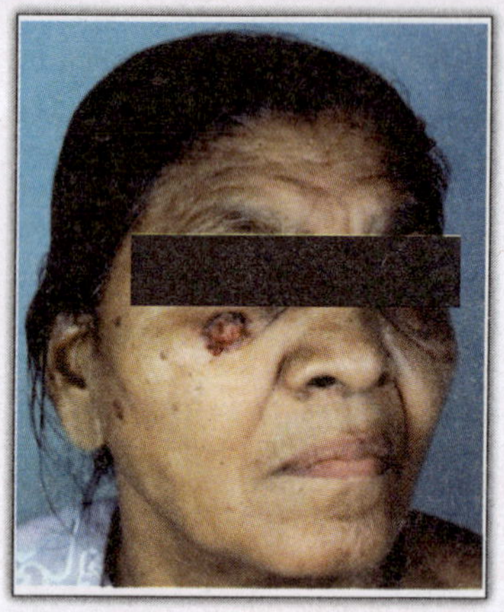

a. Marjolin's ulcer
b. Basal cell carcinoma
c. Dermatofibrosarcoma
d. Nevus

30. **A person sustained Road Traffic Accident is found lying on road and is conscious. All of following can be done for transportation of the patient EXCEPT:**
a. Strap head, chest and pelvis on spine board
b. Put him in lateral position on stretcher to prevent aspiration
c. Talk to patient while he is on board
d. Roll him on stretcher like a log roll

31. **In a School bus accident, as per the guidelines of Triage; which of the following child will you attend first on priority?**
a. Child with airway obstruction
b. Child with shock
c. Child with flail chest
d. Child with severe head injury

32. **French in Foley's Catheter refers to?**
a. Outer circumference b. Inner circumference
c. Outer diameter d. Inner radius

33. **Which of the following is not a part of Preoperative patient surgical Checklist?**
a. Oral consent b. Doctor's signature
c. Site marking d. Confirming patient identity

34. **After cholecystectomy gallbladder specimen is shown below. Identify the condition?**

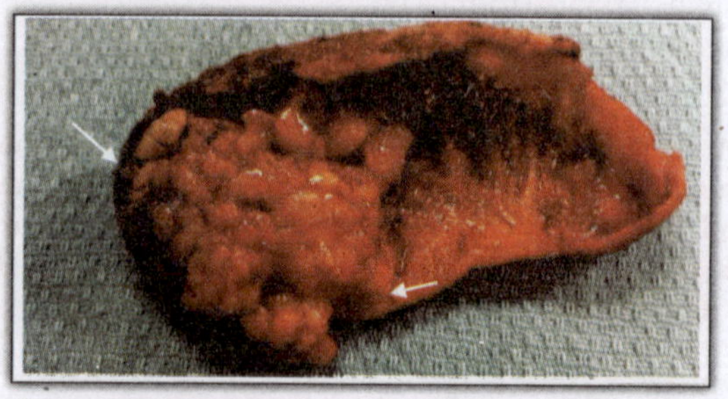

a. Cancer gallbladder b. Cholesterolosis
c. Strawberry gallbladder d. Polyps in gallbladder

35. **Most common presentation of Abdominal Desmoid tumor is?**
a. Fever b. Abdominal pain
c. Abdominal mass d. Rectal prolapse

36. **A 10 year old child with pain and mass in right lumbar region with no fever, with right hip flexed and X ray shows Spine changes. Most probable diagnosis is?**
a. Pyelonephritis
b. Psoas abscess
c. Retrocecal Appendicitis
d. Torsion of Right Undescended testis

37. **Most appropriate method of checking the patency of the ICD tube?**
a. By checking continuous air bubbles coming out of the underwater drain
b. By checking the movement of air water column in the tube during respiration
c. By checking position of the tube on chest X ray
d. By auscultation

38. **Following a blunt trauma abdomen patient had renal laceration for which he was operated. Now after 1 week patient is hemodynamically stable and asymptomatic. There after 2 days patient developed Urinoma. Patient was stable and No fever. How will you manage the patient?**
a. Percutaneous nephrostomy
b. Surgical exploration and repair
c. Urethral stenting
d. Wait and watch

39. **Best management of 4 cm size renal staghorn calculus?**
a. ESWL
b. PCNL
c. Intra renal repair surgery
d. Open pyelolithotomy

40. **Which layer involved in blister formation in a superficial partial thickness burn?**
a. Epidermis b. Dermis
c. Papillary dermis d. Reticular dermis

41. **Length of insertion of Nasogastric tube is best measured by?**
a. Tip of Nose to ear to umbilicus
b. Tip of Nose to ear to Xiphoid process
c. Mouth to ear to Umbilicus
d. Mouth to ear to midway between xiphisternum and umbilicus

AIIMS MAY 2017

42. **Kraissl's lines are?**
a. Point of maximum tension in a fracture
b. Point of tension in hanging
c. Collagen and elastin lines in stab injury
d. Relaxed tension lines in skin

43. **Pancreatic cancer has highest association with?**
a. Peutz-Jeghers syndrome
b. Hereditary pancreatitis
c. FAP
d. FAMMM syndrome

44. A 30-year-old female was admitted to casualty with history of head trauma in a RTa. Her eye opens to pain, moans, localizes towards the pain on left-hand and away from the pain on right hand, both the legs in extended posture. Calculate her GCS?

a. 3 b. 7
c. 9 d. 11

45. A 30-year-old female with history of burns involving abdomen, both limbs and back and presented after 8 hours which of the following is the formula for calculation of fluid infusion?

a. 4 mL/kg × %TBSA for first 8 hours then 2 mL/kg × %TBSA for next 16 hours
b. 2 mL/kg × %TSBA
c. 4 mL/kg × %TSBA
d. 5 mL/kg × %TSBA

46. A 21-year-old male presents with soft tissue swelling front of neck moves with deglutition and protrusion of tongue?

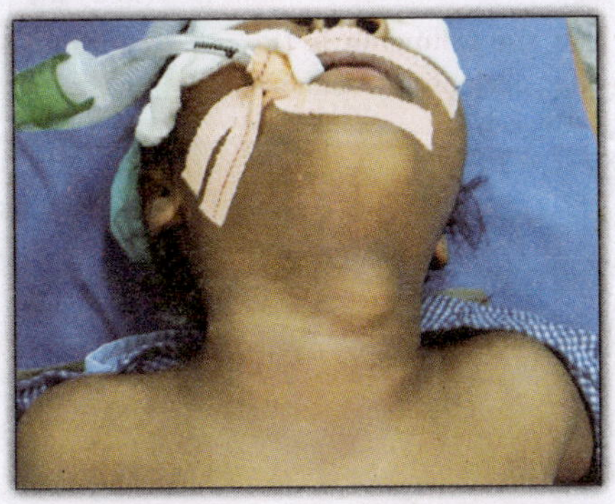

a. Thyroglossal cyst b. Branchial cyst
c. Cystic hygroma d. Cervical lymphadenopathy

47. A 18-year-old boy presented to the casualty with history of fever, abdominal pain and other features suggestive of acute appendicitis. The resident was eliciting the sign shown below. Identify the sign?

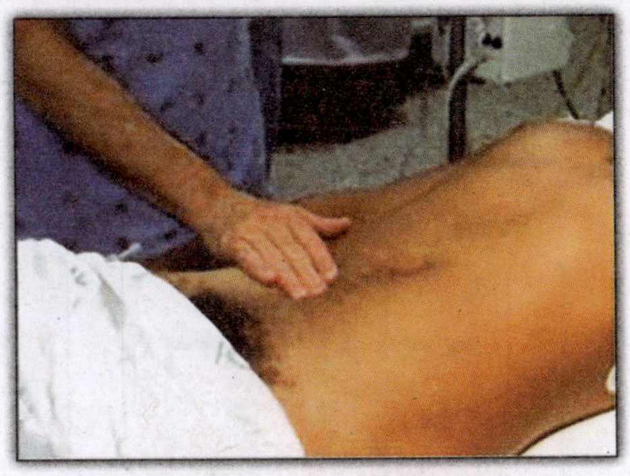

a. Rovsing's sign
b. Psoas sign
c. McBurney point tenderness
d. Ballance's sign

48. A 40-years-old female with a 2 cm nodule in the right breast and HPE proved metastatic nodule in the axilla. Best management is?

a. Quadrantectomy
b. Mastectomy with local radiotherapy
c. Patey's with adjuvant chemotherapy
d. Halsted's operation with tamoxifen

49. A 45-year-old female with history of painless breast lump measuring 6 × 5 cm in left upper outer quadrant and no axillary nodes. Core cut biopsy showed Ductal Carcinoma in situ. She underwent surgery with resection of all tumor tissue and postoperative HPE showed with DCIS with high grade necrosis with 4 mm clearance on margins. Which of the following is next step?

a. Adjuvant chemotherapy
b. Adjuvant radiotherapy
c. Adjuvant chemoradiotherapy
d. No additional treatment

50. A 30-year-old female underwent treatment for breast cancer of 1.2 × 1 cm with positive axillary nodes. She completed radiotherapy and chemotherapy and now on tamoxifen. How will you follow-up the patient?

a. Yearly bone scans
b. Routine physical examination once in 3 months for a year and annual mammogram
c. Regular checking of LFT once in 6 months
d. Follow-up with tumor markers once in 6 months

51. Most common site of post ischemic stricture?

a. Ascending colon b. Hepatic flexure
c. Splenic flexure d. Sigmoid colon

52. A 45-year-old female patient presents with bleeding per rectum and having frequency of stool refractory to treatment, upon colonoscopy multiple geographical ulcer seen, histology from lesion given. Most likely diagnosis is?

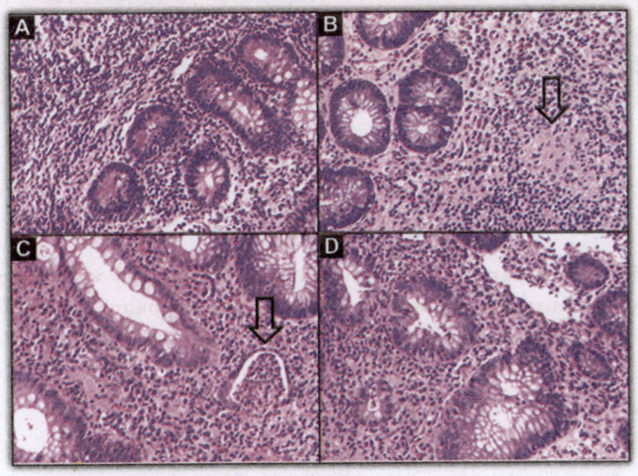

a. Pseudomembranous colitis
b. Crohn's disease
c. Adenocarcinoma of colon
d. Visceral leishmaniasis

53. A patient met with a road traffic accident with paralysis of both upper and lower limb. Patient has not passed urine and tenderness elicited in the cervical region. What will you advise?

a. The doctor should order a cervical X-ray and shift the patient from the trolley by himself
b. The doctor will instruct the radiographer to take cervical X-ray AP and lateral view without any cervical support
c. The doctor will instruct the radiographer to take cervical and chest X-ray
d. The patient should not be shifted and portable X-ray machine should be used after neck stabilisation

54. **All of the following are true regarding primary survey in a traumatized patient EXCEPT:**
 a. Cervical X-ray is part of primary survey
 b. Chest X-ray and pelvic X-ray are taken as an adjunct to primary survey
 c. CT scan is not done in hemodynamically unstable patient
 d. Chest X-ray is always done in PA view

55. **A person met with an road traffic accident and came to casualty with contusion on left anterior chest wall. His vitals are Pulse rate 90/min, BP 120/80 mm Hg, RR – 16/minute. Normal heart sounds heard but there was decreased breath sounds on left side and trachea deviated to right. Which of the following is the first line of management?**
 a. Percutaneous needle thoracocentesis
 b. Chest tube thoracocentesis
 c. Pericardiocentesis
 d. Open thoracotomy

56. **Percentage of metastatic axillary lymph nodes picked up by USG of axilla for clinically negative lymph nodes?**
 a. 10–20% b. 20–30%
 c. 30–50% d. 50–60%

57. **Which of the following is the flap shown in the picture?**

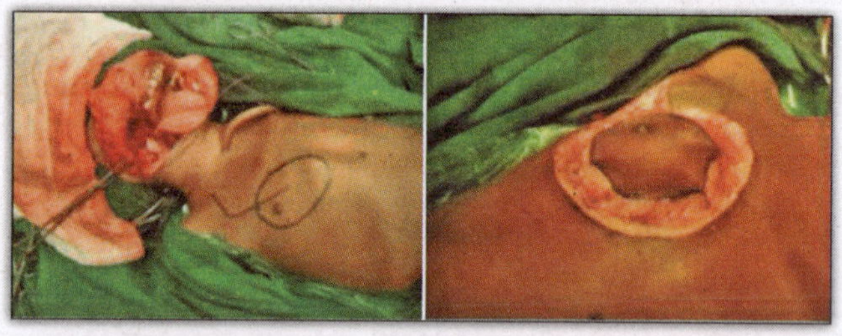

 a. Pectoral major myocutaneous flap
 b. TRAM flap
 c. VRAM flap
 d. Serratus anterior flap

58. **A 1.5-year-old child brought to the emergency with history of burns by hot water on both hands and palms. The lesion was pink, oozing and painful to air and touch. Which of the following is the best management?**
 a. Collagen dressing
 b. Paraffin gauze and dressing
 c. Excision and grafting
 d. 1% Silver sulphadiazine cream and keep wound open

59. **A 23-year-old lady with 20 weeks pregnancy with a thyroid swelling on right side. FNAC of the nodule determined papillary carcinoma thyroid. Which of the following cannot be done to treat?**
 a. I-131 radioablation
 b. Total thyroidectomy
 c. Total thyroidectomy with lymph node dissection
 d. Right lobectomy

60. **After laparoscopic cholecystectomy, drain was removed on 1st postoperative day and patient discharged. On 3rd day patient develops fever and pain abdomen. USG shows 4 × 4 cm subhepatic collection. Next step will be?**
 a. Antibiotics b. Pigtail catheter drainage
 c. Re-exploration and t-tube
 d. ERCP

AIIMS NOVEMBER 2016

61. **Which of the following is a true diverticulum of esophagus?**
 a. Zanker's diverticulum
 b. Meckel's diverticulum
 c. Parabronchial diverticulum
 d. Epiphrenic diverticulum

62. **Suture length used to close the abdominal surgical wound is?**
 a. Equal to the length of incision
 b. Twice the length of incision
 c. Four times the length of incision
 d. Five times the length of incision

63. **Which of the following is a muscle splitting incision?**
 a. Lanz incision b. Pfannensteil incision
 c. Kocher's incision d. Rutherford morrison incision

64. **Which of the following is the most common symptom of aorto-iliac occlusive disease?**
 a. Impotence
 b. Gluteal claudication
 c. Calf claudication
 d. Asymptomatic

65. **Which of the following is used for wound infection severity grading?**
 a. Glasgow score b. ASA score
 c. APGAR score d. Southampton

66. **A patient is brought with ongoing massive hematemesis, the patient is hemodynamically stable and conscious. What is the next step of management?**
 a. Put the patient in Recumbent position and maintain airway
 b. Arrange for emergency endoscopy
 c. IV fluids
 d. Observe

67. **Which of the following region in the below picture constitutes to Zone 4 retroperitoneal haemorrhage?**

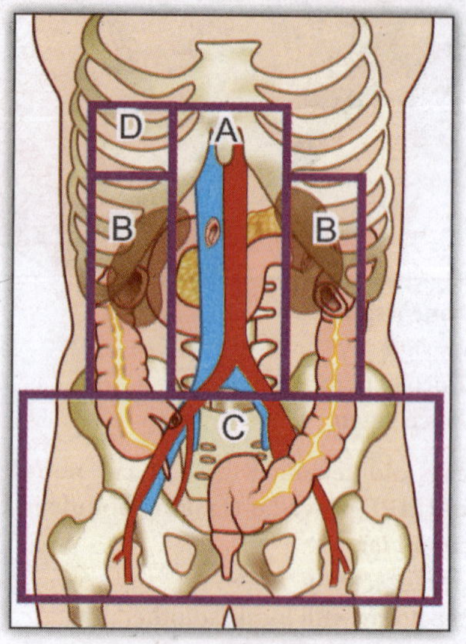

 a. A b. B
 c. C d. D

68. After a laparotomy, a woman presents with Burst abdomen. After treating the infection, the surgeon decides for resuturing. What is the suture material used?

a. 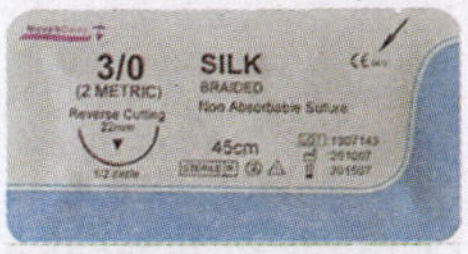

b. 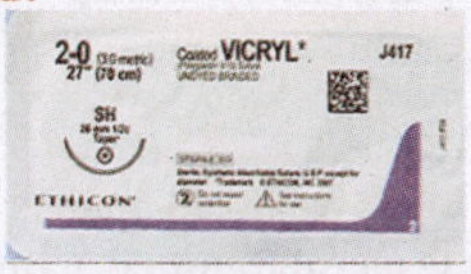

c. 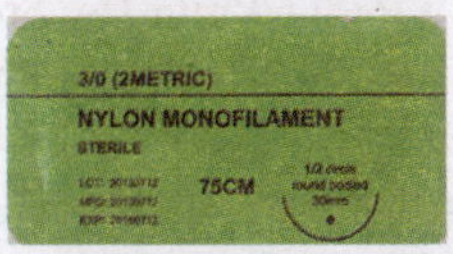

d. 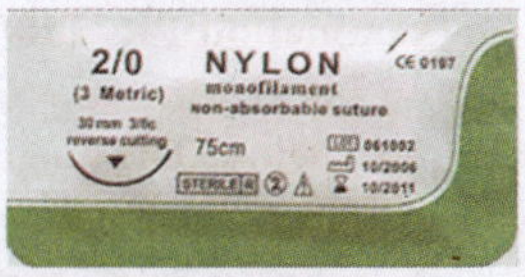

69. A patient with carcinoma right colon is undergoing right hemicolectomy. What instrument the surgeon is holding in his hand?

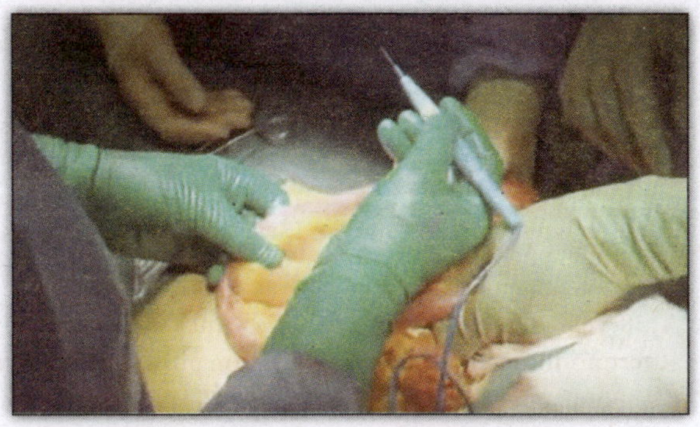

a. Harmonic scalpel
b. Bipolar cautery
c. Monopolar cautery
d. Suction

70. Identify the instrument shown in this picture?

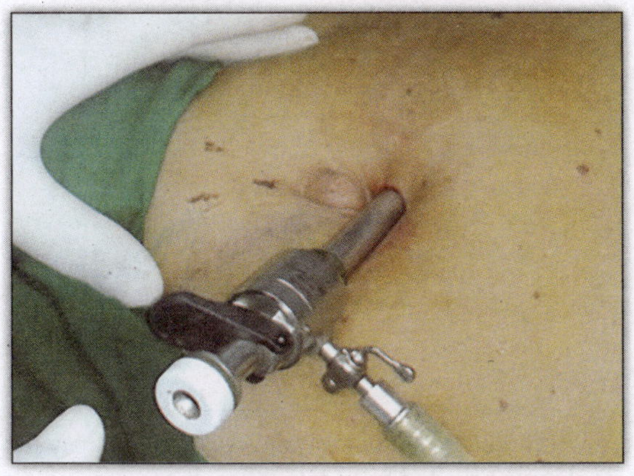

a. Laparoscopic Camera
b. Laparoscopic Port
c. Laparoscopic Trocar
d. Laparoscopic cannula

71. A 28-year-old male brought to emergency department with history of road traffic accident. He was evaluated & found to have BP-130/80 mm Hg, pulse rate - 88/min, RR -22/min. On auscultation there was decreased air entry on one side with absent breath sounds. X-ray chest is given below. Focussed assessment with sonography in trauma (FAST) was done, which was negative in all quadrants. Your most probable diagnosis is?

a. Pneumothorax
b. Rupture of esophagus
c. Flail chest due to fracture of ribs 5, 6, 7, 8 ribs
d. Normal CXR

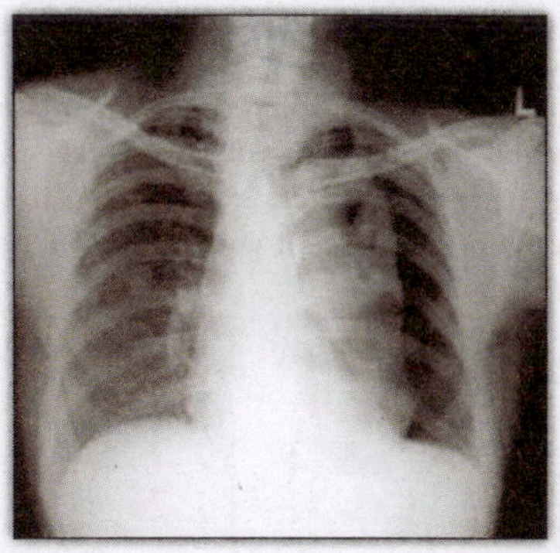

72. A 26-year-old young male met with a road traffic accident and came to the ER. On examination his BP—90/56 mm Hg, Pulse—140/min, SpO_2 86%, GCS-8. On examination the patient had multiple injuries and FAST ultrasound screening positive in all four quadrants. He was operated and the post-op pictures shown below. Your correct match to describe the following are?

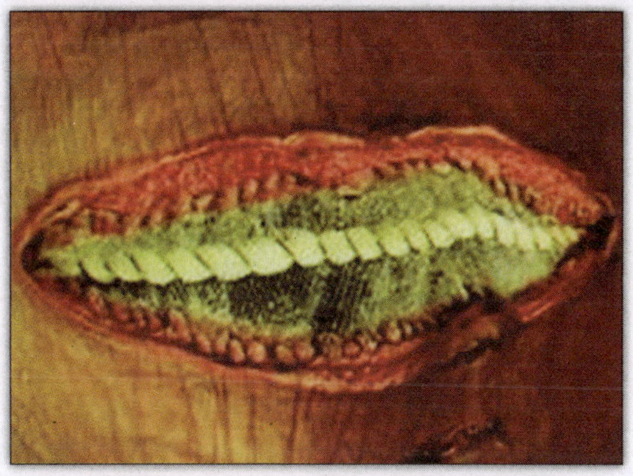

a. Abdomino-thoraco surgery, closure of abdomen
b. Abdominal laparotomy, mesh closure of abdomen
c. Damage control surgery, mesh closure of abdomen
d. Abdominoplasty primary closure of abdomen

73. After thoracic surgery with intraoperative pleural injury, right pleural collection was found and Chest drain (ICD) was placed. When should the drain be removed?

a. Partial expansion and when drain output is less than 30 mL for 2 consecutive days
b. Complete expansion and when drain output is less than 50 mL for 2 consecutive days
c. Complete expansion and when drain output is less than 200 mL for 2 consecutive days
d. Remove the drainage on 4th day irrespective of drainage

74. In a patient with obstructive jaundice cause of serum Bilirubin > 40 mg/dL can be?

a. Complete CBD obstruction
b. Long term CBD obstruction
c. Renal failure
d. Malignant obstruction

75. In Scintigraphy the gallbladder is not visualized in?

a. Acute cholecystitis
b. Chronic cholecystitis
c. Carcinoma gallbladder
d. CBD stone

AIIMS MAY 2016

76. A chief surgeon has completed performing laparotomy. He closes the abdominal wall with nylon sutures. He asks you to close skin with interrupted 3.0 nylon suture. Which of the following set of instrument you will use to perform the task entrusted on you?

a. 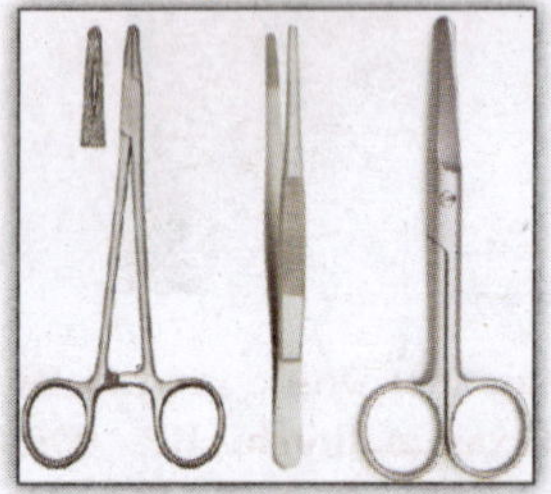

b. 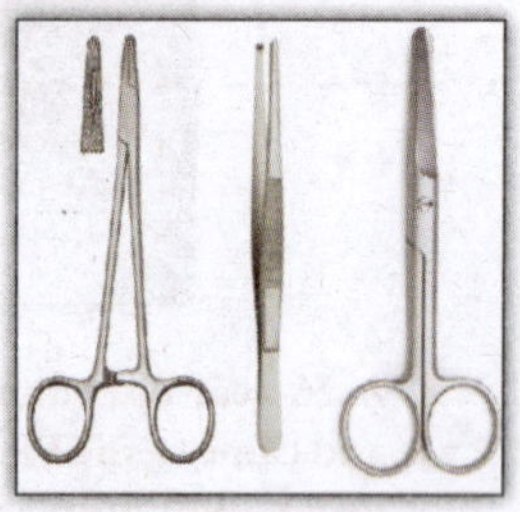

c. 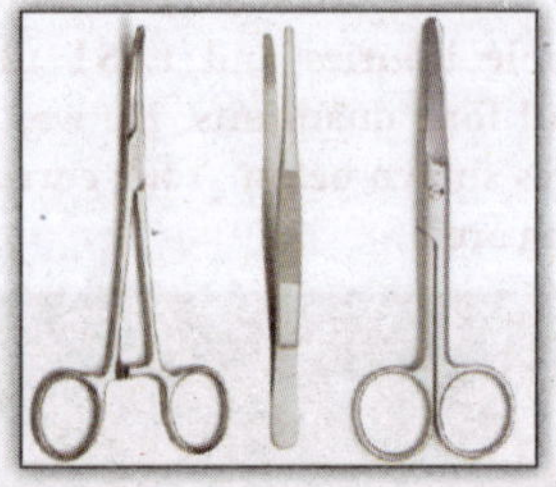

d. 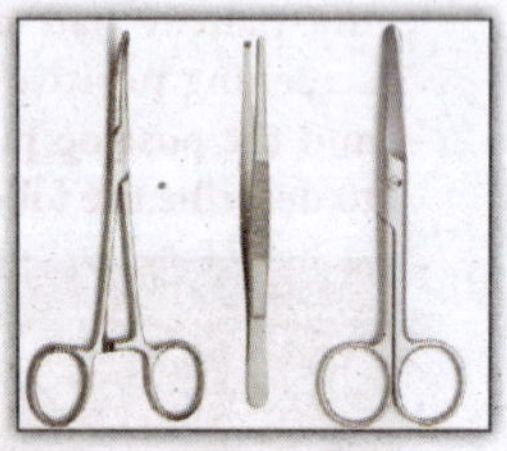

77. A consultant surgeon completed a modified radical mastectomy. He instructs the resident to close the surgical site by subcuticular sutures. Which of the following suture material you will use to close the wound?

a. 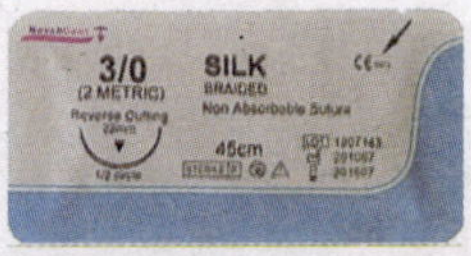

b. 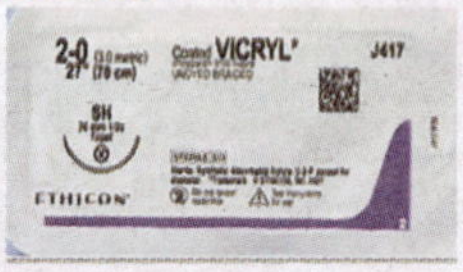

c. 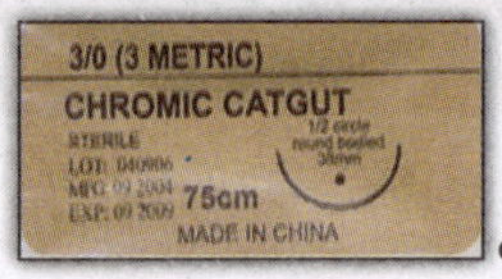

d. 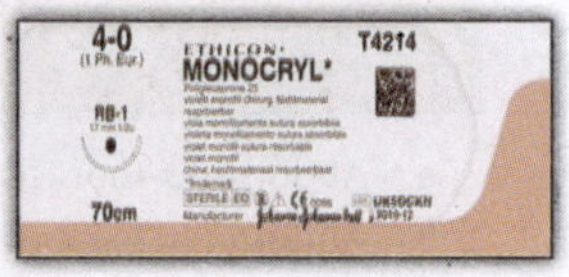

78. The consultant surgeon planned to perform a midline laparotomy for right hemicolectomy for a carcinoma caecum. You were asked to clean, paint and drape for the operation. You will clean which part of the body for this operation?

a. Nipple to mid thigh including genitalia
b. Epigastrium to pubic symphysis
c. Chin to pubic symphysis
d. Epigastrium to mid-thigh including genitalia

79. A 70-year-old presents with a lesion on the cheek. The lesion had a raised pearly edge and telengiectasia on the surface. The diagnosis is?

a. Basal cell carcinoma b. Squamous cell carcinoma
c. Wart d. Acnitic keratosis

80. After a major surgery on 3rd postoperative day, you were instructed to remove foley's. You dry to deflate and remove the catheter but you can not deflate. Your resident tries and he could not remove it either. The next step to remove catheter will be

a. Ultrasound guided puncture of balloon
b. CT guided puncture of balloon
c. Push in ether till the balloon bursts and then remove the catheter
d. Push in water till the balloon bursts and then remove catheter

81. A 2-year-old child sustained flame burn over face, both upper limb, front of abdomen and chest. Percentage of burns involved is?

a. 45% b. 54%
c. 60% d. 40%

82. A 65-year-old male came to casualty with complaints of fever, abdominal pain and episode of binge drinking. On examination PR -120/min, BP 90/60 mm Hg, SpO_2 – 88% and his creatinine was 2.4 mg/dL. CT scan of abdomen is given below. The diagnosis is?

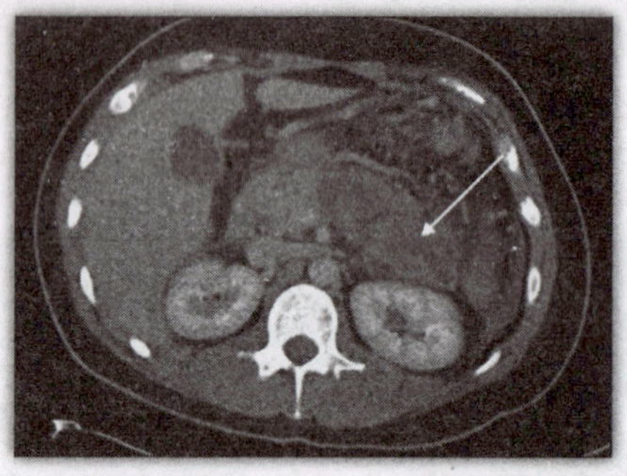

a. Acute pancreatitis b. Severe acute pancreatitis
c. Acute pyelonephritis d. Liver abscess

83. A 30-year-old male came to emergency department with severe abdomen pain. On examination pulse rate – 114/min, BP- 80/40 mm Hg with tenderness all over the abdomen. His chest X-ray was done and is shown below. The most appropriate management is?

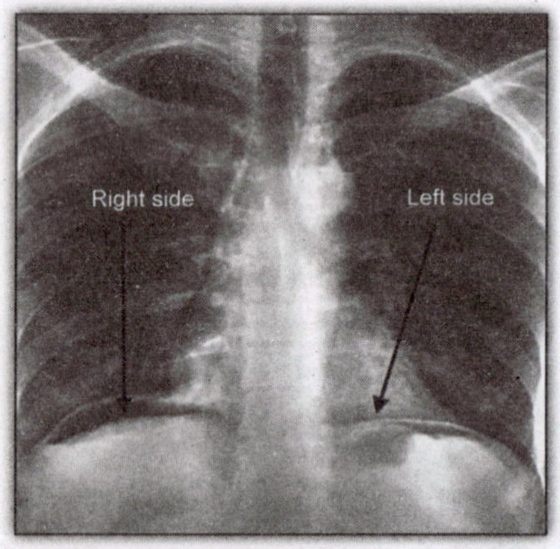

a. IV fluids and antibiotics followed by laparotomy
b. Intravenous fluid and antibiotics alone
c. IV potassium
d. Immediate laparotomy

84. Urobilinogen levels in obstructed jaundice due to gall stones will be?

a. Markedly raised b. Slightly raised
c. Completely absent d. Normal

AIIMS NOVEMBER 2015

85. In which type of Jaundice Urobilinogen is completely absent?

a. Hepatitis b. Obstructive jaundice
c. Hemolysis d. Liver failure

86. **A 45-year-old man present with obstructive jaundice with waxing and waning, pruritus and clay colored stool for 2 months. Imaging study suggestive of dilated pancreatic and bile duct. Most probable diagnosis is?**
   a. Pancreas head carcinoma
   b. Periampullary carcinoma
   c. Cholangiocarcinoma
   d. Pancreatitis

87. **Maximum and minimum score of Glasgow coma scale is?**
   a. 18 and 3 b. 18 and 0
   c. 15 and 3 d. 15 and 0

88. **Peau d' orange in carcinoma breast is due to?**
   a. Subdermal lymphatic obstruction
   b. Coopers ligament contraction
   c. Retraction of lactiferous ducts
   d. Invasion of skin with malignant cell

89. **Type of hernia that is located at site number 1 in the given picture is?**

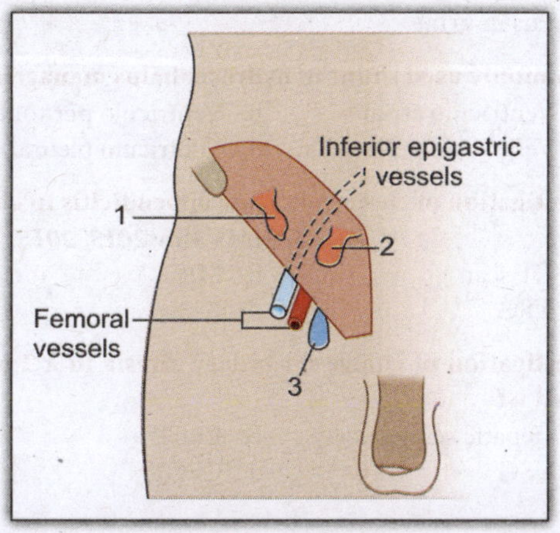

   a. Direct inguinal hernia b. Indirect inguinal hernia
   c. Femoral hernia d. Pantaloon hernia

90. **A child presents with swelling in right groin region which increases on cough impulse and is reducible. On reducing the swelling by hand a gurgling sound was heard. Which of the following is not true about the swelling?**
   a. Child has right indirect inguinal hernia
   b. Patent processes vaginal is
   c. Hernial sac contains greater omentum only
   d. Hernial sac contains intestine

91. **Which of the following is the best guide to measure fluid resuscitation in shock?** ***(AIIMS Nov. 2017, 2015)***
   a. CVP
   b. Urine output
   c. Oxygen saturation
   d. Systemic BP

92. **Regarding Meckel's diverticulum all are true EXCEPT:**
   a. 3% of population
   b. 3 inch long
   c. Remnant of distal part of vitello intestinal duct
   d. Found on Anti mesentric border
   e. 2 Foots from iliocaecal valve
   f. Pain at umbilicus

93. **Most cost effective method to prevent infection is?**
   a. Alcohol based sanitizers
   b. Hand washing
   c. Disinfectant
   d. Chemoprophylaxis

94. **Thyroid storm during surgery is due to?** ***(AIIMS Nov 2018, 2015)***
   a. Recurrent laryngeal nerve injury
   b. Inappropriate preoperative preparation
   c. Rough handling during surgery
   d. Removal of parathyroid

95. **During laparoscopic inguinal hernia repair a tacker was place below and lateral to the iliopubic tract. Post operative the patient complained of pain and loss of sensation over medial aspect of thigh. This is due to the involvement of?** ***(AIIMS Nov 2015, May 2015)***
   a. Lateral cutaneous nerve of thigh
   b. Ilioinguinal nerve
   c. Genitofemoral nerve
   d. Obturator nerve

AIIMS MAY 2015

96. **During laparoscopic inguinal hernia repair a tacker was place below and lateral to the iliopubic tract. Post operative the patient complained of pain and loss of sensation over medial aspect of thigh. This is due to the involvement of?** ***(AIIMS Nov 2015, May 2015)***
   a. Lateral cutaneous nerve of thigh
   b. Ilioinguinal nerve
   c. Genitofemoral nerve
   d. Obturator nerve

97. **In a patient with thrombocytopenia, what is the target platelet count after platelet transfusion to perform an invasive procedure?**
   a. 40,000 b. 50,000
   c. 30,000 d. 60,000

98. **Bleeding from a Mallory weiss tear occurs usually from?**
   a. Left gastric artery b. Short gastric arteries
   c. Phrenic vein d. Coronary vein

99. **In esophageal cancer prognosis is best determined by?**
   a. Age of patient b. Cellular differentiation
   c. Length of involvement d. T stage

100. **Oncotype DX test is done to decide which of the following in a breast cancer?**
   a. Chemotherapy in hormone receptor positive patients
   b. Chemotherapy in hormone receptor negative patients
   c. Hormone therapy in hormone receptor positive
   d. Herceptin in HER2 +ve

101. **A lady who is 9 week pregnant comes with a 2.5 cm mass in the upper outer quadrant of left breast. Ultrasound failed to show any abnormality. The ideal management will be to?**
   a. Palpation guided core biopsy
   b. Aspirate the cyst and reassure
   c. Call patient one month after delivery
   d. Do mammography

102. A 60-year-old lady comes with blood stained discharge from the nipple with family history of breast cancer. Next best step for her will be?

a. Ductoscopy
b. Nipple discharge cytology
c. Sono-Mammogram
d. MRI

103. Which is the best incision preferred for diaphragmatic surgery? ***(AIIMS May 2015, 2014)***

a. Circumferential
b. Radial
c. Vertical
d. Transverse

104. A pregnant lady was stabbed in the right side of the chest. She is shoulting and yelling for help on entering the casualty. On examination she has tachycardia and BP was 90/60 mm Hg. Breath sounds are decreased on the right side. What is the first consideration for her?

a. Oropharyngeal airway
b. Establish IV line and start normal saline
c. Needle decompression on right side of the chest
d. Immediate tracheostomy

105. Most commonly performed and acceptable method of bariatric surgery is?

a. Biliopancreatic division
b. Biliopancreatic division with ileostomy
c. Laparoscopic gastric banding
d. Roux-en-Y procedure

106. Physiological changes in laparoscopy include all EXCEPT:

a. Increases PCWP
b. Increased ICP
c. Decreased FRC
d. Increased pH

107. A 3-year-old child comes with hydrocoele of the hernia sac. Management will include?

a. Herniotomy
b. Herniorrhapy
c. Only observation
d. Operate at 5 years

108. All are true about functional division of liver EXCEPT:

a. Based on portal vein and hepatic vein
b. Divided into 8 segments
c. Three major and three minor fissures
d. 4 sectors

109. In a child surgery was done for Biliary stricture with hepatojejunal anastomosis, post operative bilirubin level after 2 weeks was 6 mg/dL from a preoperative level 12 mg/dL. The reason for this could be?

a. Normal lowering of bilirubin takes time
b. Delta bilirubin
c. Anastomotic stricture
d. Mistake in lab technique

110. A patient with Steroid resistant ITP underwent Laparoscopic splenectomy. Patient got fever on 3rd postoperative day. Next investigation is likely to reveals?

a. Left lower lobe consolidation
b. Port site infection
c. Intra abdominal collection
d. Pus in urine

111. Commonly used shunt in hydrocephalus management?

a. Ventriculo atrial
b. Ventriculo peritoneal
c. Ventriculo pericardial
d. Ventriculo pleural

112. Investigation of choice for acute appendicitis in children is? ***(AIIMS May 2015, 2013, Nov 2014)***

a. CT scan
b. MRI
c. USG
d. X-ray

113. Investigation of choice for biliary atresia in a 2 month old infant is?

a. Hepatic scintigraphy
b. ERCP
c. USG
d. CECT

AIIMS NOVEMBER 2018

1. Ans. (b) Concentric method

Ref: Guidelines for the early detection and screening of breast cancer, Cairo, World Health Organization (http://applications.emro.who.int/dsaf/dsa701.pdf)

The breast examination can be done using vertical strip, wedge section, and/or concentric circle detection methods.

- **Radial spoke or Wedge technique:** The wedge section technique was developed as some women find the circular movement of the hand easier to use during the breast self-examination. In this method, the breast is divided into wedges, moving the palmar pads of the fingers towards the center of the breast or the nipple. Both breasts are examined wedge by wedge in this manner until completely covered.
- **Vertical strip method:** With the vertical strip method the woman should start in the underarm area of the breast, moving the fingers downward slowly until she reaches the area below the breast. The fingers are then moved slightly towards the middle and the process begins again, this time moving the hand upwards over the breast. This process continues up and down until the whole surface of the breast and underarms is examined. Both breasts should be examined.
- **Concentric circle method:** In this method, the woman uses a circular motion starting with a small circle around the nipple area to feel the breast. The circle is widened as the woman moves over the surface of the breast. The breast, upper chest and underarm area are fully examined through this circular motion. As with other methods, both breasts should be fully examined.

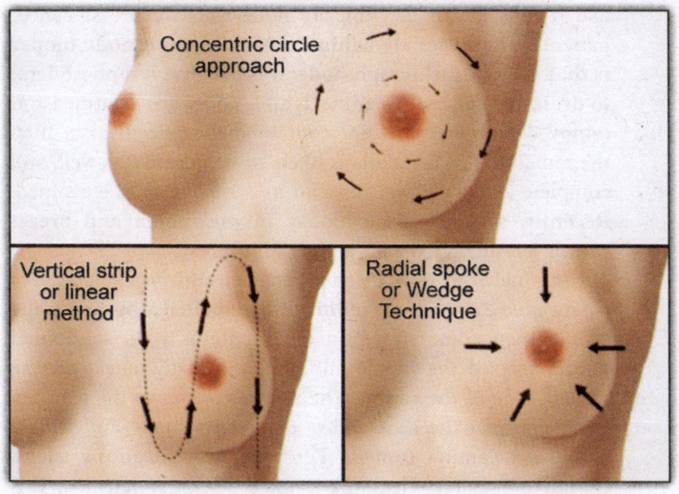

Fig: Different techniques of clinical breast exam

2. Ans. (c) Puckering

Ref: Bailey 26th ed page 812, 816, Sabiston 18th ed ch 34

Conspicuous means clearly visible; obvious or showy.

We found no direct text quoting this statement however our inference goes in favour of Puckering. Both Nipple retraction and Peau d orange are seen in both Malignant and Benign conditions while Puckering is seen in only underlying breast cancer.

Option (A)

Flattening or actual inversion of the nipple can be caused by fibrosis in certain benign conditions, especially subareolar duct ectasia.

Option (B)

Peau d' orange (French- skin of an orange; orange peel appearance) is due to dermal edema caused by obstruction of the superficial cutaneous lymphatics by the tumor cells. Occasionally, the same phenomenon is seen over a chronic abscess where the infiltrated skin is tethered by the sweat ducts it cannot swell, leading to an appearance like orange skin.

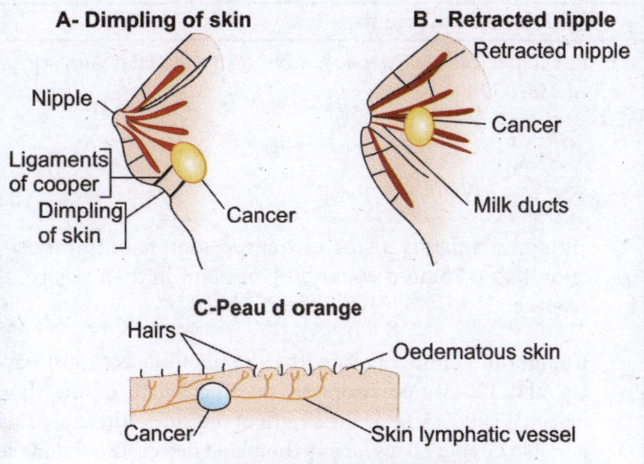

A - Due to pull by lig of cooper
B - Due to retraction of milk ducts
C - Due to lymphatic obstruction

3. Ans. (c) Rough handling during surgery

Ref: Sabiston 18th ed ch 36, Stoelting's coexisting Diseases 7th Ed page 461, Harrison 19th ed page 2297

Thyroid storm during surgery is due to release of large amount of thyroid hormone into the circulation during manipulation of the gland. Preoperative preparation is a preventive measure but the cause and trigger is still the manipulation of the gland. **Thyrotoxic crisis or thyroid storm** is rare and presents as a life threatening exacerbation of hyperthyroidism, accompanied by fever, delirium, seizures, coma, vomiting, diarrhea and jaundice. The mortality rate due to cardiac failure, arrhythmia, or hyperthermia is as high as 30%, even with treatment. *Thyrotoxic crisis is usually precipitated by acute illness (e.g. stroke, infection, trauma, diabetic ketoacidosis), surgery (especially on the thyroid), or radioiodine treatment of a patient with partially treated or untreated hyperthyroidism.*

Management requires intensive monitoring and supportive care, identification and treatment of the precipitating cause, and measures that reduce thyroid hormone synthesis.

- Large doses of **propylthiouracil** (500–1000 mg loading dose and 250 mg every 4 h) should be given orally or by nasogastric tube or per rectum; the drug's inhibitory action on T4 → T3 conversion makes it the anti thyroid drug of choice.
- If not available, **methimazole** can be used in doses up to 30 mg every 12 h
- One hour after the first dose of propylthiouracil, stable **iodide** is given to block thyroid hormone synthesis via the Wolff-Chaikoff effect (the delay allows the antithyroid drug to prevent the excess iodine from being incorporated into new hormone). A saturated solution of potassium iodide (5 drops KI every 6 h) or, where available, ipodate or iopanoic acid (500 mg per 12 h) may be given orally. Sodium iodide, 0.25 gm IV every 6 h, is an alternative but is not generally available.
- **Propranolol** should also be given to reduce tachycardia and other adrenergic manifestations (60-80 mg PO every 4 h; or 2 mg IV every 4 h)

4. Ans. (a) Rhomboid flap

Ref: Bailey 26th ed page 408, 409, SRB Manual of Surgery 4th ed 346, 350

NOTE

Rhomboid flap is a type of transposition flap. Transposition flap is rotated about a pivot point into an adjacent defect

Rhomboid (Limberg) flap: The rhomboid defect must have 60- and 120-degree angles so that the length of the short diagonal is the same as the length of the sides. There are four possible Limberg flaps for any rhomboid defect. The rhomboid excision and Limberg flap are one example of a flap technique for complete removal of the site of disease and subsequent primary tissue closure. The disadvantage of the flap techniques include the complexity of the procedures; the necessity for inpatient hospitalization, typically less than a weeks. Recurrences in 5% of cases.

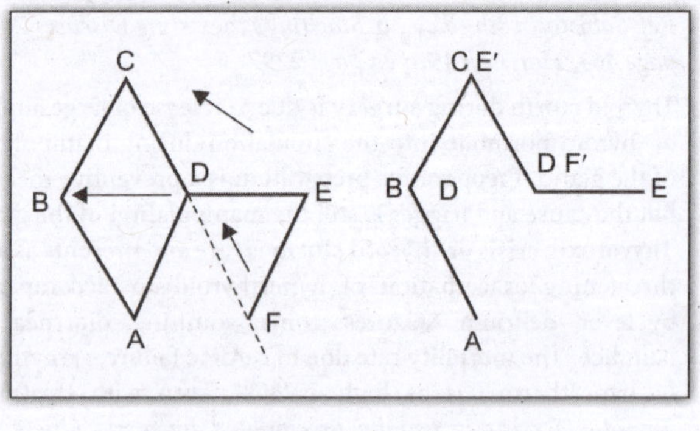

Fig: Line diagram of Limberg flap

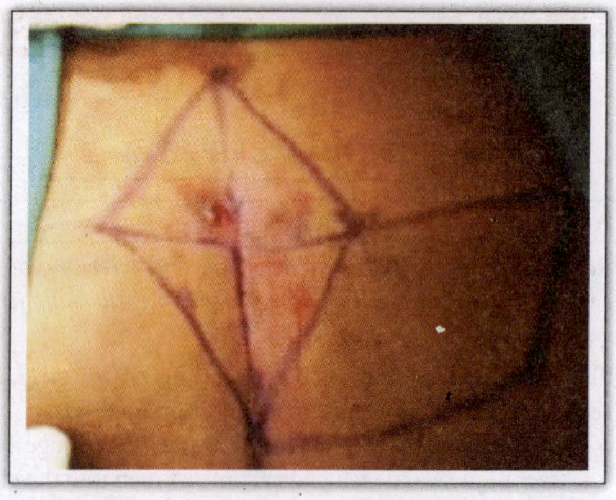

Fig: Preoperative markings for Rhomboid (Limberg) flap

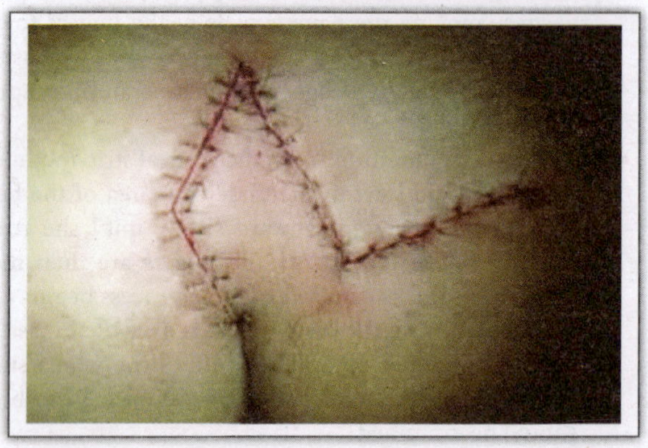

Fig: Postoperative picture of Rhomboid (Limberg) flap.

5. Ans. (c) Sentinel lymph node biopsy

Ref: Mastery of Surgery page 489, 506, Bailey 26th ed page 136, 799, 814

The aim of sentinel lymph node biopsy is to avoid complete axillary dissection in clinically node-negative breast cancer patients. **The rationale behind sentinel lymph node biopsy is that the sentinel lymph node(s) is the first lymph node(s) to drain the cancer.** If sentinel lymph nodes are identified and removed and these do not contain metastatic disease, then the remainder of the axilla is likely to be negative as well, and complete axillary dissection and its sequelae can be avoided. **Recently, sentinel node biopsy in melanoma and breast cancer has attracted a great deal of interest.**

The sentinel node is localised peroperatively by the injection of patent **blue dye and/ or radioisotopelabelled albumin** in the breast. The recommended site of injection is in the subdermal plexus around the nipple although some still inject on the axillary side of the cancer. The marker passes to the primary node draining the area and is detected visually and with a hand-held gamma camera. Peropererative diagnosis allows completion axillary clearance if nodal disease is detected. This may be achieved with frozen-section analysis, touch imprint cytology (TIC) or by molecular methods.

Indications for sentinel lymph node biopsy or axillary node sampling include:

- Operable breast cancer (T1, T2)
- Clinically node-negative

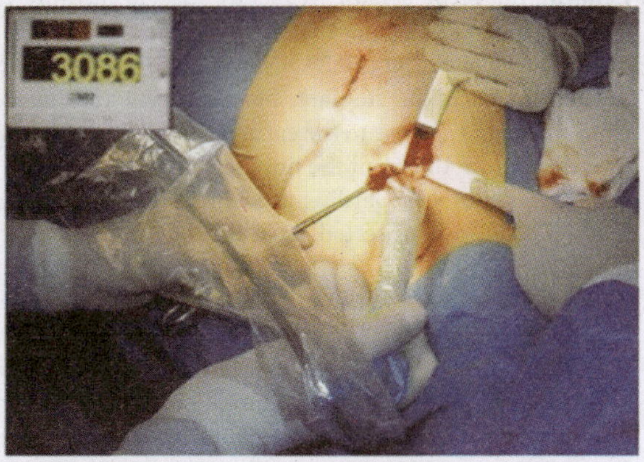

© Follacchio GA et al J. Exp. Clin. Cancer Res. (2015)

Fig: Intraoperative radio-guided localization and excision of sentinel node: Performing axillary mapping using a gamma probe to identify the location of the projection of the sentinel node in the axilla

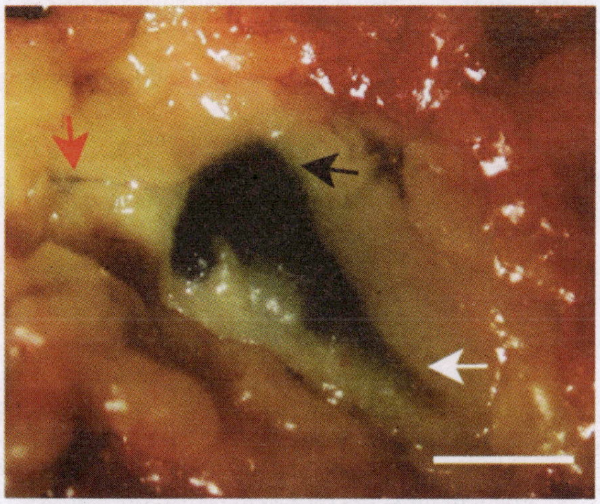

Fig: A black-stained SLN (as indicated by black arrow) with afferent lymph vessel (as indicated by white arrow) and efferent lymph vessel (as indicated by red arrow)

6. Ans. (c) Cecum

Ref: Bailey's 25th Ed pg 1197

Emergency laparotomy is performed to surgically manage intestinal obstruction.

If the site of obstruction is unknown, adequate exposure is best achieved by a midline incision. Assessment is directed to:

- The site of obstruction : small or large intestine
- The nature of the obstruction
- The viability of the gut.
- **Identification and assessment of the caecum is the best initial manoeuvre.**
- **If it is collapsed, the lesion is in the small bowel** and may be identified by careful retrograde assessment. A **dilated caecum indicates large bowel obstruction.**
- To display the cause of obstruction, distended loops of small bowel should be displaced with care and covered with warm moist abdominal packs.

7. Ans. (a) Orange

Ref: SRB's Surgical Operations: Text & Atlas - Page 170

The name comes from the designer, **Frederic Foley**, a surgeon working in Boston, Massachusetts in the 1930s. The French scale or French gauge system is commonly used to measure the size (outside diameter) of a catheter). It is most often abbreviated as Fr, but can often abbreviated as FR or F. The outer diameter of the catheter in millimeters can be determined by dividing the French size by 3; that is **1 F = 1/3 mm outer diameter**. The standard male catheter length of **41-45 cm** can be used for males and females, but a shorter female length of **25 cm** can be more comfortable and discrete for some women

Change Frequency

- Latex Foley catheter: 4 weekly change
- Silicone Foley catheter: 8–12 week change

Two Way Foley's Catheter (A): It is a flexible self retaining indwelling catheter that is often passed through the urethra and into the bladder. Side channel is used to inflate the balloon so that it is kept indwelling and main channel is to hook the drainage bag. Balloon capacity is typically 5–50 mL (5 mL for retaining catheter, 30–50 mL for hemostasis)

Three-Way Catheters (B): Also called haemostatic catheters, these are generally thicker catheters with an extra channel to be used to flush the bladder. Through this tube, it is possible to inject water (i.e. NaCl 0.9%) into the bladder to be able to flush it continuously in order to clean the bladder of blood cloths or other debris, for instance after prostate surgery. These catheters are often of a larger diameter (20-24 Fr.) to allow for large chunks of debris to pass through it.

- Following a transurethral resection of the prostate, a large (24 Fr.) three-way Foley catheter with 30 cc balloon is used to maintain hemostasis
- Used for bladder irrigation/lavage and clot removal.

Indications for Urethral Catheterization

- Acute and chronic urinary retention.
- Maintain a continuous outflow of urine for patients with voiding difficulties, as a result of neurological disorders that cause paralysis or loss of sensation affecting urination.
- Need for accurate measurements of urinary output in critically ill patients.
- Perioperative use for selected surgical procedures.
- Patients undergoing urological surgery or other surgery on contiguous structures of the genitourinary tract.
- Anticipated prolonged duration of surgery.
- Need for intra-operative monitoring of urinary output.
- To assist in healing of open sacral or perineal wounds in incontinent patients.
- Patient requires prolonged immobilisation (e.g. potentially unstable thoracic or lumbar spine, multiple traumatic injuries such as pelvic fractures).
- To allow bladder irrigation/lavage. (3 way catheter)
- To facilitate continence and maintain skin integrity (when conservative treatment methods have been unsuccessful).
- To improve comfort for end of life care if needed.
- Management of intractable incontinence.

Contraindications for Urethral Catheterization

- Acute prostatitis
- Suspicion of urethral trauma

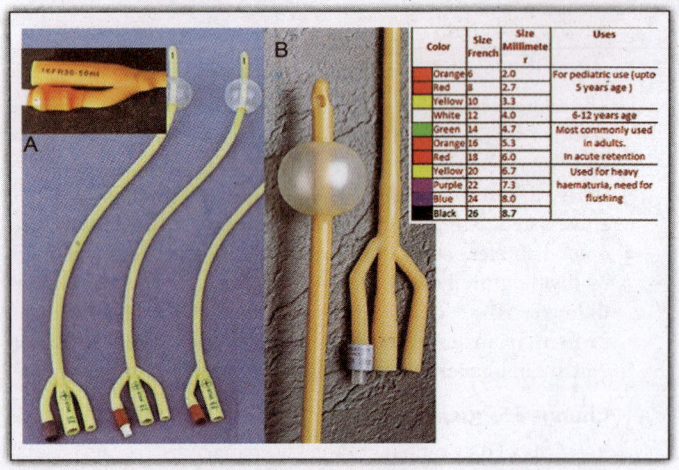

Color	Size French	Size Millimeter	Uses
Orange	6	2.0	For pediatric use (upto 5 years age)
Red	8	2.7	
Yellow	10	3.3	
White	12	4.0	6-12 years age
Green	14	4.7	Most commonly used in adults.
Orange	16	5.3	
Red	18	6.0	In acute retention
Yellow	20	6.7	Used for heavy haematuria, need for flushing
Purple	22	7.3	
Blue	24	8.0	
Black	26	8.7	

Fig: Foley's catheter parts and sizes

8. Ans. (a) Sitting with neck flexed

Ref: SRB's Surgical Operations: Text & Atlas -By Sriram Bhat M Page 171, Shackleford's Surgery of the Alimentary Tract 8th Ed Pg 665

Nasogastric (NG) intubation is one of the commonly performed procedures in the Emergency Department. Its use as a conduit into the stomach.

Nasogastric Tube (Ryles):

Indications/ Uses:

- To decompress stomach during upper abdominal surgeries
- To decompress stomach in intestinal obstruction
- To decompress stomach post operative
- For gastric lavage (14-18 French Catheter is typically used for suction, while enteral feeding tubes may be smaller 8 French).
- For administration of medications or enteral feeding - when the patient is unable to swallow (8 French)
- To monitor gastric bleeding

Contraindications:

- Skull base fractures
- Facial fractures
- Obstructed airway
- Oesophageal varices
- Clotting disorder

Positioning: Place patient in sitting position with neck flexed slightly and head of bed elevated to 45°. Flexion of the neck may facilitate passage of the tube into the esophagus and avoid endotracheal insertion

Length: *The method most frequently used to measure correct length of the NG tube prior to insertion is the distance from nose to ear to xiphisternum (NEX).* Estimate the length of the tube needed to reach the stomach by measuring the tube either from the tip of the nose to the earlobe and down to the xiphoid process or from the tip of the nose to the umbilicus.

Controversy exists regarding measurement of the length of the NG tube to be inserted. Two most common methods of measurement are:

A. From the nose tip to the earlobe and then to the end of the xiphoid process (NEX)

B. From the nose tip to the earlobe and then to a point midway between Xiphoid process and umbilicus.

NG Tube in Children: The placement of a NG tube in children is often difficult. Their large tonsils and adenoids may hinder the passage. These tissues are soft, easily injured, and may bleed as the NG tube is passed. The tongue, large by comparison with adults, may push into the oropharynx and impede passage of the NG tube. Their nostrils and nasal passage are quite small and limit the size of NG tube that may be passed.

How to confirm its placement in stomach?

- Greenish grey fluid on aspiration confirms that the tube is in stomach
- Inject 50 mL of air into the tube and listen for gurgling sound in the epigastrium
- pH readings should be between 1 and 5.5 for feeding to commence safely
- Chest X-ray confirmation of placement is mandatory prior to instilling material such as medications or tube feedings down an NG tube

Size:

- <u>*NG tube (for adult patients)*</u> - 14-18 French
- <u>*NG tube (for pediatric patients)*</u> - In pediatric patients, the correct tube size varies with the patient's age; to find the correct size (in French), add 16 to the patient's age in years and then divide by 2, so that for an 8-year-old child, for example, the correct size is 12 French ([8 + 16]/2 = 12)

9. Ans. (d) DVT

Ref: Paul Marino's ICU book 4th Ed Ch 6 Pg 113

The device shown in the picture is a Pneumatic compression device used in DVT prophylaxis

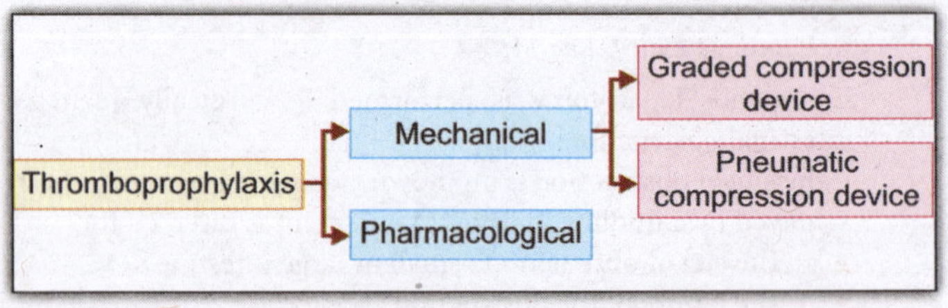

Mechanical Thromboprophylaxis		
	Graded Compression Stockings/TED stockings (Thromboembolism deterrent)	**Intermittent Pneumatic Compression**
Device	Stocking	**Inflatable bladder** around the lower extremities and connected to a pneumatic pump
Pressure at ankle	18 mm Hg external pressure	35 mm Hg external compression

Contd...

Mechanical Thromboprophylaxis		
Pressure at thigh	8 mm Hg external pressure	20 mm Hg external compression
Gradient	10 mm Hg	15 mm Hg
Mechanism	10 mm Hg pressure gradient acts as a driving force for venous outflow from the leg	Repeated inflation and deflation creates a pumping action that further augments venous outflow from the legs
Duration	Continuous	Intermittent
Advantages	Relatively cheap Decreases incidence of DVT by around 50% when used alone Mobility not affected	More effective. Can be used alone for thromboprophylaxis in the early period following craniotomy. Favored method of mechanical prophylaxis used in the ICU
Disadvantages	Least effective method of thromboprophylaxis, never used as sole means of prevention in critically ill patients	The inflatable bladders restrict mobility and can macerate the skin Repeated inflation and deflation of the bladders is often annoying for awake patients.
	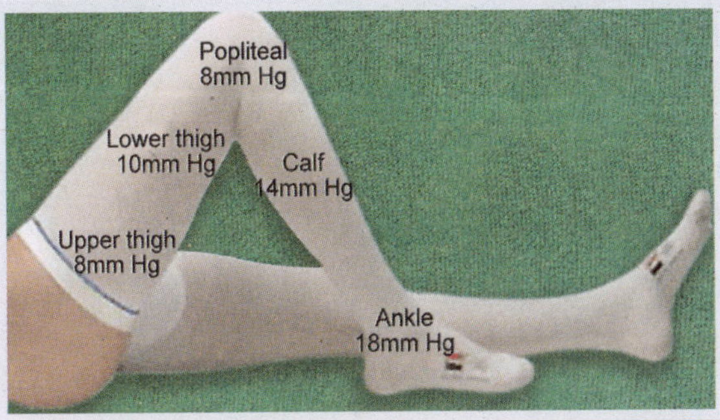	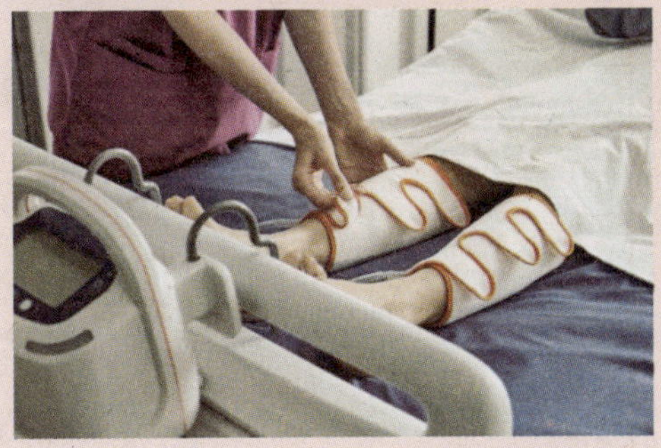

10. Ans. (d) Dermatome

Ref: Bailey 26th ed page 407, Practical Plastic Surgery by Zol B. Kryger 140, 148, 454

The instrument shown in the picture is a Dermatome used for harvesting Skin grafts.

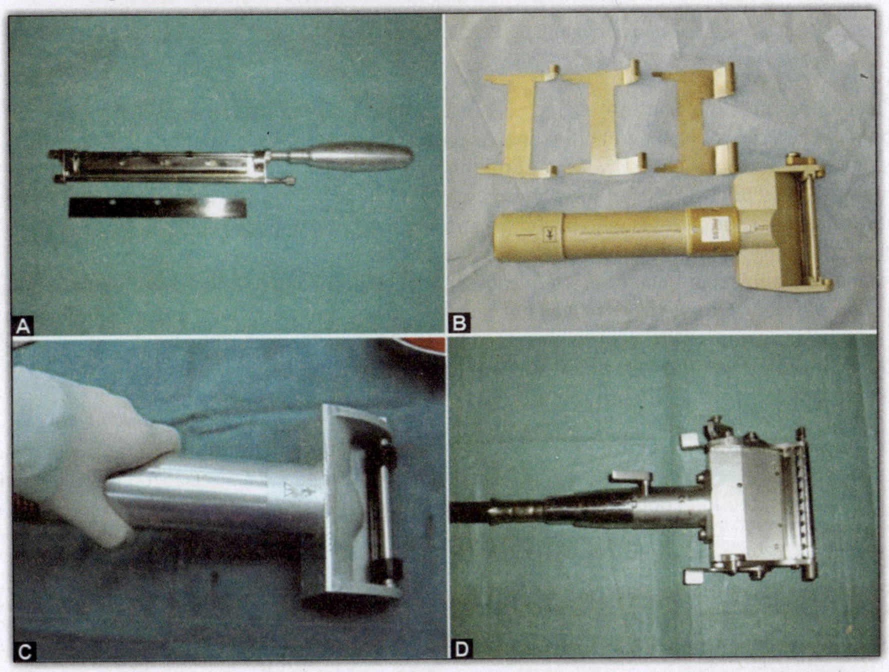

Fig: The most popular tools for skin graft harvesting and grafting. **(A)** Humby knife; **(B)** Humeca Battery operated dermatome; **(C)** Padgett Dermatome; **(D)** Zimmer air dermatome

Skin Graft Harvesting Tools are:

- Free-hand knives
- Various types of dermatomes
- Drum (manually operated)
- Powered dermatomes (Electric or air);
- Battery operated Davol dermatome
- Humeca Battery operated dermatome
- Padgett dermatome
- Zimmer air dermatome

11. Ans. (b) Chemoport

Ref: Totally Implantable Venous Access Devices by Isidoro Di Carlo, Roberto Biffi Pg 38

The instrument shown in the given picture is chemoport

Chemo Port

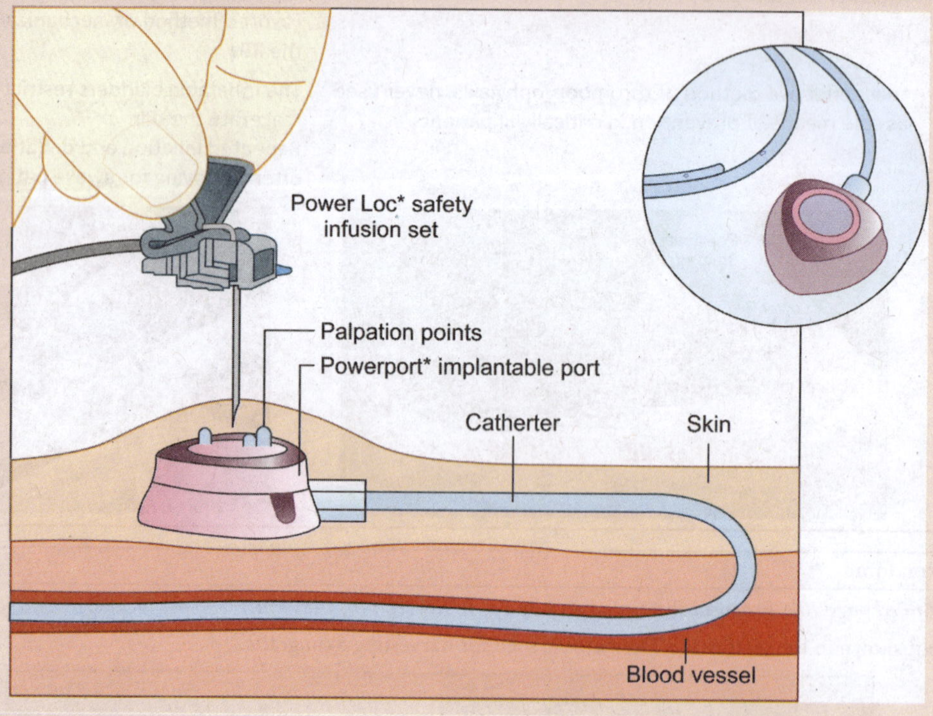

Indications:

- Principally indicated for intravenous infusates that cannot be administered through peripheral veins, damaged peripheral veins that can no longer accept an indwelling needle, and/or patients and treating practitioners who strongly prefer easy and safe venous access (Similar to external Central venous catheter.
- Totally implantable access ports are used for patients who will need central venous access for an extended period of time (3 to 6 months or longer) or for patients who prefer an unobtrusive subcutaneous device
- Cancer patients undergoing chemotherapy are good candidates for implantation because
  - There are many vesicant/irritant chemotherapy agents that can induce tissue necrosis if extravasation occurs;
  - Long-term chemotherapy frequently damages peripheral veins so that peripheral access is difficult;
  - A safe and convenient venous access route is needed for long-term chemotherapy regimens;
  - Blood products, fluids for volume expansion, and/or parenteral nutrition are often administered
  - Frequent blood sampling for therapeutic monitoring

Advantages over External Central Venous Catheter:

- Less Frequent Catheter Care
- Lower Risk of Catheter-related Infections and Catheter-related Thrombosis
- Fewer Restrictions on Patient Activities;
- Less Obvious and Better Cosmetic Appearance

Disadvantages of implantable ports include:

- Need for a Specialized Needle (Non-coring Needle)
- Possible Extravasation of Infusate Due to Inadequate Puncture
- Need for Minor Surgical Procedure.

12. Ans. (b) 9

Ref: Bailey 26th Ed Pg 321, Schwartz 10th ed page 168 – 170, Harrison 19th ed page 260

- The GCS is E3V_TM6

- In intubated patients, since it is not possible to assess verbal response, "T" is added as subscript.
- Best possible score in intubated patient- 10
- Worst possible score in intubated patient - 2
- In the given question Eye opening score is 3 and Motor score is 6, hence total Score is 9.

The Glasgow Coma Scale Score[a]

		1	2	3	4	5	6
Eyes (same for adults & pediatric)		No eye opening	Opens to painful stimuli	Opens to speech	Opens spontaneously	N/A	N/A
Verbal	**Pediatric**	No verbal response	Inconsolable, agitated	Inconsistently inconsolable, moaning	Cries but consolable, inappropriate interactions	Smiles, orients to sounds, follows objects, interacts	N/A
	Adult	No sounds	Un intelligible sounds	Inappropriate words	Confused	Oriented	
Motor	**Pediatric**	No motor response	Extension to pain (decerebrate response)	Abnormal flexion to pain (decorticate response)	Withdraws from pain	Withdraws from touch	Moves spontaneously or purposefully
	Adult	No motor response	Extensor posturing	Flexor posturing	Withdraws from pain	Localizes to pain	Obeys command

[a]Add the three scores to obtain the Glasgow Coma Scale (GCS) score, which can range from 3 to 15. Add "T" after the GCS if intubated and no verbal score is possible. For these patients, the GCS can range from 3T to 10T.

NOTE

- Glasgow Coma Scale (GCS) score ranges from 3 to 15. But in intubated patients (no verbal score is possible), the GCS can range from 3T to 10T (T stands for intubation)
- Pediatric Glasgow coma scale (PGCS) applies to child less than 2-years-old

13. Ans. (a) IV crystalloid 2 liters within 2 minutes

Ref: ATLS 10th edition 2018 updates, Miller's 8th Ed Pg 2438

- Patients with trauma are prone to hypocoagulability. Administration of large quantities of crystalloids will cause further dilution of coagulation factors. Hence, early transfusion of blood products is advocated.
- Disadvantages of aggressive volume resuscitation during Early Resuscitation:
- Increased blood pressure
- Decreased blood viscosity
- Decreased hematocrit
- Decreased clotting factor concentration
- Greater transfusion requirement
- Disruption of electrolyte balance
- Direct immune suppression
- Premature reperfusion
- Increased risk for hypothermia
- The ATLS guidelines have been updated in 2018. Following are the salient features:

ATLS 2018 Guidelines - Salient Features

Initial Assessment:	Clinicians can quickly assess A, B, C, and D in a trauma patient (10-second assessment) by identifying themselves, asking the patient for his or her name, and asking what happened. An appropriate response suggests that there is no major airway compromise (i.e., ability to speak clearly), breathing is not severely compromised (i.e., ability to generate air movement to permit speech), and the level of consciousness is not markedly decreased (i.e., alert enough to describe what happened).

Contd...

ATLS 2018 Guidelines - Salient Features	
AIRWAY	**Airway maintenance with restriction of cervical spine motion** Assess the airway to ascertain patency Establish a definitive airway if there is any doubt about the patient's ability to maintain airway integrity. Supplemental oxygen must be administered to all severely injured trauma patients. While assessing and managing a patient's airway, avoid excessive movement of the cervical spine. Based on the mechanism of trauma, assume that a spinal injury exists until it has been excluded by appropriate radiographic adjuncts and clinical evaluation. When airway management is necessary, the cervical collar is opened, and a team member manually restricts motion of the cervical spine. Drug-assisted intubation is indicated in patients who need airway control, but have intact gag reflexes, especially in patients who have sustained head injuries.
BREATHING	Oxygenated inspired air is best provided via a tight fitting oxygen reservoir face mask with a flow rate of at least 10 L/min.
CIRCULATION	• Rule out Non haemorrhagic causes of shock. • External hemorrhage identified and controlled during the primary survey using direct manual pressure • **A bolus of 1 L of an isotonic solution (20 mL/kg for children weighing less than 40 kg)** to achieve an appropriate response in an adult patient. If unresponsive to initial crystalloid therapy, early blood transfusion is indicated. (See charts below). • Adequate resuscitation generates a urine output of: • 0.5 mL/kg /hr → Adults • 1 mL/kg/hr → Children > 1 yr age • 2 mL/kg/hr → <1 yr age • Massive transfusion → > 10 units of pRBCs within the first 24 hours of admission or more than 4 units in 1 hour • Damage control resuscitation → Most commonly 1:1:1 ratio of Packed RBCs:FFP: Platelets • Calcium administration • Early administration of Tranexamic acid (within 3 hours) • Identification and management of coagulopathy using point of care technologies like Thromboelastography (TEG) if available.

Responses to Initial Fluid Resuscitation[a]

	Rapid response	Transient response	Minimal or no response
Vital signs	Return to normal	Transient Improvement recurrence of decreased blood pressure and increased heart rate	Remain abnormal
Estimated blood loss	Minimal (<15%)	Moderate and ongoing (15%-40%)	Severe (>40%)
Need for blood	Low	Moderate to high	Immediate
Blood preparation	Type and cross match	Type-specific	Emergency blood release
Need for operative intervention	Possibly	Likely	Highly likely
Early presence of surgeon	Yes	Yes	Yes

[a]Isotonic crystalloid solution, up to 1000 mL in adults; 20 mL/kg in children

Contd...

ATLS 2018 Guidelines - Salient Features	
DISABILITY (Neurologic Evaluation)	• Evaluation of GCS

Glasgow Coma Scale (GCS)

Original Scale	Revised Scale	Score
Eye Opening (E)	Eye Opening (E)	4
Spontaneous	Spontaneous	3
To Speech	To sound	2
To pain	To pressure	1
None	Non-testable	NT
Verbal Response (V)	Verbal Response (V)	5
Oriented	Oriented	4
Confused conversation	Confused	3
Inappropriate words	Words	2
Incomprehensible sounds	Sounds	1
None	None	NT
	Non-testable	
Best Motor Response (M)	Best Motor Response (M)	6
Obeys commands	Obeys commands	5
Localizes pain	Localizing	4
Flexion withdrawal to pain	Normal flexion	3
Abnormal flexion (decorticate)	Abnormal flexion	2
Extension (decerebrate)	Extension	1
None (Flaccid)	None	NT
	Non-testable	

GCS Score = (E[4] + V[5] + M[6]) = Best possible score 15; worst possible score 3.
* If an area cannot be assessed, no numerical score is given for that region, and it is considered "non-testable".

EXPOSURE	• Hypothermia can be present when the patient arrives, or it may develop quickly in the ED if the patient is uncovered and undergoes rapid administration of room-temperature fluids or refrigerated blood. • Aggressive measures are to be taken to prevent the loss of body heat and restore body temperature • Use of a high-flow fluid warmer to heat crystalloid fluids to 39°C (102.2°F) recommended. When fluid warmers are not available, a microwave can be used to warm crystalloid fluids, but it should never be used to warm blood products.
Adjuncts to Primary Survey with Resuscitation	Continuous ECG, pulse oximetry, carbon dioxide (CO2) monitoring, and assessment of ventilatory rate, arterial blood gas (ABG) blood lactate, x-ray examinations (e.g., chest and pelvis), FAST, extended focused assessment with sonography for trauma (eFAST), and Diagnostic Peritoneal Lavage (DPL). Urinary And Gastric Catheters. Pulse rate, blood pressure, pulse pressure, ventilatory rate, ABG levels, body temperature, and urinary output reflect the adequacy of resuscitation.
SPECIFIC SYSTEMS:	
Chest trauma	• 8 cm over the needle catheter (preferred over 5 cm catheter) for chest tube placement. Chest tube size now decreased to 28-32F (from 36-40 F) • To avoid excessively medial placement of chest tube → **insert in 5th intercostal** space slightly anterior to mid-axillary line. • Use of eFAST for diagnosis of pneumothorax

Contd...

ATLS 2018 Guidelines - Salient Features

Abdominal and Pelvic trauma

Palpation of prostate gland no longer recommended for urethral injury
Preperitoneal packing added to algorithm

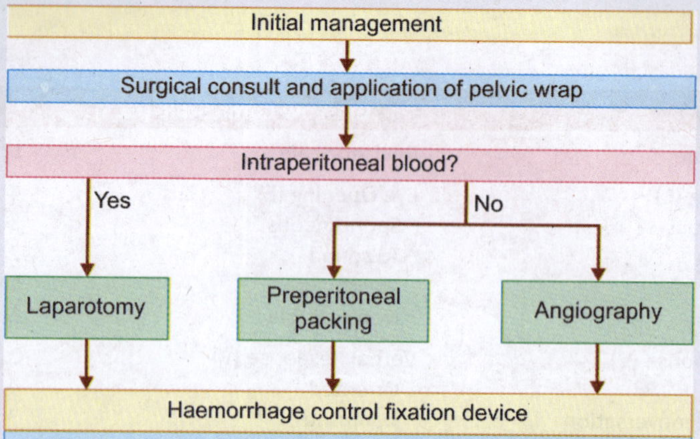

Pelvic fractures and hemorrhagic shock management algorithm.

Head trauma

- GCS
  13-15 → Mild Brain Injury
  9-12 → Moderate Brain Injury
  3-8 → Severe Brain Injury
- Seizure prophylaxis
- Guidelines for anticoagulation reversal have been added

Spinal cord injury

- Restriction of spinal motion (as against "immobilization")
- Canadian C-spine rule
- Backboard awareness: Quickly evaluate patients with or without neurological
- Deficits (e.g., quadriplegia/tetraplegia or paraplegia) and remove them from the backboard as soon as possible. A patient who is allowed to lie on a hard board for more than 2 hours is at high risk for pressure ulcers.

Musculoskeletal

Weight based IV antibiotic regime

Thermal injuries

Titration of fluids to urine output

Burn Resuscitation Fluid Rates and Target Urine Output by Burn Type and Age

Category of burn	Age and weight	Adjusted fluid rates	Urine output
Flame of Scald	Adults and older children (≥ 14 years old))	2mLLR × KG × % TBSA	0.5 mL/kg/hr
	Children (<14 years old)	3mLLR × kg × % TBSA	1 mL/kg/hr
	Infants and young children (≤30 kg)	3mLLR × kg × % TBSA Plus a sugar-containing solution at maintenance rate	1 mL/kg/hr
Electrical Injury	All ages	4mLLR × kg × % TBSA until urine clears	1-1.5 mL/kg/hr until urine clears

Abbreviation: LR, Loctated Ringer's solution, TBSA, total body surface area

Paediatric trauma

- Limiting Crystalloid administration
- Common causes of deterioration in intubated patients: "Don't be a DOPE" (D for dislodgement, O for obstruction, P for pneumothorax, E for equipment failure)
- Pediatric Emergency Care Applied Research Network (PECARN) Criteria for Head CT and to safely rule out presence of clinically important traumatic brain injuries among pediatric head injury patients without the need for CT imaging, including those that would require neurosurgical intervention.

Contd...

ATLS 2018 Guidelines - Salient Features	
Geriatric	Lower threshold for imaging
Pregnancy	Indication of amniotic fluid leak is vaginal pH of >4.5
Transfer to definitive care	• Specific mention of avoiding CT in primary hospital • Avoid procedures that do not change plan of care • SBAR template for communication (Situation, Background, Assessment, Recommendation)

Signs and Symptoms of Hemorrhage by Class

Parameter	Class I	Class II (mild)	Class III (moderate)	Class IV (severe)
Approximate blood Loss	<15%	15-30%	31-40%	>40%
Heart rate	↔→↑←↕	↔/↑	↑	↑/ ↑↑
Blood pressure	↔	↔	↔/↓	↓
Pulse pressure	↔	↓	↓	↓
Respiratory rate	↔	↔	↔/↑	↑
Urine output	↔	↔	↓	↓↓
Glasgow Coma Scale score	↔	↔	↓	↓
Base deficit	0 to -2 mEq/L	-2 to -6 mEq/L	-6 to -10 mEq/L	-10 mEq/L or Less
Need for blood products	Monitor	Possible	Yes	Massive Transfusion Protocol
Base excess is the quantity of base (HCO_3^-, in mEq/L) that is above or below the normal range in the body. A negative number is called a base deficit and indicates metabolic acidosis.				

AIIMS MAY 2018

14. Ans. None

Ref: Maingot 11th ed Ch 46, Skandalakis' Surgical Anatomy Chapter 9

Recall Bias

If Boundaries was not asked in the exam and Relationship with structures was asked then Option (C) Medial umbilical ligament medially, Testicular vessels laterally and peritoneal fold inferiorly will become a correct answer.

NOTE

Options was provided as set of 3 and all options contained Medial Umbilical ligament as one of the boundary. Since Medial umbilical ligament is not mentioned as any of the boundary of triangle of doom in any standard text of Journal, it's likely that this was a dummy question and was cancelled post exam.

The Triangle of Doom is defined by Vas deferens (round ligament in females) medially, Gonadal vessels laterally and peritoneal reflection inferiorly with apex at internal/ deep ring. Within this triangle are: external iliac vessels, deep circumflex iliac vein, genital branch of the genitofemoral nerve, and the femoral nerve (deep).

The Triangle of Pain is formed by the iliopubic tract (Inguinal ligament) inferolaterally and the gonadal vessels superomedially. The contents of this imaginary triangle include several nerves, such as lateral femoral cutaneous, anterior femoral cutaneous, femoral branch of genitofemoral, and femoral nerve. Also known as **"Electrical hazard zone"**. Electrocautery should not be used in this region.

Circle of Death is formed by the common iliac artery, internal and external iliac arteries, obturator artery, aberrant obturator artery, and inferior epigastric artery. The venous counterparts are similar in name, course, and position.

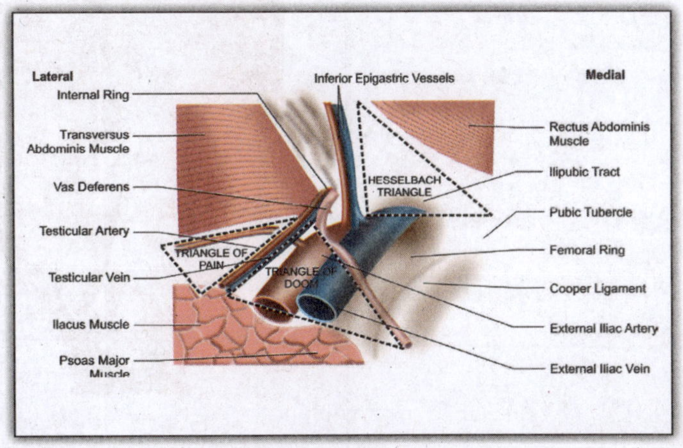

Fig: Triangle of pain and doom

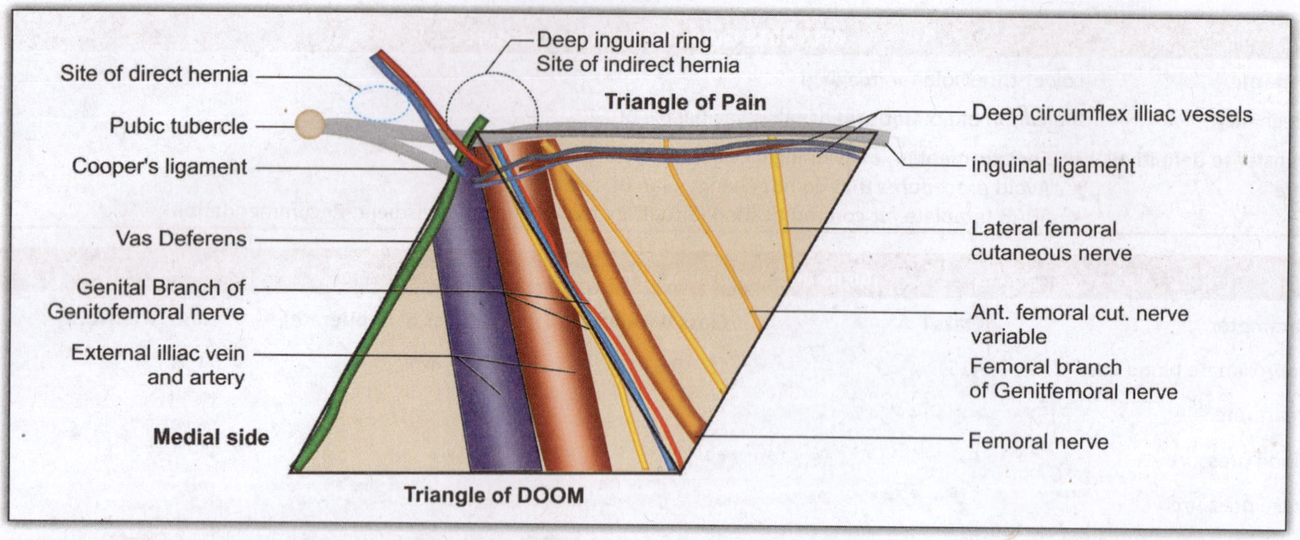

Fig: Quadrangle of pain and doom on right side

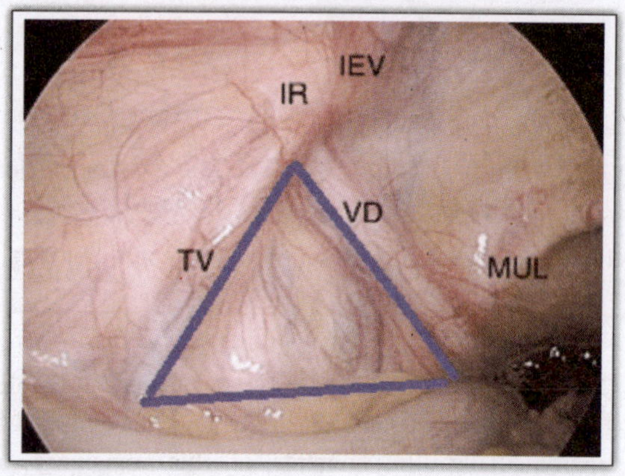

Fig: Laparoscopic view of Triangle of Doom of Left Side: MUL = Medial umbilical ligament, VD = Vas deferens, TV = Testicular vessels, IR = Inferior/ Deep Ring, IEV = Inferior epigastric vessels

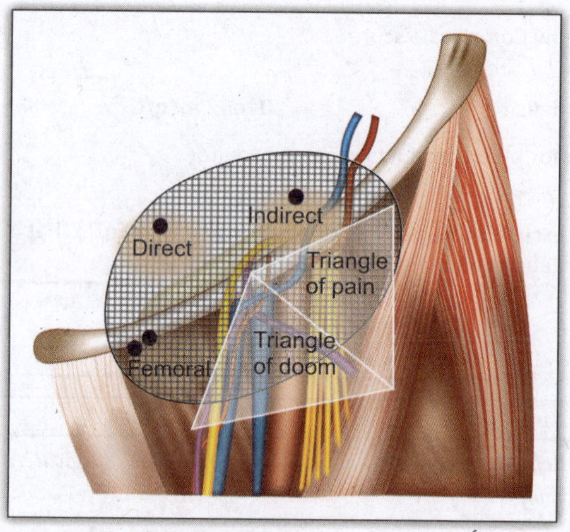

Fig: Laparoscopic hernia repair: Fixation of mesh is avoided below the red line (Triangle of Doom and Pain)

Clinical Importance of triangle of Doom and triangle of Pain is that in Laparoscopic hernia surgery the mesh fixation should avoid these regions.

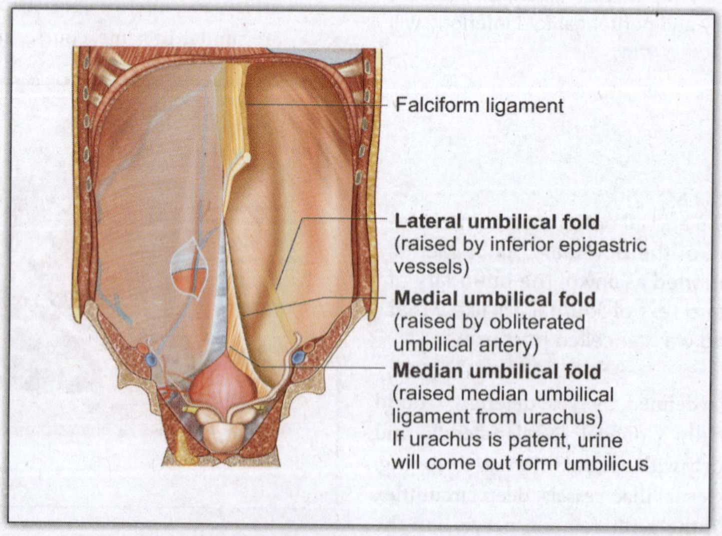

Fig: Peritoneal folds of anterior abdominal wall

15. Ans. (b) Cystine

Ref: Smith's General Urology 17th Ed Pg 253

Cystine stones are typically resistant to ESWL. They frequently require endoscopic or percutaneous approach.

Types of Renal Stones

	Calcium stones (oxalate >> phosphate)	Triple phosphate stone (magnesium ammonium ± calcium phosphate) (struvite)	Uric acid	Cystine	Others or unknown
Percentage of all Stones	70	15–20	5–10	1–2	±5
Causes	**Idiopathic hypercalciuria** (50%) Hypercalciuria and hypercalcemia (10%) Hyperoxaluria (5%) Enteric (4.5%) Primary (0.5%) Hyperuricosuria (20%) Hypocitraturia No known metabolic abnormality (15% to 20%)	Formed largely after infections by bacteria (e.g., ***Proteus*** & some staphylococci) that convert urea to ammonia. The resultant alkaline urine causes the precipitation of magnesium ammonium phosphate salts. These form some of the largest stones the so-called ***staghorn calculi*** are almost always a consequence of infection.	Associated with hyperuricemia (Gout, Leukemia) Associated with hyperuricosuria **50% of uric acid stones are idiopathic**; unexplained tendency to excrete urine of pH below 5.5 may predispose to uric acid stones, because uric acid is insoluble in acidic urine	*Cystine stones* are caused by **Autosomal recessive genetic defects** in the renal reabsorption of amino acids, including cystine, leading to cystinuria. Stones form at low urinary pH.	Indinavir therapy
Crystals in urinalysis	Calcium oxalate dihydrate- Envelope shaped, Calcium Oxalate monohydrate- Dumbbell shaped, Calcium phosphate- rectangular	**Coffin lid shaped**	Yellowish crystals of varying size & shape	Hexagonal	
Radiopacity	Radiopaque	Radiopaque	Radiolucent	Radiopaque	Indinavir stones are Radiolucent

Footnote:
- Stone formation is enhanced by a deficiency in inhibitors of crystal formation in urine. The list of such inhibitors is long, including pyrophosphate, diphosphonate, citrate, glycosaminoglycans, osteopontin, and a glycoprotein called nephrocalcin
- Suspected uric acid stones can be treated by alkalinization of urine to keep pH >7.0, for spontaneous dissolution by 3 months.
- Cystine stones are typically resistant to ESWL. Require medical or surgical approach
- Indinavir stones are the only stones that can not be picked by NCCT.
- Uric acid stones are not picked by plain X ray but can be picked by NCCT. Urine pH < 6.5 is suspicious of Uric acid stone

16. Ans. (b) Bladder exotrophy

Ref: Bailey's 25th Ed Pg 1714

Exstrophy Epispadias Complex

Entities that constitute the exstrophy-epispadias complex.

- **Cloacal exstrophy:** Omphalocele-exstrophy of the bladder-imperforate anus-spinal defect (OEIS) complex is a rare constellation of clinical abnormalities
- **Classic bladder exstrophy:** Due to incomplete closure of inferior part of anterior abdominal wall. Usually associated with separation of pubic bones. Bladder exstrophy is around four times more frequent than cloacal exstrophy
- **Superior vesical fissure:** an uncommon variant of classic bladder exstrophy called superior vesical fissure. Small bilobed urinary bladder with a normal urethra
- **Male epispadias**
- **Female epispadias**

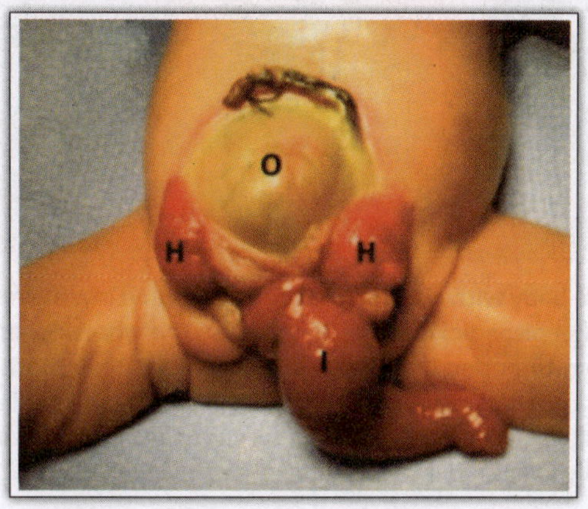

Fig: Patient with cloacal exstrophy showing the O = omphalocele, H= hemibladders, I = **"Elephant trunk sign"** representing the intussuscepted ileum.

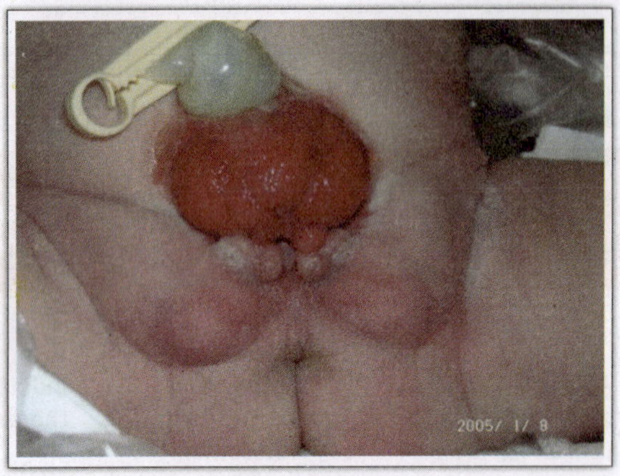

Fig: Newborn girl with classic bladder exstrophy. Notice the open urethral plate, bifid clitoral halves, and anterior displacement of the vaginal orifice. In females, a completely split clitoris can be seen next to the open urethral plate. The vaginal opening appears narrow and is placed anteriorly on the perineum. As the anus is ventrally positioned as well, the perineum is shortened.

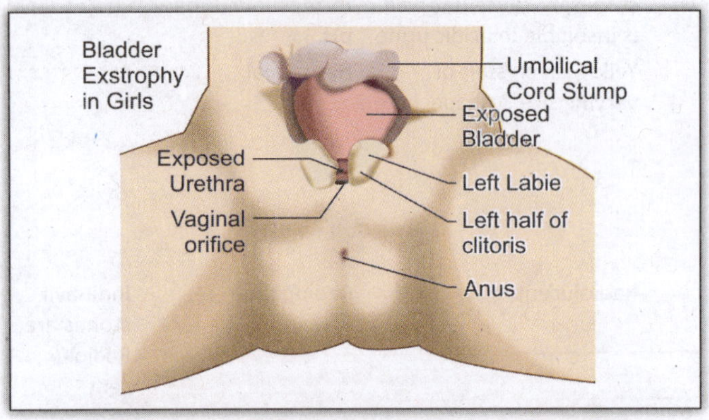

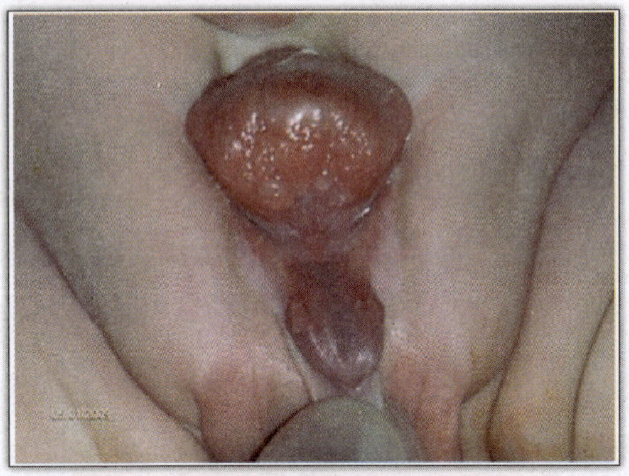

Fig: Male baby with classical bladder exstrophy: In male newborns, an open (= epispadic) urethral plate covers the whole dorsum of the penis from the open bladder to the glandular grove. Both corpora cavernosa are located beneath the urethral plate. The penis appears shorter than normal and dorsally curved. The normal-sized testes are usually located in the scrotum

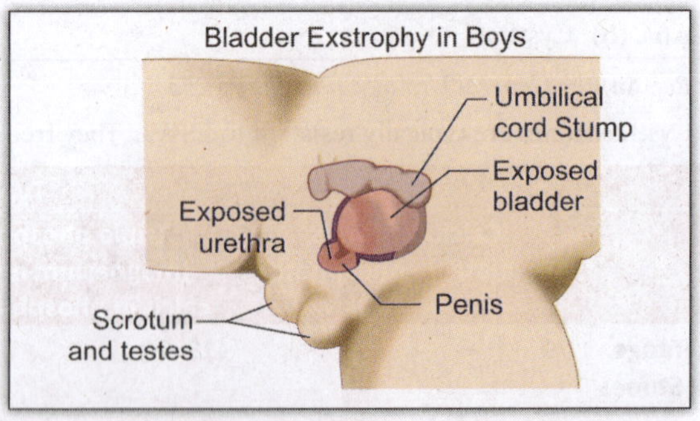

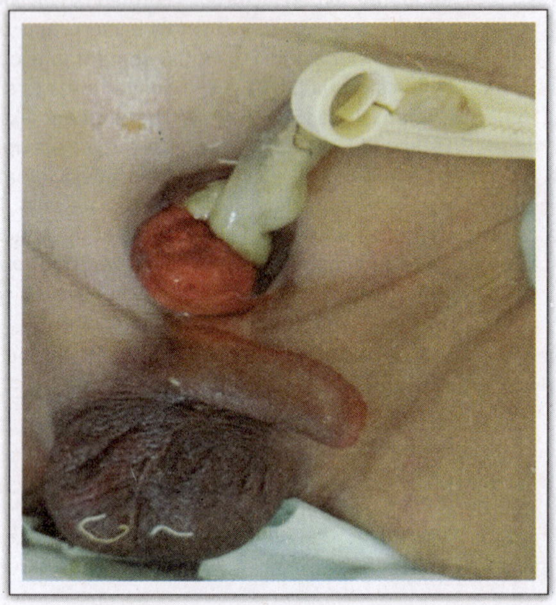

Fig: Male baby with Superior vesical fissure: variant of classic bladder exstrophy called superior vesical fissure. Small bilobed urinary bladder protruding through anterior abdominal wall with a normal urethra and penis

17. Ans. (c) In OT

Ref: Sabiston 20th Ed page 417, Bailey 26th ed page 20, Mastery of surgery 5th ed page 123

(See table of "Damage Control Surgery" in AIIMS Nov 2016 General Surgery) (see page no. 969-970)

Sequence of steps: **Stage 1; Patient selection (ER)→Stage 2; Control of haemorrhage and contamination (OT) → Stage 3; Resuscitation continued in ICU→ Stage 4; Definitive surgery (OT)→ Stage 5; Abdominal closure (ICU)**

18. Ans. (a) Sitting with neck flexed

Ref: SRB's Surgical Operations: Text & Atlas - By Sriram Bhat M Page 171, Shackleford's Surgery of the Alimentary Tract 8th Ed Pg 665

Repeat AIIMS Nov 2018 General Surgery (See for explanation) (see page no. 928)

19. Ans. (a) Sentinel lymph node biopsy

Ref: Mastery of Surgery 6th Ed Pg 591-594, Bailey 26th ed page 136, 799, 814

NOTE

Similar question on Sentinel Lymph node biopsy is asked in AIIMS NOV 2018 (See for explanation), where gamma camera is shown. In this question dye is seen injecting.

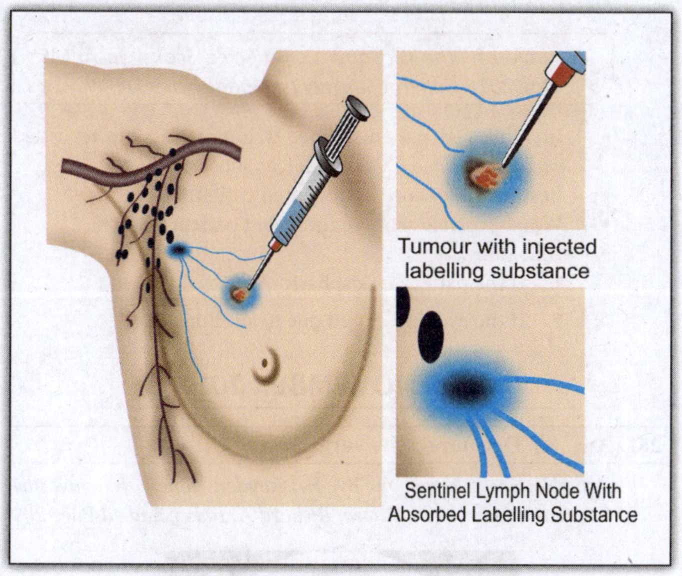

Fig: Sentinel Lymph node biopsy illustration

20. Ans. (a) Tension pneumothorax

Ref: Bailey's 25th Ed Pg 290, Harrison 19th Ed Pg 1719, ATLS 2018 Updates

See Table of "Chest Trauma" in AIIMS Nov 2016 Surgery (see page no. 969)

- Hypotension, tachycardia with a history of RTA decreases the likelihood of this being a case of pleural effusion and hydrothorax.
- Now, distended neck veins suggest the presence of increased intrathoracic pressure. It could also suggest a cardiac tamponade, especially in the setting of hypotension.
- The resonant chest is the biggest clue, it points towards pneumothorax. A pneumothorax with haemodynamic instability is a tension pneumothorax, and needs immediate treatment.

21. Ans. (a) Basal cell carcinoma

Ref: Holland Frei Cancer Medicine 8, Volume 8 By Donald W. Kufe 8th Ed Pg 505; Robin's 9th Ed Pg 1155-1157

Patterns of Neoprastic Spread for Common Human Malignancias

Neoplasms	Hematogenous	Lymphatic	Local infiltration (expressed as local recurrence)
Adenocarcinoma			
Breast	++++	+++	++
Endometrium	+	++	+
Ovary	++	+++	++++
Stomach	++++	++++	+++
Pancreas	++++	++++	+++
Colon	+++	+++	+
Kidney	++	++	++
Prostate	+++	+++	+++
Liver	+	+	++++
Epidermal carcinoma			
Lung	++++	+++	++
Oropharynx	++	+++	+++
Larynx	+	+++	++
Cervix	+	++++	+++
Transitional cell carcinoma			
Bladder	++	+++	++++
Cutaneous neoplasm			
Squamous cell carcinoma	+	++	+
Melanoma	+++	+++	++
Basal cell carcinoma	0	0	+
Sarcoma			
Bone	++++	+	+
Soft tissue	++++	+	+++
Brain neoplasm	0	0	++++

Key: Does not occur; o, <1%; +, 1-5%; ++, 15-+++0%; 3, 30%; ++++, 50%

22. **Ans. (b) T2 N0 M0**

Ref: Bailey's 26th Ed Pg 709

Tumor size >2 cm but < 4cm → T2

No evidence of lymph node spread or metastasis → N0M0

Hence, the stage is T2N0M0.

The TNM Staging System

Primary Tumor (T)	
TX	Primary tumor cannot be assessed
TO	No evidence of primary tumor
Tis	Carcinoma *in situ*
T1	Tumor <2 cm in greatest dimension
T2	Tumor >2 but <4 cm
T3	Tumor >4 cm but <6 cm
T4	Tumor invades adjacent structures, e.g. mandible, skin
Regional Lymph Nodes (N)	
NX	Regional lymph nodes cannot be assessed
N0	No regional lymph node metastasis
N1	Metastasis in a single ipsilateral lymph node <3 cm in greatest dimension
N2a	Metastasis in a single ipsilateral lymph node >3 cm but not more than 6 cm
N2b	Metastasis in multiple ipsilateral lymph nodes, non >6 cm in greatest dimension
N2c	Metastasis in bilateral or contralateral lymph nodes, none >6 cm in greatest dimension
N3	Metastasis in any lymph node >6 cm
Distant Metastasis	
M0	No evidence of distant metastasis
M1	Evidence of distant metastasis

23. **Ans. (c) 30-40%**

Ref: Miller's 8th Ed Pg 1832, Sabiston 20th Ed Pg 50

Classification of Hemorrhage

Parameter	Class I	Class II	Class III	Class IV
Blood loss (mL)	<750	750–1500	1500–2000	>2000
Blood loss (%)	<15	15–30	30–40	>40
Heart rate (bpm)	<100	>100	>120	>140
Blood pressure	Normal	Orthostatic	Hypotension	Severe hypotension
CNS symptoms	Normal	Anxious	Confused	Obtunded
Pulse pressure	Normal or increase	Decrease	Decrease	Decrease
Respiratory/year	15-20 bpm	20-30 bpm	30-40 bpm	35 bpm
Urine output (mL/ hour)	30	20-30	5-10	Negligible
Fluid replacement (3-1 rule)	Crystalloid	Crystalloid	Crystalloid + Blood	Crystalloid + Blood

Contd...

24. **Ans. (b) E2 VT M3**

Ref: Bailey 26th Ed Pg 321, Schwartz 10th ed page 168 – 170, Harrison 19th ed page 260

See table of "The Glasgow Coma Scale Score" in AIIMS Nov 2018 General Surgery (see page no. 931)

- In intubated patients, since it is not possible to assess verbal response, "T" is added as subscript.
- Best possible score in intubated patient- 10
- Worst possible score in intubated patient - 2
- Also know:
  - If the patient is dysphasic- V_D
  - If the eyes are closed due to swelling: E_C

AIIMS NOVEMBER 2017

25. **Ans. (c) Decompressive surgery**

Ref: Netter's Neurology By H. Royden Jones, Jr., Jayashri Srinivasan, Gregory J. Allam, Richard A. Baker 2nd ed Page 209

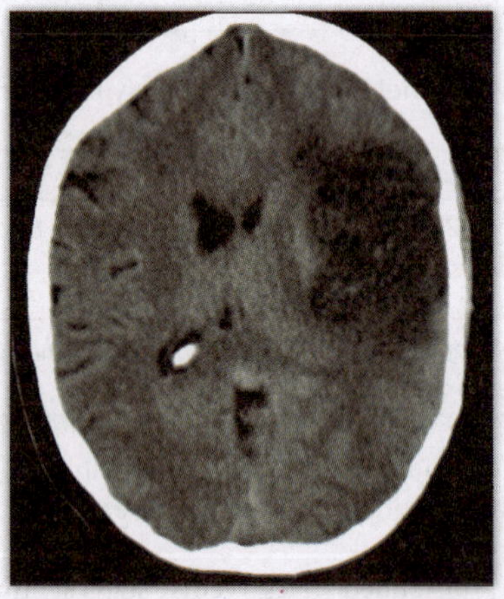

Fig: CT brain showing Edema/ heatoma in Middle cerebral artery territory compressing the ventricles

The patient is having a low GCS, with CT showing significant edema in the Middle Cerebral Artery territory (at least >50%) and compressed ventricle. In such cases brain herniation is impending and need to be referred for decompressive neurosurgery.

NOTE

The only independent radiologic predictor of fatal brain swelling was involvement of >50 percent of the MCA territory on head CT

The **STATE criteria** may be useful

- Score – GCS<8
- Time <48 h
- Age < 60 yrs
- Territory infarct > 150 cm^3 or >50% MCA territory
- Expectancy of life is high

26. Ans. (b) Urine output

Ref: Bailey 26th ed page 17, British Journal of Anesthesia

Shock Monitoring

The minimum standard for monitoring of the patient in shock is continuous heart rate and oxygen saturation monitoring, frequent non-invasive blood pressure monitoring and hourly urine output measurements. Most patients will need more aggressive invasive monitoring, including central venous pressure and invasive blood pressure monitoring

Bailey states "Ultimately, the goal of treatment is to restore cellular and organ perfusion. Ideally, therefore, monitoring of organ perfusion should guide the management of shock. The best measures of organ perfusion and the best monitor of the adequacy of shock therapy remains the urine output"

Monitoring of Patient in Shock	
Minimal	**Additional modalities**
ECG	Central venous pressure
Pulse oximetry	Invasive blood pressure
Blood pressure	Cardiac output
Urine output	Base deficit and serum lactate

Central Venous Pressure

Patients whose state of shock is not rapidly corrected with a small amount of fluid should have central venous pressure monitoring and continuous blood pressure monitoring through an arterial line. Low CVP always means hypovolemia, but high CVP can signify either over expansion of blood volume or cardiac failure. There is no 'normal' central venous pressure (CVP) for a shocked patient, and reliance cannot be placed on an individual pressure measurement to assess volume status. Some patients may require a CVP of 5 cm H_2O, whereas some may require a CVP of 15 cm H_2O or higher. Further, ventricular compliance can change from minute to minute in the shocked state, and CVP is a poor reflection of end diastolic volume (preload). **CVP measurements should be assessed dynamically as response to a fluid challenge.** A fluid bolus (250– 500 mL) is infused rapidly over 5–10 minutes. The normal CVP response is a rise of 2–5 cm H_2O which gradually drifts back to the original level over 10–20 minutes. **Patients with no change in their CVP are empty and require further fluid resuscitation.** Patients with a large, sustained rise in CVP have high preload and an element of cardiac insufficiency or volume overload.

Resuscitation requires appropriate fluid management and is dependent on the cause of shock and the time course of the illness. For example, in hypovolaemic shock with a low CVP, fluid replacement is required. In contrast, in cardiogenic shock due to left-sided heart failure (i.e. with a raised CVP), diuretic therapy with fluid restriction may be indicated. To complicate matters further, cardiogenic shock due to right-sided heart failure (i.e. also with a raised CVP) may require fluid administration to ensure adequate filling of, and cardiac output from, the left side of the heart! The time course of the disease is also important. For example, at the onset of septic shock, fluid replacement is essential, but, if acute respiratory distress syndrome develops later, fluid restriction is necessary to prevent pulmonary oedema.

(Ref: Oxford Desk Reference: Acute Medicine edited by Richard Leach, Kevin Moore, Derek Bell)

27. Ans. (c) Heart Rate/Mean Arterial pressure

Ref: Sabiston 20th Ed Page 52

- Shock Index is defined as Heart rate divided by Systolic BP.
- Shock Index is known as hemodynamic stability indicator in Shock cases.
- Modified Shock Index (MSI) includes Diastolic BP also and defined as heart rate divided by

Mean Arterial Pressure

- MAP= Systolic Pressure+ (2 X Diastolic Pressure) divided by 3
- High MSI indicates- Hypodynamic state
- Low MSI indicates- Hyperdynamic state
- MSI is better indicator than SI to predict the mortality in shock

28. Ans. (c) 11

Ref: Bailey 26th Ed Pg 321

This is a pretty straightforward question.

EVM score = Eye opening 2+ Verbal 3 + Motor 6 = 11

(See Details of Glasgow COMA SCOE in Surgery AIIMS Nov 2018) (see page no. 931)

29. Ans. (b) Basal cell carcinoma

Ref: Harrison 19th ed page 500, Schwartz 9th ed chapter 16

Basal cell cancer (BCC) or Rodent Ulcer often occurs on the face above a line joining the angle of the mouth and the ear lobe.

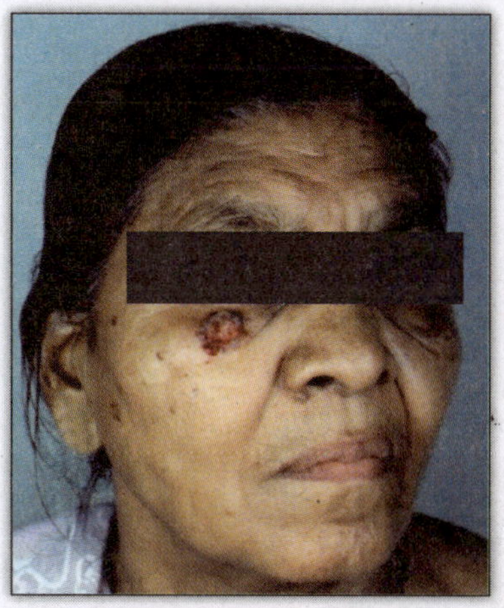

© Patidar S (Baroda Skin Clinic)

Fig: Basal cell carcinoma: Indurated ulcer with raised margins over right infraorbital region due to Basal cell carcinoma. Basal cell cancer (BCC) or **Rodent Ulcer** often occurs on the face above a line joining the angle of the mouth and the ear lobe. There are 5 common clinical subtypes of basal cell carcinoma (BCC)

BCC Clinical Subtype					
Subtype	**Site**	**Growth**	**Lesion**	**Color**	**Surface**
Solid or Nodular (60-80%) 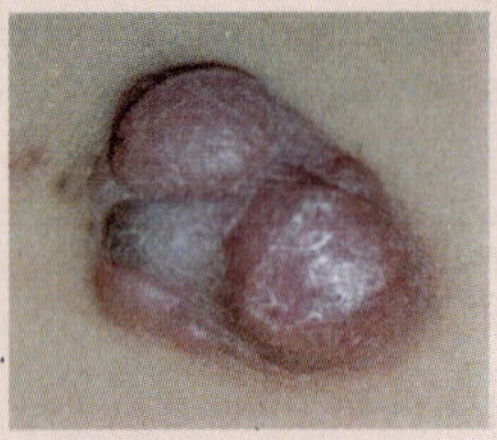	Face	Slow	Nodule	Skin translucent	Telangiectasia
Rodent ulcer 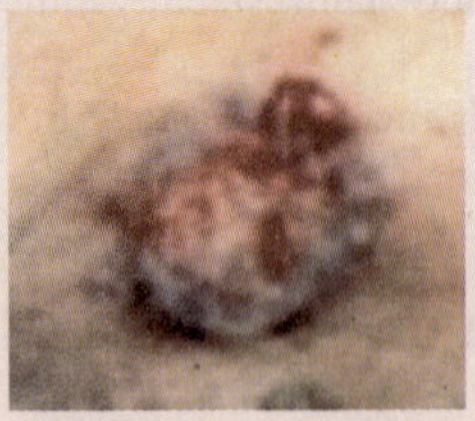	Face	Faster	Central ulcer, rolled borders	Translucent necrotic, Red	Telangiectasia
Pigmented 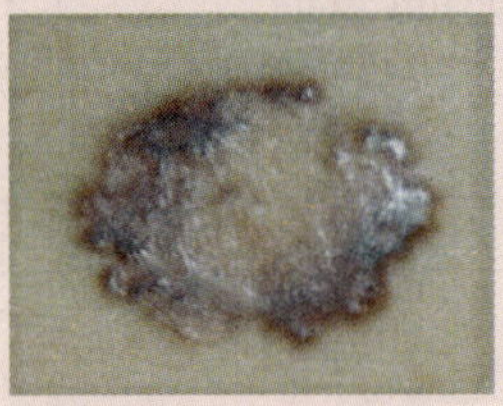	Face	Slow	Nodule	Brown	Telangiectasia
Adenocystic 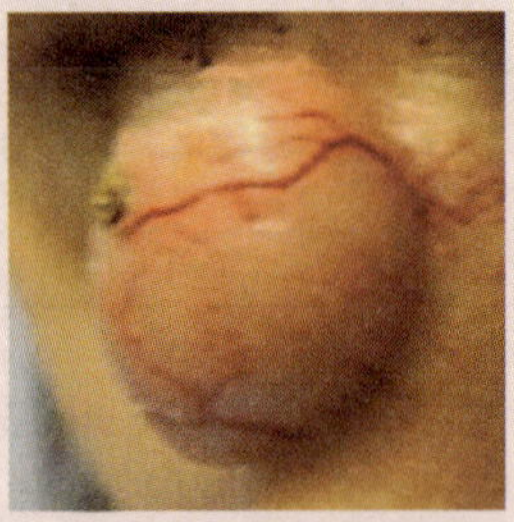	Face	Slow	Lobulated cyst + rolled edges	Erythomatous/ + squamous	Telangiectasia
Superficial 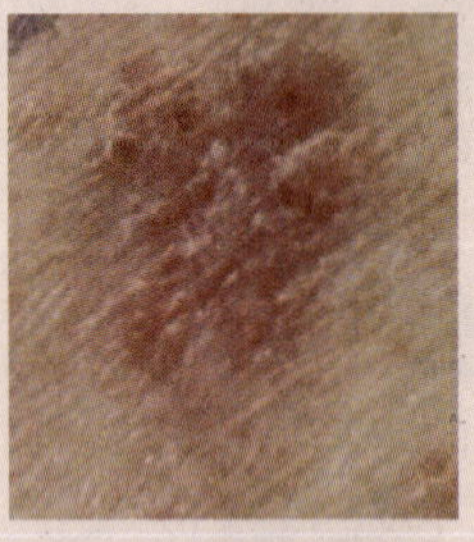	Trunk, Limbs	Slow	Plaque, pearly border	Red scaly	Well defined
Morphoeic (2-6% of BCC) 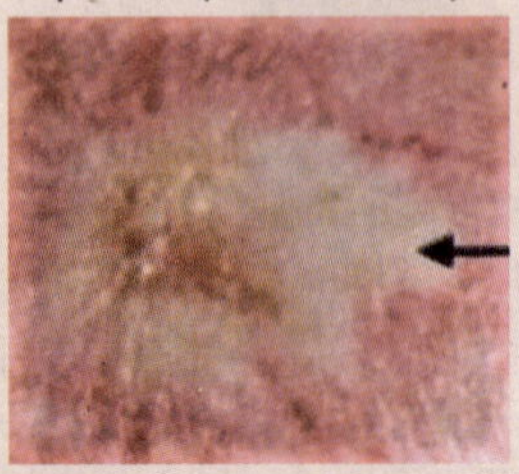	Face	Slow	Scar like plaque	Yellowish	Undefined
Metatypical or Basosquamous	Face	Rapid	Plaque + Metastasis	Yellowish	Undefined Telangiectasia

Risk Categories of BCC		
	Low risk BCC	High risk BCC
Site		Mid face, Ear region
Size	< 2 cm	> 2 cm
Histology	Non Basosquamous	Basosquamous/ Metatypical
Course	Primary	Recurrent
Immunity	Normal	Compromised

30. Ans. (b) Put him in lateral position on stretcher to prevent aspiration

Ref: Sabiston 20th edition page 415, Bailey 26th ed page 304, 330

All polytrauma patients should be considered to sustain Cervical spine injury unless proven otherwise. I.e. Full spine precautions must be observed until it is confirmed that the patient's vertebral column is intact, either by physical examination and clinical findings or by radiologic confirmation when warranted.

- The cervical spine is stabilized by fitting the patient with a hard cervical collar
- A patient with a spinal injury should be strapped to a spine board and the head fixed to the board with tape.

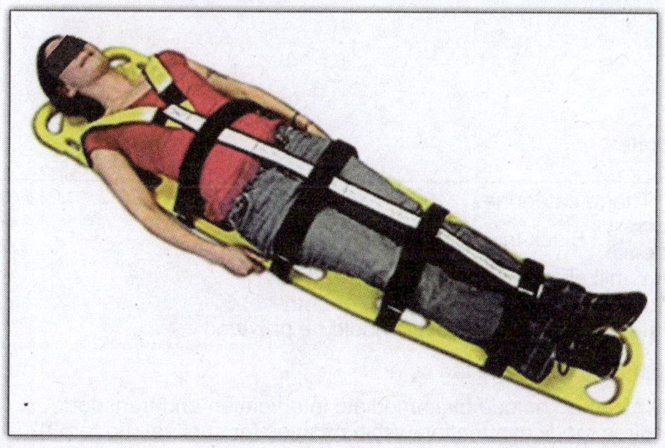

- The thoracic, lumbar, and sacral segments of the spine are protected by maintaining the patient in the supine position at all times by strapping on spine board.
- If the patient is to be moved, strict log roll technique is used. Percussion and auscultation should be performed on both the front and back of the chest wall after log rolling. Once the patient has been evaluated anteriorly, a log roll should be performed to inspect the back. A total of 5 people are required to perform spinal Log roll

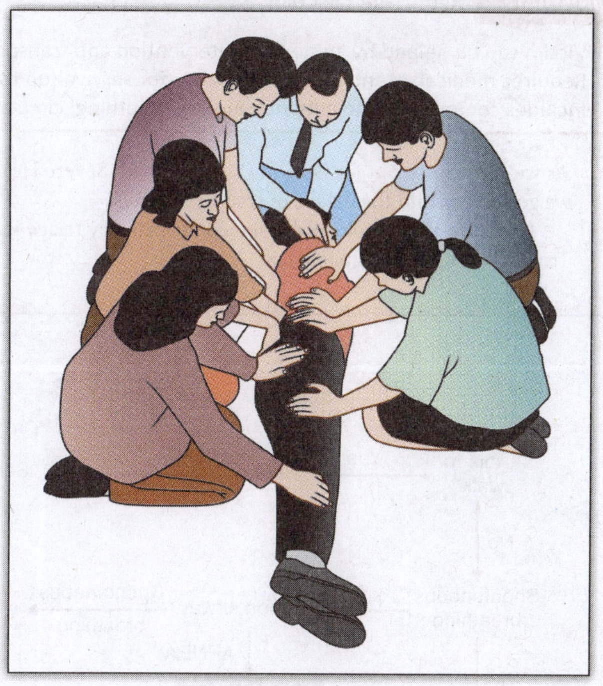

31. Ans. (a) Child with airway obstruction

Ref: Miller's 8th Ed Pg 2476, Trauma: Resuscitation, Perioperative Management, and Critical Care by William C. Wilson, Pg 73

The options in this question are very close. See division into triage groups below:

Triage Groups in Mass Casualty Incidents		
With the aid of triage tags or colored flags, the patients are sorted into four groups.		
Triage tag	**Assessment of treatments needed**	**Types of injuries**
Green (minor)	Minor injuries with no immediate need of treatment Psychologic support is needed Patients can walk	Wounds Minor fractures
Yellow (delayed)	Urgent treatment is needed No vital threat is present	Fractures, joint injuries Amputation, major blood loss Burns
Red (immediate)	Vital threat is immediate	Respiratory insufficiency, shock Brain trauma Burns with immediate vital threat Abdominal trauma
Black (expectant)	Patients are dead or moribund	Respiratory arrest, cardiac arrest Head injuries with dismal prognosis

Triage Categories

EXPECTANT Black triage tag color	**DELAYED** Yellow Triage Tag Color
• Victim unlikely to survive-given severity of injuries, level of available care, or both • Palliative care and pain relief should be provided	• Victim's transport can be delayed • Includes serious and potentially life-threatening injuries, but status not expected to deteriorate significantly
IMMEDIATE Red Triage Tag Color	**MINOR** Green Triage Tag Color
• Victim can be helped by immediate intervention and transport • Requires medical attention within minutes for survival(up to 60) • Includes compromises to patient's Airway, Breathing, circulation	• Victim with relatively minor injuries • Status unlikely to deteriorate over day • May be able to assist in own care: "Walking Wounded"

As we can see, except for Option (D) Child with Severe Head injury; all other options fall under the red, that is, immediate group. Now, we go further into the details of triage protocols.

There are a few protocols designed for primary triage in adults and paediatric patients. The protocols for adults are START (Simple Triage And Rapid Treatment).

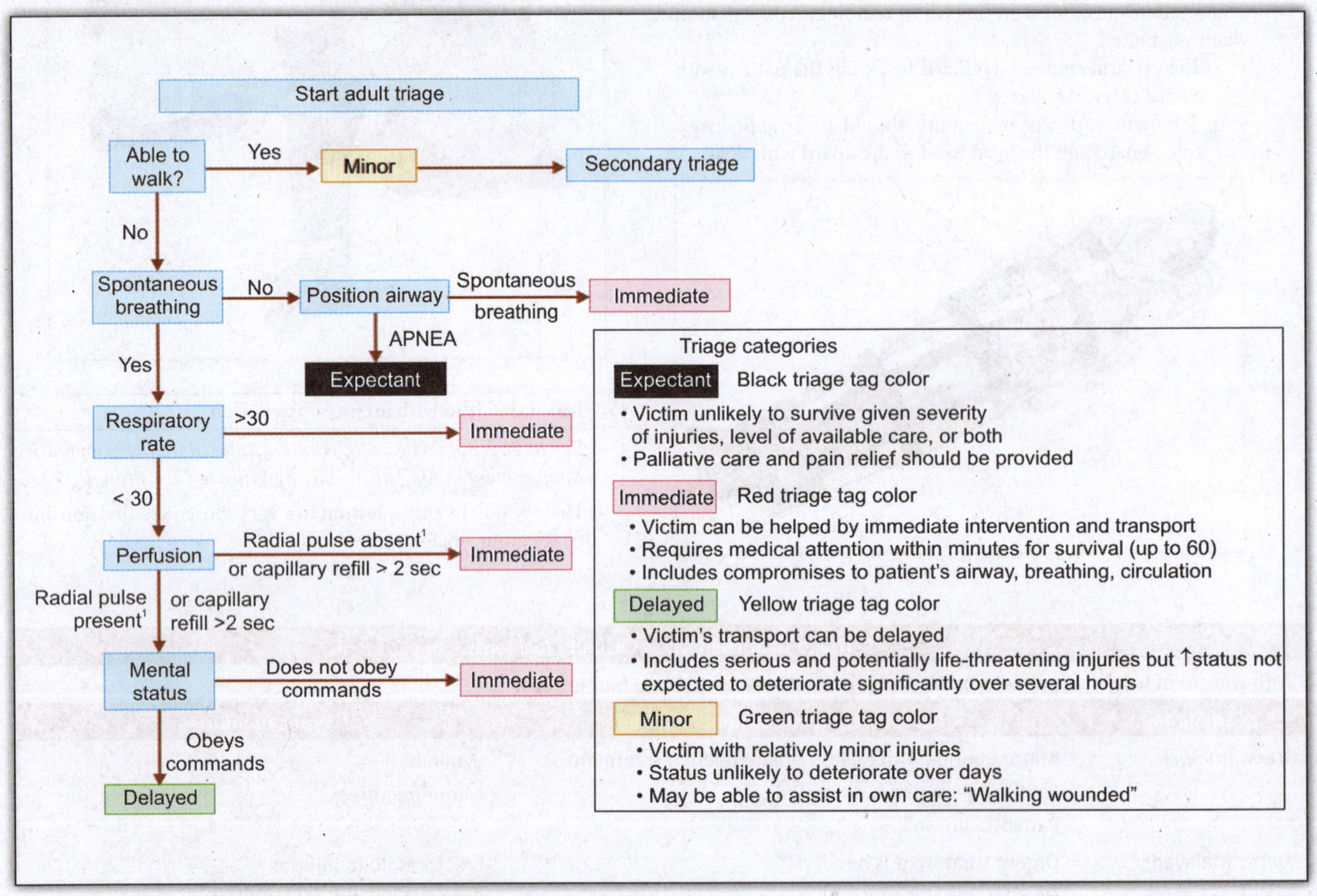

The protocols for paediatric patients are JumpSTART, Paediatric trauma tape (PTT). JumpSTART is one of the most common protocols.

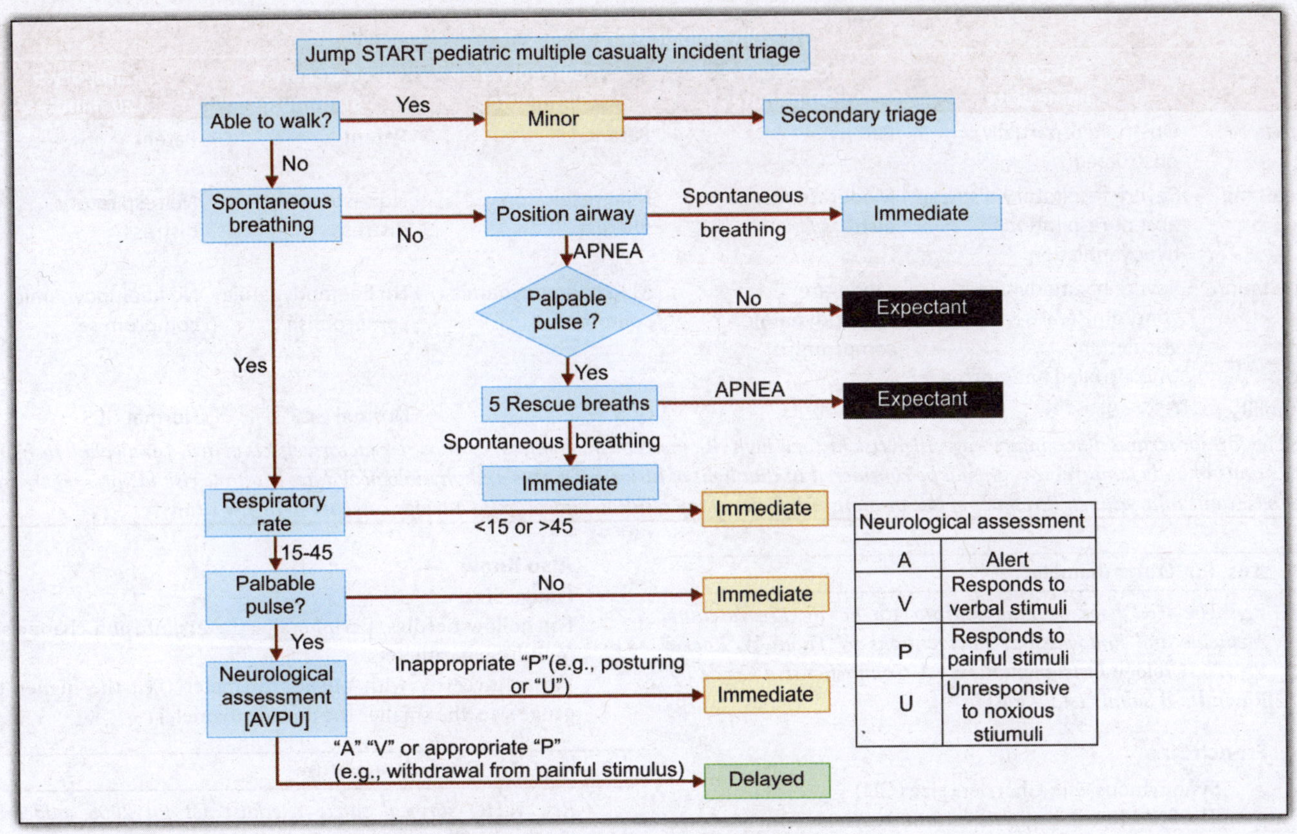

There is an algorithm for secondary triage, that is, after arrival in the hospital.

It involves categorisation of patients into 3 categories: ones who will survive despite no treatment, those who will not survive despite treatment, and those who may survive with immediate treatment. Obviously, the last group is given top priority.

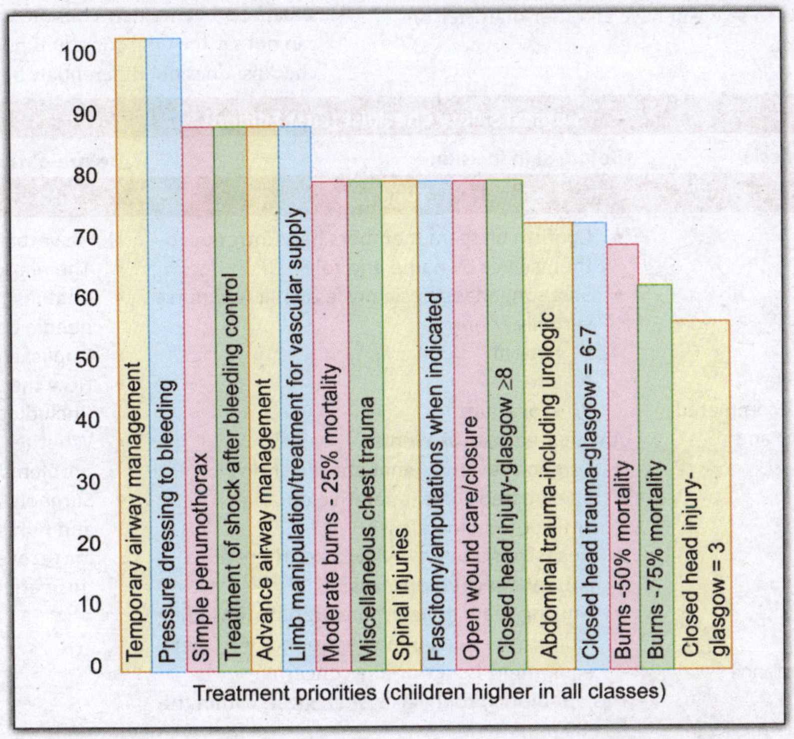

Physiological Predictors					
	Category 1 Immediate	Category 2 30 minutes	Category 3 30 minutes	Category 4 60 minutes	Category 5 120 minutes
Airway	Obstructed/partially obstructed	Patent	Patent	Patent	Patent
Breathing	Severe respiratory distress/ absent respiration/ hypoyentilation	Moderate respiratory distress	Mild respiratory distress	No respiratory distress	No respiratory distress
Circulation	Severe haemodynamic conpromise/absent criculation Uncontrolled haemorrhage	Moderate haemodynamic compromise	Mild haemodynamic compromise	No haemodynamic compromise	No haemodynamic compromise
Disability	GSC < 9	GCS 9–12	GCS > 12	Normal GCS	Normal GCS
Risk factors for serious illness injury - age, high risk history, high risk mechanism of injury, cardiac risk factors, effects of drugs or alcohol, rash and alterations in body temperature - should be considered in that light of history of events and physiological data. Multiple risk factors = increased risk of serious injury/illness. Presence of one or more risk factors may result in allocation to a triage category of higher acuity.					

32. Ans. (c) Outer diameter

Ref: The ICU book by Paul Marino 4th Ed Pg 17; Vascular Medicine and Endovascular Interventions by Thom W. Rooke Pg 126; Urology Instrumentation - A Comprehensive Guide by Ravindra B Sabnis 1st Ed Pg 116

French Size

- Synonymous with Charriere size (CH)
- The French scale begins at zero, and each increment of one French unit represents an increase of ⅓ (0.33) millimeter in outer diameter: i.e.,
- **French size × 0.33 = outside diameter (mm).**
- E.g: 5 French units in size will have an outer diameter of 5 × 0.33 = 1.65 mm.

Also Know

Gauge Size

For hollow needles, peripheral catheters,infusion channels of multilumen catheters.

Varies inversely with outside diameter (i.e., the higher the gauge size, the smaller the outside diameter)

33. Ans. (b) Doctor's signature

Ref: WHO surgical safety checklist 1st Ed 2008 guidelines; Textbook of Anesthesia for Postgraduates By TK Agasti Pg 313

"Informed consent is essential in the preoperative checklist. Verbal consent may be accepted in life threatening or emergency situations but written consent is always preferable" Hence we can not say the Oral consent is not a part of checklist. The WHO checklist does not differentiate between types of consent.

Surgical Safety Checklist (First Edition)		
Before induction of anaesthesia	**Before skin incision**	**Before patient leaves operating room**
Sign in	**Time out**	**Sign out**
• Patient has confirmed ▪ Identity ▪ Site ▪ Procedure ▪ Consent • Site marked/not applicable • Anaesthesia safety check completed • Pulse oximeter on patient and functioning Does patient have a: Known allergy? • No • Yes Difficult airway/aspiration risk? • No • Yes, and equipment/assistance available Risk of > 500 mL blood loss (7 mL/kg in children)? • No • Yes, and adequate intravenous access • And fluids planned	• Confirm all team members have introduced themselves by name and role • Surgeon, anaesthesia professional And nurse verbally confirm ▪ Patient ▪ Site ▪ Procedure Anticipated critical events • Surgeon reviews: what are the critical or unexpected steps, operative duration, anticipated blood loss? • Anaesthesia team reviews: are there any patient-specific concerns? • Nursing team reviews: has sterility (including indicator results) been confirmed? Are there equipment issues or any concerns? Has antibiotic prophylaxis been given within the last 60 minutes? • Yes • Not applicable Is essential imaging displayed? • Yes • Not applicable	Nurse verbally confirms with the team: • The name of the procedure recorded • That instrument, sponge and needle counts are correct (or not Applicable) • How the specimen is labelled (Including patient name) • Whether there are any equipment problems to be addressed • Surgeon, anaesthesia professional and nurse review the key concerns for recovery and management of this patient

34. Ans. (d) Polyps in Gallbladder

Ref: Sternberg's surgical pathology 5th ed page 1614, Bailey 26th ed page 1108

Gallbladder polyp is the best possible answer. Gallbladder cancer is mostly a Histopathological diagnosis and from gross specimen it is difficult to ascertain as Gallbladder cancer. Moreover it can develop in Gallbladder Polyps, Stones etc. Also in gallbladder cancer specimen mostly Radical Cholecystectomy with segmental Liver resection is given in history (Mostly but not necessarily)

NOTE

Gallbladder pathologies are often seen mixed rather isolated. Example stone with cholesterolosis, stone with polyp, Polyp with carcinoma etc .

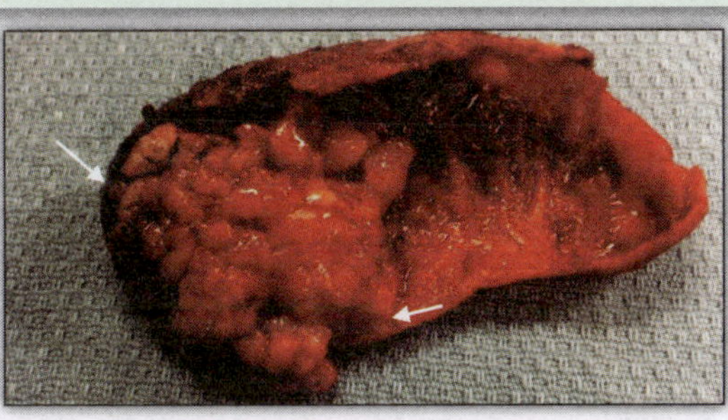

Fig: Gallbladder polyps: Gross photo showing a sessile polypoid mass (yellow arrows) located at the fundic region of the opened gallbladder

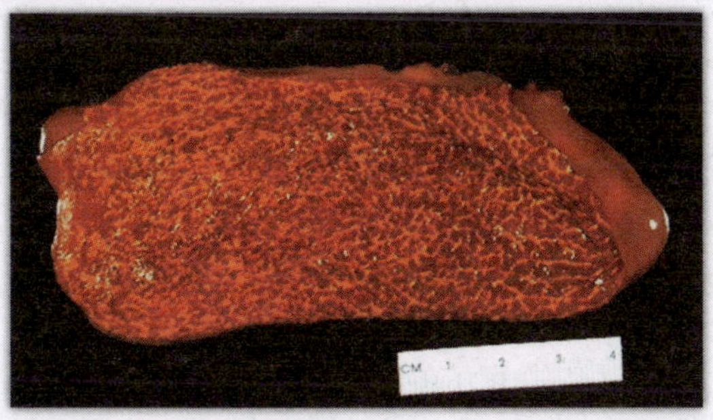

Fig: Gallbladder cholesterolosis/ Strawberry Gallbladder: The appearance of the gallbladder mucosa seen here is consistent with cholesterolosis (containing cholesterol crystal deposits). Microscopically, the mucosa in cholesterolosis of the gallbladder contains many foamy macrophages which produce the grossly visible strawberry-like appearance.

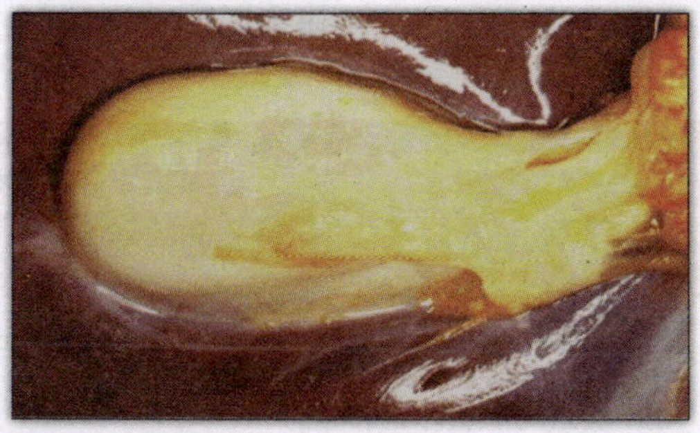

Fig: Porcelain gallbladder: This is a gross appearance of the gallbladder termed "porcelain gallbladder" because the wall and surfaces of the gallbladder are hard and tan-white like a porcelain vase. This is one end result of chronic cholecystitis.

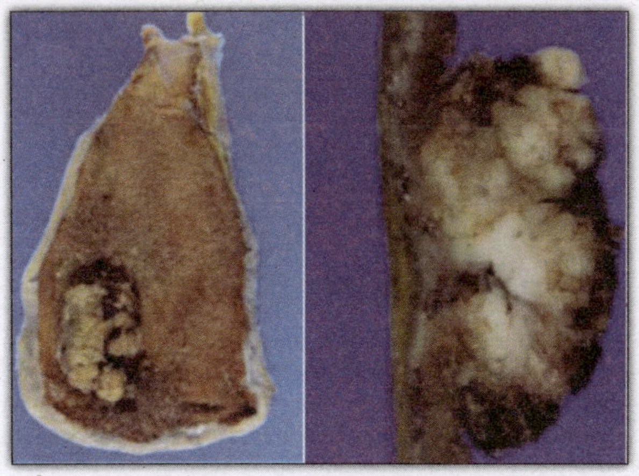

© Kawasaki Y (Japan)

Fig: Gallbladder cancer: Macroscopic appearance of the gall-bladder mass located in the fundus. Tumor infiltration to the muscularis layer is evident macroscopically in the cut section side view. Adenocarcinomas are divided into infiltrative (65%), papillary (15%), and colloid (10%) subtypes. Nearly 60% of carcinomas originate in the fundus, 30% in the body, and 10% in the neck

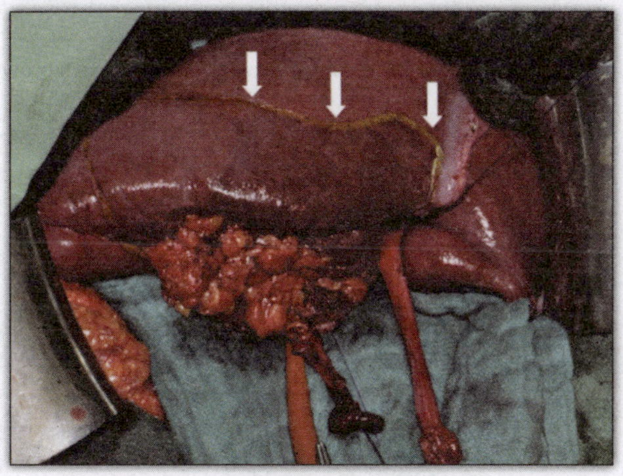

© Scheingraber S (Germany)

Fig: Gallbladder cancer infiltrating the liver: En bloc resection of the tumor mass with liver segments IVb and V. Arrows demonstrate demarcation of segment IVb after round ligament approach

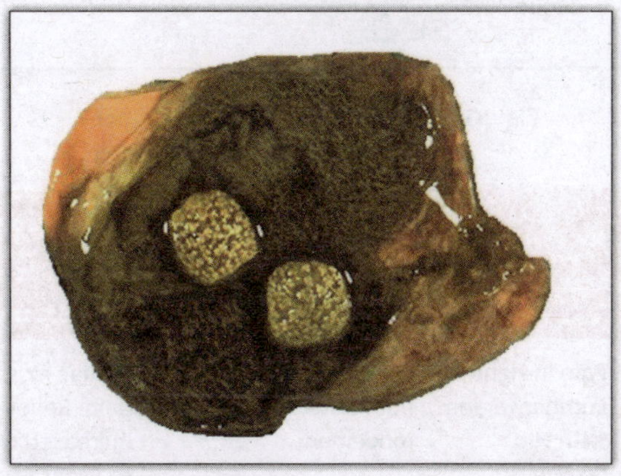

Fig: Gallbladder Cholesterol stones: Two composite cholesterol gallstones are seen here with a yellowish green appearance

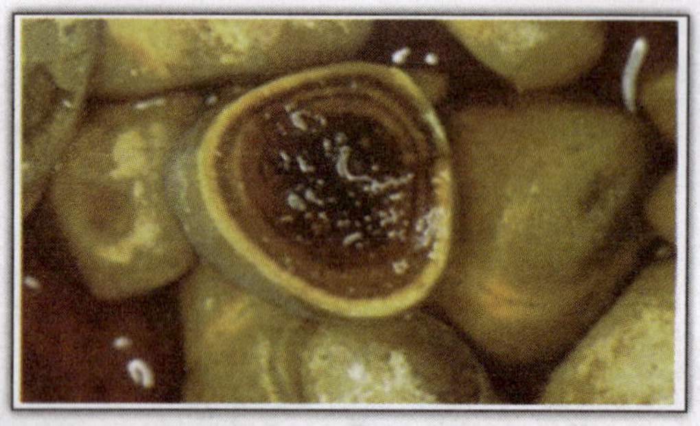

Fig: Gallbladder Mixed stones: Yellow tan faceted mixed gallstones are present. These Gallstones consist of a mixture of cholesterol, bilirubin, and calcium. These stones are squared off (faceted) because they sat together. Hint: if you find one faceted stone, there is probably at least one more somewhere else.

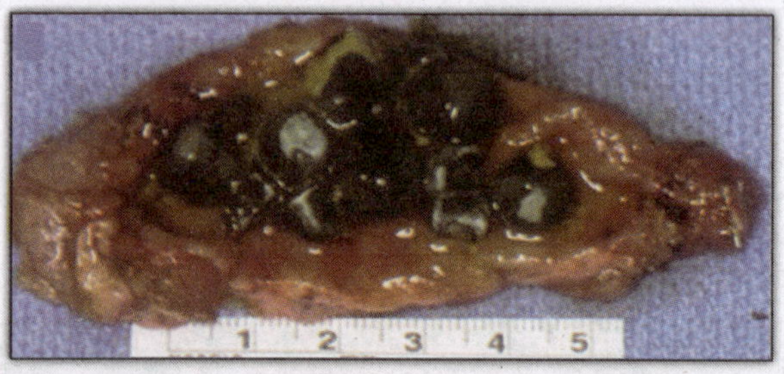

Fig: Gallbladder Pigment stones: These are black or dark brown pigmented hard stones.

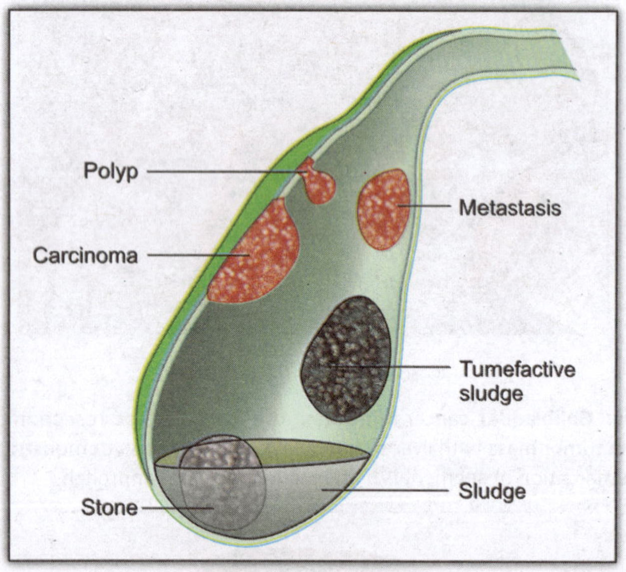

Fig: Gallbladder pathologies Illustration

35. Ans. (c) Abdominal mass

Ref: Sabiston 20th ed Page 765, 1073, Devita 10th ed page 1485 Schwartz 9th edn Page 1065

Desmoid Tumor

A desmoid tumor is a tumor arising in the musculoaponeurotic structures of the abdominal wall, especially below the level of the umbilicus. It is a completely unencapsulated fibroma and is so hard that it creaks when it is cut.

Aetiology

About 80% of cases occur in women, many of whom have borne children, and the neoplasm occurs occasionally in scars of old hernial or other abdominal operation wounds. Consequently, trauma, for example the stretching of the muscle fibres during pregnancy or possibly a small haematoma of the abdominal wall, appears to be an aetiological factor. They can occur in cases of familial adenomatous polyposis (FAP).

Clinical features: Patients with desmoid tumors present with a painless enlarging mass. Local symptoms may arise from compression of adjacent organs or neurovascular structures. Magnetic resonance imaging (MRI) provides information regarding the extent of the disease and its relationship to intra-abdominal organs.

Treatment

Unless the tumor is excised widely, with a surrounding margin of at least 2.5 cm of healthy tissue, recurrence commonly takes place. After removal of a large tumor, repair of the defect in the abdominal wall by nylon mesh is required. These tumors are moderately radiosensitive. (Intraperitoneal desmoids are best left alone when possible.)

36. Ans. (b) Psoas Abscess

Ref: Bailey 26th ed Page 985, SRB Manual of Surgery 4th ed page 769

This question is based on the clinical judgement and differential diagnosis of Right Lumbar mass and pain. Site of pain and Mass are often overlapping into different regions of the abdomen and can not be relied upon completely. Hip flexed attitude is given that means hip extension is painful, this points towards Appendicitis irritating Psoas muscle or Psoas Abscess. No fever points towards non infectious pathology or Cold abscess. Psoas Cold abscess is the best fit in this case.

	Pyelonephritis	Psoas abscess	Retrocaecal appendicitis	Torsion of right undescended testis
Age	Any	83% under 30 years	Young	Young
Pain in right Lumbar region with Hip flexion	Loin/Lumbar pain not related to Hip movement	Rt Iliac fossa, Back/Lumbar pain. Relieved on Hip flexion, Increased on extension due to Psoas muscle spasm	Rt Iliac fossa/Lumbar pain. Relieved on Hip flexion, Increased on extension due to Psoas muscle spasm.	RIF pain not related to Hip movement

Contd...

	Pyelonephritis	Psoas abscess	Retrocaecal appendicitis	Torsion of right undescended testis
Age	Any	83% under 30 years	Young	Young
Mass in right Lumbar region	Lumbar Lump	Lump RIF/LIF smooth, non mobile, not moving with respiration. ***Non tender locally in Cold abscess***	Lump RIF	Undescended testis can present as Lumbar, Iliac fossa, Inguinal mass
Fever	Present	Present (Absent in Cold abscess)	Present	Absent (uncommon)
Spine change on X-ray	Lumbosacral scoliosis with concavity to the right	Spine may show Gibbus, Tenderness, Paraspinal spasm and restricted movement.	Lumbosacral scoliosis with concavity to the right	No spine changes

NOTE

Swellings that are cross fluctuant

1. Ranula
2. Psoas abscess
3. Compound palmar ganglion
4. Bilocular hydrocele

37. Ans. (b) By checking the movement of air water column in the tube during respiration

Ref: Bailey 26th edition Page 355

The chest tube is connected to a closed chest drainage system, which allows for air or fluid to be drained, and prevents air or fluid from entering the pleural space. The system is airtight to prevent the inflow of atmospheric pressure. This chamber has a one-way valve that allows air to exit the pleural cavity during exhalation but does not allow it to re-enter during inhalation due to the pressure in the chamber. The water-seal chamber must be filled with sterile water and should be checked regularly. **The water in the water-seal chamber should rise with inhalation and fall with exhalation (this is called tidaling), which demonstrates that the chest tube is patent.** Continuous bubbling may indicate an air leak, and newer systems have a measurement system for leaks the higher the number, the greater the air leak.

ICD Monitoring

Drainage collection chamber	Underwater seal chamber	Assessment and Management of Air leak
Tidaling	**Bubbling**	
Yes	Yes	Indicates patient air leak (pneumothorax)
No	No	Indicates lung re expansion or obstruction by kinks or clots
No	Yes	Indicates possible connection or system air leak
Yes	No	Observed with pneumonectomy or decreased lung compliance

Contd...

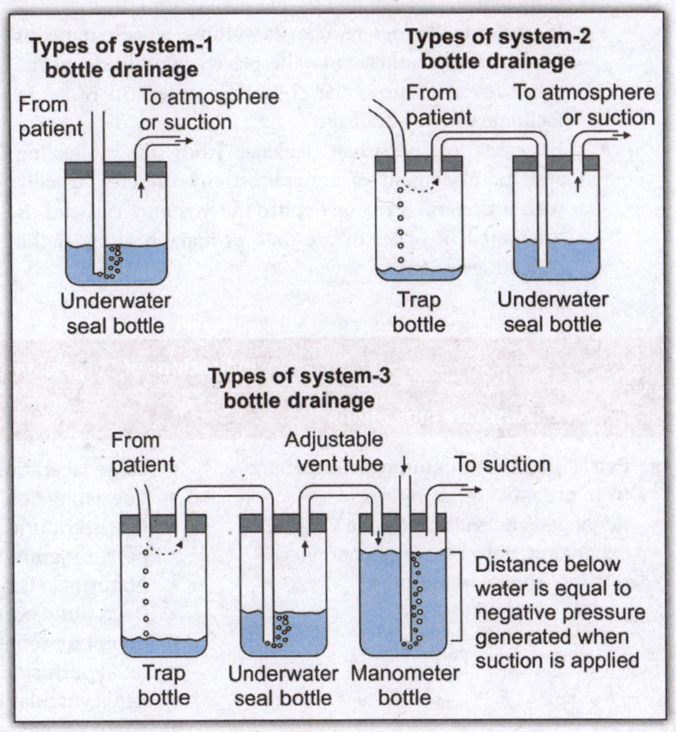

38. Ans. (d) Wait and Watch

Ref: Smith Urology page 17th ed page 125, Sabiston 20th ed page 2091

Campbell 10th ed page 1178- Persistent urinary extravasation can result in urinoma, perinephric infection, and even renal loss. These patients are initially administered systemic antibiotics and carefully observed with appropriate antibiotics. ***In a high percentage, the extravasation resolves spontaneously. Should it persist, placement of an internal ureteral stent often corrects***

the problem. A nonoperative approach with careful observation usually results in a functional renal unit. Perinephric abscess rarely occurs after renal injury, but persistent urinary extravasation and urinoma are the typical precursors. Percutaneous drainage offers a good initial method of management of perinephric abscess, followed by surgical drainage if necessary.

Extravasating urine is collected near the urinary tract and may manifest as:

- Free fluid, also called urinary ascites, if the fascial planes are disrupted (less frequently in renal tears)
- Acute spread to local tissues
- Encapsulated fluid collection surrounding by a fibrous capsule resulting from chronic tissue irritation by urine (urinoma)

Treatment

- Small urinomas can reabsorb spontaneously. Should it persist, placement of an internal ureteral stent often corrects the problem
- If urinoma is larger or if the patient developed septic fever, drainage is Mandatory. The drainage catheter can be positioned under US or CT guidance in the most dependent portion of a urinoma. Percutaneous techniques of catheter drainage eliminate the need for open surgical revision in most cases. Insertion of a small (6–10F) catheter (with numerous side holes) is usually sufficient.
- If urinoma do not reduce its volume, a percutaneous nephrostomy catheter may be placed in addition to the other to decompress the collecting system in order to facilitate urinary drainage
- In cases of persistent leakage from the collecting system, placement of a nephrostomy catheter, usually with a ureteral stent or nephroureterostomy catheter, is warranted in order to promote primary healing of the collecting system.
- If hemodynamically unstable, surgical exploration and repair is warranted.
- When surgical exploration for renal trauma is indicated, it is recommended to use a transabdominal approach and early exploration of the renal hilum and vasculature before exploring the retroperitoneum

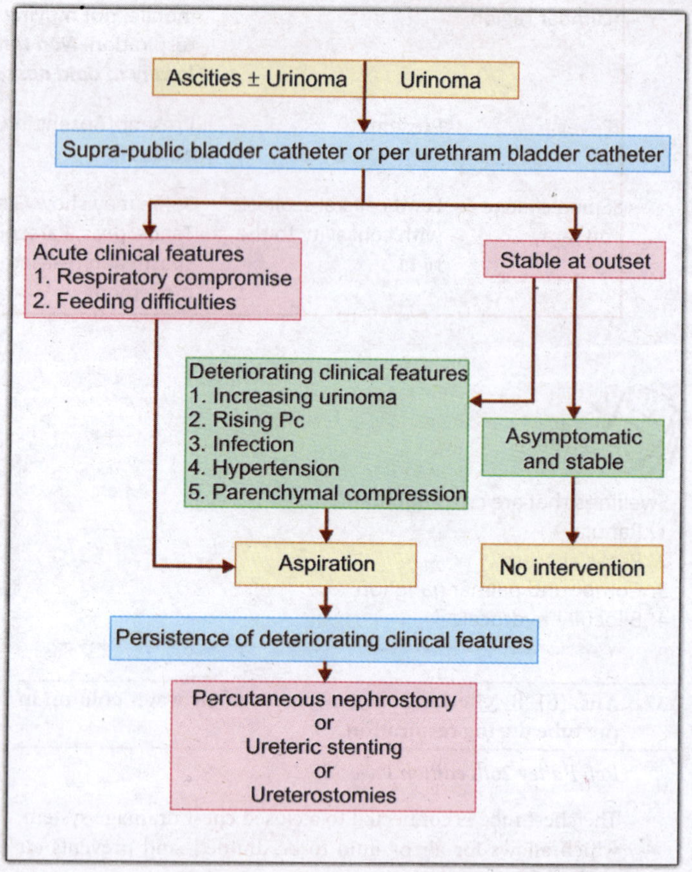

Indications of Surgical Intervention in Renal Trauma

Absolute indications	Relative indications
• Persistent, life-threatening hemorrhage from probable renal injury • Renal pedicle avulsion (grade V injury) • Expanding, pulsatile, or uncontained retroperitoneal hematoma	• Large laceration of the renal pelvis or avulsion of the ureteropelvic junction • Coexisting bowel or pancreatic injuries • Persistent urinary leakage, postinjury urinoma, or perinephric abscess with failed percutaneous or endoscopic management • Abnormal intraoperative one-shot IV urogram • Devitalized parenchymal segment with associated urine leak • Complete renal artery thrombosis of both kidneys or of a solitary kidney when renal perfusion appears preserved • Renal vascular injuries after failed angiographic management • Renovascular hypertension

39. Ans. (b) PCNL

Ref: Campbell 10th ed page 1364, Smith Urology 17th ed page 114, Bailey 26th ed page 1294

Latest treatment of large Staghorn calculus is "Sandwich technique"- Using both PCNL and ESWL, but it must be reviewed as primary PCNL only as per Campbell Urology

Campbell states: "The use of multiple endourologic techniques for the treatment of patients with staghorn stones is referred to as combination therapy or **"sandwich therapy."** The most frequently used multimodal regimen consisted of a primary percutaneous stone debulking by PCNL followed by ESWL of any inaccessible, residual infundibulo calyceal stone extensions or fragments. After ESWL a secondary percutaneous procedure (PCNL) is performed. These various stages are usually separated by 1 or 2 days. ***Stone-free rates for combined therapy are similar to those obtained by PNL alone or by open surgery.*** The management of patients with staghorn stones by a combined approach must be viewed as primarily percutaneous in nature, with ESWL being used only as an adjunct to minimize the number of access points required"

Treatment Modalities for Nephrolithiasis				
Treatment	**Indications**	**Advantages**	**Limitations**	**Complications**
Extracorporeal shock wave lithotripsy (ESWL)	Mainly used for renal and proximal ureteral stones <2 cm	Minimally invasive Outpatient procedure	Requires spontaneous passage of fragments, Less effective in patients with morbid obesity or hard stones	Ureteral obstruction by stone fragments, Perinephric hematoma
Ureteroscopy	Ureteral stones	Definitive Outpatient procedure	Invasive, May be difficult to clear fragments, Commonly requires postoperative ureteral stent, laser fiber is passed through the scope, and energy is delivered to fragment the calculus	Ureteral stricture or injury
Ureterorenoscopy	Renal stones <2 cm	Definitive Outpatient procedure	Same as above	Ureteral stricture or injury
Percutaneous nephrolithotomy (PCNL)	Mainly used for Renal stones >2 cm (including Staghorn calculus) Proximal ureteral stones >2 cm	Definitive	Invasive (various energy sources (laser, ultrasound) are used to fragment large renal calculi)	Bleeding Injury to collecting system, Injury to adjacent structures

Footnote:
- ***Ninety-five percent of stones 4 mm or smaller in size pass spontaneously***. Patients may be given up to 4 weeks to pass a partially obstructing stone without permanent renal damage.
- Smaller stones **(up to 6 mm)** may cause severe symptoms, such as flank pain and nausea, but typically pass without intervention beyond supportive care.
- Calculi **≥7 mm** are more likely to become impacted or to have a prolonged passage through the ureter. For this reason, intervention at the time of presentation is preferred for larger stones (except cases where the calculus is in the very distal ureter)
- Stone removal is indicated for stones with a **diameter between 6-7 mm** but can be delayed and shall be tailored as per needs.

40. Ans. (c) Papillary dermis

Ref: Bailey 26th ed page 390

Degree of Burn Injuries					
Degree		**Level of injury**	**Clinical features**	**Treatment**	**Outcome**
1st degree burns		Limited to the epidermis	Skin is **painful and red,** There are **no blisters**. Heal spontaneously in **3 to 4 days**	Epidermal (1st degree) burnsrequire only symptomatic treatment.	
2nd degree burns	Superficial partial thickness burns	**Limited to the dermal layers** of the skin, involve the **papillary dermis**	They appear **red**, warm, edematous, and **blistered**, often with denuded, moist, mottled red or pink epithelium.	Tetanus prophylaxis Cleaning (e.g., with chlorhexidine gluconate)	Epithelialization in 7–21 days
			Blanch to touch, very **painful**. Such burns frequently arise from brief contact with hot surfaces, liquids, flames, or chemicals.Heal in **7–14 days**	Topical agent (e.g., 1% silver sulfadiazine) Sterile gauze dressingc Physical therapy Splints as necessary	Hypertrophic scar rare Return of full function
	Deep partial thickness burns	**Limited to the dermal layers** of the skin,involve the **reticular dermis** and thus can damage some dermal appendages (e.g., nerves, sweat glands, or hair follicles).	Blisters present, **do not blanch to touch**, Less sensitive to pain, but remain **painful to pinprick,** hairs may be easily plucked out. Heals in **21–60 days (Some says 14 to 35 days)** , Hypertrophic scar common	As for superficial partial-thickness burns Early surgical excision and skin grafting an option	Epithelialization in 21–60 days in the absence of surgery Hypertrophic scar common Earlier return of function with surgical therapy

Contd...

Degree of Burn Injuries					
Degree		Level of injury	Clinical features	Treatment	Outcome
Full-thickness burns	3rd degree burns	Involve **all layers of the skin and some subcutaneous tissue**, all the skin appendages, including hair follicles and sweat and sebaceous glands, and sensory fibers for touch, pain, temperature, and pressure are destroyed	Blisters may be absent, Painless, insensate dry surface that may appear either white and leathery or charred and cracked, with exposure of underlying fat	As for superficial partial-thickness burns Wound excision and grafting at earliest feasible time	Functional limitation more frequent Hypertrophic scar mainly at graft margins
	4th degree burns	Also involve **fascia, muscle, and bone.** They often result from prolonged contact with thermal sources or high electrical current.	Same as above, Deep structures like muscles and bones are also visible.		

Only definitive method of differentiating superficial and deep partial-thickness burns is by length of time to heal
* Some textbooks have not mentioned Fourth degree burns separately

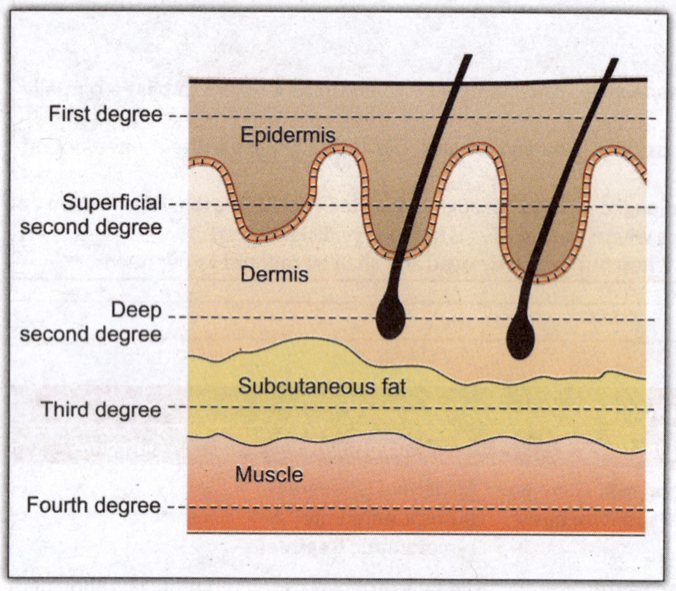

41. Ans. (b) Tip of Nose to ear to Xiphoid process

Ref: Emergency Medicine Procedures 2nd ed by Eric F. Reichman ch 58

Nasogastric (NG) intubation is one of the commonly performed procedures in the Emergency Department. Its use as a conduit into the stomach. The method most frequently used to measure correct length of the NG tube prior to insertion is the distance from nose to ear to xiphisternum (NEX). Estimate the length of the tube needed to reach the stomach by measuring the tube either from the tip of the nose to the earlobe and down to the xiphoid process or from the tip of the nose to the umbilicus.

Controversy exists regarding measurement of the length of the NG tube to be inserted. Two most common methods of measurement are:

- From the nose tip to the earlobe and then to the end of the xiphoid process (NEX)
- From the nose tip to the earlobe and then to a point midway between Xiphoid process and umbilicus.

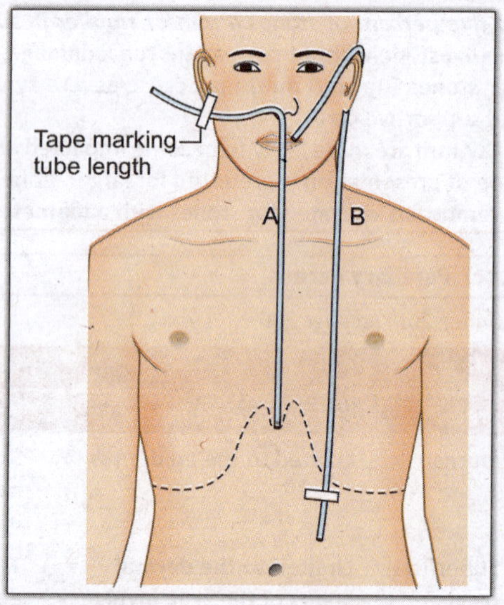

Fig: Two methods of NG tube insertion

NG Tube in children: The placement of a NG tube in children is often difficult. Their large tonsils and adenoids may hinder the passage. These tissues are soft, easily injured, and may bleed as the NG tube is passed. The tongue, large by comparison with adults, may push into the oropharynx and impede passage of the NG tube. Their nostrils and nasal passage are quite small and limit the size of NG tube that may be passed.

AIIMS MAY 2017

42. Ans. (d) Relaxed tension lines in skin

Ref: Grabb and Smith's Plastic Surgery 7th page 1 – 3

This question refers to the cutaneous lines meant for incision in plastic surgery so as to avoid scarring. The three best line systems known are:

Line Systems in Plastic Surgery	
Line	**Description**
Langer's line	**Langer's lines**, sometimes called **cleavage lines**, are topological lines drawn on a map of the human body. They were described by Karl Langer who studied these lines by producing wounds with a spike on fresh cadaver. He investigated directional variations in the mechanical and physical properties of skin and produced a series of diagrams depicting lines of cleavage in the skin and showed that the orientation of these lines correspond to the natural orientation of collagen fibers in the dermis, and are generally parallel to the orientation of the underlying muscle fibers. Wounds against langer Lines generally have poor cosmetic outcome. These lines represent skin tension in rigor mortis but frequently do not relate to the lines of choice in making elective incisions. Indeed Langer's lines often run at right angles to the RSTLs in the face.
Kraissl's lines	Kraissl's lines are essentially exaggerated wrinkle lines obtained by studying the loose skin of elderly faces whilst contracting the muscles of facial expression. These lines for the most part correspond to RSTLs, but slight variation exists on the face, especially on the lateral side of the nose, the lateral aspect of the orbit, and the chin. ***Kraissl's lines coincides with wrinkle lines***, although not always, and tend to be perpendicular to the muscle action.
Borge's Relaxed skin tension lines	Tension is present in all directions in the skin but mainly in one direction, which follows the relaxed skin tension lines (RSTLs) first described by Borges. Relaxed skin tension lines (RSTLs) are those which correspond to the directional pull (which forms furrows) when the skin is relaxed: they do not always correspond to wrinkle lines. The tension across the RSTL is constant even during sleep but can be altered (increased, decreased or abolished) by underlying muscle contraction. The direction of the RSTLs can be determined by pinching the skin in different directions. Pinching at right angles to the RSTLs will result in fewer and higher furrows than pinching parallel to these lines

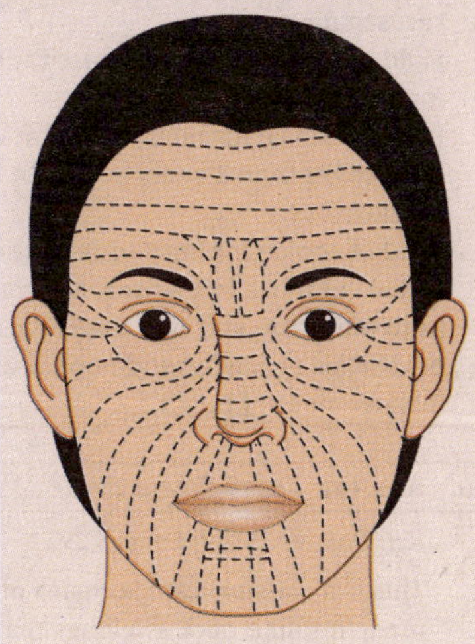

43. Ans. (a) Peutz-Jeghers syndrome

Ref: Sabiston 20th Ed Pg 1541-1543, Robbins 9th ed page 593

Name	Defect	Risk of pancreatic cancer
Peutz-Jeghers syndrome	STK11 gene mutation	100 fold increased risk
Hereditary pancreatitis	Mutation in cationic trypsinogen PRSS1 gene	50 fold increased risk
Cystic fibrosis	CFTR gene mutation	30 fold increased risk
FAMMM syndrome	CDKN2A gene mutation	20 fold increased risk
Hereditary breast and ovarian cancer	BRCA 2 gene mutation	10 fold increased risk
Lynch syndrome	MLH1 gene mutation	8 fold increased risk
FAP	APC gene mutation	4 fold increased risk
Familial pancreatic cancer	Unknown gene	18 fold increased risk

44. Ans. (c) 9

Ref: Bailey 26th ed page 312, Schwartz 10th ed page 168–170

See table of Glasgow Coma Scale Score in Surgery AIIMS Nov 2018

E = Eye opening = Eye opens to pain = 2
V = Verbal = Moans = Unintelligible sounds = 2
M = Motor = Localizes towards pain on left is M5 and withdrawal on right is M4 (best score is taken so M5) = 5
So total GCS score = 2 + 2 + 5 = 9 (Moderate head injury)

45. Ans. (c) 4 mL/kg × %TSBA

Ref: Bailey 26th ed page 390 – 392, Sabiston 20th ed page 513 – 514, http://dghs.gov.in/WriteReadData/userfiles/file/Practical_handbook-revised_Karoon.pdf

Option (A) is designed to confuse you. One that 4 mL/kg × BSA% is divided into 2 halves, one half for first 4 hours and another half for next 16 hours from the time of burn. Secondly 8 hours have already passed so that calculation will exceed 24 hours and should not be applied. Hence simply 4 mL/kg × TBSA% should be the answer.

The most commonly used fluid resuscitation formula for burns is Parkland formula.

Resuscitation Formulas			
Formula	**Crystalloid volume**	**Colloid volume**	**Free water**
Parkland Brooke	4 mL/kg per % TBSA burn (1/2 in first 8 hours and another 1/2 in next 16 hours)	None	None

Contd...

Resuscitation Formulas			
Formula	**Crystalloid volume**	**Colloid volume**	**Free water**
Brooke	1.5 mL/kg per % TBSA burn	0.5 mL/kg per % TBSA burn	2.0 L
Galveston (pediatric)	5000 mL/m² burned area + 1500 mL/m² total area	None	None

Footnote:
- In children with burns over 10% TBSA and adults with burns over 15% TBSA, consider the need for intravenous fluid resuscitation.
- Fluid of choice for burn resuscitation in first 24 hours is Ringer lactate
- Fluid of choice for burn resuscitation in children below 20 kg or younger than 2 years in first 24 hours is Ringer lactate with 5% dextrose
- Fluid of choice for burn resuscitation after 24 hours is colloids
- If oral fluids are to be used, salt must be added.
- Both mafenide and silver sulfadiazine have antibacterial properties against pseudomonas and are used in management of burns.

46. Ans. (a) Thyroglossal cyst

Ref: Bailey's 25th Ed page 729

This is a classical case scenario of Thyroglossal cyst. There are many midline neck swellings that moves with deglutition but only one out of them also moves with protrusion of tongue.

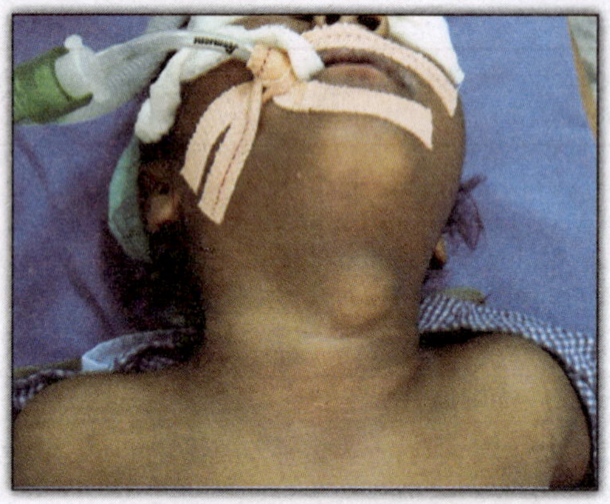

© MedEasy, Dr Prashant Bharadwaj

Fig: Thyroglossal cyst

Thyroglossus Cyst	
Embryology	• The thyroid gland descends early in fetal life from the base of the tongue towards its position in the lower neck with the isthmus lying over the second and third tracheal rings. • At the time of its descent, the hyoid bone has not been formed and the track of the descent of the thyroid gland is variable, passing in front, through or behind the eventual position of the hyoid body.

Contd...

Thyroglossus Cyst	
	• Thyroglossal duct cysts represent a persistence of this track and may therefore be found anywhere in or adjacent to the midline from the tongue base to the thyroid isthmus. Rarely, a thyroglossal cyst may contain the only functioning thyroid tissue in the body.

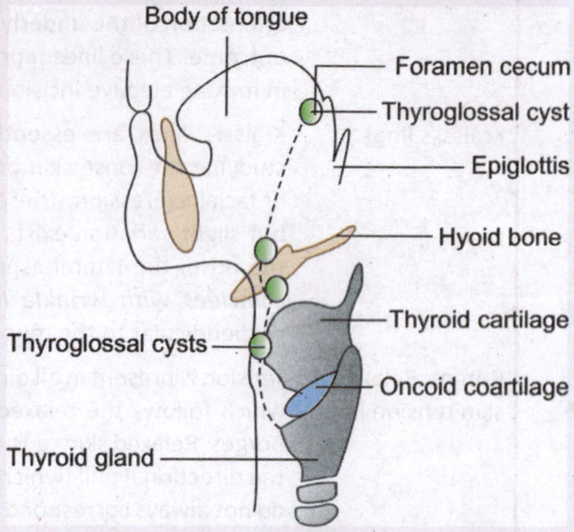

Clinical features	• The cysts almost always arise in the midline but, when they are adjacent to the thyroid cartilage, they may lie slightly to one side of the midline. • Classically, the cyst moves upwards on swallowing and with tongue protrusion, but this can also occur with other midline cysts such as dermoid cysts, as it merely indicates attachment to the hyoid bone. • Thyroglossal cysts may become infected and rupture onto the skin of the neck presenting as a discharging sinus. Although they often occur in children, they may also present in adults, even as late as the sixth or seventh decade of life.
Treatment	Treatment must include excision of the whole thyroglossal tract, which involves removal of the body of the hyoid bone and the suprahyoid tract through the tongue base to the vallecula at the site of the primitive foramen caecum, together with a core of tissue on either side. This operation is known as ***Sistrunk's operation*** and prevents recurrence, most notably from small side branches of the thyroglossal tract.

47. Ans. (c) McBurney point tenderness

Ref: Bailey 26th ed page 1202 – 1203, Schwartz 10th ed page 1243-48, Sabiston 20th ed page 1297 - 1302

Options A, B, and C are related to acute appendicitis

Option (D) Ballance's sign is fixed dullness on the left flank with shifting dullness in the right flank. This is seen in rupture of spleen.

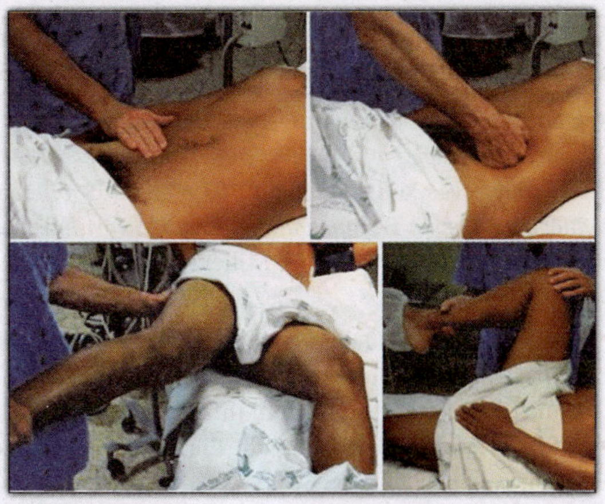

Fig: Signs of Appendicitis: The sequence of abdominal discomfort and anorexia associated with acute appendicitis is pathognomonic. The pain is described as being located in the periumbilical region initially and then migrating to the right lower quadrant. Rectal and pelvic examinations are most likely to be negative. However, if the appendix is located within the pelvis, tenderness on abdominal examination may be minimal, whereas anterior tenderness may be elicited during rectal examination

a. **Blumberg sign:** The exact location of the tenderness is directly over the appendix, which is most commonly at McBurney's point (located one third of the distance along a line drawn from the anterior superior iliac spine to the umbilicus).
b. **Rovsing's sign:** Pain in the right lower quadrant during palpation of the left lower quadrant
c. **Psoas sign:** Pain on extension of the right hip (typical of a retrocecal appendix)
d. **Obturator sign:** Pain on internal rotation of the hip (suggesting a pelvic appendix)
e. **Dunphy's sign:** Any movement, including coughing, may cause increased pain. (Not shown in picture)

48. Ans. (b) Mastectomy with local radiotherapy

Ref: NCCN Guidelines version 2.2017, Schwartz 9th ed ch 17

Metastatic axillary lymph node is a Early Invasive Breast Cancer (Stage I, IIA, or IIB) breast cancer and shall not be treated with BCS (Breast conservative surgery. Quadrantectomy being one of the BCS is hence ruled out. Mastectomy with radiotherapy is the management of choice in such a case.

Schwartz 9th ed states **"NSABP B-06 compared total mastectomy to lumpectomy with or without radiation therapy in the treatment of women with stage I and II breast cancer. After 5- and 8-year follow-up periods, the disease-free, distant disease-free, and overall survival rates for lumpectomy with or without radiation therapy were similar to those observed after total mastectomy. However, the incidence of ipsilateral breast cancer recurrence (in-breast recurrence) was higher in the lumpectomy group not receiving radiation therapy"**.

49. Ans. (d) No additional treatment

Ref: Sabiston 20th ed page 851-855, Schwartz 10th ed page 536-538, NCCN guidelines for breast cancer version 2.2017

For pure DCIS, margins of at least 2 mm are associated with a reduced risk of ipsilateral breast tumor recurrence (IBTR) relative to narrower negative margin widths in patients receiving WBRT. The routine practice of obtaining negative margin widths wider than 2 mm is not supported by the evidence. DCIS with microinvasion (defined as no invasive focus >1 mm in size) should be considered as DCIS when considering the optimal margin width. The optimal margin width for treatment with excision alone is unknown, but should be at least 2 mm. Some evidence suggests lower rates of IBTR with margin widths wider than 2 mm.

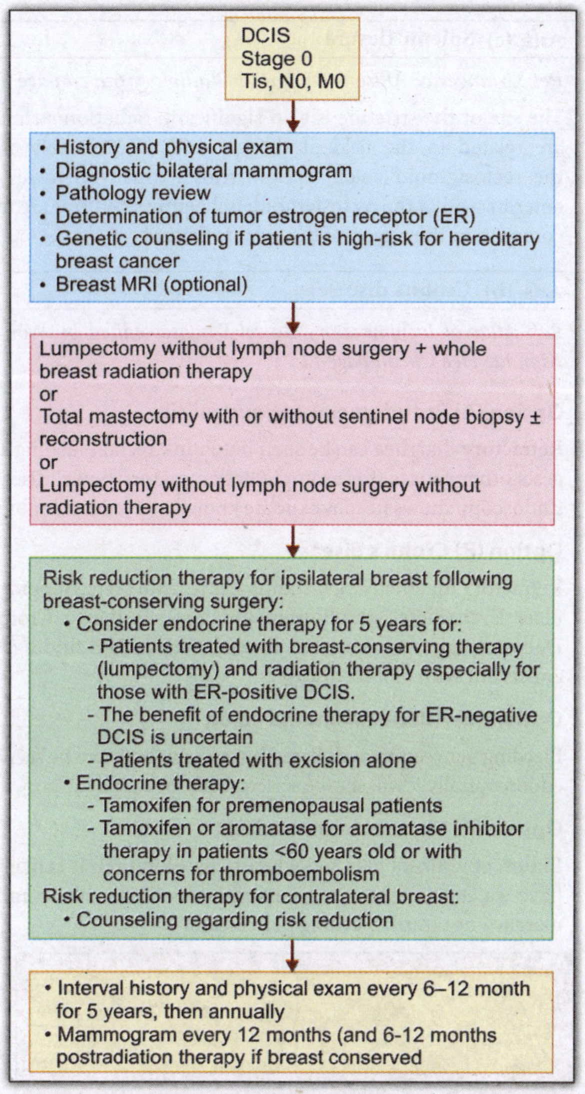

50. Ans. (b) Routine physical examination once in 3 months for a year and annual mammogram

Ref: MD Anderson Handbook of Surgical Oncology 5th ed page 71 - 72, NCCN guidelines for breast cancer, 2016, Bailey and Love, 26th ed page 816

Follow-up of invasive Breast Cancer Patient Includes:

- History and physical exam 1–4 times per year as clinically appropriate for 5 years, then annually
- Periodic screening for changes in family history and referral to genetic counseling as indicated
- Educate, monitor, and refer for lymphedema management
- Mammography every 12 months
- Routine imaging of reconstructed breast is not indicated

- In the absence of clinical signs and symptoms suggestive of recurrent disease, there is no indication for laboratory or imaging studies for metastases screening
- Women on tamoxifen: annual gynecologic assessment every 12 months if uterus present
- Women on an aromatase inhibitor or who experience ovarian failure secondary to treatment should have monitoring of bone health with a bone mineral density determination at baseline and periodically there after

51. Ans. (c) Splenic flexure

Ref: Grainger & Allison's Diagnostic Radiology 6th ed page 699

The site of the stricture is also significant: radiation strictures are related to the field of therapy and so invariably affect the rectosigmoid colon; endometriosis usually involves the anterior wall of the rectosigmoid; ischaemic strictures are most common in the region of the splenic flexure.

52. Ans. (b) Crohn's disease

Ref: Atlas of Inflammatory Bowel Diseases edited by Won Ho Kim, Jae Hee Cheon page 11

Option (A) Pseudomembranous colitis

Refractory diarrhea can be seen but Frank rectal bleeding suggests other causes (for example, inflammatory bowel disease). Endoscopy shows fibrous exudate known as Pseudomembrane.

Option (B) Crohn's disease

Refractory diarrhea and bleeding per rectum seen. Geographic ulcer is characteristically seen (but not specific to Crohn's). Deep serpiginous ulcer seen on endoscopy. HPE findings are consistent with Cohn's disease.

Option (C) Adenocarcinoma colon

Bleeding per rectum and altered bowel habit both can be seen but endoscopically it will show a scricture like or exophytic growth.

Option (D) Visceral leishmaniasis

Endoscopy shows pale and whitish discoloration. It is likely to have watery diarrhea (possibly with blood), i.e. blood mixed diarrhea not frank bleeding per rectum.

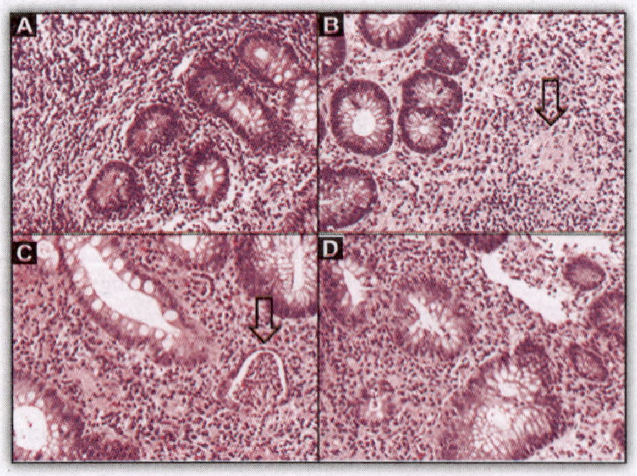

Fig: Crohn's disease HPE: Histopathology of lower GI biopsies demonstrating Crohn's disease. (A) Terminal ileum showing mild active ileitis, with lymphocytic and neutrophilic infiltration into glands (B) Chronic active colitis with **granuloma formation** (arrow) in the ascending colon. (C, D) Descending colon with chronic active colitis with **crypt abscess** (arrow) formation (C) and cryptitis (D).

53. Ans. (d) The patient should not be shifted and portable X-ray machine should be used after neck stabilisation.

Ref: Sabiston Textbook of Surgery, 20th edition; pg. 420 – 421, Schwartz Principles of Surgery, 10th edition; pg. 197 – 198, Bailey and Love, 26th edition; pg. 303 & 327 – 330; Emergency Management of the Trauma Patient: Cases, Algorithms, Evidence edited by Mark Bisanzo, Pg 5; Miller's Anaesthesia 8th Ed Pg 2183, 2184

- According to ATLS guidelines, standard practice dictates that all victims of blunt trauma be assumed to have an unstable cervical spine until this condition is ruled out.
- Stabilization is achieved with the help of a rigid collar, a soft collar is of no use.
- **Miller's 8th Ed Pg 2183-2184 states that:**

"The once standard 'three views' (with their inherent difficulties and substantial false-negative rates) have been supplanted by CT scanners that allow rapid, thin-slice evaluation, with sagittal reconstruction. A large meta-analysis concluded that 'modern multislice helical CT alone is sufficient to rule out traumatic, unstable cervical spine injuries.' However, some remain concerned that CT may fail to identify ligamentous injuries that would be evident on magnetic resonance imaging (MRI). With respect to a conscious patient who has not yet undergone complete radiologic evaluation, several clinical surveys have confirmed that patients who are alert, non-intoxicated, and free of significant distracting injuries invariably have pain, midline tenderness, limitation of voluntary movement, or neurologic signs if they have a cervical spine fracture."

- In most centers, a **standard trauma series** is performed on each patient. This series of **plain X-rays consists of a lateral c-spine, a supine anteroposterior (AP) chest X-ray, and an AP pelvis**. This is especially true in the age of the readily available CT scan for stable patients. The trauma series remains important in patients who are too unstable to go to CT scan.
- The NEXUS score is one of the scores designed to take decision regarding imaging of patients with suspected C-spine injury.

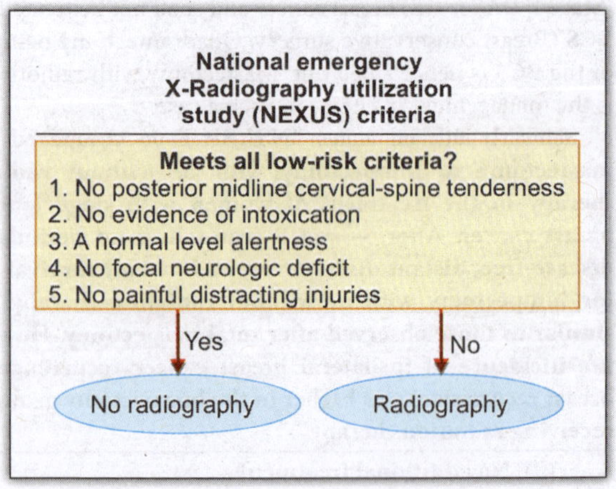

- We can thus conclude that our patient requires imaging for sure.
- The lateral c-spine has a variable sensitivity, given an adequate film (i.e., visualization of the C7-T1 junction),

the sensitivity is better. This study is probably unnecessary in most cases where the patient is alert and with a normal neurologic exam. In stable cases, the patient can go to CT scan for c-spine imaging if necessary. **The exceptions are those patients with severe neck pain or deformity; and also haemodynamically unstable patients.** Similarly, **patients with altered mental status or those with neurologic deficits should have a lateral c-spine X-ray immediately in the trauma bay. A lateral cervical spine X-ray that demonstrates an injury is an important finding, whereas a negative or inadequate film does not exclude cervical spine injury.**

- X-rays should be used judiciously and should not delay patient resuscitation.
- The **AP chest film** (since the patient is supine) and AP pelvis may provide information that can guide resuscitation of the patient with blunt trauma.
- Chest X-rays may detect potentially life-threatening injuries that require treatment and pelvic films may demonstrate fractures of the pelvis that indicate the need for early blood transfusion.
- These films can be taken in the resuscitation area, usually with a portable X-ray unit, but should not interrupt the resuscitation process.
- Thus, although CT scan is a better modality as compared to X-rays if the patient is stable, our patient has a high suspicion of cervical spine injury and thus, must not be transported repeatedly. In such a case, X-ray offers a portable option advantage.

54. Ans. (d) Chest X-ray is always done in PA view

Ref: Sabiston Textbook of Surgery, 20th edition; pg. 413 – 417, Schwartz Principles of Surgery, 10th edition; pg. 161 and 173, ATLS guidelines, 9th edition; pg. 6-9 and 13.

Let us go Through the Options

Option (A) Cervical X-ray is part of primary survey and Option (B) Chest X-ray and pelvic X-ray are taken as an adjunct to primary survey
True.
All three form a part of primary survey.
See Figure in AIIMS General Surgery AIIMS Nov 2014 for details of primary and secondary survey.
Option (C) CT scan is not done in hemodynamically unstable patient
True.
See previous question.
Option (D) Chest X-ray is always done in PA view
False.
Patient with trauma are in supine position. Hence, PA view of chest X-ray will not be feasible. An AP view is thus accepted.

55. Ans. (b) Chest tube thoracocentesis

Ref: Schwartz 10th ed page 163 – 164, Bailey 26th ed page 353 – 355, ATLS guidelines 2016, Rosen's Emergency Medicine - Concepts and Clinical Practice By John Marx, Ron Walls, Robert Hockberger 8th ed page 218

See table of CHEST TRAUMA in Surgery AIIMS NOV 2016 (see page no. 969)

Tension pneumothorax and open pneumothorax can be differentiated based on one striking difference. Hypotension is seen in tension pneumothorax. Hence, this is a case of open pneumothorax not tension pneumothorax. Tension pneumothorax is managed by emergency needle decompression while open pneumothorax is managed by tube thoracostomy. Hence the answer here is tube thoracostomy (Chest tube drain).

56. Ans. (d) 50–60%

Ref: Schwartz Principles of Surgery 10th ed page 527 & 531

PET can detect axillary lymph node involvement with higher sensitivity in patients with higher nodal stages: 41% in pN1, 67% in pN2, and 100% in pN3. USG is 41.2% sensitivity and 93% specificity for detecting metastatic axilla (Ref: Breast Imaging: The Requisites By Debra Ikeda, Kanae Kawai Miyake 3rd ed Page 446)

57. Ans. (a) Pectoralis major myocutaneous flap

Ref: Schwartz principles of surgery 10th edition; pg.1872 – 1875, Sabiston Textbook of surgery 20th edition; pg. 1953 -1954

The picture shown is of PMMC (Pectoralis major myocutaneous flap)

Uses of PMMC Flap Reconstruction

- Buccal mucosa—alveolus reconstruction
- Tongue for hemiglossectomy, total and extended glossectomy as a single flap or in combination with other flaps
- **Oropharynx reconstruction:** Muscle only for small defects and composite flap for complex defects
- **Larynx–pharynx reconstruction:** As patch or tube reconstruction after laryngectomy and pharyngectomy. For salvage laryngectomy
- **Neck–parotid reconstruction:** For large skin cover after composite resection involving the skin
- **Salvage surgery:** Reconstruction of choice for majority of salvage surgery
- In resource constrained setup it is reconstruction of choice for majority of defects.

Limitations of PMMC Flap

- Reach not enough for maxilla and skull base defects
- Difficult to cover defects above the zygoma
- Flaps drags down in some cases due to its weight

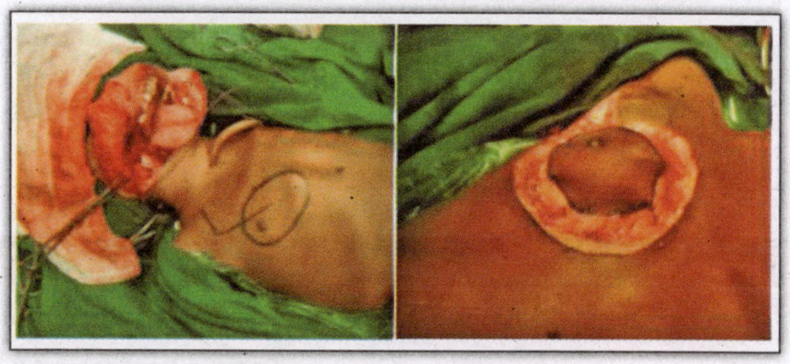

© Qureshi SS, Ahmed QG, Yadav PS (TMH MUMBAI)

Fig: Pectoralis Major Myocutaneous Flap (PMMC): Intraoperative photograph showing the skin paddle of PMMC and its suturing to the surgical defect

58. Ans. (b) Paraffin gauze and dressing

Ref: Bailey 26th edition; page 392 – 394, Kirk General Surgical Operations 6th ed page 548, http://www.rch.org.au/clinicalguide/guideline_index/Burns/

Burn wound dressings serve three purposes:

- They absorb drainage
- They provide protection and a measure of isolation from the environment
- They decrease wound pain

Option (A)

Collagenase is the most commonly employed enzymatic debriding agent currently commercially available in the United States. It is slow acting, requiring several days to one week to adequately debride or heal intermediate-depth partial thickness wounds.

Option (B)

Sterile liquid paraffin reduces crusting. Superficial burns and covered by paraffin dressing gauze followed by bulky absorptive dressing to leave it unchanged for 1 week or it get soaked. Subsequently twice per week until the wound is healed. (Kirks)

Option (C)

Excision and skin grafting is the last resort of the burns management often for large area burns and in late stages in cases of contractures. Tangential shaving (excision) of the dead tissue is done until we observe punctate bleeding in deep burns before grafting not superficial burns.

Option (D)

Silver sulfadiazine (1%) is the most commonly used burn wound dressing applied once or twice daily and can be soothing. SSD and related agents should not be used in women who are pregnant or breastfeeding or in infants younger than two months old.

Management of Burns

Superficial burns	Deep dermal burn	Full thickness burn
• Clean the burn wound and remove the roof of all blisters. • Expose superficial bums of the face but apply sterile liquid paraffin to reduce crusting. • For burns of perineum, clean these and expose but apply silver sulfadiazine cream. Nurse the patient without dressings on a sterile sheet on air or water bed. • Cover superficial buns of other areas with two layers of paraffin gauze and a bulky absorptive dressing. Leave this dressing for 1 week unless it becomes soaked, whereupon you should change it. Change the dressing at 1 week and subsequently twice per week until the wound is healed.	• Tangentially shave with a graft knife between 2nd and 5th day. • Continue to shave until you observe punctate bleeding from the surface. • Achieve haemostasis with immure and apply a split skin graft. • Re-dress at 4 days. • When fully healed, apply a pressure garment for 6 months or longer if necessary, to minimize hypertrophy & contracture of the resulting scars. • Treat areas that are not healed at 3 weeks as full-thickness burns.	**Escharotomy:** • Note the areas of full thickness burns that are circumferential around digit, limb or trunk. If the viability of the distal pan is jeopardized, or if respiration is hindered, as with partial circumferential burns of the chest wall, carry out an escharotomy. • Give IV dose of diazepam. • Incise along the full length of full thickness burn. • Repeat the longitudinal escharotomy at different sites of the circumference until satisfactory perfusion of the distal part. • Dress the wounds with paraffin gauze or silver sulfadiazine **Grafting:** • Identify site of grafting not >20% BSA • Identify donor site of skin graft. • Excise the chosen area of full-thickness burn till bed consists of viable tissue. • Harvest a split skin graft and mesh it to expand. • Apply the mesh graft to the burn wound site and dress with several layers of paraffin gauze and an absorbent dressing. • Re-dress after 4 days. • Do not excise further burn until the donor site has healed and is ready for reharvesting, or another donor site is available.

Burns Classification According to Causes

Thermal	Flame	Damage from superheated, oxidized air
	Scald	Damage from contact with hot liquids
	Contact	Damage from contact with hot or cold solid materials
Chemical		Contact with noxious chemicals
Electric		Conduction of electrical current through tissues

Burns Depth Assessment			
Depth	**Cause**	**Surface/color**	**Pain sensation**
Superficial	Sun, flash, minor scald	Dry, minor blisters, erythema, brisk capillary return	Painful
Superficial partial thickness - (superficial dermal)	Scald	Moist, reddened with broken blisters, brisk capillary return	Painful
Deep partial thickness - (deep dermal)	Scald, minor flame contact	Moist white slough, red mottled, sluggish capillary return	Painless
Full thickness	Flame, severe scald or flame contact	Dry, charred whitish. Absent capillary return	Painless

59. Ans. (a) I-131 radioablation

Ref: Sabiston 20th ed page 903-908, Schwartz 10th ed page 1543 – 1548, Bailey 26th ed page 766 – 768; 25th Ed pg 788

The key to the answer lies in the fact that the patient is pregnant.

According to Bailey 25th Ed Pg 788

"Radio iodine is absolutely contraindicated during pregnancy because of the risk to the fetus."

Ideally, the patient being pregnant, should not be undergoing surgical procedures. However, as the surgery is a cancer surgery, it will be classified as "time-sensitive" and essential surgery and cannot be postponed till the end of pregnancy. The risks associated with anaesthesia are risk of transplacental transfer of anaesthetic drugs, risk of termination of pregnancy, preterm labor and so on. Following is the algorithm to be followed under such circumstances:

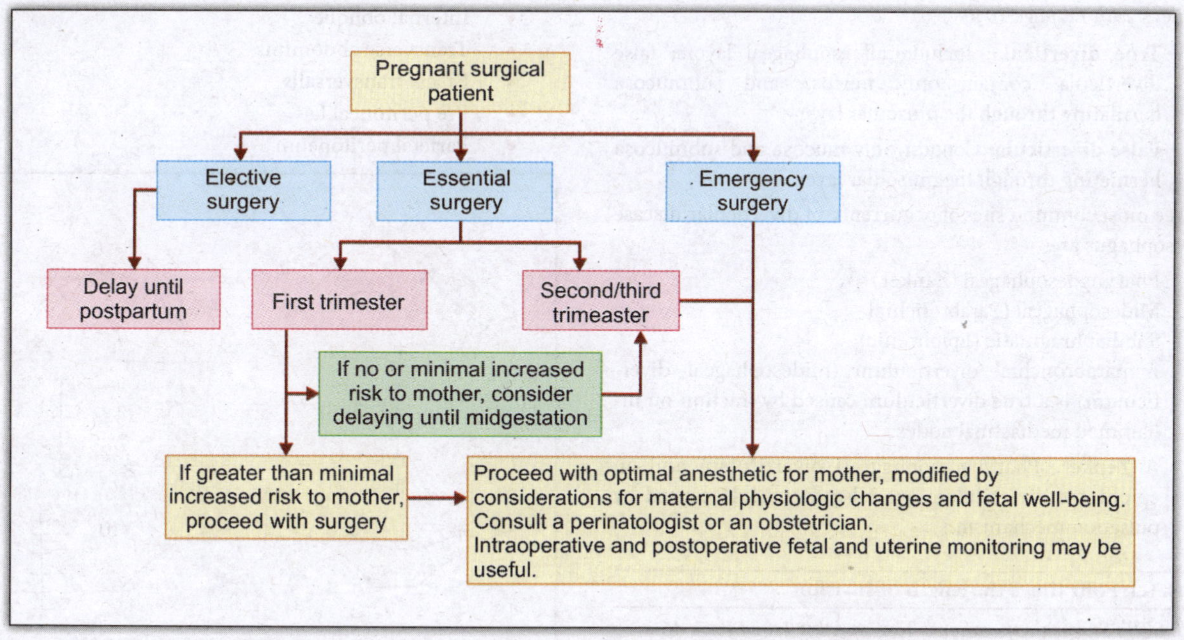

Hence, it is relatively safe to consider this patient for surgery since she is already in her 2nd trimester.

60. Ans. (a) Antibiotics, (b) Pigtail catheter

Ref: Sabiston Textbook of Surgery, 20th ed; pg. 1501 – 1504

Laparoscopic cholecystectomy is the preferred and most widely used method of removal of the gallbladder in patients with symptomatic cholelithiasis. Bile leaks after laparoscopic cholecystectomy represent a spectrum of extrahepatic biliary duct injuries, and range in severity from minor cystic duct (CD) leaks to complete transection of the common bile duct (CBD). Once a bile duct leak or injury is identified, the principles of management are well defined and include effective drainage of intra-abdominal collections and detailed cholangiographic evaluation of the biliary system. ***If no drain is in situ USG guided Pigtail catheter drainage is idealy be done first.***

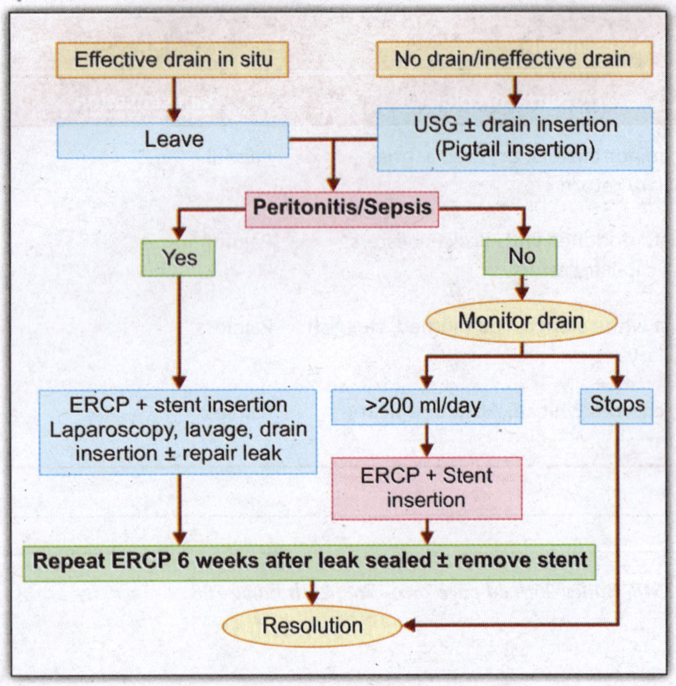

AIIMS NOVEMBER 2016

61. Ans. (c) Parabronchial diverticulum

Ref: Cummings 5th ed page 974, Sabiston 20th ed page 1019, Bailey's 25th Ed page 1040

- **True diverticula:** Include all esophageal layers; false diverticula: contain only mucosa and submucosa herniating through the muscular layer
- **False diverticula:** Contain only mucosa and submucosa herniating through the muscular layer.

Three most common sites of occurrence of diverticular disease of esophagus are:

1. Pharyngoesophageal (Zanker)
2. Midesophageal (Parabronchial
3. Subdiaphragmatic (Epiphrenic)

- A parabronchial diverticulum (midesophageal diverticulum) is a true diverticulum caused by traction on inflammed mediastinal nodes.
- A Zenker (Pharyngoesophageal) diverticulum and an epiphrenic diverticulum are false diverticula caused by pulsation mechanism.

62. Ans. (c) Four times the length of Incision

Ref: SRB's Surgical Operations: Text & Atlas 1st ed Page 46

Jenken's Rule

It has been estimated that for abdominal wall closure the length of the suture material should be at least 4 times the length of the wound. The closure technique involves taking 1 cm bites, 1 cm apart

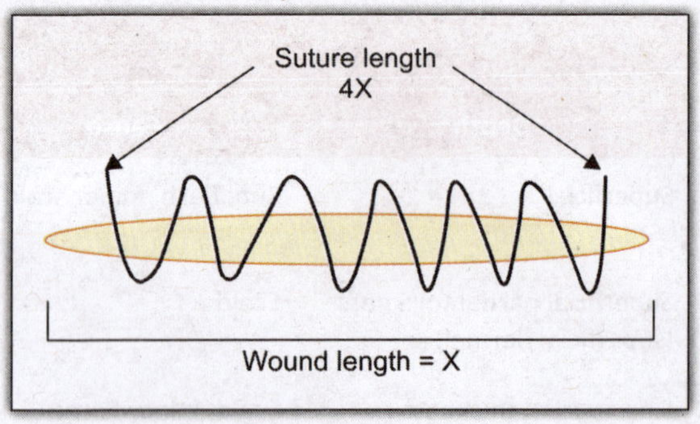

63. Ans. (a) Lanz incision

Ref: Farquharson 10th Ed page 214, Kirk's General Surgical Operations By Richard Novell, Daryll Baker, Nicholas Goddard 6th ed page 94

The **Gridiron** (Right angled to Spino-umbilical line at Mc Burney's point) and **Lanz incisions** (Transverse incision at McBurney's point) are muscle-splitting incisions which are the incisions of choice for open appendicectomy. The Lanz incision is more generous and involves more muscle cutting.

Layers encountered in muscle splitting incision of open appendectomy are: (FAQ)

- Skin
- Subcutaneous fat
- Scarpa's fascia
- External oblique aponeurosis
- Internal oblique
- Transverse abdominis
- Fascia transversalis
- Pre peritoneal fat
- Parietal peritoneum

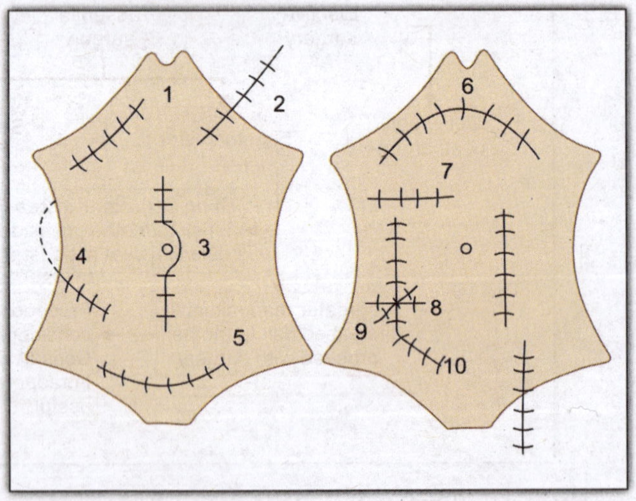

Fig: Commonly used abdominal incision: 1 = Kocher; 2 = Thoracoabdominal; 3 = Midline; 4 = Lion (Muscle splitting); 5 = Pfannenstiel; 6 = Gable; 7 = Transverse Muscle splitting; 8 = Lanz (Muscle splitting); 9 = Gridiron (Muscle splitting); 10 = Rutherford Morrison (Muscle cutting); 11 = Paramedian; 12 = McEvedy

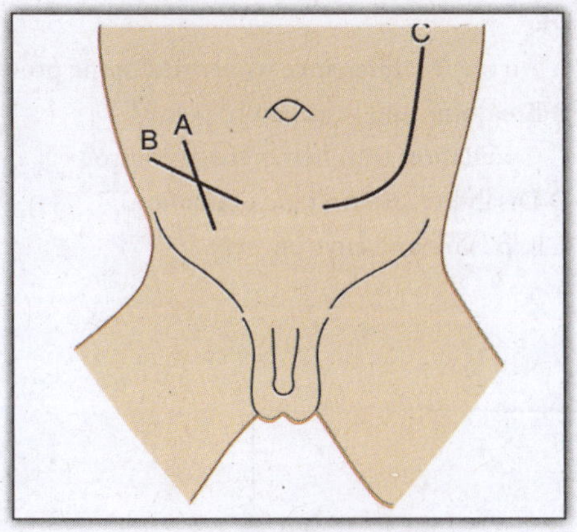

Fig: Incision of open appendectomy; A = Gridiron; B = Lanz; C = Rutherford Morrison (Shown on left side for clarity)

64. Ans. (b) Gluteal claudication

Ref: Rutherford Vascular Surgery 6th ed ch 1

Patients with arterial occlusive disease of more proximal (aortoiliac) distribution usually suffer from buttock and thigh claudication, although a significant number also complain of calf claudication. Buttock and thigh claudication does not usually produce the severe cramping muscular pain experienced in the calf. The sensation is more of an "aching" discomfort associated with weakness. These patients may even deny the existence of pain per se, complaining only that the hip or thigh "gives out" or "tires" after they have walked a certain distance. Patients with osteoarthritis of the hip or knee may complain of similar extremity discomfort that is also brought on by exercise; however, important differentiating factors for osteoarthritis are as follows:

- The amount of exercise causing their symptoms is variable.
- The pain does not disappear as promptly with rest.
- The pain varies in severity from day to day, frequently in association with changes in weather conditions or physical activity.

65. Ans. (d) Southampton

Ref: Bailey & Love's Short Practice of Surgery 26th ed Page 54, SRB's Manual of Surgery 5th ed Page 36

There are scoring systems for the severity of wound infection, which are particularly useful in surveillance and research. Examples are the Southampton and ASEPSIS systems

Southampton Wound Grading System

Grade		Appearance
0		Normal healing
I		Normal healing with mild bruising or erythema
	IA	Some bruising
	IB	Considerable bruising
	IC	Mild erythema
II		Erythema plus other signs of inflammation

Contd...

Southampton Wound Grading System

Grade		Appearance
	IIA	At one point
	IIB	Around sutures
	IIC	Along wound
	IID	Around wound
III		Clear or haemoserous discharge
	IIIA	At one point only (<2 cm)
	IIIB	Along wound (>2 cm)
	IIIC	Large volume
	IIID	Prolonged (>3 days)
Major Complications		
IV		Pus
	IVA	At one point only (<2 cm)
	IVB	Along wound (>2 cm)
V		Deep or severe wound infection with or without tissue breakdown; haematoma requiring aspiration

The asepsis wound Score

Criterion	Points
Additional treatment	**0**
• Antibiotics for wound infection	**10**
• Drainage of pus under local anaesthesia	**5**
• Debridement of wound under general anaesthesia	**10**
Serous discharge	Daily 0–5
Erythema	Daily 0–5
Purulent exudate	Daily 0–10
Separation of deep tissues	Daily 0–10
Isolation of bacteria from wound	10
Stay as inpatient prolonged over 14 days as result of wound infection	5

66. Ans. (a) Put the patient in recumbent position and maintain airway

Ref: Miller's Anaesthesia 8th Ed Pg 2425; Schwartz principles of surgery 8th ed, ch 6, AHA 2015 Guidelines Update for Cardiopulmonary Resuscitation and Emergency Cardiovascular Care

In case of hemodynamically stable patient, airway is to be maintained first

Initial assessment of a trauma patient includes the following elements:

- Preparation
- Triage
- Primary survey (ABCDEs)
- Resuscitation
- Adjuncts to primary survey and resuscitation
- Consideration of the need for patient transfer
- Secondary survey (head-to-toe evaluation and patient history)

- Adjuncts to the secondary survey
- Continued post resuscitation monitoring and reevaluation
- Definitive care

ATLS emphasizes the **ABCDE mnemonic**—Airway, Breathing, Circulation, Disability, and Exposure.

Primary Survey

- Life-threatening injuries are identified
- Simultaneously **resuscitation** is begun

ABCDE

- **A** Airway Maintenance w/Cervical spine protection
- **B** Breathing and ventilation
- **C** Circulation with hemorrhage control
- **D** Disability (Neurologic evaluation)
- **E** Exposure and environment

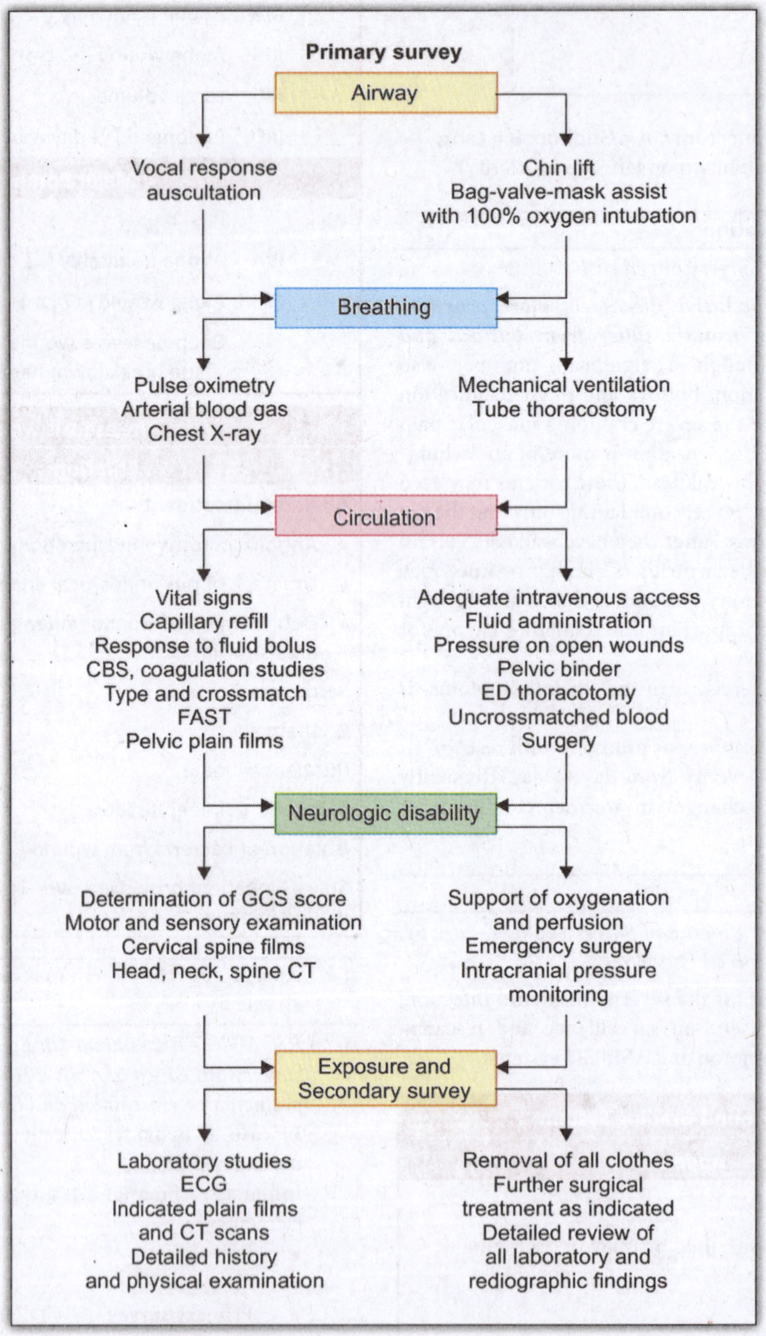

The **secondary survey** does not begin until the primary survey (ABCDEs) is completed, resuscitative efforts are underway, and the normalization of vital functions has been demonstrated.

Secondary Survey				
Item to assess	**Establishes/Identifies**	**Assess**	**Finding**	**Confirm by**
Level of consciousness	• Severity of head injury	• GCS score	• 8, Severe head injury • 9–12, Moderate head injury • 13–15, Minor head injury	• CT scan • Repeat without paralyzing agents
Pupils	• Type of head injury • Presence of eye injury	• Size • Shape • Reactivity	• Mass effect • Diffuse brain injury • Ophthalmic injury	• CT scan
Head	• Scalp injury • Skull injury	• Inspect for lacerations and skull fractures • Palpable defects	• Scalp laceration • Depressed skull fracture • Basillar skull fracture	• CT Scan
Maxillofacial	• Soft-tissue injury • Bone injury • Nerve injury • Teeth/mouth injury	• Visual deformity • Malocclusion • Palpation for crepitation	• Facial fracture • Soft-tissue injury	• Facial-bone X-ray • CT scan of facial bones
Neck	• Laryngeal injury • C-spine injury • Vascular injury • Esophageal injury • Neurologic deficit	• Visual inspection • Palpation • Auscultation	• Laryngeal deformity • Subcutaneous emphysema • Hematoma • Bruit • Platysmal penetration • Pain, tenderness of c-spine	• C-spine X-ray or CT • Angiographyduplex exam • Esophagoscopy • Laryngoscopy
Thorax	• Thoracic-wall injury • Subcutaneous emphysema • Pneumothorax shemothorax • Bronchial injury • Pulmonary contusion • Thoracic aortic disruption	• Visual inspection • Palpation • Auscultation	• Bruising, deformity, or paradoxical motion • Chest-wall tenderness, crepitation • Diminished breath sounds • Muffed heart tones • Mediastinal crepitation • Severe back pain	• Chest X-ray • CT scan • Angiography • Bronchoscopy • Tube thoracostomy • Pericardiocentesis • TE ultrasound
Abdomen/ Flank	• Abdominal-wall injury • Intraperitoneal injury • Retroperitoneal injury	• Visual inspection • Palpation • Auscultation • Determine path of penetration	• Abdominal-wall pain/ tenderness • Peritoneal irritation • Visceral injury • Retroperitoneal organ injury	• DPL/ultrasound • CT scan • Laparotomy • Contrast GI X-ray studies • Angiography
Pelvis	• Genitourinary (GU) tract injuries • Pelvic fracture(s)	• Palpate symphysis pubis for widening • Palpate bony pelvis for tenderness • Determine pelvic stability only once • Inspect perineum • Rectal/vaginal exam	• GU tract injury (hematurial) • Pelvic fracture • Rectal, vaginal, and/or perineal injury	• Pelvic X-ray • GU contrast studies • Urethrogram • Cystogram • IVP • Contrast-enhanced CT
Spinal cord	• Cranial injury • Cord injury • Peripheral nerve(s) injury	• Motor response • Pain response	• Unilateral cranial mass effect • Quadriplegia • Paraplegia • Nerve root injury	• Plain spine X-rays • CT scan • MRI
Vertebral column	• Column injury • Vertebral instability • Nerve injury	• Verbal response to pain, lateralizing sings • Palpate for tenderness • Deformity	• Fracture versus dislocation	• Plain X-rays • CT scan • MRI

Contd...

Secondary Survey				
Item to assess	**Establishes/Identifies**	**Assess**	**Finding**	**Confirm by**
Extremities	• Soft-tissue injury • Bony deformities • Joint abnormalities • Neurovascualr defects	• Visual inspection • Palpation	• Swelling, bruising, pallor • Malalignment • Pain, tenderness, crepitation • Absent/diminished pulses • Tense muscular compartments • Neurologic deficits	• Specific X-rays • Doppler examination • Compartment pressures • Angiography

NOTE

Except for cardiac arrest scenarios, the "A-B-C" (Airway-Breathing-Circulation) rather than "C-A-B" sequence is followed for management.

67. Ans. (d) D

Ref: Rutherford's Vascular Surgery page 2433, Oxford Textbook of Vascular Surgery by Matt Thompson Pg 202

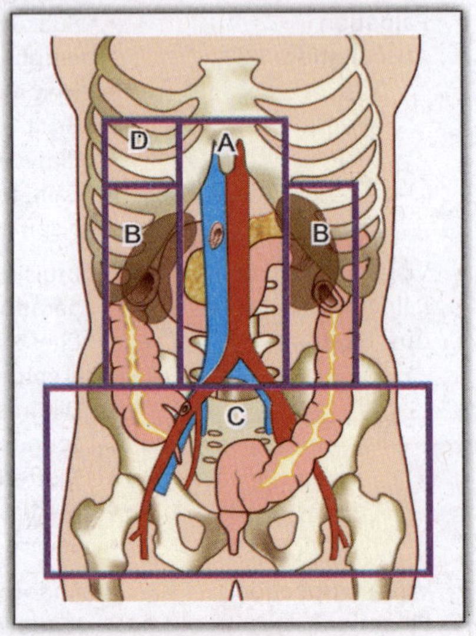

Fig: Zones of Abdomen trauma

Retroperitoneal Hemorrhage Zones		
A = Zone 1 (Central)	Aorta and Vena cava	Midline retroperitoneum extending from the aortic hiatus to the sacral promontory. This zone is subdivided into • **Supramesocolic area:** contains the suprarenal aorta and its major branches (celiac axis, superior mesenteric artery [SMA], and renal arteries), the supramesocolic inferior vena cava (IVC) with its major branches, and the superior mesenteric vein (SMV). • **Inframesocolic area** contains the infrarenal aorta and IVC.
B = Zone 2 (Lateral)	Renal vessels	(Left and right), which includes the kidneys, the paracolic gutter, and the renal vessels
C = Zone 3 (Pelvic)	Iliac vessels	Which includes the pelvic retroperitoneum and contains the iliac vessels
D= Zone 4	Portal vein and retro hepatic vena cava.	Perihepatic area, which contains the hepatic artery, the portal vein, the retrohepatic IVC, and the hepatic veins

Footnote:

- Nunn et al. proposed first anatomic division of the retroperitoneal space into **three zones** for description and decision making in the treatment of retroperitoneal injury. Zone 4 was added later and hence its not shown normally in the diagrams
- The major abdominal vasculature is located in the retroperitoneum, and thus injuries may present with contained retro-peritoneal hematomas rather than free bleeding
- Zone 3 predominates in blunt trauma (70%), whereas zone 2 is the most commonly seen in penetrating injury (50%). Retroperitoneal hematomas are associated with morbidity of up to 60% and mortality from 13% to 40%

68. Ans. (d) Nylon, Monofilament, Nonabsorbable, Reverse cutting

Ref: Maingot's 11th ed ch 4

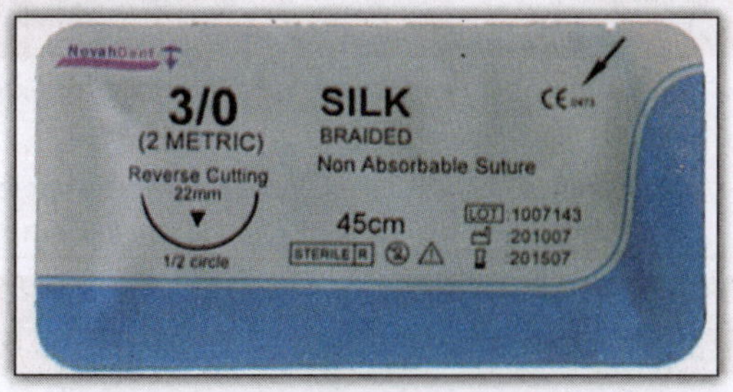

Fig: Mersilk in reverse cutting needle

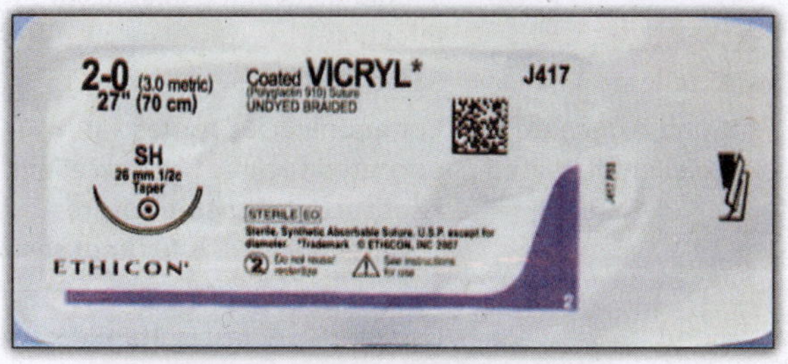

Fig: Vicryl in round body needle

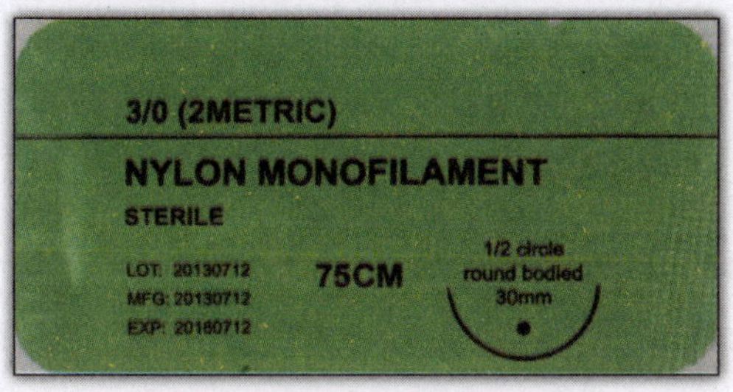

Fig: Nylon in round body needle

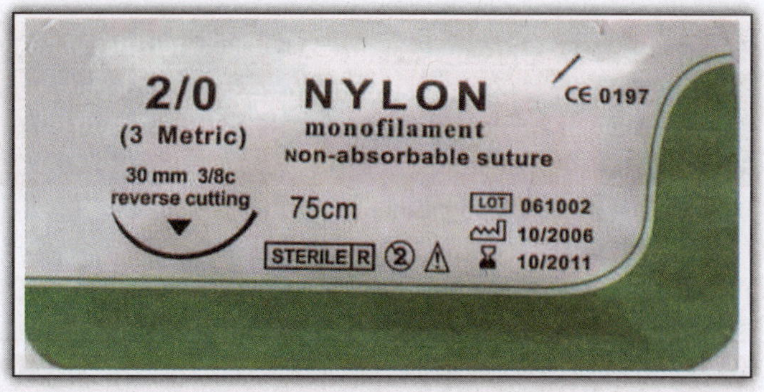

Fig: Nylon in reverse cutting needle

Considering 3 points below a Nylon or Prolene suture with cutting needle is used for Burst abdomen/Wound dehiscence.

1. High strength is required mostly under tension hence synthetic non absorbable mateial is used.
2. Monofilament material have less chances of infection than polyfilament (Braided) material.
3. Resuturing is done by mass closure hence skin penetration is required, hence cutting needle is used.

Maingot Says

"Resuturing should be performed using a strong monofilament nonabsorbable suture such as polypropylene. There are several technical considerations when closing such a wound, such as whether to use continuous or interrupted sutures, and whether or not to use retention sutures. Continuous closure has the theoretical advantages of evenly distributing the tension along the length of the wound and being quicker to perform. However, the tissue at the site of dehiscence is often weakened, and if one of the sutures cuts through the fascia the wound will open. There may therefore be a benefit in closing the fascia with interrupted sutures."

Characteristics of Absorbable Suture Materials

Suture (trade name)	Manufacturing process	Effective strength (d)	Complete absorption (d)	Absorption profile		Application
				Tissue reactivity	Handling	
Surgical gut	Collagen from sheep intestine submucosa	4–10	70	High	Poor	Used for quick-healing mucosa
Chromic gut	Catgut treated with chromic acid	10–14	90	Moderate	Poor	Used for quick-healing mucosa
Polyglycolic acid (Dexon)	Synthetic monofilament or braided	14–21	60–120	Minimal	Good	Subcutaneous sutures, mucosa, ligation of vessels
Polyglactic acid (Vicryl)	Synthetic braided, lubricated with polyglactin 370; undyed or purple	20–30	60–90	Minimal	Excellent	Subcuticular and subcutaneous sutures
Monocryl (poliglecaprone 25)	Synthetic, monofilament, made of copolymer of glycolide and epsilon caprolactone.	Best knot strength in absorbable sutures	90 days	Minimal (Less eactive than Vicryl)	Excellent	Indicated for use in general soft tissue approximation, but not for use in CVS, CNS, microsurgery or ophthalmic surgery

Contd...

Suture (trade name)	Manufacturing process	Effective strength (d)	Complete absorption (d)	Absorption profile		Application
				Tissue reactivity	Handling	
Polydioxane (PDS)	Monofilament polyester	40–60	180	Minimal	Good	Used for extended support
Polyglyconate (Maxon)	Synthetic monofilament	40–60	180–210	Minimal	Excellent	More supple than polydioxane

Characteristics of Absorbable Suture Materials

Suture (trade name)	Manufacturing process	Tissue reactivity	Handling	Application
Silk	Braided; derived from cocoon of silkworm larva	High	Excellent	Vessel ligation; high capillarity; should be avoided in areas prone to infection
Cotton	Braided	High	Excellent	Same as silk
Polyester	Braided terephthalate (Dacron), polyethylene (Mersilene), coated with Teflon (Tevdek), silicone (Ti-Cron), polybutilate (Ethibond)	Minimal	Good if uncoated; excellent if coated	Commonly used for fascia; uncoated sutures have excellent knot security; coated sutures require five throws for knot security
Nylon	Synthetic polyamide monofilament or braided	Minimal	Good	Used for skin, fascia; requires five throws for knot security
Polypropylene (Prolene, Surgilene)	Plastic monofilament	Minimal	Good	High elasticity; commonly used for skin closure and vascular anastomoses; requires five throws
Polybutester (Novofil)	Plastic monofilament copolymer	Minimal	Good	Very high elasticity; used when tissue swelling is present
Steel	Alloy monofilament	None	Poor	Retention sutures, bone

Characteristics of Nonabsorbable Suture Materials

69. Ans. (c) Monopolar cautery

Ref: SRB's Surgical Operations: Text & Atlas - Page 568

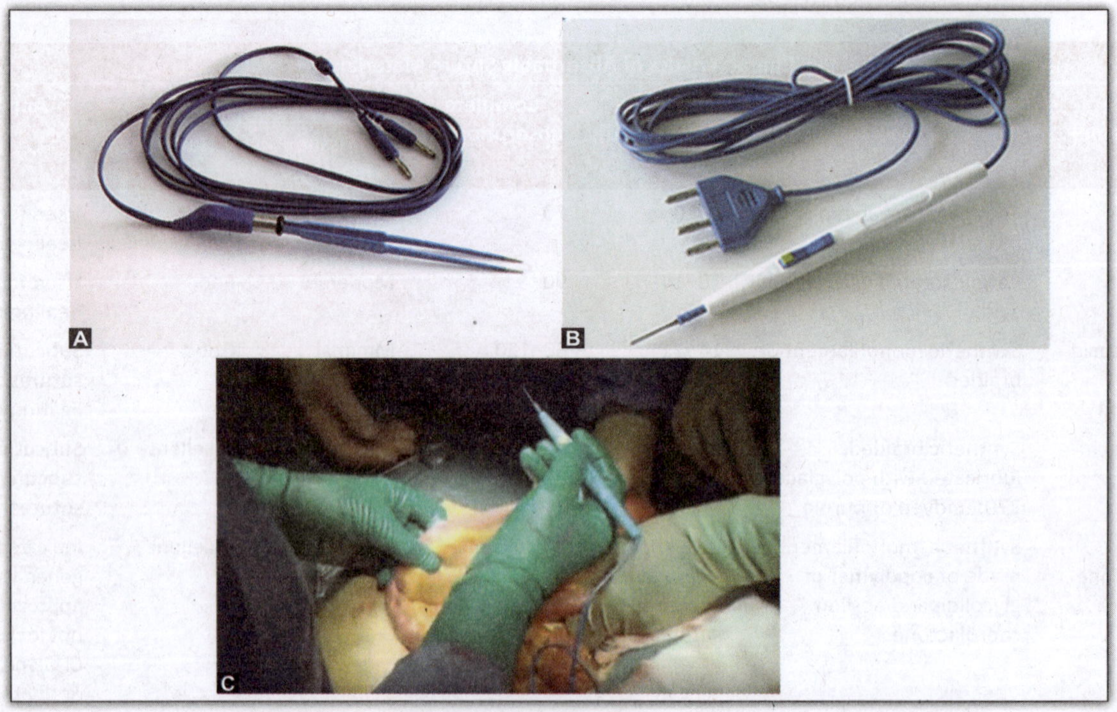

Fig: **(A)** Bipolar diathermy; **(B)** Monopolar diathermy; **(C)** Monopolar diathermy intraoperative

Principles of Diathermy:

The effects of electricity on tissue: At low frequencies alternating current (a.c.) causes a dangerous shock but with frequencies above 20kHz, muscular contraction stops, pain stops and the only detectable effect, is heat generation within the tissue. The heating is produced because of the Joule effect. At high frequencies, the body can be modelled as a resistor, instead of the capacitive+resistive elements as happens in low frequencies. Thus, the heating energy is:

$$E = I^2 RT$$

- Where **E** is the energy in Joules
- **I** is the current through the skin in Amperes
- **R** is the resistance of your body in Ohms
- **T** is the time in seconds

Types of Diathermy:

There are two main types of diathermy Monopolar and Bipolar. Polarity refers to the number of electrode poles at the site of application

Types of Diathermy

	Monopolar	Bipolar
Power	High power generator (400 W)	Low power generator (50 W)
Electrodes	One hand held electrode and one plate electrode (70 cm sq)	2 electrodes in pair of forceps
Uses	Cutting and coagulation	Coagulation only
Adjacent tissue	Should be careful about adjacent tissue	Adjacent tissue is never damaged
Contraindications	Artificial valves, Pacemakers	
Adverse effects	Plate electrode burns	

Monopolar cautery vs Bipolar cautery

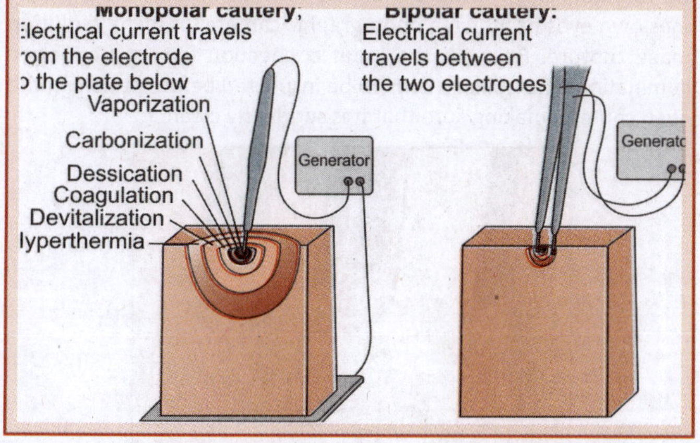

70. Ans. (d) Laparoscopic cannula

Ref: Textbook of Practical Laparoscopic Surgery By R. K. Mishra, RK Mishra page 79

The given picture shows first trocar in place with obturator removed and pneumoperitoneum CO_2 gas supply in place. Hence idealy after removal of obturator the trocar assembly is incomplete and shall be called as cannula. In case cannula is not provided in the options, Trocar can be marked.

There are lot of confusion Regarding terms used in Laparoscopic instrumentations because many terms are used interchangeably even in standard text books.

To simplify and summarize:

- **Trocar assembly** includes cannula, seal and obturator. Sometimes obturator alone is called trocar.
- **Port** is the point of entry in the skin from which a trocar enters. Sometimes cannula is wrongly called as port.

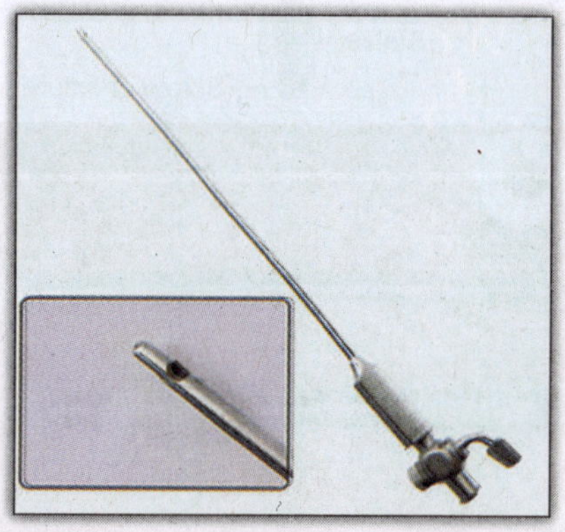

Fig: A Veress needle is a spring-loaded needle used to create pneumoperitoneum for laparoscopic surgery. It was first developed in 1932 by Janos Veres, a Hungarian internist working with tuberculosis patients. Raoul Palmer introduced the use of the Veress needle in laparoscopy to establish a pneumoperitoneum.

Two methods are used for establishing abdominal access during laparoscopic procedures.

1. **Hasson technique:** The first, direct puncture laparoscopy, begins with the elevation of the relaxed abdominal wall with two towel clips or a well-placed hand.
2. **Veress needle:** A small incision is made in the umbilicus, and a specialized spring-loaded (Veress) needle is placed in the abdominal cavity

Modern needles are **12 to 15 cm long** and external diameter of 2 mm. The outer cannula consists of a beveled needle point for cutting through tissues of the abdominal wall. A spring-loaded, inner stylet is positioned within the outer cannula. This inner stylet has a dull tip to protect any viscera from injury by the sharp, outer cannula. Direct pressure on the tip—as when penetrating through tissue—pushes the dull stylet into the shaft of the outer cannula. When the tip of the needle enters a space such as the peritoneal cavity, the dull, inner stylet springs forward. Carbon dioxide is then passed through the Veress needle to inflate the space, creating a pneumoperitoneum

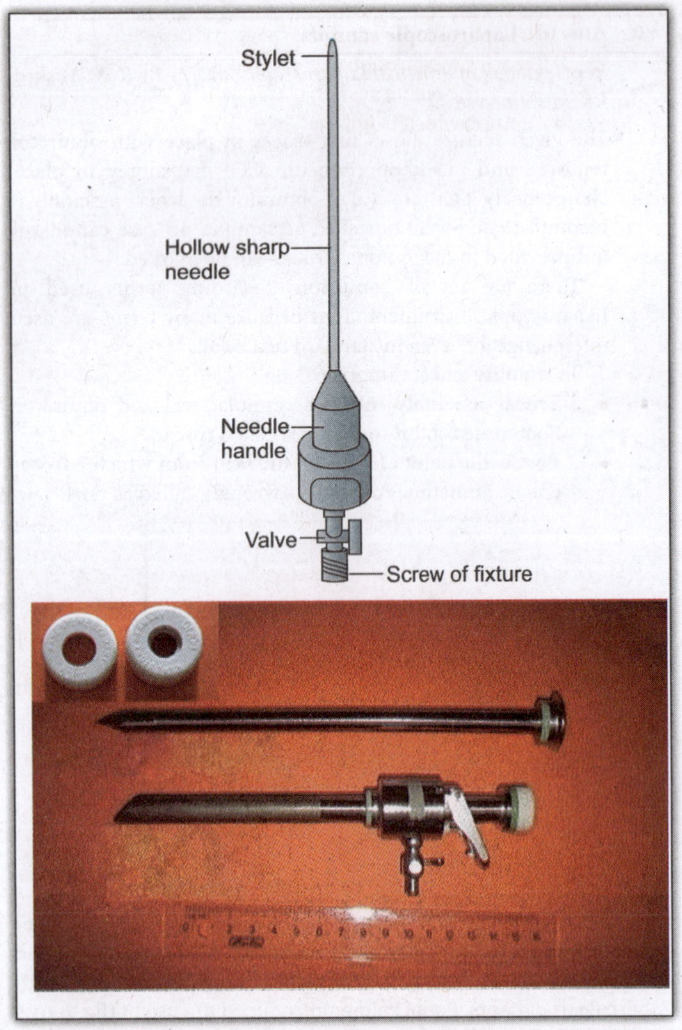

Fig: Laparoscopy Trocar Assembly: Trocar assembly includes Cannula (below in the picture), Seal (with cannula and insat) and Obturator (Above in the picture).

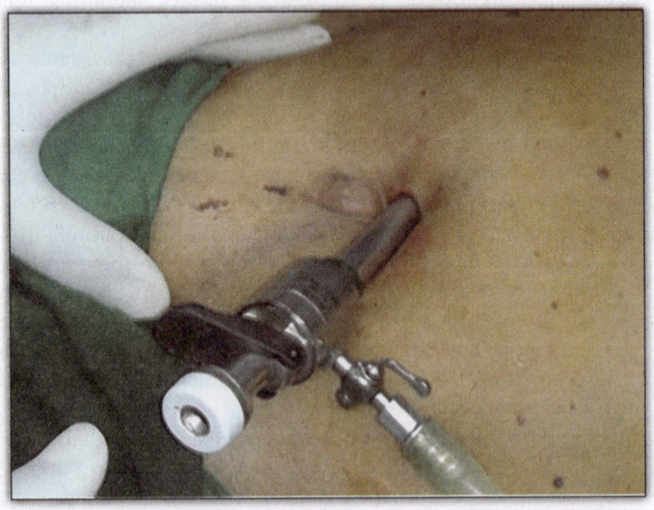

Fig: First trocar in place: The given picture shows first trocar in place with obturator removed and pneumoperitoneum CO_2 gas supply in place

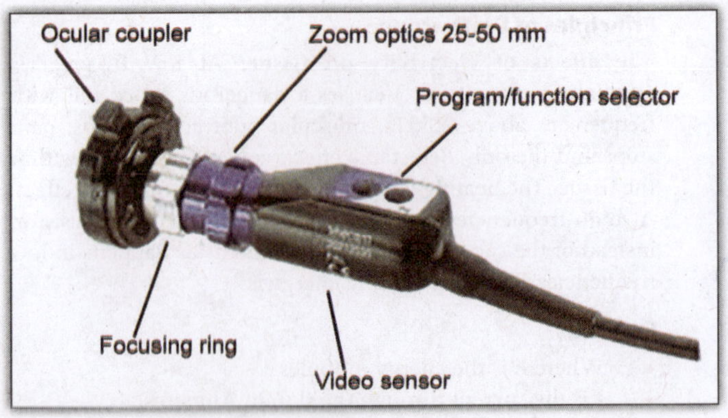

Fig: Laparoscopic Camera (Labelled)

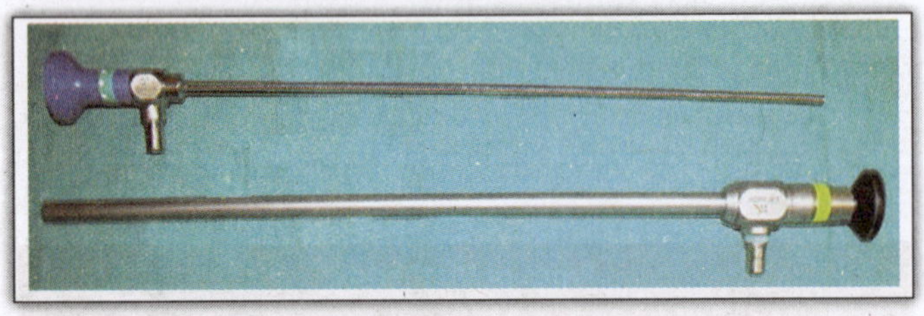

Fig: Laparoscope 5 mm above and 10 mm below: Laparoscopes vary in their physical dimensions; however, the most practical sizes are the **5 and 10 mm** diameters and 15-30 cm in length. Laparoscope are straight but can be angled.

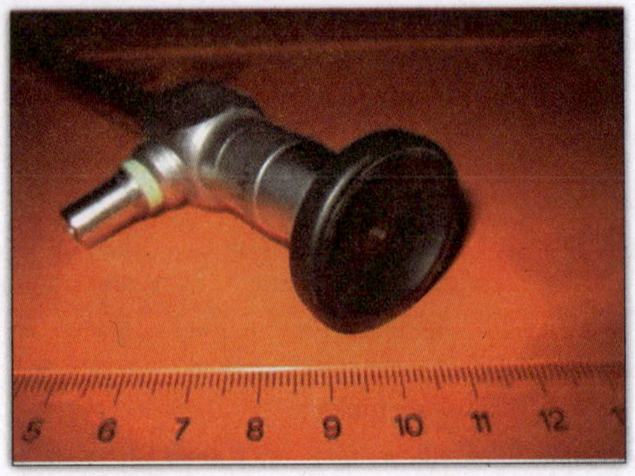

Fig: Ocular of Laparoscope: The proximal end is the head or the ocular; this is where the video camera is attached for display on the monitor. This is where one can view the tissue directly with ones own eyes or attach a photographic camera for high-resolution image capture. Below is the input connection for the fiber-optic illumination. The ocular needs to be inspected before attaching the video camera, making sure that it is spotlessly clean

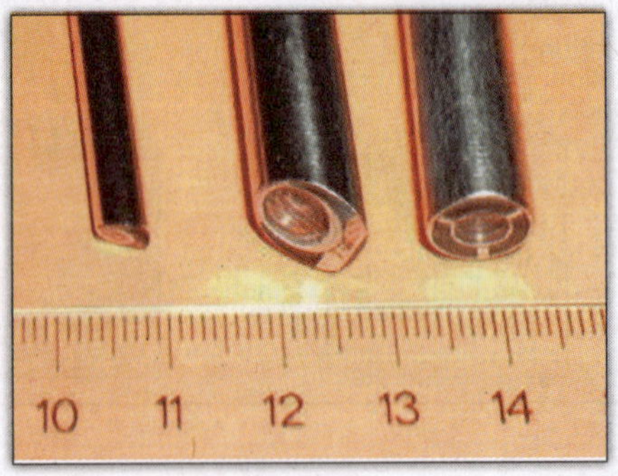

Fig: Tip of Laparoscope: Laparoscopic tip can be 0 degrees or 30 degrees (most common- center of picture). Angulations increases the field of vision.

71. Ans. (a) Pneumothorax

Ref: Rosen's Emergency Medicine - Concepts and Clinical Practice By John Marx, Ron Walls, Robert Hockberger 8th ed page 218

(See Radiological features of Pneumothorax in AIIMS Nov 2017 Radiodiagnosis) (see page no. 1123)

Hint to Diagnosis

- Decreased air entry is seen in pneumothorax, flail chest and esophageal rupture.
- Absent breath sounds is seen with pneumothorax characteristically. In flail chest and esophageal rupture Breath sound can be decreased not absent.
- Epigastric tenderness on USG probe is seen in esophageal rupture, which is not seen here.
- Chest X-ray is characteristic of pneumothorax.
- Vital signs differentiate a tension pneumothorax from a simple pneumothorax; each can have similar signs, symptoms, and examination findings, but hypotension qualifies the pneumothorax as a tension pneumothorax.

Chest Trauma

	Physical exam	Investigations	Management
Tension pneumothorax • A clinical diagnosis • One-way valve causing accumulation of air in pleural space	• Respiratory distress, tachycardia, distended neck veins, cyanosis, asymmetry of chest wall motion • Tracheal deviation • Percussion hyperresonance • Unilateral absence of breath sounds, hypotension	• Non-radiographic diagnosis	**Emergent needle decompression** by large bore IV needle, 2nd ICS mid clavicular line, followed by **Tube thoracostomy (chest tube insertion)** in 5th ICS, anterior axillary line
Open pneumothorax • Air entering chest from wound rather than trachea	Same as above except hypotension	• **ABG's:** Decreased pO_2 • CXR is characteristic	• Air-tight dressing sealed on 3 sides • **Tube thoracostomy (chest tube insertion)** • Surgery
Esophageal injury	• Usually penetrating trauma (pain out of proportion to degree of injury), decreased breath sound	• CXR: mediastinal air (not always) • Esophagram (Gastrograffin) • Flexible esophagoscopy	• Early repair (within 24 hours) improves outcome but all require repair
Flail Chest • Free-floating segment of chest wall due to > 4 rib fractures, each at 2 sites • Underlying lung contusion (cause of morbidity and mortality)	• Paradoxical movement of flail segment • Palpable crepitus of ribs • Decreased air entry on affected side	• **ABGs:** Decreased pO_2, increased pCO_2 • **CXR:** Rib fractures, lung contusion	• O_2 + fluid therapy + pain control • Judicious fluid therapy in absence of systemic hypotension • Positive pressure ventilation • +/– intubation and ventilation
Ruptured Diaphragm	Blunt trauma to chest or abdomen (e.g. high lap belt in MVC)	• **CXR:** Abnormality of diaphragm/lower lung fields/NG tube placement. • **CT scan & endoscopy:** Sometimes helpful for diagnosis	Laparotomy for diaphragm repair and because of associated intra-abdominal injuries

72. Ans. (c) Damage control surgery, mesh closure of abdomen

Ref: Mastery of Surgery 6th Ed Pg 591-594, Bailey 26th ed page 136, 799, 814

The patient is having tachycardia, hypotension, low saturation and 4 quadrant FAST is positive so basically the patient is hemodynamically unstable and cannot survive a full blown surgery. The patient needs to be treated by step wise approach called as damage control surgery.

Types of Temporary Abdominal Closure (TAC)

- Towel-clipping of skin edges (Simplest and fastest)
- Open packing of abdomen
- Zipper closure
- Wittmann patch (overlapping Velcro-like sheets)
- Synthetic mesh closure
- Silastic (plastic bag) closure (also known as the Bogotá Bag)
- Vaccum assisted device (VAC) closure

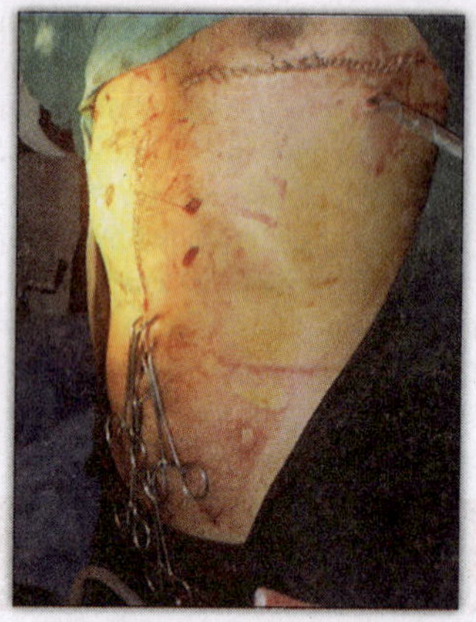

Fig: Towel clip closure

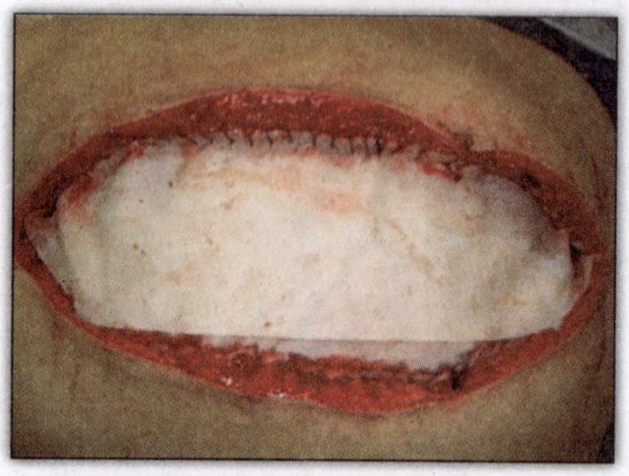

Fig: Wittmann patch (overlapping Velcro-like sheets)

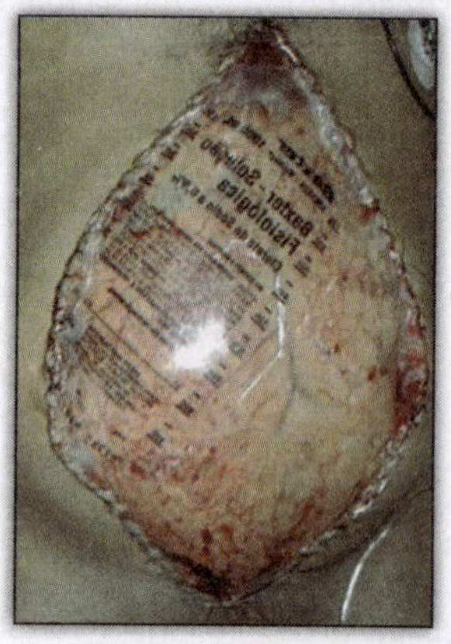

Fig: Bogota technique using a presterilized, soft 3-L IV bag

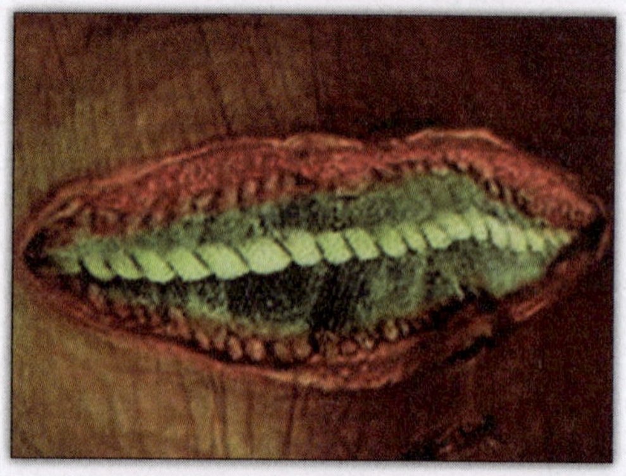

Fig: Polypropylene mess closure

Damage Control Surgery

This concept of tailoring the operation to match the patient's physiology and staged procedures to prevent physiological exhaustion is called 'damage control surgery'. The term "**damage control**" was coined by the United States Navy during World War II; whereby the continued functioning of a damaged ship is ensured above conducting complete repairs, which would prevent a rapid return to battle. Following major injury, protracted surgery in the physiologically unstable patient with the "**deadly triad**" the combination of hypothermia, acidosis and coagulopathy – carries a very high mortality rate

Deadly Triad

Hypothermia	Acidosis	Coagulopathy
• Clinically important if less than 37°C for more than 4 hours • Can lead to cardiac arrhythmias, decreased cardiac output, increassed systemic vascular resistance • Can induce and exacerbate coagulopathy by inhibition of clotting cascade reaction	• Uncorrected haemorrhagic shock leads into inadequate cellular perfusion, anaerobic metabolism and the production of lactatic acid • Interferes with blood clotting mechanisms and promotes coagulopathy and blood loss	• Hypothermia, acidosis and the consequences of massive blood transfusion all lead to the development of a coagulopathy • Platelet dysfunction at low temperature • Activation of the fibrinolytic system • Haemodilution following massive resuscitation

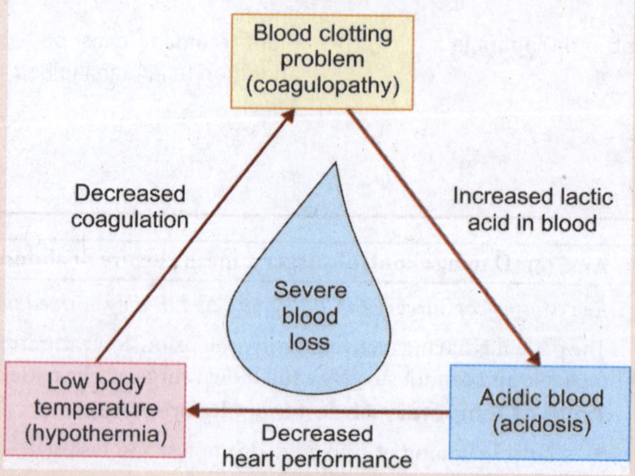

Principles of damage control surgery	• Control haemorrhage • Prevention contamination • Avoid further injury • Nothing else

Indications for Damage Control Surgery	
Anatomical	Inability to achieve haemostasis Complex abdominal injury, e.g. liver and pancreas Combined vascular, solid and hollow organ injury, e.g. aortic or caval injury Inaccessible major venous injury, e.g. retrohepatic vena cava Demand for non-operative control of other injuries, e.g. fractured pelvis Anticipated need for a time-consuming procedure
Physiological (decline of physiological reserve)	Temperature < 34ºC pH < 7.2 Serum lactate > 5 mmol/L [N (Normal) < 2.5 mmol/L Prothrombin time (PT) > 16 s Partial thromboplastin time (PTT) > 60 s >10 units blood transfused Systolic blood pressure < 90 mm Hg for > 60 minutes
Environmental	Operating time > 60 minutes Inability to approximate the abdominal incision Desire to reassess the intra-abdominal contents (directed relook)

The Stages of Damage Control Surgery	
Stage 1: Patient selection	• The decision that damage control surgery is required should be made at the earliest opportunity, preferably in the emergency department or at the beginning of the operation. • Patient selection is based on indications • Prehospital and emergency department times should be minimized • BTLS • FAST- Focused assessment with sonography in trauma • No unnecessary investigations • Rapid transport to the operating room without repeated attempts to restrore circulating volume as they require operative control of haemorrhage
Stage 2: Control of haemorrhage and control of contamination	• The initial surgical focus is haemorrhage control, which is followed by control and limitation of contamination • This is achieved using a range of abbreviated techniques including simple ligation of bleeding vessels, shunting of major arteries and veins, drainage, temporary stapling off of bowel, and therapeutic packing.
	• The management of liver injuries can be summarized as 'the four Ps': ▪ Push ▪ Pringle ▪ Plug ▪ Pack • External fixation • Do not insist on anatomical reposition, but on fracture stabilisation • Following the above the abdomen is closed in a temporary fashion using a sheet of plastic (e.g. Opsite) over the bowel, an intermediate pack to allow suction, and a further sheet of adherent plastic drape to the skin to form a watertight and airtight seal. Suction is applied to the intermediate pack area to collect abdominal fluid. This technique is known as the **"Vacpac"** or **"Opsite sandwich"** • The best situation is closure of the abdominal fascia, or, if this cannot be achieved, then skin closure only. Occasionally, mesh closure can be used, with skin grafting over the mesh and subsequent abdominal wall reconstruction
Stage 3: Resuscitation continued in the intensive care unit	• As soon as control has been achieved the patient is transferred from the operating theatre to the intensive care unit where resuscitation is continued; the aim of this is the correction of hypothermia, acidosis and coagulopathy. • The resuscitation is individualized through repeated point of care testing in the operating room of haemoglobin level, acidosis (pH and lactate) and clotting, and is therefore directed towards the early delivery of biologically active colloids, clotting products, recombinant factor VIIa and whole blood in order to buy time. • Following this, further physiological investigation or radiological intervention can be carried out.

Contd...

The Stages of Damage Control Surgery	
Stage 4: Definitive surgery	• The team should aim to perform definitive anastomosis, vascular reconstruction and closure of the body cavity within 24–72 hours of injury; however, this must be individualized to the patient, the response to critical care resuscitation • Definitive orthopedic surgery can be done 5-10 days after trauma • Undue haste and a premature return to theatre will convert a definitive second operation into a second damage control procedure and result in further physiological insult for the patient; however, undue delay may increase the risk of intra-abdominal sepsis and the progression of previously unrecognized injuries. • Primary repair with end-to-end anastomosis undertaken • Copious washout should be performed and the abdomen closed • Internal fixation of fractures
Stage 5: Abdominal closure	The abdomen is closed as soon as possible, bearing in mind the risks of ACS.
• Sequence of steps: **ER → OR → ICU → OR → ICU**	

73. Ans. (c) Complete expansion and when drain output is less than 200 mL for 2 consecutive days

Ref: With text

The timing of chest tube removal in regard to drainage volume has been investigated by Younes and colleagues in a prospective randomized trial. There was no major difference in the rate of fluid accumulation and need for thoracocentesis between groups of drainage amounts of 50 mL/day, 150-mL/day, or 200 mL/day, respectively. Using the threshold of daily drainage of less than 200 mL could lead to quicker removal of the chest tube, reducing hospitalization time. **This study demonstrated that chest tube removal was safe if drainage is less than 200 mL per day**. (Ref: Evidence-Based Practice of Critical Care Saunders- Elsevier By Clifford S. Deutschman, Patrick J. Neligan Page 568)

Studies suggest <2 mL/kg/day or <200 mL/day (whichever is less) may be appropriate for chest tube removal **(Ref: The 5-Minute Anesthesia Consult -by Nina Singh Radcliff Page 219)**

NOTE

Per day or 24 hours apart is equivalent to 2 consecutive days

74. Ans. (c) Renal failure

Ref: Rush University Review of Surgery 5th ed Page 319, SRB Manual of surgery 4th ed page 752

In obstructive jaundice, serum bilirubin level will not go beyond 40 mg%. At this point raised intrabiliary pressure (Normal is 12-22 cm of H_2O) to 25 cm of H_2O, blocks the formation of bilirubin and secretion of cholesterol and bile acids completely. Maximum production of bilirubin per day possible is 250 mg%. Normal maximum excretion of bilirubin by kidney per day is 210 mg%. So maximum possible raise of serum bilirubin is 40 mg% in obstructive jaundice.

Situations in which even higher bilirubin levels can be found include renal insufficiency, hemolysis, hepatocellular disease, and rarely, a bile duct hepatic vein fistula.

75. Ans. (a) Acute cholecystitis

Ref: Core Radiology By Jacob Mandell Cambridge University Press page 572

Tc99 Iminodiacetic acid analogs are used to image the biliary system. Regardless of the tracer, its typically called as HIDA scan

In acute cholecystitis, the gallbladder is not visible as there is no filling of the gallbladder with bile containing the radioisotope due to the edema at the neck of gallbladder and cystic duct

HIDA Protocol

- NPO for 6 hours
- Cholecystokinen (CCK 0.02 μg/kg) is to be given to empty gallbladder befoe Radiotracer is administered.
- Dynamic imaging of right upper quadant stats immediately after Radiotracer is administered.
- As soon as gallbladder is visualized, acute cholecystitis is ruled out.
- If gallbladder is not visualized in 1 hour, morphine 0.04 mg/kg (max 4 mg) and imaging to be continued for 3 min more.
- If patient is allergic to morphine or any other contraindication to morphine then Imaging for 4 hours
- Normal HIDA scan- Liver is visible in 5 min, GB is visible in 15 minutes, tracer in intestine ensures patent CBD.

AIIMS MAY 2016

76. Ans. (b) Needle holding forceps, Toothed dissecting forceps, Mayo's forceps

Ref: Practical Medical Procedures at a Glance -By Rachel K. Thomas Page 37

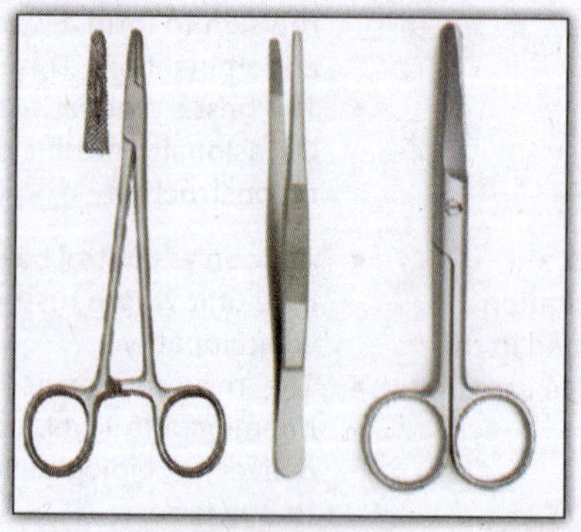

Fig: Option (A) Needle holding forceps, Non toothed dissecting forceps, Mayo's scissors

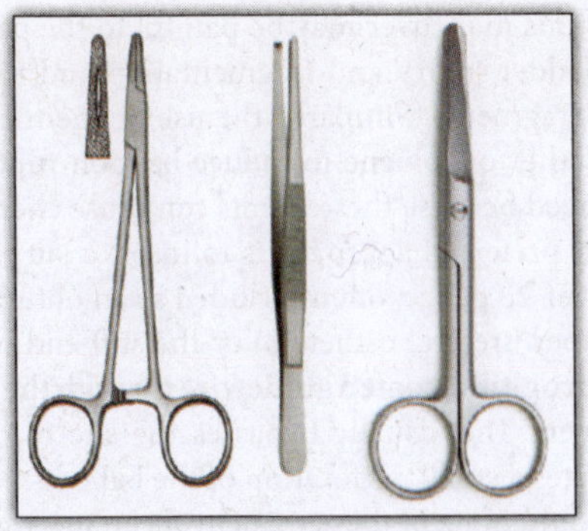

Fig: Option (B) Needle holding forceps, Toothed dissecting forceps, Mayo's scissors

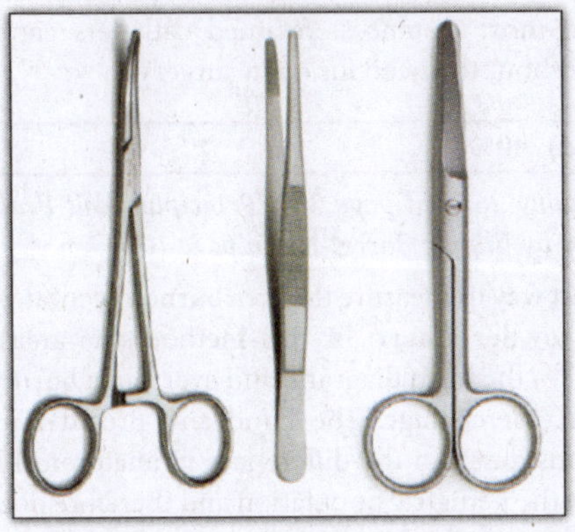

Fig: Option (C) Haemostatic forceps, Non toothed dissecting forceps, Mayo's scissors

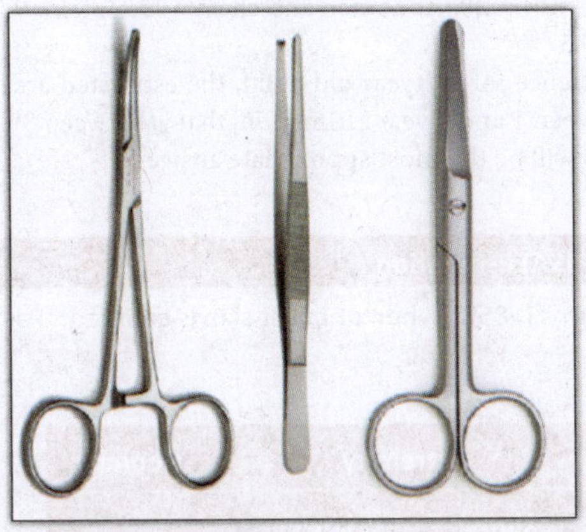

Fig: Option (D) Haemostatic forceps, Toothed dissecting forceps, Mayo's scissors

For skin closure following instruments/materials are used:

- Needle holder
- Toothed Forceps (For grasping the wound's edge)
- Scissors to cut sutures after knotting
- Suture material

NOTE

There are two suture cutting scissors. One is for Intraoperative suture cutting (Mayo's Scissors) and another is for Post operative suture cutting after healing (Heath suture cutting forceps)

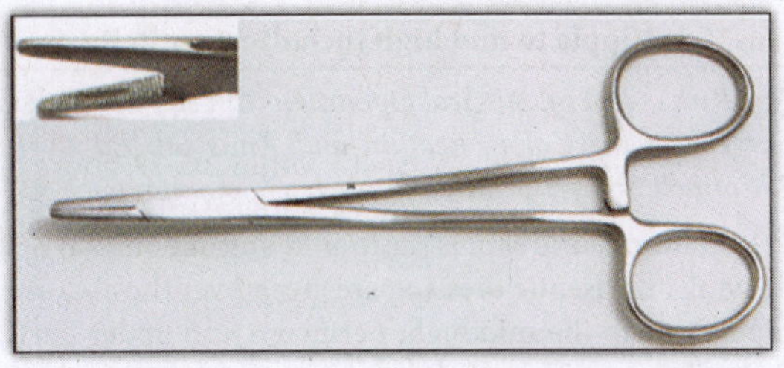

Fig: Needle Holding forceps

- Blades having criss cross or transverse serrations fo needle holding
- Blade length is smaller than haemostatic foceps
- Blade have a central groove unlike Haemostatic forceps
- Modified box joint

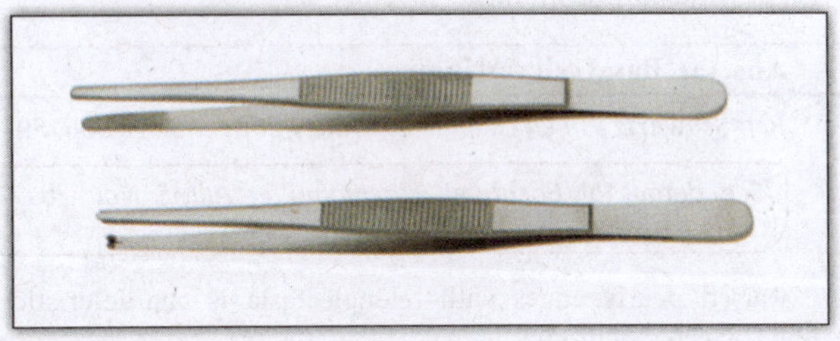

Fig: Dissecting/Thumb forceps: Lower = Toothed dissecting forceps for holding skin margins, Fascia, Aponeurosis etc. Upper = Non toothed Dissecting forceps for holding delicate soft tissue

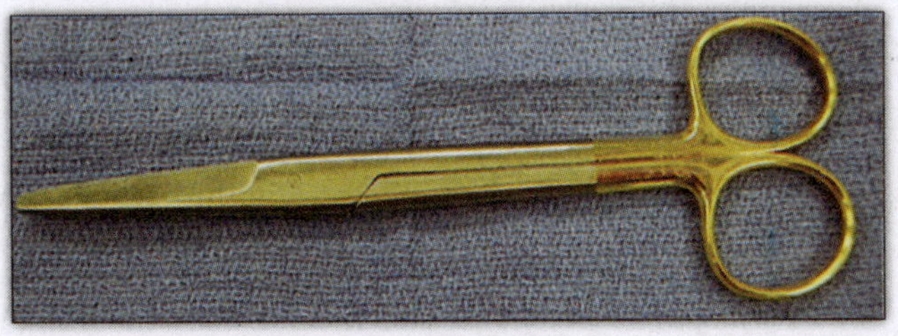

Fig: Mayo's scissors

- AKA- Suture cutting scissors
- Hemi blunt ends (tips), a feature that differentiate it from other surgical scissors
- Straight blade Mayo's scissors are used in suture cutting
- Curved blade Mayo's scissor is used for cutting tough body structures like rectus sheath, linea alba, aponeurosis etc
- During appendectomy curved Mayo's scissors are used to split internal onlique and transverse abdominis
- Rarely used for dissection of tissues

77. Ans. (d) Monocryl

Ref: Mastery of Surgery by Fischer 5th ed page 553

See Details of Suture Material in AIIMS NOV 2016 Surgery (see page no. 965-966)

In breast surgery closure is by interrupted 3-0 Monocryl in the deep dermis, and running 4-0 Monocryl subcuticular sutures for skin

- Monocryl is less reactive than Vicryl with less tendency to "spit" due to foreign body reactions
- Monocryl has best knot strength in all absorbable sutures.

78. Ans. (a) Nipple to mid high including genitalia

Ref: Kirk's General Surgical Operations 6th ed Page 38, Operative Surgery of the Colon, Rectum and Anus 6th Ed By P Ronan O'Connell, Robert D. Madoff, Michael Solomon page 345

Preparation of the skin is same as in any abdominal operation. Shaving and aseptic dressing are given over the abdomen from nipple line to the midthigh, perineum and upper part of both thighs in case of Lower abdomen/Anorectal operations.

Parts Preparation Differ for Different Sites

- Neck—from chin to nipple line
- Abdomen—from nipple line to mid thigh
- Chest—from chin to umbilicus
- Foot—from toes to inguinal region
- Hands—from fingers to axilla

79. Ans. (a) Basal cell carcinoma

Ref: Schwartz 9th ed chapter 16, Bailey 26th ed page 580, 591

(See details of Basal cell carcinoma in AIIMS Nov 2017 Surgery) (see page no. 941)

Raised pearly edges with telengiectasia is characteristic of Basal cell carcinoma.

BCC is usually a slow growing, locally invasive malignant tumor of pluripotential epithelial cells arising from basal cell layer of epidermis and hair follicles, hence affecting the pilosebaceous skin

80. Ans. (a) Ultrasound guided puncture of balloon

Ref: Campbell Urology 10th ed page 182

Campbell states "If the balloon remains inflated, the problem is along the catheter's inflation lumen or in the balloon itself. Although over inflation of the balloon has been described in an attempt to rupture the balloon, we do not recommend it because this maneuver may be painful to the patient and may cause bladder injury and fragmentation and retention of the balloon fragments. Similarly, the use of chemical instillations such as ether or toluene to induce balloon rupture should be discouraged because these agents can cause chemical cystitis.

- Our preferred approach is to insert a **surgical steel wire** (24 or 28 gauge; often included as an obturator for small-caliber ureteral catheters) or the stiff end of a 0.035-inch **hydrophilic-coated guidewire** through the valve inflation lumen. This usually bypasses the site of obstruction or creates a small perforation of the balloon.
- Should none of these maneuvers be successful, the use of **ultrasound-guided needle puncture** can be conducted with a long spinal needle (22 gauge) using either a transrectal, transvaginal, or suprapubic surface probe. In most instances, retained catheters can be removed without the need for open surgery.

81. Ans. (d) 40%

Ref: Bailey 26th ed page 389, Principles And Practice Of Burn Surgery by Juan P. Barret-Nerín page 10

The best way to measure the area burned accurately is the **Lund and Browder Chart**. In this method, the areas burned are plotted in the burn diagram, and every area burned is assigned an exact percentage. The Lund and Browder method takes into consideration the differences in anatomical location that exist in the pediatric population and therefore does not over or underestimate the burn size in patients of different ages.

For 1-4 year old child

Face (Front) = 6.5%, Both upper limb (Front and back) = (10 + 10) = 20, Abdomen and chest = 13. Total = 9.5 + 13 + 20 = 39.5

Hence for a 2 year old child, the estimated area should be between 1 and 4 year estimation, that is between 39.5%. Hence 40% will be the most appropriate answer.

Percentage of Body Surface Area (BSA) Estimation

For Small & very large burns: If <15% of total surface area or very large burns (>85%, when unburnt skin is counted). Palm of patient's hand equals 1% of BSA. For medium sized burns, it is inaccurate.

A. For Large areas: Wallace rule of nines

	Head and Neck	Trunk		Extremity		Genital
		Anterior	Posterior	Upper	Lower	
Adult	9	18	18	9	18	1
Infant	18	18	18	9	14	–

B. For burns in children: In children younger than 3 years old, the head accounts for a larger relative surface area and should be taken into account when estimating burn size. Diagrams such as the **Lund and Browder chart** give a more accurate accounting of the true burn size in children. It is the **most accurate method** and can also be used for adults

Contd...

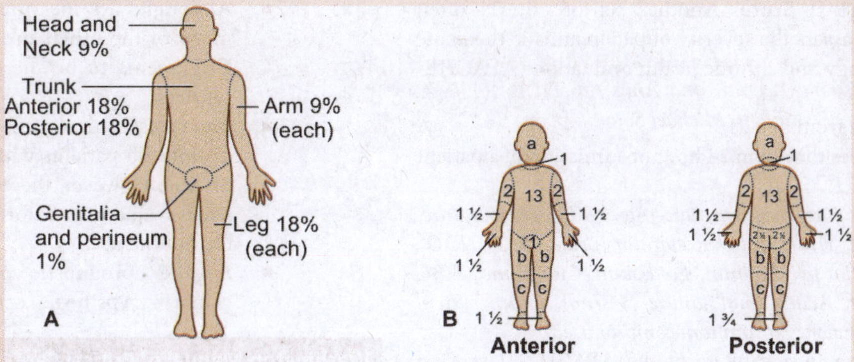

Relative percentage of body surface area (% BSA) affected by growth

Age	0–1	0–4	5–9	10–14	15
A–½ of head	9 ½%	8 1/2%	6 ½%	5 ½%	4 ½%
B–½ of one thigh	2 ¾%	3 1/4%	4%	4 ¾%	4 ¼%
C–½ of thigh	2 ½%	2 1/2%	2 ¾%	3%	3 ¼%

82. Ans. (b) Severe acute pancreatitis

Ref: Schwartz 9th ed chapter 33, Sabiston 18th ed chapter 55, The Washington Manual of Critical Care by Marin Kollef page 418

This question is based purely on CT severity scoring system. Other information are fillers and does not fits into any severity scoring systems. CTSI has become the gold standard for detecting and assessing the severity of pancreatitis. CT scanning is routinely performed on patients who are suspected of harbouring severe pancreatitis, regardless of their Ranson's or APACHE scores. The numerical CTSI is the sum of the Balthazar grade points and pancreatic necrosis grade points. Maximum score 10 (>6 indicates severe pancreatitis)

Atlas of Gastroenterology by Tadataka Yamada Part 2 Page 520
Table 45.7 Classification of Mild and Severe Pancreatitis

Model	Mild pancreatitis	Severe pancreatitis
Hematocrit (%)	Normal	44%
Ranson's score	0–1	>3
APACHE-II	1–6	>8
Glasgow score	0	>2 (3 or more)
CRP at 48 hours	25–100 mg/dL	>
IL-6	Normal	2–7 pg/mL
Urine TAP	<15 nmol/l	>37 nmol/l
CTSI & MRIS	1–3	>6

Assessment of Severity of Pancreatitis

An early discrimination between mild edematous and severe necrotizing forms of the disease is of the utmost importance to provide optimal care to the patient. Several predictors of severity, including early prognostic signs, serum markers, and CT scans, are commonly used for this purpose.

- **Early Prognostic Signs**
  - Ranson Score: In 1974, Ranson identified a series of prognostic signs for early identification of patients with severe pancreatitis. Out of these 11 objective parameters, five are measured at the time of admission, whereas the remaining six are measured within 48 hours of admission.
    - If the number of positive Ranson signs is <2, expected to have a mild attack with little morbidity and a mortality rate of less than 1%.
    - With 3 or 4 positive Ranson's criteria, the mortality rate may reach 15%, and half of patients may need to be treated in an intensive care unit.
    - With 5 to 6 or signs will require intensive care
    - The mortality rate increases to >50% (may reach 90%) when there >7 positive Ranson signs.

Ranson's Prognostic Signs of Pancreatitis

Criteria for acute pancreatitis not due to gallstones	
At admission	During the initial 48 hours
Age >55 years	Hematocrit fall >10 points
WBC >16,000/mm³	BUN elevation >5 mg/dL
Blood glucose >200 mg/dL	Serum calcium <8 mg/dL
Serum LDH >350 IU/L	Arterial PO_2 <60 mm Hg
Serum AST >250 U/dL	Base deficit >4 mEq/L
	Estimated fluid sequestration >6 L
Criteria for acute gallstone pancreatitis	
At admission	During the initial 48 hours
Age >70 years	Hematocrit fall >10 points
WBC >18,000/mm³	BUN elevation >2 mg/dL
Blood glucose >220 mg/dL	Serum calcium <8 mg/dL
Serum LDH >400 IU/L	Base deficit >5 mEq/L
Serum AST >250 U/dL	Estimated fluid sequestration >4 L

Abbreviations: AST, aspartate transaminase; BUN, blood urea nitrogen; LDH, lactate dehydrogenase; PO_2, partial pressure of oxygen; WBC, white blood cell count.

- **APACHE-II Score**: Another set of criteria often used to assess the severity of pancreatitis is the *a*cute *p*hysiology *a*nd *c*hronic *h*ealth *e*valuation (APACHE-II) score.
  - Score from 0 to 71
  - Applies to with in 24 hour of admission of a patient to ICU
  - *Takes into consideration- Age, GCS, Temperature, MAP, Heart rate, Respiratory rate, FiO_2, PaO_2, Arterial pH, Sodium, Potassium, Creatinine, WBC count, Acute renal failure (yes/no), organ system insufficiency or immonocompromised.*
  - The main advantage of the APACHE-II scoring system is the immediate assessment of the severity of pancreatitis.
  - A score of eight or more at admission is usually considered indicative of severe disease
- **Glasgow criteria:** The Glasgow criteria are valid for both gallstone and alcohol induced pancreatitis, whereas the Ranson score is only for alcohol induced pancreatitis. If a patient scores 3 or more it indicates severe pancreatitis and the patient should be transferred to ITU. It is scored through the mnemonic, PANCREAS:
  - P – PaO_2 <8kPa
  - A – Age >55 years old
  - N – Neutrophilia - WCC >15 × 10(9)/L
  - C – Calcium <2 mmol/L
  - R – Renal function, Urea >16 mmol/L
  - E – Enzymes: LDH >600 iu/L; AST >200 iu/L
  - A – Albumin <32 g/L (serum)
  - S – Sugar: blood glucose >10 mmol/L
- **BISAP score:**
  - Bedside index of severity in acute pancreatitis is a new prognostic scoring system as accurate as other scoring systems.
  - Calculated with in 24 hour
  - Scored on a scale of 0 to 5
  - Score of >3 or more indicates severe pancreatitis

  1. BUN > 25
  2. Impaired Mental Status
  3. Systemic inflammatory response (>2 criteria)
  4. Age > 60 years
  5. Pleural effusion on CT

- **Biochemical markers**
  - Although serum enzymes such as amylase and lipase are helpful in the diagnosis of pancreatitis, these have no prognostic value.
  - Severalrecentresearchstudieshavesuggestedadditional markers that may have prognostic value, including acute phase proteins such as C-reactive protein (CRP> 150 mg/dl at 48 hours of onset od symptoms is and independent predictor of severity and is the most accurate indicator of severe pancreatitis, along with an impaired general condition and CECT findings), $alpha_2$-macroglobulin, polymorphonuclear neutrophil–elastase, alpha1-antitrypsin, and phospholipase A2.
  - Although CRP measurement is commonly available, many of the others are not. Therefore, at this time, CRP seems to be the marker of choice in clinical settings.
  - The measurement of IL-6 has recently been shown to distinguish patients with mild or severe forms of the disease. However, these tests have to undergo large-scale evaluations before they can be recommended for routine use.
  - Another prognostic marker under evaluation is urinary–trypsinogen activation peptide (TAP).

Washington Manual of Critical Care 2ND ED Table 50.3 Single factor on admission associated with severe acute pancreatitis

- Hematocrit > 44%
- Obesity
- CRP > 150 mg/dL
- Albumin < 2.5 mg/dL
- Calcium < 8.5 mg/dL
- Early hyperglycemia

- **Computed tomography severity score (CTSI):** CT scanning with bolus IV contrast has become the gold standard for detecting and assessing the severity of pancreatitis. Currently, IV (bolus) contrast-enhanced CT scanning is routinely performed on patients who are suspected of harbouring severe pancreatitis, regardless of their Ranson's or APACHE scores. **Maximum score 10 (> 6 indicates severe pancreatitis)**. The numerical CTSI has a maximum of ten points, and is the sum of the Balthazar grade points and pancreatic necrosis grade points:

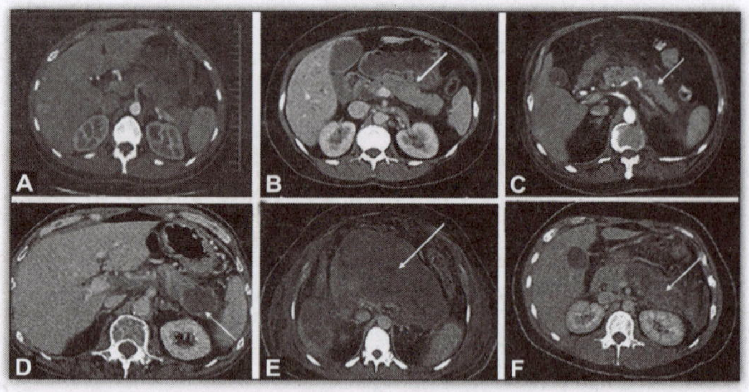

Fig: Balthazar CT score of Pancreatitis: (A) Normal CT Abdomen: Balthazar Grade, **(B) Balthazar Grade B:** Focal/ diffuse enlargement of pancreas (arrow), **(C) Balthazar Grade C:** Peripancreatic inflammation (arrow), **(D) Balthazar Grade D:** Fluid collection at single location (arrow), **(E) Balthazar Grade E:** Gas bubbles (arrow), **(F) Pancreatic necrosis** > 50%, 6 points

Computed Tomography Severity Score (CTSI)

Balthazar grade	Appearance on CT	CT grade points
Grade A	Normal CT	0 points
Grade B	Focal or diffuse enlargement of the pancreas	1 point
Grade C	Pancreatic gland abnormalities and peripancreatic inflammation	2 points

Contd...

Grade D	Fluid collection in a single location	3 points
Grade E	Two or more fluid collections and / or gas bubbles in or adjacent to pancreas	4 points
Necrosis Score		
Necrosis score		**Points**
No necrosis		0 points
0 to 30% necrosis		2 points
30 to 50% necrosis		4 points
Over 50% necrosis		6 points

83. Ans. (a) IV fluids and antibiotics followed by laparotomy

Ref: Bailey 26th ed page 1171

Gas under the right diaphragm is characteristic of intestinal perforation. Under the left diaphragm Gastric shadow is visible which is normal. Patient is Hemodynamically unstable and hence cannot be taken to the Laparotomy immediately. Patient needs to be Optimized first with IV fluids, NG tube and Antibiotics before taking to the Laparotomy and repair.

- Before the 1980s, duodenal perforation due to peptic ulcer disease was the most common form of small bowel perforation. Today, iatrogenic injury incurred during GI endoscopy is the most common cause of small bowel perforation
- CT scanning is the most sensitive test for diagnosing duodenal perforations

84. Ans. (c) Completely absent

Ref: Harrisons 19th ed page no 280, Algappan Manual of Practical Medicine 4th edition page 308, Sherlock's Diseases of the Liver and Biliary System 12th Ed page 210

Indirect repeat Surgery AIIMS NOV 2015 (Role reversal between Option and Question "In which type of Jaundice Urobilinogen is completely absent"?)

Urobilinogen

Urobilinogen is produced by bacterial breakdown of bilirubin excreted in bile into the bowel. It is partly absorbed in the bowel and undergoes hepatobiliary recirculation. The fraction that is not cleared by the liver enters the general circulation and is partly excreted in urine.

Increased Urobilinogen	Decreased Urobilinogen
• Excessive bilirubin production (e.g. in cases of hemolysis or absorption of hematoma) • Inefficient hepatic clearance of the reabsorbed urobilinogen (e.g. in patients with cirrhosis or at some stages of hepatitis) • Excessive exposure of bilirubin to intestinal bacteria (e.g. constipation or bacterial overgrowth).	Near complete biliary obstruction (e.g. carcinoma of the pancreas) or severe cholestasis (e.g. in early stages of viral hepatitis).

Standard clinical tests for urobilinogen do not distinguish between normal and low urinary urobilinogen levels.

Furthermore, urobilinogen excretion can be reduced, normal, or elevated in patients with hepatitis as noted above. Tubular reabsorption and instability of the pigment in acid urine can also influence results. Because of these complexities, tests for urinary urobilinogen are usually not useful in the differential diagnosis of liver diseases.

Types of Jaundice			
Features	**Prehepatic or hemolytic**	**Hepatic or hepatocellular**	**Posthepatic or obstructive**
Mechanism	Increased Bilirubin production	Hepatocellular failure	Bile duct obstruction
Common cause	Haemolysis	Virus, drugs, alcohol	Ca pancreas, gallbladder
Onset	Rapid	Gradual	Gradual
Symptoms	Anemia, fever	Anorexia, nausea, vomiting, Distaste	Recurrent abdominal colic, fluctuating jaundice
Skin	Mild yellow	Orange	Greenish yellow
Urine	Colorless (absent bile pigment)	High colored	Dark colored (Presence of Bile pigment)
Uobilinogen	++	+	Absent
Pruritus	Nil	+	+++
Bradycadia	Nil	Rare	+
Stool	Normal	Pale	Clay colored
Serum bilirubin	Unconjugated	Both conjugated and unconjugated	Conjugated
AST and ALT	Normal	Grossly elevated	Slightly elevated
Serum alkaline phosphatase	Normal	Slightly elevated	Grossly elevated
GGT	Normal	Normal or Increased	Increased

Contd...

Types of Jaundice			
Features	**Prehepatic or hemolytic**	**Hepatic or hepatocellular**	**Posthepatic or obstructive**
5' Nucleotidase	Normal	Normal or Increased	Grossly Increased
Serum albumin	Normal	Decrease	Normal
Prothrombin time	Normal	Increased	Normal
Coomb's test	Positive	–	–
Osmotic fragility	Increased	–	–
Spleen	++	+/–	–
Gallbladder	Not palpable	Not palpable	Not palpable

Central Features of the Common Types of Acute Jaundice				
	Gallstones in common bile duct	**Carcinoma in port-ampullary region**	**Acute viral hepatitis**	**Cholestatic drug jaundice**
Antecedent history	Dyspepsia, previous attack	Nil	Contacts, injections, transfusion or nil	Taking drug
Pain	Constant epigastric, billary colic or none	Constant epigastric, back or none	Ache over liver or none	None
Pruritus	±	+	Translate	+
Rate of development of jaundice	Slow	Slow	Rapid	Rapid
Type of jaundice	Fluctuates or persistent	Usual but not always	Rapid onset, slow fall with recovery	Variable, usually mild
Weight loss	Slight to moderate	Progressive	Slight	Slight
Examination Diathesis	Frequently female, obese	Over 40 year old	Young usually	Often older female, psychotic
Depth of jaundice	Moderate	Deep	Variable	Variable, rash sometimes
Ascites	0	Rarely with metastases	If severe and prolonged	0
Liver	Enlarged, slightly tender	Enlarged, not tender	Enlarged and tender	Slightly enlarged
Palpable gallbladder	0	+ (sometimes)	0	0
Tender gallbladder area	+	0	0	0
Palpable spleen	0	Occasionally	About 20%	0
Temperature	↑	Not usually	↑ onset only	↑ onset
Investigations Leucocytes count	↑ or normal	↑ or normal	↓	Normal
Differential leukocytes	Polymorphs ↑	–	Lymphocytes↑	Eosinophilia at onset
Faeces Color	Intermittently pale	Pale	Variable, light to dark	Pale
Occult blood	0	±	0	0
Urine: urobilin (ogen)	+	Absent	– Early + Late	– Early
Serum bilirubin (μmol/l)	Usually 50–170	Steady rise to 250–500	Varies with severity	Variable
Serum alkaline phosphatase (times normal)	>3×	>3×	<3×	>3×
Serum aspartate transaminase (times normal)	<5×	<5×	>10×	>5×
Ultrasound and CT	Gallstones + dilated duct	Dilated ducts + mass	Splenomegaly	Normal

AIIMS NOVEMBER 2015

85. Ans. (b) Obstructive Jaundice

Ref: Harrisons 19th ed page 280, Algappan Manual of Practical Medicine 4th edition page 308, Sherlock's Diseases of the Liver and Biliary System 12th Ed page 210

Indirect repeat Surgery AIIMS MAY 2016 (Role reversal between Option and Question "Urobilinogen levels in Obstructed Jaundice due to gall stones will be?)

See previous question for explanation

86. Ans. (b) Periampullary carcinoma

Ref: Maingot 11th ed ch 41, Practicals And Viva In Surgery By Ghosal page 94

Waxing and Waning course of Jaundice is characteristically seen in Periampullay carcinoma. Tumor increases in size in duodenal lumen and necrosis occurs in the tumor, as a result some portion of tumor is sloughed out and obstruction is relieved and Jaundice wanes. At the time of sloughing there is hemorrhage so Melaena occurs. Again tumor increases in size and obstructs the ampulla, leading to waxing of jaundice

Periampullary cancers include a group of malignant neoplasms arising in the pancreas or in or near the ampulla of Vater. They are usually discovered because of obstructive jaundice or pain

Periampullary carcinoma includes

- Carcinoma of Head of pancreas near ampulla (2–3 cm) 40-60%-most common
- Carcinoma of Ampulla of vater - 20–40%
- Distal Bile duct carcinoma- 10%
- Duodenal carcinoma, near Ampulla - 10%

Differential Diagnosis of Obstructive Jaundice					
	Obstructive Jaundice				
	Periampullary carcinoma	Carcinoma head of pancreas	CBD stones	Cholangitis	Carcinoma gallbladder
Jaundice	Waxing waning	Progressive	Progressive (less than malignant disease)	Intermittent as part of Chacot's triad	+ Pota hepatis LN hartmann pouch on mouth
Melena	++	No	No	–	–
Gallbladder	Palpable, cyctic, globular	Palpable, cyctic	Non palpable	–	+ Hard, firm
Pain	Painless or dull aching epigastric	Painless	Colicky pain, radiates to back, shoulder, right chest followed by Dull aching	Intermittent as part of Charcot's triad	Colicky initially followed by dull aching later
Fever	–	–	+ with chills and Rigors	+ intermittent as part of charcot's triad	–

87. Ans. (c) 15 and 3

Ref: Bailey 26th Ed Pg 321, Schwartz 10th ed page 168 – 170, Harrison 19th ed page 260

Teasdale and Jennett published the Glasgow Coma Scale (GCS) in the Lancet in 1974 as an aid in the clinical assessment of post traumatic unconsciousness. The original GCS has three components: eye (E), verbal (V) and motor (M) response to external stimuli. The best or highest responses are recorded. The scale consisted of 14 points, but was later adapted to 15, with the division of the motor category 'flexion to pain' into two further categories

NOTE

- Glasgow Coma Scale (GCS) score ranges from 3 to 15. But in intubated patients (no verbal score is possible), the GCS can range from 3T to 10T (T stands for intubation)
- Pediatric Glasgow coma scale (PGCS) applies to child less then 2 years old

The Glasgow Coma Scale Score[a]							
		1	2	3	4	5	6
Eyes (same for adults & pediatric)		No eye opening	Opens to painful stimuli	Opens to speech	Opens spontaneously	N/A	N/A
Verbal	**Pediatric**	No verbal response	Inconsolable, agitated	Inconsistently inconsolable, moaning	Cries but consolable, inappropriate interactions	Smiles, orients to sounds, follows objects, interacts	N/A
	Adult	No sounds	Un intelligible sounds	Inappropriate words	Confused	Oriented	
Motor	**Pediatric**	No motor response	Extension to pain (decerebrate response)	Abnormal flexion to pain (decorticate response)	Withdraws from pain	Withdraws from touch	Moves spontaneously or purposefully
	Adult	No motor response	Extensor posturing	Flexor posturing	Withdraws from pain	Localizes to pain	Obeys command

[a] Add the three scores to obtain the Glasgow Coma Scale (GCS) score, which can range from 3 to 15. Add "T" after the GCS if intubated and no verbal score is possible. For these patients, the GCS can range from 3T to 10T.

Classification of Head Injury Severity	
Classification	**Range of glasgow coma scale score**
Mild	GCS ≥13
Moderate	9 ≤ GCS ≤12
Severe	GCS ≤8

88. Ans. (a) Subdermal lymphatic obstruction

Ref: Bailey 26th ed page 812, 816

Recall Bias

Some people recalled that one option was Skin edema. In that case Skin or dermal edema is the most appropriate answer.

Peau d' orange (French-skin of an orange; orange peel appearance) is due to dermal edema caused by obstruction of the superficial cutaneous lymphatics by the tumor cells. Occasionally, the same phenomenon is seen over a chronic abscessWhere the infiltrated skin is tethered by the sweat ducts it cannot swell, leading to an appearance like orange skin.

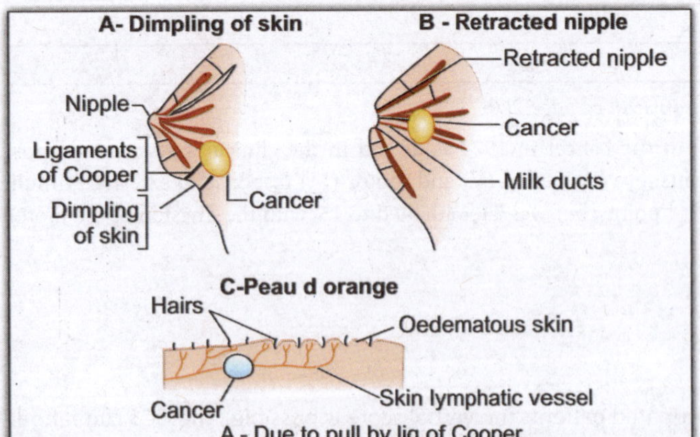

A - Due to pull by lig of Cooper
B - Due to retraction of milk ducts
C - Due to lymphatic obstruction

89. Ans. (b) Indirect inguinal hernia

Ref: Bailey 26th ed page 955

This question is based on the anatomy of Hesselbach's triangle and the hernias of Inguinal Region

Legends:

- Indirect inguinal hernia
- Direct inguinal hernia
- Femoral hernia

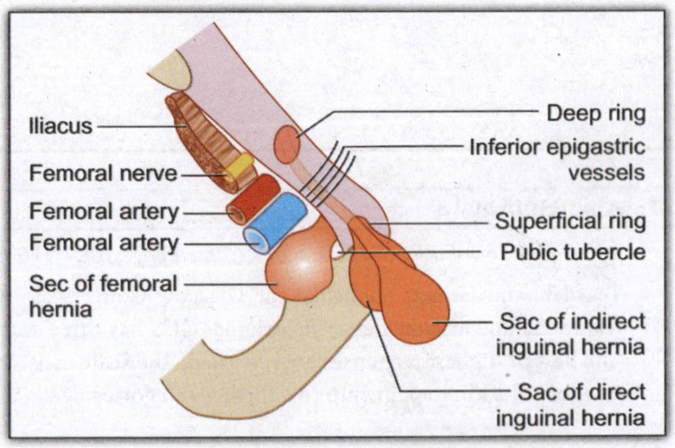

An indirect hernia is lateral as its origin is lateral to the inferior epigastric vessels. It is also oblique as the hernia passes obliquely from lateral to medial through the abdominal muscle layers. Direct inguinal hernia enters through medial half of weak posterior wall (Hesselbach's triangle) and becomes superficial through superficial inguinal ring

Hasselbach's Triangle

- **Medial border:** Lateral margin the rectus sheath, also called linea semilunaris
- **Superolateral border:** Inferior epigastric vessels
- **Inferior border:** Inguinal ligament, sometimes referred to as Poupart's ligament

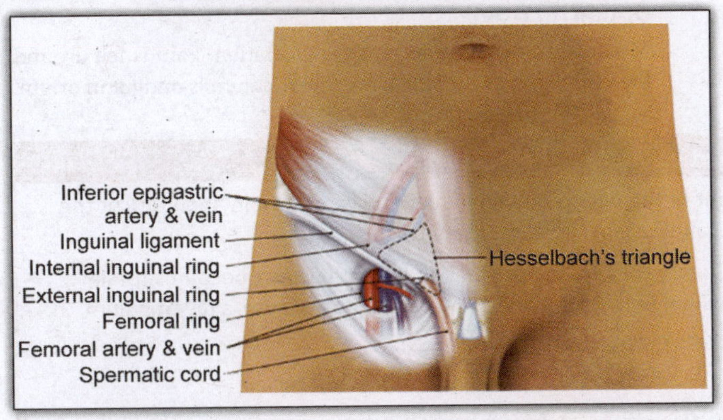

90. Ans. (c) Hernial sac contains greater omentum only

Ref: Bailey 26th ed page 955, Schwartz 9th ed ch 37

This is a case of Congenital Inguinal hernia.

The first lines of the practice of surgery 7th ed By Samuel Cooper Page 574; **In young children, the congenital hernia more frequently contains intestine than omentum, because in them the latter part is very short.**

Bailey says: The congenital inguinal hernia is known as indirect, oblique or lateral while the acquired hernia is called direct or medial

Schwartz says: Congenital hernias, which make up the majority of pediatric hernias, can be considered an impedance of normal development, rather than an acquired weakness. During the normal course of development, the testes descend from the intra-abdominal space into the scrotum in the third trimester. Their descent is preceded by the gubernaculum and a diverticulum of peritoneum, which protrudes through the inguinal canal and ultimately becomes the processus vaginalis. Between 36 and 40 weeks, the processus vaginalis closes and eliminates the peritoneal opening at the internal inguinal ring. Failure of the peritoneum to close results in a ***patent processus vaginalis (PPV)*** and thus explains the high incidence of indirect inguinal hernias in preterm babies. It should be noted that the processus vaginalis continues to close as the child ages, with most closing within the first few months of life. Children with congenital indirect inguinal hernias will present with a PPV; however, its presence does not necessarily indicate an inguinal hernia

91. Ans. (b) Urine output

Ref: Bailey 26th ed page 17, British Journal of Anesthesia

Shock Monitoring

The *minimum standard for monitoring of the patient in shock is continuous heart rate and oxygen saturation monitoring, frequent non-invasive blood pressure monitoring and hourly urine output measurements.* Most patients will need more aggressive invasive monitoring, including central venous pressure and invasive blood pressure monitoring.

Bailey states "Ultimately, the goal of treatment is to restore cellular and organ perfusion. Ideally, therefore, monitoring of organ perfusion should guide the management of shock. **The best measures of organ perfusion and the best monitor of the adequacy of shock therapy remains the urine output."**

Monitoring of Patient in Shock	
Minimal	**Additional modalities**
ECG	Central venous pressure
Pulse oximetry	Invasive blood pressure
Blood pressure	Cardiac output
Urine output	Base deficit and serum lactate

Central Venous Pressure

Patients whose state of shock is not rapidly corrected with a small amount of fluid should have central venous pressure monitoring and continuous blood pressure monitoring through an arterial line.

Low CVP always means hypovolemia, but high CVP can signify either over expansion of blood volume or cardiac failure.

There is no 'normal' central venous pressure (CVP) for a shocked patient, and reliance cannot be placed on an individual pressure measurement to assess volume status. Some patients may require a CVP of 5 cm H_2O, whereas some may require a CVP of 15 cm H_2O or higher. Further, ventricular compliance can change from minute to minute in the shocked state, and CVP is a poor reflection of end diastolic volume (preload). **CVP measurements should be assessed dynamically as response to a fluid challenge.** A fluid bolus (250–500 mL) is infused rapidly over 5–10 minutes. The normal CVP response is a rise of 2–5 cm H_2O which gradually drifts back to the original level over 10–20 minutes. **Patients with no change in their CVP are empty and require further fluid resuscitation.** Patients with a large, sustained rise in CVP have high preload and an element of cardiac insufficiency or volume overload.

Resuscitation requires appropriate fluid management and is dependent on the cause of shock and the time course of the illness. For example, in hypovolaemic shock with a low CVP, fluid replacement is required. In contrast, in cardiogenic shock due to left-sided heart failure (i.e. with a raised CVP), diuretic therapy with fluid restriction may be indicated. To complicate matters further, cardiogenic shock due to right-sided heart failure (i.e. also with a raised CVP) may require fluid administration to ensure adequate filling of, and cardiac output from, the left side of the heart! The time course of the disease is also important. For example, at the onset of septic shock, fluid replacement is essential, but, if acute respiratory distress syndrome develops later, fluid restriction is necessary to prevent pulmonary oedema. **(Ref: Oxford Desk Reference: Acute Medicine edited by Richard Leach, Kevin Moore, Derek Bell).**

92. Ans. (a) 3% of population; (b) 3 inch long; (c) Remnant of distal part of vitello intestinal duct

Ref: Maingot 11th ed ch, Bailey 26th ed page 1169, Sabiston 19th ed page 1268 -1270, Schwartz 9th Ed Ch 28, Sutton 7th Ed Pg 631

Recall Bias

More than 4 options are recalled. Hence we will be discussing all recalled options

Option (A) False

A Meckel's diverticulum is a persistent remnant of the vitellointestinal duct and is present in about 2% of the population.

Option (B) False

Meckel's diverticulum is classically 5 cm long (2 inches).

Option (C) False

Meckel's diverticulum represents the remnant of the proximal part of the intestino-vitelline duct.

Option (D) True

Meckel's is found on the antimesenteric side of the ileum

Option (E) True

Meckel's diverticulum is 60 cm (2 foot) from the ileocaecal valve.

Option (F) True

Meckel's may present as chronic ulceration. Pain is felt around the umbilicus, as the site of the diverticulum is midgut in origin.

Meckel's Diverticulum	
Definition	A Meckel's diverticulum is a persistent remnant of the vitellointestinal duct and is present in about 2% of the population. It is the most common congenital anomaly of the alimentary tract
Embryology	In fetal life the umbilicus is connected to the gut by the vitellointestinal duct. Further duct becomes totally obliterated and vanishes. The bowel end (Proximal end) of the duct may persist as a Meckel's diverticulum.

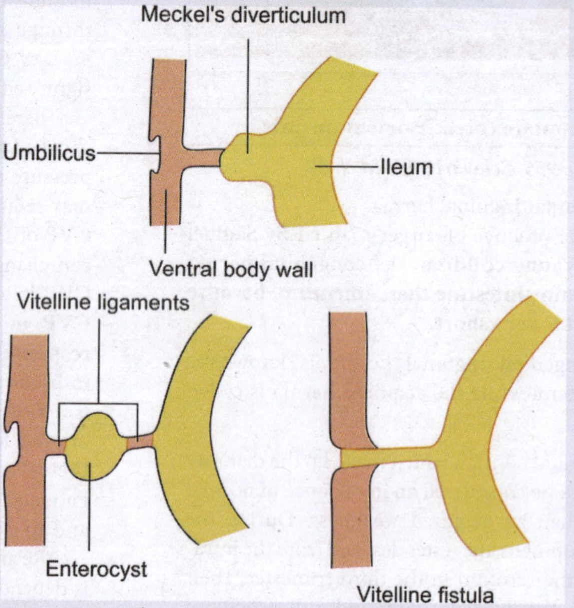

Epidemiology	Present in 2% population
Anatomy	• It is found on the antimesenteric side of the ileum, commonly at 60 cm **(2 foot) from the ileocaecal valve** and is classically 5 cm long **(2 Inches)** • A Meckel's diverticulum contains all three coats of the bowel wall and has its own blood supply.
Clinical features	In around **20% of cases**, the mucosa of a Meckel's diverticulum contains heterotopic epithelium of gastric, colonic or pancreatic type. • Vast majority of Meckel's diverticula are **asymptomatic** unless associated complications • **Haemorrhage:** If gastric mucosa is present, peptic ulceration can occur and present as painless maroon rectal bleeding or melaena. Most common presentation in children • **Diverticulitis:** Present in 20% of patients with symptomatic Meckel's diverticula, is associated with a clinical syndrome that is indistinguishable from acute appendicitis, although if perforation occurs the presentation may resemble a perforated duodenal ulcer. • **Intussusception:** A Meckel's can be the lead point for ileoileal or ileocolic intussusception. • **Chronic ulceration:** Pain is felt around the umbilicus, as the site of the diverticulum is midgut in origin. • **Intestinal obstruction:** A band between the apex of the diverticulum and the umbilicus. Most common presentation in adults • **Perforation.** • **Neoplasms**, most commonly carcinoid tumors, are present in 0.5 to 3.2% of symptomatic Meckel's diverticula that are resected.

Contd...

Meckel's Diverticulum	
Diagnosis	Most Meckel's diverticula are discovered incidentally on radiographic imaging, during endoscopy, or at the time of surgery. In the absence of bleeding, Meckel's diverticula rarely are diagnosed before the time of surgical intervention. **Meckel's diverticulum is infrequently visualised on contrast studies, even when carefully sought, and scintigraphic techniques are more useful for diagnosis.** • Plain radiography, barium studies, angiography, computed tomography (CT), ultrasonography, and scintigraphy all play complementary roles in the diagnosis of the complications of Meckel diverticulum. • **Radionuclide scans (99mTc-pertechnetate) can be helpful in the diagnosis of Meckel's diverticulum; this test is, however, positive only when the diverticulum contains associated ectopic gastric mucosa that is capable of uptake of the tracer. The accuracy of radionuclide scanning is reported to be 90% in pediatric patients but less than 50% in adults.** • The diagnosis is notoriously difficult and remains a continuing challenge for the radiologist. • In all imaging modalities, findings of Meckel diverticulum are nonspecific.
	• **Most Meckel diverticula are diagnosed during surgery or autopsy, with imaging playing a secondary role.** • **The most sensitive technique is scintigraphy, and various modifications to imaging techniques have been devised to improve sensitivity**. Ultrasonography and CT are improving and can help in making an anatomic diagnosis. • **Diagnosis of ectopic gastric mucosa using $^{99}Tc^{m}$-pertechnetate:** Meckel's diverticulum. $^{99}Tc^{m}$-pertechnetate scintigraphy images showing focal area of intense abnormal tracer accumulation in the hypogastrium appearing at the same time as gastric mucosal uptake, this pattern is characteristic of Meckel's diverticulum. The Tc-99 is taken up by gastric mucosa (hence positive in the region of stomach- black areas in the picture). A black area is also seen in the region of the intestines. it signifies **ectopic gastric mucosa, suggestive of Meckel's diverticulum.**
Management	When found in the course of abdominal surgery, a Meckel's can safely be left alone provided it has a wide mouth and is not thickened. **Meckel's diverticulectomy**: A broad-based Meckel's diverticulum should not be amputated at its base and invaginated (as for an appendix), as there is the risk of stricture and of leaving heterotopic epithelium behind. It is safer simply to excise the diverticulum, either by resecting it and suturing the defect at its base, or with a linear stapler-cutter.

MNEMONIC **RULE OF 2 =** Occurs in 2 per cent of patients, 2 inches (5 cm long), 2 feet (60 cm) from the ileocaecal valve, 20 per cent heterotopic epithelium

93. Ans. (b) Hand washing

Ref: Bailey 26th ed page 51, 62

Hand washing is the simplest and most effective measure to prevent infection.

Scrubbing

'Scrubbing up' is the process of washing the hands and arms prior to donning a gown and gloves, to minimise the microbial loads on parts of the surgical staff that might come into contact with the patient.

- Time spent scrubbing varies from unit to unit but as a general rule surgeons in training should usually start scrubbing before, and finish after, the senior surgeon.
- Excessive time or vigour in scrubbing may cause breakdown of the skin with an increased risk of infection. As a result, some centers are now adopting the use of water-free, spirit-based antiseptic solutions.
- All sterile team members should perform the hand and arm scrub before entering the surgical suite. The basic principle of the scrub is to wash the hands thoroughly, and then to wash from a clean area (the hand) to a less clean area (the arm).
- There are two methods of scrub procedure. One is a numbered stroke method, in which a certain number of brush strokes are designated for each finger, palm, back of hand, and arm. The alternative method is the timed scrub, and each scrub should last from three to five minutes, depending on facility protocol.

Scrub Technique

- You should not scrub if you have an open wound or an infection. (Uninfected cuts or abrasions can be covered after a routine scrub-up process by applying a sterile clear dressing before gloving)
- All jewellery on the hands should be removed.
- If hands are visibly soiled, wash hands with a plain soap before surgical hand preparation
- A theatre hat, mask and eye protection should be fitted so that no hair is exposed and you are protected from splashback.
- Artificial nails are prohibited
- Before starting, ensure that your facemask is comfortable and secure (this is non-sterile so cannot be adjusted once you are scrubbed)
- A sterile scrubbing brush and nail cleaner are used for 1–2 min to remove dirt from under the nails and from deep creases in the skin. Keep natural nails short (tips less than 0.5 cm long)

- When performing surgical hand antisepsis using an antimicrobial soap, scrub hands and forearms for the length of time recommended by the manufacturer, 2 to 5 min. Long scrub times (e.g. 10 min) are not necessary
- When using an alcohol-based surgical hand rub product with sustained activity, follow the manufacturer's instructions. Apply the product on dry hands only. Do not combine surgical hand scrub and surgical hand rub with alcohol-based products sequentially. After application of the alcohol-based product, allow hands and forearms to dry thoroughly before donning sterile gloves
- Surgical hand antisepsis should be performed using either an antimicrobial soap or an alcohol-based hand rub. The hands are then washed systematically, paying special attention to the clefts between the fingers. This should be carried out on at least two further occasions, extending up the forearms to just below the elbows. After applying disinfectant, the arms are washed from distal to proximal, with hands up and elbows flexed to avoid/minimise any contamination from the more proximal 'unclean' areas.
- Following the final rinse the hands and arms should be raised to face level, away from the body. This allows water to drop from the elbows.
- The hands and arms should be dried using a sterile towel for each side. Drying with each towel should start with the fingers and work across the hand and up the arm. The towel should then be discarded
- The first scrub up of the day, therefore, should take about 5 min from start to drying.
- If the surgeon stays within the theatre suite and there are no significant external contacts or contamination, subsequent scrub up will be shorter, with no need for the use of the nail cleaner or brush.
- If the scrubbing procedure is interrupted, e.g. by touching the tap, the scrubbing procedure should be restarted.

Surgical Hand Preparation Technique Using Alcohol Based Hand Rub (ABHR)

- Put approximately 5 mL (3 doses) of alcohol-based hand rub in the palm of your left hand, using the elbow of your other arm to operate the dispenser
- Dip the fingertips of your right hand in the hand rub to decontaminate under the nails (5 seconds).
- Smear the hand rub on the right forearm up to the elbow. Ensure that the whole skin area is covered by using circular movements around the forearm until the hand rub has fully evaporated (10-15 seconds). Repeat for opposite hand and arm
- Put approximately 5 mL (3 doses) of alcohol-based handrub in the palm of your left hand, using the elbow of your other arm to operate the distributor. Rub both hands in the same time up to the wrists. Repeat for opposite hand and arm
- Cover the whole surface of the hands up to the wrist with alcohol-based hand rub, rubbing palm against palm with a rotating movement.
- Rub the back of the hands up to the wrist with alcohol-based handrub, rubbing palm against palm with a rotating movement.
- Rub the back of the left hand, including the wrist, moving the right palm back and forth and vice-versa.
- Rub palm against palm back and forth with fingers interlinked.
- Rub the thumb of the left hand by rotating it in the clasped palm of the right hand and vice versa.
- When the hands are dry, sterile surgical clothing and gloves can be donned.

94. Ans. (c) Rough handling during surgery

Ref: : Sabiston 18th ed ch 36, Stoelting's coexisting Diseases 7th Ed page 461, Harrison 19th ed page 2297

Repeat AIIMS Nov 2018 (See for explanation) (see page no. 925)

95. Ans. (c) Genitofemoral nerve

Ref: Schwartz 9th ed page ch 37, Gray's 41st ed page 1096

Both Lateral cutaneous nerve and Genitofemoral nerve can be injured luring Laparoscopic hernia repair. Genitofemoral nerve injury causes loss of sensation on medial side while Lateral cutaneous nerve causes loss of sensation of Lateral side of thigh.

In laparoscopic inguinal surgery, the iliopubic tract is an important anatomic feature. Lateral to the spermatic vessels, and ***immediately below the fibers of the iliopubic tract, are the genital and femoral branches of the genitofemoral nerve, the femoral nerve and the lateral femoral cutaneous nerve.*** Consequently, clips placed below the iliopubic tract and lateral to the femoral vessels may cause temporary or permanent neuralgias, involving one or more of the nerve branches mentioned above. (Ref: Annibali R, Fitzgibbons RJ. Surgical anatomy of the inguinal region and lower abdominal wall: the laparoscopic perspective. 80 Annual Clinical Congress, American College of Surgeons, Chicago, 1994)

The femoral branch of the genitofemoral nerve is found lateral to the genital branch and is seen leaving the retroperitoneum underneath the iliopubic tract. Also found laterally, and sometimes in association with the femoral branch of the genitofemoral nerve, is the lateral cutaneous nerve of the thigh. After emerging from the lateral edge of the psoas muscle, it, too, leaves the retroperitoneum inferior to the iliopubic tract to innervate the anterolateral skin of the thigh. The ***femoral nerve is not routinely seen during laparoscopic inguinal hernia repair*** (Schwartz 9th ed page ch 37)

Being able to palpate a spiral tacker with the surgeon's other hand avoids placement of spiral tacks below the iliopubic tract, thereby ***avoiding injury to the lateral cutaneous nerve of the thigh or the femoral branch of the genitofemoral nerve.*** (Schwartz 9th ed page ch 37)

Laparoscopically, the lateral femoral cutaneous nerve and the genital and femoral branches of the genitofemoral nerve are at risk when placing lateral fixation tacks below the iliopubic tract, yet the lateral femoral cutaneous nerve may too be affected by mesh entrapment. Such ***injury to the lateral femoral cutaneous nerve will lead to meralgia paresthetica, a "pins and needles" sensation over the lateral aspect of the thigh.*** It also may be associated with a specific paresthesia known as formication (Schwartz 9th ed page ch 37)

Genitofemoral Nerve

The **genitofemoral nerve** originates from the **L1 and L2** ventral rami and is formed within the substance of psoas major.

- **Motor supply:** The genitofemoral nerve innervates **cremaster** via the genital branch.
- **Cutaneous supply:** The genitofemoral nerve innervates the skin of the **scrotum** in males or **mons pubis and labium majus** in females via the genital branch, and the **anteromedial skin of the thigh** via the femoral branch.

Nerve	Segment	Innervated Muscles	Cutaneous Branches
Iliohypogastric	T12-L1	Transversus abdominis, Abdominal internal oblique	Anterior cutaneous ramus, lateral cutaneous ramus
Ilioinguinal	L1		Anterior scrotal nerves in males, anterior labial nerves in females
Genitofemoral	L1, L2	Cremaster in males	Femoral ramus, genital ramus
Lateral femoral cutaneous (A.K.A Lateral cutaneous nerve of thigh)	L2, L3		Lateral femoral cutaneous is direct branch of lumbar plexus (Entrapment causes ***Meralgia paraesthetica; pain and paraesthesia on the anterolateral aspect of the thigh***)
Femoral	L2-L4	Anterior division: Sartorius, Pectineus Posterior division: iliacus, psoas, Quadriceps femoris	Intermediate cutaneous nerve of thigh (Br of ant division; L2-L3) Medial cutaneous nerve of thigh (Br of ant division; L2-L3) Saphenous nerve (Br of post division; L3-L4)

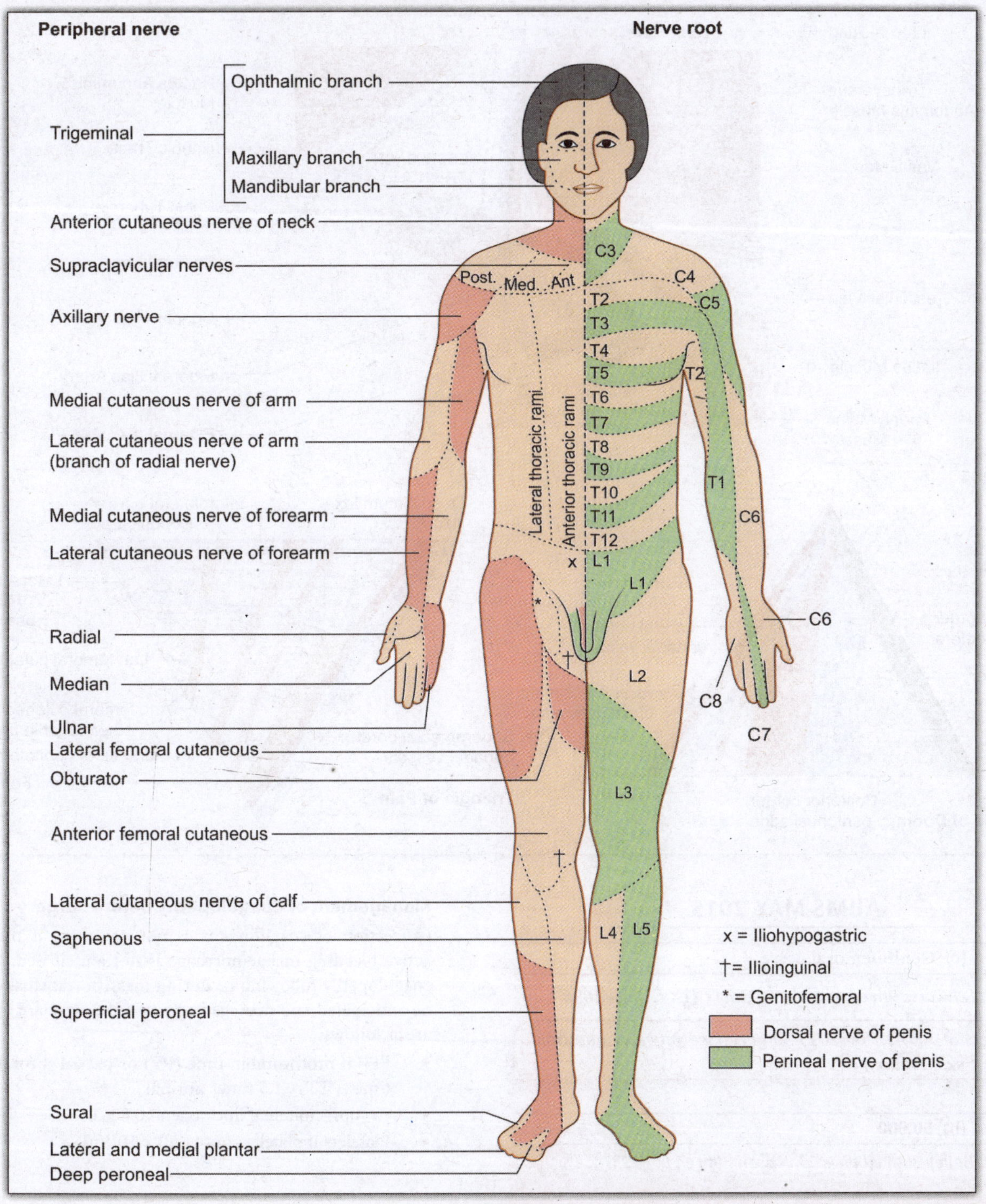

The posterior perspective has also resulted in the characterization of important areas to avoid. Basic knowledge of the boundaries of these triangles allows one to avert the dangers associated with injury to their contents

- **Triangle of doom:** The triangle of doom is bordered medially by the vas deferens and laterally by the vessels of the spermatic cord, thereby pointing its apex superiorly. The contents of the space include the external iliac vessels, deep circumflex iliac vein, femoral nerve, and genital branch of the genitofemoral nerve
- **Triangle of pain:** The triangle of pain can be conceptualized as the space bordered by the iliopubic tract and gonadal vessels. The structures within this space include nerves such as the lateral femoral cutaneous, femoral branch of the genitofemoral, and femoral.
- **Circle of death:** The circle of death is a vascular continuation formed by the common iliac, internal iliac, obturator, aberrant obturator, inferior epigastric, and external iliac vessels.

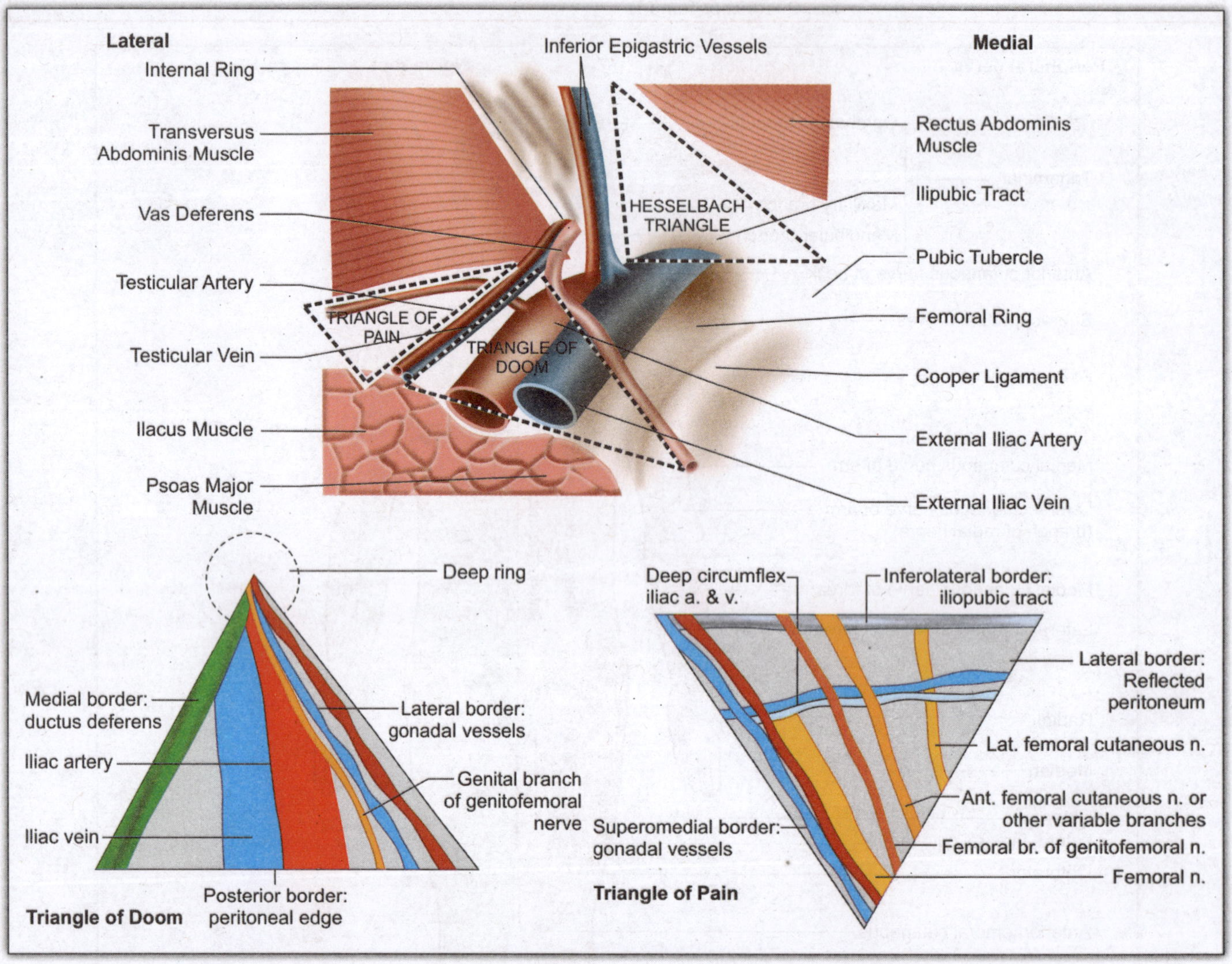

AIIMS MAY 2015

96. Ans. (c) Genitofemoral nerve

Ref: Schwartz 9th ed page ch 37, Gray's 41st ed page 1096

Repeat AIIMS Nov 2015 Surgery (See previous question for explanation)

97. Ans. (b) 50,000

Ref: Bailey 26th ed page 23, Nelson 20th ed page 2374

Management of Coagulopathy Before Surgery

Correction of coagulopathy is not necessary if there is no active bleeding or haemorrhage is not anticipated. However, coagulopathy following or during massive transfusion should be anticipated and managed aggressively. Standard guidelines are as follows:

- FFP if prothrombin time (PT) or partial thromboplastin time (PTT) >1.5 times normal
- Cryoprecipitate if fibrinogen <0.8 g/L
- Platelets if platelet count $<50 \times 10^9$/mL

98. Ans. (a) Left gastric artery

Ref: Bailey 26th ed page 994 Sabiston 19th ed page 1167, Schwartz9th ed page 875, 941, Harrison 19th ed page 277

Mallory-Weiss Syndrome

- It is seen in adults with severe prolonged vomiting, causing longitudinal tear in the mucosa of stomach at and just below the cardia, leading to severe haemate mesis.
- Violent vomiting often may be due to migraine or vertigo or following a bout of alcohol.
- Presents with severe vomiting and later haemate mesis, with features of shock.
- It is common in 1 o'clock position.
- Almost 90% of Mallory Weiss tears are located on the gastric side of the gastroesophageal junction.
- A bleeding **left gastric artery**, associated with a Mallory–Weiss tear, can be seen on arteriogram as well.

99. Ans. (d) T stage

Ref: Bailey 26th ed page 1004-1013, Sabiston 19th ed page 1049-1064, Robbin's 9th ed page 758

Long-term survival after esophagectomy depends on a number of factors, such as the depth of tumor invasion (T stage), the number of involved lymph nodes, and the location of the tumor in the esophagus. The prognosis is better for tumors of the cervical esophagus and for those located at the GEJ than for tumors located in the thoracic esophagus. The impact of the type of resection performed on long-term survival remains a subject of debate.

Detailed images of the esophageal wall by EUS make it the most accurate modality available for determination of the depth of tumor invasion (T) before treatment. The same definition of the esophageal wall is not offered by computed tomography (CT). A thickened esophageal wall, the principal CT finding in esophageal carcinoma, is not specific for esophageal carcinoma and lacks the definition required to distinguish T1, T2, and T3 tumors. In differentiation of T3 from T4 tumors, EUS is superior to CT.

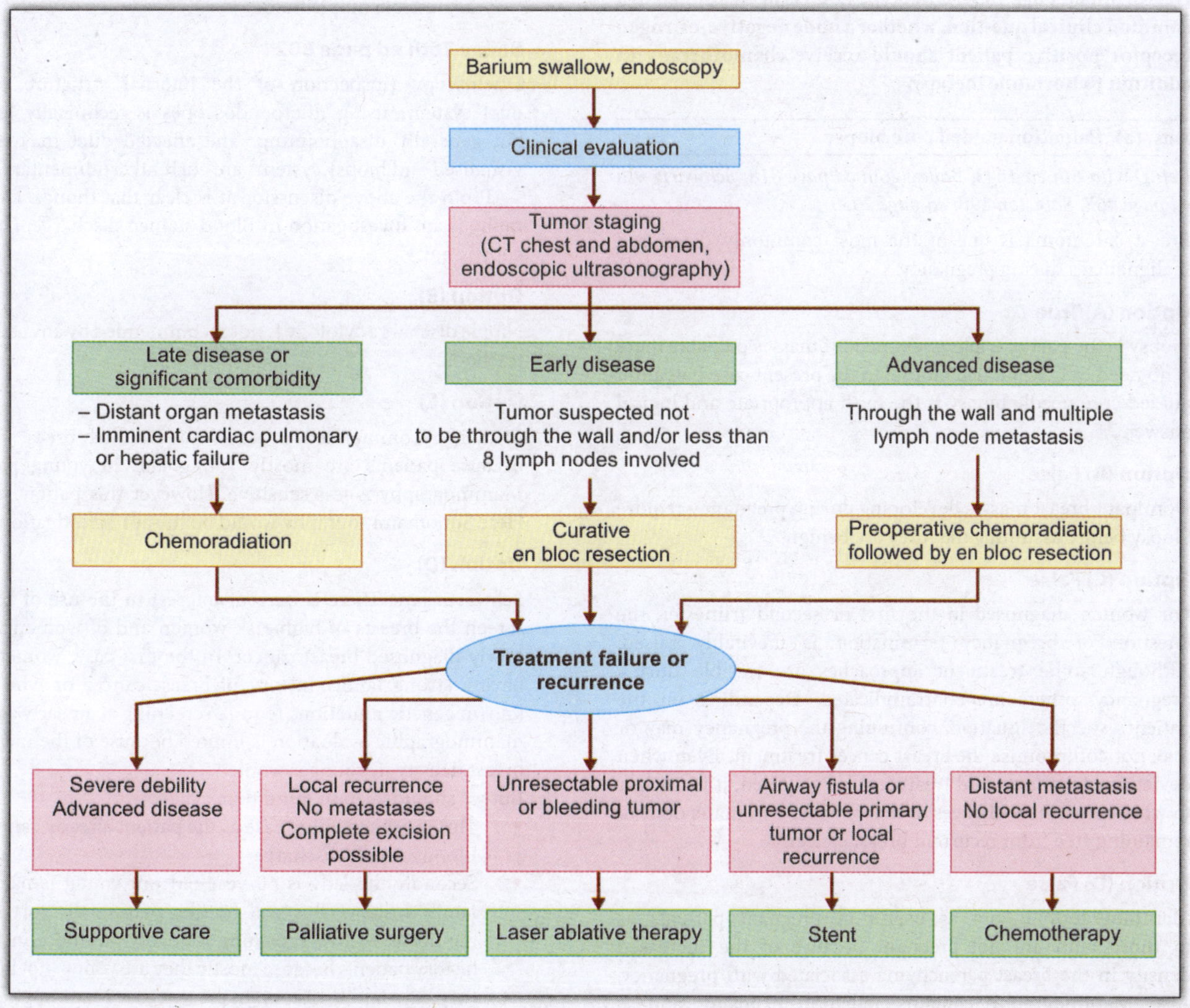

100. Ans. (a) Chemotherapy in hormone receptor positive patients

Ref: Devita 8th ed page 559, 778, Harrison 19th ed page 528, 101e.8

Harrison says; Commercial diagnostic tests, such as **Mamma-print and Oncotype DX** for breast cancer, are available to help the patients and their physicians make treatment decisions

Devita says; In newly diagnosed patients with **node-negative, estrogen-receptor positive breast cancer, the Oncotype DX assay can be used to predict the risk of recurrence in patients treated with tamoxifen.** The precise clinical utility and appropriate application for other multiparameter assays, such as the MammaPrint assay, the Rotterdam Signature, and the Breast Cancer Gene Expression Ratio are under investigation.

Oncotype DX candidate gene panel was first evaluated in NSABP B-20, wherein women with hormone receptor-positive, node-negative breast cancer were randomized to tamoxifen with or without CMF chemotherapy.

From the above discussion it appears that Hormone therapy in Hormone receptor positive is the answer but Giving hormone therapy in Hormone.

Receptor positive patient is no rocket science and nothing to be a clinical question that confuses a clinician. Not read following lines from Devita.

Devita 8th ed Page 1634; Oncotype DX has been applied to a common clinical question, whether a node negative, estrogen receptor positive patient should receive chemotherapy in addition to hormone therapy.

101. Ans. (a) Palpation guided core biopsy

Ref: Devita 8th ed 1643, Bailey 26th ed page 818, Schwartz 9th ed page 467, Sabiston 19th ed page 2035

Breast carcinoma is one of the most commonly diagnosed malignancies during pregnancy.

Option (A) True

Biopsy is the part of triple assessment. If mass is palpable there is no need of USG guided biopsy. In the present case Palpation guided core needle biopsy is the most appropriate and logical answer.

Option (B) False

Dominant breast masses developing during pregnancy require biopsy before assuming that they are benign.

Option (C) False

For women diagnosed in the first or second trimester, the question of pregnancy termination is inevitably raised. Although some treatment approaches are feasible during pregnancy, others are contraindicated. Depending on the patient's specific situation, continuing the pregnancy may or may not compromise the breast cancer treatment. Even when deviations from standard treatment are required, it is unclear to what extent such changes or delays affect a woman's odds of remaining free from recurrent breast cancer.

Option (D) False

Mammography is not as useful in pregnant patients as in those who are not pregnant because of the increased density in the breast parenchyma associated with pregnancy. Also Mammography contains radiation exposure and is contraindicated in pregnancy, especially 1st trimester.

102. Ans. (c) Sono Mammogram

Ref: Sabiston 19th ed page 832, Bailey 26th ed page 799-801

Option (A)

NOTE

Ductoscopy and Ductography are different entity

The primary indication for **ductography** is nipple discharge, particularly when the fluid contains blood. Radiopaque contrast media is injected into one or more of the major ducts and mammography is performed

Mammary ductoscopy is an endoscopic technique that allows for direct visualization and sampling of intraductal lesions. Ductoscopy provides a way to directly visualize and sample or excise lesions in the mammary ducts. The indications for performing a ductoscopy include:

- Pathologic nipple discharge from a single duct orifice (bloody or high-volume clear fluid)
- Known breast lesions (atypical ductal hyperplasia [ADH], ductal carcinoma in situ [DCIS], or invasive cancer) with expressible nipple fluid

Bailey 26th ed page 802

Ductoscopy (inspection of the internal structure of the duct system) using microendoscopes is technically feasible but generally disappointing. The affected duct may not be visualised and biopsy systems are currently rudimentary.

From the above discussion it is clear that though Ductography is apt investigation in Blood stained discharge, Ductoscopy is not.

Option (B)

Nipple discharge cytology is not recommended by any standard textbook.

Option (C)

MRI is recommended in cases of Familial breast cancer because patients are mostly young and in young patients Mammography is less sensitive. However this patient is Old. Here Sonomammography would be the apt investigation.

Option (D)

Schwartz says; There is current interest in the use of MRI to screen the breasts of high-risk women and of women with a newly diagnosed breast cancer. In the first case, women who have a strong family history of breast cancer or who carry known genetic mutations require screening at an early age, but mammographic evaluation is limited because of the increased breast density in younger women.

But we should keep in mind that

- This is not screening case as the patient already came with Bloody nipple discharge
- Secondly the lady is 60 year old not young female with family history. This will be like putting the cart before the horse. MRI is screening modality of choice in family history patients because mostly they are young, not because they have family history. In present case Mammography or Sono-Mammography will be good and cheaper.

103. Ans. (a) Circumferential

Ref: General Thoracic Surgery By Thomas W. Shields, Joseph LoCicero, Carolyn E. Reed, Richard H. Feins 7th ed page 692, Skandalakis' Surgical Anatomy Ch 8

Incisions on the diaphragm should be made to avoid injury to major branches of Phrenic nerve. Most satisfactory access is provided by the circumferential incision at the periphery of the diaphragm, which permits excellent exposure of the upper abdominal contents from the thorax and vice versa, with little or no possibility of phrenic nerve or any of its branch injury

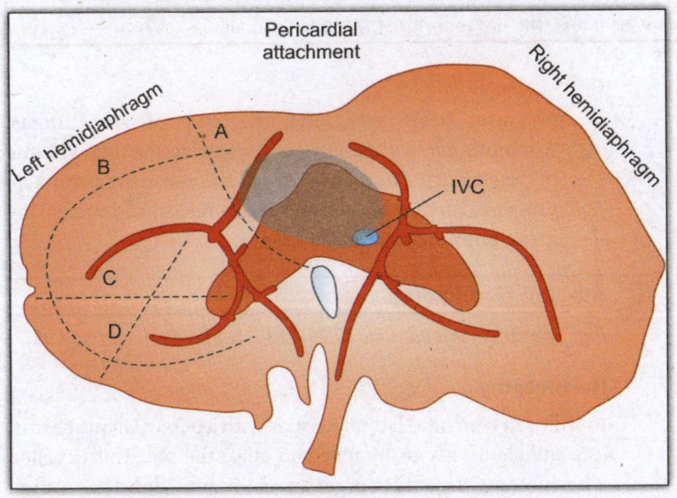

Fig. Dashed lines indicate incisions that will avoid phrenic nerves. **A.** The diaphragmatic component of a combined abdominothoracic incision extending down into the esophageal hiatus. **B.** Circumferential incision. **C, D,** Incisions extending from lateral (midaxillary) and posterior costal areas into the central tendon.

104. Ans. (c) Needle decompression on right side of the chest

Ref: Bailey 26th ed page 354, Sabiston 19th ed page 1599

The patient is suffering from Tension Pneumothorax. (Different case scenaio of Tension Pneumothorax was asked in Surgery AIIMS Nov 2013)

See table of Chest Trauma in Surgery AIIMS Nov 2016 (see page no. 969)

The diagnosis of tension pneumothorax is implied by respiratory distress and hypotension in combination with any of the following physical signs in patients with chest trauma: tracheal deviation away from the affected side, lack of or decreased breath sounds on the affected side, and subcutaneous emphysema on the affected side. Patients may have distended neck veins due to impedance of the superior vena cava, but the neck veins may be flat due to systemic hypovolemia. Vital signs differentiate a tension pneumothorax from a simple pneumothorax; each can have similar signs, symptoms, and examination findings, but **hypotension qualifies the pneumothorax as a tension pneumothorax.**

Schwartz Says

Although immediate needle thoracostomy decompression with a 14-gauge angiocatheter in the second intercostal space in the midclavicular line may be indicated in the field, tube thoracostomy should be performed immediately in the ED before a chest radiograph is obtained

Sabiston Says

Emergent needle decompression for tension pneumothorax is carried out on the affected side by placing an 18-gauge needle or angiocatheter into the hemithorax at the midclavicular line in the second anterior intercostal space. This emergency maneuver relieves the tension created within the thorax. It does not treat the pneumothorax; subsequent chest tube insertion is required.

105. Ans. (d) Roux-en-Y procedure

Ref: Sabiston 19th ed page 363, Schwartz 9th ed page 932, Harrison 19th ed page 2398

Maingot 11th ed ch 52 States

- Roux-en-Y gastric bypass is the most commonly performed procedure in the United States and accounts for 80–85% of procedures performed
- BPD had a higher percentage of excess weight loss (70%) than other bariatric procedures

Indications for Bariatric Surgery
BMI >40 kg/m^2 or BMI >35 kg/m^2 with an associated medical comorbidity worsened by obesity
Failed dietary therapy
Psychiatrically stable without alcohol dependence or illegal drug use
Knowledgeable about the operation and its sequelae
Motivated individual
Medical problems not precluding probable survival from surgery

Classification of Bariatic Sugery

Restrictive	Malabsorptive	Combined restrictive and malabsorptive
Laparoscopic adjustable gastric banding (LAGB) Sleeve gastrectomy (SG) Vertical banded gastroplasty (VBG)	Biliopancreatic diversion (BPD) Jejunoileal bypass (JIB)	Roux-en-Y gastric bypass (RYGB-Largely restrictive) BPD with duodenal switch (DS) - Largely malabsorptive

Weight Loss and Reduction in Comorbidities after Bariatric Surgery					
	Gastric banding	Gastroplasty	Gastric bypass	BPD or DS	Total
EWL (Excess weight loss)	47%	68%	62%	70%	61%
Mortality	0.1%[a]	0.1%[a]	0.5%	1.1%	NR
Resolution of DM	48%	72%	84%	99%	77%
Resolution of hyperlipidemia	59%	74%	97%	99%	79%
Resolution of hypertension	43%	69%	68%	83%	62%
Resolution of sleep apnea	95%	78%	80%	92%	86%

Abbreviations: BPD, biliopancreatic diversion; DS, duodenal switch; EWL, excess weight loss; NR, not reported; DM, diabetes mellitus

106. Ans. (d) Increased pH

Ref: Bailey 26th ed page 94, Morgan's 5th Ed Pg 542, Laparoscopic Surgery: A Colloquium by Ronald C. Merrell Pg 289

- The hallmark of laparoscopy is the creation of a pneumoperitoneum with pressurized CO_2. The resulting increase in intraabdominal pressure displaces the diaphragm cephalad, causing a decrease in lung compliance and an increase in peak inspiratory pressure. Atelectasis, **diminished FRC,** ventilation/perfusion mismatch, and pulmonary shunting contribute to a decrease in arterial oxygenation.
- Increased Intraabdominal pressure leads to **increased ICP**.
- The high solubility of CO_2 increases systemic absorption by the vasculature of the peritoneum. This, combined with smaller tidal volumes because of **poor lung compliance,** leads to increased arterial CO_2 levels and **decreased pH.**
- A head-down (Trendelenburg) position if required causes a cephalad shift in abdominal viscera and the diaphragm. FRC, total lung volume, and pulmonary compliance will be further decreased.
- Peritoneal insufflation induces alterations of hemodynamics, characterized by decreases of cardiac output, elevations of arterial pressure, and increases of systemic and **pulmonary vascular resistances.**
- Pulmonary Capillary wedge pressure (PCWP) is a measure of left atrial filling pressures. In response to insuffiation there is an increase in central venous pressure (CVP), pulmonary capillary wedge pressure (PCWP), mean arterial pressure (MAP), and systemic vascular resistance (SVR), with a concomitant decrease in cardiac index and ejection fraction. These changes suggest a systolic ventricular dysfunction in the face of the acute rise in afterload. When the patient is positioned in Trendelenburg position, there is a further increase in CVP, PCWP, and MAP, but a decrease in SVR along with an increase in cardiac index and ejection fraction. This suggests increased preload facilitates ventricular function and reverses some of the changes caused by insufflation. In the final phase—release of pneumoperitoneum—there is a decrease in CVP, PCWP.
- Hemodynamic changes are accentuated in high-risk cardiac patients
- Hypercarbia, if allowed to develop, will stimulate the sympathetic nervous system and thus increase blood pressure, heart rate, and the risk of arrhythmias. Attempting to compensate by increasing the tidal volume or respiratory rate will increase the mean intrathoracic pressure, further hindering venous return and increasing mean pulmonary artery pressures.

107. Ans. (a) Herniotomy

Ref: Sabiston 19th ed page 1120-1126, Bailey 26th ed page 957

Herniotomy

In children who have lateral hernias with a persistent processus, it is sufficient only to remove and close the sac. This is called a herniotomy. In adult surgery, herniotomy alone has a high recurrence rate and some form of muscle strengthening is added (herniorrhaphy). **Congenital hydroceles are treated by herniotomy if they do not resolve spontaneously**.

Herniotomy is performed via an inguinal skin crease incision, opening Scarpa's fascia and then the external oblique. The cremaster is cut and, through an initially small opening, the cord grasped and gently delivered. The vas and vessels are separated from the sac which is then divided and proximally ligated.

108. Ans. (a) Based upon portal vien and hepatic vein

Ref: Grays 40th ed page 1165, 1178, Sabiston 19th Ed page 1413-1417, Schwartz 9th ed page 1095, Bailey 26th ed page 1065-1067

Anatomical division of liver into right and left lobes of liver (not functional anatomy of 8 segments) is based on portal vein and hepatic vein

Option (A)

(Grays) Functional anatomy of the liver is based on the distribution of portal venous branches in the parenchyma.

Option (B)

Grays 41st ed page 1162; Current understanding of the functional anatomy of the liver is based on Couinaud's division of the liver into eight (subsequently nine, then later revised back to eight) functional segments, based on the distribution of portal venous branches in the parenchyma.

Option (C)

Grays 41st ed page 1162; Knowledge of the fissures of the liver is essential for understanding liver surgery. Three major fissures (main, left and right portal fissures), not visible on the surface, run through the liver parenchyma and contain the three main hepatic veins. Three minor fissures (umbilical, venous and fissure of Gans) are visible as physical clefts of the liver surface. The fissure of Gans is also known as Rouvière's sulcus or the incisura hepatis dextra. Accessory fissures are rare.

Option (D)

Grays 41st ed page 1162; The liver is divided into four portal sectors by the four main branches of the portal vein.

Lobar Anatomy of the Liver

- The liver is divided into right and left lobes determined by portal and hepatic vein branches.
- Briefly, a plane without any surface markings running from the gall-bladder to the left side of the IVC (known as the *portal fissure, or Cantlie's line*) divides the liver into right and left lobes.
- The right lobe is further divided into anterior and posterior segments.
- The left lobe is divided into a medial segment (also known as the *quadrate lobe*) that lies to the right of the falciform ligament and umbilical fissure and a lateral segment lying to the left. This system, although anatomically more correct, is only sufficient for mobilization of the liver and simple hepatic procedures. It does not describe the more intricate and functional segmental anatomy that is essential to understand before pursuing complex hepatobiliary surgery.

Functional Anatomy of Liver

- The functional anatomy of the liver is composed of eight segments, each of which is supplied by a single portal triad (also called a *pedicle*) composed of a **portal vein, hepatic artery, and bile duct. These segments are further organized into four sectors that are separated by scissurae containing the three main hepatic veins.**
- This system was originally described in 1957 by Woodsmith and Goldburne as well as Couinaud and defines hepatic anatomy as it is most relevant to surgery of the liver.
- The main scissura contains the middle hepatic vein, which runs in an anteroposterior direction from the gallbladder fossa to the left side of the vena cava and divides the liver into right and left hemi-livers. **The line of the main scissura is also known as *Cantlie's line.***
- The right liver is divided into an anterior (segments V and VIII) and posterior (segments VI and VII) sector by the right scissura, which contains the right hepatic vein. The right portal pedicle, composed of the right hepatic artery, portal vein, and bile duct, splits into right anterior and posterior pedicles that supply the segments of the anterior and posterior sectors.
- The left liver has a visible fissure along its inferior surface called the ***umbilical fissure.*** The ligamentum teres (containing the remnant of the umbilical vein) runs into this fissure. The falciform ligament is contiguous with the umbilical fissure and ligamentum teres. The umbilical fissure is *not* a scissura, does not contain a hepatic vein, and in fact, contains the left portal pedicle (triad containing the left portal vein, hepatic artery, and bile duct), which runs in this fissure, branching to feed the left liver. The left scissura runs posterior to the ligamentum teres and contains the left hepatic vein. The left liver is split into an anterior (segments III and IV) and posterior (**segment II—the only sector composed of a single segment**) sector by the left scissura.
- **The caudate lobe (segment I)** is the dorsal portion of the liver and embraces the IVC on its posterior surface and lies posterior to the left portal triad inferiorly and the left and middle hepatic veins superiorly. The main bulk of the caudate lobe is to the left of the IVC, but inferiorly, it traverses between the IVC and left portal triad, where it fuses to the right liver (segments VI and VII). **This part of the caudate lobe is known as the right portion or the caudate process.** The left portion of the caudate lobe lies in the lesser omental bursa and is covered anteriorly by the gastrohepatic ligament (lesser omentum) that separates it from segments II and III anteriorly. The gastrohepatic ligament attaches to the ligamentum venosum (sinus venosus remnant) along the left side of the left portal triad.

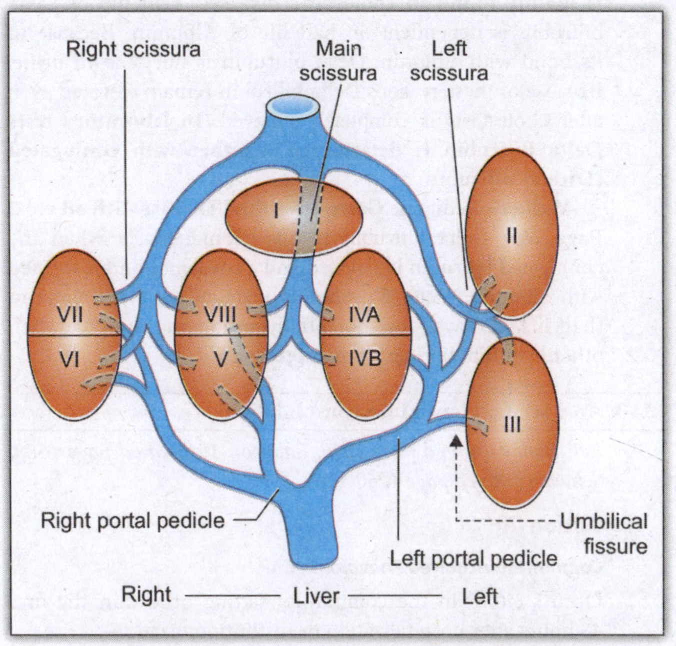

Schematic demonstrating the segmental anatomy of the liver. Each segment receives its own portal pedicle (triad of portal vein, hepatic artery, and bile duct). The eight segments are illustrated, and the four sectors, divided by the three main hepatic veins running in scissurae, are shown. The umbilical fissure (not a scissura) is shown to contain the left portal pedicle.

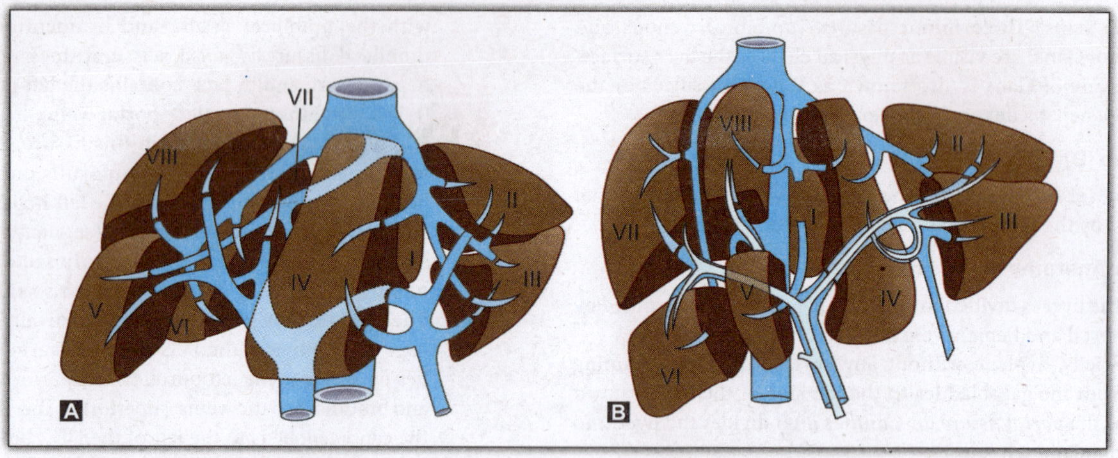

Fig. Segmental anatomy of the liver as seen at laparotomy in the anatomic position (A) and in the ex vivo position (B).

109. Ans. (b) Delta bilirubin

Ref: Harrison 19th ed page 280

Delta-bilirubin is a novel form of bilirubin first noticed when the sum of conjugated and unconjugated bilirubin was less than the total bilirubin concentration when measured by high-performance liquid chromatography. **This form of Bilirubin is mainly found in cholestatic diseases.** Half life of Delta bilirubin is dependent on half life of Albumin. Because of its bond with albumin, Delta bilirubin is not seen in urine. Because of these reasons Delta bilirubin remain elevated even after cholestasis is completely relieved. **In laboratory tests Delta Bilirubin is determined together with conjugated (Direct) Bilirubin.**

Walker's Pediatric Gastrointestinal Disease -5th ed vol 2 Page 767; Delta bilirubin results spontaneously when the conjugated bilirubin is elevated and a covalent bond is formed with albumin. Delta bilirubin is metabolized with albumin (half-life -22 days), thus potentially prolonging jaundice when other liver function tests are improving.

110. Ans. (a) Left lower lobe consolidation

Ref: Bailey 26th ed page 1096, Sabiston 19th ed ed page 1558, Schwartz 9th ed page 1260-1262

Option (A)

Community-Acquired Pneumonia CAP

Occurs either in the community setting or within the first 48 hours after hospitalization or institutionalization.

Hospital Acquired Pneumonia HAP

It is defined as a new pneumonia (not present on admission) that occurs 48 hours or more after admission to a hospital.

In people whose spleen is removed or does not function properly, the most common cause of sepsis is infection with a bacterium called **Streptococcus pneumoniae** also known as the pneumococcus. Experts recommend that people without a functional spleen have certain vaccinations to reduce the risk of sepsis. Although these vaccines do not prevent all infections with pneumococcus, H. influenzae type B (Hib), and meningococcus, they can protect most people and reduce the severity of infection in others. When possible, vaccines should be given at least two weeks before planned surgical removal of the spleen. The vaccine should be given 14 or more days after emergency removal of the spleen (e.g. due to trauma)

Bailey states

Post-splenectomy septicaemia may result from Streptococcus pneumoniae, Neisseria meningitides, Haemophilus influenzae and Escherichia coli. The risk is greater in the young patient, in splenectomised patients treated with chemoradiotherapy and in patients who have undergone splenectomy for thalassaemia, sickle cell disease and autoimmune anaemia or thrombocytopenia.

Option (B)

Port site infection is nothing but surgical site ingfection that occurs from 4-8 postoperative days.

Option (C)

Although abdominal abscess/collection is a cause of postoperative fever, it is usually occurs 7-10 days after surgery.

Option (D)

UTI is most commonly acquired Nosocomial infection. It usually occurs after postoperative day 3 often accompanied by dysuria and low grade fever.

Postoperative Fever

It is defined as a temperature >38°C (100°F) on 2 consecutive postoperative days, or >39°C (102.2°F) on any 1 postoperative day. However, most febrile postoperative patients are not infected, and indeed a significant proportion of infected patients may not be febrile, depending on the definition of *fever.* Because fever is common in the absence of infection, it is important to consider causes of postoperative fever other than infection and to make a presumptive diagnosis before instituting antibiotic treatment. ***Fever in the first 3 days after surgery most likely has a noninfectious cause.***

Only two important infectious causes of fever are likely in the first 36 hours after laparotomy. The first is an injury to bowel with intraperitoneal leakage, which is characterized by marked hemodynamic changes—first tachycardia and then hypotension and falling urine output. The other early cause of fever and infection is an invasive soft tissue infection beginning in the wound and caused either by β-hemolytic streptococci or by clostridial species (**most commonly *C. perfringens***).

Causes of Postoperative Fever			
Immediate (within hours)	**Acute (within first week)**	**Subacute (1–4 weeks out)**	**Delayed (>1 month)**
Trauma (including surgery)/ cytokine release Medications Malignant hyperthermia, Neuroleptic malignant syndrome, Toxic shock syndrome Transfusion reaction Necrotizing fasciitis Infection, thrombosis, or other non infectious cause present prior to surgery Aspiration chemical pneumonitis (Mendelson syndrome)	Surgical site infection (after 48 hours) Pneumonia UTI IV catheter infection Thrombophlebitis **Non infectious:** MI, DVT/PE, CVA/SAH, hematoma, pancreatitis, EtOH withdrawal, gout, bowel ischemia, TTP, hyperthyroidism, adrenal insufficiency, transfusion or Drug reaction, inflammatory reaction to implanted hardware, etc.	Surgical site infection Thrombophlebitis/DVT/PE Central venous catheter related infections. Antibiotic associated diarrhoea (C. difficile) Drug reaction Nosocomial or other infection: Pneumonia, UTI, IV catheter, intra abdominal abscess, sinusitis, otitis media, osteomyelitis, endocarditis, cholecystitis (can be acalculous) etc	Post cardiotomy syndrome Viral infections like Hepatitis, CMV, HIV Implant infection SSI due to coagulase negative staph, Infective endocarditis

Wound infection is the most common cause of postoperative fever overall

Watch for surgery specific causes: meningitis after neurosurgery, toxic shock after nasal or vaginal packing, parotitis after oral surgery, rejection after transplant surgery, fat emboli after orthopedic surgery, infected hardware, etc.

111. Ans. (b) Ventriculo peritoneal

Ref: Bailey 26th ed page 608, Nelson 20th ed page 2817

Hydrocephalus describes an increase in CSF volume and ventricular enlargement, ofte resulting in symptoms of raised ICP. It may be due to physical blockage (obstructive hydrocephalus) or due to failure of normal reabsorption (communicating hydrocephalus).

Investigation

- **CT scan** is a first-line investigation to demonstrate hydrocephalus
- **Lumbar Puncture** can confirm raised ICP and relieve it temporarily, but only after review of the CT to exclude a mass lesion or obstructive hydrocephalus, which might lead to 'coning' at LP

Management

Acute hydrocephalus is a surgical emergency

- **External ventricular drains (EVDs)** are an effective temporary measure to relieve hydrocephalus. Most commonly they are inserted freehand to the right of midline, anterior to the coronal suture, so that the catheter tip rests adjacent to the foramen of Monro in the lateral ventricle. The catheter is then connected to a drain set such that CSF drains when the ventricular pressure exceeds a threshold typically set at 10–20 mm Hg.
- **Ventriculoperitoneal (VP)** shunting comprises insertion of a ventricular catheter, which may be antibiotic impregnated, into the frontal or occipital horn of the lateral ventricle, while a distal catheter is tunnelled subcutaneously to the abdomen. Ventriculoatrial and ventriculopleural shunting is also possible. The major complications of shunting are occlusion (characterized by headache, papilledema, emesis, mental status changes) and bacterial infection (fever, headache, meningismus), usually caused by Staphylococcus epidermidis.

112. Ans. (c) USG

Ref: Nelson 20th ed page 1889-1891, Gore and Levine textbook of gastrointestinal radiology 3rd ed page 2282, CT and MRI of whole body by John R Haaga, 5th Ed., Ch. 30

Appendicitis is one of the most common causes of acute abdomen

Gold standard is CT scan but the best investigation is USG.

Nelson Mentions

Ultrasound is usually utilized for diagnostic accuracy in the evaluation of acute appendicitis and has demonstrated >90% sensitivity and specificity in pediatric centers experienced with the technique. The ultrasound criteria for appendicitis include wall thicken ≥6 mm, luminal distention, lack of compressibility, a complex mass in the RLQ, or an appendicolith. The visualized appendix usually coincides with the site of localized pain and tenderness. Findings that suggest advanced appendicitis on ultrasound include asymmetric wall thickening, abscess formation, associated free intraperitoneal fluid, surrounding tissue edema, and decreased local tenderness to compression. The main limitation of ultrasound is an inability to visualize the appendix, which is reported in up to 20% of cases. **A normal appendix must be visualized to exclude appendicitis by ultrasound.** Certain conditions predictably decrease the sensitivity and reliability of ultrasound for appendicitis, including obesity, bowel distention, and pain, which interferes with the exam. **Major advantages of ultrasound include its easy availability, rapid method, low cost, and freedom from need for patient preparation and ionizing radiation.** Ultrasound can be particularly helpful in adolescent girls, a group with a high negative appendectomy rate (normal appendix found at surgery), because of its ability to evaluate for ovarian pathology without ionizing radiation. A diagnostic or normal ultrasound exam eliminates the need for CT and should be considered the first exam in a center experienced with the technique.

Although the clinical diagnosis is usually made on the basis of history, physical examination, and laboratory data, **ultrasound with its lack of ionizing radiation should be the investigation of choice in young patients and children.**

The technique used is known as **graded compression** and uses the **linear probe** (high frequency).

Findings supportive of the diagnosis of appendicitis on ultrasound include:

- Aperistaltic, noncompressible, dilated appendix (>6 mm outer diameter)
- Appendicolith
- Distinct appendiceal wall layers
- Echogenic prominent pericaecal fat
- Periappendiceal fluid collection
- **Target appearance** (axial section)

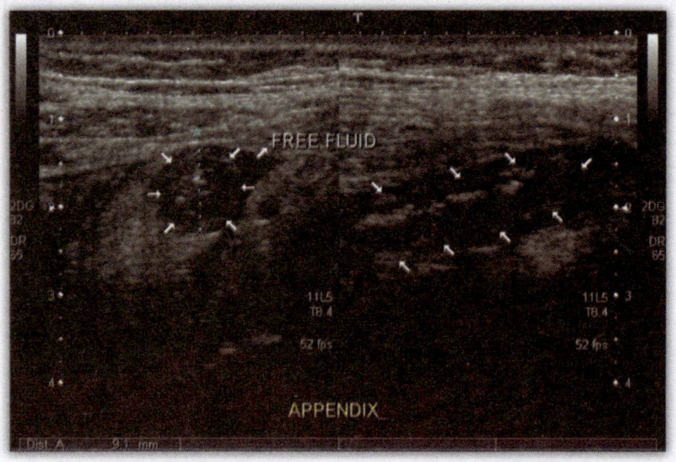

Fig: The above figure is the ultrasound image in acute appendicitis giving the typical target appearance in the first image and a blind ending loop in second image

Option (A) CT Scan

Had been the gold standard imaging study for evaluating children with suspected appendicitis, but carries the significant negative effects of radiation exposure and increased costs. It should be used only in carefully selected patients and always observing the reduced radiation dosage recommendations for children.

CT is highly sensitive and specific for diagnosing acute appendicitis. Features in typical cases of acute appendicitis include an abnormal appendix, periappendiceal inflammation, and changes in the cecal apex. Changes in the cecal apex include focal cecal apex thickening, an **arrowhead sign**, and a **cecal bar**.

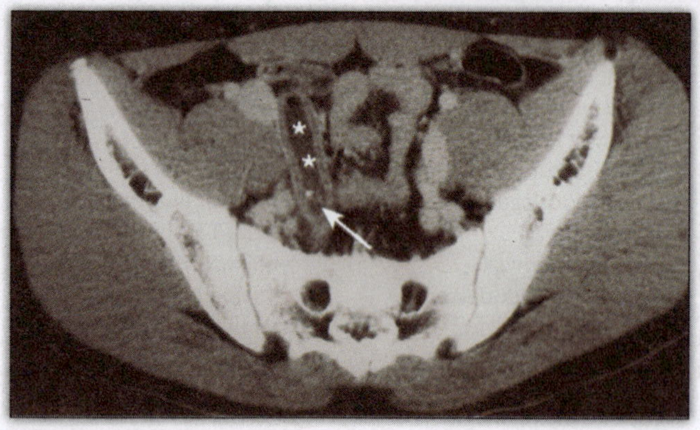

Fig: Acute appendicitis. The appendix (*asterisks*) is dilated with a thickened wall owing to mural edema. A small appendicolith (*arrow*) is also seen

113. Ans. (a) Hepatic scintigraphy

Ref: Bailey 26th ed page 121, 1104, Nelson 20th ed page 1928-1936, Ghai 8th ed page 328

USG is done to check of choledocholithiasis, perforation of the bile duct, or other structural abnormalities of the biliary tree such as a choledochal cyst. It can also help to look for spleen and any other vascular malformations. In biliary atresia **"triangular cord sign"** is seen. Liver echogenicity is also seen.

Hepatic scintigraphy with technetium-labeled iminodiacetic acid derivatives is a sensitive but not specific test for biliary atresia. But is more specific than USG hence choice of answer. However first investigation to be done will be USG being easily available and also non-invasive. Most valueable procedure is liver biopsy.

Orthopedics

15

AIIMS NOVEMBER 2018

1. Sprengel's deformity is associated with all EXCEPT: *(AIIMS Nov 2018, Nov 2017)*

a. Dextrocardia b. Klippel Feil Syndrome
c. Diastematomyelia d. Congenital scoliosis

2. Earliest sign of compartment syndrome of leg?

a. Loss of pulse
b. Change in skin color
c. Tingling and numbness
d. Pain on passive stretching of toes

3. Identify the deformity in the given picture?

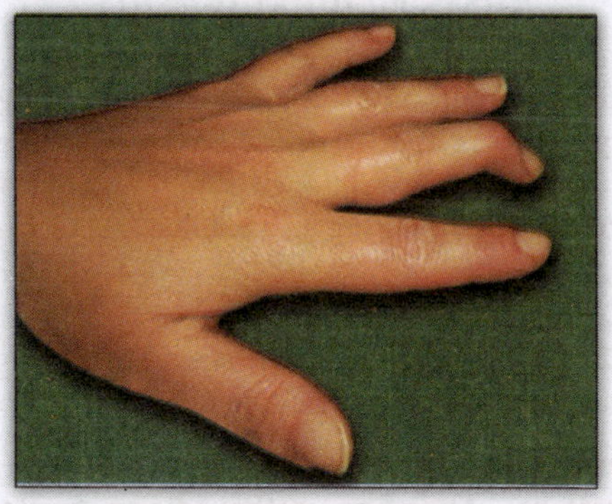

a. Swan neck deformity b. Boutonniere deformity
c. Mallet finger d. Jersey finger

4. An 8-year-old child presents with fever and wound with discharging pus from right thigh for 4 months. Given below is the X-ray. Identify the marked structure?

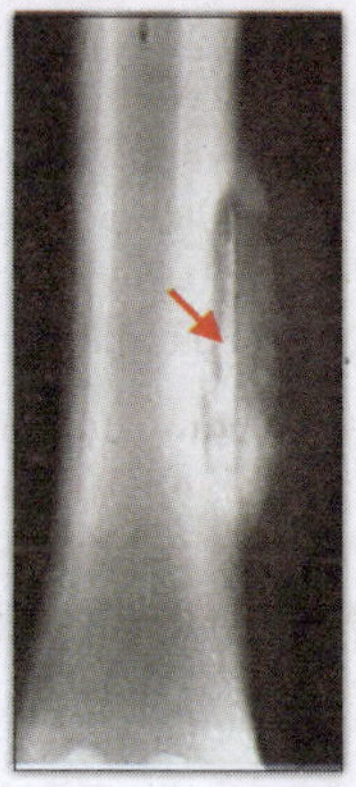

a. Cloacae b. Woven bone
c. Involucrum d. Sequestrum

5. Patellar Clunk syndrome is interposition of hypertrophied scar tissue at ?

a. Superior pole of patella and impinging on femoral component during flexion
b. Superior pole of patella and impinging on femoral component during extension
c. Inferior pole of patella and impinging on femoral component during flexion
d. Inferior pole of patella and impinging on femoral component during extension

6. This is the x ray of a 7-year-old child. Identify the deformity?

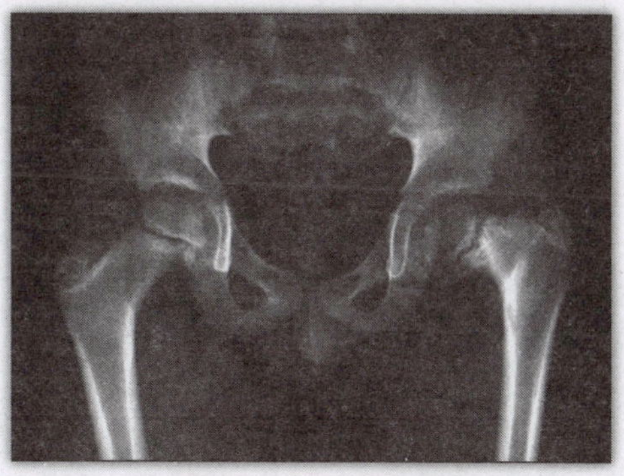

a. Coxa vara b. Coxa valgus
c. Coxa magna d. Coxa saltans

7. Identify the lytic lesion at end of radius in the given X-ray?

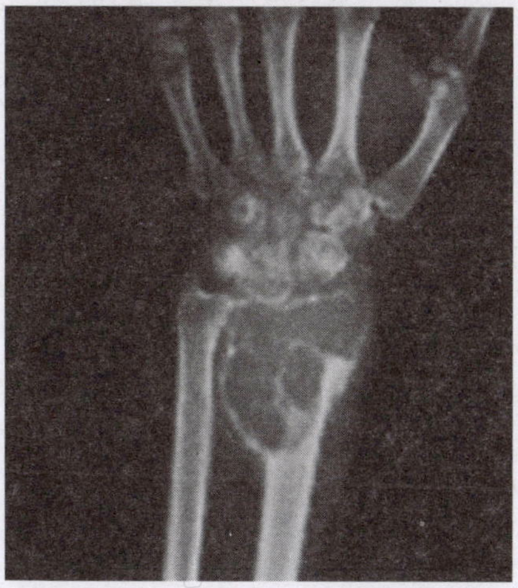

a. GCT b. Osteoclastoma
c. Aneurysmal bone cyst d. Osteosarcoma

AIIMS MAY 2018

8. A 60-year-old female presenting with small joints of hand involved with sparing of distal interphalangeal joint. History of morning stiffness involving knees was present. Most likely diagnosis is?

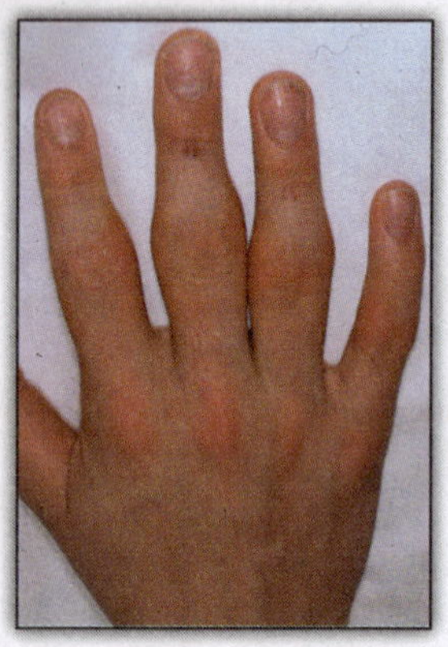

a. Rheumatoid Arthritis
b. Osteoarthritis with Heberden nodes
c. CRPS (Complex regional pain syndrome) due to trauma
d. Synovitis fibrosis

9. A patient comes with hip flexion deformity. Which of the following is the clinical test to make diagnosis?

a. Trendelenburg test
b. Thomas test
c. Allis test
d. Ober's test

10. A child image is given below, identify the deformity?
(AIIMS May 2018, Nov 2016)

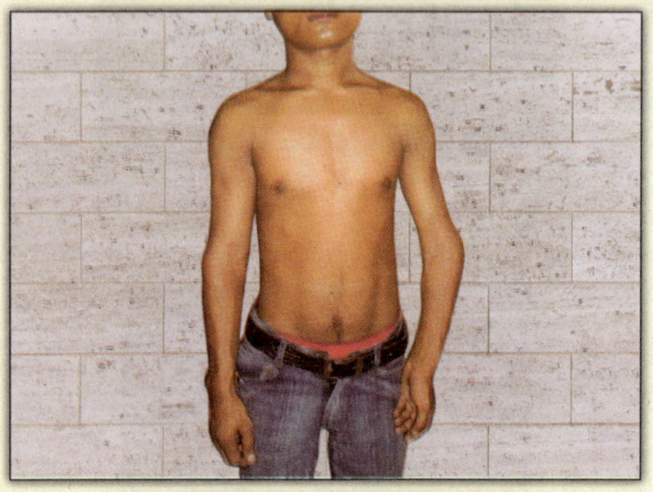

a. Fracture medial condyle of Humerus
b. Fracture lateral condyle of Humerus
c. Supracondylar fracture
d. Intercondylar fracture

11. A patient with Supracondylar fracture is unable to flex the thumb. Which of the following nerve is likely to be injured?

a. Superficial branch of ulnar nerve
b. Deep branch of ulnar nerve
c. Anterior Interosseous nerve
d. Posterior Interosseous nerve

12. A 55-year-old presents with severe backache for 10 days and urinary incontinence with history of intervertebral disc prolapse. There is no h/o fever or weight loss. What is the likely diagnosis?

a. Pott's spine
b. Multiple myeloma
c. Cauda equina syndrome
d. Bone metastasis

13. A patient sustained leg injury in a RTA, X-ray knee was done as given below. What will be the best management?
(AIIMS May 2018, May 2017, Nov 2016)

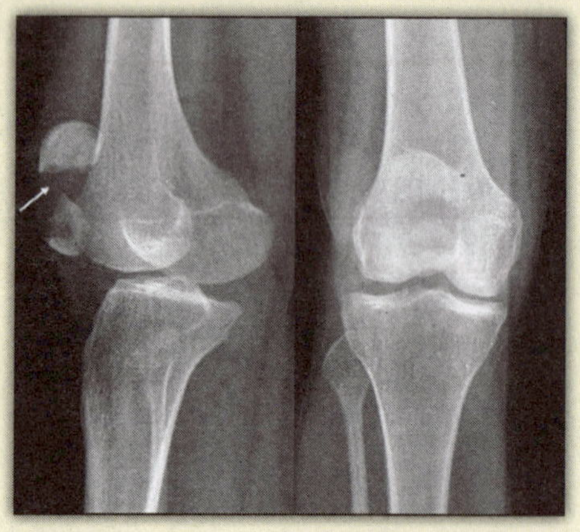

a. K wire
b. Patellectomy
c. Compression plate
d. Tension Band wiring

AIIMS NOVEMBER 2017

14. A patient presents with both bone fracture of right forearm. A pop cast was applied and NSAIDs was given for pain. One week later he developed symptoms of compartment syndrome. The attending nurse should check first?

a. Check pulse
b. Check finger for colour change
c. Dressing for odour and discharge
d. Pain in spite of analgesics

15. A patient with history of RTA comes in emergency department. Attending orthopedician writes Gustilo's Type IIIB for his both bones fracture in lower limbs injury. According to Gustilo Anderson Classification what is correct?

a. Open fracture, wound of size < 1 cm in length without extensive soft-tissue damage, flaps or avulsions
b. Open fracture, wound between 1 and 10 cm in length without extensive soft-tissue damage, flaps or avulsions
c. Open fracture, limb wound of size > 10 cm with extensive soft tissue damage and periosteal stripping
d. Open fracture with extensive soft tissue damage laceration and avulsion injury, regardless of size of wound

16. A patient comes with complaint of lower limb weakness. Examiner places one hand under the patient heel and patient is then asked to raise his other leg against downward resistance. What is the test being performed?

a. Hoover's test
b. Mc Bride test
c. Waddell's test
d. O'Donoghue's test

17. **A 20-year-old boy with history of fall on outstretched hand comes with tenderness in anatomical snuff box. X-ray picture is shown below. Identify the pathology?**

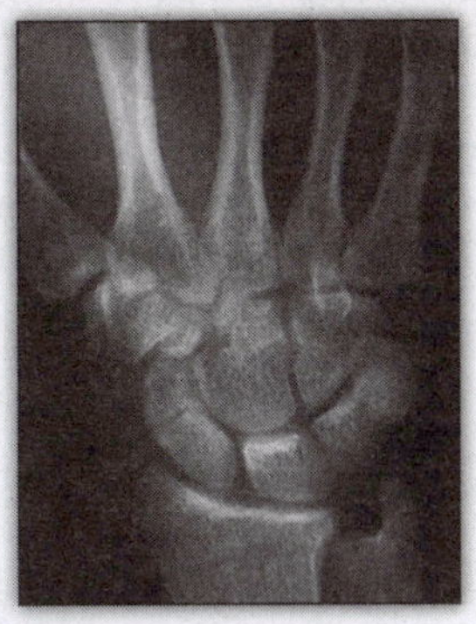

a. Scaphoid fracture
b. Trans scaphoid perilunate dislocation
c. Distal radius fracture
d. Hamate fracture

18. **Glucosamines are used in treatment of?**
a. Diabetes
b. Cataract
c. Arthritis
d. Glaucoma

19. **Sprengel's deformity is associated with all EXCEPT:** *(AIIMS Nov 2018, Nov 2017)*
a. Dextrocardia
b. Klippel Feil syndrome
c. Diastematomyelia
d. Congenital scoliosis

20. **A Young bodybuilder on long term steroid use is suffering from hip pain on rest for past 6 months. His X-ray revealed destruction of articular surface of femoral head with the presence of subchondral cyst and positive crescent sign. His MRI is suggestive of Marrow edema. What is your diagnosis?**
a. Tuberculosis of Hip
b. Fracture neck of Femur
c. Osteochondroma of Femur
d. Avascular necrosis of femoral head

21. **Which of the following fracture classification system is used for the fracture of the given picture?**

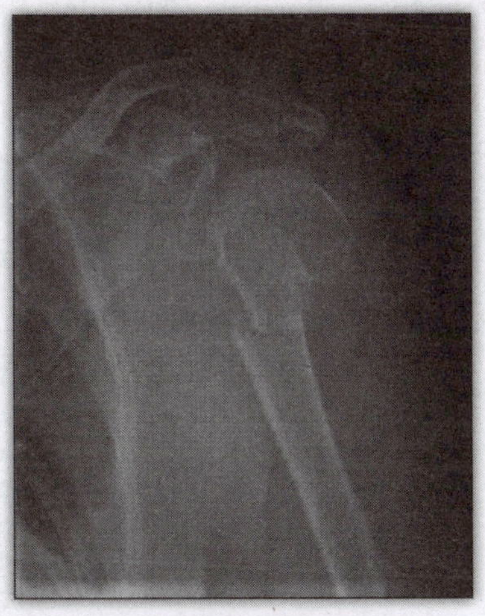

a. Garden type 3 proximal humerus
b. NEER type 3 proximal humerus
c. Schatzker's type 3 proximal humerus
d. Gustilo's type 3 proximal humerus

AIIMS MAY 2017

22. **A 23-year-old boy badminton player sustained injury on left ankle, he was immobilized for 3 months, the cast was removed and patient was able to walk normally. Later, he complained of pain and swelling in the left calf, left ankle and foot. His mother massaged him for 30 minutes. After a while he developed acute onset of breathlessness and was brought to emergency and died. Most likely cause of death is?**
a. Fat embolism
b. Pulmonary thromboembolism
c. Pneumonitis
d. Acute MI

23. **A patient with fracture of hip dies 2 days after admission. Most likely cause is?**
a. Fat embolism
b. Pulmonary hypertension
c. Post traumatic MI
d. Hypovolemic shock

24. **In the given picture which movement of hip is tested?**

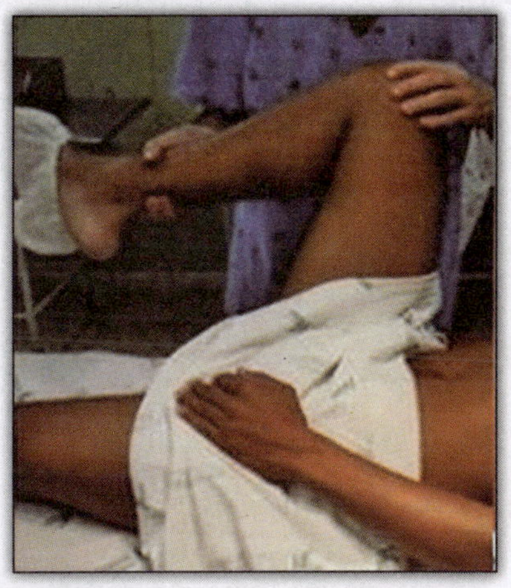

a. Abduction
b. Adduction
c. Internal rotation
d. External rotation

25. **Hand to knee gait in polio due to weakness of which muscle?**
a. Gluteus maximus
b. Gluteus medius
c. Soleus gastrocnemius
d. Quadriceps

26. **Haglund deformity is associated with?**
a. Knee
b. Elbow
c. Ankle
d. Wrist

27. **March fracture following stress is seen in________of second metatarsal?**
a. Shaft
b. Base
c. Neck
d. Head

28. A patient came with complaints of inability to move his 4th and 5th digit, cannot hold pen and he was not able to hold paper between fingers. Which of the following site given below is the probable cause of injury to the nerve in question?

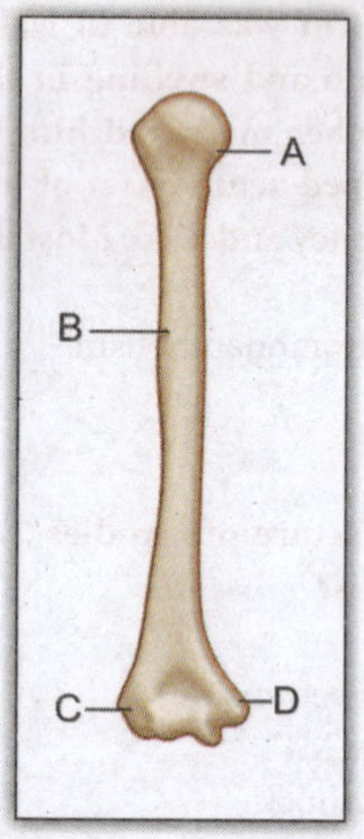

a. Medial epicondyle
b. Surgical neck of humerus
c. Spiral groove
d. Lateral condyle

29. A patient sustained leg injury in a RTA, X-ray knee was done as given below. What will be the best management?

(AIIMS May 2018, May 2017, Nov 2016)

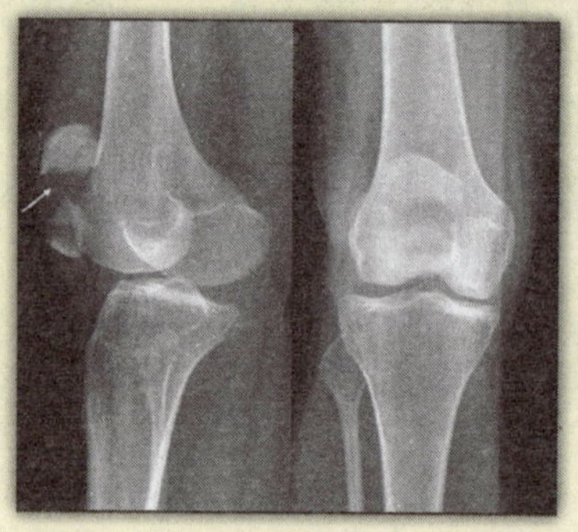

a. K wire
b. Patellectomy
c. Compression plate
d. Tension band wiring

30. A middle aged women with history of back pain came to OPD. On examination she was positive for schober test. Her Sclera, nose and ears were hyperpigmented. Most likely diagnosis is?

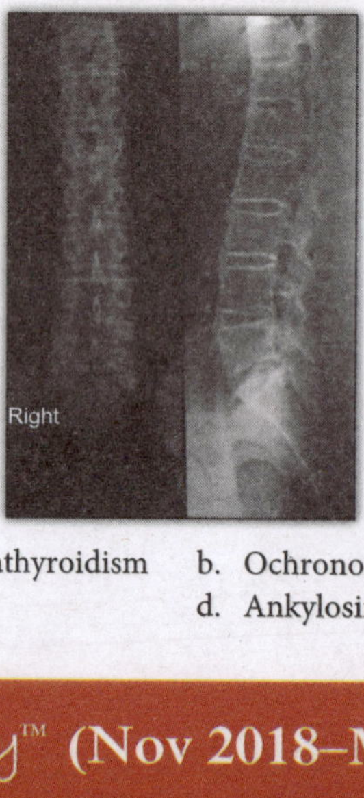

a. Hypoparathyroidism
b. Ochronosis
c. Fluorosis
d. Ankylosing spondylitis

31. Which of the following is true regarding Galeazzi fracture dislocation?

a. Interosseous membrane tear with triangular fibrocartilage complex (TFCC) tear and radial shaft fracture
b. Interosseous membrane tear + Radial shaft fracture
c. Radial collateral ligament tear with interosseous membrane tear with radial shaft fracture
d. Interosseous membrane tear with triangular fibrocartilage complex (TFCC) tear and ulnar shaft fracture

32. Which of the following image is of bone holding forceps?

a. 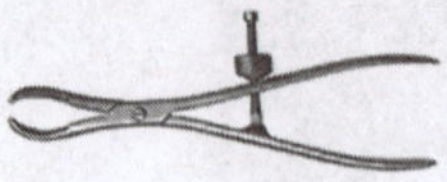

b. 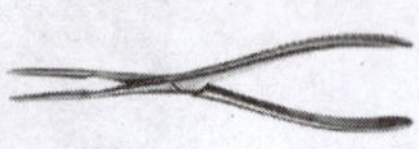

c. 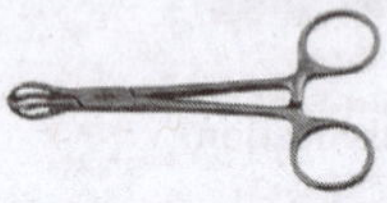

d. 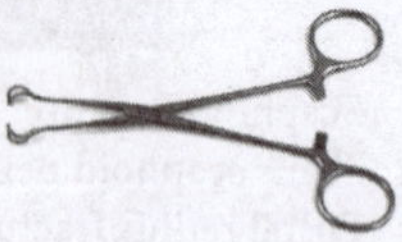

33. A 14-year-old boy fell on outstretched hand, X-ray is as shown below. Which of the following vascular structure is most commonly injured?

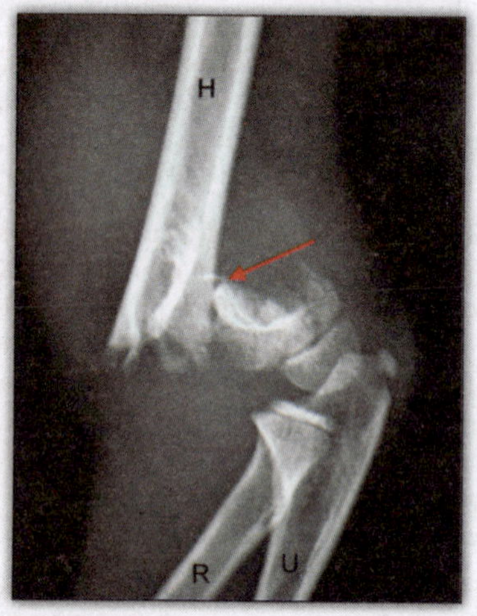

a. Brachial artery
b. Cephalic vein
c. Radial artery
d. Ulnar artery

34. An elderly patient slipped in bathroom and sustained injury over hip. X-ray is shown below. Attitude of her limb will be?

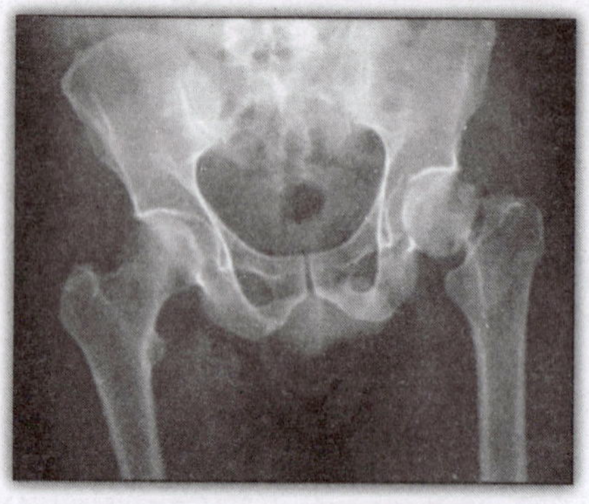

a. Shortened and externally rotated
b. Shortened, externally rotated and abducted
c. Shortened, internally rotated and adducted
d. Lengthened and internally rotated

35. Most common sequelae of shoulder dislocation in young adult is?
a. Recurrent dislocation
b. Rotator cuff tear
c. Adhesive capsulitis
d. Subcapsular tendinitis

AIIMS NOVEMBER 2016

36. Cartilage formation following fracture is favoured by?
a. Rigid immobilization
b. Compressor plate
c. Necrosed bone end
d. Movements at fracture site

37. A child image is given below, identify the deformity?
(AIIMS May 2018, Nov 2016)

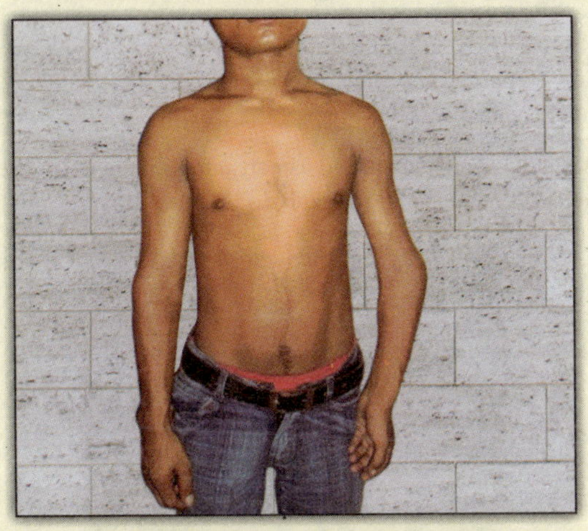

a. Fracture medial condyle of humerus
b. Fracture lateral condyle of humerus
c. Supracondylar fracture
d. Intercondylar fracture

38. A patient sustained leg injury in a RTA, X-ray knee was done as given below. What will be the best management?
(AIIMS May 2018, May 2017, Nov 2016)

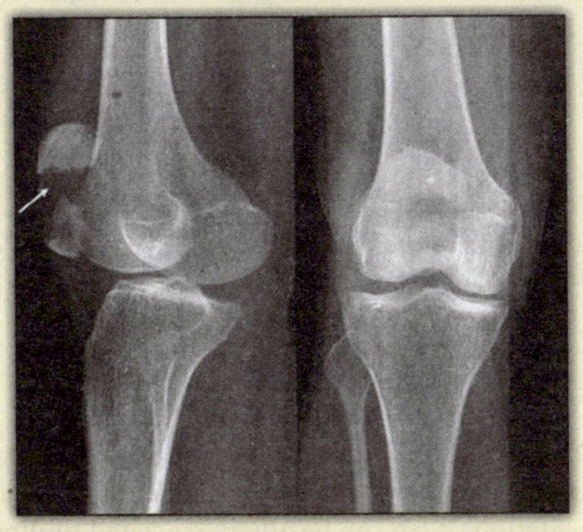

a. K wire
b. Patellectomy
c. Compression plate
d. Tension band wiring

39. Which of the following best describes the lesion in the picture?

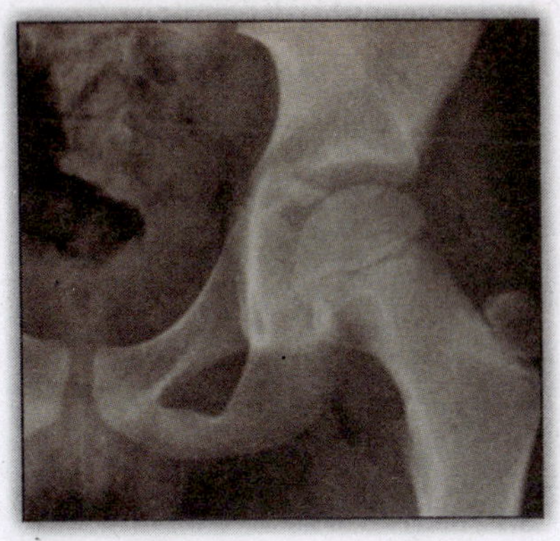

a. Ewing sarcoma
b. Chronic osteomyelitis
c. Osteosarcoma
d. Callus formation

40. A patient comes with history of trauma and attitude of limb is shown in picture below, what is the most appropriate diagnosis?

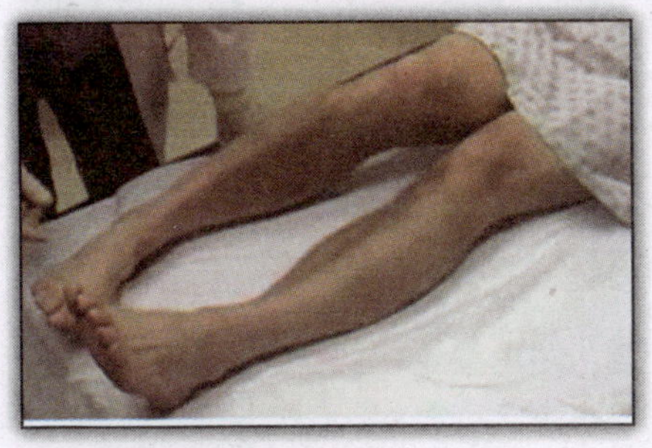

a. Anterior dislocation of hip
b. Posterior dislocation of hip
c. Superior dislocation of hip
d. Inferior dislocation of hip

AIIMS MAY 2016

41. The picture given below shows a hand following a nerve injury. Identify the nerve?

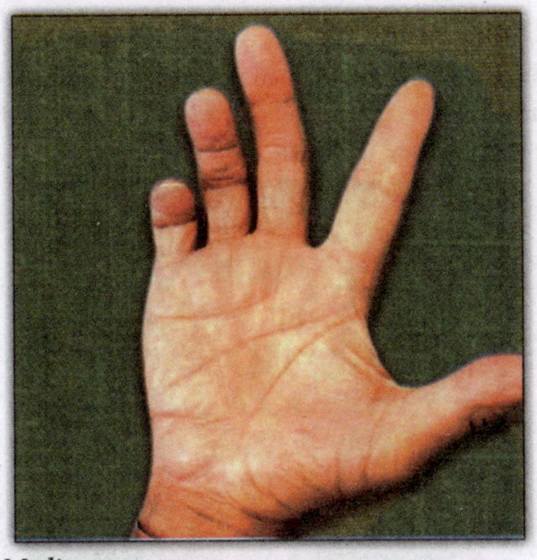

a. Median nerve
b. Ulnar nerve
c. Radial nerve
d. Musculocutaneous nerve

42. **A child presented with deformity as shown in the picture below. The most probable diagnosis is?**

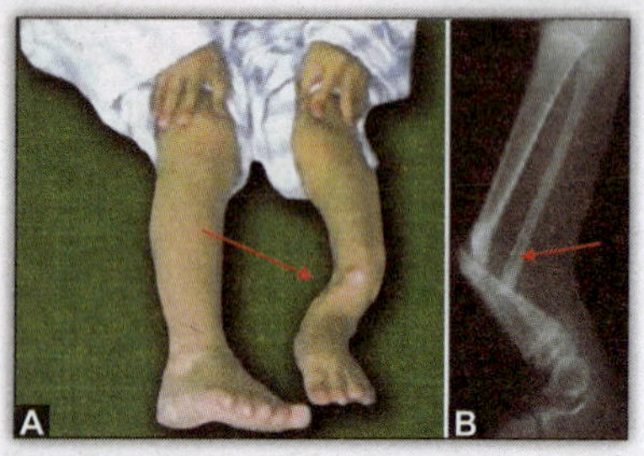

a. Fibular hemimelia
b. Tibial hemimelia
c. Pseudoorthorosis of tibia
d. Medial Angulation of tibia

43. **The below is X-ray pelvis of 1-year-old baby. All of the following tests will be positive EXCEPT:**

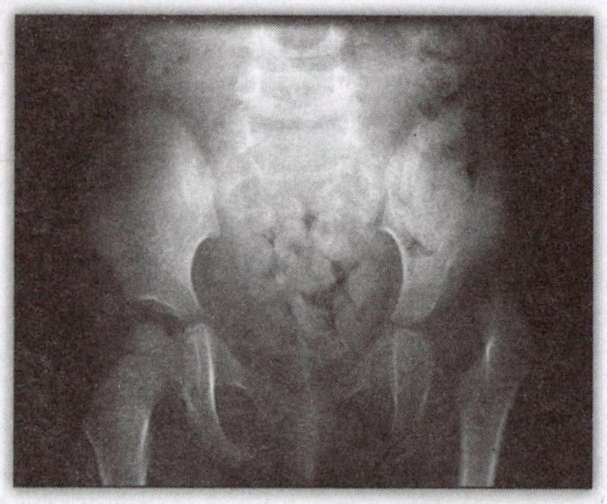

a. Narath test
b. Ortolani test
c. Gaenslen test
d. Barlow test

44. **Which fracture is shown in the X-ray below?**

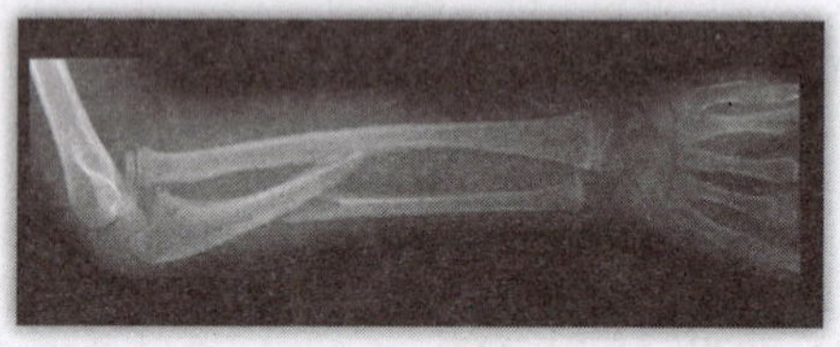

a. Monteggia fracture
b. Coles fracture
c. Galeazzi fracture
d. Smith fracture

45. **A 30-year-old male with complaint of pain and swelling in right shoulder. X-ray shoulder of the patient is given below. The most probable diagnosis is?**

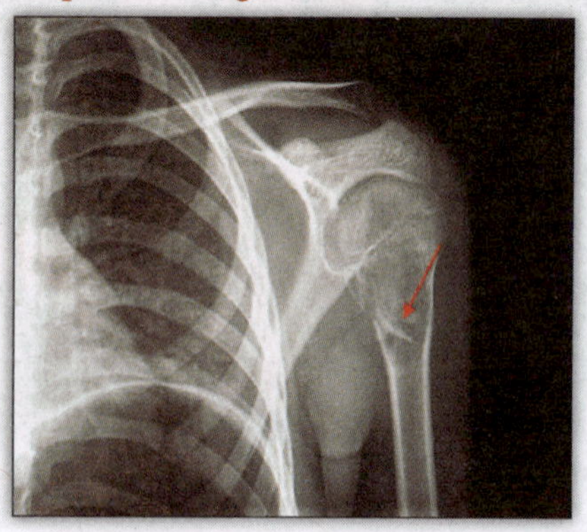

a. Simple bone cyst
b. Ewing's sarcoma
c. Giant cell tumor
d. Adamantinoma

46. **A 25-year-old male had early morning backache and stiffness presents to Orthopaedics OPD. X-ray is shown below. What is most probable diagnosis?**

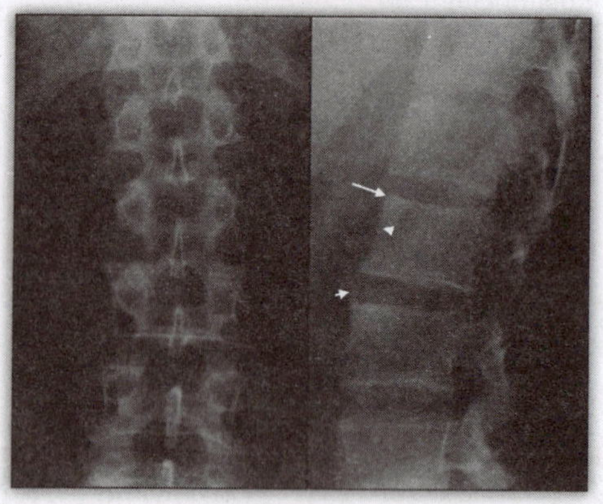

a. Rheumatoid arthiritis
b. Ankylosing spondylitis
c. Hyperparathyroidism
d. Pagets disease

47. **A 24-year-old sustained the fracture shown in the X-ray below. The nerve most likely to be injured is?**

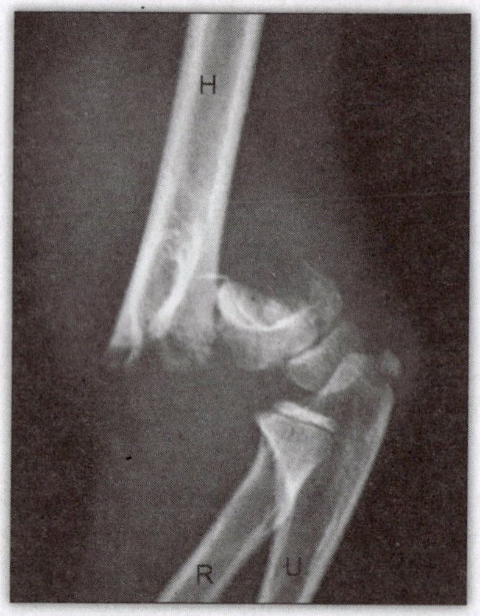

a. Ulnar nerve
b. Median nerve
c. Radial nerve
d. Musculocutaneous nerve

AIIMS NOVEMBER 2015

48. **Axillary nerve injury is seen in all EXCEPT:**

a. Surgical neck humerus fracture
b. Dislocation of shoulder joint
c. Improper use of crutches
d. Intramuscular injection

49. **A 25-year-old male had early morning backache and stiffness. Pain and stiffness is relieved by warm water fomentation. What can be other associated finding?**

a. Swelling of proximal interphalangeal joint
b. Limited chest expansion
c. Nodule in olecranon
d. Dupuytren's contracture

50. A 10-year-old girl presents to orthopedic OPD with deformity as shown below. Which fracture causes this deformity?

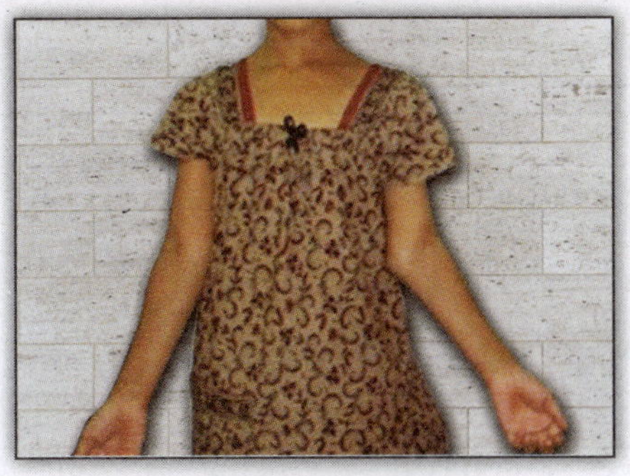

a. Medial epicondyle fracture of humerus
b. Lateral epicondyle fracture of humerus
c. Supracondylar fracture of humerus
d. Fracture shaft of humerus

51. A child presented with pain in forearm following trauma. Identify the pathology in the X-ray film of?

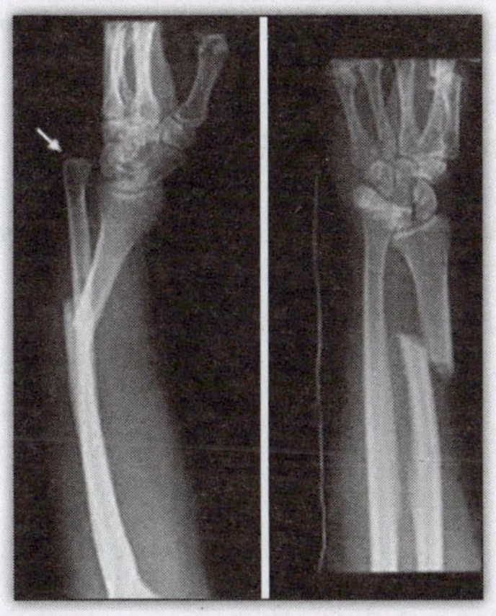

a. Cole's fracture b. Smith's fracture
c. Galeazzi's fracture d. Barton's fracture

52. Identify the deformity shown in picture below.

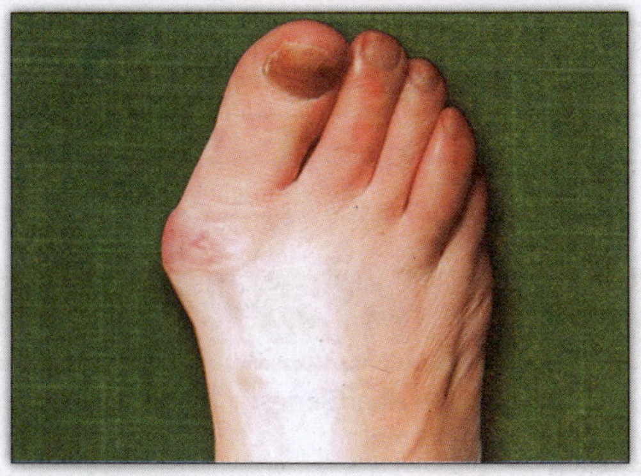

a. Hallux varus
b. Hallux valgus
c. Forefoot adduction deformity
d. Rheumatoid nodule

53. An adolescent aged patient with pain in knee region with radiolucent lytic areas in the upper tibial on X-ray as shown below. What is the most probable diagnosis?

a. Gaint cell tumor b. Simple bone cyst
c. Adamantinoma d. Ewing's sarcoma

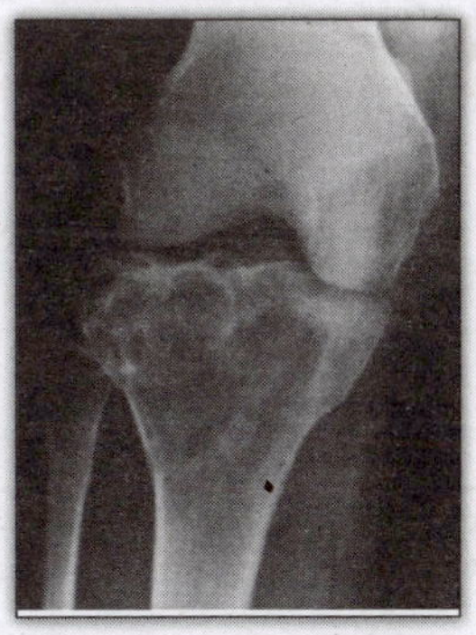

54. Identify the test being performed in the image below?

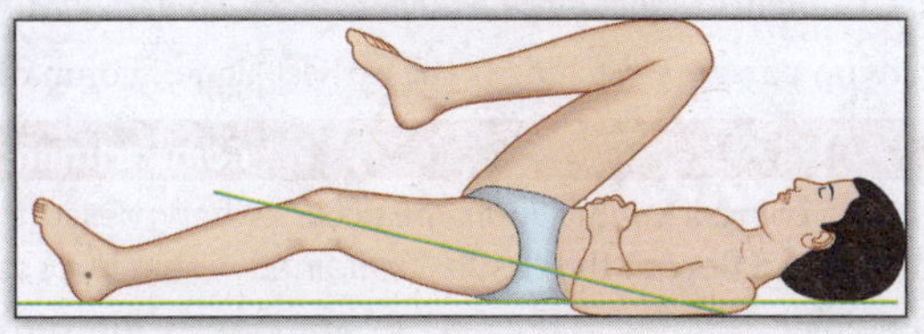

a. Trendelenburg's test b. Thomas test
c. Smith test d. Narath test

AIIMS MAY 2015

55. Judet view for?
a. Pelvis b. Calcaneum
c. Scaphoid d. Spine

56. Investigation of choice for stress fracture is?
a. MRI b. CT
c. Bone scan d. X-ray

57. Shenton line is seen in?
a. Hip joint b. Pelvis
c. Shoulder d. Knee

58. Jersey finger is caused by rupture of?
a. Extensor digiti minimi
b. Flexor digitorum superficialis
c. Flexor digitorum profundus
d. Extensor indicis

59. Traction not used in lower limb?
a. Gallows b. Bryant
c. Dunlop d. Perkin

60. Removal of vertebral disc can be done by all approaches EXCEPT:
a. Laminotomy b. Laminectomy
c. Laminoplasty d. Hemilaminectomy

61. Which of the following is seen in osteoporosis?
a. Normal calcium, decreased ALP
b. Decreased calcium, increased ALP
c. Normal calcium, normal ALP
d. Decreased calcium, decreased ALP

62. A 42-year-old man is diagnosed to have irreparable tear of the rotator cuff. Treatment of choice will be?
a. Tendon transfer
b. Reverse shoulder replacement
c. Total shoulder replacement
d. Acromioplasty

ANSWERS WITH EXPLANATIONS

AIIMS NOVEMBER 2018

1. Ans. (a) Dextrocardia

Ref: Apley's 9th ed page 181, Nelson's 18th Ed Ch 680; Paediatric Orthopedics by Jan Douwes Visser Pg 25

"Dextrocardia is not associated with Sprengel Deformity"

Repeat AIIMS Nov 2017 Orthopedics (See for explanation) (see page no. 1015)

2. Ans. (d) Pain on passive stretching of toes

Ref: Campbell's Operative Orthopaedics by Frederick M Azar, 13th Ed Pg 3724

Pain on passive stretching is the earliest sign of compartment syndrome

Compartment Syndrome and Volkmann's Ischemia	
Acute compartment syndrome occurs when pressure rises within a confined space in the body, resulting in a critical reduction of the blood flow to the tissues contained within the space	
Etiology	• **Fracture is the most common cause of compartment syndrome.** The most common fracture associated with acute compartment syndrome in adults is tibial diaphyseal fracture followed by supracondylar fracture of humerus. • The second most common cause of acute compartment syndrome is soft tissue injury, which added to tibial diaphyseal fracture makes up almost two thirds of the cases. • Adolescence younger patients are at more risk of compartment syndrome • **Deep flexor muscles, flexor digitorum profundus are most commonly involved** in Volkman's ischemic contracture.
Clinical features	1. Pain out of proportion to physical examination findings 2. Pain on passive stretching: 1st sign 3. Pressure increased 4. Pallor/may also be pink 5. Pulseness 6. Paresthesia 7. Paralysis
Indications of fasciotomy	1. Pain with passive motion 2. Pain out of proportion to the injury 3. Clinical signs such as demonstrable motor or sensory loss 4. Compartment pressures greater than 35 mm Hg (slit or wick catheter technique) or greater than 40 mm Hg (needle technique) 5. Interrupted arterial circulation to the extremity for more than 4 hours

3. Ans. (c) Mallet finger

Ref: Campbell 12th Ed Pg 1370

Type III fractures of the distal phalanx produce a "mallet" finger.

Ligament Injuries of Finger				
	Description	History/physical exam	Work-up/findings	Treatment
Boutonniere Deformity	• Extensor tendon (central slip injury) at PIP ruptures, lateral bands slip volar and flex PIP • Associated with RA 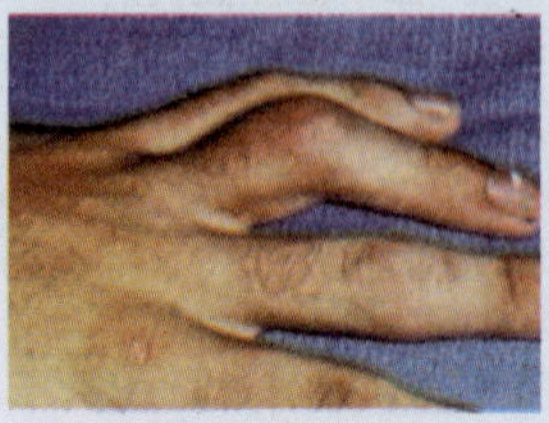	**Hx:** Hand trauma PE: PIP flexed, no active extension, DIP extended	**XR:** Hand series: Normal	• Splint PIP in extension, DIP free • Reconstruct central slip and bands • **Severe:** Fusion or arthroplasty

Contd...

Ligament Injuries of Finger	Description	History/physical exam	Work-up/findings	Treatment
Jersey Finger	Flexor digitorum profundus (FDP) tendon injury by forceful extension on a flexed digit, typically in an athlete grabbing opponent's jersey. (Also called a Zone 1 Flexor tendon injury). Occur mostly in rugby/football. Occurs most commonly in the ring finger (75%). 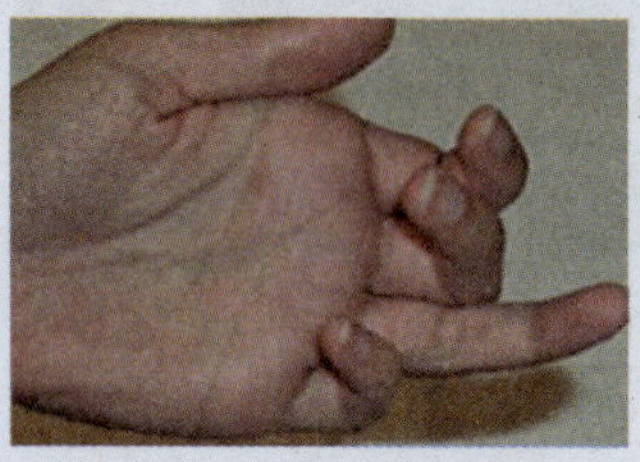	**Hx:** Extension injury, 1/2 pain. PE: FDS: 1 sublimis test FDP: 1 profundus test	**XR:** Rule out fracture (1/2 avulsion fracture)	• Primary repair • Older patient: DIP fusion
Mallet Finger	**AKA: baseball, dropped, dolphin finger** • Hyperflexion Extensor digitorum tendon injury of the fingers at DIP • FDP unopposed so DIP flexes	**H/O:** Hyperflexion injury of Extensor digitorum, usually occurs when a ball, while being caught, hits an outstretched finger **Exm:** Cannot extend DIP, minimal pain & swelling, hyperextended PIP Jt	X-ray: 1/2 avulsion fracture	• **Constant splint** (DIP only) for 8 weeks followed by 4 wks night only splint • Operative treatment is considered only if there is a large fragment (>50%) & subluxation of DIP.
Swan Neck Deformity	• FDS rupture/volar plate injury • Lateral bands subluxes dorsally, PIP hyperextends & DIP flexes 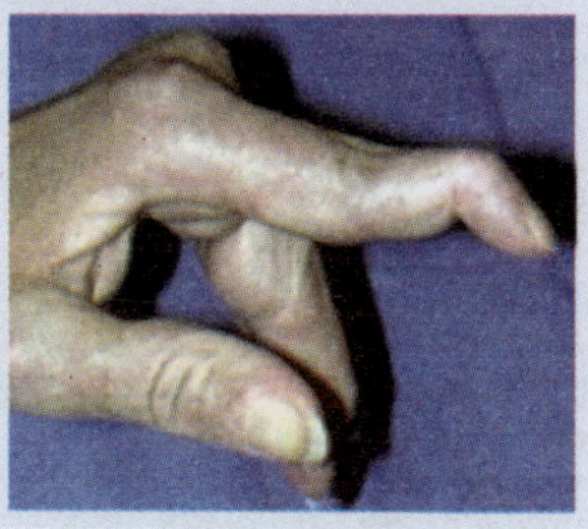	**Hx:** Trauma, RA, spastic **PE:** PIP hyperextended, DIP flexed	XR: Hand series	• **Early:** Splint • **Late:** Surgical repair (individualize each case)
Gamekeeper's Thumb	**- AKA; SKIER'S THUMB** - Ulnar collateral ligament tear of the thumb metacarpo phalangeal joint • **Mechanism:** forceful radial deviation or fall on extended thumb causing hyperabduction 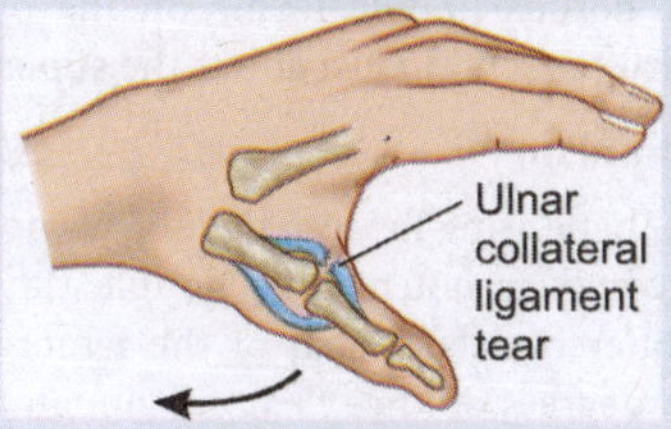	**H/O:** Trauma. Pain & swelling. EXM: Partial rupture: Only the ligament proper is torn and the thumb is unstable in flexion but stable in full extension because the palmar plate is intact. Complete rupture, both ligament proper & palmar plate are torn & thumb is unstable in all positions	**XR:** 1/2 avulsion fracture. Stress view shows injury	• **Incomplete:** Splint 2–4 weeks, avoid pinch for 6–8 weeks • **Complete:** Surgical repair (treat Stener lesion; proximal end of torn ligament gets trapped in front of the adductor pollicis aponeurosis)

4. Ans. (d) Sequestrum

Ref: Campbell 12th Ed Pg 706, 731

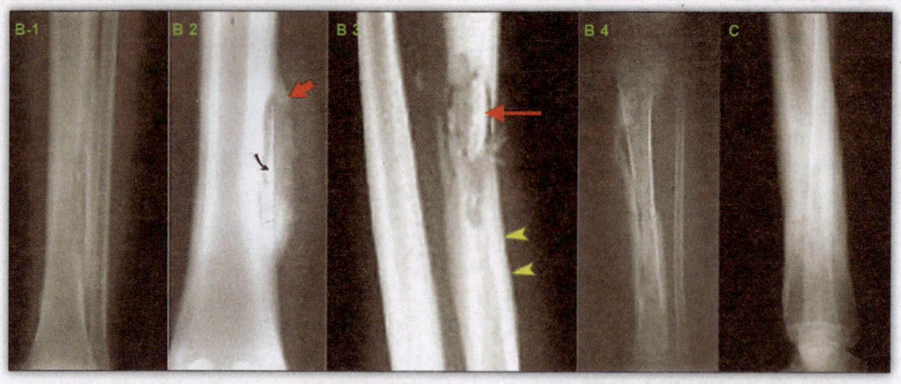

Fig: Different stages of chronic osteomyelitis on X-rays

Chronic Osteomyelitis X-ray: Jones et al. described a classification of chronic hematogenous osteomyelitis in children in which three main types are identified based on radiographic appearance:

Jones Classification of Chronic Hematogenous Osteomyelitis in Children

Class		Explanation	Example X-ray
Type A		Brodie abscess (Subacute osteomyelitis)	Solitary circumscribed oval cavity surrounded by a zone of sclerosis A1 = Upper end of tibia A2 = Femur AP view A3 = Femur frog leg view
Type B (sequestrum involucrum)	B1	Localized cortical sequestrum	Localised cortical sequestrum of tibia
	B2	Sequestrum with normal structural involucrum	Sequestrum (black arrow) with normal structural involucrum (white arrow) of proximal humerus
	B3	Sequestrum with sclerotic involucrum	Sequestrum (white arrow) with sclerotic involucrum (black arrow head) of radius
	B4	Sequestrum without/Inadequate structural Involucrum	Sequestrum without/inadequate structural involucrum of tibia
Type C		Sclerotic	Sclerotic tibia

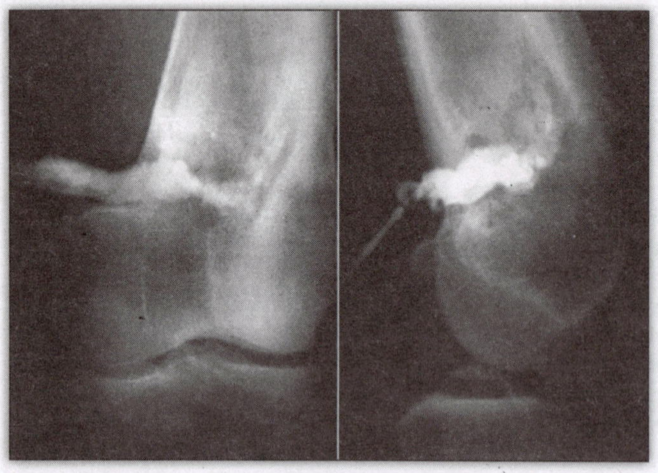

Fig: Sinogram in Chronic osteomyelitis: AP and Lateral roentgenograms of a sinogram in with chronic osteomyelitis that tracks into the intramedullary cavity

5. Ans. (b) Superior pole of patella and impinging on femoral component during extension

Ref: Campbell 12th Ed Pg 428

Patellar Clunk Syndrome is a patellofemoral complication of Total knee arthroplasty.

Anatomy

It has been described in association with posterior-stabilized knee arthroplasties.

A fibrous nodule forms on the posterior surface of the quadriceps tendon just above the **superior pole of the patella**.

Mechanism

Note that during flexion, the fibrous nodule enters the femoral intercondylar notch. This nodule can become entrapped in the intercondylar notch of the femoral prosthesis and at 30 to 45 degrees of knee flexion, enough tension is developed so as to cause the knee to pop or "clunk **as the knee is actively extended.**

Causes

- Proximal placement of the patellar button so that it overhangs the cut surface of the patella is one possible cause, as the prominent button could impinge on the quadriceps tendon, with resultant fibrous tissue proliferation.
- Femoral component design is another possible cause. Early posterior-stabilized components with a relatively high, sharp femoral sulcus also could impinge on the quadriceps tendon because they allow the patellar component to fall into the notch with lesser degrees of flexion.

Treatment

- The recommended treatment for this condition is arthroscopic debridement of the nodule. Arthrotomy and nodule excision are reserved for patients with recurrence after arthroscopic treatment or in the setting of loose or malpositioned patellar components that may require revision.
- A limited synovectomy of the posterior surface of the quadriceps tendon as a prophylactic measure for this condition when performing a posterior-stabilized arthroplasty has also been suggested.

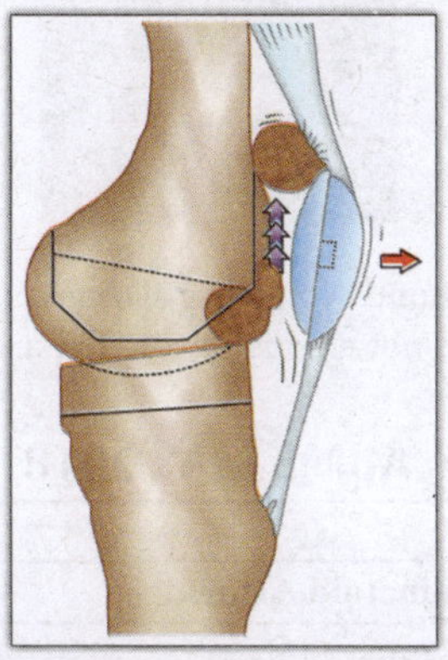

Fig: Patellar clunk syndrome

6. Ans. (a) Coxa vara

Ref: Apley's 9th ed page 508

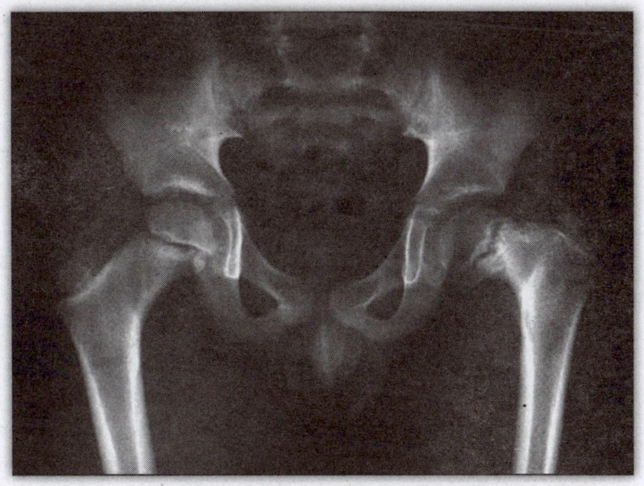

Fig: The given picture shows reduced angle of inclination or Neck shaft angle on left side. Hence Coxa Vara

Option (C) Coxa magna is the asymmetrical, circumferential enlargement and deformation of the femoral head and neck.

Neck Shaft angle/Angle of Inclination: This is the angle formed by the longitudinal axis of the femoral shaft and the line drawn along the axis of the femoral neck, which passes through the center the femoral head. At birth this angle measures about 140 to 150 degrees. Primarily because of the loading across the femoral neck during walking, this angle usually reduces to its normal adulthood value of about ***125 degrees***. The normal range of the neck-shaft angle is between 125° and 140°. If the angle is either larger or smaller than this range, it is defined as coxa valga or coxa vara, respectively

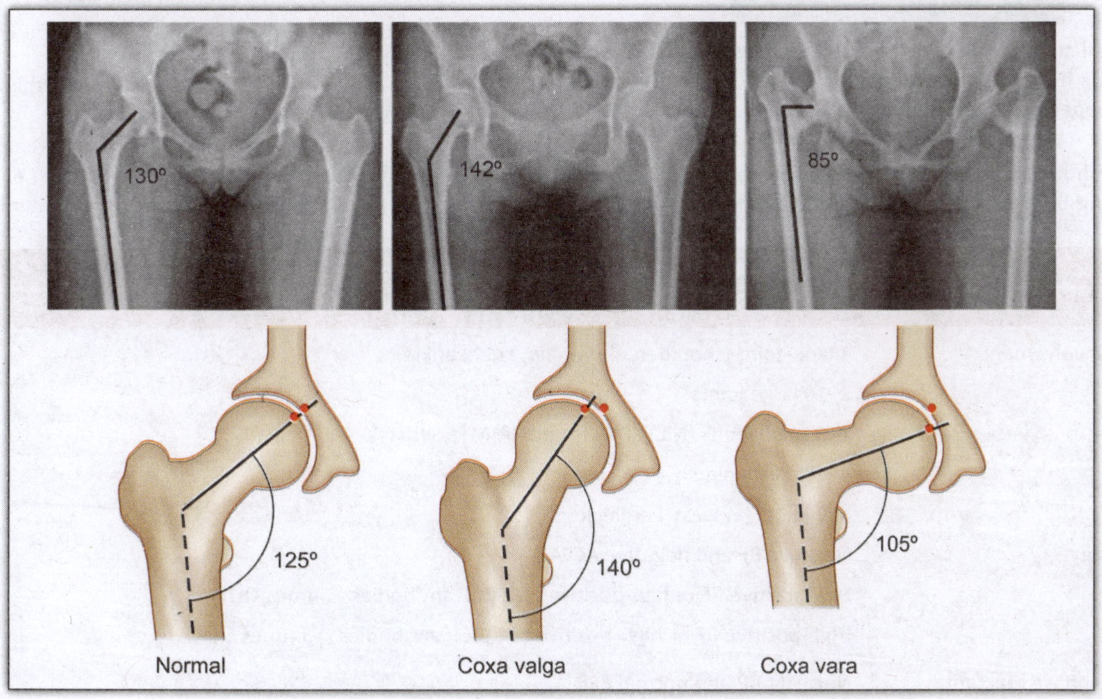

Figs A to C: **(A)** Normal angle of inclination; **(B)** Coxa vara; and **(C)** Coxa valga

A change in the normal angle of inclination is referred to as either coxa vara or coxa valga.

- **Coxa vara** (Latin coxa, hip, + vara, to bend inward) describes an angle of inclination markedly <125 degrees
- **Coxa valga** (Latin valga, to bend outward) describes an angle of inclination markedly >125 degrees.

7. Ans. (a) GCT, (B) Osteoclastoma

Ref: With text

NOTE

Both GCT and Osteoclastoma were provided in the options

Option (A) & (B): Giant-cell Tumor (Osteoclastoma)

Which represents 5% of all primary bone tumors and appears in mature bone, most commonly in the distal femur, proximal tibia, proximal humerus and distal radius, though other bones also may be affected. It is hardly ever seen before closure of the nearby physis and characteristically it extends right up to the subarticular bone plate.

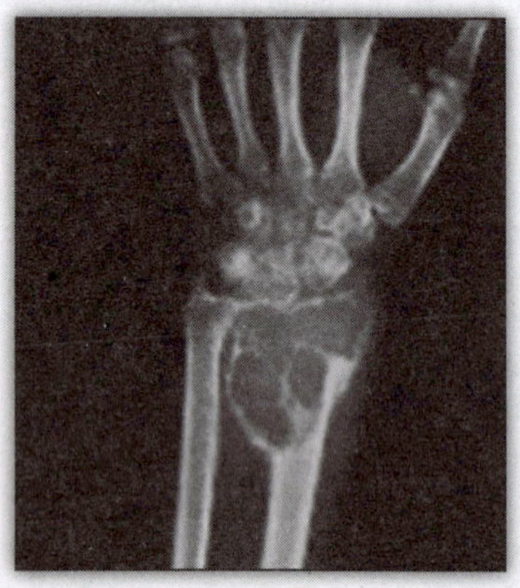

Fig: Giant cell tumor: The expansile and lytic lesion of the distal radius extends from the distal diaphysis to the subchondral bone. Hardly ever appears before epiphysis has fused, the pathognomonic feature is that it extends right up to the subarticular bone plate

X-rays show a radiolucent area situated eccentrically at the end of a long bone and bounded by the subchondral bone plate. The center sometimes has a **soap-bubble appearance** due to ridging of the surrounding bone. ***The appearance of a 'cystic' lesion in mature bone, extending right up to the subchondral plate, is so characteristic that the diagnosis is seldom in doubt.*** (Ref: Apley 9th ed page 202)

Option (C)

In an adult an aneurysmal bone cyst may be mistaken for a giant-cell tumor but, unlike the latter, it usually does not extend right up to the articular margin. While GCT always abuts against the joint margin. **(Ref: Apley 9th ed page 201)**

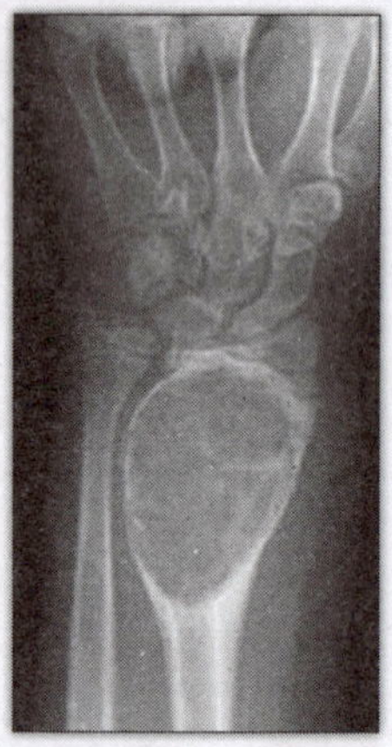

Fig: Aneurysmal Bone cyst: Expansile cystic lesion of the lower end of Radius not extending into the articular margin

AIIMS MAY 2018

8. Ans. (a) Rheumatoid Arthritis

Ref: Harrison's 19th Ed Pg 2136

Clinical features of rheumatoid arthritis are:

- Early morning joint stiffness lasting more than 1 h that eases with physical activity.
- The earliest involved joints are typically the small joints of the hands and feet.
- The initial pattern of joint involvement may be monoarticular, oligoarticular (≤ 4 joints) or polyarticular (>5 joints), usually in a symmetric distribution.

Classification Criteria for Rheumatoid Arthritis

		Score
Joint involvement	1 large joint (shoulder, elbow, hip, knee, ankle)	0
	2–10 large joints	1
	1–3 small joints (MCP, PIP, Thumb IP, MTP, wrists)	2
	4–10 small joints	3
	>10 joints (at least 1 small joint)	5
Serology	Negative RF and negative ACPA	0
	Low-positive RF or low-positive anti-CCP antibodies (3 times ULN)	2
	High-positive RF or high-positive anti-CCP antibodies (>3 times ULN)	3
Acute-phase reactants	Normal CRP and normal ESR	0

Contd...

Classification Criteria for Rheumatoid Arthritis		
		Score
	Abnormal CRP or abnormal ESR	1
Duration of symptoms	<6 weeks	0
	6 weeks or more	1
Note: • Patients with a score of ≥ 6 have "definite" rheumatoid arthritis • Abbreviations: ▪ RF- Rheumatoid factor ▪ ACPA- Anti Citrullinated Protein Antibody ▪ CRP- C Reactive protein ▪ RA- Rheumatoid arthritis ▪ ESR- Erythrocyte Sedimentation Rate		

9. Ans. (b) Thomas test

Ref: Campbell's 13th Ed Pg 1398

- The presence of a hip flexion contracture is determined by the Thomas test.
- Thomas test detects hip flexion contracture by extending affected hip while contralateral hip is held flexed, flattening and immobilizing lumbar spine.
- **Method:** With the patient supine, both hips are flexed maximally, thus flattening any lumbar lordosis. The legs are then alternatively brought into extension with any residual flexion contracture noted while the pelvis and lumbar spine are held stationary by keeping the contralateral hip flexed.

Tests For Hip Joint		
Test	Description	Diagram
Trendelenberg test	• Weakness of the hip abductor is tested • Positive for hip abductor weakness when the pelvis sags more than 2 cm during single-leg stance on the limb tested • Positive in superior gluteal nerve injury, weakness of abductors of the hip joint	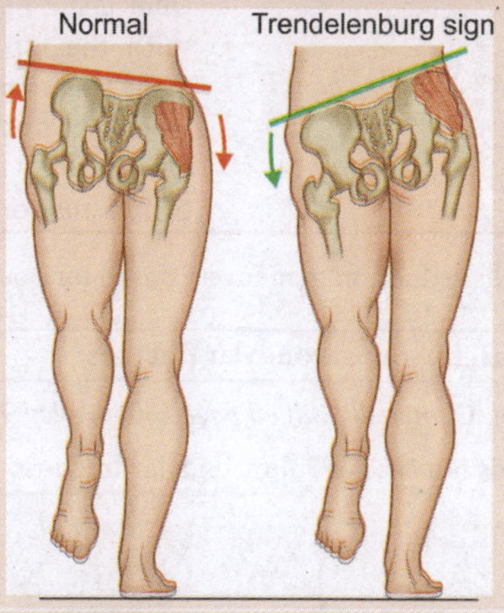
Thomas test	• The presence of a hip flexion contracture is determined by the Thomas test. • With the patient supine, both hips are flexed maximally, thus flattening any lumbar lordosis. • The legs are then alternatively brought into extension with any residual flexion contracture noted while the pelvis and lumbar spine are held stationary by keeping the contralateral hip flexed.	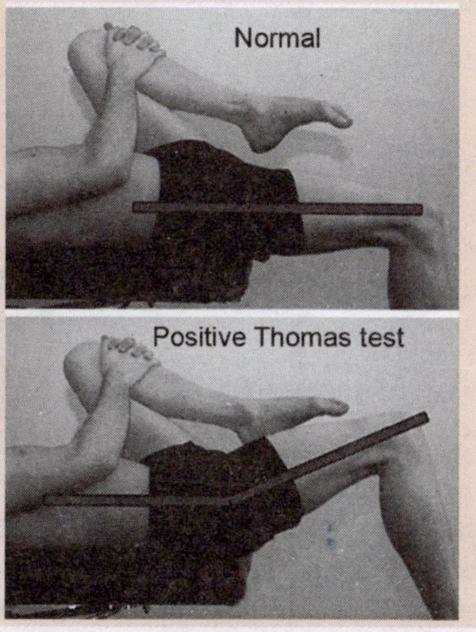

Contd...

Tests For Hip Joint		
Test	**Description**	**Diagram**
FADIR test or anterior impingement test (Flexion ADduction Internal Rotation)	• Performed by flexing the hip to 90 degrees, adducting across the midline, and maximally internally rotating the hip • Hips with symptomatic anterior impingement are limited in internal rotation and are painful with this maneuver. • With anterior impingement, patients have distinctly more pain with the FADIR test than with other extremes of rotation	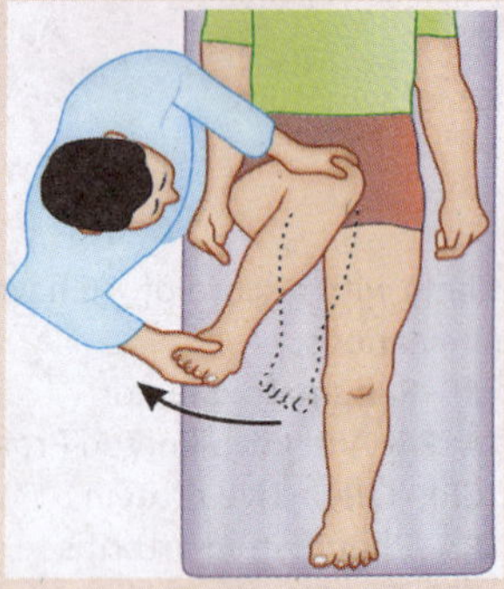
FABER test Flexion, ABduction, and External Rotation (Patrick's test)	• Performed to evaluate pathology of the hip joint or the sacroiliac joint. • Leg is flexed and the thigh abducted and externally rotated	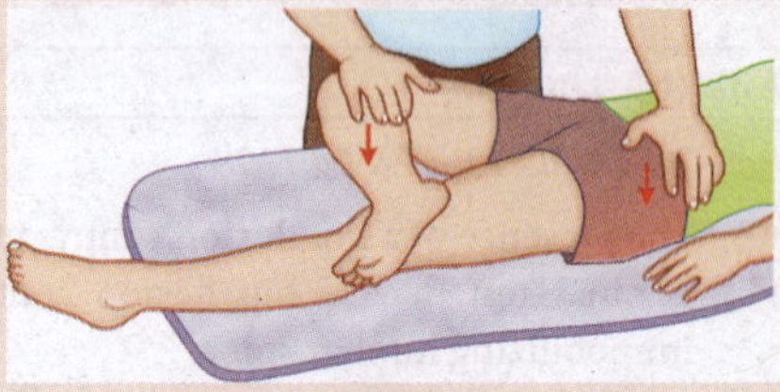
Ober test	• The Ober test is performed with the patient in the lateral position by abducting the patient's hip with the knee flexed and then letting the hip fall into adduction. • A delay in adduction due to gravity is a positive Ober test. • With the hip extended past neutral, a positive Ober test signifies tightness of the iliotibial band, whereas a positive Ober test with the hip in neutral flexion/extension is indicative of a gluteus medius contracture or tendinopathy.	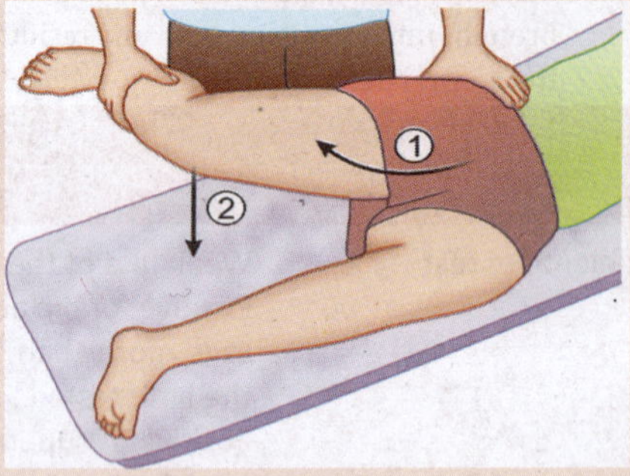

Allis reduction maneuver is used for posterior hip dislocation.

10. Ans. (c) Supracondylar fracture

Ref: Campbell 12th ed page 1404, Apley 9th ed page 757, Maheshwari 4th ed page 93

This is a case of Supracondylar fracture

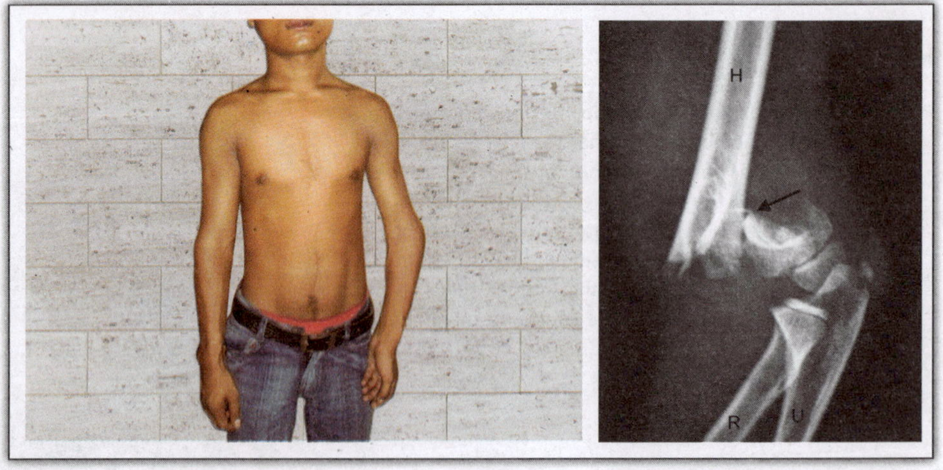

Figs A and B: (A) Cubitus varus ('GUN-STOCK' DEFORMITY): The deformity is *most obvious when the elbow is extended and the arms are elevated.* The most common cause is malunion of a supracondylar fracture. The deformity can be corrected by a wedge osteotomy of the lower humerus but this is best left until skeletal maturity; **(B) Supracondylar fracture** radiograph showing extension type injury with posterior displacement of the distal segment

Supracondylar Fracture of Humerus	
Age group	Most common in children and elderly patients, but it may occur at any age
Mechanism	Flexion type or an extension type, depending upon the **displacement of the distal fragment** of bone • **Posterior angulation or displacement or Extension type (95 per cent of all cases)** suggests a hyperextension injury, usually due to a fall on the outstretched hand and is stable only in significant flexion. • **Anterior angulation or displacement or flexion type** is produced by a fall on the flexed elbow and is relatively stable in extension
Classification	**Gartland classification** is useful for determining appropriate treatment for supracondylar fractures: • **Type I:** undisplaced • **Type II:** displaced with intact posterior cortex • **Type III:** is a completely displaced fracture (although the posterior periosteum is usually still preserved, which will assist surgical reduction).
Clinical features	Pain, swelling, S shaped deformity, Loss of anatomical landmark, signs of neurovascular injury can accompany and should be checked.
Adequacy of reduction	**Baumann angle** usually is considered the angle formed by the intersection of a line perpendicular to the long axis of the humeral shaft and the physeal line of the lateral condyle; reported **normal values range from 9 to 26 degrees**. A common rule of thumb is that a Baumann angle of at least 10 degrees is acceptable 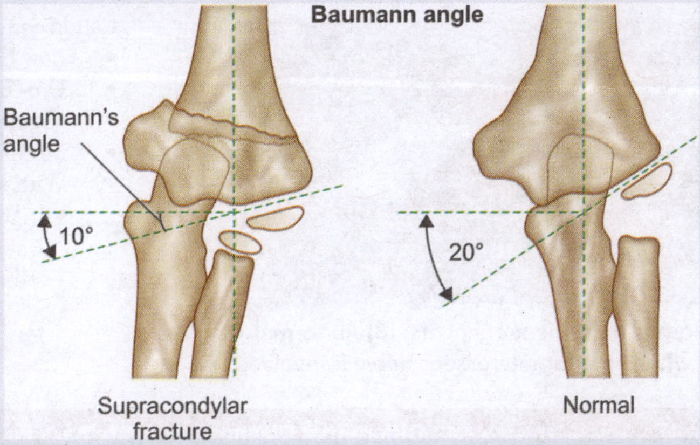
Treatment	• Side-arm skin traction for Type 1 injury **(Dunlop traction)** • Overhead skeletal traction for Type 1 injury • **CRPP** (closed reduction percutaneous pinning) for type 2 injury • **ORIF** (open reduction and internal fixation) for type 3 injury. Performed emergently (<8 hours) or urgently (≤24 hours) or after the swelling has decreased, but not later than 5 days after injury because the possibility of myositis ossificans apparently increases after that time
Early Complications	• **Brachial artery injury** (earlier 5%, now a days < 1%) - perform angiography, or Doppler • Compartment syndrome (uncommon) • **Nerve injury:** Most commonly ***median nerve (particularly the anterior interosseous branch)***. Most nerve injuries are associated with type III displaced supracondylar fractures. The radial nerve lies posterolateral to the supracondylar fractures thus less commonly involved. Ulnar nerve which is posteriorly located is uncommonly injured. Conclusion: **MEDIAN > ULNAR > RADIAL** • **Neuropraxia**—is reported to occur in 3% to 22%
Late complications	• **Malunion** • **Cubitus varus** (carrying angle <5 degrees) and Cubitus valgus (carrying angle > 15 degrees) **(Cubitus varus AKA Gun stock deformity is far more common)**. Cubitus varus is the most common angular deformity that results from supracondylar fractures in children. The most common cause is malunion of a supracondylar fracture. • **Cubitus valgus**, although mentioned in the literature as causing tardy ulnar nerve palsy, rarely occurs and is more often caused by nonunion of lateral condylar fractures. • **Tardy ulnar nerve palsy** (Not due to supracondylar fracture per se but its complication as valgus) • Elbow stiffness and myositis ossifficans
Management of cubitus varus	Three basic types of osteotomies have been described: A medial opening wedge osteotomy with a bone graft, an oblique osteotomy with derotation, and a lateral closing wedge osteotomy (easiest, safest and most stable osteotomy)

NOTE

Baumann angle is different from Carrying angle. Carrying angle is a small degree of cubitus valgus, formed between the axis of a radially deviated forearm and the axis of the humerus. The normal carrying angle of the elbow is 5–15 degrees of valgus; anything more than this is regarded as a valgus deformity.

11. Ans. (c) Anterior interosseous nerve

Ref: Textbook of Orthopaedics, Trauma and Rheumatology E-Book By Raashid Luqmani 2nd Ed Pg 122

- Anterior interosseus nerve is a motor branch of median nerve. It supplies flexor pollicis, flexor digitorum profundus and pronator quadratus.
- Since flexor pollicis is affected due to injury to anterior interosseus nerve, the patient is unable to flex the thumb. The patient is unable to do **"OK" sign**.

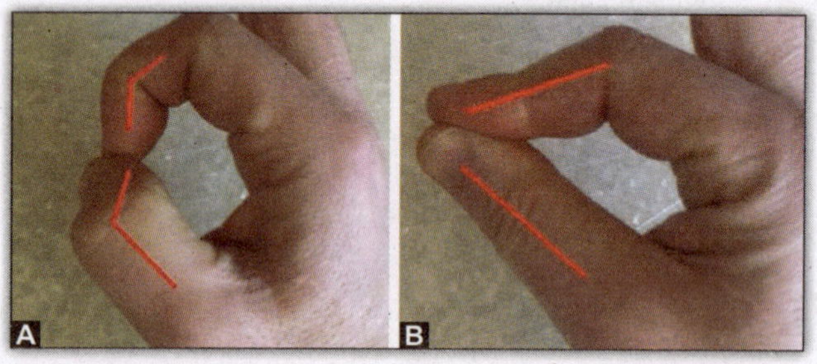

Figs A and B: (A) Normal movement of fingers; **(B)** Abnormal movement of fingers when anterior interosseus nerve is involved

Some Fracture Dislocations and Associated Nerve Injuries	
Fracture	**Nerve**
Anterior shoulder dislocation	Axillary/ Brachial dislocation
Diaphyseal fracture of humerus	Radial nerve injury
Supracondylar fracture	Anterior interosseus nerve/ Radial/Median
Hip dislocation/Posterior wall acetabular fractures	Sciatic nerve
Knee dislocation	Peroneal

12. Ans. (c) Cauda equina syndrome

Ref: Apley's 9th Ed Pg 246, 480

Cauda equina syndrome consists of a spectrum of:

- Low back pain
- Uni- or bilateral sciatica
- Saddle anaesthesia
- Motor weakness in the lower extremities
- With variable rectal and urinary symptoms
  - Absence of history of weight loss and fever in the above question points towards a non malignant diagnosis.

Differential Diagnosis of Acute Back Pain					
Disease of condition	**Patient age (years)**	**Location of pain**	**Quality of pain**	**Aggravating or relieving factors**	**Signs**
Back strain	20–40	Low back, buttock, posterior thigh	Ache, spasm	Increased with activity or bending	Local tenderness, limited spinal motion
Acute disc herniation	30–50	Low back to lower leg	Sharp, shooting, or burning pain; paresthesia in leg	Decreased with standing; increased with bending or sitting	Positive straight leg raise test, weakness, asymmetric reflexes
Osteoarthritis or spinal stenosis	30–50	Low back to lower leg; often bilateral	Ache, shooting pain "pains and needles" sensation	Increased with walking, especially up an incline; decreased with sitting	Mild decrease in extension of spine; may have weakness or asymmetric reflexes
Spondylolisthesis	Any age	Back, posterior thigh	Ache	Increased with activity or bending	Exaggeration of the lumbar curve, palpable "step off" (defect between spinous processes), tight hamstrings
Ankylosing spondylitis	15–40	Sacroiliac joints, lumbar spine	Ache	Morning stiffness	Decreased back motion, tenderness over sacroiliac joints
Infection	Any age	Lumbar spine, sacrum	Sharp pain, ache	Varies	Fever, percussive tenderness, neurologic signs, or fever
Malignancy	>50	Affected bone(s)	Dull ache, throbbing pain; slowly progressive	Increased with recumbency or cough	May have localized tenderness, neurologic signs, or fever

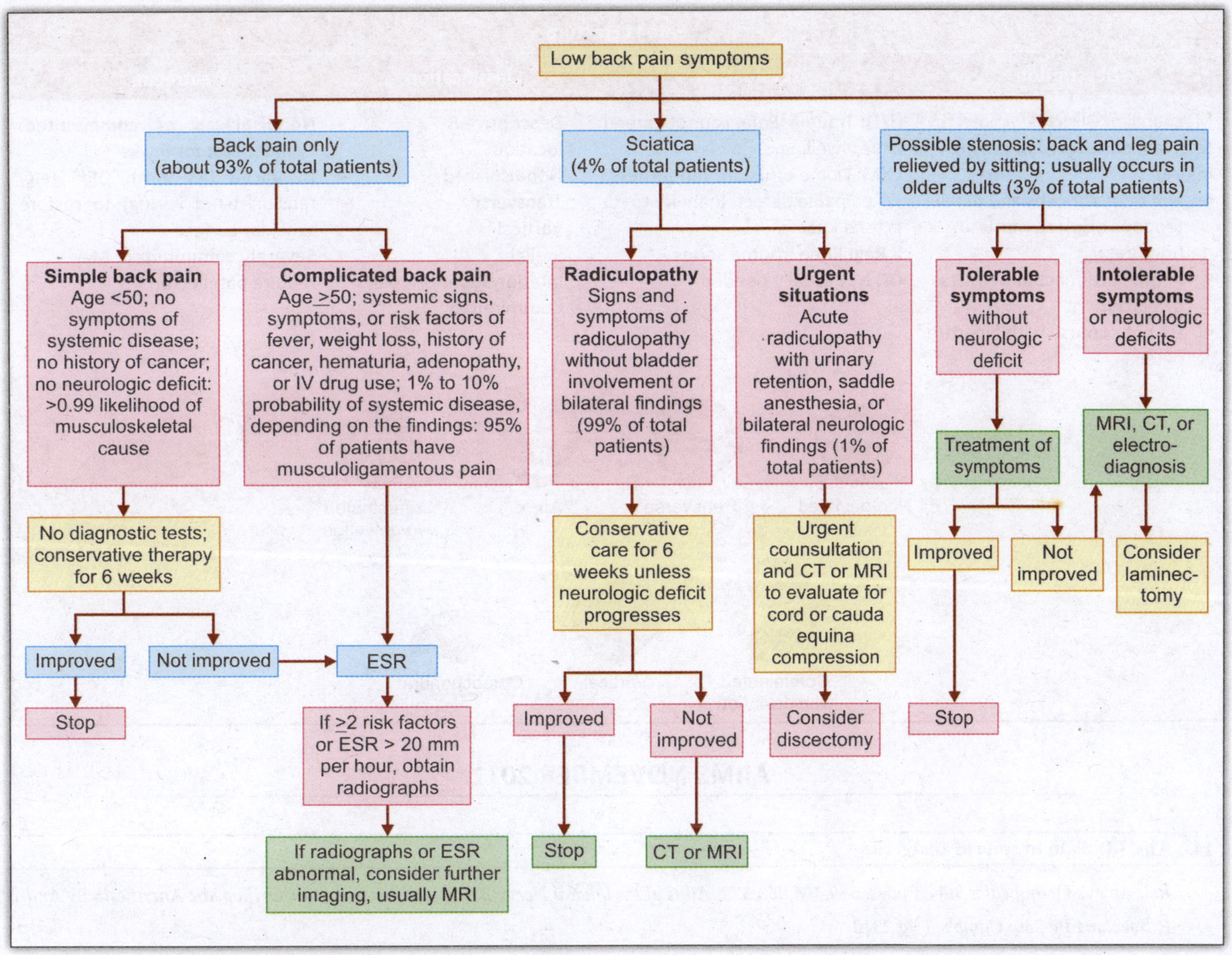

13. Ans. (d). Tension band wiring

Ref: Apley 9th ed page 702, 887

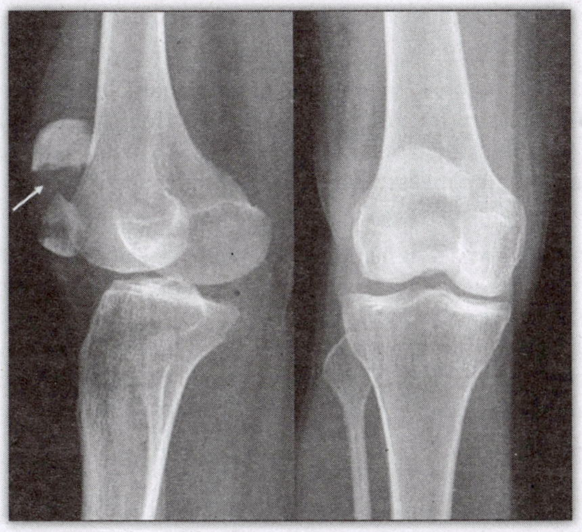

Fig: The lateral and AP radiograph of knee shows a displaced transverse fracture of patella, the treatment of which should be Tension band wiring

- The lateral and AP radiograph of knee shows a displaced transverse fracture of patella, the treatment of which should be Tension band wiring (TBW). Although K Wire is a part of TBW, the whole process of TBW is to be applied to achieve stability of the fragments.
- Cerclage and tension-band wires are essentially loops of wire passed around two bone fragments and then tightened to compress the fragments together. When using cerclage wires, make sure that the wires hug the bone and do not embrace any of the close lying nerves or vessels.
- Both techniques are used for **patellar fractures**: the tension-band wire is placed such that the maximum compressive force is over the tensile surface, which is usually the convex side of the bone
- **Displaced transverse fracture:** The lateral expansions are torn and the entire extensor mechanism is disrupted. Operation is essential. Through a longitudinal incision the fracture is exposed and the patella repaired by the tension-band principle. The fragments are reduced and transfixed with two stiff K-wires; flexible wire is then looped tightly around the protruding K-wires and over the front of the patella

Patella Fracture			
Description	**Evaluation**	**Classification**	**Treatment**
Mechanism: Direct & indirect: (e.g. fall, dashboard or kicking injury) • Pull of quadriceps and patella tendons displace most fractures • If intact, retinaculum resists displacement • Do not confuse with bipartite patella	**H/O:** Trauma, Pain, cannot extend knee, swelling. **EXM:** Dome effusion. Tenderness, +/- palpable defect. Inability to extend knee. **X Ray:** Knee trauma series **CT:** Not usually needed	Descriptive & location: Nondisplaced Transverse Vertical Stellate Inferior/superior pole Comminuted	• **Nondisplaced or comminuted:** cylinder cast for 6 wks • **Displaced (>3 mm):** ORIF (e.g. tension band wiring) to restore articular surface • **Severely comminuted:** May require patellectomy

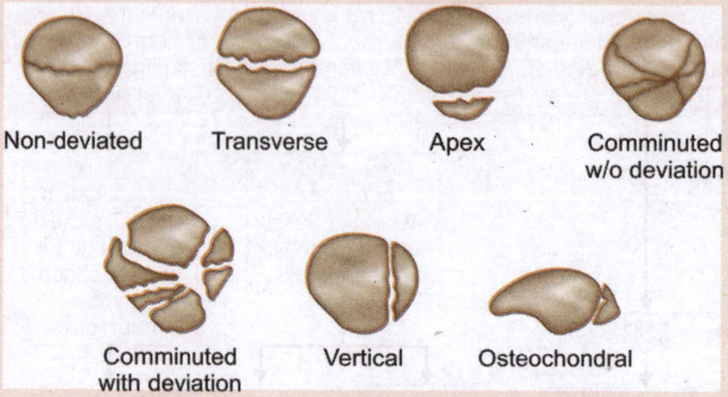

AIIMS NOVEMBER 2017

14. Ans. (d) Pain in spite of analgesics

Ref: Apley's Orthopedics 9th ed page: 339,496,563,572, Atlas of Peripheral Nerve Blocks and Anatomy for Orthopedic Anesthesia By André P. Boezaart Pg 230; Campbell Pg 2312

Pain out of proportion to that expected with the injury is the most important and the first symptom of compartment syndrome and hence should be checked first.

Compartment Syndrome	
Definition	Elevation of the interstitial pressure in a closed osteofascial compartment that results in microvascular compromise.
Common causes	Fracture is the most common cause of compartment syndrome. The most common fracture associated with acute compartment syndrome in adults is **tibial diaphyseal** fracture followed by **supracondylar fracture of humerus**. **Soft tissue injury, which added to tibial diaphyseal fracture makes up almost two thirds of the cases.** **Adolescent younger patients are at more risk.**
Types	**Acute compartment syndrome:** fractures, soft tissue, trauma, arterial injury, limb compression during altered consciousness, burns, intravenous fluid extravasation and anticoagulants, acute exertional compartment syndromes **Chronic exertional compartment syndrome:** Due to recurrence of increased pressure,commonly in the anterior or deep posterior compartment of the leg. Exercise can increase muscle volume by 20%, causing an increase in pressure in a noncompliant compartment
Pathophysiology	Increased tissue pressure, decreased capillary blood flow, and local tissue necrosis caused by oxygen deprivation. Significant muscle necrosis can occur with normal blood flow if intracompartmental pressure is increased to more than 30 mm Hg for longer than 8 hours. Higher pressures cause greater compromise of neuromuscular viability in shorter periods of time.

Contd...

Compartment Syndrome	
Clinical features	Tightness of the involved compartment Pain with passive motion of the muscles passing through the compartment Pain out of proportion to that expected with the injury (most important, first symptom). Hypoesthesia or paresthesia (tested with pinprick, light touch, two-point discrimination). Paralysis of muscle groups affected by the acute compartment syndrome is recognized as being a late sign.
	Palpable swelling in the compartment affected may be a further sign of compartment syndrome Peripheral pulses and capillary return may be present and are usually absent if artery is involved or at late presentation
Investigations	**Compartment Pressure level measurement:** Adequate evaluation not possible, altered neurological function by vascular injuries, continuous epidural anesthesia, peripheral nerve injury, or tourniquet palsy. **Invasive Devices:** pressure monitor, arterial line manometer, Whitesides three-way stopcock apparatus, wick monitor. **Non invasive:** Ultrasonography to measure submicrometer displacement of the fascia wall caused by volume expansion of the muscle compartment, which is related to changes in intramuscular pressure; Infrared imaging to determine temperature differences between the proximal and distal skin surfaces
Treatment	In isolated limb injuries, splitting of the cast and underlying padding can decrease compartment pressure by as much as 50% to 85%. Any circular constrictive bandages also should be released. Positioning of the limb is important; placing the limb at the level of the heart produces the highest arteriovenous gradient. On the other hand, elevation of the Limb decreases arterial inflow without significantly increasing venous outflow, thus increasing local ischemia. If symptoms do not resolve within 30 to 60 minutes after appropriate treatment, pressure measurement should be repeated and, if results are equivocal, fasciotomy is indicated.

15. Ans. (c) Open fracture, limb wound of size > 10 cm with extensive soft tissue damage and periosteal stripping

Ref: Campbell 13th ed page 2563

Gustilo and Anderson Open Fracture Classification

Gustilo Type	I	II	IIIA	IIIB	IIIC
Images	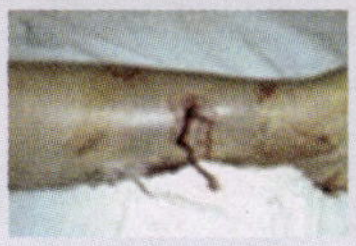	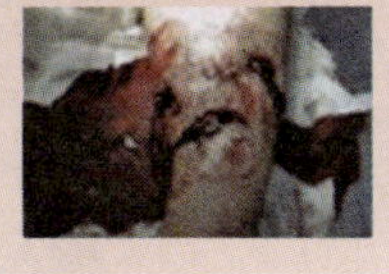	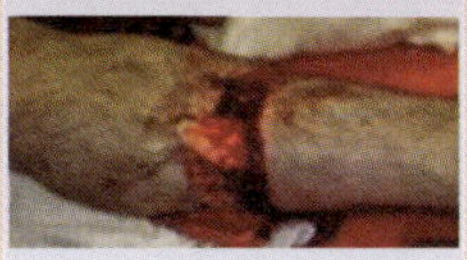	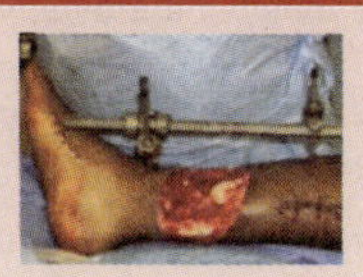	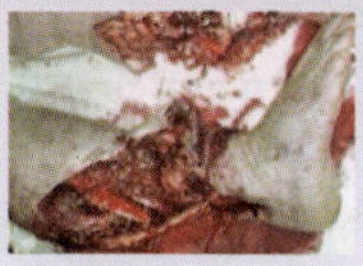
Energy	Low energy	Moderate	High	High	High
Wound Size	< 1 cm	> 1 cm	>10 cm	>10 cm	>10 cm
Soft Tissue	Minimal	Moderate	Extensive	Extensive	Extensive
Contamination	Clean	Moderate contamination	Extensive	Extensive	Extensive
Fracture Pattern	Simple fracture pattern with minimal comminution	Moderate comminution	Severe comminution or segmental fractures	Severe comminution or segmental fractures	Severe comminution or segmental fractures
Periosteal Stripping	No	No	Yes	Yes	Yes
Skin Coverage	Local coverage	Local coverage	Local coverage including	Requires free tissue flap or rotational flap coverage	Typically requires flap coverage
Neurovascular Injury	Normal	Normal	Normal	Normal	Exposed fracture with arterial damage that requires repair

16. Ans. (a) Hoover's test

Ref: Neurologic Emergencies edited by Latha Ganti, Joshua N. Goldstein page 198, Neurology and Trauma by Randolph W. Evans 2nd ed page 648

Hoover's Sign: An important test of motor examination is to perform Hoover's test (Hoover 1908). This is probably the best known and touted as one of the more reliable signs to assess conversion type paresis or plegia. In brief it involves two steps:

- **Hip extension:** In patients with functional weakness, a discrepancy can be observed between their voluntary hip extension (which is often weak) and their involuntary hip extension when the opposite hip is being flexed against resistance (which should be normal).
- **Hip flexion:** The opposite test, in which hip flexion in the weak leg is tested while the examiner's hand is held under the good heel. The absence of downward pressure in the good leg indicates a lack of effort transmitted to either leg.

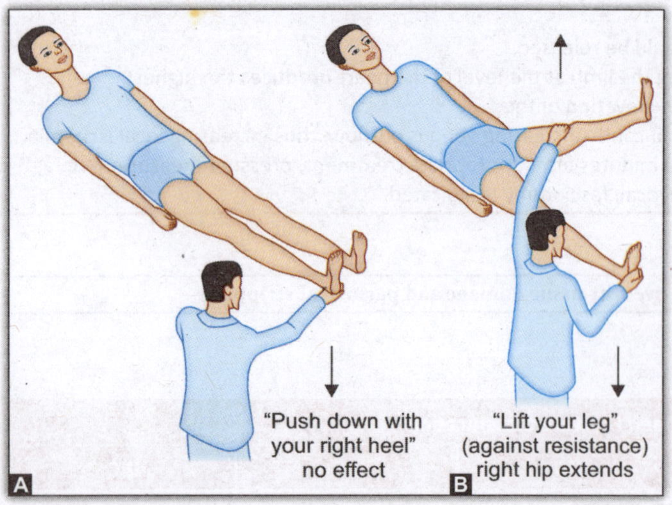

Figs A and B: **(A)** Hip extension is weak when tested directly; **(B)** Hip extension is normal when asked to flex opposite hip

False-positive Hoover's signs can occur with cortical neglect, hip pain, and multiple sclerosis. However, Hoover's sign does not differentiate conversion disorder from feigning, simulated weakness, or malingering.

Tests in Orthopaedics for Malingering

- **Hoover's test** is used to check for malingering in patients presenting with lower limb weakness. It relies on the fact that all individuals, extend their hip when flexing the contralateral hip against resistance. Hold the supine patient's heels off the table and ask them to raise one leg. If this is easy, the test is negative, if difficult, the patient will push the contralateral leg towards the table to assist raising the leg. Lack of downward pressure from the contralateral leg is a positive sign of malingering.
- **Mankopf's test:** Palpation of a painful area should increase the pulse rate by at least 5 per cent and absence of this finding is a positive behavioural sign.
- **O'Donoghue's manoeuvre:** Patients with true physiological pain have a greater passive range of motion than active so, it is a positive behavioural sign if the patient's active range of motion is greater.
- **McBride's test:** Also as know the patient to stand on one leg while raising the opposite knee to the chest. This should lessen low back pain. A reported increase in pain, or a refusal to do the test, is a positive behavioural sign.
- **Burn's test:** Also as know the patient to kneel on a chair and touch the floor-those with true back pain or sciatica should be able to do this but those with non-organic back pain usually cannot.

17. Ans. (a) Scaphoid fracture

Ref: Apley 9th ed page 386, 396, 780

Scaphoid fracture: The scaphoid is potentially the most unstable of all the carpal bones. As the wrist flexes and extends, so does the scaphoid bone; the lunate and triquetrum follow passively. Tenderness in the anatomical snuffbox is typical of a scaphoid injury. Pain X-ray shows a gap between the scaphoid and lunate (the **Terry-Thomas sign**; Named after British comedian Terry Thomas' midline diastema. The actor Terry Thomas with the trademark gap between his front teeth) and rotation of the scaphoid. If the scaphoid is flexed, it will look foreshortened and the tubercle may appear as a dense 'ring' in the bone. A true lateral view is examined to assess the relative alignment of the distal radius, the lunate, capitate and scaphoid. In a normal wrist, the articular surfaces of the radius, lunate and capitate are parallel. Following a fracture of the scaphoid or rupture of the scapholunate ligament (scapholunate dissociation), the lunate no longer passively follows the scaphoid. The scaphoid tends to flex and the lunate assumes its default position of extension (dorsal tilt). **(Ref Apley 9th ed page 395)**

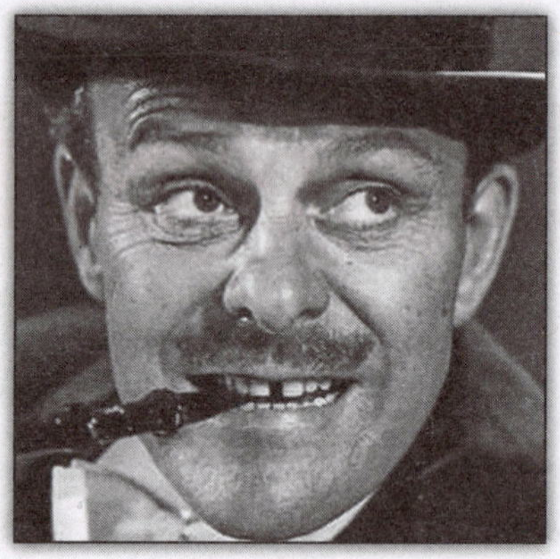

Fig: British comedian Terry Thomas' with midline diastema

Option (B)

Around 60% of perilunate dislocations are associated with a scaphoid fracture which is then termed a trans-scaphoid perilunate dislocation

Diagnosis Based on Site of Tenderness in Orthopedics

Site	Diagnosis
Tip of radial Styloid	De Quervain's disease
Anatomical snuffbox	Scaphoid fracture
Base of first metacarpal	Carpo-metacarpal osteoarthritis
Over the lunate	Kienböck's disease
Just distal to the head of the ulna	Triangular fibrocartilage complex

Mayfield Classification of Carpal Instability AKA: Perilunate Instability Classification (Carpal Dislocations)		
Stage I	Scapholunate dissociation (rotatory subluxation of the scaphoid)	Disruption of the scapholunate ligament with resultant Terry Thomas sign exacerbated in clenched fist views
Stage II	Perilunate dislocation	The lunate remains normally aligned with the distal radius, and the remaining carpal bones are dislocated (almost always dorsally) the capitolunate joint is disrupted, and the lunate projects through the space of Poirier 60% are associated with scaphoid fractures
Stage III	Midcarpal dislocation	Triquetrolunate interosseous ligament disruption or triquetral fracture neither the capitate or the lunate is aligned with the distal radius
Stage IV	Lunate dislocation	Dorsal radiolunate ligament injury dislocation of the lunate in a palmar direction tipped teacup appearance

18. Ans. (c) Arthritis

Ref: With Text

Osteoarthritis of the knee initial management of most patients should be nonoperative and may include physical therapy, bracing, orthoses, ambulatory aids, NSAIDs, glucosamine, chondroitin, intraarticular injections of a steroid or hyaluronic acid, and analgesics. **(Ref: Campbell 12th ed page 468)**
New forms of medication have been introduced in recent years, particularly the oral administration of glucosamine and intra-articular injection of hyalourans. **(Ref: Apley 9th ed page 573)**

NOTE

Glucosamine and/or chondroitin sulfate or hydrochloride should not be prescribed for patients with symptomatic osteoarthritis of the knee. Level I Grade A recommendation

19. Ans. (a) Dextrocardia

Ref: Apley's 9th ed page 181, Nelson's 18th Ed Ch 680; Paediatric Orthopedics by Jan Douwes Visser Pg 25

"Dextrocardia is not Associated with Sprengel Deformity"

- Sprengel deformity, or congenital elevation of the scapula, is a disorder of development that involves a high scapula and limited scapulothoracic motion.
- The scapula originates in early embryogenesis at a level posterior to the 4th cervical vertebra, but descends during development to below the 7th cervical vertebra. Failure of this descent, either unilateral or bilateral, is the Sprengel deformity.
- The severity of the deformity depends on the location of the scapula and associated anomalies.
- The scapula in **mild cases** is rotated, with a palpable or visible bump corresponding to the superomedial corner of the scapula in the region of the trapezius muscle. Function is generally good.
- In **moderate cases**, the scapula is higher on the neck and connected to the spine with an abnormal omovertebral ligament or even bone. Shoulder motion, particularly abduction, is limited.
- In **severe cases**, the scapula is small and positioned on the posterior neck, and the neck may be webbed.
- The majority of patients have associated anomalies of the musculoskeletal system, especially in the spine (including **Klippel-Feil anomaly** with congenital cervical vertebral fusions, making spinal evaluation important.

Treatment

- In mild cases, treatment is generally unnecessary, although a prominent and unsightly superomedial corner of the scapula can be excised.
- In more severe cases, surgical repositioning of the scapula with rebalancing of parascapular muscles can significantly improve both function and appearance.
- An operation to bring the scapula inferiorly to near its normal position is ideally attempted soon after 3 years of age, because the operation becomes more difficult as the child grows. In older children, an attempt to bring the scapula inferiorly to its normal level can injure the brachial plexus.
- Green described surgical release of muscles from the scapula along with excision of the supraspinatus portion of the scapula and any omovertebral bone.
- The scapula is moved inferiorly to a more normal position, and the muscles are reattached.
- Woodward described transfer of the origin of the trapezius muscle to a more inferior position on the spinous processes.

Woodward Procedure is Preferred Since

- The muscles are incised farther from the scapula, which lowers the risk of formation of a scar keloid that may fix the scapula in poor position;
- A larger mobilization is possible; and
- The postoperative scar is not as thick as with Green's procedure

20. Ans. (d) Avascular necrosis of femoral head

Ref: Apley 9th ed page 94, 102

Avascular Necrosis of Femoral Head

Etiology

- Trauma is the major cause of AVN.
- Avascular necrosis has also been associated with steroid use, alcohol abuse, Gaucher's disease, hemoglobinopathies, and in patients subject to severe changes in barometric pressure, such as deep sea divers.

Presentation

- Pain is the most common feature. Pain in groin on internal rotation and patient walks with an antalgic (limping) gait.
- Thigh wasting and 1–2 cm shortening
- Hip moves into external rotation on passive flexion: also known as Sector Sign positivity.

- Bilateral in 80% patients with steroid use and 50% of idiopathic cases.

Investigations: MRI is investigation of choice. Later X-ray appearances are usually pathognomonic; however, once bone destruction occurs the X-ray changes can be mistaken for those of OA. The cardinal distinguishing feature is that in osteonecrosis the 'joint space' (articular cartilage) is preserved in the face of progressive bone collapse and deformity, whereas in OA articular cartilage loss precedes bone destruction.

Treatment

- Management of AVN depends on **the age of the patient, size of the lesion, and stage of the disease.**
- In the **elderly** who develop AVN following a hip fracture, **total hip arthroplasty** is the treatment of choice. In **younger patients** with idiopathic AVN, determining the size of the lesion is important as this has a direct influence on the prognosis.
- The **size** is best determined by MRI.
- **Small lesions** (less than 15% of the femoral head) may **resolve without treatment. Large lesions** (greater than 50% of the femoral head) tend to progress to collapse of the head and **secondary osteoarthritis**, despite treatment. For intermediate-sized lesions, a number of treatment options have been proposed.
- **A classification based on the location of the lesion also has prognostic significance.** If the lesion is **medial** in the head, then progression is rare; if it is lateral in the head the prognosis is worst. The more proximal the fracture more are chances of AVN and non union
- **Subcapital > Transcervical > Basal > Intertrochanteric**
- Treatments range from simple decompression of the femoral head to lower the intraosseous pressure, to bone grafting of the involved area
- There have been a number of osteotomies described whose purpose is to remove the affected area of the femoral head from the weight-bearing axis of the hip

21. Ans. (b) NEER type 3 proximal humerus

Ref: Apley 9th ed page 744, Campbell 12th ed page 2839

Even if you dont know the details of the fracture classification systems in the options, if you know which classification system is for proximal humerus, the question will be solved.

Option (A)

Garden classification is used for femoral neck fractures

Option (C)

Schatzker classification is used for Tibial Plateau fractures

Option (D)

Gustilo classification is used for open fractures

Option (B)

The most widely accepted classification of Proximal humerus fracture is that of Neer (1970) who drew attention to the four major segments involved in these injuries: *the head of the humerus, the lesser tuberosity, the greater tuberosity and the shaft.* Neer's classification distinguishes between the number of displaced fragments, with ***displacement defined as > 45 degrees of angulation or > 1 cm of separation or both.*** Thus, however many fracture lines there are, if the fragments are undisplaced it is regarded as a one-part fracture. If the fragments are undisplaced it is regarded as a one-part fracture; if one segment is separated from the others, it is a two-part fracture; if two fragments are displaced, that is a three-part fracture; if all the major parts are displaced, it is a four-part fracture.

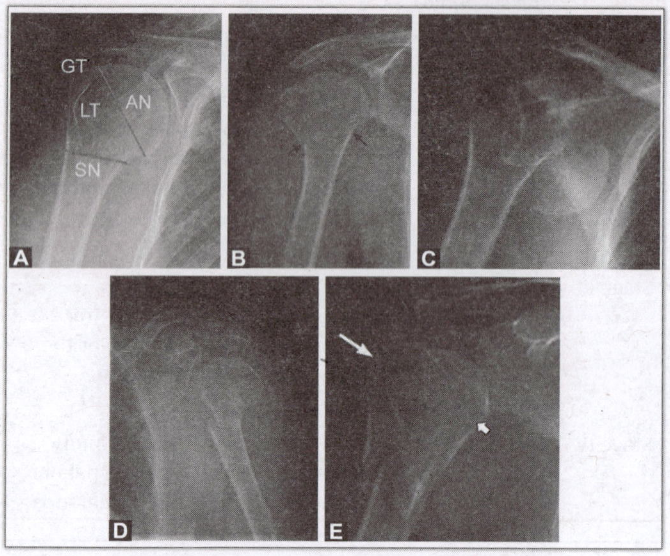

Figs A to E: (A) Normal Proximal Humerus X-ray: AN = Anatomical neck, GT = Greater tuberosity, LT = Lesser tuberosity, SN = Surgical neck; **(B) Type I- Minimal displacement:** Fracture of greater tuberosity and surgical neck but no displacement and no angulation; **(C) Type II- Anatomical neck 2 part NEER fracture; (D) Surgical neck 2 part NEER fracture:** Surgical neck is displaced more than 1 cm from the humeral head; **(E) Type IV- 2 Greater Tuberosity part NEER fracture: Greater tuberosity** (long arrow) is displaced more than 1 cm from the humeral head (short arrow) which remains at anatomic position

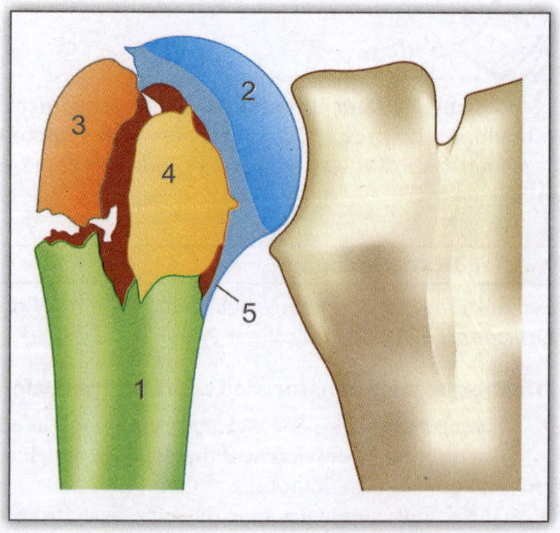

Fig: Fractures of the proximal humerus. Diagram of a fractured proximal humerus, showing the four main fragments, two or more of which are seen in almost all proximal humeral fractures. 1 = shaft of humerus; 2 = head of humerus; 3 = greater tuberosity; 4 = lesser tuberosity

Neer Classification of Proximal Humerus Fracture		
	Type	Subtype
I	Minimal displacement	1-part
II	Anatomical neck	2-part
III	Surgical neck	2-part
IV	Greater tuberosity	2, 3, or 4-part
V	Lesser tuberosity	2, 3, or 4-part
VI	Fracture dislocation	Anterior - 2, 3, 4-part, or articular surface involvement Posterior - 2, 3, 4-part, or articular surface involvement

AIIMS MAY 2017

22. Ans. (b) Pulmonary thromboembolism

Ref: Bailey 26th ed page 913–918, Schwartz 10th ed page 918–922, Harrison's 19th Ed page 1634

NOTE

This case was widely published in many English daily on 2nd May 2017, the news report states that "The autopsy confirmed that the clot, measuring 5 × 1 cm, got dislodged due to the massage and travelled to the lungs"

This is a case of sudden death, out of the options Fat embolism, pulmonary thromboembolism and acute MI, all three can cause sudden death.

Let us see hints in the question now:

- Acute breathlessness favours diagnosis of pulmonary thromboembolism or fat embolism more than acute MI
- Since there is a history of immobilisation, diagnosis of pulmonary thromboembolism is more likely.

If we review the chain of events in the question. The patient developed ankle trauma followed which a cast was given and patient was immobilised. If it were a case of fat embolism, the onset of symptoms of breathlessness are after manipulation of injury. In this case, immobilisation of three months led to formation of thrombus in deep venous system which got dislodged when the mother tried to massage the area. Pain and swelling in the calf region are indicative of DVT.

Pulmonary Thromboembolism

Deep vein thrombosis (DVT) and pulmonary embolism are frequent complications after major abdominal and orthopedic procedures.

Risk Factors for Pulmonary Thromboembolism

- Factor V leiden mutation
- Deficiency of Protein C and S
- Hyperhomocysteinemia
- Antiphospholipid antibody syndrome
- Cancer, systemic arterial hypertension, chronic obstructive pulmonary disease, long-haul air travel, air pollution, obesity, cigarette smoking, eating large amounts of red meat, oral contraceptives, pregnancy, postmenopausal hormone replacement, surgery, and trauma.

Pathophysiology

- When venous thrombi are dislodged from their site of formation, they embolize to the pulmonary arterial circulation or, paradoxically, to the arterial circulation through a patent foramen ovale or atrial septal defect. About one-half of patients with pelvic vein thrombosis or proximal leg DVT develop PE, which is often asymptomatic
- The most common gas exchange abnormalities are hypoxemia (decreased arterial PO_2) and an increased alveolar-arterial O_2 tension gradient, which represents the inefficiency of O_2 transfer across the lungs. Anatomic dead space increases because breathed gas does not enter gas exchange units of the lung. Physiologic dead space increases because ventilation to gas exchange units exceeds venous blood flow through the pulmonary capillaries

Other Factors

- Increased pulmonary vascular resistance
- Impaired gas exchange due to increased alveolar dead space
- Alveolar hyperventilation
- Increased airway resistance
- Decreased pulmonary compliance

Progressive right heart failure is the usual cause of death from PE

Evaluation

- For patients who have DVT, the most common history is a cramp in the lower calf that persists for several days and becomes more uncomfortable as time progresses. For patients who have PE, the most common history is unexplained breathlessness.
- In evaluating patients with possible VTE, the initial task is to decide on the clinical likelihood of the disorder. Patients with a low likelihood of DVT or a low-to-moderate likelihood of PE can undergo initial diagnostic evaluation with d-dimer testing alone (see "Blood tests") without obligatory imaging tests. If the d-dimer is abnormally elevated, imaging tests are the next step.

Imaging Tests for Pulmonary Thromboembolism

Computed tomography of the chest with intravenous contrast is the principal imaging test for the diagnosis of PE. Multidetector-row spiral CT acquires all chest images with 1 mm of resolution during a short breath hold. This generation of CT scanners can image small peripheral emboli. Sixth-order branches can be visualized with resolution superior to that of conventional invasive contrast pulmonary angiography. The CT scan also obtains excellent images of the RV and LV and can be used for risk stratification along with its use as a diagnostic tool.

- **V/Q scans:** Lung scanning has become a second-line diagnostic test for PE, used mostly for patients who cannot tolerate intravenous contrast. Small particulate aggregates of albumin labeled with a gamma-emitting radionuclide are injected intravenously and are trapped in the pulmonary capillary bed. The perfusion scan defect indicates absent or decreased blood flow, possibly due to PE. The diagnosis of PE is very unlikely in patients with normal and nearly normal scans but is about 90% certain in patients with high-probability scans.

- **Echocardiography:** Transesophageal echocardiography when CT scanning facilities are not available or when a patient has renal failure or severe contrast allergy that precludes administration of contrast despite premedication with high-dose steroids. This imaging modality can identify saddle, right main, or left main PE.

Transthoracic echocardiography rarely images thrombus directly. The best-known indirect sign of PE on transthoracic echocardiography is McConnell's sign: Hypokinesis of the RV free wall with normal motion of the RV apex.

- **Pulmonary angiography:** Chest CT with contrast (see above) has virtually replaced invasive pulmonary angiography as a diagnostic test. Invasive catheter-based diagnostic testing is reserved for patients with technically unsatisfactory chest CTs and those in whom an interventional procedure such as catheter-directed thrombolysis or embolectomy is planned. A definitive diagnosis of PE depends on visualization of an intraluminal filling defect in more than one projection. Secondary signs of PE include abrupt occlusion ("cut-off") of vessels, segmental oligemia or avascularity, a prolonged arterial phase with slow filling, and tortuous, tapering peripheral vessels.

Algorithm for diagnostic imaging

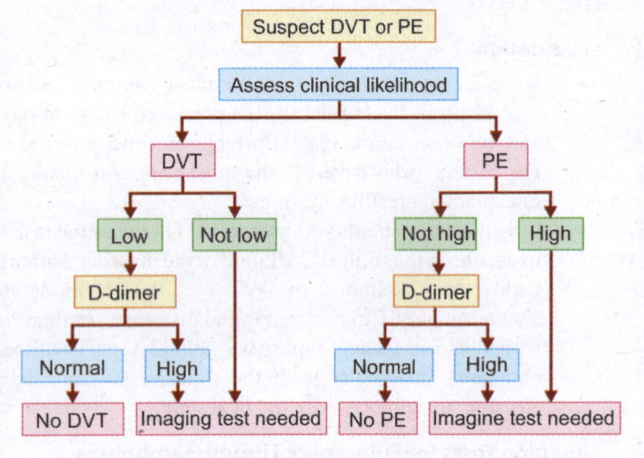

Important Chest X-ray Signs of Pulmonary Thromboembolism

A normal or nearly normal chest X-ray often occurs in PE. Well-established abnormalities include focal oligemia (Westermark's sign), a peripheral wedge-shaped density above the diaphragm (Hampton's hump), and an enlarged right descending pulmonary artery (Palla's sign).

The management of Pulmonary thromboembolism has been discussed in AIIMS Medicine May 2016.

23. Ans. (a) Fat embolism

Ref: Apley's 9th Ed page 681

Compare this question to the question on pulmonary thromboembolism asked in same paper to test your knowledge of both the differential diagnosis. There is sudden death after the history of trauma, which favours the diagnosis of fat embolism over pulmonary thromboembolism. Although both MI and hypovolemic shock can be cause of death, but history of fracture favours the diagnosis of fat embolism.

FAT Embolism

- Fat embolism is a common phenomenon following limb fractures.
- Circulating fat globules larger than 10 µm in diameter occur in most adults after closed fractures of long bones and histological traces of fat can be found in the lungs and other internal organs.
- A small percentage of these patients develop clinical features similar to those of ARDS; this was recognized as the fat embolism syndrome long before ARDS entered the medical literature.
- The source of the fat emboli is probably the bone marrow, and the condition is more common in patients with multiple fractures

Clinical features:

- Early warning signs of fat embolism (usually within 72 hours of injury) are a slight rise of temperature and pulse rate.
- In more pronounced cases there is breathlessness and mild mental confusion or restlessness.
- Pathognomonic signs are petechiae on the trunk, axillae and in the conjunctival folds and retinae.
- In more severe cases there may be respiratory distress and coma, due both to brain emboli and hypoxia from involvement of the lungs. The features at this stage are essentially those of ARDS.

Investigations:

- There is no infallible test for fat embolism; however, urinalysis may show fat globules in the urine and the blood PO_2 should always be monitored; values below 8 kPa (60 mm Hg or less) within the first 72 hours of any major injury must be regarded as suspicious.
- A chest X-ray may show classical changes in the lungs.

Management:

- Management of severe fat embolism is supportive.
- Symptoms of the syndrome can be reduced with the use of supplemental high inspired oxygen concentrations immediately after injury and the incidence appears to be reduced by the prompt stabilization of long-bone fractures.
- Intramedullary nailing is not thought to increase the risk of developing the syndrome.
- Fixation of fractures also allows the patient to be nursed in the sitting position, which optimizes the ventilation–perfusion match in the lungs.

24. Ans. (c) Internal rotation

Ref: Apley's 9th Ed page 515

NOTE

The picture provided in the examination was not the perfect demonstrative picture of the tests of internal or external rotation. The picture in the examination was very similar to Obturator sign which is a clinical use of internal rotation of hip: Pain on internal rotation of the hip (suggesting a pelvic appendix). Further we have included classical pictures of all the tests in the explanation below

The assessment of hip movements is difficult because any limitation can easily be obscured by movement of the pelvis.

Thus, even a gross limitation of extension, causing a fixed flexion deformity, can be completely masked simply by arching the back into excessive lordosis. Fortunately it can be just as easily unmasked by performing Thomas' test.

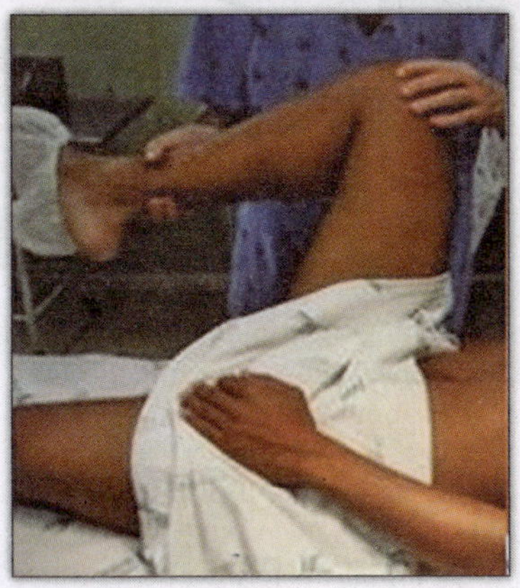

Fig: Obturator sign: Pain on internal rotation of the hip (suggesting a pelvic appendix)

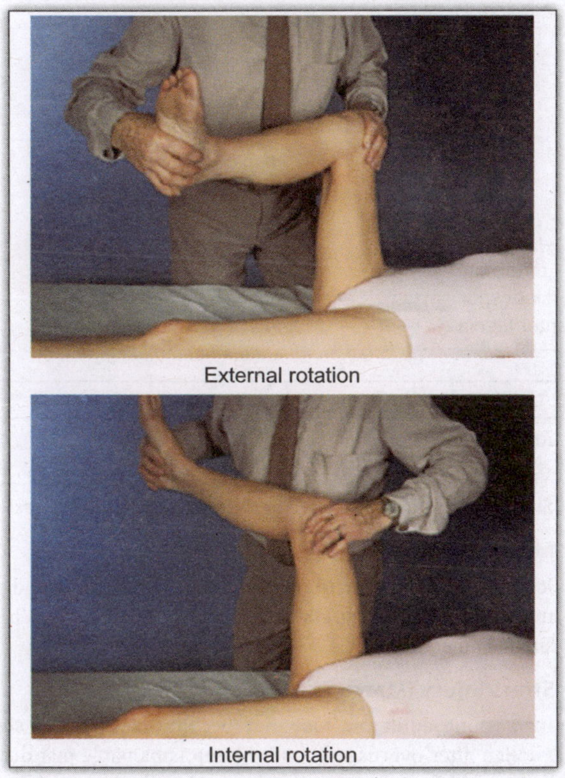

Fig: Rotation of hip joint: To test rotation both legs, lifted by the ankles, are rotated first internally (medially) and then externally (laterally); the patellae are watched to estimate the amount of rotation. Rotation in flexion is tested with the hip and knee each flexed 90 degrees. If internal rotation is full with the hip extended, but restricted in flexion, this suggests pathology in the anterosuperior portion of the femoral head, probably avascular necrosis (the so-called 'sectoral sign'). However, in a young person, pain on internal rotation with the hip flexed may indicate a torn acetabular labrum. Internal rotation is checked by rotating the foot laterally in flexion position of hip and knee joint. Range of motion is 40 degrees. External rotation is checked by rotating the foot medially. Normal range of motion is 45 degrees

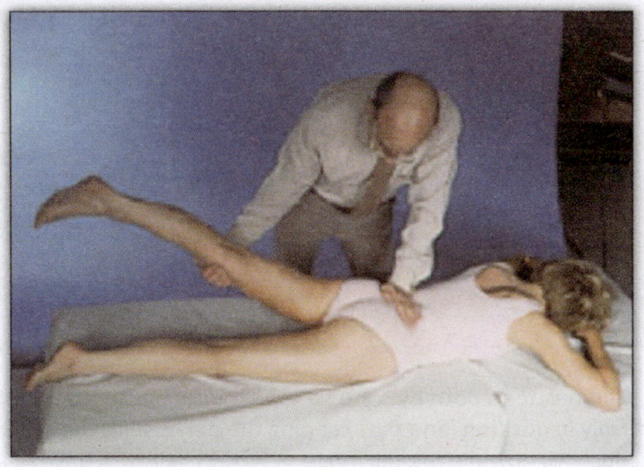

Fig: Extension: In prone position, stabilize hip with one hand the extend the hip joint. Range of motion is 10–20 degrees

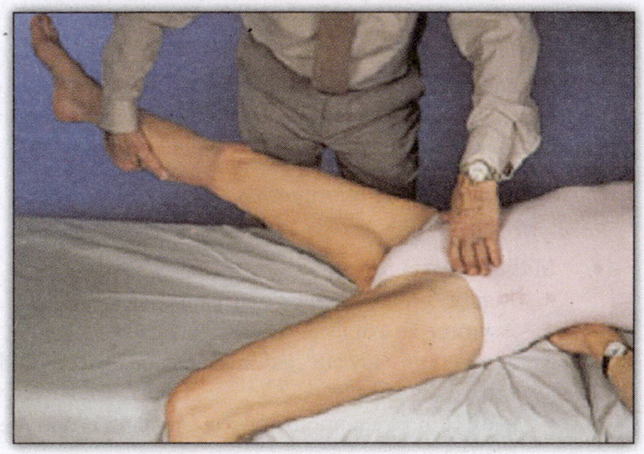

Fig: Testing Abduction: When testing abduction the pelvis must be prevented from tilting sideways. This is achieved by placing the 'sound' hip (the hip opposite to the one being examined) in full abduction and keeping it there. A hand is placed on one iliac crest to detect the slightest movement of the pelvis. Then, after checking that the anterior superior iliac spines are level, the affected joint is moved gently into abduction. The normal range is about 40 degrees

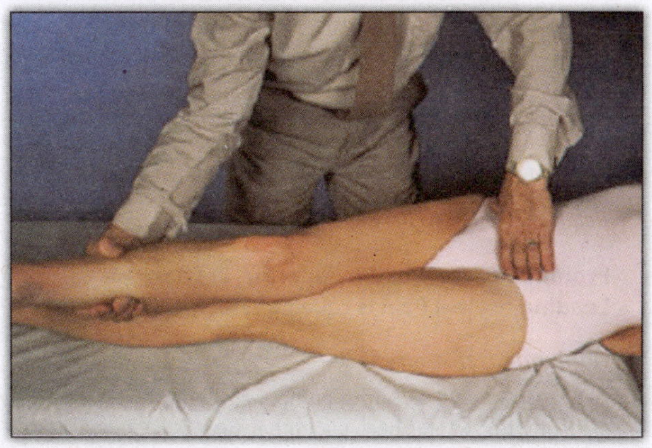

Fig: Testing Adduction: Adduction is tested by crossing one limb over the other; the pelvis must be watched and felt to determine the point at which it starts to tilt. The normal range of adduction is about 30 degrees

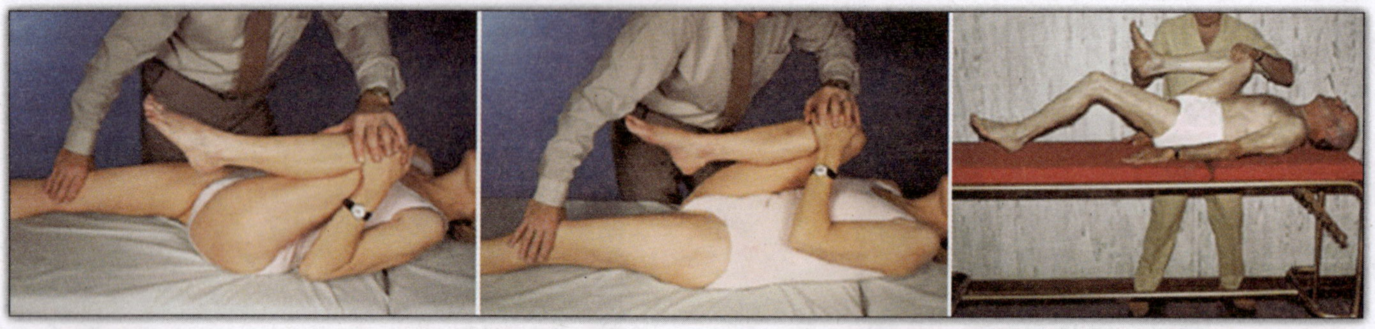

Fig: Thomas test: Both hips are flexed simultaneously to their limit, thus completely obliterating the lumbar lordosis; holding the 'sound' hip firmly in position (and thus keeping the pelvis still), the other limb is lowered gently; with any flexion deformity the knee will not rest on the couch Meanwhile the full range of flexion will also have been noted; the normal range is about 130 degrees

25. Ans. (d) Quadriceps

Ref: Textbook of Orthopedics: With Clinical Examination Methods in Orthopedics by John Ebnezar P- 358

Hand to knee gait is typically seen in polio in which the person places on hand on the knee to walk to prevent it from buckling due to quadriceps paralysis

Muscles Involved in Poliomyelitis

Paralytic Polio

- **In the early stage:**
  - Rigidity and tenderness of neck muscles
  - Asymmetric paralysis
  - Most commonly affected muscle is quadriceps and it is partially affected
  - Muscle most commonly affected in hand is opponens pollicis
  - Bulbar polio results in paralysis of respiratory and cardiovascular centers
- **Post polio residual paralysis**
  - Wasting, paralysis and deformity of lower limb muscles
  - **Deformity at hip:** Flexion, abduction and external rotation
  - **Deformity at knee:** Triple deformity of flexion, posterior subluxation and external rotation
  - **Foot:** Equinovarus is most common deformity followed by equino-valgus, calcaneo-valgus, calcaneo-varus
  - **Upper limb:** Shoulder and elbow muscles

26. Ans. (c) Ankle

Ref: Campbell 11th Ed Ch 85

Prominence of Posterosuperior Portion of Calcaneus Leading to Heel Pain is called as Haglund Deformity

Haglund's Deformity

- Also known as pump bump, achillodynia, retrocalcaneal bursitis, winter heel, cucumber heel
- This is due to a bony prominence or enlargement seen on the posterosuperior portion of calcaneus leading to retro calcaneal bursitis.
- This deformity usually occurs in younger individuals between 20–30's
- Chronic irritation by ill fitting shows leads to retrocalcaneal bursitis
- Treatment initially is to wear better fitting shoes
- Surgical intervention is required in other cases to remove the bony prominence

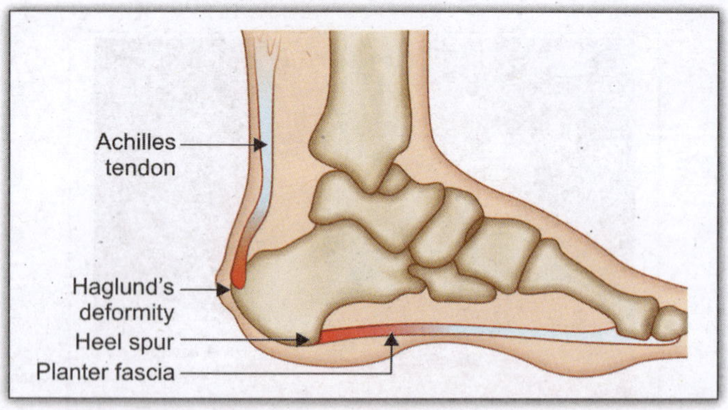

27. Ans. (c) Neck

Ref: With text

Various textbook gives conflicting views between neck and Shaft of 2nd metatarsal. We are hereby reviewing the text.

March Fracture

It typically occurs in the shaft or neck of second and third metatarsals due to aggressive prolonged (Anatomy by Vishram singh 2nd ed page 325)

Stress Injury (March Fracture)

In a young adult the foot may become painful and slightly swollen after overuse. A tender lump is palpable just distal to the ***midshaft of a metatarsal bone***. Usually the **second metatarsal** is affected, especially if it is much longer than an 'atavistic' first metatarsal. (Apley 9th ed page 932). Here the site of lump is states not the site of fracture, hence we cannot rely completely.

Military recruits in their first few weeks of training also are vulnerable to so-called march fractures. Patients often note the gradual onset of pain directly over the second metatarsal neck region 2 to 4 weeks after beginning a running or aerobics program. (Ref: Campbell 12th ed page 4201) Here also site of pain is given not the site of fracture, but comparing between site of pain and site of lump, site of pain is more reliable for localizing the site of fracture.

Metatarsal stress fractures are common in distance runners and ballet dancers. The second metatarsal NECK is the most likely site for stress fracture, but all metatarsals are susceptible. **(Ref: Rockwood & Green's Fractures in Adults, 6th Edition, Chapter 21)**

28. Ans. (a) Medial epicondyle

Ref: Apley's 9th Ed page 303

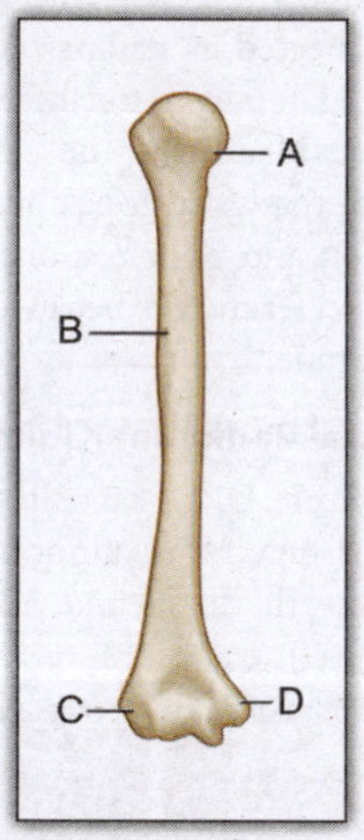

Legends of Plate

A = Neck of humerus - Axillary nerve injury
B = Shaft of humerus - Radial nerve injury
C = Lateral epicondyle - Tardy Ulnar nerve palsy
D = Medial epicondyle - Ulnar nerve palsy

The inability to hold paper between 4th and 5th finger indicates ulnar nerve injury. Ulnar is usually injured at the level of medial epicondyle, therefore it is the answer of choice here.

Ulnar Nerve Injury

Injuries of the ulnar nerve are usually either near the wrist or near the elbow, although open wounds may damage it at any level.

Clinical Features

Low Lesions

- These are often caused by cuts on shattered glass. There is numbness of the ulnar one and a half fingers. The hand assumes a typical posture in repose – the claw hand deformity – with hyperextension of the metacarpophalangeal joints of the ring and little fingers, due to weakness of the intrinsic muscles.
- Hypothenar and interosseous wasting may be obvious by comparison with the normal hand. Finger abduction is weak and this, together with the loss of thumb adduction, makes pinch difficult. *The patient is asked to grip a sheet* of paper forcefully between thumbs and index fingers while the examiner tries to pull it away; powerful flexion of the thumb interphalangeal joint signals weakness of adductor pollicis and first dorsal interosseous with overcompensation by the flexor pollicis longus (Froment's sign). Entrapment of the ulnar nerve in the pisohamate tunnel (Guyon's canal) is often seen in long-distance cyclists who lean with the pisiform pressing on the handlebars. Unexplained lesions of the distal (motor) branch of the nerve may be due to compression by a deep carpal ganglion or ulnar artery aneurysm.

High Lesions

- These occur with elbow fractures or dislocations. The hand is not markedly deformed because the ulnar half of flexor digitorum profundus is paralysed and the fingers are therefore less 'clawed' (the 'high ulnar paradox'). Otherwise, motor and sensory losses are the same as in low lesions.
- 'Ulnar neuritis' may be caused by compression or entrapment of the nerve in the medial epicondylar (cubital) tunnel, especially where there is severe valgus deformity of the elbow or prolonged pressure on the elbows in anaesthetized or bed-ridden patients. It is important to be aware of this condition in patients who start complaining of ulnar nerve symptoms some weeks after an upper limb injury; one can easily be misled into thinking that the nerve lesion is due to the original injury!

Treatment

- Exploration and suture of a divided nerve are well worthwhile, and anterior transposition at the elbow permits closure of gaps up to 5 cm. While recovery is awaited, the skin should be protected from burns. Hand physiotherapy keeps the hand supple and useful.
- If there is no recovery after nerve division, hand function is significantly impaired. Grip strength is diminished because the primary metacarpophalangeal flexors are lost, and pinch is poor because of the weakened thumb adduction and index finger abduction. Fine, coordinated finger movements are also affected. Metacarpophalangeal flexion can be improved by extensor carpi radialis longus to intrinsic tendon transfers (Brand), or by looping a slip of flexor digitorum superficialis around the opening of the flexor sheath (Zancolli procedure). Index abduction is improved by transferring extensor pollicis brevis or extensor indicis to the interosseous insertion on the radial side of the finger.

29. Ans. (d) Tension band wiring

Ref: Apley 9th ed page 702, 887

Repeat AIIMS MAY 2018 Orthopedics (See for explanation) *(see page no. 1011)*

30. Ans. (b) Ochronosis

Ref: Apley Orthopedics 9th ed page 82

This is a case of Alkaptonuria, a rare, heritable disorder characterized by the appearance of homogentisic acid in the urine, dark pigmentation of the connective tissues **(ochronosis)** and calcification of hyaline and fibrocartilage.

- Asymptomatic until the third or fourth decade when they present with **pain and stiffness of the spine** and (later) larger joints.
- Dark pigmentation of the ear cartilage and the sclerae, and clothes may become stained by **homogentisic acid** in the sweat.
- X-rays reveal **narrowing and calcification of the intervertebral discs** at multiple levels, and spinal osteopo-

rosis. At a later stage the large peripheral joints may show chondrocalcinosis and severe osteoarthritis.

- **Positive schober's test:** This indicates limitation of range of movement of lumbar spine.

Schober test

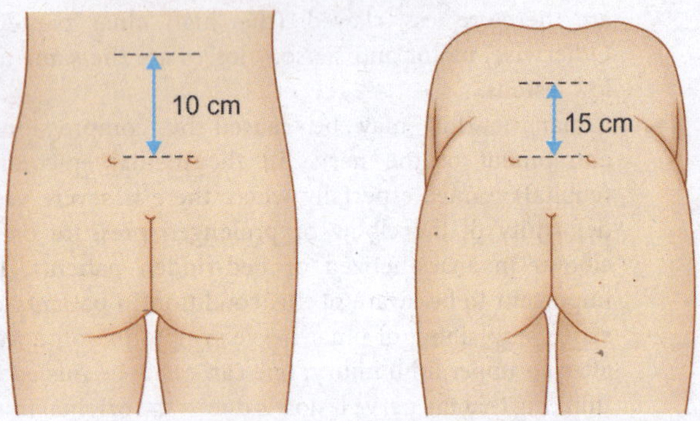

The Schober test detects reduced flexion. With the patient standing, mark the skin overlying the fifth lumber spinous process (usually at the level of the posterior superior iliac spine or the dimple of Venus) and also 10 cm above. On forward flexion, this should increase to >15 cm.

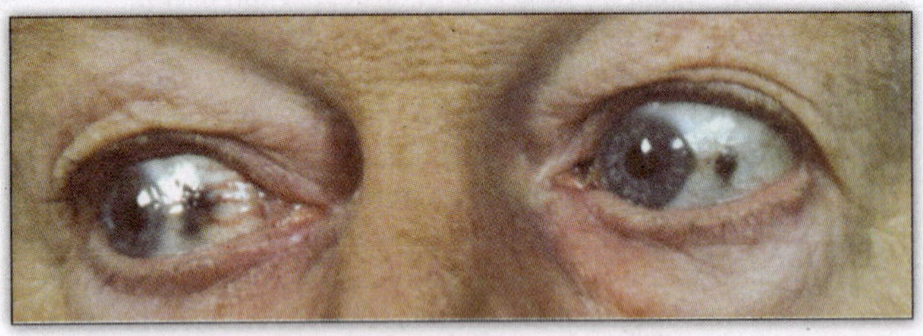

Fig: Bluish-black pigmentations on several parts of the sclera due to Alkaptonuria (also known as ochronosis)

All the options given can show positivity of Schober's test. But only ochronosis leads to deposition of pigmentation in connective tissue of eyes, ears, nose, intervertebral discs.

- Ochronosis is the bluish black discoloration of certain tissues, such as the ear cartilage and the ocular tissue, seen with alkaptonuria, a metabolic disorder. Additionally, ochronosis can occasionally occur from exposure to various substances such as phenol, trinitrophenol, resorcinol, mercury, picric acid, benzene, hydroquinone, and antimalarials.
- Deficiency of the enzyme **homogentisic acid oxidase** leads to accumulation of homogentisic acid, which is deposited in connective tissue and excreted in the urine. On standing the **urine turns dark (hence the name, alkaptonuria)**; cartilage and other connective tissues are stained grey – a condition referred to as ochronosis. Clinical problems arise from degenerative changes in articular cartilage with the development of osteoarthritis, and from calcification of the intervertebral discs.

31. Ans. (a) Interosseous membrane tear with triangular fibrocartilage complex (TFCC) tear and radial shaft fracture

Ref: Apley's 7th Ed page 790, Fractures and Injuries of the Distal Radius and Carpus: The Cutting Edge By David J. Slutsky, A. Lee Osterman P- 231

Galeazzi fracture is fracture of distal radius (between middle 1/3rd and distal 1/3rd) with disruption and dislocation of distal radioulnar joint. It is associated with tearing of interosseus membrane and the triangular fibrocartilage complex.

Components of Distal Radioulnar Joint (DRUJ)

The distal radius and ulna are linked to each other by the interosseous membrane, the capsule of the DRUJ and the triangular fibrocartilage complex (TFCC). The triangular fibrocartilaginous plate is connected as its apex to the base of the ulnar styloid process and laterally to the inferomedial ridge of the radius. Its outer fibers blend with those of the ligaments around the ulnar aspect of the wrist. It has been proposed that major cause of dislocation and poor response to conservative management in Galeazzi fracture is because of injury to TFCC and intraosseus membrane.

Stablisers of Distal Radioulnar Joint

Intraosseus membrane, DRUJ capsule, triangular fibrocartilage complex, pronator quadratus, ulnocarpal ligament, extensor carpi ulnaris subsheath, dorsal and volar radio ulnar ligament are stablisers of DRUJ.

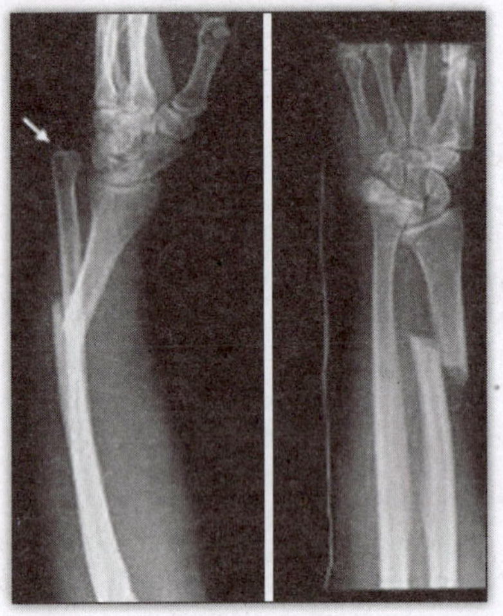

Fig: The X-ray shows a fracture of the distal radius and distal radioulnar joint dislocation typically seen in Galeazzi fracture

Galeazzi Fracture	
Mechanism of injury	This injury was first described in 1934 by Galeazzi. The usual cause is a ***fall on the hand; probably with a superimposed rotation force.*** The radius fractures in its **lower third and the inferior radio-ulnar joint** subluxates or dislocates.
Site and components	Fracture of distal radius (between middle 1/3rd and distal 1/3rd) with disruption and dislocation of distal radioulnar joint. It is associated with tearing of interosseus membrane and the triangular fibrocartilage complex. It has been proposed that major cause of dislocation and poor response to conservative management in Galeazzi fracture is because of Injury to TFCC and intraosseus membrane.

Contd...

Galeazzi Fracture	
Clinical features	More common than Monteggia. **Prominence or tenderness over the lower end of the ulna is the striking feature**. It may be possible to demonstrate the instability of the radio-ulnar joint by 'balloting' the distal end of the ulna **(the 'piano-key sign')** or by rotating the wrist. It is important also to test for an ulnar nerve lesion, which may occur.
X-ray	A transverse or short oblique fracture is seen in the lower third of the radius, with angulation or overlap. The distal radio-ulnar joint is subluxated or dislocated **(better demonstrated in lateral view)**
Treatment	The important step is to restore the length of the fractured bone. In children, closed reduction is often successful; in adults, reduction is best achieved by open operation and compression plating of the radius. An X-ray is taken to ensure that the distal radio-ulnar joint is reduced • *If the distal radio-ulnar joint is reduced and stable:* No further action is needed. The arm is rested for a few days, then gentle active movements are encouraged. The radio-ulnar joint should be checked, both clinically and radiologically, during the next 6 weeks. • *If the distal radio-ulnar joint is reduced but unstable*: The forearm should be immobilized in the position of stability (usually supination), supplemented if required by a transverse K-wire. The forearm is splinted in an above-elbow cast for 6 weeks. If there is a large ulnar styloid fragment, it should be reduced and fixed. • *If the distal radio-ulnar joint is irreducible* This is unusual. Open reduction is needed to remove the interposed soft tissues. The triangular fibrocartilage complex (TFCC) and dorsal capsule are then carefully repaired and the forearm immobilized in the position of stability (again, usually supination, supported by a wire if needed) for 6 weeks.

32. Ans. (a)

Ref: Practical Orthopedics By John Ebnezar page 339, Maheshwari 5th ed page 372, SRB's Surgical Operations: Text & Atlas page 116

NOTE

In examination the picture were marked with Green, Red, Orange and Blue colour arrows etc, and Options were given in colour arrows. Answer was Orange arrow

Now they have entered into the domain of orthopedics instruments, expect some picture based questions on this topic in future AIIMS exams.

Bone Holding Forceps

There are different types of Bone holding forceps, Each with curved and straight models.

A. **Lane's Bone holding forceps without Ratchet:** for holding femur and tibia. Like all other instruments designed by lane, this instrument is also long. Kern bone holding forceps is similar to Lane except that it is shorter than Lane.
B. **Lane's Bone holding forceps without Ratchet:**
C. **Fergusson's Bone holding forceps:** AKA Lion tooth bone holding forceps.
D. **AO Type forceps:** For radius and ulna, Self retaining
E. **Burn's bone holding forceps:** Used for radius, ulna and fibula. Blades are triangular, curved and serrated with pointed tip. Catch lock mechanism for locking.

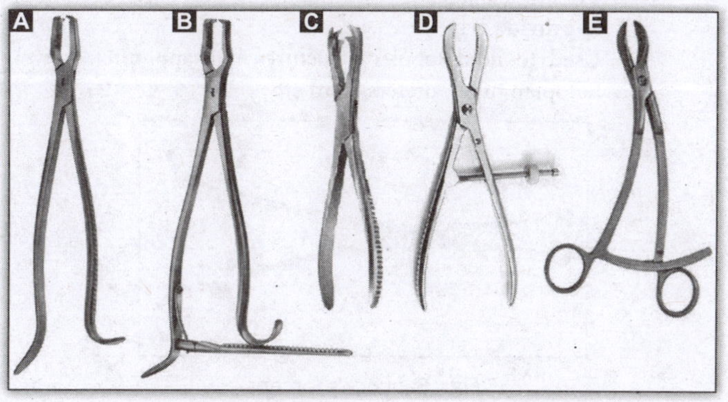

Sequestrum Holding Forceps

A forceps with small, powerful teeth used for extracting necrotic or sharp fragments of bone from surrounding tissue. It has a stout blade with thick transverse serrations with a groove in the middle without a ratchet. Sequestum should be formed before removal, hence X-ray is mandatory.

Uses: Used to remove sequestrum in osteomyelitis.

Two types: Straight (left) and curved (right)

NOTE

The instrument appears like the crocodile bone holding forceps, but does not have a catch to prevent crushing of the sequestrum

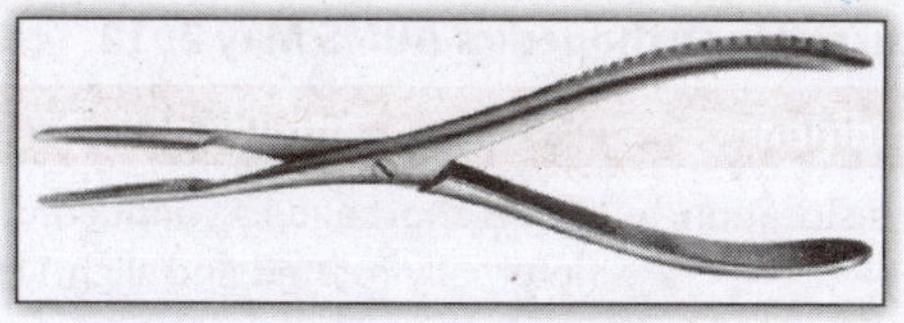

Fig: Sequestrum holding forceps

Lane's Tissue Forceps

- It is short, thick, bulkier and heavy
- It has finger bows, shaft with catch, box joint and blades
- Blades are small compared to shaft, and are curved with fenestrations to accommodate bulky tissue

- The tip of blade have single sharp tooth on one side and groove on other side
- Used to hold bulky and slippery tissue like fat and breast tissue
- Can also be used as towel clip

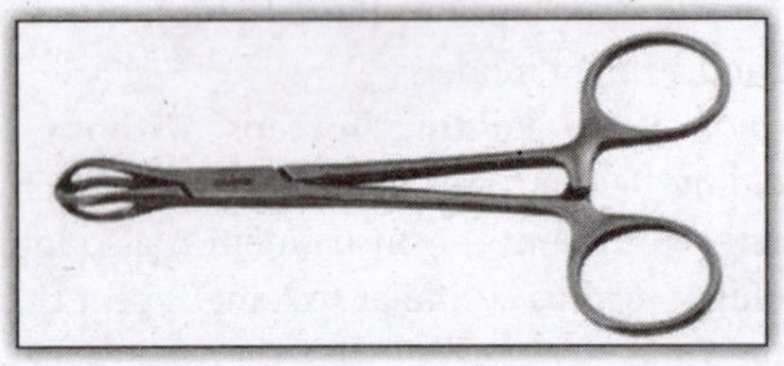

Fig: Lane's tissue forceps

Babcock's Tissue Forceps

- Light and non traumatic instrument having finger bows, shaft with catch, box joint, and blades
- Terminal part of blades are curved with triangular fenestrated to hold delicate structures
- Tip of the blades are non traumatic with small serrations to provide grip
- Used to hold tubular structures like appendix, bowel, fallopian tubes, ureters, cord etc

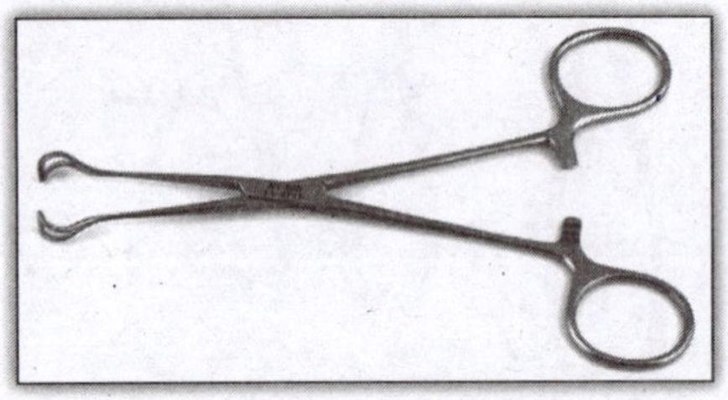

Fig: Babcock's forceps

33. Ans. (a) Brachial artery

Ref: Apley's 9th Ed, P- 779

The radiograph is showing a supracondylar fracture

See Details of Supracondylar Fracture in AIIMS May 2018 Orthopedics (see page no. 1008-1009)

34. Ans. (a) Shortened and externally rotated

Ref: Apley's 9th Ed page 848

From X-ray it is clear that there is a fracture neck of femur. The femoral neck is the most common site of fractures in the elderly. The attitude of limb in fracture neck of femur is shortened and externally rotated.

Garden Classification of Fracture Neck of Femur is Discussed in Orthopedics AIIMS May 2012

Condition	Attitude of limb
Posterior dislocation of hip	Leg is short and lies adducted, internally rotated and slightly flexed
Anterior dislocation of hip	The leg lies externally rotated, abducted and slightly flexed. It is not short, because the attachment of rectus femoris prevents the head from displacing upwards
Fracture neck of femur	Leg is shortened and externally rotated

Fracture Neck of Femur

Risk factors: Osteoporosis, osteomalacia, diabetes, stroke (disuse), alcoholism and chronic debilitating disease. In addition, old people often have weak muscles and poor balance resulting in an increased tendency to fall. Post menopausal women, whites > black.

Mechanism of injury: Minor fall in old age. Fall from height with multiple trauma in younger age

Pathology: Fracture neck of femur are prone to avsacular necrosis and slow union because of following factors

- By tearing the retinacular vessels the injury deprives the head of its main blood supply;
- Intra-articular bone has only a flimsy periosteum and no contact with soft tissues which could promote callus formation; and
- Synovial fluid prevents clotting of the fracture haematoma.

Transcervical fractures are, by definition, intracapsular.

- Stage I: Incomplete (so called abducted or impacted)
- Stage II: Complete without displacement.
- Stage III: Complete with partial displacement—the fragments are still connected by the posterior retinacular attachment; the femoral head trabeculae are no longer in line with those of the innominate bone.
- Stage IV: Complete with full displacement—the proximal fragment is free and lies correctly in the acetabulum so that the trabeculae appear normally aligned with those of the innominate.

Complications

Avascular necrosis: 30% of displaced fractures and 10% of undisplaced fractures

Non union: 30% of all fractures

Osteoarthritis

Treatment

Non operative treatment

- Garden I and II, undisplaced fractures in patients with dementia
- Old and undisplaced garden I fracture

Operative treatment accurate reduction, internal fixation and early mobility

- All displaced fractures
- All fractures in young

35. Ans. (a) Recurrent dislocation

Ref: Campbell 12th ed page 2289

Complications of Shoulder Dislocation

- **Recurrent dislocation:** Younger the patient, more is chance for dislocation. It is the most common complication
- Damage to the nerves originating with the brachial plexus occurs in 5% to 14% of shoulder dislocations. The axillary nerve and musculocutaneous nerve are most commonly injured. Most injuries are a neuropraxia, and a full recovery is typical.

Rotator cuff tears are common in patients older than 40 years with an anterior dislocation. If good ranges of motion and strength have not returned within 3 to 4 weeks after the injury, visualization of the rotator cuff with magnetic resonance imaging (MRI) or ultrasound is indicated.

36. Ans. (d) Movement at fracture site

Ref. Campbell's Operative Orthopaedics By S. Terry Canale, James H. Beaty 12th ed page 2597, Apley ed 9th ed page 690

Healing by callus, though less direct (the term 'indirect' could be used) has distinct advantages: it ensures mechanical strength while the bone ends heal, and with increasing stress the callus grows stronger and stronger (an example of Wolff's law). With rigid metal fixation, on the other hand, the absence of callus means that there is a long period during which the bone depends entirely upon the metal implant for its integrity.

Fracture Healing

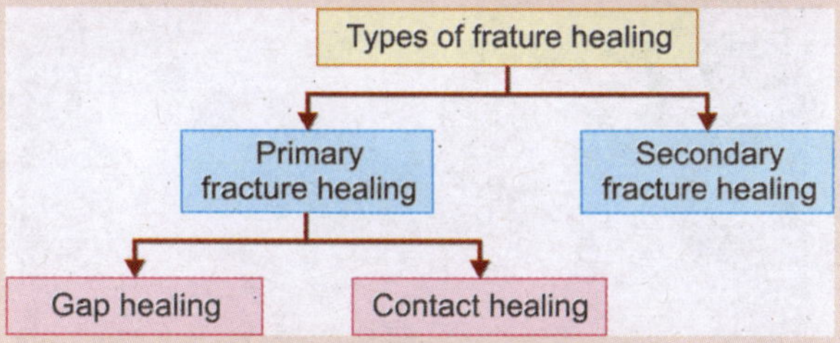

Primary bone healing is the type of healing in which callus is not formed and required rigid stabilization with or without compression of the bone ends. Secondary bone healing occurs when there is no rigid fixation and hence there is callus formation.

Factors Afffecting Fracture Healing

Systemic/General factors

- Age (healing is faster in children)
- Infection (slows healing)
- Pre-existing abnormal bone (slows healing)
- Nutrition and general health
- **Hormonal factors:** Growth hormone, Corticosteroids (microvascular osteonecrosis), thyroid, estrogen, androgen, calcitonin, PTH, prostaglandins
- **Diseases:** Diabetes, anemia, neuropathies, tabes
- Vitamin deficiencies, A, C, D, K
- **Drugs:** Nonsteroidal anti-inflammatory drugs (NSAIDs), anti-coagulants, factor XIII, calcium channel blockers (verapamil), cytotoxins, diphosphonates, phenytoin, sodium fluoride, tetracycline, nicotine, alcohol
- Systemic growth factors
- Environmental temperature
- Central nervous system trauma

Local factors

- Proximity of bone ends (displacement delays healing)
- Bone loss (Inverse relation)
- Soft tissue interposition (delays healing)
- Intra-articular fracture (delays healing)
- Ischemic fracture ends (delays healing)
- **Type of Bone:** Cancellous (spongy) bone > Cortical (compact) bone
- **Abnormal bone:** Radiation necrosis, infection, tumor or other pathological condition
- **Interfragmentary movement:** Rigid fixation limits interfragmentary movement, hence limits callus formation and healing. Flexible fixation allows interfragmentary movements and hence callus formation and healing.
- Denervation
- **Factors depending on injury:** Degree of local damage, Compound fracture, comminution of fracture, velocity of injury, Low circulatory levels of vitamin K1
- **Factors depending on treatment:** Extent of surgical trauma, Implant-induced altered blood flow, degree and kind of rigidity of internal or external fixation, Degree, duration, and direction of load-induced deformation of bone and soft tissues, extent of contact between fragments, Factors stimulating posttraumatic osteogenesis (bone grafts, bone morphogenetic protein, electrical stimulation, surgical technique, intermittent venous stasis
- **Factors associated with complications:** Infection, venous stasis, metal allergy.

37. Ans. (c) Supracondylar fracture

Ref: Campbell 12th ed page 1404, Apley 9th ed page 757, Maheshwari 4th ed page 93

Repeat AIIMS MAY 2018 Orthopedics (See for explanation) (see page no. 1008)

38. Ans. (d) Tension band wiring

Ref: Apley 9th ed page 702, 887

Repeat AIIMS MAY 2018 Orthopedics (See for explanation) (see page no. 1021)

39. Answer. (b) Chronic osteomyelitis

Ref. Yochum And Rowe's Essentials Of Skeletal Radiology 3rd ed page 1204

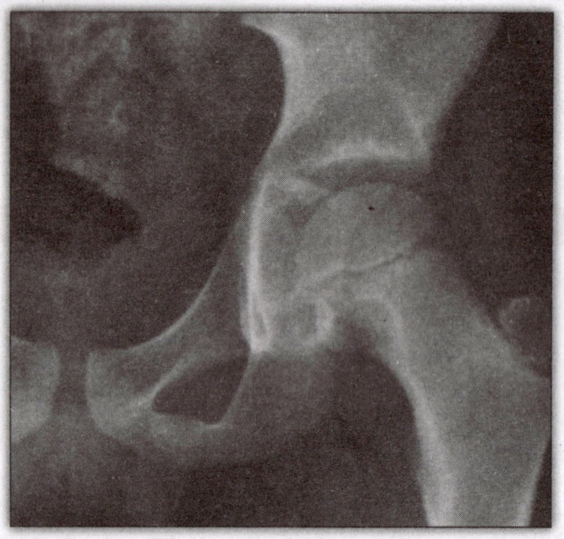

Fig: The given picture is of Brodie's Abscess a type of chronic osteomyelitis as per Jone's classification. Solitary circumscribed oval cavity surrounded by a zone of sclerosis

Ewing's sarcoma mimicks acute osteomyelitis both clinically and radiologically. However the radiological similarities are mostly between Ewing and Acute osteomyelitis (not chronic osteomyelitis)

Metaphyseal region of the bone is most commonly involved in osteomyelitis (depending on the age as mentioned in the table) and osteosarcoma. Callus formation indicates a healing fracture. The table below helps us to differentiate the three main entities Ewing's, osteomyelitis and osteosarcoma.

	Ewing's sarcoma	Acute osteomyelitis	Chronic osteomyelitis	Osteosarcoma
Age group	10–20 years	Any age (most common 2–12 years)	Any age (most common 2–12 years)	Primary osteosarcoma: 10–20 years Secondary osteosarcoma: elderly
Site	Diaphyseal Femur (MC site)	**Neonates:** Metaphysis and Epiphysis **Children:** Metaphysis **Adults:** Epiphysis and Subchondral regions. Femur (MC site)	**Neonates:** Metaphysis and Epiphysis **Children:** Metaphysis **Adults:** Epiphysis and subchondral regions. Femur (MC site)	Metaphyseal and it can extend into epiphysis and diaphysis. Femur (MC site)
Radiological features	**Permeative pattern (MC). Onion skin periosteal reaction, sclerosis.** Less commonly Codman's triangle, Sunburst or spiculated periosteal reaction.	Regional osteopenia. **Periosteal reaction/ thickening (periostitis). Codman's triangle.** Focal bony lysis or cortical loss. Endosteal scalloping. Loss of bony trabecular architecture. New bone apposition eventual peripheral sclerosis	Formation of a **sequestrum, involucrum or cloaca**	Medullary and cortical bone destruction. Permeative or moth-eaten appearance. **Sunburst type periosteal reaction. Codman triangle.** Less commonly lamellated (onion skin) reaction. Soft-tissue mass tumor matrix ossification/calcification giving ill-defined **fluffy or cloud-like** appearance or rings and arcs of chondroid lesions.

40. Ans. (b) Posterior dislocation of hip

Ref: Apley's 9th ed page 843

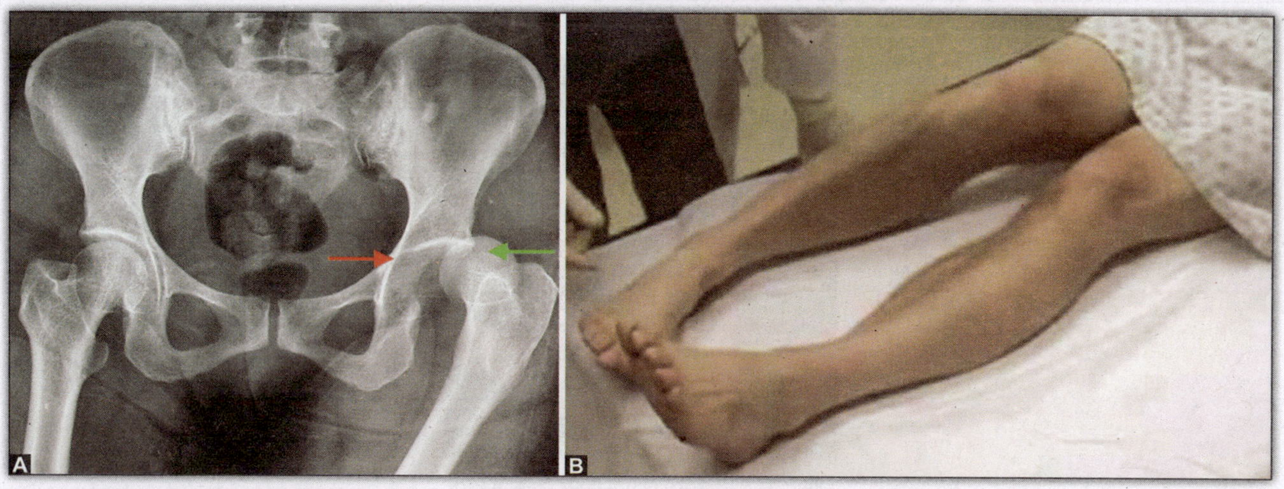

Figs A and B: (A) Posterior Dislocation of Hip: In the AP film the femoral head is seen out of its socket and above the acetabulum. The Right femoral head (white arrow) lies superior (and posterior) to the acetabulum (Red arrow). No Pelvic fracture is seen; **(B)** Position of limb in Posterior dislocation of hip: Typical attitude of the limb is **Flexion, Adduction, Internal rotation (FADIR)**

Hip Dislocation		
Description	**Evaluation**	**Treatment**
• High energy trauma (ESP Motor Vehicle Accident-dashboard injury or significant fall.) • Orthopaedic emergency • Multiple associated injuries +/– fractures, (e.g. femoral head & neck)	• H/O: Trauma. Severe pain, cannot move thigh/hip. • Pain (esp. with motion), good neurovascular exam • X-ray: AP pelvis, frog lateral (Femoral head is different size) Also femur & knee series • CT: Rule out fracture or bony fragments	Early reduction essential, then repeat X-ray & neurologic exam **Posterior I:** Closed reduction & abduction pillow **Posterior II-V:** • Closed reduction (open if irreducible) • ORIF fracture or excise fragment **Anterior:** Closed reduction, ORIF if necessary.

Classification		
Anterior	**Posterior**	**Central**
Epstein classification	Thompson classification	Not a true dislocation
10% hip dislocation	Most common (85-90%), 10% associated with sciatic nerve injury	Although this is called 'central dislocation', it is really a fracture of the acetabulum.
• Superior (A, B, C) • Inferior (A, B, C) A. No associated fracture B. Femoral head fracture C. Acetabular fracture	• Simple, no posterior fragment • Simple, large posterior fragment • Comminuted posterior fragment • Acetabular fracture • Femoral head fracture	Head of femur is felt in Per rectal examinations
No shortening, may be true lengthening of limb	Shortening of limb	Shortening of limb
Abducted, flexed, externally rotated leg	Adducted, flexed, Internally rotated leg	Adducted or abducted, externally or internally rotated depending on the extent of penetration into the pelvis

Complications: Osteonecrosis (AVN) reduced risk with early reduction; Sciatic nerve injury (posterior dislocations); Femoral artery & nerve injury (anterior dislocations); instability & recurrence; osteoarthritis; Heterotopic ossification

Vascular sign of narath is positive in posterior dislocation of hip joint. Due to posterior dislocation, the hip joint falls on the femoral artery, and this causes feeble or absent femoral pulse.

41. Ans. (b) Ulnar nerve

Ref: Apley 9th ed page 10

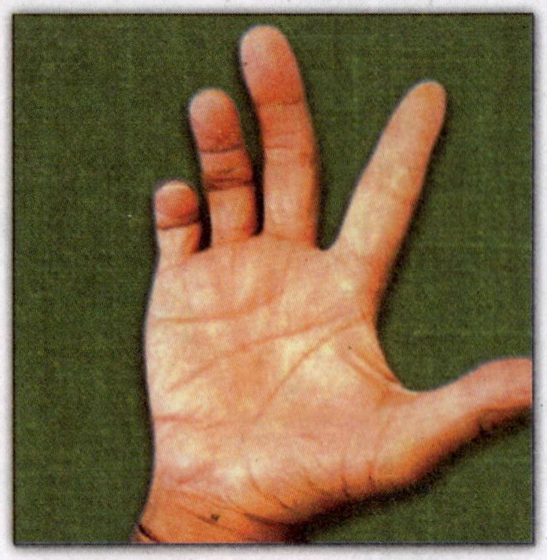

Fig: The picture is of Ulnar claw hand

Brachial Plexus Nerve Lesions		
Nerve (Segment)	**Motor deficit(s)**	**Sensory deficits**
Long thoracic (C 5,6,7)	**Winged Scapula**- *Serratus anterior*	None
Suprascapular (C 5,6)	Hard to start shoulder abduction - *Supraspinatus*	None
Axillary (C 5, 6)	Difficult abducting arm to horizontal - *Deltoid* Loss of shoulder roundness - Deltoid	Lateral side of arm below point of shoulder
Musculocutaneous (C 5, 6, 7)	Very weak flexion of elbow joint- *Biceps & Brachialis* Weak supination of radioulnar joint -*Biceps*	Lateral forearm
Radial (C 5 - T1)	Low lesions are usually due to fractures or dislocations at the elbow, or to a local wound. Wrist extension is preserved	Posterior lateral & arm; dorsum of hand
	High lesions occur with fractures of the humerus or after prolonged tourniquet pressure. There is an obvious ***Wrist drop***, due to weakness of the radial extensors of the wrist, as well as inability to extend the metacarpophalangeal joints or elevate the thumb.	Sensory loss is limited to a small patch on the dorsum around the **anatomical snuffbox.**
	Very high lesions may be caused by trauma or operations around the shoulder. More often, though, they are due to chronic compression in the axilla; this is seen in drink and drug addicts who fall into a stupor with the arm dangling over the back of a chair (**'Saturday night palsy'**) or in thin elderly patients using crutches (**'crutch palsy'**). In addition to weakness of the wrist and hand, the triceps is paralysed and the triceps reflex is absent.	Posterior lateral & arm; dorsum of hand
Median C 5 - T1) at elbow	Pronation of radioulnar joints-Pronator teres & quadratus **Bishop/Benediction Hand/Pope's Blessings Hand** (When the patient tries to make a fist, they are *unable to flex the index and middle fingers* while the ring & index fingers flexdue to loss of lateral lumbrical action 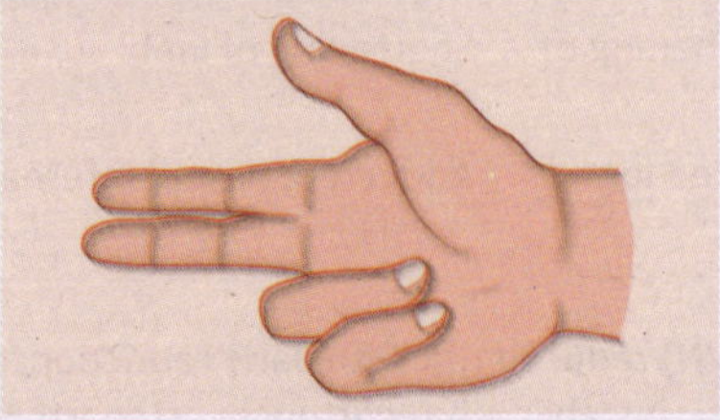 Weak wrist flexion - *Fl. carpi radialis* Weakened opposition of thumb - *thenar muscles*	Radial portion of palm; palmar surface & tips of radial 3½ digits
	Ape hand- Thumb hyper extended and adducted - *thenar muscles*	

Contd...

Brachial Plexus Nerve Lesions		
Nerve (Segment)	**Motor deficit(s)**	**Sensory deficits**
	"Papal Hand" Loss of flexion of I.P. joints of thumb & fingers 1 & 2 - *Fl. pollices longus ; Fl. digit. superficialis, Fl. digit profundus*	
Median (C 5 - T1) at wrist	**Ape/Simian hand deformity (MC):** Thumb hyper extended and adducted (unopposable thumb like an ape), Weakened opposition of thumb due to week thenar. Seen at rest 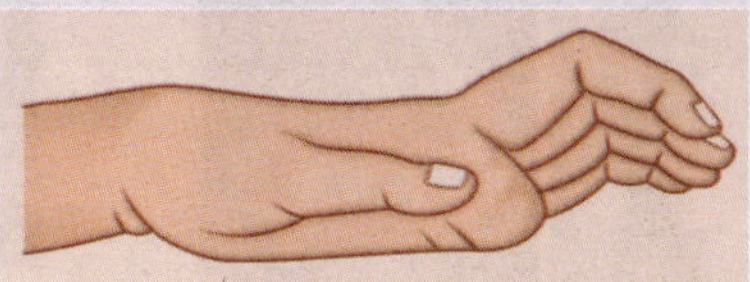	Palmar surface & tips of radial 3½ digits including thumb
Ulnar (C 8, T1) at elbow	**"Ulnar Claw hand" (AKA 'intrinsic minus' hand)**- Loss of flexion/ hyperextension of 4th& 5th MCP joints and loss of extension (i.e. Flexion) of IP joints. Due to paralysis of palmar and dorsal interossei and medial 2 lumbricals. Typical presentation at rest. Wasted hypothenar eminence and loss of adduction of thumb. Similar to the hand of benediction except that ulnar claw is seen at rest while benediction hand is seen while trying to make fist 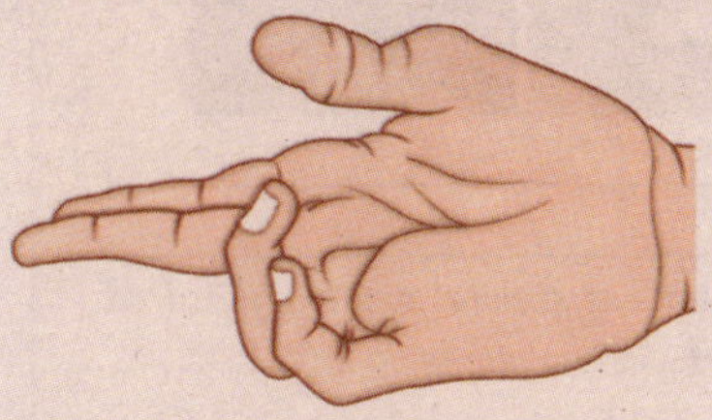	Ulnar and dorsal aspect of palm and of ulnar 1½ digits
	Ulnar paradox: In lesion of the ulnar nerve at the elbow, in addition to the muscles of the hand medial half of flexor digitorum profundus (FDP) & flexor carpi ulnaris are also paralysed. The ulnar claw will develop as before, but with one key difference. There will not be any flexion of the ring and little fingers. Now the ulnar claw only consists of hyperextension at the MCP joints, giving a less evident claw hand. This is known as the 'ulnar paradox'. The worse injury, lesion at elbow, looks less serious than a lesion at the wrist. Ulnar nerve injury of elbow is more prominent when patient is asked to make a fist.	
Ulnar (C 8, T1) at wrist	**"Ulnar Claw hand" (AKA 'intrinsic minus' hand)**—Loss of flexion/ hyperextension of 4th& 5th MCP joints and loss of extension (i.e. Flexion) of IP joints. Due to paralysis of palmar and dorsal interossei and medial 2 lumbricals. Typical presentation at rest. Wasted hypothenar eminence and loss of adduction of thumb. Unlike ulnar nerve injury at elbow, the FDP is spared and hence Clawing is more prominent.	
	Note: Dupuytren's contracture: This typically involves the little and ring fingers and can mimic a claw hand, but the metacarpophalangeal joint is flexed and the contracted fingers cannot passively be extended. Palpation of the Dupuytren's tissue in the palm confirms the diagnosis.	
Combined median & ulnar nerve palsy at wrist	**Full claw hand** with thenar and hypothenar flattening, and thumb adduction and flexion. **[AKA- Simian hand or Ape Hand (true)]**	Palm and digits

42. Ans. (c) Pseudoorthorosis of tibia

Ref: Apley 9th ed page 692

Congenital tibial pseudoarthrosis of the tibia describes abnormal bowing that can progress to a segment of bone loss simulating the appearance of a false joint. Overall, 10% of patients with NF1 are diagnosed with tibial pseudoarthrosis

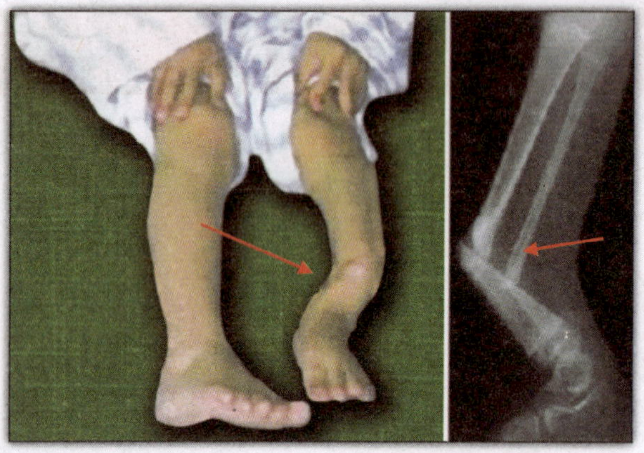

43. Ans. (c) Ganselan test

Ref: Yochum and rowe's essentials of skeletal radiology 3rd ed page 235, Apley 9th ed page 354

The X-ray is consistent with developmental dysplasia of hip (DDH)

The tests useful to diagnose DDH are:

- Ortolani's test:
- Barlow's test:
- Vascular sign of Narath: is positive in posterior dislocation of hip joint. Due to posterior dislocation, the hip joint falls on the femoral artery, and this causes feeble or absent femoral pulse.
- Galeazzi sign or Allis test
- Telescopy test

Ganselan Test

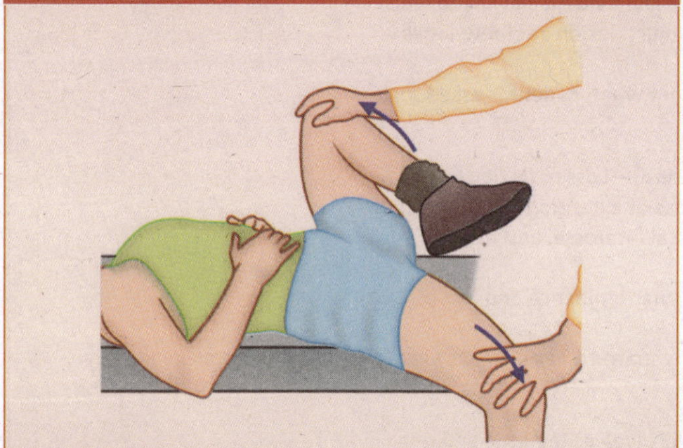

The test can help **distinguish between lumbar spine involvement and SI joint** dysfunction. The patient lies supine, close to the side of the examination table. The examinerv allows the near leg to hang over the side of the table, and instructs the patient to actively flex the other leg to his or her chest and hold it; stabilising the patient, the examiner applies pressure to the near leg, forcing it into hyperextension. Pain implies SI joint dysfunction.

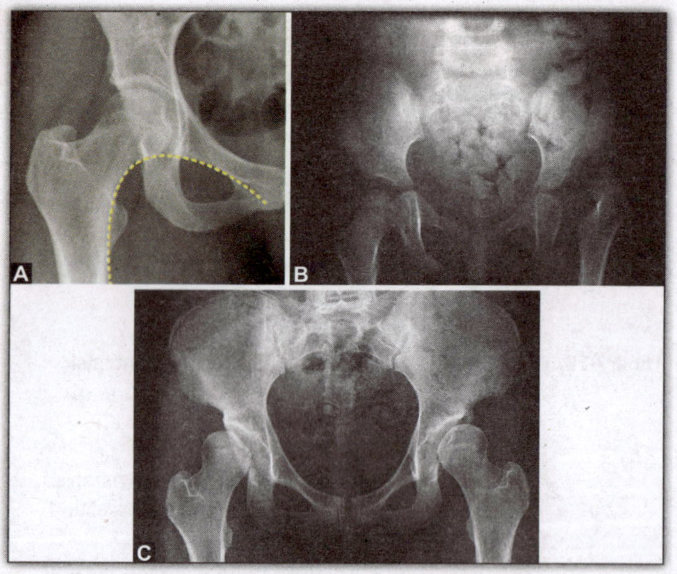

Figs A to C: **(A)** Figure shows the normal shenton line: Shenton line is an imaginary line drawn along the inferior border of the superior pubic ramus (superior border of the obturator foramen) and along the inferomedial border of the neck of femur. This line should be continuous and smooth. Interruption of the Shenton line can indicates: 1. Developmental dysplasia of the hip (DDH), 2. Fractured neck of femur; **(B)** Unilateral DDH; **(C)** Bilateral DDH

DDH–X-rays: Numerous radiographic measurements have been used to assist in the evaluation of DDH (a typical radiographic evaluation is described in the image below). From an anteroposterior radiograph of the hips, a horizontal line (Hilgenreiner line) is drawn between the triradiate epiphyses. Next, lines are drawn perpendicular to the Hilgenreiner line through the superolateral edge of the acetabulum (Perkin line), dividing the hip into four quadrants. The proximal medial femur should be in the lower medial quadrant, or the ossific nucleus of the femoral head, if present (usually observed in patients aged 4 to 7 months), should be in the lower medial quadrant.

- The acetabular index is the angle between the Hilgenreiner line and a line drawn from the triradiate epiphysis to the lateral edge of the acetabulum. Typically, this angle decreases with age and should measure less than 20 degrees by the time the child is 2-years-old. The angle should not exceed 30°
- The acetabular roof Shenton line is an imaginary line drawn along the inferior border of the superior pubic ramus (superior border of the obturator foramen) and along the inferomedial border of the neck of femur. This line should be continuous and smooth.
- Von Rosen's lines: with the hips abducted 45° the femoral shafts should point into the acetabula. In each case the left side is shown to be abnormal.

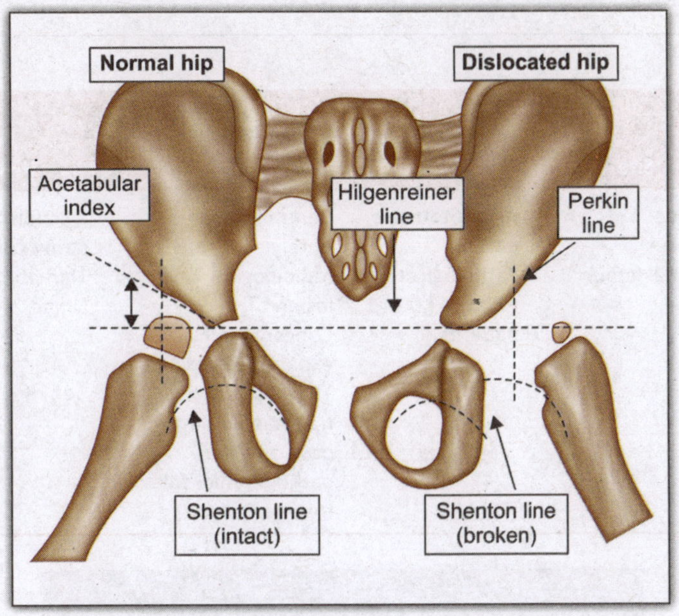

44. Ans: (a) Monteggia fracture

Ref: Apley 9th ed page 774

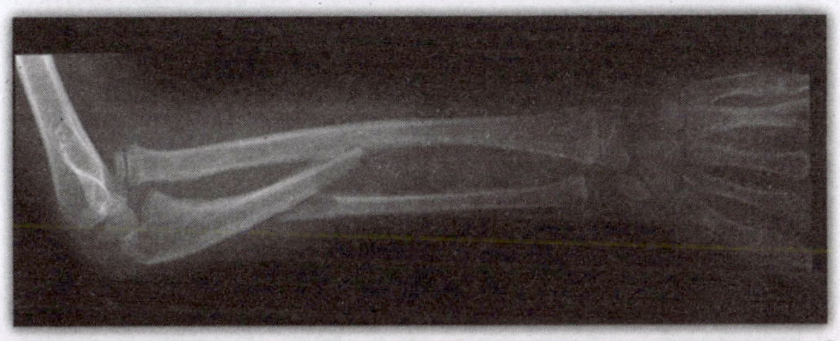

Monteggia Fracture Dislocation	
Definition	Fracture of proximal/shaft of ulna with anterior angulation of ulna and anterior dislocation of radial dead. In less common type the angulation and dislocation is posteriorly
Mechanism of injury	Direct blow or fall on outstretched hand
Clinical features	Pain and tenderness on lateral side of elbow. Dislocated head of radius is masked by swelling. Ulnar deformity is visible
	Bado classification: (Based on radial head location): • **Anterior (Most common)** • Posterior • Lateral • Anterior with associated both bone fracture
X-ray	Fracture of upper third of ulna with forward bowing Forward dislocation of radial head
Treatment	Ulna: ORIF (plates/screws) Radial head: Closed reduction (open if irreducible or unstable) Peds: Closed reduction & cast.

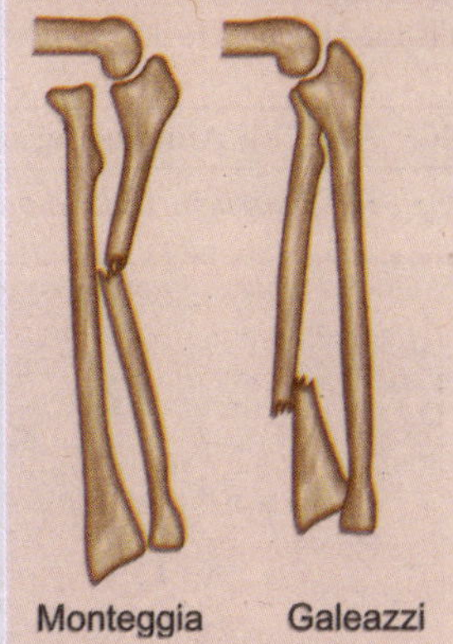

45. Ans. (a) Simple bone cyst

Ref: Apley 9th ed page 200-201

Unicameral bone cyst					
Demography	**Site**	**Presentation**	**Imaging**	**Histology**	**Treatment**
1st–2nd Decades, M:F 2 : 1	Proximal humerus Proximal femur	**Asymptomatic unless** Pathological fracture (2/3 rd patients)	Centrally located, purely radiolucent lesion Concentrically expands cortex. Thinned cortical fragmen falls into base of lesion, pathognomic **"fallen fragment sign"**	Cyst filled with **straw-colored fluid** Thin fibrovascular Lining	Observation Aspiration/injection (steroids, bone marrow, bone graft substitute, sclerosant) Curettage

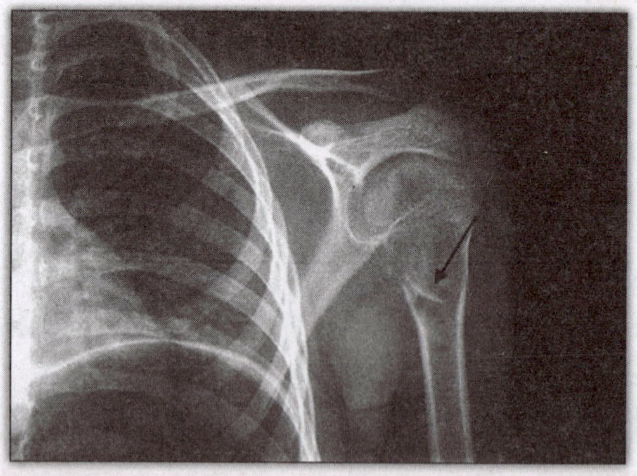

Fig: Simple/Unicameral bone cyst: Centrally located, purely radiolucent lesion, Concentrically expands cortex. Thinned cortical fragmen falls into base of lesion, pathognomic **"fallen fragment sign"**

46. Ans. (b) Ankylosing spondylitis

Ref: Harrison 19th ed page 2170, Apley 9th ed page 66

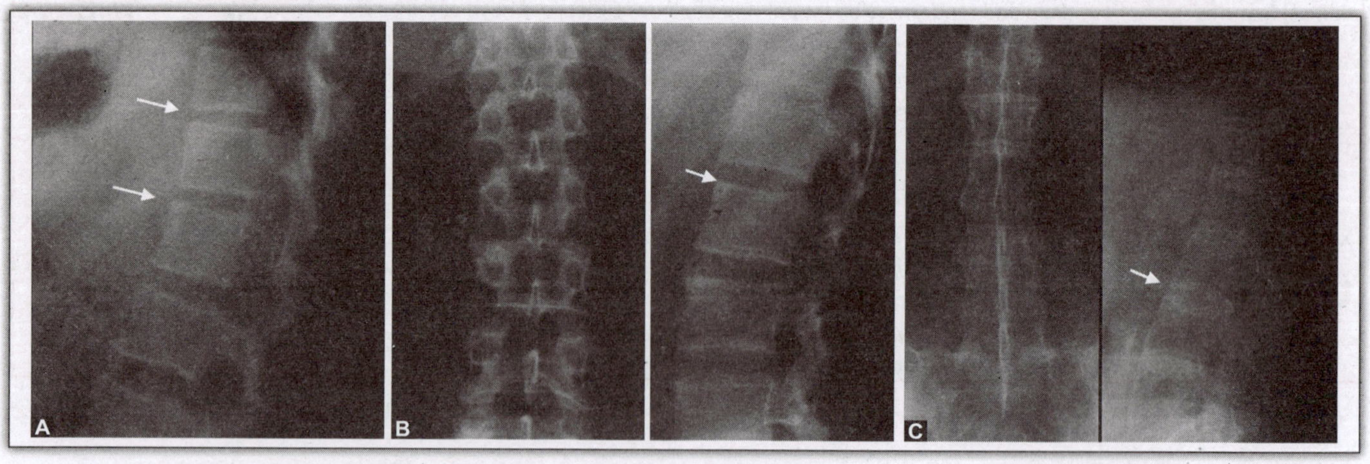

Figs A and B: (A) Ankylosing Spondylitis: Lateral view of the thoracolumbar region showing slight abnormalities in the form of slight vertebral squaring (arrows); **(B) Ankylosing Spondylitis:** Frontal and lateral view of the lumbar spine showing bridging syndesmophytes (arrows); **(C) Ankylosing Spondylitis:** Frontal and lateral view of the lumbar spine showing fusion of several vertebral bodies (arrow)

Ankylosing Spondylitis	
Ankylosing spondylitis (AS) is an inflammatory disorder of unknown cause that primarily affects the axial skeleton; peripheral joints and extraarticular structures are also frequently involved.	
Ankylosing spondylitis, Reiter's disease and psoriatic arthritis characteristically test negative for rheumatoid factor; they have been grouped together as the 'seronegative spondarthritides'. The term *axial spondyloarthritis*, coming into common use, includes early or mild forms that do not meet classical criteria for AS	
Age of onset	15 and 25 years
Genetic marker	HLA B 27 in 95% cases **HLA-B27 is associated with AS and Aortic Root Dilatation with AR**
Clinical features	**Sacroiliitis** is often the earliest manifestations of AS. The initial symptom is usually dull pain, insidious in onset, felt deep in the lower lumbar or gluteal region, accompanied **by low-back morning stiffness of up to a few hours'** duration that improves with activity and returns following inactivity The most specific findings involve **loss of spinal mobility, with limitation of anterior and lateral flexion and extension of the lumbar spine and of chest expansion.**
Posture	In established cases the posture is typical: ***Loss of the normal lumbar lordosis, increased thoracic kyphosis*** and a forward thrust of the neck; upright posture and balance are maintained by standing with the hips and knees slightly flexed, and in late cases these may become fixed deformities. Spinal movements are diminished in all directions, but loss of extension is always the earliest and the most severe disability. It is revealed dramatically by the **'wall test':** The patient is asked to stand with his back to the wall; heels, buttocks, scapulae and occiput should all be able to touch the wall simultaneously.
Extraskeletal manifestations	General fatigue and loss of weight are common. **Acute anterior uveitis** (most common extraskeletal manifestation 25–40%); it usually responds well to treatment but, if neglected, may lead to permanent damage including **glaucoma**. Other extraskeletal disorders, such as **aortic valve disease**, carditis and **pulmonary fibrosis** (apical), are rare and occur very late in the disease. **Chest expansion**, which should be at least 7 cm in young men, is often markedly decreased. About 10% of patients meeting criteria for AS have **psoriasis.**
X-ray	The cardinal sign – and often the earliest–**is erosion and fuzziness of the sacroiliac joints.** The earliest vertebral change is flattening of the normal anterior concavity of the vertebral body ('squaring'). Later, ossification of the ligaments around the intervertebral discs produces delicate bridges **(syndesmophytes)** between adjacent vertebrae. Bridging at several levels gives the appearance of a **'bamboo spine'** **SASSS = Stoke Ankylosing Spondylitis Spine Score:** Anterior and posterior changes in the lumbar spine Grade 0: Normal findings. Grade 1: Erosion, sclerosis and/or squaring. Grade 2: Syndesmophytes. Grade 3: Total ankylosis.
Special investigations	The ESR and CRP are usually elevated during active phases of the disease. **HLA-B27** is present in 95% of cases. Serological tests for rheumatoid factor are usually negative.
Management	All management of AS should include an exercise program designed to maintain posture and range of motion. Nonsteroidal anti-inflammatory drugs (NSAIDs) are the first line of pharmacologic therapy for AS. Anti TNF alpha drugs are being tried.

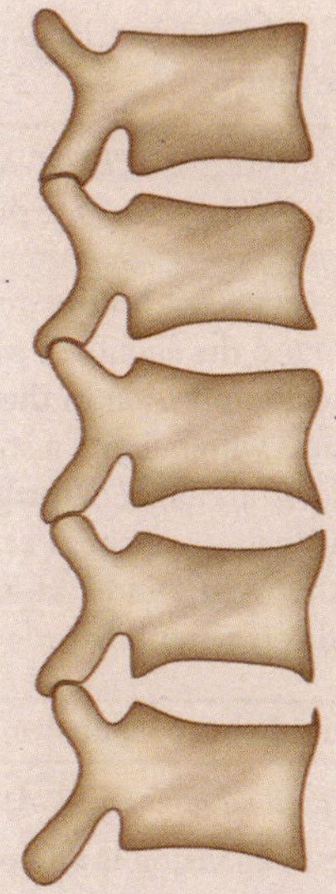

47. Answer: (b) Median nerve

Ref: Apley 9th ed page

The radiograph is showing a supracondylar fracture

See Details of Supracondylar fracture in AIIMS MAY 2018 Orthopedics (see page no. 1008-1009)

The nerve most likely to get damaged is anterior interosseous branch of median nerve

Fracture/Dislocation Associated Nerve Injuries	
Fracture/dislocation	**Nerve injured**
Anterior dislocation of shoulder	Axillary or circumflex humeral nerve
Inferior dislocation of shoulder	Axillary nerve
Fracture surgical neck of humerus	Axillary nerve
Fracture shaft of humerus	Radial nerve
Fracture supracondylar of humerus	Anterior interosseous branch of median nerve
Elbow dislocation	Ulnar nerve
Lateral condyle of humerus fracture	Tardy ulnar nerve palsy
Medial condyle of humerus fracture	Ulnar nerve
Monteggia fracture–dislocation	Posterior-interosseous
Lunate dislocation, Volkman's contracture	Median nerve
Hip dislocation	Sciatic nerve
Knee dislocation	Common peroneal nerve
Tibial plateau fracture, neck of fibula fracture	Common peroneal nerve

AIIMS NOVEMBER 2015

48. Ans. (c) Improper use of crutches

Ref: Apley 9th ed page 282

Improper use of Crutches leads to radial nerve palsy not Axillary nerve injury

See Table of BRACHIAL PLEXUS NERVE LESIONS in AIIMS MAY 2016 Orthopedics (see page no. 1028-1029)

Radial nerve very high lesions may be caused by trauma or operations around the shoulder. More often, though, they are due to chronic compression in the axilla; this is seen in drink and drug addicts who fall into a stupor with the arm dangling over the back of a chair ('Saturday night palsy') or in thin elderly patients using crutches (**'crutch palsy'**). In addition to weakness of the wrist and hand, the triceps is paralysed and the triceps reflex is absent.

49. Ans. (b) Limited chest expansion

Ref: Harrison 19th ed page 2170, Apley 9th ed page 66

Decreased chest expansion is one of the extraskeletal manifestation of Ankylosing Spondylitis, which is frequently asked in AIIMS examinations

See Table of Ankylosing Spondylitis MAY 2016 Orthopedics (see page no. 1032-1033)

50. Ans. (b) Lateral epicondyle fracture of humerus

Ref: Apley's 9th ed page 371

The clinical picture and picture is consistent with Cubitus Valgus.

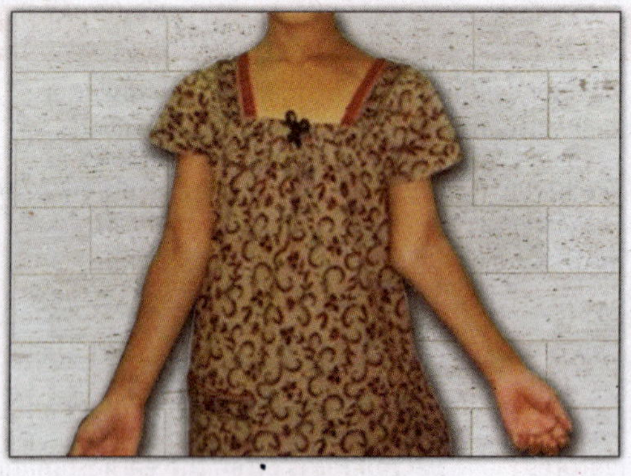

Cubitus Valgus

The normal carrying angle of the elbow is 5–15 degrees of valgus; anything more than this is regarded as a valgus deformity, which is usually quite obvious when the patient stands with arms to the sides and palms facing forwards. The commonest cause is longstanding **non-union of a fractured lateral condyle**; the deformity may be associated with marked prominence of the medial condylar outline. The importance of cubitus valgus is the liability to delayed ulnar palsy; years after the causal injury the patient notices weakness of the hand, with numbness and tingling of the ulnar fingers. The deformity itself needs no treatment, but for delayed ulnar palsy the nerve should be transposed to the front of the elbow. Great care is needed in performing the operation. Excessive dissection of the nerve or rough handling can impair nerve function.

Varus and valgus deformities (cubitus varus and cubitus valgus) are usually the result of trauma around the elbow. By far the best way to demonstrate a varus deformity is to ask the patient to lift his or her arms sideways to shoulder height; in this position the deformity becomes much more obvious, the arm taking on the appearance of a rifle butt (gunstock deformity

Carrying angle (normal 5°-15°)	Negative (<5°)	**Cubitus varus:** Physeal damage (e.g. malunion supracondylar fracture)
	Positive (>15°)	**Cubitus valgus:** Physeal damage (e.g. lateral epicondyle fracture)

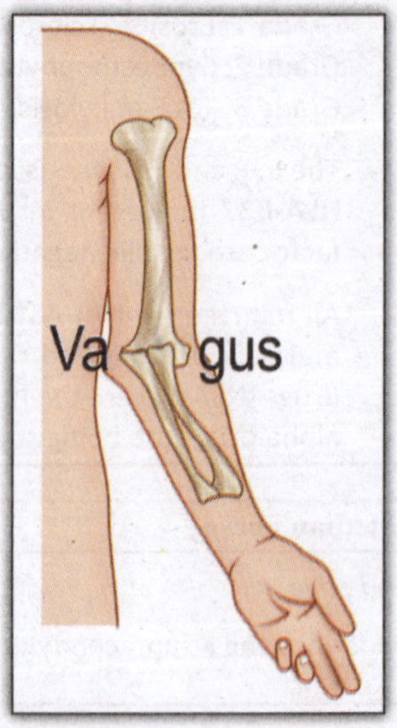

51. Ans. (c) Galeazzi's fracture

Ref: Apley's 9th ed page 790

The X-ray shows a fracture of the distal radius and distal radio-ulnar joint dislocation typically seen in Galeazzi fracture

See Details of Galeazzi Facture in AIIMS MAY 2017 Ortho (see page no. 1022-1023)

52. Ans. (b) Hallux valgus

Ref: Apley's 9th ed page 603-604

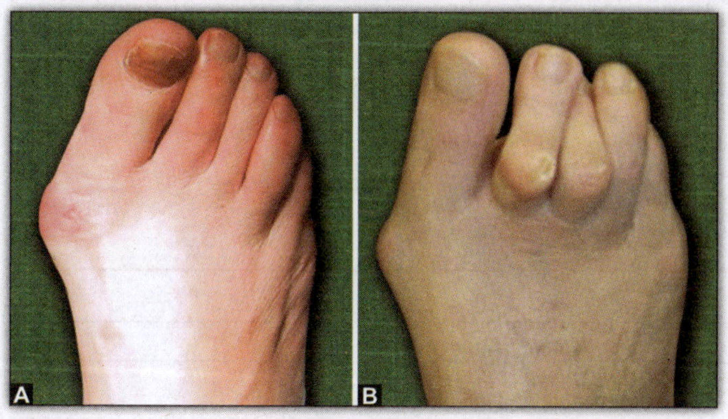

Figs A and B: (A) Hallux Valgus deformity; **(B)** Hallux Valgux with Hammer toe deformity of 2nd and 3rd toe

Hallux Valgus (Bunion)

Hallux valgus (lateral deviation of the great toe) is not a single disorder, as the name implies, but a complex deformity of the first ray that frequently is accompanied by deformity and symptoms in the lesser toes.

Hallux abductus (or hallux valgus) angle: The angle created by the bisection of the longitudinal axis of the hallux and the longitudinal axis of the first metatarsal. Historically, a hallux abductus (HA) angle of greater than 15 degrees was considered abnormal, but such deformities are not always symptomatic, and some cases of an HA angle greater than 15 degrees occur naturally due to the shape of the articular surfaces involved. Contemporary research suggests an ***HA angle of 20 degrees or greater is abnormal***. If the **valgus angle of the first metatarsophalangeal joint exceeds 30 to 35 degrees,** pronation of the great toe usually results.

Intermetatarsal (IM) angle: The angle determined by the bisection of the longitudinal axes of the first and second metatarsals. An IM angle less than 9 degrees is considered normal.

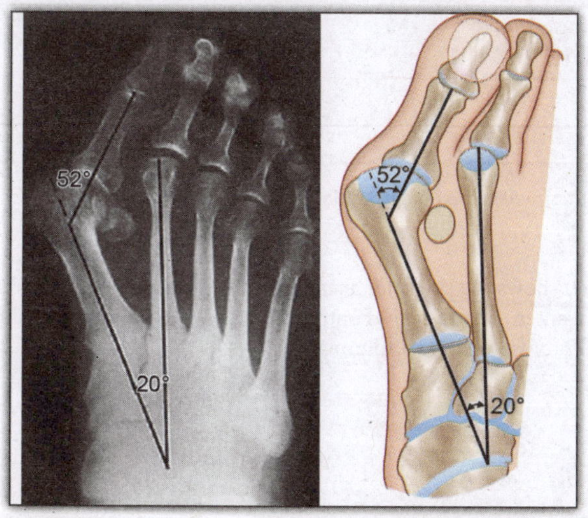

The valgus posture of the great toe frequently causes a **hammer toe–like deformity of the second toe**. In addition, the splaying of the forefoot makes the wearing of shoes more difficult; with shoes that have a narrow toe box, corns often develop, as does bursal hypertrophy over the medial eminence of the first metatarsal head **(bunion)**. Amputation of the second toe frequently is followed by severe hallux valgus because the great toe tends to drift toward the third to fill the gap left by amputation.

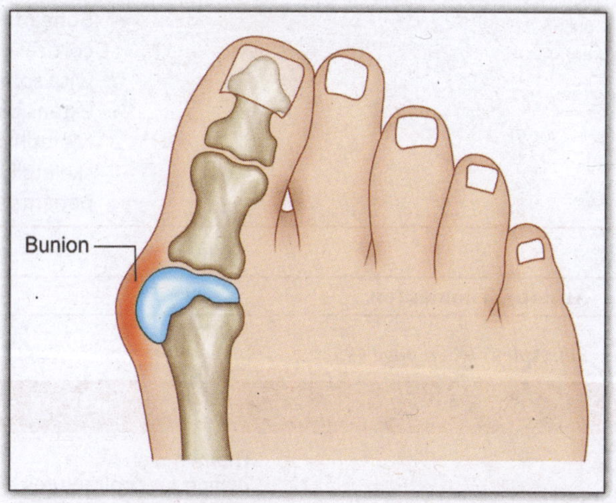

Hallux valgus complex. Note increase in intermetatarsal angle, lateral dislocation of sesamoids, subluxation of first metatarsophalangeal joint (leaving metatarsal head uncovered), and pronation of great toe associated with marked hallux valgus.

53. Ans. (a) Gaint cell tumor

Ref: Apley's 9th ed page 203

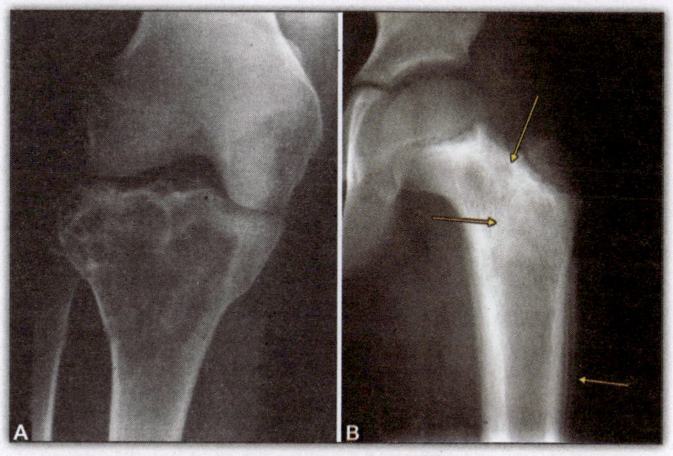

Figs A and B: (A) Giant cell tumor: Radiograph of proximal tibia with characteristic Soap bubble appearance; **(B) Ewing sarcoma:** Femur is most common location. Involves Diaphysis. Top arrow indicates reactive sclerosis, Middle arrow indicates **Permeative reaction (Most common pattern),** Lower arrow indicates Onion skin periosteal reaction. Permeative pattern is poorly demarcated with multiple small irregular holes suggestive aggressive process. Acute osteomyelitis mimics Ewing's sarcoma clinically and radiologically

Giant Cell Tumor						
Demography	**Site**	**Presentation**	**Imaging**	**Histology**	**Treatment**	**Comments**
20–40 yrs F> M	Eccentrically located in epiphysis, Distal femur Proximal tibia Distal radius	Pain Pathological fracture (10%–30%)	Purely radiolucent (no matrix formation) Usually no rim of reactive bone Abuts subchondral Bone may exhibit cortical destruction with soft tissue extension Metaphyseal in skeletally immature patients	Multinucleated **giant** cells in sea of mononuclear cells Nuclei of mononuclear cells identical to nuclei of giant cells	Extended curettage Resection if residual bone stock inadequate Consider radiation for spinal/ sacral tumors Resection of pulmonary metastases	3% incidence of **benign pulmonary metastases**

54. Ans. (b) Thomas test

Ref: Apley's 9th ed page 495

Thomas Test

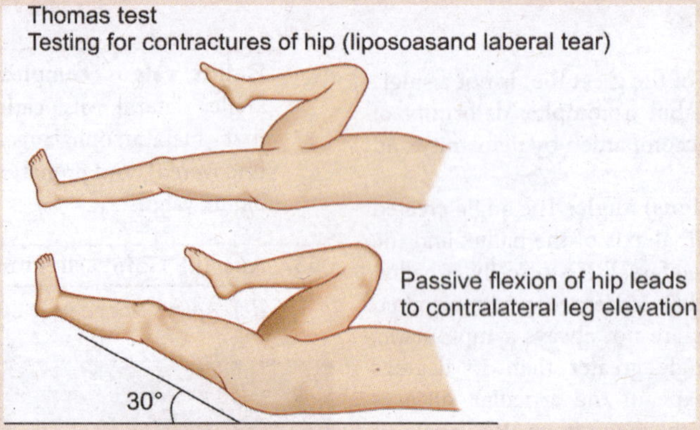

The assessment of hip movements is difficult because any limitation can easily be obscured by movement of the pelvis. Thus, even a gross limitation of extension, causing a **fixed flexion deformity.**

Procedure: The patient lying supine, maximally flex both hips simultaneously thus completely obliterating the lumbar lordosis; holding the 'sound/normal hip firmly in position (and thus keeping the pelvis still), the other limb is lowered gently. The angle between the femur and examining table is the residual flexion and represents the flexion contracture or **fixed flexion deformity.** The normal range is about **130 degrees.**

AIIMS MAY 2015

55. Ans. (a) Pelvis

Ref: Yochum and Rowe's Essentials of skeletal radiology 3rd ed page 85, Maheshwari 5th ed page 38, 369

Judet Views

Two views are taken of one hip. Elevating the hip by 45° (anterior oblique) shows the posterior acetabular margin, superior pubic ramus attachment to the anterior acetabulum (anterior column), and obturator foramen. Elevating the contralateral hip by 45° (posterior oblique) shows the iliac wing, posterior acetabulum, and its fusion with the ischial ramus (posterior column).

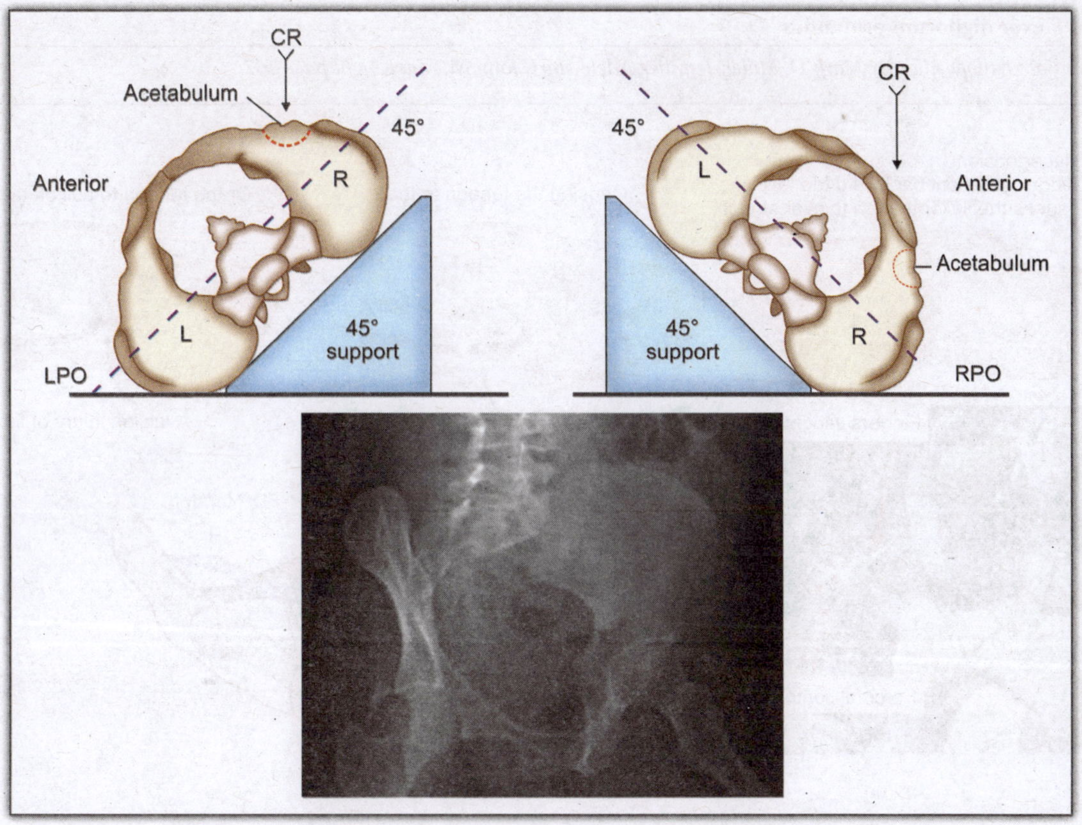

56. Ans. (a) MRI

Ref: Apley 9th ed page 724, MRI of Musculoskeletal system: 5th ed ch 8

- **Stress fractures and insufficiency fractures** are common in the **foot and ankle.**
- **Stress fracture** is related to repetitive stress to normal bone structure.
- **Insufficiency fractures** occur when normal stress is applied to abnormal bone.
- In the foot, stress fractures most commonly involve the **second through fourth metatarsal shafts and necks.**
- **Metatarsal bases** are more commonly involved in **ballet dancers.**
- Navicular and base of the fifth metatarsal may also be involved.
- Stress response is the first stage of stress fractures.
- **Edema, hyperemia, and increased osteoclastic activity in the involved region show a poorly defined area of signal abnormality on MRI** with low signal intensity on T1- and high signal intensity on T2-weighted or STIR sequences. Over time, a linear fracture line may be evident, especially in the navicular and calcaneus.
- **MRI is more sensitive and specific than radionuclide scans**, particularly in the elderly or osteopenic population.
- **Plain radiographs (X-rays) have poor sensitivity** in detecting stress fractures, as positive findings may take months to appear.
- The appearance on **CT is similar to plain radiograph.**
- **Bone scans can show evidence of stress fracture within a few days** upon onset of symptoms. It is represented as a focus of increased radioisotope activity ('hot spot') due to increased bone turnover at the site of new bone formation.

57. Ans. (a) Hip joint

Ref: Yochum and rowe's essentials of skeletal radiology 3rd ed page 235, Apley 9th ed page 354

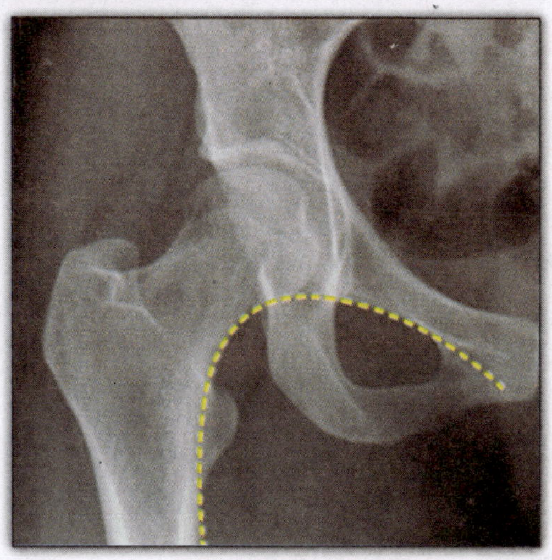

Fig: Shows the normal Shenton line: Shenton line is an imaginary line drawn along the inferior border of the superior pubic ramus (superior border of the obturator foramen) and along the inferomedial border of the neck of femur. This line should be continuous and smooth. Interruption of the Shenton line can indicates:

- Developmental dysplasia of the hip (DDH)
- Fractured neck of femur

58. Ans. (c) Flexor digitorum profundus

Ref: Essential Orthopaedics By Mark D. Miller, Jennifer Adele Hart, John M. MacKnight page 367

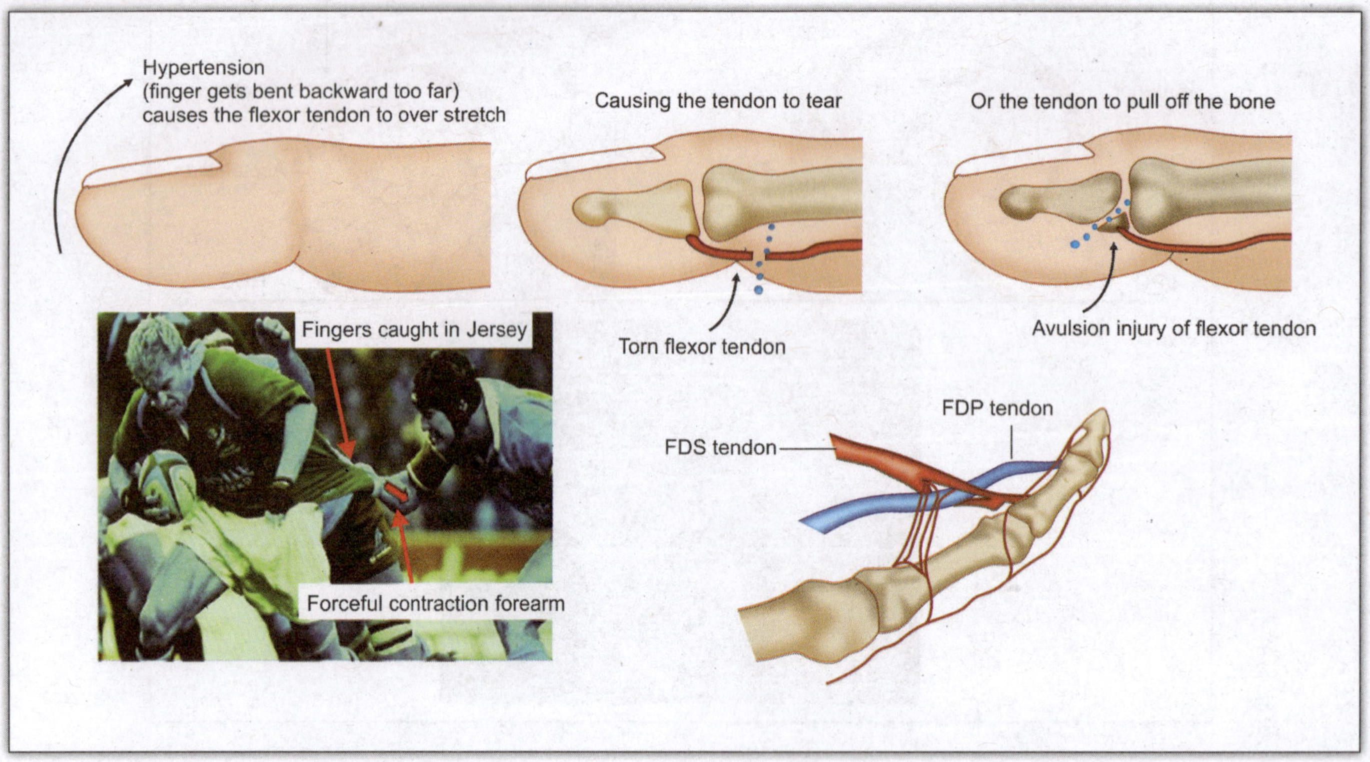

Leddy Parker Classification

The basic classification system is called the Leddy Parker Classification, and it has 3 types.

- **Type 1** is the **worst**, the tendon retracts all the way to the palm and it needs to be treated with **surgery within a week** because when the tendon moves so far out of position, its nutritional supply is disrupted
- **Type 2** injury occurs when the tendon retracts to the PIP (the middle finger joint). It still needs to be treated in a few weeks before excessive scar tissue forms around the tendon and prevents it from being stretch back out to its normal length.
- **Type 3** injury is the **avulsion type fracture**, which should also be repaired, but the piece of bone acts like an anchor and prevents the tendon from drifting. The tendon hardly retracts at all.

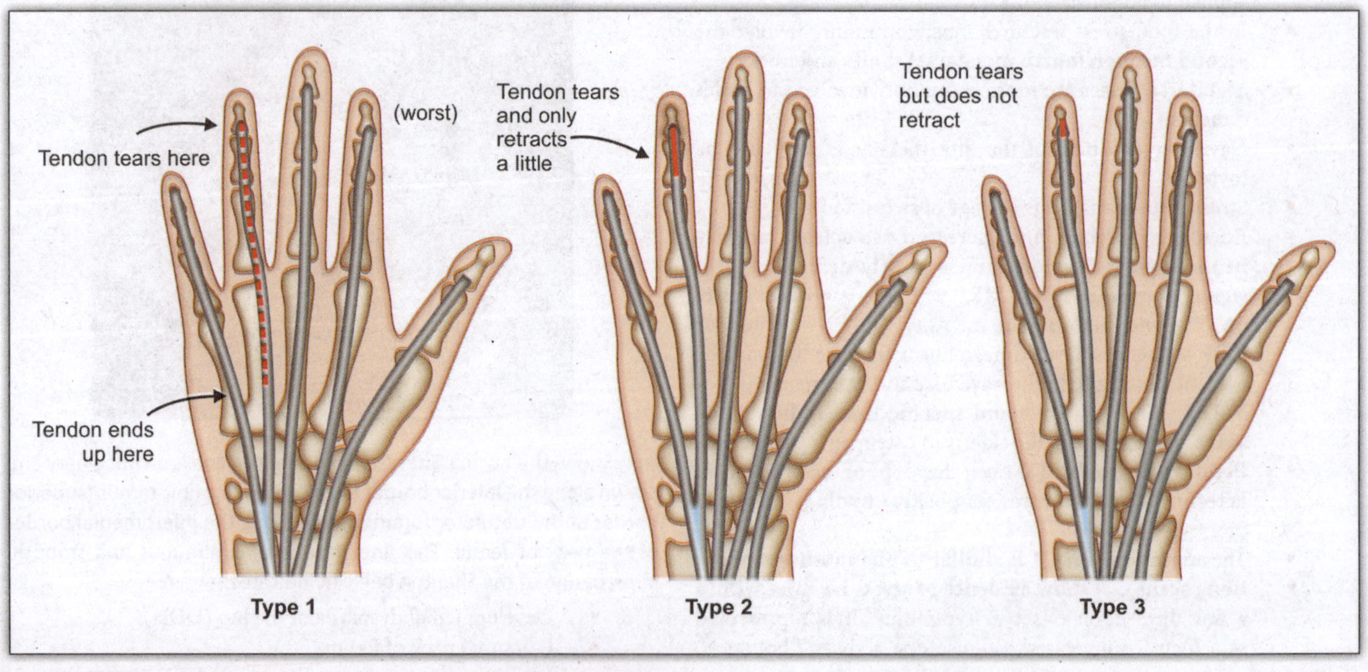

Ligament Injuries of Finger				
	Description	**History/Physical Exam**	**Work-Up/Findings**	**Treatment**
Boutonniere deformity	• **Extensor tendon** (central slip injury) at PIP ruptures, lateral bands slip volar and flex PIP • Associated with RA	Hx: Hand trauma PE: PIP flexed, no active extension, DIP extended	XR: Hand series: normal	• Splint PIP in extension, DIP free • Reconstruct central slip and bands • Severe: Fusion or arthroplasty
Jersey finger	**Flexor digitoum pofundus (FDP)** tendon injury by forceful extension on a flexed digit, typically in an athlete grabbing opponent's jersey. (also called a Zone 1 Flexor tendon injury). Occur mostly in rugby/football. Occurs most commonly in the ring finger (75%).	Hx: Extension injury, 1/2 pain. PE: FDS: 1 sublimus test FDP: 1 profundus test	XR: Rule out fracture (1/2 avulsion fracture)	• Primary repair • Older patient: DIP fusion
Mallet finger	AKA: **Baseball, dropped, dolphin finger** Hyperflexion **Extensor digitorum tendon injury** of the fingers at DIP • FDP unopposed so DIP flexes	History of **Hyperflexion** injury of Extensor digitorum, usually occurs when a ball, while being caught, hits an outstretched finger Exm: Cannot extend DIP, minimal pain & swelling, hyperextended PIP Jt	X-ray: 1/2 avulsion fracture	• **Constant splint** (DIP only) for 8 weeks followed by 4 weeks night only splint • Operative treatment is considered only if there is a large fragment (>50%) & subluxation of DIP.
Swanneck deformity	• FDS rupture/volar plate injury • Lateral bands subluxes dorsally, PIP hyperextends & DIP flexes	Hx: Trauma, RA, spastic PE: PIP hyperextended, DIP flexed	XR: Hand series	• Early: Splint • Late: Surgical repair (individualize each case)
Gamekeeper's thumb	AKA; **SKIER'S THUMB** **Ulnar collateral ligament** tear of the thumb metacarpo phalangeal joint Mechanism: forceful radial deviation or fall on extended thumb causing **hyperabduction** 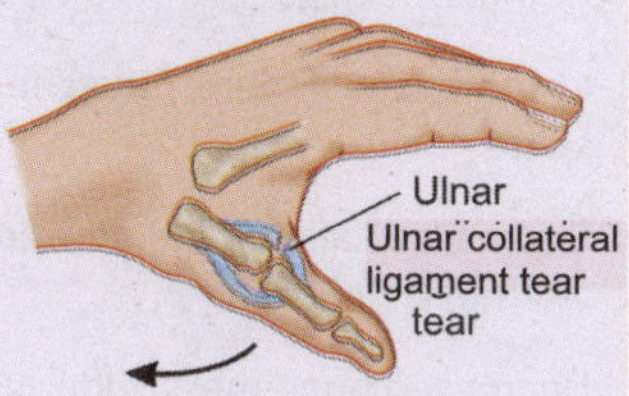	History of: Trauma. Pain & swelling. EXM: **Partial rupture:** only the ligament proper is torn and the thumb is unstable in flexion but stable in full extension because the palmar plate is intact. **Complete rupture**, both ligament proper & palmar plate are torn & thumb is unstable in all positions	XR: 1/2 avulsion fracture. Stress view shows injury	• Incomplete: Splint 2–4 weeks, avoid pinch for 6–8 weeks • Complete: Surgical repair (treat **Stener lesion**; proximal end of torn ligament gets trapped in front of the adductor pollicis aponeurosis)

59. Ans. (c) Dunlop

Ref: Textbook of Orthopedics by John Ebnezar 4th ed page 66

Dunlop or Modified Dunlop Skin Traction

This type of traction is occasionally useful for the management of supracondylar humeral fractures. Place the patient supine and suspend the arm in skin traction with the shoulder abducted and slightly flexed. In addition, slightly flex the elbow. Modification of this type of traction provides counteraction on the humerus, which can be achieved with the arm over the edge of the bed and counterweight suspended from a felt cuff over the humerus, or with a felt cuff over the forearm pulling laterally with the elbow flexed. Two disadvantages of dunlop traction are that it cannot be applied over skin injuries and that elevation of the humeral fracture above the level of the heart is not possible with this method.

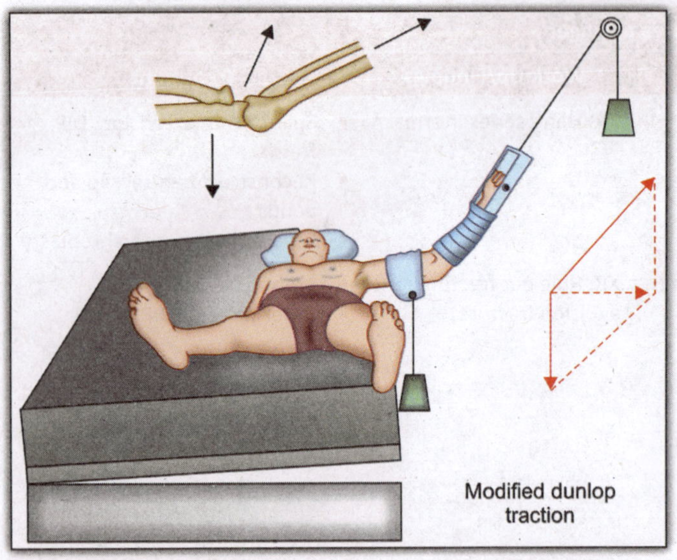

Traction Systems and Uses	
Russel's traction	Trochanteric traction (fracture shaft of femur)
Buck's traction	Conventional skin traction
Perkin's traction	Fracture shaft of femur in adults
90-90 traction	Fracture shaft of femur in children
Gallow's traction	Fracture shaft of femur in children <2 years
Byrants traction	Fracture shaft of femur in children <2 years
Agnes Hunt traction	Correction of hip deformity
Well leg traction	Correction of abduction or adduction deformity of hip
Dunlop traction	Supracondylar fracture of humerus
Smith traction	Supracondylar fracture of humerus
Calcaneal traction	Open fractures of ankle or leg
Metacarpal traction	Open forearm fracture
Head halter traction	Cervical spine injuries
Crutchfield traction	Cervical spine injuries
Halo pelvic traction	Scoliosis

60. Ans. (c) Laminoplasty

Ref: Current Diagnosis and Treatment in Orthopedics, 2nd ed., New York: McGraw-Hill, 2000, page 199–201, Maheshwari 5th ed page 257

"In laminoplasty, the lamina is reattached in a fashion that expands the spinal canal and decompresses the spinal cord"

There are several types of decompression surgery:

- **Laminectomy** is the removal of the entire bony lamina, a portion of the enlarged facet joints, and the thickened ligaments overlying the spinal cord and nerves.
- **Laminotomy** is the removal of a small portion of the lamina and ligaments, usually on one side. Using this method the natural support of the lamina is left in place, decreasing the chance of postoperative spinal instability. Sometimes an endoscope may be used, allowing for a smaller, less invasive incision.
- **Foraminotomy** is the removal of bone around the neural foramen—the space between vertebrae where the nerve root exits the spinal canal. This method is used when disc degeneration has caused the height of the foramen to collapse, resulting in a pinched nerve. It can be performed with a laminectomy or laminotomy.
- **Laminoplasty** is the expansion of the spinal canal by cutting the laminae on one side and swinging them open like a door. It is used only in the cervical area.

61. Ans. (c) Normal calcium, normal ALP

Ref: Apley 9th ed page 131, Harrison 19th ed page 2493

Osteoporosis can be defined as a decrease in the quantity of bone per unit volume that is sufficient to compromise its mechanical function. The bone tissue is mineralized normally, but there is not enough of it to preserve the normal skeletal architecture.

Metabolic Disorders of Bone	
Hypercalcemia	**Symptoms:** Constipation, nausea, abdominal pain, confusion, stupor, coma
1° hyperparathyroidism	Increased urine calcium, decreased serum phophate, "**brown tumors**" result
2° hyperparathyroidism	Malignancy #1, Multiple Endocrine Neoplasm (MEN) syndromes
Hypocalcemia	**Symptoms:** Hyper reflexia, tetany +Chvostek's/Trousseau's sign, papilledema, prolonged QT interval
1° hypoparathyroidism	Hair loss, vitiligo
Renal osteodystrophy	Chronic renal failure, "Rugger jersey" spine
Rickets/osteomalacia	Decreased/failed mineralization, vitamin D deficiency
Osteoporosis	Decreased bone mass, elderly
Scurvy	Vitamin C deficiency results in defective collagen
Osteopetrosis	Increased bone density due to reduced osteoclast activity
Paget's disease	Simultaneous osteoblast and osteoclast activity results in dense, but more brittle bones

Characteristic of Major Metabolic Disorders of Bone				
Features	**Osteomalacia (soft bone disease)**	**Osteoporosis**	**Osteopetrosis Marble bone/brittle bone/ albert's schonberg**	**Osteogenesis imperfects**
Associated with	Vitamin D metabolism, hypoparathyroidism, CRF	Postmenopausal women due to ↓ estrogen level, smoking	AD (AR form is rare)	**AR** form is fatal
Mechanism	Amount of Ca^{++} accretion per unit bone matrix is deficient in adults.	Bone resorption >Bone formation. Matrix and minerals both are lost over time	Loss of ruffled border of osteoclast- ↓bone resorption, bone overgrowth	Mutation in type-I collagen.
Pathogenesis	Osteoid formation is normal but defect in mineralization of bone matrix (Qualitative)	Bone quality normal (matrix mineral ratio normal) but ↓in quantity (amount)	Pathological # are frequent as the bones are weak and brittle	Defective collagen synthesis.
Histopathology	↑in thickness of osteoid seams	Thin trabeculae that have normal calcification, normal osteoblast and osteoclast.		Woven bone
Clinical feature		m/c affect: Long cancellous bone.	Obliteration of medullary cavity- Anemia, pancytopenia, hepatosplenomegaly.	Thin translucent blue sclera, Laxity of joint ligaments, deafness due to otosclerosis, abnormal teeth.
X-ray	Washed out bone on X-ray (loss of trabeculae) ↓ Looser's zone (visible at NOF) ***Milkman #/Pseudo #*** ***Tri-radiate pelvis*** ***Protrusion acetabuli***	m/c site – compression # of vertebrae at D_{12} - L_1 level. D-L spine is the m/c site of weakness. ***Codfish vertebrae***	Chalky white bone deposits, ↑ radio opacity of bones. ***Sandwich vertebrae*, *Bone within bone appearance*, *Rugger jersey spine in type-2,*** Meta and diaphysis wide in long bones- ***Erlenmeyer flask deformity***	Multiple # in infant is characteristics but healing is normal
Laboratory	25 (OH) vit-D is ↓. Which is most sensitive and earliest marker for nutritional osteomalacia. ↑↑ALP	Normal serum level of Ca^{++}, PO_4^-, ALP and PTH.	Level of serum Ca^{++}, ALP is Normal = (in adult). May be ↓Ca^{++}, ↓ PO_4^- = (in children) ↑Acis phosphatase	

62. Ans. (a) Tendon transfer

Ref: Campbell Operative Orthopedics page 2230- 2235 table 46-3, Apley 9th ed page 348, Manual of Orthopaedics Swiontkowski, Marc F.; Stovitz, Steven D 6th Ed page 227

This is a controversial question with confusion between option (a) Tendon transfer and Option (b) Reverse shoulder replacement. *Conclusion to the discussion below is that since arthropathy is not given in the question it is grade V tear and Tendon transfer is preferred over Reverse Shoulder replacement. In case of Irreparable rotator cuff tear with arthropathy (grade VI tear), Reverse shoulder replacement is preferred.*

Introduction

The **rotator cuff muscles (supraspinatus, infraspinatus, and teres minor)** plus the subscapularis and the long head of the biceps are very important dynamic stabilizers of shoulder. Pain in the mid-range of abduction suggests a minor rotator cuff tear or supraspinatus tendinitis; pain at the end of abduction is often due to acromioclavicular arthritis. An acute rotator cuff tear can be difficult to repair if not detected within the first 6 weeks postinjury. Rotator cuff tears are common in patients older than 40 years with an anterior dislocation. Acute tears of the rotator cuff are rare and occur mainly in individuals younger than 40 years old who have a history of significant trauma. Attritional tears of the rotator cuff are more common and occur in older individuals.

Apley Says

Massive full thickness tears that cannot be reconstructed are treated by subacromial decompression and debridement of degenerate cuff tissue; the relief of pain may allow reasonable abduction of the shoulder by the remaining muscles. Other methods to reconstruct irreparable tears in the younger patient include **supraspinatus advancement, latissimus dorsi transfer, rotator cuff transposition, fascia lata autograft and synthetic tendon graft.**

Campbell Says

Occasionally, despite the surgeon's best efforts and the use of all techniques of mobilization, some tears are so large or retracted, or both, that an anatomical repair is impossible. In this situation, several options are available, none of which is ideal. The two repair options are **nonanatomical repair or partial repair.** Muscle transfers or slides are another option. The final option is simple débridement. Partial repair has been shown to be superior to débridement, tendon transfers, and tendon augmentation procedures for the treatment of massive irreparable rotator cuff tears.

Option (A)

Tendon transfers for the treatment of irreparable rotator cuff tears may involve transfer of rotator cuff tendons or other muscle-tendon units. Cofield described subscapularis tendon. For anterosuperior tears involving the subscapularis and the supraspinatus, transfer of the pectoralis major has been described. For posterosuperior tears involving the infraspinatus and supraspinatus, the latissimus dorsi has been transferred (Campbell)

Grades of Rotator Cuff Pathology with Indications for Use of Extracellular Matrix in Repair

Grade	Tear characteristic	Current treatment	Outcome
I	Partial thickness tear (<50 % of articular or basal surface)	Arthroscopic decompression, debridement or repair with acrominoplasty	95% healing with repair
II	Partial thickness tear (>50% of articular or basal surface)	Arthroscopic decompression/ débridement or repair with acromioplasty	40% failure within 5 years with débridement only; 95% heal when repaired
III	Small to medium tear (<3 cm, 1 tendon)	Arthroscopic repair	Moderate failure rate (5%-10% re-tear rate; 85% pain free but > 50% with reduced function)
IV	Large, massive tear (3-5 cm, 2-3 tendons); repairable	Open or arthroscopic repair	Moderate failure rate (≥30% re-tear rate, 85% pain free but function reduced)
V	Large, massive tear (3-5 cm, 2-3 tendons); not repairable (unable to reappose to tuberosity with low tension)	Open or arthroscopic attempt at repair, muscle/ tendon transfer, débridement, and/or partial repair	High failure rate (≥50% re-tear and/or low outcome scores)
VI	Massive, retracted irreparable tear with intra-articular pathology	Open reverse total shoulder replacement (aggressive)	Adequate, but limited function

Contd...

Option (B)

End-stage rotator cuff disease leads to an entity known as cuff tear arthropathy. Due to a massive rotator cuff tear, normal humeral head depression of the supraspinatus is lost and the unopposed deltoid pull leads to superior subluxation and shearing forces across the glenoid. **A reverse total shoulder replacement works better for people with cuff tear arthropathy because it relies on different muscles to move the arm.** In a healthy shoulder, the rotator cuff muscles help position and power the arm during range of motion. A conventional replacement device also uses the rotator cuff muscles to function properly. In a patient with a large rotator cuff tear and cuff tear arthropathy, these muscles no longer function. The reverse total shoulder replacement relies on the deltoid muscle, instead of the rotator cuff, to power and position the arm. (Campbell)

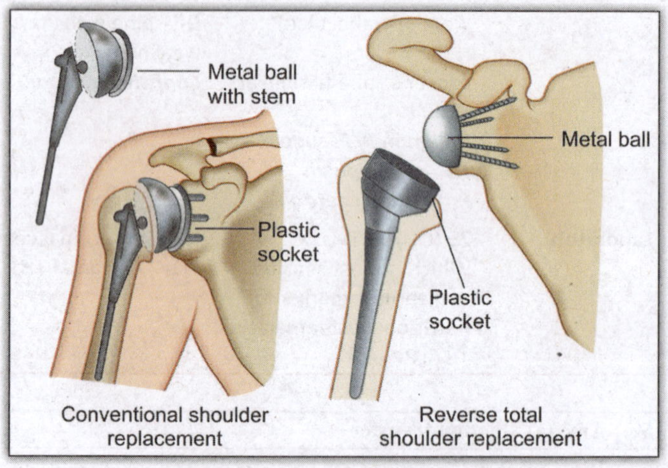

Also Know

MRI has shown 80% to 97% sensitivity in detecting full-thickness rotator cuff tears. For the assessment of partial tears, the sensitivity is 67% to 89%. Arthrography is useful for detecting rotator cuff tears and some larger Bankart lesions found with anterior instability. It is now usually combined with CT or MRI. For identifying rotator cuff partial tears, MRA has been shown to be more sensitive and specific than MRI alone, a sensitivity of 91° and a specificity of 93° have been reported.

Dermatology

16

AIIMS NOVEMBER 2018

1. A 28-year-old lady with asymptomatic pearly dome-shaped small nodules on forehead since 2 months as shown in the picture. Her 2 year old daughter also has similar lesion. What is the most probable causative agent? ***(AIIMS Nov 2018, 2015)***

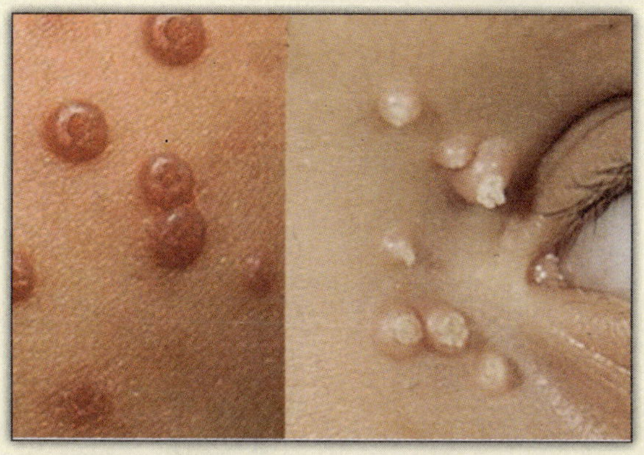

a. HHV 6
b. Coxsackie
c. Pox virus
d. Papilloma virus

2. A patient with history of bullae involving >30% BSA along with rashes all over body with erosions of the lips and other mucosa for few days. What can be the triggering factor of this condition?

a. Drug induced
b. Idiopathic
c. Bacterial infections
d. Viral infections

3. Identify the following skin condition in this histopathology slide? ***(AIIMS Nov 2018, May 2017)***

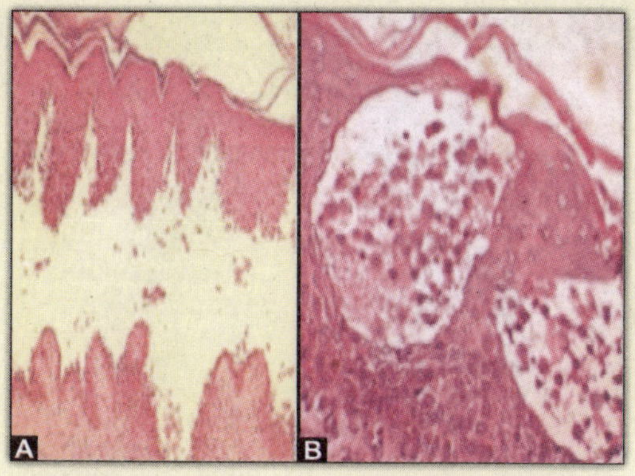

a. Lepromatous leprosy
b. Pemphigus vulgaris
c. Mycosis fungoides
d. TEN

4. What is the management for the case in the given image?

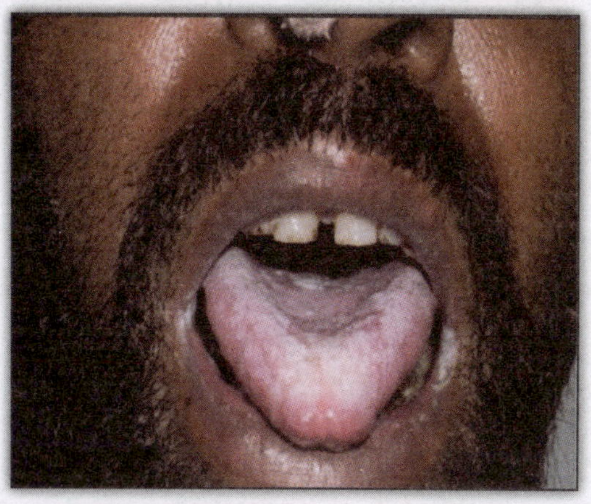

a. Dapsone plus steroids
b. Stop smoking and screen for carcinoma
c. Vitamin supplements
d. Antifungals treatment for oral candidiasis

5. Patients with rashes in groin region as shown in the figure below. Which of the following cannot be the cause?

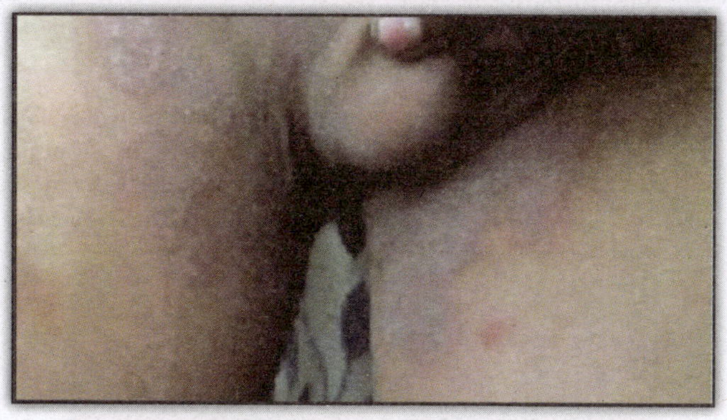

a. Aspergillus
b. Microsporum
c. Epidermophyton
d. Trichophyton

6. Patients with 1 year history of painful nodulocystic acne. What is drug of choice for the case?

a. Topical clindamycin
b. Oral isotretinoin
c. Topical adapalene
d. Oral doxycycline

7. A child patient comes to OPD with history of black central arch rashes on his body. What is your diagnosis?

a. Meningococcemia
b. Dengue hemorrhagic fever
c. Leptospirosis
d. Scrub typhus

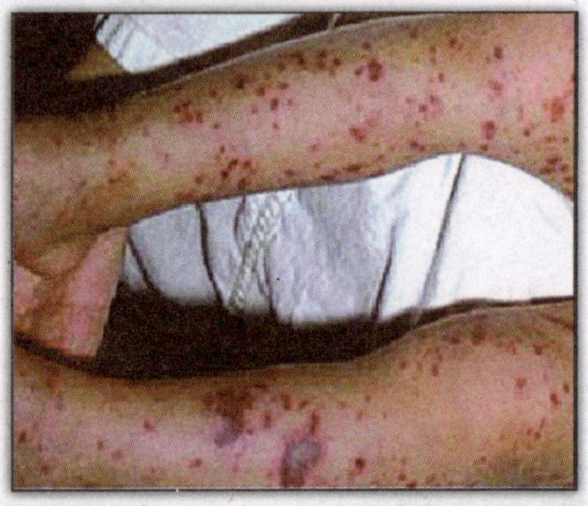

AIIMS MAY 2018

8. In Neuritic leprosy most common nerve used to take biopsy is?

a. Sural nerve
b. Ulnar Nerve
c. Superficial branch of radial nerve
d. Median nerve

9. Contact induced dermatitis is due to presence of which metal in cement?

a. Nickel
b. Chromium
c. Zinc
d. Iron

10. Which of the following antifungal drug is developing drug resistance and has not been prescribed for tinea cruris and tinea corporis since last 2 years?

a. Griseofulvin
b. Terbinafine
c. Itraconazole
d. Voriconazole

11. A male patient with history of fever joint pain develops rash and hyperpigmentation over the nose as shown in the image, after 5 days of taking NSAIDs. Most likely diagnosis is: ***(AIIMS May 2018, Nov 2017)***

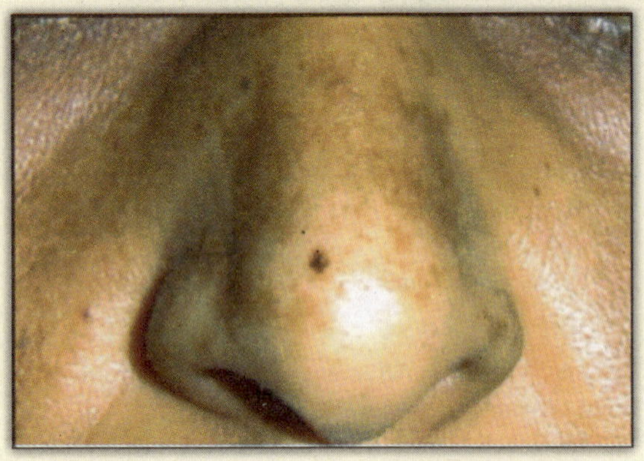

a. Melasma
b. Fixed drug eruption
c. Dengue fever
d. Chikungunya fever

AIIMS NOVEMBER 2017

12. Which of the following is least like to cause the lesion shown in the given picture?

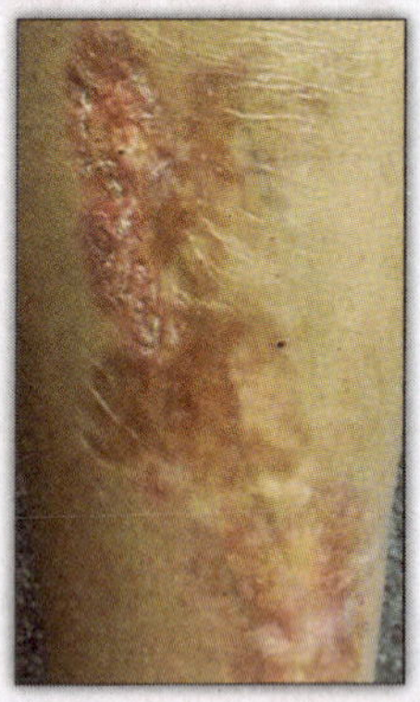

a. Diabetes mellitus
b. Necrobiosis lipoidical
c. Hypothyroidism
d. Hyperthyroidism
e. Sarcoidosis

13. Maximum numbers of desmosomes are seen in which layer of skin marked in the given picture?

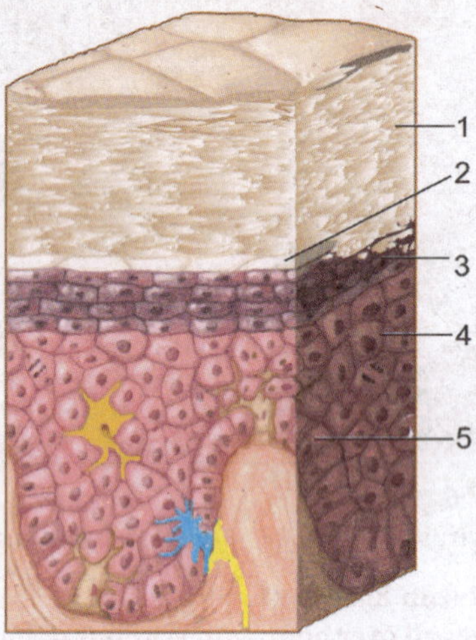

a. 1
b. 2
c. 3
d. 4

14. A male patient with history of fever joint pain develops rash and hyperpigmentation over the nose as shown in the image, after 5 days of taking NSAIDs. Most likely diagnosis is: ***(AIIMS May 2018, Nov 2017)***

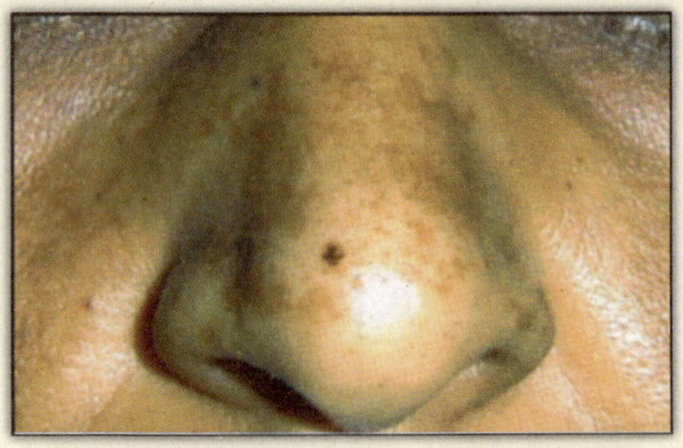

a. Melasma
b. Fixed drug eruption
c. Dengue fever
d. Chikungunya fever

15. Which of the following is likely to cause the lesions seen in the pictures below:

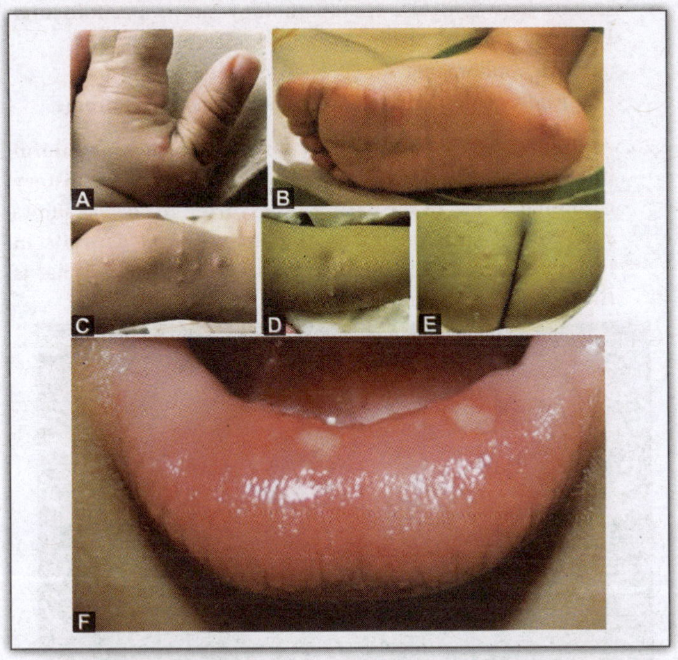

a. Pox virus
b. HHV 7 virus
c. Coxsackie virus
d. Varicella virus

AIIMS MAY 2017

16. A 12-year-old child presents with 4 hypopigmented lesions of on back and on front of left arm with loss of sensation. What should be the treatment of this child?

a. Rifampicin 600 mg once a month + dapsone 100 mg daily + clofazimine 300 mg once a month and 50 mg daily
b. Rifampicin 600 mg once a month + dapsone 100 mg daily
c. Rifampicin 450 mg once a month + dapsone 50 mg daily + clofazimine 150 once a month + 50 mg alternate days
d. Rifampicin 450 mg once a month + dapsone 50 mg daily + clofazimine 150 mg once a month + 50 mg daily

17. A 30-year-old lady comes with a 2 month history of non-scarring patchy alopecia on the left side. There was no scaling or erythema. Most likely diagnosis is:

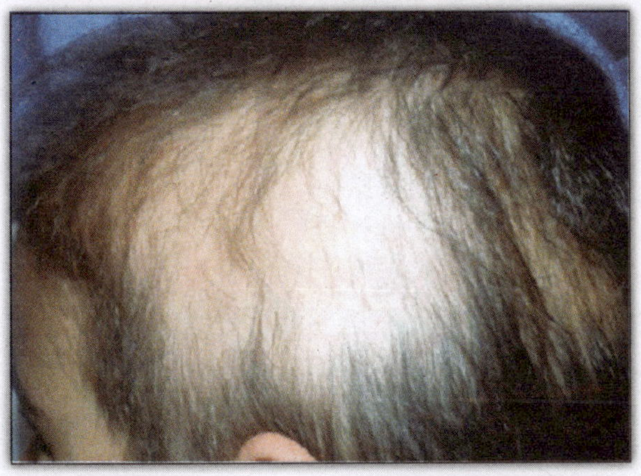

a. Alopecia areata
b. Trichotillomania
c. Telogen effluvium
d. Androgenetic alopecia

18. A child with itching and erythema over the patchy hair loss as shown in the picture. Which of the following will aid in the diagnosis?

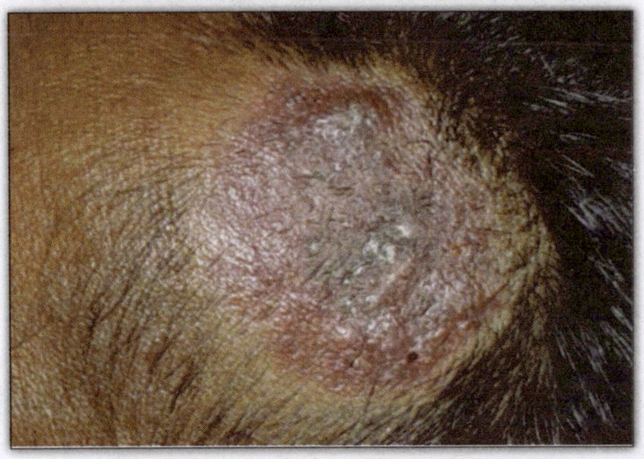

a. KOH mount
b. Slit skin smear
c. Tzanck smear
d. Gram stain

19. A child had hyperpigmented patch with hair on cheek since birth. Most likely diagnosis is:

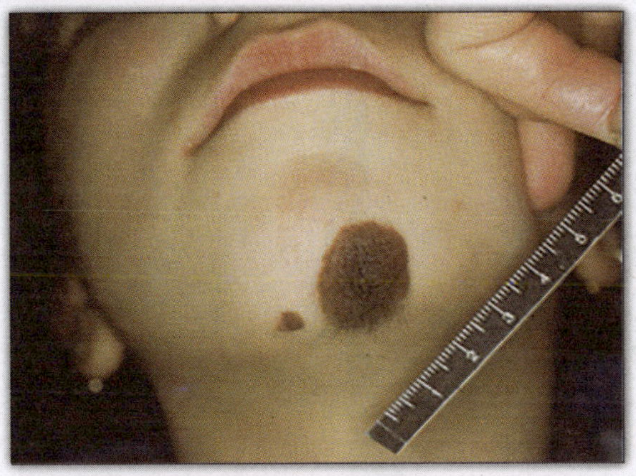

a. Congenital melanocytic nevus
b. Hematoma
c. Verrucous epidermal nevus
d. Melanoacanthoma

20. Identify the following skin condition in this histopathology slide: ***(AIIMS Nov 2018, May 2017)***

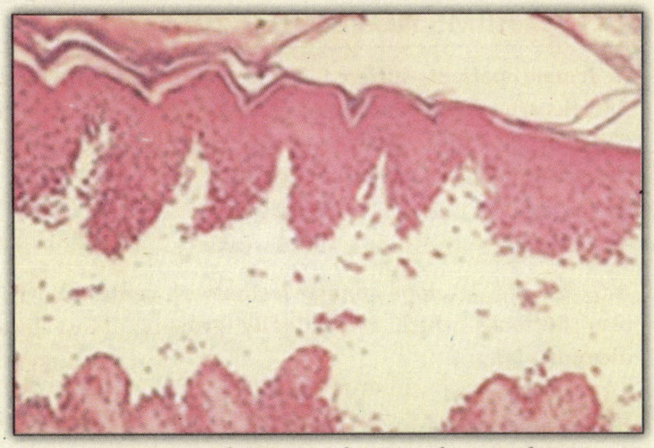

a. Lepromatous leprosy
b. Pemphigus vulgaris
c. Mycosis fungoides
d. TEN

21. A patient presents with skin and oral lesions. Immunofluorescence picture is shown below. All are true EXCEPT:

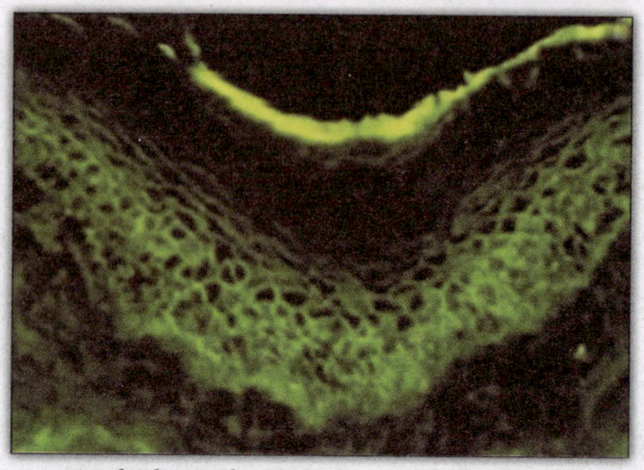

a. Antibodies to desmoglein 1
b. Antibodies to desmoglein 3
c. Antibodies to hemidesmosomes
d. IgG antibodies on immunofluorescence

22. A 12-year-old comes with red, itchy exudative lesions in cubital fossa, popliteal fossa and neck. What is most likely diagnosis?

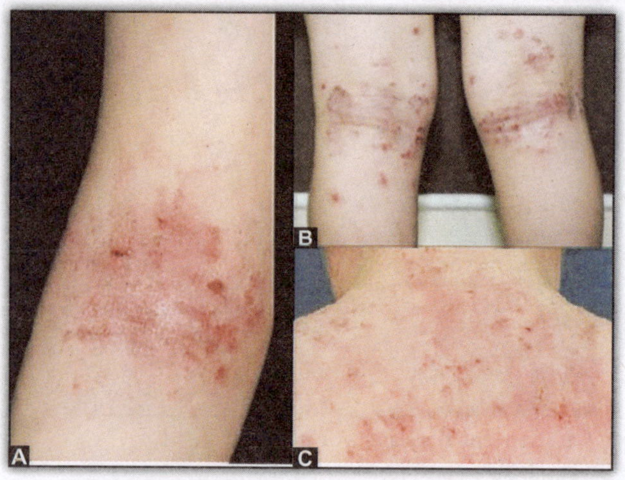

a. Dermatitis herpetiformis
b. Pemphigus
c. Psoriasis
d. Atopic dermatitis

AIIMS NOVEMBER 2016

23. A female patient suffered from exanthematous rashes 4 weeks after being started on phenytoin and valproate for epilepsy. After how many days of restarting the drug, will the exanthematous rash occur again?

a. 1 day
b. 1 week
c. 2 weeks
d. 4 weeks

24. A 5-year-old develops annular lesion with central scarring over buttocks which is gradually growing. Most likely diagnosis is?

a. Tinea corporis
b. Annular psoriasis
c. Discoid lupus erythematosus
d. Lupus vulgaris

25. A patient presents with areas of loss of hair over occipital and temporal areas with nonscarring, empty follicle and blood in few hair follicles. Histopathology shows perifollicular lymphocytic infiltration. Most likely diagnosis is?

a. Trichotillomania
b. Alopecia areata
c. Androgenic alopecia
d. Loose Anagen syndrome

26. A middle aged female patient comes with recurrent painful blisters over oral mucosa and genital area. She gives history of similar lesion in the past. A biopsy from the lesion shows subprabasal split on histopathology and IgG deposits in immunofluorescence microscopy as shown below. What is the most likely diagnosis?

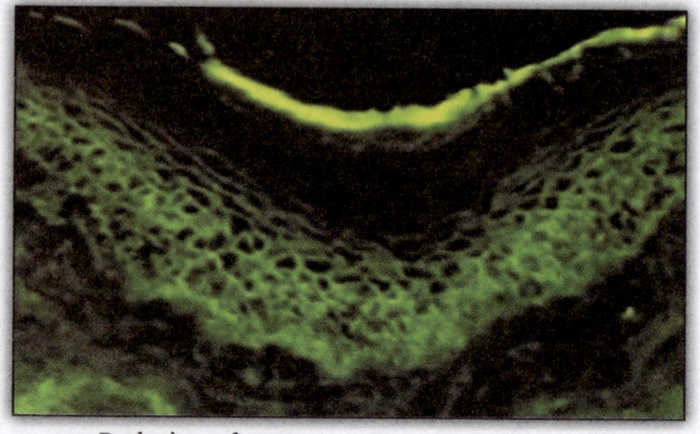

a. Beçhet's syndrome
b. Pemphigus vulgaris
c. Lupus vulgaris
d. Dermatitis herpetiformis

27. Nail hyperpigmentation is seen in all EXCEPT:

a. Cyclophosphamide
b. Chlorpromazine
c. Amiodarone
d. Chloroquine

28. A 24-year-old male presented with following lesion on his genitalia, following intercourse with multiple sexual partners, and multiple times. Which human papilloma virus is the causative agent?

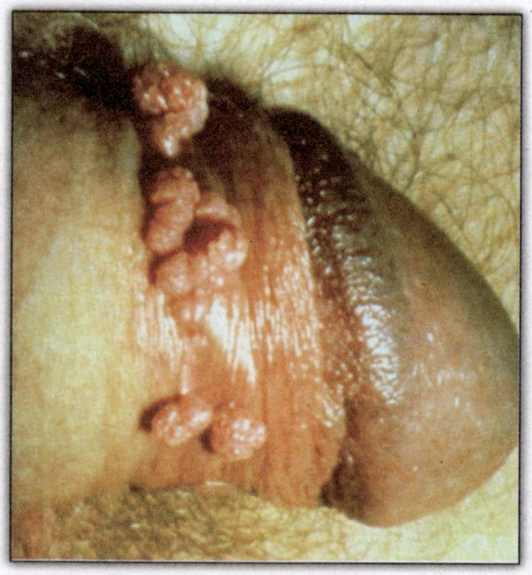

a. HPV 6, 11
b. HPV 16, 18
c. HPV 31, 33
d. HPV 35, 45

AIIMS MAY 2016

29. A 10-year-old child presented to dermatology OPD with multiple small papules on face for last 3 months. Skin biopsy was done and sent for histopathology as shown below. What is your diagnosis?

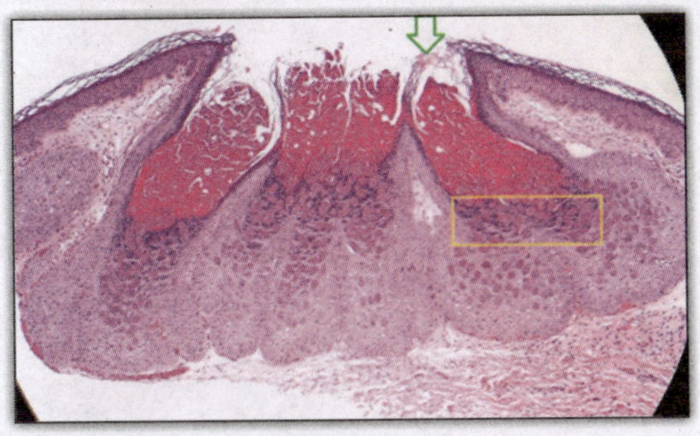

a. Squamous cell carcinoma
b. Molluscum contagiosum
c. Herpes simplex infection
d. Squamous papilloma with central ulceration

30. A 35-year-old factory worker developed itchy, annular scaly plaques in both groins. The lesion healed temporarily to topical steroids but continue to extend at the periphery. The most likely diagnosis is:

a. Annular lichen planus
b. Granuloma annulare
c. Tinea cruris
d. Erythema annulare centrifugum

31. A 40-year-old farmer has itchy erythematous popular lesions on face, neck and V area of chest. The lesions were aggravated during summer and reduced during winter. The most appropriate investigation to arrive at a diagnosis is:

a. IgE levels in blood
b. Skin biopsy
c. Patch test
d. Serology

32. A 22-year-old women developed small itchy wheals and rash after physical exertion, on sun exposure, on eating spicy food and on anger. Most likely diagnosis is? ***(AIIMS May 2016, Nov 2012)***

a. Chronic idiopathic urtricaria
b. Photodermatitis
c. Solar urtricaria
d. Cholinergic urtricaria

33. A 45-year-old patient had multiple hypo-aesthtic and mildly erythematous patches on his trunk and extremities. His both ulnar and lateral popliteal nerves were thickened. The most probable diagnosis is:

a. Borderline lepromatous leprosy
b. Borderline tuberculoid leprosy
c. Borderline leprosy
d. Lepromatus leprosy

34. A 35-year-old male presents with bald patches and with no scars. The patches are well demarcated with broken hair at the edges. What is most probable diagnosis?

a. Alopecia areata
b. Androgenic alopecia
c. DLE
d. Telogen effluvium

AIIMS NOVEMBER 2015

35. A 35-year-lady presents with bilateral buccal reticulate white streaks as shown, pain and burning sensation on eating spicy food. There is no history of tobacco chewing but shows amalgamated 3rd molar tooth is present. What is most likely cause?

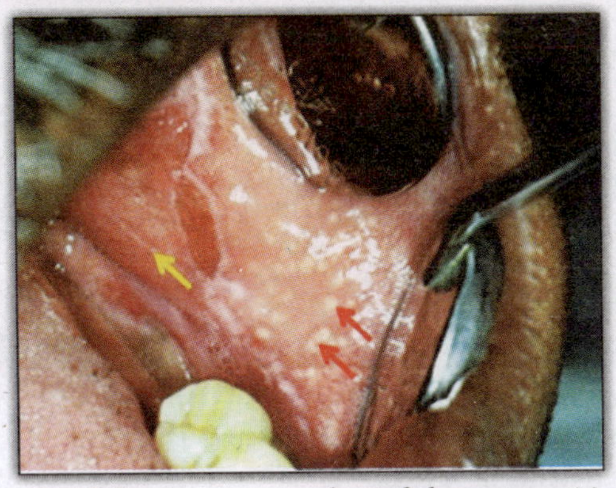

a. Candida
b. Aphthous stomatitis
c. Lichen planus
d. Leukoplakia

36. Oral candidiasis presents with white patch in all EXCEPT:

a. Acute pseudomembranous candidiasis
b. Chronic atrophic candidiasis
c. Chronic hyperplastic candidiasis
d. Chronic mucocutaneous candidiasis

37. A 20-year-old patient with neurocysticercosis develops fever followed by generalized peeling of skin and mucous membrane sparing palms and soles followed by hyperpigmentation, starting one month after taking medications for seizures. What is the most probable diagnosis?

a. SJS
b. TEN
c. Fixed drug eruption
d. Pemphigus vulgaris

38. A 28-year-old lady with asymptomatic pearly doam shaped small nodules on forehead since 2 months as shown in the picture. Her 2 year old daughter also has similar lesion. What is the most probable causative agent? ***(AIIMS Nov 2018, 2015)***

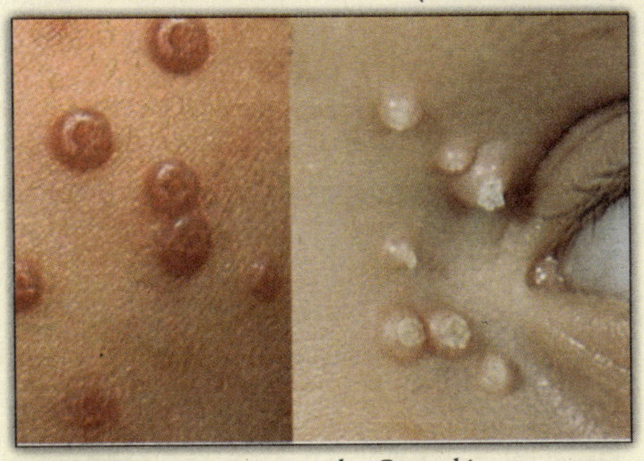

a. HHV 6
b. Coxsackie
c. Pox virus
d. Papilloma virus

39. What is treatment of choice of nodulocystic acne in a young boy with oily skin?

a. Oral isotretinoin
b. Topical retinoic acid
c. Topical steroid
d. Systemic antibiotic

40. **An athletic Male with itchy lesion at groin as shown below, causative agent can be all EXCEPT:**

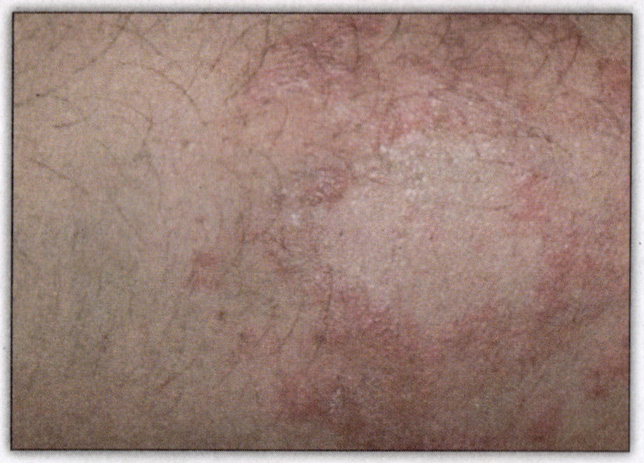

a. Trichophyton
b. Microsporum
c. Epidermophyton
d. Aspergillus

41. **A young male presented with a hypo anesthetic patch on right forearm. On examination there is ulnar nerve thickening. Skin biopsy of hypo pigmented patch is given below. What is the most probable diagnosis?**

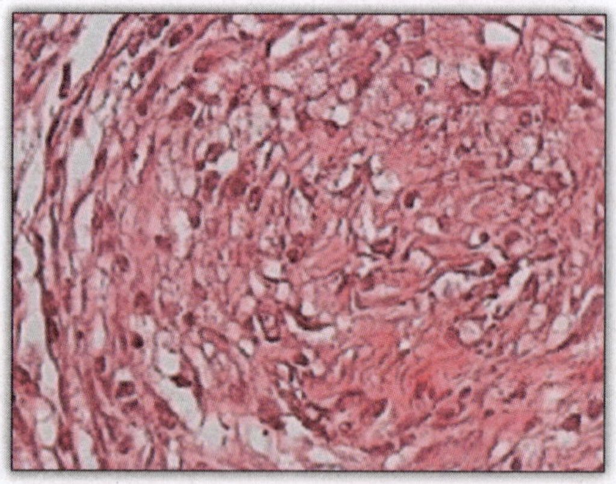

a. TT leprosy   b. LL leprosy
c. Lymphoma   d. Histiocytosis

42. **A 18-year-female with hypopigmented patchs in both ankles as shown below. What is not used for treatment?**

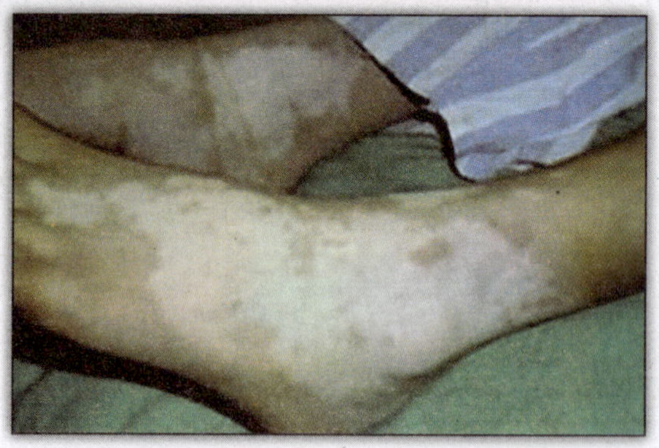

a. Topical clobetasol   b. Topical tretinoin
c. Topical tacrolimus   d. Topical methoxsalen

AIIMS MAY 2015

43. **A young boy came with similar lesions shown below over elbows and shaft of penis. Diagnosis?**
(AIIMS May 2015, 2014)

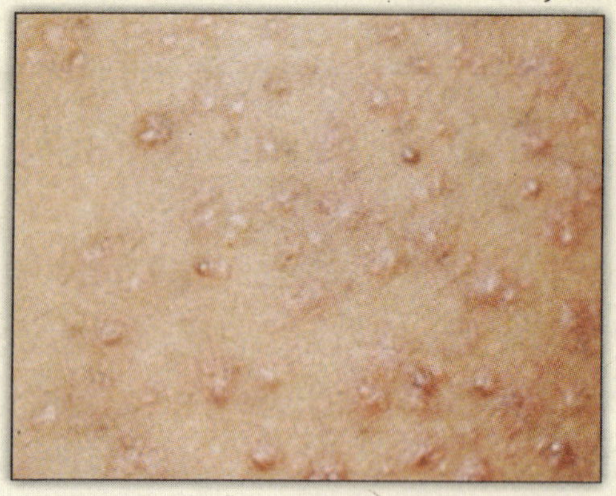

a. Lichen nitidus   b. Lichen planus
c. Scabies   d. Lichen scrofulosorum

44. **The patient came with history of bullae involving >30% body surface area as shown in the picture and erosions of the lips for the past 7 days. What is most probable regarding the etiology?**

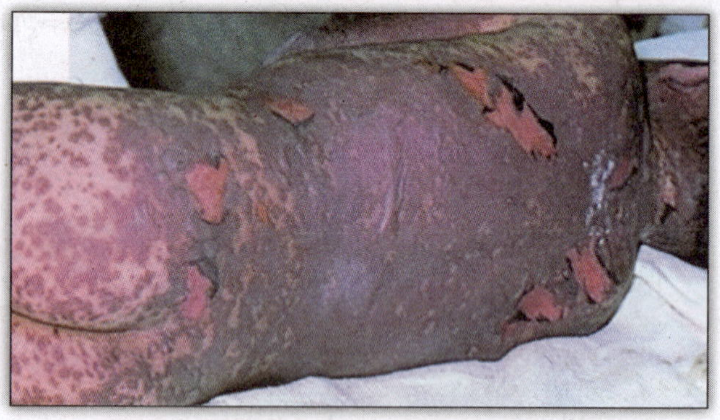

a. Drugs   b. Bacterial infection
c. Viral infection   d. Malignancy

45. **A 7 months pregnant lady with diabetes comes with lesions all over the body, mainly tunk as in the picture below. Which of these drugs is the appropriate treatment?**

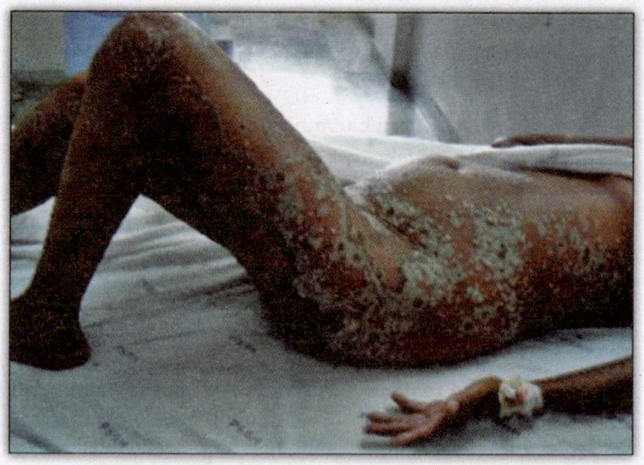

a. Cyclosporine   b. Azathioprine
c. Methotrexate   d. Retinoids

46. A 65-year-old male presented with Itchy tense blisters are seen on normal looking skin as well as urticarial plaques, as seen in the figure. What is the diagnosis?

(AIIMS May 2015, Nov 2014)

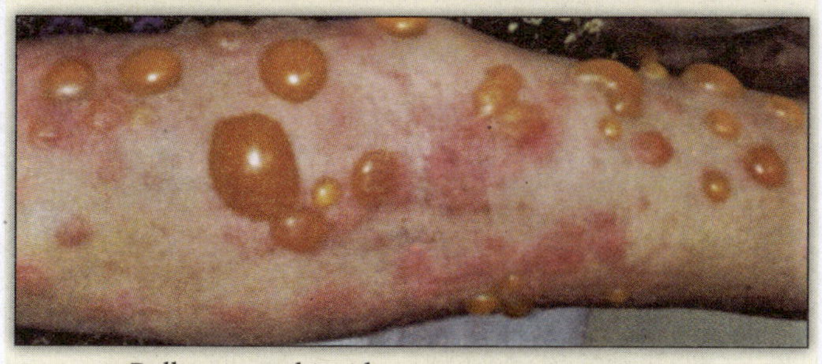

a. Bullous pemphigoid
b. IgA pemphigus
c. Dermatitis herpetiformis
d. Pemphigus vulgaris

47. A 50-year-old man from Bihar comes with juicy looking papules over face and back of neck as shown in picture below which were hypopigmented and with no hypoesthesia or nerve thickening. History of prolonged fever in childhood was present. Diagnosis?

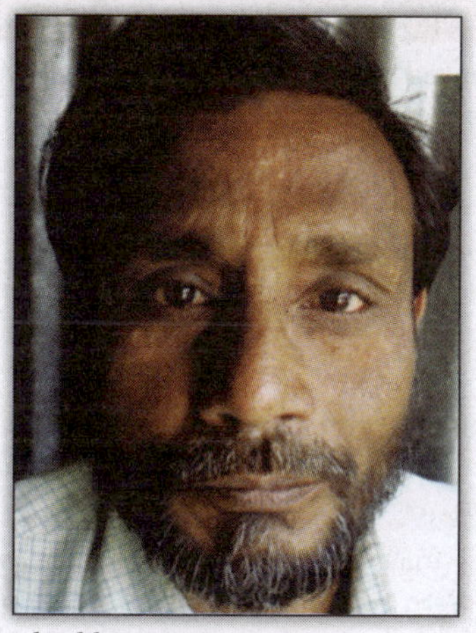

a. Tuberculoid leprosy
b. Post-kala-azar dermal leishmaniasis
c. Lepromatous leprosy
d. Mycosis fungoides

48. A 25-year-old girl presented with erythromatous papule on the face as shown in the picture below with flushing on sun exposure and increasing with emotional disturbance. Most likely diagnosis is: ***(AIIMS May 2015, Nov 2014)***

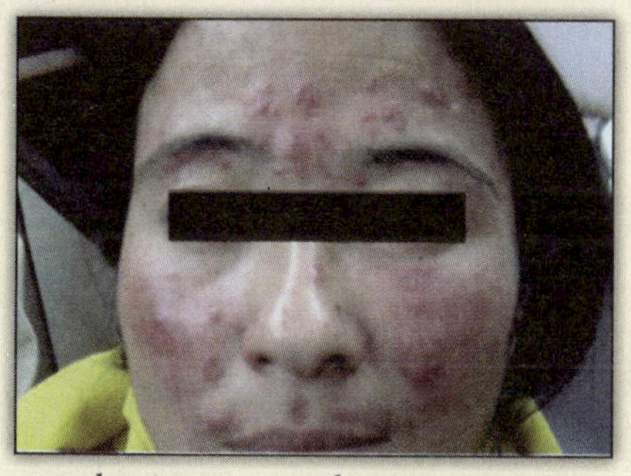

a. Acne vulgaris
b. Acne rosacea
c. SLE
d. DLE

49. A man with leprosy came with multiple lesion of the skin as shown below. What is the correct classification of this lesion?

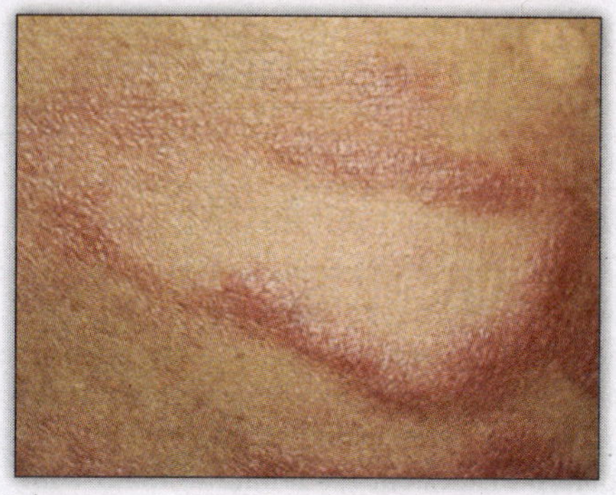

a. LL leprosy
b. BL leprosy
c. BT leprosy
d. BB leprosy

50. A patient presented with vesicle on shin. Microscopy on Tzanck smear showed giant cells causative agents is?

a. Vaccinia virus
b. Varicella zoster virus
c. Mycobacterium
d. Molluscum contagiasum

51. A young boy came with unilateral white skin lesion with leucotrichia, as shown in the picture below. What is the diagnosis?

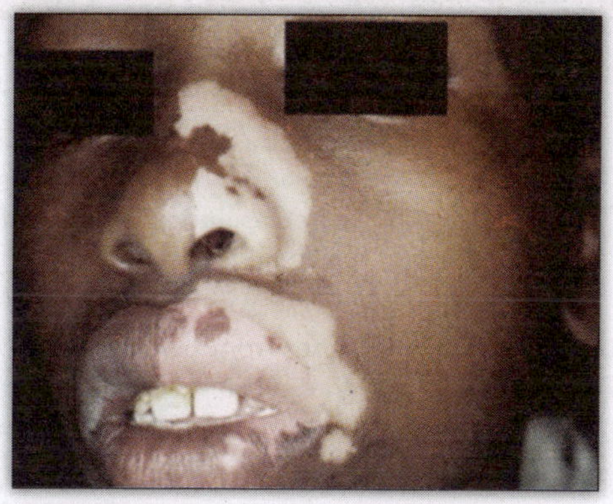

a. Segmental vitiligo
b. Piebaldism
c. Focal vitiligo
d. Waardenburg syndrome

52. A lady came with complaints of a bluish lesion over left side of forehead and left eye. An irregular bluish lesion is seen over the left superior conjunctiva as shown below. What is the diagnosis?

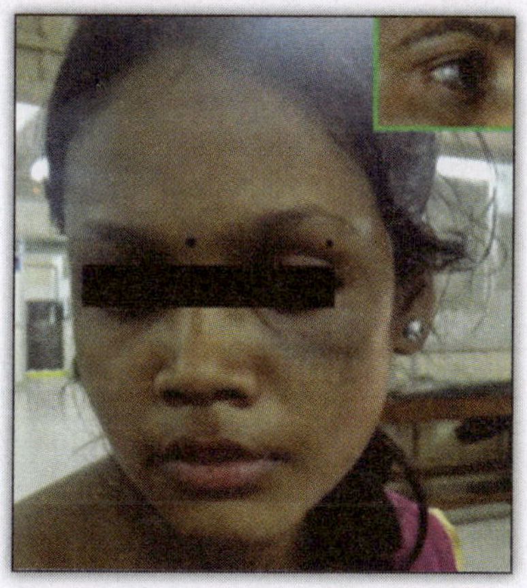

a. Nevus of Ota
b. Nevus of Ito
c. Becker's nevus
d. Mongolian spot

AIIMS NOVEMBER 2018

1. Ans. (c) Pox Virus

Ref: Bolognia 11th Ed page 1501

This condition is molluscum contagiosum. The clues in the question are typical presence of pearly white papules. If you notice the image properly, some of them show a central umbilication, which is also a typical feature of molluscum contagiosum and by history of presence in immediate family members, indicate contagious nature. Molluscum contagiosum is caused by Pox group of viruses.

Option (A) Herpes Virus:

Herpes virus infections of the skin are generally characterized by vesicular eruptions.

Option (B) Coxsackie:

Coxsackie virus also presents with papulovesicular eruptions on knees, buttocks and around the mouth.

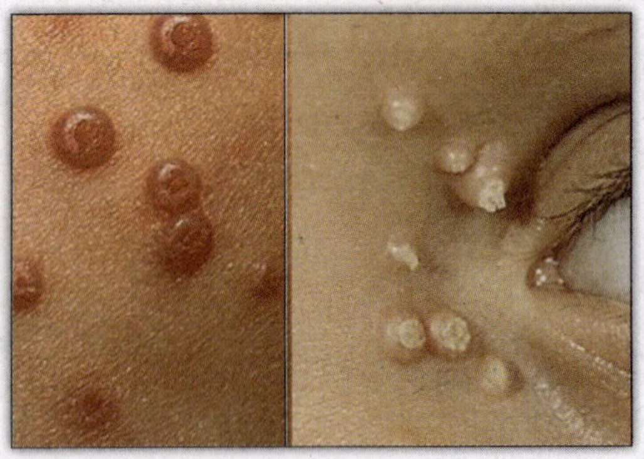

Fig: Lesions of molluscum contagiosum: Dome shaped, grouped pink/skin colored or pearly, with central umblication/pore of papules which are asymptomatic. Enlarging slowly it may reach a diameter of 5–10 mm in 6–12 weeks. (and by history of presence in immediate family members, indicate contagious nature)

Molluscum Contagiosum	
Etiology	Molluscum contagiosum (MC) is a viral infection of skin caused by molluscum contagiosum virus (MCV), a DNA virus belonging to the Poxviridae family and the genera of Molluscipoxvirus.
Mode of transmission	Either by direct skin-to-skin contact or indirectly by fomites. Rare under the age of 1 year, perhaps due to maternally transmitted immunity and a long incubation period. In hot countries, where children are lightly dressed and in close contact with one another and where the personal hygiene may be poor, spread within a household is not uncommon. Genital lesions in adults are probably transmitted through sexual contact.
Incubation period and progress	Varies from 2 weeks to 6 months. A lesion starts as a tiny papule and progresses to a size of 5–10 mm in 6–12 weeks. Small lesions may join to form a plaque ('agminate form').The number also varies from very few to innumerable. The presence of numerous lesions in an adult suggests immunosuppression.
Clinical features	Discrete, dome-shaped, umbilicated, waxy papules. They may be skin colored, pink or white. A central punctum is visible in all well-formed lesions. The distribution is influenced by the mode of infection, the type of clothing and the climate. In children, lesions are usually distributed on the axillae, sides of trunk, lower abdomen, thighs and face. In young adults and adolescents, genital lesions are usually due to sexual transmission.
Treatment	
In most cases, the lesions resolve spontaneously over a period of 6–9 months; rarely do they persist for several years. Resolution is heralded by inflammation, suppuration and crusting.	
Physical treatment	Cryotherapy using liquid nitrogen. Curettage or diathermy can be done for large lesions. Pulsed dye laser can also be considered for recalcitrant lesions.
Chemical treatment	Phenol Cantharidine 40% silver nitrate paste Topical wart paints, containing 15%–20% salicylic acid in collodion or acrylate base Potassium hydroxide 10% solution Topical therapy with 0.5% podophyllotoxin Imiquimod cream Nitric oxide Cidofovir
Systemic treatment	Oral cimetidine Cidofovir

2. Ans. (a) Drug induced

Ref: Bolognia 3rd Ed page 319

This is a typical description of Toxic epidermal necrolysis

From the clinical picture now it's quite evident that the diagnosis is TEN, because

- Acute history of few days
- Involvement of mucosal membranes and generalized rash
- Involvement of more than 30% BSA
- Bullae formation

The most common cause of TEN are drug reactions, hence the answer is (A)

Severe acute bullous disorders which can lead to widespread involvement of body are either due to infections or due to drug reactions. The diseases causing this kind of a picture are following:

- Erythema multiforme (EM)
- Steven Johnson syndrome (SJS)
- Toxic epidermal necrolysis (TEN)
- To answer this question we need to have a crisp understanding of these entities because It has now become clear that Stevens-Johnson syndrome (SJS) and toxic epidermal necrolysis (TEN) are variants within a continuous spectrum of adverse drug reactions, whereas erythema multiforme (EM) is a distinct disorder with different clinical signs and precipitating factors, e.g. herpes simplex virus (HSV) infections.

Medications Most Frequently Associated with Stevens–Johnson Syndrome and Toxic Epidermal Necrolysis

Allopurinol
Aminopenicillins Amithiozone (thioacetazone), Antiretroviral drugs, especially NNRTIs Barbiturates
Carbamazepine
Chlormezanone, Phenytoin anticonvulsants Lamotrigine
Phenylbutazone
Piroxicam
Sulfadiazine
Sulfadoxine
Sulfasalazine Trimethoprim–sulfamethoxazole

EM- SJS- Ten Complex

Clinical criteria allow the distinction of both forms of EM from SJS/TEN in the vast majority of patients. These clinical criteria are as follows: (1) the type of elementary skin lesion; (2) the distribution of skin lesions (topography); (3) the presence or absence of overt mucosal lesions; and (4) the presence or absence of systemic symptoms

	EM minor	EM major	Stevens-Johnson syndrome (SJS)	SJS/TEN overlap syndrome	Toxic epidermal necrolysis (TEN), or Lyell's syndrome
Common cause	Infection	Infection	Medication	Medication	Medication
Type of skin lesions	Typical targets • ± Papular atypical targets	Typical targets • ± Papular atypical targets • Occasionally bullous lesions	Dusky red lesions, Flat atypical targets (Targetoid lesion with 2 zones)	Dusky red lesions, Flat atypical targets (Targetoid lesion with 2 zones)	Poorly delineated erythematous plaques, Epidermal detachment, Dusky red lesions, Flat atypical targets (Targetoid lesion with 2 zones)
Distribution	Extremities (especially elbows, knees, wrists, hands), face	Extremities, face	Trunk and face; Isolated lesion **Confluence (+)** on face and trunk	Trunk and face; Isolated lesions. **Confluence (++)** on face and trunk	Tunk and face; Isolated lesions are rare. **Confluence (+++)** on face, trunk, and elsewhere
%BSA involved in detachment	<10%	<10%	**<10%.** The skin lesions progress to epidermal necrosis and sloughing.	***10-30%***	**>30%.** The skin lesions progress to **full-thickness epidermal necrosis.**
Mucosal involvement	Absent or mild	Severe	**Mucosal membranes are affected in 92 to 100 percent of patients, usually at two or more distinct sites (ocular, oral, and genital)**	Mucosal involvement seen	Severe: **Mucous membranes are involved in nearly all cases**
Systemic symptoms	Absent	Present	Present	Present	Present

Contd...

Prodrome	Nil	Mild if any	It is characterized by a **prodrome of malaise and fever**, followed by the rapid onset of erythematous or purpuric macules and plaques.	Prodrome of upper respiratory tract symptoms, fever and painful skin	TEN also begins with a prodrome of fever and malaise, although temperatures are typically higher than those seen with SJS, often **exceeding 39 degrees Celsius.**
Progression to TEN	No	No	Yes	Yes	--
Precipitating factors	Herpes simplex virus Other infectious agent	Herpes simplex virus, Mycoplasma pneumoniae, Other infectious agents Rarely drugs	Drugs, Occasionally Mycoplasma pneumoniae, Rarely immunizations	Drugs, Occasionally Mycoplasma pneumoniae, Rarely immunizations	Drugs, Occasionally Mycoplasma pneumoniae, Rarely immunizations
Mortality	Rare	Rare	1- 5%	Between SJS & TEN	25- 35 %

Footnote:

- Currently, TEN and SJS are considered to be two ends of a spectrum of severe epidermolytic adverse cutaneous drug reactions, differing only by their extent of skin detachment
- Drugs are assumed or identified as the main cause of SJS/TEN in most cases, but **Mycoplasma pneumoniae and Herpes simplex virus** infections are well documented causes alongside rare cases in which the etiology remains unknown.
- TEN and SJS usually occur **7–21 days** after initiation of the responsible drug
- The medications most frequently incriminated are allopurinol, nonsteroidal anti-inflammatory drugs, antibiotics and anticonvulsants
- Historically, these three presentations were considered to form a spectrum from mild to fulminatingly severe cases. *More **recently, there has been a re-evaluation of this concept and a tendency to consider erythema multiforme minor and major as part of one spectrum**, often related to infections (especially herpes virus) and perhaps on occasion to drug reactions.*
- On this basis SJS and TEN are separable from erythema multiforme and are more closely linked to drug sensitivities, and may be regarded as severe variants of a single disease.
- Exfoliation is due to extensive death of **keratinocytes via apoptosis;** the latter is mediated via the cytotoxic secretory protein granulysin and interaction of the death receptor–ligand pair Fas–FasL
- Optimal medical management of SJS and TEN requires early diagnosis, immediate discontinuation of the causative drug(s), and rapid initiation of supportive care and specific therapy
- Specific therapies that have the potential to selectively block keratinocyte apoptosis, such as high- dose **IVIg,** may provide added benefit over supportive care alone.

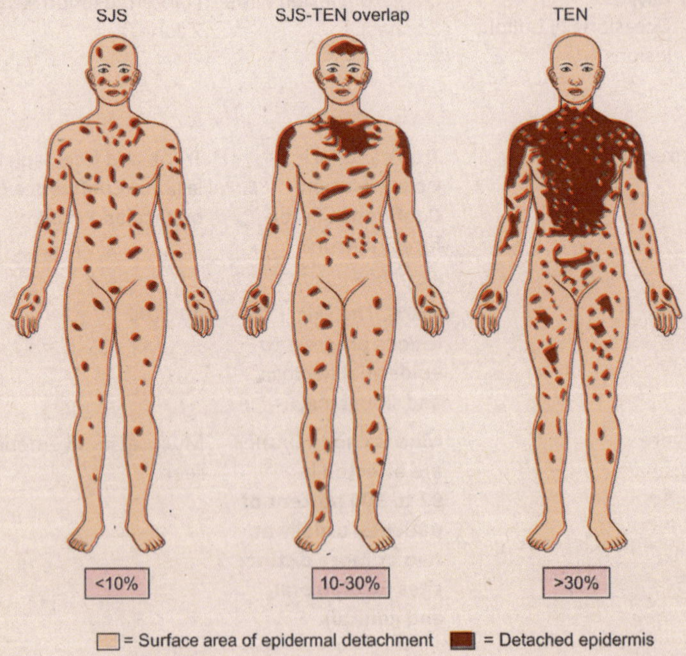

SJS – Stevens-Johnson syndrome TEN – Toxic epidermal necrolysis

3. Ans. (b) Pemphigus vulgaris

Ref: Lever's Histopathology of the Skin 3rd ed Page 190, Rook's 8th Ed page 40.2

The color plate in the question is showing an intraepidermal blister and row of tombstone appearance which is typical of Pemphigus Vulgaris

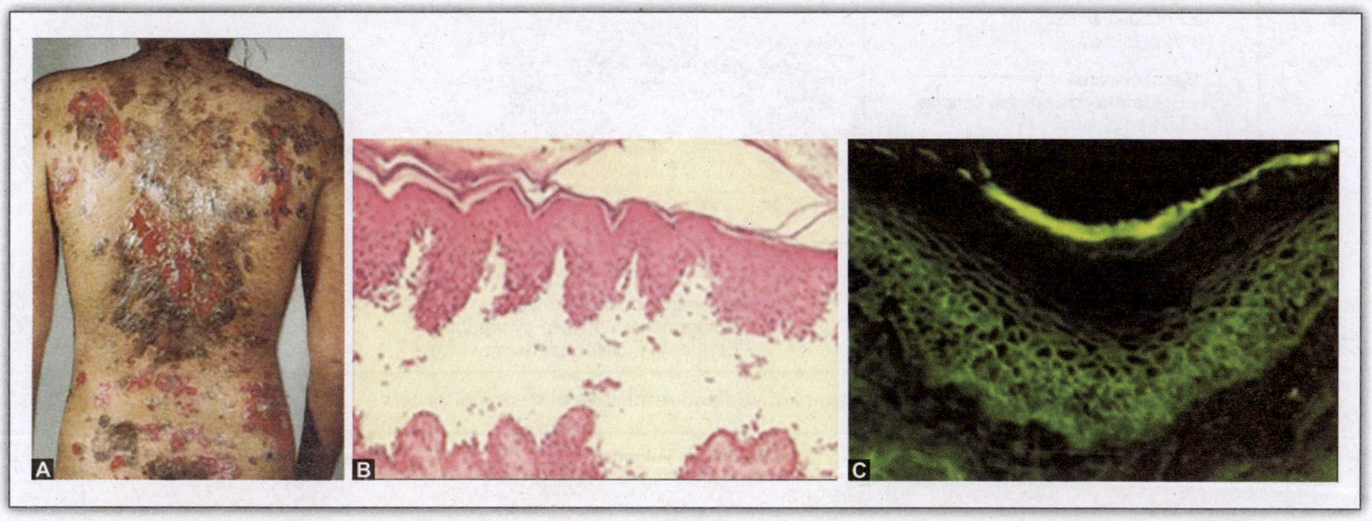

Figure Legends

a. **Pemphigus vulgaris (PV):** Patients suffering from mucocutaneous pemphigus vulgaris (PV) usually have flaccid blisters and erosions on the trunk with crusts and hyperpigmentation accompanied by mucosal ulcerations in the mouth

b. **Pemphigus vulgaris histopathology:** Suprabasal acantholysis (cleft); **C1;** In PV, the epidermal cleavage plane is located in the deep epidermis, usually right above the basal layer (Suprabasal cleft). A single layer of basal keratinocytes remains attached to the basement membrane as a **"Row of tombstones"** appearance. In PF, epidermal splitting occurs between granular layers (subcorneal blisters within the epidermis)

c. **Pemphigus vulgaris immunohistochemistry:** Direct immunofluorescence showing granular deposits of immunoglobulin lgG3 and C3 in intracellular space **(fish net pattern)**

Classification of Bullae	
Intraepidermal	
Subcornea	Subcorneal pustular dermatosis
Granular cell layer	Pemphigus foliaceus and erythematosus Bullous ichthyosiform erythroderma Subcorneal pustular dermatosis Staphylococcal scalded skin syndrome Bullous impetigo
Spinous layer	Familial benign pemphigus
Suprabasal	Pemphigus vulgaris Acantholytic disorders like Hailey-Hailey disease, Darier's disease and Grover's disease (transient acantholytic dermatosis)
Basal layer	Epidermolysis bullosa simplex Toxic epidermal necrolysis Erythema multiforme Lupus erythematosus Lichen planus
Sub Epidermal Bullae (Dermoepidermal Junction)	
Lamina lucida	Bullous and cicatricial pemphigoid, pemphigoid (herpes) gestationalis, dermatitis herpetiformis, thermal burns
Lamina densa	Bullous SLE, epidermolysis bullosa dystrophica, epidermolysis bullosa aquisita, porphyria cutanea tarda

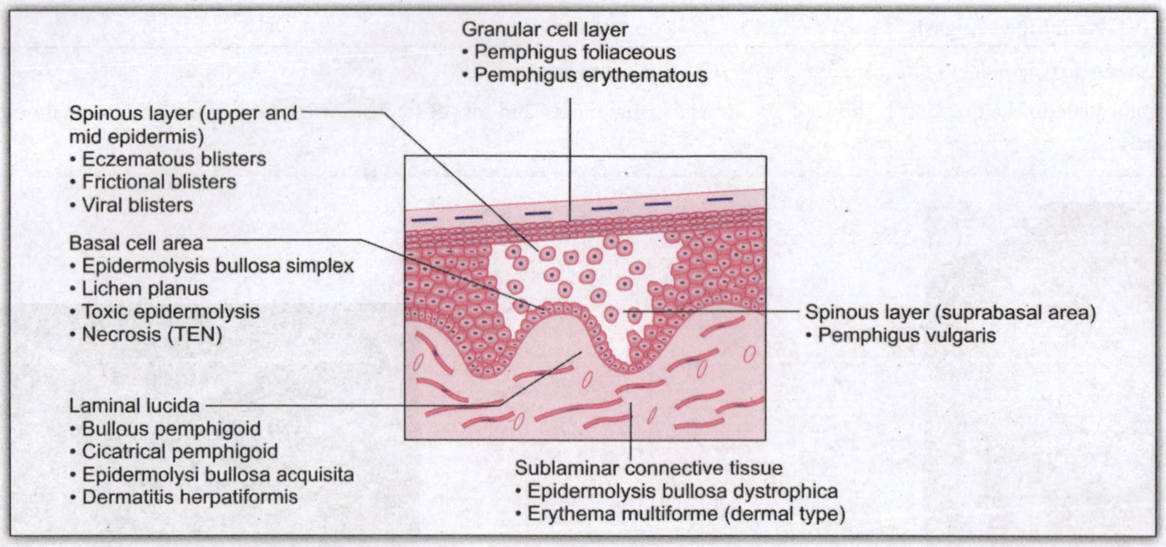

Fig: Different layers of skin and respective blistering disorders

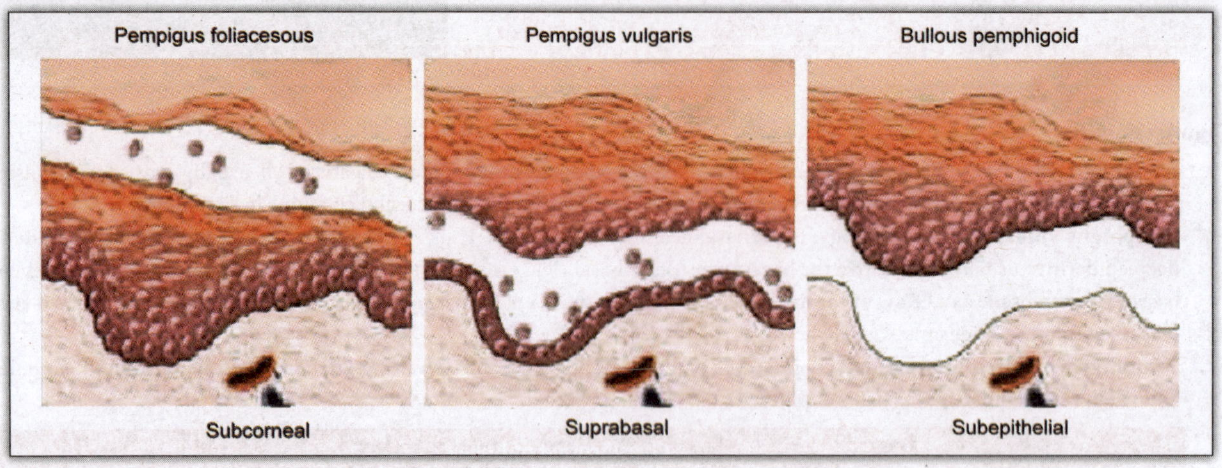

Fig: Different types of pemphigus and skin layers involved

4. Ans. (d) Antifungal for oral candidiasis

Ref: Roxburgh's 17th ed 43, 98, 241, 277

This is a case of oral candidiasis. However, lets rule out the options.

a. Dapsone and steroids: These would be typically given in a case of Behçet's disease which is manifested by recurrent oral aphthous ulcers, genital ulcers and other systemic manifestations. The picture doesn't show oral ulcers, but a whitish patch on the tongue.

b. Stop smoking and screen for carcinoma: This would typically be seen in the setting of leukoplakia or erythroplakia. Clinically, leukoplakia may appear as a uniformly white plaque (homogeneous leukoplakia) or as white flecks or fine nodules on an atrophic erythematous base (speckled or verrucous leukoplakia), the latter with a greater malignant potential. Other pointers to malignant change are presence of a nodule, erosion or ulceration within the lesion, induration or hardness at the periphery, and location on the anterior floor of the mouth and undersurface of the tongue. Although the picture may resemble leukoplakia, in absence of specific biopsy findings, leukoplakia would only be a diagnosis of exclusion, if this clinical picture doesn't fit in with any other options

c. Vitamin supplements: Vitamin supplements are generally given for glossitis due to riboflavin deficiency which presents with loss of papillae or bald tongue, but not whitish patch on tongue

d. Antifungal treatment for oral candidiasis: This is a picture of oral candidiasis, hence antifungals will be treatment of choice. We will discuss oral candidiasis in more details in the text

Whitish Lesions of Tongue

Local	Systemic
Materia alba	Candidiasis
Candidiasis	Lichen planus
Frictional keratosis	Lupus erythematosus
Smoker's keratosis	Papillomas (some)
Idiopathic keratosis	Hairy leukoplakia (mainly human immunodeficiency virus disease)
Carcinoma	Syphilitic keratosis
Burns (including snuff and cocaine)	Chronic renal failure
Skin grafts	Inherited lesions (e.g. white-sponge nevus)
Leukoplakia	

Of this list commonly asked topics in exams would be oral candidiasis, leukoplakia, oral lichen planus. Hence, we will discuss them in more details.

Oral Candidiasis

Up to 50% of the healthy population harbor *Candida albicans* as an oral commensal. Carriage is more common in cigarette smokers. *Candida* resides particularly on the posterior dorsum of the tongue.

Healthy neonates, who have yet to develop immunity to *Candida* species, may develop thrush. In other patients, predisposing factors include antibiotic or corticosteroid use, xerostomia and severe T-cell immune defects associated with immunosuppression (e.g. given to prevent graft rejection in organ transplantation) or immunodeficiencies such as leukemia or HIV disease.

The following forms of oral candidiasis have been described:

1. **Acute pseudomembranous candidiasis (Oral thrush):** It is the most common type and is produced by the colonization of *Candida* species. It is characterized by curdy white patches covered by a pseudomembrane over the gums, teeth, cheeks and palate. On removal, the membrane reveals an erythematous base. The disease can extend to the esophagus or pharynx and may cause ulceration. There is a significant association between maternal vaginal candidiasis and neonatal oral thrush. It is also a common feature in patients with AIDS. About 5%–10% of hospitalized, debilitated and elderly patients may be affected by oral thrush Immunosuppression, diabetes mellitus and malignancies are other predisposing factors. Coincident oral herpes simplex may also occur.
2. **Chronic pseudomembranous candidiasis:** The lesions are similar to the acute type but are more persistent. Such a manifestation is seen in immunocompromised patients.
3. **Acute atrophic candidiasis**: It is characterized by the marked pain and by the presence of a denuded atrophic inflamed membrane commonly over the dorsum of the tongue. It is especially associated with antibiotic therapy or corticosteroids.
4. **Chronic hyperplastic candidiasis (Candidal leukoplakia):** It presents as a very persistent, firm, irregular white plaque present commonly over the cheeks or tongue surrounded by an erythematous margin. Other areas like the lips and floor of the mouth may be involved. The plaque, unlike oral thrush, cannot be removed easily. Smokers are more prone to develop this type of oral candidiasis. A malignant change may develop. It may clear with prolonged anticandidal therapy.
5. **Median rhomboid glossitis:** It is an acquired condition where the dorsum of the tongue shows a diamond shaped area with loss of papillae. It may be a true invasion by *Candida albicans* or a developmental abnormality invaded secondarily by *Candida albicans*.
6. **Chronic atrophic candidiasis (Denture stomatitis, denture sore mouth):** The condition is often confined to the upper denture bearing areas, i.e. the palate and gums. It is characterized by dusky-red, sharply defined patches at the denture margin. The epithelium is often shiny and atrophic. Sometimes marked edema can be present. Secondary papillomatosis and angular cheilitis may be associated.
7. **Angular cheilitis (Perlèche):** It is characterized by erythema, maceration, fissuring and soreness at the angles of the mouth. The predisposing factors include poor nutritional status, habitual lip licking, depth of folds (e.g. elderly people with sagging of commissures), poorly fitting dentures and malocclusion.

Topical antifungals are the first line of treatment for uncomplicated oral candidiasis.

They include:

1. Nystatin suspension (4–6 lakh U q.i.d.) held in the mouth for 5 minutes and then swallowed,
2. Nystatin oral tablets 1 lakh U q.i.d. dissolved slowly in the mouth,
3. Clotrimazole troches 10 mg 1 tab dissolved in mouth 5 times per day,
4. Gentian violet 1%–2%,
5. Chlorhexidine rinses,
6. Ketoconazole 2% cream, and
7. Amphotericin gel.

For reinfection, unresponsive and chronic cases, systemic therapy is indicated:

1. Ketoconazole 200 mg/day for 1–2 weeks,
2. Fluconazole 50–100 mg/day for 1 week, or
3. Itraconazole 100 mg/day for 3 weeks

Differential diagnosis of white oral lesions
White lesions that can be scraped off
Allergic reactions (e.g. due to cinnamon aldehyde in toothpastes or mouthwashes)
Chemical (e.g. aspirin, silver nitrate, hydrogen peroxide, and sodium hypochlorite) or thermal burns
Diphtheria
Pseudomembranous candidiasis White coated tongue
White lesions that cannot be scraped off
Actinic cheilitis
Carcinoma in situ/Squamous cell carcinoma
Cheek chewing
Darier's disease
Dyskeratosis congenita
Frictional keratosis (white plaque with a rough, frayed surface due to mechanical irritation, e.g. rough or maladjusted dentures)
Hyperplastic candidiasis
Hereditary benign intraepithelial dyskeratosis Leukoedema
Leukoplakia
Lichen planus
Linea alba
Lupus erythematosus
Nicotine stomatitis (nonpremalignant white lesion on the palate in heavy smokers and those with a long history of drinking extremely hot beverages)
Oral lichen planus
Oral submucous fibrosis
Pachyonychia congenita
Secondary syphilis
Tobacco pouch keratosis (premalignant white lesion in the area of tobacco contact, most commonly the anterior mandibular vestibule)
Uremic stomatitis (adherent white plaques as a manifestation of uremia)

5. Ans. (a) Aspergillus

Ref: Roxburgh's 17th ed page 40

Tinea Cruris

Tinea cruris or groin ringworm is very itchy and is for the most part a disorder of young men. Well-defined, itchy, red scaling patches occur asymmetrically on the medial aspects of both groins. These gradually extend down the thigh and on to the scrotum unless treated. **T. rubrum and E. floccosum** are the causative fungi.

Trichophyton, Microsporum and Epidermophyton species are responsible for this group of dermatophyte infections. Trichophyton rubrum, T. mentagrophytes and Epidermophyton floccosum are the most common causes of dermatophyte infection in humans.

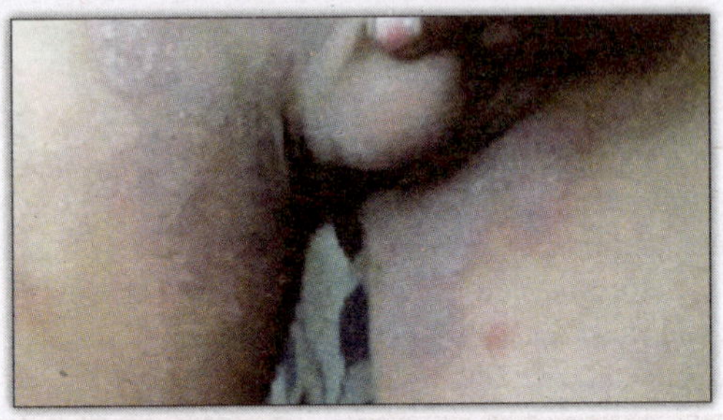

Fig: Ringworm of the groin (tinea cruris)

6. Ans. (b) Oral isotretinoin

Ref: Roxburgh 17th ed page page 159

The treatment of acne is guided by its severity. Nodulocystic acne is a severe variant of Acne, where first line of treatment is oral isotretinoin.

Acne vulgaris is a chronic inflammatory disease of the pilosebaceous follicles, characterized by comedones, papules, pustules, nodules, and often scars.

Clinical Features:

Comedones: The comedo is the primary lesion of acne. It may be seen as a flat or slightly elevated papule with a dilated central opening filled with blackened keratin (open comedo or blackhead). Closed comedones (whiteheads) are usually 1 mm yellowish papules that may require stretching of the skin to visualize. Macrocomedones, which are uncommon, may reach 3–4 mm in size.

Papules: The papules and pustules are 1–5 mm in size, and are caused by inflammation, so there is erythema and edema.

Nodules and cysts: Papules may enlarge, become more nodular, and coalesce into plaques of several centimeters that are indurated or fluctuant, contain sinus tracts, and discharge serosanguinous or yellowish pus.

Acne affects primarily the face, neck, upper trunk, and upper arms. On the face it occurs most frequently on the cheeks, and to a lesser degree on the nose, forehead, and chin. The ears may be involved, with large comedones in the concha, cysts in the lobes, and sometimes pre and retroauricular comedones and cysts. On the neck, especially in the nuchal area, large cystic lesions may predominate.

Age of Presentation:

- Acne typically begins at puberty and is often the first sign of increased sex hormone production.
- Acne may also begin in 20–35 year old women who have not experienced teenage acne.
- Neonatal acne is a common condition that develops a few days after birth.

Pathogenesis: The four major factors involved in the etiology of acne are:

1. Seborrhea
2. Comedo formation (comedogenesis)
3. Colonization of the intrafollicular duct with P. acnes
4. Inflammation.

Acne vulgaris is exclusively a follicular disease, with the principle abnormality being comedo formation. It is produced by the impaction and distension of the follicles with a keratinous plug in the lower infundibulum. The keratinous plug is caused by hyperproliferation and abnormal differentiation of keratinocytes of unknown causes.

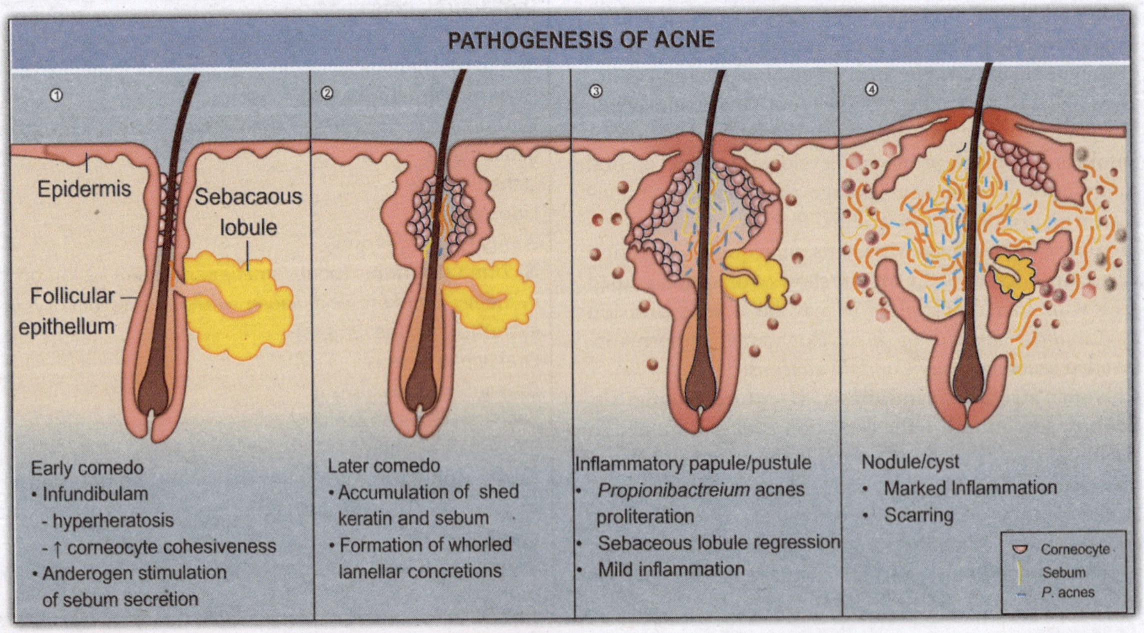

Grading of severity of acne		
Mild acne	Moderate acne	Severe acne
• Comedones • Few papules	Predominantly papules and pustules Few nodules >0.5-1 cm	• Predominantly nodules • Cysts • Acne conglobata

7. Ans. (a) Meningococcemia

Ref: Roxburgh's 17th ed page 86, Ananthanarayan 9th ed page 232

Similar Question was asked in Microbiology AIIMS MAY 2016 with same color plate but the format of the question was different.

The development of crops of purple purpuric papules with darker and occasionally crusted central areas and sometimes pustules is seen in the course of subacute bacterial endocarditis, gonococcemia and meningococcemia

AIIMS MAY 2018

8. Ans. (a) Sural nerve

Ref: Green's Operative Hand Surgery By Scott W. Wolfe, page 109; Procedural Dermatosurgery By Biju Vasudevan 1st Ed page 275

- In pure neuritic leprosy, it is difficult to arrive at a diagnosis due to absence of cutaneous lesions. In such cases, nerve biopsy is the gold standard for diagnosis of neuritic leprosy.
- Usually, a cutaneous nerve like sural nerve or radial cutaneous nerve is used for nerve biopsy in pure neuritic leprosy.
- Sural nerve is the most preferred site for biopsy in peripheral neuropathies as well as Hansen's disease (leprosy) because:
  - It is a purely sensory nerve.
  - Resulting sensory loss is confined to a small area in the dorsolateral part of the foot.
  - Easy to identify and access at the lateral malleolus.
  - It has been extensively studied.
- **Neuropathy in leprosy:**
  - The nerves suffer a triple blow from *M. leprae*: infective neuropathy, immunologic neuropathy, and compressive neuropathy (intraneural and extraneural compression)
  - The ulnar, median, and radial nerves, usually in that order, are affected in the upper extremity in 70% of active and relapsing cases of leprosy.
  - A thickened sensory nerve that would leave minimal functional deficit (superficial radial, sural, supraclavicular) is preferred for nerve biopsy.
  - The bacteria preferentially infect nerves in the cooler parts of the body: The fine terminal dermal nerves, small subcutaneous nerves, and superficially located large nerve trunks.
  - Sensory loss almost always precedes motor loss because superficial dermal nerve damage precedes deeper nerve trunk damage.
  - Nonmyelinated and thinly myelinated fibers are affected before myelinated fibers.

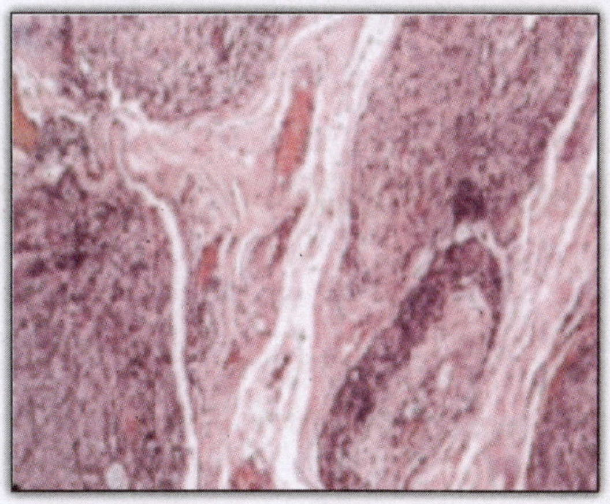

Fig: Endoneurial inflammation in pure neuritic leprosy

9. Ans. (b) Chromium

Ref: Rook's Textbook of Dermatology, 8th Edition, page 26.34

This question is based upon occupational contact dermatitis.

Contact dermatitis is the most common occupational dermatosis; irritant contact dermatitis accounts for over 2/3 of all cases while the remaining are due to allergic contact hypersensitivity.

Occupational contact dermatitis may manifest as cumulative irritant, allergic or photocontact dermatitis. The hands are the most common sites affected (80%–90% of cases) along with other exposed parts. Dust and vapors affect the face and neck. Dermatitis of the feet and legs is more often seen in miners and cement workers.

A large number of industrial chemicals and substances can cause dermatitis. Some of them are irritants, some sensitizers and a few are both. Though noxious agents vary from country to country and from time to time, substances that commonly produce occupational contact dermatitis are metals, rubber chemicals, resins, soldering fluxes, cutting fluids, solvents, soaps and detergents, foodstuffs, and plants.

Common allergens in occupational contact dermatitis	
Metals: Metals and metallic salts are common occupational skin sensitizers as they are used in many industrial processes. Chromium, nickel, cobalt and mercury salts are common sensitizers.	
Chromium and chromate	**Hexavalent chromate is often the commonest occupational allergen in industrialized countries. The commonest cause of allergic contact dermatitis from chromate is cement because hexavalent chromate is present in cement as an impurity.** Other sources of chrome allergy are leather apparel, welding fumes, cutting fluids, and electroplating fluids. Some green pigments used in dyes and paints contain chromate salts and some of these pigments are used in TV picture tubes, army uniforms, offset printing inks, and paints. Other sources are anti-rust paints, galvanized iron sheets, magnetic tapes, and matches.
Nickel	**It is used in the making of alloys and its salts are used in electroplating processes.** More females than males are sensitized and the allergy is more often non-occupational. Sources of occupational nickel contact dermatitis are electroplating fluids and instruments used in the electronic industry. **Hairdressers have a high risk of developing nickel allergy** due to use of nickel-plated equipment such as scissors, metallic trays, curlers, and clippers.
Mercury	Mercury and mercuric salts may cause allergic dermatitis in **dentists and dental technicians.**

Other allergens causing occupational contact dermatitis	
Rubber chemicals	Latex from the rubber tree seldom causes allergy in the manufacture of rubber.
Resins	Resins are extensively used in industries especially the electronics and electrical industries.
Epoxy resins	Epoxy resins are commonly used resins and are also common sensitizers. They are used in the manufacture of electronic chips, circuit boards, electrical insulators, domestic adhesives, tables, chairs, paints, and moulds.
Acrylic resins	There are various types of acrylic resins. They are used in the manufacture of sealants in electronic and electrical components, textile and leather furnishings, latex paints, coating for automobiles, orthopedic implants, dentures and bone cement.
Polyurethane resins	These consist of various di- and polyisocyanate compounds. They are used as surface coating agents, adhesives (in paints, foams, printing films), insulators (in refrigerators and ovens), in the manufacture of soft tyres, furniture, light aircraft as well as in the repair of cushion material boats and furniture.
Formaldehyde resins	These include phenol, para-tertiary butyl phenol, urea, and melamine formaldehyde resins. Phenol formaldehyde resins are used in the manufacture of electrical components and laminates; para-tertiary butyl phenol formaldehyde resins as adhesives for leather, cloth or wood products; urea formaldehyde resins as adhesives for plywood and other wood products; and melamine formaldehyde resins for the manufacture of dinner ware, food containers, and also for impregnating textiles
Colophony	**Colophony is the most commonly used natural resin.** It is obtained from the pine tree and is used in adhesives, printing inks, soldering flux and for impregnating papers and electrical cables. Contact hypersensitivity to colophony is well known and is commonly nonoccupational (sticking plaster). The commonest occupational cause of colophony allergy is soldering flux, used in electrical and electronic industries.
Cutting fluids	Cutting fluids provide lubrication and cooling for metal working operations. The fluids may be neat oils or water based. Sensitization may occur to many of the components, but is especially common to the biocides, followed by corrosion inhibitors and coupling agents. Amongst the biocides, formaldehyde releasers (e.g. Dowicide, Grotan HD, Grotan BK, Bronopol, Forcide 78, Bazkid 80) are the most common sensitizers.
Solvents	Commonly used solvents include alcohols, formalin, kerosene, toluene, xylene, benzene, ethers, ketones, amines, and chlorinated hydrocarbons. Occupational dermatitis from solvents commonly occurs in the transport, metal/engineering, and electronic industries, where solvents are usually used for degreasing. Painters and carpenters, who use solvents to dilute paints and lacquers as well as to remove stains from the skin, can also develop dermatitis. Solvents are amongst the most common causes of occupational dermatitis. They primarily produce irritant dermatitis, but solvents like formalin and turpentine may cause ACD. Common sites of involvement are the hands and fingers, though airborne contact dermatitis affecting the face and neck can also occur.
Soaps and detergents	They are used by almost all factory workers for skin cleaning and also frequently by workers in the cleaning, food and hotel industries, and hairdressers. They contain several skin irritants including alkalis, enzymes, emulsifiers, and solvents. Fragrances and biocides are skin sensitizers.
Plants and woods	Foresters, gardeners, horticulturists, florists, timber workers, and furniture makers can develop dermatitis from plants and woods due to chemical resins secreted by them. Hair, spines, and wood dust can cause mechanical injury to the skin. Plants known to cause dermatitis are Parthenium, chrysanthemum (Compositae), poison ivy and poison oak (Anacardiaceae), Primula obconica (Primulaceae). Common types of wood that cause allergic contact dermatitis are mahogany, oak, pine, rose wood, satin, and teak wood.

10. Ans. (b) Terbinafine

Ref: http://aac.asm.org/content/61/7/e00115-17.full, https://www.ncbi.nlm.nih.gov/pubmed/29577447

- This question has become very relevant in today's era. Superficial dermatophytosis has become resistant to common antifungals
- However sensitivity testing for antifungals is far more difficult than bacterial infections. Although Dermatologists in practice would know the answer straight away, that superficial dermatophytosis are now developing resistance to terbinafine, it is equally difficult to do in vitro tests to identify the same. However, now microbiological research is documenting resistance of superficial dermatophytes to terbinfaine.

"In the last few years, infections caused by dermatophytes along with a concomitant increase in the number of difficult to treat cases have increasingly been recogniszd, indicating that dermatophytosis remains a challenging public health problem. The majority of infections are caused by Trichophyton rubrum and Trichophyton mentagrophytes complex. Terbinafine, an allylamine antifungal used orally and topically is considered to be a first-line drug in the therapy of dermatophyte infections. Terbinafine resistance has been predominantly attributed to point mutations in the squalene epoxidase (SQLE) target gene a key enzyme in the ergosterol biosynthetic pathway leading to single amino acid substitutions. Here, we report the largest series of 20 terbinafine-resistant Trichophyton interdigitale isolates obtained predominately from cases of tinea corporis/cruris in three hospitals in Delhi, India exhibiting elevated MICs (4 to ≥32 μg/mL) to terbinafine and all harboring single-point mutations Leu393Phe or Phe397Leu in the SQLE gene. In 12 (60%) *T. interdigitale* isolates, the Phe397Leu substitution was observed, whereas in the remaining 8 (40%) isolates the substitution Leu393Phe was reported for the first time in T. interdigitale. Furthermore, 10 susceptible *T. interdigitale* isolates (0.125-2 μg/mL) had a wild-type genotype. Remarkably, considerably high terbinafine resistance rate of 32% was observed among 63 T. interdigitale isolates identified by sequencing of the internal transcribed spacer region. This high level of terbinafine resistance of Indian dermatophyte isolates is worrisome warranting antifungal susceptibility testing and mutation analysis for monitoring this emerging resistance."

11. Ans. (d) Chikungunya fever

Ref: Tropical Dermatology E-Book By Steven K Tyring, Omar Lupi, Ulrich R Hengge, P- 148, Andrew's diseases of skin 11th Ed page 404

This is a total googly question by AIIMS

Approach to this Question: The clues in the question are of history of fever with rash and joint pains. It points out towards a viral fever with rash. Therefore both dengue and chikungunya are a possibility. We can rule out melasma because melasma doesn't have an acute onset. Although they tried to confuse you with giving history of NSAID intake, but we know the progression of fixed drug eruption. It generally happens on the same spot, starts with a bullous eruption which leaves a hyperpigmentation thereafter. The common sites are Glans penis >> Lips. Therefore even fixed drug eruption is ruled out. Now coming to the two confusing options, dengue and chikungunya. Dengue classically presents with morbilliform rash and petechial or ecchymotic eruption. Hence, chikungunya is both the answer of exclusion and answer of selection.

Cutaneous Manifestations of Chikungunya Fever

Chikungunya (CHK) is an acute onset, mosquito-borne viral disease characterized by high fever, predominant musculoskeletal symptoms, and skin rash. The etiological agent is a RNA virus that belongs to the *alphavirus* genus of the family *Togaviridae.* The disease is transmitted to humans by the bite of infected ***Aedes mosquito;*** two species namely *Aedes aegypti* and *Aedes albopictus*. These mosquitoes generally bite throughout daylight hours with peaks of activity in the early morning and late afternoon. Approximately 4–7 days after the mosquito bite, patients display acute symptoms of painful polyarthralgia, high fever, myalgia, and headache. *Mucocutaneous involvement tends to be a prominent and significant finding in the acute phase of infection.* A host of mucocutaneous manifestations, occurring in 30–50% of all cases of Chikungunya infection, have been described. *Few of these are very characteristic and specific, and thus help in distinguishing the infection from its close differential of dengue fever and other viral febrile illnesses.*

- **Generalized morbilliform maculopapular rash** with normal islands of intervening skin and characteristically sparing the face has been the most commonly (30–55%) reported manifestation. The rash develops within 3–4 days of the onset of fever and tends to subside in about a week without any sequel.
- **Skin hyperpigmentation** is the next most commonly encountered finding. It occurs in the form of centrofacial pigmentation predominantly involving the nose (Chick sign). It is, the most commonly described pigmentation developing during the acute phase of the disease and helps in the retrospective diagnosis of infection.

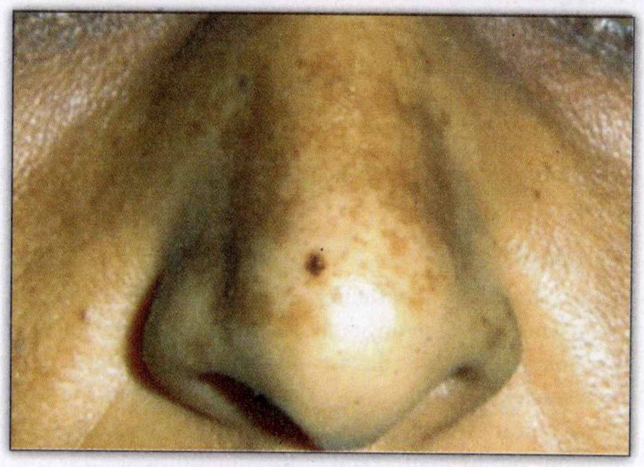

Fig: Chick sign: Skin hyperpigmentation of nose in dengue

- Nonhealing ulcers and **genital ulcers** on the scrotum, vulva, and groins may occur.
- Vascular response in the form of facial flushing, erythema, and edema of ear lobules resembling Milian's ear sign, erythema of striae in females have been described
- Infants younger than 12 months tend to have different spectrum of skin lesions that include acrocyanosis and symmetrical superficial vesicolobullous lesions.
- Subepidermal blisters and TEN like symptoms.

AIIMS NOVEMBER 2017

12. Ans. (c) Hypothyroidism

Ref: Hall's Manual of Skin as a Marker of Underlying Disease - Page 158, 159, 201, 329, Mosby's Color Atlas and Text of Dermatology page 262

Recall Bias

More than 4 options were recalled for this question. All are discussed below.

This question is based on dermatological manifestations of systemic diseases. **"Myxedema in Hypothyroid is Periorbital not Pretibial like Hyperthyroid"**

Option (A)

Diabetic dermopathy is a constellation of well-demarcated, hyperpigmented, atrophic depressions, macules, or papules located on the anterior surface of the lower legs that is usually found in patients with DM. It is the most common cutaneous marker of DM. Other cutaneous markers of DM are loss of hair over the legs, acrochordons, pruritus, acanthosis nigricans, ichthyosis, cutaneous amyloidosis, syringoma, callosity, and brittle nails.

Option (B)

Necrobiosis lipoidica (NL); also known as necrobiosis lipoidica diabeticorum) is a fairly distinct clinical entity that, although not the most common, is the best recognized cutaneous marker of diabetes mellitus. It may be seen outside of the setting of diabetes mellitus, although up to three-quarters of patients with NL have or will have diabetes mellitus. Necrobiosis lipoidica is a chronic granulomatous dermatosis characterized by one or more yellow-brown, telangiectatic plaques with central atrophy and raised violaceous borders, typically in the pretibial regions.

Option (C)

In **Hypothyroidism** the predominant cutaneous symptom is Pale, cold, dry coarse, hyperkeratotic skin, followed by hair loss and puffy edema. Myxedema in hypothyroid is periorbital (nonpitting).

Option (D)

Hyperthyroidism patients have warm, moist, erythematous skin. Many develop onycholysis and scalp hair loss. In addition patients with Grave's disease develops Pretibial myxedema and Acropachy. Myxedema can occur anywhere in the body but most commonly at pretibial location and is characterized by non pitting thickening and induration of the skin.

Option (E)

Sarcoidosis: Cutaneous lesions of sarcoidosis are classified as specific (Noncaseating granulomas) and non specific lesions (Erythema Nodosum). It is seen as localized lesion of scalp or as a manifestation of systemic disease. These lesions ranges from brownish red to violaceous papule and plaque that blanch on diascopy revealing "Apple jelly" color. The lesions are most commonly seen in the head and neck region however the lesion may occur anywhere. There are case reports of Cutaneous Sarcoidosis mimicking Necrobiosis lipoidica-like skin lesions on both shins.

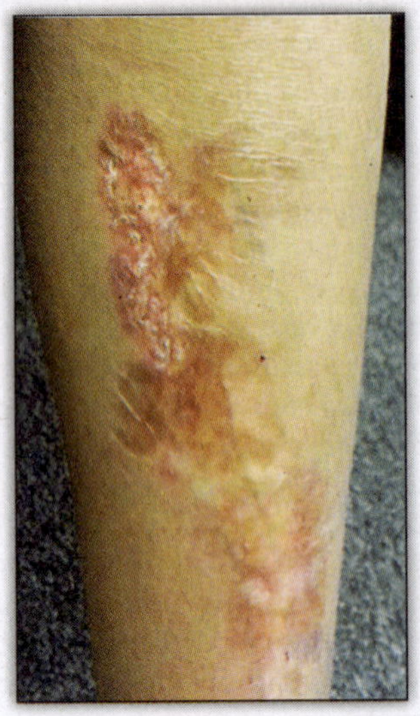

© Pathak R, Karmacharya P

Fig: Necrobiosis lipoidica (NL; also known as necrobiosis lipoidica diabeticorum) is a fairly distinct clinical entity that, although not the most common, is the best recognized cutaneous marker of diabetes mellitus. It may be seen outside of the setting of diabetes mellitus, although up to three-quarters of patients with NL have or will have diabetes mellitus. Necrobiosis lipoidica is a chronic granulomatous dermatosis characterized by one or more yellow-brown, telangiectatic plaques with central atrophy and raised violaceous borders, typically in the pretibial regions

Differential Diagnosis of Necrobiosis Lipoidica:

- Diabetic dermopathy is a constellation of well-demarcated, hyperpigmented, atrophic depressions, macules, or papules located on the anterior surface of the lower legs that is usually found in patients with DM. It is the most common cutaneous marker of DM. Other cutaneous markers of DM are loss of hair over the legs, acrochordons, pruritus, acanthosis nigricans, ichthyosis, cutaneous amyloidosis, syringoma, callosity, and brittle nails.
- Hyperthyroidism: Patients with hyperthyroidism have warm, moist, erythematous skin may develop onycholysis and scalp hair loss. In addition patients with Grave's disease develops pretibial myxedema and Acropachy. Myxedema can occur anywhere in the body but most commonly at pretibial location and is characterized by nonpitting thickening and induration of the skin.
- Sarcoidosis: Cutaneous lesions of sarcoidosis are classified as specific (Noncaseating granulomas) and nonspecific lesions (Erythema Nodosum). It is seen as localized lesion of scalp or as a manifestation of systemic disease. These lesions ranges from brownish red to violaceous papule and plaque that blanch on diascopy revealing "Apple jelly" color. The lesions are most commonly seen in the head and neck region however the lesion may occur anywhere. There are case reports of Cutaneous Sarcoidosis mimicking Necrobiosis lipoidica—like skin lesions on both shins.

13. **Ans. (d)** 4

Ref: Lookingbill and Marks' Principles of Dermatology By James G. Marks, Jeffrey J. Miller 6th ed page 3

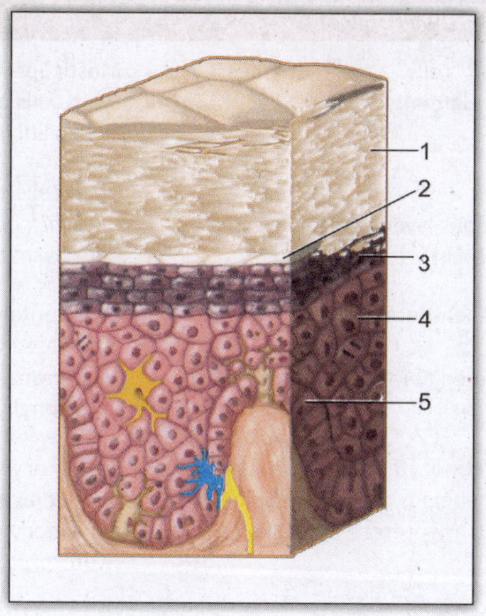

Figure Legends

1. Stratum corneum
2. Stratum lucidum
3. Stratum granulosum
4. Stratum spinosum
5. Stratum basale

Stratum spinosum (Marked as 4) derives its name from spines or intercellular bridges that extends between the keratinocytes, composed of Desmosomes and visible on Light Microscopy.

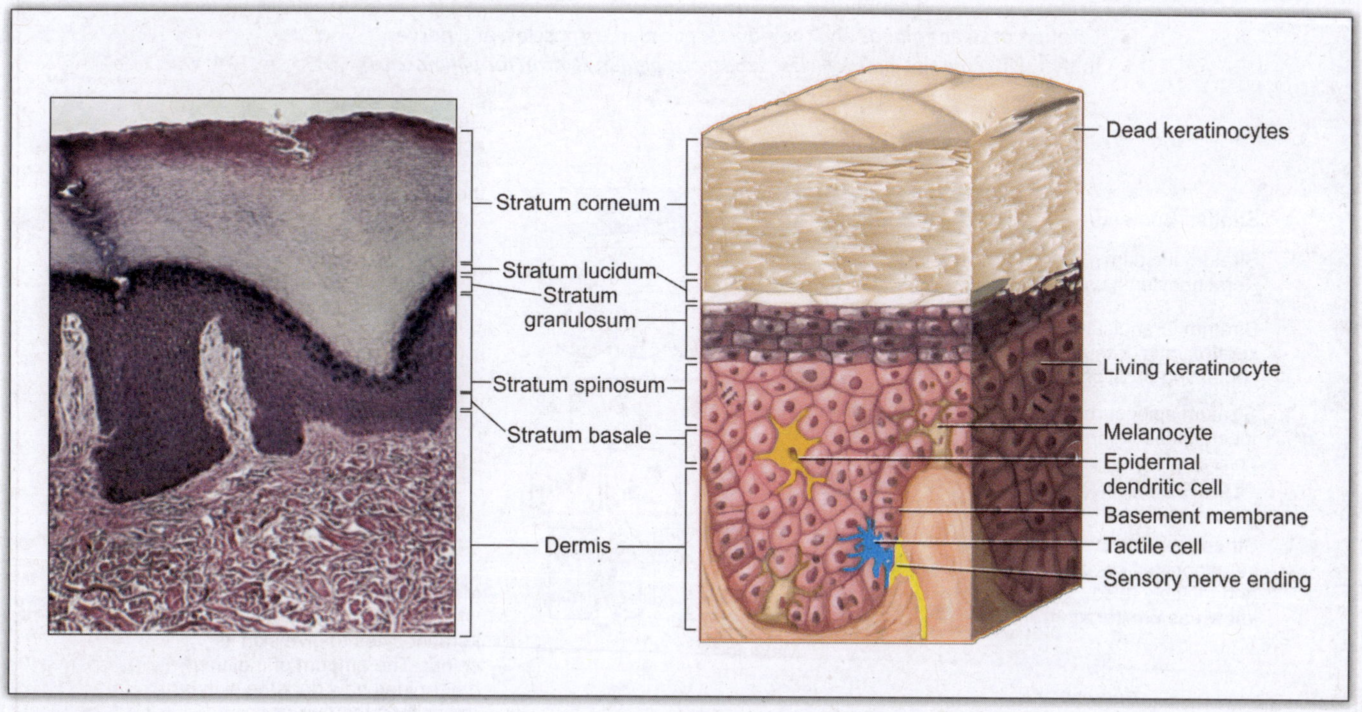

Fig: Histology of skin layers with comparative illustration

Histology of Skin

	Layer	Cells	Comments
Epidermis	Stratum corneum	• Many flattened, dead "cells", called squames, packed with keratin filaments	• Most superficial layer of epidermis • Dead cells containing Keratin with hard protein envelop. Intracellular lipid
	Stratum lucidum	• Dead cells • Indistinct homogeneous layer of keratinocytes, present only in thick skin	• Dead cells containing dispersed Keratohyalin • Cells *lack nuclei* and organelles • Cytoplasm is packed with keratin filaments and eleidin
	Stratum granulosum	• Flattened nucleated keratinocytes arranged in 3 to 5 layers • Keratinocytes contained Keratin and Profilliggrin	• Cells contain many coarse keratohyalin granules associated with tonofilaments • Membrane-coating (waterproofing) granules occasionally present
	Stratum spinosum	• Several layers of keratinocytes (called "*prickle cells*"). Keratinization begins at Stratum Spinosum • Langerhans cells also are present in this layer	• Keratinocytes are mitotically active, especially in the deeper layers. • Keratinocytes contain membrane-coating (waterproofing) granules
	Stratum basale (germinativum)	• Keratinocytes are mitotically active • *Melanocytes* & *Merkel cells* also present	• Deepest layer of epidermis, composed of a single layer of tall cuboidal keratinocytes
Dermis	Papillary layer	• Superficial thin layer of connective tissue that interdigitates with epidermal ridges of the epidermis. • Forms dermal papillae where *Meissner corpuscles* and *capillary loops* may be found. • Contains delicate collagen *(type I and type III)* fibers. • Contains anchoring fibrils *(type VII collagen)*, microfibrils (fibrillin) & elastic fibers.	
	Reticular layer	• Extensive part of the dermis, lying deep to the papillary layer • Contains thick bundles of collagen *(type I)* fibers & elastic fibers • *Arteries*, veins, and *lymphatics* are present • Location of *sweat glands* and their ducts, pacinian corpuscles, and nerves. • In thin skin, contains *hair follicles, sebaceous glands, & arrector pili muscles*	

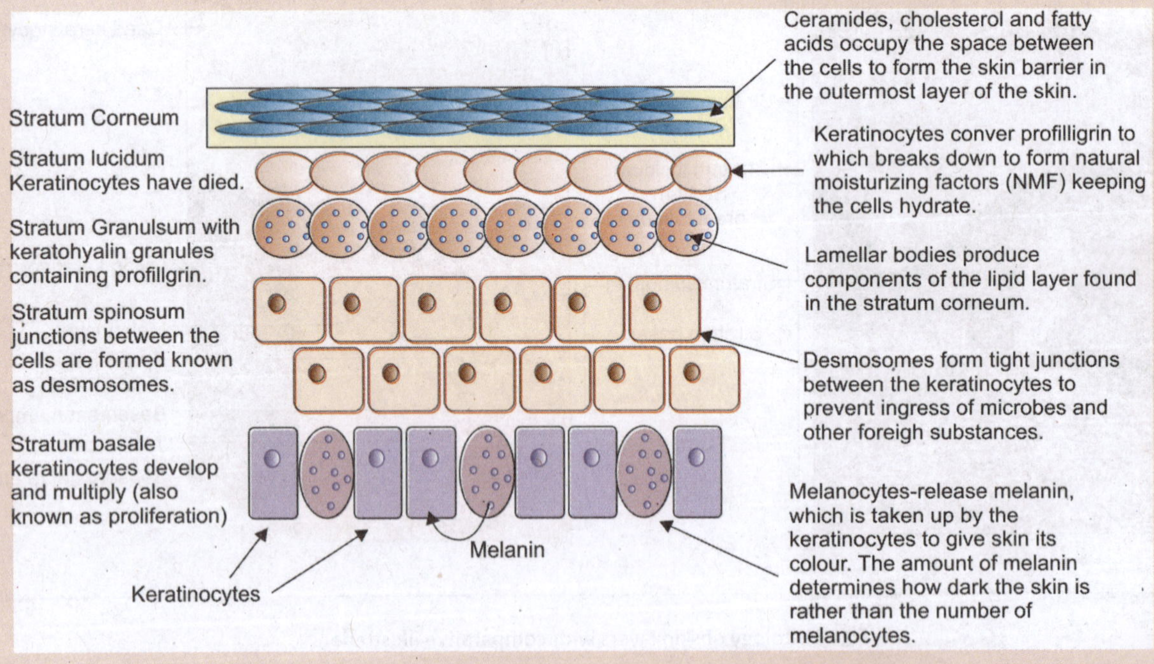

14. Ans. (d) Chikungunya fever

Ref: Tropical Dermatology E-Book By Steven K Tyring, Omar Lupi, Ulrich R Hengge, P- 148, Andrew's diseases of skin 11th Ed page 404

Repeat AIIMS May 2018 Dermatology (See for explanation) (see page no. 1059)

15. Ans. (c) Coxsackie virus

Ref: Color Textbook of Pediatric Dermatology by William L. Weston, Alfred T. Lane, Joseph G. Morelli 4th ed Page 136

Let us first try to understand the basic lesions here. What we see are multiple, vesicles on palms, soles and mouth of a child and some of them have a background erythema. Bearing that in mind let us try to rule out the options.

Option (A)

Pox viruses: The orthopoxviruses include variola, vaccinia, monkeypox, cowpox, buffalopox, and Cantagalo and Aracatuba. The parapoxviruses are primarily zoonotic, and include orf, paravaccinia, bovine papular stomatitis, deerpox, and sealpox. Tanapox is the sole yata poxvirus to cause human disease. Variola are small pox is eradicated. Buffalo pox, cowpox, orf present as solitary painful lesions which are mostly papule or nodule at site of inoculation in animal handlers with secondary ulceration and crusting. Therefore option A is ruled out.

Option (B)

HHV7: Causes erythematous discrete macules, hence that option is also ruled out.

Option (D)

Varicella or chicken pox virus: Vesicles with erythematous base are seen in varicella but are located majorly on trunk, face and oral mucosa. Here the distributions of lesions go against the diagnosis of varicella.

Option (C)

Skin diseases caused by coxsackie viruses

- **Herpangina:** Vesicular eruptions in pharynx and posterior oropharynx (caused by A8, A10, A16)
- **Hand Foot Mouth disease:** Hand foot and mouth disease (HFMD) was first described in Canada in 1957 by Robinson and Alsop et al coined the term hand,foot and mouth disease 1959. An abrupt onset of scattered papules that progress to oval or linear vesicles in an acral distribution should suggest hand-foot-and-mouth disease
- **Etiology:** Hand foot and mouth disease is most frequently caused by Coxsackie virus A—16 and less commonly by other Coxsackie viruses (A5,A7, A 9, A10, B1, B3, and B5). Transmission is mainly via fecal oral contact and less commonly by respiratory droplets. During epidemics, transmission can occur via mother to fetus. Children from 2-10 years are commonly affected. Incubation period ranges from 2-5 days and virus shedding lasts up to 5 weeks.

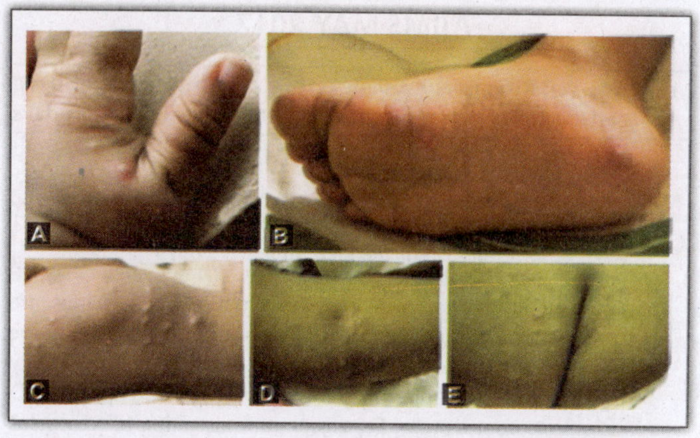

Figs A to E: Multiple eruptions over the hand, feet, knee, elbow and buttocks: Multiple eruptions on the hands and feet are asymptomatic red papules that quickly become small, gray, 3–7 mm vesicles surrounded by a red halo. They are often oval, linear, or crescentic, and run parallel to the skin lines on the fingers and toes. Especially in children who wear diapers, vesicles and erythematous, edematous papules may occur on the buttocks. Treatment is supportive, with the use of oral topical anesthetics

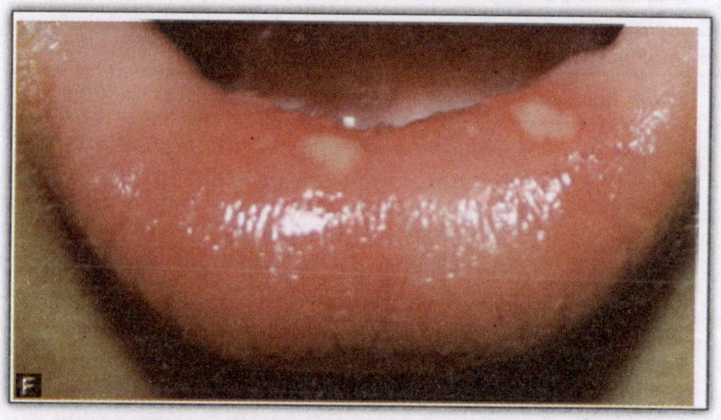

Fig: (F) Oral ulcers on the labial mucosa of lower lip: In 90% of cases oral lesions develop; these consist of small (4–8 mm), irregular shape, rapidly ulcerating vesicles surrounded by a red areola on the lower lip, buccal mucosa, tongue, soft palate, and gingiva. The lower lip was edematous. Lesions are self-limiting and heals without scarring

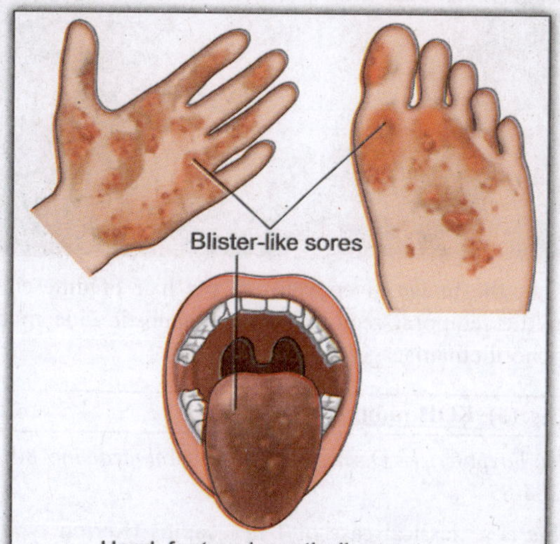

Hand, foot and mouth disease

AIIMS MAY 2017

16. Ans. (c) Rifampicin 450 mg once a month + dapsone 50 mg daily + clofazamine 150 once a month + 50 mg alternate days

Ref: KDT 6th Ed page 753, IADVL 2nd Ed page 2084

See Details of LEPROSY REGIMEN in AIIMS NOV 2018 Community Medicine (see page no. 563)

Since all lesions are with loss of sensation, and lesions are spread on both front and back of arm, more than one nerve are expected to be affected hence, this is a case of multibacillary leprosy in a 12-year-old child. This question is based upon WHO classification of leprosy. For easier administration of treatment of leprosy by field workers WHO classified leprosy in two forms. A patient is classified according to his presenting complaints

Paucibacillary form	Multibacillary form
• 1-5 skin lesions • Single nerve thickening • Slit skin smear negative	• >5 skin lesions • >1 nerve thickening • Slit skin smear positive at any site

17. Ans. (b) Trichotillomania

Ref: Rook's Dermatology 9th ed page 86.17-86.1

See Table of Differential Diagnosis of ALOPECIA in AIIMS NOV 2016 Dermatology (see page no. 1073)

Let us understand how to approach this kind of a question. Whenever a patchy alopecia is suggested in the question, the next thing to find is if it is scarring or nonscarring alopecia.

For purpose of exams, if nonscarring patchy alopecia is given in the question, there are two differentials only which have to kept in mind. They are alopecia areata or trichotillomania.

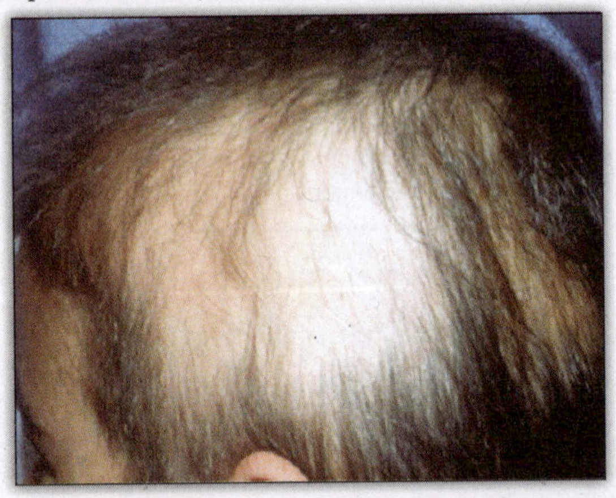

In the image given you can see hair of different length on the temporal region. It is a diagnostic clue in favor of trichotillomania.

18. Ans. (a) KOH mount

Ref: Fitzpatcrick's Dermatology in general medicine, 8th ed page 2284-85

This is a classical case of Tinea capitis (Kerion type). Since tinea capitis is a dermatophytic infection, investigation of choice here will be KOH mount.

See AIIMS NOV 2014 Dermatology for Details of KOH Mount (see volume II)

Tineas are dermatophyte infections of the skin. From top to bottom, left to right: fungal infections of (a) hair (tinea capitis); (b) face (tinea capitis/ringworm); (c) arm (tinea corporis); (d) close-up of ringworm; (e) torso with concentric rings (tinea imbricata/tinea corporis); (f) groin (tinea cruris); (g) toe webbing (tinea pedis); (h) foot (tinea pedis/"moccasin" type); and (i) nails (onyciomycosis).

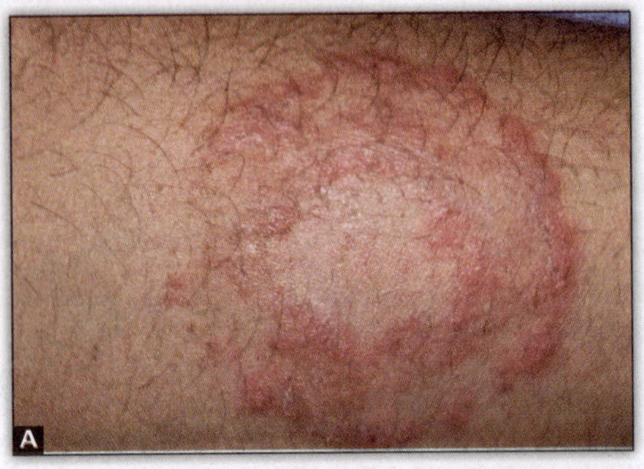

Source: Public Health Image Library (PHIL, http://phil.cdc.gov/phil/home.asp)

Fig: (A) Tines cruris: The itchy lesion in picture is a typical dermatophyte infection, and its known Jock's itch or Tinea cruris. It is also known as Dhobi's itch. Although prevalent worldwide, tinea cruris is more common in tropical regions. It is more common in young (18–25 years) males. It may be more common in men than in women probably because tinea pedis (with which tinea cruris is frequently associated) is more prevalent in men, males perspire more than females, anatomical differences (greater areas of occlusive skin where the scrotum is in contact with the thigh), and clothing differences. Tinea cruris is frequently recurrent; factors favoring recurrence are high environmental temperature and sweating, and the wearing of athletic supporters or shorts that produce chafing in the groins. In obese persons, there is constant mechanical irritation of apposed surfaces, decreased aeration, increased sweating, and difficulty in maintaining hygiene and inspecting the area involved

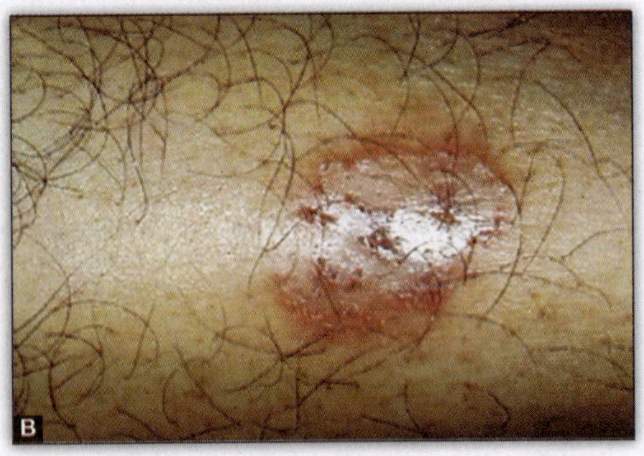

© Sentamilselvi G, Janaki C, Murugusundram S

Fig: (B) Tinea Corporis with intralesional papules suggestive of hair invasion

Subject-wise MCQs and Answers with Explanations

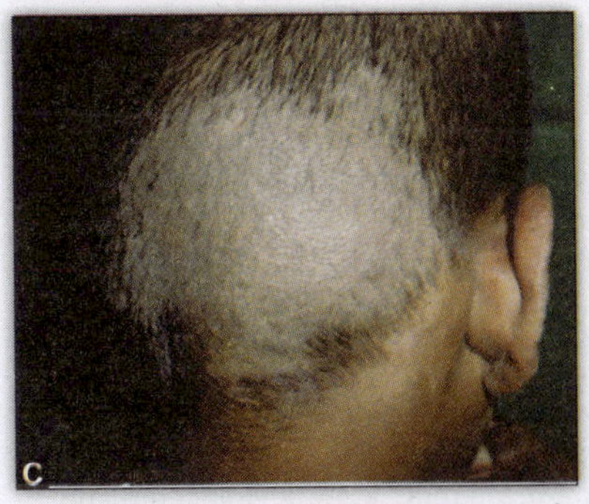

© Sentamilselvi G, Janaki C, Murugusundram S

Fig: (C) Tinea Capitis Black Dot Type with Tinea facei involving the pinna

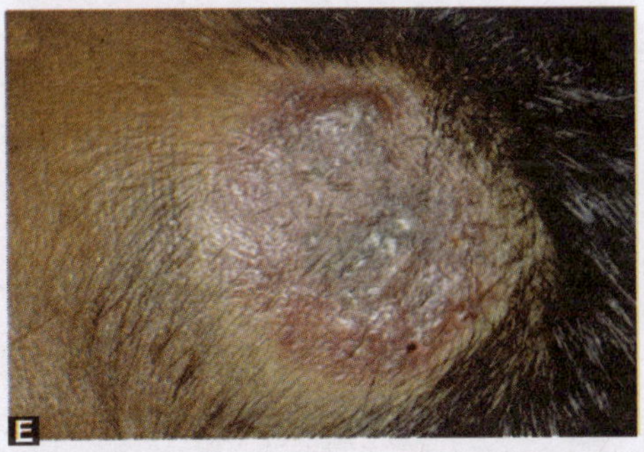

© Sentamilselvi G, Janaki C, Murugusundram S

Fig: (E) Tinea Capitis Kerion

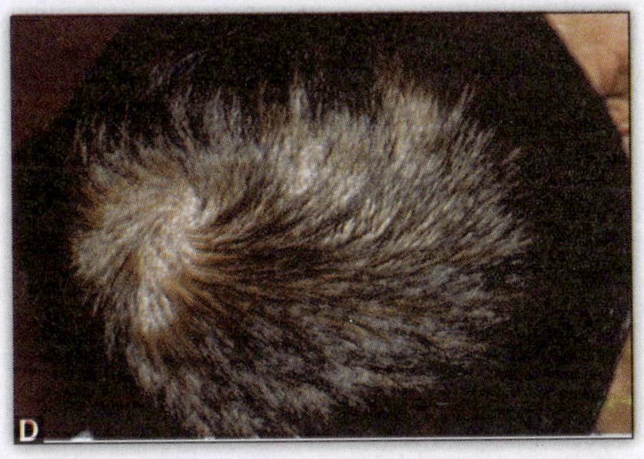

© Sentamilselvi G, Janaki C, Murugusundram S

Fig: (D) Tinea Capitis Grey Patch Type

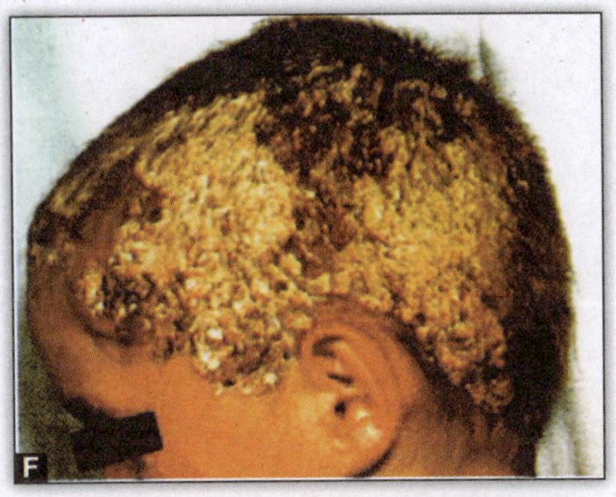

Fig: (F) Tinea Capitis Kerion

Dermatophyte

- Group of filamentous fungi which affect only the superficial keratinized layers of the skin
- Classified into three genera: Trichophyton, Microsporum, Epidermophyton
- In cultures on **Sabroud's agar** they form characteristic hyphae and two types of sexual Apores, microconidia and macroconidia
- Differentiation of species is dependent upon macroconidia
- Trichophyon species infect skin, nails and hair. **T. rubrum is the most common specie affecting human beings**
- Epidermophyton species affect skin and nails but not the hair. Only one specie is known: E. floccosum
- Laboratory investigation: Scrapings are taken from the edge of the lesion mixed with 10% KOH on a slide, after placing a cover slip and the preparation heated to bring about a clearing. They are seen under microscope for septate hyphae.
- Wood's lamp may also be useful

Skin disease	Location of lesions	Clinical features	Fungi most frequently responsible
Tinea corporis (ringworm)	Nonhairy, smooth skin.	Circular patches with advancing red, vesiculated border and central scaling. Pruritic.	All dermatophytes can cause. *M/C = T. rubrum*
Tinea imbricate	Subtype of tinea corporis	Concentric rings are seen	*T. circinata*
Tinea pedis[1] (**Athlete's foot**)	Interdigital spaces on feet of persons wearing shoes.	Acute: itching, red vesicular. Chronic: itching, scaling, fissures.	*T. rubrum,* *T. mentagrophytes,* *E. floccosum*
Tinea cruris (Ringworm of the groin/**Dhobie itch**/Eczema marginatum **Jock's itch**)	Groin	Erythematous scaling lesion in intertriginous area. Pruritic.	*T. rubrum (M/C),* *T. mentagrophytes,* *E. floccosum*

Contd...

Tinea capitis (Mainly seen in children, MC mycosis of children)	Scalp hair. Classification according to the size and the location of the spore • **Endothrix:** fungus inside hair shaft. • **Ectothrix:** Fungus on surface of hair.	**Inflammatory variety:** • **Kerion:** It is rare & presents with boggy swelling on scalp of a child which is indurated and studded with broken hair and pustules. Lymphadenopathy is commonly seen. It heals with scarring.	T. verrucosum and T. mentagrophytes
		• **Favus:** Presents with a yellow cup shaped crust composed of dense mat of mycelia and epithelial debris. Called scutulum due to its shield like shape.	The most common cause of favus is T. schoenleinii. At times, T. violaceum and M. gypseum
		Non-inflammatory variety: • **Gray patch tinea:** Presents as papules which spreads to involve all hair in its path, multiple such partial hairless patches showing numerous broken hair and dandruff like scaling. This type of tinea capitis is usually observed in epidemics in schools • **Black dot tinea capitis** is an endothrix type of infection. Hair shaft breaks at the level of scalp and remnant of hair appears as black dot.	Microsporum audouinii.
Tinea barbae **(Barber's itch)**	Moustache and beard area of face	Edematous, erythematous lesion.	*T. mentagrophytes*
Tinea Faciei	Non hair bearing areas of face		T. mentagrophytes and T. rubrum
Tinea unguium (onychomycosis)	Nail. (Toe nail more common than finger nail)	Nails thickened or crumbling distally; discolored; lusterless. Usually associated with tinea pedis.	All dermatophytes. But Most commonly *T. rubrum, T. mentagrophytes, E. floccosum*
Dermatophytid **(id reaction)**	Usually sides & flexor aspects of fingers & Palm. Any site	Pruritic vesicular to bullous lesions. Most commonly associated with tinea pedis.	No fungi present in lesion. May become secondarily infected with bacteria.

[1]May be associated with lesions of hands and nails (onychomycosis)

Dermatophyte Involvement

	Skin	**Hair**	**Nails**
Trichophyton	√	√	√
Microsporum	√	√	
Epidermophyton	√		√

Tinea Unguium (Onychomycosis)

Distal and lateral subungual onychomycosis	**Most common type**. The most common etiologic agent is T. rubrum. Toenails > fingernails. It starts by invasion of the stratum corneum of the hyponychium of the distal nail bed or the lateral nail fold. Subsequently, the infection moves proximally in the nail bed and invades the ventral surface of the nail plate. Subungual hyperkeratosis and splinter hemorrhages are seen.
White superficial onychomycosis	**Second most common type:** Primarily invasion of the dorsal surface of the nail plate. It is usually caused by Trichophyton mentagrophytes and is characterized by well circumscribed powdery white patches away from the free edge of the nail.

Contd...

Proximal subungual onychomycosis	**Least common** variant of onychomycosis. It is most commonly caused by T. rubrum; other causes are T. mentagrophytes and T. tonsurans. The first clinical sign is a whitish to brownish area on the proximal part of the nail plate. This rare type is an early indicator of **HIV infection** and is also associated with peripheral vascular compromise.
Total dystrophic	End point of all the types.

19. Ans. (a) Congenital melanocytic nevus

Ref: Bulognia Dermatology 3rd Ed page 1873

This is classic congenital melanocytic nevus. Dermatology is a visual science and this image should be imprinted on mind as congenital melanocytic nevus.

However let us rule out the options.

Option (B) Hematoma

It is not present at birth, it does not show hypertrichosis and resolves with time.

Option (C) Verrucous epidermal nevus

It is not hyperpigmented, it has a warty surface and follows blaschko's lines.

Option (D) Melanoacanthoma

It is present in elderly above 40, as hyperpigmented verrucous plaques on face and trunk. Hence ruled out.

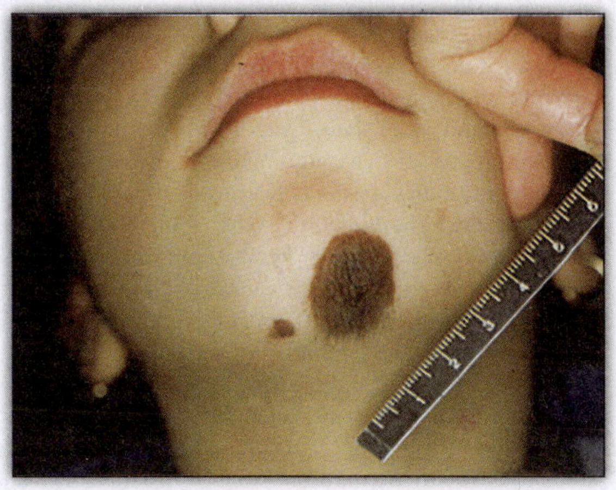

Fig: Congenital Melanocytic Nevus

Congenital Melanocytic Nevus	
Incidence	Congenital nevi are found in about 1% of newborn infants
Size	On the basis of the size, they are categorized as small CMN (diameter less than 1.5 cm), medium-sized CMN (between 1.5 and 19.9 cm) and large or giant CMN (20 cm or greater).
Clinical features	They are usually solitary. The growth of a congenital nevus is very rapid and disproportionate to the growth of the particular body area in the first six months of age. In adults, the nevus remains static unless there is infection, trauma or development of malignancy. Small and medium nevi appear as hyperpigmented macules, solitary or multiple, at birth. Their growth is gradual and the **nevi darken, appear raised and develop coarse hair**, often in a spurt during puberty. Large CMN (also called giant, garment nevi or bathing trunk nevi) are commonly situated on the back and thighs, but may involve the arms or legs. Smaller satellite lesions are also found in the vicinity as well as at a distance from the main nevus The nevi become larger, darker and more rugose as the child grows and develop a warty surface and nodules. The hairs become coarse like terminal hair and are often concentrated in the center.
Special forms	Cerebriform CMN in scalp, Neurocutaneous CMN associated with melanotic tumors of meninges
Malignant transformation	They can have potential of **malignant transformation**. High risk for giant congenital melanocytic nevus, Clinically, changes such as sudden appearance of nodules, very dark pigmentation (especially in fair-skinned individuals), itching, pain, bleeding or ulceration should arouse the suspicion of malignant melanoma
Histopathology	The classic histological features of congenital nevi after the neonatal period are: 1. Presence of nevus cells in the reticular dermis 2. Extension of nevus cells in the collagen bundles in a single row ('Indian file' appearance), sheets or combinations 3. Higher concentration of nevus cells around blood vessels, nerves and adnexal tissues

20. Ans. (b) Pemphigus vulgaris

Ref: Lever's Histopathology of the Skin 3rd ed page 190, Rook's 8th Ed page 40.2

The color plate in the question is showing an intraepidermal blister and row of tombstone appearance which is typical of Pemphigus Vulgaris

See Dermatology AIIMS NOV 2018 for Details of Pemphigus Vulgaris (see page no. 1053)

21. Ans. (c) Antibodies to hemidesmosomes

Ref: Bolognia 3rd ed page 495, Lever dermatopathology 10th ed page 273

See Details of Pemphigus Vulgaris in AIIMS NOV 2018 Dermatology (see page no. 1053)

- The diagnosis here is straightforward. It is a case of Pemphigus vulgaris. It is evident from history of oral lesions and characteristic fishnet appearance of indirect immunofluorescence. However, this time they have gone ahead and asked about autigens involved in pemphigus.
- Pemphigus is an autoimmune disease where the autoantibodies are directed against antigens located in the epidermis. The individual cells of the epidermis, called keratinocytes, contain keratin intermediate filaments (KIF) in their cytoplasm and are tightly bound to each other by sophisticated structures called desmosomes. In pemphigus, the desmosomes are disrupted, and cells become rounded and separate (acantholysis).
- Desmosomes are disk-like structures at which the plasma membranes of two adjacent keratinocytes attach. Ultrastructurally, the desmosome appears as a disc-shaped organelle that is shared by two neighboring keratinocytes, each providing half of the structure.
- The structure includes an electron dense region called the desmosomal plaque that rests on the plasma membrane of the keratinocyte; on its inner side the plaque provides attachment to KIF. The dense material between the plasma membrane of the two keratinocytes constitutes the desmoglea. Desmosomes contain desmosomal cadherins (desmogleins and desmocollins) as transmembrane components, and desmoplakin and plakoglobin as cytoplasmic components. Cadherins are calcium ion dependent cell adhesion molecules that show homophilic adhesion (i.e. a cadherin molecule of one cell binds to the same molecule on another cell). In addition, a few other desmosomal proteins have been identified: plakophilins, envoplakin, periplakin and plectin.

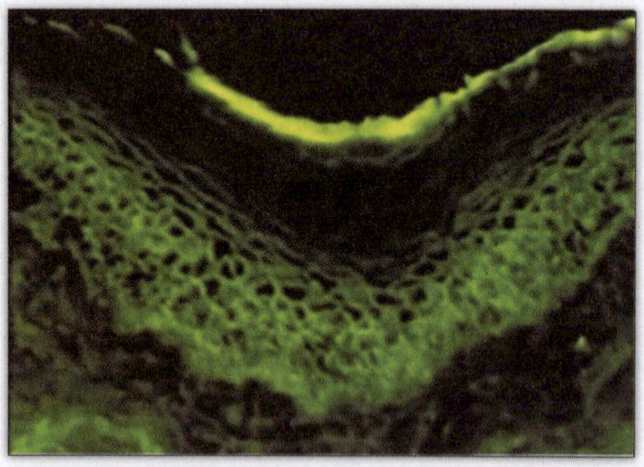

Fig: Pemphigus Vulgaris Immunohistochemistry: Direct immunofluorescence showing granular deposits of immunoglobulin IgG3 and C3 in intracellular space (fish net pattern)

Target Antigens in Pemphigus

Disease	Autoantibodies	Antigens
Pemphigus vulgaris Mucosal-dominant type Mucocutaneous type	IgG IgG	Desmoglein 3 Desmoglein 3, 1
Pemphigus foliaceus	IgG	Desmoglein 1
Paraneoplastic pemphigus	IgG	Desmoglein 3, 1, Plectin, Desmoplakin I, Desmoplakin II, BPAG1, Envoplakin, Periplakin, A2ML1
Drug-induced pemphigus	IgG	Desmoglein 3, 1
IgA pemphigus Subcorneal pustular dermatosis type	IgA	Desmocollin 1

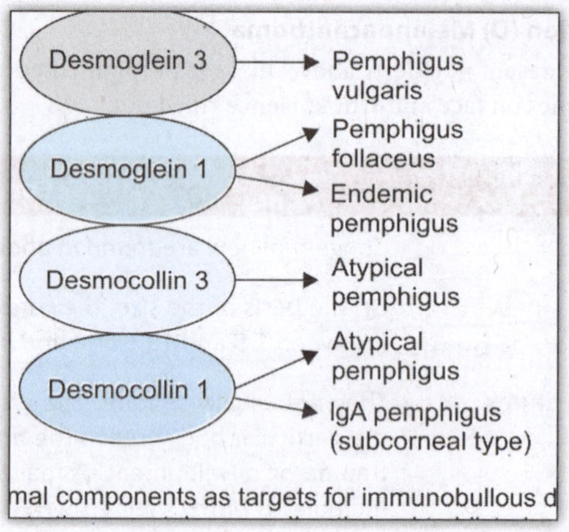

Desmosomal components as targets for immunobullous diseases. Antibodies to these proteins may directly lead to blistering skin and mucous membrane disorders

Also of importance to know here is to know desmosome compensation theory since the level of questions is rising every year in AIIMS.

Desmosomes Compensation Theory

The sites of blisters in pemphigus vulgaris and foliaceus are explained logically by the desmoglein compensation theory: Dsg1 and Dsg3 compensate for each other when they are coexpressed in the same cell. While patients with pemphigus foliaceus have only anti-Dsg1 IgG autoantibodies, individuals with the mucosal-dominant type of pemphigus vulgaris have only anti-Dsg3 IgG autoantibodies. Those with the mucocutaneous type of pemphigus vulgaris have both anti- Dsg3 and anti-Dsg1 IgG autoantibodies. Of note, the intraepithelial expression pattern of Dsg1 and Dsg3 differs between the skin and mucous membranes. In the skin, Dsg1 is expressed throughout the epidermis, but more

Contd...

Desmosomes Compensation Theory

intensely in the superficial layers whereas Dsg3 is expressed in the lower portion of the epidermis, primarily in the basal and parabasal layers. In contrast to the skin, Dsg1 and Dsg3 are expressed throughout the squamous layer of mucosa, but Dsg1 is expressed at a much lower level than Dsg3.

When sera contain only anti-Dsg1 IgG (which interferes with the function of Dsg1), blisters appear only in the superficial epidermis of the skin because that is the only area in which Dsg1 is present without coexpression of Dsg3. In the unaffected deep epidermis, the presence of Dsg3 compensates for the loss of function of Dsg1. Although the anti-Dsg1 IgG binds to mucosa, no blisters are formed, because of the coexpression of Dsg3. Thus, sera containing only anti-Dsg1 IgG cause superficial blisters in the skin without mucosal involvement, as is seen in patients with pemphigus foliaceus.

When sera contain only anti-Dsg3 IgG, they are inefficient in producing cutaneous blisters because coexpressed Dsg1 compensates for the impaired function of Dsg3, resulting in no, or only limited, skin lesions. However, in the mucous membranes, Dsg1 cannot compensate for the impaired Dsg3 function because of its low expression. Therefore, sera containing only anti-Dsg3 IgG cause oral erosions without apparent skin involvement, as is seen in patients with the mucosal-dominant type of pemphigus vulgaris.

When sera contain both anti-Dsg1 and anti-Dsg3 IgG, they interferewith the function of both Dsg1 and Dsg3, resulting in extensive blisters and erosions of the skin as well as the mucous membranes, as is seen in patients with the mucocutaneous type of pemphigus vulgaris. It is not clear why splits appear just above the basal layer instead of the whole epithelium falling apart. However, it is speculated that cell–cell adhesion in the basal and parabasal layers might be weaker than in other parts of the epithelium because there are fewer desmosomes. In addition, autoantibodies, which penetrate from the dermis, might have better access to the lower part of the epithelia.

22. Ans. (d) Atopic dermatitis

Ref: Fitzpatrick's Dermatology in general medicine, 8th edn. Pg: 165

Let's Discuss Option Wise

Option (A) Dermatitis herpetiformis

Presents in elderly individuals with small vesicles, pustules, papules and excoriation with extreme pruritus mainly on elbows, knees, buttocks, sacrum, shoulders, posterior hairline and scalp. Thus this option is ruled out on basis of age of the patient and distribution of lesions.

Option (B) Pemphigus

It mainly presents with flaccid bullae that rupture easily in elderly people with oral erosions. Hence this diagnosis is also ruled out.

Option (C) Psoriasis

It presents with silvery micaceous, scaly plaques mainly on knees, elbows, extensor aspects of limbs. Hence the option is also ruled out.

Option (D) Atopic Dermatitis

This is the answer in this question. Hints that favor diagnosis. The age of patient is pediatric age group, flexural preponderance, red itchy lesions favor an eczematous pathology.

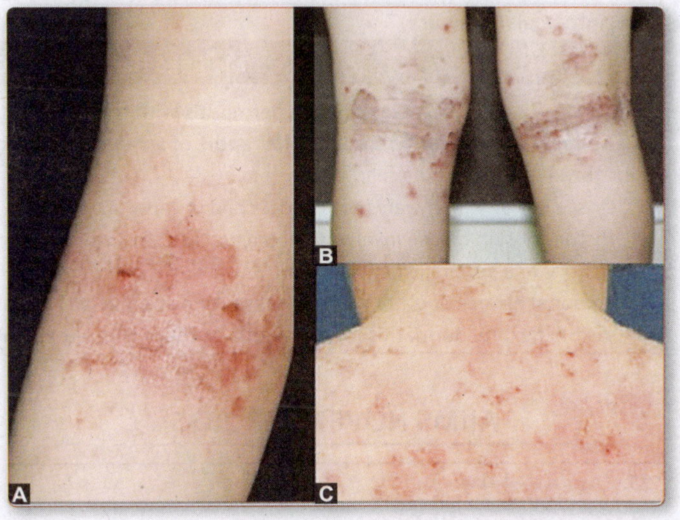

Fig: Atopic dermatitis (which is synonymous with atopic eczema) is an itchy, chronic, or chronically relapsing, inflammatory skin condition. The rash is characterized by itchy papules (occasionally vesicles in infants) which become excoriated and lichenified, and typically have a flexural distribution. The eruption is frequently associated with other atopic conditions in the individual or other family members.

Hanifin and Rajka Criteria of Atopic Dermatitis
3 major and 3 minor criteria need to be fulfilled

Major Criteria

1. Pruritus.
2. Typical morphology and distribution (flexural lichenification or linearity in adults and facial and extensor involvement in infants and children).
3. Chronic or chronically relapsing dermatitis.
4. Personal or family history of atopy (asthma, allergic rhinitis, or atopic dermatitis).

Contd...

Minor or Less Characteristic Features

1. Xerosis
2. Ichthyosis, palmar hyperlinearity or keratosis pilaris.
3. Immediate (type 1) skin test reactivity.
4. Elevated serum IgE.
5. Early age of onset.
6. Tendency toward cutaneous infections (esp. Staph. Aureus and HSV infection)/impaired cell mediated immunity.
7. Tendency toward nonspecific hand or foot dermatitis.
8. Nipple eczema
9. Cheilitis.
10. Recurrent conjunctivitis.
11. Dennie–Morgan infraorbital folds (bilateral symmetrical folds formed by two additional creases beneath the eyelids).
12. Keratoconus (conical cornea resulting from degenerative changes, leading to the cornea being pushed outwards due to intraocular pressure).
13. Posterior and anterior subcapsular cataracts (small opacities and translucent globules seen in the lens at the pole in front of the posterior or anterior capsule).
14. Orbital darkening (bluish to grayish periorbital pigmentation, possibly following chronic rubbing).
15. White dermographism/delayed blanch (development of a delayed white line on firm stroking of the skin, instead of the usual red line seen normally).
16. Facial pallor/facial erythema.
17. Pityriasis alba.
18. Anterior neck folds.
19. Itch when sweating.
20. Intolerance to wool or lipid solvents.
21. Perifollicular accentuation.
22. Food intolerance.
23. Course influenced by environmental/emotional factors.

Modified Hanifin Rajka Criteria of Atopic Dermatitis

In order to qualify as a case of atopic dermatitis with the UK diagnostic criteria, the child must have:

- **An itchy skin condition (or parental report of scratching or rubbing in a child)**

Plus three or more of the following:

1. Onset below age 2 years (not used if child is under 4 years)
2. History of skin crease involvement (including cheeks in children under 10 years)
3. History of a generally dry skin
4. Personal history of other atopic disease (or history of any atopic disease in a first degree relative in children under 4 years)
5. Visible flexural dermatitis (or dermatitis of cheeks/forehead and outer limbs in children under 4 years)

AIIMS NOVEMBER 2016

23. Ans. (a) 1 day

Ref: Andrew's 11th Ed page 119

Recall Bias

We particularly confirmed from students that neither the term "Post Herpetic Neuralgia" was provided in the question, nor it was framed as a case scenario of Post herpetic neuralgia. Some students got confused and recalled it as Post Herpetic neuralgia.

Drug Hypersensitivity Syndrome

- Phenytoin is known to cause a cutaneous drug reaction called as Drug Hypersensitivity syndrome
- Drug hypersensitivity syndrome (DHS) is an adverse idiosyncratic drug reaction characterized by a triad of fever, skin eruption, and internal organ involvement, and can be life threatening.
- Drugs most commonly associated with DHS include the aromatic anticonvulsant agents phenytoin, carbamazepine, and phenobarbital (which are cross-reactive), when it has been called the anticonvulsant hypersensitivity syndrome.
- DHS occurs most frequently on first exposure to the drug, with initial symptoms starting 1 to 6 weeks later. In patients with a history of DHS, re-exposure to the offending agent may cause development of symptoms within 1 day. DHS is not related to the dose or the serum concentration of the drug.

Clinical Features of DHS

- A mild to high fever ranging from 38°C to 40°C, and malaise, which can be accompanied by pharyngitis and cervical lymphadenopathy, are the presenting symptoms in most patients.
- A generalized exanthem occurs in approximately 85% of patients, usually simultaneously with the appearance of the fever or shortly thereafter. It often progresses from a macular erythema, which starts on the face, upper trunk, and upper extremities, to a dusky reddish and confluent papular rash that is pruritic. It can further progress to exfoliative dermatitis.
- Edema is a hallmark of DHS, particularly in a facial distribution.
- Atypical lymphocytosis with a subsequent prominent eosinophilia may occur during the initial phases of the reaction in up to 30% of patients.
- Liver abnormalities, presenting as elevated transaminases, alkaline phosphatase, prothrombin time, and bilirubin, are present in approximately 50% of patients; in some patients, development of severe hepatitis with jaundice may occur.
- Other organs, such as the kidney (interstitial nephritis, vasculitis), central nervous system (encephalitis, aseptic meningitis), or the lungs (interstitial pneumonitis, respiratory distress syndrome, vasculitis), may less commonly be involved.

Drug Reaction with Eosinophilia and Systemic Symptoms (DRESS Syndrome)
The characteristic (and according to some authors) diagnostic features of DRESS include: • Rash developing late (>3 weeks) after the inciting medication is started. It often occurs with the first exposure to the medication. • Long-lasting symptoms (>2 weeks) after the discontinuation of the causative drug. • Fever (over 38°C). • Multiorgan involvement. • Eosinophilia (>1500 absolute eosinophilia). • Lymphocyte activation (lymphocytosis, atypical lymphocytosis, lymphadenopathy). • Frequent reactivation of herpes viruses HHV-6, HHV-7, EBV, and cytomegalovirus.

Drugs associated with drug hypersensitivity syndrome	Drugs causing exanthematous eruption
Allopurinol Antibacterial agents [sulfonamides and related drugs (dapsone and sulfasalazine), minocycline, nitrofurantoin] Anticonvulsants (carbamazepine, lamotrigine, phenobarbital, phenytoin) Antiretroviral agents (indinavir, nevirapine) Terbinafine	Penicillin Ampicillin Sulfonamides Gentamycin Barbiturates Digitalis Phenothiazines NSAIDs Isoniazid Phenytoin Carbamazepine

24. Ans. (d) Lupus vulgaris

Ref: Rook's 9th ed page 4.19, Rook 8th ed page 31.11

The cinching clue in the question is central scarring and location on buttocks which are hallmark of lupus vulgaris

Let us rule out the options

Option (A) Tinea corporis

Although Tinea corporis occurs over gluteal region and is annular but it shows central clearing and never shows scarring.

Option (B) Annular psoriasis

It will be present with scaling and never scarring.

Option (C) Discoid lupus erythematosus

Although it can be annular with central scarring, it also presents with scales, pigmentation and is more common on sun exposed sites like face. In India Lupus is common below the Umbilicus.

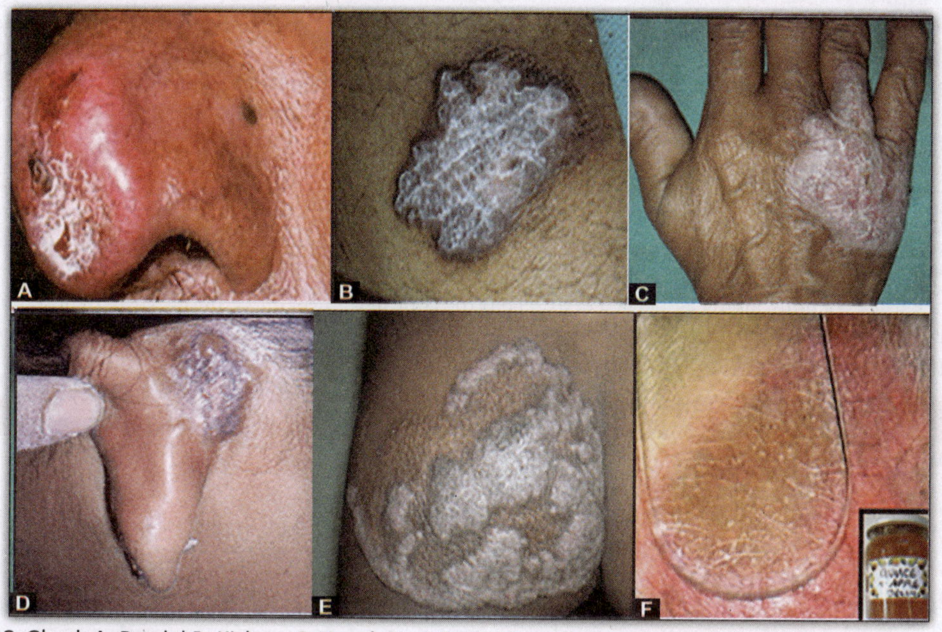

Credit: Pic A; Dwari BC, Ghosh A, Paudel R, Kishore P, Nepal, Pic B-E; Dr Mary Thomas, Dr Meryl Antony

Figs A to F: Lupus vulgaris: **(A)** Erythematous plaque type of lupus vulgaris on the dorsum of the nose; **(B)** Psoriasiform lupus vulgaris: Solitary plaque with silvery scaling; **(C)** Erythematous plaque type of lupus vulgaris on the dorsum of the hand; **(D)** Nodular lupus vulgaris on the retroauricular area; **(E)** Giant plaque of lupus vulgaris on the gluteal region; **(F)** Diascopy: Pressing a glass slide on the lesion conpresses the blood out of the small vessels. Diascopy is of particular value in detecting granulomatous nodule which have a translucent brownish color known as Apple jelly nodules (e.g. Lupus vulgaris, Sarcoidosis of skin). Note: It is not the Nodule shape of consistency which but the color on blanching which name it as Apple Jelly Nodule. Apple jelly color can be seen in insat for the reference

Cutaneous TB Classification		
Host immunity	**Method of inoculation**	**Disease**
Naive host	Direct inoculation	Tuberculous chancre (primary inoculation)
Multibacillary: Low host immunity		
	Contiguous spread	Scrofuloderma
	Autoinoculation	Orificial TB
	Hematogenous spread	Acute miliary TB, TB gumma
Paucibacillary or high host immunity		
	Direct inoculation	Tuberculosis verrucosa cutis, lupus vulgaris
	Hematogenous	Lupus vulgaris
Tubeculids		Lichen scrofulosorum, papulonecrotic tuberculid, erythema induratum of bazin

Lupus vulgaris:

- Most common form of cutaneous TB in India
- Most common site: In India it is **buttock > thigh > legs**, worldwide it is **face** (particularly around nose)
- **Clinical forms:** Psoriasiform, plaque, Nodular, ulcerative, vegetative, popular and tumor like
- Lupus vulgaris in advanced stages may show similarity with scarring lesions of DLE. Whereas fresh lesions of lupus vulgaris are characterized by reddish brown macule and papule of soft friable consistency and soft erythematous Nodule. A few surrounding nodules may appear and later coalesce to form a soft plaque
- Extension of the plaque is a slow process; gradually it becomes infiltrated and may show scaling. In the classical descriptions of lupus vulgaris, the presence of yellowish brown **apple-jelly nodules** at the edge of a plaque is often seen on diascopic examination
- The edges of the lesion gradually extend in some areas and heal with **atrophic central scarring.** Sometimes causing considerable tissue destruction over many years. The plaque is characterized by evidence of healing and atrophic scarring in some areas interspersed between areas of activity giving a **wolf bitten appearance** (Hence the name Lupus, Latin for wolf)
- Lupus vulgaris has a tendency to ulcerate, which is very uncommon in DLE
- Pigmentation is absent in lupus vulgaris which is common in DLE
- Mutilation of acral sites like nose and earlobes is a common feature of both Lupus vulgaris and DLE
- Lupus vulgaris of ear lobule is called **Turkey Ear** (Named after Istanbul, Turkey)

Scrofuloderma:

- Scrofuloderma results from the involvement and breakdown of the skin overlying a contiguous tuberculosis focus. This is usually a lymph gland, an infected bone or joint, or a lacrimal gland or duct.
- A bluish-red nodule overlying the infected gland or joint breaks down to form undermined ulceration with granulating tissue at the base. Numerous fistulae may intercommunicate beneath ridges of a bluish skin. Progression and scarring produce irregular adherent masses, densely fibrous in places and fluctuant or discharging in others. Excessive granulation tissue may give rise to fungating tumors. After healing, characteristic puckered scarring marks the site of the infection.

25. Ans: (a) Trichotillomania

Ref: Rook 8th Ed page 55.4

All the options are causes of nonscarring alopecia. Let us review the clinical features of common causes of nonscarring alopecia. Perifollicular lymphocytic infiltration is characteristic of Alopecia Areata but seen in both Alopecia Areata and Trichotillomania. However Perifollicular hemorrhage is seen only in Trichotillomania.

Causes of Alopecia	
Causes of scarring alopecia	
Lichen planus	Traction alopecia
DLE	Kerion, Favus (Tinea capitis, Herpes zoster)
Dermatomyositis	Tertiary syphilis
Radiodermatitis	Incontinentia pigmenti
Mechanical trauma	Ichthyosis
Postoperative (e.g. flap necrosis)	Epidermolysis bullosa
Burns	Central centrifugal cicatricial alopecia
Accidental alopecia	Acne keloidalis
Dermatitis artefacta	Acne necrotica
Scleroderma	Chronic graft-versus-host disease

Contd...

Causes of Alopecia
Causes of nonscarring alopecia
Androgenic alopecia Telogen effluvium (Surgery, vitamin and mineral def, anemia, weight loss, drugs) Anagen effluvium (Due to chemotherapy) Trichotillomania Alopecia areata Alopecia steroids (due to dandruff) Moth eaten alopecia (Top hairs spared, secondary syphilis)

Classical features of different types of nonscarring alopecia for purpose of exams and this question are as follows in the table?

Differential Diagnosis of Alopecia

	Androgenetic alopecia	Telogen effluvium	Alopecia areata	Trichotillomania
Clinical features	Males with decreased hair density over bitemporal and vertex of scalp; females with mid frontoparietal scalp involvement (widened hairpart, Christmas tree' pattern) but preservation of anterior hair line	Nonscarring alopecia with diffuse shedding of hair typically involving entire scalp, often due to a trigger. Triggers include pregnancy (typically 2–3 months after delivery), fever, chronic illness or severe stressor, diet or starvation, hypothyroidism, certain medications	Presents with round to oval alopecic non-scarring patches on scalp, 'exclamation mark' hairs; different patterns include patchy (most common), reticular, diffuse with generalized thinning, alopecia totalis (loss of entire scalp hair), alopecia universalis (loss of scalp and body hair), ophiasis pattern (band-like hair loss at periphery of temporal/occipital scalp). May have nail involvement (pitting most common)	Non-scarring alopecia due to habitual hair pulling typically in young girls, may be classified as obsessive compulsive disorder Presents with alopecia of varying lengths of broken hair in localized area over scalp, eyebrows, or eyelashes
Type of hairs seen on scalp	**Miniaturized hair, vellus hair, Thin hair**	**Telogen hairs**	**Exclamation mark hairs**	**Broken hair of different length are seen**
Trichogram	Increase in the proportion of follicles in telogen, which is probably consequent upon a shortened anagen phase	On trichogram or phototrichogram, more than 20%, and at times more than 50%, of hairs are found to be of the telogen type. On histopathology, the number of telogen hair follicles is substantially increased. The normal terminal: Vellus ratio of 7:1 is preserved in telogen effluvium (cf. AGA in which the terminal: Vellus ratio is <4:1).	Trichogram reveals a "mixed" telogen-dystrophic pattern and yellow dots on dermoscopy	
Histology	Vellus hair, telogen hairs, no inflammation	On histopathology, the number of telogen hair follicles is substantially increased.	A perifollicular lymphocytic infiltrate in a **"swarm of bees"** pattern is characteristic of the acute stage of the disease	Deformed hair shafts (trichomalacia), empty follicles, pigmented hair casts in follicles, ± perifollicular infiltrate or fibrosis, perifollicular hemorrhages

26. Ans: (b) Pemphigus vulgaris

Ref: Lever's Histopathology of the Skin 3rd ed Page 190

See Details of Pemphigus Vulgaris in AIIMS NOV 2018 Dermatology (see page no. 1053)

27. Ans. (c) Amiodarone

Ref: Rook's 8th Ed page 65.14

Drugs Causing Nail Hyperpigmentation (melanonychia and usually longitudinally multiple bands)		
Chemotherapeutic causes of melanonychia	**Other drug/agent-related causes of melanonychia**	
• Bleomycin sulfate	• Amodiaquine	• Mepacrine
• Busulfan	• Amorolfine	• Mercury
• **Cyclophosphamide**	• Arsenic	• Minocycline
• Dacarbazine	• **Chloroquine**	• Melanocyte-stimulating hormone
• Daunorubicin hydrochloride	• **Chlorpromazine (Blue grey)**	• Polychlorinated biphenyl (PCB)
• Doxorubicin	• Clofazimine	• Phenytoin
• Etoposide	• Clomipramine	• Phenothiazine
• 5-Fluorouracil	• Corticotropin	• Psoralen
• Hydroxyurea	• Cyclines	• Roxithromycin
• Imatinib (Diffuse)	• Diquat	• Steroids
• Melphalan hydrochloride	• Fluconazole	• Sulfonamide
• Methotrexate	• Fluoride	• Tetracycline
• Nitrogen mustard	• Gold salts	• Thallium
• Nitrosourea	• Ibuprofen	• Timolol
• Tegafur	• Ketoconazole	• Zidovudine
	• Lamivudine	

Drugs and their Effects on Nails	
ACE inhibitors	Captopril Onycholysis, Losartan Chromonychia, clubbing (reversible)
Antifungal	Ketoconazole: Longitudinal pigmented bands, splinter hemorrhages Itraconazole: Accelerated nail growth, longitudinal beading Fluconazole: Increased nail growth, longitudinal melanonychia
Aspirin	Purpura of the nail bed
AZT	Blue lunulae, diffuse hyperpigmentation of the nail plates, longitudinal or transverse melanonychia, paronychia, slow growth
Beta-blockers	Thickening and discoloration of nail plates, nail pits, Beau's lines, pterygium inversum unguis
Calcium channel blockers	Nail dystrophy
Cancer chemotherapy	Diffuse hyperpigmentation of nail plates, longitudinal and transverse melanonychia, transverse leukonychia, Mees' lines, transverse loss of nail plate, Beau's lines, onycholysis, nail shedding, subungual hyperkeratosis, paronychia, nail dystrophy, slow growth
Carbamazepine	Onychomadesis, longitudinal melanonychia
Cephalexin	Periungual inflammation, nail shedding
Chloroquine	Blue purple transverse nail bed pigmentation
Chloramphenicol	Onycholysis, photo-onycholysis
Cloxacillin	Nail shedding
Clofazimine	Brownish discoloration of the nail plates (reversible), subungual hyperkeratosis, onycholysis
Cyclosporine	Transverse leukonychia, nail pitting, increased nail growth
EGFR inhibitors	imatinib, PRIDE syndrome (paronychia), pyogenic granuloma-like lesions of the nail folds sorafenib, sunitinib, gefitinib, cetuximab
Fluoroquinolones	Photo-onycholysis, Beau's lines, subungual hemorrhages
Ibuprofen	Longitudinal melanonychia
Lamivudine	Paronychia, pseudopyogenic granuloma, longitudinal melanonychia
Mepacrine	Brownish discoloration of the nail beds, pitting, ridging or shedding of the nails
OCP	Increased nail growth, nail loss, photo-onycholysis in patients of porphyria cutanea tarda
Penicillamine	Absent lunulae, onychoschizia, longitudinal ridges, elkonyxis. Beau's lines, yellow nail syndrome
Phenytoin	(Use in pregnancy) Hypoplasia, anonychia or nail dystrophy in the newborn
Phenolphthalein	Nail plate ridges, blue lunulae

Contd...

Drugs and their Effects on Nails	
Psoralens	Photo-onycholysis, pain, splinter hemorrhages, longitudinal melanonychia, proximal nail plate pigmentation, Beau's lines, subungual hematomas
Salbutamol	Periungual erythema
Sirolimus	Chronic onychopathy, periungual infection
Sulfonamide (including dapsone)	Onycholysis, Beau's lines, partial leukonychia, slow growth, fixed drug eruption of periungual hypersensitivity tissues
Tetracycline	Photo-onycholysis, splinter hemorrhages, painful nails, nail pigmentation (with minocycline)
Thiazide diuretics	Onycholysis
Quinine	Photo-onycholysis
Vitamin A toxicity (Retinoids)	Brittle nails, thinning, softening, shedding, Beau's lines, onychoschizia, onychomadesis, elkonyxis, medial nail dystrophy, chronic (sometimes painful), paronychia, transverse leukonychia, 'curly' nails

28. Ans. (a) HPV 6, 11

Ref: Rook's Textbook of Dermatology 9th ed Page 56

This is typically a case of genital warts which is a sexually transmitted disease caused by HPV 6 and 11.

Genital wart/condyloma acuminatum: These lesions are soft, pink, pedunculated papilliferous masses (cauliflower like) with finger-like peduncles and an irregular surface. They are usually seen on moist, partially keratinized epithelium such as the preputial cavity, urinary meatus, labia minora, introitus, vagina, cervix, anus, an anal canal, but may affect intertriginous areas as well (groin, perineum, and anal area). Genital warts are a sexually transmitted infection (STI).

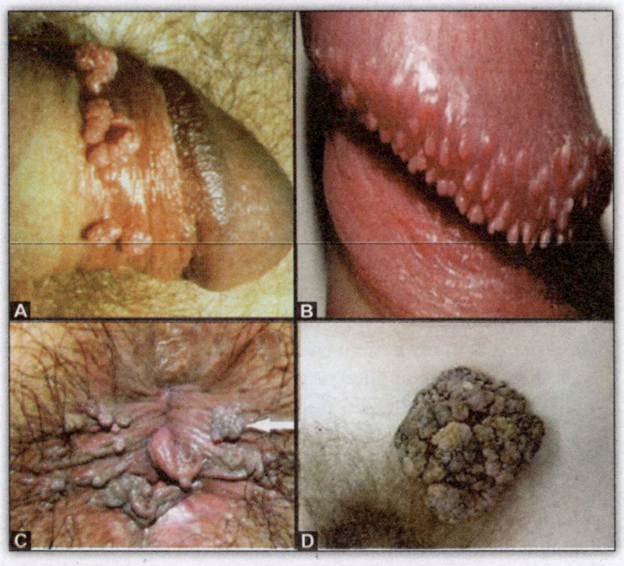

Fig: (A) Condyloma acuminatum or genital wart of the foreskin and shaft of penis; **(B)** Condyloma acuminatum or genital wart of the glans of penis; **(C)** Condyloma acuminatum or genital wart of the anal verge; **(D)** Buschke-Lowenstein tumor; Giant condyloma caused by human papillomavirus types 6 or 11 is a very rare variant. First described by Buschke and Löwenstein in 1925. Slow-growing, locally destructive verrucous plaque that typically appears on the penis but may occur elsewhere in the anogenital region

Etiology: The virus that causes genital warts is called human papilloma virus (HPV). Not all types of HPV cause genital warts. Most cases of infection with HPV cause no visible symptoms. Around 90% of all cases of genital warts are caused by two strains of the virus, type 6 and type 11. Genital warts are usually flat, papular, or pedunculated growths on the genital mucosa. Patients with visible warts may be infected simultaneously with oncogenic "high risk" HPVs such as types 16 and 18, which mostly give rise to subclinical lesions associated with intraepithelial neoplasia (IN) and anogenital cancer.

Recommended Regimens for External Genital Warts

Patient-Applied:
Podofilox 0.5% solution or gel OR
Imiquimod 5% cream OR
Sinecatechins 15% ointment
Provider–Administered:
Cryotherapy with liquid nitrogen or cryoprobe. Repeat applications every 1–2 weeks. OR
Podophyllin resin 10%–25% in a compound tincture of benzoin OR
Trichloroacetic acid (TCA) or Bichloroacetic acid (BCA) 80%–90% OR
Surgical removal either by tangential scissor excision, tangential shave excision, curettage, or electrosurgery.

AIIMS MAY 2016

29. Ans. (b) Molluscum contagiosum

Ref: Sternberg pathology 5th ed page 978, Bolognia 11th Ed page 1501

The clinical picture and histopathology is consistent with Molluscum contagiosum

See Details of Molluscum Contagiosum and Pox Virus in AIIMS Nov 2018 Dermatology (see page no. 1050)

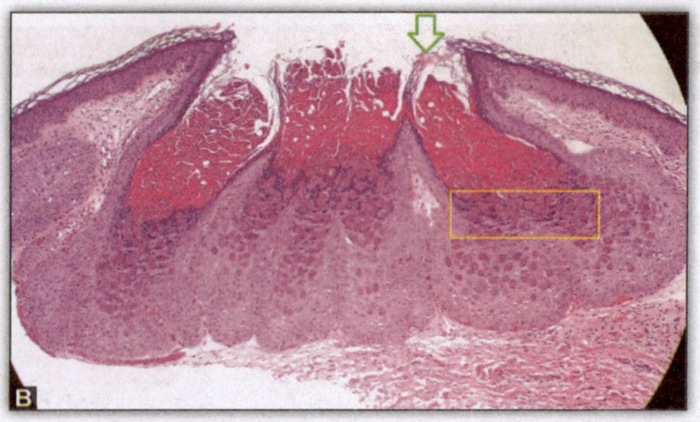

Fig: Histopathology of molluscum contagiosum:

- Pear shaped nodules of epidermis growing into the dermis as a closed packed lobule which on the surface appears as volcanic micro craters (green downwards arrow) separated by the epidermal lips of the crater.
- *Epidermal acanthosis*; increased thickness of surrounding epidermis (yellow rectangle)

30. Ans. (c) Tinea cruris

Ref: IADVL Textbook 2nd Ed page 262

See Details of Tinea cruris in AIIMS MAY 2017 Dermatology (see page no. 1064-1065)

31. Ans. (c) Patch test

Ref: Rook's 8th Ed page 26.93

This is a case of photo allergic contact dermatitis. Following clues in the question help us arrive at the diagnosis

- **Farmer by occupation:** Susceptible to both sunlight and allergans which are distributed in environment
- **Lesion morphology:** Itchy popular lesions indicate an allergic reaction
- **Location:** V area of neck and face indicate sun exposed site and localization indicate role of sunlight
- Increase in summer again indicate role of certain allergens which may be more common in summers and of sunlight

Let's Rule Out Options

Option (A) IgE Levels

Although it may point towards an allergic cause, but won't pinpoint photoallergic reaction of sensitizing agent.

Option (B) Skin Biopsy

The major use of a skin biopsy in photodermatoses is to differentiate PLE from lupus erythematosus, and Actinic Reticuloid from mycosis fungoides. It has no role in photo-allergic dermatoses.

Option (C) Patch Test

This test is diagnostic for photoallergic contact dermatitis.

Option (D) Serology

These are especially useful in the diagnosis of porphyrias and systemic lupus erythematosus.

To Establish the Diagnosis of a Photodermatosis

The diagnosis of a photodermatosis is based on the history and clinical examination and is further confirmed by pathologic examination of the lesions, phototests and photopatch tests.

- History is an important clue to the diagnosis of a photodermatoses. Many patients are able to relate their disease to light exposure.
- The distribution of the rash is of paramount importance in making a diagnosis of photodermatoses. The rash is most often sharply demarcated and limited to the light exposed parts of the body like the forehead, bridge of the nose, upper cheeks, chin, rims of ears, back, sides and 'V' of the neck, upper chest, dorsa of hands and feet, and extensor (actually dorsolateral) aspects of arms, and depending on the attire, sometimes on the lower extremities. Characteristically, sparing occurs under the hair fringe, below the eyebrows, on the upper eyelids, below the nose, the lower lip and below the chin, behind the earlobes, and in the web spaces of the fingers. The depths of the skin folds are invariably spared.
- Though the morphology of the primary and secondary skin lesion is not always pathognomonic, some guess to the diagnosis can be made by the following findings:
  - Patients with PLE present with itchy, often eczematous plaques.
  - Patients with photosensitive lichenoid eruption present with small shiny, often hypopigmented papules.
  - Patients with hydroa vacciniforme develop papules surmounted with vesicles leading to varioliform scars.
  - Patients with solar urticaria develop pruritic evanescent wheals, which sometimes become confluent.
  - Subacute lupus erythematosus is characterized by nonitchy, scaly, erythematous edematous malar plaques.
  - Patients with erythropoietic protoporphyria complain of a severe burning sensation initially with no visible features, i.e. the symptoms are out of proportion to the signs.

Patch Test

Patch testing is the gold standard for identification of a contact allergen to diagnose Photoallergic contact dermatitis. Because it was impractical to test unlimited number of allergens, standardized panels of allergens have been designed. Although standardized panels, which include relatively few of all known allergens & many patients need additional testing. The patches of chemicals are applied as for ordinary patch testing, except that they are applied in duplicate and both sets are covered with an opaque material. Only one set of tests is read at 48 hours (to indicate the presence of ordinary contact dermatitis or a primary irritant reaction) and then irradiated with 5–15 J/m^2 of UVA. The irradiated side is covered again and at 96 hours both sides are evaluated.

Day Zero

The first appointment will take about half an hour. Tiny quantities of 25 to 150 materials in individual square plastic or round aluminum chambers are applied to the upper back. They are kept in place with special hypoallergenic adhesive tape. The patches stay in place undisturbed for 48 hours.

Day 2

At the second appointment, Patch test results should be read at 2 days unless discomfort occurs earlier. Since 30% of reactions are negative at 2 days, additional reading(s) should be performed at 4, and sometimes 7 days after the initial application, depending on the allergen.

Day 4

These marks must still be visible at the third appointment, usually two days later (4 days after application) to rule out false positive and to give extra time for false negatives.

32. Ans. (d) Cholinergic urticaria

Ref: Roxburgh 17th ed page 71-75; Fitzpatrick's 6th ed page 1181-1203; Rooks 7th ed page 47.1-47.29

The question states that there is urticarial on exposure to sunlight. Both solar and cholinergic urticarias are physical urticarias. Other provocative symptoms like emotions and spicy food points towards Cholinergic Urticaria. Also to differentiate these urticarias, provocation tests are performed.

Cholinergic urticarial	Solar urticarial
Cholinergic urticaria is a very distinctive type in which characteristic small wheals appear in association with sweating. It accounts for about 5% of urticaria, and lesser degrees are common in adolescents. Whealing occurs on stimulation of sweating, whether induced by a rise in core temperature, emotion or gustatory stimuli.	Wheals develop at the site of exposure within minutes of visible, long- or short-wave ultraviolet radiation and usually fade within 2 hours
Raising the core body temperature by 0.7–1.0°C by: • Exercise in a hot environment until sweating • Hot bath (42°C) for 15 minutes induce itching within minutes, with widespread small wheals. In an individual patient, either method may be more successful. In exercise-induced anaphylaxis, only the exercised induced challenge will be positive.	Exposure to sunlight or solar simulator induces redness, itching wheals at site of exposure within a few minutes lasting less than 1 hour. Exposure to a monochromator can determine the individual wavelengths that induce whealing

33. Ans. (a) Borderline lepromatous leprosy

Ref: IADVL Textbook, 2nd Ed, P- 2032

Lets Discuss Option Wise

Option (B) Borderline Tuberculoid

The lesions are well-defined infiltrated plaques whose number varies from 3 to 10. The margins may be well defined and raised in a part of the lesion, flat and vague in another. They have a tendency for a break in borders and the development of satellite lesions.

Option (C) Mid borderline

It is characterized by widespread bilateral but asymmetrical erythematous infiltrated plaques with a punched out or annular appearance. The plaque is depressed in the center and has a sharp inner edge and a sloping outer border.

Option (D) Lepromatous

The initial lesions are bilaterally symmetrical macules. Initially there may not be any loss of sensation. With progression lesions become shiny papules and nodules which are infiltrated and may be located on ear lobed and give lion faced appearance. The nerves may become bilaterally thickened and also anesthetic.

From this description we can rule out that this is not a case of either three. Now let us look at borderline lepromatous leprosy

- Tendency towards symmetrical spread as evident by macules all over trunk and extremities
- Bilateral involvement of nerves
- The lesions may be multiple annular erythematous plaques or macules which show hypoanesthesia.

Ridley-Jopling Classification of Leprosy

The Ridley-Jopling classification is based on clinical (Skin and nerve involvement), histopathological, bacteriological (bacteriological/morphological index in skin and nasal smear), and immunological (lepromin test) parameters. It is mainly based on histopathology, reflecting the immunological status of an individual patient and consists of a 5-group system

	Tuberculoid leprosy (TT)	Borderline tuberculoid (BT)	Borderline borderline (BB)	Borderline lepromatous (BL)	Lepromatous leprosy (LL)
Hypopigmentation	+	+	+	+	+
No. of lesions	<3	3–10	Numerous but countable	Numerous & uncountable	Numerous & uncountable
Symmetry	Unilateral asymetrical	Unilateral asymetrical	Bilateral but asymetrical	Bilateral & symetrical	Bilateral & symetrical
Anhydrosis, sensory loss & hair loss	Complete loss	Impaired	Decreased	Slightly decreased	Normal
Types of lesion	Macules or plaques (0.5–30 cm).	Plaques	Plaques	Macular, annular plaques or nodule	Early macules and late nodules

Contd...

Lesion	Mostly single (or 2–3) Asymmetrical and usually unilateral. Erythematous, raised edges central flattening. Loss of sensation hair and sweeting, the surface is dry, rough, and irregular, and the lesions feel firm on palpation. Thickened nerves may be palpable	Most common presenting form of leprosy. Well defined infiltrated plaques. Margins raised or flat well defined or vague in parts. The surface is dry and anhidrotic. Lesions may also be hypopigmented, slightly erythematous macules	Features of both TT & LL. Widespread bilateral but asymmetrical erythematous infiltrated plaques with a punched out or annular appearance. Plaque is ***depressed in the center and has a sharp inner edge and sloping outer border***. Lesions are of varied sizes, bizarre shapes with irregular borders and may have **geographic appearance.**	Lesions tend to be more widespread than BB but are not as symmetrical as in lepromatous leprosy. The nodular or punched out plaques lesions. Diffuse infiltration of pinna and eyebrows seen in LL start making their appearance in BL leprosy.	**Early Macules**: numerous, small (<2 cm), bilaterally symmetrical, smooth, shiny, ill-defined macules, hypopigmented, erythematous or coppery. **Late Nodules:** macules enlarge and coalesce. The lesions are bilaterally symmetrical and smooth surfaced with sloping edges. If a patient is not treated at this stage, the skin becomes more infiltrated and assumes a **waxy appearance.**
Satellite lesion	Absent	Present	Absent	Absent	Absent
Site	Any site but preferable sites are face, lateral or dorsal aspects of the extremities, and the buttock	Any site	Any site.	More at the sites of LL	Face including nose, ear. Nose: **saddle nose,** epistaxis, Anosmia, discharge, **Larynx**: hoarseness, stridor, asphyxia, tongue and palate, neuritis, iritis, orchitis. Deformity & ulceration of hands, feet,
Sensations	Anesthetic macule	Anesthesia is less severe than TT	Anesthesia is less than BT	Anesthesia is often absent	Sensations of touch and pain (pin-prick) are usually unimpaired
Nerve thickening	Thick or tender nerve trunks and nerve to lesion	Thickened or tender or both	Thickened or tender or both	Thickened or tender or both	Multiple thickened nerves
Lepromin test	+++	++ or +	Variable + or –	—	—
Cutaneous nerve	Destroyed/swollen	Cellular infiltrate	Cellular infiltrate	Infiltrate	Cutaneous nerve preserved
Granuloma	Compact/ tuberculoid granuloma eroding epidermis	Tuberculoid granuloma but less well defined	Diffuse epithelioid granuloma	Granuloma composed of lymphocytes & macrophage	Thin epidermis, flat rete ridges, diffuse lepoma of foamy macrophages, plasma cells & lymphocytes
Acid fast bacilli	AFB are not found except in areas of caseation	AFB may still be found in the nerve	AFB are easily detectable and numerous	AFB = as numerous as in LL	AFB are seen in large numbers in macrophages, nerves & skin appendages
Grenz zone (clear zone b/n epidermis & dermis)	Absent	Present	Present	Present	Present

Contd...

Slit smear (AFB)	No AFB	Nil to scanty	Moderate	Many	Numerous + globi
Lepra reactions	Lepra I	Lepra I	Lepra I	Lepra I & II	Lepra II
ENL				ENL+	ENL+
Comments		Satellite lesion	Punched out lesion, Inverted saucer lesion, Swiss chease pattern lesion	Onion peel appearance of nerves	Leonine facies, Oil paint appearance on face, Onion peel appearance of nerves, Most infectious stage

Indian classification
- Tuberculoid
- Borderline tuberculoid
- Mid borderline
- Borderline lepromatous
- Lepromatous
- Pure neuritic type

WHO classification
- For treatment purposes, in 1982, the who study group on chemotherapy of leprosy for control programs classified leprosy into two types: paucibacillary (PB) (including the tuberculoid, indeterminate, and borderline tuberculoid forms), and multibacillary (MB) (including lepromatous, borderline lepromatous, and midborderline forms)
- Pure neuritic has not been classified
- A simple classification based on the number of lesions has been recommended for use by field workers: 1–5 lesions as paucibacillary, and 6 or more as multibacillary leprosy
- All slit skin smear positive cases are MB

34. Ans. (a) Alopecia areata

Ref: Rook's 8th Ed page 66.13

The clinical picture of a male presenting with non scaring patchy bald spots is consistent with Alopecia areata.

See Table of Differential Diagnosis of Alopecia in AIIMS Nov 2016 Dermatology (see page no. 1073)

AIIMS NOVEMBER 2015

35. Ans. (c) Lichen planus

Ref: Rook dermatology 8th ed page 41.1

Clues in the Question are

- **Bilateral reticulate white streaks** is very characteristic of **wickham's striae** seen in lichen planus.
- Dental amalgams are known to predispose to lichen planus

Symptoms of burning on intake of spicy food can occur in all the mentioned options, so let's rule out the options.

Option (A) Oral Candida

The characteristic sign of this condition is a sharply defined patch of creamy, crumbly, curd like white pseudomembrane, which, when removed, leaves an underlying erythematous base. This membrane consists of desquamated epithelial cells, fibrin, leukocytes and fungal mycelium that attaches it to the inflamed epithelium. Present in preterm babies, immunocompromised conditions such as AIDS.

Option (B) Recurrent Aphthous Stomatitis (RAS)

It is characterized by recurring episodes of ulcers, typically from childhood or adolescence, each lasting from 1 to about 4 weeks before healing. Aphthae typically are multiple round or ovoid ulcers with a circumscribed margin, erythematous halo and a yellow or grey floor.

Option (D) Leukoplakia

The World Health Organization defines leukoplakia as a white patch or plaque on the mucosa that cannot be rubbed off and that is not recognized as a specific disease entity, which implies a diagnosis of exclusion (e.g. of LP, candidosis). The term is also used irrespective of the presence or absence of epithelial dysplasia, although there is a small malignant potential to some keratoses. Leukoplakia is common in adults: around 1% are affected, although some populations show higher prevalences. Most cases are seen in the 50–70 age group.

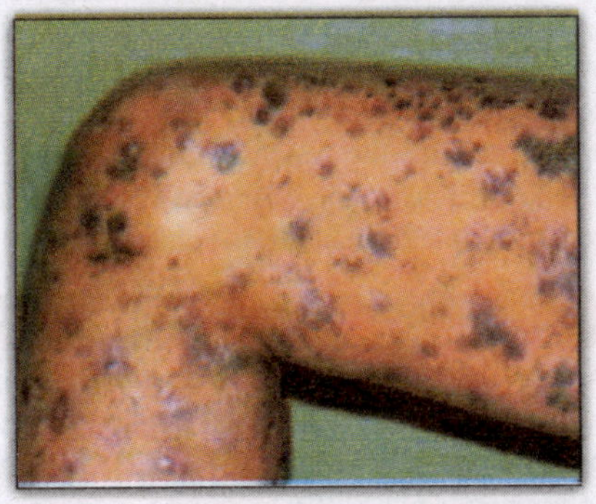

Fig: Typical plaques of lichen planus: Pruritic, Polygonal, Purple (Violaceous), Plain (flat) topped papule and Plaque (Mnemonic 5P)

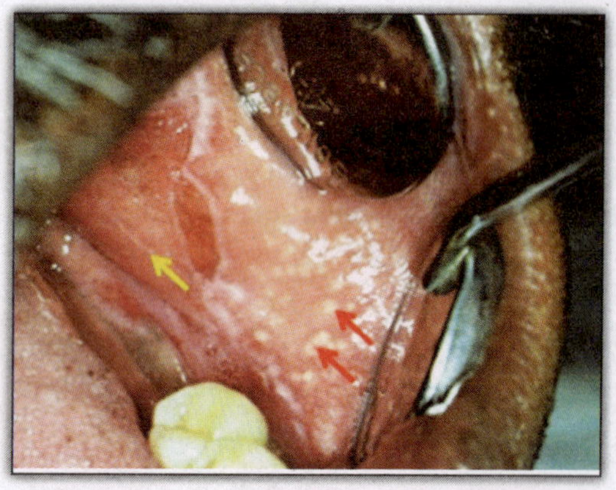

Fig: Wickham Striae in Lichen Planus of left buccal mucosa: Note the while lacy pattern AKA- Wickham striae posteriorly (yellow line) and the Fordyce granules anteriorly (red arrow), which appears as a small yellow nodule

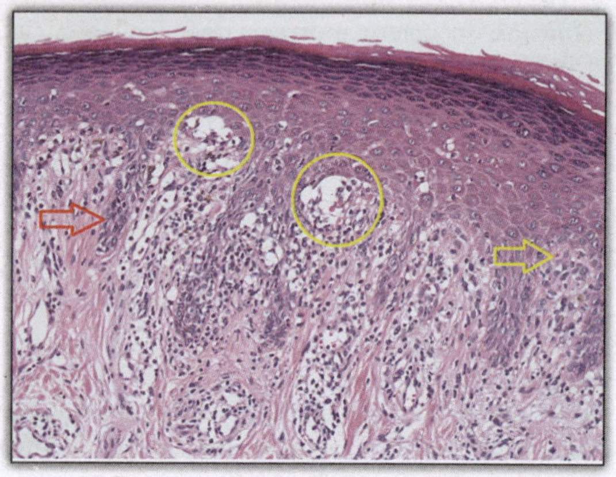

Fig: Histopathology of Lichen Planus

- The primary features are hyperkeratosis without parakeratosis, focal increases in the granular cell layer, irregular acanthosis with a **"sawtooth" appearance of Rete Ridges** (Red arrow), Basal epidermal liquefactive degeneration and a band-like lymphocytic infiltrate at the dermal– epidermal junction.
- Apoptotic or dyskeratotic keratinocytes (also referred to as **Civatte, hyaline or cytoid bodies**) are usually present in the basal layer (Yellow arrow tip)
- Subepidermal Lichenoid Band due to deposition of lymphocytes and histiocytes
- Vacuolar changes within the basal cell layer may become confluent and result in small separations between the epidermis and the dermis (called **"Max-Joseph spaces"** - yellow circles). There is often incontinence of pigment with multiple dermal melanophages.

Lichen Planus

Lichen planus (LP), is self-limiting, papulosquamous prototype of lichenoid dermatoses, is an idiopathic inflammatory disease of the skin and mucous membranes. Classic LP pruritic, polygonal, purple (Violaceous), plain (flat) topped papule and plaque (Mnemonic 5P) that favor the extremities.

Contd...

Lichen Planus	
Pathogenesis	LP represents T-cell-mediated autoimmune damage to basal keratinocytes that express altered self-antigens on their surface. CD8 cell is the major effector cell
Etiology	• **Unknown but associated with** ▪ **HCV**: In several case–control studies, the prevalence of HCV (3.4–38%) was 2 to 13.5-fold higher in patients with LP than in control. Of the various types of LP, it is the oral form that is most commonly viewed as a manifestation of HCV infection ▪ Vaccines ▪ *H. pylori* bacteria ▪ **Contact allergens:** Dental amalgams, heavy metals ▪ Drugs ▪ Autoantigens
Cutaneous	Typical plaques of lichen planus: pruritic, polygonal, purple (Violaceous), plain (flat) topped papule and Plaque (Mnemonic 5P). Although the Koebner phenomenon (i.e. isomorphic response) is commonly seen in LP, excoriations and impetiginization are unusual. Face is generally spared.
Oral mucosal	• Oral LP can appear in at least seven forms, which occur separately or simultaneously: atrophic, bullous, erosive, papular, pigmented, plaque-like and reticular. • The most common and characteristic form of oral LP is the **reticular.** It is characterized by slightly raised whitish linear lines in a lace-like pattern **"Wickham's striae"** or in rings with short radiating spines. This form is usually asymptomatic and the most common site of involvement is the **buccal mucosa**; lesions are often bilateral and symmetric. • Gingival involvement is common, and oral LP affecting the gingivae exclusively is seen in approximately 10% of cases. It typically presents as chronic desquamative gingivitis
Types	Hypertrophic, atrophic, guttate (eruptive), annular, linear, vesiculobullous, follicular or lichen planopilaris, ulcerative (erosive), lichen planus pigmentosus, actinic or lichen planus subtropicus, lichen planus pemphigoides
Nail	Pterygium (diagnostic), onychorrhexis, thinning
Genital	Annular shaped genital mucosal lesion
Scalp	Scarring alopecia
Treatment	Steroid is the mainstay of treatment

36. Ans. (b) Chronic atrophic candidiasis

Ref: Rook's 8th Ed page 69.88

"Chronic atrophic candidiasis, also known as chronic erythematous candidiasis appears as raw red lesion, not whit patchy lesion"

Oral Candidiasis

- Up to 50% of the healthy population harbor *Candida albicans* as an oral commensal. Carriage is more common in cigarette smokers. Candida resides particularly on the posterior dorsum of the tongue.
- Infection is likely to result from xerostomia, local disturbance in salivary flora such as occurs during broad-spectrum antimicrobial treatment, or depressed immune responses.
- Of the several clinical presentations of oral candidiasis, only **thrush, candida leukoplakia and chronic mucocutaneous candidiasis present as white lesions; the other types, acute and chronic atrophic candidiasis, are red.**

Type of Candidiasis and Predisposing Factors	
Acute pseudomembranous candidiasis (thrush)	Any local: Dry mouth, antimicrobial. General: Corticosteroids, leukemia, HIV
Acute atrophic candidiasis ('antibiotic mouth: antibiotic sore mouth)	Any Broad-spectrum antibiotics or corticosteroids
Erythematous candidiasis	Any, HIV especially
Chronic atrophic candidiasis (denture-related stomatitis)	Adults denture wearing, especially at night
Chronic hyperplastic candidosis (candidal leukoplakia)	Usually middle-aged or elderly tobacco smoking, denture wearing, immune defect
Median rhomboid glossitis	Third or later decades Tobacco smoking, denture wearing, HIV
Chronic mucocutaneous candidosis	Usually first decade often immune defect; rarely endocrinopathy

37. Ans. (b) TEN

Ref: Bolognia 10th Ed, page 356

Recall Bias

Most of the recallers believe that this was not an image based question. Few were of the opinion that it was an image based question. Anyways we have provided a Pictures for future Image based question.

See table of "EM- SJS- TEN COMPLEX" in AIIMS NOV 2018 Dermatology (see page no. 1051)

This is a case of drug reaction due to anti convulsant. Since there is history of wide spread skin peeling, it is most likely to be a case of Toxic epidermal necrolysis (TEN)

Clues are:

- Temporal course with the drug (time lag after drug intake)
- Widespread skin peeling
- Sparing of palms and soles
- Non recurrent nature of lesions, hence unlikely to be fixed eruption.

Fixed Drug Reaction	
Adverse drug reaction appearing soon after ingestion of offending drug (30 minutes to 8 hours, average 2 hours). Reoccurs at fixed site again and again In previously sensitized individuals	
Lesion	Mucocutaneous junction (**Lip, glans**). Glans is the MC site. Begins as a red patch that soon evolves to an iris or target lesion similar to erythema multiforme Occurs ***repeatedly at the same site*** (Fixed) Mostly **solitary** but can be multiple (mostly <6) Usually asymptomatic. Symptomatic on erosion Macule → papule → vesicle → bullae → erosion **Heals by Hyperpigmentation**
Offending Drugs	
NSAIDS	Aspirin, Paracetamol, Ibuprofen, Oxyphenbutazone, Phenazone, Metamizole
Antibiotics	**Sulfonamides (Cotrimoxazole, Dapsone), TETRACYCLINE**, Penicillins, Ampicillin, Amoxicillin, Erythromycin, Fluconazole, Fluoroquinolones, Nystatin, Griseofulvin, Arsenicals, Mercury, PAS, Thioacetazone, Quinine, **Metronidazole**
Barbiturates and tranquil-lizers	Barbiturates, Chloral Hydrate, Opium, Benzodiazepine, Dextromethorphan, Anticonvulsants
Phenolphtha-lein and related	**Phenolphthalein**, Codeine, Hydrazine, Oleoresins
Miscellaneous	Sympathomimetics, Sympatholytics, Food Flavors, Magnesium Hydroxide, Hyoscine,

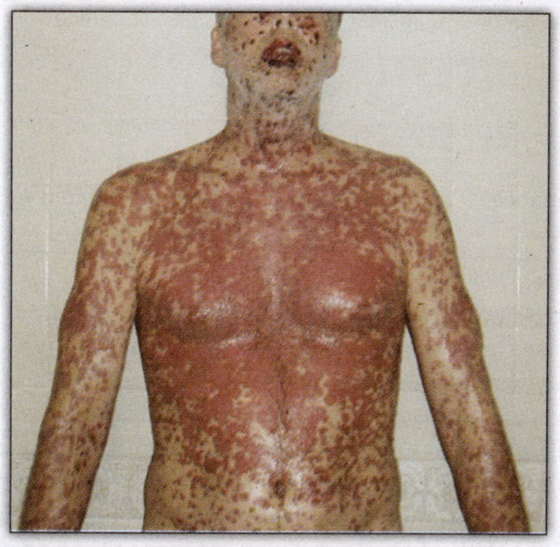

Fig: Stevens-Johnson Syndrome Note there is no exploitation of epidermis. Targetoid lesions on the trunk of patient, as well as the mucosal involvement on the lips

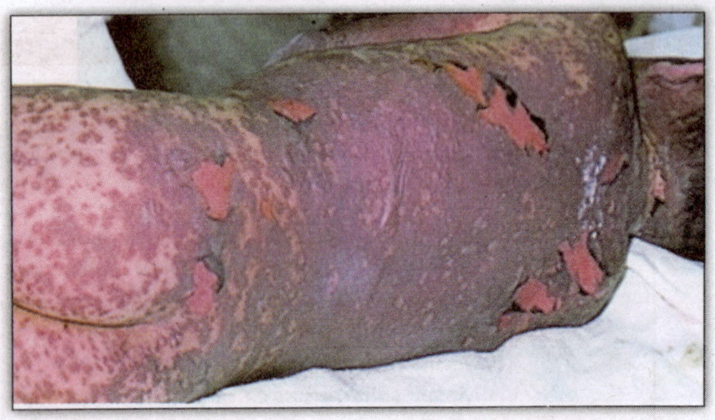

Fig: Toxic Epidermal Necrolysis The initial bullae have coalesced, leading to extensive exfoliation of the epidermis. Scattered apoptotic keratinocytes in the basal and suprabasal layers of the epidermis immediately. In later stages: sub-epidermal cleavage covered with confluent necrosis of the whole epidermis. There is a thrifty/ mild perivascular inflammatory infiltrate, especially consisting of lymphocytes. Immunopathology: variable numbers of lymphocytes (CD 8+) and epidermal macrophages, lymphocytes (CD4 +) in the papillary dermis.

38. Ans. (c) Pox virus

Ref: Bolognia 11th Ed page 1501

Repeat AIIMS NOV 2018 Dermatology (See for explanation) (see page no. 1082)

This condition is molluscum contagiosum. The clues in the question are typical presence of pearly white papules. If you notice the image properly, some of them show a central umbilication, which is also a typical feature of molluscum contagiosum and by history of presence in immediate family members, indicate contagious nature. Molluscum contagiosum is caused by Pox group of viruses.

39. Ans. (a) Oral isotretinoin

Ref: Rook's 8th Ed page 42.33

The question states nodulocystic acne which is a severe form of acne, in a young boy with oily skin. Therefore the drug of choice is oral isotretinoin.

General Guidelines for Treatment of Acne

	Mild acne (No comedones, no inflammatory lesions, some papules and/or pustules)		Moderate acne (Many inflammatory papules, pustules, 1–2 nodules and/or scarring)		Severe acne (>2 nodules, cysts, abscesses, bridging scars)
	Comedonal	**Papular pustular**	**Papular/pustular**	**Nodular**	**Nodular/conglobate**
1st choice	Topical retinoid	Topical retinoid + topical antimicrobial	Oral antibiotic + topical retinoid ± BPO	Oral antibiotic + topical retinoid ± BPO	Oral isotretinoin
2nd choice	Alternate topical retinoid or azelaic acid or salicylic acid	Alternate topical antimicrobial + alternate topical retinoid Or azelaic acid	Alternate oral antibiotic + alternate topical retinoid ± BPO	Oral isotretinoin or Alternate oral antibiotic + alternate topical retinoid ± BPO/azelaic acid	High-dose oral antibiotic + topical retinoid + BPO
Alternative for females	See 1st choice	See 1st choice	Oral antiandrogen + topical retinoid/azelaic acid ± topical antimicrobial	Oral antiandrogen + topical retinoid ± oral antibiotic ± alternate antimicrobial	High-dose oral antiandrogen + topical retinoid ± alternate topical antimicrobial
Maintenance therapy	Topical retinoid	Topical retinoid + BPO			

Footnote:

- **Benzoyl peroxide** gel has a potent bacteriostatic effect, with a reduction in lesion count as early as after 4 days of application. It also reduces the size and number of comedones present and inhibits sebum secretion.
- **Salicylic acid** penetrates into the sebaceous gland and has comedolytic and anti-inflammatory effects. It can be used as adjunctive therapy and is used in cleansers, toners, masks, and peels.
- **Azelaic acid** has antimicrobial, anti-inflammatory and comedolytic activity and it is relatively non-irritating.
- **Topical retinoids** may be used for correcting abnormal follicular keratinization leading to microcomedones. They include:
  - **Tretinoin** not only corrects follicular keratinization but also thins the stratum corneum, which may potentiate the penetration of other topical agents. It can be irritating to the skin but this can be minimized by the correct method of application.
  - **Adapalene** is nonphotodegradable and nonphototoxic and can be used simultaneously with benzoyl peroxide due to its milder irritation potential.

Contd...

- **Tazarotene** 0.05% gel has a higher potential for irritation that can be minimized when applied as short contact therapy. It is suitable for individuals with oily skin.
- **Topical antibacterials** may be used for the initial several weeks of therapy along with topical retinoids or benzoyl peroxide especially when pustules are present.
- **Oral antibiotics** like doxycycline, minocycline, and azithromycin have antibacterial and anti-inflammatory actions. However, if there is no response after adequate antibacterial therapy or if recurrence is prompt and troublesome after stoppage, sebostatic agents may be used.
- **Sebostatic agents:**
  - Hormonal therapy may be used in unresponsive young women not desiring conception.
  - Isotretinoin is also sebostatic and is usually used in men but can be administered to women if adequate care is taken to prevent pregnancy

40. Ans. (d) Aspergillus

Ref: Neena Khanna 4th ed page 285

See details of Dermatophytes in AIIMS MAY 2017 Dermatology (see page no. 1065)

The itchy lesion in picture is a typical dermatophyte infection, and its known **Jock's itch** or Tinea cruris. It is also known as **Dhobi's itch**. Since it is a dermatophyte infection, it cannot be caused by Aspergillus.

41. Ans. (a) TT Leprosy

Ref: IADVL 2nd Ed page 2033

The clinical picture and histopathology picture is consistent with tuberculoid leprosy.

See Table of "Ridley Jopling Classification of Leprosy" in AIIMS MAY 2016 Dermatology for Clinical Correlation (see page no. 1077)

Hints in the question:
- Solitary/single patch
- Anesthetic patch
- Ulnar nerve thickening

Microscopy: All sites of involvement have granulomatous lesions closely resembling those found in tuberculosis, and bacilli are almost never found, hence the name "paucibacillary" leprosy. The *presence of granulomas and absence of bacteria reflect strong T-cell immunity.*

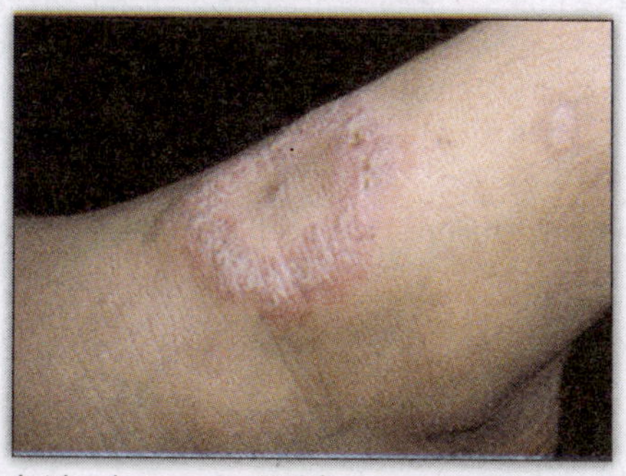

Fig: Tuberculoid leprosy (TT)/ paucibacillary Morphology: Tuberculoid leprosy begins with localized flat, red skin lesions that enlarge and develop Saucer right up (side up) lesion: Annular lesion with indurated elevated hyperpigmented margins and depressed pale centers (central healing). Sharp outer edge and vague inner edge that slopes towards the center of the lesion. Neuronal involvement dominates tuberculoid leprosy. Nerves become enclosed within granulomatous inflammatory reactions and, if small (e.g., the peripheral twigs), are destroyed

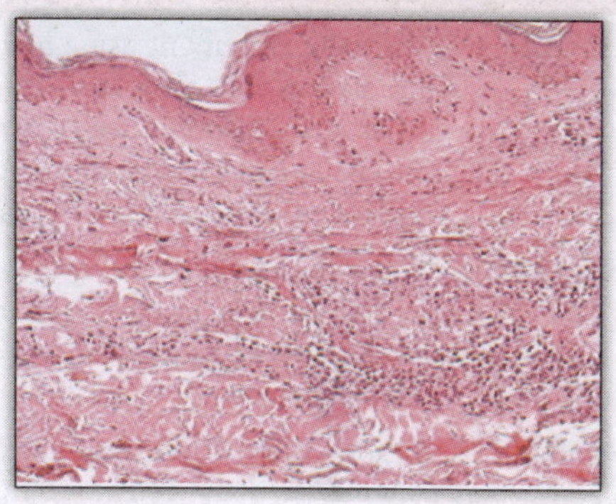

Fig: Granulomatous inflammation in the dermis is composed of epithelioid cells surrounded by T cells

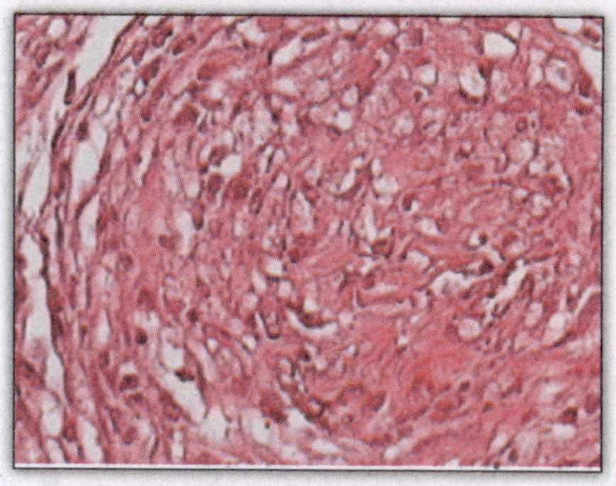

Fig: Granuloma in tuberculoid leprosy, showing foamy histiocytes arranged in a concentric pattern

42. Ans. (b) Topical tretinoin

Ref: IADVL 2nd ed page 760

The diagnosis is straight forward. Depigmented macules on skin. It is a case of vitiligo.

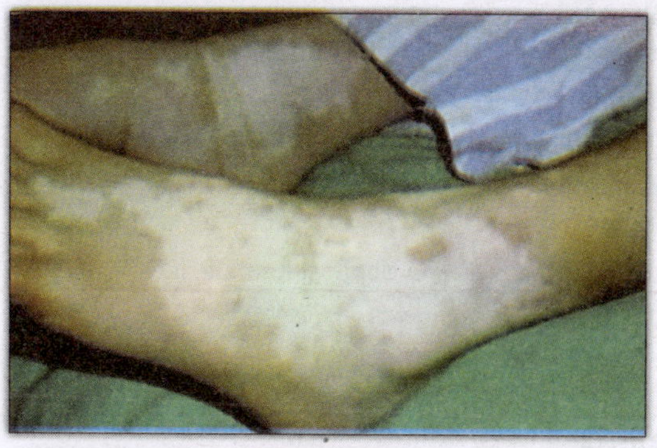

Fig: Vitiligo

Vitiligo versus Leprosy		
	Vitiligo	**Leprosy**
Lesion	Depigmented, no change in texture, non scaly	Hypopigmented, infiltrated and raised, scaly
Hair in the patch	Depigmentated	Number may be decreased
Sensation	No loss	May be impaired
Nerve	No thickening	May be thickened

Treatment Options for Vitiligo	
Psoralen and UVA therapy	Topically, treatment using a combination of psoralen derivatives or other photosensitizing agent, followed by irradiation with long wave ultraviolet light constitutes photochemotherapy. When it uses the psoralen group of drugs with long wave UV irradiation (320–400 nm wavelength), then it is called as PUVA therapy. It is called PUVASOL therapy when sun exposure is utilized as the source of UVA. 5-Methoxypsoralen and 8-methoxypsoralen are naturally occurring whereas 4,5,8 trimethylpsoralen (TMP) is synthetic.
Topical PUVA therapy	As a general rule, if the vitiligo macule is less than 6 sq. cm in size, usually 0.1% can be applied weekly followed 2–3 hours later by solar UVA irradiation for 30 to 60 seconds. The time of exposure can be generally increased by 30 seconds per sitting and the frequency to biweekly or triweekly sittings until the patch becomes slightly erythematous.
Oral PUVA therapy	Oral psoralen therapy should preferably be with long-term TMP administration. The treatment is begun with 0.6 mg/kg/body weight (40 mg for a patient of 70 kg body weight) of TMP ingested with food 2 hours before sun exposure, preferably between 11 am and 1 pm. Initially the exposure should be for 5 minutes availing approximately 3 joule/sq. cm of UVA. The exposure time is gradually increased until erythema beginning about 12–18 hours after exposure, and maximal at 48 hours is achieved after each exposure, with twice a week treatment
Narrow band UVB	Narrow band UVB therapy is now considered the treatment of choice for stable vitiligo. Narrow band fluorescent bulbs of Philips TL-01, each of 100 W with an emission spectrum of 311 nm, are used.
Excimer Laser	The 308-nm xenon chloride excimer laser is an effective and safe modality for the treatment of chronic stable vitiligo, with good results achieved in a relatively short duration of time
Khellin with UVA exposure	
Phenylalanine with UVA exposure	
Calcipotriol with PUVA therapy	Calcipotriol is a vitamin D analogue that could act in vitiligo by playing a role in calcium regulation by 1,25 dihydroxy vitamin D3 receptors on melanocytes and/or by the regulation of defective calcium homeostasis.
Other agents	Topical application of pseudocatalase and calcium chloride with short-term suberythemogenic UVB
Topical corticosteroids	With the current view of vitiligo as an autoimmune disorder, a number of corticosteroid preparations in different forms and routes (topical, intralesional and oral) have been used in the treatment of vitiligo with encouraging results. Topical corticosteroids have virtually become the first line of treatment for patients with a few localized lesions. Potent fluorinated corticosteroids yield results when used for a period of 2 to 4 months, but side effects may develop, in which case treatment needs to be interrupted.
Topical calcineurin inhibitors	The use of topical calcineurin inhibitors (viz. tacrolimus and pimecrolimus) has been advocated considering the autoimmune hypothesis of vitiligo pathogenesis
Basic fibroblast growth factor	
Placental extract preparation	
Other oral therapy	Cyclophosphamide, levamisole. azathioprine, oral corticosteroids, oral cyclosporine, azathioprine

AIIMS MAY 2015

43. Ans. (a) Lichen nitidus

Ref: Rook's 8th Ed page 41.21-41.23, Fitzpatrick's 8th Ed page 312-316

Repeat May 2014 (Without picture and option D was Molluscum contagiosum)

Please note the classical description, multiple, shiny, discrete, pin shaped (read small) papules in a young boy on typical location of shaft of penis, dorsal surface of hands and forearms. This description fits classically with Lichen nitidus

Lets Rule Out the Options.

Option (B) Lichen Planus

Typically flat topped, violaceous, pruritic, papules and plaques seen on the flexor surface of arms and extensor surface of limbs.

Option (C) Scabies

Intensely itchy excoriations and burrows seen on the anterior surface of wrist, web spaces, genitals. The burrows may look like papules, but they are not shiny.

Option (D) Lichen Scrofulosorum

Rare tuberculid that presents as a lichenoid eruption of minute papules in children and adolescents with tuberculosis. The lesions are usually asymptomatic, closely grouped, skin-colored to reddish-brown papules, often perifollicular and are mainly found on the abdomen, chest, back, and proximal parts of the limbs.

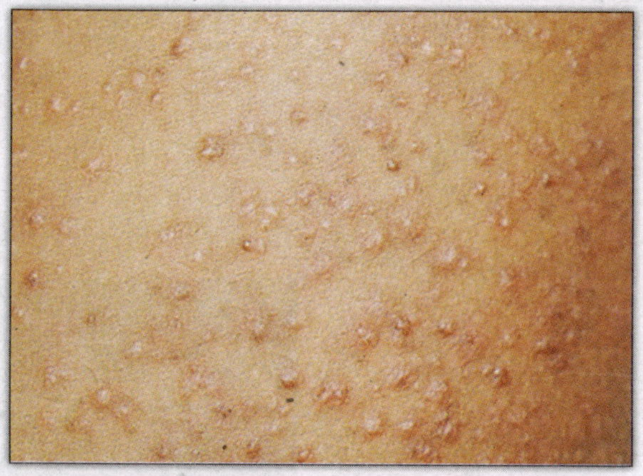

Fig: Shiny discrete pin head sized papules seen in lichen nitidus

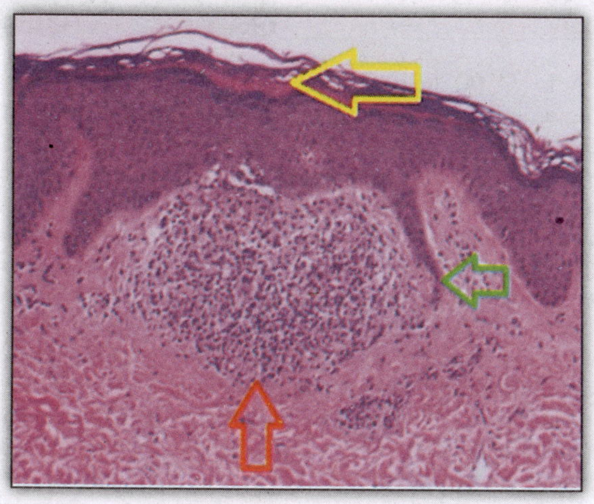

Fig: Histology of lichen nitidus showing parakeratosis (yellow arrow), well-defined granuloma (red arrow) nfiltrate composed of lymphocytes, epithelioid cells and occasional Langhans giant cells, enclosed by hyperplastic rete ridges (Green arrow) giving the appearance of "claw clutching a ball" on scanning magnification (H and E, ×40). Similar resemblance can be seen in histology of early lesions of juvenile xanthogranuloma (JXG) and lichenoid eruptive histiocytoma. Occasionally, micropapular lichen planus and tuberculoid leprosy may show such appearance, although with shorter "claws."

Lichen Nitidus (LN)	
Lichen nitidus (LN) is an idiopathic lichenoid dermatosis clinically characterized by a monomorphic eruption of asymptomatic, minute, skin-colored papules	
Children and young adults are the usual sufferers	
Usual sites: Common sites of involvement are the forearm, penis (glans and shaft), buttocks, lower abdomen & chest. Some cases may have a generalized distribution.	Description of lesions Individual lesions of LN are flesh-colored, pinpoint to pinhead-sized, flat to dome-shaped, shiny, discrete papules
Other features: Koebnerization may be present. The lesions are usually asymptomatic, but rarely mild to intense pruritus may be associated. Healing occurs without scarring or pigmentary changes.	
Types: Linear, spinous, vesicular, follicular, perforating, hemorrhagic and actinic	
Mucous membrane is spared, i.e. Wickham Striae is not seen. (Note; Mucous membrane is involved in Lichen Planus)	

44. Ans. (a) Drugs

Ref: Bolognia 3rd Ed, P- 355, Neena khanna 4th ed page 83

There are two hints in the question which leads us to the diagnosis

- >30% body surface involvement
- History of bullae
- Erosions of the lips

The diagnosis of this condition is toxic epidermal necrolysis.

See table of "EM- SJS- TEN COMPLEX" in AIIMS NOV 2018 Dermatology (see page no. 1051)

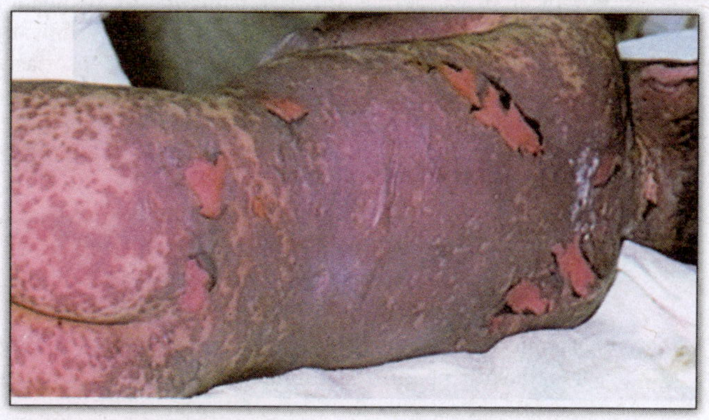

Fig: Toxic epidermal necrolysis. The initial bullae have coalesced, leading to extensive exfoliation of the epidermis. Scattered apoptotic keratinocytes in the basal and suprabasal layers of the epidermis immediately. In later stages: sub-epidermal cleavage covered with confluent necrosis of the whole epidermis. There is a thrifty/mild perivascular inflammatory infiltrate, especially consisting of lymphocytes. Immunopathology: variable numbers of lymphocytes (CD 8+) and epidermal macrophages, lymphocytes (CD4 +) in the papillary dermis.

45. Ans. (a) Cyclosporine

Ref: Bolognia 3rd Ed page 2242, IADVL 2nd Ed page 1054, Roxburgh's 18th ed page 148-150, Fizpatrick 7th ed page 959-960

The clinical picture is consistent with pustular psoriasis of pregnancy AKA impetigo herpitiformis.

Cyclosporine is the drug of choice in pregnancy. As retinoids, PUVA and Methotrexate are contraindicated in pregnancy, cyclosporine and/or steroid is used. Localized disease is treated by topical steroid while generalized disease is treated by systemic steroid. Systemic steroid should be avoided in routine care of Psoriasis, because the disease requires progressively higher dose and withdrawal of steroid is associated with relapse into more severe forms.

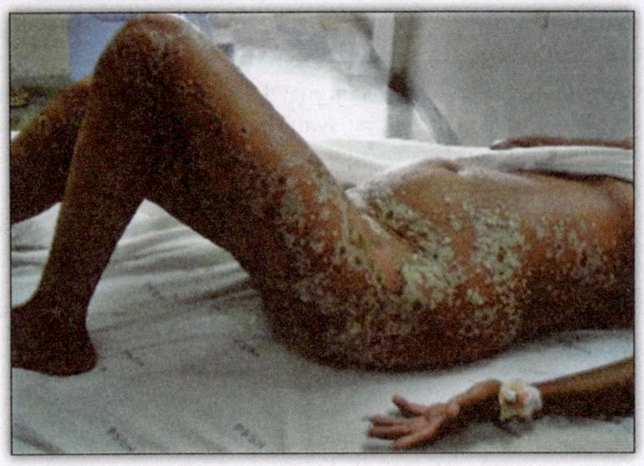

Impetigo Herpetiformis

Erythematous, scaly, figurative lesions, with pustules on the periphery on the trunk in pregnancy is consistent with Impetigo herpetiformis. It is a rare dermatosis of pregnancy with typical onset during the last trimester of pregnancy and rapid resolution in the postpartum period. Clinically and histologically, it is consistent with pustular psoriasis. This similarity has led some authors to name the disease "the pustular psoriasis of pregnancy.

Treatment Modalities for Pustular Psoriasis

- **Oral retinoids:** Drug of choice. It is teratogenic and hence absolutely contraindicated in pregnant women
- **Cyclosporine:** Second line treatment for pustular psoriasis. Cyclosporine is not teratogenic, and it is classified as a pregnancy prescribing category C drug. Use during pregnancy should be considered only in exceptional patients for whom the potential benefits of cyclosporine therapy dramatically outweigh the risks.
- **Oral corticosteroids:** Used in pustular psoriasis. They are pregnancy category C.

Use of corticosteroids in psoriasis: Although dramatic in short-term effectiveness, they are not recommended for psoriasis because of their toxicity and the propensity of the disease to recur in a more severe form on cessation of therapy. However it is used in

- Erythrodermic psoriasis
- Severe generalized plaque psoriasis
- Acute exacerbation while changing to other agents or waiting for them to take effect
- Both corticosteroids and ciclosporin can be used in pustular psoriasis in pregnancy.

46. Ans. (a) Bullous pemphigoid

Ref: Rook's 8th Ed, page. 40.26

The clinching point in the question are itchy tense blisters on normal skin and urticarial plaques. The tense blister is seen in sub epidermal blistering disorder.

Bolognia says, ***characteristically, bullous pemphigoid is an intensely pruritic eruption with widespread blister formation. In early stages, or in atypical variants of the disease, only excoriated, eczematous or urticarial lesions (either localized or generalized) are present.***

Rook's 8th Ed says, ***Bullous pemphigoid commonly starts with itching and a non-specific rash on the limbs that may be either urticaria-like or occasionally eczematous and rarely may simulate vesicular eczema. Blisters may arise on erythematous and on normal skin and may be associated with dermal edema. The blisters are tense and dome shaped, obtaining a diameter of many centimeters.***

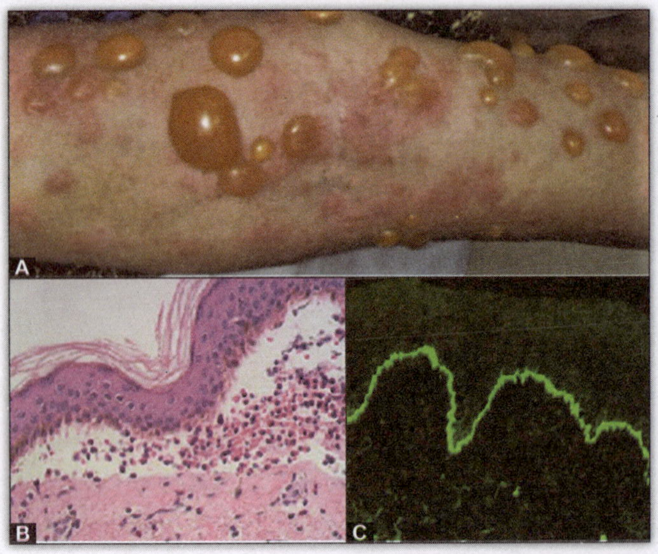

Figs A to C: (A) Bullous Pemphigoid clinical picture: intensely pruritic eruption with widespread blister formation. Erythematous plaques covered with large, tense blisters with clear fluid, located symmetrically on the flexural site of the upper limbs, the trunk, the cervical region and the lower limbs, an erosion of 2-3cm diameter on the anterior thorax covered by hematic crust, erythematous plaques with clearly defined edges, covered with pearly white scales, located in the sacral region; hypochromic plates located on the posterior sites of the upper limbs and the lower limbs, atrophic skin covered by fine scales on the lower limbs; **(B)** Bullous Pemphigoid Histopathology: There is a subepidermal blister and a superficial, perivascular infiltrate predominantly of eosinophils and neutrophils. There are numerous eosinophils within the blister cavity. The adjacent epidermis is irregularly hyperplastic with prominent hypergranulosis and compact orthokeratosis; **(C)** Bullous pemphigoid - direct immunofluorescence: Homogenous, linear deposition of IgG in the basement membrane at desmoepithelial junction

47. Ans. (b) Post-kala-azar dermal leishmaniasis

Ref: Harrison's 19th ed page 1391

Although from the first look, this looks like a case of lepromatous leprosy, but normal sensation and no thickened nerves go against the diagnosis.

Case: A 50-year-old man from Mymensingh district, Bangladesh, presented with a 3-month history of nonpruritic, painless hypopigmented papules, and plaques, beginning on the face and subsequently spreading to the forearms, torso, and legs. Fifteen months before the onset of skin lesions, the patient had visceral leishmaniasis (kala-azar), successfully treated with 30 intramuscular injections of sodium stibogluconate (SSG). Polymerase chain reaction showed Leishmania donovani DNA in a buffy coat specimen.

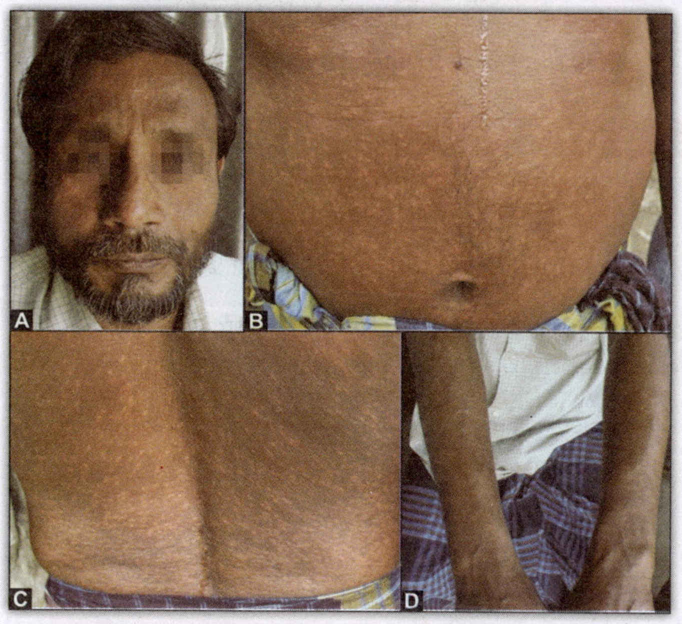

Figs A to D : This is a case of post-kala-azar dermal leishmaniasis: **(A)** The patient has hypopigmented papules and plaques over the face, most concentrated on forehead, peri-orally and on the cheeks, common areas of involvement for post-kala-azar dermal leishmaniasis (PKDL); **(B)** Hypopigmented papules on the abdomen; **(C)** Hypopigmented papules are seen on the back. The lesions are roughly symmetrical, a common characteristic of post-kala-azar dermal leishmaniasis (PKDL), and are painless and non- pruritic; **(D)** The patient has hypopigmented papules and plaques on both forearms. The absence of sensorineural changes helps to distinguish post-kala-azar dermal leishmaniasis (PKDL) from leprosy, which commonly presents with hypopigmented macules or patches associated with hypoesthesia or anesthesia, and neural thickening

Cutaneous Lieshmaniasis	
Types	• Old world cutaneous leishmaniasis (syn. oriental sore, biska button, delhi boil, baghdad boil) • Disseminated cutaneous leishmaniasis (syn. leishmaniasis cutis diffusa leproid, cheloid leishmaniasis, leishmaniasis cutanea pseudolepromatosa) • American cutaneous and mucocutaneous leishmaniasis • Visceral leishmaniasis (syn. kala-azar) and post-kala-azar dermal leishmaniasis (syn. dermal leishmanoid)

Contd...

Cutaneous Lieshmaniasis	
Infectious agent and vector	L. major, L. tropica, L. aethiopica, and L. infantum. Vector : Infected sandfly P. papatasii and P. sergenti
Reservoir	Humans, canines of the dog family, rodents. In India, the zoonotic reservoir is the desert gerbil.
Clinical features	**Cutaneous leishmaniasis**: The skin is the usual site of entry for the promastigotes. Nodules which may ulcerate with crateriform or cribriform scar. Satellite lesions present. Sporotrichoid spread present. Distribution of lesions on exposed sites. **Visceral leishmaniasis,** also known as kala-azar, is characterized by irregular bouts of fever, substantial weight loss, swelling of the spleen and liver, and anemia (which may be serious). If the disease is not treated, the fatality rate in developing countries can be as high as 100% within 2 years
Diagnosis and treatment	Demonstration of parasite on smear Leishmanin test Histopathology showing amastigotes Culture on NNN Medium

Post-Kala-Azar Dermal Lieshmaniasis	
Infectious agent	L. infantum (Mediterranean area, Middle East, Northern Africa, and China), L. chagasi (South America), and L. donovani (India, East Africa, and parts of China).
Reservoir	For L. infantum and L. chagasi, the reservoir is usually dogs and other canines, whereas in L. donovani the reservoir is man.
Vector	P. argentipes
Clinical features	Post-kala-azar dermal leishmaniasis (PKDL) is a complication of visceral leishmaniasis (VL) in areas where Leishmania donovani is endemic; it is characterized by a hypopigmented macular, maculopapular, and nodular rash usually in patients who have recovered from VL. Two types of morphological lesions are usually seen, the early hypopigmented macules and the later nodular lesions. It usually appears 6 months to 1 or more years after apparent cure of the disease but may occur earlier or even concurrently with visceral leishmaniasis especially in the Sudan. PKDL heals spontaneously in the majority of cases in Africa but rarely in patients in India. It is considered to have an important role in maintaining and contributing to transmission of the disease particularly in interepidemic periods of VL, acting as a reservoir for parasites. Systemic features may be seen. Generalized lymphadenopathy may be seen.
Diagnosis	Histopathology of skin may show the amastigote and clinch the diagnosis or may help to differentiate it from the other conditions such as leprosy, fungal infections, leucoderma, syphilis, yaws, and keloid.

48. Ans. (b) Acne rosacea

Ref: Rooks 8th ed page 43.1- 43.10, Roxburgh 18th ed page 172-178, Bolognia 2nd Ed, P- 595

Repeat AIIMS Nov 2014 (One option was different; photodermatitis in place of DLE)

The given image can lead to two main differentials; Acne vulgaris and Acne rosacea. However the clinching points which favor the diagnosis of Acne rosacea are exacerbation on sweating, sun exposure and emotional disturbance.

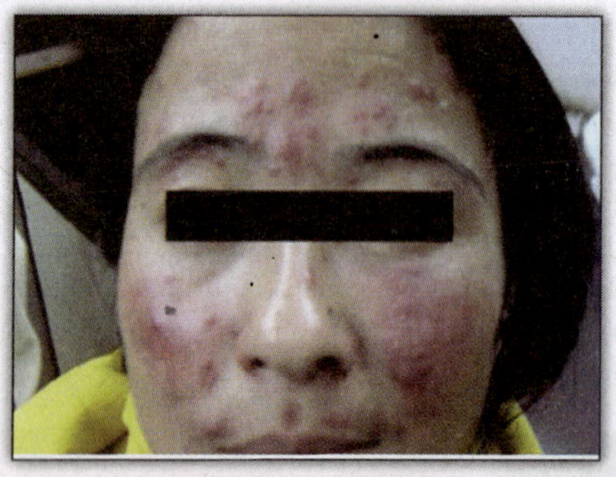

© MedEasy © Dr Ishad Aggarwal IPGIMER Kolkata

Acne Rosacea

- Chronic inflammatory condition of facial pilosebaceous units with increased vascular hyperreactive
- Common in fair-skinned patients with peak in the third to fifth decade
- Presents with easy flushing and gradual reddening of complexion
- Exacerbating factors may include particular foods (especially spicy), alcoholic beverages, UV exposure, hot weather, warm beverages, and exercise.
- ***Unlike Acne vulgaris, Acne rosacea are exacerbation on sweating, sun exposure and emotional disturbance etc.***

Histology	Early lesions with dilated blood and lymphatic vessels; later lesions show lymphectasia, perivascular and perifollicular lymphohistiocytic infiltrate, ± poorly organized granulomas, dermal fibrosis, sebaceous gland hyperplasia, ± Demodex folliculorum mites within infundibula.	
Type	**Predominant Feature**	
Erythematotelangiectatic	• Persistent centrofacial erythema • Flushing • Telangiectasias • Skin sensitivity	
Papulopustular	• Persistent centrofacial erythema • Papules • Pustules/papulopustules • Overlap with other subtypes may occur	
Phymatous	Thickened, nodular skin • Prominent pores • Can affect nose (rhinophyma, most common), chin (gnathophyma), forehead (metophyma), ears (otophyma), eyelids (blepharophyma) • May be associated with other features of rosacea or occur in isolation	
Ocular	• Dry, gritty sensation • Blepharitis • Conjunctivitis • Chalazion and hordeolum • Keratitis, episcleritis, scleritis, iritis (rare)	
Treatment	**Skin care regimen**	Sunscreen, moisturizer containing humectant, avoid cosmetics and toners and harsh exfoliation, avoid triggers
	Topical therapy	Metronidazole or azelaic acid best for inflammatory lesions, sodium sulfacetamide/sulfur
	Oral therapy	Tetracyclines, macrolides, isotretinoin
	Lasers	Pulsed-dye laser or intense pulsed light
	Surgical ablation	Phymatous lesions

49. Ans. (d) BB leprosy

Ref: IADVL textbook of Dermatology 1st ed page 2034, Neena khanna 4th ed page 266

Option (B)

The skin lesions of the BL subgroup resemble the LL form, tending to occur in a large number, but not so symmetrical and with loss of sensation in some areas.

Option (C)

The skin lesions of the BT subgroup resemble the TT form in terms of appearance and loss of sensitivity, but they occur in a larger number and are smaller. Nerve thickening tends to be irregular, less intense and appears in a larger number.

Option (D)

The presence of erythematous plaques with **fading outer borders, clear inner borders, and hypopigmented oval center (foveal spot) is suggestive of the BB subgroup.** BB leprosy is the immunologic midpoint in the fascinating clinical spectrum of the granulomatous disease. It is the most unstable and uncommon form. These patients upgrade or downgrade to a more stable clinical form at the earliest. Cutaneous lesions are characteristically annular plaques with sharp interior and exterior borders. Large plaques with islands of clinically normal skin within the plaques give rise to a **"Swiss cheese" appearance.** Lesions are numerous but are asymmetrical.

NOTE

Determining the type of leprosy is not based on clinical features alone. It involves the histological, bacteriological and immunological facets too, and these objectives seemed to have been met with in Ridley-Jopling classification.

See Table of "RIDLEY-JOPLING CLASSIFICATION OF LEPROSY" in AIIMS MAY 2016 Dermatology for Clinical Correlation (see page no. 1077)

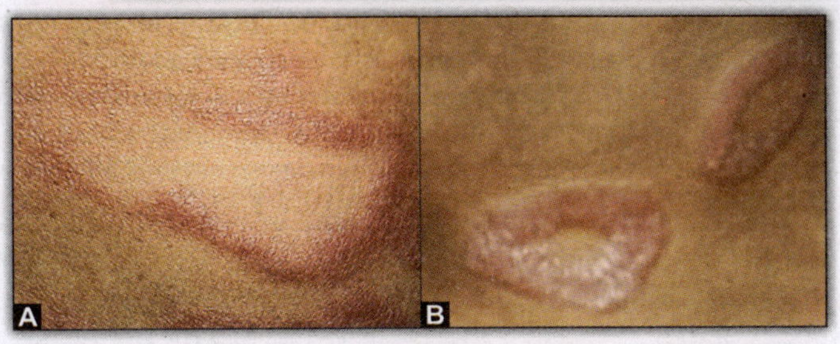

Figs A and B: Borderline Leprosy: (A) The presence of erythematous plaques with ***fading outer borders, clear inner borders, and hypopigmented oval center (foveal spot) is suggestive of the BB subgroup***. BB leprosy is the immunologic midpoint in the fascinating clinical spectrum of the granulomatous disease. It is the most unstable and uncommon form. These patients upgrade or downgrade to a more stable clinical form at the earliest. Cutaneous lesions are characteristically annular plaques with sharp interior and exterior borders. Large plaques with islands of clinically normal skin within the plaques give rise to a **"Swiss cheese"** appearance. Lesions are numerous but are asymmetrical. **(B)** Total Annular lesion: with both inner and outer edges being sharp and clear cut consistent with BB Leprosy

Type of lesion	Top view	Side view	Seen in
Saucer right up (side up) lesion: Annular lesion with a sharp outer edge and vague inner edge that slopes towards the center of the lesion	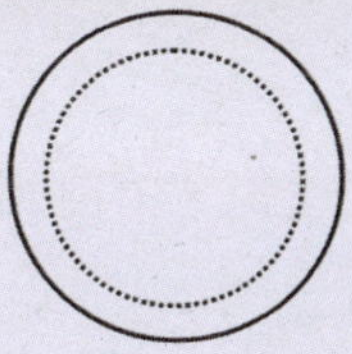	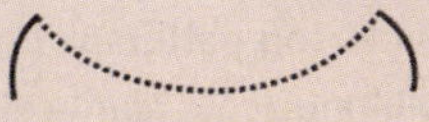	TT, BT Leprosy
Punched out lesion/Swiss cheese: Annular lesion with sharp central punch with clear inner but vague and sloping outer edges	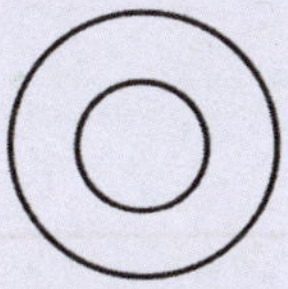	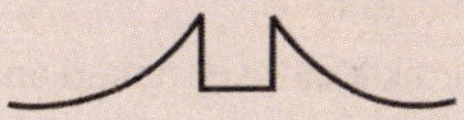	BB Leprosy
Total Annular lesion: With both inner and outer edges being sharp and clear cut	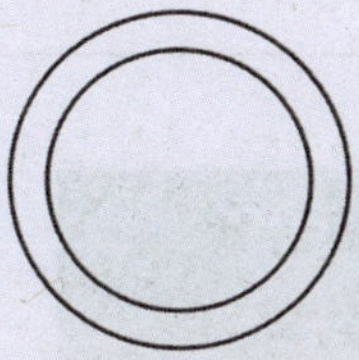		BB Leprosy
Inverted saucer lesion: A dome shaped lesion with central infiltration and gradual peripheral sloping	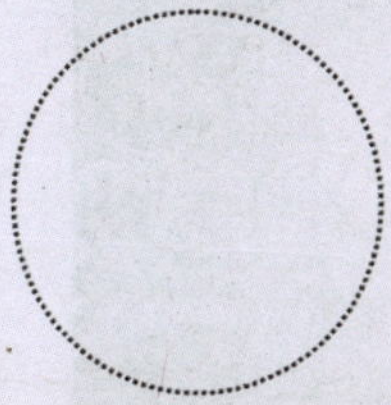	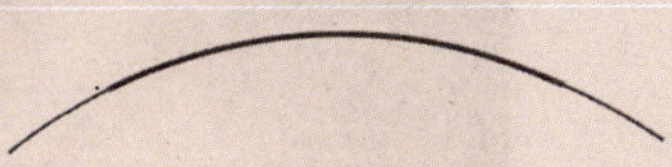	BL Leprosy
	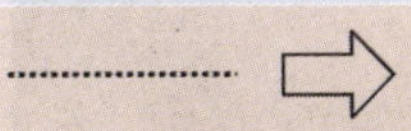	Ill defined/Sloping edges	
	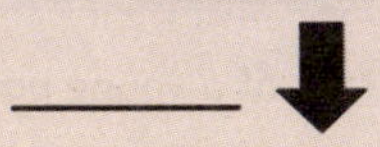	Well-defined edges	

50. Ans. (b) Varicella zoster virus

Ref: IADVL Textbook of Dermatology 1st Ed page 110, Harrison 18th ed page 394

Tzanck Smear

Tzanck test: This test is done in vesicular and bullous lesions. An early lesion is chosen, deroofed, and the excess fluid is gently blotted with gauze. The floor of the blister is then scraped gently with a scalpel blade and the material so obtained is spread on a glass slide and stained. **Tzanck smear can be stained by a variety of methods, most commonly by Giemsa stain.** Quick staining can be done by Hemacolory or Diff-Quiky within 1 minute. Other stains used are hematoxylin and eosin, Wright, methylene blue, Papanicolaou and toluidine blue. Care must be taken to avoid even minimal bleeding while scraping

Findings on Tzanck Smear in Various Dermatoses

Genodermatoses	
Hailey-Hailey disease	Multiple acantholytic cells.
Darier disease	**"Corps ronds" and "grains."** "Corps ronds" are isolated keratinocytes with a round shape and an acidophilic cytoplasm, which is retracted from the nucleus and denser peripherally ("mantle cells"). The grains are seen as small, hyaline, acidophilic ovoid bodies resembling pomegranate seeds
Immunobullous disease	
Pemphigus vulgaris	Very useful for the diagnosis of PV, particularly in the early stages of oral pemphigus. It reveals multiple acantholytic cells. A typical Tzanck cell is a large round keratinocyte with a hypertrophic nucleus, hazy or absent nucleoli, and abundant basophilic cytoplasm. Sertoli rosettes and streptophytes is also seen
Pemphigus vegetans	Acantholytic cells with eosinophils
Bullous pemphigoid	No acantholytic cell, many inflammatory cells
Staphylococcal scalded skin syndrome	Dyskeratotic acantholytic cells with no inflammatory cells
Toxic epidermal necrolysis	Necrotic basal cells, leucocytes, fibroblasts
Infective	
Leishmaniasis	Leishman Donovan bodies and wright cells
Molluscum contagiosum	Hnderson-patterson bodies
Herpes viruses (HSV, VZV, EBV, CMV)	Multinucleate giant cells **(Tzanck cell)**
Cutaneous tumors	
Basal cell carcinoma	Clusters of basaloid cells
Squamous cell carcinoma	Isolated atypical squamous cells
Pagets disease	Paget cells
Erythroplasia of queyrat	Poikilocytosis, naked and clumped nucleus
Histiocytosis X	Atypical langerhan cells
Mastocytoma	Mast cells with metachromatic granules

51. Ans. (a) Segmental vitiligo

Ref: Rooks 8th ed page 58.39- 58.51, Fitzpatrick 7th ed page 624-625.

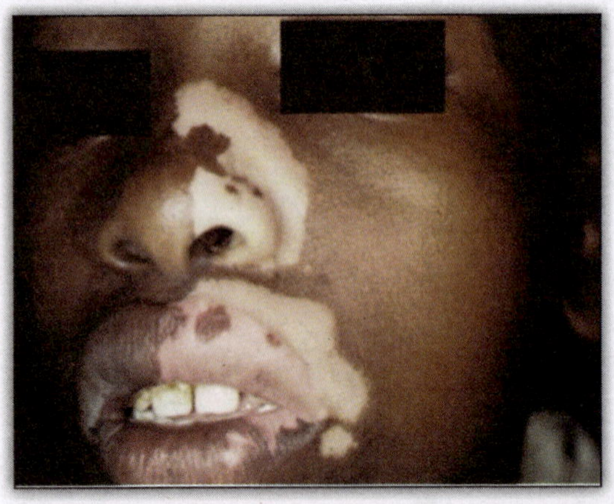

Fig: This is a case of unilateral (segmental) vitiligo affecting one side of the face of a young boy. Note that the depigmentation does not correspond to a dermatome

Vitiligo		
Vitiligo is an acquired disorder characterized by circumscribed depigmented macules and patches that result from a progressive loss of functional melanocytes.		
Prevalence	• 0.5–2% of the general population worldwide • 3%–4% in India	
Clinical features	• The most common presentation of vitiligo is totally **amelanotic** (i.e. milk- or chalk-white) macules or patches surrounded by normal skin. The lesions characteristically have discrete margins, and they can be round, oval, irregular or linear in shape. • The borders are usually convex, as if the depigmenting process were "**invading**" the surrounding normally pigmented skin. • Lesions enlarge centrifugally over time, and the rate may be slow or rapid. Vitiligo macules and patches range from millimeters to centimeters in diameter and often vary in size within areas of involvement. • The incidence of body leukotrichia varies from 10% to >60%, as follicular melanocytes are often spared in vitiligo. • One of the manifestations of vitiligo is the **isomorphic Koebner phenomenon** (IKP), characterized by the development of vitiligo in sites of trauma (e.g. a laceration, burn or abrasion).	

Classification	Two major forms are generally recognized:
	• Segmental
	• **Non-segmental form**, also called **vitiligo vulgaris**
	  ▪ **Localized:**
	    ♦ **Focal:** One or more macules in one area, but not clearly in a segmental distribution
	    ♦ **Unilateral/segmental:** One or more macules involving a unilateral segment of the body; lesions usually stop abruptly at the midline
	    ♦ **Mucosal:** Mucous membranes alone
	  ▪ **Generalized:**
	    ♦ **Vulgaris:** Scattered patches that are widely distributed
	    ♦ **Acrofacial:** Distal extremities and face
	    ♦ **Mixed:** Various combinations of segmental, acrofacial and/or vulgaris
	  ▪ **Universal:** Complete or nearly complete depigmentation	

Clinical variants and other features	• **Vitiligo ponctué:** Multiple small (confetti-like), discrete a melanotic macules, sometimes superimposed upon a hyperpigmented macule. • **Inflammatory vitiligo:** Vitiligo with raised inflammatory borders. • **Blue vitiligo:** Vitiligo develops in areas already affected by post inflammatory hyperpigmentation. • Trichrome vitiligo: Hypopigmented zone between normal and totally depigmented skin. The intermediate zone (with intermediate melanocytes) does not have a gradation of color from white to normal, but rather a fairly uniform hue. • In **quadrichrome vitiligo**, a fourth darker color is present at sites of perifollicular repigmentation. • **Pentachrome vitiligo** with five shades of color (black, dark brown, medium brown [unaffected skin], tan and white) has also been described.	
Associated disorders	**Autoimmune disorders:** Pernicious anemia, Addison's disease, Graves' disease, hyperthyroidism, hypothyroidism, thyroiditis, hyperparathyroidism, DM. Internal malignancy, antibodies against adrenal, thyroglobulin, and gastric parietal cell antigens have been detected. Gastritis, gastric carcinoma, and IgA deficiency are other associations occasionally reported	
Poor prognostic factors	• Lesions on the so-called resistant sites, such as bony prominences, non-fleshy areas, non-hairy areas and mucosal areas. They comprise the sides of the ankles, front of the wrists, back of the elbows, dorsum of feet and hands, palms, soles, nipples and areola. • The greater the percentage of associated white hair, the worse the prognosis. • Extensive long-standing disease. • Associated ailments, especially systemic ones. • Heredofamilial background. • Old age. • Iatrogenic factors, including injudicious administration of topical and systemic medicines, particularly photo-chemotherapeutic agents.	
Psoralen and PUVA	Psoralen	Photosensitizing agent which is a fluoro coumarin derivative. Natural: 8 methoxy-psoralen and 5 methoxypsoralen. Synthetic: 4,5,8 trimethylpsoralen
	Photochemotherapy	Topically, treatment using a combination of psoralen derivatives or other photosensitizing agent, followed by irradiation with long wave ultraviolet light

Contd...

Vitiligo		
	PUVA therapy	Topical psoralen + UVA (320-400 nm)
	PUVASOL	Topical psoralen + sun exposure as source of UVA
	Oral PUVA	Oral psoralen (0.6 mg/kg/body TMP, 0.3 mg/kg/body weight 8-MOP) + UVA
	Narrow band UVB	311 nm
	Excimer laser	308 nm Xenon chloride laser
	Calcipotriol + PUVA	
	Khellin + UVA	
	Phenylalanine + UVA	
Topical therapy	Topical corticosteroids	First line of treatment for patients with a few localized lesions
	Calcineurin inhibitors	Tacrolimus (0.03%, 0.1%)
	Basic fibroblast factor	
	Placental extracts	
Oral therapy	Corticosteroids	Oral mini pulse, ACTH + Corticosteroids
	Immunosuppressants	Azathioprine, cyclophosphamide, levamisole
Surgical treatment	Used mainly for stable vitiligo. Punch excision and grafting, mini punch grafting, split skin grafting, Thiersch grafting, non melanocyte cultured suspension, cultured melanocyte transplant	
Others	Cosmetic camouflaging, bleaching	

52. Ans. (a) Nevus of Ota

Ref: Bolognia 3rd Ed page 1858, Neema khanna 4/e, p 355

The clinical picture is characteristic of Nevus of Ota.

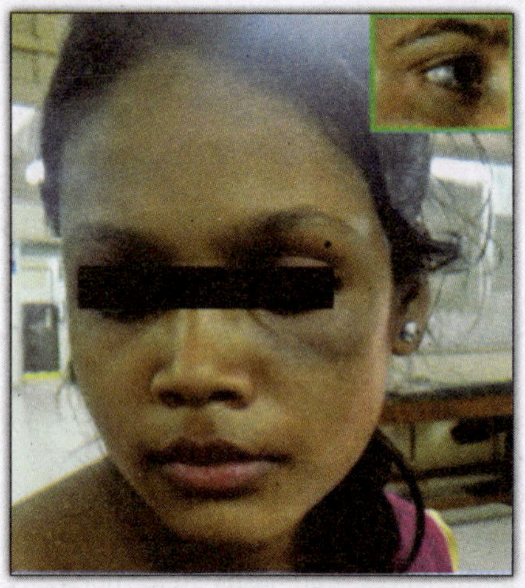

Fig: A lady came with complaints of a bluish lesion over left side of forehead and left eye. A irregular bluish lesion is seen over the left superior conjunctiva. This is a clinical picture of Nevus of Ota.

Nevus of Ota

- Nevus of Ota is a persistent, somewhat speckled, macular, slate brown or bluish hyperpigmentation in the distribution of the ophthalmic and maxillary division of the trigeminal nerve.
- It is commonly unilateral.
- It affects females more frequently than males and mostly presents at birth
- Very rarely, the area supplied by the mandibular division of the trigeminal nerve may also be involved.
- Various shades of pigmentation (black, blue-back, slate blue, purple, purplish-brown or brown) have been observed.
- Hyperpigmentation of the sclera, cornea, iris, retina, fundus, optic nerve, extraocular muscles, retrobulbar fat, orbit, hard palate, pharynx, nasal mucosa, buccal mucosa, tympanic membrane of the affected side may also be present.
- The blue to blue–gray color in nevus of Ota is due to melanin-producing melanocytes in the dermis

Also Know

- **Nevus of Ito:** Nevus of Ito differs from nevus of Ota primarily in its area of involvement; the former corresponds to the distribution of the posterior supraclavicular and lateral cutaneous brachial nerves (which encompasses the supraclavicular, scapular and deltoid regions). The clinical and histologic picture is the same as in nevus of Ota.
- **Hori's nevus:** Acquired nevus of Ota-like macules (Hori's nevus) is characterized by bilateral blue–gray to gray–brown macules of the zygomatic area (less often the forehead, upper outer eyelids and nose).

Psychiatry

17

AIIMS NOVEMBER 2018

1. A 40-year-old male was hospitalized with a psychiatric disorder which had worsened for a past few days. Patient asks the nurse to call his wife who is in the same room . When he sees wife he starts beating her up in the ward and says that she is the nurse who gave him wrong medications last night and is trying to poison him. What's the diagnosis?

(AIIMS Nov 2018, 2017)

a. Fregoli syndrome b. Capgras syndrome
c. Othello's syndrome d. Subjective doubles

2. SPIKES protocol is used for?

a. Communication with patients
b. Breaking bad news
c. Consent
d. Triage

3. An individual with a known psychiatric disorder or on treatment and is not a minor can chose to decide the caretaker and the course of treatment according to mental health act. This is called?

a. Advance directive
b. Treatment directive
c. Mental will
d. Future directive

4. Provision of mental health Act 2017 based WHO mental action gap are all EXCEPT:

a. Human rights
b. Communication regarding care and career
c. Screening family members
d. Social support

AIIMS MAY 2018

5. Which of the following is not a feature of atypical depression?

a. Variable mood responding to positive stimuli
b. TCA better than SSRI and MAO
c. Increased sleep
d. Heaviness of body

6. Most common symptom associated with adult Obsessive compulsive disorder?

a. Sexual
b. Aggressive
c. Pathological doubt
d. Need of symmetry

7. A person who is shy and prefers social isolation, is emotionally cold and prefers to stay alone. He has no hallucination of delusion. Which personality disorder he is suffering from?

a. Schizoid personality disorder
b. Paranoid personality disorder
c. Emotionally unstable personality disorder
d. Antisocial personality disorder

8. Which of the following is not an adverse effect of escitalopram?

a. Sialorrhea b. Vivid dreams
c. Nausea d. Anorgasmia

AIIMS NOVEMBER 2017

9. A schizophrenic patient on 5 mg haloperidol developed inner restlessness and urge to move. Most likely diagnosis is?

a. Tardive dyskinesia b. Rabbit syndrome
c. Akathisia d. Acute dystonia

10. A software professional after taking up new job is feeling guilty, hopeless and not able to concentrate on work. His symptoms started 3 years back when he started college. Most likely diagnosis is?

a. Cyclothymia b. Dysthymia
c. Depression d. Adjustment disorder

11. A 40-year-old male was hospitalized with a psychiatric disorder which had worsened for a past few days. Patient asks the nurse to call his wife who is in the same room. When he sees wife he starts beating her up in the ward and says that she is the nurse who gave him wrong medications last night and is trying to poison him. What's the diagnosis?

(AIIMS Nov 2018, 2017)

a. Fregoli syndrome b. Capgras syndrome
c. Othello's syndrome d. Subjective doubles

12. A middle aged male says he's the most valuable person in the world and his relatives and neighbours are jealous of him and plotting against him. His wife says otherwise and says that he was perfectly normal and behaving like this only recently. What delusion is he suffering from?

a. Delusion of grandeur
b. Delusion of persecution
c. Both Delusion of grandeur, persecution
d. Delusions of grandiose, persecution and reference

AIIMS MAY 2017

13. **Mutism and akinesis in a person, who appears awake and even alert, is best described as?**
(AIIMS May 2017, AIPG 2006)
a. Oneiroid state b. Stupor
c. Twilight state d. Delirium

14. **Which of the following mood stabilizers has anti-suicide properties?**
a. Lithium b. Carbamazepine
c. Valproate d. Lamotrigine

15. **A 20-year-old female has thoughts of cutting her fingers, she plans and imagines doing it but never actually does it. She says she is not having any guilt of having such thought. And also says the thoughts are distressing her and she is unable to control them. The thoughts vanish either by ending with a seizure or automatically subsides on its own. Which of the following is the cause?**
a. Obsession b. Thought insertion
c. Forced thinking d. Crowding of thoughts

AIIMS NOVEMBER 2016

16. **Which of the following is not a component of Polysomnography is?**
a. EEG
b. EOG
c. Intra arterial CO_2 assessment
d. Pulse oxymetry

17. **A place was hit by an earthquake. An old lady was rescued but she lost her house and everything in it, because of which she started having anxiety, fear, palpitation and inability to sleep. Her condition improved on offering help. Consider the following:**
A. Normal acute stress response
B. Projection is the defense mechanism
C. Treatment with Fluoxetine
D. Psychotherapy is required
a. A and C are correct b. A, B and C are correct
c. A and D are correct d. All are correct

18. **A patient with history of repeated hand washing, repeated checking for daily 3 hours interfering day to day activity. Which of the following is true?**
A. Repression and reaction formation are defense mechanism
B. Drug of choice are SSRI's
C. Risperidone can be used to augment the action of SSRI
D. Desensitization is the Psychotherapy of choice
a. A and B are correct b. B and C are correct
c. B, C and D are correct d. All are true

19. **Arrange the following components of Maslow's hierarchy of needs from fundamental to most evolved in order?**
a. Safety, self actualization, belonging, physiological need, self esteem
b. Physiological needs, safety, belonging, esteem, self actualization
c. Safety, physiological needs, self actualization, belonging-self-esteem
d. Self actualization, physiological needs, safety, belonging-self esteem

20. **The court has decided that the accused needs psychiatric evaluation. Many discrepancies were found between alleged symptoms and objective findings. The suspicion should point maximum towards?**
a. Malingering b. Factitious disease
c. Dissociative fugue d. Antisocial behavior

AIIMS MAY 2016

21. **A 41-year-old presented to emergency with intense "ghabraahat", palpitation, tremor, sweating and impending doom. Which of the following can be done in emergency to rule out organic cause of anxiety?**
a. Haemoglobin b. Blood sugar levels
c. T3, T4 d. ECG

22. **All of the following are true about obsession EXCEPT:**
a. Continues to persist despite resistance
b. May be present in schizophrenia
c. Disorder of content of thought
d. Ego dystonic

23. **MMSE examination is used for evaluation of?**
a. Thought b. Mood and effect
c. Cognition d. Insight

24. **Semantic memory includes all of the following EXCEPT:**
a. Words b. Events
c. Rules d. Languages

25. **In a patient with psychiatric disorder, the personal history does not include?**
a. Occupation history b. Academic history
c. Food preference d. Marital history

AIIMS NOVEMBER 2015

26. **A young girl with history of getting medications prescribed by psychiatrist for depression, presents with altered sensorium and hypotension. ECG shows QRS widening and right axis deviation >120° in terminal part. What should be the management?**
a. Hemodialysis
b. IV Flumazenil
c. IV Sodium bicarbonate
d. Physostigmine

27. **A 33-year-old male of bipolar disorder with 5 episodes of mania and 1 episodes of depression in last 8 years has done well under mood stabilizers. As he tapered down the drugs, which of the following intervention is best to improve the drug compliance?**
a. Supportive psychotherapy
b. Cognitive behavioural therapy
c. Insight oriented psychotherapy
d. Psychoeducation

28. **A 12-year-old boy diagnosed with controlled schizophrenia with no family history, well maintained on Risperidone 3 mg since last 2 months. How long should the treatment be continued?**
a. 3 months b. 12 months
c. 2 years d. 5 year

29. A 32-year-old pregnant female with manic episode for 2 weeks; with previous history of 3 episodes of mania and 4 episodes of depression in 5 years. What is the drug of choice?

a. Lithium
b. Clonazepam
c. Haloperidol
d. Promethazine

30. Pervasive developmental disorder includes all EXCEPT:

a. Impairment in cognition
b. Impairment in attention
c. Stereotype repetitive behavior
d. Impaired social interaction

31. Forgetting unpleasant feelings is called as?

a. Isolation
b. Repression
c. Dissociation
d. Suppression

32. Cognitive triad of depression includes all EXCEPT:

a. Feeling of guilt
b. Feeling of hopelessness
c. Feeling of helplessness
d. Feeling of worthlessness

AIIMS MAY 2015

33. Shy, avoidant personality comes under which cluster?

a. A
b. B
c. C
d. D

34. Which of the following is not a part of catatonia?

a. Akathisia
b. Ambivalence
c. Ambitendency
d. Akinesia

35. A young patient presents with a history of eye blinking and grunting which has now increased so much so that it disturbs his routine activity and social life making him depressed. He will be benefited by?

a. Carbamazepine
b. Methylphenidate
c. Imipramine
d. Risperidone

36. A patient with psychosis who is given haloperidol IM, develops irrelevant talks, inability to move his eyes, tremor and rigidity. Which drug should be used intravenously for immediate management?

a. Promethazine
b. Lorazepam
c. Resperidone
d. Diazepam

37. A woman comes to the psychiatrist with history of spending a lot of time in washing her hands. She is distressed about it but says that she cannot stop the practice and spends a lot of time on it. This has started affecting her social life as well. What is the best mode of treatment in her?

a. Cognitive-behavioral therapy
b. Exposure and response prevention
c. Systemic desensitization
d. SSRI

38. Feeling of uncertainty and excessive sense of responsibility is seen in?

a. Generalized anxiety disorder
b. Obsessive compulsive disorder
c. Phobia
d. Personality disorder

39. Key symptom of alcohol withdrawal is?

a. Visual hallucinations
b. Sleep disturbance
c. Tremor
d. Muscle cramps

40. A smoker is worried about the side effects of smoking. But he does not stop smoking thinking that he smokes less as compared to others and takes a good diet. This thinking is called as?

a. Cognitive behavior
b. Self protection
c. Self exemption
d. Distortion

AIIMS NOVEMBER 2018

1. Ans. (a) Fregoli's syndrome

Ref: Kaplan 11th ed page 1134

Repeat AIIMS Nov 2017 Psychiatry (See for explanation) (see page no. 1099)

2. Ans. (b) Breaking bad news

Ref: Oxford textbook of palliative care 5th ed page 295

The SPIKES Protocol was first reported by Baile WF, Buckman R, Lenzi R, Glober G, Beale EA, Kudelka AP. SPIKES—a six-step protocol for delivering bad news: application to the patient with cancer. The oncologist. 2000 Aug 1;5(4):302-11

SPIKES - The Six-Step Protocol for Delivering Bad News This acronym helps to memorise the steps and consider their elements **STEP 1:** SETTING UP the Interview **STEP 2:** Assessing the Patient's PERCEPTION **STEP 3:** Obtaining the Patient's INVITATION **STEP 4:** Giving KNOWLEDGE and Information to the Patient **STEP 5:** Addressing the Patient's EMOTIONS with empathic responses **STEP 6:** Strategy and Summary

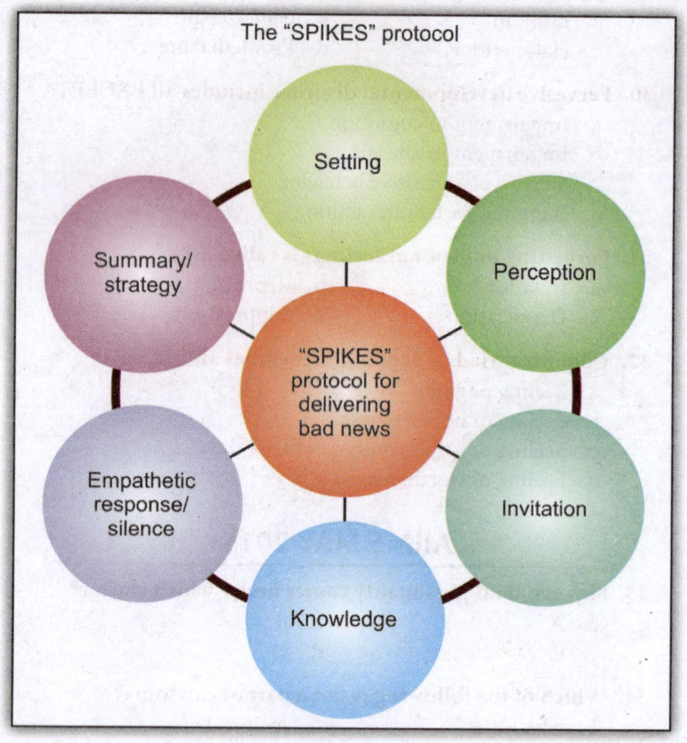

Fig: This model was modified in 2005 to P-SPIKES

Acronym	Steps	Aim of the interaction	Preparations Questions or Phrases
P	Preparation	Mentally prepare for the interaction with the patient	Review what information needs to be communicated Plan how you will provide emotional support. Rehearse key steps and phrases in the interaction.
S	Setting of the interaction	Ensure the appropriate setting for a serious and emotionally charged discussion	Ensure patient, family and appropriate social supports are present
P	Patient's perception and preparation	Begin the discussion by establishing the baseline and whether the patent and family can grasp the information Ease tension by having the patient and family contribute.	Start with open-ended questions to encourage participation. Possible phrases to use: • What do you understand about your illness? • When you first had symptom X, what did you think it might be? • What did Dr. X tell you when he sent you here? • What do you think is going to happen?
I	Invitation and Information needs	Discover what information needs the patient and/or family have and what limits they want regarding the bad information	Possible phrases to use: • If this condition turns out to be something serious, do you want to know? • Would you like me to tell you the full details of you condition? • If not, then who would you like me to talk to?
K	Knowledge of the condition	Provide the bad news or other information to the patient and/ or family Sensitively.	Do not just dump the information on the patient and family. Interrupt and check that the patent and family are understanding. Possible phrases to use: • I feel badly to have to tell you this, but... • Unfortunately, the tests showed... • I'm afraid the news is not good...

Contd...

Acronym	Steps	Aim of the interaction	Preparations Questions or Phrases
E	Empathy and exploration	Identify the cause of the emotions-e.g., poor prognosis Empathize with the patient and/ or family's feeling Explore by asking open-ended questions.	Strong feelings in reaction to bad news are normal. Acknowledge what the patient and family are feeling. Remind them such feelings are normal, even if frightening. Give them time to respond. Remind patient and family you won't abandon them. Possible phrases to use: I imaging this is very hard for you. You look very upset. Tell me how you are feeling. I wish the news were different. I'll do whatever I can to help you.
S	Summary and strategic planning	Delineate for the patient and the family the next steps including additional tests or interventions.	It is the unknown and uncertain that increase anxiety. Recommend a schedule with goals and landmarks. Provide your rationale for the patient and/or family to accept (or reject)

3. Ans. (a) Advance directive

Ref: http://www.prsindia.org/uploads/media/Mental%20 Health/Mental%20Healthcare%20Act,%202017.pdf

Mental health care Act 2017: Chapter III: Advance Directive, says

Every person who is not a minor, shall have a right to make an advance directive in writing, specifying any or all of following, namely

1. How he wished to be cared
2. How he wished not to be cared
3. Whom he wants to appoint as nominated representatives, in order of preference.

4. Ans. (c) Screening family members

Ref: http://www.prsindia.org/uploads/media/Mental%20 Health/Mental%20Healthcare%20Act,%202017.pdf

The mental health care act 2017 consists of 16 chapters and 126 sections. The cornerstone of this act has remained human rights based on the UNCRPD 2006 (United Nations Convention on Rights of Persons with Disabilities, 2006). In it,

Chapter I: Preliminary, consists of section 1 and 2, talks about various nomenclatures.

Chapter II: Mental illness and capacity to make mental healthcare and treatment decisions, consists of section 3 and 4, talks about how to determine mental illness as per international standards(ICD by WHO) and capacity of every individual to make decision about his/her mental health care and treatment choices.

Chapter III: Advance Directive, consists of section 5 to 13 (total 9), talks about how every person wishes and not wishes to be cared for and treated for a mental illness; Determination of mental illness **(Option B here).**

Chapter IV: Nominated Representative, consists of section 14 to 17(total 4) talks about selection of a representative by every person as a future career **(Option B here).**

Chapter V: Rights of person with mental illness, consists of section 18 to 28 (total 11), talks about various rights every person shall have under this law. **(Option A here)**

Chapter VI: Duties of appropriate government, consists of section 29 to 32 (total 4).

Chapter VII: Central Mental Health Authority, consists of section 33 to 44 (total 12).

Chapter VIII: State Mental Health Authority, consists of section 45 to 56 (total 12).

Chapter IX: Finance, Audit and Account, consists of section 57 to 64 (total 8).

Chapter X: Mental Health Establishments, consists of section 65 to 72 (total 8) talks about how to run any mental health setup.

Chapter XI: Mental Health Review Board, consists of section 73 to 84, talks about establishing a regulatory body, which will be conducted under State Authority.

Chapter XII: Admission, treatment and Discharge, consists of section 85 to 99.

Chapter XIII: Responsibilities of other agencies, consists of section 100 to 106. (Talks about role of various social supports, like police magistrate etc, option D here).

Chapter XIV: Restriction to discharge functions by professionals not covered by profession, consists single section of 106.

Chapter XV: Offenses and Penalties, consists of section 107, 108, 109.

Chapter XVI: Miscellaneous, consists of section 110 to 126.

AIIMS MAY 2018

5. Ans. (b) TCA better than SSRI and MAO

Ref: DSM 5 specifiers for depression with atypical features (present both in depressive disorder and bipolar disorders.

Atypical depression characteristics are

1. Mood reactivity
2. Interpersonal rejection sensitivity
3. Reverse vegetative signs (increase sleep + appetite)
4. Leaden paralysis (heaviness of body)

Better response to MAO-I comparing to TCA/SSRI is a persistent finding of atypical depression.

6. Ans. (c) Pathological doubt

Ref: Kaplan Saddock Synopsis 11th edition page 422

Most common pattern obsession of contamination (followed by washing/ compulsive avoidance of the object) > pathological doubt(followed by compulsion of checking) > intrusive thoughts(without compulsions) > need for symmetry (compulsion of slowness)

So, among the given options, pathological doubt is the best choice.

7. Ans. (a) Schizoid personality disorder

Ref: ICD 10 blue book page 158

Schizoid Personality Disorder

- Few/ nil pleasurable activities
- Emotional coldness/flattened affectivity
- Limited capacity to express warmth
- Indifferent to praise/criticism
- Little interest in sexual experience
- Preference to solitary activity
- Preoccupation with fantasy and introspection
- Lack of friends
- Insensitive to social norm/conventions

8. Ans. (a) Sialorrhea

Ref: Essential Psychopharmacology, Prescriber's guideline: Stephen Stahl page 175, Katzung 13th Ed Pg 524-525, Goodman Gilman 13th Ed Pg 272-273

Gastrointestinal Side Effects of Escitalopram

1. Decreased appetite
2. Nausea
3. Diarrhea
4. Constipation
5. Dry mouth

AIIMS NOVEMBER 2017

9. Ans. (c) Akathisia

Ref: Maudsley 10th ed page 97, Lishman Psychiatry 4th ed page 746

This question is based on the Neurological side effects of Neuroleptic drugs

See table of NEUROLOGICAL SIDE EFFECTS OF NEUROLEPTIC DRUGS in Psychiatry AIIMS MAY 2015

Option (A)

Tardive dyskinesia: Most serious adverse effect. Tardive dyskinesia is a delayed effect of antipsychotics; it rarely occurs until after 6 months of treatment. The disorder consists of abnormal, involuntary, irregular choreoathetoid movements of the muscles of the head, limbs, and trunk

Option (B)

Rabbit syndrome: A rare movement disorder that can appear late in chronic treatment with antipsychotic agents is perioral tremor, often referred to as the "Rabbit syndrome" because of the peculiar movements that characterize it. Rabbit syndrome shares many features with parkinsonism, because the tremor has a frequency of about 3 to 5 Hz, and often responds favorably to anticholinergic agents and removal of the offending agent.

Option (C)

Akathisia: A subjectively unpleasant state of inner restlessness where there is a strong desire or compulsion to move (e.g. foot stamping, constantly crossing/uncrossing legs/rocking from foot to foot/constantly pacing up and down. Akathisia = inner sense of restlessness + objective evidence of same

Option (D)

Acute Dystonia: Uncontrolled muscle spasms, e.g: eyes rolling upwards (oculogyric crisis) head and neck twisted to the side(torticollis)

10. Ans. (b) Dysthymia

Ref: Kaplan Sadock synopsis 11th ed page 382, ICD 10 Blue book page 107

Symptoms suggestive of depressive cognition; hopelessness, guilt, cognitive symptom of poor concentration, however continuous, duration more than 2 years, never remitted, also does not currently fulfill the criteria for recurrent depressive disorder. (ICD 10 Blue book page 107)

Persistent depressive disorder (Dysthymia) as mentioned in DSM 5 (300.4) is a consolidation of DSM-IV-defined chronic major depressive disorder and dysthymic disorder.

DSM 5 Criteria

A. Depressed mood for most of the day, for more days than not, as indicated by either subjective account or observation by others, for at least 2 years.

> **NOTE**
>
> In children and adolescents, mood can be irritable and duration must be at least 1 year.

B. Presence, while depressed, of two (or more) of the following: 1. Poor appetite or overeating. 2. Insomnia or hypersomnia. 3. Low energy or fatigue. 4. Low self-esteem. 5. Poor concentration or difficulty making decisions. 6. Feelings of hopelessness.

C. During the 2-year period (1 year for children or adolescents) of the disturbance, the individual has never been without the symptoms in Criteria A and B for more than 2 months at a time.

D. Criteria for a major depressive disorder may be continuously present for 2 years.

E. There has never been a manic episode or a hypomanic episode, and criteria have never been met for cyclothymic disorder.

F. The disturbance is not better explained by a persistent schizoaffective disorder, schizophrenia, delusional disorder, or other specified or unspecified schizophrenia spectrum and other psychotic disorder.

G. The symptoms are not attributable to the physiological effects of a substance (e.g., a drug of abuse, a medication) or another medical condition (e.g., hypothyroidism).

H. The symptoms cause clinically significant distress or impairment in social, occupational, or other important areas of functioning.

Cyclothymia: Persistent instability of mood, involving numerous periods of mild depression and mild elation, not fulfilling criteria of bipolar affective disorder or recurrent depressive disorder.

11. Ans. (a) Fregoli's syndrome

Ref: Kaplan 11th ed page 1134

Capgras/fregoli comes under DMS or Delusional Misidentification Syndrome. The most confusing/puzzling part is to remember or differentiate between Capgras vs Fregoli

Delusional Misidentification Syndrome

Most prominent ones are

- Capgras syndrome (or, Capgras-type misidentification):
- Fregoli's syndrome (or Fregoli-type misidentification)
- Delusion of reduplication etc (the other ones are really rare).

Always remember, Capgras is hypoidentification, where Fregoli is Hyperidentification. Hypoidentification is possible with the patient when patient less identifies an well-known person to him, and believes the well-known person to be an imposter/or, 'though looking like a known one, actually an imposter). whereas, in Hyperidentification, the patient over-identifies strangers to be a known one. or, will think a known person has changed appearance and has come as imposter/'looking like an imposter, but actually a known one'. and u can also remember Fregoli's syndrome was actually named after a Italian actor (Leopoldo Fregoli) who was famous for his disguised/changed appearance, means, same person, but different facial appearance/impersonating.

12. Ans. (c) Both delusion of grandeur, persecution

Ref: Kaplan and sadock 11th ed page 3637

Both delusions of grandeur (inappropriately inflated self esteem, seems primary here), and persecution ('the whole world is against me', seems secondary to delusion of Grandiosity here)

Delusion	False belief, based on incorrect inference about external reality, that is firmly held despite objective and obvious contradictory proof or evidence and despite the fact that other members of the culture do not share the belief.
Delusion of persecution	False belief of being harassed or persecuted; often found in litigious patients who have a pathological tendency to take legal action because of imagined mistreatment. **Most common delusion.**
Delusion of control	False belief that a person's will, thoughts, or feelings are being controlled by external forces.
Delusion of grandeur	Exaggerated conception of one's importance, power, or identity.
Delusion of infidelity	False belief that one's lover is unfaithful. Sometimes called pathological jealousy
Delusion of reference	False belief that the behavior of others refers to oneself or that events, objects, or other people have a particular and unusual significance, usually of a negative nature; derived from idea of reference, in which persons falsely feel that others are talking about them (e.g., belief that people on television or radio are talking to or about the person).

Contd...

AIIMS MAY 2017

13. Ans. (b) Stupor

Ref: Ahuja Textbook of psychiatry 10th Ed Pg 59

Akinesis (no movement) with mutism but with evidence of relative preservation of conscious awareness is called stupor. It is one of the features of retarded catatonia. The term akinetic mutism originated with Cairns and colleagues. They described a young woman who, although appearing wakeful, became mute and rigidly motionless when a craniopharyngiomatous cyst expanded to compress the walls of third ventricle and frontal lobe.

Option (A) Oneiroid State

Oneiroid schizophrenia: Described first by Mayer-gross, this is a subtype of schizophrenia with an acute onset, clouding of consciousness, disorientation, dream-like states (oneiroid means 'dream'), and perceptual disturbances with rapid shifting.

Option (B) Stupor

It is an imprecise term for:

- State of decreased reactivity to stimuli
- Unresponsiveness with immobility
- Mutism but retention of consciousness & often with open eyes that follows external objects.

Option (C) Twilight State

Describes disturbed consciousness with hallucinations. Appears as waking dreams that portray desires, wishes or fears in a direct or symbolic way. A transitory disturbance of consciousness during which many acts, sometimes very complicated may be performed without the subjects conscious volition and without any remembrance of them.

Option (D) Delirium

According to ICD 10, diagnosis of delirium must include impairment of consciousness and attention (on a continuum from clouding to coma; reduced ability to direct, focus, sustain, and shift attention), global disturbance of cognition, psychomotor disturbances, disturbance of sleep-wake cycle, and emotional disturbances.

14. Ans. (a) Lithium

Ref: With text

Kaplan's 10th Ed page 492 says: **"Clinical studies have shown that lithium reduces the incidence of suicide in patients with bipolar I disorder sixfold or sevenfold."**

Trends in Neurochemistry Research By Robert Milton Coleman- Page 169: **Initial treatment of BPD includes** lithium or valproic acid or SSRI such as bupropion, sertraline, citalopram and escitalopram. One advantage of lithium salt is that it also possesses an anti-suicidal effect.

15. Ans. (c) Forced thinking

Ref: Lishman's organic psychiatry Pg 321, 335

NOTE

Crowding of thoughts is a component of forced thinking but not vice versa. Provided the symptoms end with epilepsy, Forced thinking is best suited.

- One of the clues to diagnosis is by the thoughts vanishing in seizure.
- Forced thinking (FT) is a rare epileptic phenomenon which is usually seen in patients with temporal as well as frontal lobe epilepsy. It is a comparatively often found type of psychic seizure. ***This type of psychic aura is called 'forced thinking,' characterized by recurrent intrusive thoughts, ideas, or crowding of thoughts.***
- It is an autonomous appearance of a fixed thought induced by seizure activities.
- Patients may experience distortion of thoughts such as forced thinking, which describes a feeling of being compelled to think about a specific topic or word; or crowding of thoughts, which describes a feeling of racing, disorganised thoughts.
- Subtle but disturbing changes in the quality of perception are reported, including derealisation and depersonalisation, distortions in the perception of time and changes in the significance of objects.
- These latter are often impossible for patients to describe but may involve a sense that a specific object in their environment seems changed and has a heightened but mysterious personal relevance.
- The seizures of prefrontal origin are characterized by forced actions, forced thinking and motor "automatism followed by brief duration of seizure activity less than 1 minute or some time less than few seconds after that thoughts subside by its own.

Ruling Out Other Options

Option (A) Obsession

There is no guilt, no compulsion no attempt to stop these thoughts.

Option (B) Thought Insertion

Seen in schizophrenia. There is no description that thoughts were inserted by some external agency. Also thoughts were subsided by episode of seizures

Option (C) Crowding of Thoughts

Were also seen in schizophrenia, as no history of delusion, hallucination, etc. mentioned plus patient experience the thoughts were too fast, excessive in amount, unexplainable [patient is not able to explain the type/kind of thought] patient can anatomically locate the location of thoughts—being crowded in back of my head and being controlled by some outside agency.

AIIMS NOVEMBER 2016

16. Ans. (c) Intra arterial CO_2 assessment

Ref: Ganong 24th ed page 274, Guyton 12th ed page 764

Polysomnography (PSG), a type of sleep study, is a multi-parametric test used in the study of sleep and as a diagnostic tool in sleep medicine. The PSG monitors many body functions including brain **(EEG)**, eye movements **(EOG)**, muscle activity or skeletal muscle activation **(EMG)** and heart rhythm **(ECG)** during sleep. After the identification of the sleep apnea, the breathing functions such as respiratory airflow and respiratory effort indicators were added along with **peripheral pulse oximetry.**

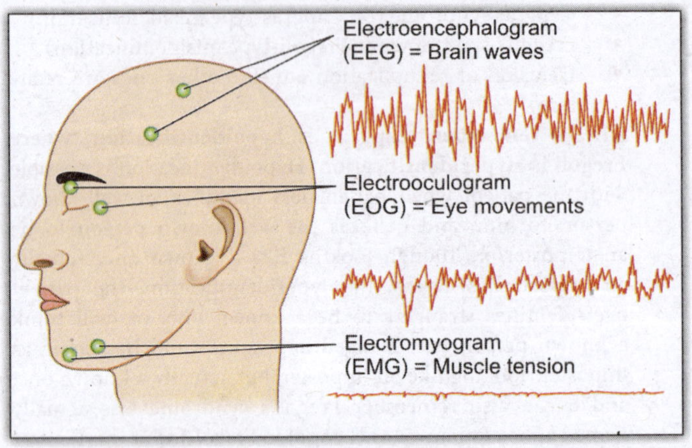

17. Ans. (c) a and d are correct

Ref: Kaplan 10th ed page 580, Niraj Ahuja 7th Ed Pg 111

This is a case of Acute stress disorder

Acute Stress Disorder

- The text revision of the fourth edition of Diagnostic and Statistical Manual of Mental Disorders (DSM-IV-TR) defines a disorder that is similar to PTSD called acute stress disorder, which occurs earlier than PTSD (within 4 weeks of the event) and remits within 2 days to 4 weeks. If symptoms persist after that time, a diagnosis of PTSD is warranted.
- According to ICD-10, in this disorder there is an immediate and clear temporal relationship between an exceptional stressor (such as death of a loved one, natural catastrophe, accident, rape) and the onset of symptoms. The symptoms show a mixed and changing picture. This disorder is more likely to develop in presence of physical exhaustion and in extremes of age. It is also more commonly seen in female gender and people with poor coping skills.
- The symptoms range from a 'dazed' condition, anxiety, depression, anger, despair, overactivity or withdrawal, and constriction of the field of consciousness. The symptoms resolve rapidly (within few hours usually), if removal from the stressful environment is possible. If the stress continues or cannot be reversed, the resolution of symptoms begins after 1–2 days and is usually minimal after about three days.

- The treatment consists of removal of the patient from the stressful environment and helping the patient to 'pass through' the stressful experience. IV or oral benzodiazepines (such as diazepam) may be needed in cases with marked agitation.
- First-line treatment for **acute stress disorder** (ASD) is trauma-focused cognitive-behavioral **therapy** (CBT), which has been shown to reduce the likelihood of subsequently developing PTSD.
- SSRIs should be started 3 to 4 weeks after exposure to a trauma in patients with no improvement in their acute stress response. The initiation of an SSRI should be at a low dose with gradual titration upward toward antidepressant doses.

18. Ans. (b) b and c are true

Ref: Kaplan 10th ed page 608, Niraj Ahuja 7th Ed Pg 95-98, Shorter Oxford Textbook of Psychiatry 6th Ed page 203

Statement a; Repression and reaction formation are defense mechanism

- **Isolation of affect:** By this defense mechanism, ego removes the affect (isolates the affect) from the anxiety-causing idea. The idea is thus weakened, but remains still in the consciousness. The affect however becomes free and attaches itself to other neutral idea(s) by symbolic associations. Thus, these neutral ideas become anxiety-provoking and turn into obsessions.
- This happens only when isolation of affect is not fully successful (incomplete isolation of affect). When it is fully successful, both the idea and affect are repressed and there are no obsessions.
- **Undoing:** This defense mechanism leads to compulsions, which prevent or undo the feared consequences of obsessions.
- **Reaction formation** results in the formation of obsessive compulsive personality traits rather than.

Regression is not a Defense Mechanism in OCD

Conditions	Defense Mechanisms Used
Obsessive-compulsive personality disorder	Rationalization, isolation, intellectualization, reaction formation, and undoing
Panic disorder	Reaction formation, undoing, somatization, and externalization
Phobias	Displacement, projection, and avoidance
Agoraphobia	Repression, displacement, avoidance, and symbolization
PTSD	Denial, minimization, splitting, projective disavowal, dissociation, and guilt
Delusional disorder	Projection, reaction formation, denial
Dysthymic disorder	Reaction formation
Hypomania	Denial
Bulimia nervosa	Introjective and projective
Factitious disorders	Repression, identification with the aggressor, regression, and symbolization
Foster care children	Denial, splitting, projection, and introjection

Statement b - True; Drug of choice are SSRI's.

Statement c - True; OCD shows clinically significant improvement after Risperidone augmentation to SRI treatment.

Statement d - False; Desensitization is the psychotherapy of choice. The principal behavioral approaches in OCD are exposure and response prevention. Desensitization is one of the psychotherapies used but is not the therapy of choice.

Desensitization is the behavior therapy of choice for phobias.

Methods of Behavior Therapy		
Systematic Desensitization* Developed by Wolpe	Based on the behavioral principle of counter conditioning, whereby a person overcomes maladaptive anxiety elicited by a situation or an object by approaching the feared situation gradually, in a psychophysiological state that inhibits anxiety. It consists of three steps: relaxation training, hierarchy construction and desensitization of the stimulus.	Phobias, OCD, Sexual disorders, Anxiety disorder
Therapeutic-Graded Exposure*	Similar to systematic desensitization, except that relaxation training is not involved and treatment is usually carried out in a real-life context. Patients afraid of cats, for example, might progress from looking at a picture of a cat to holding one.	Phobias
Flooding*	Flooding (sometimes called implosion) is similar to graded exposure in that it involves exposing the patient to the feared object in vivo; however, there is no hierarchy.	Specific phobias, PTSD, OCD
Participant Modeling	Patients learn a new behavior by imitation, primarily by observation, without having to perform the behavior until they feel ready.	Specific phobias, agoraphobia
Exposure and response prevention*	The **"Exposure"** in ERP refers to confronting the thoughts, images, objects and situations that make a person with OCD anxious. The **"Response Prevention"** in ERP refers to making a choice not to do a compulsive behavior after coming into contact with the things that make a person with OCD anxious.	OCD, Phobias

Contd...

Methods of Behavior Therapy		
Aversion Therapy*	When a noxious stimulus (punishment) is presented immediately after a specific behavioral response, theoretically, the response is eventually inhibited and extinguished. The negative stimulus is paired with the behavior, which is thereby suppressed.	Alcohol abuse, paraphilias and other behaviors with impulsive or compulsive qualities
Positive Reinforcement#	When a behavioral response is followed by a generally rewarding event, such as food, avoidance of pain, or praise, it tends to be strengthened and to occur more frequently than before the reward.	Promote desirable behaviour,
Token economy#	Based on the principle of secondary reinforcement. Tokens are given in exchange for desirable or acceptable behaviours. These can then be exchanged for primary (or direct) reinforcements, such as sweets or extra outings	Promote desirable behaviour, particularly in an institutional setting.

#Based on **operant conditioning**—a form of learning in which behavioral frequency is altered through the application of positive and negative consequences.

*Based on **classical conditioning**.

19. Ans. (b) Physiological needs, Safety, Belonging, Esteem, Self actualization

Ref: A Theory of Human Motivation By A. H. Maslow Ch1

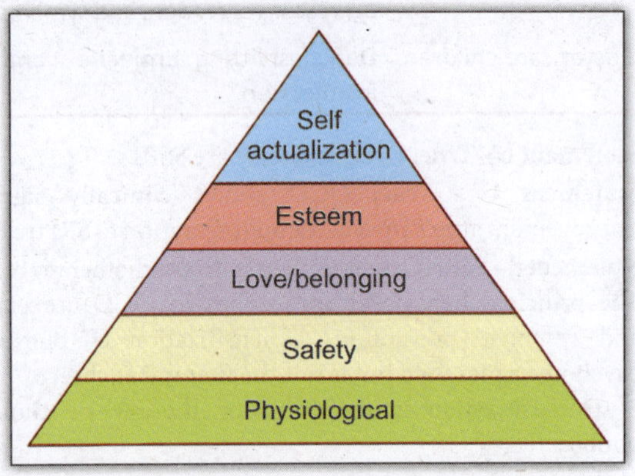

The pyramid of needs, also called **Maslow's pyramid,** offers a model to define the needs of human beings, from the most basic functions (eating, sleeping, etc.) to the more fulfilling (self-improvement, practicing art or sports, etc.). Maslow was a psychologist, but his model, summarized by a pyramid, has been used in economics and the world of business. It offers a simple and effective way of identifying the different needs. These needs must be considered within the overall pyramid, not as successive stages.

20. Ans. (a) Malingering

Ref: Kaplan's 10th ed page 658

Persons with **factitious disorder** fake illness. They simulate, induce, or aggravate illness, often inflicting painful, deforming, or even life-threatening injury on themselves or those under their care. Unlike **malingerers who have material goals**, such as monetary gain or avoidance of duties, patients with factitious disorder undertake these tribulations primarily to gain the emotional care and attention that comes with playing the role of the patient.

- A fundamental stance in psychiatric interviewing is recognizing that what is being heard may not be the literal truth.
- The unreliability of memory and the vagaries of psychopathology through which a patient's narrative is processed distort and falsify.
- At times, patients lie consciously with the explicit intent of deceiving the therapist. The purpose may be secondary gain (in this case, most probably to escape punishment), in which case the person is malingering.
- **Malingering is not a mental disorder** in the revised fourth edition of the Diagnostic and statistical manual of mental disorders (DSM-IV-TR).
- More rarely, a patient explicitly lies not for any obvious external advantage, but simply for whatever psychological advantage is conferred by assuming the sick role, in which case the person has a factitious disorder that is a DSM-IV-TR diagnosis.

AIIMS MAY 2016

21. Ans. (d) ECG

Ref: Kaplan 10th edition Page 628, Panic Disorder and Agoraphobia by Borwin Bandelow, Katharina Domschke, David Baldwin table 1.2

Recall Bias

Most likely this question should be in ALL EXCEPT format, in which case T3, T4 will be the best answer as the results of Thyroid profile cannot be obtained in emergency. In present format ECG is the best answer

Before initiating psychiatric treatment, a clinician should undertake a routine medical evaluation for the purposes of screening for concurrent disease, ruling out organicity, and establishing baseline values of functions to be monitored. Such an evaluation includes a medical history and routine medical laboratory tests, such as a complete blood count (CBC); hematocrit and hemoglobin; renal, liver, and thyroid function; electrolytes; and blood sugar. **(Kaplan 10th ed page 255)**

In the above paragraph Kaplan is talking about the Psychiatric disorders in general (not panic attacks only) and Lab tests and hence there is no mention of ECG.

Option (A)

Hemoglobin levels is done for assessment of anemia (anemia may be associated with depressive and psychotic disorders). Anemia is important in differential diagnosis since it is frequent in our society and many symptoms of it intersect with the symptoms of panic attack. It can be marked if ECG is not provided in the option.

Option (B)

In absence of history of diabetes under anti diabetic medications, hypoglycemia is rare. However, random blood sugar is the simplest and fast test to be done in emergency. It can be marked as answer if ECG is not provided in the option or if patient is on antidiabetic medications.

Option (C)

Thyroid function test can be done to rule out hyperthyroidism but thyroid function test is not done in emergency at the results takes time.

Option (D)

Many of the symptoms of panic disorder are cardinal features of cardiovascular disease. ECG is both helpful to rule out cardiac cause and it can be done in emergency.

Secondary Causes of Panic Disorder

Differential diagnosis	Symptoms	Tests
Cardiac arrhythmias	Irregular heart beats	ECG
Angina pectoris	Chest pain anxiety, dyspnea	ECG, Nitroglycerine test
Myocardial infarction	Sudden chest pain, dyspnea, palpitation, sweating, anxiety	ECG, biomarkers of MI
Syncope	Dizziness, fainting, nausea	Portable ECG, tilt table test
Pulmonary embolism	Dyspnea, chest pain, choking	CT pulmonary angiography
Vestibular dysfunction	Dizziness, somnolence, nausea, vomiting, anxiety	Caloric reflex test, Electronystagmiography, Videonystagmography
Hypoglycemia	Tachycardia, tremor, anxiety sweating, Dizziness, GI complaints	Blood glucose levels
Hyperthyroidism	Anxiety, tachycardia, palpitation, sweating, dyspnea	Thyroid profile (Mainly TSH)
Hyperkalemia	Palpitation, arrythmia, paresthesia	Potassium concentration
Insulinoma	Tremor, sweating, syncope, palpitation, tachycardia	Glucose, C peptide

Contd...

Secondary Causes of Panic Disorder

Differential diagnosis	Symptoms	Tests
Pheochromocytoma	Anxiety, tachycardia, hypertension, tremor, headache, sweating, hot flush	Catecholamines, clonidine suppression test

22. Ans. (c) Disorder of content of thought

Ref: Fish's Clinical Psychopathology 3rd ed page 36

Obscessive Compulsive Disorder

- Obsession are disorder of possession of thought.
- Obsessive-compulsive disorder (OCD) is represented by a diverse group of symptoms that include intrusive thoughts, rituals, preoccupations, and compulsions.
- These recurrent obsessions or compulsions cause severe distress to the person.
- The obsessions or compulsions are time-consuming and interfere significantly with the person's normal routine, occupational functioning, usual social activities, or relationships.
- A patient with OCD may have an obsession, a compulsion, or both.
- An obsession is a recurrent and intrusive thought, feeling, idea, or sensation. In contrast to an obsession, which is a mental event, a compulsion is a behavior.
- Specifically, a compulsion is a conscious, standardized, recurrent behavior, such as counting, checking, or avoiding.
- A patient with OCD realizes the irrationality of the obsession and experiences both the obsession and the compulsion as ego-dystonic (i.e., unwanted behavior).
- Although the compulsive act may be carried out in an attempt to reduce the anxiety associated with the obsession, it does not always succeed in doing so.
- The completion of the compulsive act may not affect the anxiety, and it may even increase the anxiety. Anxiety is also increased when a person resists carrying out a compulsion.
- OCD-schizophrenia can be present when DSM criteria for both are present.

23. Ans. (c) Cognition

Ref: Kaplan 10th ed page 1351

"The most widely used test of current cognitive functioning is the Mini-mental state examination (MMSE), which assesses orientation, attention, calculation, immediate and short-term recall, language, and the ability to follow simple commands. The MMSE is used to detect impairments, follow the course of an illness, and monitor the patient's treatment responses. It is not used to make a formal diagnosis. The maximal MMSE score is 30. Age and educational level influence cognitive performance as measured by the MMSE."

Mini Mental State Examination Questionnare		
Category	**Possible points**	**Description**
Orientation to time	0–5	Year, month, date, day of the week, and season
Orientation to place	0–5	5 items in their address
Registration	0–3	Examiner names 3 objects (eg Banana, umbrella and bicycle) Patient asked to repeat (1 point for each correct).
Attention and calculation	0–5	Serial subtraction of 7 from 100, Continue 5 times: 100 93 86 79 65 Alternative: "Spell WORLD backwards." (D-L-R-O-W)
Recall	0–3	Ask for names of 3 objects learned earlier. Banana, umbrella and bicycle
Language	0–8	Naming a pencil and a watch, following slang, following the 3 steps, following 3 staged command, and writing 1 full sentence
Complex commands	1	**Varies. Can involve drawing figure shown. (Interlocking pentagons)** All 10 angles must be present and two must intersect. 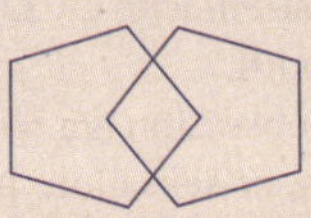
Total	0–30	

Interpretation of MMSE Score	
MMSE Score	**Cognitive function**
26–30	May be normal
21–25	Mild/Early
11–20	Moderate
0–10	Severe

24. Ans. (b) Events

Ref: CTP 9th edition Pg 666

- Declarative memory depends on medial temporal and midline diencephalic structures along with large portions of the neocortex. **This system provides for the rapid learning of facts (semantic memory) and events (episodic memory).**

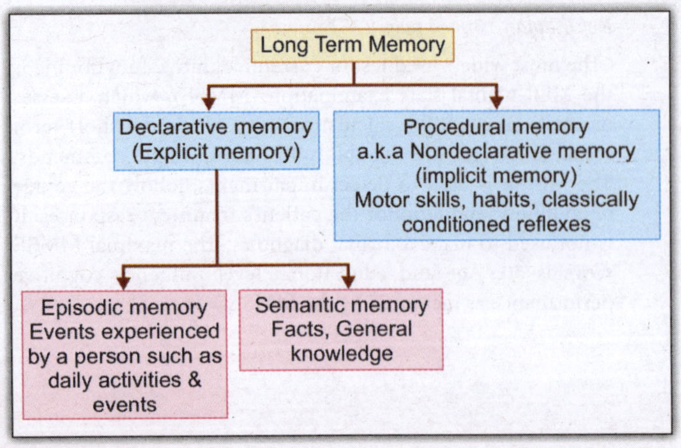

- Nondeclarative memory depends on several different brain systems. Habits depend on the neocortex and the neostriatum, and the cerebellum is important for the conditioning of skeletal musculature, the amygdala for emotional learning, and the neocortex for priming.
- Declarative memory and nondeclarative memory differ in important ways. Declarative memory is phylogenetically more recent than nondeclarative memory.
- In addition, declarative memories are available to conscious recollection.
- The flexibility of declarative memory permits the retrieved information to be available to multiple response systems.
- Nondeclarative memory is inaccessible to awareness and is expressed only by engaging specific processing systems.
- Nondeclarative memories are stored as changes within these processing systems—changes that are encapsulated such that the stored information has limited accessibility to other processing systems.
- Semantic memory, which concerns general knowledge of the world, has often been categorized as a separate form of memory. Facts that are committed to memory typically become independent of the original episodes in which the facts were learned.

25. Ans. (c) Food preference

Ref: CTP 9th ed Page 894

- The developmental and social history (personal history) reviews the stages of the patient's life.
- It is an important tool in determining the context of psychiatric symptoms and illnesses and may, in fact, identify some of the major factors in the evolution of the disorder.
- Frequently, current psychosocial stressors will be revealed in the course of obtaining a social history. It can often be helpful to review the social history chronologically to ensure all information is covered.
- Any available information concerning prenatal or birthing history and developmental milestones should be noted.
- For the large majority of adult patients such information is not readily available and when it is it may not be fully accurate. Childhood history will include childhood home environment including members of the family and social environment including the number and quality of friendships.
- A detailed school history including how far the patient went in school and how old they were at that level, any special education circumstances or learning disorders, behavioral problems at school, academic performance, and extracurricular activities should be obtained.
- Childhood physical and sexual abuse should be carefully queried.
- Work history will include types of jobs, performance at jobs, reasons for changing jobs, and current work status. The nature of the patient's relationships with supervisors and co-workers should be reviewed.
- The patient's income, financial issues, and insurance coverage including pharmacy benefits are often important issues.
- Military history, where applicable, should be noted including rank achieved, combat exposure, disciplinary actions, and discharge status.

- Marriage and relationship history including sexual preferences and current family structure should be explored. This should include the patient's capacity to develop and maintain stable and mutually satisfying relationships as well as issues of intimacy and sexual behaviours.
- Current relationships with parents, grandparents, children, and grandchildren are an important part of the social history. Legal history is also relevant, especially any pending charges or lawsuits.
- The social history also includes hobbies, interests, pets, and leisure time activities and how this has fluctuated over time. It is important to identify cultural and religious influences on the patient's life and current religious beliefs and practices. In a number of surveys it has been noted that religious beliefs are a very important part of people's lives, but this area is often not explored in psychiatric evaluations nor even in ongoing psychiatric treatment.

AIIMS NOVEMBER 2015

26. Ans. (c) IV Sodium bicarbonate

Ref: Nelson 20th Ed page 462, Harrison 19th ed page 172

- The girl was getting treatment for depression. SSRI and TCA are used in treating depression. Among these toxicity of TCA will cause ALOC, hypotension and arrhythmia, which will be rapidly progressive develop features of the anticholinergic toxidrome, including delirium, mydriasis, dry mucous membranes, tachycardia, hyperthermia, urinary retention, and slow GI motility.
- CNS toxicity can include lethargy, coma, myoclonic jerks, and seizures.
- Sinus tachycardia is the most common cardiovascular manifestation of toxicity; however, patients can develop widening of the QRS complex, premature ventricular contractions, and ventricular arrhythmias.
- Refractory hypotension is a poor prognostic indicator and is the most common cause of death in TCA overdose.

Altered Mental Status

TCA-poisoned patients can become deeply comatose relatively quickly, so careful and prompt attention to the airway and placement of an endotracheal tube is of paramount importance. The airway should be secured prior to any GI decontamination efforts.

Widened QRS on the ECG

TCAs (along with other agents such as diphenhydramine, cocaine, etc) will block the fast sodium channels on the myocardial cells, slowing the upstroke of the QRS complex. Because the effect on sodium channels is greatest within the 1st 6 hours, frequent ECGs (i.e., every 20–30 minutes) during this time frame are important. As the QRS approaches 160 msec, the chance of the patient developing monomorphic ventricular tachycardia rises to 30%. ***Sodium, usually in the form of sodium bicarbonate, is the antidote of choice.*** Indications for sodium bicarbonate include a QRS duration ≥110 msec, ventricular dysrhythmias, and hypotension. Multiple bolus doses of sodium bicarbonate, 1–2 mEq/kg each, may be needed to narrow the QRS to <110 msec. Some authors prefer to then place the patient on an infusion of sodium bicarbonate, but this may not be necessary if careful attention is paid to the QRS after the initial doses and repeat bolus dosing is provided as needed during those 1st 6–12 hours. Hypertonic (3%) saline and/or lipid emulsion therapy may be beneficial in refractory cases.

Hypotension

A direct acting vasopressor, such as norepinephrine or epinephrine, is the agent of choice. Boluses of intravenous crystalloid fluids should be used with caution to prevent fluid overload.

Seizures

Likely a result of the anticholinergic effects of TCAs, seizures are relatively common, typically brief, and should be treated with agents the work on the γ-aminobutyric acid receptor complex in the brain. Benzodiazepines are the agent of choice. Asymptomatic children should receive appropriate decontamination and be observed with continuous cardiac monitoring and serial ECGs for at least 6 hours. If any manifestations of toxicity develop, the child should be admitted to a monitored setting. Children who remain completely asymptomatic with normal serial ECGs may be candidates for discharge after 6 hours of close observation.

27. Ans. (d) Psychoeducation

Ref: CTP 9th ed Page 1837

"**Psychoeducation** is now clearly established as an effective treatment in combination with pharmacotherapy for the prevention of recurrences of bipolar disorder."

A primary function of a therapist when working with a person with bipolar disorder is that of psychoeducation. Psychoeducation, when delivered in a group setting, has been shown to delay time to affective relapse, when compared to a control nonspecific group intervention. Psychoeducation seeks to inform the patient as to the cyclical, recurrent nature of bipolar disorder and stresses the benefits of adherence to medication recommendations. Psychoeducation reinforces to the patient the biologic basis of bipolar disorder and helps ameliorate shame related to behaviors influenced by mood episodes. Patients are taught that bipolar disorder is a chronic condition, similar in some ways to diabetes and hyper-tension that requires lifestyle changes, as well as frequent monitoring and **consistency in medication compliance.** Consequences of affective episodes are explored, seeking to bolster the motivation of the individual to remain in treatment. Psychoeducation appears to be most useful when delivered to a more euthymic patient.

28. Ans. (c) 2 years

Ref: Maudsley 11th edition page 60

A placebo-controlled study showed that when no active prophylactic treatment is given, 57% of first-episode patients have relapsed at 1 year. After 1–2 years of being well on antipsychotic medication, the risk of relapse remains high (figures of 10–15% per month have been quoted), but this area is less well researched. Although the current consensus is that antipsychotics should be prescribed for 1–2 years after a first episode of schizophrenia, Gitlin et al found that withdrawing antipsychotic treatment in line with this consensus led to a relapse rate of almost 80% after 1 year medication free and 98% after 2 years. Other studies in first-episode patients have found that discontinuing antipsychotics increases the risk of relapse five-fold and confirmed that only a small minority of patients who discontinue remain well 1–2 years later.

29. Ans. (c) Haloperidol

Ref: Maudsley 11th ed page 435

Recommendations for the Treatment of Psychosis in Pregnancy

- Patients with a history of psychosis who are maintained on antipsychotic medication should be advised to discuss a planned pregnancy as early as possible.
- Be aware that drug-induced hyperprolactinaemia may prevent pregnancy. Consider switching to alternative drug.
- Such patients, particularly if they have suffered repeated relapses, are best maintained on antipsychotics during and after pregnancy. This may minimise foetal exposure by avoiding the need for higher doses, and/or multiple drugs should relapse occur.
- There is most experience with **chlorpromazine** (constipation and sedation can be a problem), **trifluoperazine, haloperidol, olanzapine** and **clozapine** (gestational diabetes may be a problem with both SGAs). If the patient is established on another antipsychotic, the most up-to-date advice should always be obtained. Experience with other drugs is growing and a change in treatment may not be necessary or wise.
- NICE recommends avoiding depot preparations and anticholinergic drugs in pregnancy.
- A few authorities recommend discontinuation of antipsychotics 5–10 days before anticipated delivery to minimise the chances of neonatal effects. This may, however, put mother and infant at risk and needs to be considered carefully. Antipsychotic discontinuation symptoms can occur in the neonate (e.g. crying, agitation, increased suckling). Some centres used mixed (breast/bottle) feeding to minimise withdrawal.

With SGAs, discontinuation may not be necessary or desirable.

30. Ans. (a) Impairment in cognition

Ref: Kaplan 10th edition page 1192

- Pervasive developmental disorders include several that are characterized by impaired reciprocal social interactions, aberrant language development, and restricted behavioral repertoire. More than two thirds of children with autistic disorder have mental retardation, although it is not required for the diagnosis.
- Autistic disorder, the best known of these disorders, is characterized by sustained impairment in comprehending and responding to social cues, aberrant language development and usage, and restricted, stereotypical behavioral patterns.
- Short attention span, poor ability to focus on a task, insomnia, feeding and eating problems, and enuresis are also common among children with autism.
- Autistic spectrum disorders include autism, Asperger's, Pervasive Developmental Disorder NOS (not otherwise specified).

DSM V Diagnostic Crtieria for Autism

- Persistent deficits in social communication and social interaction across multiple contexts, as manifested by the following, currently or by history (examples are illustrative, not exhaustive; see text):
- Deficits in social-emotional reciprocity, ranging, for example, from abnormal social approach and failure of normal back-and-forth conversation; to reduced sharing of interests, emotions, or affect; to failure to initiate or respond to social interactions.
- Deficits in nonverbal communicative behaviors used for social interaction, ranging, for example, from poorly integrated verbal and nonverbal communication; to abnormalities in eye contact and body language or deficits in understanding and use of gestures: to a total lack of facial expressions and nonverbal communication.
- Deficits in developing, maintaining, and understanding relationships, ranging, for example, from difficulties adjusting behavior to suit various social contexts; to difficulties in sharing imaginative play or in making friends; to absence of interest in peers.

Specify Current Severity

Severity is based on social communication impairments and restricted, repetitive patterns of behavior.

- Restricted, repetitive patterns of behavior, interests, or activities, as manifested by at least two of the following, currently or by history (examples are illustrative, not exhaustive; see text):
- Stereotyped or repetitive motor movements, use of objects, or speech (e.g. simple motor stereotypies, lining up toys or flipping objects, echolalia, idiosyncratic phrases).
- Insistence on sameness, inflexible adherence to routines, or ritualized patterns of verbal or nonverbal behavior (e.g. extreme distress at small changes, difficulties with transitions, rigid thinking patterns, greeting rituals, need to take same route or eat same food every day).
- Highly restricted, fixated interests that are abnormal in intensity or focus (e.g. strong attachment to or preoccupation with unusual objects, excessively circumscribed or perseverative interests).
- Hyper- or hyporeactivity to sensory input or unusual interest in sensory aspects of the environment (e.g. apparent indifference to pain/temperature, adverse response to specific sounds or textures, excessive smelling or touching of objects, visual fascination with lights or movement).

Specify Current Severity

- Severity is based on social communication impairments and restricted, repetitive patterns of behavior
- Symptoms must be present in the early developmental period (but may not become fully manifest until social demands exceed limited capacities, or may be masked by learned strategies in later life).

Contd...

- Symptoms cause clinically significant impairment in social, occupational, or other important areas of current functioning.
- These disturbances are not better explained by intellectual disability (intellectual developmental disorder) or global developmental delay. Intellectual disability and autism spectrum disorder frequently co-occur; to make comorbid diagnoses of autism spectrum disorder and intellectual disability, social communication should be below that expected for general developmental level.

Note:

- Individuals with a well-established DSM-IV diagnosis of autistic disorder, Asperger's disorder, or pervasive developmental disorder not otherwise specified should be given the diagnosis of autism spectrum disorder. Individuals who have marked deficits in social communication, but whose symptoms do not otherwise meet criteria for autism spectrum disorder, should be evaluated for social (pragmatic) communication disorder.
- Specify if:
- With or without accompanying intellectual impairment
- With or without accompanying language impairment
- Associated with a known medical or genetic condition or environmental factor
- (Coding note: Use additional code to identify the associated medical or genetic condition.)
- Associated with another neurodevelopmental, mental, or behavioral disorder
- (Coding note: Use additional code[s] to identify the associated neurodevelopmental, mental, or behavioral disorder[s].)
- With catatonia associated with autism spectrum disorder to indicate the presence of the comorbid catatonia.

31. Ans. (b) Repression

Ref: Kaplan 10th edition page 206

Option (A) Isolation

Splitting or separating an idea from the affect that accompanies it but is repressed.

Option (B) Repression

Expelling or withholding from consciousness an idea or feeling. Primary repression refers to the curbing of ideas and feelings before they have attained consciousness: secondary repression excludes from awareness what was once experienced at a conscious level. The repressed is not really forgotten in that symbolic behavior may be present. This defense differs from suppression by effecting conscious inhibition of impulses to the point of losing and not just postponing cherished goals. Conscious perception of instincts and feelings is blocked in repression.

Option (C) Dissociation

Temporarily but drastically modifying a person's character or one's sense of personal identity to avoid emotional distress.

Option (D) Suppression

Consciously or semiconsciously postponing attention to a conscious impulse or conflict. Issues may be deliberately cut off, but they are not avoided. Discomfort is acknowledged but minimized.

32. Ans. (a) Feeling of guilt

Ref: Kaplan 10th ed Page 534

Cognitive Theory of Depression/Cognitive Triad of Beck

According to cognitive theory, depression results from specific cognitive distortions present in persons susceptible to depression. Those distortions, referred to as depressogenic schemata, are cognitive templates that perceive both internal and external data in ways that are altered by early experiences.

Aaron Beck postulated a cognitive triad of depression that consists of:

Views about the self: "A negative self-precept;

About the environment: "A tendency to experience the world as hostile and demanding, and

About the future: The expectation of suffering and failure.

Therapy consists of modifying these distortions.

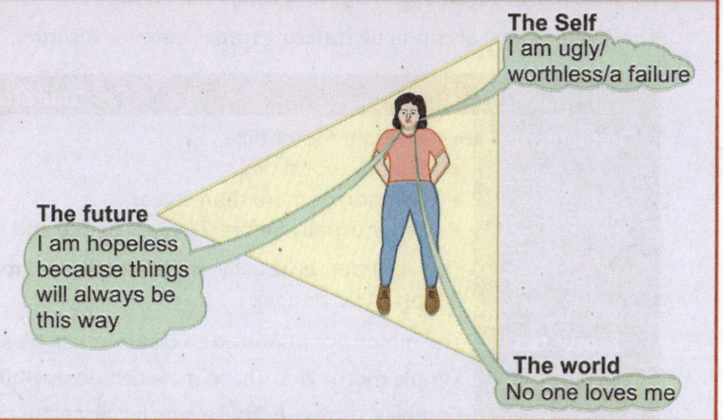

AIIMS MAY 2015

33. Ans. (c) C

Ref: Kaplan 10th edition page 791; DSM V criteria

A **personality disorder** is an enduring pattern of inner experience and behavior that deviates markedly from the expectations of the individual's culture, is pervasive and inflexible, has an onset in adolescence or early adulthood, is stable over time, and leads to distress or impairment.

Personality disorder subtypes classified in DSM-V-TR are:

- **Schizotypal, Schizoid and Paranoid (Cluster A):** Cluster A includes three disorders with odd, aloof features, such as paranoid, schizoid, and schizotypal.
- **Narcissistic, Borderline, Antisocial and Histrionic (Cluster B):** Cluster B includes four disorders with dramatic, impulsive, and erratic features, such as borderline, antisocial, narcissistic and histrionic.
- **Obsessive-Compulsive, Dependent and Avoidant (Cluster C):** Cluster C includes three disorders sharing anxious and fearful features, such as avoidant, dependent, and obsessive-compulsive.

34. Ans. (a) Akathisia

Ref: Kaplan 10th ed page 477, Niraj Ahuja 7th Ed Pg 62

Akathisia is the subjective feeling of restlessness and a common extra pyramidal side effect of antipsychotic medication.

The classic feature of the catatonic type is a marked disturbance in motor function; this disturbance may involve stupor, negativism, rigidity, excitement, or posturing. Sometimes, the patient shows rapid alteration between extremes of excitement and stupor. Associated features include stereotypies, mannerisms, and waxy flexibility. Mutism is particularly common.

Features of Catatonia	
Mutism	Complete absence of speech
Rigidity	Maintenance of a rigid posture against efforts to be moved
Negativism	An apparently motiveless resistance to all commands and attempts to be moved, or doing just the opposite
Posturing	Voluntary assumption of an inappropriate and often bizarre posture for long periods of time
Stupor	Akinesis (no movement) with mutism but with evidence of relative preservation of conscious awareness
Echolalia	Repetition, echo or mimicking of phrases or words heard
Echopraxia	Repetition, echo or mimicking of actions observed
Waxy flexibility	Parts of body can be placed in positions that will be maintained for long periods of time, even if very uncomfortable; flexible like wax
Ambitendency	Due to ambivalence, conflicting impulses and tentative actions are made, but no goal directed action occurs, e.g. on asking to take out tongue, tongue is slightly protruded but taken back again
Other signs	Like mannerisms, stereotypies (verbal and behavioral), automatic obedience (commands are followed automatically, irrespective of their nature) and verbigeration (incomprehensible speech)

35. Ans. (d) Risperidone

Ref: Maudsley 11th ed Page 346, Niraj Ahuja 6th Ed page 181

The above patient seems to be suffering from Tourette's disorder.

Tourette's Disorder	
Characteristic	• Multiple motor tics. • Multiple vocal tics. • Duration of more than 1 year. • Onset usually before 11 years of age and almost always before 21 years of age. The disorder is usually more common (about three times) in males and has a prevalence rate of about 0.5 per 1000 people.
Motor tics	The motor tics in Tourette's disorder can be simple or complex. **Simple motor tics:** These may include **eye-blinking**, grimacing, shrugging of shoulders, tongue protrusion. **Complex motor I:** These are facial gestures, stamping, jumping, hitting self, squatting, twirling, echokinesis (repetition of observed acts), copropraxia (obxene acts). Motor tics are often the earliest to appear, beginning in the head region and then progressing downwards. These are later followed by the vocal tics.

Contd...

Tourette's Disorder	
Vocal Tics	The vocal tics Tourette's disorder can also be simple or complex. **Simple vocal tics:** Simple vocal tics include coughing, barking, throat-clearing, sniffing, clicking. **Complex vocal Sim:** These include some very characteristic, though not always present, symptoms of Tourette syndrome. For example, echolalia (repetition of heard phrases), palilalia (repetition of heard words), coprolalia (use of obscene words), and mental coprolalia (thinking of obscene words). Obsessions and Compulsions are often the associated symptoms. These are usually the last symptoms to appear.
Treatment	Pharmacotherapy is usually the preferred mode of treatment. The drug of choice is haloperidol (in small doses), though low doses of risperidone and olanzapine have also been used recently. SSRIs (like fluoxetine) have been used for the treatment of co-morbid obsessive compulsive symptoms. In the resistant cases or in case of severe side-effects, pimozide or clonidine can be used under expert supervision. Behavior therapy can sometimes be used, as an adjunct. Clonidine has been shown in open studies to reduce the severity and frequency of tics but in one study this effect did not seem to be convincingly larger than placebo. Adverse effects of antipsychotics may outweigh beneficial effects in the treatment of tics and so it is recommended that clonidine is tried first. Antipsychotics may, however, be more effective than clonidine in alleviating tics in some individuals. Risperidone has been shown to be more effective than placebo in a small (N = 34), randomised study.

36. Ans. (a) Promethazine

Ref: Kaplan 10th ed page 926, KDT 7th ed page 444, Goodman and Gilman's 11th Ed Table 18-4

Neurological Side Effects of Neuroleptic Drugs

	Acute dystonia	Akathisia	Parkinsonism	Tardive dyskinesia	Neuroleptic malignant syndrome
	Early	**Intermediate**	**Intermediate**	**Late (tardive)**	**Any**
Onset	Within 7 days of therapy or ↑ dose	Within 3 months of therapy or ↑ dose	Within 3 months of therapy or ↑ dose	>3–6 months (↓dose may unmask dyskinesia)	Anytime during therapy (↑ dose or high potency drugs)
Incidence	15–20% with typical neuroleptics, 5% with atypical	20%	30%	5% per year of therapy i.e. 50% in 10 years	0.5% (20–30% mortality)
Mechanism	Unclear, dopamine hypofunction at basal ganglia	D2 receptor blockage in mesocortical pathway	D2 receptor blockage at striatum	D2 receptor blockage at striatum	Idiosyncratic, relative depletion of dopamine in CNS
Risk factors	Male, young, mental retardation, history of ECT, dose elevation	Elderly, female, mental retardation, Iron deficiency, affective disorders, dose elevation	Elderly, Females, dementia, underlying parkinsonism, AIDS, dose elevation	Elderly, female, history of ECT, substance abuse, iron deficiency, mental retardation, mood disorder, organic brain damage, anticholinergic dose decrease	Male, young, dose elevation
Symptoms	Slow, irregular, continuous contractions, oculogyric movements of tongue, torticollis, trismus, abnormal posture, blepharospasm	Uncontrolled restlessness, pacing, compulsive foot taping, rocking movement, adversity to stand still, rapid alternation of standing and sitting	R = Rigidity A = Akinesia (MC) T = Tremor (atypical-coarse, not pill rolling, late) Rabbit syndrome = Lip and perioral tremors	Most serious adverse effect. Rapid, irregular, continuous or intermittent contractions, orofasciolingual or limb/trunkal, ↑by stress activity	Life threatening F = Fever E = Encephalopathy V = Vitals unstable E = Elevated CPK, WBC R = Rigidity

Contd...

Neurological Side Effects of Neuroleptic Drugs					
	Acute dystonia	Akathisia	Parkinsonism	Tardive dyskinesia	Neuroleptic malignant syndrome
Treatment	Antiparkinsonian agents are diagnostic and curative Anti-cholinergics: Benzatropine, promethazine or hvdroxyzine i.m. clears the reaction within 10-15 minutes. Antihistaminics: Diphenhydramine	Reduce dose and/or change antipsychotic. **Propranolol= doc**, central anticholinergic may reduce the intensity in some cases	Antiparkinsonian agents Anticholinergics may be useful as monotherapy in early, untreated Parkinson's or as adjunct therapy to patients already on levodopa Antihistaminics: Amantadine, Diphenhydramine	No established treatment, discontinue or replace the antipsychotic agent and then eliminate all drugs with central anticholinergic Action, lithium and carbamazepine for psychosis, BZD: buspirone for dyskinesia	Stop neuroleptic immediately; dantrolene or bromocriptine may help; antiparkinsonian agents not effective anticholinergics are of no help.

37. Ans. (b) Exposure and response prevention

Ref: Kaplan 10th ed page 610

See table of Methods of Behavior Therapy in Psychiatry AIIMS Nov 2016 (see page no. 1101-1102)

Although few head-to-head comparisons have been made, behavior therapy is as effective as pharmacotherapies in OCD, and some data indicate that the beneficial effects are longer lasting with behavior therapy. Many clinicians, therefore, consider behavior therapy the treatment of choice for OCD. Behavior therapy can be conducted in both outpatient and inpatient settings. **The principal behavioral approaches in OCD are exposure and response prevention**.

38. Ans. (b) Obsessive compulsive disorder

Ref: Anxiety Disorders in Adults: A Clinical Guide by Vladan Starcevic 2nd ed Pg 239

In very broad terms, obsessional **self-doubt** pertains to a person's recurrent and tormenting feeling that something about him or her is "not right." This feeling may refer to various aspects of the person's personality, behavior, thinking, physical appearance, or health. Self-doubt is often associated with uncertainty as to whether the person has done something or not. This uncertainty and inflated sense of responsibility often lead to checking compulsions. They may serve several purposes: alleviating distress or anxiety, **"making sure"** that there is no reason for further doubting, abolishing uncertainty, and *reassuring oneself that one will not be held responsible in case of an accident or other mishap*. The latter is particularly evident when checking is future-oriented.

39. Ans. (c) Tremor

Ref: Kaplan 10th ed page 390

The classic sign of alcohol withdrawal is tremulousness, although the spectrum of symptoms can expand to include psychotic and perceptual symptoms (e.g. delusions and hallucinations), seizures, and the symptoms of delirium tremens (DTs), called alcohol withdrawal delirium in DSM-IV-TR. Tremulousness (commonly called the shakes or the jitters) develops 6 to 8 hours after the cessation of drinking, the psychotic and perceptual symptoms begin in 8 to 12 hours, seizures in 12 to 24 hours, and DTs during 72 hours, although physicians should watch for the development of DTs for the first week of withdrawal.

Withdrawal Symptoms				
	Alcohol	Cocaine	Opioid	Nicotine
Craving	+++	+++	+++	+++
Mood	Anxiety or psychomotor agitation	Dysphoric/ Depressed mood	Dysphoric mood	Dysphoric/ Depressed mood
Sleep	Insomnia	Hypersomnolence	Insomnia	Insomnia
Tremor	+++			
Appetite	Decreased (Anorexia)	Increased		Increased
Autonomic hyperactivity	Sweating, Tachycardia (>100), hypertension, hyper reflexia, diaphoresis, hyperthermia, and muscle fasciculations		Tachypnea, hyper reflexia, tachycardia, hypertension, sweating, hyperthermia	No (infact there is decreased heart rate)

Contd...

Withdrawal Symptoms				
	Alcohol	**Cocaine**	**Opioid**	**Nicotine**
GIT	Nausea or vomiting		Diarrhea, cramping, nausea, vomiting	
Hallucinations	Transient visual, tactile, or auditory hallucinations or illusions		Sensory distortions or hallucinations (e.g. transient visual, tactile, or auditory)	
Seizures	Grand mal seizures	Single event. MC substance abuse related to seizures		
Others			COLD TURKEY (Piloerection and Rhinorrhea), Hyperalgia, joint and muscle aches. Pupillary dilation, photophobia, Yawning	Irritability, frustration, or anger Headache, poor concentration

Footnote:
Physical dependence is absent in LSD and are very mild in cannabis.
Physical and psychological withdrawals are mild in Cannabis, Ecstacy, phencyclidine, amphetamines.

40. Ans. (c) Self exemption

Ref: Kaplan 10th ed page 270

NOTE

Self exempting is a belief not defense mechanism per se. If denial (a defense mechanism) is provided in the option it is the best answer, more so if defense mechanism is particularly asked in the question.

Self-Exempting Beliefs/Risk Minimizing Belief

Smokers are prone to deny their risk of developing smoking-related diseases or rationalize the health consequences of smoking behavior in order to reduce cognitive dissonance (mental stress discomfort). "self-exempting beliefs" is also known as risk-minimizing beliefs or **risk denial** towards smoking hazards.

Delusional projection, psychotic denial, distortion, and splitting belong to the narcissistic mechanisms of defense and it is not always possible to differentiate between them.

- **Denial:** i.e. not believing the truth. Smokers may refuse to admit that he/she is at risk of Lung cancer even though he/she knows that smoking causes Lung cancer.
- **Distortion** is a defense mechanism where an individual is grossly reshaping external reality to suit inner needs.

Radiodiagnosis & Radiotherapy

18

AIIMS NOVEMBER 2018

1. A young female with history of renal calculi complaints of bone pain and abdominal cramps. On investigation multiple fractures were discovered and Serum calcium and PTH was raised. Which of the following will be the best investigation to arrive at a definitive diagnosis?

(AIIMS Nov 2018, May 2017)

a. FDG PET
b. SestaMIBI
c. USG
d. CT

2. What is the name of the procedure given in this radiograph?

a. Myelography
b. Angiography
c. Fluoroscopy
d. Neurography

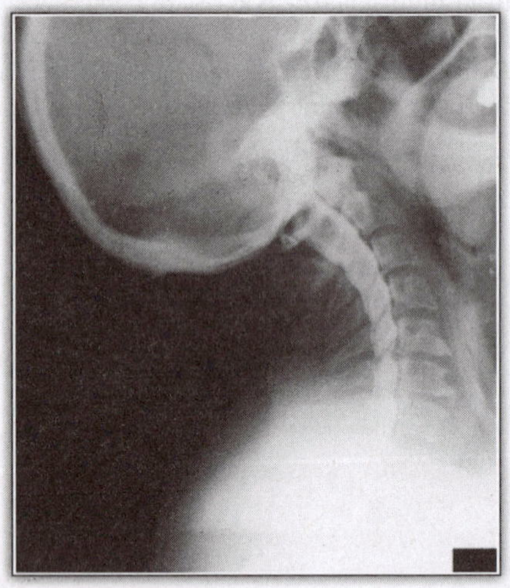

3. Empty thecal sac sign on MRI is seen in?

a. Discitis
b. Arachnoiditis
c. Vertebral osteomyelitis
d. Tethered cord syndrome

4. Which of the following investigation does not have any ionizing radiation?

a. Mammography
b. Angiography
c. CT Scan
d. MRI

5. Patient admitted with complaints of abdominal pain. Plain X-ray abdomen erect showed the following findings. What is your diagnosis? ***(AIIMS Nov 2018, May 2017)***

a. Eventration of diaphragm
b. Diaphragmatic hernia
c. Pneumoperitoneum
d. Pneumothorax

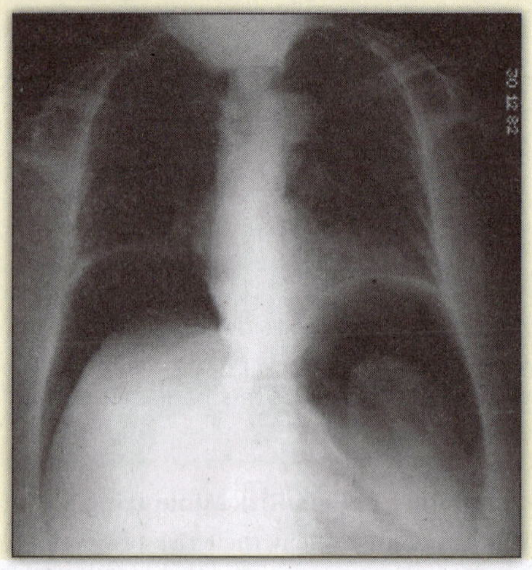

6. What is the diagnosis of the given radiograph?

a. Cervical rib
b. Costochondritis
c. Fracture of left 2nd rib
d. Spondylolisthesis of C5 over C6

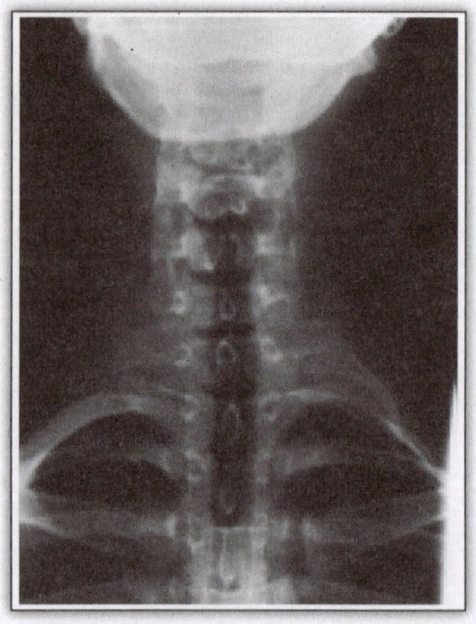

AIIMS MAY 2018

7. A middle aged female patient with history of cholelithiasis, presented with vomiting and abdominal pain, abdominal radiograph showed Rigler triad. Which of the following is not a component of Rigler's triad?

a. Pneumobilia
b. Small bowel obstruction
c. Ectopic gall stone
d. Large bowel obstruction

8. A 50-year-old male presented in the emergency with high BP 160/100 and heart rate of 120/min. A CECT is done which is given below. What is the management of the given condition?

a. Start Beta Blockers
b. Shift to OT for repair
c. Low molecular weight heparin
d. Vitamin K inhibitors

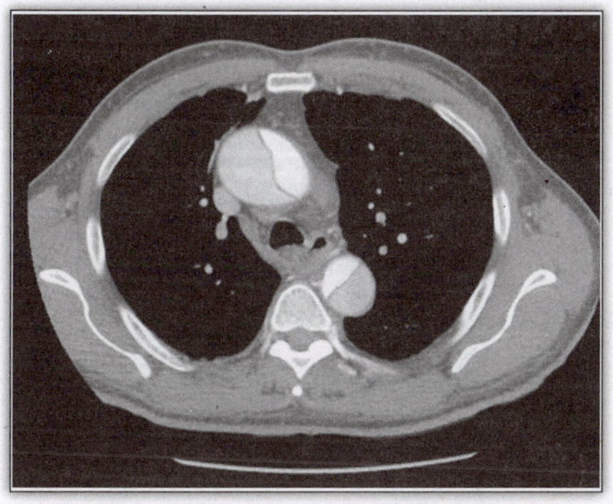

9. Characteristic of venous blood flow of lower limb in Duplex Doppler is?

a. Monophasic
b. Biphasic
c. Triphasic
d. Non phasic

AIIMS NOVEMBER 2017

10. Most likely diagnosis as per the given image is?

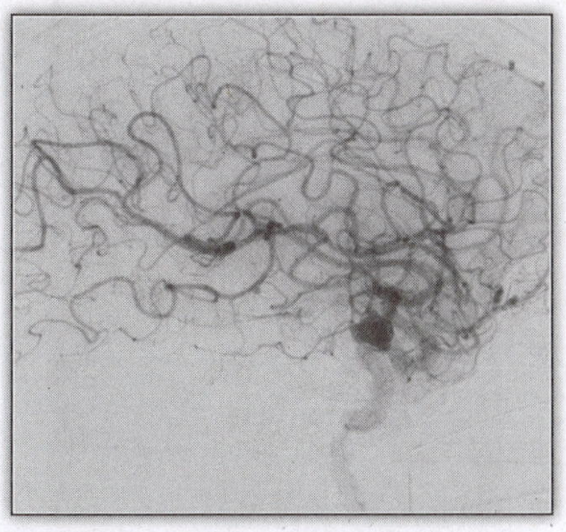

a. Carotid cavernous fistula
b. Pseudoaneurysm of Internal carotid artery
c. Tumor blush of Angiofibroma
d. Extensive head and neck Hemangioma

11. A 30 year old male comes with sudden onset breathlessness and right pleuritic chest pain. Chest X-ray shows?

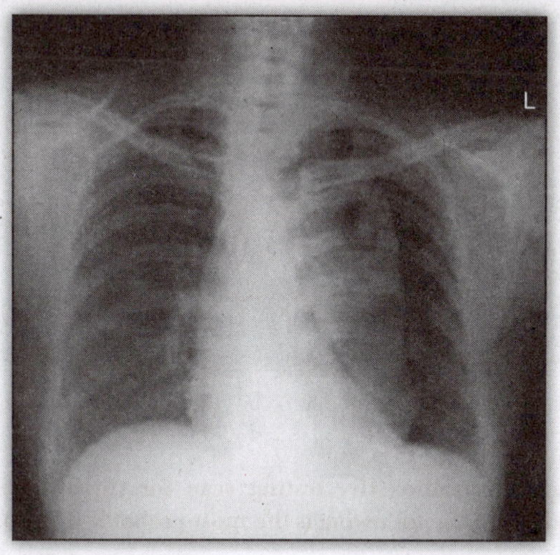

a. Pulmonary embolism
b. Pneumothorax
c. Pleural effusion
d. Hydropneumothorax

12. All of the following are 18-FDG positive on PET scan EXCEPT:

a. Large neuroendocrine tumour
b. Typical carcinoid
c. Atypical carcinoid
d. Small cell carcinoma

AIIMS MAY 2017

13. A young female with history of renal calculi complaints of bone pain and abdominal cramps. On investigation multiple fractures were discovered and serum calcium and PTH was raised. Which of the following will be the best investigation to arrive at a definitive diagnosis?

(AIIMS Nov 2018, May 2017)

a. FDG PET
b. Sestamibi
c. USG
d. CT

14. A 65-year-old male banker came for an ultrasound to renew his medical insurance. On right kidney, a complex cyst was found, the picture of the CT scan is shown, the cyst is solid exophytic encroaching on the adjacent structure. On ultrasound complex renal cyst. Most likely diagnosis is?

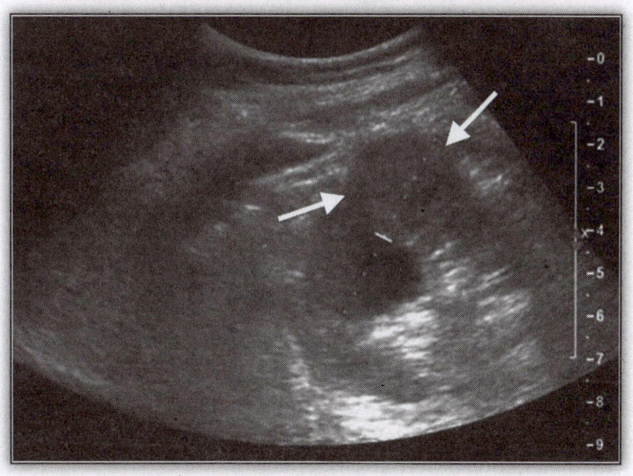

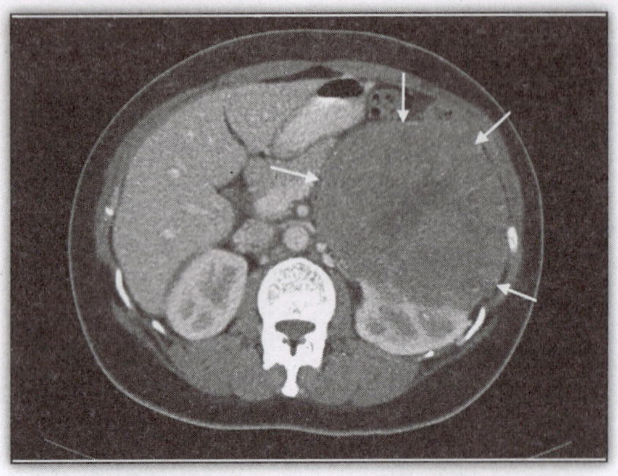

a. Renal cell carcinoma b. Angiomyolipoma
c. Parapelvic cyst d. Renal cyst

15. Below is radioactive testing scan for thyroid pathology. Which of the following is the most probable diagnosis?

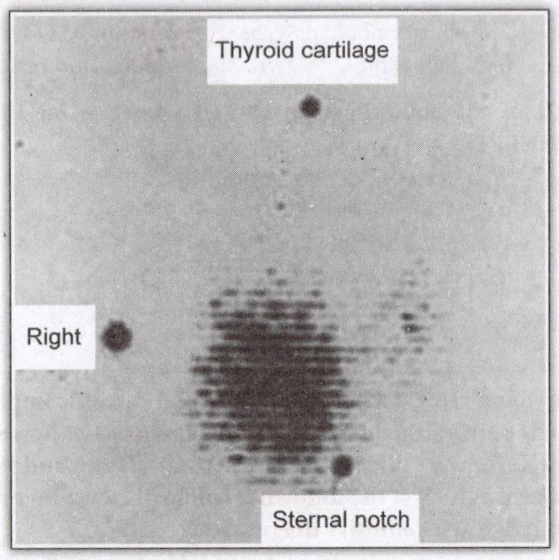

a. Lateral aberrant thyroid b. Hypersecretory adenoma
c. Grave's disease d. Papillary carcinoma of thyroid

16. Which of the following is not seen in the following chest X-ray?

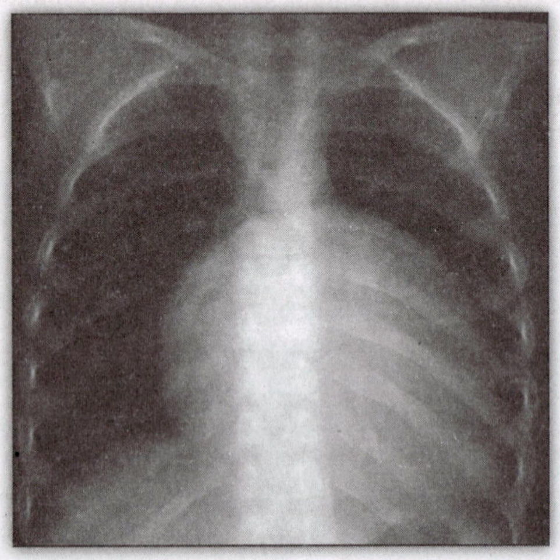

a. Right atrial enlargement
b. Narrow vascular pedicle
c. Decrease pulmonary blood flow
d. Pulmonary venous hypertension

17. A 20-year-old male presented with fever, cough and mucopurulent sputum. His WBC count was-28000/dl. The chest X-ray was as follows. Sputum smear should show which organism?

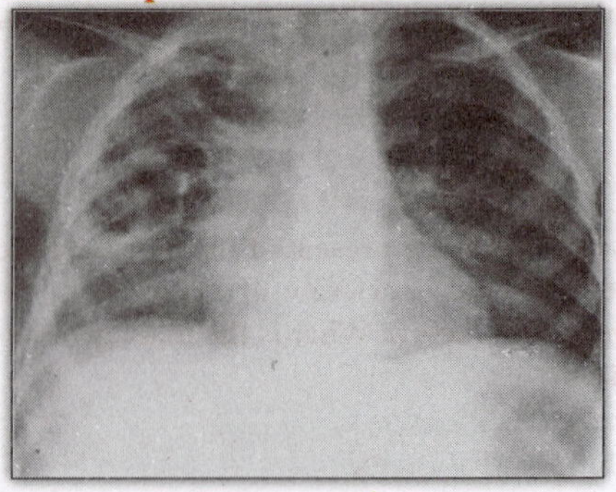

a. Staphylococcus aureus. b. Streptococcus pneumoniae
c. Chlamydia trachomatis d. Aspergillus fumigatus

18. Patient admitted with complaints of abdominal pain. Plain X-ray abdomen erect showed the following findings. What is your diagnosis? ***(AIIMS Nov 2018, May 2017)***

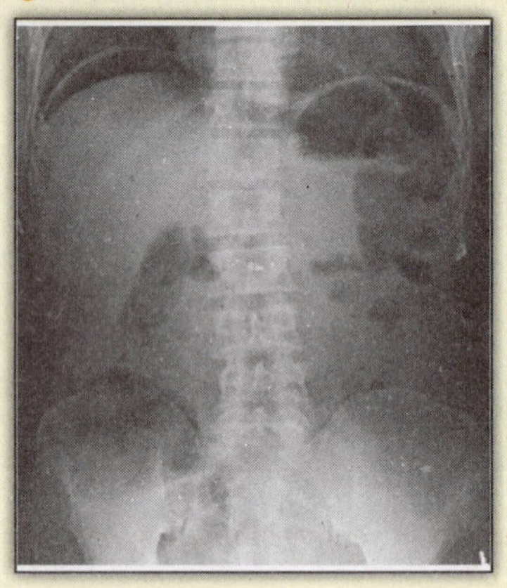

a. Eventration of diaphragm
b. Diaphragmatic hernia
c. Pneumoperitoneum d. Pneumothorax

19. A patient presented with fever and pain abdomen. He gives history of loose stools more than 7 times a day for several months. Abdominal X-ray is shown below. What is the most probable diagnosis?

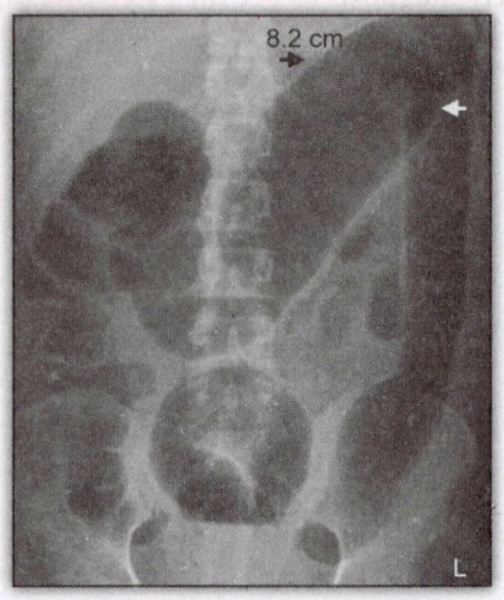

a. Pneumatosis intestinalis b. Toxic megacolon
c. Pseudomembranous colitis
d. Adenocarcinoma of colon

AIIMS NOVEMBER 2016

20. What is the diagnosis from X-ray wrist of this child?

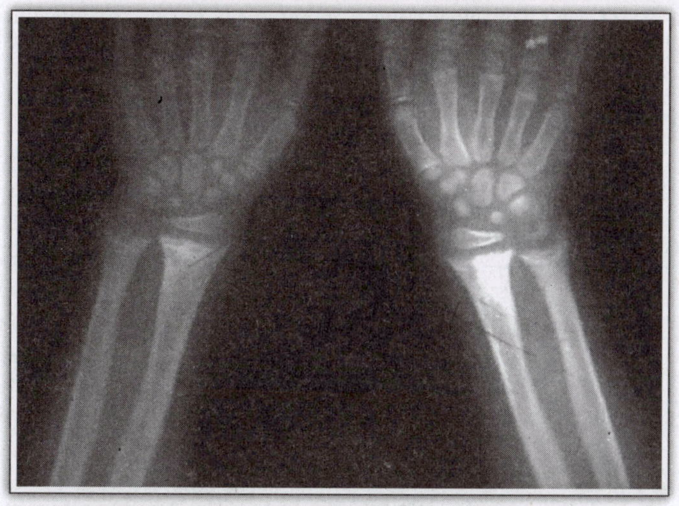

a. Colles fracture
b. Scaphoid dislocation
c. Rickets
d. Chronic osteomyelitis

21. A child comes with history of pain in right hip and difficulty in walking. X-ray hip was done as seen in the picture. Which of the following is most likely diagnosis?

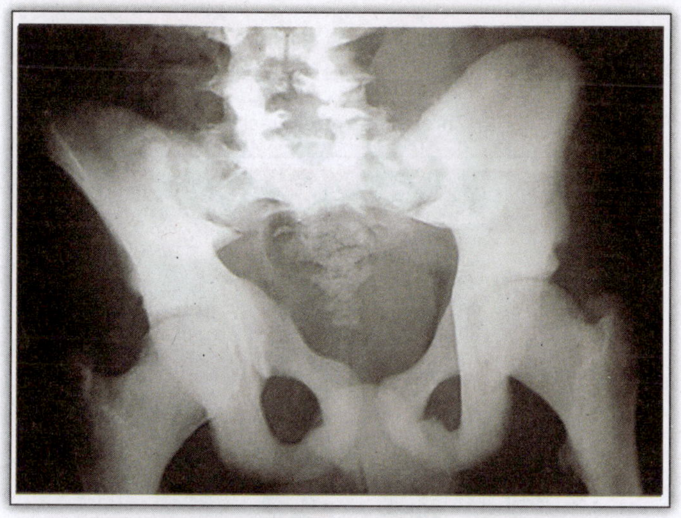

a. Osteopetrosis
b. Osteoporosis
c. Osteopoikilocytosis
d. Osteogenesis imperfecta

AIIMS MAY 2016

22. A patient is receiving pelvic external beam radiation for metastatic endometrial carcinoma. Which of the following organs in the field is most radiosensitive?

a. Ovary
b. Bladder
c. Vagina
d. Rectum

AIIMS NOVEMBER 2015

23. A patient presented with low back pain, X-ray lumbar spine is shown below. Identify the pathology in the given X-ray of spine?

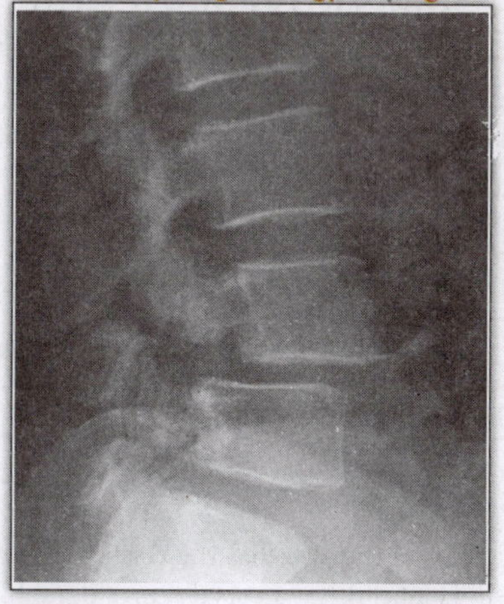

a. Spondylosis
b. Spondylolysis
c. Spondylolisthesis
d. Ankylosis

24. A patient with no history of chest trauma presents with history of fever and dyspnea. Chest X-ray is shown below. What is most likely diagnosis?

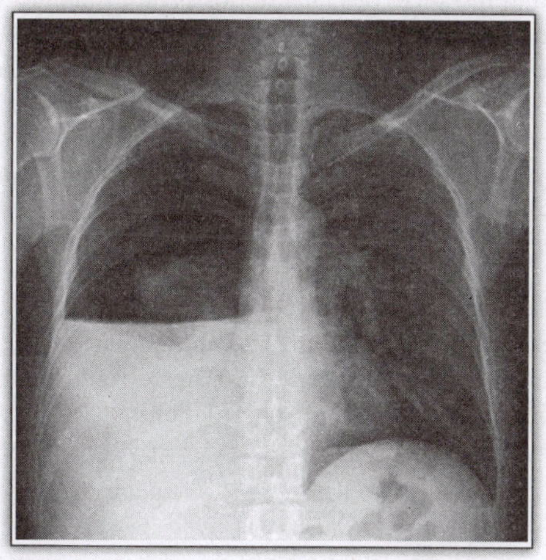

a. Pleural effusion
b. Peumothorax
c. Hydropneumothorax
d. Lung abscess

AIIMS MAY 2015

25. Patient with history of tachyarrhythmias is on implantable cardioverter defibrillator. He develops shock. Best method to know the position and integrity of ICD is to do?
(AIIMS May 2015, Nov 2012)

a. Contract CT
b. MRI
c. USG
d. Plain radiograph

26. Best non invasive investigation to check for viability of myocardium is?

a. Echocardiogram
b. FDG-18 PET CT
c. MIBG scintigraphy
d. Thallium scintigraphy

27. Expansion of the contrast space in myelography is seen in?

a. Intramedullary tumor
b. Extramedullary intradural tumor
c. Spinal dysraphism
d. Extradural tumor

AIIMS NOVEMBER 2018

1. Ans. (b) SestaMIBI

Ref: Grainger and Allison's Diagnostic Radiology 5th ed vol 2 ch 71

This is a case of Parathyroid adenoma causing Hyperparathyroidism

Repeat AIIMS May 2017 Radiodiagnosis (See for explanation) *(see page no. 1124)*

2. Ans. (a) Myelography

Ref: Chapman and Nakielny's Guide to radiological procedure 6th ed page 304, 308

In the figure, we can see that the cervical spinal cord appears enhanced. Hence, this is a cervical myelograph.

Uses: CT and MRI have replaced myelography as the primary method for investigating suspected disc prolapse. The main remaining uses of myelography are in patients with claustrophobia or who are otherwise not suitable for MRI. Myelography also allows a dynamic assessment of the spinal canal in instances of spinal stenosis and instability

Contrast: The early oil-based media were diagnostically poor and led to arachnoiditis. The early water-soluble media were very toxic and also led to arachnoiditis and the first intrathecal contrast medium with acceptably low toxicity was **metrizamide**, a non-ionic dimer. ***Iohexol and iopamidol are non-ionic monomers licensed for intrathecal use and the ones most commonly used currently.***

Limitations of Myelography

Myelography can not visualize entrapment of the nerve root lateral to the termination of the nerve root sheath. It is thus unable to detect lateral disc herniations.

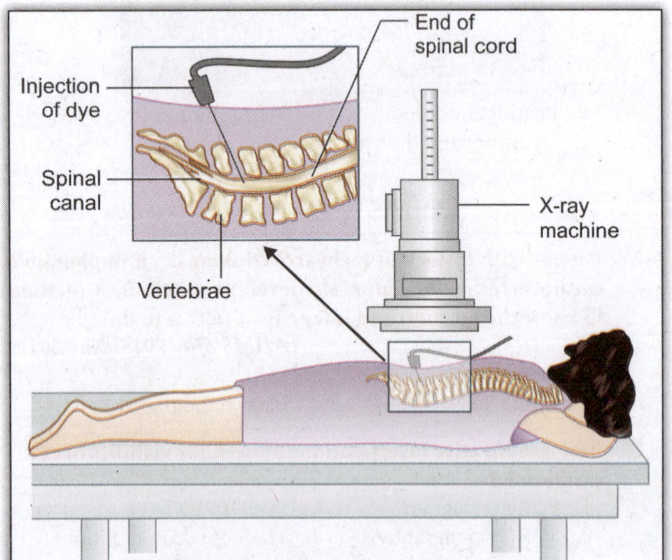

A myclogram requires the injection of dye into the spinal canal under x-ray guidance. The dye is usually injected in the lower back region (lumbar) and in some cases, in the neck (cervical) area

Cervical myelography: Contrast medium injected into the thecal sac by lumbar puncture and then run up to the cervical spine, or by direct cervical puncture at C1/2.

Radiographic views: After needle withdrawal, two AP radiographs are obtained with the tube angulated cranially and caudally, in turn, along with both oblique views once again with cranial and caudal tube tilt.

3. Ans. (b) Arachnoiditis

Ref: Grainger 6th ed pg 1371

Arachnoiditis - nerve roots are peripherally distributed, irregularly thickened and clumped together, often stuck to the dura, resulting in an empty thecal sac sign. Intrathecal soft tissue mass with a broad dural space representing a large group of matted lymph nodes is also seen.

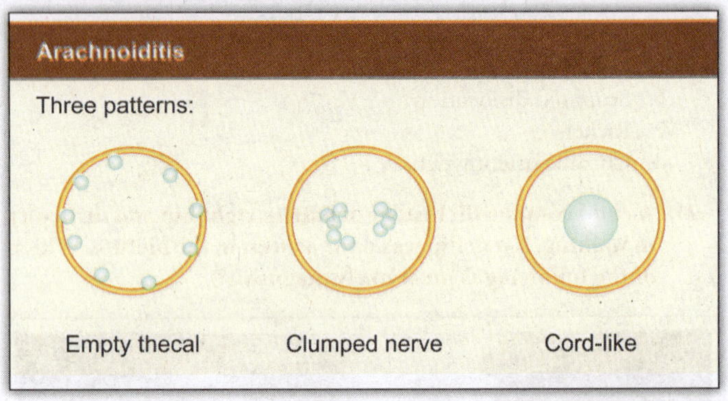

Fig: Three patterns of arachnoiditis

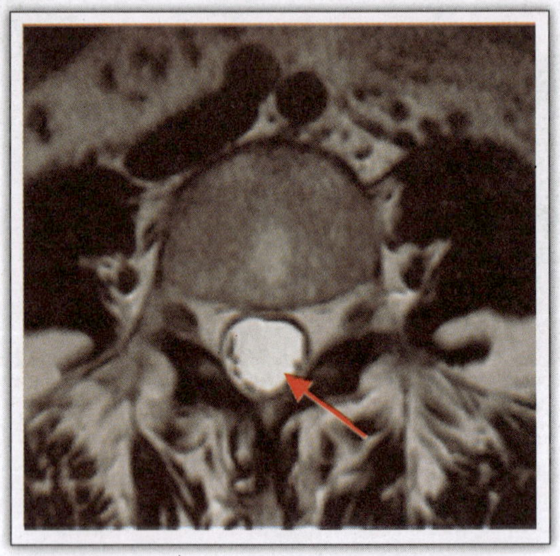

Fig: Empty Thecal sac sign seen in arachnoiditis.

4. Ans. (d) MRI

Ref: Magnetic Resonance Imaging of Congenital Heart Disease -Mushabbar A. Syed, Raad H. Mohiaddin Springer page 39

MRI like ultrasound, does not use any ionizing radiation, thus avoiding the risk of carcinogenesis

Ionizing and Non Ionizing Radiations			
Radiation	**Typical Frequency (per sec)**	**Typical Energy (kJ/mol)**	**Type of radiation**
Particles			*Ionizing radiation*
α-particles		4.1×10^8	
β-particles		1.5×10^7	
Electromagnetic radiation			
Cosmic rays	6×10^{21}	2.4×10^9	
Y-rays	$3 \times 10^{20} s^{-1}$	1.2×10^8	
X-rays	3×10^{17}	1.2×10^5	
Ultraviolet	3×10^{15}	1200	*non-ionizing radiation*
Visible	5×10^{14}	200	
Infrared	3×10^{13}	12	
Microwaves	3×10^9	1.2×10^{-3}	
Radio waves	3×10^7	1.2×10^{-5}	

5. Ans. (c) Pneumoperitoneum

Ref: Grainger and Allison's Diagnostic Radiology 5th ed ch 29 The X-ray abdomen (in question) (erect) shows presence of gas under the right dome of diaphragm suggestive of pneumoperitoneum.

Pneumoperitoneum

The most common cause is a perforation of the abdominal viscus—most commonly, a perforated ulcer, although a pneumoperitoneum may occur as a result of perforation of any part of the bowel; other causes include a benign ulcer, a tumor, or trauma.

X-ray signs of Pneumoperitoneum are

a. **Gas under diaphragm:** The above X-ray abdomen (erect) shows presence of gas under the right dome of diaphragm suggestive of pneumoperitoneum. **The erect chest radiograph is superior to the erect abdominal view for the demonstration of free intra-abdominal gas since, in the erect abdominal view, the X-ray beam is passing through any free gas under the diaphragm at an oblique angle.** CT is superior to plain radiographs in detecting minute quantities of pneumoperitoneum

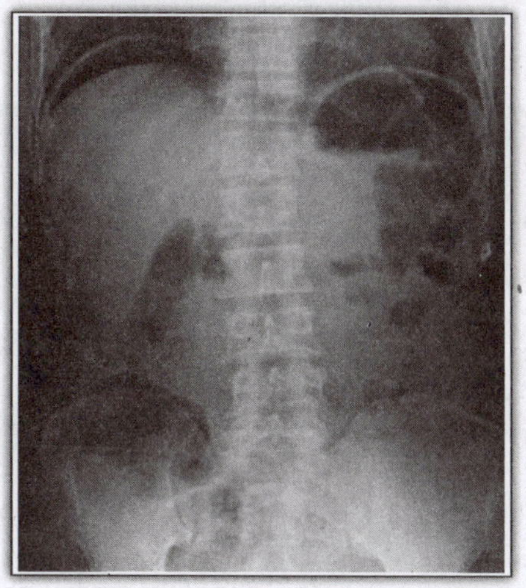

Fig: Pneumoperitoneum- gas under the diaphragm

b. **Doges cap sign** refers to free air in Morrison's pouch. Morrison's pouch is normally a potential space between the right kidney and the liver. This is a particularly difficult sign of pneumoperitoneum for several reasons. Firstly, it may be the only sign of pneumoperitoneum and may be very subtle. Secondly, it can be easily misinterpreted as gas in the duodenum. The Italian Doges wore this distinctively shaped cap. Gas in Morrison's pouch is only loosely shaped like a Doges cap and should not be taken too literally. Gas in Morrison's pouch on supine Radiographs may have the following features

- Triangular in shape
- Concave medial border
- Positioned inferior to the right 11th rib
- Positioned superior to the right kidney

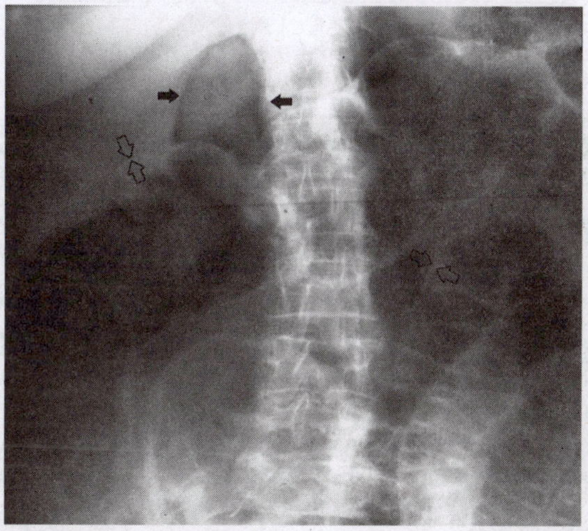

Fig: Doges cap sign

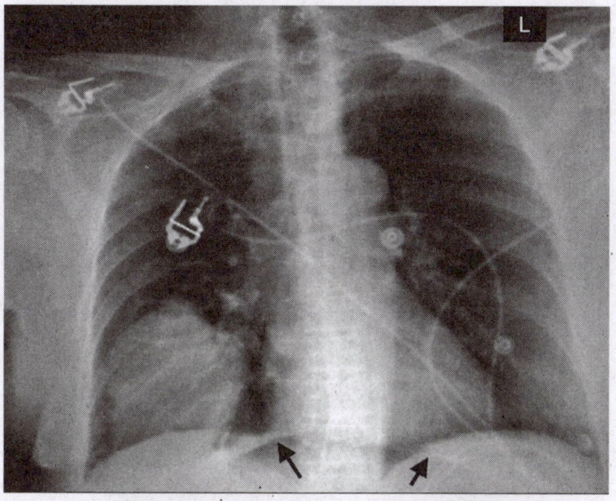

Fig: Cupola sign: Air accumulates underneath the central tendon of the diaphragm in the midline

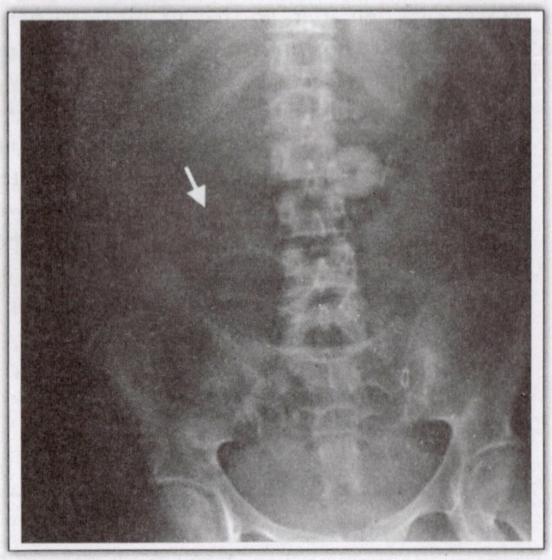

Fig: Rigler's sign (double wall sign) is seen when air is present on both sides of the intestine

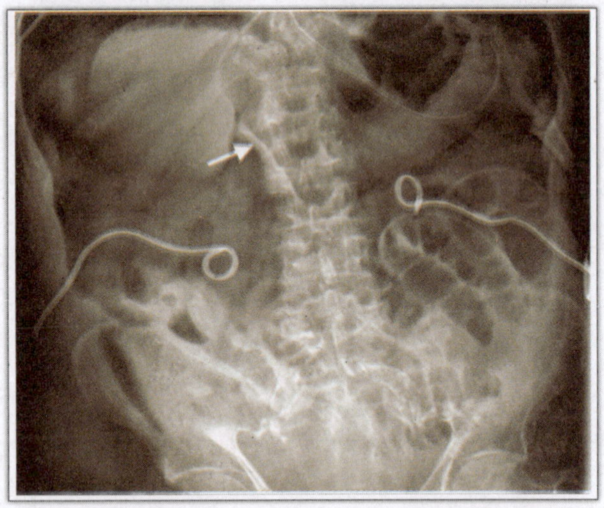

Fig: Falciform ligament sign in which falciform ligament is outlined with air in a supine patient with free abdominal gas

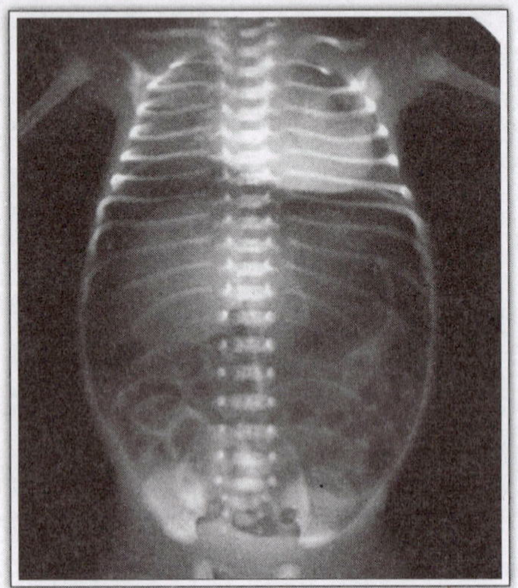

Fig: Football sign is seen in massive pneumoperitoneum, where the abdominal cavity is outlined by gas from a perforated viscus

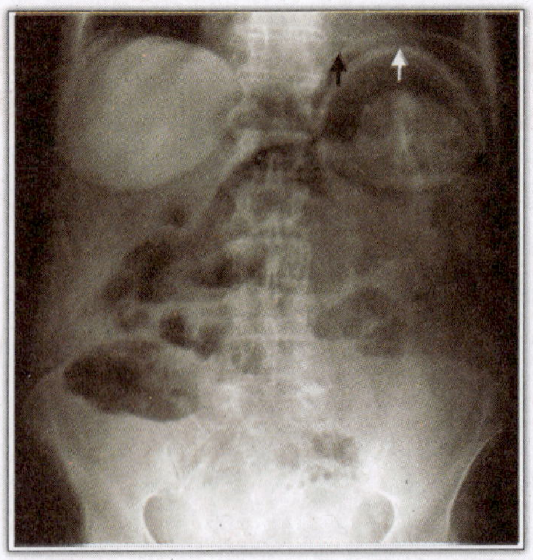

Fig: Double bubble sign is an appearance of subdiaphragmatic gas under the left hemidiaphragm in which there are two collections of overlapping gas, one of these collections is subdiaphragmatic free gas and the other is normal gas within the fundus of the stomach

6. Ans. (a) Cervical rib

Ref: Sutton 7th ed page 432, 1109, 1120

Cervical RIB

Cervical ribs have an incidence of 1-2% and are usually bilateral but frequently asymmetrical. The supplementary rib usually arises from the seventh cervical vertebra, rarely from the sixth and very rarely from the fifth. Ribs slope downward from the neural arch in the cervical spine but upward in the thoracic spine. Cervical ribs vary greatly in size and shape and clinical symptoms hear little relation to the radiographic abnormality. A large cervical rib may be asymptomatic.

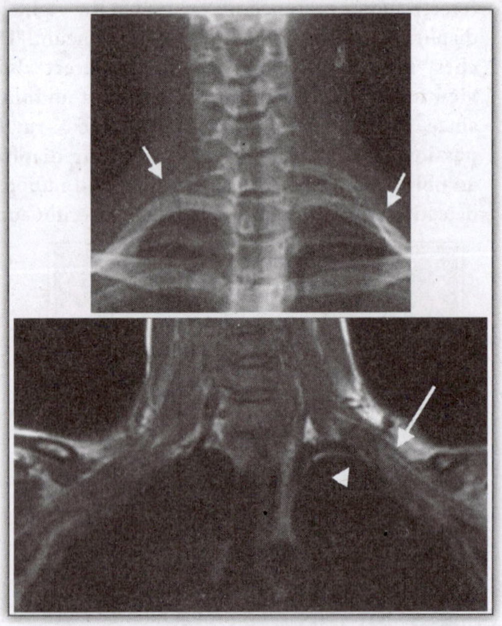

Curtesy: Dahlin LB et al- J Brachial Plex Peripher Nerve Inj (2009)

(A) Frontal radiograph showing bilateral cervical ribs, shorter on the right side. The lateral end of the cervical ribs is marked with arrows. (B) MRI T1-weighted coronal image showing the cervical rib (arrow head, B) with its pseudoarthrotic bony formation that lifts up the brachial plexus (long arrow).

AIIMS MAY 2018

7. Ans. (d) Large bowel obstruction

Ref: Rapid review of Radiology Shahid Hussain page 41, Bailey 26th ed page 1183

NOTE

Do not get confused with Rigler's sign. In pneumoperitoneum the presence of free intraperitoneal air outlines the bowel so that both sides of the bowel wall can be seen. This is called as Rigler's sign

Rigler's triad is a triad of small bowel obstruction (86%), pneumobilia (69%) and ectopic gallstones (25%). It is diagnostic of Gallstone ileus. Often, however, the gallstone is not seen on plain film since the stones frequently have a predominant composition of cholesterol with little calcification.

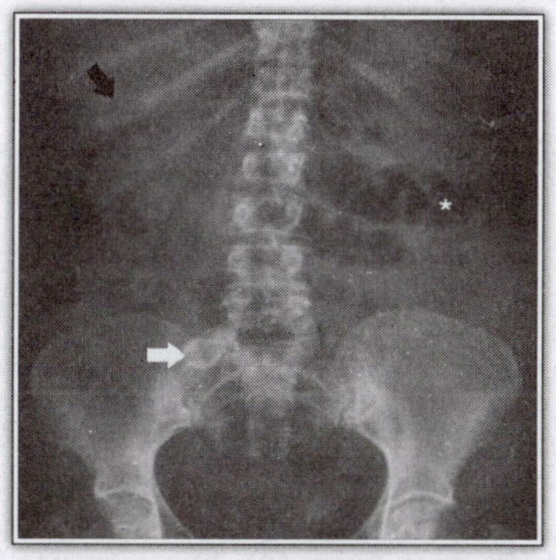

Fig: Plain X-ray erect abdomen demonstrating Rigler's triad. Pneumobilia (air in biliary tract- black arrow), Gallstone in terminal ileum (white arrow) and dilated small bowel suggestive of obstruction (astrerisk)

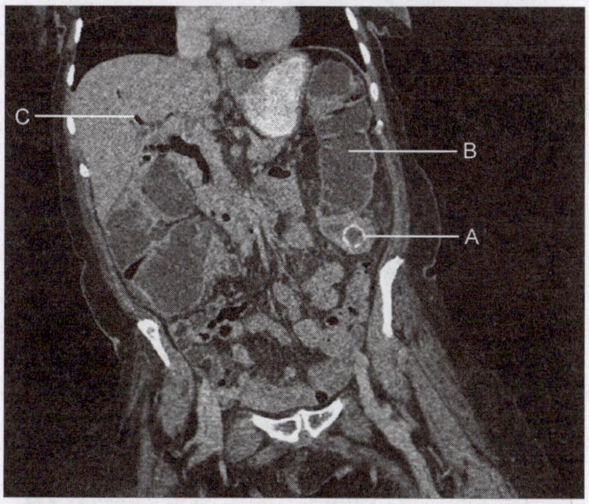

Fig: CECT abdomen (Coronal) demonstrating Rigler's triad. (A) Ectopic gallstone within the descending colon, (B) Small bowel obstruction seen as intestinal dilation proximal to the impacted gallstone, (C) pneumobilia secondary to a cholecystoenteric fistula

8. Ans: (b) Shift to OT for repair

Ref: Sabiston 20th Ed Pg 1746-1747

This is a case of Dissecting aortic aneurysm. Both Ascending and descending aorta ae involved hence Surgical repair needs to be done.

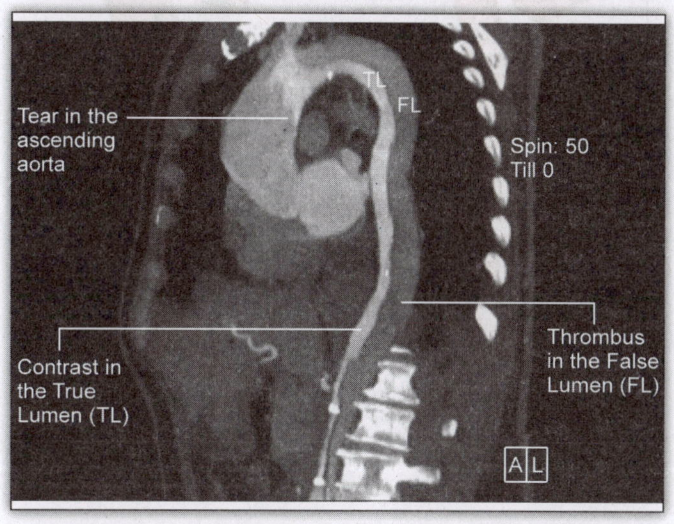

Fig: Aortic dissection from the ascending aorta extending to the bifurcation of the common iliacs

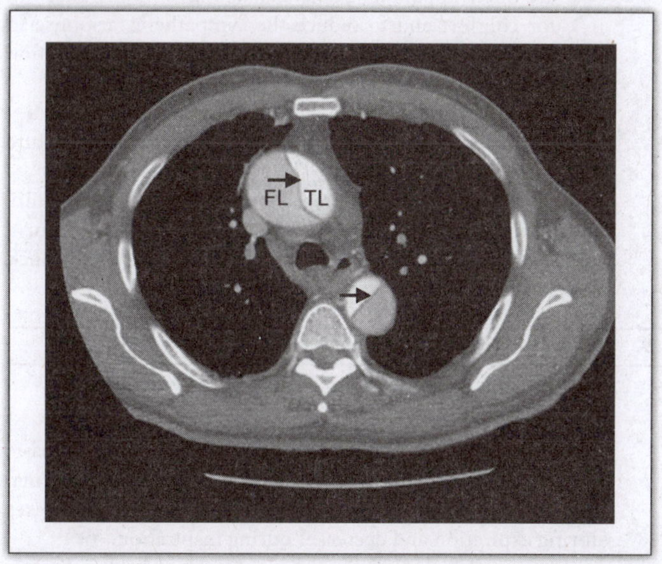

Fig: Aortic dissection the arrows demonstrate the intimal flaps in both the ascending aorta (anterior) and the descending aorta (posterior). TL is the true lumen as this has contrast within it whilst the darker false lumen (FL) does not

Stanford Classification

There are 4 different classifications of aortic dissection and the commonest one used is the Stanford classification dividing them into:

- **Type A dissection** involves the ascending aorta and/or the arch
- **Type B dissections** involve only the descending aorta and occur distal to the origin of the left subclavian artery.

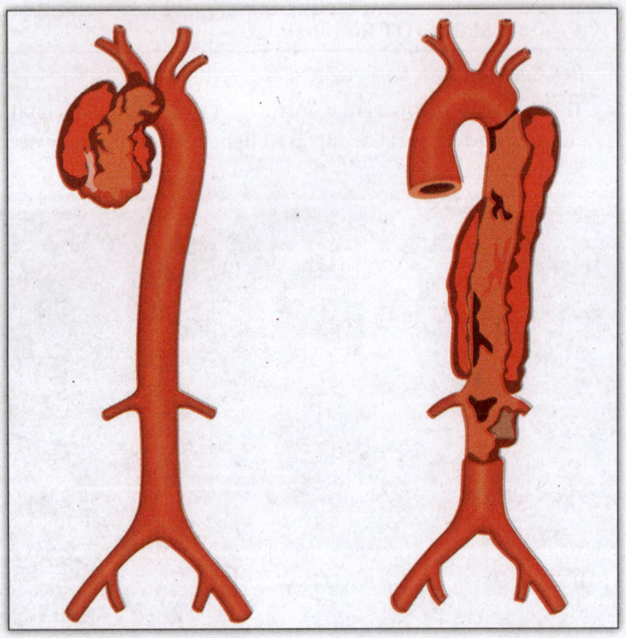

Fig: Stanford classification of Aortic dissection

Management

- **General principles:** Patients with suspected dissection are often in pain and opiate analgesia is important both for comfort and to reduce the sympathetic response to pain which itself can cause progression of the dissection process.

Definitive treatment depends upon the type of dissection:

Type A dissections require open surgery to prevent rupture into the pericardial sac.

Type B dissections are managed medically but may require endovascular stenting if the patient has persistent pain, a rapidly expanding aortic diameter, or malperfusion of branch vessel organs.

9. Ans. (a) Monophasic

Ref: Introduction to vascular Ultrasonography by Zwiebel 5th ed Page 66

Venous flow in the lower extremities is normally Monophasic with modulations due to respiration. That is in the normal study, the Doppler signal of the lower extremity veins increases during expiration and decreases during inspiration.

In arteries, each cycle of cardiac activity produces a distinct "wave" on the Doppler frequency spectrum that begins with systole and terminates at the end of diastole.

- **Low pulsatility (Monophasic)** is indicated by broad systolic peaks and persistent forward flow throughout diastole. Low pulsatility waveforms are also **monophasic**, meaning that flow is always forward and the entire waveform is either above or below the Doppler spectrum baseline (depending on the orientation of the ultrasound transducer). (e.g., the internal carotid artery).
- **Moderate pulsatility (Biphasic)** is indicated by tail, sharp and narrow systolic peaks and relatively little diastolic flow (e.g., the external carotid artery). Examples of moderate pulsatility are found in the external carotid artery and the superior mesenteric artery (during fasting).
- **High pulsatility (Triphasic/ Multiphasic)** is characterized by narrow systolic peaks, flow reversal early in diastole and absence of flow late in diastole. This is ***Classic triphasic pattern*** with, the first phase (1) is systole, the second phase (2) is brief diastolic flow reversal and the third phase (3) is diastolic forward flow. Triphasic flow is seen in normal extremity arteries at rest.

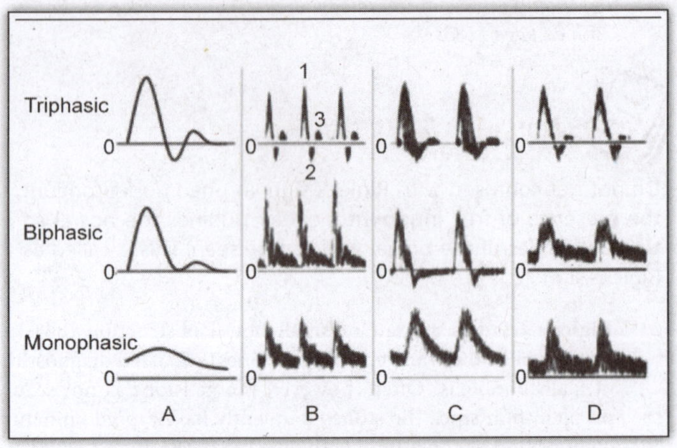

Fig: Possible waveform illustrations characterized as triphasic, biphasic and monophasic

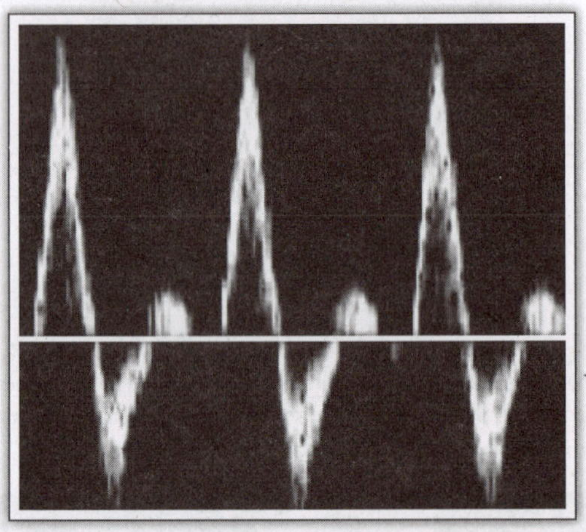

Fig: Triphasic (pulsed Doppler) waveform depicted with forward flow in systole, reverse flow (late systole/early diastole) and forward flow (late diastole)

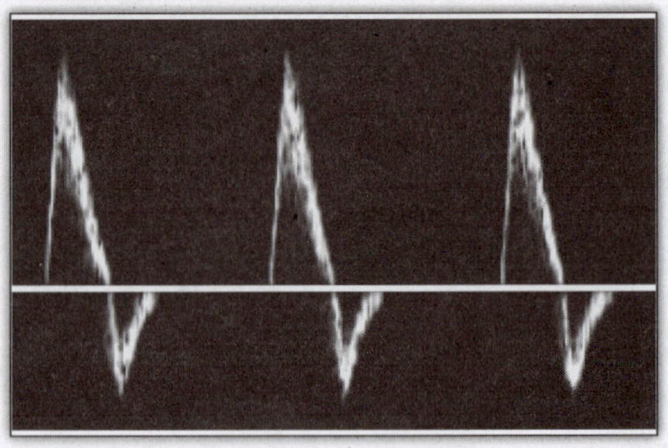

Fig: High-resistant, biphasic (pulsed Doppler) waveform depicted with forward flow in systole and reverse flow (late systole/early diastole), without a forward flow in late diastole

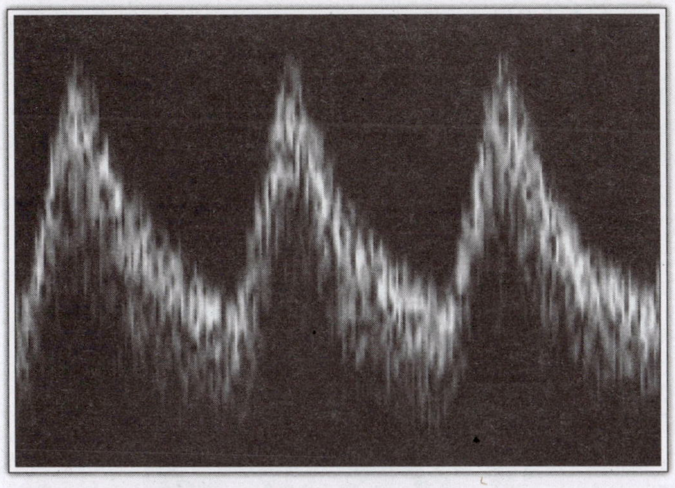

Fig: Low-resistant (Monophasic) waveform with a single phase, slow acceleration and deceleration

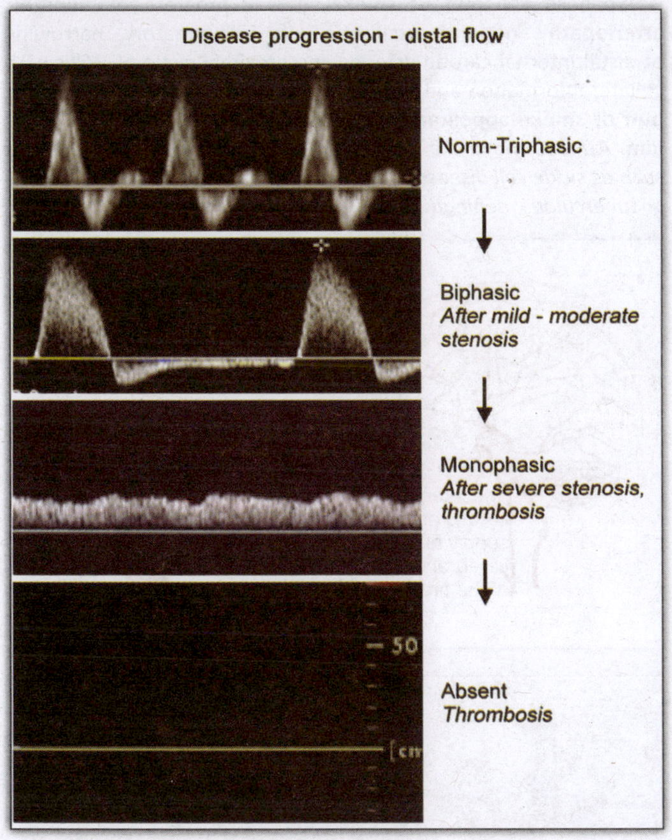

Fig: **Doppler flow in disease status**

AIIMS NOVEMBER 2017

10. Ans. (b) Pseudoaneurysm of Internal carotid artery

Ref: Grainger 5th ed ch 70, Diagnostic and intervention radiology by Thomas J. Vogl , Wolfgang Reith , Ernstn J. Rummeny page 419, Head and Neck Vascular Anomalies: A Practical Case-Based Approach By Gresham T. Richter, James Y. Suen P-177

- The given image is of Digital subtraction Angiography (DSA) of Pseudoaneurysm of Internal Carotid artery

Clue: Even if you don't know about digital substraction angiography , it is very easy to identify that this plate in question shows a vascular structure with contrast. There is one dilated structure in the middle which most likely looks like an aneurysmal dilatation.

False aneurysms, also known as a pseudoaneurysm, is when there is a breach in the vessel wall such that blood leaks through the wall but is contained by the adventitia or surrounding perivascular soft tissue. The risk of rupture is higher than that of a true aneurysm of comparable size due to poor support of the aneurysm wall and thus false aneurysms generally require treatment.

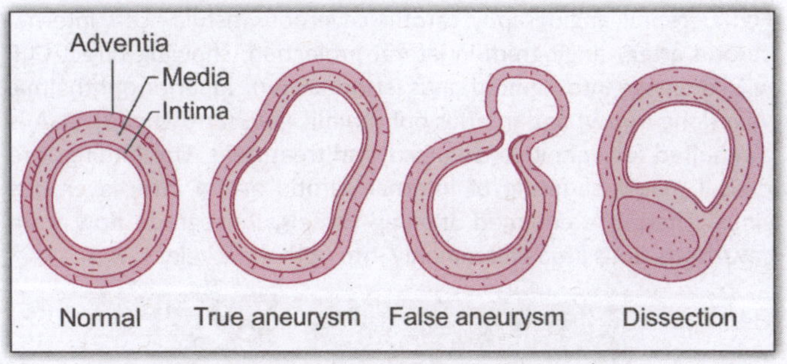

Option (A)

Carotid cavernous fistula findings are typical. Rapid shunting of Internal carotid artery into cavernous sinus. There are enlarged draining vessels. Retrograde flow from cavernous sinus, most commonly into ophthalmic veins

Option (C)

Tumor blush is enhancement of tumour after administration of contrast. There is no tumour enhancement seen in the picture

Option (D)

DSA of hemangioma would show pooling of contrast , tumour blush and flow voids . None of which is seen here

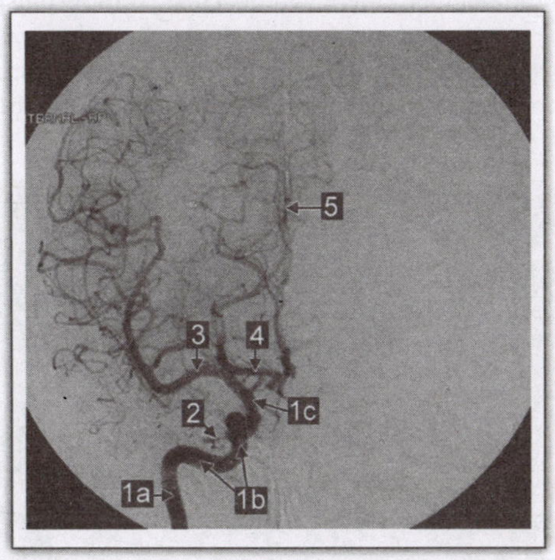

Fig: **Normal Cerebral arteriogram-AP arterial phase:** 1- Internal carotid artery (ICA), 1a-Cervical ICA, 1b-ICA in carotid canal and cavernous sinus, 1c-Carotid siphon, 2-Opthalmic artery, 3-Middle cerebral artery, 4- Anterior cerebral artery, 5-Pericallosal artery

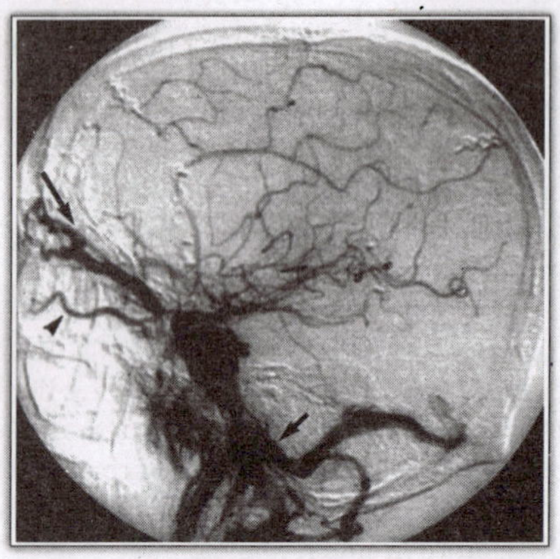

Fig: Cerebral angiography carotid cavernous fistula- Left internal carotid artery angiogram in lateral projection, showing direct CCF with drainage into sigmoid sinus (short arrow), superior ophthalmic vein (long arrow) and inferior ophthalmic vein (arrowhead). DSA is a required for definitive diagnosis and treatment. The findings are typical. Rapid shunting of Internal carotid artery into cavernous sinus. There are enlarged draining vessels. Retrograde flow from cavernous sinus , most commonly into opthalmic veins

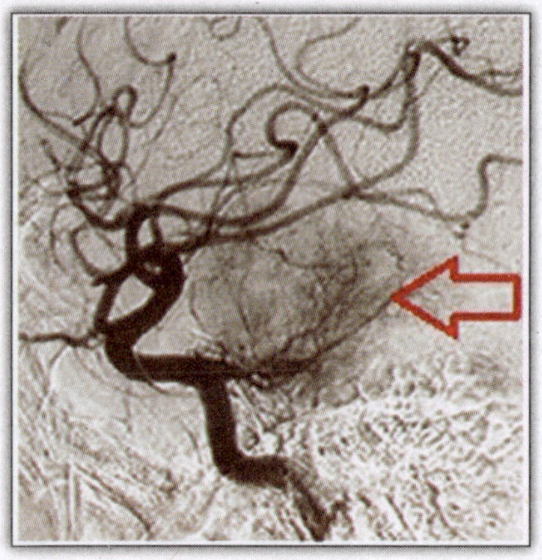

Fig: Cerebral angiography hypervascular tumor blush, due to angiofibroma supplied predominantly by branches of the right meningohypophyseal trunk from the right internal carotid artery (ICA). Tumor blush is enhancement of tumour after administration of contrast

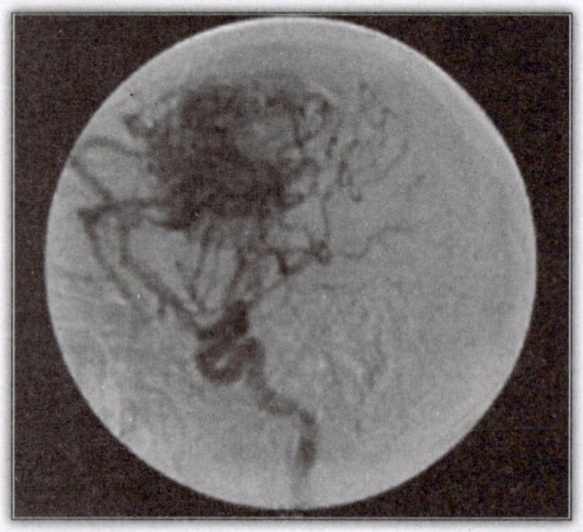

Fig: Cerebral angiography- cerebral proliferative angiopathy (CPA)- left internal carotid artery injection showing diffuse proliferative angiogenesis with feeders supplied from branches of left anterior cerebral artery and left middle cerebral artery

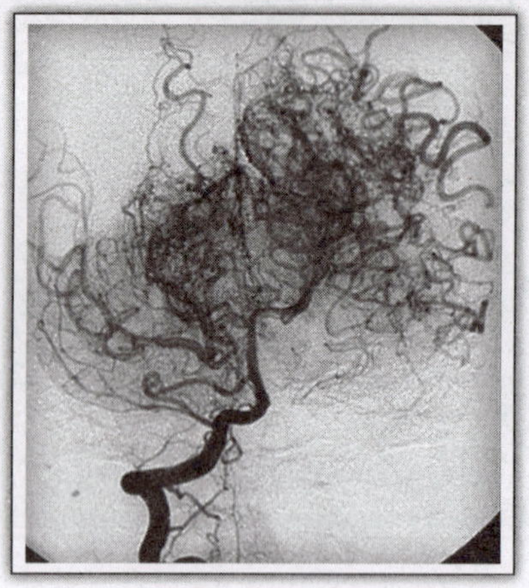

Fig: Cerebral angiography Moyamoya disease: Moya moya is Japanese for **'puff of smoke',** it is a progressive **idiopathic arteriopathy** non-atherosclerotic, non-inflammatory narrowing of distal internal carotid arteries and proximal circle of Willis with collateral formation and the net like vessels give the characteristic **puff of smoke appearance.** Mainly seen in Japan and the Pacific Rim. *A moya moya-like pattern may be found in other conditions such as sickle cell disease, Down's syndrome, previous radiotherapy or tuberculous meningitis and Type 1 neurofibromatosis*

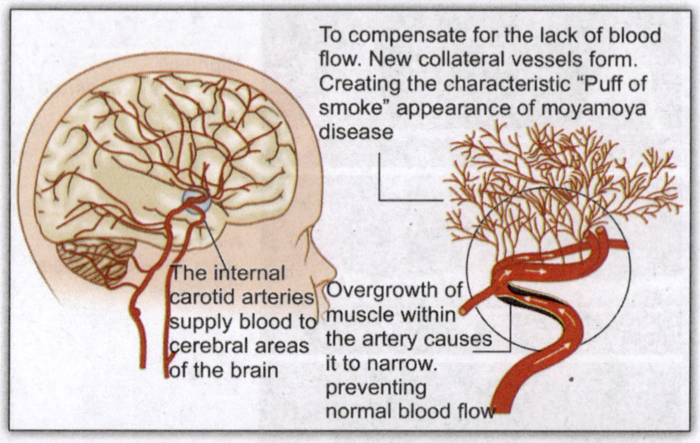

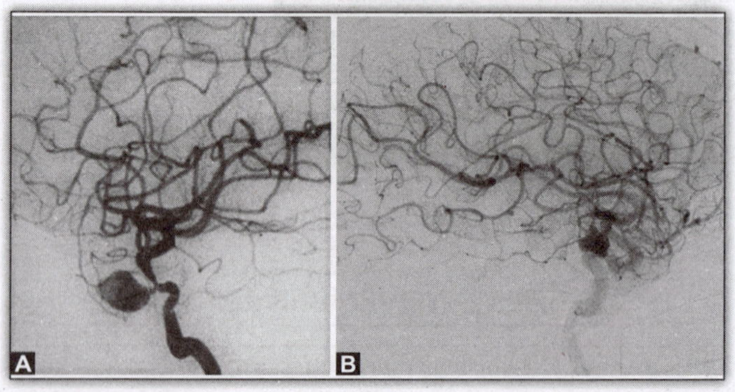

Figs A and B: Cerebral angiography ICA Pseudoaneurysm: Irregular pseudo-aneurysm at the cavernous part of the internal carotid artery. A patent pseudoaneurysm sac has the appearance of a focal outpouching from the artery of origin. On CTA a thrombosed pseudoaneurysm or thrombosed false lumen appears as an eccentric and usually smooth filling defect in or adjacent to the true lumen

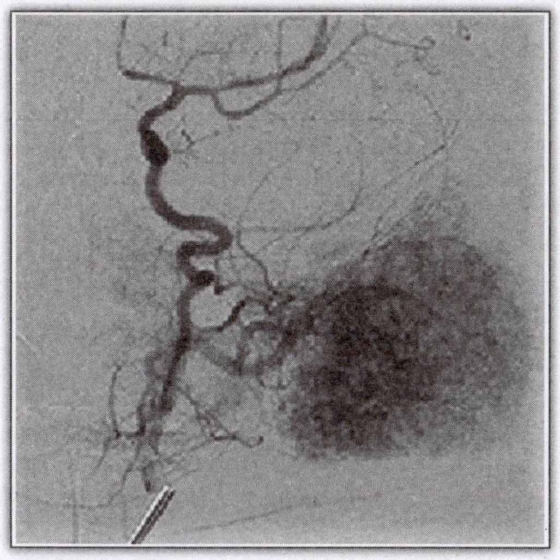

Fig: DSA of hemangioma would show pooling of contrast, tumor blush and flow voids

11. Ans. (b) Pneumothorax

REF: Rosen's Emergency Medicine - Concepts and Clinical Practice By John Marx, Ron Walls, Robert Hockberger 8th ed page 218

Given Chest X-ray is characteristic of Left Pneumothorax

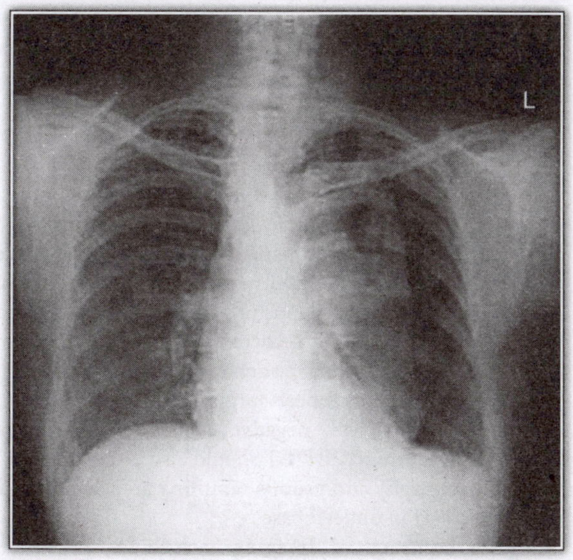

Fig: Left pneumothorax: Pneumothorax refers to the presence of gas (air) in the pleural space and on chest X-ray

Radiological Features of Pneumothorax

- Simple pneumothorax: Visceral pleural edge visible (thin sharp white line) with dark area lacking vascular markings laterally. Loss of volume on the affected side (e.g. raised hemidiaphragm). A small pneumothorax may not be visualized on a standard inspiratory film. An expiratory film may be of benefit.
- Tension pneumothorax—this is a clinical and not a radiological entity. Radiological signs are similar to simple pneumothorax.
- Associated mediastinal shift to the opposite side is seen.
- Pneumothorax may be difficult to visualize on frontal films, particularly on supine films. Look for increased lucency over the costophrenic recess (the **deep sulcus sign**).

12. Ans. (b) Typical carcinoid

Ref: Grainger Allison 6th ed page 352

18-FDG is negative or weakly on PET scan for typical carcinoids because of lower rate of metabolism and low differentiation of cells. Hence its use in typical carcinoids is of limited importance. Therefore large cell neuroendocrine tumours of lung , small cell and non small carcinomas and atypical carcinoids show higher uptake compared to typical carcinoids **(Ref: Clinical Management of Neuroendocrine Tumors of the Lung, By Pier Luigi Filosso p- 287)** 18FDG PET may not be very useful for adenocarcinoma, small carcinoids <1cm and typical carcinoids of lung because of poor metabolic rates of the cells. **(Ref: Diagnostic Imaging: Nuclear Medicine E-Book By Paige A Bennett, Umesh D Oza page 420)**

This question is based upon functional and metabolic imaging in oncology. The uses of functional imaging in current cancer practice include

- Detection of malignancy, particularly if the primary site is unknown
- Differential diagnosis of lesions found on anatomic imaging studies
- Tumor grading
- Disease staging
- Assessing for recurrence
- Therapeutic monitoring

[18F]fluorodeoxyglucose–positron emission tomography (FDG-PET) and proton magnetic resonance spectroscopy (MRS) are used in routine clinical practice for oncology.

Positron Emission Tomography (PET)

PET is the most sensitive functional imaging technique used in clinical practice, with the ability to quantify processes that occur at subnanomolar concentrations. The basic principle is that a biological substance is labeled with a radiotracer which can emit positron. It is then infused in the body. Certain tissues take up the molecule and PET scanner detects the location of molecule in the body as the tracer decays.

Radionuclides most commonly used include 11C, 13N, 15O and 18F, all of which are isotopes of atoms that are found in molecules of biologic importance (11C, 13N and 15O) or that can be substituted without significant disruption of molecular structure (18F)

FDG is the mainstay of PET oncologic imaging. As with all radiopharmaceuticals, distribution of FDG throughout the body obeys the tracer principle: It is administered in such small amounts (<10 μg) that while portraying the pathway of interest, it leaves that pathway completely intact. There is no pharmacologic or toxic effect. Neoplastic cells undergo accelerated glycolysis, even under aerobic conditions, a phenomenon known as the Warburg effect.

That metabolic difference between normal and cancer cells is exploited in FDG-PET imaging. Increased levels of glucose transporters and hexokinase and decreased levels of glucose-

6-phosphatase contribute to the relatively increased glucose metabolism of cancer cells. 8 Unlike glucose, because FDG lacks a hydroxyl group at the 2 position, it cannot undergo further metabolism (phosphorylation) and remains trapped within the cell. Therefore rapidly dividing highly metabolically active cells tend to accumulate FDG. Area of hypermetabolism is seen as "hot spot"

Increased uptake FDG in tumor is because of

- Elevated levels of GLUT
- Elevated levels of hexokinase
- Increased rates glycolysis

Clinical applications: FDG-PET is superior to anatomic imaging for a variety of tumors and indications. Notable is that PET can identify metastatic deposits in lymph nodes that are still small (<1 cm) and considered benign by computed tomography (CT). In contrast, PET may recognize large masses, such as post therapy fibrotic tissue, as benign if minimal FDG uptake is demonstrated. The most serious limitation to tumor detection with PET is that increased FDG uptake can also be demonstrated in inflammatory tissue.

- PET has proved capable of differentiating high- and low-grade brain tumors, of assessing prognosis in patients with brain tumors and may be useful in guiding stereotactic brain biopsy.
- PET is the most accurate noninvasive technique for detecting and staging lung cancer
- PET has changed surgical management in 28% of patients with colorectal cancer by identifying resectable or unresectable metastasis not identified on clinical examination or CT. PET is of higher sensitivity than is CT arterial portography (80% to 90%) in detecting intrahepatic metastases.
- PET has not proved as useful for breast cancer as for lung cancer, primarily owing to lower glucose utilization in the breast and background activity from concurrent mastopathy
- Anatomic complexity in the head and neck region, particularly after surgery, renders PET evaluation of this area a boon to therapeutic monitoring. Tumors as small as 4 mm have been detected in the head and neck with PET.
- PET has been successfully applied to detecting subclinical involvement of lymph nodes in melanoma

AIIMS MAY 2017

13. Ans. (b) SestaMIBI

Ref: Grainger and Allison's Diagnostic Radiology 5th ed vol 2 ch 71

This is a case of parathyroid adenoma causing hyperparathyroidism.

Classical signs and symptoms of hypercalcemia & primary hyperparathyroidism is summarized as **Mnemonic:**

- **Stones** (Kidney stones, renal dysfunction and failure)
- **Bones** (Bone pain, pathological fracture)
- Abdominal **goans** (Anorexia, constipation, nausea, vomiting, peptic ulcer, pancreatitis)
- Psychiatric **moans** (fatigue, confusion, anxiety, psychosis, depression)

Localisation of abnormal parathyroid gland can be done by the following imaging modalities:

- **Ultrasound**: Parathyroid adenomas typically appear as oval, well-defined anechoic or hypoechoic masses posterior to the thyroid gland. They tend to be of the order of 10 mm in diameter but can grow to a very large size (4–5 cm). As glands become larger, they are more likely to be multilobulated and to contain echogenic areas, cysts and calcifications. There are several problems in the localization of parathyroid adenomas by US. Retropharyngeal, retro-oesophageal and mediastinal parathyroid glands, which account for 5–15% of all glands, are not easily accessible by US. An exophytic thyroid nodule can be indistinguishable from a parathyroid nodule on ultrasound.
- **Computed tomography** does not have any advantage over ultrasound in detecting an adenoma located in a normal parathyroid site, but is very useful for detecting abnormalities lying in sites inaccessible to ultrasound, such as behind the trachea, in the mediastinum, or in an undescended inferior parathyroid gland in the carotid sheath.
- **Magnetic resonance imaging** is increasingly being used for localizing abnormal parathyroid glands. Parathyroid adenomas typically are isointense to muscle on T1-weighted images and of high signal intensity on T2-weighted images.
- **Radionuclide imaging with ^{201}Tl or ^{99m}Tc-MIBI**, using a subtraction technique whereby the image of the thyroid gland as shown by ^{99m}Tc or ^{123}I is removed, is a noninvasive technique for tumour localization. ^{99m}Tc-MIBI can also be used on its own to detect adenomas; early (15 min post injection) and delayed (90 min post injection) images are acquired for this purpose. ^{99m}Tc-MIBI is more sensitive than ^{201}Tl in preoperative data acquisition and in patients undergoing reoperation. Cumulative analysis of ^{99m}Tc-MIBI scintigraphy in patients with hyperparathyroidism demonstrates a sensitivity of 90% for single adenomas, 55% for abnormal glands in patients with multiglandular disease and 75% for recurrent hyperparathyroidism; the specificity for primary adenomas has been shown to be 98%. In patients where surgical re-exploration is being planned, but with negative conventional scintigraphy, **^{11}C-methionine PET/CT** should also be considered.
- **Angiography and venous sampling** are usually used as a last resort in difficult cases.
- **The accuracy of imaging techniques in localizing parathyroid disease.**
- There is great variation in the reported accuracy of imaging techniques in the localization of parathyroid disease. The overall sensitivity for identifying parathyroid adenomas with ^{99m}Tc-sestamibi ranges from 80% to 95%, which is significantly higher than that of ^{201}Tl. The specificity is high at 91–98%.
- Modern US using high-resolution (7.5–10 MHz) probes is only slightly less sensitive than nuclear medicine; the highest reported sensitivity for identifying an adenoma is 82%. The specificity, however, is high, ranging from 78% to 100%.
- The sensitivity of CT in identifying parathyroid adenomas is similar to that of US, with specificities ranging from 92% to 95%.
- The results for MRI are similar to those for CT.

14. Ans. (a) Renal cell carcinoma

Ref: Grainger & Allison's Diagnostic Radiology, 5th ed CH 39, Campbell Walsh Urology 11 th ed page 1306-1308, 1316 – 1322

NOTE

The pictures are representational. In examination smaller mass was seen on the CT compared to this picture.

The majority of simple renal cyst are asymptomatic and is incidentally found by ultrasound. Simple cysts are the most common renal masses. Most are clinically insignificant, being discovered incidentally at autopsy or on imaging studies. "Simple" renal cysts are well-marginated, thin walls with no enhancement of the cyst. They can be diagnosed on ultrasound, CT, or MRI. A cystic lesion in the kidney that deviates from the typical "simple" cyst appearance should be viewed with suspicion and may warrant further imaging to exclude other renal cystic lesions, particularly variants of **renal cell carcinoma**.

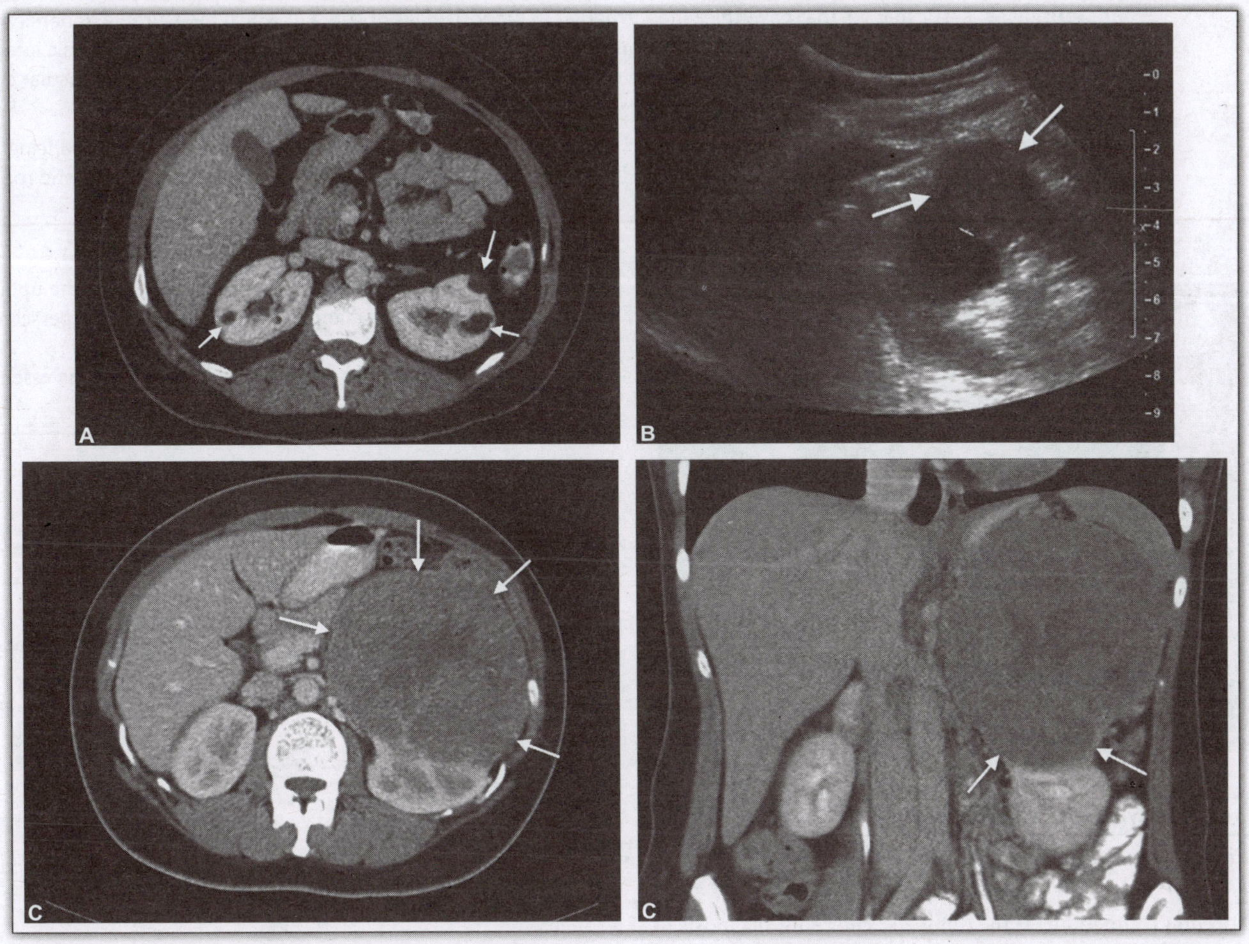

Figs A to C: A. Renal angiomyolipoma: Most lesions involve the cortex and demonstrate macroscopic fat (less than -20 HU). The tumours are hypodense (dark) due to fat content; **B. USG kidney:** The renal cell carcinoma is identified as a rounded mass extending off the posterior kidney (arrows). Note the dark area next to the mass, which represents a renal cyst. **C.** Transverse and coronal CT. This patient presented with a huge left upper pole mass (arrows). One of the helpful imaging signs is called the 'claw sign', where a small claw-like parenchyma from the organ extends around the tumour, as indicated by the yellow arrows on the coronal CT. This allowed us to correctly predict that the tumour was arising from the left kidney

The **Bosniak classification system** of renal cystic masses divides renal cystic masses into five categories based on imaging characteristics on contrast-enhanced CT. It is helpful in predicting a risk of malignancy and suggesting either follow up or treatment.

Bosniak Renal Cyst Classification System

Category	Description
I	A **benign simple cyst** with a hairline-thin wall that does not contain septa, calcifications, or solid components. It measures water density and does not enhance **(percentage malignant: ~0%)**

Contd...

Bosniak Renal Cyst Classification System	
Category	**Description**
II	A benign cyst that may contain a **few hairline-thin septa** (< 1mm in thickness) in which "perceived" enhancement may be present. **Fine calcification** (not measurable) or a short segment of slightly thickened calcification may be present in the wall or septa. Uniformly high-attenuation lesions **<3 cm** (so-called high-density cysts) that are well marginated and do not enhance are included in this group. Cysts in this category do not require further evaluation. **(Percentage malignant: ~0%)**
IIF ("F" for follow-up)	Cysts that may contain **multiple hairline-thin septa** or minimal smooth thickening of their wall or septa. **Perceived enhancement** of their septa or wall may be present. Their wall or septa may contain **calcification that may be thick and nodular**, but no measurable contrast enhancement is present. These lesions are generally well marginated. Totally intrarenal, nonenhancing, high-attenuation renal lesions **>3 cm** are also included in this category. These lesions require follow-up studies to prove benignity. **(Percentage malignant: ~5%)**
III	**"Indeterminate"** cystic masses that have thickened irregular or smooth walls or septa in which measurable enhancement is present. These are surgical lesions and although some will prove to be benign (e.g., hemorrhagic cysts, chronic infected cysts and multilocular cystic nephroma), some will be malignant, such as cystic renal cell carcinoma and multilocular cystic renal cell carcinoma. **(Percentage malignant: ~55%)**
IV	These are clearly **malignant cystic masses** that can have all the criteria of category III, but also contain enhancing soft tissue components adjacent to, but independent of, the wall or septa. These lesions include cystic carcinomas and require surgical removal. **(Percentage malignant: ~100%)**

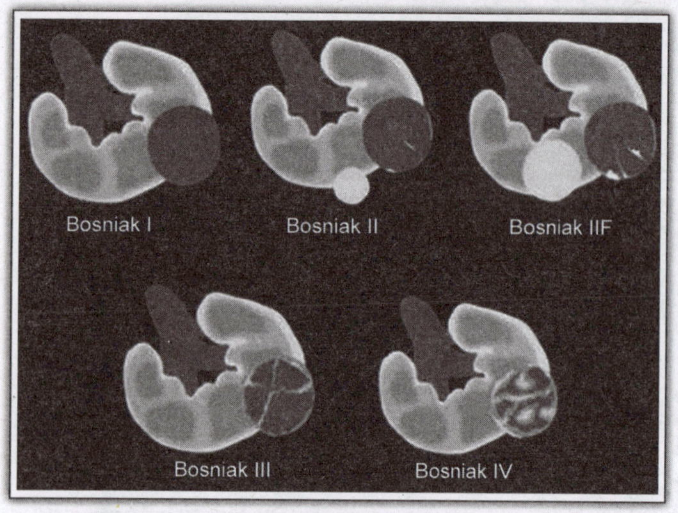

15. Ans. (b) Hypersecretory adenoma

Ref: Grainger & Allison's Diagnostic Radiology 5th ed ch 7, Essentials of Nuclear Medicine imaging. Fred A Milter. Page. 605

Tc 99m (Technetium) is the isotope of choice for diagnosis of thyroid disorders as it is cheap, involves less radiation, less time 20 minutes and ^{99m}Tc half life is 6 hours.

NOTE

Only absolute indication in modern days is autonomous toxic nodule in toxic thyroid showing hot nodule.

Interpretation of the Scan

- Right lobe uptakes the isotope tracer while lift lobe does not
- There is no ectopic thyroid tissue hence lateral aberrant thyroid and retrosternal extension can be ruled out
- There is one single hot nodule suppressing the uptake of the remaining gland, hence Toxic nodule/Hypersecretory adenoma
- There is no cold nodule hence malignancy is essentially ruled out

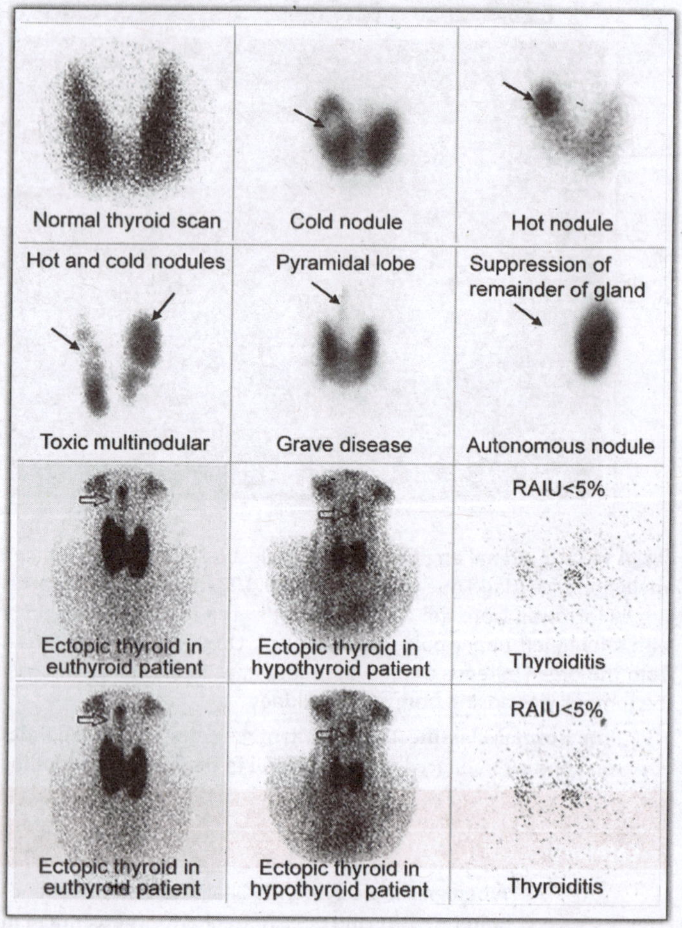

16. Ans. (d) Pulmonary venous hypertension

Ref: Grainger and Allison's Diagnostic Radiology 5th ed ch 23

This is a CXR of Ebstein's anomaly with box shaped heart. It presents with pulmonary oligemia (decreased pulmonary blood flow) not pulmonary plethora (increased pulmonary blood flow) or pulmonary hypertension. (See table of Pulmonary Oligemia Vs Plethora in Radiodiagnosis AIIMS NOV 2013)

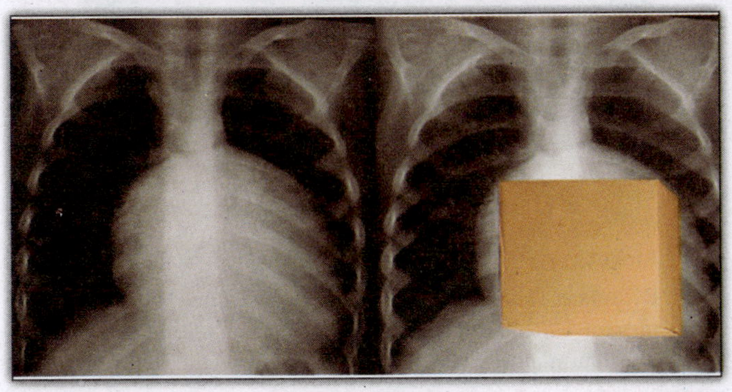

Fig: Ebstein anomaly CXR: Show massive cardiomegaly with decreased pulmonary flow best depicts the **box-shaped heart**, an appearance caused by enlargement of the right atrium and hypoplasia of the pulmonary trunk. Elongated and enlarged right atrium may result in an elevated apex

- Ebstein's anomaly is a congenital abnormality of the tricuspid valve.
- The septal and mural leaflets are more apically placed than normal i.e. if the tricuspid septal attachment lies more than 1.5 cm "beneath" the apex than mitral septal attachment, this can be considered Ebstein anomaly (in adults, the measurement is 2 cm), resulting in a malfunctioning, regurgitant tricuspid valve and atrialization of the proximal right ventricle.
- The consequence is gross right atrial enlargement and raised right atrial pressure. The anomaly is usually associated with an ASD and there is thus right-to-left shunting at the atrial level and subsequent cyanosis.
- Ultimately, Ebstein's anomaly results in gross enlargement of the cardiac contour with a prominent curved right atrial border on the plain chest radiograph.

17. Ans. (a) Staphylococcus aureus

Ref: Grainger and Allison's Diagnostic Radiology; 5th ed ch 15

Chest X-ray shows right sided pneumonia with the presence of pulmonary infiltrates and characteristic multiple air filled spaces (**pneumatoceles**). Pneumatocoeles are intrapulmonary air-filled cystic spaces which may contain air-fluid levels. **Staph aureus** is the most likely organism to present in this fashion.

Staph. aureus pneumonia occurs in debilitated hospitalized or institutionalized patients and less frequently as a community-acquired infection. It is usually acquired by aspiration from the upper respiratory tract. Chest radiographs typically demonstrate heterogeneous opacities in a scattered multifocal and bilateral distribution. **Pleural effusion or empyema and cavitation** are common; air bronchograms are unusual. **Pneumatoceles** may form, particularly in children.

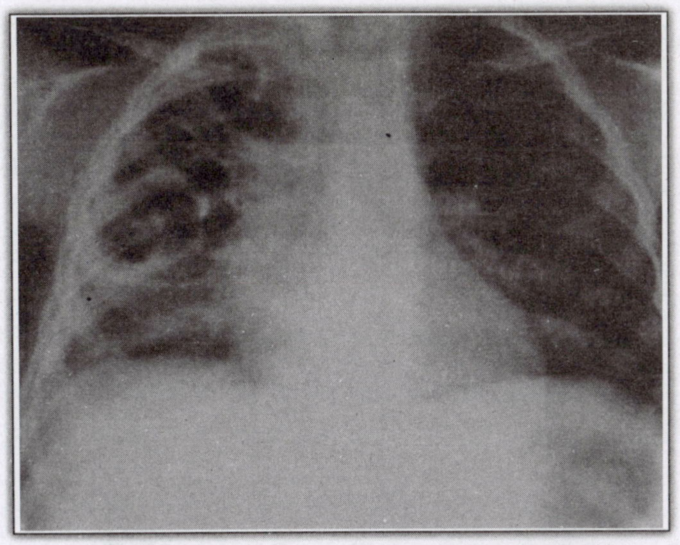

Fig: Right sided pneumonia with the presence of pulmonary infiltrates and characteristic multiple air filled spaces (pneumatoceles)

Causes of Pneumatocoele

- ***Pneumonia:*** *(Staphylococcus aureus (most common), Streptococcus pneumoniae, Haemophilus influenzae, Escherichia coli*, Group A streptococci, *Klebsiella pneumoniae*, Adenovirus, Primary pulmonary tuberculosis).
- Trauma: usually blunt trauma
- Positive pressure ventilation, especially in preterm neonates
- Hydrocarbon ingestion

18. Ans. (c) Pneumoperitoneum

Ref: Grainger and Allison's Diagnostic Radiology 5th ed ch 29

Repeat AIIMS Nov 2018 Radiodiagnosis (See for explanation) (see page no. 1117)

The above X-ray abdomen (erect) (in questions) shows presence of gas under the right dome of diaphragm suggestive of pneumoperitoneum.

19. Ans. (b) Toxic Megacolon

Ref: Grainger & Allison's Diagnostic Radiology 5th ed ch 33

As the patient has a history of diarrhea from several months and X-ray of abdomen shows dilated large gut loop so the diagnosis is toxic megacolon which is a complication of ulcerative colitis.

- **Toxic megacolon** is complication that can be seen in both types of inflammatory bowel disease (more commonly in ulcerative colitis) and less commonly in infectious colitis. Chemical mediators such as nitric oxide and interleukins are thought to play a pivotal role in its pathogenesis.
- **Radiographic features:** The colon (typically transverse colon) becomes dilated to at least 6 cm (usually greater). There is additional loss of haustral markings, with pseudopolyps often extending into the lumen. Thumbprinting from mucosal oedema may be present.

There may be signs of pneumoperitoneum if dilatation has progressed to cause perforation.

- **Intramural bowel gas (pneumatosis intestinalis)** is presence of gas within the wall of the bowel. Intramural gas can be seen in intestinal ischaemia and eventually bowel infarction. Gas in the bowel wall in the neonatal period is diagnostic of necrotising enterocolitis.
- Gas tracks along the bowel wall, appearing as either linear (usually submucosal) or rounded cystic collections (usually subserosal).

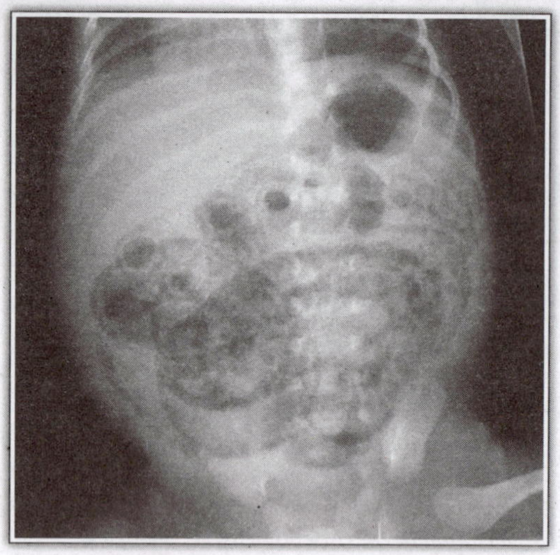

Fig: Pneumatosis intestinalis

AIIMS NOVEMBER 2016

20. Ans. (c) Rickets

Ref: Yochum and Rowe's Essentials of Skeletal Radiology 3rd ed page 1516

The above X-ray shows splaying, fraying and cupping of metaphysis which are characteristic appearance of rickets

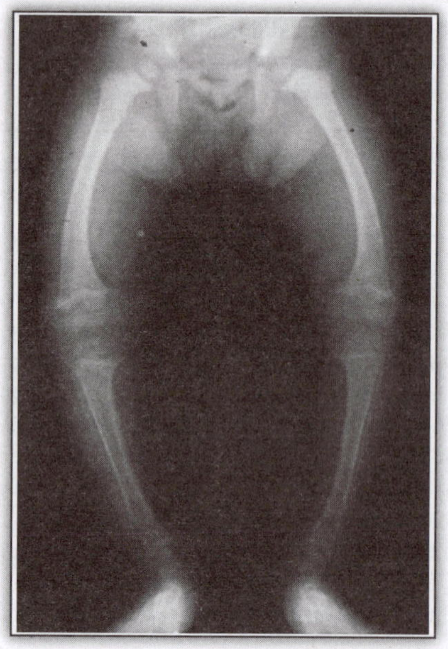

Fig: Rickets of lower limbs

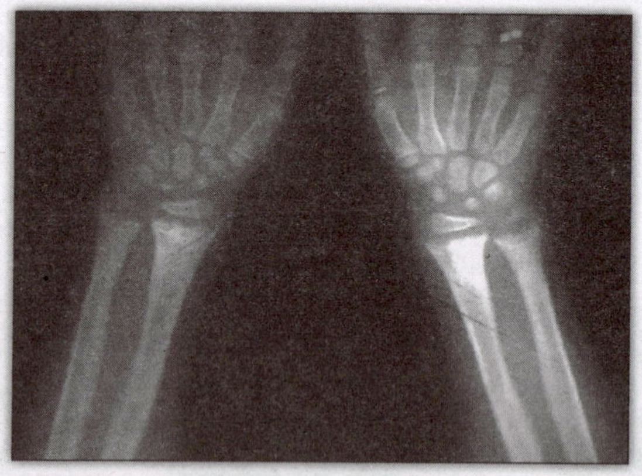

Fig: Rickets of upper limbs

Rickets

Rickets is a softening of bones in children due to deficiency or impaired metabolism of vitamin D, magnesium, phosphorus or calcium, potentially leading to fractures and deformity.

Types

- Nutritional rickets
- Vitamin D Resistant rickets
- Vitamin D Dependent rickets (Type I & Type II)
- Congenital rickets

Signs and Symptoms

- Bone pain or tenderness
- Axial widening of metaphysis aka **Fraying of metaphysis (first sign of rickets)**
- **Metaphyseal fraying**: Normally metaphysis meets growth plate as a smooth line of sclerosis known as zone of provisional calcification. Serrated metaphyseal ends seen in rickets is known as fraying.
- **Metaphyseal cupping** refers to the inward bulging of the metaphysis.
- During infancy and early childhood, the long bones show the greatest deformity, both at the cartilage-shaft junctions and in the diaphyses resulting in characteristic bowing deformities of the arms and legs.
- Dental problems
- Muscle weakness (rickety myopathy or **"floppy baby syndrome"** or "slinky baby" (such that the baby is floppy or slinky-like)
- Increased tendency for fractures (easily broken bones), especially greenstick fractures
- Skeletal deformity
  - Toddlers: **Bowed legs (genu varum)**
  - Older children: **Knock-knees (genu valgum)** or "windswept knees"
  - Cranial, pelvic and spinal deformities (such as lumbar lordosis)
- Growth disturbance
- Hypocalcaemia (low level of calcium in the blood)
- Tetany (uncontrolled muscle spasms all over the body)
- **Craniotabes** (soft skull)
- Costochondral swelling (aka "rickety rosary" or **"rachitic rosary"**)
- Harrison's groove
- **Double malleoli sign** due to metaphyseal hyperplasia

- Widening of wrist raises early suspicion, it is due to metaphyseal cartilage hyperplasia.

Diagnosis

- Blood tests: Serum calcium may show **low levels of calcium, serum phosphorus may be low and serum alkaline phosphatase may be high.**
- Arterial blood gases may reveal metabolic acidosis
- An X-ray or radiograph of an advanced sufferer from rickets tends to present in a classic way: **bow legs or Genu Varum** (outward curve of long bone of the legs) and a deformed chest. Changes in the skull also occur causing a distinctive **"square headed" appearance**. These deformities persist into adult life if not treated. Long-term consequences include permanent bends or disfiguration of the long bones and a curved back.
- **Reappearance of the zone of provisional calcification is the most important sign of healing rickets.**

21. Ans. (a) Osteopetrosis

Ref: Yochum and Rowe's Essentials of Skeletal Radiology 3rd ed vol. 1 page 770

The below X-ray of the pelvis shows generalised increase in bone density or generalised sclerosis characteristic of osteopetrosis also known as **Albers-Schönberg disease, osteosclerosis, marble bones and chalk bones.**

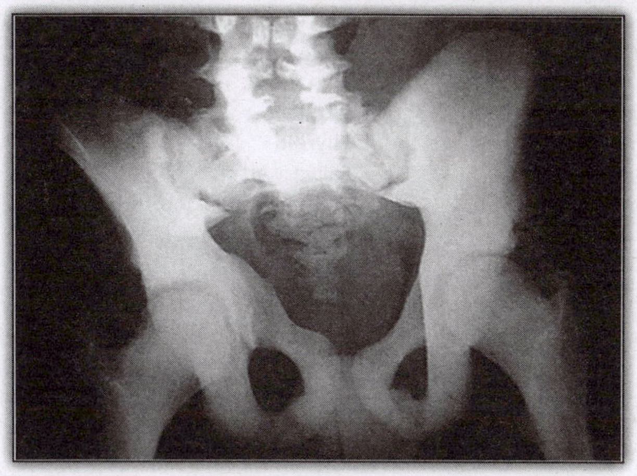

Fig: Osteopetrosis: Diffuse osteosclerosis (increased bone density), Cortical thickening with medullary cavity being replaced

	Osteopetrosis (Albers Schonberg disease/osteo-sclerosis/Marble bones/chalk bones)	Osteopoikilosis or Osteopoikilocytosis	Osteogensis imperfecta (Brittle bone disease)	Osteoporosis
Pathology	Defective osteoclasts. i.e. osteoclasts fail to resorb bone. Bones become thick & dense	Benign, autosomal dominant sclerosing dysplasia of bone	Defective collagen I production involving the connective tissue & bones	Reduction in bone mineral density
X-ray	• Diffuse osteosclerosis • Cortical thickening with medullary involvement • **Erlenmeyer flask deformity** • **Bone within bone appearnce, Sandwich vertebrae**	Multiple punctate sclerotic **bone islands** or foci of compact bone located in cancellous bone around the joint. Particularly in the pelvis, metaphyses and epiphyses of long bones, tarsals and carpals. Long axis of lesion is along the long axis of bone. May be mistaken for sclerotic metastases but osteopoikilosis is **symmetrical, periarticular** and the lesions are uniform in size	• Severe osteoporosis. Most common affect appendicular skeleton, especially lower limbs, but upper limbs and skull may be involved • Excessive bone malleability and plasticity • Deformed (overtubulated) bones • Cortical thinning • Hyperplastic callus • **Wormian bones** • **Codfish vertebrae**	• More than 30–50% bone loss is required to appreciate decreased bone density and **Looser's zone (Pseudofracture)** • Vertebral osteoporosis manifests as: pencilling of vertebrae, loss of cortical bone (**picture frame vertebra**) and trabecular bone (**ghost vertebra**), compression fractures and vertebra plana • Loss of trabeculae in proximal femur

AIIMS MAY 2016

22. Ans. (a) Ovary

Ref: Introduction to Radiobiology by Maurice Tubiana Page 115

Among the options provided, ovary is the most radiosensitive

Radiosensitivity of Tissue and Organs			
Very high	**High**	**Intermediate**	**Low**
Bone marrow (most) Gonads (Ovaries and Testis) Growing cartilage/Growth plate/Epiphysis Breast (Prepubescent) Optic lens	Skin Growing muscles/bones Brain Spinal cord Pituitary Thyroid Salivary gland Stomach, small intestine, colon, rectum Liver, lung, heart, kidney Cornea	Adult bone Adult cartilage Oral mucosa Esophagus Urinary bladder	Pancreas Uterus Vagina Adrenals

- The brain (except the brainstem) can withstand up **to 6,000 cGy** before the risk for necrosis begins to rise.
- Cord radiation tolerance is limited by transient myelitis, demyelination and necrosis. With 4,500 cGy the risk of these is approximately 5%.
- Susceptibility of various phases of cell cycle to radiation is: **G2M > G2 > M > G1 > Early S > Late S**
- In terms of lethality of radiations: Human fetus is most sensitive in first three weeks (after conception to implantation)
- In terms of radiation induced damage the fetus is most sensitive from 8-15 weeks.
- A dose > 5,1 Gy before 18 weeks causes 100% fetal mortality
- Radiation induced congenital abnormalities are maximum from: day 18 to day 45

AIIMS NOVEMBER 2015

23. Ans. (c) Spondylolisthesis

Ref: Youchum and Rowe's Essentials of Skeletal Radiology vol 1, 3rd ed page 463, Apley 9th ed page 484

The picture shown is consistent with Beheaded Scotty dog sign of Spondylisthiosis.

Spondylolisthesis is the forward displacement of a vertebra, especially the fifth lumbar vertebra, most commonly occurring after a fracture.

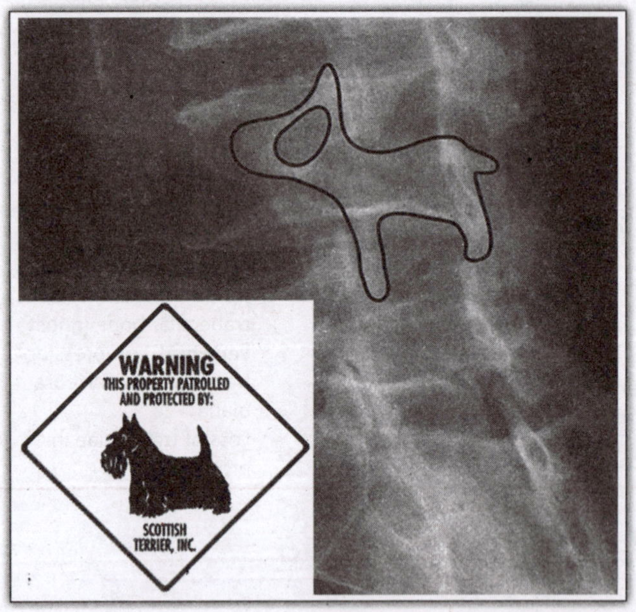

Fig: Normal vertebra with **Scottish dog sign** (without collor and without beheading). The scotty dog sign refers to the normal appearance of the lumbar spine when seen on oblique radiograph. It is important to remember the body parts of the dog corrosponding to the parts of vertebra as shown in the figure below

- The **transverse process** being the nose
- The **pedicle** forming the eye
- The **inferior articular facet** being the front leg
- The **superior articular facet** representing the ear
- The **pars interarticularis** (the portion of the lamina that lies between the facets) equivalent to the neck of the dog.

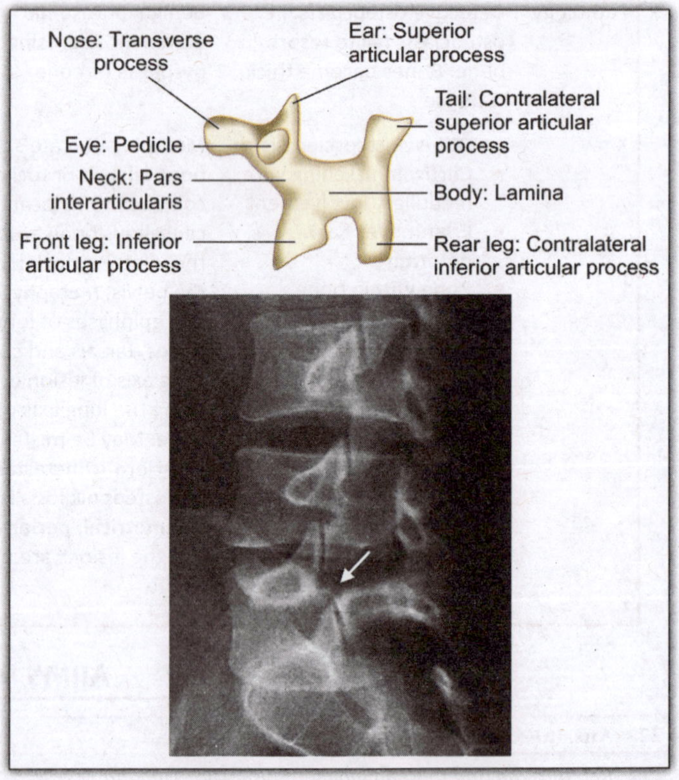

Fig: Spondylolysis is seen as a broken neck or a collar on the 'Scotty dog' (arrow). Oblique X-ray views of the lumbar spine showing the 'Scotty dog' figure, the ear of which is the superior articular process, the eye is the pedicle, the nose is the transverse process, the neck is the pars interarticularis and the front limb is the inferior articular process. If spondylolysis is present, the **pars interarticularis**, or the neck of the dog, will have a defect or break. It often looks as if the dog has a collar around the neck. Spondylolysis is a defect in the pars interarticularis of the neural arch, the portion of the neural arch that connects the superior and inferior articular facets. It is commonly known as pars interarticularis defect or more simply as pars defect

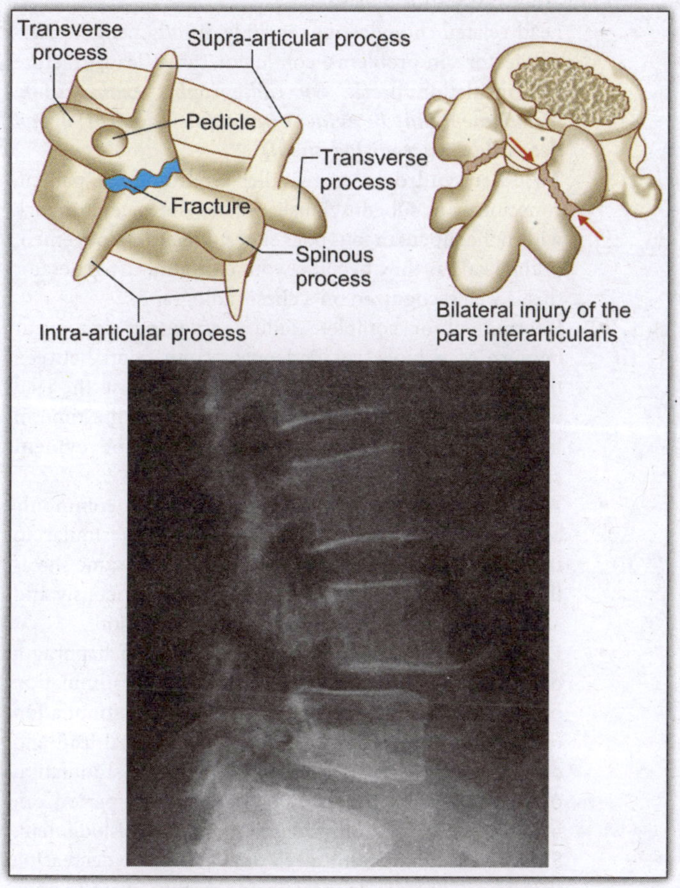

Fig: In spondylolisthesis the defect in pars interarticularis is seen as if the **Scotty dog is beheaded** in the oblique view, it is also known as Terrier sign

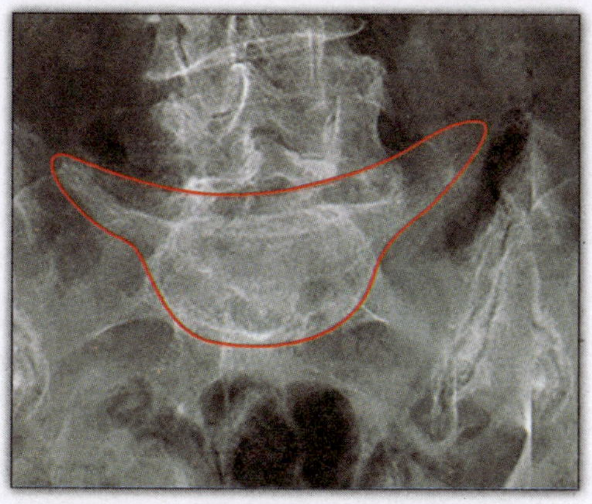

Fig: Inverted napoleon hat sign is seen on anterior posterior radiograph indicating spondylolisthesis of L5 over S1

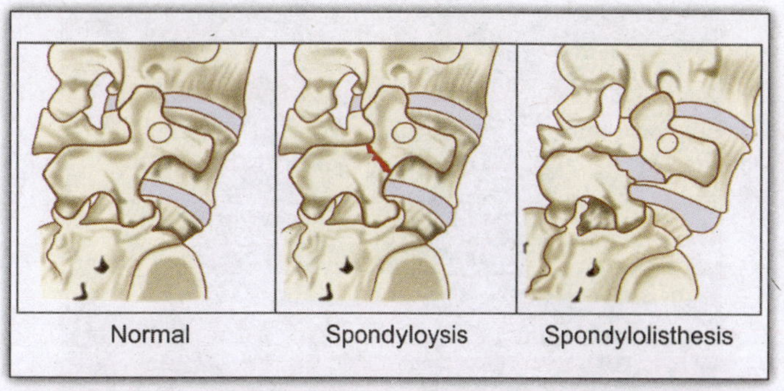

Spondylolisthesis Grades	
Grade 1	0–25% of vertebral body has slipped forward
Grade 2	20–50%
Grade 3	50–75%
Grade 4	75–100%
Grade 5	100%, Vertebral body completely fallen off (i.e., spondyloptosis)

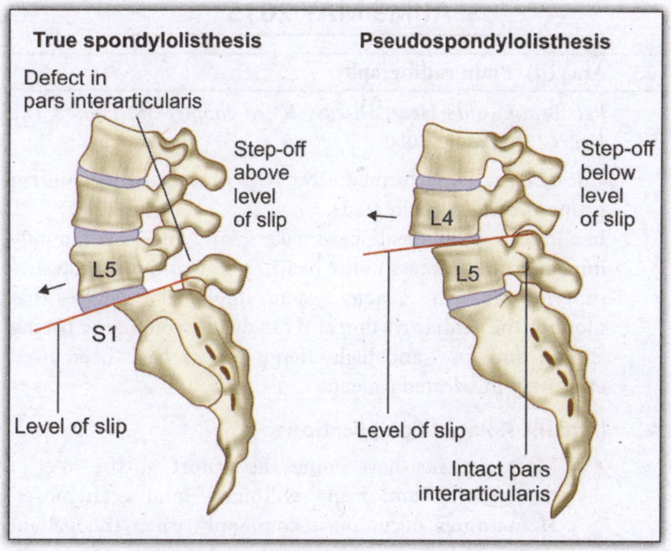

24. Ans. (c) Hydropneumothorax

Ref: Sutton 7th ed vol 1 page 92

Hydropneumothorax is a term given to the concurrent presence of a pneumothorax as well as a hydrothorax (i.e. air and fluid) in the pleural space. On an erect chest radiograph, recognition of hydropneumothorax is classically shown as an air-fluid level. On the supine radiograph, this may be more challenging where a sharp pleural line is bordered by increased opacity lateral to it within the pleural space may sometimes suggest towards the diagnosis.

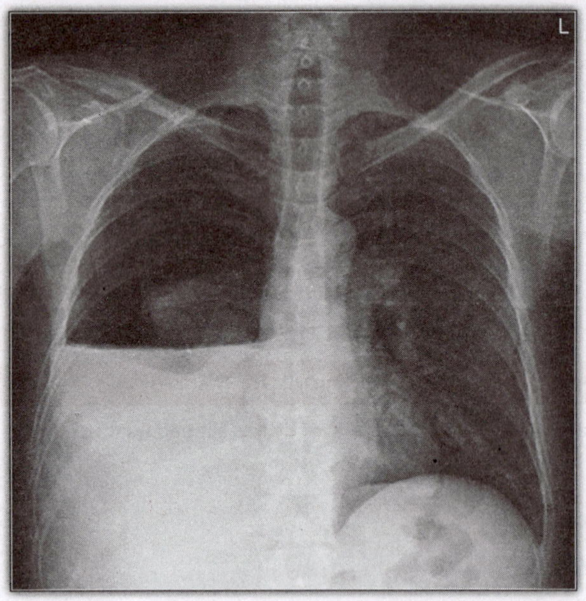

Fig: Right hydropneumothorax

AIIMS MAY 2015

25. Ans. (d) Plain radiograph

Ref: Braunwald's Heart Disease 9th ed chapter 38, Hurst's The Heart 13th ed page 1050

Chest X-ray is performed after ICD placement to confirm proper position of the leads.

In adults, permanent pacemakers are most commonly implanted with access to the heart by way of the subclavian–superior vena cava venous system. Implantable devices that monitor the cardiac rhythm and can deliver competing pacing stimuli and low- and high-energy shocks have been used effectively in selected patients.

Implant-Related Complications

- Most patients have some discomfort at the site of the incision and many will have mild ecchymoses. **Hematomas** occur most commonly when the patient is taking clopidogrel or when heparin or heparin equivalents are used in the early postimplantation period. Most hematomas resolve without evacuation
- Complications of **subclavian puncture** include traumatic **pneumothorax and hemopneumothorax**, inadvertent arterial puncture, **air embolism, arteriovenous fistula, thoracic duct injury, subcutaneous emphysema and brachial plexus injury.**
- A pacing lead can also be placed in the left ventricle by passing it across an unsuspected atrial or ventricular septal defect or patent foramen ovale. **LV lead placement should be recognized by a posteriorly positioned lead on lateral fluoroscopy.** A right bundle branch block pattern during ventricular pacing should raise suspicion of LV pacing.
- Patients should be made aware of the potential for **lead perforation**. Although **cardiac tamponade** is the most dramatic outcome from perforation, asymptomatic ventricular perforation can occur. Signs can include elevation of pacing or sensing thresholds, right bundle branch block pattern from a lead placed in the right ventricle, intercostal muscle or diaphragmatic contraction, **friction rub, pericarditis, or pericardial effusion.**

Lead-Related Complications

- Lead-related complications include dislodgment, header-connector pin problems, conductor/cable (lead) fracture and insulation break. ***On radiographic examination, dislodgment may be evident (macrodislodgment) or not detectable (microdislodgment).***
- **Twiddler syndrome:** In twiddler syndrome, the patient, consciously or subconsciously, rotates the generator pack within the subcutaneous pocket, resulting in dislodgement of the leads as they become wound around the generator this is well recognized on a chest radiograph.
- Intermittent or complete failure of output can occur because of a loose or inadequate connection between the lead and connector block, usually because the lead was incorrectly connected to the header at the time of implantation. **The poor connection may be evident radiographically.**
- **Acute device proarrhythmia** presents most commonly as ventricular extrasystoles morphologically similar to the paced beats because they originate at the same site as the paced beats. They usually resolve spontaneously and almost never require pharmacologic suppression.
- **Extracardiac stimulation** usually involves the diaphragm or the pectoral or intercostal muscles. Usually stimulation of the left hemidiaphragm by the RV lead) or stimulation of the phrenic nerve on the right by the atrial lead and on the left by the LV lead. Diaphragmatic stimulation occurring during the early postimplantation period can be due to either microdislodgment or macrodislodgment. Stimulation can be minimized or alleviated by decreasing the voltage, but an adequate pacing margin of safety must be maintained after the output parameters are decreased. If the problem cannot be resolved by reprogramming, lead repositioning will be required.

Device System Infection

- **Erosion** is an uncommon complication that usually occurs because of an indolent infection, although it may also be the result of a device pocket that is too small for the pulse generator, particularly in a thin patient.
- The incidence of infection after initial device implantation should be less than 1%. Preoperative antibiotics reduce the incidence of infection.
- The most common clinical presentation is **localized pocket infection**; sepsis is uncommon. Many infectious agents can be responsible, but early infections are **most commonly caused by Staphylococcus aureus,** are aggressive and are often associated with fever and systemic symptoms.
- **Late infections commonly caused by Staphylococcus epidermidis** are more indolent, usually without fever or systemic manifestation.

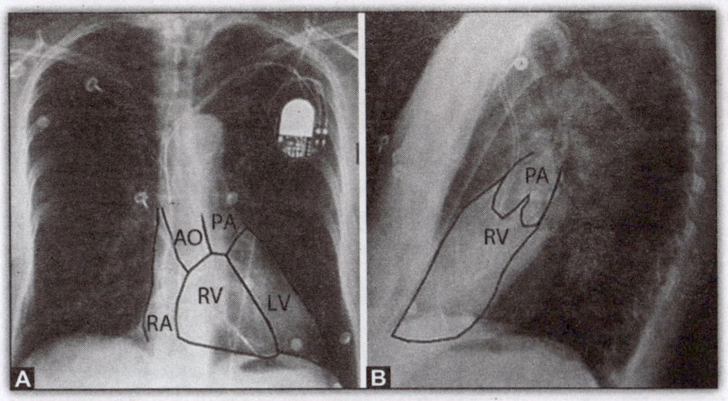

Figs A and B Normal cardiac anatomy; Frontal (A) and lateral (B) chest radiographs show the aorta (AO in a), left ventricle (LV in a), main pulmonary artery (PA), right atrium (RA in a) and right ventricle (RV)

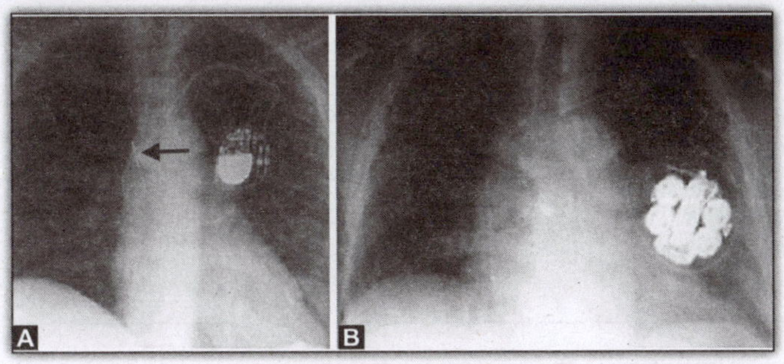

Figs A and B Lead displacement; (A) Frontal chest radiograph shows a dual-chamber pacemaker with the right atrial lead (arrow) dislodged into the superior vena cava; (B) The above radiograph shows coiling of the leads known as **Twiddler syndrome**

26. Ans. (b) FDG-18 PET CT

Ref: Harrison's 19th ed page 270 e4, Braunwald's Heart Disease 9th ed chapter 17

PET has traditionally been regarded as the gold standard technique for the assessment of myocardial viability. The positron-emitting tracer F-18 fluorodeoxyglucose (FDG) assesses myocardial glucose metabolism and is an indicator of myocardial viability. Because uptake is heterogeneous in normal myocardium in the fasting state, oral glucose loading or a combination of insulin and glucose infusions is used to enhance myocardial uptake. The SPECT radiopharmaceuticals, 201Tl and 99mTc isonitriles, require an intact (viable) cell membrane for uptake and also provide an assessment of myocardial viability in addition to perfusion. However, PET identifies ischemic or hibernating myocardium in 10–20% of regions otherwise classified as fibrotic (infarcted) by SPECT perfusion tracers.

FDG is a glucose analogue used to image myocardial glucose use with PET. After injection of 5 to 10 mCi, FDG rapidly exchanges across the capillary and cellular membranes. It is phosphorylated by hexokinase to FDG-6-phosphate and not metabolized further or used in glycogen synthesis. Because the dephosphorylation rate of FDG is slow, it becomes trapped in the myocardium, permitting PET or SPECT imaging of regional glucose use. FDG uptake may be increased in hibernating but viable myocardium and FDG uptake in asynergic myocardial regions with reduced blood flow at rest has become a scintigraphic marker of hibernation.

Before considering the tests for myocardial viability it is important to understand few terms.

- **Stunned myocardium:** It refers to a state in which there is wall dysfunction but the perfusion (resting and stress) is normal.
- **Myocardial ischemia:** It refers to a state in which there is decreased perfusion on stress but normal perfusion during rest (seen a reversible perfusion defect). These patients will significantly benefit from treatment.
- **Hibernating myocardium:** In this the myocardium shows decreased perfusion on both stress and resting phase (seen as fixed defect) but the myocytes are viable and will benefit from revascularization; see: hibernating myocardium.
- **Myocardial infarct:** In this there is absent perfusion on both stress and resting phase (seen as fixed defect) and the myocytes are not viable.

Imaging Techniques for Myocardial Viability

	Comments	Imaging technique	Half life	Comments
Thallium 201	Myocardial perfusion imaging	SPECT	72 hours	• Excessive radiation dose • Redistribution may occur • Single injection for stress and resting phase
99mTc-Sestamibi SPECT	Myocardial perfusion imaging	SPECT	6 hours	• Less radiation dose • No redistribution • Separate injections for stress and resting phase
18 FDG [18F- Fluoro-2-Deoxyglucose]	Myocardial viability and Inflammation imaging	PET	110 minutes	• Based on the fact that myocardium utilizes glucose for metabolism when under effect of ischemia (hence the ischemic myocardium will show greater uptake than normal cells) • Under normal circumstances, it utilizes fatty acids for energy • Non-viable myocardium will not show any uptake

Contd...

Imaging Techniques for Myocardial Viability				
	Comments	**Imaging technique**	**Half life**	**Comments**
Cardiac MR perfusion imaging	Myocardial perfusion imaging	MR		• No ionising radiation exposure • Dynamic imaging with gadolinium for perfusion • Delayed imaging for viability assessment
Computed tomography myocardial perfusion imaging	Myocardial perfusion imaging	CT		• Single phase or dynamic perfusion imaging during stress and rest • Coronary arteries can be assessed at the same time

NOTE

Diagnostic quality of FDG imaging is critically dependent on hormonal milieu and substrate availability. Most clinical FDG studies are performed after 50 to 75 g of glucose loading in the form of oral dextrose approximately 1 to 2 hours before the FDG injection to increase glucose metabolism, to increase FDG uptake and to improve image quality. Although 90% of FDG images are of diagnostic quality in non-diabetic patients, the quality of FDG images after glucose loading alone is less certain in patients with clinical or subclinical diabetes, as the increase in plasma insulin levels may be attenuated, tissue lipolysis may not be inhibited and free fatty acid levels may remain high. Standardization schemes to optimize FDG image quality in diabetic patients include (1) intravenous insulin injections after glucose loading, (2) hyperinsulinemic-euglycemic clamping and (3) use of nicotinic acid derivative.

27. Ans. (b) Extramedullary intradural tumor

Ref: Sutton's 6/e page 254, Harrison 18th ed page 3382, Osborn's Neuroradiology 1/e, p 587

Expansion of the contrast filled space i.e., the subarachnoid space, is seen in any intramedullary, extradural lesion like meningioma.

Spinal Tumors		
Extramedullary (Outside the Spinal Canal)		**Intramedullary**
Extradural (Outside dura)	**Intradural (In subarachnoid space)**	**Always intradural (with in spinal cord)**
50% of the spinal tumours are extradural	40% are intradural extramedullary	10% are intradural intramedullary
Displacement or compression of the spinal cord, but they result in narrowing of both the ipsilateral and the contralateral subarachnoid spaces	Displace the cord away from the tumor, widening the ipsilateral subarachnoid space, narrowing the contralateral subarchnoid space	Fusiform enlargement of the cord, circumferential narrowing of the adjacent subarachnoid space
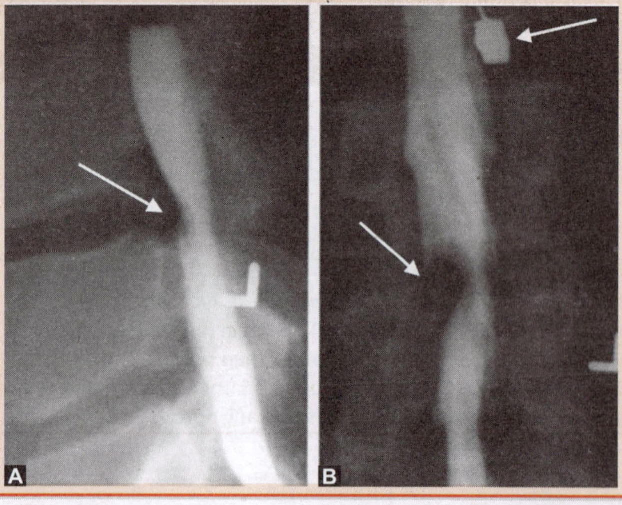	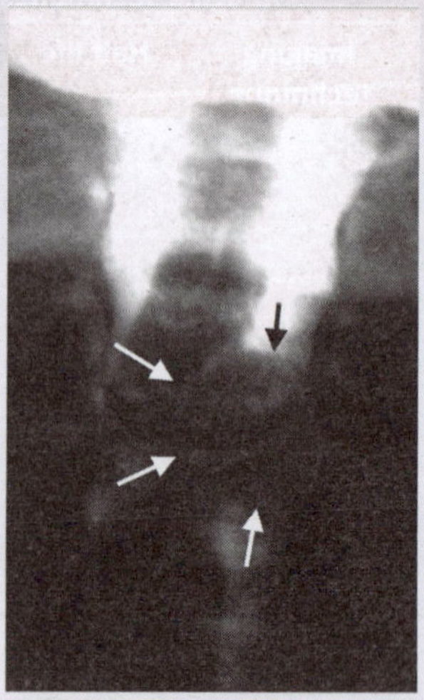	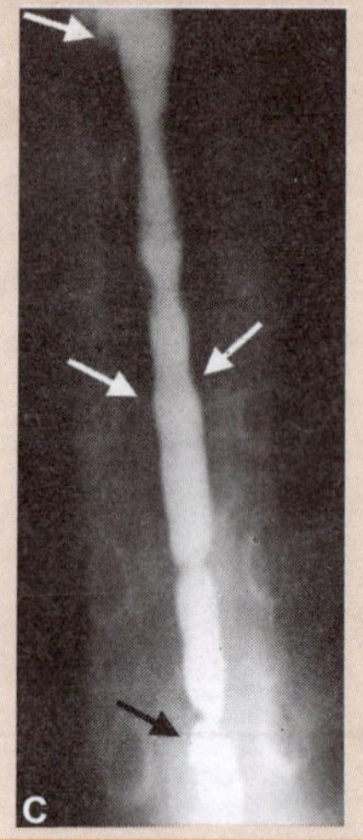

Contd...

Feathered appearance	Meniscus sign, widening of ipsilateral subarachnoid space	Widening of the cord, trouser leg appearance
Metastasis Osteoblastoma Osteochondroma Chondrosarcoma Giant cell tumor Myeloma, neuroblastoma Ganglioneuroma, lymphoma	Metastasis Nerve sheath tumors; Schwannoma, Neurofibroma Meningioma, subdural empyema	Ependymoma Astrocytoma Teratoma, infarct, Hematoma, Hemangioblastoma

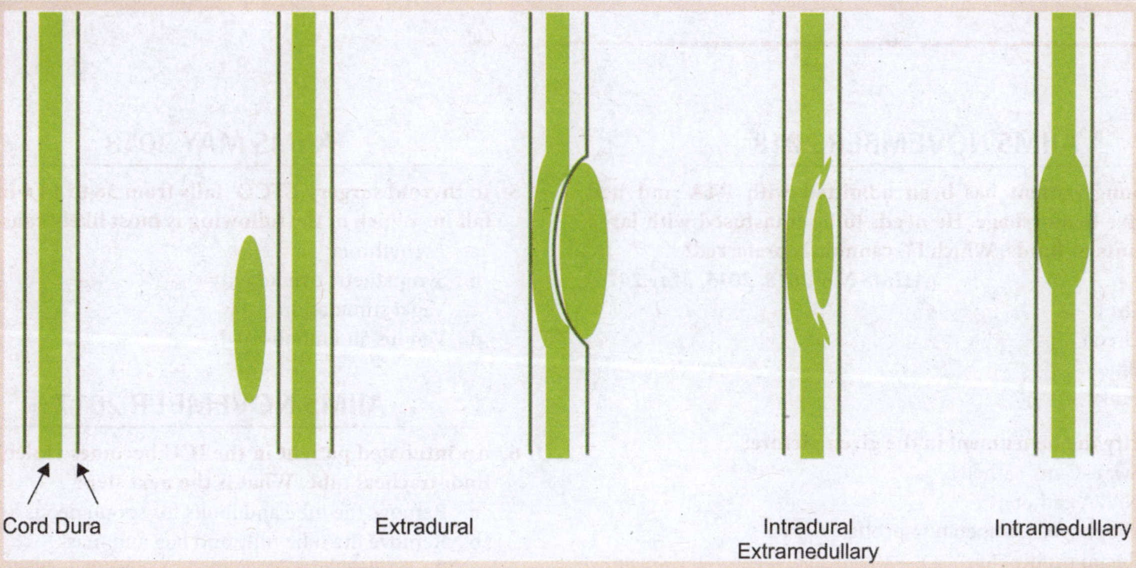

Anesthesia

19

AIIMS NOVEMBER 2018

1. A young patient has been admitted with RTA and had massive hemorrhage. He needs to be transfused with large amounts of fluids. Which IV cannula is preferred?
(AIIMS Nov 2018, 2015, May 2016)

a. Grey
b. Green
c. Blue
d. Pink

2. Identify the instrument in the given picture:

a. Swan-Ganz catheter
b. NAVA catheter
c. Esophageal temperature probe
d. Rectal probe

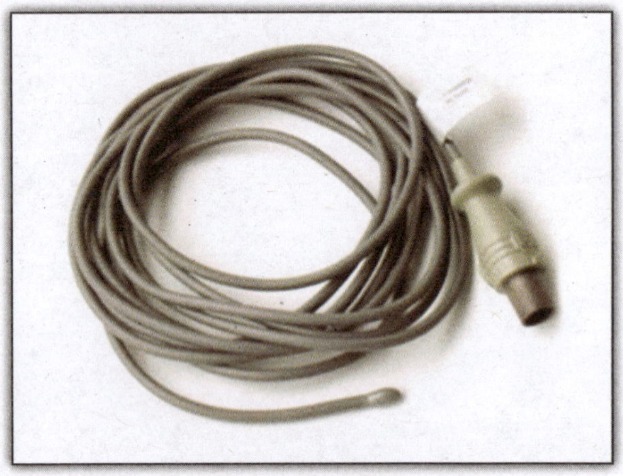

3. Which of the following statements is correct regarding difference between adult and child resuscitation?

a. Ventricular dysrhythmias are uncommon in children
b. Infant myocardium more refractory to hypoxia because of congenital heart disease.
c. More ventilation to be given compared to chest compression
d. Dissolved aortic oxygen concentration is more in pre attack state.

4. First reflex to appear after spinal shock is:

a. Bulbocavernosus reflex
b. Abdominal reflex
c. Plantar reflex
d. Cremasteric reflex

AIIMS MAY 2018

5. In thyroid surgery $ETCO_2$ falls from 38 to 14 with a sudden fall in. Which of the following is most likely cause?

a. Arrhythmia
b. Sympathetic overactivity
c. Vagal stimulation
d. Venous air embolism

AIIMS NOVEMBER 2017

6. An intubated patient in the ICU becomes violent, pulls out Endotracheal tube. What is the next step?

a. Remove the tube and looks for spontaneous breathing
b. Remove the tube fully and bag and mask
c. Re-intubate
d. Do back physiotherapy to remove secretions

7. Which of the following drug used for intravenous induction of anesthesia?

a. Dexmedetomidine
b. Lorazepam
c. Bupivacaine
d. Neostigmine

8. Which is the correct sequence?

a. Assess the patient's response, call for help, check carotid pulse, start CPR
b. Check carotid pulse, start CPR, call for help, defibrillate
c. Defibrillate, assess response, check carotid pulse, maintain airway
d. Start CPR, call for help, defibrillate, check pulse

9. Mask that can deliver maximum O_2?

a. Nasal prongs
b. Oxygen mask
c. Venturi mask
d. Face mask with a reservoir

10. What is the recommended duration of preoxygenation before intubation?

a. 3 min
b. 4 min
c. 5 min
d. 6 min

11. Least susceptible nerve fibers to local anesthetics is:

a. A alpha
b. A delta
c. B
d. C

12. Color of 22 Gauge IV cannula is?

a. Grey
b. Green
c. Blue
d. Pink

13. Which of the following is considered balanced resuscitation?
a. Giving colloids and crystalloids ratio of 1:1
b. Maintaining pH by ensuring acid base are balanced
c. Maintaining permissible hypotension to avoid bleeding
d. Maintaining airway Breathing and circulation

14. During resuscitation of a septic shock patient, Norepinephrine was given. How would you assess that patient is responsive to norepinephrine?
a. Reduced renal perfusion and reduced urine output
b. Increased mean arterial pressure
c. Tachycardia d. Bradycardia

AIIMS MAY 2017

15. All of the following are true regarding the procedure performed with the instrument shown below EXCEPT:

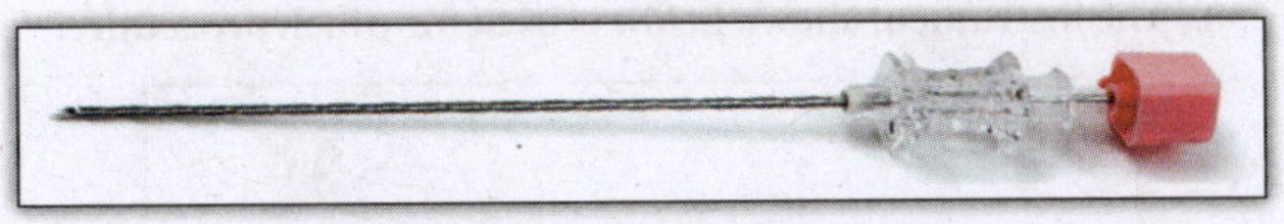

a. Absolutely contraindicated in coagulation disorder
b. Done in lateral recumbent position
c. Bevel of needle faces upwards
d. Breath holding not required

AIIMS NOVEMBER 2016

16. A chronic smoker underwent laparoscopic abdominal surgery under general anesthesia induced with fentanyl and propofol. The following $EtCO_2$ graph was observed intraoperatively. What is your probable diagnosis?

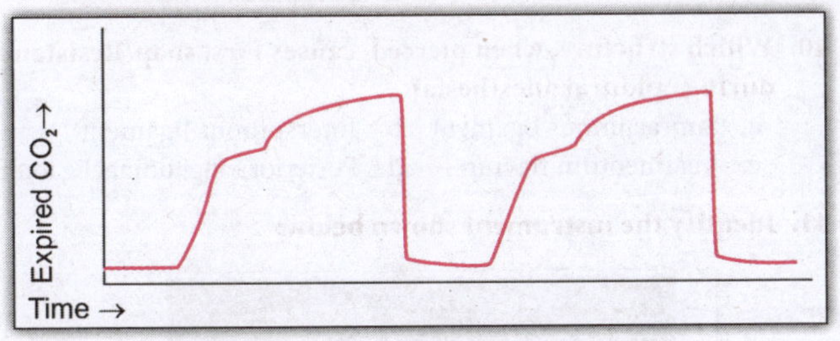

a. Rebreathing b. Bronchospasm
c. Endobronchial intubation
d. Leak in the sample line

17. An inotropic drug is to be infused at the rate of 10 μg/kg/min. In a 5 mL vial 200 mg of drug is present. 2 vials of the drug diluted in 250 mL of normal saline is prepared for infusion. If 16 drops = 1 mL, what must be the drop rate for a 80 kg patient?
a. 8 drops/min b. 16 drops/min
c. 20 drops/min d. 22 drops/min

18. Why 100% oxygen has to be given to a patient after recovery from N_2O anesthesia?
a. 2nd gas effect b. Diffusion hypoxia
c. Both d. None

19. Best route of drug administration during resuscitation of neonate?
a. Endotracheal b. Umbilical artery
c. Umbilical vein d. Intraosseous

20. On giving epidural anesthesia xylocaine with epinephrine was injected. Within 3 minutes the patient had hypotension. Most probable reason for this:
a. Systemic toxicity of drug
b. Drug injected in subarachnoid space
c. Vasovagal shock d. Anaphylaxis

21. During laryngoscopy and intubation, which of the following is not performed: (AIIMS Nov 2016, 2003)
a. Flexion of neck
b. Extension of head at atlanto-occipital joint
c. The laryngoscope is lifted upwards levering over the upper incisors
d. In a straight blade laryngoscope, epiglottis is lifted up by the tip

22. A nonresponsive patient is brought to emergency department with no proper history. What will be your first step?
a. Check carotid pulse b. Check responsiveness
c. Start CPR d. Defibrillator

23. What is the ratio of chest compression and ventilation for all ages done by single rescuer?
a. 30:1 b. 15:1
c. 30:2 d. 10:1

AIIMS MAY 2016

24. All of the following act on neuromuscular junction EXCEPT:
a. Pipercuronium b. Dantrolene sodium
c. Succinylcholine d. Mivacurium

25. Allergic reactions occurring during the immediate perioperative period is due to administration of:
a. Local anesthetics b. Neuromuscular blockers
c. Opioids d. Induction agents

26. Which of the following is not true regarding rapid sequence intubation (RSI) in a cardiac patient:
a. Simultaneous administration of an induction and neuromuscular blocking agents
b. Preoxygenate the patient with 100% oxygen for 3 minutes before intubation
c. Induction should be done with thiopentone and succinylcholine for muscle relaxant
d. Cricoid pressure is applied till endotracheal tube has been secured with a cuff

27. A 46-year-old male was given a subarachnoid block using 12 mg of bupivacaine by anesthetist. After 10 minutes of administration the BP dropped to 72/44 mm Hg and heart rate was 52/min. The level of block was found to be at T6. What is the reason for bradycardia in this patient?
a. Bezold-Jarisch reflex
b. Bain bridge reflex
c. Reverse bainbridge reflex
d. Blockade of cardiac accelerator nerve fibers

28. A sevoflurane vaporizer can accurately deliver the dose of an anesthetic agent which resembles it in which of the following property?
a. Blood gas partition co-efficient
b. Vapor pressure
c. Oil gas partition co-efficient
d. Molecular weight

29. The relation of age and MAC requirements are represented correctly in which of the following:

a. Neonates > adults > infants
b. Infants > neonates > adults
c. Infants > adults > neonates
d. Adults > infants > neonates

30. A drug that undergoes Hoffmann elimination is:

a. Atracurium b. Vecuronium
c. Pancuronium d. Mivacurium

31. A patient with diarrhea and severe dehydration requires rapid infusion of IV fluids. Which color of cannula will you prefer? *(AIIMS May 2016, Nov 2015)*

a. Grey b. Green
c. Blue d. Pink

AIIMS NOVEMBER 2015

32. In case of massive bleeding during surgery which size of IV cannula is used? *(AIIMS May 2016, Nov 2015)*

a. 16 G b. 20 G
c. 22 G d. 24 G

33. A patient was in surgery when following capnography picture was noticed. What is the next most appropriate step?

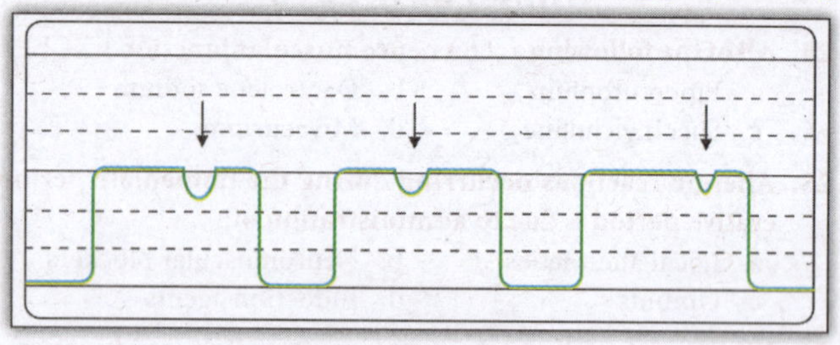

a. Administer skeletal muscle relaxant
b. Check for anesthetic machine connections
c. Check endotracheal tube position
d. Change soda lime container

34. Tip of cuff of LMA placed over? Point marked as A in the device shown in the picture is placed over:

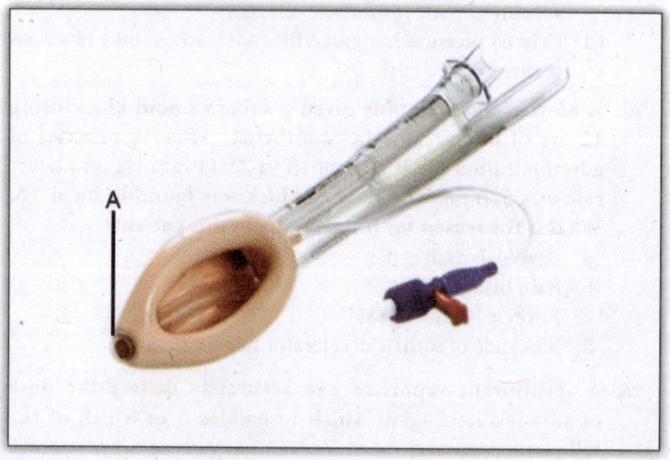

a. Above esophagus
b. Above epiglottis
c. Above vocal cords
d. Above thyroid cartilage

35. What is true about medical oxygen cylinder?

a. Black body white shoulder
b. Black body grey shoulder
c. Grey body white shoulder
d. Grey body black and white shoulder

36. Ideal site for measuring temperature during anesthesia?

a. Rectum b. Tympanic membrane
c. Pulmonary artery d. Lower end of esophagus

37. A pregnant female presents with lacenta previa, bleeding and systolic BP of 85 mm Hg, induction and maintenance of anesthesia for cesarean section is done by:

a. Ketamine followed by intubation and GA
b. Propofol followed by intubation and GA
c. Thiopentone followed by muscle relaxant
d. Epidural with bupivacaine

38. The instrument shown below is used for which procedure:

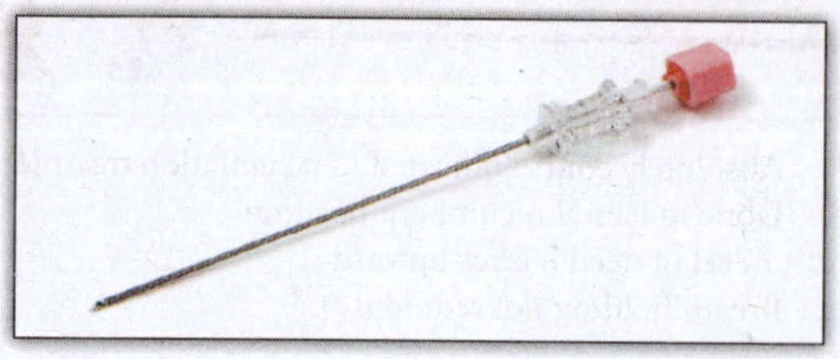

a. Bone marrow aspiration b. Lumbar puncture
c. Pleural biopsy d. Suction

39. Which anti-cholinergic drug is most commonly used pre-anesthetic medication?

a. Glycopyrrolate b. Neostigmine
c. Propantheline d. Atropine

40. Which structure, when pierced, causes First snap/Resistance during epidural anesthesia?

a. Supraspinous ligament b. Interspinous ligament
c. Ligamentum flavum d. Posterior longitudinal ligament

41. Identify the instrument shown below:

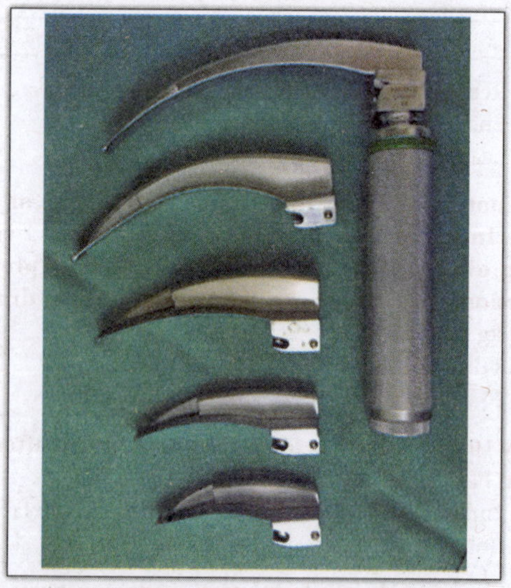

a. Straight blade high pressure laryngoscope
b. Curved blade laryngoscope
c. Macintosh laryngoscope
d. LMA

AIIMS MAY 2015

42. Which of these anesthetic agents is contraindicated in a patient with coronary artery disease with pulse rate of 48/min, low BP and decreased myocardial contractility in on Echo?

a. Ketamine b. Dexmedetomidine
c. Etomidate d. Fentanyl

43. Which of the following muscle relaxant can be used in a patient with high bilirubin of 6 mg/dL and serum creatinine of 4.5 mg/dL?

a. Vecuronium b. Atracurium
c. Pancuronium d. Mivacurium

44. Which anesthetic agent can cause pain on IV administration?

a. Thiopentone
b. Propofol
c. Ketamine
d. Midazolam

45. Which of the following combinations can be used for day care surgery?

a. Remifentanil, Midazolam, Propofol
b. Fentanyl, Midazolam, Thiopentone sodium
c. Morphine, Midazolam, Propofol
d. Morphine, Ketamine, Diazepam

ANSWERS WITH EXPLANATIONS

AIIMS NOVEMBER 2018

1. Ans. (a) Grey

Ref: Oxford American Handbook of Clinical Examinations and Practical Skills by Elezabeth Burns Ch 18, Bailey 25th ed page 291

Same question regarding rapid infusion of IV fluid was asked in many sessions of AIIMS exams in different language. Be it Massive hemorrhage in RTA or Intraoperative or be it Diarrhoea; the concept is rapid infusion and answer remains the same.

ACLS guidelines recommend securing IV access by two large bore cannula (14–16 G) in patient needed resuscitation

In case of a massive bleeding or severe dehydration, we would like to resuscitate the patient with rapid infusion of IV fluids. This can be effectively achieved with a higher gauge cannula. Always remember, higher the Gauge, smaller the cannula.

Cannula Sizes and Color Codes

Color Code	Gauge (G)	External Dia (mm)	Length (mm)	Flow Rate (ml/min)	Uses
Red	14	2.2	32	325	For emergency use (e.g: shock)
Grey	16	1.7	50	196	For use in large blood transfusions and emergency use (Shock)
Green	18	1.3	45	96	Suitable for IV fluids and smaller blood transfusions
Pink	20	1.1	33	61	Suitable for the majority of patients that require IV fluids
Blue	22	0.9	25	36	For difficult hand veins - elderly patients with fragile veins. May be used in slightly older children
Yellow	24	0.7	19	22	Used commonly in pediatric patients

Size and flow data may vary to some extent with the manufacturer

MNEMONIC to remember the color codes of IV cannula in increasing order of caliber - Rahul Gandhi Grows Pink Before Yelling (for Red, Grey, Green, Pink, Blue, Yellow)

NOTE

- These values may differ amongst different manufacturers.
- The larger the gauge size, the smaller the diameter. This is because the gauge size denotes how many cannulas of that size will fit into a tube of fixed diameter. E.g. 22 cannulas of 22 G will fit into the tube of fixed diameter

2. Ans. (c) Esophageal temperature probe > (D) Rectal probe

Ref: Dorsh 5th Ed Pg 863

NOTE

The same temperature probe can be used for measuring temperature through esophagus as well as rectum. We have chosen the answer to be esophageal temperature probe since the description is more specific than "rectal probe".

Types of Temperature Probes

Infrared Thermometer

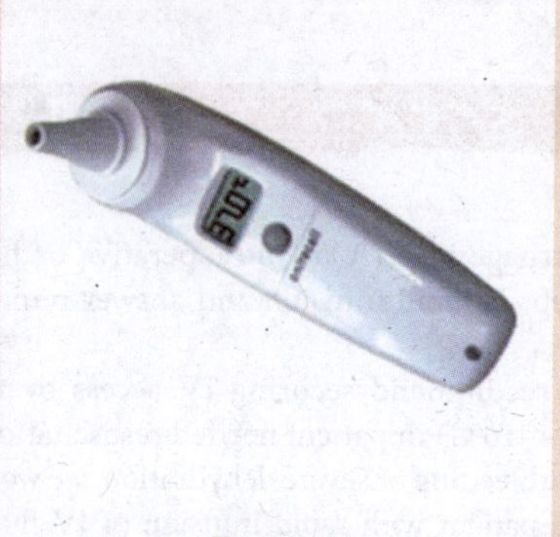

Ear canal

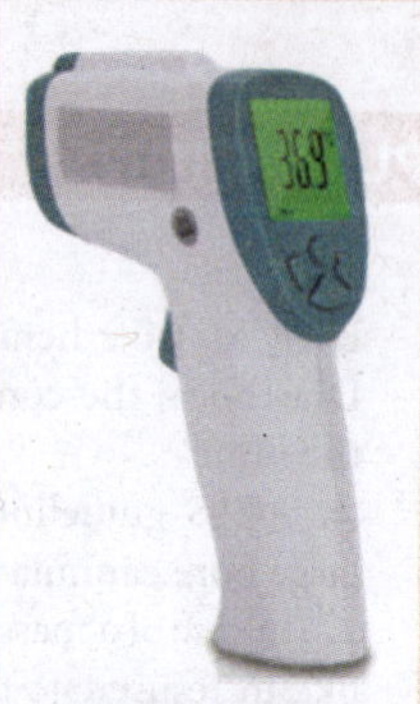

Usually forehead

Esophageal Temperature

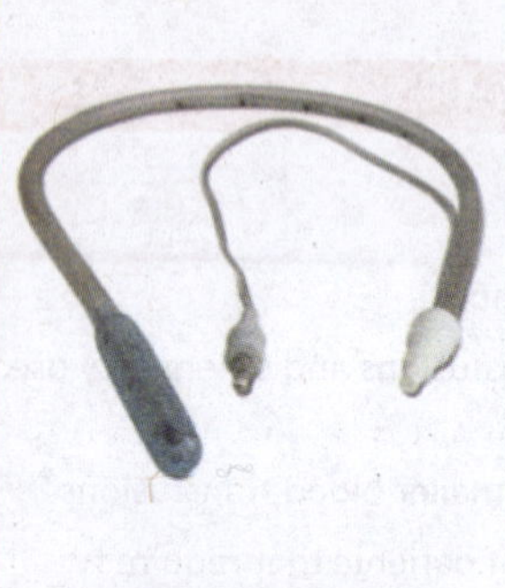

Esophageal stethoscope/ temperature probe

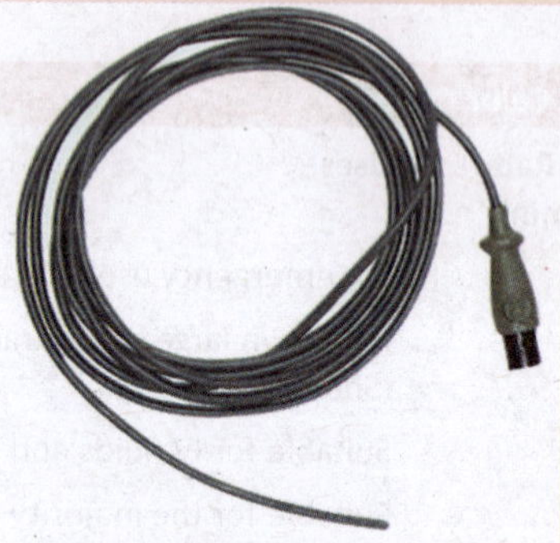

Esophageal temperature probe

Note: The esophageal probe can be used to measure oral, nasopharyngeal as well as rectal temperature too.

Urinary Bladder Temperature Sensor

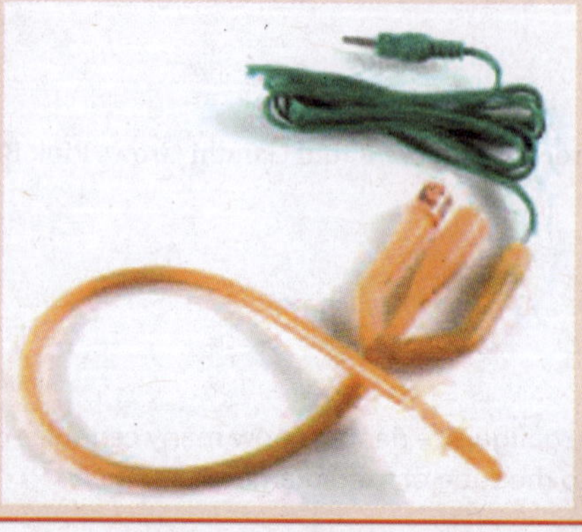

Contd...

Tympanic Membrane Temperature Probe

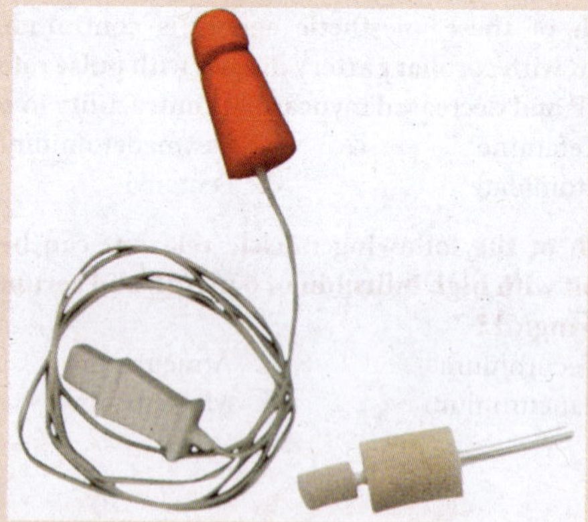

Fig: Types of tympanic probes

Note: It is designed in such a way so as to seal the auditory canal completely proximally, while the distal end is designed in an atraumatic way to avoid damage to the tympanic membrane.

Swan-Ganz Catheter

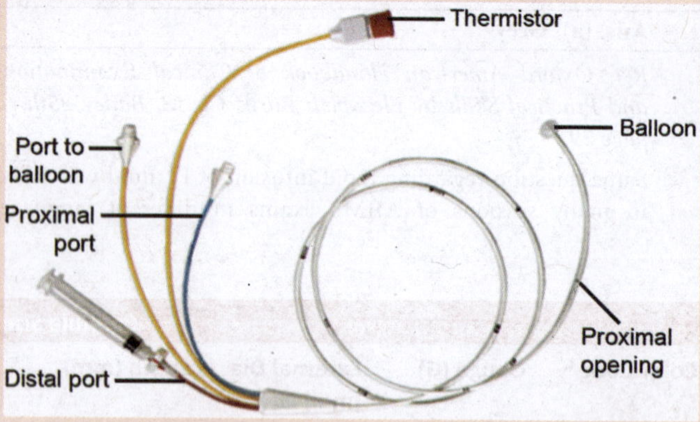

About Neurally Adjusted Ventilatory Assist (NAVA)

- During normal respiration, a spontaneous breath begins with an impulse generated by the respiratory centers in the brain. This impulse is then transmitted via phrenic nerves and electrically activates the diaphragm, leading to a muscle contraction.
- The diaphragm contracts into the abdominal cavity, which leads to a descending movement, creating a negative alveolar pressure and an inflow of air.
- The signal that excites the diaphragm is proportional to the integrated output of the respiratory center in the brain and controls the depth and cycling of the breath.
- The electrical discharge of the diaphragm is captured by a special catheter fitted with an array of electrodes (the Edi catheter) and visualized on the ventilator screen. This is Edi, the electrical activity of the diaphragm.
- The Edi catheter is placed in the esophagus much like an ordinary feeding tube. With NAVA, the Edi is used to deliver ventilation in time with and in proportion to the diaphragm activity.
- The advantages are fewer periods of over- and under-assist, Improved patient-ventilator synchrony, reduced sedation, improved comfort scores, improved sleep quality. It is believed to improve weaning.

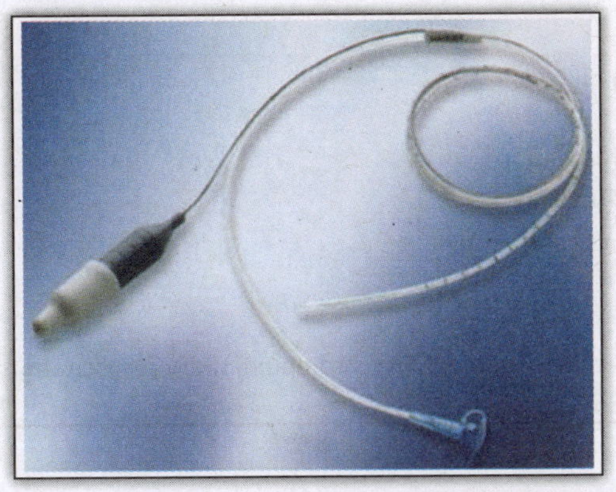

3. Ans. (b) Infant myocardium more refractory to hypoxia because of congenital heart disease.

Ref: Miller's 8th Ed Pg 2857

Relative hypoxia is normal in utero and infant hearts tolerate hypoxia better than adult hearts do, thus infant myocardium more refractory to hypoxia because of congenital heart disease.

Option (A) Ventricular Dysrhythmias are Uncommon in Children

Miller's 8th Ed Pg 2877 says:

"Pediatric VF or VT has been an underappreciated pediatric problem. Recent studies indicate that VF and VT (i.e., shockable rhythms) occur in 27% of in-hospital cardiac arrests at some time during the resuscitation. In a population of PICU patients, as many as 41% of arrests were associated with VF or VT. According to the NRCPR database, 10% of children with in-hospital cardiac arrest had an initial rhythm of VF/VT. **In all, 27% of the children had VF/VT at some time during the resuscitation**...

The treatment of choice for short-duration VF is prompt defibrillation.

In general, the mortality rate increases by 7% to 10% per minute of delay to defibrillation. Because VF must be considered before defibrillation can be provided, early determination of the rhythm by electrocardiography is critical. **An attitude that VF is rare in children can be a self-fulfilling prophecy with a uniformly fatal outcome**"

Hence, Option (A) is incorrect.

Option (B) Infant Myocardium more Refractory to Hypoxia Because of Congenital Heart Disease

- Fetal myocardial metabolism differs from that of adults. Relative hypoxia is normal in utero and infant hearts tolerate hypoxia better than adult hearts do.
- This difference may be due in part to high concentrations of glycogen in fetal myocardial tissue and to the ability to use anaerobic metabolism more effectively.
- Because of the high glycogen stores and the ability to use anaerobic metabolism efficiently, the fetal or newborn heart is relatively resistant to hypoxia and can be resuscitated more easily if oxygenation and perfusion are reestablished reasonably quickly.

Hence, Option (B) is correct

Option (C) More Ventilation to be given Compared to Chest Compression

- In infants and children, asphyxial cardiac arrest is more common than cardiac arrest from a primary cardiac event; therefore, ventilation may have greater importance during resuscitation of children
- The asphyxial nature of the majority of pediatric cardiac arrests necessitates ventilation as part of effective CPR. In case of 2 rescuers, a 15:2 ratio has been suggested in the pediatric algorithm.
- Thus, although more importance has been given to ventilation in pediatric scenarios, the number of chest compressions per cycle is still more than the number of breaths to be given.

Option (D) Dissolved Aortic Oxygen Concentration is more in Pre Attack State

Children often show minimal signs and symptoms till the last minute. Hence, the pre-arrest phase (see Table below) is essential in screening for such patients who may be in impending respiratory or cardiac failure. Obviously, such patients will not have a high aortic oxygen concentration since they are already in a compromised physiological state.

Hence, Option (D) is incorrect.

Phases of Cardiac Arrest and Resuscitation	
Pre-arrest phase (protect)	Optimize patient monitoring and rapid emergency response Recognize and treat respiratory failure or shock to prevent cardiac arrest
Arrest (no-flow) phase (preserve)	Minimize interval to BLS and ACLS Organize response with clear leadership Minimize interval to defibrillation, when indicated
Low-flow (CPR) phase (resuscitate)	Push hard, push fast Allow full chest recoil Minimized interruptions in compressions Avoid overventilation Titrate CPR to optimize myocardial blood flow (coronary perfusion pressures and exhaled CO2) Consider adjuncts to improve vital organ perfusion during CPR Consider ECMO if standard CPR/ALS not promptly successful

Contd...

Postresuscitation phase	
Short-term	Optimize cardiac output and cerebral blood flow Treat arrhythmias, if indicated Avoid hyperglycemia, hyperthermia, hyperventilation Debrief to improve future responses to emergencies
Long-term rehabilitation (regenerate)	Early intervention with occupational and physical therapy Bioengineering and technology interface Possible future role for stem cell transplantation
ACLS, advanced cardiac life support; ALS, advanced life support; BLS, basic life support; CPR, cardiopulmonary resuscitation; ECMO, extracorporeal membrane oxygenation	

4. Ans. (a) Bulbocavernosus reflex

Ref: Bailey's 26th Ed Pg 329

- Spinal shock refers to a temporary dysfunction of the spinal cord, with a loss of reflexes and sensorimotor function caudal to the level of injury.
- It is manifested by absence of anal wink and bulbocavernosus reflexes and by flaccid paralysis. It is a temporary phenomenon and recovers usually in 24 to 48 hours even in severe injuries. There is no specific treatment for spinal shock
- When spinal shock starts to resolve the bulbocavernosus reflex returns.
- The anal and bulbocavernosus reflexes both depend on intact sacral reflex arcs
- The bulbocavernosus reflex is a contraction of the anal sphincter felt with the examining finger in response to squeezing the glans penis. (In females, clitoris is used for eliciting this reflex)
- The anal reflex is an externally visible contraction of the anal sphincter in response to perianal pin prick (anal wink).
- The appearance of reflex cord activity (bulbocavernosus, anal and plantar) without the presence of any motor or sensory activity indicates cord transection.

AIIMS MAY 2018

5. Ans. (d) Venous air embolism

Ref: SRB's Surgical Operations: Text & Atlas 2nd Ed by Sriram Bhat Pg 499

In the above question, there is a sudden drastic fall in ET CO_2.

Changes in End-tidal Carbon Dioxide ($ETCO_2$)

Increased $ETCO_2$	Reduced $ETCO_2$
Decreased alveolar ventilation • Reduced respiratory rate • Reduced tidal volume • Increased equipment dead space	**Increased alveolar ventilation** • Increased respiratory rate • Increased tidal volume
Increased CO_2 production • Fever • Hypercatabolic state	**Reduced CO_2 production** • Hypothermia • Hypocatabolic state
Increased inspired pCO_2 • Rebreathing • CO_2 absorber exhausted • External source of CO_2	**Increased alveolar dead space** • Reduced cardiac output • Pulmonary embolism • High positive end expiatory pressure during intermittent positive-pressure ventilation
	Sampling error • Inadequate tidal volume • Water blocking sampling line • Air entrainment into sampling line

- During thyroid surgery, the head end of the table is elevated to improve venous return. This reduces venous congestion in the neck and decreases oozing in the surgical field. Around 15 degree head up position can be achieved by placing pillows or towel rolls beneath the shoulder. Neck is extended.
- However, as the neck is at a higher level than the heart, there is a chance of air embolism.
- Thus, veins should be ligated securely and then cut.
- Any doubtful air in internal jugular vein should be aspirated immediately.

AIIMS NOVEMBER 2017

6. Ans. (a) Remove the tube and looks for spontaneous breathing

Ref: Critical Care Medicine: Perioperative Management by Michael James Murray 2nd Ed Pg 469; AACN Protocols for Practice: Care of Mechanically Ventilated Patients by Suzanne M. Burns 2nd Ed Pg 28

In the ICU patients are sedated enough to "tolerate" the endotracheal tube (this is a very noxious stimulus) and at the same time breathe spontaneously. In such conditions, the patient may sometimes get violent and try to remove the tube. Let us also go option wise and discuss the possible scenarios:

Option (A) Remove the Tube and Look for Spontaneous Breathing

- **In the operation theater:** During extubation while waiting for the patient to breathe satisfactorily. If the patient removes tube, most commonly he is capable of maintaining spontaneous respiration.
- **During weaning from ventilator:** In these conditions sedation is generally stopped and the patient is trying to maintain respiration with some help from the ventilator. This is a common outcome and we see if the patient is breathing comfortably spontaneously and maintaining saturation, there is no need to supplement respiration/re- intubate.

Option (B) Remove the Tube Fully and Bag and Mask

This is done when we doubt the ability of the patient to breathe spontaneously given his medical condition. We do not want the patient to desaturate and hence we support his ventilation. However, the bag and mask ventilation will have to be coordinated with the patient's inspiration and there are high chances of incoordination, resulting in lesser benefit and patient discomfort.

Option (C) Re-intubate

When the patient is not likely to maintain his airway/ respiration. We also have to keep in mind the possible complications of reintubation like higher risk of nosocomial pneumonia, increased risk of mortality.

Option (D) Do Back Physiotherapy to Remove Secretions

This is obviously not the immediate next step. Physiotherapy and secretion removal will depend on the decision to intubate and wean later.

All said and done, Option (A) and Option(C) both look like the next logical step. Looking for spontaneous ventilation and assessment of breathing pattern may not be as harmful as accepting reintubation as a rule of thumb in ICU patients, given the complications associated with reintubation.

Hence Option (A) should be the next logical step. Not all self extubations require reintubation.

7. Ans. (b) Lorazepam > (a) Dexmedetomidine

Ref: Miller's 8th Ed Pg 2620; Clinical Anesthesia by Paul G. Barash 6th Ed Table 18.2

Let us go through the options:

Option (A) Dexmedetomidine and Option (B) Lorazepam

Both Dexmedetomidine (alpha-2 receptor agonist) and lorazepam (barbiturate) are primarily used as sedative agents, however both have been used as an adjunct to induction of anesthesia.

The deciding factor between these 2 options can be the fact that dexmedetomidine has been approved by FDA for sedation earlier in ICU setting and recently in operation theaters as well and its use for induction of anesthesia and in operation theaters accounts for its off label use.

Option (C) Bupivacaine

Bupivacaine is a local anesthetic and cannot be used in induction of general anesthesia. It is cardiotoxic and must not be given intravenously.

Option (D) Neostigmine

Neostigmine is an anticholinesterase and is used for reversal of action of nondepolarizing muscle relaxants.

Following are the general set of steps followed during administration of general anesthesia:

- **Premedication:** Premedication traditionally refers to the administration of medications to relieve anxiety before surgery. However, the term encompasses any medication given in the preoperative period and therefore includes prophylactic analgesia and antiemesis agents, as well as drugs used to promote gastric emptying or counteract acid secretions. Commonly used drugs are: Midazolam (0.02-0.03 mg/kg), Opioids, Metoclopramide, Glycopyrrolate, H_2 receptor blockers like Ranitidine
- **Induction:** Maybe Intravenous (more common) or inhalational (with agents like ether- uncommon, sevoflurane, halothane). The intravenous agents are Propofol (2 mg/kg), Thiopentone (3–5 mg/kg), Midazolam (in higher doses- 0.1–0.2 mg/kg), Ketamine (1–2 mg/kg), etomidate (0.2 mg/kg)
- **Maintenance:** With inhalational agents like nitrous oxide, halothane, isoflurane, desflurane, sevoflurane along with opioids, muscle relaxants (if necessary) and most importantly, oxygen.
- **Emergence:** May include reversal (most commonly with neostigmine and glycopyrrolate if a muscle relaxant has been used); extubation if an endotracheal tube or an airway device has been used. Basically, it involves stoppage of anesthetic agents to bring the patient back to wakefulness. Adequate analgesia and antiemesis should be ensured for smooth recovery and minimum discomfort to the patient.
- **Postoperative care:** Involves monitoring of the vitals, further analgesic and antiemetic agents if necessary.

Induction Characteristics and Dosage Requirements for the Currently Available Sedative-Hypnotic Drug

Drug name	Induction Dose (mg/kg)	Onset (sec)	Duration (min)	Excitatory activity	Pain on injection	Heart rate	Blood pressure
Thiopental	3–6	<30	5–10	+	0 – +	↑	↓
Methohexital	1–3	<30	5–10	++	+	↑↑	↓
Propofol	1.5–2.5	15–45	5–10	+	++	0–↓	↓↓
Midazolam	0.2–0.4	30–90	15–30	0	0	0	0/↓

Contd...

Induction Characteristics and Dosage Requirements for the Currently Available Sedative-Hypnotic Drug							
	Induction						
Drug name	Dose (mg/kg)	Onset (sec)	Duration (min)	Excitatory activity	Pain on injection	Heart rate	Blood pressure
Diazepam	0.3–0.6	45–90	15–30	0	+/+++	0	0/↓
Lorazepam	0.03–0.06	60–120	60–120	0	++	0	0//↓
Etomidate	0.2–0.3	15–45	3–12	+++	+++	0	0
Ketamine	1–2	15–45	3–12	+++	+++	0	0
Ketamine	1–2	45–60	10–20	+	0	↑↑	↑↑

0, none; +, minimal; ++, moderate; +++ severe; ↓, decrease; ↑, increase.
From white PF. Textbook of Intravenous Anesthesia. Baltimore, Williams and Wilkins, 1997, pp. 27-46 and 77-92.

8. Ans. (a) Assess the patient's response, call for help, check carotid pulse, start CPR

Ref: 2015 American Heart Association Guidelines Update for Cardiopulmonary Resuscitation and Emergency Cardiovascular Care

See table of Anesthesia ADULT CARDIAC ARREST - BASIC CARDIAC LIFE SUPPORT (BCLS) in AIIMS NOVEMBER 2016

9. Ans. (d) Face mask with reservoir

Ref: Ward's Anesthetic equipment Page 207-219

Oxygen Delivery Devices			
Criteria	Subtypes	Description	Examples
Performance of the device	Fixed	Controlled FiO_2	Venturi mask
	Variable performance	No control on FiO_2. The oxygen concentration delivered to the upper airway varies with the phase and pattern of respiration (as well as the selected oxygen ow rate)	Nasal prongs, Face mask
Flows delivered by the device	Low flow	Deliver O_2 at flows that are less than the patient's inspiratory flow rate leading to air entrainment	Nasal prongs, Face mask
	High flow		Venturi mask
Degree of Dependency	Low dependency	Spontaneous breathing. Supplemental oxygen alone is sufficient to correct hypoxia.	Nasal prongs, standard facemasks
	Medium dependency	Spontaneous breathing. Supplemental O_2 plus degree of respiratory assistance required.	Continuous Positive Airway Pressure (CPAP) mask and equipment
	High Dependency	Unreliable or absent breathing. Supplemental O_2 and full respiratory support required	Involves use of intensive operating theater or non-invasive ventilators
Low dependency devices can be further classified as:			
Low dependency devices	No capacity	No capacity for O_2 storage	Nasal prongs
	Low capacity	<100 mL capacity	Facemasks for children, tracheostomy masks (70-100 mL)
	Medium capacity	Capacity 100–250 mL	Standard adult facemasks (175-200 mL)
	High capacity	Capacity 250–2500 mL	Facemask with reservoir bag
	Very high capacity	Capacity >2500 mL)	Oxygen tent

Contd...

Footnote:

- Air is only entrained into a facemask when the patient's inspiratory flow rate exceeds the oxygen supply rate.
- To achieve a FiO_2 near 1.0 (100% oxygen) by providing sufficient oxygen flow alone, rates in excess of 60 l min^{-1} would be required (in order to exceed the patient's peak inspiratory flow rate) which is impractical. Increasing mask size simply increases the risk of rebreathing CO_2.
- A large amount of oxygen delivered to the facemask is lost to the atmosphere whenever the patient's inspiratory flow rate is (a) less than the oxygen supply rate and (b) during exhalation.
- High-capacity masks are designed to store some of this wasted oxygen in a reservoir bag (usually of >1 L volume) attached to the facemask, thus providing a higher FiO_2.
- With these devices, oxygen flows directly into the reservoir bag, which fills during exhalation and whenever the patient's inspiratory flow rate is less than the flow rate of delivered oxygen.
- **Following are flow rates and predicted FiO_2 with Facemask with reservoir bag:**

O_2 flow rate L/min	No valves	One way valve
3	0.5–0.65	0.45–0.6
6	0.6–0.75	0.6–0.75
9	0.65–0.80	0.65–0.80
12	0.7–0.85	0.7–0.85
15	0.75–0.9	0.75–0.9

10. Ans. (a) 3 min

Ref: Miller's 8th Ed page 1653, Anesthesia Tutorial of the Week (ATOTW) 297 by World Federation of Societies of Anesthesiologists – Apnoea and Pre-oxygenation dated 04/10/2013

In between induction of general anesthesia and securing the airway, there is a period of time called **apnea time**. This is the time when we attempt intubation/ventilation. It obviously follows that during this time the patient is using reserve oxygen in the lungs. If the intubation/ventilation is difficult, we need more reserve so that the patient can survive the apnea time without significant desaturation. Hence comes the concept of preoxygenation.

Preoxygenation

Why?

- Preoxygenation, the process of replacing nitrogen in the lungs with oxygen, provides an increased length of time before hemoglobin desaturation occurs in a patient with apnea. This lengthened ***apnea time*** provides an improved margin of safety while the anesthesiologist secures the airway and resumes ventilation.
- With the induction of anesthesia, hypoxemia can quickly develop as a result of hypoventilation or apnea in combination with decreases in functional residual capacity (FRC) attributable to the supine position, muscle paralysis and the direct effects of the anesthetic agents themselves.
- *Adequate preoxygenation is essential when mask ventilation after the induction of anesthesia is contraindicated (e.g.: Rapid sequence induction) or anticipated to be difficult, when intubation is anticipated to be difficult and in patients with a smaller FRC (i.e., patients who are obese or pregnant).*
- ***Because difficulty with airway management can unexpectedly occur, routine preoxygenation before induction of general anesthesia is recommended.***

Method

- Preoxygenation is typically performed via a facemask attached to either the anesthesia machine or a Mapleson circuit. To ensure adequate preoxygenation, 100% oxygen must be provided at a flow rate high enough to prevent rebreathing (10 to 12 L/min) and no leaks around the facemask must be present.
- *An end-tidal concentration of oxygen greater than 90% is considered to maximize apnea time.*

Tidal volume ventilation through the facemask for 3 minutes, which *allows the exchange of 95% of the gas in the lungs* → MOST EFFECTIVE

OR

4 VITAL CAPACITY breaths over 30 seconds→ not as effective as the tidal volume method but MORE RAPID

OR

8 VITAL CAPACITY breaths over 60 seconds has been shown to be more effective.

- Head-up positioning has been shown to improve the quality of preoxygenation in both obese and non- obese patients. The use of noninvasive positive-pressure ventilation (PPV) for preoxygenation also prolongs apnea time.

11. Ans. (d) C

Ref: With Text

- For susceptibility to Local Anesthesia Physiology books like Ganong gives a sequence of: **C > B > A**
- Older editions of Anesthesia books however give a sequence of: **B > C > A** (In general, for the nerve fibers of similar type; the larger the fiber, the more resistant it is to the local anesthetic. The size principle fails when myelinated fibers is compared with unmyelinated fibers. Smaller nerves are more sensitive to the local anesthetics due to their relatively high membrane surface area to axon unit volume ratio. E.g. B fibers are most sensitive to local

anesthetic blockage. Amongst the sensory nerve which conducts the cold temperature sensation are blocked most readily. (*Ref: Cousins and Bridenbaugh's Neural Blockade in Clinical Anesthesia and Pain Page 100*)

- Miller 8th edition clarifies all previous controversies and gives a sequence of: **$A\delta > A\delta > A\beta > A\alpha > B > C$**
- Myelin greatly increases the speed of nerve conduction by insulating the axolemma from the surrounding conducting salt medium and forcing the "action current" generated by an impulse to flow through the axoplasm to the nodes of Ranvier, which are periodic interruptions in the myelin sheath where the active impulse is regenerated (Miller)
- Small-diameter axons, such as C fibers, are often stated to be more susceptible to local anesthetic block than larger diameter fibers are. However, when careful measurements are made of single-impulse annihilation in individual nerve fibers, exactly the opposite differential susceptibility is noted **(Miller 8th ed page 1039)**
- Small myelinated axons (A gamma motor and A delta sensory fibers) are the most susceptible to impulse annihilation. Next in order of block are the large myelinated (A alpha and A beta) fibers and the least susceptible are the small, nonmyelinated C fibers. In fact, in this last group, impulses in the slowest conducting population are the most resistant to local anesthetic. The widespread notion that local anesthetics block the smallest fibers first or most is thus clearly wrong. **(Miller 8th ed page 1037)**

Relative Susceptibility of Mammalian A, B and C Nerve Fibers to Conduction Block Produced by Various Agents

	Most Susceptible	Intermediate	Least Susceptible
Hypoxia	B	A	C
Pressure	A	B	C
Local anesthetics	A	B	C

12. Ans. (c) Blue

Ref: Oxford American handbook of clinical examinations and Practical skills by Elezabeth Burns Ch 18, Bailey 25th ed page 291

See details of IV Cannula in AIIMS Nov 2018 Anaeshtesia (see page no. 1139)

13. Ans. (c) Maintaining permissible hypotension to avoid bleeding

Ref: ATLS guidelines 9th edition Page 72, 75; Miller's 8th Ed Pg 2435

"Balancing the goal of organ perfusion with the risks of rebleeding by accepting a lower-than-normal blood pressure has been termed "controlled resuscitation," "balanced resuscitation," "hypotensive resuscitation," and "permissive hypotension." The goal is the balance, not the hypotension. Such a resuscitation strategy may be a bridge to, but is not a substitute for, definitive surgical control of bleeding".

"Early administration of pRBCs, plasma and platelets and minimizing aggressive crystalloid administration in these patients may result in improved survival. This approach has been termed balanced, hemostatic or damage control resuscitation".

- In trauma patients, intravascular volume is lost to hemorrhage, uptake by ischemic cells and extravasation into the interstitial space. Administration of IV fluids will predictably increase cardiac output and arterial blood pressure in a hypovolemic trauma patient.
- The ATLS curriculum advocates rapid infusion of **1- 2 L of warmed isotonic crystalloid solution** in any hypotensive patient, with the goal of restoring normal arterial blood pressure.
- Conversely, fluid administration during active hemorrhage may be counterproductive.

Risks of Aggressive Volume Replacement during Early Resuscitation

- Increased blood pressure
- Decrease blood viscosity
- Decrease hematocrit
- Decrease clotting factor concentration
- Greater transfusion requirement
- Disruption of electrolyte balance
- Direct immune suppression
- Premature reperfusion
- Increased risk for hypothermia

- Early resuscitation is complex because the risks associated with aggressive intravascular volume replacement, including the potential for exacerbating hemorrhage and thus prolonging the crisis, must be weighed against the risk for hypoperfusion and ischemia.
- In trauma patients with massive hemorrhage, packed cell:FFP: Platelets ratio is 1:1:1

14. Ans. (b) Increased Mean Arterial Pressure

Ref: Miller's 8th ed page 367

- Norepinephrine acts at alpha and beta receptors, but it is typically used for its potent alpha agonism.
- **Peripheral vasoconstriction increases arterial blood pressure and may cause reflex bradycardia.**
- Venous return is increased by the powerful venoconstriction. Cardiac output is frequently unchanged or decreased; oxygen consumption is markedly increased.
- It is frequently the pressure of last resort in supporting systemic vascular resistance. It is used in septic shock to maintain mean arterial pressure.
- Because of its short half-life of 2.5 minutes, continuous infusion is preferred. Whereas less than 2 μg/minute (30 ng/kg/minute) may uncover the effects of beta1-adrenergic stimulation, the usual infusion rates of greater than 3 μg/minute (50 ng/kg/minute) elicit peripheral vasoconstriction from alpha-adrenergic stimulation.
- An increase in arterial pressure increases renal perfusion and hence urine output.

Surviving Sepsis Bundle

To be Completed within 3 Hours of Time of Presentation*:

- Measure lactate level
- Obtain blood cultures prior to administration of antibiotics
- Administer broad spectrum antibiotics
- Administer 30 mL/kg crystalloid for hypotension or lactate ≥4 mmol/L

* "Time of presentation" is defined as the time of triage in the emergency department or, if presenting from another care venue, from the earliest chart annotation consistent with all elements of severe sepsis or septic shock ascertained through chart review.

To be Completed within 6 Hours of Time of Presentation:

- Apply vasopressors (for hypotension that does not respond to initial fluid resuscitation) to maintain a mean arterial pressure (MAP) ≥65 mm Hg
- In the event of persistent hypotension after initial fluid administration (MAP < 65 mm Hg) or if initial lactate was ≥4 mmol/L, re-assess volume status and tissue perfusion and document finding. Re-measure lactate if initial lactate elevated.

Document findings mean:

Either

- Repeat focused exam (after initial fluid resuscitation) by licensed independent practitioner including vital signs, cardiopulmonary, capillary refill, pulse and skin findings. Or two of the following:
- Measure CVP
- Measure $ScvO_2$
- Bedside cardiovascular ultrasound
- Dynamic assessment of fluid responsiveness with passive leg raise or fluid challenge

AIIMS MAY 2017

15. Ans. (a) Absolutely contraindicated in coagulation disorder

Ref: Miller's 8th Ed page 1699, Harrison 19th edition page 443e-2

The picture seen above is that of Quincke's cutting needle which is used for lumbar puncture

NOTE

Modern disposable single use Lumbar puncture needle was given

Let us go through the options one by one:

Option (A) False

According to Miller's Anaesthesiology 8th Ed, Coagulopathy is a Relative contraindication to lumbar puncture.

Option (B) True

Lumbar puncture can be done in lateral as well as sitting position. Prone position has also been described for the same.

Option (C) True

Bevel of needle faces upwards.

According to Miller's 8th Ed Pg 1712: The incidence of post dural puncture headache is less when the needle bevel is placed in the long axis of the neuraxis, parallel to dural fibers, i.e. bevel faces laterally in sitting position, while it faces upwards in lateral position.

For further details regarding post dural puncture headache, see Anesthesia AIIMS Nov 2013.

Relationship Amongst Variables and Postspinal Puncture Headache

Factors that can increase the incidence of headache after spinal puncture

Age: Younger, more frequent

Sex: Females > Males

Needle size: Larger > Smaller

Needle bevel: Less when the needle bevel is placed in the long axis of the neuraxis

Pregnancy: More when pregnant

Dural punctures: More with multiple punctures

Factors that do not increase the incidence of headache after spinal puncture

Insertion and use of catheters for continuous spinal anesthesia

Timing of ambulation

Option (D) True

Breath holding not required. Breath holding during lumbar puncture can only help in ensuring cooperation of the patient by helping him to cope with the sudden pain due to needle prick, since it acts as a distraction. It is certainly not an essential part of lumbar puncture. The opening pressure of the cerebrospinal fluid (CSF) is recorded while the patient is reclining with the legs extended, the neck straight and the head at the same level as the spine and breathing normally (not during Valsalva maneuver or breath holding) (Ref: Blueprints Neurology by Frank W. Drislane 4th ed Page 8)

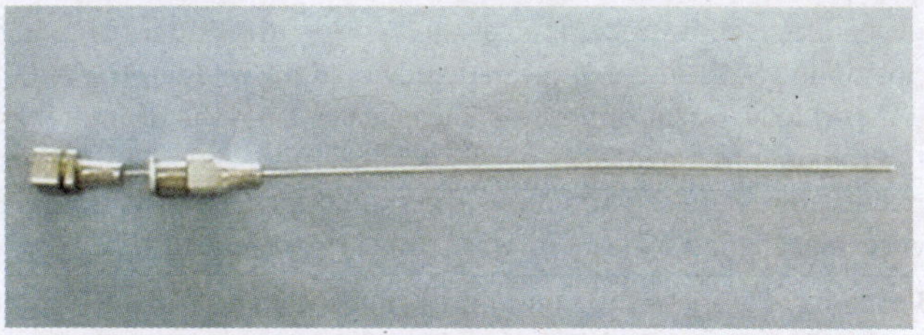

Fig: Lumbar puncture needle metallic

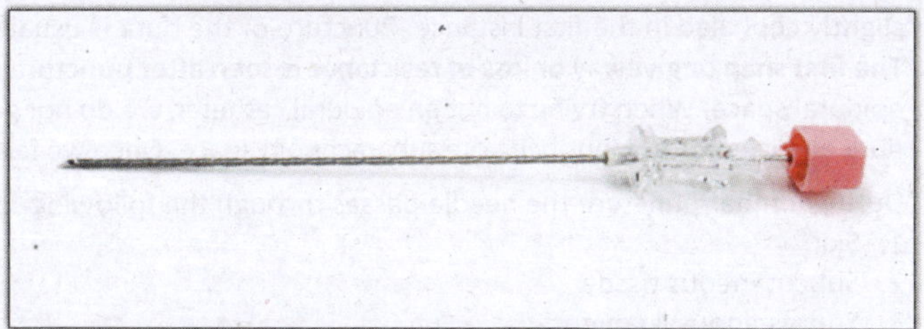

Fig: Lumbar puncture needle (single use)

Points of identification: Thin slender, steel needle with stillate, having gauge No: 22-24

Lumbar Puncture

Indications:

1. For the diagnosis of various types of Meningitis.
2. CSF pressure study
3. Spinal anesthesia
4. Myelography
5. Intrathecal administration of the drugs
6. Sub-Arachnoid hemorrhage
7. CNS Malignancy
8. Demyelinating diseases
9. Guillain-Barré syndrome
10. Unexplained Coma

Precaution: Patients with an altered level of consciousness, a focal neurologic deficit, new-onset seizure, papilledema, or an immunocompromised state are at increased risk for potentially fatal cerebellar or tentorial herniation following LP. Neuroimaging should be obtained in these patients prior to LP to exclude a focal mass lesion or diffuse swelling

Contraindications:

Absolute contraindications: patient refusal, patient's inability to maintain stillness during the needle puncture and raised intracranial pressure, which may theoretically predispose to brainstem herniation.

Relative contraindications intrinsic and idiopathic coagulopathy, skin or soft tissue infection at the proposed site of needle insertion, severe hypovolemia; and lack of anesthesiologist experience.

Legal contraindication: The often-cited relative contraindication of preexisting neurologic disease (e.g., lower extremity peripheral neuropathy) is not usually based on medical criteria but rather on legal considerations

Complications:

1. CSF leakage
2. Infections
3. Injury to spinal cord, paralysis
4. Patients with coagulation defects including thrombocytopenia are at increased risk of post-LP spinal subdural or epidural hematomas, either of which can produce permanent nerve injury and/or paralysis.

Patient positioning:

1. The lateral decubitus position is the most commonly used because it allows easier administration, less dependent on assistant and allow more accurate measurement of the opening pressure.
2. The sitting position when low lumbar and sacral levels of sensory anesthesia are adequate for the surgical procedure (perineal and urologic operations), or when obesity or scoliosis makes identification of midline anatomy difficult in the lateral position
3. The prone position should be chosen when the patient is to be maintained in that position during the surgical procedure (rectal, perineal, or lumbar procedures) .

The procedure should be performed on a firm surface; if the procedure is to be performed at the bedside, the patient should be positioned at the edge of the bed and not in the middle. The patient is asked to lie on his or her side, facing away from the examiner and to "roll up into a ball." The neck is gently anteflexed and the thighs pulled up toward the abdomen; the shoulders and pelvis should be vertically aligned without forward or backward tilt.

Site of puncture: The spinal cord terminates at approximately the L1 in adults and L3 in infacts Although the spinal cord ends at the lower border of L1 in adults, the subarachnoid space continues to S2. LP is therefore performed at or below the ***L3–L4 interspace.*** A useful anatomic guide is a line drawn between the posterior superior iliac crests, which corresponds closely to the level of the L3–L4 interspace. The interspace is chosen following gentle palpation to identify the spinous processes at each lumbar level. A line joining both iliac crests **(Tuffier's line)** passes across the spine of L4 and is a reliable landmark for locating the L3/4 interspace, which is usually easily defined and is the one most often used. or sometimes the L4-5 space.

Note: The incidence of post dural puncture headache is less when the **needle bevel is placed in the long axis of the neuraxis, parallel to dural fibers-** i.e., bevel faces laterally in sitting position, while it faces upwards in lateral position.

Procedure: Sterilize the skin over the lumbar spine and raise a skin weal with lidocaine 1% over the appropriate interspace. Inject 2–3 mL more lidocaine into the subcutaneous tissue. Insert the needle or introducer in the midline in slightly cephalad angle (15 degrees) Feedback from the needle tip will monitor the progress of the needle through the supraspinous and interspinous ligaments, the ligamentum flavum and sometimes the dura mater. If bone is contacted, withdraw the needle to the subcutaneous tissue and redirect slightly cephalad in the first instance. Puncture of the dura is usually obvious and when the stylet is removed CSF should flow freely.

The first snap or giveway or loss of resistance is seen after puncture of ligamentum flavum. This first loss of resistance is used for identifying epidural space. When trying to put an epidural catheter, we do not go any further in. The second loss of resistance is due to puncture of the dura and is used for identifying the subarachnoid space. Once we feel the second giveway, we withdraw the stylet and look for CSF.

During lumbar puncture the needle passes through the following structures in that sequence

1. Skin
2. Subcutaneous tissue
3. Supraspinous ligament
4. Interspinous ligament
5. Ligamentum flavum (First snap/loss of resistance)
6. Dura matter
7. Arachnoid matter
8. Subarachnoid space (Target)

Contd...

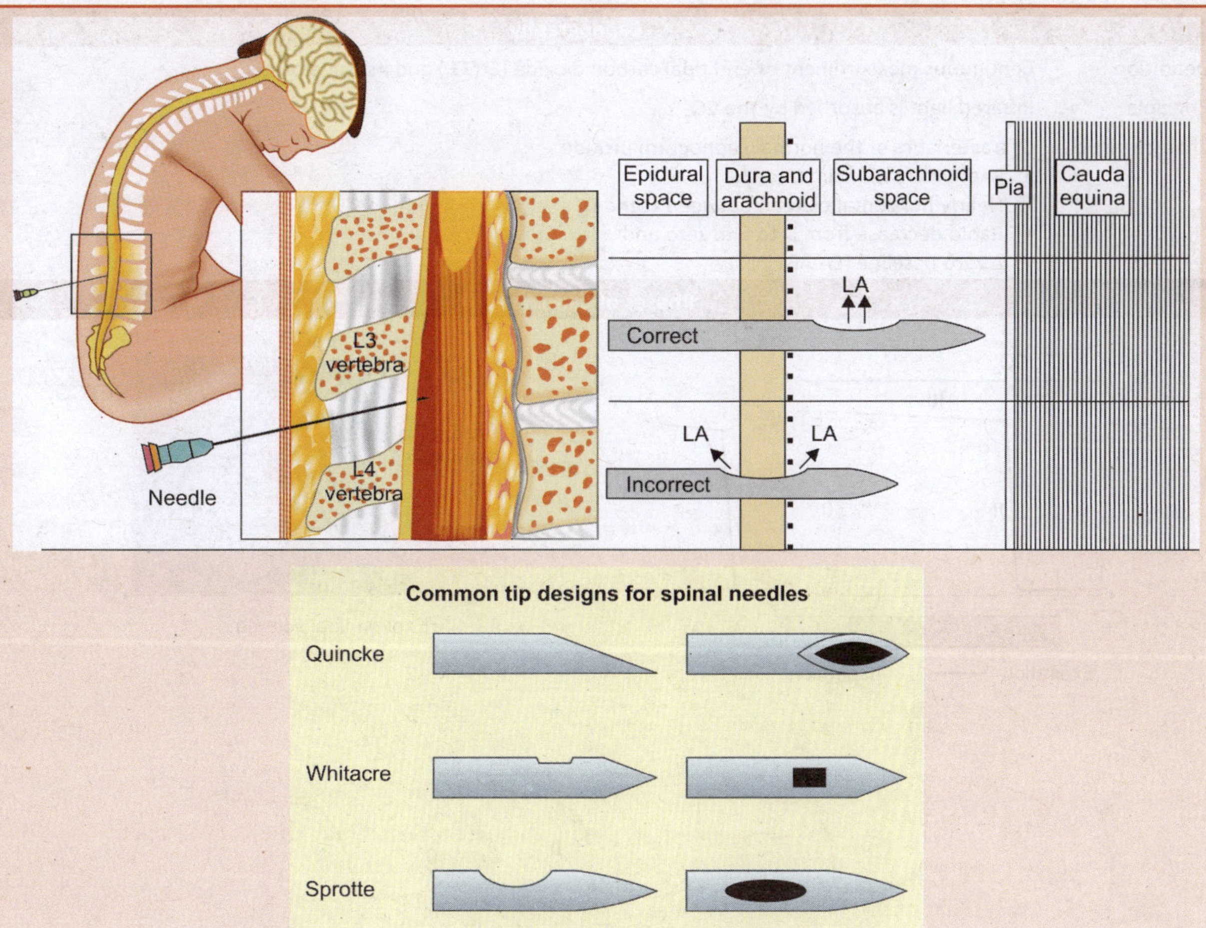

AIIMS NOVEMBER 2016

16. Ans. (c) Endobronchial intubation

Ref: Dorsh 5th Ed Ch 22, www.capnography.com (Dr Bhawani Shankar Kodai, Poineer of Capnography)

Recall Bias

We firmly confirmed it with students that

1. Waveform was not touching the baseline which is a fault in the question as ideally waveform of endobronchial intubation should be touching the baseline. But since the source of this picture made this waveform through illustrations and they are not the real capnographs, we shall consider it as practically touching the baseline for the purpose of this question.
2. There were no values in the graph.
3. It was leak in the sample line and not leak of expiratory valve as option (D). Leak of sample line and endobronchial intubation both show dual/bifid/biphasic waveforms which are extremely difficult to distinguish except that the Leak of sample line also shows dual plateau.
4. Smoker and laparoscopic surgery was particularly mentioned in the question.

Note

- This question is a very confusing one, since the above capnograph has an element of each of the options, but is not a classical picture of any of them.
- Elective endobr anchial intubation is done with a smaller tube and hence shows normal capnograph. It is only accidental endobroanchial intubation which shows the above waveform.
- Accidental endobronchial intubation can be classical or partial. Classical endobronchial intubation will show a biphasic waveform or a waveform similar to the bronchospasm or COPD.
- The prime reason of taking option (c) as answer is that the exact picture was asked in the exam and it is the first picture you see on googling endobronchial intubation capnogram, where it is given as partial endobronchial intubation (Not classical) (from the website http://www.derangedphysiology.com). At another place the same picture is given as tube at Carina.

Now let us first discuss capnography and details of a capnogram in greater detail:

Capnography	
Definition	Continuous measurement of end tidal carbon dioxide ($EtCO_2$) and its waveform
Principle	Infrared light is absorbed by the CO_2
Characteristic	Characteristics of the normal capnogram include • Rapid increase from B to C • Nearly horizontal plateau between C and D • Rapid decrease from D to E to zero and • A zero baseline (EA AB)

Phases of Capnography

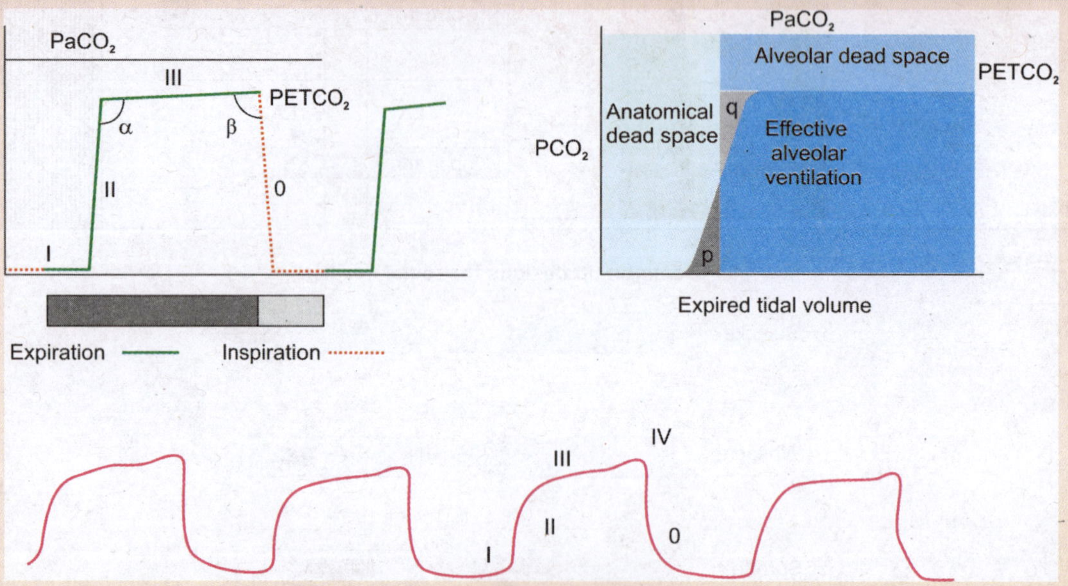

Phase I (Inspiratory baseline)	*EA* in the graph. It is the **latter part of inspiration or beginning of expiration**, during which the CO_2 level remains at zero.
Phase II (Expiratory upstroke)	*BC* in the graph. Represents **mixing of dead space with alveolar gas** i.e. the emptying of connecting airways and the beginning of the emptying of alveoli. As exhalation continues, gas from alveoli in regions with relatively short conducting airways appears and mixes with dead space gas from regions with relatively long conducting airways, resulting in an increasing CO_2 level.
Phase III (Alveolar plateau)	*CD* in the graph. Shows the **alveolar plateau.** Because of uneven emptying of alveoli, the slope continues to rise gently. Point D shows the best approximation of alveolar CO_2 (end of expiration, beginning of inspiration).
Phase IV (Inspiratory downstroke)	*DE* in the graph. As the patient inhales, CO_2-free gas enters the patient's airway and the CO_2 level abruptly falls to zero at the onset of inspiration.

Uses of Capnography

1. **Surest confirmatory sign of endotracheal intubation**, as esophageal intubation will leads to zero $EtCO_2$
2. Intraoperative **displacement or blockage of ET** tube will also leads to zero $EtCO_2$
3. In **malignant hyperthermia** $EtCO_2 > 100$ mm Hg
4. In **pulmonary embolism** there is sudden fall of $EtCO_2$
5. In cardiac arrest also $EtCO_2$ falls to zero
6. **Cardiac arrest:** In intubated patients, failure to achieve an $EtCO_2$ of greater than 10 mm Hg by waveform capnography after 20 minutes of CPR may be considered as one component of a multimodal approach to decide when to end resuscitative efforts, but it should not be used in isolation.

Let us now go through the options and compare/contrast with the capnograph in the question:

Option (a) Rebreathing

Figure 1 is the picture asked in the question, while Figure 2 is the classical picture of rebreathing. In both the instances, the baseline appears elevated (Phase 1). Thus, there is some element of rebreathing in the figure asked. However, we cannot miss the pattern in phase 3 of Figure 1 (Biphasic waveform), which is not present during rebreathing (Fig. 2). Thus, this figure is not classical of rebreathing.

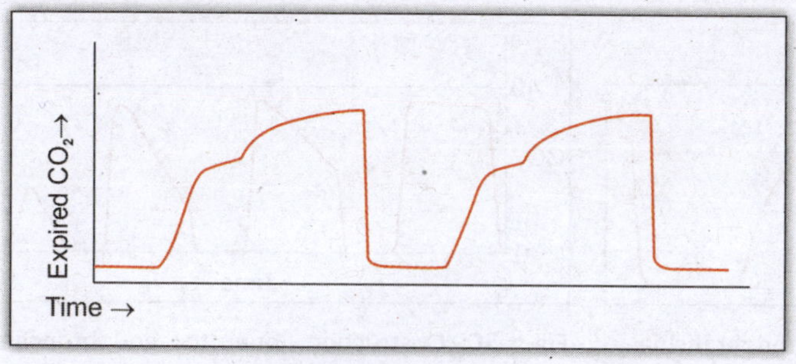

Fig. 1:

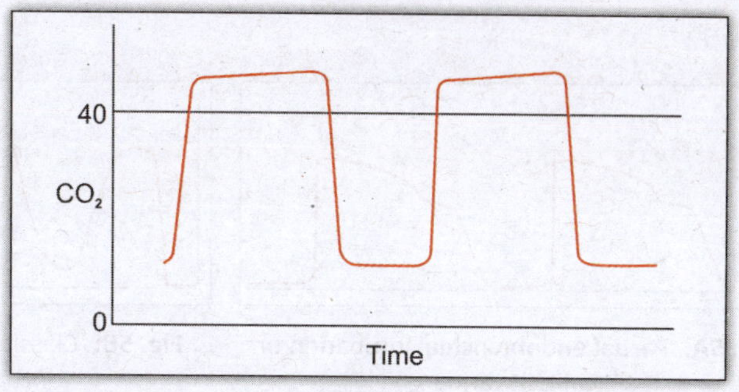

Fig. 2:

Option (b) Bronchospasm

(For D/D and treatment of bronchospasm, see explanation in AIIMS Nov 2013).

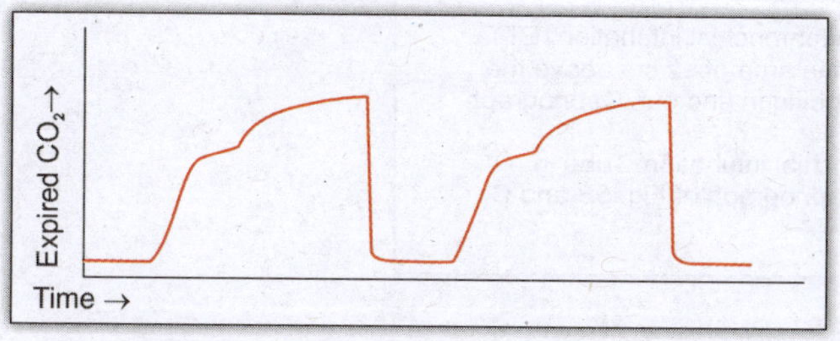

Fig. 1:

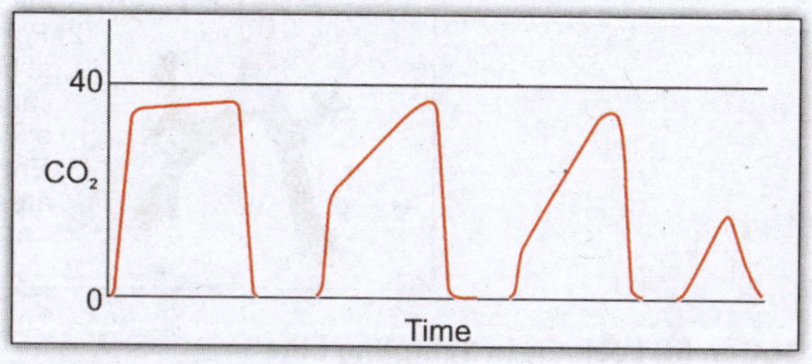

Fig. 3:

Figure 3 indicates classical bronchospasm due to the upsloping of **phase 3 (shark fin appearance)** seen in the graph. Figure 1 is not classical of Bronchospasm. Given the history in the question, the patient is a chronic smoker and hence his airways will be hyperreactive and prone to bronchospasm. But Biphasic/Dual waveform is not seen in bronchospasm. However, one possibility is that the graph can be likened to a curare cleft, which indicates that the patient is breathing, indicating a possible light plane of anesthesia. Thus, it could mean that the patient's light plane has stimulated a bronchospasm, hence making this pattern a combination of ***bronchospasm (Fig. 3) + curare cleft (Fig. 4),*** but that will be too hypothetical and is not mentioned independently in any standard reference. Hence, we would not like to consider this as answer.

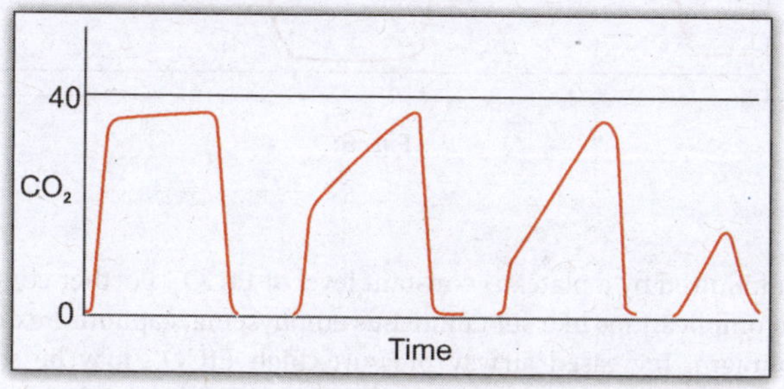

Fig. 3:

+

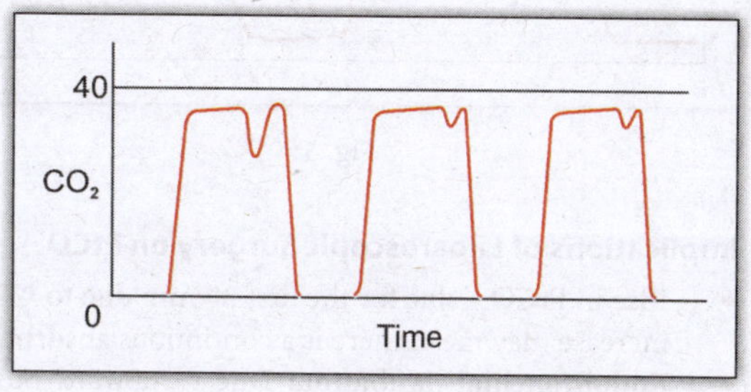

Fig. 4:

Option (c) Endobronchial Intubation

The characteristic features of capnogram in endobronchial intubation are dependent on the extent of endobronchial intubation. Classically it can be seen as **Dual/Bifid/Biphasic waveform.** Note the cleft reaching but not touching the baseline however the complete waveform touches the baseline) or it may be seen as Partial Endobronchial intubation. Occasionally, it may be like the one seen in COPD/Bronchospasm (Shark fin appearance).

The creation of a pneumoperitoneum and the Trendelenburg position, both of which are used to improve visualization, are associated with cephalad movement of the diaphragm. This may increase the risk of endobronchial intubation.

In present case, if the endobronchial intubation is such that the tube is partially in the bronchus, which can happen due to peritoneal insufflation (Laparoscopic surgery) causing upward movement of diaphragm and lungs, leading to slipping of the tube further into the right bronchus, thereby causing only partial lung isolation. This can lead to differential emptying of both lungs, the right lung preferentially empties representing the first part of the dual waveform seen. This is followed by emptying of the left lung which is slower due to obstruction to airflow.

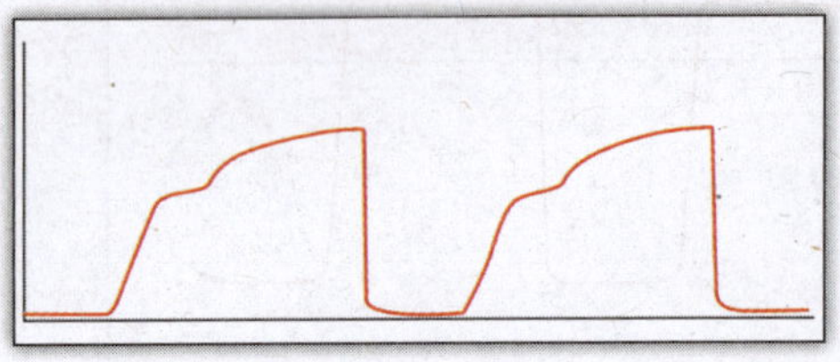

Fig. 5A: Partial endobranchial intubation or tube at carina

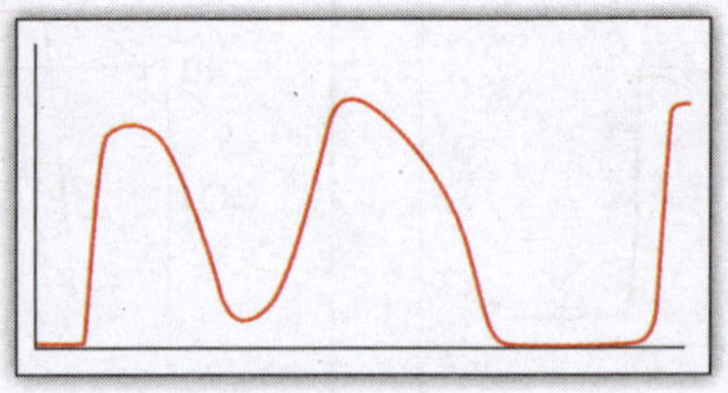

Fig. 5B: Classical endobranchial intubation

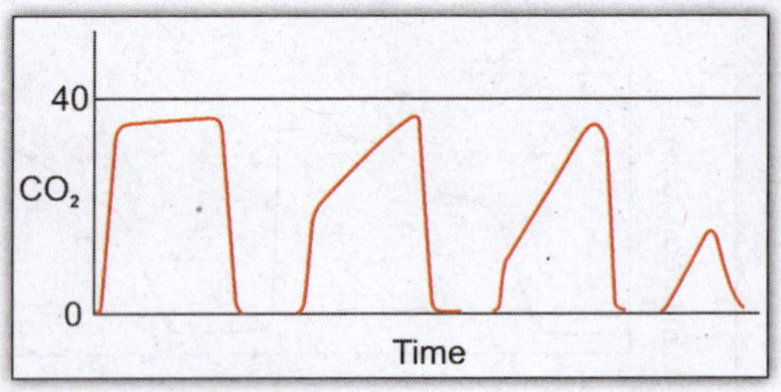

Fig. 5C: Obstruction due to endobronchial intubation causing similar waveform as in COPD or bronchospasm

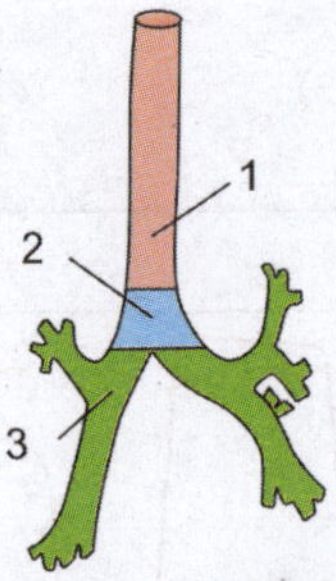

(1) Endotracheal intubation: ETT tip >2 cm above the carina and below the level of the larynx
(2) Partial endobronchial intahation: ETT at borderline area of ≤2 cm above the carina or going in and out. Capnograph of Fig 5A
(3) Endobronchial intubation: Tube in area 3. Capnograph of Fig. 5B and C

Option (d) Leakage in Sampling Line

Figure 6 represents leak in sample line. This diagram is extremely similar to the one asked in the question as both have dual/biphasic waveforms. The difference is that the waveform of Figure 1 has slopes not plateau while Figure 6 (Leak in sampling line) has **dual plateau**.

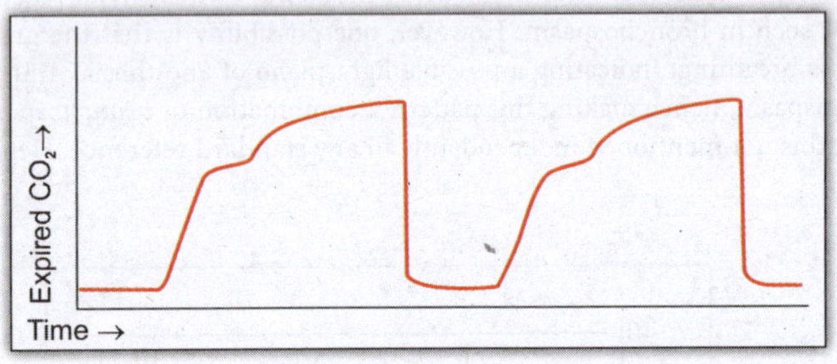

Fig. 1:

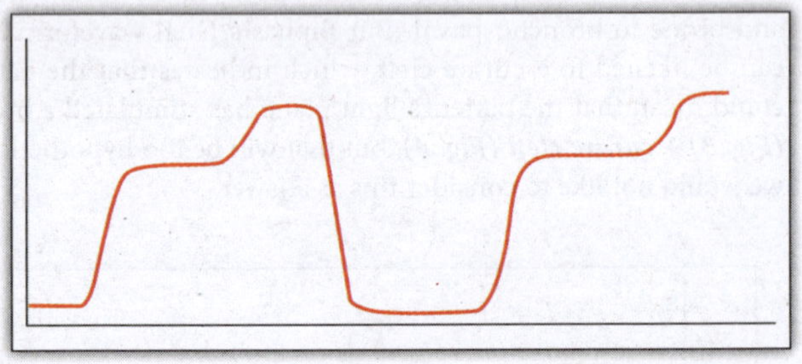

Fig. 6:

Implications of Laparoscopic Surgery on $EtCO_2$

- Rise in $EtCO_2$ value for the first 30 min due to CO_2 insufflation followed by a plateau- constant level of $EtCO_2$. Further continuous increase may mean there is a continuous absorption of CO_2 in complications like subcutaneous emphysema, capnothorax etc.
- **Endobronchial intubation:** Due to upward pushing of diaphragm. Increased airway pressure, high $EtCO_2$, may be shark-fin appearance of $EtCO_2$, but capnography is a poor tool for diagnosis. Is usually associated with desaturation, but hemodynamically stable. Best is to confirm clinically by auscultation and reduced unilateral air entry
- CO_2 embolism - sudden drop in $EtCO_2$ along with hypotension
- Pneumothorax - raised airway pressures, hypotension, desaturation, hyperresonance, decreased air entry
- Bronchospasm- Shark fin pattern, raised airway pressures, may precipitate desaturation, diagnosis by clinical confirmation by auscultation. Bronchospasm may be precipitated during any surgery in a light plane of anesthesia

Some Important Capnography

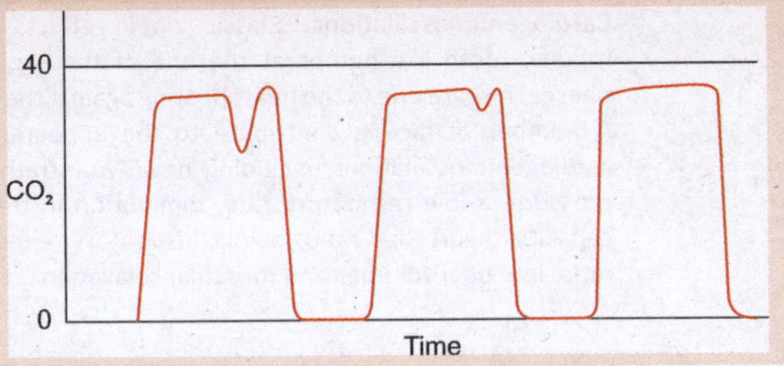

Curare cleft or notch, which is seen during spontaneous ventilation. As the muscle relaxant is repeated, the curve becomes normal in shape. **The cleft is caused by a lack of synchronous action between the intercostal muscles and the diaphragm, most commonly caused by inadequate muscle relaxant**. Depth of the cleft is proportional to the degree of muscle paralysis. Also is seen in patients with cervical transverse lesions, flail chest, hiccups and pneumothorax and when a patient tries to breathe during mechanical ventilation.

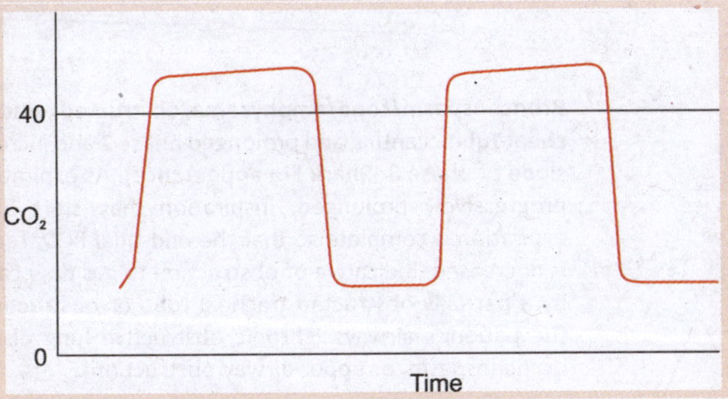

Rebreathing: The baseline is elevated and the waveform is normal in shape. Caused by an incompetent expiratory valve or **exhausted absorbent in the circle system;** insufficient fresh gas flow to a Mapleson system; problems with the inner tube of a Bain system; deliberate addition of CO_2 to the fresh gas; or in some cases, an incompetent inspiratory valve. This is normal in rebreathing circuits such as **Mapleson D or bain circuit.**

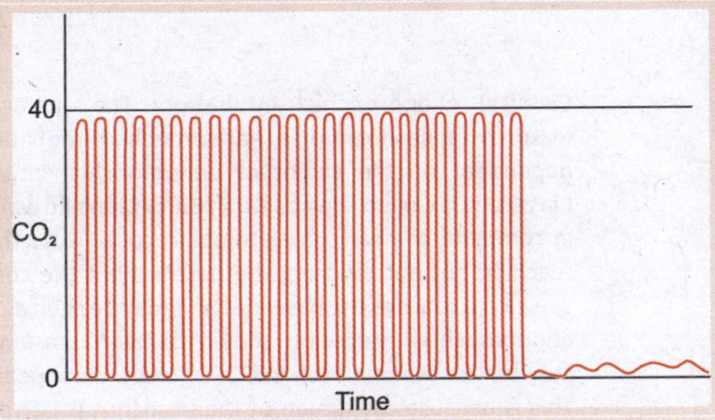

Extubation: A sudden drop of end tidal CO_2 to zero is usually caused by an acute event relating to the airway, such as **extubation**, esophageal intubation, **complete breathing system disconnection,** ventilator malfunction, or a totally obstructed tracheal tube. It may also be the result of a plugged gas sampling tube.

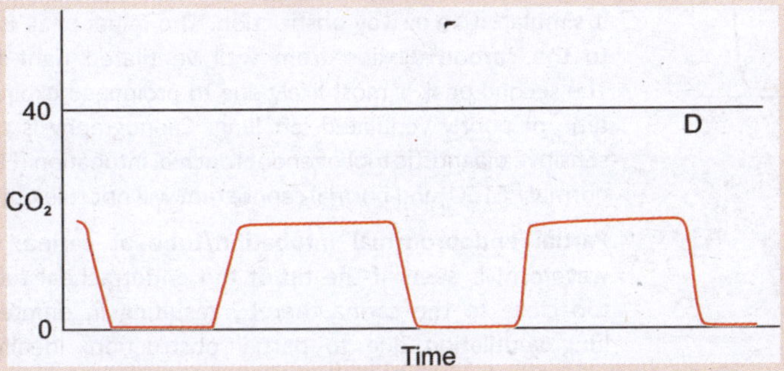

Hyperventilation: Low end-tidal CO_2 with a good alveolar plateau may be the result of hyperventilation or an increase in dead space ventilation. Comparison of $PETCO_2$ with $PaCO_2$ is necessary to distinguish these two conditions.

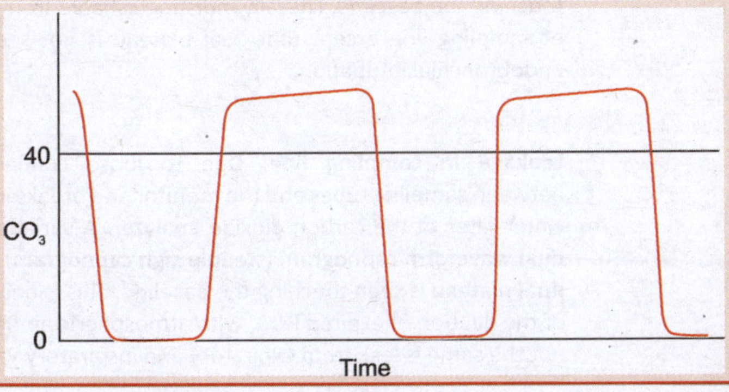

Hypoventilation: Elevated end-tidal CO_2 with good alveolar plateau may be caused by hypoventilation or increased CO_2 delivery to the lungs.

Contd...

Some Important Capnography

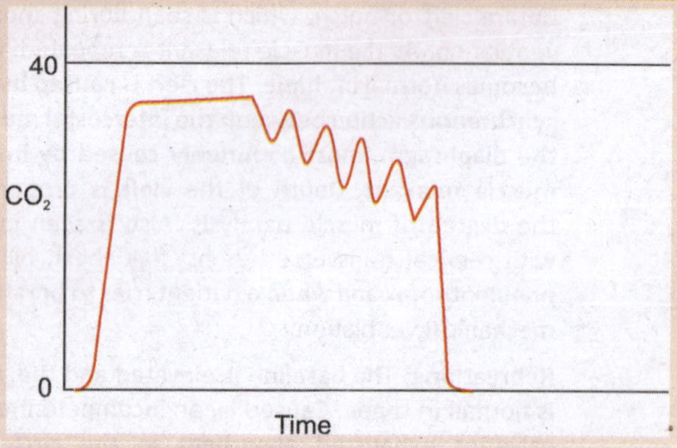

Cardiogenic oscillations: Classic ripple effect; small, regular, tooth like humps at the end of the expiratory phase. They are due to the heart beating against the lungs. A number of factors contribute to the appearance of cardiogenic oscillations, including negative intrathoracic pressure, a low respiratory rate, diminution in the vital capacity: heart size ratio, a low inspiratory: expiratory ratio, low tidal volumes and muscular relaxation.

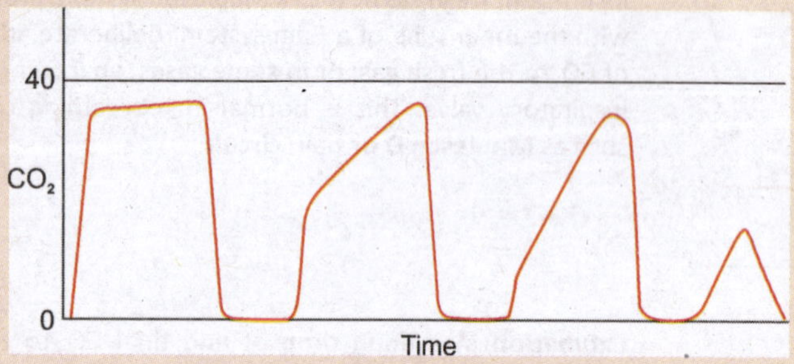

Bronchospasm/copd/emphysema/obstructed endotracheal Tube: Slanting and prolonged phase 2 and increased slope of phase 3 (**Shark Fin appearance**). As expiration is progressively prolonged, inspiration may start before expiration is complete so that the end-tidal PCO_2 reading is decreased. Indicative of obstruction to gas flow caused by a partially obstructed tracheal tube or obstruction in the patient's airways (chronic obstructive lung disease, bronchospasm, or upper-airway obstruction).

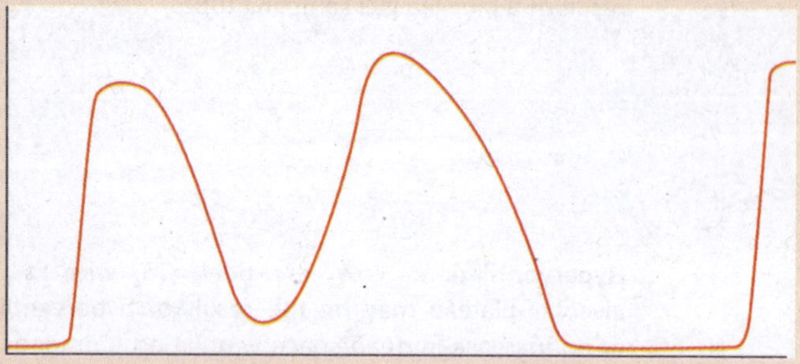

Classical endobronchial intubation: The characteristic features of capnogram in endobronchial intubation are dependent on the extent of endobronchial intubation. Classically it can be seen as **Dual/Bifid/Biphasic waveform** in complete or near complete obstruction. Note the cleft reaching but not touching the baseline but the complete waveform touches the baseline) or it may be seen as partial endobronchial intubation shown below. Occasionally, it may be like the one seen in COPD (Shark fin appearance). This is because the lumen of the bronchus is narrow and it simulated an airway obstruction. The initial peak is due to the carbon dioxide from well ventilated right lung. The second peak is most likely due to prolonged expiratory time of poorly ventilated left lung. Capnography is not a sensitive diagnostic tool of endobronchial intubation (EBI). A normal $PETCO_2$ and normal capnogram will not rule out EBI.

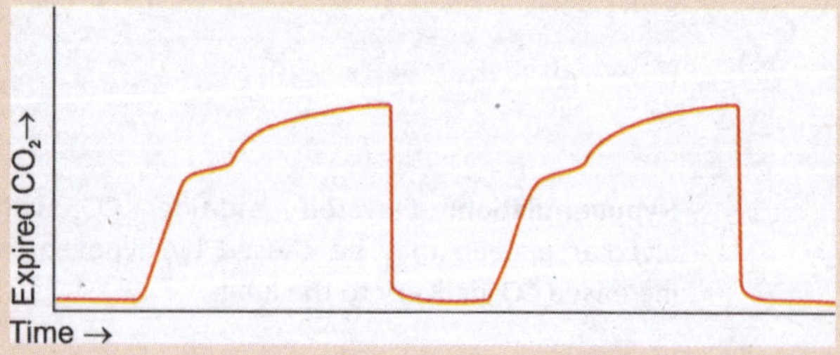

Partial endobronchial intubation/tube at carina: Dual waveform is seen. If the tip of the endotracheal tube is too close to the carina thereby resulting in differential lung ventilation due to partial obstruction. Ideally its touching the baseline. Literally indistinguishable from leak of sampling line except that dual plateau is not seen in endobronchial intubation.

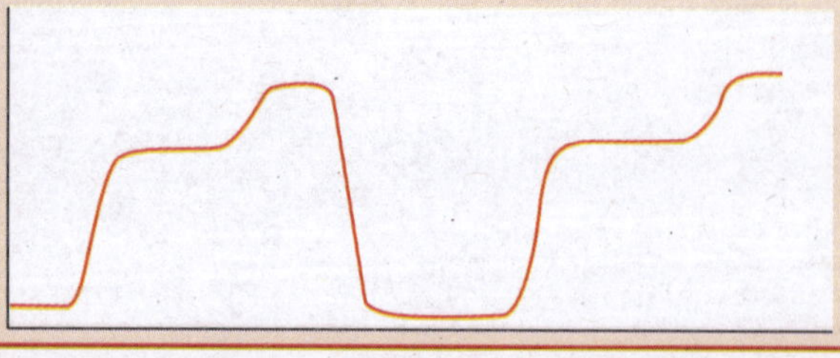

Leakage in sampling line: Due to loose connection between sampling tubes and the monitor and breaks in the water filter of the carbon dioxide analyzer. A variation of **dual waveform capnogram (steeple sign capnogram)** with **dual plateau** is seen touching the baseline. This is because of the dilution of expired PCO_2 with atmospheric air. This is not the same is leak from expiratory and inspiratory valve.

Contd...

Some Important Capnography

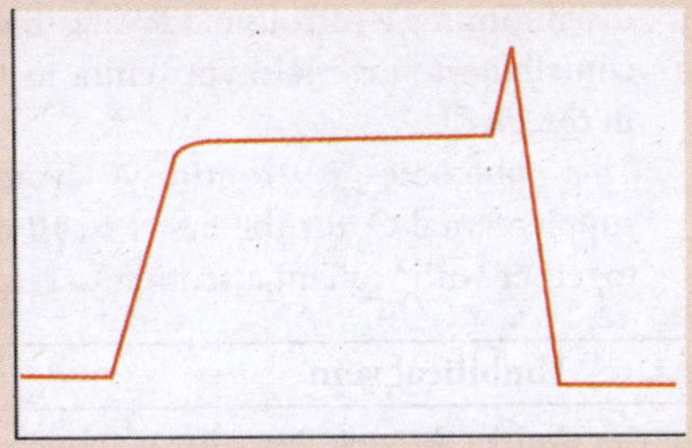	Slit in the sampling tube can result in a **Pig tail** capnogram or **Tail up** capnogram. This is a variant of above graph. Note the elevation from the baseline which will help to differentiate from next capnograph.
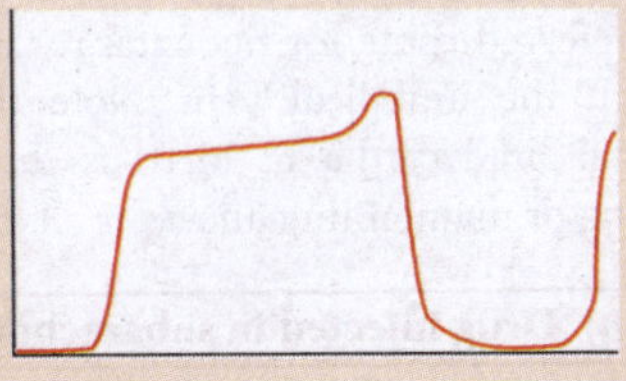	A terminal upswing at the end of phase 3, known as **phase 4**, can occur in pregnant subjects, obese subjects during anesthesia and IPPV and low compliance states.
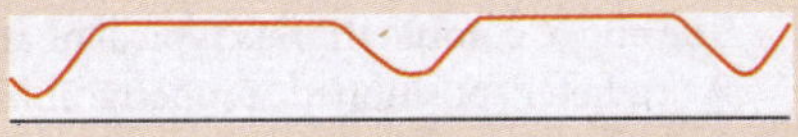	**Expiratory valve leak:** The capnogram shows prolonged phase II as well as slanting of descending limb of inspiratory segment. The expiratory unidirectional valve leak allowing previously exhaled gases, high in CO_2, to be rebreathed with each inspiration. Rebreathing causes elevation from the baseline
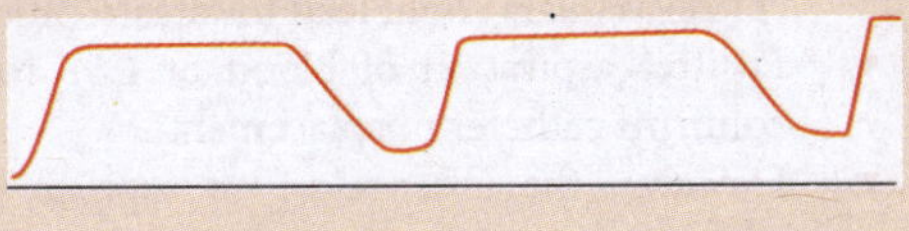	**Inspiratory valve leak:** An incompetent inspiratory valve will allow exhaled CO_2-containing gas to enter the inspiratory limb of the circuit during expiration. During the next inspiration, the CO_2-containing gas in the inspiratory limb enters the patient, extending the expiratory alveolar plateau (phase III-plateau) of the time capnogram. Rebreathing causes elevation from the baseline.
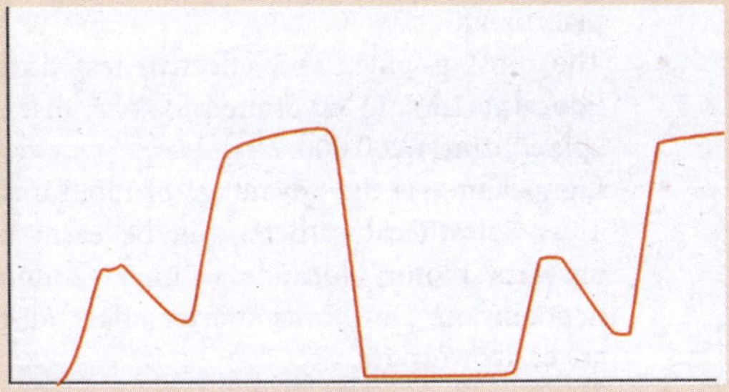	**Severe kyphoscoliosis:** Dual waveform appearance. Kyphoscoliosis resulted in a compression of the right lung. The compressed right lung was poorly ventilated and was relatively hypercapnic, whereas the left lung was hyperventilated and was relatively hypocapnic. Under these circumstances, relatively hypocapnic gas from well ventilated, low airway resistance lung reached the CO_2 analyzer first causing first distinct low peak and relatively hypercapnic gas from poorly ventilated, high airway resistance lung reached the CO_2 analyzer last causing second distinct high peak.
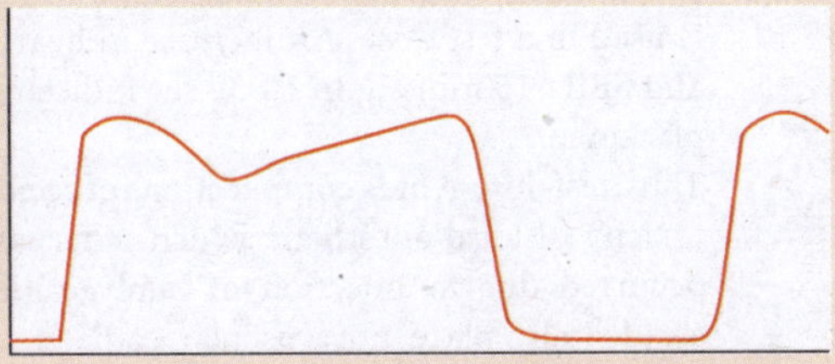	**One lung transplantation: Dual wave form variant.** The first peak in phase III is from the transplanted normal lung, whereas the second peak is from the native disease lung.

Footnote:

1. In nonaccidental/elective one lung ventilation or dual lung ventilation the tube lumen size is smaller and compatible to the bronchus, hence in elective endobronchial intubation the capnograph looks normal and similar to the endotracheal intubation
2. Causes of dual waveform (Bifid or Biphasic) are:
   - **Leakage in sampling line:** Loose connection between sampling tubes and the monitor and breaks in the water filter of the carbon dioxide analyzer
   - **Pathological:** Severe kyphoscoliosis
   - **Iatrogenic:** Partial endobronchial intubation (Tube at carina)
   - Following one lung transplantation

17. Ans. (a) 8 drops/min

Ref: Dosage Calculations by Gloria D. Pickar Pg 331

This question is purely calculation based. However, this is an important calculation since one must know how to set the drip rate when you do not have an infusion pump. This must done meticulously and units (microgram or milligram, per minute or per hour) must not be missed.

200 mg in 1 vial, 200 × 2 = 400 mg in 2 vials

Now let us calculate the concentration of the infusate that we have prepared

400 mg in 250 mL NS

But, 400 mg = 4,00,000 micrograms (1 mg = 1000 micrograms)

Thus, each mL contains 4,00,000/250 = 1600 micrograms/mL

Now, the infusion rate is 10 mcg/kg/min = 800 mcg/min

Thus we have to give 800/1600 = 0.5 mL/min

16 drops = 1 mL, Therefore, 8 drops/min = 0.5 mL/min

Alternative ways in which this question can be asked:

- **Calculate drip rate in a microdrip set**
  Micro drip sets are specially designed for in pediatrics where more fine tuning is important
  Here, 60 drops = 1 mL
  In that case, the answer would be 30 drops/min
  (**Note:** Most books mention drop factor as 60 for micro drip, while some mention 64. In that case answer would be 32.)
- **Calculate the infusion rate on an infusion pump/syringe pump**
  Commonly, syringe pumps may have a setting where you have to calculate infusion rate in mcg/kg/**hour. (Note: some may have a setting for/min as well. Do read the question very carefully)**
  So, our infusion rate is 800 mcg/min that gives 48000 mcg in 60 min or 48000 mcg/hr or 48 mg/hr
  Our concentration is 1600 mcg/mL or 1.6 mg/mL
  That is we have to give at an infusion rate of 48/1.6 = 30 mL/hr

Easier Way

From the first calculation, our infusion rate is 0.5 mL/min, Thus, in 60 minutes we have to give 0.5 × 60 = 30 mL/hr

18. Ans. (b) Diffusion hypoxia

Ref: Miller's 8th Ed page 656, 3401

To see details of Second gas effect, see explanation in AIIMS Nov 2013 (see volume II)

- Diffusion hypoxia refers to the rapid diffusion of nitrous oxide into alveoli at the end of a nitrous oxide anesthetic.
- During the initial 5 to 10 minutes after discontinuation of anesthesia, the flow of N_2O from blood into the alveoli can be several liters per minute, resulting in dilution of alveolar oxygen.
- Nitrous oxide dilutes the alveolar gas and produces a transient decrease in PAO_2 and $PaCO_2$.
- In a patient breathing room air, the resulting decrease in PAO_2 can produce arterial hypoxemia, whereas decreased $PaCO_2$ can depress the respiratory drive.
- The combined effects of respiratory depression from anesthesia, reduced alveolar PCO_2 and reduced alveolar PO_2 can result in hypoventilation and oxyhemoglobin desaturation.
- In the absence of supplemental oxygen administration, diffusion hypoxia can persist for 5 to 10 minutes after discontinuing a nitrous oxide anesthetic; therefore, it may contribute to arterial hypoxemia in the initial moments in the PACU.
- This outcome is routinely avoided by providing supplemental O_2 for the first 1 to 10 minutes of recovery, together with vigilant attention to respiration.

19. Ans. (c) Umbilical vein

Ref: Chestnut's Obstetric Anesthesia 5th ed page 178

The preferred route for neonatal resuscitation is intravenous, through the umbilical vein. Note that most of the times neonatal bradycardia at birth is due to hypoxia and that securing or maintaining airway is all that is required.

20. Ans. (b) Drug injected in subarachnoid space

Ref: Shnider and Levinson Anesthesiology for obstetrics 4th ed Page 134

- The above combination is typical of an epidural test dose.
- A catheter positioned properly in the epidural space can provide excellent surgical anesthesia, postoperative analgesia and labor analgesia.
- Inadvertent placement of the catheter into the cerebrospinal fluid (CSF) (intrathecal) or an epidural vein (intravascular) could lead to catastrophic complications.
- Positive aspiration of blood or CSF from the catheter confirms catheter misplacement.
- However, the absence of an aspirate cannot rule out whether or not the catheter is actually in the epidural space.
- An epidural test dose involves injecting local anesthetic to determine accidental intravenous or intrathecal catheter placement.
- The most popular and effective test dose is 3 mL of lidocaine 1.5% (3 cc diluted to 4 cc, discard 1 cc) with epinephrine 1:200 000.
- Lignocaine has the advantage of rapid onset and offset. Thus, intrathecal catheter can be easily identified but onset of motor blockade within 1-2 min, along with hypotension. Due to its shorter offset, all these changes are easily worn off.
- The purpose of adrenaline is to detect intravascular placement. 5 mcg/cc adrenaline (total 15 mcg adrenaline) is used in a test dose. An increase in heart rate >10 bpm and SBP >15 mm Hg in 10-30 sec indicates intravascular placement.
- Thus, test dose avoids complications of accidental systemic toxicity of local anesthetic which otherwise would have occurred due to injection of bupivacaine through the accidentally place intravascular catheter. Also, if larger doses of Bupivacaine were given without confirming with test dose in an accidental intrathecal catheter, the result would be catastrophic.

Other Options

Option (A) Systemic Toxicity of the Drug

Systemic toxicity of lignocaine is primarily neurotoxic and later cardiotoxic. The patient should manifest perioral tingling, numbness, seizures etc.

Option (C) Vasovagal Shock

Note that the epidural has already been inserted, the painful part is over. There is no reason why a patient should have vasovagal collapse at this point of time.

Option (D) Anaphylaxis

Unlikely. Anaphylaxis would be associated with other symptoms like rashes, breathing difficulty. Also, we have given adrenaline along with xylocaine.

21. Ans. (c) The laryngoscope is lifted upwards levering over the upper incisors

Ref: Miller's 8th Ed Pg 1666, 1667

Preparation and Positioning

- Preparation for DL includes proper patient positioning, adequate preoxygenation and ensuring the availability and proper functioning of all necessary equipment—laryngoscopes, tracheal tubes, tube stylets, an empty syringe for inflating the tracheal tube cuff, a suction apparatus and the essential equipment for mask ventilation, including an oxygen source.
- Adequate preparation is of the utmost importance; as with any airway procedure, the first attempt should be the best attempt.
- For direct laryngoscopy (DL) to be successful, a line of sight from the mouth to the larynx must be achieved.
- The classical model used to describe the anatomic relationships necessary to achieve this involves the **alignment of three anatomic axes— oral, pharyngeal and laryngeal**.
- Positioning the patient in the **sniffing position** approximates this alignment.
- **Cervical flexion**
  (35 degrees; accomplished by a **7- to 9-cm elevation of the head on a firm cushion**; patients with shorter necks may require less head elevation) **aligns the pharyngeal and laryngeal axes.**
  Patients who are obese often require elevation of the shoulders and upper back to achieve adequate cervical flexion, which can be accomplished by placing the patient in the ***ramped*** **position (HELP position-Head elevated laryngoscopy position)** using either a specialized device, such as the **Troop Elevation Pillow or folded blankets.** Confirming horizontal alignment of the external **auditory meatus with the sternal notch** is useful for ensuring optimal head elevation in both obese and nonobese patients.
- **Maximal head extension: At the atlanto-occipital joint brings the oral axis closer into alignment.** Adequate cervical flexion also facilitates maximal atlanto-occipital extension, which provides optimal alignment of the oral and pharyngeal axes (the primary determinant for quality of laryngeal view) and enhanced mouth opening.

Technique

- The laryngoscope is a handheld instrument consisting of a blade attached to a handle containing a light source. Most are reusable and made of steel, although disposable, plastic versions are available.
- The curved blade and the straight blade are the two basic types of laryngoscope blades available for DL; multiple variations of both styles exist.
- The Macintosh is the most commonly used curved blade (larger flange, generally considered less likely to cause dental damage), whereas the Miller is the most commonly used straight blade (esp. in patients with a short thyromental distance; provide a better view of the glottis in patients with a long, floppy epiglottis). In general, the Macintosh is most commonly used for adults, whereas the straight blades are typically used in pediatric patients.
- Both are designed to be held in the left hand and both have a flange on the left side that is used to retract the tongue laterally. Each type of blade has its benefits and drawbacks and is associated with its own technique for use.
- The technique for laryngoscopy consists of the opening of the mouth, inserting the laryngoscope blade, positioning of the laryngoscope blade tip, applying a lifting force exposing the glottis and inserting a tracheal tube through the vocal cords into the trachea.
- Mouth opening is best achieved using the ***scissors*** **technique**; the right thumb pushes caudally on the right lower molars while the index or third finger of the right hand pushes on the right upper molars in the opposite direction.
- **The Macintosh blade is inserted in the right side of the mouth and the flange is used to sweep the tongue to the left.** Once the laryngoscope has been inserted in the mouth, the right hand can be used to ensure that the upper lip is not impinged between the laryngoscope and the upper incisors. The blade is advanced along the base of the tongue until the epiglottis is visualized; the tip of the blade is then advanced further and positioned in the vallecula.
- **A force oriented at a 45° angle up and away from the laryngoscopist indirectly lifts the epiglottis by placing tension on the hyoepiglottic ligament, exposing the glottic structures.**
- ***The tip of the blade should not be lifted by using the laryngoscope as a lever, rocking back on the upper incisors, which can damage the teeth and provides an inferior view of the glottis.***
- **A properly oriented vector of force is achieved by using the anterior deltoid and triceps, not by radial flexion of the wrist.**
- Passage of the ETT is facilitated by an **anterior angulation of the tip,** which can be accomplished by shaping the ETT with a malleable stylet into a ***hockey stick*** **shape, with approximately a 60° angle formed 4 to 5 cm from the distal end,** or by accentuating the natural anterior curvature of the ETT by inserting the tip into the 15-mm connector, forming a circle, for several minutes before performing DL.
- **The Miller laryngoscope blade** is inserted using the **paraglossal technique.**
- This method provides maximal tongue control and avoids contact of the laryngoscope with the maxillary incisors.
- The laryngoscope is inserted lateral to the tongue and carefully advanced along the paraglossal gutter between the tongue and tonsil. Application of continued moderate lifting force to the laryngoscope handle helps maintain lateral displacement of the tongue and reduces contact with the maxillary teeth.

- As the laryngoscope is advanced, the epiglottis comes into view and the tip of the laryngoscope is passed **posterior to the epiglottis. The optimal position of the tip of the straight laryngoscope is in the midline of the posterior surface of the epiglot tis, close to the anterior commissure of the vocal cords.**
- This position achieves good control of the epiglottis and facilitates the passage of the tracheal tube. The direction of force applied to the handle is the same as when using the Macintosh blade.
- The use of external laryngeal manipulation can improve the laryngeal view.
- **Backward, upward, right- ward pressure (the BURP maneuver)** on the thyroid cartilage is most commonly used.
- **Optimal external laryngeal manipulation (OELM)** is achieved when the laryngoscopist uses his or her right hand to guide the position and pressure is exerted by an assistant's hand on the larynx.

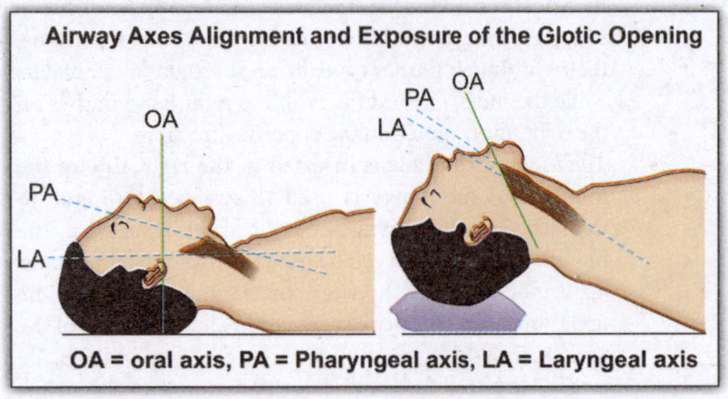

Fig: Sniffing position and alignment of axes

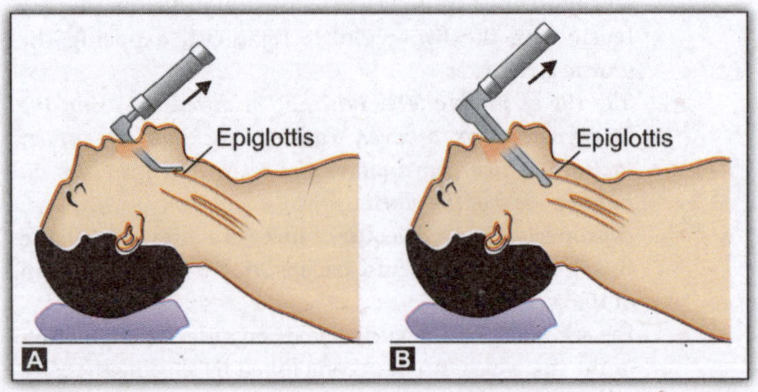

Fig: Placement of laryngoscope; **A.** Macintosh blade—anterior to epiglottis; **B.** Miller blade—posterior to epiglottis

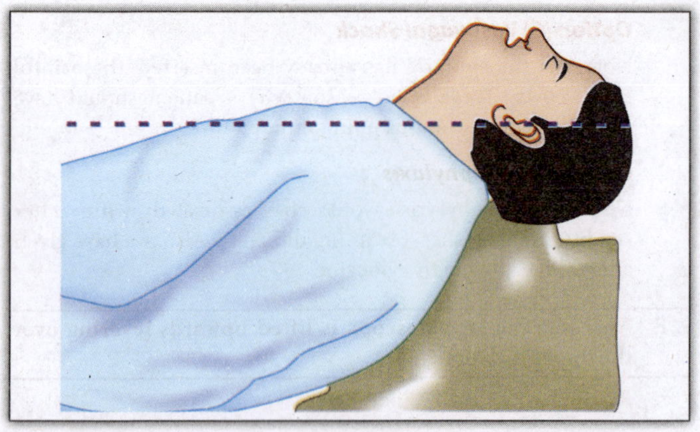

Fig: HELP position. Head elevated laryngoscopy position. Observe the line joining external auditory meatus and sternal notch

22. Ans. (b) Check responsiveness

Ref: AHA 2015 Guidelines Update for Cardiopulmonary Resuscitation and Emergency Cardiovascular Care

However, most recallers think that first step was asked, some recallers think that next step not the first step was asked. In later case it can be presumed that the examiner specifically wants to know the next step after checking responsiveness, hence checking carotids will become the answer.

Recall Bias

The first step according to the 2015 guidelines is to verify scene safety, however since the patient has been brought to the emergency department, there is no question of scene safety here. Please note that the patient's response has to be rechecked by the healthcare provider himself when he first reaches the site.

Scenario 1

Patient brought to the casualty by layman and informed that the patient was unresponsive: This is the most common scene in our country where the patient is brought by a relative or a layman to the casualty. Obviously, when informed that a patient is unresponsive, on reaching the scene, the qualified medical officer must check if the patient is indeed unresponsive. This involves calling out to the patient once loudly, if unresponsive (this hardly takes any time), second step is activated emergency services with defibrillator. Third step is check for pulse and respiration simultaneously for 10 seconds and then proceed accordingly.

Basic life support sequence guidelines as per AHA 2015 are given below:

Step	Lay Rescuer not Trained	Lay Rescuer Trained	Healthcare Provider
1	Ensure scene safety.	Ensure scene safety.	Ensure scene safety.
2	Check for response.	Check for response.	Check for response.
3	Shout for nearby help. Phone or ask someone to phone 9-1-1 (the phone or caller with the phone remains at the victim's side, with the phone oil speaker).	Shout for nearby help and activate the emergency response system (9-1-1, emergency response). If someone responds, ensure that the phone is at the side of the victim if at all possible.	Shout for nearby help/activate the resuscitation team; can activate the resuscitation team at this time or after checking breathing and pulse.

Step	Lay Rescuer not Trained	Lay Rescuer Trained	Healthcare Provider
4	Follow the dispatcher's instructions.	Check for no breathing or only gasping; if none, begin CPR with compressions.	Check for no breathing or only gasping and check pulse (ideally simultaneously). Activation and retrieval of The AED/ emergency equipment by either the lone healthcare provider or by the second person sent by the rescuer must occur no later than immediately after the check for no normal breathing and no pulse identifies cardiac arrest.
5	Look for no breathing or only gasping, at the direction of the dispatcher.	Answer the dispatcher's questions and fallow the dispatcher's instructions.	Immediately begin CPR and use the AED/defibrillator when available.
6	Follow the dispatcher's instructions.	Send the second person to retrieve an AED, if one is available.	When the second rescuer arrives, provide 2-person CPR and use AED/defibrillator.

AED indicates automated external defibrillator. and CPR, cardiopulmonary resuscitation.

Scenario 2

Healthcare professional (HCP) has initiated CPR and you have been called for help: In this situation, when one reaches the scene of arrest and the CPR has already been initiated, you will not re-assess the consciousness of the patient, assuming that the first steps have already been taken care of by the attending HCP and you have to provide advanced care as per the guidelines.

A. Adult Basic Life Support (BLS)

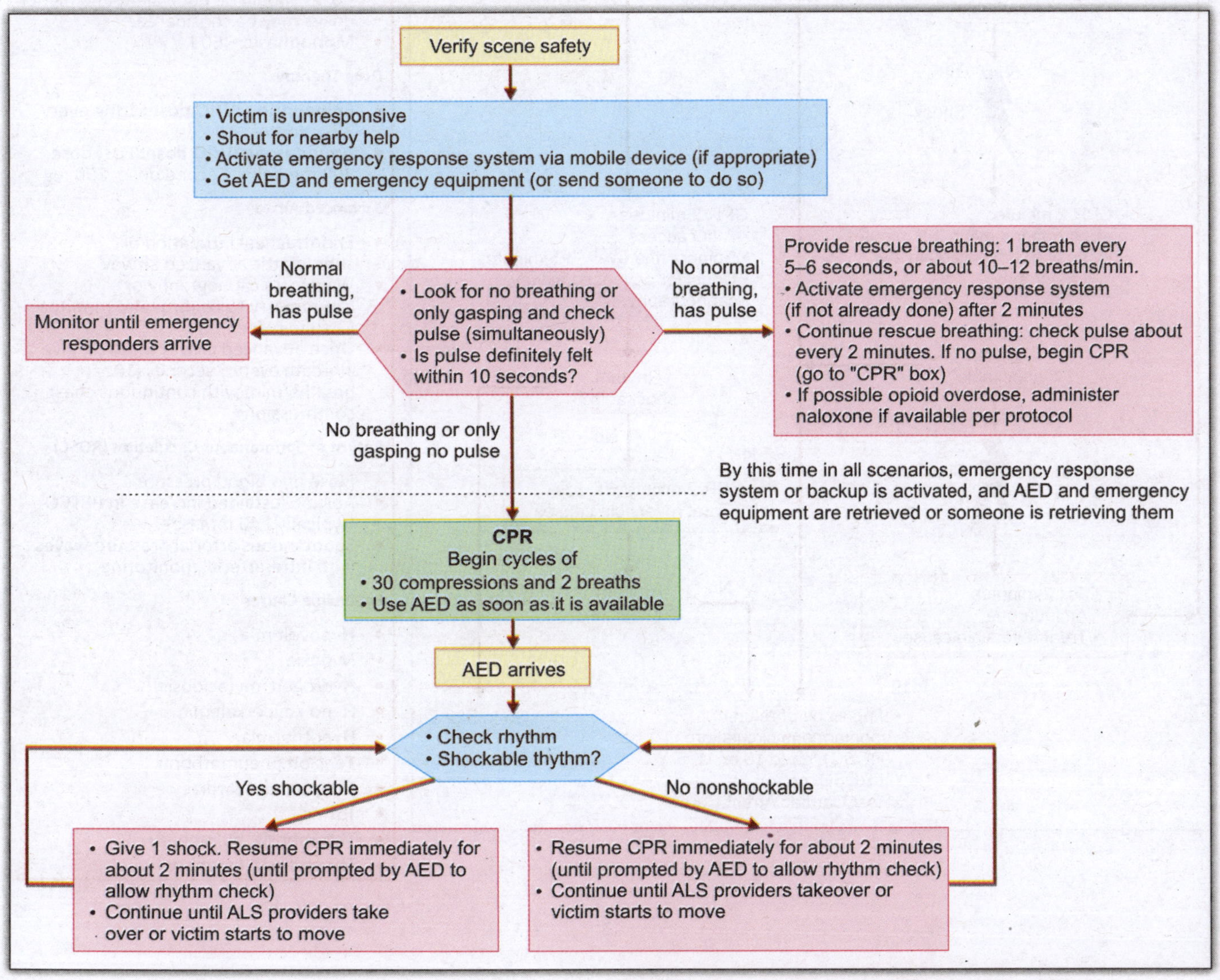

B. Advanced Cardiac Life Support

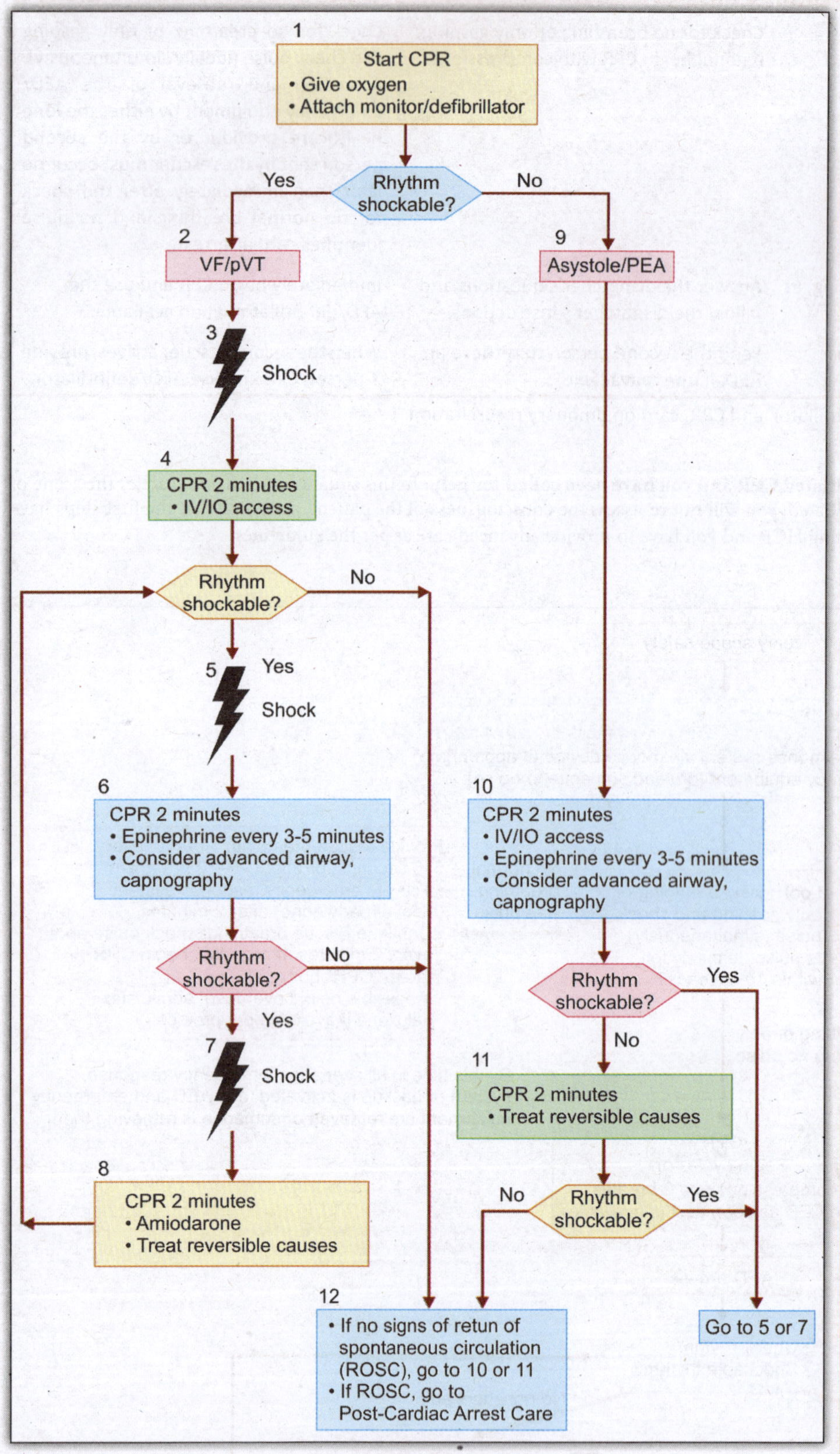

CPR Quality

- Push hard (at least 2 inches [5 cm]) and fast (100-120/min) and allow complete chest recoil.
- Minimize interruptions in compressions.
- Avoid excessive ventilation.
- Rotate compressor every 2 minutes, or sooner if fatigued.
- If no advanced airway, 30:2 compression-ventilation ratio.
- Quantitative waveform capnography
  - If $PEtCO_2$ <10 mm Hg, attempt to improve CPR quality.
- Intra-arterial pressure
  - If relaxation phase (diastolic) pressure <20 mm Hg, attempt to improve CPR quality.

Shock Energy for Defibrillation

- **Biphasic:** Manufacturer recommendation (e.g. initial dose of 120-200 J); if unknown, use maximum available. Second and subsequent doses should be equivalent and higher doses may be considered.
- **Monophasic:** 360 J

Drug Therapy

- **Epinephrine IV/IO dose:** 1 mg every 3-5 minutes
- **Amiodarone IV/IO dose:** First dose: 300 mg bolus, Second dose: 150 mg.

Advanced Airway

- Endotracheal intubation or supraglottic advanced airway
- Waveform capnography or capnometry to confirm and monitor ET tube placement
- Once advanced airway in place, give 1 breath every 6 seconds (10 breaths/min) with continuous chest compressions

Return of Spontaneous Circulation (ROSC)

- Pulse and blood pressure
- Abrupt sustained increase in $PETCO_2$ (typically ≥40 mm Hg)
- Spontaneous arterial pressure waves with intra-arterial monitoring

Reversible Causes

- Hypovolemia
- Hypoxia
- Hydrogen ion (acidosis)
- Hypo-/hyperkalemia
- Hypothermia
- Tension pneumothorax
- Tamponade, cardiac
- Toxins
- Thrombosis, pulmonary
- Thrombosis, coronary

C. Pediatric BLS – Single Rescuer

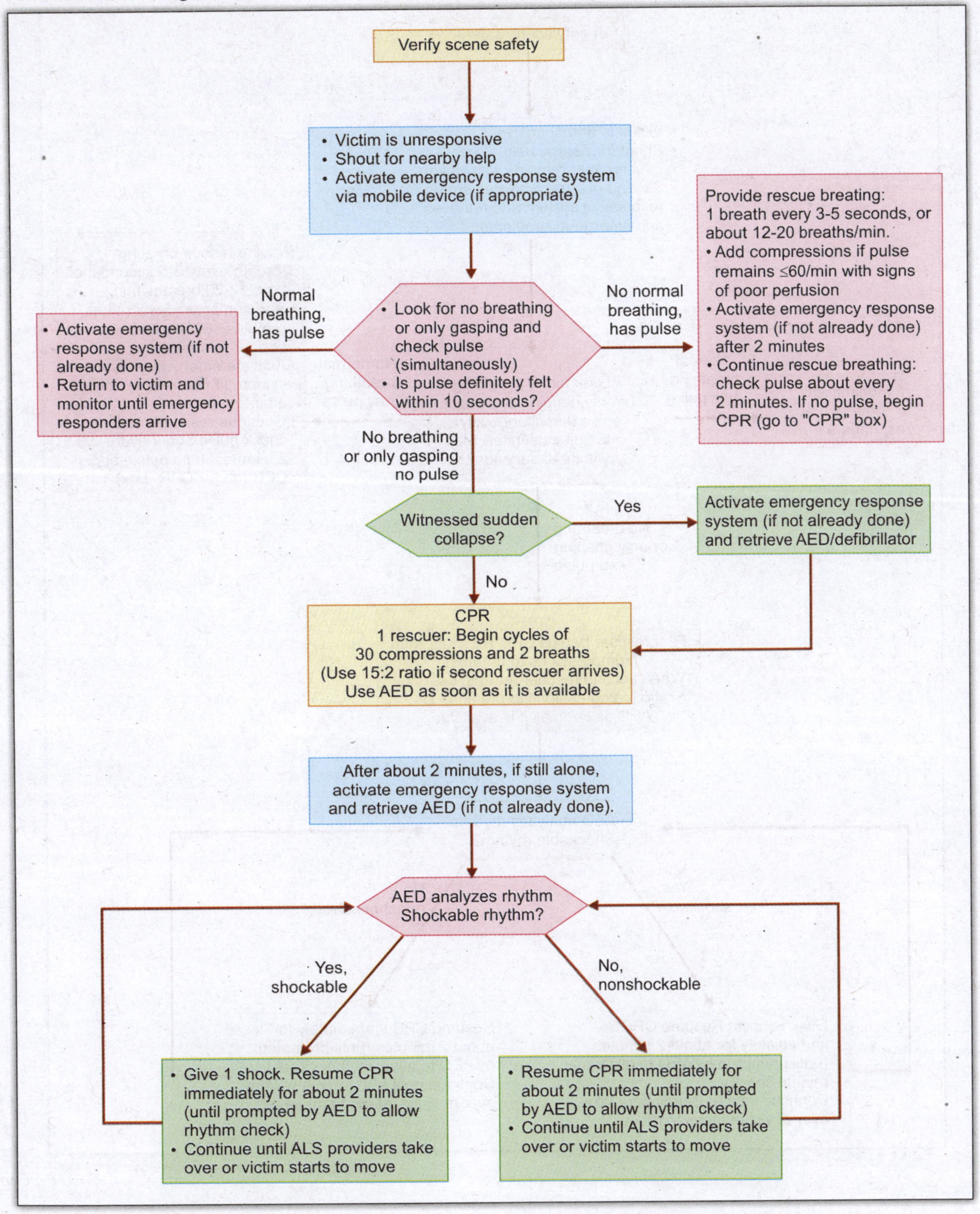

D. Pediatric Basic Life Support – 2 or More Rescuers

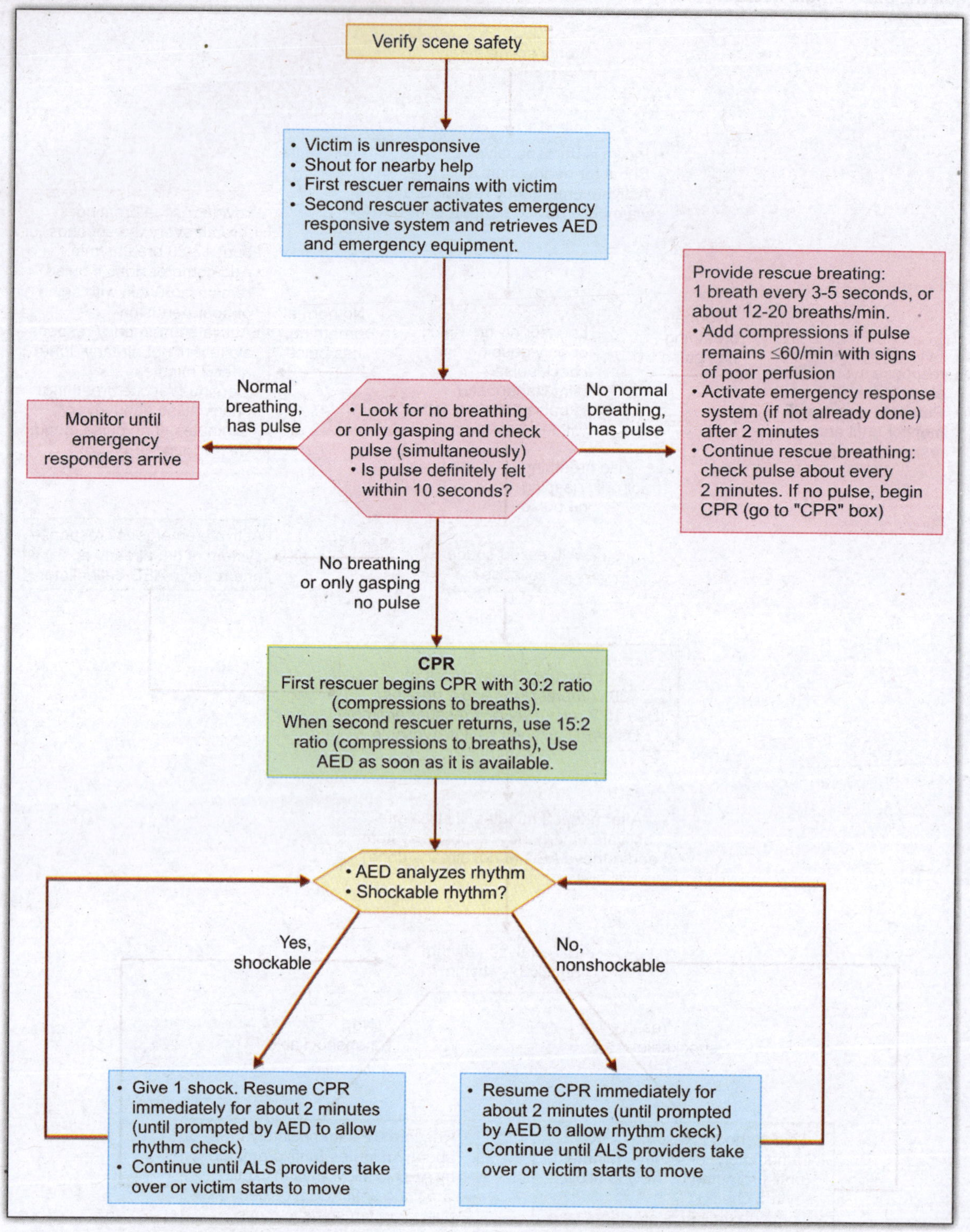

Contd...

E. Neonatal Resuscitation Algorithm

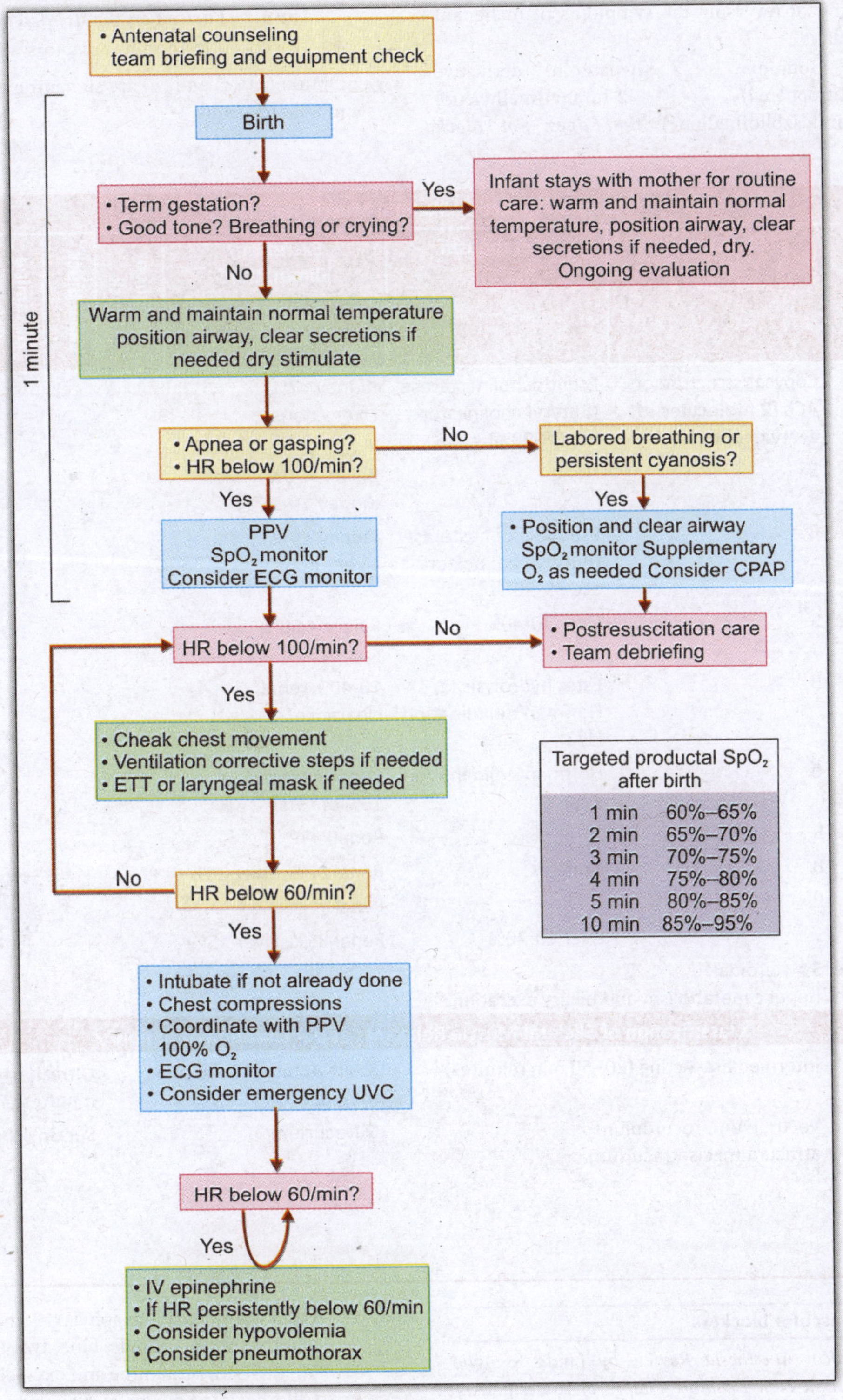

23. Ans. (c) 30:2

Ref: AHA 2015 Guidelines Update for Cardiopulmonary Resuscitation and Emergency Cardiovascular Care

See previous question for details of CPCR

AIIMS MAY 2016

24. Ans. (b) Dantrolene sodium

Ref: Miller's Anesthesia 8th Ed page 1291, KDT 6th ed page 339, 347

- Dantrolene is the only medication that has been shown to be effective in reversing the symptoms of malignant hyperthermia
- Dantrolene sodium is a hydantoin derivative (1-[[[5-(4-nitrophenyl)- 2-furanyl]methylene] imino]-2,4-imidazolidinedione) ***that does not block neuromuscular transmission but causes muscle weakness by direct action on the striated muscle cell.***
- It acts on Ryanodine receptors within the muscle.

Option (a), (c) and (d) are all neuromuscular blockers/skeletal muscle relaxants.

Peripherally Acting Skeletal Muscle Relaxants

Muscle relaxant	Structure[1]	Metabolism	Excretion/ Elimination[2]	Ganglion Block	Vagal Block	Histamine Release	Onset (min)	Duration (min)
Succinylcholine (Depolarizing)	Copycat structure of ACh **(2 molecules of acetylcholine)**	Pseudocholinesterase (Butyryl cholinesterase 98-99%)	Kidney <2%, Liver - none				1–1.5	5–8
Rocuronium	S	None	Biliary >70%, Kidney 10-25%)				1–2	30–60
Mivacurium	B	Pseudocholinesterase (Butyrylcholinesterase 95-99%)	Kidney <5%, Liver - none				2–4	12–18
Vecuronium	S	Liver 30-40%	Biliary = 60%, Kidney = 40%				2–4	60–90
Atracurium	B	Ester hydrolysis (2/3) Hoffman's elimination (1/3)	10-40% renal clearance				2–4	30–60
Cisatracurium	B	Hoffman's elimination 77%	Renal clearance is 16% of total				2–4	30–60
Pipracurium	S		Renal				2–4	80–100
D-tubocurarine	B	None	Renal 80%, Liver 20%	++	+	+++	4–6	80–120
Doxacurium	B		Renal				4–6	90–120
Pancuronium	S	Liver 10-20%	Renal 85%, Liver 15%	+	+		4–6	120–180

[1] B = benzylisoquinoline; S = steroidal.
[2] Biliary excretion means hepatic metabolism and biliary excretion

Classification of Skeletal Muscle Relaxants as per Duration of Action

Long-Acting (>50 minutes)	Intermediate-Acting (20–50 min minutes)	Short-Acting (15–20 min minutes)	Ultrashort-acting (<10–12 min minutes)
Pancuronium, Pipecuronium, Tubocurarine Metocurine, Doxacurium, Gallamine, Alcuronium	Vecuronium, rocuronium, atracurium, cisatracurium	Mivacurium	Succinylcholine gantacurium

25. Ans. (b) Neuromuscular blockers

Ref: Essential Clinical Anesthesia Review by Linda S. Aglio Ch 44, Australian and New Zealand College of Anaesthetists. ANZAAG-ANZCA Anaphylaxis Management Guidelines Version 1.1; 2013

- Risk factors for anaphylaxis include a history of atopy, drug or food allergy, multiple operations, systemic mastocytosis and hereditary angioedema.
- Common perioperative triggers of anaphylaxis include neuromuscular blocking agents, antibiotics (most commonly beta-lactam antibiotics) and latex.
- Less commonly, anaphylaxis may be provoked by chlorhexidine, colloids, blue dyes (isosulfan, patent blue V), heparin, protamine and oxytocin.
- Chlorhexidine can be found in many products such as skin preparations and wipes, lubricant gels and impregnated central venous lines and hence all the above should be avoided in patients with documented chlorhexidine allergy.
- It is rare for opioids or hypnotic agents (barbiturates, propofol, etomidate) to be the source of anaphylaxis.
- **The neuromuscular blocking agents most commonly associated with anaphylaxis are rocuronium and suxamethonium.**

- Anaphylaxis occurs due to IgE sensitization towards the quarternary ammonium groups in the neuromuscular blocking agents.
- Cross-reactivity with other nondepolarizing neuromuscular blocking agents is also highest with rocuronium and suxamethonium.

Treatment

The drug of choice for anaphylaxis is adrenaline.

The α1 agonist effect of adrenaline causes vasoconstriction, which decreases mucosal edema and hypotension. Its β1 agonist effect increases inotropy of the heart while its β2 agonism decreases mediator release and enhances bronchodilation.

The immediate management of anaphylaxis is to stop the suspected trigger, secure the airway, give high flow oxygen and administer adrenaline in titrated doses with close hemodynamic monitoring..

Grades of Anaphylaxis (Ring and Messmer Grading Scale)

Grade	Summary	Specific signs and symptoms
Grade 1	Generalized mucocutaneous signs	Erythema urticaria angioedema
Grade 2	Multi-organ manifestations	Mucocutaneous signs bronchospasm Hypotension
Grade 3	Severe life-threatening multi-organ manifestations	Arrhythmia cardiovascular collapse bronchospasm can have cutaneous signs
Grade 4	Cardiopulmonary arrest	Cardiac arrest

Dose of Adrenaline in Anaphylaxis

Grade of Anaphylaxis	Adult dose	Child dose
Grade 1-2	5–20 micrograms IV	1–5 micrograms/kg IV
Grade 3	100-200 micrograms IV	5-10 micrograms/kg IV
Grade 4	1 milligram IV	0.01 milligram/kg IV
If intravenous access not available	10 micrograms/kg IM (maximum 500 micrograms)	<12 years old: 300 micrograms IM <6 years old: 150 micrograms IM

26. Ans. (c) Induction should be done with thiopentone and succinylcholine for muscle relaxant

Ref: Miller's Anesthesia 8th edition page 1655, Continuing Education in Anesthesia, Critical Care and Pain | Volume 5 Number 2 2005, http://www.uptodate.com/contents/induction-agents-for-rapid-sequence-intubation-in-adults

Option (A)

RSI is the *virtually simultaneous administration of a sedative and a neuromuscular blocking agent* to render a patient rapidly unconscious and flaccid in order to facilitate emergent endotracheal intubation and to minimize the risk of aspiration. Multiple studies confirm the high-success rate of RSI using the combination of a sedative and a paralytic drug (Uptodate). This is correct for both cardiac and noncardiac patients

Option (B)

Step 1 in RSII is preoxygenation with 100% oxygen, 3 minutes tidal volume breaths, 4 vital capacity breaths or until the expired oxygen fraction is >85%. This option is correct in both cardiac and noncardiac patient

Option (C)

Historically, a 'classical' RSI has employed thiopental as an induction agent and succinylcholine for neuromuscular block. However there are many variants like for example in cardiac patients Etomidate is preferred over thiopental (see table below).

Hence, this option is correct for noncardiac patient and false for cardiac patients.

Option (D)

Cricoid pressure is applied before the loss of consciousness subsequent to injection of the induction agent till tube position and adequate seal are confirmed. This option is true for both cardiac and noncardiac patient.

Rapid Sequence Induction and Intubation (RSII)

Rapid-sequence induction of anesthesia and intubation (RSII) of the trachea is a specialized method of IV induction commonly used when a frequent ***risk for gastric regurgitation and pulmonary aspiration of gastric contents is present***. If not performed properly, or if the patient is unable to be intubated very rapidly (2 minutes or less), the patient could suffer extreme morbidity from hypoxia, hypercapnia or acidosis, or even death. The goal is to achieve optimal intubating conditions rapidly to minimize the length of time between the loss of consciousness (LOC) and securing of the airway with a cuffed ETT.

MNEMONIC = 4 P

- **Preoxygenation**—with 100% oxygen, **3 minutes tidal volume breaths**, 4 vital capacity breaths **or until the expired oxygen fraction is >85%**
- **Push the sedative:** an induction dose of IV anesthetic (***without face mask ventilation***) e.g. Etomidate, midazolam or ketamine. And ***apply cricoid pressure before the loss of consciousness*** subsequent to injection of the induction agent.
- **Paralyze**—followed by 1 to 1.5 mg/kg of IV suxamethonium, or vecuronium or rocuronium
- **Placement of tube**—and the trachea is intubated with **cuffed ET tube** without attempts at positive pressure ventilation. ***Intubation within 60 to 90 seconds*** must be considered acceptable. After tube position and adequate seal are confirmed the cricoid pressure may be released.

Contd...

Indications	• Patients with a full stomach (i.e., when NPO guidelines have not been observed) • Bowel obstruction • Pregnant, starting in the second trimester • Poorly controlled GERD, presence of a nasogastric tube • Morbid obesity • Diabetic gastroparesis • RSII is also a useful induction technique when ventilation via a mask is predicted to be difficult, but intubation is not, such as with an edentulous, bearded patient with an otherwise reassuring airway examination
Choice of induction agent	• **Thiopental** provides rapid loss of consciousness at a predictable dose (3–7 mg/kg) with a clearly defined end-point. It is noticeably quicker than both etomidate and propofol. However, it has a longer duration of action and its side effects are potentially life-threatening. Thiopental has a relatively high rate of anaphylaxis. • **Etomidate** has the major advantage of cardiovascular stability, so it is useful for the induction of anesthesia in patients with severe cardiovascular disease. However, the slow speed of onset and potential adrenal suppression limit its use. These disadvantages outweigh the benefits gained through its cardiovascular stability in the majority of patients. • **Ketamine:** During emergency anesthesia where there is circulatory collapse, ketamine should be considered.
Choice of neuromuscular blocking agent	• **Succinylcholine** has been the agent of choice for neuromuscular block. (1 to 2 mg/kg) • When succinylcholine is contraindicated or its side effects are undesired, RSII can be accomplished using nondepolarizing NMBDs **(rocuronium 1.0 to 1.2 mg/kg or vecuronium 0.3** mg/kg); these doses provide adequate intubating conditions in less than 90 seconds. • **Rocuronium** has a more rapid onset than previous non-depolarizing blockers and is proposed as an alternative agent for RSI. However, the duration of action of rocuronium is much longer than that of succinylcholine. The current development of a new non-depolarizing neuromuscular blocking agent reversal agent, **Sugammadex** (ORG-25969), may provide a safe method of antagonism allowing safer use of rocuronium for RSI. • **Sugammadex** may be the most exciting drug in clinical neuromuscular pharmacology in the last 50 years. The combination of rocuronium and sugammadex could replace succinylcholine for rapid-sequence induction of anesthesia and completely eliminate residual paralysis in the postanesthetic recovery room. Sugammadex (ORG 25969) is the first selective relaxant binding agent (su refers to sugar and gamadex refers to the structural molecule gamma-cyclodextrin). A modified γ-cyclodextrin, sugammadex is a new type of reversal agent.
Cuff specification	• Low-volume high pressure cuffs provide better protection against aspiration and not high-volume low pressure, since the latter cuff may develop folds through which aspiration can occur.
Cricoid pressure	• Cricoid pressure, eponymously referred to as the **Sellick maneuver** after the physician who first described it, involves the application of pressure at the cricoid ring to occlude the upper esophagus, thereby preventing the regurgitation of gastric contents into the pharynx. • The recommended force to be applied is **10 Newtons (N)** while the patient is awake, increased to 30 N after LOC. • Cricoid pressure is applied **before the loss of consciousness** subsequent to injection of the induction agent. • ***Cricoid pressure is to be applied till tube position and adequate seal are confirmed*.**
Controversies in cricoid pressure	• Opponents point to studies showing that cricoid pressure results in a decrease in lower esophageal sphincter tone, potentially increasing the risk for regurgitation and to magnetic resonance imaging (MRI) studies showing that cricoid pressure does not, in fact, result in compression of the esophagus, but rather a lateral displacement. • Worsens laryngeal visualization during direct laryngoscopy, potentially lengthening the time to intubation and increasing the risk of pulmonary aspiration and can result in occlusion of the subglottic airway, resulting in difficulty with intubation of the trachea or ventilation via a mask. On the other hand, advocates argue that properly applied cricoid pressure is effective in reducing the risk of aspiration and that reports of problems are due to incorrect application. The authors of a recent MRI study of cricoid pressure argue that the position of the esophagus is irrelevant because the effectiveness of cricoid pressure is due to occlusion of the hypopharynx. • In general, because of the relatively infrequent risk of application of cricoid pressure, its use is encouraged for RSII unless glottic visualization proves difficult, *in which case it can be easily released.*
Modified cricoid pressure technique	• The use of mask ventilation in conjunction with cricoid pressure. • Patients at risk for rapid development of hypoxemia (e.g., patients who are obese, pregnant, or critically ill; pediatric patients) • In emergent situations during which preoxygenation cannot be satisfactorily completed or when a longer time to acceptable intubating conditions is required because of the use of standard doses of nondepolarizing NMBDs. • Although the effect of positive pressure ventilation with cricoid pressure applied in terms of gastric insufflation of air is not definitively known, gentle PPV (inspiratory pressure <20 cm water [H_2O]) in conjunction with cricoid pressure may be acceptable in these clinical scenarios.

27. Ans. (a) Bezold-Jarisch reflex

Ref: Miller's Anesthesia 8th Ed Pg 1970

This is a highly controversial topic which is still debated. Even most of the Subjèct experts are not sure of the Answer. (A) Bezold-Jarisch reflex and (C) Reverse bain bridge reflex both have been implicated for bradycardia in spinal anesthesia and there are references to support both. However, if one have to choose a answer, we would rather go for (A) Bezold-Jarisch reflex because it is more widely describes, first to be conceptualized and more popular one. Now read following description:

The sympathectomy produced by spinal anesthesia induces hemodynamic changes. The block height determines the extent of sympathetic blockade, which determines the amount of change in cardiovascular parameters. However, this relationship cannot be predicted. **Hypotension and bradycardia** are the most common side effects seen with sympathetic denervation. Risk factors associated with hypotension include hypovolemia, preoperative hypertension, high sensory block height, obesity, combined general and spinal anesthesia and addition of phenylephrine to the local anesthetic. Hypotension occurs in about 33% of the non-obstetric population.

Option (A)

The concept of depressor reflexes originating in the heart was introduced by von Bezold in 1867 and was later revived by Jarisch. The Bezold–Jarisch reflex overlaps with vasovagal syncope. It was initially described as a bradycardic response to injection of various alkaloid compounds and later found to be mediated by chemoreceptors in the heart. The term has now come to include reactions triggered by cardiac mechanoreceptor activation and it has been used to describe perioperative bradycardia with hypotension. (**Ref: Oxford Journals Medicine and Health BJA Volume 86, Issue 6Pp. 859-868**)

The Bezold-Jarisch reflex (BJR) has been implicated as a cause of bradycardia, hypotension and cardiovascular collapse after central neuraxial anesthesia and in particular spinal anesthesia. The BJR is a cardio-inhibitory reflex and consists of the triad of symptoms, bradycardia, hypotension and coronary vasodilatation, seen after intravenous injection of Veratrum alkaloids in animals.

The Bezold-Jarisch reflex may be a possible cause of profound bradycardia and circulatory collapse after spinal anesthesia, especially in the presence of hypovolemia, when a small end-systolic left ventricular volume may trigger a mechanoreceptor-mediated bradycardia.

- The Bezold-Jarisch reflex responds to noxious ventricular stimuli sensed by chemoreceptors and mechanoreceptors within the left ventricular wall by inducing the triad of hypotension, bradycardia and coronary artery dilatation.
- The activated receptors communicate along unmyelinated vagal afferent type C fibers.
- These fibers reflexively increase parasympathetic tone.
- Because it invokes bradycardia, the Bezold-Jarisch reflex is thought of as a cardioprotective reflex. This reflex has been implicated in the physiologic response to a range of cardiovascular conditions such as myocardial ischemia or infarction, thrombolysis, or revascularization and syncope.
- Natriuretic peptide receptors stimulated by endogenous ANP or BNP may modulate the Bezold-Jarisch reflex. Thus, the Bezold-Jarisch reflex may be less pronounced in patients with cardiac hypertrophy or atrial fibrillation.

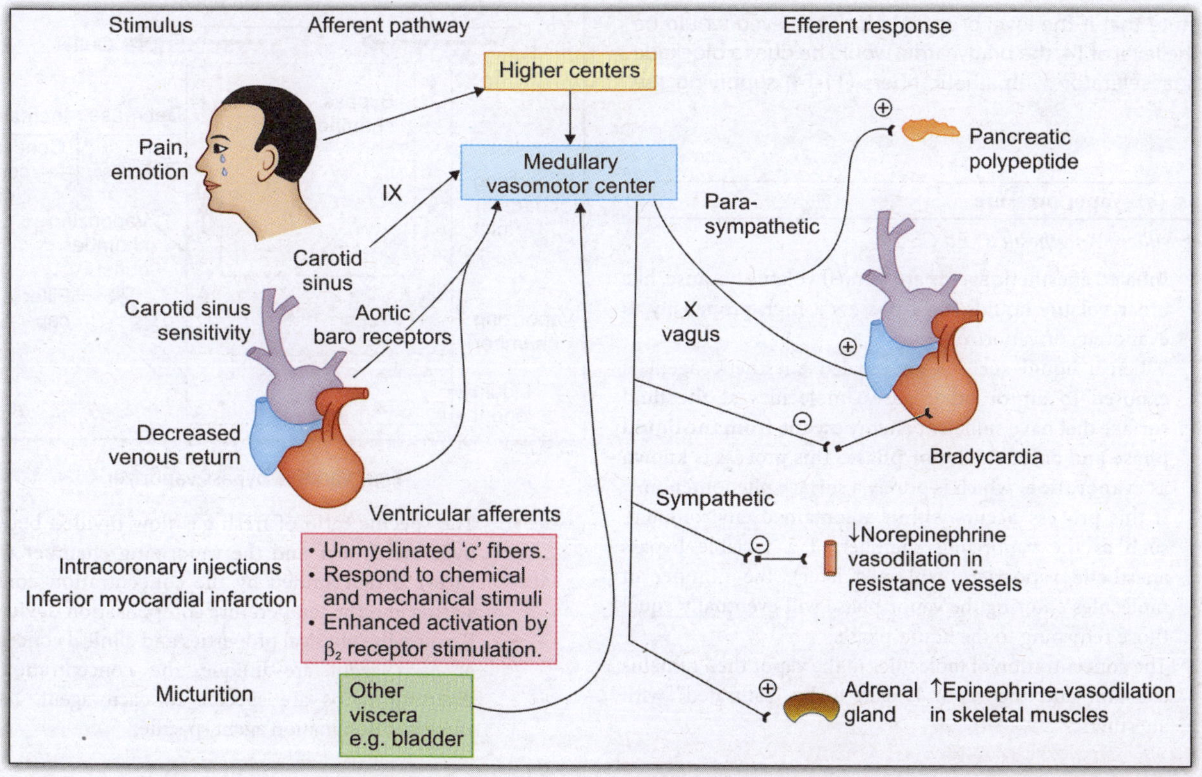

Option (B) Bainbridge Reflex

The Bainbridge reflex is elicited by stretch receptors located in the right atrial wall and the cavo atrial junction. An increase in right-sided filling pressure sends vagal afferent signals to the cardiovascular center in the medulla. These afferent signals inhibit parasympathetic activity, thereby increasing the heart rate. Acceleration of the heart rate also results from a direct effect on the SA node by stretching the atrium. The changes in heart rate are dependent on the underlying heart rate before stimulation.

Option (C) Reverse Bainbridge Reflex

A "reverse" Bainbridge reflex has also been proposed to explain the decreases in heart rate observed under conditions in which venous return is reduced, such as during spinal and epidural anesthesia, controlled hypotension and severe hemorrhage.

Option (D)

The mechanism responsible for bradycardia is not clear. Blockade of sympathetic cardioaccelerator fibers originating from T 1-4 spinal segments is often suggested as the cause. The fact that bradycardia is more common with high blocks supports this mechanism. However, significant bradycardia sometimes occurs with blocks that are seemingly to low to block cardioaccelerators. Diminished venous return has also been proposed as a cause of bradycardia during spinal anesthesia. Intracardiac stretch receptors have been shown to reflexively decrease heart rate when filling pressures fall. The presence of bradycardia does not always indicate that cardioaccelerator fibers are blocked. Bradycardia can be manifested when right atrial pressure is decreased because of reduced venous return (Ref: **Barash – Clinical Anesthesia 6th Ed page 946)**

NOTE

Please note that if the level of spinal block achieved would be above the level of T4, the bradycardia would be due to blockade of cardioaccelerator sympathetic fibers (T1-T4) supplying the heart.

28. Ans. (b) Vapor pressure

Ref: Miller's Anesthesia 8th Ed Ch 29

- Inhaled anesthetic agents are termed volatile because, like other volatile liquids, they possess a high propensity to evaporate, or vaporize.
- When a liquid such as an inhaled anesthetic agent is exposed to air or other gases, molecules at the fluid surface that have sufficient energy **escape from the liquid phase and enter the vapor phase**. This process is known as **evaporation**, which is purely a surface phenomenon.
- If this process occurs within a contained environment, such as the vaporizing chamber of a variable bypass anesthetic vaporizer (explained later), the number of molecules entering the vapor phase will eventually equal those returning to the liquid phase.
- The concentration of molecules in the vapor then remains constant and the vapor is said to be "saturated" with anesthetic.
- At this point of evaporative equilibrium, the anesthetic molecules in the vapor phase are bombarding the walls of the container and creating a partial pressure known as **the saturated vapor pressure, or simply vapor pressure.** Substances with a high propensity to evaporate generate higher vapor pressures.
- We must note that the question refers to the ***dose of the anesthetic agent delivered*** rather than the effect on the body is being referred to in the above question, hence options (A) Blood gas partition co-efficient and (C) Oil gas partition co-efficient are ruled out, since they determine patient related effects like onset and offset of action.
- The modern day vaporizers are variable bypass vaporizers.
- When volatile anesthetic agents evaporate, their resultant saturated gas concentrations greatly exceed those used clinically, so these concentrations must be diluted to safe ranges.
- *Variable bypass* refers to the method of carefully regulating the concentration of vaporizer output by diluting gas fully saturated with anesthetic agent with a larger flow of gas.
- Basic vaporizer components include a vaporizer inlet port (fresh gas inlet), the concentration control dial, the bypass chamber, the vaporizing chamber, the vaporizer outlet port and the filling assembly. **A concentration control dial determines the ratio of gas that flows through the bypass chamber and the vaporizing chamber and a temperature-compensating device further adjusts that ratio. Vaporizer concentration control dials are labeled to set vaporizer output in terms of volume percent (v/v%) and the vaporizers are calibrated at sea level.**

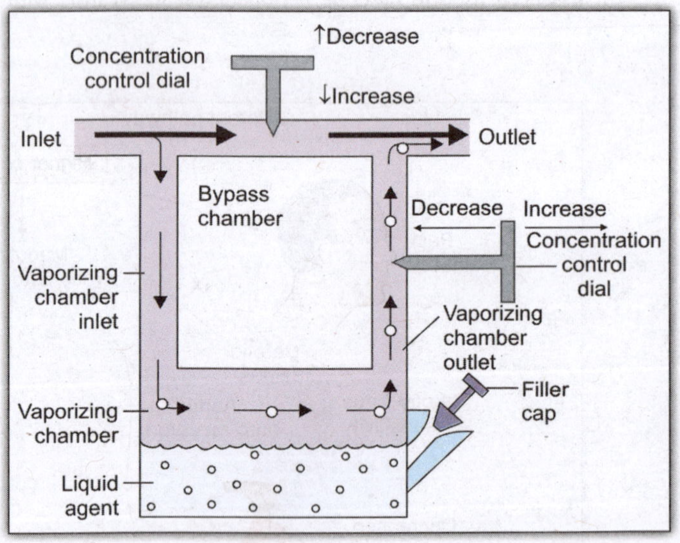

Fig: Variable bypass vaporizer

- The specific ratio of fresh gas flow divided between the bypass chamber and the vaporizing chamber (**splitting ratio**) is determined by the concentration control dial setting and the temperature compensation device.
- Because the physical properties and clinical concentrations of each agent are unique, the concentration-specific diverting ratios are specific to each agent, hence the vaporizer designation agent specific.

- When describing the proportion of a single gas in a sample containing a mixture of gases, we can refer to the individual gas in terms of its partial pressure (mm Hg) or by its percentage by volume relative to the sum volume of the all the gases present, which is known as volume percent or volume-volume percent (v/v%).
- The volume that a gas occupies at a given temperature and pressure is related to the number of molecules of gas present, **not the size (type) of the molecules.** Hence, option (D) Molecular weight is also ruled out.
- Different anesthetic agents have different saturated vapor pressures at a given temperature. Therefore, the partial pressure exerted by the vapor in a mixture of gases will be different. Hence, splitting ratios are agent-specific and vaporizers cannot be interchanged **unless 2 vapors have the same vapor pressure.**
- Note that the effect of the anesthetic agent in the body depends on the partial pressure and not the volume percent.

29. Ans. (b) Infants > Neonates > Adults

Ref: Miller's anesthesia 8th Ed Pg 2764

Anesthetic requirement is smaller for preterm than for term neonates and smaller for term neonates than for 3-month old. Infants have a higher MAC than that of older children or adults; the reasons for these age-related differences in MAC are not known.

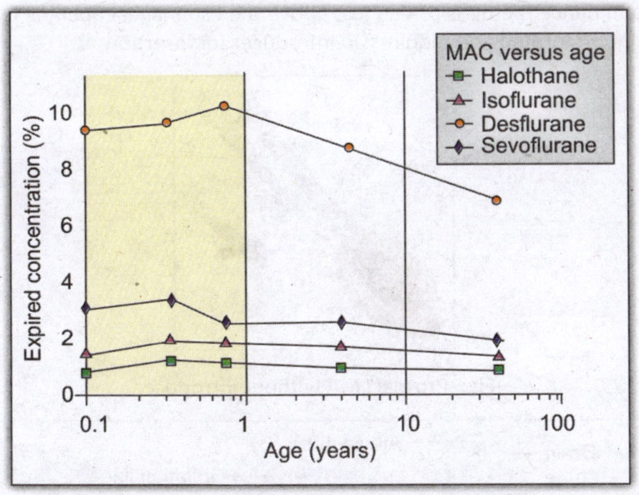

Fig: The minimum alveolar concentrations (MACs) of four commonly used inhaled anesthetics are plotted versus age. MAC is highest in infants 3 to 6 months of age.

30. Ans. (a) Atracurium

Ref: Miller 8th ed page 976

See table of Peripherally Acting Skeletal Muscle Relaxants in Anesthesia AIIMS May 2016 (see page no. 1164)

31. Ans. (a) Grey

Ref: Oxford American handbook of clinical examinations and Practical skills by Elezabeth Burns Ch 18, Bailey 25th ed page 291

See table of IV Cannula in AIIMS Nov 2018 Anesthesia (see page no. 1139)

Same question regarding rapid infusion of IV fluid was asked in many sessions of AIIMS exams in different language. Be it Massive hemorrhage in RTA or Intraoperative or be it Diarrhea; the concept is rapid infusion and answer remains the same.

ACLS guidelines recommend securing IV access by two large bore cannulae (14–16 G) in patient needed resuscitation. In case of a massive bleeding or severe dehydration, we would like to resuscitate the patient with rapid infusion of IV fluids. This can be effectively achieved with a higher gauge cannula. Always remember, higher the Gauge, smaller the cannula.

AIIMS NOVEMBER 2015

32. Ans. (a) 16 G

Ref: Oxford American handbook of clinical examinations and Practical skills by Elezabeth Burns Ch 18, Bailey 25th ed page 291

See table of IV Cannula in AIIMS Nov 2018 Anesthesia (see page no. 1139)

Same question regarding rapid infusion of IV fluid was asked in many sessions of AIIMS exams in different language. Be it Massive hemorrhage in RTA or Intraoperative or be it Diarrhea; the concept is rapid infusion and answer remains the same.

ACLS guidelines recommend securing IV access by two large bore cannulae (14- 16 G) in patient needed resuscitation. In case of a massive bleeding or severe dehydration, we would like to resuscitate the patient with rapid infusion of IV fluids. This can be effectively achieved with a higher gauge cannula. Always remember, higher the Gauge, smaller the cannula.

33. Ans. (a) Administer skeletal muscle relaxant

Ref: Miller 7th ed page 1427, Understanding Anesthesia Equipment by Jerry A. Dorsch 5th Ed Ch 22

See table of Capnography and table of some Important Capnography in Anesthesia AIIMS Nov 2016 (see page no. 1153 to 1155)

The cleft in the capnograph is due to patients own respiratory efforts due to inadequate muscle relaxants. The next most appropriate is to increase the muscle relaxant.

A good alveolar plateau greatly increases the chances that the end-tidal reading is a reliable estimate of the alveolar level. The angle between the end of Phase III and the descending limb of the capnogram is called the beta angle. Normally, it is approximately 90°. The angle will be increased with rebreathing. Another possible cause of an increased beta angle is a prolonged response time compared with the respiratory cycle time, particularly in children. The angle will be decreased if the slope of Phase III is increased.

34. Ans. (a) Above esophagus

Ref: Miller 7th ed page 1584, Understanding Anesthesia Equipment by Jerry A. Dorsch 5th Ed Ch 17

The device shown in the picture is Proseal LMA which has internal drainage (gastric) tube which is lateral to the airway tube and ends at the tip of the mask for aspiration of gastric contents in the event of passive regurgitation and hence the tip is placed just above the esophageal opening

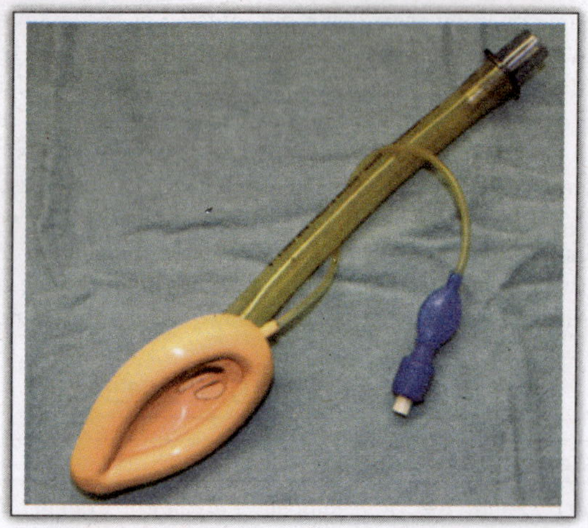

Fig: LMA classic

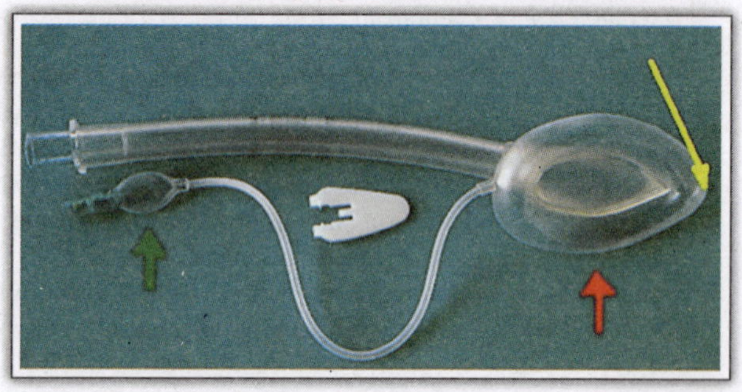

Fig: LMA unique

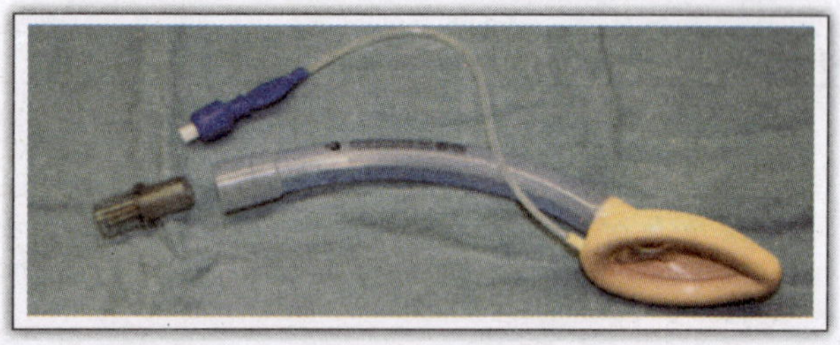

Fig: LMA classic excel is adapted for intubating through LMA. Clue for identification—The connector is detachable so as to facilitate intubation

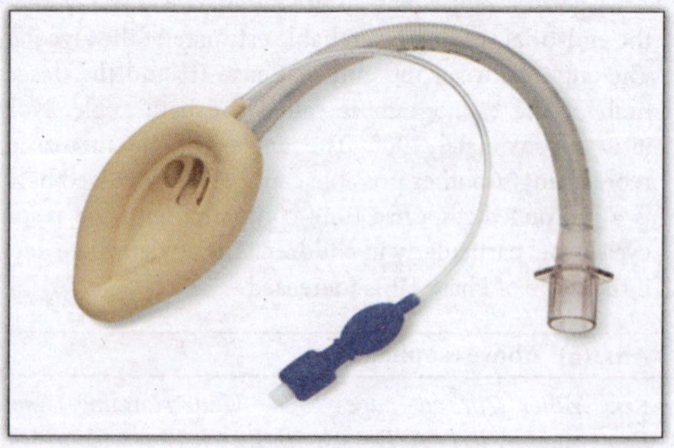

Fig: Flexible LMA has a wire reinforced tube to avoid kinking on flexion

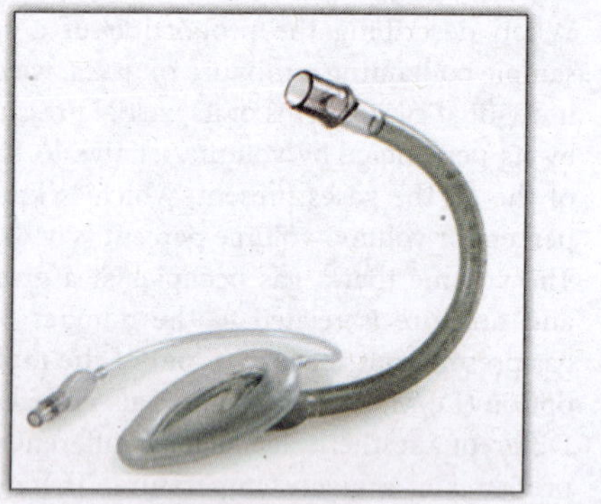

Fig: Flexible LMA (Single use)

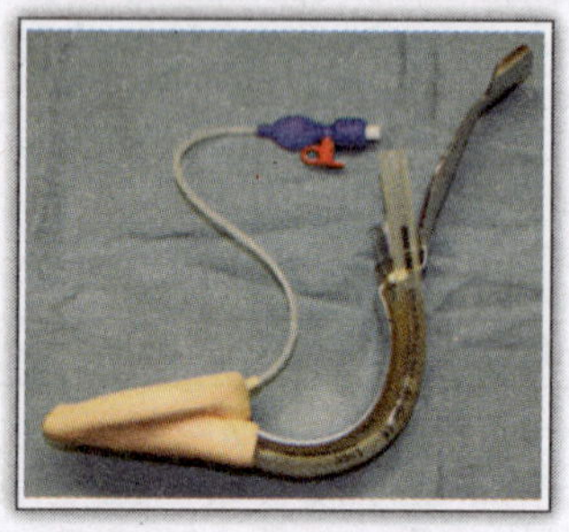

Fig: PROSEAL LMA with introducer: The device shown in the picture is PROSEAL LMA which has internal drainage (gastric) tube which is lateral to the airway tube and ends at the tip of the mask for aspiration of gastric contents in the event of passive regurgitation and hence the tip is placed just above the esophageal opening It is not preformed and requires an introducer for insertion.

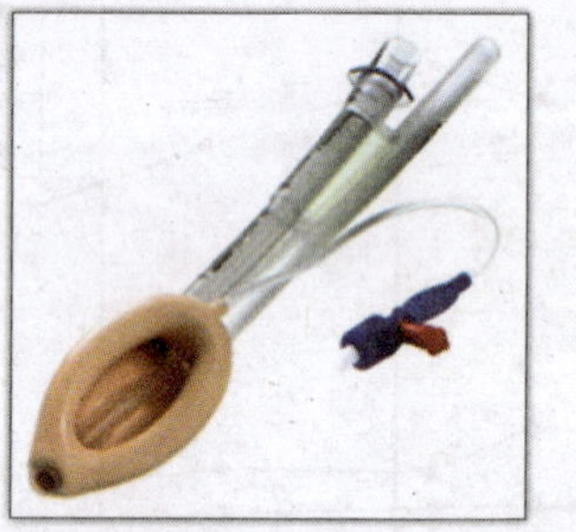

Fig: Proseal LMA without introducer

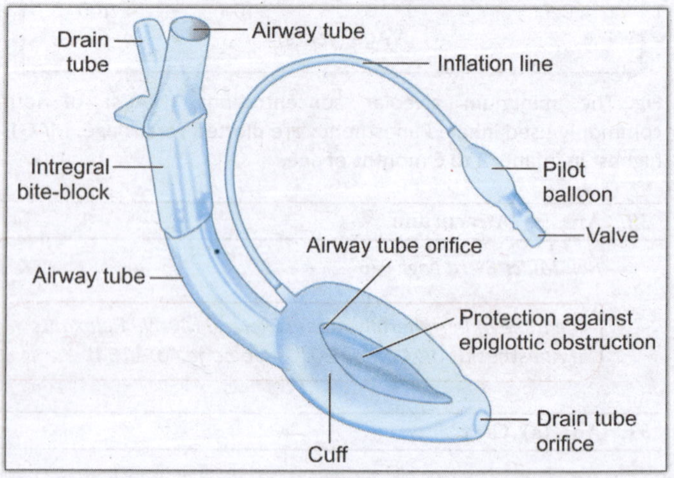

Fig: LMA supreme: Preformed 2nd generation LMA with gastric port above the airway tube

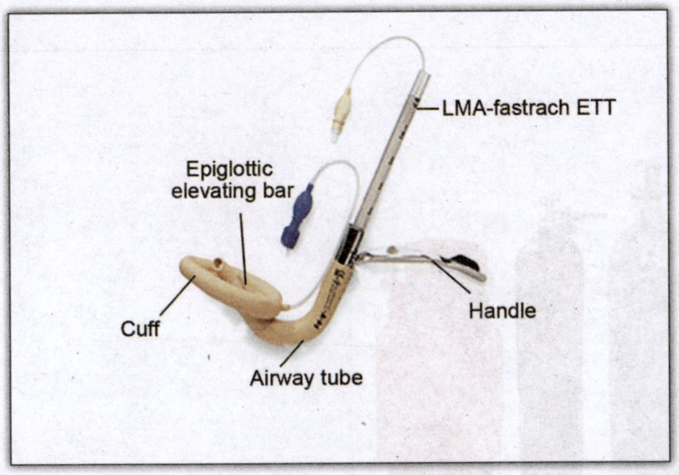

Fig: Intubating LMA/LMA Fastrach: Especially designed for intubation through LMA with a special Endotracheal tube that comes as a part of the kit. It has a metal handle attached to the LMA to help maneuver the tube

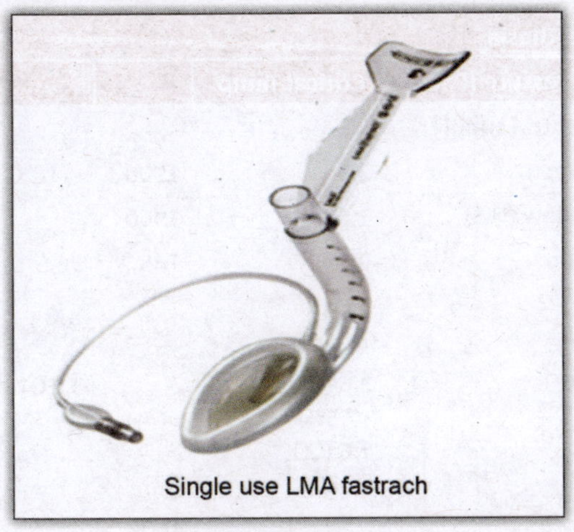

Fig: Single use LMA fastrach/intubating LMA

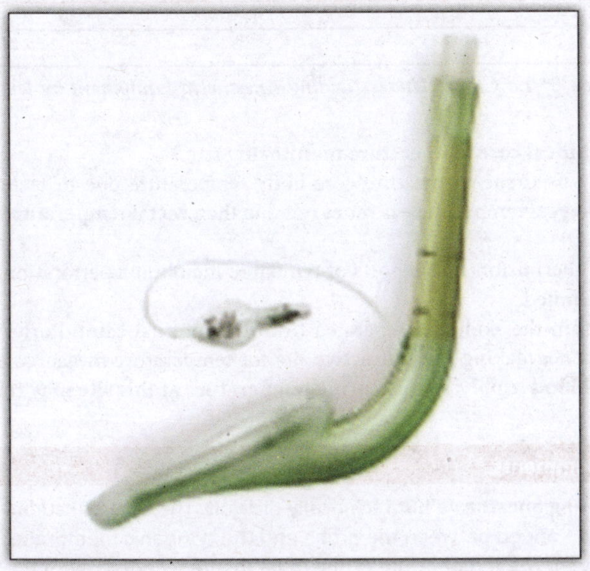

Fig: Ambu LMA: Clue for identification—Looks like classic LMA in a Preformed form and is green color

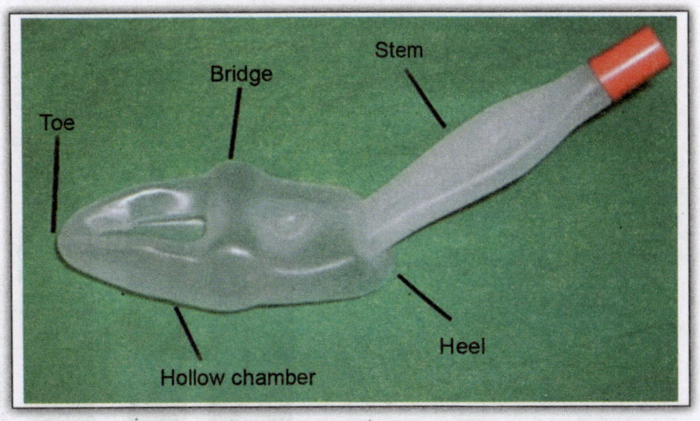

Fig: SLIPA-Streamlined liner of pharyngeal airway (SLIPA): Cuffless device. Slipper shaped. Size determined by distance between thyroid cornuae

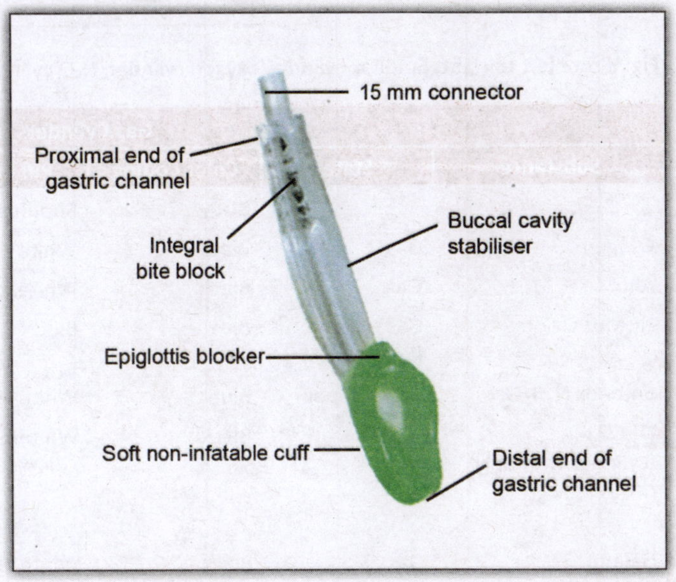

Fig: IGel: Cuffless. Made of thermoplastic elastomer. Contorts to the airway anatomy

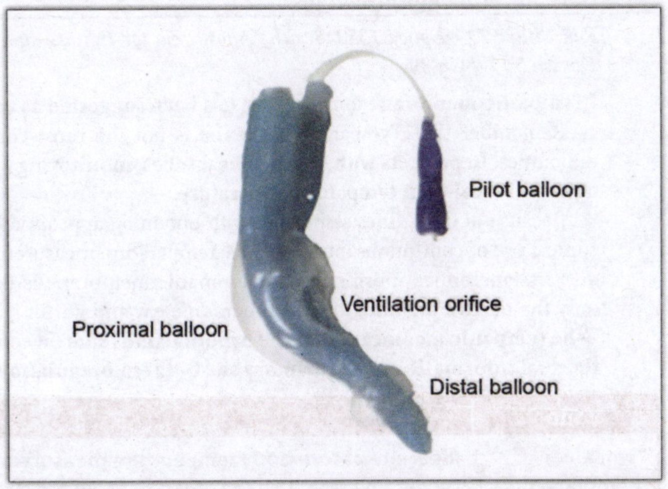

Fig: Elisha airway device has 3 separate channels for gastric tube, ventilation and fiberoptic intubation. Endotracheal tube can be inserted through fiberoptic intubation

35. Ans. (a) Black body white shoulder

Ref: Wylie Churchill-Davidson's A Practice of Anesthesia 7th Edition Pg 471

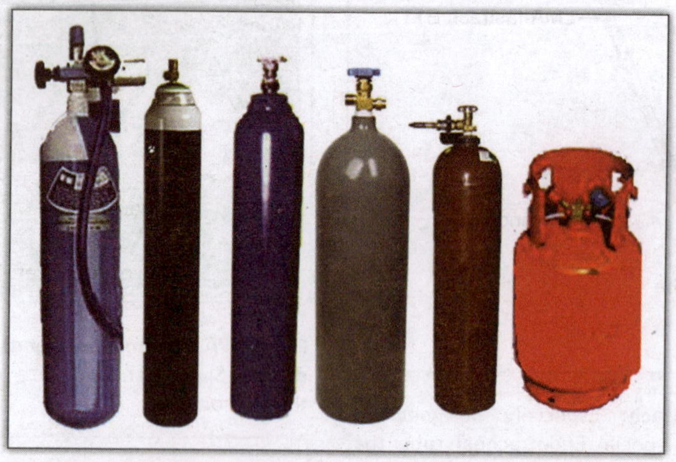

Fig: From left to right: Entonox cylinder, oxygen cylinder, N_2O cylinder, CO_2 cylinder (pure), helium cylinder, cyclopropane cylinder

Gas Cylinders Used in Anesthesia							
Substance	**State**	**Color Coding**	**Pin Index**	**Pressure (PSIG)**	**Critical Temp.**		
		Body	**Shoulder**	**Central supply**			
Oxygen	Gas	Black	White	Green	2,5	1900	-118°C
AIR	Gas	Black	White/black	Yellow (U.S)	1,5	1900	
Nitrous Oxide	Gas + Liquid (below 98°F)	Blue	Blue	Blue	3,5	745	36.5°C
Entonox N_2O/O_2	Gas & Vapor	Blue	White /Blue	NA	7		
O_2-CO_2 (cylinder with only CO_2 is fully grey)		Black	White/Grey	NA	2,6 (CO_2 <7.5%) 1,6 (CO_2 >7.5%)		31°C (for CO_2)
Helium	Gas	Black	White/Brown	NA		1600	
Cyclopropane		Orange	Orange	NA	3,6		

36. Ans. (b) Tympanic membrane

Ref: Miller 7th ed page 1550, Smith's Anesthesia for Infants and Children 8th Ed Ch 59, Understanding Anesthesia Equipment by Jerry A. Dorsch 5th Ed Ch 29.

"Tympanic-membrane temperature has been suggested as the most ideal core temperature monitoring site."

Remember that Tympanic membrane is not the most commonly used site to measure core body temperature due to technical difficulties. **In patients with endotracheal tubes, monitoring of esophageal temperature is more reliable than rectal temperature and more practical than tympanic temperature.**

Because of difficulties associated with obtaining appropriate-sized thermistors and reports of tympanic membrane perforation, the clinical use of continuous intraoperative temperature measurement is limited.

"The anatomical position of the tympanic membrane is deep within the skull and separated from the internal carotid artery by only the narrow air-filled cleft of the middle ear and a thin shell of bone, making it an attractive site for temperature measurements. **"The tympanic membrane and the hypothalamus share a common blood supply, so measuring temperature at this site may reflect thermal information at the primary site of thermoregulation."**

Site	Comments
Tympanic membrane	**Ideal site of core body temperature measurement during anesthesia** but technically difficult. The external auditory canal to be sealed by the probe to allow the air column trapped between the probe and the tympanic membrane to reach a steady-state temperature. It is not necessary for the temperature probe to be in direct contact with the tympanic membrane Disadvantage – Chances of tympanic perforation

Contd...

Site	Comments
Naso-pharyngeal	Tip needs to be placed in the posterior nasopharynx close to the soft palate. Disadvantage—using the probe with an uncuffed endotracheal tube that has a moderate to large air leak may lead to falsely low readings.
Esophageal	**Most commonly used site of core body temperature measurement during anesthesia**, Tip of the probe is placed in the distal third of the esophagus at the point where the heart sounds are the loudest Disadvantage – Site may not be exact, cold water and high flows may cause erroneous readings.
Axillary	The tip of the thermometer is carefully placed over the axillary artery and the arm is closely adducted Disadvantage—malpositioning of the probe may result in unreliable estimates of core temperature. Infusion of cool solutions at high flow rates in small children on the ipsilateral side of the thermometer probe may result in falsely low temperature readings.
Rectal temperature	Disadvantage—Probe's insulation by feces, its exposure to cooler blood returning from the legs, the influence of an open abdominal cavity during laparotomy, or irrigations of the bladder or the abdomen with either cold or warm solutions. Relative contraindications are inflammatory bowel disease, neutropenia and/or thrombocytopenia and the need to irrigate the bowel or bladder.
Bladder	Considered to be one of the most accurate methods of measuring core temperature. Its precision has been demonstrated to be identical to pulmonary-artery-temperature monitoring as long as urinary output is high; however, when urinary output is normal or less than normal, this site may become inaccurate in reflecting central temperature
Pulmonary artery catheter	***Gold standard for core temperature measurement in noncardiac surgery***. Because of its invasive nature, its use—particularly in the pediatric population—has been limited to special situations, such as in critically ill children.

37. Ans. (a) Ketamine followed by intubation and GA;
(c) Thiopentone followed by muscle relaxant

Ref: Miller's Anaesthesiology 8th Ed Pg 2345, William's 24th ed page 518, KDT 7th ed page 376

- Caesarean section is preferably done under spinal anesthesia. General anesthesia is avoided in pregnant patients, as the drugs used during general anesthesia are likely to cause depression of respiration in the baby and also, pregnant patients are considered to be full stomach and difficult intubation.
- However, there are a few select cases like fetal distress, maternal compromise where general anesthesia is indicated.
- General anesthesia is very commonly administered as rapid sequence induction with thiopentone and succinyl choline.
- Maintenance is by oxygen, nitrous oxide and minimal inhalational agents like isoflurane and sevoflurane, since MAC >1 is associated with uterine atony.
- Sedative agents like midazolam and fentanyl are mostly avoided till the delivery of the baby.

In the above case, patient is likely to have lost a lot of blood due to placenta previa and hence is hypotensive. The patient will keep losing blood till the baby is out. Low systolic BP means the fetus is likely to suffer due to decreased uteroplacental circulation. Also, the mother is likely to be compensating the BP by catecholamine release and hence is likely to crash her BP after spinal anesthesia or even general anesthesia due to sympatholysis. Now, let us consider the options one by one.

Option (A) Ketamine followed by GA and Intubation

Ketamine (1-2 mg/kg) is known to have sympathomimetic effects and raises blood pressure. This followed by GA and intubation (Assuming muscle relaxant has been given, however not mentioned in the option) seems like a good option to maintain blood pressure even after induction of anesthesia. However, we must remember that in hypovolemic patients there is maximal vasoconstriction, ketamine in these cases is not likely to cause further vasoconstriction but causes myocardial depression instead. Thus, it is mandatory to resuscitate with fluids and blood even if we are using ketamine for induction.

Option (B) Propofol followed by Intubation and GA

Propofol is known to cause profound hypotension and also depression of baroreceptor reflex, preventing compensation of hypotension by tachycardia. Hence, use of Propofol for this patient is out of question.

Option (C) Thiopentone followed by Muscle Relaxant

Thiopentone (3–5 mg/kg) is generally preferred in induction of pregnant patients since it causes lesser disturbances in hemodynamics (to avoid hypotension and uteroplacental compromise in pregnant patients) and also lower doses produce no significant neonatal effects providing induction to delivery time is <5 minutes, (while doses of >8 mg/kg produce neonatal depression).

However, in this particular case, where systolic BP is 85 mm Hg, even the lesser hypotension caused by Thiopentone can have significant adverse effects. Thus, Thiopentone would not be our first choice for induction, although this method can be used with adequate fluid resuscitation and lower doses of Thiopentone followed by muscle relaxant.

However, we certainly require intubation in pregnant patients once they lose their consciousness since they are considered full stomach and are likely to aspirate. Intubation has not been mentioned in this option.

Option (D) Epidural with Bupivacaine

Epidural is considered to induce lesser hypotension as compared to spinal anesthesia, since we give titrated doses of bupivacaine in the epidural space, as against single shot of profound sympatholysis in the intrathecal space. However, we must understand that epidural bupivacaine will still cause hypotension, by neuraxial blockade and sympatholysis. Also, if we intend to give only epidural anesthesia, the time for onset of action is at least 30 minutes. This case is clearly an emergency and wasting 30 crucial minutes could be detrimental.

The examiner most likely wants to stress on the point that ketamine should be used in hypotensive patients, thus we accept this as our option of choice.

Ideal option of choice would have been induction with Etomidate (0.3 mg/kg), which is cardiostable and has minimal effects on hemodynamics, followed by muscle relaxant succinylcholine and then intubation.

38. Ans. (b) Lumbar puncture

Ref: Miller's Anaesthesiology 8th Ed Pg 1699

NOTE

Modern disposable single use Lumbar puncture needle was given

See details of Lumbar Puncture in AIIMS MAY 2017 Anesthesia (see page no. 1147-1148)

39. Ans. (a) Glycopyrrolate

Ref: Miller's Anesthesia 8th Ed Pg 378

- The addition of a muscarinic anticholinergic drug to anesthetic premedication for decreasing secretions and preventing harmful vagal reflexes was mandatory in the era of ether anesthesia, but **it is less important with modern inhaled agents**.
- Routine preoperative use of these drugs as antisialagogues continues in some pediatric and otorhinolaryngologic cases, along with administration of ketamine or when fiberoptic intubation is planned.
- Atropine has a tertiary structure that easily crosses the blood-brain barrier. CNS effects have been seen with the relatively large doses (1–2 mg). In contrast, one of the synthetic antimuscarinic drugs, **glycopyrrolate, does not cross the blood-brain barrier** because of its quaternary structure and has gained popularity for this use.
- **Atropine and glycopyrrolate both can be used as premedication.** However, Glycopyrrolate is the more frequently used premedication used, amongst the handful situations where premedication is actually used. Earlier, Atropine was administered in neonates who have a higher vagal tone. However, this is not frequently practiced.

40. Ans. (c) Ligamentum flavum

Ref: Fundamentals of Anesthesia, Tim Smith Colin Pinnock Ted Lin, 3rd Ed page 118, Gray's Anatomy 40th ed page 729.

See details of Lumbar Puncture in AIIMS MAY 2017 Anesthesia (see page no. 1147-1148)

41. Ans. (c) Macintosh laryngoscope

Ref: Understanding Anesthesia Equipment by Dorsch 5th Ed Ch 18

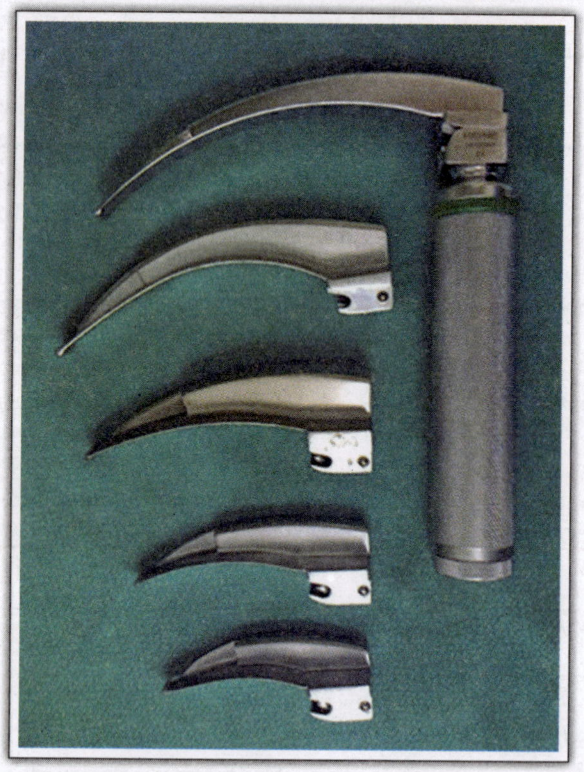

Fig: Laryngoscope handle with an assortment of Macintosh blades (Most commonly used) (large adult, small adult, pediatric, infant and neonate). Curved blades

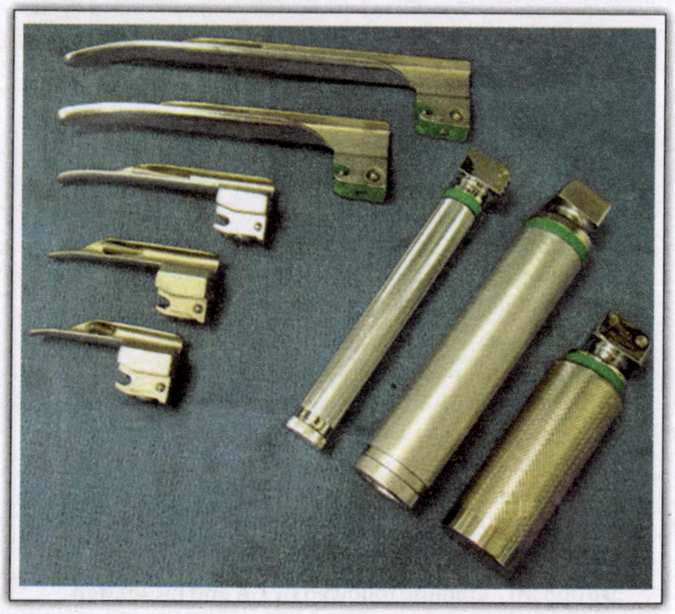

Fig: Laryngoscope handles with an assortment of Miller blades (large adult, small adult, pediatric, infant and neonate). Straight blades

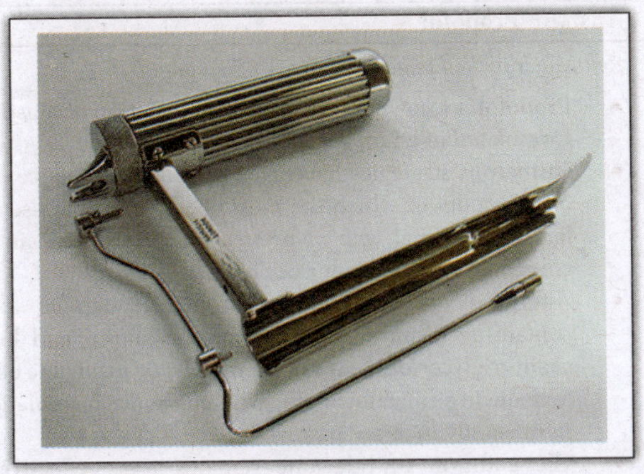

Fig: Magill laryngoscope with the light carrier detached. Magill's blades (minimum or no blind area) are used in infants. Straight blades

NOTE

- Upper incisors are commonly injured during Laryngoscopy
- Laryngoscope blades are available in 0 to 5 sizes, Size 0 is used in Infants while Size 5 is used in Large adults. Miller blade is also available in 00, 0, 1, 2, 3, 4
- Straight blades are often preferred in infants as the epiglottis is larger, soft and floppy as cartilaginous framework is not yet developed. The epiglottis is inclined at 45 degrees to the glottis. The larynx in more anterior and high up in the neck opposite to C3 C4 vertebral body. In this case the straight blades are places behind or posterior to epiglottis, where it is lifted out of the way of vocal cords (epiglottis is "included").

Direct Laryngoscopy	
Technique	• Direct laryngoscope is held in nondominant hand so as to keep dominant hand free for instrumentation or surgery • Neck position in laryngoscopy: Extension of atlanto-occipital joint, flexion of cervical spine "SNIFFING THE MORNING AIR" position. • Mouth opening using the scissors technique. This is accomplished by placing the thumb on the lower teeth and the index finger on the upper teeth. • Initial blade insertion is from the left side as the mouth is scissored open and the blade is then directed initially from left to right to position the blade flange ultimately toward the left side of the patient's mouth on complete insertion of the blade • The blade is advanced carefully and directed in a midline approach until the epiglottis is visualized. After the soft palate tissue and tongue are lifted in a direction along the axis of the laryngoscope handle and the glottic opening is exposed, a tracheal tube can be inserted using the right hand and advanced from the right corner of the patient's mouth and through the vocal cords • The laryngoscope should never be hinged at the incisors while lifting.
Diagnostic indications in ENT	• When indirect laryngoscopy is not possible as in infants and young children and the symptomatology points to larynx and/or hypopharynx, e.g. hoarseness, dyspnoea, stridor and dysphagia. • When indirect laryngoscopy has not been successful, e.g. due to excessive gag reflex or overhanging epiglottis obscuring a part of the complete view of the larynx. • To examine hidden areas of: Hypopharynx: Base of tongue, valleculae and lower part of pyriform fossa. Larynx: Infrahyoid epiglottis, anterior commissure, ventricles and subglottic region. • To find the extent of growth and take a biopsy.
Therapeutic indications in ENT	• Removal of benign lesions of larynx, e.g. papilloma, fibroma, vocal nodule, polyp or cyst. • Removal of foreign bodies from larynx and hypopharynx. • Dilatation of laryngeal strictures.
Contraindications	• Diseases or injuries of cervical spine. (Video laryngoscope may be used) • Limited mouth opening where the laryngoscope cannot be introduced
Caution	• Highly stimulates the sympathetic system hence to be carefully used in patients with heart disease, raised Intracranial pressure etc. If essential, a quick laryngoscopy (,15 seconds) maybe done or adjuvants which lower BP or heart rate can be used during laryngoscopy e.g: esmolol
	• Loose teeth

AIIMS MAY 2015

42. Ans. (b) Dexmedetomidine

Ref: Miller's 8th ed page 854, KDT 7th ed page 384

Dexmedetomidine is an alpha 2 agonist and causes a decrease in central sympathetic outflow. Hence, it causes bradycardia and hypotension. Thus, we would like to avoid this agent in the given scenario of pre-existing hypotension and bradycardia in a patient with coronary artery disease, in whom hypotension should be prevented in order to maintain cardiac perfusion increased workload. Also, the sympathetic system might be maintaining the BP in the above patient and sympatholysis may cause profound hypotension.

About other options:

Option (A) Ketamine

Ketamine causes increased central sympathetic discharge and hence increases BP as well as heart rate. This patient is a known case of coronary artery disease. Increase in heart rate will cause increased myocardial oxygen demand, as well as increased BP will cause increased myocardial afterload. These changes will cause increased load on the heart and may precipitate ischemia. However, in the setting of hypotension, bradycardia, Ketamine may be given in such a patient and certainly preferred over the option Dexmedetomidine.

Option (C) Etomidate

Etomidate is a very cardiostable drug and can be used for induction in this scenario.

Option (D) Fentanyl

Fentanyl is an agent known to cause bradycardia and thus may cause decrease in Cardiac Output (Cardiac output = Heart Rate X Stroke Volume), especially if the patient is in pain. However, it causes lesser hemodynamic instability as compared to Dexmedetomidine and thus fentanyl can be given in titrated doses.

43. Ans. (b) Atracurium

Ref: Miller's Anaesthesiology 8th ed. Ch 34, Table – 34-7

See Table of Peripherally Acting Skeletal Muscle Relaxants in Anesthesia AIIMS May 2016 (see page no. 1164)

Atracurium undergoes Hoffman's elimination as well as degradation by esterases and thus is not dependent on kidneys for elimination. Hence, it can be safely given in patients with renal disease.

Anesthetics Safe in Renal Failure	
Inhalational	Desflurane, Halothane, Isoflurane
Intravenous	Propofol Barbiturates: Thiopental, Methohexital
Opioids	Remifentanil, Fentanyl, Sulfentanil
Muscle relaxants	Atracurium, Cisatracurium (Best), Mivacurium, Rocuronium (with caution)

44. Ans. (b) Propofol

Ref: Miller's 7th ed page 2622, KDT 6th ed page 375

- Propofol is known to cause pain on injection because it is formulated in an oil based preparation
- Numerous strategies have been proposed to reduce pain on injection, of which the most effective are the use of a large antecubital vein or pretreatment with lidocaine in conjunction with venous occlusion.
- Alternative preparations of propofol, such as those containing bisulfite or comprising medium- and long-chain triglycerides, have had a modest or negligible effect in reducing injection pain, whereas some formulations significantly increase pain.
- The addition of lidocaine remains more effective at reducing pain than the choice of propofol formulation.

NOTE

- Drugs causing pain on IV injection: Propofol, Etomidate
- Thiopental causes severe pain on intra Arterial injection.

45. Ans. (a) Remifentanil, Midazolam, propofol

Ref: Morgan's 3rd ed page 173, 884, Miler's 8th ed page 726

Ambulatory/Day Care Anesthesia	
Agents	• Anxiolytic and sedation: Midazolam • Induction agent of choice: Propofol • Muscle relaxant: Mivacurium (skeletal muscle relaxant of choice), succinylcholine (postoperative myalgia is a disadvantage) • Inhalation agents: Isoflurane, sevoflurane, desflurane • TIVA (total Intravenous anesthesia): Propofol, Remifentanil/Alfentanil/Sufentanil
Switch technique	• Induction by propofol, maintenance with sevo/ isoflurane, rapid emergence with Propofol
Agents with a short duration of action are preferred for daycare procedures, so that the patient has minimal residual effects and can be discharged safely on the same day.	